Textbook of
Pediatrics

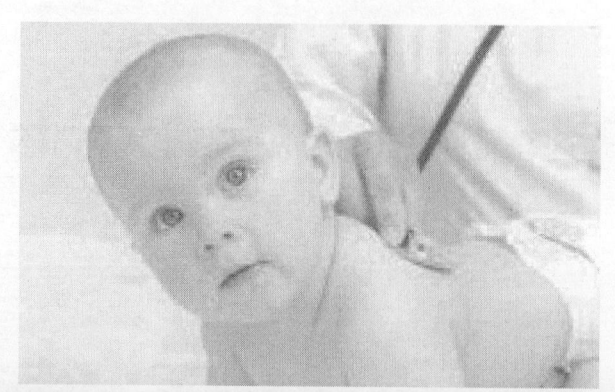

Textbook of Pediatrics

GP Mathur
MD (Ped), MD (Med), DCH, FIAP, FIMSA

Commonwealth Medical Fellow
Former Professor and Head
Department of Pediatrics, GSVM Medical College
Kanpur (UP), India
Professor and Head, Department of Pediatrics
Nepal Medical College, Kathmandu, Nepal

Sarla Mathur
MD (Ped), DCH

Certificate Course in Advance Medicine (UK)
Former Professor and Head, Department of Pediatrics
GSVM Medical College, Kanpur (UP), India
Professor, Department of Pediatrics
Nepal Medical College, Kathmandu, Nepal

MMA Faridi
MD, DCH, MNAMS, FIAP

Professor and Head, Department of Pediatrics
University College of Medical Sciences and Guru Teg Bahadur Hospital
Dilshad Garden, Delhi, India

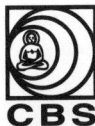

CBS Publishers & Distributors Pvt Ltd

New Delhi • Bengaluru • Chennai • Kochi • Mumbai • Pune
Hyderabad • Kolkata • Nagpur • Patna • Vijayawada

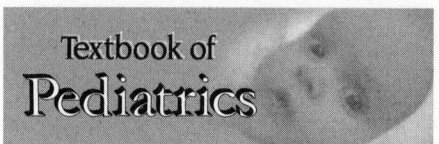

ISBN: 978-81-239-2471-7

First Edition: 2015

Published by Satish Kumar Jain and produced by Varun Jain for

CB3 Publishers & Distributors Pvt Ltd

4819/XI Prahlad Street, 24 Ansari Road, Daryaganj, New Delhi 110 002, India.

Ph: 23289259, 23266861, 23266867   Fax: 011-23243014   Website: www.cbspd.com
                                                                      e-mail: delhi@cbspd.com; cbspubs@airtelmail.in.

Corporate Office: 204 FIE, Industrial Area, Patparganj, Delhi 110 092

Ph: 4934 4934   Fax: 4934 4935   e-mail: publishing@cbspd.com; publicity@cbspd.com

Branches

- **Bengaluru:** Seema House 2975, 17th Cross, K.R. Road,
  Banasankari 2nd Stage, Bengaluru 560 070, Karnataka
  Ph: +91-80-26771678/79   Fax: +91-80-26771680   e-mail: bangalore@cbspd.com
- **Chennai:** No. 7, Subbaraya Street, Shenoy Nagar, Chennai 600 030, Tamil Nadu
  Ph: +91-44-42032115, M: 09500090969   Fax: +91-44-42032115   e-mail: chennai@cbspd.com
- **Kochi:** 36/14 Kalluvilakam, Lissie Hospital Road, Kochi 682 018, Kerala
  Ph: +91-484-4059061-65   Fax: +91-484-4059065   e-mail: kochi@cbspd.com
- **Mumbai:** 83-C, Dr E Moses Road, Worli, Mumbai-400018, Maharashtra
  Ph: +91-22-24902340/41   Fax: +91-22-24902342   e-mail: mumbai@cbspd.com
- **Pune:** Bhuruk Prestige, Sr. No. 52/12/2+1+3/2 Narhe, Haveli
  (Near Katraj-Dehu Road Bypass), Pune 411 041, Maharashtra
  Ph: +91-20-64704058, 64704059, 32392277   Fax: +91-20-24300160   e-mail: pune@cbspd.com

Representatives

- **Hyderabad** 0-9885175004   • **Kolkata** 0-9831437309, 0-9051152362
- **Nagpur**   0-9021734563   • **Patna**   0-9334159340   • **Vijayawada** 0-9000660880

Printed at Magic International Pvt.Ltd., Greater Noida

to

_____

*all those
who promote the well-being
of
neonates, infants, children
and the youth
throughout the world*

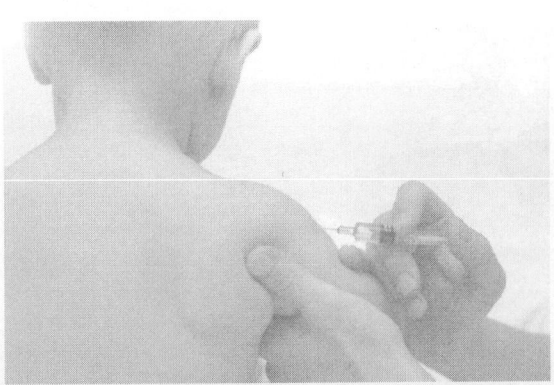

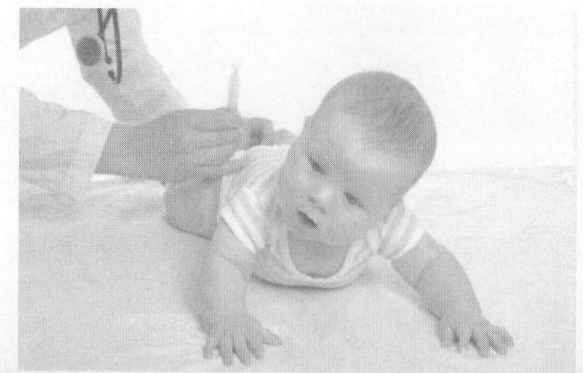

Foreword

Health of children shapes the future of the country. The true measure of nation's standing is how well it attends to its children because health matters both in and itself—as a measure of direct determinant of physical and mental health, longevity, and consequently the productivity of the society and the nation. The primary and basic factors are nutrition, physical and mental health, protection from communicable diseases, and then to undertake required therapeutic measures in the hands of competent pediatricians. The players in the field to give their contribution could be governmental agencies, parental factors but most important is a pediatrician who is required to be trained in a medical institution/hospital and has access to affordable world-class, comprehensive textbook on the subject.

I congratulate Prof GP Mathur for filling this gap by providing a comprehensive and yet concise textbook which has largely been directed to the specific needs of students studying pediatrics at undergraduate and postgraduate levels and for family physicians. The book covers all essential aspects of the subject in 40 chapters written by the leading specialists in their respective fields.

The well-illustrated book covers wide aspects of pediatric practice, starting from neonates to adolescents, emphasizing preventive, therapeutic, and related social and psychological aspects. Special care has been taken to deal with common and often ignored problems related to ophthalmology, otorhinolaryngology, dermatology, and psychiatry. Further, a CD accompanies the book to facilitate teaching and learning process as well as for presentation in lectures and seminars as illustrations. I can imagine the hard work and dedication by Prof GP Mathur and his team which has evolved in the form of a very useful textbook.

Prof KC Singhal
Vice Chancellor
NIMS University
Jaipur, Rajasthan, India
Mob. +91 9784737000
E-mail : kcsinghal@yahoo.co.in

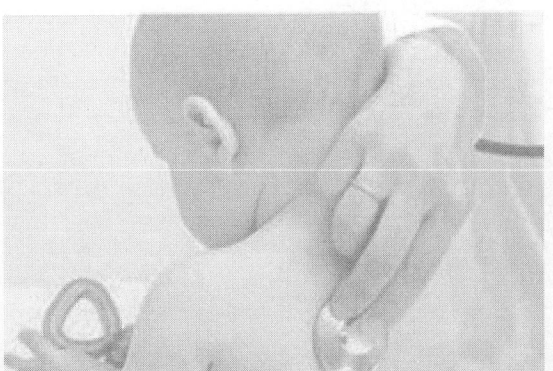

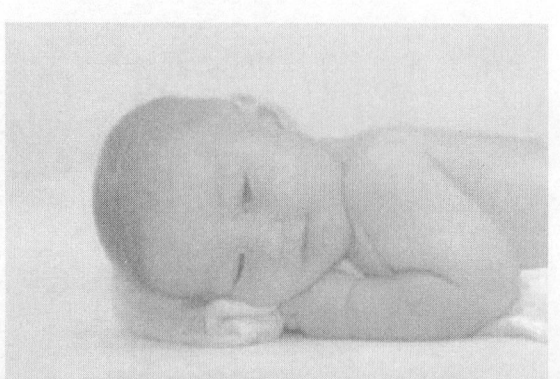

Preface

*T*extbook of Pediatrics covers the text in 40 chapters to provide comprehensive and latest information regarding various aspects of children diseases and problems of child health. The first edition represents the "state-of-the-art" on the care of the normal and ill neonate, child, and adolescent by presenting both evidence-based medicine as well as astute clinical experiences from leading national and international authors.

This edition of *Textbook* attempts to provide essential information that the medical students, house staff, practitioners, and other care providers involved in pediatric health care need to understand to effectively address the biologic, psychologic, and social problems that the children and youth may face. The accompanying CD provides clinical photographs, radiographs, algorithms, and nutritional and other relevant information to enhance learning and also support teaching. Our goal is to be comprehensive, yet concise and reader-friendly, embracing both the new advances in science as well as the time-honored art of pediatric practice. Although, to an ill child and his/her family and physician, even the rarest disorder is of central importance, all health problems cannot possibly be covered with the same degree of detail in one general textbook of pediatrics. Thus, leading articles and subspecialty texts are referred and should be consulted when more information is desired.

It reminds us how Prof RS Dayal, Prof BN Das Gupta, Prof JR Srivastava, Prof PM Udani and Prof OP Ghai have encouraged us that there is need to write book on pediatrics to promote scientific management of pediatric problems faced by the postgraduate students, pediatricians and general practitioners. Prof (Dr) Shekhar Babu Rizyal, Principal, Nepal Medical College, Kathmandu, Nepal, has been a source of encouragement to us. The editors are grateful to Prof (Dr) KC Singhal, Vice Chancellor, NIMS University, Jaipur, Rajasthan, for writing the Foreword to the book, highlighting its special features.

The outstanding value of the *Textbook* is due to its expert and authoritative contributors. We are all indebted to these dedicated authors for their hard work, knowledge, thoughtfulness, and good judgment. We are grateful to our fellow colleagues and residents of the department of pediatrics for their help in completing the book. Our sincere appreciation also goes to Mr YN Arjuna, Senior Vice President—Publishing, Editorial and Promotion, Mrs Ritu Chawla, Manager, Mrs Jyoti Kaur and Mr Neeraj Prasad of CBS Publishers & Distributors, for having been instrumental in ensuring the high quality of publication of this edition. We have all worked hard to produce this edition that will be helpful to those who provide care for children and youth and those desiring to know more about children's health worldwide.

Last but not the least, we especially wish to thank our families for their patience and understanding without which this textbook would not have been possible.

We welcome comments concerning omissions and errors, healthy reviews regarding content and critical thoughts and suggestions for future editions. These may be emailed to *drgpmathur2004@yahoo.co.in*

GP Mathur
Sarla Mathur
MMA Faridi

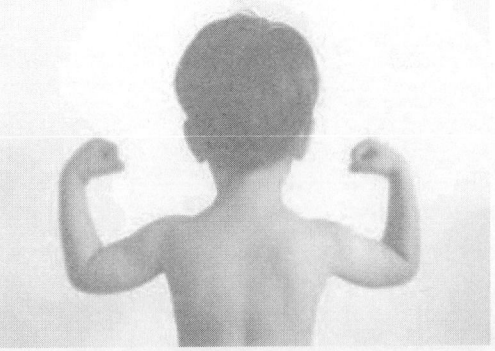

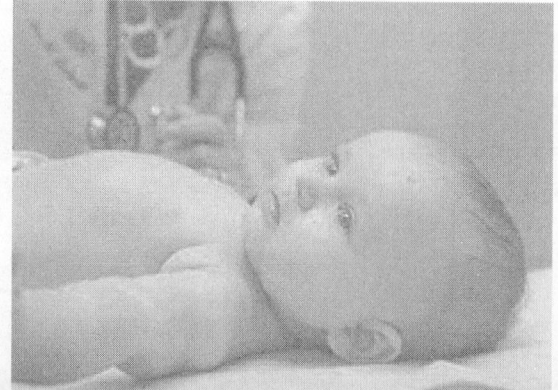

Contributors

B Adhisivam MBBS, DCH, DNB (Ped)
Assistant Professor of Pediatrics
Department of Pediatrics
Jawaharlal Institute of Postgraduate Medical
Education and Research (JIPMER)
Pondicherry, India

EE Afiadigwe MBBS, FWACS
Consultant Otorhinolaryngologist
Nnamdi Azikiwe University Teaching Hospital
Nnewi Anambra State, Nigeria

Kamran Afzal MBBS, MD (Ped)
Associate Professor
Department of Pediatrics
Jawaharlal Nehru Medical College, AMU
Aligarh, India

Shazia Afzal MBBS, DCH
Child Specialist
Inamdar Multispeciality Hospital
Fatima Nagar, Pune 411040, India

Anil Agarwal MBBS, MS (Ortho)
Specialist and Head
Department of Paediatric Orthopaedics
Chacha Nehru Bal Chikitsalaya
(Affiliated to Maulana Azad Medical College)
Geeta Colony, Delhi, India

Rachna Agarwal MBBS, MD (Obstetrics and Gynaecology)
Associate Professor
Department of Obstetrics and Gynaecology
University College of Medical Sciences and
Guru Teg Bahadur Hospital, Dilshad Garden
Delhi, India

Puneet Aggarwal MBBS, MD
Consultant Dermatologist
Nirmal Kaya Skin Clinic
E4/16, Krishna Nagar, Delhi, India

Sanjeev Aggarwal MBBS, MD (PGIMER), DNB (Ped)
Consultant Pediatrician and Neonatologist
Delhi, India

(Surg Cdr) Abhay I Ahluwalia MBBS, MD, DNB, DM (Endocrinology)
Associate Professor of Medicine
Armed Forces Medical College
Pune 411040, India

Satinder Aneja MBBS, MD (Ped)
Director-Professor and Head
Department of Pediatrics
Lady Hardinge Medical College and
Kalavati Saran Children Hospital, New Delhi, India

Akash A Bang MBBS, MD (Ped), DNB (Ped)
Lecturer in Pediatrics
Mahatma Gandhi Institute of Medical Sciences
Sewagram, Wardha, Maharashtra, India

Shikha Bansal MBBS, MD, DNB, MNAMS
Consultant Dermatologist
Shanti Gopal Hospital, Indirapuram (UP), India

MS Bhatia MBBS, MD, MNAMS
Professor and Head
Department of Psychiatry
University College of Medical Sciences and
Guru Teg Bahadur Hospital, Dilshad Garden, Delhi, India

Sushmita N Bhatnagar MBBS, MS, MCh (Ped Surg), MPhil (Hosp Admin)
Associate Professor and Incharge Unit-II
Department of Pediatric Surgery
Jerbai Wadia Childrens' Hospital, Lower Parel
Mumbai, India

Sanjay Chattree MBBS, MD, DCH
Senior Consultant
Department of Paediatrics and Neonatology
Jaipur Golden Hospital, Delhi, India

Alkesh Chaudhary MBBS, MS, FMRF
Specialist in Vitreo-Retinal Diseases
Consultant, Eye Surgeon
MD Eye Care and Laser Centre
M-165, Greater Kailash, Part II, Delhi, India

Zia Chaudhuri MBBS, MS, DNB, MNAMS, FRCS (Glasgow)
Associate Professor
Department of Ophthalmology
Maulana Azad Medical College and
Guru Nanak Eye Center
Delhi, India.

Anuradha Chugh MBBS, DOMS
Consultant, Eye Surgeon
MD Eye Care and Laser Centre
M-165, Greater Kailash, Part II, Delhi, India

Rajeshwar Dayal MBBS, MD (Ped), FAMS, FIAP, DNB, DCH (London)
Professor and Head, Department of Pediatrics
SN Medical College, Agra (UP), India

Pooja Dewan MBBS, MD
Lecturer, Department of Pediatrics
University College of Medical Sciences and
Guru Teg Bahadur Hospital, Dilshad Garden, Delhi, India

Jyoti Dhawan MBBS, MD
Consultant Dermatologist
Vardaan Skin Clinic, Sector 24, Rohini, Delhi, India
All India Institute of Medical Sciences
Ansari Nagar, Delhi, India

Geetika Dheer MBBS, MD
Assistant Professor
Department of Pediatrics, Christian Medical College
Ludhiana (Punjab), India

Anjan Dhua MBBS, MS, MCh (Pediatric Surgery)
Assistant Professor
Department of Pediatric Surgery
PGIMER and Dr. RM Lohia Hospital
New Delhi, India

Debashis Dutt MBBS, MD
Professor, Department of Epidemiology
All India Institute of Hygiene and Public Health
(Allh and PH)
110, Chittaranjan Avenue
Kolkata (West Bengal), India

KE Elizabeth MBBS, PhD, MD (Paed), DCH, FIAP
Consultant in Nutrition and Genetics
Professor in Paediatrics, SAT Hospital
Govt. Medical College
Trivandrum, India

Clement C Ezechukwu MBBS, FWACP (Paed)
1993 Heinz Fellow of the British Paediatric Association
Associate Professor, Department of Paediatrics
Faculty of Medicine, College of Health Sciences
Nnamdi Azikiwe University, Nnewi Campus
Anambra State, Nigeria

MMA Faridi MD, DCH, MNAMS, FIAP
Professor and Head, Department of Pediatrics
University College of Medical Sciences and
Guru Teg Bahadur Hospital
Dilshad Garden, Delhi, India

Neerja Goel MBBS, MD (Obstetrics and Gynaecology)
Professor, Department of Obstetrics and Gynecology
University College of Medical Sciences and
Guru Teg Bahadur Hospital
Dilshad Garden, Delhi, India

Mridula Goswami BDS, MDS (Pediatric and Preventive Dentistry)
Professor and Head, Department of Pediatric Dentistry
Maulana Azad Institute of Dental Sciences
Delhi, India

Anshul Grover MBBS, DGO, DNB
Specialist, Department of Obstetrics and Gynecology
Hindu Rao Hospital, Delhi, India

Chander Grover MBBS, MD, DNB, MNAMS
Lecturer, Department of Dermatology and STD
University College of Medical Sciences and
Guru Teg Bahadur Hospital, Dilshad Garden, Delhi, India

Divesh Gulati MBBS, MS (Ortho), MCh (Orthopedics), USAIM
Associate Consultant Orthopaedics
Sant Parmanand Hospital, Civil Lines, Delhi, India

Sheffali Gulati MBBS, MD, MAMS, FIMSA
Additional Professor, Chief Incharge
Child Neurology Division
Department of Pediatrics, All India Institute of Medical
Sciences, Ansari Nagar
Delhi, India

Anupam Gupta MBBS, MD (Physical Medicine and Rehabilitation)
Assistant Professor, Department of Psychiatric and
Neurological Rehabilitation
National Institute of Mental Health and
Neurosciences (NIMHANS)
Bangalore, India

Bindiya Gupta MBBS, MD (Obstetrics and Gynaecology)
Senior Research Associate, Department of
Obstetrics and Gynecology
University College of Medical Sciences and
Guru Teg Bahadur Hospital
Dilshad Garden, Delhi, India

Devendra K Gupta MBBS, MS, MCh, FICS, FAMS, FRCS (Glasgow)
DSc (Honoris Causa)
President-Elect, World Federation of
Association of Pediatric Surgeons
Vice Chancellor, KGMU (CSMMU), Lucknow (UP), India

Lipy Gupta MBBS, MD
Senior Resident, Department of Dermatology and STD
University College of Medical Sciences and
Guru Teg Bahadur Hospital, Dilshad Garden, Delhi, India

Neerja Gupta MBBS, MD (Pediatrics), DM (Medical Genetics)
Pool Officer
Genetics Unit, Department of Pediatrics
All India Institute of Medical Sciences
Ansari Nagar, Delhi, India

Pratima Gupta MBBS, MD (Microbiology), MAMS, CAFE, FHM
Professor and Head, Department of Microbiology
Himalayan Institute of Medical Sciences
Jolly Grant, Dehradun (Uttaranchal), India

Sunil Kumar Gupta MBBS, MD
Professor, Department of Dermatology
Dayanand Medical College, Ludhiana (Punjab), India

Sunil Kumar Gupta MBBS, MD (Ped), PhD (Environmental Sciences)
Consultant Pediatrician and Neonatologist and
Scientist of Environmental Medicine
(including Environmental Health)
Krishna Ram Hospital and Research Centre and
Shree Krishna Ram Charitable Hospital
Jaipur, India

Pankaj Hari MBBS, MD (Ped)
Additional Professor
Division of Pediatric Nephrology
Department of Pediatrics
All India Institute of Medical Sciences
Ansari Nagar, Delhi, India

KS Jacob MBBS, MD, MRCPsych, PhD
Professor and Head
Department of Psychiatry
Christian Medical College, Vellore, India

Divya Jain MBBS, MS, DNB
Senior Resident
Department of Ophthalmology
Maulana Azad Medical College and
Guru Nanak Eye Center, Delhi, India.

Sandhya Jain MBBS, MD (Obstetrics and Gynaecology)
Assistant Professor
Department of Obstetrics and Gynecology
University College of Medical Sciences and
Guru Teg Bahadur Hospital, Dilshad Garden, Delhi, India

Tarsem Jindal MBBS, MD, FIAP, FIAMS
Senior Consultant and Head
Department of Paediatrics and Neonatology
Jaipur Golden Hospital, Delhi, India

Mathew John MBBS, MD, DM, DNB
Consultant Endocrinologist
Kerala Institute of Medical Sciences
Assistant Professor of Dr Somervell Memorial Medical
College, Karakonam, Thiruvananthapuram, India

Madhulika Kabra MBBS, MD (Pediatrics)
Professor, Genetics Unit, Department of Pediatrics
All India Institute of Medical Sciences
Ansari Nagar, Delhi, India

Umesh Kapil MBBS, MD, DNB
Professor Public Health Nutrition
Human Nutrition Unit
All India Institute of Medical Sciences
Ansari Nagar, Delhi, India

Deepshikha Khanna MBBS, MD
Senior Resident, Department of Dermatology and STD
University College of Medical Sciences and
Guru Teg Bahadur Hospital
Dilshad Garden, Delhi, India

Vandana Khare MBBS, MD (Pathology)
Consultant Pathologist
Pushpwati Singhania Research Institute
Delhi, India

Gibby Koshy M Trop Paed (UK)
Postgraduate Research Assistant
Child and Reproductive Health Research Group
Liverpool School of Tropical Medicine
Pembroke Place, Liverpool, United Kingdom

Sriram Krishnamurthy MBBS, MD (Pediatrics)
Assistant Professor, Department of Pediatrics
Jawaharlal Institute of Postgraduate
Medical Education and Research (JIPMER)
Pondicherry, India

Arun Kumar MSc (Medical Biochemistry), PhD (Medical Biochemistry)
Assistant Professor
Department of Biochemistry College of Medicine and
JNM Hospital
West Bengal University of Health Sciences (JNM Hospital
Campus)
Kalyani, Nadia (West Bengal), India

Navneet Kumar MBBS, MS (ENT), DNB
Lecturer, Department of ENT
Christian Medical College, Ludhiana (Punjab), India

Praveen Kumar MBBS, MD (Ped)
Professor, Department of Pediatrics
Lady Hardinge Medical College, Delhi, India

Vivek Kumar MBBS, MD, DNB
Senior Consultant Cardiologist and
Head—Community Outreach Programme
Escorts Heart Institute and Research Centre, Delhi, India

Shaveta Kundra MBBS, MD
Assistant Professor
Department of Pediatrics, Christian Medical College
Ludhiana (Punjab), India

Manabu Kurokawa PhD (Medicine)
Microbiologist and Sr. Researcher
Department of Microbiology, Kobe Institute of Health
Chuo-ku, Kobe 650-0046, Japan

KP Kushwaha MD (Ped), FIAP
Chief of Training, BPNI
Principal, BRD Medical College
Gorakhpur (UP), India

Rakhi Kusumesh MS (Ophthalmology)
Senior Resident, Dr RP Centre for Ophthalmic Sciences
All India Institute of Medical Sciences
Ansari Nagar, Delhi, India

S Mahadevan MBBS, MD, PhD, MNAMS
Professor Pediatrics and Professor (Academic)
Jawaharlal Institute of Postgraduate Medical Education
and Research (JIPMER)
Pondicherry, India

Rupesh Masand MBBS, MD (Ped)
Assistant Professor, Department of Pediatrics
NIMS Medical College and Hospital
NIMS University, Jaipur (Rajasthan), India

Anuj Narayan Mathur MBBS, MD (Ophthalmology)
Chief Medical Officer, School Health Services
Shahdara South Zone
Municipal Corporation of Delhi (MCD)
Delhi, India

GP Mathur MD (Ped), MD (Med), DCH, FIAP, FIMSA
Commonwealth Medical Fellow
Former Professor and Head
Department of Pediatrics, GSVM Medical College
Kanpur (UP), India

Professor and Head, Department of Pediatrics
Nepal Medical College, Kathmandu, Nepal

Sarla Mathur MD (Ped), DCH
Certificate Course in Advance Medicine (UK)
Former Professor and Head, Department of Pediatrics
GSVM Medical College, Kanpur (UP), India
Professor, Department of Pediatrics
Nepal Medical College, Kathmandu, Nepal

Sumit Mathur MBBS (Hon), DLO
ENT Specialist, C-1/5A, Mayur Vihar, Phase-3, Delhi, India.

Shilpa Mehta MBBS, MD (Dermatology)
Resident, Internal Medicine
John Stroger Hospital of Cook County
Chicago, USA

Sumita Mehta MBBS, DNB, MICOG
Specialist, Department of Obstetrics and Gynecology
University College of Medical Sciences and
Guru Teg Bahadur Hospital, Dilshad Garden
Delhi, India

Shalini Mohan MS (Ophthalmology)
Lecturer, Department of Ophthalmology
GSVM Medical College, Kanpur (UP), India

Anup Mohta MBBS, MS, MCh, MAMS
Professor and Head, Department of Pediatric surgery
Chacha Nehru Bal Chikitsalaya (Affiliated to Maulana
Azad Medical College)
Geeta Colony, Delhi, India

Sharmila (Banerjee) Mukherjee MBBS, MD (Ped)
Assistant Professor, Department of Pediatrics
Lady Hardinge Medical College
Delhi, India

Madhumita Nandi MBBS, MD (Ped)
Assistant Professor of Pediatrics
In-Charge Pediatric Nephrology Clinic
Department of Pediatric Medicine
Institute of Postgraduate Medical Education and
Research, Kolkata (West Bengal), India

Manish Narang MBBS, MD (Pediatrics)
Lecturer, Department of Pediatrics
University College of Medical Sciences and
Guru Teg Bahadur Hospital, Dilshad Garden
Delhi, India

Kazuo Ono PhD (Medicine), DMSc
Professor, Faculty of Health and Culture
Kobe Tokiwa College, 2-6-2 Otani-cho Nagata-ku
Kobe 653-0838, Japan

(Surg Lt Cdr) Rajesh Pandey MBBS
Resident Medicine
Armed Forces Medical College, Pune, India

Upasna Pandit MBBS, MD (Obstetrics and Gynaecology)
Senior Resident
Department of Obstetrics and Gynaecology
University College of Medical Sciences and
Guru Teg Bahadur Hospital
Dilshad Garden, Delhi, India

Deepika Pandhi MBBS, MD
Reader, Department of Dermatology and STD
University College of Medical Sciences and
Guru Teg Bahadur Hospital
Dilshad Garden, Delhi, India

AK Patwari MBBS, MD, DCH, MNAMS, FIAP, FAMS
Research Professor, International Health
Center for Global Health and Development
School of Public Health, Boston University, USA

Resident Faculty and Coordinator
CGHD India Country Program, New Delhi, India

Piyush Prasad MBBS, MD (Pediatrics), DCH (UK)
Diplomat CH (Cal), FICMCH
Consultant Pediatrician
Prasad Children's Hospital and Research Centre
1/210 A, Professor's Colony, Agra (UP), India

Ramesh Prasad MBBS, MD (Ped), FRCP (Edin), DCH (Lond), MD
(Medicine), FRCP (Glasgow) DCH (Agra)
Former Professor and Head
SN Medical College, Agra
Consultant Pediatrician
Prasad Children's Hospital and Research Centre
1/210 A, Professor's Colony, Agra (UP), India

Jyotsna Punj MBBS, MD (Anesthesiology)
Associate Professor
Department of Anesthesiology and Critical Care
All India Institute of Medical Sciences
Ansari Nagar, Delhi, India

Shiba Kumar Rai PhD (Med), DMSc
Professor, Department of Microbiology
Nepal Medical College
National Institute of Tropical Medicine
Public Health Research, Narayan Gopal Chowk
Shankha Marg, Kathmandu, Nepal

Sandeep Rawal MBBS, MD
Consultant, Department of Pediatrics and Neonatology
Jaipur Golden Hospital, Delhi, India

Manoranjitham S MSc (N)
Professor in Nursing
Head of Psychiatric Nursing Department
College of Nursing, Christian Medical College
Vellore, India

Tapas Kumar Sabui MBBS, MD, DCH
Associate Professor, Department of Pediatrics
In-Charge Pediatric Rheumatology Clinic
NRS Medical College, Kolkata (West Bengal), India

Bela Sachdeva MBBS, DCH, DNB (Ped)
DIP. Child Psychology (Oxford)
PG DIP. Hosp. and Health Management
Senior Consultant (Pediatrics)
Dharamshila Cancer Hospital (Visiting Consultant)
Hospital and Health Administrator
E-166, Sec 21, Jalvayu Vihar, Noida (UP), India

Debopam Samanta MBBS, MD (Ped)
Pediatric Neurology Fellow
University of Virginia Medical Centre
Charlottesville, Virginia, USA

Ram Samujh MBBS, MS, FRCS (Ireland), MCh (Ped. Surgery)
Additional Professor of Pediatric Surgery
Department of Pediatric Surgery
Advanced Pediatric Center
Postgraduate Institute of Medical
Education and Research, Chandigarh, India

Nishanath Sanalkumar MBBS, MD, ABIM (Internal Medicine)
ABIM (Endocrinology), Consultant
Endocrinology and Diabetes
Kerala Institute of Medical Sciences
Thiruvananthapuram, India

Kabir Sardana MBBS, MD, DNB, MNAMS
Assistant Professor
Department of Dermatology and STD
Maulana Azad Medical College and
Associated Lok Nayak Hospital
Bahadur Shah Zafar Marg, Delhi, India

Yogesh Kumar Sarin MBBS, MS, Dip NB, MCh (Pediatric Surgery),
MNAMS, MBA (HCA), FICS, FIAS, FIMSA
Professor and Head
Department of Pediatric Surgery
Maulana Azad Medical College and
Associated Lok Nayak Hospital
Bahadur Shah Zafar Marg, Delhi, India

Neha Sareen BSc, MSc
Research Scientist
Department of Gastroenterology and Human Nutrition
All India Institute of Medical Sciences
Ansari Nagar, Delhi, India

Rogina JS Savarimuthu MSc (N)
Junior Lecturer in Nursing
Departmental Sister In-Charge of
Child and Adolescent Unit
College of Nursing, Christian Medical College
Vellore, India

Sidharth Kumar Sethi MBBS, MD (Ped)
Fellow, Pediatric Nephrology
Division of Pediatric Nephrology
Department of Pediatrics, All India Institute of
Medical Sciences
Ansari Nagar, Delhi, India

Reena Sharma MBBS, MD
Department of Dermatology and STD
University College of Medical Sciences and
Guru Teg Bahadur Hospital
Dilshad Garden, Delhi, India

Ritu P Sharma MSc, PhD (Food and Nutrition)
Assistant Professor
Government College of Home Science
Chandigarh, India

Sanjib Kumar Sharma MBBS, MD (Medicine)
Associate Professor
Department of Medicine, In-Charge Dialysis Division
BP Koirala Institute of Health Sciences, Dharan, Nepal

Shilpa Sharma MS, MCh, DNB
Senior Research Associate
Department of Pediatric Surgery
All India Institute of Medical Sciences
Ansari Nagar, New Delhi, India

Alpana Singh MBBS, MD (Obstetrics and Gynaecology)
Lecturer, Department of Obstetrics and Gynecology
University College of Medical Sciences and
Guru Teg Bahadur Hospital
Dilshad Garden, Delhi, India

Tejinder Singh MBBS, MD, DNB, FIAP
PG Dip Higher Education
Masters Distance Education
Professor and Head, Department of Pediatrics
Vice Principal and Program Director
CMCL-FAIMER Regional Institute
Convener-MCI Nodal Center for Faculty Development
Program In-Charge, PGDMCH (IGNOU)
Christian Medical College, Ludhiana (Punjab), India

Archana Singal MBBS, MD, MNAMS
Professor, Department of Dermatology and STD
University College of Medical Sciences and
Guru Teg Bahadur Hospital
Dilshad Garden, Delhi, India

PK Singhal MBBS, MD (Ped)
Former Assistant Professor, Department of Pediatrics
All India Institute of Medical Sciences
Delhi, India

Senior Consultant
Indraprastha Apollo Hospital
Delhi, India

Arvind Sinha MBBS, MS, MCh (Pediatric Surgery)
Assistant Professor and In-Charge
Department of Pediatric Surgery
Himalayan Institute of Medical Sciences, Jolly Grant
Dehradun, India

Mala Sinha MS (Obst and Gynaec), MS (Plastic Surgery)
Ex. Head, Department of Plastic Surgery
Patna Medical College, Patna
S-104, Udaigiri Bhawan, Budh Marg
Patna (Bihar), India

Shalini Sinha MBBS, MS, MCh (Ped Surg)
Assistant Professor, Department of Pediatric Surgery
Maulana Azad Medical College and
Associated Lok Nayak Hospital, New Delhi, India

Sidharth Sonthalia MBBS, MD
Senior Resident
Department of Dermatology and STD
University College of Medical Sciences and
Guru Teg Bahadur Hospital
Dilshad Garden, Delhi, India

Shruti Srivastava MBBS, MD
Lecturer, Department of Psychiatry
University College of Medical Sciences and
Guru Teg Bahadur Hospital
Dilshad Garden, Delhi, India

SP Srivastava MBBS, MD (Ped), DHA, FIAMS, FIAP, MCh Fellow (UK), FIMSA, FAAP (USA)
Dr BC Roy Award of Medical Council of India
Retd. Professor and Head
Department of Upgraded Pediatric Department
Patna Medical College, Patna
S-104, Udaigiri Bhawan, Budh Marg
Patna (Bihar), India

Amar Taksande MBBS, MD
Fellowship in Pediatric Cardiology
Associate Professor
Department of Pediatrics, MGIMS, Sevagram
Wardha (Maharashtra), India

Satyendra Tewari MBBS, MD, DM, FACC, FSCAI, FCSI, FICC
Consultant Interventional Cardiologist and
Additional Professor
Department of Cardiology
Sanjay Gandhi Postgraduate Institute of Medical Sciences
Lucknow (UP), India

Satish Kamtaprasad Tiwari MBBS, MD (Ped), LLB
Associate Professor, Department of Pediatrics
Medical College, Amravati (Maharashtra), India

Anurag Tomar MBBS, MD (Ped)
Associate Professor, Department of Pediatrics
NIMS Medical College and Hospital, NIMS University
Jaipur (Rajasthan), India

Swati Tomar MBBS, MS (Ophth)
Associate Professor, Department of Ophthalmology
NIMS Medical College and Hospital
NIMS University, Jaipur (Rajasthan), India

VN Tripathi MBBS (Hon), MD (Ped), MNAMS, FIAP, FICMCH, FAAP (Hon)
Principal and Dean
Government Medical College
Ambedkar Nagar (UP), India

M Vanathi MBBS, MD
Associate Professor, Department of Ophthalmology
Dr Rajendra Prasad Institute of Medical Sciences
All India Institute of Medical Sciences
Ansari Nagar, Delhi, India

Saurabh Varshney MBBS, MS (ENT), MAMS, MIAO, DHA, DBA, PGDMLS, FCCP
Vice Principal (Undergraduate) State Nodal Officer (Uttarakhand)
Professor and Head, Department of ENT
Himalayan Institute of Medical Sciences
Jolly Grant; Doiwala, Dehradun (Uttarakhand), India

Mahesh Verma BDS, MDS (Prosthetic Dentistry)
Director-Principal
Maulana Azad Institute of Dental Sciences, Delhi, India

SK Verma MBBS, MD (AIIMS), FIAFM, FICFMT
Professor, Department of Forensic Medicine
University College of Medical Sciences
Dilshad Garden, Delhi, India

Amit Vij MBBS, MD
Consultant Dermatologist
Max Hospital, Noida (UP), India

Sangeeta Yadav MBBS, MD (Ped)
Director-Professor
In-Charge Division of Pediatric and
Adolescent Endocrinology
Department of Pediatrics, Maulana Azad
Medical College and Associated LN Hospital, Delhi, India

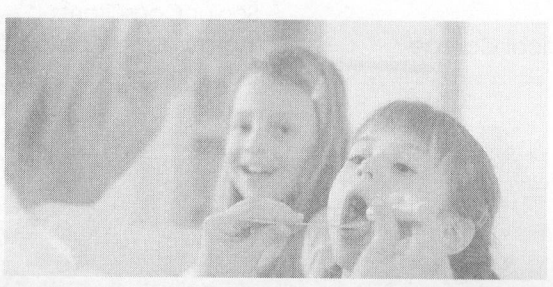

Contents

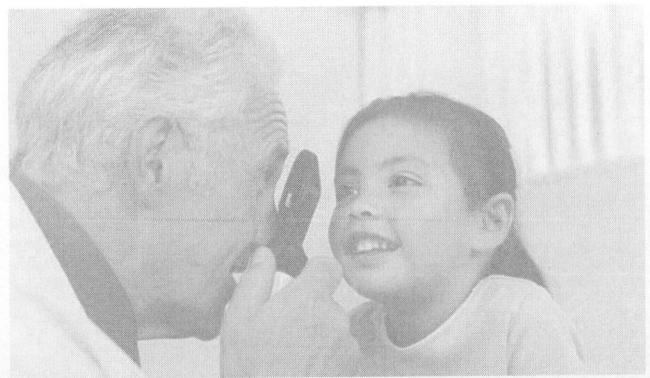

1 The Field of Pediatrics

1.1 INTRODUCTION

The word pediatrics is derived from Greek words pais or paido which means child and iatria which means healing (medical treatment). Pediatrics (pe"de-at'riks; the branch of medicine dealing with children diseases) is concerned with the health of infants, children and adolescents, their growth and development; so that they have opportunity to achieve full potential as adults. Children are among the most vulnerable or disadvantaged in society, and thus their needs should be given special attention. Pediatrics deals with growing individuals: Newborn to adolescence. As mother and child is one unit, pediatricians are interested in the perinatal problems and training the mother to look after the baby especially advice regarding breastfeeding immediately afterbirth in collaboration with the obstetricians who have major role to play. At the time of delivery if the pregnant woman is Rh −ve, hepatitis B +ve, VDRL +ve or HIV +ve or suffering with illness, e.g. eclampsia, diabetes mellitus, heart disease, or undergoing for cesarian section (CS) pediatrician should be available well in time to look after the newborn.

Pediatricians also help future parents especially if there is family history of chromosomal or metabolic disorders, e.g. Duchenne muscular dystrophy, thalassemia, Down syndrome, diabetes mellitus.

As the subject of pediatrics deals with growth, periods of growth are presented in Table 1.1.

Teenager—A boy or girl is to his or her teens aged between 13 and 19 years. Teens means the numbers 13 to 19.

Juvenile—It means young person; juvenile court—where children are tried; juvenile delinquency—lawbreaking by young people; juvenile delinquent—young offender.

Puberty—The period marked by the beginning of secondary sex characteristics; stage at which a person becomes physically able to become a parent; maturing of the sexual functions.

Behrman RE. Overview of Pediatrics. In: Behrman RE, Kliegman RM, Jenson HB (eds). *Nelson Textbook of Pediatrics.* 17th edn. Philadelphia: Saunders, 2004; 1–6.

Needlman RD. Growth and development. In: Behrman RE, Kliegman RM, Jenson HB (eds). *Nelson Textbook of Pediatrics.* 17th edn. Philadelphia: Saunders, 2004; 23–66.

Table 1.1: Periods of growth (age periods)	
Before birth	
Embryonic period	Beginning from first week
Fetal period	Begins from 9 weeks
Afterbirth	
Newborn	First 28 days
Infant	First yr
Toddler	Second yr
Preschool yrs	2–5 yrs
Early school yrs (Middle-childhood)	6–11 yrs
Adolescence	10–20 yrs
Early adolescence	10–13 yrs
Middle adolescence	14–16 yrs
Late adolescence	17–20 yrs

1.2 HISTORY AND EXAMINATION

History Taking

History should be taken from the mother (more reliable), father, caregiver, and from children. Important additional points listed in Box 1.1 in history taking must be considered.

On the basis of history try to analyze the differential diagnosis and think which system/systems is involved. Examine first the system involved. Before going for systemic examination do the general examination including the measurements.

History taking in a patient in the pediatric age group is similar to that of an adult patient with some important additions. Information is usually obtained from the parents, but a grown-up child may be able to add some more points.

As usual the name, age, sex, address, present complaints, history of present illness (HOPI), treatment history, past illness, family history, social and occupational history etc., are to be noted. But also note in a pediatric case history mentioned in Box 1.1

Some special information in family and social history gives significant clues to the diagnosis of many diseases in infancy and childhood. These are family composition, presence of consanguinity; stillbirth, miscarriages or abortions; health of other sibs; any one in the family has or had any disease (congenital, heredo-familial or acquired); financial status of the family; food habits; housing, traditions. Also take history of adverse reactions to drugs and vaccination.

Physical Examination

In the examination of children, the rigid rules as for examining adult patients should not be applied. A friendly manner, slow and easy approach and soft voice facilitate examination. The infant should be examined as he/she allows; heart and lungs examination when he is quiet, mouth and eyes when open. It is always better to examine the child with clothes off but many children do not like removable of all clothes. Undressing the child, when essential, should better be performed by the mother. Babies

below 6 mo of age and most school-going children can be examined on the table, but those between 6 mo and 3 to 4 yr, secured in the mother's lap or over her shoulder, cooperate quite well during examination. Sudden touch with the cold metal of the stethoscope or even a cold hand startles the infant, crying ensues and makes the examination difficult. Examination of a part like the throat, ear or rectum, likely to be associated with pain and discomfort should be performed in the end. In a non-cooperative child if the examiner feels that it is important to proceed with the examination, he should do so in an orderly systemic manner in the hope that the child will accept the inevitable. In general, more information is usually obtained by careful inspection than from any other method of examination (Boxes 1.2 and 1.3).

The procedures for examining different systems are mentioned in the chapters on the respective systems. Whatever may be the technique of approach the findings must be recorded systematically according to the standard clinical method. The height, weight and head circumference of the child should be recorded and compared with the standard chart.

Box 1.1: Important additional points to be considered in history taking

Antenatal, natal (birth history), postnatal

Developmental milestones

Infant feeding and nutrition

Immunization

Schooling

Adverse reaction to *vaccination* and drugs

Box 1.2: Pre-requisites for examination of a child

Welcome the parents and the child

Talk to the parents and observe the child

Let him/her be adjusted with the environment

While talking to parents offer the child to fiddle with the toy/stethoscope/pen/measuring tape

Examine the child with warm hands

Examine the child, which is comfortable to the child, parents and the examiner

Start examination from feet

Tickle the sole

Box 1.3: Suggested scheme for examination of infants and young children

Observe Listen Play Palpate

Infants and young children are comfortably examined in the lap of the mother

Feet

Hands and pulse

Face

Head

Neck

Abdomen

Chest

Neurological examination

Genitalia, groin, anus

Other invasive clinical tests—nose, ear, throat, teeth (number, caries), funduscopy

Multiple measurements at intervals give information regarding the pattern of growth that cannot be obtained by single measurements.

Student should have:
- Stethoscope
- Measuring tape
- Patella hammer
- Tuning fork
- Torch
- Growth charts

In the ward following items should be available for taking measurements:
- Weighing machines: Adult and infant weighing machines
- Measuring height: Stadiometer
- Measuring length: Infantometer
- Blood pressure (BP) instrument with different sizes of cuff (3, 5, 7, 12, 18 cm cuff). BP varies with the age of the child and is closely related to height and weight. BP in the legs with the cuff technique is about 10 mm Hg higher than that in the arms. For lower extremity BP determination, the stethoscope is placed over the popliteal artery.

Measurements will provide information about growth and development; milestones and school performance will tell the mental and cognitive development.

General Outline of a Case Examination

- History taking
- Physical examination

General examination includes vital signs (pulse, blood pressure (BP), respiratory rate, and temperature), general signs (pallor, cyanosis, clubbing, edema, hydration, lymphadenopathy) and measurements (weight, head circumference [including anterior and posterior fontanels], height/length including upper and lower segments, span, and other measurements such as chest circumference, abdominal circumference, mid-arm circumference)

- Local examination for example in case of swelling
- Systemic examination
- Provisional diagnosis (consider differential diagnosis; require hospitalization, admit)
- Provisional treatment if needed or wait for the laboratory reports
- Laboratory investigations
- Diagnosis and treatment based on laboratory reports
- Treatment

General (including nursing care, nutrition, and guidelines to parents—general; special to a particular disease)

- Specific
- Local
- Prognosis
- Follow-up (to come for checkup, but should come immediately if there is deterioration in condition or reaction to drugs/vaccination)

Needlman RD. Growth and development. In: Behrman RE, Kliegman RM, Jenson HB (eds). Nelson Textbook of Pediatrics. 17th edn. Philadelphia: Saunders, 2004; 23-66.

1.3 RIGHTS OF THE CHILD

Declaration of the Rights of the Child

Proclaimed by General Assembly resolution 1386 (XIV) of 20 November 1959

Whereas the peoples of the United Nations have, in the Charter, reaffirmed their faith in fundamental human rights and in the dignity and worth of the human person, and have determined to promote social progress and better standards of life in larger freedom,

Whereas the United Nations has, in the Universal Declaration of Human Rights, proclaimed that everyone is entitled to all the rights and freedoms set forth therein, without distinction of any kind, such as race, colour, sex, language, religion, political or other opinion, national or social origin, property, birth or other status,

Whereas the child, by reason of his physical and mental immaturity, needs special safeguards and care, including appropriate legal protection, before as well as afterbirth,

Whereas the need for such special safeguards has been stated in the Geneva Declaration of the Rights of the Child of 1924, and recognized in the Universal Declaration of Human Rights and in the statutes of specialized agencies and international organizations concerned with the welfare of children,

Whereas mankind owes to the child the best it has to give, *Now therefore,*

The General Assembly

Proclaims this Declaration of the Rights of the Child to the end that he may have a happy childhood and enjoy for his own good and for the good of society the rights and freedoms herein set forth, and calls upon parents, upon men and women as individuals, and upon voluntary organizations, local authorities and national Governments to recognize these rights and strive for their observance by legislative and other measures progressively taken in accordance with the following principles:

Principle 1: The child shall enjoy all the rights set forth in this declaration. Every child, without any exception whatsoever, shall be entitled to these rights, without distinction or discrimination on account of race, colour, sex, language, religion, political or other opinion, national or social origin, property, birth or other status, whether of himself or of his family.

Principle 2: The child shall enjoy special protection, and shall be given opportunities and facilities, by law and by other means, to enable him to develop physically, mentally, morally, spiritually and socially in a healthy and normal manner and in conditions of freedom and dignity. In the enactment of laws for this purpose, the best interests of the child shall be the paramount consideration.

Principle 3: The child shall be entitled from his birth to a name and a nationality.

Principle 4: The child shall enjoy the benefits of social security. He shall be entitled to grow and develop in health; to this end, special care and protection shall be provided both to him and to his mother, including adequate prenatal and postnatal care. The child shall have the right to adequate nutrition, housing, recreation and medical services.

Principle 5: The child who is physically, mentally or socially handicapped shall be given the special treatment, education and care required by his particular condition.

Principle 6: The child, for the full and harmonious development of his personality, needs love and understanding. He shall, wherever possible, grow up in the care and under the responsibility of his parents, and, in any case, in an atmosphere of affection and of moral and material security; a child of tender yr shall not, save in exceptional circumstances, be separated from his mother. Society and the public authorities shall have the duty to extend particular care to children without a family and to those without adequate means of support. Payment of State and other assistance towards the maintenance of children of large families is desirable.

Principle 7: The child is entitled to receive education, which shall be free and compulsory, at least in the elementary stages. He shall be given an education, which will promote his general culture and enable him, on a basis of equal opportunity, to develop his abilities, his individual judgment, and his sense of moral and social responsibility, and to become a useful member of society.

The best interests of the child shall be the guiding principle of those responsible for his education and guidance; that responsibility lies in the first place with his parents.

The child shall have full opportunity for play and recreation, which should be directed, to the same purposes as education; society and the public authorities shall endeavour to promote the enjoyment of this right.

Principle 8: The child shall in all circumstances be among the first to receive protection and relief.

Principle 9: The child shall be protected against all forms of neglect, cruelty and exploitation. He shall not be the subject of traffic, in any form.

The child shall not be admitted to employment before an appropriate minimum age; he shall in no case be caused or permitted to engage in any occupation or employment which would prejudice his health or education, or interfere with his physical, mental or moral development.

Principle 10: The child shall be protected from practices, which may foster racial, religious and any other form of discrimination. He shall be brought up in a spirit of understanding, tolerance, friendship among peoples, peace and universal brotherhood, and in full consciousness that his energy and talents should be devoted to the service of his fellow men.

International Rights

Children are now recognized as having their own human rights. These are laid down in the United Nations Convention on the Rights of the Child, which has been ratified by all members of the United Nations excluding the USA and Somalia. Implications of the convention include the involvement of children in clinical decision-making and in issues of consent (Box 1.4).

Universal Children's Day is celebrated on 20th November to focus the right of every child as mentioned in Box 1.5. **Let us say no to child labour.**

Box 1.4: Summary of the United Nations Convention on the Rights of the Child (1989)

1. *Survival rights*
   The child's right to life and to the most basic needs—food, shelter and access to health care
2. *Developmental rights*
   To achieve their full potential—education, play, freedom of thought, conscience and religion. Those with disabilities to receive special services
3. *Protection rights*
   Against all forms of abuse, neglect, exploitation and discrimination
4. *Participation rights*
   To take an active role in their communities and nations.

Every child has the right to:
Play with colors
Sing rhymes
Read stories
Wear school uniform
Sit infront of a black board
Experience childhood

Source: Hindustan Times, New Delhi on Friday, November 20, 2009.

Declaration of the Rights of the Child, Proclaimed by General Assembly resolution 1386(XIV) of 20 November 1959.

Published in Hindustan Times, New Delhi on Friday, November 20, 2009.

1.4 HEALTH PROBLEMS ASSOCIATED WITH THE USE OF COMPUTER

Working for hr on a computer is now a fact of life. But there are certain risks involved with prolonged computer use. Most people including children and adolescents who sit for hr in front of a computer experience some discomfort or pain. Many people who spend part of their time in front of a computer screen suffer from visual and non-visual problems, which are listed in Box 1.6.

What Causes the Problems Occur?

Simply stated, there are two divisions where the problems lie. The first deals with the issue of ergonomics. Specifically, how do you improve the compatibility between the individual and computer by improving the lighting, the office furniture, the quality of the screen image and the basic comfort of the workstation?

The second division deals with how you improve the individual. It deals with those people who need to wear bifocals. Bifocals that are conventionally prescribed for normal reading activity many times do

Box 1.6: Symptoms related to computers

Non-visual problems
• Headaches
• Pains developing in the neck and shoulder area
• Carpal tunnel syndrome
• Back pain
Visual problems
• Blurred vision while viewing the monitor
• Increased blur at distance, particularly at night
• Problems focusing from distance to near or vice versa
• Increased sensitivity to bright light or fluorescent light
• Increased dry eye syndrome

not work well while sitting in front of a screen. There are two reasons for this. The first deals with the fact the computer screen is usually at a different height than the normal reading level, usually significantly higher. The second deals with the distance of the screen from the individual. Usually the distance of the screen is further than normal reading distance.

SEVEN POINT CHECKLIST

This seven point checklist can help to recognize and avoid the most common health problems (Box 1.7).

Contact stress: Contact stress refers to the pressure that is put on different parts of the body whilst in a relatively fixed position. Wrist and hand problems are common with computers. For example, 'floating' your hand over the mouse for long periods leads to strain on the ligaments in the back of the hand and the wrist. The sensation is not unlike gripping a pen for long periods. Leaning wrists against hard surfaces such as the edge of the desk leads to similar problems. Health problems may occur as a result of high repetition of hand movements, forceful typing, or having bent wrists whilst using the keyboard. Carpal tunnel syndrome is a painful condition that affects the wrists and hands following pressure to the median nerve. Numbness may also be experienced in one or both hands and even the simplest of tasks involving the hands becomes a painful and sometimes impossible activity. Attention to posture, light keyboard actions and mouse movement and simple regular exercise can help to prevent problems. If problems do arise it is important to stop and seek medical assistance. In extreme cases surgery may be required to relieve symptoms, but rest, coupled with remedial exercise, is the most likely medical intervention.

Organizing your work: Organizing your work can help prevent computer-related health problems. Think about the nature and pattern of your work. If you have to undertake repetitive tasks with the computer try, where possible, to vary these with other activities. Do not be tempted to sit at the computer during breaks

Box 1.7: Seven point checklist to recognize the most common health problems

C ontact stress
O rganisation
M onotony
P osture
U ncomfortable environment
T etchiness
E xercise

T etchiness: *Tetchy* bad-tempered and irritable (from old French *teche* 'blotch, fault')

(coffee and lunch breaks); much better to step out for some fresh air. Think carefully before accepting overtime or agreeing to take on extra work, or forcing the pace to try and finish the work you have. The more work you accept the more it may be assumed you can cope. There are times you may need to assert your rights in order to keep a balance in your life.

Computer monotony: Any task that involves staring at a computer screen, no matter how exciting or interesting, leads to physical fatigue. The most common physical complaints are eye strain and problems with vision (blurring and itching being typical). Headaches also occur due to prolonged staring at a screen. Remember to look away from the screen when you don't need to use it. Check that the light levels are comfortable and that you are not dealing with screen-reflected glare from windows or lighting. Some people find glare-reducing screens useful. If you experience repeated headaches you should visit your doctor.

Posture: Bad posture is enemy number one. You should be able to reach the keyboard and mouse whilst bending your elbows at 90 degrees, with your shoulders relaxed. If you are stretching, this could cause problems. Your back should be straight and the top of the monitor should be just below eye level. If your monitor is to the left or right of your keyboard you are putting strain on your neck. Long periods of time at the computer often lead to pain in the lumbar region of the back. Neck and shoulder problems also result from poor seating and the poor organization of equipment on the desk (stretching for the telephone or files, etc.).

Uncomfortable computer environments: Poor lighting levels or screening, poor air circulation, noise and equipment issues all contribute to an uncomfortable work setting. The attitude of colleagues affects the atmosphere of work. A good combination of environmental and relationship factors are necessary to help avoid stress.

Working with a computer a fact of life: Working for hr with a computer is now a fact of life. Whether it is an aspect of your work or whether you use computers just for fun, there are certain risks involved with prolonged computer use. The seven point checklist can help to recognize and avoid the most common health problems. Many people who spend part of their time in front of a computer screen suffer from visual and nonvisual problems. Some people do not have any problems. Both children and young adults and individuals using bifocals must discuss first with eye care professionals for symptoms.

Mathur GP, Khare V, Mathur S. Computer related health problems. In: Mathur GP, Mathur Sarla (eds). *Current Trends in Pediatrics*. Vol 3. Delhi: Academa Publishers, 2007; 457–61.

Olitsky SE, Hug D, Smith LP. Disorders of vision. In: Kliegman RM, Behrman RE, Jenson HB, Stanton BF (eds). *Nelson Textbook of Pediatrics*. 18th edn. Vol 2. Philadelphia: Saunders, 2007; 2573–76.

Raskin NH. Headache. In: Braunwald E, Fauci AS, Kasper DL, Hauser SL, Longo DL, Jameson JL (eds). *Harrison's Principles of Internal Medicine*. 15th edn. Vol I. New York: McGraw-Hill, 2001; 85–94.

1.5 MEDICAL ETHICS

The practice of medicine has been an art since ancient days. In the ancient days the physicians were supposed to maintain highest standard of professional conduct uninfluenced by motives of profit. The doctors were considered almost as God or an angel by the society. Keeping this in mind, the ethical guidelines were framed. The Hippocratic Oath, which is now almost 25 centuries old, was based on these basic principles of service to humanity. The medical ethics is not a mere academic exercise but affects routine patient care.

The present scenario: In today's world the circumstances have totally changed. The money power has resulted in soaring expectations. The respect for human life is decreasing. The relationship of faith and trust is changing into that of disbelief and hate relationship. The medicolegal cases are gradually increasing. The overall impact is that the doctor–patient relationship is in doldrums. The financial considerations are more important than the health of the patient and the honor and the traditions of medical profession.

Reasons for unethical acts: The increasing unethical practices in medical profession are multi-factorial in origin. Doctors have succumbed to the marketing practices of pharmaceutical companies; they accept commissions for referrals; have misused technologies for personal gain; have issued irrational prescriptions, etc.

Ethical dilemmas: There are many situations where physicians are in ethical dilemmas because of typical behavior of patients, relatives or colleagues, etc. As per the article 21 of Constitution of India every individual has his own life and he can lead it as per his own wishes within the framework of the law. Thus, not only ethically but also legally an individual has right to decide whether to live or not to live. Probably because of this only it is said that an individual can refuse any type of trial or treatment on his body. A doctor cannot force any treatment or clinical research trials on individuals against his/her will. The right to die has also been extensively discussed time and again.

The paradox is such that in one situation an individual is not interested in living because of chronic, untreatable, end-stage disease resulting in poor quality of life; but law and ethics says that any life cannot be terminated. As against this there are recommendations to give death penalty by injecting lethal drugs. These individuals are not interested in death; in fact they want to live. Should they be given another chance? The important ethical issue and dilemma in such situation is that, should a doctor get involved in killing an individual only because it has been ordered by law. Is it ethical for the physicians to get involved in **'Judicial killing'**? Can law ask doctors to do an unethical act? Why an individual then can't ask for "mercy killing" when he is not interested in living painful, poor quality life?

Another ethical consideration that is important is whether to divulge the secret information about the patient. Can we do this, especially with life-threatening diseases like malignancy, HIV, etc? There can be cases in consumer courts for hiding or revealing such **"double edged information"**.

One of the codes of conduct for doctors is not to use touts or agents for procuring patients. In today's commercialized practice, we come across not only the agents of doctors but also the increasing trends of "cut practice". The decline started when specialist began treating patient according to the dictates of the referring general practitioners. There are many general practitioners who survive only on the "referral fee" and accumulate a huge amount of money by way of commission. The very fact that the doctors who do not give or take 'cuts' are a minority nowadays speaks badly enough of our noble profession.

The effects of unethical practices: The influence of the pharmaceutical industry on the medical profession cannot be denied. There is definite increase in the cost of medicines, which must be borne by the patients. It often leads to the unscientific use of expensive, hazardous medicines. As a result, the profession is discredited. Patients have lost their faith in profession. The practitioner is seen as a trader, not as a professional. While technologies may have enhanced doctors' medical skills and capabilities, they lose out on clinical skills by becoming dependant on technology. Unfortunately, this dependence is governed by market pressures and not by scientific practice. Technology has become the means to make more money faster—more often than not, through its misuse. Sex selection and determination are classic examples of the unethical use of medical technology and knowledge. Sometimes unethical practice also gets involved in criminal activities as has happened in organ transplantations.

Tiwari SK. Legal aspects in medical practice. *Indian Pediatr* 2000;37:961–6.

Tiwari SK, Baldwa M. Medical negligence. In: Gupte S (Ed). *Recent Advances in Pediatrics*. New Delhi: Jaypee Brothers, 2004; 14:311–29.

Tiwari SK, Baldwa M. What is medical negligence. In: Baldwa M, Tiwari S, Shah N (eds). Legal problems in day-to-day pediatrics practice. 1st edn. Hyderabad: Paras Publishing, 2005;16–49.

1.6 SEX EDUCATION

Sex education means, learning, understanding, acquiring and implementing the knowledge related to sexual behavior and reproduction of living organisms. Thus, it automatically includes various issues related to natural or unnatural practice of sexual acts. The information regarding use of contraceptives, prevention of unwanted pregnancy, protection from STD's including HIV is imparted.

Spectrum/course material: The material may include:
a. Information related to human physiology, anatomy, growth and development, physical and mental changes during puberty, sexual intercourse, pregnancy, etc.
b. Issues related with relationships between friends, relatives and members of opposite sex. An insight that marital relationship is much more and beyond sexual relationship and also includes mental and emotional aspects.
c. Issues of personality development, exchange of thoughts, decision-making and to work with reasoning and responsibility.
d. Information regarding sexually transmitted diseases, contraceptive measures, HIV and AIDS, etc.
e. The course material should also include, information regarding sexual abuse, abstinence, when and how to "Say No".
f. The information related to our ancient cultural, religious, social and community thoughts, beliefs and concepts along with their importance in the present circumstances/scenario.

How to give: Sex education can be improved drastically by developing five approaches:
1. Targeted training and support for teachers
2. Peer-led sex education by teenagers
3. Story-based scenarios to promote applied learning
4. Local development of educational materials
5. Use of trained sexual health professionals to address learning needs of pupils, teachers, and parents.

The different methods of propagating the knowledge can be utilized like:
1. Organizing workshops for the beneficiaries,

2. Panel discussions with eminent experts in the field as panelist,
3. Question and Answer sessions,
4. Group Discussions,
5. Actual training or demonstration from flip charts, posters, booklets, and
6. Establishing "Teen Clubs" or "Teen Clinics".

Role of parents: The parents must take interest and help the adolescents specially when there is crisis. The parents must answer child's sex related queries using simple language, which the child can understand. There is no need to get embarrassed while satisfying child's curiosity. The mothers should be friendly with girls in and around puberty so as to explain the physical and emotional changes in her daughter. The mother must be secure and confident of her own femininity.

Tiwari SK, Chaturvedi P. Adolescent Sexuality; In: Gupte S (editor) Recent advances (vol.15) New Delhi, Jaypee Brothers 2005; 400–17.

1.7 LEGAL ISSUES IN PEDIATRIC PRACTICE

In this era where the doctors are becoming specialist and super specialist, the medical faculty has evolved from noble profession to commercial profession. There have been many turbulent changes in the society. This has not spared even doctor–patient relationship. These rapid changes in the medical field have even strained the age-old good relations between the patient and the treating physician or surgeon. In today's situation this relationship is strained resulting in increasing number of legal problems. Bringing the doctors under the ambit of Consumer Protection Act has further marginalized this relationship. The legal cases of medical negligence are rising because of the ease with which cases can be launched in consumer court. A doctor should treat the patient to the best of his knowledge, skill, care and judgment.

What is pediatric age? There is no statutory or legal age limit of child/adolescence. The word "Child" has not been defined precisely either in the constitution or the General Clauses Act. This word is not identical with the word "minor". The definitions vary from Acts to Acts. According to Indian Majority Act, 1875 a child means 18 yr unless it falls in the category of specified exceptional case, in which case it is 21 yr. According to The Children Act, 1960 a child means a boy who has not attained the age of 16 yr or a girl who has not attained the age of 18 yr. The Indian Academy of Pediatrics recommends that a pediatrician should continue to examine and treat children upto 18 yr of age. According to American Academy of Pediatrics, adolescent means up to 10–19 yr of age.

Who is pediatrician? A Pediatrician or "Child Specialist" means a doctor who has specialized in managing a child. As per the Indian Medical Council (Professional conduct, Etiquette and Ethics) Regulation, April 2002; the Clause 7.20 says that, a physician shall not claim to be specialist unless he has a special qualification in that branch. According to, Supreme Court (Poonam Varma v. Ashwin Patel; AIR 1996 SC 2111), the **right to practice**, in any particular system of medicine, is dependant upon registration which is permissible only if qualification, and that too, a recognized qualification, is possessed by a person in that system. A person who does not have knowledge of a particular system of medicine but practices in that system is **a quack** and a mere pretender to medical knowledge or skill, or to put it differently, a charlatan. Supreme Court in its various other judgments had made it clear that the medical practitioners should practice within the scope of ones qualifications and skills.

Dos in pediatric practice?. We must accept the changes and challenges in the practice of medicine. Do right things and have a clear conscience. Communicate in compassionate and sensitive way with the patient or relatives. Finances and bills should be explained properly. Maintain proper records including refusals for investigations or treatment. Attend regularly and personally, whether a patient or a case in CPA. Take due cognizance and reply in time. Inform the insurance company. Continue follow-up treatment of the patient. Take the help of a legal, medicolegal expert while filing the reply. Produce affidavits of colleagues and ask for expert witness whenever necessary. Give references relevant to case and demand cross-examination. Update not only your knowledge and skill but also that of your staff. Update the facilities and instruments. Attend workshops, conferences, CMEs, etc. Stay calm; avoid surprises, anger, panic and self-doubt. Inform police whenever necessary. Have a valid informed consent for the treatment. Preserve the documents, records especially in medicolegal, controversial or complicated cases. Give guarded prognosis. Adjust the doses of drugs according to weight especially in children with renal/hepatic disorders. The pathological or radiological tests shall be advised in writing. Insist for post-mortem examination if the cause of death cannot be ascertained. Record the history of drug allergy. If the patient was examined hurriedly, ask him to come for review next day. If the diagnosis is not confirmed, mention **"diagnosis under review"**. Explain treatment modalities whenever required especially in complicated cases. Give/write instructions in comprehensive local language. In case of any deviation from standard practice, mention the reasons. When you are not sure, consult your senior, colleague or specialist. Refer to higher center whenever necessary.

Don'ts for pediatricians. Do not ignore or disrespect the courts. Neglect your duties as doctor. Volunteer to handover the documents unless specifically asked for. Rely entirely on your advocates. Give unnecessary details. Get panicky or frightened simply because there is case in consumer forum. Use vague or nonspecific terminology. Behave in a rude, rough or inhuman manner. Avoid communicating with patients or relatives. Hesitate in consulting your senior or colleagues especially in difficult cases. Over-prescribe or under-prescribe. Do not prescribe without examining the patient. Do not accept substitutes. Exceed your level of competence or field of specialization. Do not be overconfident. Talk lose about your colleagues, may be that you would have done same thing at that moment making an error of judgment. You never know under what circumstances this had happened. Manipulate or tamper with the documents. Do unlawful or unethical acts. Experiment with patients. Issue false or bogus certificates. Certificate was issued on request is no defense. Neglect the treatment while completing legal formalities especially in serious or emergency situation. Do not allow modern diagnostic tests to substitute your clinical acumen. Over investigate.

Tiwari S K. Legal aspects in medical practice. *Indian Pediatr* 2000; 37: 961–6.

Tiwari SK, Baldwa M. Medical Negligence. *Indian Pediatr* 2001; 38: 488–95.

Tiwari SK, Baldwa M. Doctors and Criminal Law. *Indian Pediatr* 2002; 39:1119–25.

1.8 GUIDING PEDIATRICIANS IN CHILD CARE

The art of medicine has gradually became medical science and ultimately ended in commerce. The age-old doctor–patient relationship is gradually becoming a buyer–seller relationship. This has not only prompted the Government, but also legal luminaries to bring the medical service under Consumer Protection Act, thus giving a legal sanction to commercialization of health services. This has resulted in gradually increasing legal tussles/battles between patients and the doctors/hospitals. Hence, we have to be very careful, vigilant and updated in our practice.

Establishment of clinic/hospital: Establishment of clinic/hospital is like dream come true for any medical graduate after a lengthy and hectic medical curriculum. The clinic/hospital must be neat, clean, tidy and well-equipped as per the need of the patient.

Communication skills: The communication skills that are learned in medical schools and that are practiced throughout a medical career go a long way in facilitating the excellent care of the patient throughout the length of the doctor–patient relationship.

Doctor–patient relationship: A healthy ongoing doctor–patient relationship based on mutual trust is vital for providing effective and quality patient care.

Quality care: The quality care is not synonymous with costly care. Quality means identifying and completely satisfying customers needs profitably. It means, doing it right, the first time and every time.

Duties of doctors: Every doctor has some basic things to do as he approaches a patient. He must *listen* to patient (take proper history) and *examine* him carefully. A doctor has to *attend* the patient and give *diligent care*, once he decides to treat the patient. He must *explain* the relevant facts related to the illness and give *proper medicines*. Doctors must have average, recent *knowledge and equipment's* in possession, as per his specialty. The practitioners must be able to *foresee* the complications and *refer* the patient at proper time. Some of the illnesses are self-limiting, while others are progressive. Some of the illnesses have mild progression while others have fulminant course irrespective of treatment. Hence, in any illness doctors should have foreseeability. The treating doctor must be able *to foresee* common complications, diagnose and treat them at proper time. If the doctor misses this it may amount to negligence. If the complications are too remote then it is not negligence. Doctors must maintain a proper *record* of their patients.

Rights of doctors: As doctors have duties, they also have some rights. A doctor has right to *turn away* a patient before starting treatment but he should provide minimal basic care especially in emergency. He has a right to select *the drugs* from wide range of options available, supported by standard medical practice. A doctor can select *the investigations and method of treatment* depending upon various factors and obtain written refusal in case patient does not want to do as advised. He *can delegate* the powers to properly trained personals or colleagues, usually with the willingness of patient. The better alternative to the practitioners is to start group practice so that one of the regular consultants is always available. Doctor can decide regarding *visits, fees* to be charged, etc. and to maintain the patient's *record* including its secrecy in certain specific situations.

History taking and examination: The duty or care starts with proper listening to patient's history. Once the history is over the attending doctor must carefully examine the patient for various signs related to the suspected diagnosis. Missing of important signs may itself result in wrong or missed diagnosis ultimately resulting in improper treatment.

Sometimes the diseases (metabolic, genetic) are so uncommon or their manifestations are so atypical that it is really very difficult to diagnose them with routinely available facilities or investigations. It is always better to refer cases to higher center where the rare and latest investigations may be done to confirm the diagnosis.

Telephonic consultations: It is a common practice to advice treatment on phone. It is better to avoid telephonic consultations. The doctors can collaborate with colleagues nationally and internationally. This may create legal implications in the future.

Investigations: If it is not possible to diagnose the illness clinically, help of investigations should be taken. Those investigations, which are necessary according to the presenting symptoms and signs, must be advised. Do not advice unnecessary investigations. If patient does not do the suggested investigations, this becomes a contributory negligence on the part of the patient or relatives.

Diagnosis of the complications: Some of the illnesses are self-limiting, while others are progressive. Some of the illnesses have mild progression while others have fulminant course irrespective of treatment. Hence, in any illness doctors should have foreseeability. If the doctor misses this it may amount to negligence. If the complications are too remote then it is not negligence.

Rational drug therapy: The importance of rational drug therapy is widely accepted in practice of medicine. A doctor must use his knowledge and qualification in managing a patient with minimal drugs. As a qualified pediatrician we must prevent the misuse of antibiotics, multivitamins, steroids, artificial and commercial foods/breast milk substitutes, etc. There is need for following evidence-based standard protocols.

Delegation of duties: A doctor can delegate his duties to a qualified and competent junior, assistant, partner, nursing staff or laboratory assistant. In such situation it is the responsibility of the person to whom the duty was delegated. The person delegating the duty cannot be held negligent if something untoward happens. If the staff to whom, the duty is delegated is unqualified or incompetent, then it is the liability of the doctor delegating such duty. If the qualified staff makes a mistake then the doctor may not be held directly responsible.

Special situations: One needs to respond to the parent's/patient's expression about their illness in a concerned and respectful way. Most of aggrieved patients complain that they were never given time to explain their problems and things were not explained to them in a proper manner. The pediatrician should be an educator about disease, death and grief.

a. *Diagnosis in emergency situation:* In the practice of medicine, many times we have to tackle the emergency situation. In such situation the clinical features may not be very obvious to suggest a particular diagnosis. Proper history may not be available especially if the patient is unconscious or distressed. At the same time, sufficient time may not be there to go in for investigations.

b. *Serious patient:* In pediatric practice one has to learn and manage parents in addition to managing a child patient. The condition of the child should be explained in simple language. Use the words cautiously, as the parents may hang onto the words subsequently. Deliver the news preferably with a loved one or family member. Explain in detail the disease process. The prognosis should be guarded and the statements shall be balanced. A hint about the seriousness and probable outcome may be offered. The pediatrician should avoid giving estimates of survival lengths, even when these are explicitly asked for. The more serious the illness and not improving, the more we must talk to parents. Be as reassuring and effective as possible. Respond to the parent's/patient's emotions of anger and grief with empathy. Reassure them that you welcome a second opinion. Refrain from picking faults with our colleagues or their treatment.

c. *Death of a child:* Somebody has rightly said, that if we lose the parent, the past is lost, if we lose a spouse, the present is lost, but if we lose a child then the future is lost. Hence, it is one of the devastating experiences in the life of any parent and needs lot of emotional support. Preferably, the information should be delivered by, a senior person responsible for the care of the child. It is beneficial to inform 2–3 close relatives if available. Do not announce the death suddenly. Inform that the child is deteriorating and we are doing our best (for about half to one hour). Try to ensure and offer help to ease the situation.

Consent: The consent is obtained after explanation and reasonable understanding of facts and not by hiding facts or misrepresentation of facts. Consent should be taken in writing. The consent should preferably be taken in presence of witnesses (two from patient side and two from hospital side). Sometimes a child is brought to pediatricians by neighbors (parents of child are immediately not available for consent). In such situations if it is genuine and real emergency, the child can be managed even without consent. The neighbor's consent cannot have legal validity.

Documents: Documents are the property of hospitals and should be produced on written requests only. Documents are confidential of patients and should be released with his consent. A well-maintained document may be helpful in most of the cases of negligence. Documents should be: Clean, Complete, Chronological, Comprehensive, and Correct and without manipulations.

Ethical issues in practice: So as to maintain purity and sanctity of the art of healing, the Fathers of Medicine had laid down a code of conduct for the physicians. These ethical guidelines were framed keeping in mind that the art of healing is a mission for service in human life. The physicians must work with nobility and dignity for the welfare of human beings. The purity in life as well as in medical profession was of utmost importance. The aim was "never do harm to anyone". The painful paradox is that, in today's lavishing health care, we may also be exposing the patients to a potential hazard. Many irrational drugs or drug combinations are pumped in pharmaceutical market. Nevertheless, the ethical duty of a physician is to promote the patient's best interests.

Health education programs: The medical practitioners must actively participate in various health education programs (nutritional programs, programs on immunization) to control and prevent disease related morbidity and mortality in children. The various government, semi-government and NGOs can be involved in such health education programs.

Group practice: It is difficult for us to find time in discharging our family, social and other such liabilities. Hence, need of the hour is to start group practice. The advantages of group practice includes:

a. Duty can be delegated to equally competent colleagues.
b. The "second opinion" is easily available.
c. Different sub-specialties may be developed under one roof.

d. Need for referral is decreased.
e. Decreases the stress and strain of managing a hospital.
f. Scientific and academic knowledge can be updated regularly.

Professional insurance: Indemnity means 'to make good the loss sustained by the insurer'. The doctor's indemnity policy provides insurance protection to the doctors against their legal liability to pay damages arising out of their negligence in the performance of professional duties. The insured includes the policy-holder and his qualified assistants or employees named in the proposal. The professional indemnity may not protect from legal problems but it may turn out to be a protector for financial losses. Thus, it gives mental peace over and above financial relief. While signing a contract for professional indemnity, hospital insurance or risk management one must read in between the lines.

If there is a case in Consumer Court: Take due cognizance of the case and give reply in time. Try to explain misunderstandings, misrepresentation in written statement. Attend personally with or without your lawyer. The answers should be brief, clear and comprehensive. Produce affidavits of colleagues and ask for expert's witness whenever necessary. Give references relevant to the case and demand cross-examination. As far as possible always ask for counter compensation. Do not ignore or disrespect court.

What to do?

Do right things rather than doing things rightly. For sound sleep no pillow is as soft as a clear conscious. Follow and adhere to morality and natural rules and various laws. Have a good rapport with patients, their relatives and others. Update your knowledge regarding recent developments, research, instruments, etc. Fight for your rights.

Liben S, Pediatric Palliative Care: The care of Children with Life-limiting Illness. In: Behrman RE, Kliegman RM, Jenson HB (eds). *Nelson Textbook of Pediatrics.* 17th edn. Philadelphia: Saunders, 2004; 143–8.

2 ◆ Growth and Development

2.1 INTRODUCTION

The understanding of growth and development helps to monitor children's progress, to identify delays or abnormalities in development and to counsel parents and prescribe treatment. By monitoring children and families, one can also observe the inter-relationship between physical growth and cognitive, motor and emotional development. Growth means an increase in mass of protoplasm brought about by an increase in size of individual cells, an increase in number of cells or both. Growth is a process rather than a static quality. Development means gradual change from lower to a higher state. It specifies maturation of functions. In the process of the growth and development in children virtually every organ and physiologic process undergoes a predictable sequence of structural and functional changes, or both, which makes the science different till he/she attends adulthood. By monitoring children and families over time, pediatricians have the unique opportunity to observe how the process of growth and development are interrelated: the enlargement of head, trunk, and limbs; the progressive increases in strength and ability to control large and small muscles; the development of social relatedness, thought, and language; and the emergence of personality. The growth and development from conception to adolescence can be arbitrarily divided into eight stages as follows:

1. *Before birth:*
   • Embryonic period, and
   • Fetal period
2. *Afterbirth:*
   • Newborn

   • First year
   • Second year
   • Preschool years (2–5 yrs)
   • Middle childhood (6–11 yrs)
   • Adolescence (10–20 yrs).

Factors that Influence Growth and Development

Development is not solely determined by the intrinsic (genetics) and extrinsic (environment) factors, though they play important role in the development of the child. Height, for example, is a function of a child's genetic environment (biologic), personal habits of eating (psychologic), and access to nutritious food (social). Biologic, psychologic, and social factors combine to shape development and will be discussed separately to understand each class of influence separately.

a. *Biologic influences:* Biological influences on development include genetics, *in utero* exposure to teratogens, postpartum illnesses, exposure to hazardous substances and maturation.
   1. Heredity accounts for half of the variance in IQ and in other personality traits such as sociability and desire for novelty.
   2. Prenatal exposure to teratogens such as mercury and alcohol effects on development. High level of ingestion of alcohol during pregnancy will result in fetal alcohol syndrome including deficiency of length, weight and head circumference, facial abnormalities, cardiac defects (primarily septal defects), joint and limb abnormalities, delayed development and mental retardation.

3. Postpartum illnesses such as meningitis and traumatic brain injury and exposure to hazardous substances affect growth and development.

4. Chronic illness can affect growth and development either directly or through changes in parenting or peer experiences.

5. Physical and neurologic maturation propels children forward and sets lower limits for the emergence of most abilities. The age at which children walk independently is similar around the world, despite differences in child rearing practices.

6. Maturation brings about hormonal changes in addition to physical changes in size, body proportions, and strength. Sexual differentiation both somatic and neurologic begins *in utero*. Behavioral effects of testosterone may be evident in young children and continue to be salient throughout life.

7. Temperament refers to a child's characteristic style of responding, and is clinically useful in two ways. First, it can help parents understand and accept the characteristics of their children without feeling responsible for having caused them. Second, behavioral and emotional problems often develop when there is conflict between temperamental characteristics of children and parents.

b. *Psychological influences:* During first year of life 'basic trust' is established through the mother's consistent responsiveness to her child's needs. Children progress optimally at all stages of development when they have adult caregivers pay attention to their verbal and nonverbal cues and respond accordingly.

c. *Social factors* include mother and other caregivers, family system, and birth order have influence on the development of the child.

d. *Unifying concepts:* Interaction between biologic and social factors influences growth and development of the child. Children growing up in poverty are in double developmental jeopardy, because of increased exposure to biologic risk factors such as environmental lead and undernutrition, and decreased access to corrective educational and therapeutic experiences.

Needlman RD. Growth and development. In: Behrman RE, Kliegman RM, Jenson HB (eds). *Nelson Textbook of Pediatrics.* 17th edn. Philadelphia: Saunders, 2004; 23–27.

2.2 FETAL GROWTH AND DEVELOPMENT

Most events in growth and development occur before birth. In this period there is transformation of fertilized egg into embryo and fetus, the elaboration of the nervous system, and the emergence of behavior in utero. In addition to that psychologic changes occur in the parents during the period of gestation. The uterus is permeable to adverse social and environmental influences such as maternal undernutrition; alcohol and cigarette, and drug use; and perhaps psychologic trauma. The complex interplays between these forces and the somatic and neurologic transformations occurring in the fetus influences infant behavior at birth and may affect parent child interactions throughout infancy. Milestones of prenatal development are documented in Table 2.1.

Somatic development: Intrauterine life is divided into two periods: embryonic and fetal.

Embryonic period: By 6 days postconceptual age, as implantation begins, the embryo consists of a spherical mass of cells with a central cavity, the blastocyst. By 2 wk, implantation is complete and the uteroplacentral circulation has begun; the embryo has two distinct layers, ectoderm and endoderm, and amnion has begun to form. By 3 wk, the third primary germ layer (mesoderm) has appeared, along with primitive neural tube and blood vessels. Paired heart tubes have begun to pump. During 4–8 wk, lateral folding of the embryologic plate, followed by growth at the cranial and caudal ends and the budding of arms and legs, produces a human-like shape. Precursors of skeletal muscle and vertebrae (somites) appear, along with the branchial arches that will form the mandible, maxilla, palate, external ear, and other head and neck structures. Lens placodes appear, marking the site of future eyes; the brain grows rapidly. By the end of 8 wk, as the embryonic period closes, the rudiments of all major organ systems have developed; the average embryo weighs 9 g and has a crown-rump length of 5 cm.

Fetal period: The fetal period begins from the 9th wk. Fetal somatic changes consist of increases in cell number and size and structural remodeling of several organ systems. By 10 wk the face is recognizably human. The midgut returns from the umbilical cord into the abdomen, rotating counterclockwise to bring the stomach, small intestine, and large intestine into their normal positions. By 12 wks, the gender of the external genitals becomes clearly distinguishable. Lung development proceeds with the budding of bronchi, bronchioles, and successively smaller divisions. By 20–24 wk, primitive alveoli have formed and surfactant production has begun; before that time, the absence of alveoli renders the lungs useless as organs of gas exchange. The usual lower limit of viability is 20 wk; weight 460 g; length 19 cm.

Table 2.1: Milestones of prenatal development	
Week	Developmental events
1	Fertilization and implantation: Beginning of *embryonic period*
2	Endoderm and ectoderm appear bilaminar embryo
3	First missed menstrual period; mesoderm appears trilaminar embryo; somites begin to form
4	Neural folds fuse; folding of embryo into human-like shape; arm and leg buds appear; crown-rump length 4–5 mm
5	Lens placodes, primitive mouth, digital rays on hands
6	Primitive nose, philtrum, primary palate; crown-rump length 21–23 mm
7	Eyelids begin
8	Ovaries and testes distinguishable
9	*Fetal period* begins; crown-rump length 5 cm; weight 9 g
10	External genitals distinguishable
20	Usual lower limit of viability; weight 460 g; length 19 cm
25	*Third trimester* begins; weight 900 g; length 25 cm
28	Eyes open; fetus turns head down; weight 1300 g
38	Term

The third trimester begins 25 wk. During the third trimester, weight triples and length doubles as body stores of protein, fat, iron and calcium increase.

Neurologic development: During the third week, a neural plate appears on the ectodermal surface of the trilaminar embryo. Infolding produces a neural tube that will become the central nervous system (CNS) and a neural crest that will become the peripheral nervous system. Neuroectodermal cells differentiate into neurons, astrocytes, oligodendrocytes and ependymal cells, whereas microglial cells are derived from mesoderm. By the 5th wk, the three main subdivisions of forebrain, midbrain, and hindbrain are evident. The dorsal and ventral horns of the spinal cord have begun to form, along with the peripheral motor and sensory nerves. Myelinization begins at midgestation and continues throughout the 1st yr of life. By the end of embryonic period (wk 8), the gross structure of the nervous system has been established. On a cellular level, the growth of axons and dendrites and the elaboration of synaptic connections continue at a rapid pace, making the CNS vulnerable to teratogenic or hypoxic influences.

Behavioral development: Muscle contractions first appear around 8 wk, soon followed by lateral flexion movements. By 13–14 wk, breathing and swallowing motions appear and tactile stimulation elicits graceful movements. The grasp reflex appears at 17 wk and is well developed by 27 wk. Eye opening occurs around 26 wk. By midgestation, the full range of neonatal movements can be observed. During the third trimester, fetuses respond to external stimuli with heart rate elevation and body movements. As with infants in the postnatal period, reactivity to auditory (vibroacoustic) and visual (bright light) stimuli vary depending on their behavioral state, which can be characterized as quiet sleep, active sleep, and awake. Individual differences in the level of fetal activity are commonly noted by mothers and have been observed ultrasonographically. Fetal behavior is affected by maternal medications and diet, increasing, for example, after ingestion of caffeine and may be entrained to the mother's diurnal rhythms.

Fetal movement increases in response to a sudden auditory tone, but decreases after several repetitions (habituation). If the tone changes in pitch, the movement increases again, this indicates that the fetus distinguishes between a familiar repeated tone and a novel one. The ability to habituate to repeated stimuli, a form of learning, is diminished in neurologically impaired or physically stressed fetuses. Similar responses to visual and tactile stimuli have been observed.

Psychologic changes in parents: The psychologic changes during pregnancy fall roughly into three stages. Stage 1 begins when a woman first learns that she is pregnant. Ambivalent feelings are the norm, whether or not the pregnancy was planned. Elation at the thought of producing a baby and the wish to be the perfect parent compete with fears of inadequacy and of the lifestyle changes that mothering will impose. The father-to-be faces also similar mixed feelings. Stage 2 begins with awareness of fetal movements, or quickening, at approximately 20 wk or earlier with ultrasonic visualization. The evidence that a fetus exists as a separate being often heightens a woman's feelings, both positive and negative. Parents worry about the fetus's healthy development and mentally normal. What they will do if the child is malformed? Reassurances based on ultrasonic examination or amniocentesis may not completely allay their fears, especially if they had an earlier malformed child. During stage 3, toward the end of pregnancy, a woman becomes aware of patterns of fetal activity and reactivity and begins to ascribe to her fetus an individual personality and an ability to survive independently.

Threats to fetal development: Mortality and morbidity are highest during the prenatal period. Some 30% of pregnancies end in spontaneous abortion, most often during the 1st trimester as a result of chromosomal or other abnormalities. Major congenital malformations requiring neonatal surgical intervention occur in approximately 2% of live births. Teratogens associated with gross physical and mental abnormalities include various infectious agents (toxoplasmosis, rubella, syphilis), chemical agents (mercury, thalidomide, antiepileptic medications, and ethanol), high temperature, and radiation.

2.3 THE NEWBORN (FIRST 28 DAYS AFTERBIRTH)

The newborn (neonatal) period begins at birth and includes 1st 28 days of life. The biologic and psychologic challenges facing neonates and their parents consist of establishing effective feeding routines, a predictable sleep-wake cycle and foundation for cognitive and emotional development.

Physical development: The weight of newborn infant may decrease 10% below birth weight in the first week as a result of excretion of excess extravascular fluid and possibly poor intake. Intake improves as colostrum is replaced by higher-fat milk, as infant learns to latch on and suck more efficiently, and as mothers become more comfortable with feeding techniques. Skin-to-skin contact between mothers and infants immediately afterbirth may correlate with an increased rate and longer duration of breastfeeding. Infant should regain or exceed birth weight by 2 wks age and should grow at approximately 30 g (1 oz)/day during first month.

Parenting: Parenting a newborn infant requires dedication because a newborn needs is urgent, continuous, and often unclear. Parents must attend to an infant's signals and respond emphatically. Success or failure in establishing feeding and sleep cycles determines parent's feelings of efficacy.

Interactional abilities: Soon afterbirth, neonates are alert and ready to interact and nurse. This first alert-awake period may be affected by maternal analgesics and anesthetics or fetal hypoxia. Nearsighted neonates have a fixed focal length of 8–12 inches, approximately the distance from the breast to mother's face, as well as an inborn visual preference for faces. Hearing is well developed, and infants preferentially turn toward

a female voice. These innate abilities and predictions increase the likelihood that when a mother gazes at her newborn, the baby will gaze back. The initial period of social interaction, usually lasting about 40 minutes, is followed by a period of somnolence. After that, briefer periods of alertness or excitation alternate with sleep. If a mother misses her baby's first alert-awake period, she may not experience as long a period of social interaction for several days.

Adaptation to extrauterine life: Adaptation to extrauterine life requires rapid and profound psychologic changes, including aeration of the lungs, rerouting of the circulation, and activation of the intestinal tract. To obtain nourishment, to avoid hypo- and hyperthermia, and to ensure safety, neonates react appropriately to sensory stimuli.

Underaroused infants are not able to feed and interact; overaroused infants show signs of autonomic instability, including flushing or mottling, perioral pallor, hiccupping, vomiting, uncontrolled limb movements, or inconsolable crying.

Behavioral states: Six behavioral states have been described which regulate arousal: quiet sleep, active sleep, drowsy, alert, fussy, and crying. In the alert state, infants visually fixate on objects or faces and follow them horizontally and (within a month) vertically; they also reliably turn toward a novel sound, as if searching for its source. When overstimulated they may calm themselves by looking away, yawning, or sucking on their lips or hands, thereby increasing parasympathetic activity and reducing sympathetic nervous activity. The behavioral state determines an infant's muscle tone, spontaneous movement, electroencephalogram pattern, and response to stimuli. In active sleep, for example, an infant may show progressively less reaction to a repeated heel prick (habituation), whereas in the drowsy state the same stimulus may push a child into fussing or crying.

Parents and infant mutual regulation: Parents actively participate in an infant's behavioral state regulation, alternately stimulating or soothing with the goal of prolonging the social interaction. In turn, the parents are regulated by the infant's signals, for example, responding to cries of hunger with a let down of milk (or with a bottle). Such interactions constitute a system directed toward furthering the infant's physiologic homeostasis and physical growth. At the same time, they form the basis for the emerging psychologic relationship between parent and child. Infants in the presence of the parent are associated with the pleasurable reduction of tension (as in feeding) and show this preference by calming more quickly for their mother than for a stranger.

The physician's role: Pediatric interventions to support healthy newborn development include (i) promoting optimal medical practices before, during, and after delivery; (ii) assessing parent–infant interactions; and (iii) teaching parents about their newborn's individual competencies and vulnerabilities.

2.4 THE FIRST YEAR (INFANT)

The physical growth, maturation, acquisition of competence, and psychologic reorganization occur in discontinuous (not continuous; interrupted) bursts. Physical growth parameters and normal ranges for attainable weight, length/height and head circumference can be estimated as noted in Tables 2.2 and 2.3. At about 2 mo, the emergence of voluntary (social) smiles and increasing eye contact mark a change in the parent–child relationship. Between 3 and 4 mo, the rate of growth slows to approximately 20 g/day. Early reflexes that limited voluntary movements recede. Disappearance of the asymmetric tonic neck reflex means that infants can begin to examine objects in the midline and manipulate them with both hands. Waning of the grasp reflex allows them both to hold objects and voluntarily to let them go. Increasing control of truncal flexion makes intentional rolling possible. Increasing control of the physical growth during this period is rapid; growth is rapid during first month, but slows after 6 mo. Children acquire new competences in the gross motor, fine motor, cognitive and emotional domains. Tables 2.4 to 2.7 present an overview of key developmental milestones arranged cross-sectionally. Complex skills build on simpler ones, and development in each domain affects functioning in all of the others. Due to increasing mobility and exploration of inanimate world during 6–12 mo there are advances in cognitive understanding and communicative competence and new tensions in response of attachment and separation. The ability to sit unsupported (about 7 mo) and to pivot while sitting (around 9–10 mo) provides increasing opportunity to manipulate several objects at a time. These explorations are aided by the emergence of a pincer grasp (around 9 mo). Many infants begin crawling and pulling to stand around 8 mo and walk before their first birthday either independently or in a walker. Motor achievements correlate with increasing myelinization and cerebellar growth. Tooth eruption occurs, usually starting with the mandibular central incisors. Tooth development also reflects in part skeletal maturation.

Total sleep requirements are approximately 14–16 hr/24 hrs, with about 9–10 hrs concentrated sleep at night; about 70% of infants sleep for a 6 to 8 hr stretch by age 6 mo. By 4–6 mo, the sleep electroencephalogram shows a mature pattern. However, the sleep cycle remains shorter than in adults (50–60 minutes, versus approximately 90). As a result, infants arouse to light sleep or wake frequently during the night.

Infants' wariness of strangers often makes the 9 mo examination difficult, particularly if the infant is temperamentally prone to react negatively to unfamiliar situations. Initially, the pediatrician should avoid direct eye contact with the child. Time spent talking with the parent and introducing the child to a small toy (washable toy) will make the child comfortable and will allow examination. When feasible, the examination can be continued on the parent's lap.

2.5 THE SECOND YEAR (TODDLER)

The growth and development of second year is discussed in 12–18 mo and 18–24 mo old children.

Table 2.2: Formulas for appropriate average height and weight of normal infants and children

Weight	Kilograms	(Pounds)
At birth	3.25	(7)
3–12 mo	age (mo) + 9/2	(age [month] + 11)
1–6 yrs	age (year) × 2 + 8	(age [year] × 5 + 17)
7–12 yrs	age (year) × 7 – 5/2	(age [year] × 7 + 5)
Height	*Centimeters*	*(Inches)*
At birth	50	(20)
At 1 yr	75	(30)
2–12 yrs	age (year) × 6 + 77	(age [year] × 2½ +30)

Table 2.3: Growth and caloric requirements

Age	Approx. daily weight gain (g)	Approx. monthly weight gain	Growth in length (cm/month)	Growth in head (cm/month) circumference	Recommended daily allowance (kcal/kg/day)
0–3 mo	30	2 lb	3.5	2.00	115
3–6 mo	20	1¼ lb	2.0	1.00	110
6–9 mo	15	1 lb	1.5	0.50	100
9–12	12	13 oz	1.2	0.50	100
1–3 yrs	8	8 oz	1.0	0.25	100
4–6 yrs	6	6 oz	3 cm/yrs	1 cm/yrs	90–100

1 lb = 16 oz; 1 oz = 30 g; 1 kg = 2.2 lb

Table 2.4: Developmental milestones (gross motor) during the 1st year of life and from 1 to 5 yrs of age	
Age week/month	*Developmental milestones (gross motor)*
1st 4 wks	Supine: generally flexed and a little stiff; Prone: lies in flexed attitude; turns head from side to side; head sags on ventral suspension; Reflex: Moro response active; stepping and placing reflexes
At 4 wk	Supine: tonic neck posture predominates (extension of the arm corresponding to the side of the face, while flexion develops in the contralateral extremities); head lags on pull to sitting position; Prone: legs more extended; holds chin up; turns head; head lifted momentarily to plane of body on ventral suspension
At 8 wk	Supine: tonic neck posture predominates; head lags on pull to sitting position; Prone: raises head slightly farther; head sustained in plane of body on ventral suspension
At 12 wk	Supine: tonic neck posture predominates; reaches toward and misses objects; waves at toy; Prone: lifts head and chest, arms extended; head above plane of body on ventral suspension; Sitting: head lag partially compensated on pull to sitting position; early head control with bobbing motion; back rounded; Reflex: typical Moro response has not persisted; makes defensive movements or selective withdrawal reactions
At 16 wk	Supine: symmetric posture predominates; hands in midline; reaches and grasps objects and brings them to mouth; Prone: lifts head and chest, head in approximately vertical axis; legs extended; Sitting: no head lag on pull to sitting position; head steady, tipped forward; enjoys sitting with full truncal support; Standing: when held erect, pushes with feet
At 28 wk	Supine: lifts head; rolls over; squirming movements; Prone: rolls over; pivots; crawls or creep-crawls (knobloch); Sitting: sits briefly, with support of pelvis; leans forward on hands; back rounded; Standing: may support most of weight; bounces actively
At 40 wk (approx. 9 mo)	Sits up alone and indefinitely without support, back straight; pulls to standing position; "cruises" or walks holding on to furniture; creeps or crawls
At 52 wk (12 mo, 1 yr)	Walks with one hand held (48-wk); rises independently; takes several steps
15 mo	Walks alone; crawls up stairs
18 mo	Runs stiffly; sits on small chair; walks upstairs with one hand held; explores drawers and wastebaskets
24 mo	Runs well; walks up and down stairs, one steps at a time; opens doors; climbs on furniture; jumps
30 mo	Goes up stairs alternating feet
36 mo	Rides tricycle; stands momentarily on one foot
48 mo	Hops on one foot; throws ball overhead; uses scissors to cut out pictures; climbs well
60 mo	Skips

Moro reflex: An infant symmetrically abducts and extends the arms and flexes the thumbs, followed by flexion and adduction of upper extremities

Age 12–18 mo: The growth rate slows further in the second year of life and appetite declines. "Baby fat" is decreased because of increased mobility. The abdomen is protuberant due to exaggerated lumbar lordosis. Brain growth continues, with myelinization throughout the second year. Most children begin to walk independently near their first birth day; some do not walk up to 15 mo. Early walking is not associated with advanced development in other domains. At first, infants toddle with a wide-based gait, knees bent, and arms flexed at the elbow; the entire torso rotates with each stride; the toes may point in or out, and the feet strike the floor flat. As toddlers master reaching, grasping, and releasing, and greater mobility gives them access to more and more objects, exploration increases. Parents who cannot recall any other milestone tend to remember when their child begins to walk, perhaps because the symbolic significance of walking as an act of independence. Receptive language precedes expressive. After acquiring a vocabulary of about 50 words, toddlers begin to combine them to make simple sentences.

Parents may express concern about poor intake as growth slows. The growth chart should provide reassurance.

Age 18–24 mo: Motor development is incremental at this age, with improvement in balance and agility and the emergence of running and stair climbing. Height and weight increase at a steady rate, although head growth slows slightly. Toddlers demonstrate flexibility in problem solving, for example, using a stick to obtain a toy out of reach, or figuring out how to wind a mechanical toy. Separations at bed time are often difficult, with frequent tantrums. Many children use

Table 2.5: Developmental milestones (fine motor and vision) during the 1st year of life and from 1 to 5 year of age

Age week/month	Developmental milestones (fine motor and vision)
1st 4 wks	Reflex: grasp reflex active
At 1 wk	–
At 8 wk	–
At 12 wk	Supine: reaches toward and misses objects; waves at toy
At 16 wk	Sees pellet, but makes no move to it; Supine: hands in midline; reaches and grasps objects and brings them to mouth
At 28 wk	Reaches out for and grasps large objects; transfers objects from hand to hand; grasp uses radial palm; rakes at pellet
At 40 wk (approx. 9 mo)	Grasps objects with thumb and forefinger; pokes at things with forefinger; picks up pellet with assisted pincer movement; uncovers hidden toy; attempts to retrieve dropped object; releases object grasped by other person
At 52 wk (12 mo)	Picks up pellet with unassisted pincer movement of forefinger and thumb; releases object to other person on request or gesture
15 mo	Makes a tower of three cubes; makes a line with crayon; inserts pellet in bottle
18 mo	Makes a tower of four cubes; imitates scribbling; imitates vertical stroke; dumps pellet from bottle
24 mo	Builds a tower of seven cubes (6 at 21-mo); circular scribbling; imitates horizontal stroke; folds paper once imitatively
30 mo	Tower of 9 cubes; makes vertical and horizontal strokes but generally will not join them to make a cross; imitates circular stroke; forming closed figure
36 mo	Tower of 10 cubes; imitates construction of "bridge" of 3 cubes; copies a circle; imitates a cross
48 mo	Copies bridge from model; imitates construction of "gate" of 5 cubes; copies cross and square; draws a man with 2 to 4 parts besides head; names longer of 2 lines
60 mo	Draws triangle from copy; names heavier of two weights

Grasp reflex: Normal infants grasp the object, and with attempted removal, the grip is reinforced

a special blanket or stuffed toy as a transitional object: something that functions as a symbol of the absent parent (in psychoanalytic term, the object). The most dramatic developments in this period are linguistic. Children may point at things with their index finger rather than their whole hand as though calling attention to objects not for the purpose of having them but of finding their names. After the realization that

Table 2.6: Developmental milestones (language, speech and hearing) during the 1st yr of life and from 1 to 5 yrs of age

Age week/month	Developmental milestones (language, speech and hearing)
1st 4 wks	–
At 4 wk	–
At 8 wk	–
At 12 wk	–
At 16 wk	–
At 28 wk	Polysyllabic vowel sounds formed
At 40 wk (approx. 9 mo)	Repetitive consonant sounds (mama, dada)
At 52 wk (12 mo)	A few words besides "mama," "dada"
15 mo	Jargon; follows simple commands; may name a familiar object (ball)
18 mo	10 words (average); names pictures; identifies one or more parts of body
24 mo	Puts 3 words together (subject, verb, object) to form sentences
30 mo	Refers to self by pronoun "I"; knows full name
36 mo	Knows age and sex; counts 3 objects correctly; repeats 3 numbers or a sentence of 6 syllables
48 mo	Counts 4 coins accurately; tells a story
60 mo	Names 4 colors; repeats sentence of 10 syllables; counts 10 coins correctly

Table 2.7: Developmental milestones (social, emotional and behavior) during the 1st yr of life and from 1 to 5 yrs of age

Age week/mo	Developmental milestones (social, emotional and behavior)
1st 4 wks	Visual preference for human face; Visual: may fixate face or light in line of vision; "doll's-eye" movement of eyes on turning of the body
At 4 wk	Body movements in cadence with voice of other in social contact; beginning to smile; Visual: watches person; follows moving object
At 8 wk	Smiles on social contact; listens to voice and coos; Visual: follows moving object 180 degrees
At 12 wk	Sustained social contact; listens to music: says "aah, ngah"
At 16 wk	Laughs out loud; may show displeasure if social contact is broken; excited at sight of food
At 28 wk	Prefers mother; babbles; enjoys mirror; responds to changes in emotional content of social contact
At 40 wk (approx. 9 mo)	Responds to sound of name; plays peek-a-boo or pat-a-cake; waves bye-bye
At 52 wk (12 mo, 1 yr)	Plays simple ball game; makes postural adjustment to dressing; comes when called
15 mo	Indicates some desires or needs by pointing; hugs parents
18 mo	Feeds self; seeks help when in trouble; may complain when wet or soiled; kisses parent with pucker
24 mo	Handles spoon well; often tells immediate experiences; helps to undress; listen to stories with pictures
30 mo	Helps put things away; pretends in play
36 mo	Plays simple games (in "parallel" with other children); helps in dressing (unbuttons clothing and put on shoes); washes hands
48 mo	Plays with several children with beginning of social interaction and role playing; goes to toilet alone
60 mo	Dresses and undresses; asks questions about meaning of words; domestic role-playing

words can stand for things, a child's vocabulary balloons from 10 to 15 words at 18 mo to 100 or more at 2 yr. After acquiring a vocabulary of about 50 words, toddlers begin to combine them to make simple sentences, the beginning of grammar. At this stage, toddlers understand two-step commands, such as "give me the pen and then get your ball." Children with delayed language acquisition often have greater behavior problems. Language development is facilitated when parents and caregivers use clear, simple sentences, ask questions, and respond to children's incomplete sentences and gestural communication with the appropriate words. Regular periods of looking at picture books together with the child continue to provide an ideal context for language development.

Language development is facilitated when parents and caregivers use clear, simple sentences; ask questions; and responds to children's incomplete sentences and gestural communication with appropriate words. Regular periods of looking at picture books together continue to provide an ideal context for language development. Children with delayed language acquisition often have greater behavior problems and frustrations due to problems with communication. With children's increasing mobility, physical limits on their explorations become less effective; parents should ask them not to go beyond/or climb/or run.

2.6 PRESCHOOL YEARS (2–5 YRS)

By the end of the 2nd yr somatic and brain growth slows, with corresponding decreases in nutritional requirements and in appetite. The average child gains approximately 2 kg in weight and 7 cm in height per year. The toddler's prominent abdomen flattens, and the body becomes leaner. Physical activity is at the peak. The need for sleep declines to 11–13 hr/24 hr. Visual acuity reaches 20/30 by age 3 yrs and 20/20 by 4 yrs. All 20 primary teeth have erupted by 3 yrs of age. Handedness is usually established by the 3rd year. Bowel and bladder control takes place during this period (average age is 30 mo but there is individual and cultural variations). Daytime bladder control precedes bowel control and girls precede boys. Bed-wetting is normal up to the age of 4 yrs in girls and 5 yrs in boys. Many children master toilet training with ease while for others, toilet training is troublesome. Refusal to defecate in the toilet or potty is relatively common and can lead to constipation and parental frustration.

Language development occurs most rapidly between 2 and 5 yrs of age. Vocabulary increases from 50–100 words to more than 2,000, the number of words. As a rule of thumb, between age 2 and 5 yrs, the number of words in a typical sentence equals the child's age (2 by age 2 yrs, 3 by age 3 yrs, and so on). It is important to distinguish between speech (the production of intelligible sounds) and language, which refers to the underlying mental act. Language includes both expressive and receptive functions. Receptive language (understanding) varies less in its rate of acquisition than does expressive language; therefore, it has greater prognostic importance. Language acquisition depends critically on environmental input. Key determinants include the amount and variety of speech directed toward children and the frequency with which adults ask questions and encourage verbalization. Language is a critical barometer of both cognitive and emotional development. Mental retardation may first become apparent with delayed speech at approximately 2 yrs. Child abuse and neglect is correlated with delayed language, particularly the ability to convey emotional states. Preschool language development lays the foundation for later success in school. Picture books have a special role not only in familiarizing young children with printed words but also in the development of verbal language. Reading aloud with a young child is an interactive process in which a parent focuses the child's attention on a particular picture, requests a response (by asking "What's that?"), and then gives the child feedback ("Right, it's a dog"). Parents should have a regular time each day for reading or looking at books with their children.

During the preschool period, play is marked by increasing complexity and imagination, from simple scripts replicating common experiences such as shopping and putting baby to bed (2 or 3 yrs of age) to more extended scenarios involving singular events such as going to the zoo or going on a trip (3 or 4 yrs of age) to the creation of a scenarios that have only been imagined, such as flying to the moon (4 or 5 yrs of age). Play allows children to experience mastery by solving puzzles, practicing adult roles, assuming the aggressive role rather than the victim (spanking a doll), taking on superpowers (superhero play), and obtaining things that are denied in real life. Creativity, inherent in all play, is particularly apparent in drawing, painting and other artistic activities.

Preschool children normally experience complicated feelings toward their parents that can include possessiveness toward one parent, jealousy and resentment of the other parent, and fear that these negative feelings might lead to abandonment. Curiosity about genitals and adult sexual organs is normal, as is masturbation. Excessive masturbation that interferes with a child's normal activities, acting out of sexual intercourse in doll play or with other children, extreme modesty, or mimicry of adult seductive behavior all suggest the possibility of sexual abuse or inappropriate exposure. Parents should begin to teach children about 'private' areas before school entry.

Corporal punishment is inappropriate in the modern context in which most families now live. No evidence shows that spanking per se is harmful, but regular use of corporal punishment may reflect an excessive desire for control, as well as a lack of other parenting techniques. Children mimic the corporal punishment they receive, and it is not uncommon for preschool-age children to strike their parents back.

Child Development, Hearing and Vision

The main objectives of developmental pediatrics are:
1. To help all children achieve their maximum developmental potential
2. The early detection and management of delayed development, including specific sensory impairments of hearing and vision; even where there is no specific treatment, the effects of a condition can be modified
3. To act as the entry point for the care and management of the child with special needs.

Four Areas of Development

It is useful to subdivide early child development into four functional skill areas: gross motor, fine motor and vision, language, speech and hearing, and social, emotional and behavior (Tables 2.4 to 2.7 and Figs 2.1 to 2.9).

Developmental milestones during the 1st yr of life and from 1 to 5 yrs of age are listed in Tables 2.4 (Gross motor), 2.5 (Fine motor and vision), 2.6 (Language, speech and hearing), and 2.7 (Social, emotional and behavior). Data are derived from those of Gasell (as revised by Knobloch), Shirley, Provence, Wolf, Bailey, and others. After 5 yrs the Stanford-Binet, Wechsler-Bellevue, and other scales offer the most precise estimates of developmental level. In order to have their greatest value, they should be administered only by an experienced and qualified person.

Parents naturally wish to know that their child's development is normal. Health professionals will need to decide whether the individual child is within the normal range for his age and stage of development. The range of normal is wide. This adds to the complexity of assessing child development.

Variation in rate of development. This can be demonstrated by considering the age of range for the important developmental mile stone of walking unsupported. The percentage of children who are walking unsupported is: 25% by 11 mo; 50% by walking 12 mo; 75% by 13 mo; 90% by 15 mo; 97.5% by 18 mo.

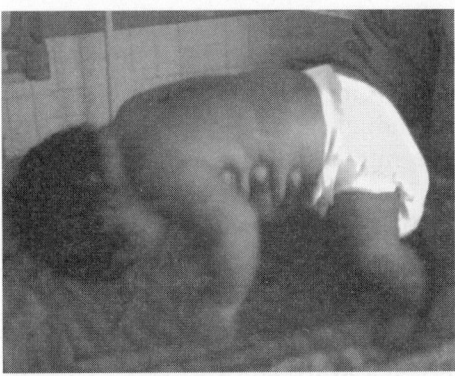

Fig. 2.1: Ventral suspension: unable to hold neck in the line with trunk at 4 wks.

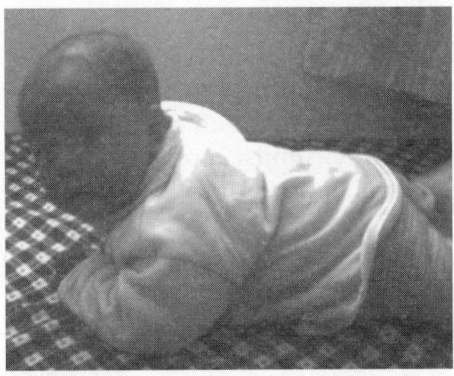

Fig. 2.2: Prone position: chest is maintained off the couch and body weight is supported on forearms in a 5-mo-old infant.

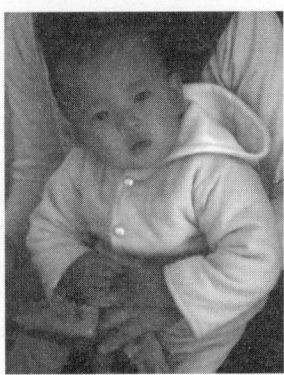

Fig. 2.3: Grasping with both hands around 5 mo of age.

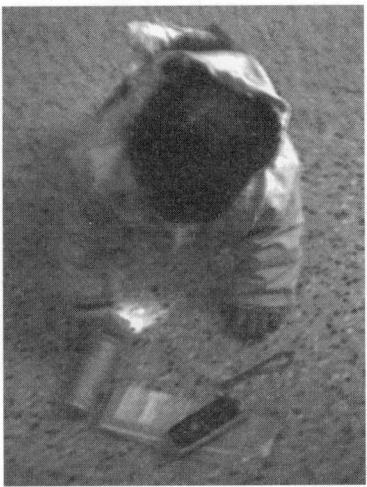

Fig. 2.4: Crawls to take torch; infant around 9 mo old.

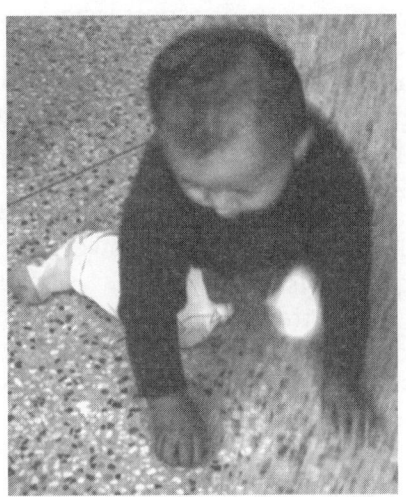

Fig. 2.5: Pincer movement: picks up pellet with unassisted pincer movement of forefinger and thumb at 12 mo of age.

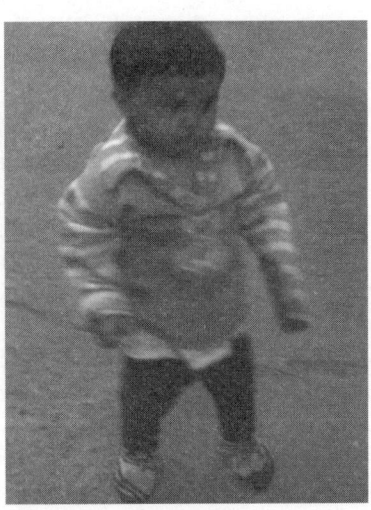

Fig. 2.6: Walk with short, uncertain steps (toddler) at 15 mo.

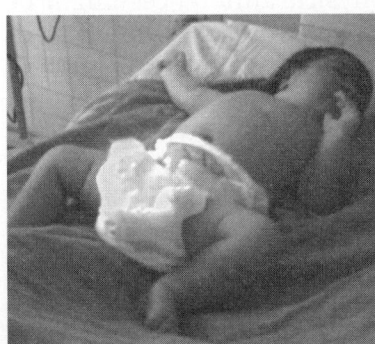

Fig. 2.7: Supine position: generally flexed.

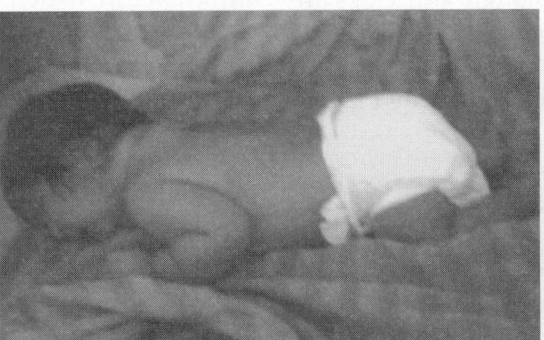

Fig. 2.8: Prone position: lies in flexed attitude turns head to one side.

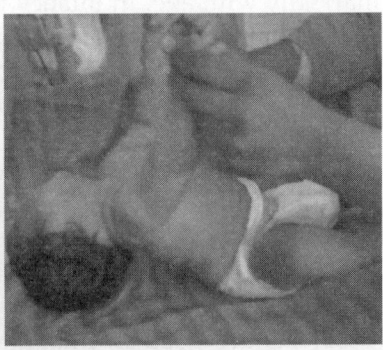

Fig. 2.9: Pulls to sit: note complete head lag in a newborn.

Variation in pattern of development. The pattern by which children reach key milestones varies, as documented by the variants in locomotor skills. Normal infants' progress from immobility to walking, but all do not do so in the same way. Whilst most achieve mobility by crawling, some bottom-shuffle and others commando crawl or creep a few just stand up and walk. The locomotor pattern (crawling, creeping, shuffling, just standing up and walking) influences the age of walking. The limit age of 18 mo for walking applies predominantly to children who have had crawling as their early mobility pattern. Children who bottom shuffle or commando crawl tend to walk later than crawlers, so that within those not walking at 18 mo there will be some children who are simply reflecting variants of normal locomotor patterns.

There is even more variation in the rate of acquisition of social skill and behavior, e.g. when children can dress themselves or toilet-trained, but the concept of limit ages still applies to determining whether a child's developmental progress is normal.

Eventual level of attainment. This depends on heredity and environment. Lack of stimulation may be associated with developmental delay, particularly in speech and language and social skills. In addition to the acquisition of skills, their quality is also important. For example, a child may attain a developmental mile stone in language, such as putting words and sentences together, but is unskilled and clumsy in trying to converse with other children and adults.

In the case of preterm infant, when assessing developmental age, it should be calculated from the expected date of delivery. This is done up to around 2 years of age, by which time the number of weeks early the child was born is no longer a significant proportion of the child's life and should cease to be counted.

Cognitive Development

Cognition refers to higher mental function. This varies markedly with age. In infancy thought processes are centered around immediate experiences at that time. The thought processes of preschool children, which have been called preoperational thought (by Piaget), are as follows:

- That they are the centre of the world
- That inanimate objects are alive and have feelings and motives
- Use of magical thinking
- that everything has a purpose. Toys and other objects are used in imaginative play as aids to thought to help make sense of experience and social relationships.

In middle school children, the dominant mode of thought is practical and orderly, tried to immediate circumstances and specific experiences. This has been called operational thought.

It is only in the mid-teens that an adult style of abstract thought (formal operational thought) begins to develop with the ability for abstract reasoning, testing hypotheses and manipulating abstract concepts.

2.7 MIDDLE CHILDHOOD (6–11 YRS)

During middle childhood (6–11 yrs), children increasingly separate from parents and seek acceptance from teachers and other adults, and from peers. The average growth during this period is 3–3.5 kg (7 lb) and 6 cm (2.5 in) per year. Growth occurs discontinuously in 3 to 6 irregularly timed spurts each year, each growth spurt lasting on average 8 wks. The head grows only 2–3 cm in circumference throughout the entire period of middle childhood, reflecting slower brain growth than before; myelinization is complete by 7 yrs of age. Body habitus (endomorphic, mesomorphic, or ectomorphic) tends to remain relatively stable throughout middle childhood. Growth of the midface and lower face occurs gradually. Loss of deciduous teeth is a sign of maturation, beginning after eruption of the 1st molars around 6 yrs of age. Replacement with adult teeth occurs at a rate of about 4 yrs. Lymphoid tissues (including tonsils and adenoids) continue to hypertrophy, often giving rise to impressive tonsils and adenoids, which may require surgical removal. Muscular strength, coordination and stamina increase progressively, as does the ability to perform complex movements such as dancing, shooting basketballs. Sedentary habits at this age are associated with increased lifetime risk of obesity and cardiovascular disease. The sexual organs remain physically immature, but there is interest in gender differences. Masturbation is common.

Fears of being "defective" can lead to avoidance of situations in which physical differences might be revealed, such as physical training, gym class, or medical examinations. Children with actual physical disabilities may face special stresses because of their difference. Girls, in particular, often worry that they are overweight, and many engage in unhealthy dieting to achieve an abnormally thin cultural ideal. Shortness, particularly in boys, may be associated with decreased educational attainment and increased risks for behavior problems.

Social and emotional development proceeds in three contexts: The home, the school, and the neighborhood. Of these, the home remains the most influential. The parent-child relationship continues to provide a secure base from which children can venture forth. The beginning of school coincides with a child's further separation from family and the increasing importance of teacher and peer relationships. The peer group exerts a profound influence on the child's personality, often including mannerisms, speaking accent, aspirations, and relationship to the law. In the neighborhood, real dangers such as busy streets, bullies, and strangers tax school-aged children's common sense and resourcefulness.

Children need unconditional support as well as realistic demands from parents, as they venture in to a world that is often frightening. Children who show unusual difficulty in separating from parents and in facing school and neighborhood challenges may be reacting to their parents' difficulty letting them go. Other parents exert excessive pressure on their children to adopt adult behaviors and achieve academic or competitive success. Children who struggle to meet such expectations may develop behavior problems or somatic symptoms such as headaches or stomachaches as a result.

Pediatricians need to be alert to children's functioning in all contexts (home, school, and neighborhood) and consider how each of those environments either supports or overwhelms the child's ability to adapt and grow. Use of the **HEADSS** mnemonic—**H**ome, **E**ducation and employment, peer **A**ctivities, **D**rugs, **S**exuality, and **S**uicide or depression can help.

Needlman RD. Growth and development. In: Behrman RE, Kliegman RM, Jenson HB (eds). *Nelson Textbook of Pediatrics.* 17th edn. Philadelphia: Saunders, 2004; 51–53.

Thompson M, Grace C, Cohen L. Best Friends, Worst Enemies. New York: Ballantine, 2001.

2.8 ADOLESCENCE (between 10 and 20 yrs of age)

Between 10 and 20 yrs of age, children undergo rapid changes in body size, shape, physiology, and psychologic and social functioning. Hormones set the development agenda in conjunction with social structures designed to foster the transition from childhood to adulthood. Adolescence proceeds across three distinct periods—early, middle, and late. Each period is marked by a characteristic set of salient biologic, psychologic, and social issues (Table 2.8). However, individual variation occurs, both in terms of the timing of somatic changes and the quality of the adolescent's experience. Gender and subculture markedly affect the developmental course, as do physical and social stressors, such as cerebral palsy or parental alcoholism.

Table 2.8: Central issues in early, middle, and late adolescence physically mature slower growth			
Variable	*Early adolescence*	*Middle adolescence*	*Late adolescence*
Age (year)	10–13	14–16	17–20 and beyond
SMR	1–2	3–5	5
Somatic	Secondary sex characteristics; beginning of rapid growth; awkward appearance	Height growth peaks; body shape and composition change; acne and odor; menarche/spermarche	Physically mature slower growth
Sexual	Sexual interest usually exceeds sexual activity	Sexual drive surges; experimentation; questions of sexual orientation	Consolidation of sexual identity
Cognitive and moral	Concrete operations; conventional morality	Emergence of abstract thought; questioning mores; self-centered	Idealism; absolutism
Self-concept	Preoccupation with changing body; self-consciousness	Concern with attractiveness; increasing introspection	Relatively stable body image
Family	Bids for increased independence; ambivalence	Continued struggle for acceptance of greater autonomy	Practical independence; family remains secure base
Peers	Same-sex groups; conformity; cliques	Dating; peer groups less important	Intimacy; possibly commitment
Relationship to society	Middle-school adjustment	Gauging skills and opportunities	Carrier decisions, e.g. drop out, college, work

SMR sexual maturity rating

Early Adolescence

Biologic development: Adrenal production of androgen (chiefly dehydroepiandrosterone sulfate (DHEAS) may occur as early as age 6 with development of underarm odor and faint genital hair (adrenarche). Levels of luteinizing hormone (LH) and follicle-stimulating hormone (FSH) rise progressively throughout middle childhood without producing any dramatic effect. The rapid changes of puberty begin with increased sensitivity of the pituitary to gonadotropin-releasing hormone (GnRH), pulsatile release of GnRH, LH, and FSH during sleep and corresponding rises in gonadal androgens and estrogens. Some children enter puberty earlier perhaps due to their increase weight and adiposity. The resulting sequence of somatic and physiologic changes gives rise to the sexual maturity rating (SMR). However, SMR stages are not perfectly synchronized (e.g., SMR 2 penis development precedes SMR 2 pubic hair by on average 1.5 years). The range of normal progress through the stages of sexual maturity is wide (Tables 2.9 and 2.10).

In girls, the first visible sign of puberty is the appearance of breast buds, between 8 and 13 yr. Menses begin 2–2½ yrs later (normal range 9–16 yrs), around the peak in height velocity. Less obvious changes include enlargement of ovaries, uterus, labia, and clitoris; thickening of endometrium and vaginal mucosa; and increased vaginal glycogen, predisposing to yeast infections.

In boys, testicular enlargement (measured by orchidometer) begins as early as 9½ yrs. Peak growth occurs when testis volumes reach approximately 9–10 cm^3 during SMR 4. Under the influence of LH and testosterone, the seminiferous tubules, epididymis, seminal vesicles, and prostate enlarge. The left testis normally is lower than the right; the opposite may be true in situs inversus. Some degree of breast hypertrophy occurs in 40–65% of pubertal boys as a result of a relative excess of estrogenic stimulation. Gynecomastia sufficient to cause embarrassment and social disability occurs in fewer than 10%. Breast swelling less than 4 cm in diameter has a 90% chance of spontaneous resolution within 3 yrs. For greater degrees of enlargement, hormonal or surgical treatment may be indicated. Obesity may exacerbate gynecomastia and should be addressed through diet and exercise.

Sexuality: Sexuality includes not only sexual behaviors but also interest and fantasies, sexual orientation, attitudes toward sex and its relationship to emotions, and awareness of socially defined roles and mores. Interest in sex increases in early puberty, ejaculation

Table 2.9: Classification of sex maturity stages in girls		
SMR stage	Pubic hair	Breasts
1	Preadolescent	Preadolescent
2	Sparse, lightly pigmented, straight, medial border of labia	Breast and papilla elevated as small mound; areola diameter increased
3	Darker, beginning to curl, increased amount	Breast and areola enlarged, no contour separation
4	Coarse, curly, abundant but amount less than in adult	Areola and papilla form secondary mound
5	Adult feminine triangle, spread to the medial surface of thighs	Mature, nipple projects, areola part of general breast contour

SMR: Sexual maturity rating
Source: Tanner JM. *Growth at Adolescence.* 2nd edition. Oxford, England: Blackwell Scientific Publications 1962

Table 2.10: Classification of sex maturity stages in boys			
SMR stage	Pubic hair	Penis	Testes
1	None	Preadolescent	Preadolescent
2	Scanty, long, slightly pigmented	Slight enlargement pink, texture altered	Enlarged scrotum
3	Darker, start to curl, small amount	Longer	Larger
4	Resembles adult type but less in quantity, coarse, curly	Larger; glans and breadth increase in size	Larger, scrotum dark
5	Adult distribution, spread to medial surface of thighs	Adult size	Adult size

SMR: Sexual maturity rating
Source: Tanner JM. *Growth at Adolescence.* 2nd edition. Oxford, England: Blackwell Scientific Publications 1962

occurs for the first time, usually during masturbation and later spontaneously during sleep. Early adolescents sometimes masturbate socially. Sexual behavior, other than masturbation is less common in early puberty. Sexual intercourse before 14 yrs of age has also been reported. Mutual sexual exploration is not necessarily a sign of homosexuality.

Cognitive and moral development: In Piagetian theory, adolescence marks the transition from concrete operational thinking characteristic of school-aged children to formal logical operations. Some early adolescents demonstrate formal thinking, others acquire the capability later, and others do not ever fully acquire it. The ability to treat possibilities as real entities may affect critical decisions, such as whether or not to have unprotected intercourse or engage in other risk-taking behavior. The development of moral thinking roughly parallels general cognitive development.

Self-concept: Self consciousness increases exponentially in response to the somatic transformations of puberty. Self-awareness at this age tends to center on external characteristics in contrast to the introspection of later adolescence. It is normal for early adolescents to scrutinize their appearance and to feel that everyone else is staring at them too. Girls, in particular, are at risk for viewing themselves as fat/out of shape may be at increased risk of depression. Severe body image distortions, such as anorexia nervosa, also tend to appear at this age.

Relationships with family, peers, and society: In early adolescence, the trend is toward separation from family and increased interest in peer activities. This shift is the renunciation of family norms of dress and grooming in favor of the peer group uniform, such as hair, clothes, and body ornamentation. Such stylistic changes frequently spark conflicts. Not all adolescents rebel, and not all parents reject such assertions of separateness as signs of insurrection. However, most adolescents continue to strive to please their parents even while they disagree on certain issues. Separation from family often involves selecting adults outside of the family as role models and developing close relationships with particular teachers or the parents of other children. Early adolescents often socialize in same sex peer groups. An early adolescent's relationship to society centers on school. The societal preoccupation with youth and sexuality generates constant exposure to sexually suggestive and explicit images. At the same time, reliable information about sexuality in general and contraception in particular, remains sparse. Ready access to pornography on the Internet may increase the risk of premature sexual activity or exploitation.

Implications for parents and pediatricians: Physical growth, body preoccupation, and sexual interest correlate with sexual maturity, whereas cognitive advancement, separation, and changes in social behavior may correlate more closely with chronological age or grade in school. Discordance between chronological age and sexual maturation may increase the stress of early adolescence. As a group, early maturing boys enjoy greater social success and self-esteem than do those who mature later. For girls, by contrast, early maturation is associated with poorer school performance and lower self-esteem. Early adolescents often have questions about the somatic and social changes they are experiencing.

Parents and children often need help differentiating between the normal discomforts of the age and truly concerning behaviors. Interest in sex sometimes heralded by the appearance of pornographic magazines, is normal; sexual intercourse in early adolescence, though fairly common, is usually a sign of developmental dysfunction.

Middle Adolescence

Biologic development: In middle adolescence growth accelerates above the prepubertal rate of 6–7 cm (3 inches) per year. In the average girl, the growth spurt peaks at 11.5 yrs at a top of velocity of 8.3 cm (3.8 inches) per yr and then slows to a stop at 16 yrs. In the average boy, the growth spurt starts later, peaks at 13.5 yrs at 9.5 cm (4.3 inches) per yr, and then slows to a stop at 18 yrs. Weight gain parallels linear growth, with a delay of several months, so that adolescents seem first to stretch and then fill out. Pubertal weight gains account for 40% of adult weight. Muscle mass also increases, followed several months later by an increase in strength; boys show greater gains in both. Lean body mass approximately 80% in the average prepubertal child, increases in boys to 90% and decreases in girls to 75% as subcutaneous fat accumulates.

Bone maturation correlates closely with SMR because epiphyseal closure is under androgenic control. Boys with SMR 3 pubic hair and SMR 4 genitals normally have their peak growth spurt ahead of them; girls at the same SMR are usually past their peaks. Widening of the shoulders in boys and of the hips in girls is also hormonally determined. Other physiologic changes include a doubling in heart size and lung vital capacity from preadolescent norms. Blood pressure, blood volume, and hematocrit rise, particularly in boys. Androgenic stimulation of sebaceous and apocrine glands results in acne and body odor. A physiologic increase in sleepiness may be mistaken for laziness.

Sexual maturation in middle adolescence occurs with the achievement of menarche in 30% of girls by SMR 3 (mean age 12–14 yrs) and in 90% by SMR 4 (mean age 13–15 yrs). Menarche usually follows approximately 1 yr after the growth spurt begins. The timing of menarche appears to be determined by genetics as well as such factors as adiposity, chronic illness, and exercise. The average age at menarche in developed countries has decreased, perhaps in response to better nutrition and less physical activity. Before menarche the uterus achieves a mature configuration, vaginal lubrication increases, and a clear vaginal discharge appears, sometimes mistaken for a sign of infection. In boys, spermarche occurs and the penis lengthens and widens.

Sexuality: Dating becomes a normative activity during middle adolescence; but dating relationships are often superficial at this stage, emphasizing attractiveness and sexual experimentation rather than intimacy. The degree of sexual activity varies widely. At age 16 yr, approximately 30% of girls and 45% of boys report having sexual intercourse, whereas 17% report petting, and some 22% report kissing as the only sexual behavior. Biologic maturation and social pressures (including religiosity) combine to determine sexual activity. Most parents discourage sexual activity, but some actually encourage it in hopes of boosting the child's popularity or of living vicariously through the child's experiences. Homosexual experimentation is common, but it does not necessarily reflect a child's ultimate sexual orientation. In addition to sexual orientation middle adolescents begin to sort out other important aspects of sexual identity, including beliefs about love, honesty, and propriety. Adolescents tend to choose one of three sexual paths: celibacy, monogamy, or polygamous experimentation. Most have some knowledge of the risks of pregnancy, acquired immunodeficiency syndrome, and other sexually transmitted diseases, but knowledge does not consistently control behavior. A minority use any contraception at first intercourse, and a fewer than 75% consistently use condoms or other effective methods.

Duru Shah and researchers of Federation of Obstetrics and Gynecological Societies of India, surveyed 3,500 young girls aged between 15 and 25 yrs from diverse socioeconomic backgrounds, in roughly 10 metros and towns. Questions about sexual activity were directed at only 2,400 girls/women in the sample who were not married. 1 in 4 (25%) was sexually active. 16% used contraception during first sexual encounter. 17% who had sex did so out of curiosity. Of the total 3,500 sample population, 41% said the media had been their only source of information about sex and contraception. 1 in 5 said their mothers had not given them any information. The mothers do not talk to their daughters' shows that people still do not talk their daughters where sex is concerned. As a result, girls indulge in it with no proper knowledge, often ending up with diseases and unwanted pregnancies.

Cognitive and moral development: Middle adolescents question and analyze extensively with the transition to formal operational thought. Questioning of moral conventions fosters the development of personal codes of ethics. An adolescent's new flexibility of thought has pervasive effects on relationships with self and others.

Self-concept: Intense feelings of inner turmoil and misery are common and may be difficult to differentiate from psychiatric illness. Girls may tend to characterize themselves and their peers according to interpersonal relationships ("I am a girl with close friends"), whereas boys as a group may focus on abilities ("I am good at sports").

Relationships with family, peers, and society: Puberty commonly results in strained relationships between adolescents and their parents. As part of separation, adolescents may become distant from parents, redirecting emotional and sexual energies toward peer relationships. As dating increases, the need to belong to same-sex groups declines. Middle adolescents often begin thinking seriously about what they want to do as adults, a question that formerly had been comfortably hypothetical. The process involves self-assessment and assessment of the opportunities available.

Implications for parents and pediatricians: Adolescents vary greatly in their rate of physical and social progress and in the resolution of central conflicts about autonomy and self-esteem. In talking to a boy, for example, one might observe that some boys are interested sexually in girls, some boys are interested in other boys, and some boys are interested in both (or neither).

Late Adolescence

Biologic development: The final stages of breast, penile and pubic hair development occur by 17–18 yrs of age in 95% of males and females. Minor changes in hair distribution often continue for several years in males, including the growth of facial and chest hair and the onset of male pattern baldness in a few.

Psychosocial development: Cognition tends to be less self-centered, with increasing thoughts about concepts such as justice, patriotism, and history. Older adolescents are often idealistic but also may be absolutist and intolerant of opposing views. Religious or political groups that promise answers to complex questions may hold great appeal. Slowing physical changes permit the emergence of a more stable body image. Sexual experimentation decreases as adolescents adopt more stable sexual identities. In contrast to the often superficial dating relationships of middle adolescence, these relationships increasingly involve love and commitment. Career decisions become pressing because an adolescent's self-concept is increasingly bound up in the emerging role in society (as student, worker, or parent).

Implications for parents and pediatricians: The crucial task of adolescence is that of establishing a stable sense of identity, including separation from family of origin, initiation of intimacy, and realistic planning for economic independence. To achieve these milestones, developmental progress is required of both adolescents and their parents. Continued difficulty in any of these areas may constitute an indication for referral for counseling.

Growth Velocity

For both sexes, growth acceleration begins in early adolescence, but peak growth velocities are not reached until SMR 3 or 4. Boys typically peak 2–3 years later than girls and continue their linear growth for approximately 2–3 years after girls have stopped. First there is increase in height (height velocity) in girls and then there will be increase in weight (weight velocity). In girls, the first visible sign of puberty is the appearance of breast buds between 8 and 13 years. Menses typically begin 2–2½ yrs later (normal range 9–16 yrs) around the peak in height velocity. Less obvious changes include enlargement of ovaries, uterus, labia and clitoris; thickening of the endometrial and vaginal mucosa; and increased vaginal glycogen. On the other hand in boys both height and weight velocity increase simultaneously. In boys the first visible sign of puberty is testicular enlargement which begins as early as 9½ year. Peak growth occurs when testis volumes reach approximately 9–10 cm^3. Under the influence of LH and testosterone, the seminiferous tubules, epididymis, seminal vesicles, and prostate enlarge. The growth spurt begins distally, with enlargement of hands and feet followed by the arms and legs and finally by the trunk and chest. This asymmetric growth gives young adolescent's awkward look. Rapid enlargement of larynx, pharynx and lungs leads to changes in vocal quality, often heralded by a period of vocal instability (voice cracking) or dysphonation. Adrenal androgens stimulate the sebaceous glands, promoting the development of acne. Elongation of the optic glove often results in nearsightedness (myopia). Dental changes include jaw growth, loss of the final deciduous teeth, and eruption of the permanent cuspids, premolars and finally molars. Orthodontic appliances may be needed.

Delemarre-van de Wall HA. Regulation of puberty. Best Pract Res Clin Psychological Metab 2002; 16: 1–12.

Lissauer T, Clayden G . Child development, hearing, and vision. In: Lissauer T, Clayden G. Illustrated Textbook of Paediatrics. 2nd edn. Edinburgh: Mosby, 2001; 21–37.

Marshall WA, Tanner JM. Variations in the pattern of pubertal changes in boys. Arch Dis Child 1970; 45:13.

Marshall WA, Tanner JM. Variations in the pattern of pubertal changes in girls. Arch Dis Child 1969; 44:291.

Needlman RD. Growth and development. In: Behrman RE, Kliegman RM, Jenson HB (eds). *Nelson Textbook of Pediatrics.* 17th edn. Philadelphia: Saunders, 2004; 53–58.

Shah Darul and researchers. New Age Morality: Twenty-five percent young girls sexually active. Hindustan Times, New Delhi, India, August 3 (Monday); 2009.

Tanner JM, Davies PSW. Clinical longitudinal standards for height and height velocity for North American children. J Pediatr 1985; 107: 317.

2.9 ASSESSMENT OF GROWTH

Growth assessment is an essential component of pediatric health surveillance. The major concerns are undernutrition, failure to thrive and obesity. Growth chart is the most powerful tool in growth assessment. The other tools include an accurate scale for weighing (Infant and Adult weighing machines), a measuring board (an infantometer for measuring length), stadiometer for taking height and nondistensible plastic measuring tape. The measurements routinely carried out include weight, height/length, and head circumference. The other measurements include measuring the lower and upper body segment; span; chest circumference; abdominal circumference; mid-arm circumference and skin fold thickness (triceps and subscapular) by Harpenden skin fold calipers. Accurate measurement of weight, height/length, and head circumference is of obvious importance. Scales should be calibrated regularly. Cloth tapes stretch and should be avoided.

Measurement: Growth must be measured accurately with attention to correct technique and accurate plotting of the data on the percentile charts. These measurements should be plotted as a simple dot on an appropriate growth percentile chart. A single growth parameter should not be assessed in isolation of the other growth parameters, e.g. a child's low weight may be in proportion to his height if he is short but abnormal if he is tall. Serial measurements are used to show the pattern and determine the rate of growth. This is helpful in diagnosing or monitoring many pediatric conditions.

Weight: It is readily and accurately determined with electronic scales but must be performed on a naked infant or a child dressed only in underclothing (Figs 2.10 and 2.11). A neonate nearly looses up to 10–12% of body weight in first few days of life, but should regain birth weight by 10 days of age, and subsequently gain approximately 30 g per day. Birth weight is doubled by 5 mo and tripled at about 1 yr. A young child's expected weight in kilogram can then be estimated from the formula: Age in years plus 4, multiplied by 2 (Age in yrs + 4 × 2).

Height: In children over 2 years of age, the standing height (Figs 2.12a and 2.12b) is measured by the stadiometer. While measuring height the child should be kept head straight, eyes and ear level; gentle upward traction on mastoid process; knees straight; barefoot, with feet flat on floor; heels touching back of board. The equipment must be calibrated regularly and maintained. Sitting height is from base of spine to top of head. Standing height or crown-heel length in infants usually correlates with weight. At birth length is approximately 50 cm increasing to 75 cm at 1 yr and 100 cm at 4 yr. Subsequently there should be an annual gain of approximately 5 cm.

The estimated target height is important to assess the child's growth potential. The correct acceptable range of height for a child is within two standard deviations of the target height percentile. A useful guide for normal range is target height ± 7 cm for girls and target height ± 8.5 cm for boys. The best way to predict the child's adult height is calculated as follows:

Boys (inches or cm)

$$= \frac{\text{Father's height (cm/inches)} + \text{Mother's height (cm/inches)}}{2} + 5\,\text{inches}\,(13\,\text{cm})$$

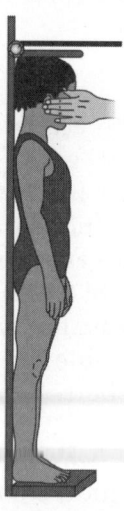

Fig. 2.12a: Measurement of height with the stadiometer; note correct standing position of the child.

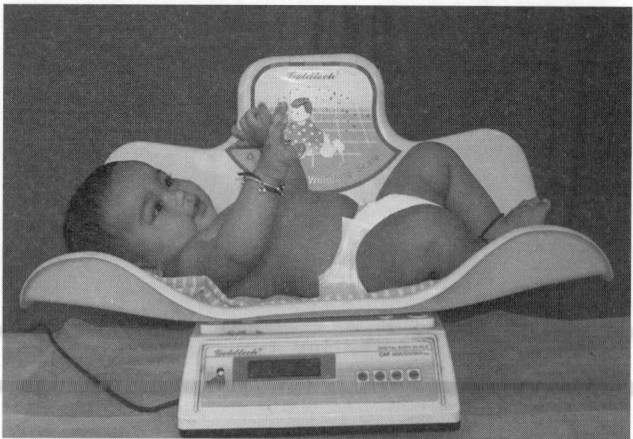

Fig. 2.10: Weight of an infant in infant weighing machine (*Courtesy:* Dr MMA Faridi).

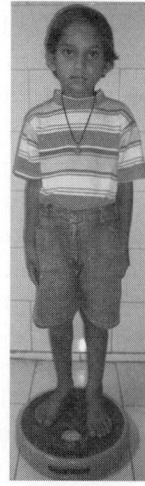

Fig. 2.11: Weight of a child in adult weighing machine (*Courtesy:* Dr MMA Faridi).

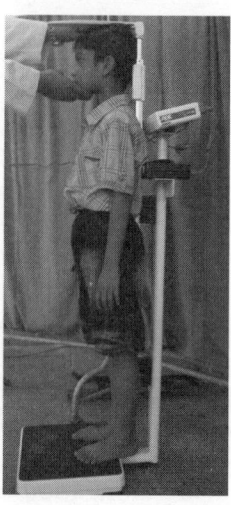

Fig. 2.12b: Height of a child (*Courtesy:* Dr MMA Faridi).

Girls (inches or cm)

$$= \frac{\text{Father's height (cm/inches)} + \text{Mother's height (cm/inches)}}{2} - 5 \text{ inches (13 cm)}$$

Most children will reach an adult height with in 4 inches (10 cm) of this estimation.

Length: In children, under 2 yrs supine length should be measured on a board (infantometer); length is measured with the help of two persons using the mother to assist. Accurate length measurement in infants can be difficult to obtain, as the legs need to be held straight and infants often dislike being held still (Figs 2.13a and b).

Body Proportions

Lower body segment: Length/height from the pubic symphysis to soles of the feet (Fig. 2.14).

Upper body segment: Length/height minus the lower body segment.

U/L ratio: 1.7 at birth; 1.3 at 3 yrs; 1.0 after 7 yrs.

High U/L ratio is seen in short limb dwarfism (e.g. achondroplasia) and in bone disorders (e.g. rickets); diminished upper segment/lower segment ratio is seen in Marfan syndrome (the arm span substantially exceeds the height (>1.05 times height); and in hypergonadotropic hypogonadism in males (primary hypogonadism) upper to lower segment ratio is considerably less than 0.9 and the proportions of the body are described as eunuchoid.

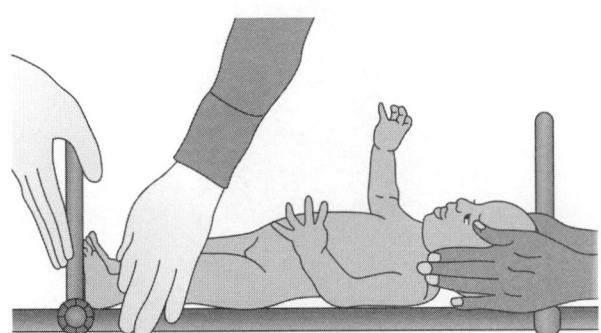

Fig. 2.13a: Measuring length of an infant with infantometer; for keeping head and feet in correct position you have take the help of another person.

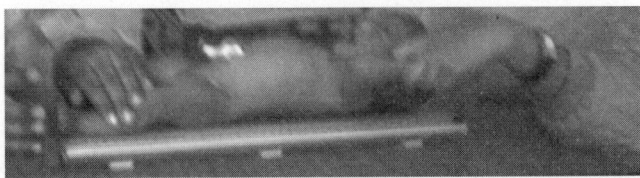

Fig. 2.13b: length of an infant.

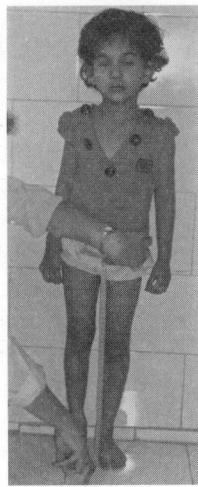

Fig. 2.14: Lower body segment (*Courtesy* Dr MMA Faridi).

Head circumference: Correct measurement of the head circumference is important. A nondistensible plastic measuring tape should be used. The tape is placed over the mid-forehead (supraorbital ridge in front) and is extended circumferentially to include the most prominent portion of the occiput in back, so that the greatest volume of the cranium is measured (Fig. 2.15). This occipitofrontal circumference is a measure of head and brain growth. The mean of three measurements is used. It is of particular importance in developmental delay or suspected hydrocephalus.

If the patient is found to have an abnormal skull, the head circumferences of the parents and siblings should also be recorded. The chances of error in the measurement of skull in the newborn are frequent and result from scalp edema, over-riding of the sutures, intravenous fluid infiltration, and the presence of a cephalohematoma. The average rate of head growth in a healthy pre-term infant is 0.5 cm in the first

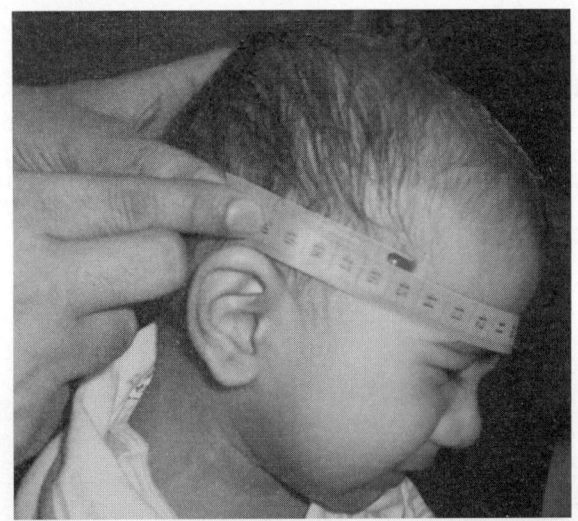

Fig. 2.15: Head circumference (*Courtesy:* Dr MMA Faridi).

2 wks, 0.75 cm during the third week, and 1 cm in the 4th wk and thereafter until the 40th wk of development. The head circumference of a term infant at birth measures 34–35 cm, increasing to 40 cm at 3 mo, 44 cm by 6 mo, and 47 cm by one year of age. The subsequent annual increase is 0.5 cm from 2 to 7 yrs and 0.3 cm from 8 to 12 yrs.

While measuring the head circumference, shape of the head, fontanels, cranial sutures, cranial defects or craniotabes should also be documented. Craniotabes is frequently associated with prematurity. Cranial bruits are most prominent over the anterior fontanel, temporal region, or the orbits and are best heard through the diaphragm of the stethoscope.

An infant has two fontanels at birth: A diamond shaped open anterior fontanel that situated at the midline at the junction of the coronal and the sagittal sutures and a posterior fontanel placed between the intersection of the occipital and parietal bones that may be closed at birth, or at the most, admit the tip of a finger. The posterior fontanel is usually closed and no palpable after the first 6 to 8 wks of life; its persistence suggests underlying hydrocephalus or the possibility of congenital hypothyroidism. The anterior fontanel varies greatly in size but the usual measurement is approximately 2 × 2 cm. The fontanel is normally slightly depressed and pulsatile and is best evaluated when an infant is held upright and is asleep or feeding. The average time of closure is 18 mo, but the fontanel may normally close as early as 9–12 mo. A bulging fontanel is a reliable indicator of increased intracranial pressure, but vigorous crying can cause a protuberant fontanel in a normal infant. A very small or absent anterior fontanel at birth may indicate premature fusion of the sutures or microcephaly, whereas a very large fontanel could be seen in many disorders listed in Box 2.1.

Three types of skull are normally observed in various communities, which is classified on the basis of cephalic index (CI): Dolichocephalic, mesaticephalic, brachycephalic (Table 2.11). Cephalic Index (CI) is defined as the ratio between breath and length of the skull expressed as below:

Box 2.1: Disorders associated with large anterior fontanel

Achondroplasia	Intrauterine growth retardation
Apert's syndrome	Kenny syndrome
Athyreosis hypothyroidism	Osteogenesis imperfecta
Cleidocranial dysostosis	Prematurity
Congenital rubella syndrome	Pyknodysostosis
Hallermann-Streiff syndrome	Russell-Silver syndrome
Hydrocephaly	13-, 18-, 21-trisomies
Hypophosphatasia	Vitamin D deficiency Rickets

$$\text{Cephalic index (CI)} = \frac{\text{Maximum breath of skull}}{\text{Maximum length of skull}} \times 100$$

Chest circumference: The chest circumference is measured at the levels of nipples, midway between inspiration and expiration, while the child is in recumbent position (Fig. 2.16). The head circumference is larger than chest circumference, becomes equal to about one year of age.

Abdominal circumference: The abdominal girth is measured at the level of umbilicus (Fig. 2.17).

Mid upper arm circumference: To measure the mid upper arm circumference (MUAC) first mark a point midway between the tip of acromion process of scapula and the olecranon of ulna, while the child

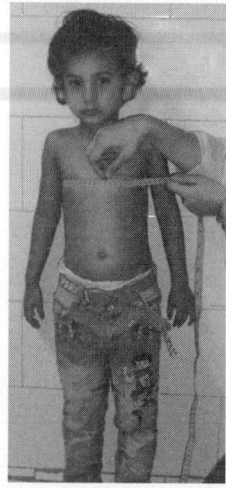

Fig. 2.16: Chest circumference (*Courtesy:* Dr MMA Faridi).

Table 2.11: Types of skull		
Types of skull	*Cephalic index (CI)*	*Race*
Dolichocephalic (long head)	70–75	Pure Aryans, Aborigines and Negroes
Mesaticephalic (medium)	75–80	Europeans and Chinese
Brachycephalic (broad, short head)	80–85	Mongolians

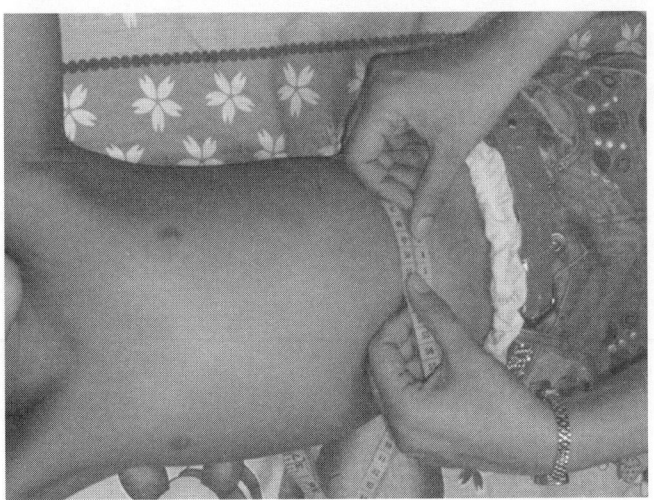

Fig. 2.17: Abdominal circumference (*Courtesy:* Dr MMA Faridi).

Fig. 2.19: Span (*Courtesy:* Dr MMA Faridi).

keeps the left arm by his side (Fig. 2.18). A mid upper arm circumference exceeding 13.5 cm is a sign of a satisfactory nutritional status; between 12.5 and 13.5 cm, it indicates mild- moderate malnutrition and below 12.5 cm severe malnutrition. Mid upper arm circumference cannot be used before the age of one year; between ages one and five years it hardly varies. MUAC yields a relatively reliable estimation of the body's mass. MUAC remains reasonably static between 15 and 17 cm among healthy because fat of early infancy is gradually replaced by muscles.

Span: Ask the child to stand against the wall. Measure the distance in the outstretched arms from the tip of middle finger from right arm to left arm (Fig. 2.19). Abnormally large span is seen in infants in patients

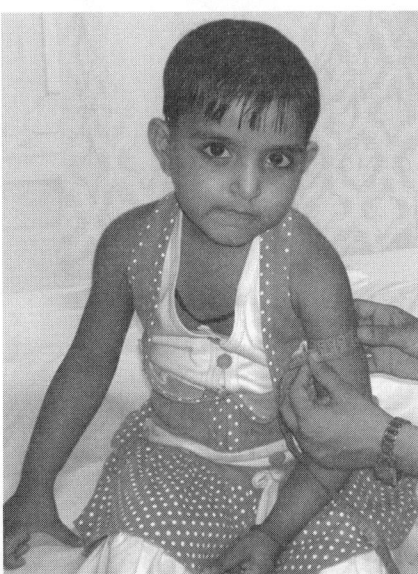

Fig. 2.18: Mid upper arm circumference (*Courtesy:* Dr MMA Faridi).

with Marfan syndrome, eunuchoidism, Klinefelter syndrome, coarctation of aorta (due to relative overgrowth of upper extremities), and in rickets with marked changes in lower extremities (bow legs).

Growth Chart

The growth chart provides most of the information needed to assess growth. If the growth measurements are recorded in a child over a period of time and are plotted on a graph, the deviation in the growth profile of the child from the normal pattern of growth for that age can be easily interpreted. This is a good tool to diagnose deviation of growth from normal. The growth charts of World Health Organization (2007 WHO reference) provide adequate information. Child growth standards based on a six months breastfeeding show that the growth is normal in infants who are breastfed for six months. Mercedes De Onis of WHO said that the new standards are based on a six months breastfeeding mandate as against the earlier norm of artificial food supplement since childbirth. The new standards are based on simultaneous studies in six countries including India. Over 300 newborns breastfed for six months in rich, educated south Delhi (India) were identified for the study and their growth was

Table 2.12: Child growth standards, based on a six months breastfeeding mandate		
Height (cm)	*Weight (kg) boys*	*Weight (kg) girls*
50	3.5	3.4
60	6.1	6.0
70	8.4	8.2
80	10.2	10.1
90	12.5	12.5
100	15.1	15.0
110	18.5	18.3

Weight-for-age: BOYS
Birth to 5 years (z-scores)

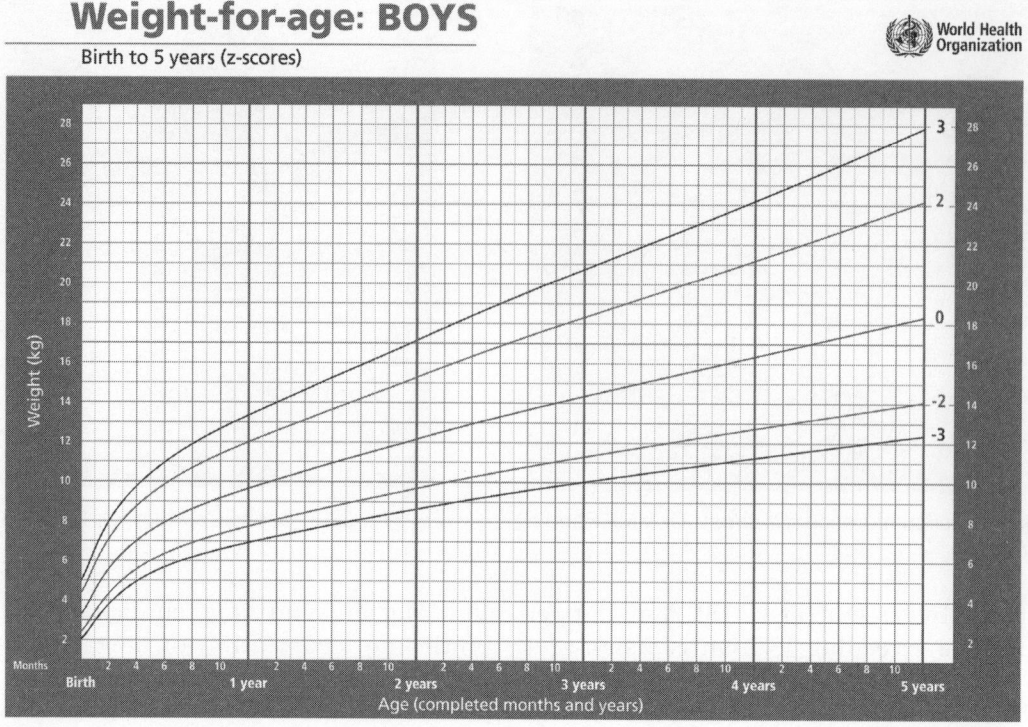

Fig. 2.20a: Weight-for-age: Boys: Birth to 5 years (z scores).

Weight-for-age: BOYS
5 to 10 years (z-scores)

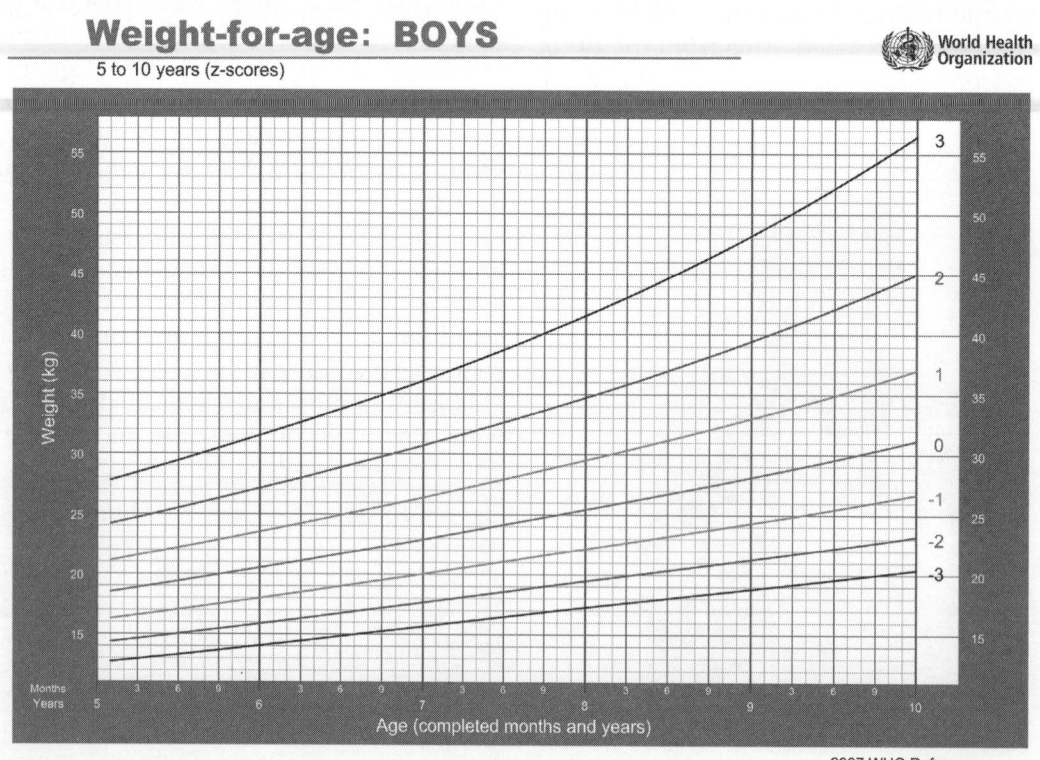

Fig. 2.20b: Weight-for-age: Boys: 5–10 years (z scores).

Weight-for-age: GIRLS
Birth to 5 years (z-scores)

World Health Organization

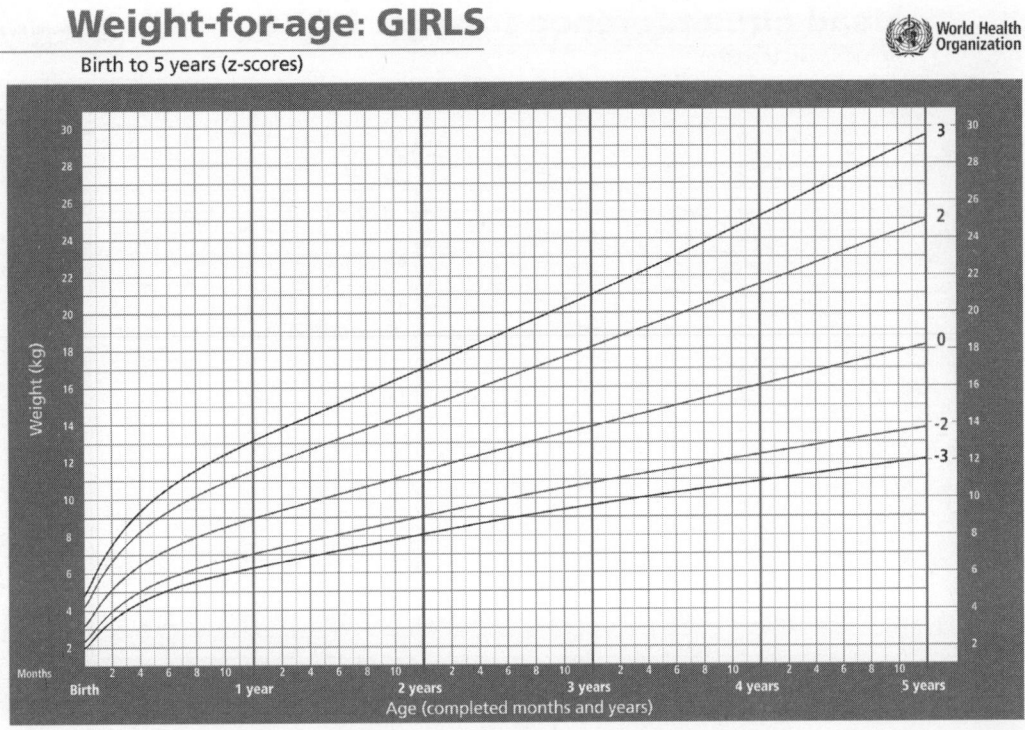

WHO Child Growth Standards

Fig. 2.21a: Weight-for-age: Girls: Birth to 5 years (z scores).

Weight-for-age: GIRLS
5 to 10 years (z-scores)

World Health Organization

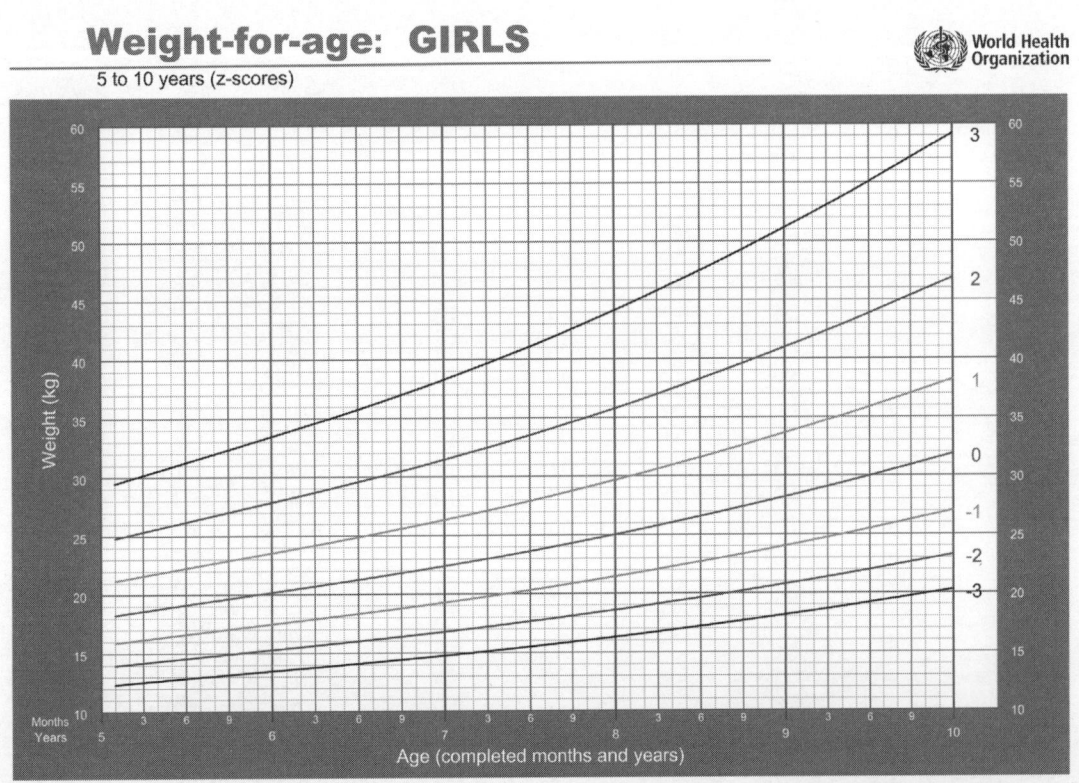

2007 WHO Reference

Fig. 2.21b: Weight-for-age: Girls: 5–10 years (z scores).

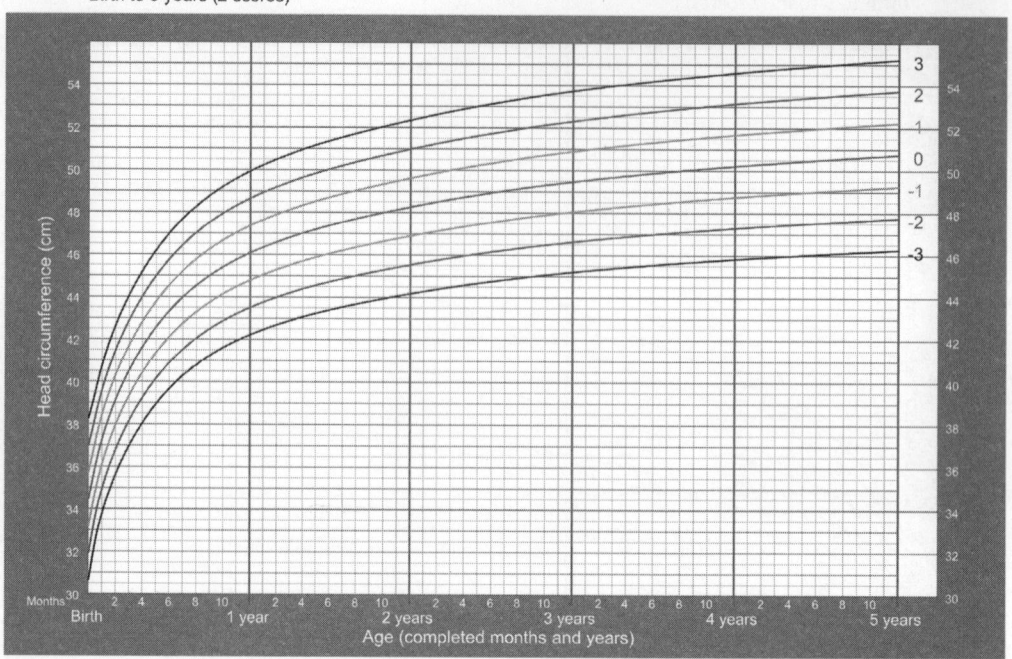

Head circumference-for-age: BOYS

Birth to 5 years (z-scores)

World Health Organization

WHO Child Growth Standards

Fig. 2.22: Head circumference-for-age: Boys: Birth to 5 years (z scores).

	Boys' weight (kg)				Length			Girls' weight (kg)		
−4 SD	−3 SD	−2 SD	−1 SD	Median	(cm)	Median	−1 SD	−2 SD	−3 SD	−4 SD
1.7	1.9	2.0	2.2	2.4	45	2.5	2.3	2.1	1.9	1.7
1.8	2.0	2.2	2.4	2.6	46	2.6	2.4	2.2	2.0	1.9
2.0	2.1	2.3	2.5	2.8	47	2.8	2.6	2.4	2.2	2.0
2.1	2.3	2.5	2.7	2.9	48	3.0	2.7	2.5	2.3	2.1
2.2	2.4	2.6	2.9	3.1	49	3.2	2.9	2.6	2.4	2.2
2.4	2.6	2.8	3.0	3.3	50	3.4	3.1	2.8	2.6	2.4
2.5	2.7	3.0	3.2	3.5	51	3.6	3.3	3.0	2.8	2.5
2.7	2.9	3.2	3.5	3.8	52	3.8	3.5	3.2	2.9	2.7
2.9	3.1	3.4	3.7	4.0	53	4.0	3.7	3.4	3.1	2.8
3.1	3.3	3.6	3.9	4.3	54	4.3	3.9	3.6	3.3	3.0
3.3	3.6	3.8	4.2	4.5	55	4.5	4.2	3.8	3.5	3.2
3.5	3.8	4.1	4.4	4.8	56	4.8	4.4	4.0	3.7	3.4
3.7	4.0	4.3	4.7	5.1	57	5.1	4.6	4.3	3.9	3.6
3.9	4.3	4.6	5.0	5.4	58	5.4	4.9	4.5	4.1	3.8
4.1	4.5	4.8	5.3	5.7	59	5.6	5.1	4.7	4.3	3.9
4.3	4.7	5.1	5.5	6.0	60	5.9	5.4	4.9	4.5	4.1
4.5	4.9	5.3	5.8	6.3	61	6.1	5.6	5.1	4.7	4.3
4.7	5.1	5.6	6.0	6.5	62	6.4	5.8	5.3	4.9	4.5
4.9	5.3	5.8	6.2	6.8	63	6.6	6.0	5.5	5.1	4.7
5.1	5.5	6.0	6.5	7.0	64	6.9	6.3	5.7	5.3	4.8
5.3	5.7	6.2	6.7	7.3	65	7.1	6.5	5.9	5.5	5.0
5.5	5.9	6.4	6.9	7.5	66	7.3	6.7	6.1	5.6	5.1
5.6	6.1	6.6	7.1	7.7	67	7.5	6.9	6.3	5.8	5.3
5.8	6.3	6.8	7.3	8.0	68	7.7	7.1	6.5	6.0	5.5
6.0	6.5	7.0	7.6	8.2	69	8.0	7.3	6.7	6.1	5.6
6.1	6.6	7.2	7.8	8.4	70	8.2	7.5	6.9	6.3	5.8
6.3	6.8	7.4	8.0	8.6	71	8.4	7.7	7.0	6.5	5.9

Table 2.13: Weight for-length reference card: Boys and Girls (below 87 cm)

(Contd.)

Table 2.13: Weight-for-length reference card: Boys and Girls (below 87 cm) (Contd.)

Boys' weight (kg)					Length			Girls' weight (kg)		
−4 SD	−3 SD	−2 SD	−1 SD	Median	(cm)	Median	−1 SD	−2 SD	−3 SD	−4 SD
6.4	7.0	7.6	8.2	8.9	72	8.6	7.8	7.2	6.6	6.0
6.6	7.2	7.7	8.4	9.1	73	8.8	8.0	7.4	6.8	6.2
6.7	7.3	7.9	8.6	9.3	74	9.0	8.2	7.5	6.9	6.3
6.9	7.5	8.1	8.8	9.5	75	9.1	8.4	7.7	7.1	6.5
7.0	7.6	8.3	8.9	9.7	76	9.3	8.5	7.8	7.2	6.6
7.2	7.8	8.4	9.1	9.9	77	9.5	8.7	8.0	7.4	6.7
7.3	7.9	8.6	9.3	10.1	78	9.7	8.9	8.2	7.5	6.9
7.4	8.1	8.7	9.5	10.3	79	9.9	9.1	8.3	7.7	7.0
7.6	8.2	8.9	9.6	10.4	80	10.1	9.2	8.5	7.8	7.1
7.7	8.4	9.1	9.8	10.6	81	10.3	9.4	8.7	8.0	7.3
7.9	8.5	9.2	10.0	10.8	82	10.5	9.6	8.8	8.1	7.5
8.0	8.7	9.4	10.2	11.0	83	10.7	9.8	9.0	8.3	7.6
8.2	8.9	9.6	10.4	11.3	84	11.0	10.1	9.2	8.5	7.8
8.4	9.1	9.8	10.6	11.5	85	11.2	10.3	9.4	8.7	8.0
8.6	9.3	10.0	10.8	11.7	86	11.5	10.5	9.7	8.9	8.1

Table 2.14: Weight-for-length reference Card: Boy and Girls (87 cm and above)

Boys' weight (kg)					Heigth			Girls' weight (kg)		
−4 SD	−3 SD	−2 SD	−1 SD	Median	(cm)	Median	−1 SD	−2 SD	−3 SD	−4 SD
8.9	9.6	10.4	11.2	12.2	87	11.9	10.9	10.0	9.2	8.4
9.1	9.8	10.6	11.5	12.4	88	12.1	11.1	10.2	9.4	8.6
9.3	10.0	10.8	11.7	12.6	89	12.4	11.4	10.4	9.6	8.8
9.4	10.2	11.0	11.9	12.9	90	12.6	11.6	10.6	9.8	9.0
9.6	10.4	11.2	12.1	13.1	91	12.9	11.8	10.9	10.0	9.1
9.8	10.6	11.4	12.3	13.4	92	13.1	12.0	11.1	10.2	9.3
9.9	10.8	11.6	12.6	13.6	93	13.4	12.3	11.3	10.4	9.5
10.1	11.0	11.8	12.8	13.8	94	13.6	12.5	11.5	10.6	9.7
10.3	11.1	12.0	13.0	14.1	95	13.9	12.7	11.7	10.8	9.8
10.4	11.3	12.2	13.2	14.3	96	14.1	12.9	11.9	10.9	10.0
10.6	11.5	12.4	13.4	14.6	97	14.4	13.2	12.1	11.1	10.2
10.8	11.7	12.6	13.7	14.8	98	14.7	13.4	12.3	11.3	10.4
11.0	11.9	12.9	13.9	15.1	99	14.9	13.7	12.5	11.5	10.5
11.2	12.1	13.1	14.2	15.4	100	15.2	13.9	12.8	11.7	10.7
11.3	12.3	13.3	14.4	15.6	101	15.5	14.2	13.0	12.0	10.9
11.5	12.5	13.6	14.7	15.9	102	15.8	14.5	13.3	12.2	11.1
11.7	12.8	13.8	14.9	16.2	103	16.1	14.7	13.5	12.4	11.3
11.9	13.0	14.0	15.2	16.5	104	16.4	15.0	13.8	12.6	11.5
12.1	13.2	14.3	15.5	16.8	105	16.8	15.3	14.0	12.9	11.8
12.3	13.4	14.5	15.8	17.2	106	17.1	15.6	14.3	13.1	12.0
12.5	13.7	14.8	16.1	17.5	107	17.5	15.9	14.6	13.4	12.2
12.7	13.9	15.1	16.4	17.8	108	17.8	16.3	14.9	13.7	12.4
12.9	14.1	15.3	16.7	18.2	109	18.2	16.6	15.2	13.9	12.7
13.2	14.4	15.6	17.0	18.5	110	18.6	17.0	15.5	14.2	12.9
13.4	14.6	15.9	17.3	18.9	111	19.0	17.3	15.8	14.5	13.2
13.6	14.9	16.2	17.6	19.2	112	19.4	17.7	16.2	14.8	13.5
13.8	15.2	16.5	18.0	19.6	113	19.8	18.0	16.5	15.1	13.7
14.1	15.4	16.8	18.3	20.0	114	20.2	18.4	16.8	15.4	14.0
14.3	15.7	17.1	18.6	20.4	115	20.7	18.8	17.2	15.7	14.3
14.6	16.0	17.4	19	20.8	116	21.1	19.2	17.5	16.0	14.5
14.8	16.2	17.7	19.3	21.2	117	21.5	19.6	17.8	16.3	14.8
15.0	16.5	18.0	19.7	21.6	118	22.0	19.9	18.2	16.6	15.1
15.3	16.8	18.3	20.0	22.0	119	22.4	20.3	18.5	16.9	15.4
15.5	17.1	18.6	22.4	22.4	120	22.8	20.7	18.9	17.3	15.6

	Table 2.15:		Head circumference-for-age: Boys: Birth to 5 years (z-score)					
Year : Month	*Months*	*−3 SD*	*−2 SD*	*−1 SD*	*Median*	*1 SD*	*2 SD*	*3 SD*
0:0	0	30.7	31.9	33.2	34.5	35.7	37.0	38.3
0:1	1	33.8	34.9	36.1	37.3	38.4	39.6	40.8
0:2	2	35.6	36.8	38.0	39.1	40.3	41.5	42.6
0:3	3	37.0	38.1	39.3	40.5	41.7	42.9	44.1
0:4	4	38.0	39.2	40.4	41.6	42.8	44.0	45.2
0:5	5	39.9	40.1	41.4	42.6	43.8	45.0	46.2
0:6	6	39.7	40.9	42.1	43.3	44.6	45.8	47.0
0:7	7	40.3	41.5	42.7	44.0	45.2	46.4	47.7
0:8	8	40.8	42.0	43.3	44.5	45.8	47.0	48.3
0:9	9	41.2	42.5	43.7	45.0	46.3	47.5	48.8
0:10	10	41.6	42.9.	44.1	45.4	46.7	47.9	49.2
0:11	11	41.9	43.2	44.5	45.8	47.0	48.3	49.6
1:0	12	42.2	43.5	44.8	46.1	47.4	48.6	49.9
1:01	13	42.5	43.8	45.0	46.3	47.6	48.9	50.2
1:2	14	42.7	44.0	45.3	46.6	47.9	49.2	50.5
1:3	15	42.9	44.2	45.5	46.8	48.1	49.4	50.7
1:4	16	43.1	44.4	45.7	47.0	48.3	49.6	51.0
1:5	17	43.2	44.6	45.9	47.2	48.5	49.8	51.2
1:6	18	43.4	44.7	46.0	47.4	48.7	50.0	51.4
1:7	19	43.5	44.9	46.2	47.5	48.9	50.2	51.5
1:8	20	43.7	45.0	46.4	47.7	49.0	50.4	51.7
1:9	21	43.8	45.2	46.5	47.8	49.2	50.5	51.9
1:10	22	43.9	45.3	46.6	48.0	49.3	50.7	52.0
1:11	23	44.1	45.4	46.8	48.1	49.5	50.8	52.2
2:0	24	44.2	45.5	46.9	48.3	49.6	51.0	52.3
2:1	25	44.3	45.6	47.0	48.4	49.7	51.1	52.5
2:2	26	44.4	45.8	47.1	48.5	49.9	51.2	52.6
2:3	27	44.5	45.9	47.2	48.6	50.0	51.4	52.7
2:4	28	44.6	46.0	47.3	48.7	50.1	51.5	52.9
2:5	29	44.7	46.1	47.4	48.8	50.2	51.6	53.0

tabulated for three years said Nita Bhandari of the Society for Applied Studies (Table 2.12). WHO child growth standards are shown in Figs 2.20 to 2.23 and Tables 2.13 to 2.16.

Each chart is composed of seven percentile curves (5th, 10th, 25th, 50th, 75th, 90th, 95th), representing the distribution of weight, length, stature, or head circumference values at each age. The percentile curve indicates the percentage of children at a given age on the X-axis whose measured value falls below the corresponding value on the Y-axis. By definition, the 50th percentile is the median, the value above (and below) which 50% of the observed values fall.

Nutritional insufficiency must be differentiated from congenital, constitutional, familial, and endocrine causes of decreased linear growth (Table 2.17). In the latter cases, the length declines first or at the same time as the weight; weight for height is normal or elevated. In nutritional insufficiency, the weight declines before the length and weight-for-height is low (unless there has been chronic stunting). In congenital pathologic short stature, an infant is born small and growth gradually tapers off throughout infancy. Causes include chromosomal abnormalities (Turner syndrome, trisomy 21), infection (TORCH [toxoplasmosis, other infections, rubella, cytomegalovirus infection, and herpes simplex] infections), teratogens (phenytoin, alcohol), and extreme prematurity. In constitutional growth delay, weight and height decrease near the end of infancy, parallel the norm through middle childhood, and accelerate toward the end of adolescence. Adult size is normal. In familial short stature, both the infants and parents are small; growth runs parallel to and just below the normal curves.

Growth charts can confirm an impression of obesity if the weight-for-height exceeds 120% of the standard (median) weight for height. The body mass index (BMI) can be calculated as weight in kilograms/(height in meters)^2 (Figs 2.24 and 2.25). If BMI is over the 95th percentile indicates "overweight," between 85th and 95th percentile is "risk of overweight," and below the 5th percentile is "underweight." BMI may not provide an accurate index of adiposity, because it does not

Table 2.16: Head circumference-for-age: Girls: Birth to 5 years (z-score)							
Year: Month	Months	-3 SD	-2 SD	-1 SD	Median	1 SD	2 SD	3 SD
0:0	0	30.3	31.5	32.7	33.9	35.1	36.2	37.4
0:1	1	33.0	34.2	35.4	36.5	37.7	38.9	40.1
0:2	2	34.6	35.8	37.0	38.3	39.5	40.7	41.9
0:3	3	35.8	37.1	38.3	39.5	40.8	42.0	43.3
0:4	4	36.8	38.1	39.3	40.6	41.8	43.1	44.4
0:5	5	37.6	38.9	40.2	41.5	42.7	44.0	45.3
0:6	6	38.3	39.6	40.9	42.2	43.5	44.8	46.1
0:7	7	39.9	40.2	41.5	42.8	44.1	45.5	46.8
0:8	8	39.4	40.7	42.0	43.4	44.7	46.0	47.4
0:9	9	39.8	41.2	42.5	43.8	45.2	45.5	47.8
0:10	10	40.2	41.5	42.9	44.2	45.6	46.9	48.3
0:11	11	40.5	41.9	43.2	44.6	45.9	47.3	48.6
1:0	12	40.8	42.2	43.5	44.9	46.3	47.6	49.0
1:1	13	41.1	42.4	43.8	45.2	46.5	47.9	49.3
1:2	14	41.3	42.7	44.1	45.4	46.8	48.2	49.5
1:3	15	41.5	42.9	44.3	45.7	47.0	48.4	49.8
1:4	16	41.7	43.1	44.5	45.9	47.2	48.6	50.0
1:5	17	41.9	43.3	44.7	46.1	47.4	48.8	50.2
1:6	18	42.1	43.5	44.9	46.2	47.6	49.0	50.4
1:7	19	42.3	43.6	45.0	46.4	47.8	49.2	50.6
1:8	20	42.4	43.8	45.2	46.6	48.0	49.4	50.7
1:9	21	42.6	44.0	45.3	46.7	48.1	49.5	50.9
1:10	22	42.7	44.1	45.5	46.9	48.3	49.7	51.1
1:11	23	42.9	44.3	45.6	47.0	48.4	49.8	51.2
2:0	24	43.0	44.4	45.8	47.2	48.6	50.0	51.4
2:1	25	43.1	44.5	45.9	47.3	48.7	50.1	51.5
2:2	26	43.3	44.7	46.1	47.5	48.9	50.3	51.7
2:3	27	43.4	44.8	46.2	47.6	49.0	50.4	51.8
2:4	28	43.5	44.9	46.3	47.7	49.1	50.5	51.9
2:5	29	43.6	45.0	46.4	47.8	49.2	50.6	52.0

Table 2.17: Severity of malnutrition: Stunting and wasting			
Grades of malnutrition	Weight-for-age* (wasting)	Height-for-age† (stunting)	Weight-for-height•
0, normal	>90	>95	>90
1, mild	75–90	90–95	81–90
2, moderate	60–74	85–90	70–80
3, severe	<60	<85	<70

Values represent percentage of median for age.

*Source: Data from Gomez F, Galvan RR, Frank S, et al. mortality in second- and third-degree malnutrition. J Trop Pediatr 1956; 2:77.

†Source: Data from Waterlow JC. Evolution of Kwashiorkor and marasmus. Lancet 1974; 2: 712.

• Source: Data from Waterlow JC. Classification and definition of protein-calorie malnutrition.BMJ 1972; 3: 566.

differentiate lean tissue and bone from fat, although it is the best clinical measure of under- and overweight. Measurement of triceps and subscapular skin fold thickness gives a better estimate of adiposity.

Other Indices of Growth

Body proportions: Body proportions follow a sequence of regular changes with development. The head and trunk are relatively large at birth, with progressive lengthening of the limbs throughout development, particularly during puberty. Proportionality can be assessed by measuring the lower body segment, defined as the length from the symphysis pubis to the floor, and the upper body segment, defined as the height minus the lower body segment (Fig. 2.14). The ratio of upper body segment divided by lower body

Table 2.18: Time of appearance in roentgenograms of centers of ossification in infancy and childhood

Boys-age at appearance*	Bones and epiphyseal centers	Girls-age at appearance*
	Humerus	
3 wk	Humerus, head	3 wk
	Carpal bones	
2 mo ± 2 mo	Capitate	2 mo ± 2 mo
3 mo ± 2 mo	Hamate	2 mo ± 2 mo
30 mo ± 16 mo	Triangular≠	21 mo ± 14 mo
42 mo ± 19 mo	Lunate≠	34 mo ± 13 mo
67 mo ± 19 mo	Trapezium≠	47 mo ± 14 mo
69 mo ± 15 mo	Trapezoid≠	49 mo ± 12 mo
66 mo ± 15 mo	Scaphoid≠	51 mo ± 12 mo
No standard available	Pisiform≠	No standard available
	Metacarpal bones	
18 mo ± 5 mo	II	12 mo ± 3 mo
20 mo ± 5 mo	III	13 mo ± 3 mo
23 mo ± 6 mo	IV	15 mo ± 4 mo
26 mo ± 7 mo	V	16 mo ± 5 mo
32 mo ± 9 mo	I	18 mo ± 5 mo
	Fingers (epiphyses)	
16 mo ± 4 mo	Proximal phalanx, 3rd finger	10 mo ± 3 mo
16 mo ± 4 mo	Proximal phalanx, 2nd finger	23 mo ± 6 mo
18 mo ± 5 mo	Proximal phalanx, 4th finger	26 mo ± 7 mo
20 mo ± 5 mo	Distal phalanx, 1st finger	32 mo ± 9 mo
23 mo ± 6 mo	Proximal phalanx, 5th finger	20 mo ± 5 mo
26 mo ± 7 mo	Middle phalanx, 3rd finger	23 mo ± 6 mo
32 mo ± 9 mo	Middle phalanx, 4th finger	26 mo ± 7 mo
18 mo ± 5 mo	Middle phalanx, 2nd finger	32 mo ± 9 mo
20 mo ± 5 mo	Distal phalanx, 3rd finger	23 mo ± 6 mo
23 mo ± 6 mo	Distal phalanx, 4th finger	26 mo ± 7 mo
26 mo ± 7 mo	Proximal phalanx, 1st finger	32 mo ± 9 mo
32 mo ± 9 mo	Distal phalanx, 5th finger	32 mo ± 9 mo
23 mo ± 6 mo	Distal phalanx, 2nd finger	23 mo ± 6 mo
26 mo ± 7 mo	Middle phalanx, 5th finger	26 mo ± 7 mo
32 mo ± 9 mo	Sesamonthid (adductor pollicis)	32 mo ± 9 mo
	Hip and knee	
Usually present at birth	Femur, distal	Usually present at birth
Usually present at birth	Tibia, proximal	Usually present at birth
4 mo ± 2 mo	Femur, head	4 mo ± 2 mo
46 mo ± 11 mo	Patella	29 mo ± 7 mo
Foot and ankle‡		

Values represent mean ± standard deviation, when applicable
*To nearest month
≠Except for the capitate and hamate bones, the variability of carpel centers is too great to make them very useful clinically
‡Standards for the foot are available but normal variation is wide, including some familial variants, so that this area is of little clinical use

segment (U/L ratio) equals approximately 1.7 at birth, 1.3 at 3 yr of age, and 1.0 after 7 yr of age. Higher U/L ratios are characteristic of short limb dwarfism (achondroplasia) or bone disorders as rickets. The lower segment is increased in comparison with the upper segment and contributes to a diminished upper segment/lower segment ratio (U/L) in Marfan syndrome and in male primary hypogonadism. The arm span substantially exceeds the height (the greatest distance between the tips of the middle finger from left to right hand with arm outspread).

Skeletal maturation: Reference standards for bone maturation facilitate estimation of bone age (Tables 2.18 and 2.19). Bone age correlates well with stage of pubertal development and can be helpful in predicting adult height in early- or late-maturing adolescents. In

Table 2.19: Model age at onset and completion of fusion in skeletal areas in adolescence		
Boys: Model age between (years)	*Area*	*Girls: Model age between (years)*
	Elbow	
13.0–13.5	Onset in humerus	11.0–11.5
15.0–15.5	Complete in ulna	12.5–3
	Foot and ankle	
14.0–14.5	Onset in great toe	12.5–13.0
15.5–16.0	Complete in tibia, fibula	14.0–14.5
	Hand and wrist	
15.0–15.5	Onset in distal phalanges	13.0–13.5
17.5–18	Complete in radius	16.0–16.5
	Knee	
15.0–15.5	Onset in tibial tuberosity	13.5–14.0
17.5–18.0	Complete in fibula	16.0–16.5
	Hip and pelvis	
15.5–16.0	Onset in greater trochanter	14.0–14.5
After 18.0	Complete in symphysis	17.5–18
	Shoulder and clavicle	
15.5–16.0	Onset in greater tubercle of humerus	14.0–14.5
After 18.0	Complete in clavicle	17.5–18.0

Table 2.20: Vital signs at various ages			
Age	*Heart rate (beats/minute)*	*Blood pressure (beats/minute)*	*Respiratory rate (breaths/minute)*
Premature	120–170*	55–75/35–45@	40–70#
0–3 mo	100–150*	65–85/45–55	35–55
3–6 mo	90–120	70–90/50–65	30–45
6–12 mo	80–120	80–100/55–65	25–40
1–3 yrs	70–110	90–105/55–70	20–30
3–6 yrs	65–110	95–110/60–75	20–25
6–12 yrs	60–95	100–120/60–75	14–22
12 yrs	55–85	110–135/65–85	12–18

*In sleep, infant heart rates may drop significantly lower, but if perfusion is maintained, no intervention is required
@A blood pressure cuff should cover approximately two thirds of the arm; too small a cuff yields spuriously high-pressure readings, and too large a cuff yields spuriously low-pressure readings
#Many premature infants require mechanical ventilatory support, making their spontaneous respiratory rate less relevant

familial short stature, the bone age is normal (comparable to chronological age). In constitutional delay, endocrinologic short stature, and undernutrition, the bone age is low and comparable to the height age. Skeletal maturation is linked more closely to sexual maturity rating than chronological age. It is more rapid and less variable in girls than in boys.

Dental development: Dental development includes mineralization, eruption, and exfoliation (*see* Chapter 27, Pediatric Dentistry). Initial mineralization begins as early as the second trimester (mean age for central incisors, 14 wk) and continues through 3 yrs of age for the primary (deciduous) teeth and 25 yrs of age for the permanent teeth. Mineralization begins at the crown and progresses toward the root. Eruption begins from the central incisors and progresses laterally. Exfoliation begins at about 6 yrs of age and continues through 12 yrs of age. Eruption of the permanent teeth may follow exfoliation immediately or may lag by 4–5 mo. Delayed eruption is usually considered when there are no teeth by approximately 13 mo of age (mean +3 SD). Common causes include hypothyroid, hypoparathyroid, familial and idiopathic. Individual teeth may fail to erupt because

Head circumference-for-age: GIRLS
Birth to 5 years (z-scores)

World Health Organization

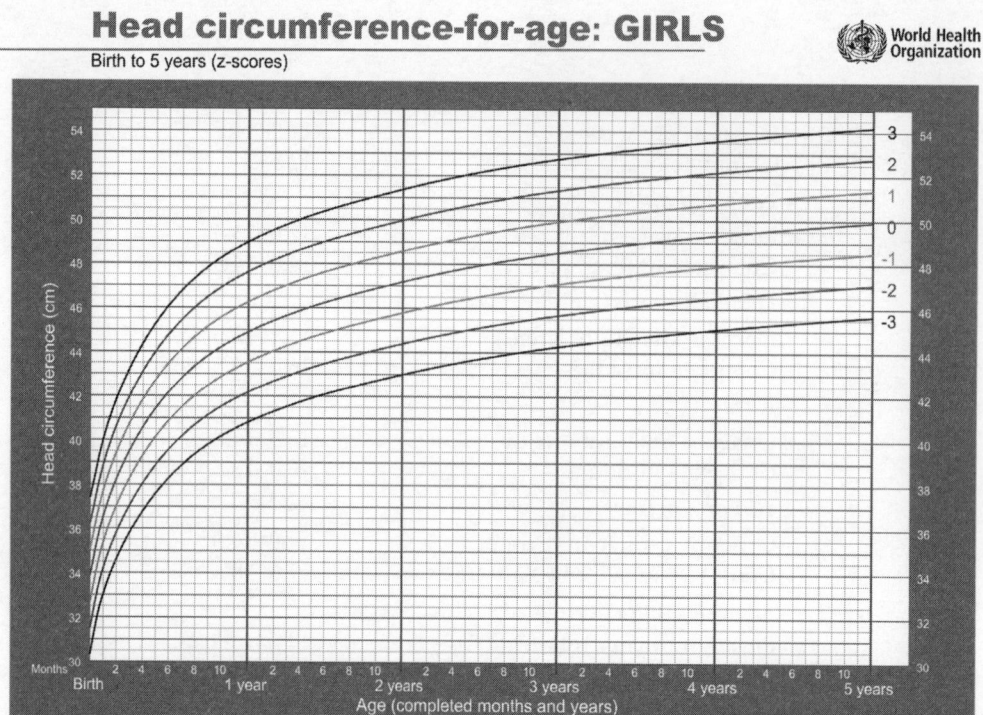

WHO Child Growth Standards

Fig. 2.23: Head circumference-for-age: Girls: Birth to 5 years (z scores).

BMI-for-age: BOYS
5 to 19 years (z-scores)

World Health Organization

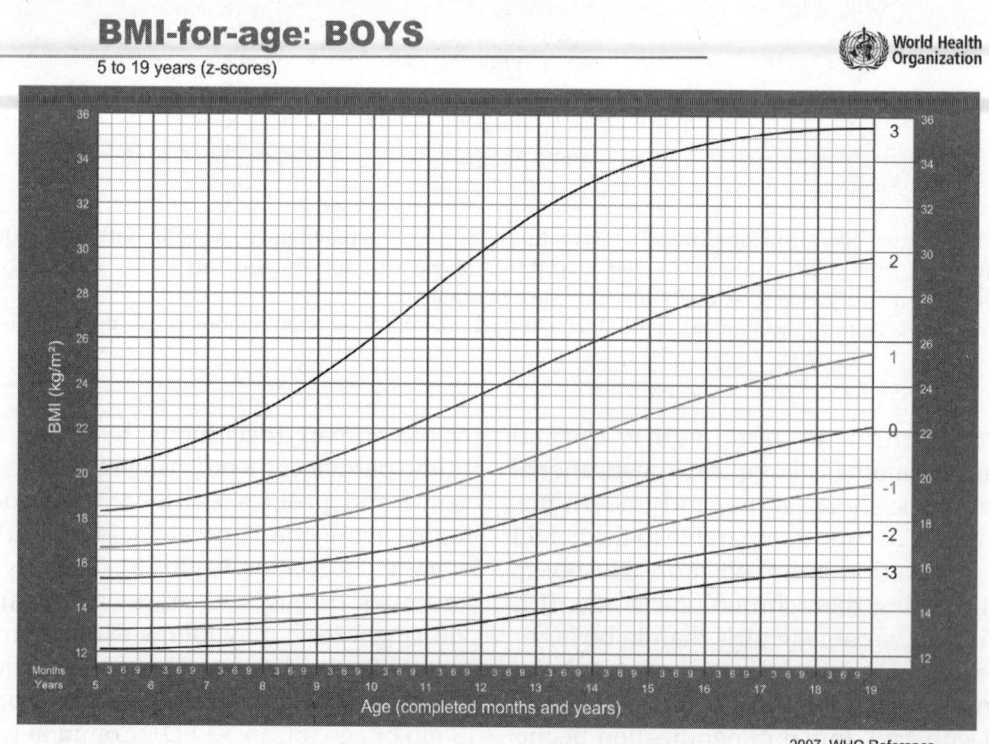

2007 WHO Reference

Fig. 2.24: Body mass index (BMI) percentiles for boys, age 5 to 19 years (z scores).

BMI-for-age: GIRLS
5 to 19 years (z-scores)

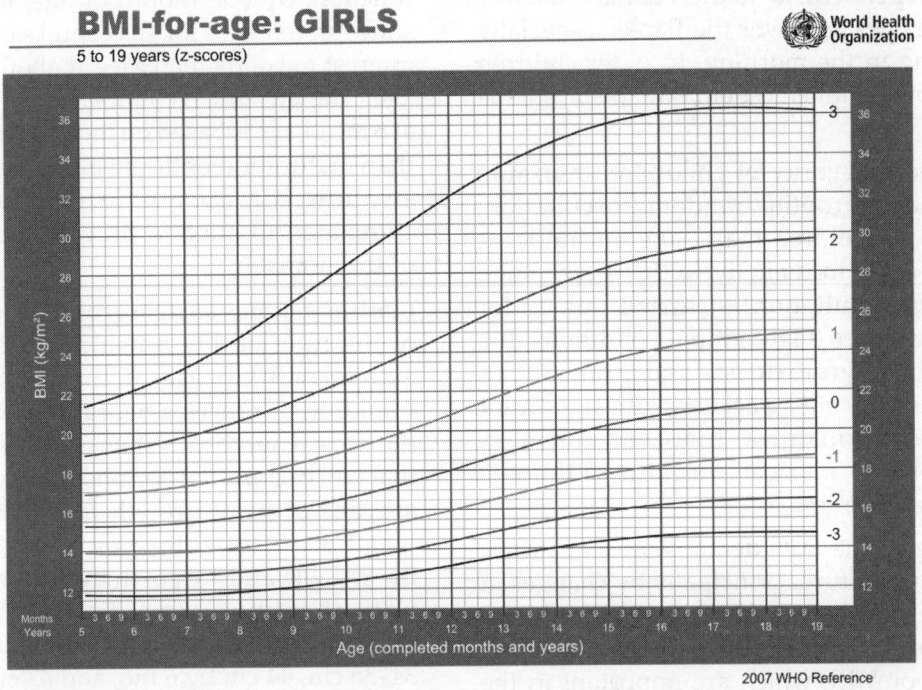

World Health Organization

2007 WHO Reference

Fig. 2.25: Body mass index (BMI) percentiles for girls, age 5–19 years (z scores).

of mechanical blockage (crowding, gum fibrosis). Causes of early exfoliation include histiocytosis X, cyclic neutropenia, trauma, and idiopathic factors. Nutritional and metabolic disturbances, prolonged illness, and certain medications (tetracycline) commonly results in discoloration or malformations of the dental enamel. A discrete line of pitting on the enamel suggests a time-limited insult.

Physiologic and structural growth: Virtually every organ and physiologic process undergoes a predictable sequence of structural and functional changes, or both, during development. Physiologic and structural changes of greater importance are discussed as follows:

1. *Respiratory system.* Respiratory rate decreases sharply during the first 2 years and then more gradually during childhood. The average respiratory rate at birth is 40/minute, 35 at 6 mo, 30 at one year; 25 at 3 yrs, 20 at 6 yrs and 14/minute at 12 yrs (Table 2.20).
2. *Paranasal sinuses.* Development of paranasal sinuses continues throughout childhood. The ethmoids, maxillary, and sphenoid sinuses are present from birth, the frontal sinuses first appear radiologically around 6 years of age. The ethmoids reach their maximum size relatively early in childhood (age 7–14 yrs); the others reach their maximum size after puberty.
3. *Cardiovascular system.* Pulse rate decreases sharply during the first 2 years and then more gradually during childhood; blood pressure rises steadily beginning at approximately 6 years of age.

Heart rate/pulse rate: The heart rate of newborn infants is rapid and subject to wide variations. The average rate ranges from 120 to 140 beats/minute and may increase to 170+ beats/minute during crying and activity, or drop to 70–90 beats/minute during sleep. As the child grows older, the average pulse rate decreases and may be as low as 40 beats/minute in athletic adolescents. The average pulse rate is 125/minute in newborn, 120 at 1–11 mo, 110 at 2 yrs, 100 at 4 to 6 yrs, 90 at 8–12 yrs, 80 at 14 yrs, 75 at 16 yrs and 70 at 18 yrs (Table 2.20).

Blood pressure: Blood pressure varies with the age of the child and is closely related to height and weight. Significant increases occur during adolescence. Exercise, excitement, coughing, crying and struggling may raise the systolic pressures of infants and children as much as 40–50 mm Hg greater than their usual levels. The blood pressure in arms is about 65/45 in the newborn, 75/50 at 1 year, 85/60 at 4 years, 95/65 at 8 years, 100/70 mm Hg at 10 years of age (Table 2.20).

Heart failure: Heart failure in infants and children usually results in some degree of hepatomegaly and occasionally splenomegaly. The sites of peripheral edema are age-dependent. In infants edema is usually seen around the eyes and over the flanks, especially after first waking in the morning. In older children and teenagers both peripheral edema and pedal edema is seen.

Innocent murmurs: Majority of childhood murmurs are innocent. During routine random auscultation, more than 30% of children may have an innocent murmur at one time in their lives; this percentage increases when auscultation is carried out under nonbasal circumstances (high out put conditions due to fever, anemia, thyrotoxicosis and pregnancy). Innocent murmurs are not associated with significant hemodynamic abnormalities. Innocent murmurs include vibratory or 'musical' murmur, pulmonic murmur and venous hum.

Electrocardiogram: The ECG demonstrates anatomic and hemodynamic features principally by changes in QRS and T-wave morphologic features. A 13-lead ECG should be performed in pediatric patients, including either lead V3R or V4R, which are important in the evaluation of right ventricular hypertrophy.

4. Lymphoid tissues develop rapidly, reaching adult size by age 6 years and continuing to hypertrophy through childhood and early adolescence before receding to adult size (Fig. 2.26).

5. The metabolism of medications and the child's response to them change rapidly in the first month of life and again in the hormonal influences in puberty. No single pattern is characteristic of all medications, and individual variation is the rule. Awareness of the possibility of changes and close monitoring are important.
Drugs in human milk—Almost all drugs are excreted in human milk.

6. Nutritional needs as well as a wide variety of biochemical and hematological values undergo marked developmental changes. For example, alkaline phosphatase level increases during period of rapid bone growth; hemoglobin has physiologic nadir at approximately 2 mo of age. The mean hemoglobin (g/dL) level is 16.8 in cord blood, 16.5 at 2 wk, 12.0 at 3 mo, 12.0 at 6 mo–6 yr, 13.0 at 7–12 yr, 14.0 in adult female, and 16.0 in adult male.

7. *Gastrointestinal system (GIT):* Swallowing and sucking: A fetus can swallow amniotic fluid as early as 12 wks of gestation, nutritive sucking in neonates first develops at about 34 wks of gestation. The coordinated oral and pharyngeal movements necessary for swallowing solids develop within the first month or two of life in term infants. Before this time solids are thrust forward by the tongue, and aspiration is a risk from poor coordination of muscle function. By one month of age, infants appear to show preferences for sweet and salty foods. Infants' interest in solids increases at about four months of age. The current recommendation to begin solids at 6 mo of age is based on nutritional concepts rather than maturation of the swallowing process. Infants swallow air during feeding and should be stimulated to burp to prevent gaseous distension of the stomach.

8. *Central nervous system growth:* During the 3rd wk of intrauterine life a neural plate appear on the ectodermal surface of the trilaminar embryo. Infolding produces a neural tube that will become the central nervous system (CNS) and a neural crest that will become the peripheral nervous system. The average of head growth in a healthy premature infant is 0.5 cm in the first 2 wks, 0.75 cm during the 3rd wk, and 1.0 cm in the 4th wk and thereafter until the 40th wk of development. The head circumference of the term infant at birth measures 34–35 cm, 44 cm by 6 mo, and 47 cm by 1 yr of age. Brain growth continues, with myelinization throughout the second year. The head grows only 2–3 cm in circumference throughout the entire period of middle childhood (6–12 yrs), reflecting slowed brain growth; myelination is complete by 7 years of age. The head grows only 2–3 cm in circumference throughout the entire period of middle childhood (6–12 yrs), reflecting slowed brain growth; myelination is complete by 7 yrs of age (Fig. 2.26).

Electroencephalogram: In young infants the EEG is dominated by generalized slow activity of so-called delta frequency, gradually during the process of maturation this is replaced by theta activity and subsequently by the alpha rhythm. Theta activity disappears last from the posterior temporal regions and the record is completely mature showing no such activity, by the age of 12–14 yrs.

9. *Somatic growth:* Periods of rapid growth: Infancy and adolescence are periods of rapid growth; high nutrient requirements for growth may be associated with voracious appetites. The physical growth during this period is rapid; growth is rapid during first six months, but slows after 6 mo. The physical growth, maturation, acquisition of competence, and psychologic reorganization occur in discontinuous (not continuous; interrupted) bursts. The weight of newborn infant may decrease 10% below birth weight in the first week but regains or exceeds birth weight by 2 wks age. The growth rate slows further in the second year of life.

By the end of the 2nd year somatic and brain growth slows, with corresponding decreases in nutritional requirements and in appetite. Growth during middle childhood occurs discontinuously in 3 to 6 irregularly timed spurts each year, each growth spurt lasting on average 8 wks (Fig. 2.26).

10. *Sexual organs growth:* The first visible sign of puberty in girls is the appearance of breast buds, between 8 and 13 years. In boys testicular enlargement begins as early as 91/2 years. At sex maturity rating 5 sexual, development is complete as seen in an adult (Fig. 2.26).

11. *Pituitary:* The anterior pituitary gland has five cell types, which produce six peptide hormones. Anterior pituitary cells are themselves controlled by neuropeptide-releasing and release-inhibiting hormones that are produced by hypothalamic neurons and play key role in the growth of an individual.

12. *Renal system:* The kidneys range in length and weight respectively, from approximately 6 cm and 24 g in a full term newborn to 12 cm or more and 150 g in an adult. The formation of nephrons (approximately 1 million nephrons) is complete at birth but functional maturation with tubular growth and elongation continues during the first decade of life. Because new nephrons cannot be formed afterbirth, progressive loss of nephrons may lead to renal insufficiency.

Mahoney CP. Evaluating the child with short stature. Pediatr Clin North Am 1987; 34: 825.

Mathers LH, Frankel LR. Stabilization of the critically ill child. In: Behrman RE, Kliegman RM, Jenson HB (eds). *Nelson Textbook of Pediatrics.* 17th edn. Philadelphia: Saunders, 2004; P279–296.

Needlman RD. Growth and development. In: Behrman RE, Kliegman RM, Jenson HB (eds). *Nelson Textbook of Pediatrics.* 17th edn. Philadelphia: Saunders, 2004; P58–62.

2.10 DEVELOPMENTAL ASSESSMENT

Developmental assessment includes early identification of problems through screening and surveillance and more definitive assessment from the developmental, social, and family history and the medical history and examination. Pediatricians should have a central role in early identification, although in practice this is not always the case. They are most effective in detecting disabilities associated with congenital or genetic abnormalities. But the problems in cognition, language, learning, and behavior are often first detected by parents or teachers.

Once a child has been identified as having a potential problem, the next step is diagnostic assessment. Pediatricians function as part of a team that may also include psychologists, educators, social workers, and other professionals. The prevalence of more common developmental disabilities are cerebral palsy (CP), visual impairment, hearing impairment, mental retardation, learning disability, behavioral disorders and attention deficit hyperactivity disorders (ADHD). The medical examination includes history, physical examination and laboratory testing. The prenatal history should include a search for potential teratogenic exposures, including radiation or medications, infectious illnesses, fever, addictive substances, and trauma. The perinatal history includes birth-weight, gestational age, Apgar scores, and any medical complications. Postnatal factors including chronic respiratory or allergic illness, recurrent otitis, head trauma, and sleep problems (particularly signs of obstructive sleep apnea) should be enquired in the history. In the physical examination growth parameters and head circumference, facial and other dysmorphology, eye findings (e.g. cataracts in various inborn errors of metabolism), and signs of neuro-cutaneous disorders (e.g. café au lait spots in neurofibromatosis, hypopigmented macules in tuberous sclerosis).

No single set of laboratory tests is indicated in all cases. Screening for hypothyroidism, phenylketonuria,

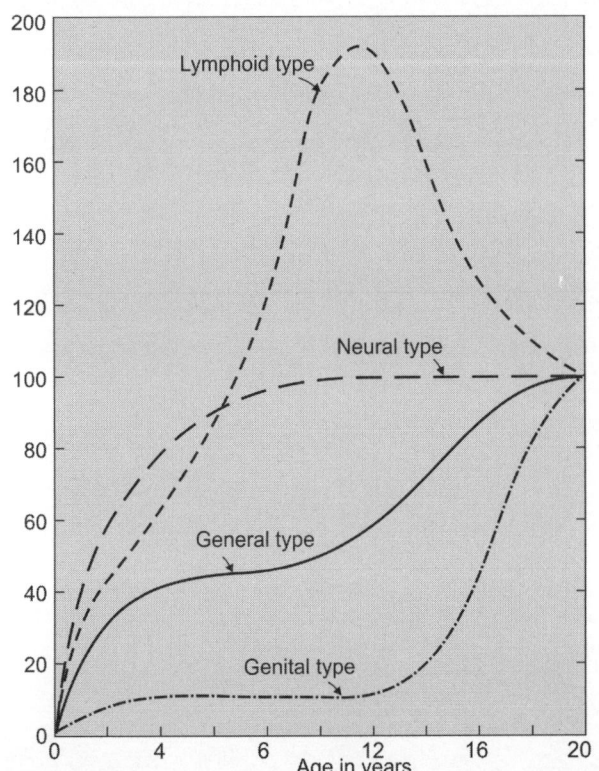

Fig. 2.26: Rate of growth of different tissues and organs (general, neural, lymphoid, and genital growth).

and other metabolic conditions in the neonatal period should be performed. Iron deficiency and lead toxicity tests should be done. Electroencephalogram and neuroimaging are not routinely indicated but should be used if there is clinical suspicion of seizure or encephalopathy or in cases of microcephaly or of rapidly expanding head circumference. The medical evaluation for mental retardation and autism should include chromosomal and biologic testing for fragile X. Ammonia and aminoacids testing may be included to screen for metabolic disease. Human immuno-deficiency virus infection must be considered in cases with progressive loss of developmental milestones and growth delay.

In neonates demonstrating their ability to track visually and turn toward sounds and their vulnerability to over stimulation is consistently associated with improvements in the infant rearing. For young children, intervention relies on parental participation. To monitor a child's progress and advise the parents, a pediatrician needs to have realistic expectations about the effectiveness of early intervention. For children who face predominantly social/environmental risk factors (e.g. poverty) strong evidence shows that early intervention can raise IQ in the short term, as well as rates of school completion, job satisfaction, and social adjustment in the long term.

Pediatricians are often called on to diagnose specific learning disabilities or attention deficit disorder in school-aged children with academic or behavioral problems or both. Vision and hearing deficits, although seldom the sole causes of school problems, must be evaluated. The interview should assess functioning in the home, the school, and the neighborhood and with peers. Definitive diagnosis usually requires a team effort. Educational testing is indicated to define areas of academic strength and weakness. Psychologic evaluation is indicated to assess emotional problems, such as depression or anxiety that may be either causes or consequences of the school problems. Assessment of the family functioning is essential. Neuropsychologic testing may be indicated to assess specific functional deficits that may cause a child to be inattentive. Pediatricians can facilitate these referrals and synthesize the information for parents and the school.

AAP Committee on Children with Disabilities: Developmental surveillance and screening of infants and young children. Pediatrics 2001; 108: 192–6.

Needlman RD. Growth and development. In: Behrman RE, Kliegman RM, Jenson HB (eds). Nelson Textbook of Pediatrics. 17th edn. Philadelphia: Saunders, 2004; 27–66.

Relier JP. Influence of maternal stress on fetal behavior and brain development. Biol Neonate 2001; 79:168–71.

Levy SE, Hyman SL. Pediatric assessment of the child with developmental delay. Pediatr Clin North Am 1993; 40:465.

3 Nutrition

3.1 NUTRITIONAL REQUIREMENTS

Nutrition may be defined as the science of food and its relationship to health. It is concerned primarily with the part played by nutrients in the body growth, development and maintenance. Nutrients are organic or inorganic complexes contained in food. Each nutrient has specific functions in the body. Most natural foods contain more than one nutrient. There are about 50 different nutrients. These nutrients may be divided into macronutrients and micronutrients. The macronutrients include proteins, fats, and carbohydrates, because they form the main bulk of food. Micronutrients are vitamins and minerals; these are required in small amounts. If the diet is deficient in one or more of these vital substances it leads to a derangement of the normal functioning of the different parts of the body, resulting in ill health, stunted growth and imperfect development. Foods are store-houses of these nutrients. There are five essential nutrients: protein, carbohydrate, fat, vitamins and minerals.

A good diet is merely a combination of foods which supply the materials vital to the body for its well-being. These dietary essentials are also known as nutrients. Normally these foods are used in formulating nutritionally adequate diets for various categories of people to meet their needs as per nutritional standards (RDA) and also for formulating special diets for therapeutic purposes (Table 3.1). In order to formulate nutritionally adequate conveniently one has to consult food group system (Table 3.2).

Balanced diet: In order to meet the nutrient needs, everyone has to eat daily at least one food item in sufficient quantity from each of the five food groups (Table 3.2). Almost all natural food-stuffs contain a mixture of different nutrients. Such a diet, in which various food stuffs are mixed in suitable proportions to carry out adequately the three functions (body

Table 3.1: Recommended dietary allowances for Indians

Group	Particulars	Body weight (kg)	Net energy (kcal/d)	Protein (g/d)	Fat (g/d)	Calcium (mg/d)	Iron (mg/d)	Vitamin A — Retinol (μg/d)	Vitamin A — β-carotene (μg/d)	Thiamine (mg/d)	Riboflavin (mg/d)	Nicotinic acid (mg/d)	Pyridoxine (mg/d)	Ascorbic acid (mg/d)	Folic acid (μg/d)	Vitamin B_{12} (μg/d)
Man	Sedentary work		2425							1.2	1.4	16				
	Moderate work	60	2875	60	20	400	28	600	2400	1.4	1.6	18	2.0	40	100	1
	Heavy work		3800							1.9	2.1	21				
Woman	Sedentary work		1875							0.9	1.1	12				
	Moderate work	50	2225	50	20	400	30	600	2400	1.1	1.3	14	2.0	40	100	1
	Heavy work		2925							1.2	1.5	16				
	Pregnant woman	50	+300	+15	30	1000	38	600	2400	+0.2	+0.2	+2	2.5	40	100	1
	Lactation															
	0–6 mo	50	+550	+25	45	1000	30	950	3800	+0.3	+0.3	+4	2.5	80	150	1.5
	6–12 mo		+400	+18						+0.2	+0.2	+3				
Infants	0–6 mo	5.4	108/kg	2.05/kg						55 μg/kg	65 μg/kg	710 μg/kg	0.1			
	6–12 mo	8.6	98/kg	1.65/kg		500		350	1200	50 μg/kg	60 μg/kg	650 μg/kg	0.4	25	25	0.2
Children	1–3 yrs	12.2	1240	22		400	12	400	1600	0.6	0.7	8	0.9		30	
	4–6 yrs	19.0	1990	30	25		18	400	2400	0.9	1.0	11		40	40	0.2–1.0
	7–9 yrs	26.9	1950	41			26	600		1.0	1.2	13	1.6		60	
Boys	10–12 yrs	35.4	2190	54		600	34	600	2400	1.1	1.3	15	1.6	40	70	0.2–1.0
Girls	10–12 yrs	31.5	1970	57			19			1.0	1.2	13				
Boys	13–15 yrs	47.8	2450	70	22	600	41	600	2400	1.2	1.5	16	2.0	40	100	0.2–1.0
Girls	13–15 yrs	46.7	2060	65	22		28			1.0	1.2	14				
Boys	16–18 yrs	57.1	2640	78	22	500	50	600	2400	1.3	1.6	17	2.0	40	100	0.2–1.0
Girls	16–18 yrs	49.9	2060	63	22		30			1.0	1.2	14				

Source: Pasricha S, Rebello LM (eds). *Some common Indian recipes and their nutritive value.* 4th edition. Hyderabad: National Institute of Nutrition, Indian Council of Medical Research, 1977; 1–128

Table 3.2: The five food groups	
Food stuff	*Main nutrient contribution*
1. Milk	
Curds, Panir (cheese), skim-milk powder	Protein
Pulses	
Dried beans and peas	Calcium
Nuts	
Meat	
Fish, poultry, eggs	Riboflavin
2. Fruits	
Orange, tomato, mango, papaya, amla, lemon juice, etc.	Carotene (vitamin A) Vitamin C
Green leafy vegetables	
Cabbage, spinach, carrot-tops, etc.	Mineral salts Iron (in leafy vegetables)
3. Other vegetables	
Brinjal, gourds, fresh beans, pumpkin, ladies finger, tinda, etc.	Vitamins and minerals (in small amounts)
4. Cereals	Carbohydrate
Rice, wheat, maize, ragi, etc.	B-Vitamins
Starchy vegetables	Protein (in cereals)
Potatoes, tapioca, yam	
5. Fats and oils	Fat (energy)
Vegetable oil, butter	Essential fatty acids
Ghee	Vitamin A (in animal fats only)
Sugar	Carbohydrate (in sugar only)
Jaggery, etc.	

Source: Pasricha S, Rebello LM (eds). *Some common Indian recipes and their nutritive value.* 4th edition. Hyderabad: National Institute of Nutrition, Indian Council of Medical Research, 1977; 1–128.

building, energy-yielding, and protective), is known as a 'Balanced Diet'. A balanced diet should provide around 60–70% of total calories from carbohydrates, preferably starch, about 10–12% from protein and 20–25% from fat. In addition, a balanced diet should provide other non-nutrients such as dietary fibre, antioxidants and phytochemicals which provide positive health benefits. The role of vegetables and fruits as a source of antioxidants is receiving considerable attention. Antioxidants restrict the damage that reactive oxygen free radicals can cause to the cell and cellular components. They are of primary biological value in giving protection from certain diseases. Some of the diseases that have their origin in deleterious free radical reactions are atherosclerosis, cancer, inflammatory joint diseases, asthma, diabetes, etc. Raw and fresh vegetables like green leafy vegetables, carrots, fresh fruits including citrus and tomato have been identified as good sources of antioxidants (free radical scavengers). Antioxidants such as vitamin C and E, beta-carotene, riboflavin and selenium protect the human body from free radical damage. Other phytochemicals such as polyphenols, flavones, etc. also afford protection against oxidant damage. Spices like turmeric, ginger, cumin and cloves are rich in antioxidants. Depending on the predominant nutrient contained, food-stuffs may be broadly classified under three heads, viz. Body-building, Protective foods, and Energy-yielding. Body-building food-stuffs are milk and milk products, meat, fish, eggs, pulses, dried beans and nuts; cereals too, contain some body building materials. The nutrients that build and renew are proteins and mineral. Some examples of protein food-stuffs are green leafy vegetables, fresh fruit, milk, meat, fish and eggs. The nutrients that carry out this protective function are chiefly the vitamins and mineral. The energy-yielding food-stuffs are chiefly cereals, sugars, fats and oils.

After 2 yrs of age, most children are eating the same foods as the rest of the family. Thus, after this age a diet based on an appropriate number of servings from the various food groups of the food guide pyramid, as modified for children older than 2 yrs of age, will provide adequate amounts of most if not all nutrients. While formulating the diet for children avoid use of too much of spices and condiments and fried foods.

Food groups	g/portion	Infants 6–12 months	Years 1–3	4–6	7–9	10–12 Girls	Boys	13–18 Girls	Boys
Cereals and millets	30	1.5	4	7	9	9	11	10	14
Pulses	30	0.5	1	1.5	2	2	2	2	2
Milk (ml)	100	5*	5	5	5	5	5	5	5
Roots and tubers	100	0.5	0.5	1	1	1	1	1	2
Green leafy vegetables	100	0.25	0.5	0.5	1	11	1	1	
Other vegetables	100	0.25	0,5	0.5	1	1	1	1	1
Fruits	100	1	1	1	1	1	1	1	1
Sugar	5	5	5	6	6	6	7	6	7
Fats and oils	5	2	4	5	5	5	5	5	5

Table 3.3: Balanced diet for infants, children and adolescents (number of portions)

*Quantity indicates top milk. For breastfed infants , 200 mL top milk is required.
One portion of pulse may be exchanged with one portion (50 g) of egg/meat/chicken/fish.
For infants introduce egg/meat/chicken/fish around 9 mo.
Cup = 200 ml; Tablespoon = 15 ml; Teaspoon = 5 ml
Source: Krishnaswamy K, Bhaskaram P, Bhat RV, et al (eds). *Dietary guidelines for Indians—A Manual.* 1st edition. Hyderabad: National Institute of Nutrition, Indian Council of Medical Research, 1998; 1–87.

Table 3.3 describes balanced diet for infants, children and adolescents.

Gopalan C, Rama Sastri BV, Balasubramanian SC, Revised and Updated by Narasinga Rao BS, Deosthale YG, Pant KC (eds). Nutritive Value of Indian Foods. Revised edn. Hyderabad: National Institute of Nutrition, Indian Council of Medical Research, 1989; 1–156.

Heird WC. Nutritional requirements. In: Behrman RE, Kliegman RM, Jenson HB (eds). Nelson Textbook of Pediatrics. 17th edn. Philadelphia: Saunders, 2004; 153–7.

Krishnaswamy K, Bhaskaram P, Bhat RV, et al (eds). Dietary guidelines for Indians—A Manual. 1st edn. Hyderabad: National Institute of Nutrition, Indian Council of Medical Research, 1998; 1–87.

Nutrient requirements and recommended dietary allowances for Indians. A report of the expert group of the Indian Council of Medical Research. 1st edn. Hyderabad: National Institute of Nutrition, Indian Council of Medical Research, 1990; 1–82.

Pasricha S, Rebello LM (eds). Some common Indian recipes and their nutritive value. 4th edn. Hyderabad: National Institute of Nutrition, Indian Council of Medical Research, 1977; 1–128.

Pasricha S. Some therapeutic diets. 5th edn. Hyderabad: National Institute of Nutrition, Indian Council of Medical Research, 1996; 1–49.

3.2 FEEDING OF INFANTS AND CHILDREN

Successful infant feeding requires cooperation between the mother and her baby, beginning with the initial feeding experience and continuing throughout the child's period of dependency. Promptly establishing comfortable, satisfying feeding practices contributes greatly to the infant's and mother's emotional well-being. Feeding time should be pleasurable for both mother and child. Mothers who are tense, anxious, irritable, easily upset, or emotionally labile are more likely to experience a difficult feeding relationship. They frequently become more comfortable and confident with appropriate guidance and support from an empathetic and experienced relative, friend, lactation consultant, or physician, which increases the likelihood of establishing successful feeding practices, not only during infancy but throughout childhood and beyond.

There is always difficulty in comparing and analyzing the data if one has not planned before hand, keeping in mind the definition of breastfeeding and complementary feeding (Table 3.4). Exclusive breastfeeding means the infant receives only breastmilk (from his/her mother or a wet nurse or expressed breastmilk) and no other liquids or complementary foods with the exception of undiluted drops or syrups consisting of vitamin and mineral supplements or medicines. Water is not permitted. Breastmilk is particularly important for preterm and low birth weight infants and those who cannot obtain sufficient breastmilk by suckling, supplements of expressed breastmilk can be given by cup.

Complementary food means any food, whether manufactured or locally prepared, suitable as a complement to breastmilk or to infant formula, when either becomes insufficient to satisfy the nutritional requirements of the infant. Such food has been variously referred to as weaning food, semi-solids or solids. These less well defined terms are now avoided in international usage.

Artificial feeding: Giving a breastmilk substitute, whether totally or partially—increases the risk of

Table 3.4: Definitions of infant feeding

Category of infant feeding	Requires that the infant receives	Allows the infant to receive	Does not allow the infant to receive
Exclusive breastfeeding	Breastmilk (including milk expressed or from wet-nurse)	Drops, syrups (vitamins, minerals, medicines)	Anything else
Predominant Breastmilk	Breastfeeding (including milk expressed or from wet-nurse) as the predominant source of nourishment	Liquids (water, and water-based drinks, fruit juice, ORS), ritual fluids and drops, syrups (vitamins, minerals, medicines)	Anything else (in particular, non-human milk, food based fluids)
Complementary feeding	Breastmilk and solid or semi-solid foods	Any food or liquid including non-human milk	-
Breastfeeding	Breastmilk	Any food or liquid including non-human milk	-
Bottle-feeding	Any liquid or semi-solid food from a bottle with nipple/teat	Any food or liquid including non-human milk. Also allows breastmilk by bottle	-

Source: WHO Global Data Bank on Breastfeeding. Breastfeeding: The best start in life. WHO Nutrition Unit, 1996

illness, poor growth and development, and malnutrition. When artificial feeding is unavoidable, families should receive the assistance necessary to give artificial feeds as safely as possible. Cup-feeding is cleaner and safer and should be advised.

Replacement feeding: The term "replacement feeding" is used to describe feeding of infants whose mothers have tested positive for HIV, and who, after counseling, choose not to breastfeed. It refers to the process of feeding a child who is not receiving any breastmilk with a diet that provides all the nutrients the child needs. During the first six months, this should be with a suitable breastmilk substitute—commercial infant formula or home-prepared formula with micronutrient supplements. After six months it should preferably be with a suitable breastmilk substitute and complementary foods made from appropriately prepared and nutrient enriched family foods, given three times a day. If suitable breastmilk substitutes are not available, appropriately prepared family foods should be further enriched and given five times a day.

Feeding during the First 6 Months of Life

Feeding should be initiated as soon afterbirth as possible, depending on the infant's ability to tolerate enteral nutrition. This will maintain normal metabolism during the transition from fetal to extrauterine life and will also promote maternal–infant bonding, most infants can start breastfeeding shortly afterbirth, almost always within 4–6 hr. Mothers who wish to initiate breastfeeding in the delivery room and continue to do so on a demand basis should be supported in doing so. If the infant is unable to tolerate

feedings, it should be withheld until the infant is carefully evaluated. If it appears that feedings must be withheld for several hours, parenteral fluids should be administered. Most infants will have established a suitable and reasonably regular schedule by one month of age. By the end of first week of life, most healthy infants will want 6–9 feedings/24 hr. Some will take enough at one feeding to be satisfied for as long as 4 hr, but others will want to be fed as often as every 2–3 hr. In general, breastfed infants prefer shorter feeding intervals than formula-fed infants. Most infants would be taking 80–90 ml per feeding by the end of the first week of life. Feeding can be considered to have progressed satisfactorily, if the infant is no longer loosing weight by the end of first week and is gaining weight by the end of the second week. Although most infants will awaken for middle-of-the-night feeding until 3–6 wks of age, some never desire this feeding and others continue to desire it well beyond 3–6 wks of age. Between 4 and 8 mo of age, many infants will loose interest in the late evening feeding and by 9–12 mo of age, most will be satisfied with 3 meals/day plus snacks. However, not all infants confirm to these general guidelines. Individual feeding needs are quite variable, and not all infants can be expected to fit the same pattern.

It is important to appreciate that infants cry for reasons other than hunger and that they do not need to be fed every time they cry. Those who awaken and cry consistently at short intervals may not be receiving enough milk, or they may have discomfort from some cause other than hunger (e.g. too much clothing; cry to gain sufficient or additional attention or to be picked up; colic; soiled, wet, or uncomfortable diapers; swallowed air ("gas"); an uncomfortably hot or cold environment; illness). Those who stop crying as soon they are picked up or held usually do not need food. Those who continue to cry when held and when food is offered should be carefully evaluated for other causes of distress. It is not desirable to allow development of habit in the infant by offering frequent, small feedings or holding and feeding to pacify all crying.

The postpartum period is a time of great anxiety and insecurity, particularly for the first-time mother who often is temporarily overwhelmed by the responsibilities of motherhood. The physician should address the questions and concerns of inexperienced or uncertain mothers shortly after birth. Ideally, these anticipatory guidance sessions should include fathers and other household members.

Breastfeeding

One of the decisions a new mother must take—ideally, sometime before the infant is born, whether the infant will be breastfed or formula-fed. Human milk is adapted to the infant's needs and is the most appropriate milk for the human infant. Breastfeeding also has practical and psychological advantages. Thus, all mothers should be encouraged to at least consider breastfeeding her baby (Table 3.5).

Advantages of breastfeeding: Breastmilk is the natural food for full-term infants during the first month of life. It is always available at the proper temperature and requires no preparation time. It is fresh and free of contaminating bacteria, and therefore, chances of having gastrointestinal disease are reduced. Although there is little if any difference in mortality rates between formula-fed and breastfed infants receiving good care, the protective effects of breastmilk against enteric and other pathogens result in less mortality. These effects are particularly important in developing

countries or any locality without a safe supply of portable water and effective methods for disposal of human waste.

Breastfeeding is associated with fewer feeding difficulties as regards to allergy and/or intolerance as compared to bovine milk. These include diarrhea, intestinal bleeding, occult melena, "spitting up," colic, and atopic eczema. Breastfed infants also appear to have a lower frequency of certain allergic and chronic diseases in later life than formula-fed infants.

Human milk contains bacterial and viral antibodies, including relatively high concentrations of secretory IgA that prevents microorganisms from adhering to the intestinal mucosa. It also contains substances that inhibit growth of many common viruses. Antibodies in human milk are thought to provide local gastrointestinal immunity against organisms entering the body via this route. They probably account at least partially, for the lower incidence of diarrhea, otitis media, pneumonia, bacteremia, and meningitis during the first year of life in infants who are breastfed exclusively vs. formula-fed for the first 4 mo of life.

Macrophages in human milk may synthesize complement, lysozyme, and lactoferrin. In addition, breastmilk contains lactoferrin, an iron-binding whey protein that is normally about one-third saturated with iron and has an inhibitory effect on the growth of *Escherichia coli* in the intestine. The lower pH of the stool of breastfed infants contributes to the favorable intestinal flora of infants fed human milk vs. formula (i.e., more bifidobacteria and lactobacilli; fewer *E. coli*), which helps protect against infections caused by some species of *E. coli*. Human milk also contains bile-salt-stimulated lipase which kills *Giardia lamblia* and *Entamoeba histolytica*. Transfer of tuberculin responsiveness by breastmilk suggests positive transfer of T cell immunity. Milk from the mother whose diet is sufficient and properly balanced will supply all the

Table 3.5: Composition: breastmilk, colostrum and cow's milk			
Constituents	*Breastmilk*	*Colostrum**	*Cow's milk*
Kcal/100 ml	67	67	67
Solids (g/ml)	13	13	12.5
Ash (minerals g/ml)	0.2	0.3	0.7
Protein (g/ml) *Total*	1.5	2.3	3.2
Casein	0.4	1.8	2.5
Whey protein	0.7	0.2	0.7
Lactalbumin	0.4	–	–
Lactoglobulin	–	0.3	–
Carbohydrate (lactose)	7	5.7	4.5
Fat	3.5	3.0	3.5
Vitamin A (µg)	60	161	23

*Colostrum (first 5 days postpartum) is deep lemon-yellow color due to increased carotenoids

necessary nutrients except, perhaps, fluoride, and after several months vitamin D.

The breastfed should receive at least 10 µg fluorides daily for the first 6 mo of life, if the water supply is not sufficiently fluoridated (≥ 0.3 ppm). If the maternal vitamin D intake is inadequate and the infant's exposure to sunlight is limited (e.g. dark-skinned infants and infants who are chronically protected from sunlight), 10 µg/24 hr of vitamin D is recommended. The iron content of human milk is somewhat low, but most normal infants have sufficient iron stores for the first 6 mo of life. Moreover, human milk iron is well absorbed. Nonetheless, after 6 mo of age, the breastfed infant's diet should be supplemented with iron-fortified complementary foods or a ferrous iron preparation. The vitamin K content of human milk also is low and may contribute to hemorrhagic disease of the newborn; parenteral administration of 1 mg of vitamin K1 at birth is recommended for all infants and this is especially important for those who will be breastfed.

The psychologic advantages of breastfeeding for mother and infant are well known. The mother is herself involved in nurturing her infant, resulting in both a feeling of being essential and a sense of accomplishment while the infant is provided with a close and comfortable physical relationship with the mother. The resumption of menstruation is no contraindication of breastfeeding. Pregnancy does not necessitate immediate cessation of nursing, but due to combined demands of supplying milk to the infant and nutrients to the developing fetus, special attention is needed for maternal nutrition.

Transmission of HIV by breastfeeding is well documented. Thus, if safe alternatives are available, breastfeeding by HIV-infected mothers is not recommended. However, in many developing countries breastfeeding may be crucial to infant survival, and therefore, the risk of HIV transmission by breastfeeding may be less than the risks of other feeding methods. The World Health Organization recommends that breastfeeding be continued, even in areas of high endemic rates of HIV infection, unless safe infant formula is readily available. Cytomegalovirus (CMV), human T cell lymphotropic virus type 1, rubella virus, hepatitis B virus, and herpes simplex virus also have been demonstrated in breastmilk. About two-thirds of seronegative breastfed infants may become infected with CMV. In term infants, this appears to be without symptoms or sequelae, but the risk of infection in preterm infants may be substantially greater. Thus, the use of fresh donor milk for feeding preterm infants is contraindicated unless the milk is known to be CMV negative. Vesicles have been noted in the mouth of infants whose mothers' milk contained herpes simplex virus. Nursing mothers with active herpes simplex lesions should feed after scrupulous hand-washing technique and should avoid nursing if there are active lesions on or near the nipple. Hepatitis B virus has been also isolated from maternal milk; the predominant means of mother–infant transmission of this virus appears to be at delivery. Active immunization of the infant within the first 24 hr of life coupled with administration of specific high-titer hepatitis B immune globulin and a follow-up active vaccination should permit the mother who is infected with hepatitis B to nurse with minimal risk to the infant. If a nursing mother acquires hepatitis B, the infant should receive the accelerated protocol of immunization. Breastmilk transmission of other viruses is rare.

Preparation of prospective mother for breastfeeding: The physician should discuss the advantages of breastfeeding to the prospective mother as early as the midtrimester of pregnancy or whenever the mother begins planning for her infant in order to promote breastfeeding. Most women, if encouraged, educated, and also protected from discouraging experiences and comments while milk secretion is becoming established, can successfully breastfeed their infants. Many mothers who are ambivalent toward breastfeeding are able to nurse successfully if reassured and supported. In order to encourage and promote exclusive breastfeeding for 1st 6 mo to enhance child survival, the Baby-Friendly Hospital Initiative (BFHI) was launched jointly by WHO and UNICEF in March, 1992. BFHI is a global effort with hospitals to provide support to the mother before, during, and after delivery so that she has a joyful breastfeeding experience. These hospitals must fully practice "ten steps to successful breastfeeding" given in a joint WHO/UNICEF document (Box 3.1). The concept of supporting mothers to breastfeed is important so that they can exclusively breastfed their infants for first 6 mo and to continue breastfeeding from 6 mo to 2 yrs along with solid foods. But promotion of breastfeeding alone is not enough to make a hospital baby-friendly. This should also include practices which will make hospital safe for newborns and their mothers such as:

i. Safe delivery practices;

ii. Proper care of the umbilical cord;

iii. Warming and temperature regulation afterbirth; and

iv. Early diagnosis and management of conditions such as absence of spontaneous breathing, aspiration, sepsis, hypoglycemia, hypocalcemia, etc.

Factors that are conducive to successful breastfeeding include good health, a proper balance of rest

Every facility providing maternity services and care for newborn infants should:

1. Have a written breastfeeding policy that is routinely communicated to all health care staff
2. Train all health care staff in skills necessary to implement this policy
3. Inform all pregnant women about the benefits and management of breastfeeding
4. Help mothers initiate breastfeeding within half-hour of birth
5. Show mothers how to breastfeed, and how to maintain lactation, even if they should be separated from their infants
6. Give newborn infants no food or drink other than breast milk, unless medically indicated
7. Practice rooming in—allow mothers and infants to remain together 24 hours a day
8. Encourage breastfeeding on demand
9. Give no artificial teats or pacifier like dummies or soothers to breastfeeding infants
10. Foster the establishment of breastfeeding support groups and refer mother to them on discharge from the hospital or clinic

and exercise, freedom from worry, early and sufficient treatment of any intercurrent disease, and adequate nutrition. If the mother's diet is adequate, she need not gain or lose weight while breastfeeding. Breast-feeding will help the uterus return to its normal size sooner and, also, may help the mother return to her pre-pregnancy weight sooner. Many women must be reassured that breast tone will be preserved by the use of a properly fitted brassiere to support the breasts, especially before delivery and during the nursing period.

Problems in Breastfeeding

Flat or short nipples which protract well do not cause difficulty in breastfeeding. By holding the breast well back on the areola using index finger on the lower side and thumb on the upper side, more breast tissue can be put into baby's mouth. It means breast is quite protractile. It will be easy for her baby to form a physiological teat.

Retracted or inverted nipples make attachment to the breast difficult. These mothers need additional support to feed their babies. Treatment should be stated early. The nipple is manually stretched and rolled out several times a day. A pump or a plastic syringe is used to draw out the nipple and the baby is then put to the breast. The plastic syringe is cut (A) and then the piston is inserted from the cut end (B).

Mother places her nipple into the syringe and gently pulls the piston (C) (Fig. 3.1).

Sore nipple: A sore nipple is caused by incorrect attachment of the baby to the breast. A baby who sucks only on the breast nipple rather than areola does not get enough milk. Therefore the baby sucks vigorously often in frustration and inflicts injury on the nipple causing soreness. Frequent washing with soap and water, pulling the baby off the breast while he is still sucking may also result in sore nipple. Candida infection of the nipple is also a cause of a sore nipple after the first few weeks. The treatment consists of correct positioning and latching of the baby to the breast. A mother would be able to feed the baby despite sore nipples if the baby is attached properly. Hind milk should be applied to the nipple after a feed and the nipple should be aired and allowed to heal in between the feeds. Mother should be advised not to wash nipple each time before/after feeding. She can clean breast and nipple once daily at time of bathing.

Breast engorgement: The milk production increases during the second or third day after delivery. If feeding is delayed or infrequent, or the baby is not well positioned at the breast, the milk accumulates in the alveoli. As the milk production increases, the amount of milk in the breast exceeds the capacity of the alveoli to store it. The breast ultimately becomes swollen, hard, warm and painful and is termed as an 'engorged breast.' Breast engorgement can be prevented by early and frequent feeds and correct attachment of the baby to the breast. Treatment consists of local warm water packs, breast massage and analgesics to the mother to relieve pain. Milk should be gently expressed to soften the breast and then the mother should be helped to correctly latch the baby to the breast.

Breast abscess: If a congested, engorged breast, an infected cracked nipple, or a blocked duct and mastitis are not treated in early stages, then an infected breast

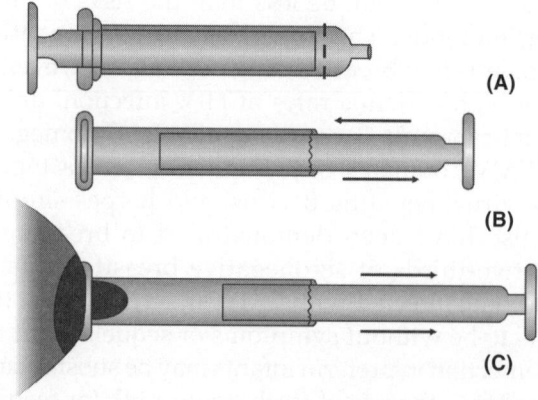

Fig. 3.1: A plastic syringe is used to draw out the nipple, if the mother has retracted or inverted nipples.

segment may form a breast abscess. The mother may also have high fever and a raised blood count. Mother should be treated with antibiotics and analgesics. The abscess should be incised and drained. Mother is advised to continue breastfeeding.

Not enough milk: This is a common complaint of the mother. First make sure that the perception of the mother regarding 'not enough milk' is correct. If the baby is satisfied and sleeping for 2–3 hours after breastfeeding and passing urine at least 6–8 hours and gaining weight, then the mother is producing enough milk.

There could be a number of reasons for 'insufficient milk' such as incorrect method of breastfeeding, supplementary feeding, bottle feeding, no night breastfeeding, engorgement of breast, any illness, painful condition, stress or insufficient sleep in the mother. Identify the possible reason and advise mother to take correct action. Advise mother to take sufficient rest and drink more fluids. Feed the baby on demand. Let the baby feed for as long as possible on each breast. Feed only at breast. Advise the mother to keep the baby with her.

Expressed breastmilk: If a mother is not in a position to feed her baby (e.g. ill mother, preterm baby, working mother, etc.), she should express her milk in a clean wide-mouthed container and this milk should be fed to her baby. Expressed breastmilk can be stored at room temperature for 6–8 hrs, in a refrigerator for 24 hrs and a freezer at –20°C for 3 mo.

Method of breastmilk expression: Ask the mother to wash her hands thoroughly with soap every time before she expresses breast milk. She makes herself comfortable and gently massages the breast. Hold the container under her nipple and areola. Place her thumb on top of the breast at least 4 cm from the tip of the nipple and the first finger on the under side of the breast opposite the thumb. Compress and release the breast tissue between her fingers and thumb a few times. If the milk does not appear, she should reposition her thumb and fingers closer to the nipple and compress and release the breast as before. Compress and release all the way around the breast, keeping her fingers the same distance from the nipple. She should never compress the nipple. The technique to express breastmilk should be taught to every mother.

Establishing and maintaining the milk supply: The most satisfactory stimulus to the secretion of human milk is regular and complete emptying of the breasts. Thus, efforts should be directed toward the early establishment of normal vigorous nursing, even during the first few days afterbirth when there appears to be little, if any, milk. Breastfeeding should begin as soon as after delivery as the conditions of the mother and the infant permit, preferably within the first hour, or so. Infants who cannot be fed on demand should be brought to the mother for feeding about every 3 hrs during the day and night. Once lactation is well established, most mothers are capable of producing more milk than their infant needs.

The maintenance of established milk secretion depends on intact hypothalamic pituitary axis regulating two hormones—prolactin and oxytocin levels. The two maternal reflexes involved in lactation are milk production reflex and milk ejection reflex. Both these reflexes involve hormones prolactin and oxytocin respectively. The three infant reflexes are rooting reflex, sucking reflex, and swallowing reflex. Rooting reflex programmes the infant to search for the nipple while gaping widely enough to take a good mouthful of breast tissue. Sucking reflex is triggered when something touches the palate. Swallowing occurs when the infant's mouth fills with milk after 2–3 sucks (swallowing reflex).

Appropriate care for tender or sore nipples should be instituted before severe pain from abrasions and cracking develops. Exposing the nipples to the air; applying pure lanolin (wool fat); avoiding soap, alcohol, and tincture of benzoin; changing disposable nursing pads lining the brassiere cups frequently; nursing more frequently; manually expressing milk; nursing in different positions; and keeping the breast dry between feedings are recommended. If nipple tenderness is sufficient to make the mother apprehensive, the milk-ejection reflex is delayed. This leads to frustration of the infant and increasingly vigorous nursing, which further injures the nipple and areolar area. Nipple shields may be helpful in these situations.

The first 2 wks after birth are crucial for establishing breastfeeding and this is the period to promote and support breastfeeding. Daily weight gains of the infant, while important for ascertaining the volume of milk produced should not be done. In addition, supplemental bottle feedings to achieve weight gain should be limited because these may compromise attempts at breastfeeding. Although the difference between breast and bottle nipples may confuse the infant, this is usually not a serious problem. It is perfectly satisfactory to have the mother squeeze by manual expression/pump her breasts and feed the breastmilk via a bottle for the 1–2 wks then, when she is relaxed and less anxious, she can attempt breastfeeding one or two times daily until mother and the infant have achieved a successful nursing routine. The additional pumping will usually increase milk production, thereby helping to ensure an adequate supply. Even after nursing is well established, it may be appropriate for the mother to pump extra milk and store it (in a freezer for up to 1 month or refrigerator for up to 24 hrs) for use when she is not available. This allows the mother some freedom, and at the same time, allows the father or other caregivers to be more involved in the infant's feeding and care. Lactation usually is not well established before the mother is discharged from the hospital, and the excitement of going home may impede an initially successful in-hospital nursing experience. One should anticipate this possibility and discuss with the mother, and to prevent discourage-ment that might produce further nursing, one may have to provide enough formula for a few comple-mentary feedings to some individual mothers.

The most important factor for successful breast-feeding is a happy, relaxed state of mind. Mothers may worry that their infants are abnormal when they cry, are drowsy, sneeze, or regurgitate milk. They are often upset by any suggestion that their milk may be lacking in quantity or quality, and they may be disturbed by the scanty supply of colostrum, nipple tenderness, and the fullness of the breasts on the fourth or fifth day after delivery. Many mothers do not feel comfortable when trying to breastfeed in an open ward, or even with another person in the room. Many mothers may worry about what is going on at home while they are in the hospital or about what is going to happen when they arrive home. The physician should provide reassurance and explanations to mothers, particularly if the infant is a first born, that minimizes worry and enhances the likelihood of successful breastfeeding. In making a support plan for individual mothers social and cultural factors should always be kept in mind.

Hygiene: Proper hygiene will help prevent irritation and infection of nipples caused by prolonged initial nursing, maceration from wetness of the nipple, or rubbing of clothing. The breasts should be washed at least once a day. If soap appears to dry the nipple and areolar area; a milder, nondrying soap should be substituted or use of soap should be temporarily discontinued. The nipple area should be kept as dry as possible. Many mothers are more comfortable wearing a properly fitted brassiere day and night. If doing so, plastic liners should be removed and a commercially available absorbent pad or clean cloth should be placed inside the brassiere to absorb any leaked milk.

Maternal diet and other factors: The breastfeeding mother's diet should contain enough calories and other nutrients to compensate for those secreted in the milk as well as for those required to produce it. A varied diet sufficient to maintain weight and providing sufficient fluid, vitamins and minerals is important. Weight reducing diets should be avoided, particularly while the infant is exclusively breastfed. Mother's diet must contain milk, but if she is allergic to milk or dislikes it, her diet should be supplemented with 1 g calcium daily. Daily fluid intake should approximately be 3 liter (3,000 ml).

Ingestion of some foods (e.g. berries, tomatoes, onions, members of the cabbage family, chocolate, spices, and condiments) by the mother may occasionally cause gastric distress or loose stools in the infant. However, no food need to be withheld from the mother unless it is known to cause, or is strongly suspected causing, distress to the infant.

Nursing mothers should not take drugs unless they are absolutely necessary. Antithyroid medications, lithium, anticancer agents, isoniazid, recreationally abused drugs and phenindione are contraindicated for the breastfeeding mother. If any of these agents or diagnostic radiopharmaceuticals, chloramphenicol, metronidazole, sulfonamides, and/or anthraquinone-derivative laxatives is required, temporary cessation of breastfeeding should be considered. Smoking cigarettes and drinking alcoholic beverages should be discouraged during breastfeeding. Breastfeeding mothers should avoid fatigue, but should exercise sufficiently to promote in them sense of physical well-being.

Technique of breastfeeding: It is important to inform the technical aspects of breastfeeding with the mother, particularly the mother who has not breastfed before (Fig. 3.2). At feeding time, the infant should be hungry, dry, and neither too cold nor too warm. He or she should be held in a comfortable, semi-sitting position to prevent vomiting with eructation. The mother, too, should be comfortable and completely at ease. The infant should be supported comfortably with the face held close to the mother's breast by one arm and hand while the other hand supports the breast, making the nipple easily accessible to the infant's mouth without obstructing nasal breathing. Offer the whole breast, not just nipple, to the baby. Wait until the baby's mouth is wide open and move him quickly onto the breast so that he takes a good mouthful of areola. He should come onto the nipple from below it, not from the top. The infant's lips should engage considerable areola as well as nipple (Figs 3.3 and 3.4). If the infant is breastfed when hungry and his or her appetite is satisfied that means the mother has adopted correct technique of breastfeeding.

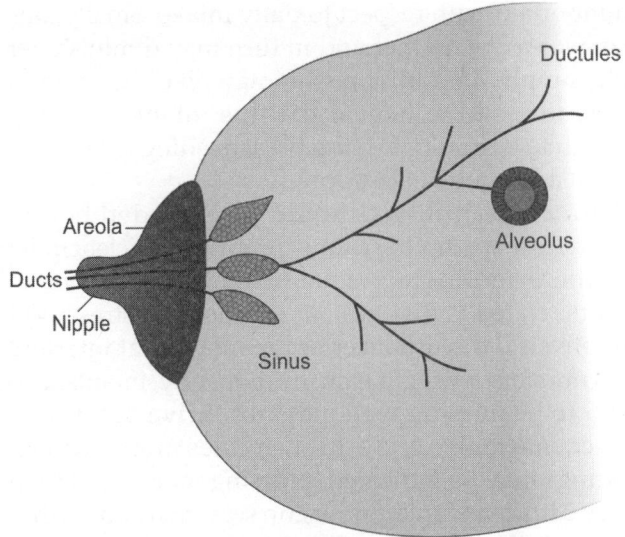

Fig. 3.2: Breast showing areola, nipple, ducts, sinus, ductules and alveolus.

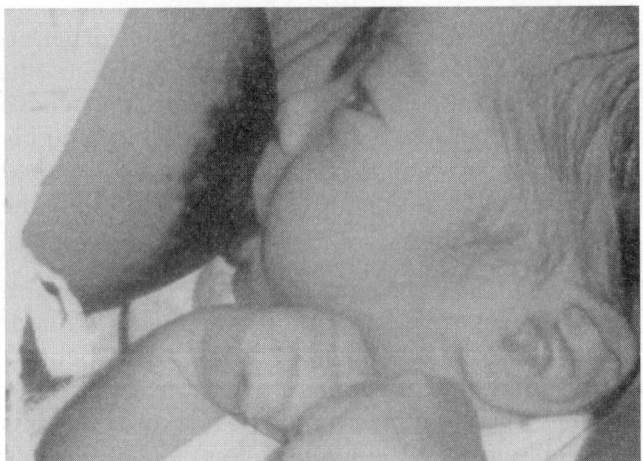

Fig. 3.3: Poor attachment (*Courtesy:* Dr Sarla Mathur).

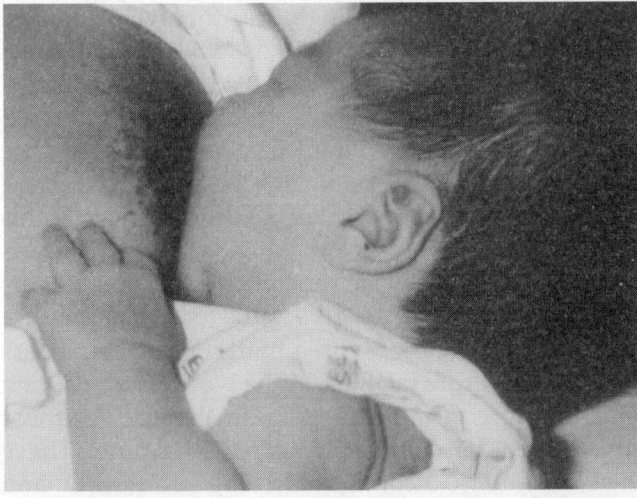

Fig. 3.4: Good attachment (*Courtesy:* Dr Sarla Mathur).

A Baby in a Good Attachment (Fig. 3.4)

- Is close to the mother, and the chin touches the breast
- Has the mouth wide open, cheeks are full
- The lower lip has turned out and you may see the tongue)
- Takes slow, deep sucks
- Causes no pain to the mother
- Mother and infant are comfortable.

Five reflexes (rooting, sucking, swallowing, milk production reflex and milk ejection reflex) and two hormones (prolactin and oxytocin) that facilitate breastfeeding are present at birth. The rooting reflex is the first to come into play. When the infant smells milk, he or she moves the head in an attempt to find the source of smell. If the cheek is touched by a smooth object (e.g. the mother's breast), the infant will turn toward that object and open his or her mouth in anticipation of grasping the nipple (i.e. rooting with the mouth for the nipple). The infant's rooting reflex brings the entire areolar area into the infant's mouth and contact of the nipple against the infant's palate and posterior tongue elicits sucking, while the buccal fat pads help keep the nipple in place. The sucking reflex is a process of squeezing the sinuses of the areola rather than simply sucking on the nipple, as is required in the bottle-feeding. Finally the milk in the infant's mouth triggers the swallowing reflex.

The breastfeeding infant's sucking results in afferent impulses to the mother's hypothalamus, and then, to both anterior and posterior pituitary. Prolactin release from the anterior pituitary stimulates milk secretion by the cuboidal cells in the acini or alveoli of the breast while secretion of oxytocin by the posterior pituitary results in contraction of the myoepithelial cells surrounding the alveoli deep in the breast, and in turn, "squeezes" milk into the larger ducts, where it is more easily available to the sucking infant. When this "let down" or milk ejection reflex functions well, milk flows from the other opposite breast as the infant begins to nurse. The milk ejection reflex is often absent or erratic during periods of pain, fatigue or emotional distress and this is considered to be a common cause of milk retention in women who are unsuccessful in breast-feeding.

Mothers should be told that if the infant is not hungry, he or she will not search for the nipple or suck. Most infants are usually sleepy for several days after birth, and hence are not avid suckers. By the third day of life when there has been some weight loss, many mothers become anxious if the mother seems uninterested in nursing. Assure the mothers that most healthy infants "wake up" and become good nursers by the 4th or 5th day of life. Infants whose mothers were sedated during labor usually suck at a lower rates and also consume less milk than infants of non-sedated mothers. Some infants will empty a breast in 5 minutes; others will nurse more leisurely, sometimes for 20 minutes or longer. Most of the milk is obtained early in the feeding (i.e. 50% in the first 2 minutes and 80–90% in the first 4 minutes). The infant should be allowed to suck until satisfied, unless the mother has sore nipples. If the infant does not "unlatch" from the breast after a reasonable period, a finger can be inserted into the corner of his or her mouth to decrease suction and facilitate removal. The infant should not be pulled from the breast. At the end of the nursing period, the infant should be held erect over the mother's shoulder or on her lap with or without gently rubbing or patting the back to assist in expelling swallowed air. This "burping" procedure often is necessary one or more times during the feeding as well as 5–10 minutes after the infant has been returned to the crib. It is an essential procedure during the early months of life but should not be overdone.

One or both breasts per feeding: The infant should empty at least one breast at each feeding; otherwise it will not be sufficiently stimulated to refill. Both breasts should be used at each feeding in the early weeks to encourage maximal milk production. After the milk supply is established the breasts may be alternated at successive feedings. Foremilk comes when breast-feeding begins is thin and watery, higher in lactose; hindmilk released after several minutes of nursing is richer in fat and calories. The infant will usually be satisfied with the amount obtained from one breast. If milk secretion becomes too great, both breasts may be offered at each feeding but incompletely emptied, there by decreasing milk production.

Determining adequacy of milk supply: If the infant is satisfied after each nursing period, sleeps 2–4 hrs between feedings, and gains weight adequately, the milk supply is sufficient. Infants who are "light sleepers" usually require considerable body contact with the mother during the first months of life, but in such cases it should not be assumed that mothers have a poor milk supply. On the other hand, if the infant nurses avidly and completely empties both breasts but appears unsatisfied afterward (e.g. does not go to sleep after nursing or sleeps fitfully and awakens after 1–2 hrs) and fails to gain weight satisfactorily, the milk supply is probably inadequate. In general weighing the infant before and after every nursing to judge the adequacy of the milk supply is neither necessary nor desirable. The amount of milk that an infant takes at single feeding ranges from one to several ounces throughout a 24 hr period and it is usually unimportant with respect to daily intake. Small gains may worry the mother and in turn may diminish her milk supply. In addition, she may give the infant a bottle to reassure herself that the infant is getting enough to eat and may stop breastfeeding even if she has an adequate milk supply.

Three possibilities should be excluded before assuming that a mother cannot produce sufficient milk: (i) errors in feeding technique; (ii) remediable maternal factors related to diet, rest, or emotional distress; and (iii) physical disturbances of the infant that interfere with nursing or weight gain. Infrequently, infants who seem to be nursing well may not thrive because of inadequate milk supply. In such cases more frequent feedings may be indicated. Nursing more often than every 2 hrs may inhibit prolactin secretion and further decrease milk production; but this is not a problem with feeding at 2 hrs intervals. Stimulation of prolactin secretion by small doses of chlorpromazine for a few days may be tried.

Expression of breastmilk: Manual expression of breast-milk is useful to relieve engorgement of the breasts. Pumping can increase milk production and relieve sore nipples because it does not cause as much nipple irritation as suckling. Breast milk can be safely stored in the freezer or refrigerator and used for feeding the infant at a later time.

Supplemental feedings: Most mothers who are returning to work plan to pump enough milk while at work to feed her infant while she is at work. Because of stress and time constrains at work, this often is not possible. These mothers should be reassured that it is acceptable to feed the infant a commercial formula during the day and continue nursing in the evening. Breast milk production will gradually decrease and the mother will not have engorge and leaking breasts. But most mothers will continue to produce enough milk for two or three feedings a day for several months. If formula or stored breastmilk is to be given after the infant has completed a breastfeeding, the warmed bottle should be available so that it can be offered immediately after the infant has been "burped." The holes in the nipples should not be so large that the infant gets this portion of food without effort; if this happens, he or she may quickly abandon any efforts to suck adequately at the mother's breast. It is, therefore, advisable to give milk (or water) with a spoon or cup and not with a bottle. Some employers provide child care facilities at the workplace enabling mothers to continue nursing successfully; others provide convenient facilities for pumping. These enable mothers to continue nursing successfully and hence should be commended and encouraged.

Weaning from breastfeeding: Most infants gradually reduce the volume and the frequency of breastfeedings between 6 and 12 mo of age after they become accustomed to solid foods and liquids by bottle and/or cup. Weaning can be initiated when mutually desired by the mother and infant by substituting commercial formula or bovine milk by bottle and/or cup for part, and subsequently for all of a breastfeeding. The breastfeedings are eventually replaced with formula or bovine milk, usually over several days, and the infant is weaned completely. If an infant takes a cup as readily as a bottle, the intermediate transfer from breast to bottle before transferring from bottle to cup can be avoided. It is advisable to continue breastfeeding for two years after introduction of solid foods and liquid (with cup) from 6 mo. These changes should be made gradually and should be a pleasant experience not a conflict, for both the mother and the infant. Praise, loving attention, and cuddling are vital to successful weaning.

When cessation of nursing is necessary at an earlier age, use of a tight breast binder and application of ice bags may help decrease milk production. Restriction of mother's fluid intake is also helpful. Small doses of estrogen for 1–2 days also may help decrease milk production at the termination of nursing.

Contraindications of breastfeeding: There are no disadvantages of breastfeeding for the healthy term infant if the mother's milk supply is ample, her diet is adequate, and she is not infected with HIV. Breastfeeding is contraindicated in infants suffering from galactosemia.

- Allergens to which the infant is sensitized can be conveyed in the milk; therefore, an attempt should be made to identify the allergen and remove it from the mother's diet but the presence of such allergens is rarely a valid reason to stop breastfeeding.
- Markedly inverted nipples may be troublesome.
- Fissuring or cracking of the nipples can usually be avoided by preventing engorgement.
- Mastitis also may be alleviated by continued and frequent nursing on the affected breast to keep it from becoming engorged, but local heat applications and antibiotics may occasionally be required.
- Acute maternal infection may contraindicate breastfeeding if the infant does not have the same infection; otherwise, there is no need to stop nursing unless the condition of either the mother or infant needs it. When the infant is unaffected, the breast may be emptied if the mother's condition permits and the milk given to the infant by bottle or cup.
- Mothers with septicemia, active tuberculosis, typhoid fever, breast cancer, or malaria should not breastfeed.

- Substance abuse and severe neurosis or psychoses are contraindication of breastfeeding.

Formula-feeding

Infants younger than 6 mo of age (e.g. rate of growth in weight and length, normality of various constituents in blood, performance of various metabolic studies, body composition) differ minimally, if at all, between infants fed human milk and infants fed on modern infant formulas. Thus, the mother who is unable or does not nurse her infant (inspite support to breastfeed) need not worry regarding the nutritional requirements of her infant if on infant formulas. Moreover, the quality of attachment and mothering and the degree of security and affection provided to breastfed infant is not different with formula-feeding.

Technique of formula-feeding: The setting for formula-feeding should be similar to that for breastfeeding, with the mother or caregiver and infant in a comfortable position, unhurried, and free from distractions. The infant should be hungry, fully awake, warm and dry. He or she should be held as though being breastfed. The nipple holes should be of a size that allows the milk to drop slowly, and the bottle should be held so that milk, not air, channels through the nipple. Bottle propping even with a "safe" holder should be avoided; this not only deprives the infant of the physical contact and security of being held but also may be dangerous, particularly for small infants who may aspirate if unattended. Otitis media is more common in infants fed with the propped bottle. The bottle of milk is customarily warmed to body temperature, but no harmful effects from feeding formula at room or even, refrigerator temperature have been demonstrated. The temperature may be tested by dropping milk onto the wrist (Box 3.2).

Eructation of air swallowed during feeding is important for avoiding regurgitation and abdominal discomfort, especially during the first 6–7 mo of life. The technique of "burping" should be the same as described for the breastfed infants. A few infants relieve themselves best after being relieved from the crib. All infants occasionally will regurgitate or "spit up" a small amount of milk after feeding and this fact mothers should know. Spitting up seems to occur more often in the formula-fed than the breastfed infant. A feeding may last from 5 to 25 minutes, depending on the age and the vigor of the infant. Because the appetite varies from one feeding to another, each bottle should contain more than the average amount taken per feeding. In no case, however, should the infant be used to take more than desired. Excess milk should be discarded.

Composition of infant formulas: The nutrient content of infant formulas must contain minimum amounts of all nutrients known or thought to be required by infants, and increasing emphasis is being placed on not exceeding a reasonable maximum content of each (regulated by the Act in most industrialized and many developing countries). Note that the minimum recommended amount of each nutrient contents of infant formulas is greater than that nutrient in human milk and hence, greater than the most recent Dietary Reference Intake for that nutrient. This, most likely reflects the perceived lower bioavailability of formula vs. human milk nutrients. Most infant formulas contain a protein source, usually a mixture of bovine milk proteins but also soy protein or a variety of hydrolyzed proteins, lactose and/or other sugars, a mixture of vegetable oils, mineral salts, and vitamins. While reconstituting the infant formula, the instructions given on the label should be strictly followed. Similarities to bovine milk from which they evolved are virtually nonexistent.

Number of feeding daily: The number of feedings required per day decreases throughout the first year of life from 8 or more shortly afterbirth to only three or four at 1 yr of age. The desired interval between feeding differs considerably among infants but, in general, ranges from 3–5 hrs during the first year of life, averaging about 4 hrs. For the first 1–2 mo feedings are taken throughout the 24 hrs period, thereafter, as the quantity of milk consumed at each feeding increases and the infant adjusts his or her demand to the family pattern of daytime activities, the infant usually sleeps for longer periods at night. As the infant develops psychologically and the relationship between the parent and infant evolves, demand feeding should gradually be replaced by a feeding regimen that accommodates the needs of the infant as well as the rest of the family.

Quantity of formula: The quantity of formula taken at a feeding varies among the infants of same age and within infants at different feedings. Rarely will an infant want more than 7–8 oz at a single feeding. The desire for formula (or breastmilk) is somewhat less during the first 2 wks of life than during the following 5–6 mo. After 6 mo of age, formula (or breastmilk) is rarely the sole source of the infant's nutrient intake. However, it remains an important source of many nutrients (e.g. calcium). It is rarely necessary to use more than 1 qt (960 ml) of formula per day. By the time the infant is taking this amount, other foods should be added to the diet. There is no advantages in ingesting more than this volume and may displace intake of other essential foods.

Infant formula vs. bovine milk: Although the current recommendations are to avoid intake of bovine milk particularly low fat or skimmed milk, before at least one year of age, but a sizable percentage of infants older than 6 mo of age are fed homogenized bovine milk rather than infant formula and almost half of these are fed low-fat or skimmed milk—often on the advice of their physician. The consequences of these practices are not known with certainty. However, infants fed bovine milk, on average, ingest roughly three times the recommended intake of protein and about 50% more sodium than the upper limit of the "safe range" of intake of this mineral but only about two-thirds of the recommended intake of iron and only half of the recommended intake of linoleic acid. Ingestion of bovine milk also increases intestinal blood loss and hence, further contributes to development of iron-deficiency anemia. The protein and sodium intakes of infants fed skimmed rather than whole bovine milk are even higher, the iron intake is equally low, and the intake of linoleic acid is very low. The most common reason for substituting low fat or skimmed milk for whole milk or formula is to reduce fat and energy intakes, the total energy intakes of infants fed skimmed milk is necessarily lower than that of infants fed whole milk or formula. It appears that infants compensate for the lower energy density of low-fat or skimmed milk by taking more of it and on/or increasing intake of other foods. Whether the high protein and sodium intakes of infants fed either whole or skimmed milk are undesirable is not known with certainty. The low iron intake, clearly, is undesirable but medicinal iron supplementation

---

Box 3.2: Feeding in not breastfed infant

- Feed the infant with animal milk or commercial infant formula
- Milk should be boiled before feeding to the baby
- To start with, milk may be diluted with an equal volume of water
- Full strength milk may be started from 4 wks of age.
- Infants fed animal milk should receive supplements of iron and vitamin C.
- About 120–180 ml of milk should be fed with one teaspoon of sugar per feed, 6–8 times over the day.
- While reconstituting the infant formula, the instructions given on the label should be strictly followed.
- The feeds should be prepared and given using a sterile cup, spoon, bottles, nipples, taking utmost care.
- Overfeeding should be avoided in artificially—fed infants to prevent obesity.
- Low-cost home-made weaning foods are preferred; commercially available preparations may be used by those who can afford them.

should prevent development of deficiency. The low intake of linoleic acid may be more problematic, because essential fatty acid deficiency in animals is associated with long-term deleterious effects on development; it is not wise to assume that biochemical essential fatty acid deficiency without clinically detectable symptoms is without consequences. The use of bovine milk in feeding the infant is important for economic as well as health reasons, particularly those with limited income, because the cost of bovine milk is considerably less than infant formula (Box 3.2).

Feeding during the Second 6 Month of Life

By 6 mo of age, the infant's capacity to digest and absorb a variety of dietary components as well as to metabolize, utilize, and excrete the absorbed products of digestion is near the capacity of the adult. Addition of other foods after 6 mo of age is recommended in addition of breastmilk/infant formula. Complementary foods given to breastfed infants or given to formula-fed infants should be introduced in a stepwise fashion beginning after 6 mo of age. Cereals, a good source of iron should be introduced first. Vegetables and fruits are introduced next, followed shortly by meats, and finally, eggs. The order in which these foods are introduced probably is not important, but only one new food should be introduced at one time, and additional new foods should be spaced by at least 3–4 days to allow detection of any adverse reactions to each newly introduced food. This is particularly important if there is a family history of food and/or other allergies. Either home-prepared or manufactured complementary or replacement foods can be used.

Feeding Problems during the First Year of Life

Underfeeding: Underfeeding is suggested by restlessness and crying, constipation, failure to sleep and failure to gain weight adequately. Weight gain may be slow or there may be an actual loss of weight. In the latter case, the skin becomes dry and wrinkled, subcutaneous tissue disappears and the infant assumes the appearance of an "old man". Deficiencies of vitamins A, B, C, and D as well as of iron and protein may be responsible for characteristic clinical manifestations. Treatment of underfeeding includes increasing nutrient intake, correcting deficiencies of vitamins and/or minerals and instructing the mother for adopting correct infant-feeding practices. If some underlying systemic disease, child abuse/neglect, or psychologic problem is responsible, specific management of these disorders is necessary.

Overfeeding: If intake is excessive, regurgitation and vomiting are the most frequent symptoms. Diets that are too high in fat delay gastric emptying, cause distension and abdominal discomfort, and may cause excessive weight gain. Diets too high in carbohydrate are likely to cause undue fermentation in the intestine, resulting in distension and flatulence as well as more rapid gain in weight than desirable. Supplementation diets rich in fats/carbohydrates are responsible for overfeeding.

Regurgitation and vomiting: Regurgitation refers to the return of small amounts of swallowed food during or shortly after eating. Regurgitation is a natural occurrence, especially during the first several months of life. It can be reduced to a negligible amount by adequate eructation of swallowed air during and after eating, by gentle handling, by avoiding emotional conflicts, and by placing the infant on the right side immediately after eating (but not for napping or sleeping). The head should not be lower than the rest of the body to avoid gastroesophageal reflux, which is common during the first 4–6 mo of life.

Vomiting is the more complete emptying of the stomach often occurring after some time after feeding. It may be associated with a variety of disturbances—some trivial and some serious.

Loose or diarrheal stools: The stool of the breast-fed infant is softer than that of the formula-fed infant. From about the 4th to 6th day of life, the stools of breastfed infants go through a transitional stage of being loose and greenish yellow and containing mucus to the typical "milk stool." Subsequently the use of laxatives or ingestion of certain foods by the mother may be temporarily responsible for loose stools in a breastfed infant. Excessive intake of breastmilk may also increase the frequency and the water content of the stool, but diarrhea should be considered infectious until proved otherwise. Formula-fed infants acquire diarrheal disturbances from over feeding during the first two weeks or so of life, too concentrated or too high in sugar content, especially lactose and contaminants. Thus, extreme care must be taken in preparation to assure that the formula or food is free of pathogens. Mild diarrheal disturbances caused by overfeeding respond quickly to temporary decrease or cessation of feeding. Withholding all solid food as well as one or several feedings and substituting boiled water or New WHO-ORS are usually all that is required.

Constipation: Constipation is practically unknown in breastfed infants receiving an adequate amount of milk and is rare in formula-fed infants receiving an adequate intake. The consistency of the stool, not its frequency, is the basis for diagnosis. Most infants have one or more stools daily, but some occasionally have a stool of normal consistency at intervals of up to 36–48 hrs. If constipation or obstipation is present from birth or shortly after birth, a rectal examination should be performed. Tight or spastic anal sphincters may occasionally be responsible for obstitation, and finger dilatation is frequently corrective. Anal fissures or cracks may also cause constipation. If irritation is alleviated, healing usually occurs quickly. Aganglionic megacolon may be manifested by constipation in early infancy; the absence of stool in the rectum on digital examination suggests its possibility, but further diagnostic work-up is indicated. Constipation may be caused by an insufficient amount of food or fluid. In some cases, it may result from diets that are high in fat or protein or deficient in bulk. Simply increasing the amount of fluid or sugar in the formula may be corrective during the first few months of life. After this age, better results are obtained by adding or increasing the amounts of cereals, vegetables, and fruits. Enemas and suppositories should never be more than temporary measures. Milk of magnesia may be given in doses of 1–2 teaspoonful but should be reserved for unresponsive or severe constipation.

Colic: Colic is a symptom complex of paroxysmal abdominal pain, presumably of intestinal origin, and severe crying. It usually occurs in infants younger than 3 mo of age. The attack of colic usually begins suddenly with a loud, more or less continuous cry. The paroxysms may persist for several hours. The face may be flushed, or there may be circumoral pallor. The abdomen is usually distended and tense. The legs may be extended for short periods but are usually drawn up on the abdomen. The feet are often cold, and the hands are usually clenched. The attack may not terminate until the infant is completely exhausted. Sometimes, passage of feces or flatus appears to provide relief. The etiology of colic usually is not apparent, but, in some infants, the attacks appear to be associated with hunger or swallowed air that has passed into the intestine. Overfeeding may also cause discomfort and distension and some foods, especially those of high carbohydrate content, may be responsible for excessive intestinal fermentation. Colic may occur in infants with intestinal allergy. Colic may mimic intestinal obstruction or peritoneal infection. Attacks commonly occur late in the afternoon or evening, suggesting that events in the household routine may be involved. Worry, fear, anger, or excitement may cause vomiting in an older child and may cause colic in an infant, and no single factor consistently accounts for colic and no treatment consistently provides satisfactory relief. Careful physical examination is important to eliminate the possibility of intussusception, strangulated hernia, or other disorders that cause abdominal pain.

Holding the infant upright or prone across the lap or on a hot water bottle or heating pad occasionally helps. Passage of flatus or fecal material spontaneously or with expulsion of suppository or enema sometimes affords relief. Sedation is occasionally indicated for a prolonged attack. Prevention of attacks should be sought by improving feeding techniques including "burping," providing a stable emotional environment, identifying possible allergic foods in the infant's or nursing mother's diet, and avoiding underfeeding or overfeeding. The fact that the condition rarely persists beyond 3 mo of age should reassure the mother.

Feeding during the Second Year of Life

By the end of the one year of life, most infants have adapted to a schedule of 3 meals a day plus two or three snacks. The mother should be given an outline of the basic daily dietary needs, and she should be aware of what to expect in terms of eating behavior as the child matures.

Reduced food intake: Towards the end of 1st yr of life, the rate of growth decreases and the child's intake, accordingly also decreases or fails to increase as rapidly as it did during the 1st yr of life. Failure to expect and recognize these changes in eating behavior often results in attempts to force feed. The child naturally rebels and feeding problems ensue. The mother should be reassured that the lack of interest in food is probably temporary and that attempts to force feed are likely to result in more severe feeding problems.

Self selection of diet: Children's likes and dislikes of particular foods become apparent after about 1 yr of age, and if possible, and practicable should be respected. The child may be permitted a wide choice of foods, as long as he or she eats adequately. Normally the child determines the quantity of a given food as well as an entire meal that will be eaten. At this age, eating habits, particularly food likes and dislikes, also may be influenced by older children in the family. Eating habits developed in the first 2 yrs of life usually persists for several years; such influences should be monitored closely.

Self feeding by infants: Infants should be permitted to participate in feeding themselves as soon as they seem physically to do so usually long before 1 yr of age. By approximately 6 mo of age, infants can hold a bottle, and within another 2–3 mo (approximately 8–9 mo), can hold a cup. Biscuits or other hand-held foods can be introduced by the age of 7–8 mo. The infant may be allowed to use a spoon as soon as it can be held and directed to the mouth, usually between 10–12 mo of age. Mothers often inhibit this important learning process because of its messiness, but it is an important aspect of the infant's overall development and should be encouraged. By the end of the second year of life, infants should be largely responsible for feeding themselves. However, because the risk of aspiration is reasonably high until approximately 4 yrs of age, infants younger than this should not be given foods that are easily aspirated (e.g. grapes, nuts, chunks of cheese and meat) unless a responsible adult is present.

Basic daily diet: Parents should be given a basic daily diet plan for the child from which, the family menu can be prepared. Daily selection from each of the food groups (gains, fruits and vegetables, meats, and dairy products) provides a balanced diet with sufficient macronutrients and micronutrients. The quantity of intake after the basic requirements have been met can usually be determined by the healthy growing child. Correcting the diet can be much more effective if reliable information is available. The older child should learn the content of a basic well-balanced diet and its importance to proper growth and good health; but this information should not be enforced rigidly.

Eating habits: Eating habits formed in the 1st and 2nd yr of life distinctly affect those of the subsequent years. Feeding difficulties frequently result from excessive parental insistence on eating and subsequent anxiety of the parents and the child if the child fails to heed this insistence.

Snacks between meals: During the 2nd year of life and for several years thereafter, snacks (milk, fruit juice, and/or cracker) may be given at either or both of the between-meal periods. However, the amount of food given as a snack should not be enough to interfere with intake at meal-times. Snacks served in child care facilities should be as nutritious as those served at home.

Vegetarian diets: Vegetable diets can supply all necessary nutrients but to do so, the vegetables and grains comprising the diet must be selected from different classes. Vegetables are high in fiber content, vitamins, and minerals. Vegetarians usually have faster gastrointestinal transit time, bulkier stools, and lower serum cholesterol levels because of the higher fiber content and less likely to develop diverticulitis and appendicitis than meat eaters. Vegetarians who consume eggs (ovovegetarians) and milk (lactovegetarians) have more choices for constructing a well-balanced diet than those who consume neither (vegan).

Vegans may develop vitamin B_{12} deficiency and because of higher fiber intake may develop trace mineral deficiencies. Nursing vegan mothers must be given supplemental vitamin B_{12} to prevent vitamin B_{12} deficiency in their breastfed infants. There also is some concern that vegetarian infants may not grow as rapidly as omnivores during the first two years of life

Feeding during Later Childhood

After 2 yrs of age, a child's diet should not differ from that of the rest of the family. All the required nutrients are supplied by a varied diet, including restriction of dietary fat to approximately 30% of the total energy intake, saturated fatty acids to less than 10% of energy, polyunsaturated fatty acids 7–8% of energy, monounsaturated fatty acids 12–13% of energy, and cholesterol to no more than 100 mg/1,000 kcal. Such diets support normal growth of children as young as 1 yr of age and implementing it after about 2 yrs of age may be easier than doing so at adolescence (Tables 3.1 and 3.3).

Although these guidelines are useful and can be used to design an appropriate diet of all children older than 2 yrs of age, the variation in energy needs among children of the same age is considerable, can vary by as much as 15–20%; level of activity is a major determinant of the amount of energy needed. As children become older and more independent, an increasing number of meals are eaten away from home, often at "fast food" restaurants where adherence to the food guidelines mentioned is difficult (solution is to limit such occasions to once or twice per week). However, the most important is that the parents understand the importance of a well-balanced diet and how best to achieve this without undue hardship for themselves or their children.

Jindal T, Chattree S. Anatomy and physiology of lactation. In: Anand RK, Kumta NB, Kushwaha KP, Gupta A (eds). The Science of Infant Feeding. New Delhi: Jaypee Brothers Medical Publishers (P) Ltd. 2002; 23–35.

Heird WC. The feeding of infants and children. In: Kliegman RM, Behrman RE, Jenson HB, Stanton BF (eds). *Nelson Textbook of Pediatrics*. 18th edn. Vol. 1. Philadelphia: Saunders, 2007; 214–25.

Lawrence RA. Breastfeeding A guide for medical profession. 3rd edn. Philadelphia: The CMV Mosby Company, 1989; 1–652.

Paul VK, Deorari AK, Agarwal R, et al. Newborn infants. In: Ghai OP, Paul VK, Bagga A (eds). *Ghai Essential Pediatrics*. 7th edn. New Delhi: CBS Publishers & Distributors Pvt Ltd, 2009; 96–159.

WHO Global Data Bank on Breastfeeding. Breastfeeding: The best start in life. WHO Nutrition Unit, 1996.

Chadha DS (ed). Packing and Labelling of Food. The Prevention of Food Adulteration Act & Rules (As on 1.10.2004). New Delhi: Confederation of Indian Industry, 2004; 80–104.

3.3 SEVERE CHILDHOOD UNDERNUTRITION (PROTEIN ENERGY MALNUTRITION)

Deficiency of a single nutrient is an example of undernutrition or malnutrition. Usually, there is deficiency of several nutrients. Protein energy malnutrition (PEM) is manifested primarily by inadequate dietary intakes of protein and energy either because the dietary intakes of these two nutrients are less than required for normal growth or because the needs for growth are greater than can be supplied by what, otherwise, would be adequate intakes for growth. However, PEM is almost always accompanied by deficiencies of other nutrients. For this reason, the term severe childhood undernutrition (SCU), which more accurately describes the condition, is preferred.

Primary malnutrition, refer, to malnutrition resulting from inadequate food intake and secondary malnutrition resulting from increased nutrient needs, decreased nutrient absorption, and/or increased nutrient losses. Both primary and secondary malnutrition occur in developing and developed countries, but primary malnutrition accounts for the major percentage of malnourished children in developing countries, whereas secondary malnutrition accounts for a higher percentage in developed countries.

Severe childhood undernutrition can be recognized in three forms—marasmus (nonedematous), kwashiorkor (edematous), and marasmic kwashiorkor (features of both disorders). Marasmus was thought to result primarily from inadequate energy intake, whereas kwashiorkor was thought to result primarily from inadequate protein intake. The three conditions have distinct clinical and metabolic features, but they also have a number of overlapping features. For example, a low plasma albumin concentration, often thought to be a manifestation of kwashiorkor, is common in children with both marasmus and kwashiorkor. The underlying causes of this spectrum of conditions are quite similar. Among these are social and economic factors such as poverty and ignorance, social factors such as food taboos, biologic factors such as maternal malnutrition and inadequate intakes of breastmilk and other foods, as well as environmental factors such as overcrowded and unsanitary living conditions.

Pathophysiology: Many of the manifestations of SCU represent adaptive responses to inadequate energy and/or protein intakes. Fat stores are metabolized first, to meet the ongoing energy requirements. Once these stores are depleted, protein catabolism provides the ongoing substrates for maintaining basal metabolism.

No specific factor is identified as to why some children develop edematous SCU and others develop nonedematous SCU, but a number of factors have been suggested:

i. The variability among infants in nutrient requirements and in body composition at the time dietary deficit incurred;

ii. Giving excess carbohydrate to a child with clinical marasmus reverses the adaptive responses to low protein intake, resulting in metabolization of body protein stores. Eventually, albumin synthesis decreases, resulting in hypoalbuminemia with edema. Fatty liver also develops secondary, perhaps, to lipogenesis from the excess carbohydrate;

iii. Aflatoxin poisoning; and

iv. The free radical damage as an important factor in the development of clinical kwashiorkor or edematous SCU, because there is low plasma concentrations of methionine, a precursor of cysteine, one of the aminoacids needed for synthesis of the major antioxidant factor, glutathione.

This possibility also is supported by lower rates of glutathione synthesis in children with edematous vs. nonedematous SCU.

Clinical manifestations: In nonedematous SCU (marasmus) initially there is failure to gain weight and irritability, followed by weight loss and listlessness until emaciation results (Table 3.6). The skin looses turgor and becomes wrinkled and loose as subcutaneous fat disappears. Loss of fat from the sucking pads of the cheeks may occur late, and the infant's face may retain a relatively normal appearance, compared with the rest of the body. Later, the face becomes shrunken and wizened (monkey facies), as a result of loss of fat from the sucking pads of the cheeks. The abdomen may be distended or flat with the intestinal pattern readily visible. There is muscle atrophy and resultant hypotonia. The temperature is usually subnormal and the pulse is slow. Infants are usually constipated but may develop starvation diarrhea with frequent small stools containing mucus.

In edematous SCU (kwashiorkor) may initially present as vague manifestations that include lethargy, apathy, or irritability. In advanced cases, there is inadequate growth, lack of stamina, loss of muscle tissue, increased susceptibility to infections, vomiting, diarrhea, anorexia, flabby subcutaneous tissues, and edema. The edema usually develops early and may mask the failure to gain weight. The liver may enlarge early or late. The edema is often present in the internal organs before it is recognized in the face and limbs.

Table 3.6: Manifestations of nonedematous (marasmus) and edematous (kwashiorkor) SCU		
Manifestations	*Nonedematous (marasmus) SCU*	*Edematous (kwashiorkor) SCU*
Edema	Absent	Present
Liver	Not enlarged	Enlarged
Dermatitis	Absent	Present with darkening of the skin in the irritated areas but not in areas exposed to sunlight, and depigmentation desquamation
Loss of subcutaneous fat	Yes (wrinkling; loss of fat from the sucking pads of the cheeks—monkey facies)	Not present (no wrinkling)
Muscle atrophy	Present	Present in advanced cases
Hair	No change	Sparse and thin, red or gray in dark-haired children
Weight loss	Marked	Present
Growth (physical, intellectual)	Retarded	Retarded

Dermatitis is common, with darkening of the skin in the irritated areas but not in areas exposed to sunlight, in contrast to pellagra. Depigmentation may occur after desquamation in these areas or it may be generalized. The hair is sparse and thin, and in dark-haired children, may become streaky red or gray. The texture is coarse in chronic disease. Eventually there is stupor, coma, and death.

Noma is a chronic necrotizing ulceration of the gingival and the cheek. It is associated with malnutrition and is often preceded by a debilitating illness (measles, malaria, tuberculosis, diarrhea, ulcerative gingivitis) in a nutritionally compromised individual. Noma presents with fever, malodorous breath, anemia, leukocytosis, and signs of malnutrition. Polymicrobial infection with *Fusobacterium necrophorum* and *Prevotella intermedia* may be inciting agents. Treatment includes local wound care, penicillin, and metronidazole as well as treatment for the underlying predisposing condition.

Treatment: Children weighing less than 60% for age with:
 i. Edema
 ii. Severe dehydration
 iii. Diarrhea
 iv. Hypothermia
 v. Shock
 vi. Systemic infection
 vii. Jaundice
 viii. Bleeding
 ix. Less than one year; or
 x. Persistent loss of appetite should be admitted for treatment in the hospital.

Children with severe wasting or edematous undernutrition should be admitted. The treatment of SCU includes three phases. Elements in the management of severe protein energy malnutrition are described in Table 3.7. The first phase (1–7 days) is a stabilization phase. During this phase, the child may have, loose motions, vomiting, dehydration, skin infection or in shock, therapy is initiated to control dehydration (oral or intravenous rehydration therapy) and antibiotics to control bacterial or parasitic infection. Depending upon the severity of dehydration, intravenous therapy, if necessary, particularly during first 24 hrs, should be started, and followed by oral rehydration therapy.

The second rehabilitation phase (wk 2–6) includes continued antibiotic therapy with appropriate changes if the initial combination was not effective and introduction of a diet providing maintenance requirements of energy and protein (~75 kcal/kg and ~1 g/kg/24 hr of protein), along with adequate electrolytes, trace minerals, and vitamins (ion not included). This phase usually lasts for an additional 7 to 10 days. If the infant is unable to take the feedings from a cup or bottle, administration of feedings by nasogastric tube rather than by the parenteral route is preferred. By the end of the second phase, any edema that was present has usually been mobilized, infections are under control, the child is becoming more interested in his or her surroundings, and his or her appetite is returning.

The third (final) phase of treatment consists primarily of feeding, and he or she should be switched gradually to a recovery diet providing up to 150 kcal/kg/24 hr and 4 g/kg/24 hr of protein. After adjustment to this diet, the child can be fed ad libitum. Once ad libitum feedings are allowed, intakes of both energy and protein can be substantial. Iron therapy usually is not started until this final phase of treatment so as to prevent binding of iron to already limited stores of transferrin, which in turn may interfere with the protein's defense mechanisms. This free iron during the early phase of treatment may exacerbate oxidant damage, precipitating clinical kwashiorkor or marasmic kwashiorkor in a marasmic child.

In developing countries, this phase is often carried out at home. However, continued hospitalization is much more effective. This allows further focus on maternal education, which is crucial for continued effective treatment as well as prevention of additional episodes.

Refeeding syndrome may complicate the acute nutritional rehabilitation of children as a result of severe hypophosphatemia during the 1st wk of starting to refeed. Serum phosphate levels of ≤0.5 mmol/L can produce weakness, rhabdomyolysis, neutrophil dysfunction, cardiorespiratory failure, arrhythmias, seizures, altered level of consciousness, or sudden death. Phosphate levels should be monitored during refeeding, and if low, phosphate should be administered during refeeding to treat severe hypophosphatemia.

Heird WC. Food insecurity, hunger and undernutrition. In: Kliegman RM, Behrman RE, Jenson HB, Stanton BF (eds). Nelson Textbook of Pediatrics. 18th edn. Vol. 1. Philadelphia: Saunders, 2007; 225–32.

World Health Organization. Management of Severe Malnutrition; A Manual for Physicians and Other Senior Health Workers. Geneva, WHO, 1999.

3.4 FAILURE TO THRIVE

Failure to thrive (FTT) is usually refer to growth below the 5th percentile or a change in growth that has crossed two major growth percentiles (from above the 75th percentile to below the 25th) in a short time. Children with FTT can be arbitrarily divided into two categories: organic FTT and nonorganic FTT (NOFTT) or psychosocial FTT(*see* Chapter 6, page-130).

Etiology: Organic FTT is due to underlying medical condition. The causes of organic FTT are numerous:

1. Various organ systems include gastrointestinal, respiratory, cardiovascular, endocrine, neurologic, and renal.
2. Infections (parasitic or bacterial infections of the gastrointestinal tract; tuberculosis, human immunodeficiency virus disease; perinatal infections).
3. Inborn errors of metabolism.
4. Malignant disorders (leukemia, lymphoma, other malignant disorders).
5. Miscellaneous (chromosomal abnormalities, congenital syndromes (fetal alcohol syndrome), lead poisoning, collagen vascular diseases).

Nonorganic Failure to Thrive (NOFTT) or psychosocial FTT occurs in a child who is usually under 5 yrs of age and has no known medical condition that causes poor growth (*see* Chapter 6, page-130). Psychosocial FTT is most often due to poverty or poor child–parent interaction. It occasionally occurs with severe stress such as child abuse (*see* Chapter 6, page-129).

Clinical manifestations: The clinical presentation of FTT ranges from failure to meet expected age norms for height and weight, to alopecia, loss of subcutaneous fat, reduced muscle mass, dermatitis, recurrent infections, marasmus, and kwashiorkor. The degree of FTT is usually measured by calculating each growth parameter (weight, height, and weight/height ratio) as a percentage of median value for age based on appropriate growth charts. For weight, mild, moderate, and severe FTT is equivalent to 75–90%, 60–74%, and less than 60% of standard, respectively. For height, the corresponding values are 90–95%, 85–89%, and less than 85%. For weight/height ratio, the values are 81–90%, 70–80%, and less than 70%. The weight-for-age percent of the standard value decreases early in the course of FTT, followed by a decrement of height-for-age. Children with chronic malnutrition often have a normal weight-for-height because both weight-and-height are reduced.

Table 3.7: Management of children with severe protein energy malnutrition	
Problem	*Management*
Hypothermia	Keep the patient warm; maintain and monitor temperature
Hypoglycemia	Monitor blood glucose; provide oral (or intravenous) glucose
Dehydration	Rehydrate carefully with oral solution containing less sodium and more potassium than standard mix
Micronutrients	Provide copper, zinc, iron, folate, multivitamins, potassium, magnesium
Infections	Administer antibiotic and antimalarial therapy, even in the absence of typical symptoms
Starter nutrition	Keep protein and volume load low
Tissue-building nutrition	Provide a rich diet
Stimulation	Prevent permanent psychosocial effects of starvation with psychomotor stimulation
Prevention of relapse	Identify causes of protein-energy malnutrition in each case; involve the family and the community in prevention

Laboratory findings: A complete blood count, lead level, and urinalysis, should be done, as these are reliable initial screening tests. Bone age is often helpful in distinguishing family short stature (bone age equivalent to chronological age) from endocrine and nutritional abnormalities (bone age is less than chronological age). Test such as thyroid function studies, tests for gastroesophageal reflux and malabsorption, organic and aminoacids, or a sweat test, should be performed if indicated by the history or physical examination.

Diagnosis: The history (including detailed dietary especially in young infants), physical examination, and observation of the parent–child interaction usually suggest the diagnosis. The latter observation, especially with feeding (weight gain in response to adequate caloric feeding) is usually helpful to the diagnosis of psychosocial FTT. Establish the causes of insufficient growth, which include: (i) failure of a parent to offer adequate calories, (ii) failure of the child to take sufficient calories, and (iii) failure of the child to retain sufficient calories. Reasons why parents or other caregivers may not offer appropriate or sufficient foods include lack of knowledge, parental depression, unusual dietary beliefs, or lack of food. Find out how the parents respond when the child cries or sleeps for prolonged periods. Children may have difficulty in swallowing if they have oral-motor dysfunction, or enlarged and recurrently infected tonsils and adenoids. Vomiting, diarrhea, and malabsorption are general causes of inadequate caloric absorption.

Treatment: Before starting treatment an understanding of all the elements that contribute to a child's growth, such as child's health and nutritional status, family issues, and the parent–child interaction. Feeding is important regardless of cause, and severity of malnutrition. For children with organic FTT, the underlying medical condition should be treated. The type of caloric supplementation (including response) depends on the specific diagnosis, medical treatment, and severity of FTT. For example, in children with renal failure, the amount of protein in the diet must be carefully monitored. For older infants and young children with psychosocial FTT, mealtimes should be approximately 20–30 min, solid foods should be offered before liquids, high calorie foods (such as butter, whole milk, cheese) should be emphasized, environmental distraction should be minimized, and children should eat with other people and not be forced fed.

Indications for hospitalization include severe malnutrition, further diagnostic and laboratory evaluation, lack of catch-up growth, and evaluation of the parent–child feeding interaction. For psycho- social FTT, hospitalization often lasts 5–10 days. For both organic and psychosocial FTT, the approach to feeding in the hospital should mimic the anticipated treatment at home before discharge.

Prognosis: FTT in the first year of life, regardless of cause is particularly ominous, because maximal postnatal brain growth occurs during the first six months of life. The brain grows as much during the first year of life as during the rest of a child's life. Approximately one-third of children with psychosocial FTT are developmentally delayed and have social and emotional problems. The prognosis for children with organic FTT is more variable, depending on the specific diagnosis and severity of FTT. Assessment and monitoring of cognitive and emotional development, with appropriate intervention, is necessary for all children with organic and psychosocial FTT.

Bauchner H. Failure to thrive. In: Kliegman RM, Behrman RE, Jenson HB, Stanton BF (eds). Nelson Textbook of Pediatrics. 18th edn. Vol. 1. Philadelphia: Saunders, 2007; 184–7.

Jolley CD. Failure to thrive. Curr Probl Pediatr Adolesc Health Care 2003; 33: 183–206.

3.5 OVERWEIGHT AND OBESITY

Obesity and overweight are terms that are commonly used interchangeably in children, but overweight is the preferred term. Overweight children are more likely to be overweight adults. Obesity is among the easiest medical conditions to recognize but most difficult to treat. Successfully preventing or treating overweight in childhood may reduce the risk of adult overweight. This may help reduce numerous problems associated with obesity.

Epidemiology: The National Health and Nutrition Examination Survey (NHANES) IV, 1999–2002, documents that 16% of children are overweight and 31% are at risk for becoming overweight or are already overweight. Initial data on the prevalence of overweight and obesity, demonstrates an obesity range of 5.6 to 24% for the children and adolescents in India. Parental obesity, particularly maternal is predictive of childhood obesity.

Pathogenesis: Overweight results from a dysregula- tion of caloric intake and energy expenditure. A complex interplay between each individual's genetic predispositions and the environment affects an intricate system that controls appetite and energy expenditure. The excess caloric intake is stored in adipose tissue, but for most individuals, there is no longer prolonged periods of reduced caloric intake, leading to a net increase in adipose tissue deposition over time.

Environmental changes: The type and cost of food has dramatically changed. The food industry through advertisement encourages people to eat convenience foods, which are relatively inexpensive and have high levels of calories, fat, and simple carbohydrates, and sodium, and low levels of fibre and micronutrients. There is increasing rise of eating snacks in between meals with many snacks being high in fat, sugar or both. The convenience of fast food, the increase in dual working parents and single-parent households, and the common practice of overscheduling children have led to fast food being a staple diet of many families. Many children consume excessive calories, with the intake of large amounts of sweetened beverages, including soda, juice and sport drinks.

An increase in sedentary activity and a lack of exercise also contribute to an increase in the prevalence of overweight. Children may watch 20 hr or more/wk television, which decreases their physical activity, exposes them to food advertising, and increase caloric intake. Other "screen time" such as video games, Internet computer use, telephone use, and home viewing of movies all may induce childhood physical activity.

Endogenous weight control mechanisms: Monitoring of "stored fuel" and short-term control of food intake (appetite and satiety) occur through neuroendocrine feedback from adipose tissue and the gastrointestinal tract to the central nervous system. Gastrointestinal hormones including cholecystokinin, glucagon-like peptide-1, and peptide YY, and vagal neuronal feedback promote satiety, whereas ghrelin stimulates appetite. Adipose tissue provides feedback regarding energy storage levels to the brain through hormonal release of leptin and adiponectin. These hormones act on the arcuate nucleus in the hypothalamus and on the solitary tract nucleus in the brainstem, and in turn, activate distinct neuronal networks. Numerous neuropeptides in the brain, including neuropeptide Y, agouti gene-related peptide, and orexin appear to be involved in appetite stimulation, whereas melanocortins and α-melanocortin-stimulating hormone are involved in satiety. The neuroendocrine control of appetite and weight is in a negative feedback system, balanced between short-term control of appetite (ghrelin, PYY) and long-term control of adiposity (leptin).

Genetics also plays important role in weight regulation. Genes appear to determine a "weight set point" that can also be considered as the protected level of stored fuel that satisfies that individual. Genetic defects in this control system manifest early onset obesity; even in early onset obesity, genetic abnormali-

ties are uncommon. Mutations in the leptin gene and a resultant leptin deficiency result in severe obesity and hyperphagia accompanied by hyperinsulinism, hypothyroidism, and immune dysfunction. Deficiency of pro-opiomelanocortin (POMC) causes early-onset obesity, adrenal insufficiency, and red hair. Genes also control resting energy expenditure (REE), which varies with ethnicity, being higher in white compared with African-American children. More than 600 genes, markers, and chromosomal regions have been associated with obesity in humans.

Diagnostic criteria for overweight: In children, the BMI percentile is used for classification because of changing adiposity during childhood (Table 3.8 and Figs 3.5 and 3.6). Children's adiposity rises in the 1st yr of life, reaches a nadir around 5–6 yrs of age, and then increases again throughout childhood. This is called the adiposity rebound. The 95th percentile BMI for a 4-yr-old is approximately 19, but it is 25 in a 13-yr-old. Consistent use of the BMI growth chart aids in early identification of children at risk for later obesity; an early obesity rebound (increase in BMI younger than 5 yrs of age) coincides with later obesity.

Clinical manifestations: In children obesity is most often associated with tall stature, slightly advanced bone age, and somewhat early puberty. Certain

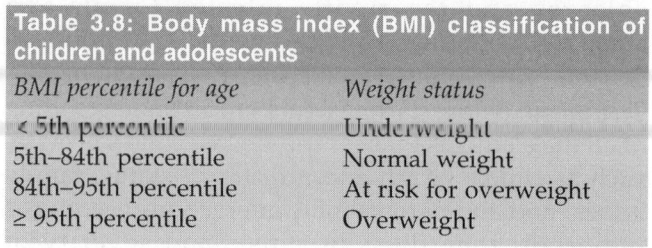

Table 3.8: Body mass index (BMI) classification of children and adolescents

BMI percentile for age	Weight status
< 5th percentile	Underweight
5th–84th percentile	Normal weight
84th–95th percentile	At risk for overweight
≥ 95th percentile	Overweight

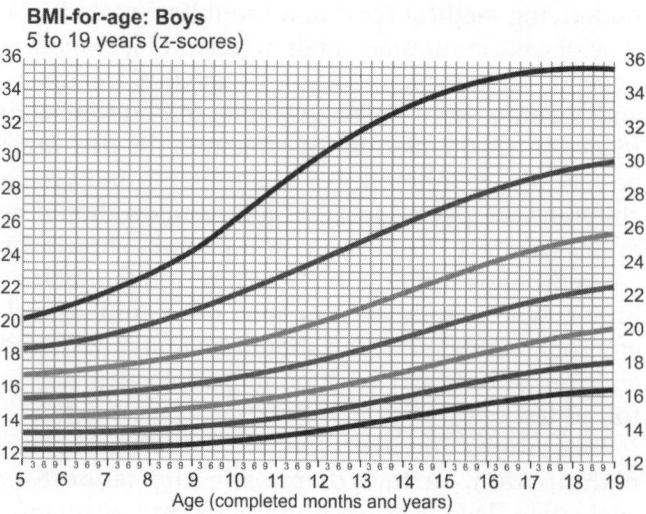

Fig. 3.5: Body mass index (BMI) for boys (age 5–19 yrs).

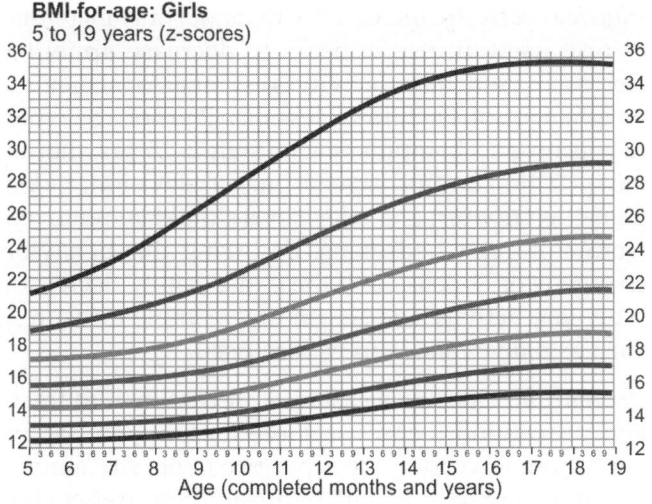

BMI-for-age: Girls
5 to 19 years (z-scores)

Age (completed months and years)

Fig. 3.6: Body mass index (BMI) for girls (age 5–19 yrs).

hormonal aberrations can result in excessive weight gain. In most patients with obesity, rapid growth in height precludes the diagnosis of hypothyroidism and hypercortisolism. By contrast hypothyroidism and cortisol excess cause delayed skeletal development, short stature, and delayed puberty. Many obese youth also have acanthosis nigricans, and is associated with

insulin resistance and a higher risk of developing type 2 diabetes. Obesity in rare instances may be associated with defects at a single genetic locus and these syndromes can usually be detected by demonstration of the typical dysmorphic features. The differential diagnosis is mentioned in Table 3.9.

Comorbidities of overweight: Comorbidities observed during childhood and adolescence includes insulin resistance, Type 2 diabetes, hypercholesterolemia, hypertriglyceridemia, metabolic syndrome, hypertension, orthopedic or musculoskeletal complications, asthma, sleep apnea, polycystic ovary syndrome, and psychosocial disorders. The metabolic syndrome (hypertension, glucose intolerance, hypertriglyceridemia, decreased high-density lipoprotein level, abdominal central obesity) is associated with an excessively high risk of cardiovascular disease. Nonalcoholic fatty liver disease (NAFLD) has been reported in 10–25% of very overweight adolescents. NAFLD is characterized by a mild increase in transaminases, a hyperechoic liver on ultrasound, and evidence of steatosis and periportal fibrosis on histologic examination; progression to liver cirrhosis may occur with time. Proteinuria caused by focal segmental glomerulosclerosis has been reported in

Table 3.9: Diseases associated with childhood obesity	
Childhood obesity diseases	*Clinical features*
Alström syndrome	Hypogonadism, retinal degeneration, deafness, diabetes mellitus
Barder-Biedl syndrome	Retinal degeneration, syndactyly, polydactyly, hypogonadism, mental retardation, autosomal recessive
Carpenter syndrome	Polydactyly, syndactyly, cranial synostosis, mental retardation
Cohen syndrome	Midchildhood-onset obesity, short stature, prominent maxillary incisors, hypotonia, mental retardation, microcephaly, decreased visual acuity
Cushing syndrome	Adrenal hyperplasia or pituitary tumor
Deletion 9q34	Early onset obesity, mental retardation, brachycephaly, prognathism, behavior and sleep disturbances
ENPP1 gene mutation	Insulin resistance childhood obesity, chromosome 6q
Fröhlich syndrome	Hypothalamic tumor
Hyperinsulinism	Pancreatic adenoma, hypoglycemia
Hypothyroidism	Delayed skeletal development and delayed puberty are more prominent features
Leptin or leptin receptor gene mutation	Early-onset severe obesity, infertility, treatable with recombinant leptin
Melanocortin 4 receptor gene mutation	Early-onset severe obesity, increased linear growth, hypephagia, hyperinsulinemia, homozygous worse than heterozygous, commonest cause of obesity
Muscular dystrophy	Late-onset obesity due in part to inactivity
Myelodysplasia	Spina bifida due in part to inactivity
Prader-Willi syndrome	Neonatal hypotonia, normal growth afterbirth, small hands and feet, mental retardation, hypogonadism, hyperphagia leading to severe childhood obesity, ghrelin paradoxically elevated
Pro-opiomelanocortin deficiency	Obesity, red hair, adrenal insufficiency
Pseudohypoparathyroidism	Variable hypocalcemia, cutaneous calcifications
Turner syndrome	Ovarian dysgenesis, lymphedema, web neck, XO chromosome

severely obese African-American adolescents. In addition to these complications that may present in adolescents, obesity in adults is associated with increased risk of malignancies and osteoarthritis.

Management: The treatment goals vary depending on the age of the child and the severity of complications from being overweight. Children are still growing, so severe caloric restriction and weight loss may be detrimental. Weight maintenance rather than weight loss is frequently a reasonable initial goal. As children grow in stature, BMI decreases. Weight loss should be done only in skeletally mature children or in those with serious complications from obesity. Weight loss should be slow (1 lb or 0.5 kg or less/wk), because more rapid weight loss requires vigorous dieting. An initial goal of a 10% reduction in weight is reasonable. Once achieved, the new weight should be maintained for 6 mo before further weight loss is attempted. The most successful approach to weight maintenance or weight loss requires substantial lifestyle changes that include increased physical activity and altered eating habits. Therapies often combine diet, exercise, behavior modification, medications, and rarely, surgery.

Pharmacologic treatment (sibutramine, orlistat topiramate, metformin) for overweight children and adolescents is reserved for those with severe medical complication along with diet and physical activity.

There is some efficacy of bariatric surgery in adolescents; the long-term safety has not been adequately studied. In the USA, the Roux-en-Y gastric bypass is one approach for weight control surgery. Less invasive procedures than the Roux-en-Y gastric by pass are available and include the adjustable gastric band that functions only by extrinsic gastric restriction.

Low-calorie diet: It is used in cases of obesity, cardiac disturbances and hypertension in overweight individuals. The diet provides less calories than total energy requirements for the day; thus it provides for depletion of body fat. This diet provides 1200 calories, 60 g protein, 30 g fat, and 170 g carbohydrates. The foods avoided while formulating the diet includes:

1. Sweets, chocolates, jiggery, jam, honey, preservers, puddings, cakes, etc.
2. Roots and tubers
3. Fried foods
4. Dried foods and nuts
5. Alcoholic drinks and soft drinks unless they contain artificial sweetening agents instead of sugar
6. Cream and free fats, and
7. Fruits like banana, custard-apple (Sharifa), dates, sapota (chiku), etc.

Physical activity: Increased activity not only increases calorie use but also appears to decrease appetite. Decreasing sedentary activity is essential for achieving weight control. In children less than 2 yrs of age avoid television and computers. Children 2–18 yrs should have <2 hrs/day of "screen time" (television, video games, computer) and televisions should be removed from children's bedrooms. Enforcing this behavior change is only possible if the entire family decreases sedentary activity and screen time. Simple measures, such as daily walks, can be discussed.

Prevention: Obesity is easier to prevent than to treat, and prevention focuses in large measure on parent education. Reversing the rapid rise in obesity among children and youth will require a comprehensive approach by schools, families, communities, industry and government.

Greydanus D, Bhave S. Obesity and Adolescents, time for increased Physical activity. Indian Pediatr 2004; 41:545–50.

Pasricha S. Some therapeutic diets. 5th edn. Hyderabad: National Institute of Nutrition, Indian Council of Medical Research, 1996; 1–49.

Skelton JA, Rudolph CD. Overweight and Obesity. In: Kliegman RM, Behrman RE, Jenson HB, Stanton BF (eds). Nelson Textbook of Pediatrics. 18th edn. Vol. 1. Philadelphia: Saunders, 2007;232–42.

3.6 VITAMIN DEFICIENCIES AND EXCESSES

Vitamins are essential organic compounds that are required in very small amounts (micronutrients) and are involved in fundamental functions in the body, such as growth, maintenance of health, and metabolism. Because our bodies cannot biosynthesize vitamins they must be supplied exogenously either as part of a well balanced diet or as supplements. Deficiency states are uncommon in developed countries, but are quite common in many developing countries. Toxicity results from excessive intakes of the fat-soluble vitamins A and D, but toxicity from excessive intakes of the water soluble vitamins is rare.

Vitamin A

Vitamin A is a generic term encompassing all β-ionone derivatives other than provitamin A carotenoids. These include retinol, retinyl ester, retinal and retinoid acid, and the vitamin A alcohol, ester, aldehyde, and acid. Retinol (Vitamin A_1) is an alcohol of high molecular weight (1 μg of retinol = 3.3 IU vitamin A). Provitamin A carotenoids is a generic term for all carotenoids (α, β, γ carotenes and cryptoxanthin; 1/6 activity of retinol) that have the biologic activity of β-carotene. They or their derivatives with vitamin A activity are required in the diets of infants, children and adults. β-carotene is partially absorbed into the intestinal lymphatics. Normal plasma values of retinol are 20–50 μg/dL in infants and 30–225 μg/dL in older children and adults.

Sources: Liver, fish liver oils, whole milk, milk fat products, egg yolk, fortified margarines; carotenoids from plants: green vegetables, yellow fruits and vegetables.

Characteristics: Fat soluble, heat stable, destroyed by oxidation, drying; bile necessary for absorption, stored in liver (vitamin content is low at birth); protected by vitamin E. Zinc is also required for mobilization.

Functions: The major role of vitamin A is in vision. The retina contains two distinct photoreceptor systems—the rods (rhodopsin), which are sensitive to light of low intensity, and the cones (iodopsin), which are sensitive to colors and to light of high intensity. Retinal is the prosthetic group of the photosensitive pigment in both. Retinoids, in addition to involvement in vision are essential for cell differentiation, activation of retinoid acid-responsive genes, and membrane stability. Vitamin A also plays a role in keratinization, cornification, bone metabolism, tooth development, placental development, growth, spermatogenesis, and mucus formation.

Vitamin A Deficiency

Clinical manifestations: Vitamin A deficiency results in ocular and extra-ocular manifestations. Ocular lesions of vitamin A deficiency develop insidiously and rarely occur before 2–3 yrs of age. The posterior segment of the eye is affected initially with impairment of dark adaptation, resulting in night blindness (nyctalopia). Later drying of the conjunctiva (xerosis conjunctivae) and cornea (xerosis corneae) occur followed by wrinkling and cloudiness of the cornea or keratomalacia leading to blindness. Dry, silver-gray plaques may appear on the bulbar conjunctiva (Bitot spots), with follicular hyperkeratosis and photophobia. WHO classification of xerophthalmia is listed in Table 3.10.

Vitamin A deficiency also may result in retardation of mental and physical growth and in apathy. Anemia with or without hepatosplenomegaly is usually present. The skin is dry and scaly and follicular hyperkeratosis may be found on the shoulders, buttocks, and extensor surfaces of the extremities. The vaginal epithelium may become cornified, and epithelial metaplasia of the urinary tract may result in pyuria and hematuria. Increased intracranial pressure with wide separation of cranial bones at the sutures may occur, but hydrocephalus, with or without paralyses of the cranial nerves, is an uncommon manifestation of vitamin A deficiency.

Table 3.10: WHO classification of xerophthalmia		
XN	:	Night blindness
X1A	:	Conjunctival xerosis
X1	:	Conjunctival xerosis with Bitot's spots
X3	:	Corneal xerosis
X3A	:	Corneal ulceration (<1/3 of cornea)
X3B	:	Corneal ulceration (>1/3 of cornea)
XS	:	Corneal scar
XF	:	Xerophthalmic fundus

Diagnosis: Dark adaptation tests may help in the diagnosis of vitamin A deficiency. Xerosis conjunctivae can be detected by biomicroscopic examination of the conjunctiva. Examination of the scrapings from the eye and vagina is also help in the diagnosis. The plasma carotene concentration is less than normal and falls quickly as compared to vitamin A.

Prevention: Infants should receive daily at least 500 μg and older children and adults 600–1500 μg of vitamin A or catotene; mothers of breastfed should be given 30,000 μg [100,000 IU] of vitamin A postpartum. Infants between 6 and 11 mo of age [30,000 μg (100,000 IU)] and older than 12 mo of age [60,000 μg (200,000 IU)] receiving water-miscible vitamin A every 4 mo, have a lower mortality associated with diarrhea and measles.

Treatment: A daily supplement of 1,500 μg of vitamin A is required for treating latent vitamin A deficiency. Xerophthalmia is treated by giving 1,500 μg/kg orally for 5 days followed by daily intramuscular injection of 7,500 μg of vitamin A in oil until recovery occurs. Morbidity and mortality rates from viral infections such as measles may be lower in nondeficient children who are given daily doses of 1,500–3,000 μg of vitamin A.

Hypervitaminosis A

Clinical manifestations: Acute hypervitaminosis A may occur in infants after ingesting 100,000 μg or more. The symptoms are nausea, vomiting, drowsiness, and, in young infants, bulging of the fontanel. Diplopia, papilledema, cranial nerve palsies, and other symptoms suggestive of brain tumor (pseudotumor cerebri) may also be present. Toxicity has been reported with supplementation during vaccination administration.

Chronic hypervitaminosis A results from ingestion of excessive doses for several weeks or months. An affected child has anorexia, pruritus, and a lack of weight gain. Irritability, limitation of motion, with tender swelling of bones, alopecia, seborrheic cutaneous lesions, fissuring of the corner of the mouth, increased intracranial pressure, and hepatomegaly also may develop. Craniotabes and desquamation of palms and soles are common. Radiographs show hyperostosis affecting several long bones, most notable at the middle of the shafts. A history of excessive ingestion of vitamin A helps to differentiate vitamin toxicity from cortical hyperostosis. In addition, serum vitamin A level is elevated. Hypercalcemia and/or liver cirrhosis may occasionally be seen.

Severe congenital malformations may occur in infants of mothers who consume large amounts of oral retinoids for treatment of acne.

Ingested carotenoids, although nontoxic, may result in yellow discoloration of the skin but not of the sclera. This disorder, carotenemia, is especially likely to occur in children with liver disease, diabetes mellitus, or hypothyroidism, and in those who have congenital absence of enzymes that convert provitamin A carotenoids.

Vitamin B Complex

Vitamin B complex includes a number of water soluble vitamins, including thiamine, riboflavin, niacin, pyridoxine, biotin, folate, vitamin B_{12}, pantothenic acid, choline and inositol. All are important constituents of enzyme systems that are closely related functionally and lack of a single factor can interrupt the entire chain of chemical processes producing diverse clinical manifestations. Diets deficient in any one of the B-complex vitamins are frequently poor sources of other B vitamins, and manifestations of several vitamin B deficiencies can usually be found in the same person. It is generally practical to treat a patient with evidence of deficiency of a specific B vitamin with the entire complex of B vitamins.

Thiamine

Thiamine (vitamin B_1; antiberiberi vitamin; aneurin) absorption from the gastrointestinal tract is excellent but may be low in those with gastrointestinal or liver disease. Fever, surgery, and/or stress increase the requirement for thiamine, but are not likely to result in deficiency. Effects of excess do not occur from oral intake of thiamine.

Sources: Liver, meat, especially pork, milk, wholegrain or enriched cereals, wheat germ, legumes, nuts

Characteristics: Water and alcohol soluble; fat insoluble; stable in slightly acid solution; labile to heat, alkali, and sulfites; polishing reduces its availability because the covering of cereal contains most of the vitamin.

Functions: It functions as a coenzyme in carbohydrate metabolism. It is also required for the synthesis of acetylcholine, and deficiency results in impaired nerve conduction. It participates in the hexose monophosphate shunt that generates nicotinamide adenine dinucleotide phosphate and pentose.

Thiamine Deficiency

Clinical manifestations: The clinical manifestations include beriberi, fatigue, irritability, anorexia, constipation, headache, insomnia, tachycardia, polyneuritis, cardiac failure, edema, and aphonia. The full-blown deficiency state is called beriberi, which is of two forms: wet beriberi and dry beriberi. The child with wet beriberi is undernourished, pale, edematous with dyspnea, vomiting and tachycardia, waxy skin and urine often contains albumin and casts. The child with dry beriberi appears plump but is pale, flabby, and listless with dyspnea, tachycardia, and hepatomegaly.

Diagnosis: There is elevated pyruvic acid in the blood. Low red blood cell transketolase and high blood or urinary glyoxylate levels are used as diagnostic indicators. Measurement of urinary thiamine excretion or excretion of its metabolites, thiazole or pyrimidine, after an oral loading dose of thiamine may help to identify the deficiency state. Clinical response to administration of thiamine also helps in making the diagnosis.

Prevention: A maternal diet containing sufficient amounts of thiamine prevents thiamine deficiency in breastfed infants. Infant formulas contain adequate thiamine. A varied diet containing fresh fruits and vegetables as well as wholegrain cereals after the period of exclusive breastfeeding or formula-feeding will provide adequate thiamine intake without supplementation.

Treatment: If a breastfed infant develops beriberi, both the mother and child should be treated with thiamine. The daily dose for children and adults, respectively, is 10 mg and 50 mg, and in the absence of gastrointestinal disturbances, oral administration is effective. However, in children with cardiac failure, thiamine should be given intramuscularly or intravenously, which is followed by dramatic improvement; but complete cure requires several weeks of treatment. The heart is not permanently damaged. Patients of beriberi should always be administered all other vitamins of the B complex, as they often have other B complex vitamin deficiencies.

Riboflavin (Vitamin B_2)

Riboflavin is essential for growth and tissue respiration; may play a role in light adaptation; required for conversion of pyridoxine to pyridoxal phosphate.

Sources: Milk, cheese, liver and other organs, meat, eggs, fish, green leafy vegetables, whole or enriched grains.

Riboflavin Deficiency

Riboflavin deficiency, without deficiencies of other members of the vitamin B-complex is rare. It is usually caused by inadequate riboflavin intake but faulty absorption may contribute in patients with biliary atresia or hepatitis and in those taking probenecid, phenothiazines or oral contraceptives. Phototherapy destroys riboflavin.

Clinical manifestations: Signs and/or symptoms of deficiency include cheilosis (perièche), glossitis, keratitis, conjunctivitis, photophobia, lacrimation, marked corneal vascularization, and seborrheic dermatitis. Superficial fissures, often covered by yellow crusts, develop in the angles of the mouth, and extend radially to the skin for distances of 1–2 cm. With glossitis, the tongue is smooth with loss of papillary structure. A normocytic, normochromic anemia with bone marrow hypoplasia is common.

Diagnosis: Useful diagnostic tests include urinary excretion of riboflavin below 30 µg/24 hrs and low levels of erythrocyte glutathionine reductase, a flavoprotein requiring flavin adenine dinucleotide (FAD).

Prevention: Deficiency is usually prevented by a diet that contains adequate amounts of milk, eggs, leafy vegetables, and lean meats.

Treatment: Treatment includes oral administration of 3–10 mg of riboflavin daily. If no response occurs within a few days, intramuscular injections of 2 mg of riboflavin in saline may be given three times a day. In addition to that child should also be given a well-balanced diet, including, supplements of other B-complex vitamins.

Niacin (Nicotinamide; Nicotinic Acid; Antipellagra Vitamin)

Niacin forms part of two cofactors, nicotinamide adenine dinucleotide and nicotinamide adenine dinucleotide phosphate, that are important in electron transfer and glycolysis. Only small losses of niacin occur in cooking.

Sources: Meat, fish, poultry, liver, wholegrain and enriched cereals, green vegetables, peanuts.

Characteristics: Water and alcohol soluble; stable to acid, alkali, light, heat, oxidation.

Functions: Essential for prevention of pellagra, B-complex deficiency syndromes.

Niacin Deficiency

Pellagra (Pellis, "skin"; nigra, "rough"), a deficiency disease, caused by a lack of niacin (nicotinic acid), affects all tissues of the body. It chiefly occurs in countries where corn (maize), a poor source of tryptophan, is a basic foodstuff.

Clinical manifestations: The early symptoms of pellagra are vague. After a long period of deficiency, the classic triad of (the 3-D) dermatitis, diarrhea, and dementia appears in pellagra cases. Children who have pellagra often have evidence of other nutritional deficiency diseases. The dermatitis of pellagra, may develop suddenly or insidiously, and may be elicited by irritants, including intense sunlight. The lesions first appear as symmetric areas of erythema on exposed surfaces resembling sun burn. The lesions are usually sharply demarcated from the healthy skin around them. The cutaneous lesions have characteristic appearance on the hands (pellagrous gloves), foot and leg (pellagrous boot), and around the neck (Casal necklace). In some cases, vesicles and bullae develop (wet type); in others, there may be suppuration beneath the scaly, crusted epidermis, and in still others the swelling may disappear followed by desquamation. The healed parts of the skin may remain pigmented.

The cutaneous lesions may be preceded by or accompanied by gastrointestinal upset including, stomatitis, glossitis, vomiting, and/or diarrhea. Swelling and redness of the tip of the tongue and its lateral margins is often followed by intense redness, even ulceration of the entire tongue and papillae.

Nervous symptoms include depression, disorientation, insomnia, and delirium.

Diagnosis: The diagnosis is made clinically on the findings of symmetric dermatitis, glossitis and gastrointestinal symptoms. Rapid clinical response to niacin is an important confirming test. N-methylnicotinamide, a normal metabolite of niacin, is almost undetectable in the urine of niacin-deficient individuals.

Prevention: A well-balanced diet containing meat, vegetables, eggs and milk provides adequate intakes of niacin.

Treatment: A well-balanced diet should be supplemented with 50–300 mg of niacin daily; in severe cases or in cases of poor intestinal absorption 100 mg may be given intravenously. Large doses of niacin are often followed by a sensation of heat as well as flushing and burning of the skin, which occurs usually within half an hour after ingestion of niacin, but not produced by nicotinamide. Large doses of niacin may cause cholestatic jaundice or hepatotoxicity. The diet should be supplemented with other vitamins, especially other

B-complex vitamins. Sun exposure should be avoided during the active phase of pellagra, and the skin lesions may be covered with soothing applications. Hypochromic anemia, if present should be treated with iron. The diet should be supervised continuously to prevent recurrence.

Pyridoxine (Vitamin B$_6$)

Vitamin B$_6$ includes pyridoxal, pyridoxine and pyridoxamine. Pyridoxine antagonists (e.g. isoniazid used in the treatment of tuberculosis), pregnancy, and drugs such as penicillamine, hydralazine, and oral progesterone-estrogen contraceptives increase the requirements for pyridoxine.

Pyridoxine toxicity: Megadoses of pyridoxine have caused neuropathy in adults.

Sources: Meat, liver, kidney, wholegrains, soybeans, nuts, fish, poultry, green vegetables.

The pyridoxine content of human milk and infant formulas is adequate. Bovine milk and cereals also are good sources of pyridoxine, but prolonged heat processing of this milk and cereal destroys it.

Characteristics: Water soluble; destroyed by ultraviolet light and by heat.

Functions: Pyridoxine is necessary for adequate functioning of the nervous system and in the formation of serotonin, metabolism of glycogen and fatty acids, and normal brain metabolism.

Pyridoxine Deficiency

Clinical manifestations: Vitamin B$_6$-dependence syndromes include vitamin B$_6$ dependent convulsions, vitamin B$_6$ responsive anemia, xanthurenic aciduria, cystathioninuria, and homocystinuria. Deficiency symptoms secondary to one of the vitamin B$_6$ dependence syndromes or inadequate intake are not as common in children as in adults. Four clinical disturbances caused by vitamin B$_6$ deficiency, include convulsions in infants, peripheral neuritis, dermatitis, and anemia.

Diagnosis: All infants with seizures should be suspected of having vitamin B$_6$ deficiency or dependence. If more common causes of infantile seizures (e.g. hypoglycemia, hypocalcemia, infection) are eliminated, 100 mg of pyridoxine should be injected. If the seizure stops, vitamin B$_6$ deficiency should be suspected, and a tryptophan loading test should be performed. In older children, 100 mg of pyridoxine may be injected while the EEG is being recorded; a favorable response of the EEG suggests pyridoxine deficiency. Erythrocyte glutamic pyruvic transaminase is low in pyridoxine deficiency.

Prevention: A daily intake of 0.3–0.5 mg of pyridoxine in an infant, 0.5–1.5 mg in a child, and 1.5–2.0 mg in an adult prevents deficiency states. Larger doses may be necessary in pyridoxine dependency.

Treatment: Convulsions due to pyridoxine deficiency should be treated with 100 mg of the vitamin given intramuscularly (IM); one dose should suffice if the diet is adequate. For pyridoxine dependent children, daily doses of 2–10 mg IM or 10–100 mg orally may be necessary.

Biotin

Biotin is used as a cofactor for enzymes involved in carboxylation reactions. In humans, there are 5 biotin-dependent carboxylases that catalyse key reactions in gluconeogenesis, fatty acid metabolism, and amino acid catabolism. It is widely distributed (yeast, animal products, synthesized in intestine), thus making a deficiency unlikely. Conditions involving deficiencies in the enzymes holocarboxylase synthetase and biotinidase that respond to treatment with biotin are described in Chapter 26, page-812.

Biotin Deficiency

Biotin deficiency is rare, because many microorganisms produce biotin. Deficiency may occur in those consuming the biotin antagonist avidin, found in raw egg white. Deficiency has been described in infants, who are exclusively on parenteral nutrition and in infants whose mothers are biotin deficient (*see* Chapter 26).

Clinical manifestations: Brawny dermatitis, orofacial lesions, alopecia, somnolence, hallucinations, hypotonia, and hyperesthesia with accumulation of organic acids are common manifestations of deficiency. Other neurologic signs may occur.

Diagnosis: Biotin deficiency is suggested by aciduria, particularly propionic and dicarboxylic acids. Response of clinical and biochemical abnormalities to biotin administration is confirmatory.

Prevention: Inclusion of biotin in parenteral nutrition infusions will prevent the most common cause of biotin deficiency in infants.

Treatment: Oral administration of 10 mg of biotin is sufficient for treatment of deficiency as well as to confirm the diagnosis of deficiency.

Folic Acid (*see* Chapter 20, page-591)

Vitamin B$_{12}$ (*see* Chapter 20, page-592)

Vitamin C (Ascorbic Acid)

Ascorbic acid is a potent reducing agent, functions in a number of enzyme systems. The need for vitamin C is increased by febrile illnesses, particularly infectious and diarrheal diseases. Iron deficiency, cold exposure, and protein depletion also increase the need of vitamin C. Cooking has destructive effect.

Characteristics: Water soluble; easily oxidized, accelerated by heat, light, alkali, oxidative enzymes, traces of copper or iron.

Functions: Integrity and maintenance of intercellular material; facilitates absorption of iron and conversion of folic acid to folinic acid; metabolism of tyrosine and phenylalanine; activity of succinic dehydrogenate and serum phosphatase in infants, not in adults.

Sources: Citrus fruits, tomatoes, berries, cantaloupe, cabbage, green vegetables.

Vitamin C Deficiency

Vitamin C deficiency results in scurvy, in which formation of collagen and chondroitin sulfate is impaired. This results in a tendency to hemorrhage, defective tooth dentin, and loosening of the teeth. Because osteoblasts cannot form osteoid, endochondrial bone formation cannot proceed; the bony trabeculae that have been formed become brittle and fracture easily. The periosteum becomes loosened and subperiosteal hemorrhage occurs, especially at the ends of the femur and tibia. Severe deficiency may result in degeneration of the skeletal muscles, cardiac hypertrophy, bone marrow depression, and adrenal atrophy.

Clinical manifestations: The usual age at onset is between 6 and 24 mo. Usually, there evidence of generalized tenderness that is particularly noticeable in the legs when the infant is picked up or when the diaper is changed. The pain results in pseudoparalysis; the legs are usually held in a froglike position with the hips and knees are semiflexed with the feet rotated outward. Edematous swelling along the shafts of the legs may be present and in some cases, a subperiosteal hemorrhage can be felt at the end of the femur. Changes in the gums most noticeable after eruption of teeth include bluish purple, spongy swellings of the mucous membrane, especially over the upper incisors. Scorbutic rosary at the costochondral junctions and depression of the sternum are other typical features; the angulation of the scorbutic heads is usually sharper than that of a rachitic rosary.

Petechial hemorrhages are often present in the skin and mucous membranes. Hematuria, melena, and orbital or subdural hemorrhages also may occur. Anemia, if present may be due to inability to utilize iron or impaired folic acid metabolism.

Diagnosis: Laboratory tests for scurvy are unsatisfactory and the diagnosis is usually based on the characteristic clinical picture, the radiographic appearance of the long bones, and a history of poor vitamin C intake. The typical radiographic changes occur at the distal ends of the long bones, particularly common in the area of the knee. The trabeculae of the shaft cannot be discerned and the bone has a ground-glass appearance. The cortex is quite thin and the epiphyseal ends of the bones are sharply outlined. The white line of Fraenkel, an irregular but thickened white line at the metaphysic, represents the zone of well-calcified cartilage. The epiphyseal centers of ossification also have a ground glass appearance and are surrounded by a white ring. The zone of rarefaction is a linear break in the bone proximal and parallel to the white line at the metaphysis. A spur or lateral prolongation of the white line may be present. Epiphyseal separation may occur along the line of destruction with either linear displacement or compression of the epiphysis against the shaft. Subperiosteal hemorrhages are not visible radiographically during the active phase of scurvy; during healing the elevated periosteum becomes calcified and the affected bone assumes a dumb-bell or club shape.

A level of zero in the ascorbic acid concentration of the white cell/platelet layer (buffy layer) of centrifuged oxalated blood indicates latent scurvy, even in the absence of clinical signs of deficiency. Saturation of the tissues with vitamin C can be estimated from the urinary excretion of the vitamin; in normal children, 80% of the test dose appears in the urine within 3–5 hrs after parentally administration of the test dose.

Differential diagnosis: Scurvy is often misdiagnosed as arthritis or acrodynia. In cases of copper deficiency the radiographic picture is very similar to that of scurvy. The pseudoparalysis of scurvy often is confused with that of syphilis; however, the latter usually occurs at an earlier age and is usually accompanied by other signs of syphilis. Henoch-Schönlein purpura, thrombocytopenic purpura, leukemia, meningitis, or nephritis may be suspected.

Prevention: Scurvy can be prevented by an adequate intake of vitamin C (e.g. by taking citrus fruits and juices). Formula-fed infants usually receive adequate amounts of ascorbic acid, provided the formula is not heated excessively. Lactating mothers should consume about 100 mg of vitamin C daily. Older children and adults need somewhat more than infants.

Treatment: The daily therapeutic dose is 100–200 mg orally or parenterally. Recovery including resumption of growth occurs early but the swelling of subperiosteal hemorrhage may not disappear for months.

Vitamin D

Two forms of vitamin D, vitamin D_2 and vitamin D_3, are produced synthetically and are available as dietary supplements. D_2-calciferol is activated ergosterol. Vitamin D_3 also is naturally present in human skin; the provitamin form, 7-dehydrocholesterol, is activated photochemically to vitamin D_3 which is then transferred to the liver. Both vitamin D_2 and vitamin D_3 are hydroxylated in the liver to 25-OH-cholecalciferol, and subsequently, in the renal cortex to 1,25-dihydroxycholecalciferol, which functions as a hormone. Receptors for 1,25-dihydroxycholecalciferol are present in most tissues, but its primary roles are facilitation of intestinal absorption of calcium and phosphorus, renal absorption of phosphorus, and possibly a direct effect on bone deposition and reabsorption of calcium and phosphorus. With the parathormone and calcitonin, 1,25-dihydroxycholecalciferol plays a major role in calcium and phosphorus homeostasis of both body fluids and body tissues.

Characteristics: Fat soluble; stable to heat, acid, alkali, and oxidation; bile necessary for absorption.

Functions: Regulates absorption and deposition of calcium and phosphorus by affecting permeability of intestinal membrane; regulates level of serum alkaline phosphatase which is concerned with calcium phosphate deposition in bones and teeth; synthesis of osteocalcin is vitamin D dependent.

Sources: Vitamin D fortified milk and margarine, fish liver oils, exposure to sunlight or other ultraviolet sources.

Vitamin D Deficiency

Vitamin D deficiency results in rickets, signifying failure to mineralize growing bone (before fusion of the epiphyses) or osteoid tissue (osteomalacia). Vitamin D deficiency rickets is still an important cause in developing countries, but rare among infants and children in industrialized countries. Nevertheless, even in developed countries, deficiency still occurs in unsupplemented dark-skinned infants, in breastfed infants of mothers who are not exposed to sunlight. Vitamin D deficiency also occurs in conditions other than inadequate intake of vitamin D include clinical entities that interfere with vitamin D absorption or metabolic conversion and activation, such as steatorrhea, hepatic, and renal diseases, or conditions that disrupt calcium and phosphorus homeostasis in other ways.

Pathophysiology: New bone formation is initiated by osteoblasts, which are responsible for matrix deposition and subsequent mineralization. Osteoblasts secrete collagen, and changes in polysaccharides, phospholipids, alkaline phosphatase and pyrophosphatase follow until mineralization occurs. Mineralization occurs in the presence of adequate calcium and phosphorus. Resorption of bone occurs when osteoclasts secrete enzymes on the bone surface, which dissolve and remove both matrix and mineral. Osteocytes covered by bone both resorb and redeposit bone. Phosphorus, calcium, fluoride, and growth hormone are known to be involved that affect bone growth. In rickets, defective bone growth results from retardation or suppression of normal epiphyseal cartilage growth and calcification.

Clinical manifestations: Rickets usually appears toward the end of the first and during the 2nd yr of life. Vitamin D deficient rickets is rare later in childhood. The softness of the skull may result in flattening and at times prominent asymmetry of the head. The anterior fontanel is larger than normal, and its closure may be delayed until after 2nd yr of life. The central parts of the parietal and frontal bones are often thickened, forming prominences, or bosses, and giving the head a box-like appearance (caput quadratum). Eruption of the temporary teeth may be delayed, and there may be defects of the enamel and extensive caries. The permanent teeth that are calcifying during the period of vitamin D deficiency may also be affected: the permanent incisors, canines and first molars almost always have enamel defects. Enlargement of the costochondral junctions may become prominent. The sternum with its adjacent cartilage appears to project forward, pigeon breast deformity, and a horizontal depression, Harrison groove develops along the lower border of the chest. As the rachitic process continues, the epiphyseal enlargement at the wrists and ankles becomes more noticeable, and bending of the softened shafts of the femur, tibia and fibula results in knock-knees (Genu valgum) and bow legs (Genu varum). Greenstick fractures may occur in the long bones, often with no clinical symptoms. Deformities of the spine, pelvis, and legs result in short stature or rachitic dwarfism. Relaxation of ligaments contributes to production of the deformities, partly accounting for knock-knees, overextension of the knee joints, weak ankles, kyphosis, and scoliosis. The muscles are poorly developed and lack tone; as a result, children do not stand or walk at the usual ages.

Diagnosis: The diagnosis of rickets is based on a history of inadequate intake of vitamin D or inadequate exposure to sunlight and the characteristic clinical signs of the condition. It is confirmed chemically and radiographic examination. The serum calcium level in children with rickets may be normal or low, serum phosphorus is less than 4 mg/dL, serum alkaline phosphatase level is elevated (normal less than 200 IU/dL) and the serum 25-hydroxychole-calciferol is low. The radiographic findings are characteristically seen in the long bones particularly in the radius and ulna. Cupping and fraying of the distal ends of the radius and ulna; double contour along the lateral outline of the radius (periosteal osteoid) is seen in active rickets. After treatment with vitamin D characteristic findings of healing rickets can be seen in serial X-rays. Above the zones of preparatory calcification (ZPC) in the rachitic metaphyses there is beginning of calcification; later ZPC are well defined and the rachitic metaphyses appear well calcified and the epiphysis of the radius has become more visible; still later ZPC, rachitic metaphyses, and the shafts have become united.

Prevention: Rickets can be prevented by exposure to ultraviolet light or by oral administration of vitamin D. Formula-fed infants and breastfed infants of mothers who have adequate exposure to sunlight receives adequate intakes of vitamin D. Breastfed infants whose mothers are not exposed to adequate sunlight, particularly those who also are protected from sunlight, dark-skinned infants, and infants born during the winter months in temperate climates also should receive a supplement of 400 IU of vitamin D daily, particularly if breastfed. Vitamin D should also be administered to pregnant and lactating mothers.

Treatment: Daily administration of 50–150 µg (1 g = 40 IU) of vitamin D_3 or 0.5–2 g of 1,25-dihydroxychole-calcerol produces healing demonstrable on roentgenogram within 2–4 wks, except in cases of vitamin D refractory rickets. Vitamin D_3 is usually adequate unless deficiency is secondary to hepatic or renal disease. A 15,000 g of vitamin D in a single dose without further therapy for several months is preferred, because rapid healing follows, possibly with earlier differential diagnosis from genetic vitamin D-resistant rickets and daily vitamin D administration is avoided. If no healing occurs the rickets is probably resistant to vitamin D.

Tetany of Vitamin D Deficiency (Infantile Tetany)

Tetany due to vitamin D deficiency occasionally accompanies rickets, particularly in infants and children with severe steatorrhea, if the serum ionized calcium concentration falls below 3–4 mg/dL. At this level, muscular irritability occurs due to loss of the inhibitory control that calcium exerts on the neuro-muscular junctions. Diagnosis is based on the combined presence of rickets, low serum calcium concentration (decreased serum phosphorus and elevated serum alkaline phosphatase levels) and symptoms of tetany.

Hypervitaminosis D

Symptoms, which develop after 1–3 mo of excessive intake of vitamin D (may be due to hypersensitivity to vitamin D), include hypotonia, anorexia, irritability, constipation, polydipsia, polyuria, and pallor. Aortic valvular stenosis, vomiting, hypertension, retinopathy, and clouding of cornea and conjunctiva may occur. Hypercalcemia and hypercalciuria occur. Proteinuria may be present and, if excessive intake continues, renal damage and metastatic calcification occur. X-rays of the long bones reveal metastatic calcification and generalized osteopetrosis.

Metastatic calcification occurs also in chronic nephritis, hyperparathyroidism and idiopathic hypercalcemia. These conditions particularly the latter two also are accompanied by hypercalcemia.

Treatment includes discontinuing vitamin D intake and decreasing calcium intake. For severely affected infants, aluminum hydroxide can be given orally.

Vitamin E

Vitamin E (α-tocopherol) is a fat-soluble antioxidant. Deficiency may occur in fat malabsorption states. Diets high in unsaturated fatty acids increase the vitamin E requirement in premature infants who absorb vitamin E poorly. Excess iron administration exaggerates signs of vitamin E deficiency.

Functions: Minimizes oxidation of carotene, vitamin A, and linoleic acid; stabilizes membranes.

Sources: Germ oils of various seeds, green leafy vegetables, nuts, legumes.

Vitamin E Deficiency

Clinical manifestations: Vitamin E deficiency has been suggested as a causative factor in the anemia of kwashiorkor, hemolytic anemia between 6 and 10 wks of age in premature infants, retinopathy of pre-maturity, increased platelet adhesiveness. Patients with malabsorption and vitamin E deficiency secondary to biliary atresia develop a degenerative, potentially reversible, neurologic syndrome consisting of cerebellar ataxia, peripheral neuropathy and posterior column abnormalities, and myopathy.

Diagnosis: Vitamin E deficiency is detected by a serum ratio of α-tocopherol to lipid of less than 0.8 mg/g and/or erythrocyte hemolysis in hydrogen peroxide of more than 10%. Blood levels should be determined 3 days after administration of vitamin E.

Prevention: 0.7 mg vitamin E/g of unsaturated fat in the diet appears adequate.

Treatment: Children with deranged fat absorption should receive more than that is given for prevention. Premature infants may be given up to 15–25 IU per day. Large oral and parenteral doses of vitamin E may prevent permanent neurologic abnormalities in children with biliary atresia or abetalipoproteinemia.

Vitamin K

Vitamin K is a naphthoquinone. The naturally occurring vitamin K is fat soluble. It is designated vitamin K_1 (K_1 is phytoquinone) to distinguish it from vitamin K_2 of bacterial origin and from synthetic naphthaquinones with vitamin K activity. The breast-milk content of vitamin K is quite low; that of bovine-milk is somewhat higher. The content of infant formulas is adequate. Suppression of intestinal bacteria by antibiotics may be responsible for vitamin K deficiency. Administration of vitamin K to a newborn infant increases concentrations of pro-thrombin, proconvertin, plasma thromboplastin component (factor IX) and Stuart-Prower factor (factor X). Large doses of synthetic vitamin K analogues, but not vitamin K_1, may result in hyperbilirubinemia and kernicterus in newborns with glucose-6-phosphate dehydrogenase deficiency and in premature infants.

Characteristics: Naturally occurring vitamin K compounds are fat soluble; stable to heat and reducing agents; labile to oxidizing agent, strong acids, alkali, light; bile salts necessary for intestinal absorption.

Functions: Prothrombin formation, coagulation factors II, VII, IX, and X and osteocalcin are vitamin K-dependent; vitamin K dependent proteins C, S, Z and M.

Sources: Green leafy vegetables, pork, liver.

Vitamin K Deficiency

Clinical manifestations: Deficiency of vitamin K or hypoprothrombinemia should be considered in all patients with a hemorrhagic disturbance. Hypopro-thrombinemia may also result from certain drugs. Dicumarol is used specifically for the production of hypoprothrombinemia in the prevention and treatment of venous thrombosis, by preventing the liver from utilizing vitamin K rather than exerting a specific effect on prothrombin. Salicylic acid, a degradation product of dicumarol, produces hypoprothrombinemia by a similar mechanism. The reduction in prothrombin resulting from salicylates, however, is mild compared with that of dicumarol. The hemorrhagic manifestations of acute rheumatic fever may be caused in some cases by large doses of salicylates; this can be reversed by vitamin K administration.

Diagnosis: Hypoprothrombinemia that is corrected by vitamin K administration establishes the diagnosis.

Prevention: All infants should receive a prophylactic dose of vitamin K at birth. The breastfed infant may benefit from additional vitamin K until the diet becomes more varied, but the formula-fed infant receives more than an adequate intake of vitamin K. Infants and children with prolonged diarrhea, as well as those who require prolonged antibiotic therapy or have steatorrhea, should receive supplemental vitamin K.

Treatment: If prothrombin deficiency is severe and hemorrhagic manifestations have appeared, 5 mg of K_1 every 24 hrs should be given parenterally. Vitamin K can be given for hypoprothrombinemia secondary to liver damage, but whole blood is usually also necessary. Oral administration of vitamin K may correct mild prothrombin deficiency; for an infant, in the doses of 1–2 mg every 24 hrs.

3.7 ANTIOXIDANTS

Antioxidants contains a mixture of beta-carotene, vitamin C and vitamin E and minerals like copper, manganese, zinc and selenium, all which have a synergistic antioxidant effect. It effectively terminates free radical activity, implicated in tissue damage. Antioxidant enzyme superoxide dismutase (SOD), catalase, and glutathione peroxidase help to catalyse the reduction of oxidants primarily inside the cell. The antioxidants exert their effect by counteracting oxidative processes that constitute to the causation of the chronic disease. Free radicals have been implicated in many diseases of childhood like kwashiorkor, rheumatoid arthritis, inflammatory bowel disease, cystic fibrosis, cancer, hepatic disorders, and neonatal disorders (retinopathy of prematurity, hypoxic ischemic encephalopathy).

"Antioxidant" means a substance which when added to food retards or prevents oxidative deteriora-tion of food and does not include sugar, cereal oils, flours, herbs, and spices. But no antioxidant other than lecithin, ascorbic acid, and tocopherol shall be added to any food.

Endogenous antioxidant mechanisms in humans can adjust their activity in relation to the changes in oxidative stress. Even though free radical mediated damage seems to be important in many pediatric diseases, supplementation with antioxidants does not have a definite role in disease prevention. Thus, the most effective disease prevention strategy regarding antioxidants is achieved by eating a wide variety of naturally occurring antioxidants. Recommended daily allowances of naturally occurring antioxidants like vitamins and minerals should be met in deficiency states such as malnutrition and liver disorders. The antioxidants are indicated in metabolic diseases, cerebrovascular disease, neurological disease, and degenerative disease of the eyes.

Heird WC. Vitamin deficiencies and excesses. In: Behrman RE, Kliegman RM, Jenson HB (eds). Nelson Textbook of Pediatrics. 17th edn. Philadelphia: Saunders, 2004; 177–90.

Chadha DS (Ed). Antioxidants. The Prevention of Food Adulteration Act & Rules (as on 1.10.2004). New Delhi: Confederation of Indian Industry, 2004; 154.

3.8 MICRONUTRIENT MINERAL DEFICIENCIES

Micronutrients include vitamins and trace elements. By definition, a trace element is <0.01% of the body weight. Trace elements have a variety of essential functions. With the exception of iron deficiency, trace element deficiency is uncommon in developed countries, but some deficiencies (iodine, fluorine, and zinc) are important public health problems in a number of developing countries. Because of low nutritional requirements and plentiful supply, deficiencies of some of the trace elements are extremely rare in humans and are typically described in patients receiving unusual diets or prolonged total parenteral nutrition without adequate delivery of a specific trace element. Excess intake of trace elements is uncommon, but it may occur due to environmental exposure or over use of supplements.

Children are especially susceptible to trace element deficiency. First, growth creates an increased demand for most trace elements. Second, some organs are more likely to sustain permanent damage due to trace element deficiency during childhood. The developing brain is particularly vulnerable to the consequences of certain deficiency states (iron, iodine). Similarly, adequate fluoride is most critical for dental health during childhood. Third, children are more prone to gastrointestinal disorders that may cause trace element deficiencies due to malabsorption.

Calcium

Function and metabolism: Structure of bone and teeth, muscle contraction, nerve irritability, coagulation of blood, cardiac action, production of milk. Absorbed from upper small intestine aided by vitamin D, ascorbic acid, lactose, acid medium; hindered by excesses of dietary oxalic acid, phytic acid, fat, fiber, phosphate. Deposited in bone trabeculas and maintained in dynamic equilibrium with body tissue

through action of parathyroid hormone, vitamin D and calcitonin. About 70% excreted in feces, 10% in urine, 15–25% retained, depending on growth rate. Serum level 9–11 mg/dL, 60% ionized. The ionized calcium concentration is the gold standard for evaluating children with calcium disorders.

Daily requirements (mg/24 hr): 0–6 mo (6 kg) 210; 7–12 mo (9 kg) 270; 1–3 yrs (13 kg) 500; 4–8 yrs (22 kg) 800.

Sources: Milk, cheese, green leafy vegetables, oysters.

Effects of deficiency (hypocalcemia): Poor mineralization of bones and teeth; osteomalacia; osteoporosis; tetany; rickets; impairment of growth.

Effects of excess (hypercalcemia): Unknown (dietary); heart block and renal stones (parenteral).

Chloride

Function and metabolism: Osmotic pressure; acid–base balance; hydrochloride in gastric juice. Readily absorbed. About 92% of intake is excreted, mainly in the urine, some in feces and sweat. Composes about 2/3 of the blood plasma anions. Blood serum level, 99–106 mEq/L; in intracellular and extracellular fluids; parallels sodium intake and output.

Daily requirements (mg/24 hr): 0–6 mo (6 kg) 180; 7–12 mo (9 kg) 300; 1–3 yr (13 kg) 350; 4–8 yr (22 kg) 500.

Sources: Table salt, meat, milk, eggs.

Effects of deficiency: Hypochloremic alkalosis may occur with prolonged vomiting or excessive sweating, with parenteral administration of glucose without saline, with excessive ACTH therapy, and with congenital alkalosis.

Effects of excess: Unknown.

Chromium

Function and metabolism: Glycemic regulation and insulin metabolism; potentiates the action of indulin. Daily requirements (mg/24 hr): 0–6 mo (6 kg) 0.2; 7–12 mo (9 kg) 5.5; 1–3 yr (13 kg) 11; 4–8 yr (22 kg) 15.

Sources: Yeast, meat

Effects of deficiency: Impaired glucose tolerance, peripheral neuropathy and encephalopathy.

Effects of excess: None known.

Cobalt

Function and metabolism: Component of vitamin B_{12} (cyanocobalamin) molecule and of erythropoietin.

Sources: Widely distributed.

Effects of deficiency: None known; hypothyroidism.

Effects of excess: Cardiomyopathy; medicinally, it may be goitrogenic or may produce cardiomyopathy.

Copper

Function and metabolism: Essential for production of red blood cells; transferrin, hemoglobin formation; absorption of iron, activities of tyrosinase, catalase, uricase, cytochrome C oxidase, 8-aminolevulinic acid dehydrase, lysyl oxidase. Absorbed with sulfur-rich proteins; transported bound to α-2-globulin as ceruloplasmin; present in erythrocytes in a labile form and more stable hemocuprein; highest concentration in liver and central nervous system (cerebrocuprein); excreted mainly via the intestinal wall and the bile; deranged metabolism in Wilson disease (hepatolenticular degeneration), and Menkes' syndrome.

Daily requirements (mg/24 hr): 0–6 mo (6 kg) 200; 7–12 mo (9 kg) 220; 1–3 yr (13 kg) 340; 4–8 yr (22 kg) 440.

Sources: Liver, oysters, meats, fish, wholegrains, nuts, legumes.

Effects of deficiency: May be cause of refractory anemia, osteoporosis, neutropenia, depigmentation and delayed bone age, bone infarctions, pseudoparalysis, ataxia.

Effects of excess: Cirrhosis, gastritis, hemolysis.

Fluorine

Function and metabolism: Tooth and bone structure. Retained when intake is above 0.6 mg/day; excreted in urine and sweat; deposited in bones as fluorapatite.

Daily requirements (mg/24 hr): 0–6 mo (6 kg) 0.01; 7–12 mo (9 kg) 0.5; 1–3 yr (13 kg) 0.77; 4–8 yr (22 kg) 1.0.

Sources: Water, sea foods, plant and animal foods (dependent on content in soil and water).

Effects of deficiency: Tendency to dental caries.

Effects of excess: Fluorosis; mottling of teeth with intake of more than 4–8 mg/24 hr (*see* Chapter 3.9, page-80).

Iodine

Function and metabolism: Constituent of thyroxine (T4) and triiodothyronine (T3).

Readily absorbed from intestine; circulates as inorganic and organic iodide; selectively concentrated about 25:1 in the thyroid gland, quickly iodized and incorporated into thyroglobulin; proteolytic enzymes release thyroxine and triiodothyronine into the blood. Excreted mainly in urine.

Daily requirements (mg/24 hr): 0–6 mo (6 kg) 110; 7–12 mo (9 kg) 130; 1–3 yr (13 kg) 90; 4–8 yr (22 kg) 90.

Sources: Iodized salt, sea food, food grown in non-goitrous areas.

Effects of deficiency: Simple goiter, endemic cretinism.

Effects of excess: Not harmful (less than 1 mg/24 hr); medicinally, may cause goiter.

Iron

Function and metabolism: Structure of hemoglobin and myoglobin for O_2 and CO_2 transport; oxidative enzymes; cytochrome C and catalase. Absorbed in ferrous form according to body need, aided by gastric juice and ascorbic acid; hindered by fiber, phytic acid, steatorrhea. Transported in plasma in ferric state bound to transferrin; stored in liver, spleen, bone marrow, and kidney as ferritin and hemosiderin; conserved and reused; minimal losses in urine and sweat; about 90% of intake excreted in stool.

Daily requirements (mg/24 hr): 0–6 mo (6 kg) 0.27; 7–12 mo (9 kg) 11; 1–3 yr (13 kg) 7; 4–8yr (22 kg) 10.

Sources: Liver, meat, egg yolk, green vegetables, whole grains, legumes, nuts.

Effects of deficiency: Anemia: Hypochromic, microcytic, growth failure.

Effects of excess: Hemosiderosis in Bantu people of Africa due to low phosphorus and high iron contents of diet. Poisoning by medicinal iron.

Magnesium

Function and metabolism: Structure of bones and teeth; activation of enzymes in carbohydrate metabolism; muscle and nerve irritability, important intracellular cation, essential in metabolic processes. Absorption is from small intestine varies with intake; some urinary excretion, but excellent renal conservation, antagonist to calcium action.

Daily requirements (mg/24 hr): 0–6 mo (6 kg) 30; 7–12 mo (9 kg) 75; 1–3 yr (13 kg) 80; 4–8 yr (22 kg) 130.

Sources: Cereals, legumes, nuts, meat, milk.

Effects of deficiency: Occurs in malabsorption and deficiency states; diabetes, may be expressed clinically as tetany; associated frequently with hypocalcemia; hypokalemia.

Effects of excess: None (dietary); toxicity from intravenous medication.

Manganese

Function and metabolism: Enzyme activation, especially superoxide dismutase; normal bone structure, carbohydrate metabolism. Poor absorption from intestine; transported in plasma; particularly high turnover rate in mitochondria; excretion mainly via the intestine in bile; competes with iron.

Daily requirements (mg/24 hr): 0–6 mo (6 kg) 0.03; 7–12 mo (9 kg) 0.6; 1–3 yr (13 kg) 1.02; 4–8 yr (22 kg) 1.5.

Sources: Legumes, nuts, wholegrain cereals, green leafy vegetables.

Effects of deficiency: Hypercholesterolemia, weight loss, decreased clotting proteins.

Effects of excess: Neurologic manifestations, cholestatic jaundice none (dietary): toxicity from chronic inhalation (encephalopathy).

Molybdenum

Function and metabolism: Component of enzymes; xanthine oxidase for conversion to uric acid and mobilization of ferritin iron in liver, liver aldehyde oxidase, sulfite oxidase.

Readily absorbed from intestine; excreted chiefly in urine, some in bile.

Daily requirements (mg/24 hr): 0–6 mo (6 kg) 2; 7–12 mo (9 kg) 3; 1–3 yr (13 kg) 17; 4–8 yr (22 kg) 22.

Sources: Legumes, grains, dark green leafy vegetables, animal organs.

Effects of deficiency: Ocular abnormalities, seizures, mental retardation, xanthinuria.

Effects of excess: Hyperuricemia and increased risk of gout.

Phosphorus

Function and metabolism: Constituent of bones and teeth; structure of nucleus and cytoplasm of all cells; acid–base balance; energy transformations and transmission of nerve impulses; metabolism of carbohydrate, protein, and fat. About 70% of intake absorbed as free phosphates; vitamin D and parathormone implicated in intestinal absorption and kidney retention; excreted in urine and feces; occurs in blood as phospholipids, organic esters, and inorganic phosphates; inorganic phosphates in blood serum of infants and children, 4–7 mg/dL; ratio of inorganic to organic phosphates in whole blood is about 1 : 20.

Daily requirements (mg/24 hr): 0–6 mo (6 kg) 100; 7–12 mo (9 kg) 275; 1–3 yr (13 kg) 460; 4–8 yr (22 kg) 500.

Sources: Milk, milk products, egg yolk, fresh foods, legumes, nuts and wholegrains.

Effects of deficiency: Rickets may develop in rapidly growing, very low birth weight babies with low intakes of both P and Ca; muscle weakness.

Effects of excess: Possibility of tetany during recovery from rickets or in newborn on formula with low Ca : P (1 : 1) ratio.

Potassium

Function and metabolism: Muscle contraction; nerve impulse conduction; intracellular osmotic pressure and fluid balance; heart rhythm. Primarily potassium is intracellular, excretion 80% in urine, some in sweat and feces; about 8% retained by growing child.

Blood serum level: 4–5.6 mEq/L.

Daily requirements (mg/24 hr): 0–6 mo (6 kg) 500; 7–12 mo (9 kg) 700; 1–3 yr (13 kg) 1000; 4–8 yr (22 kg) 1400.

Sources: All foods.

Effects of deficiency: In starvation or in such pathologic conditions as diarrhea, diabetic acidosis. ACTH excess; muscle weakness, anorexia, nausea, abdominal distention, nervous irritability, drowsiness, confusion, tachycardia; drowsiness, confusion, tachycardia; deficiency exaggerates effects of sodium.

Effects of excess: Heart block of serum level of 10 mEq/L; important in Addison disease, renal failure, or administration of potassium-containing salts.

Selenium

Function and metabolism: Cofactor of glutathione peroxidase in tissue respiration.

Daily requirements (mg/24 hr): 0–6 mo (6 kg) 15; 7–12 mo (9 kg) 20; 1–3 yr (13 kg) 20; 4–8 yr (22 kg) 30.

Sources: Sea foods, meat, wholegrain, garlic.

Effects of deficiency: Kashin cardiomyopathy, arthritis. Kashin cardiovascular disease, myositis.

Effects of excess: Alopecia, nail abnormalities, garlic odor to breath.

Sodium

Function and metabolism: Osmotic pressure; acid–base balance; water balance; muscle and nerve irritability. Readily absorbed from intestine; excreted chiefly in urine (98%); parallels chloride intake; renal excretion controlled by ACTH; extracellular cation, but small amount in muscle and cartilage; blood serum level 135–145 mEq/L.

Daily requirements (mg/24 hr): 0–6 mo (6 kg) 120; 7–12 mo (9 kg) 200; 1–3 yr (13 kg) 225; 4–8yr (22 kg) 300.

Sources: Table salt, fresh foods, milk, eggs, sodium compounds as baking soda and powder, glutamate, seasonings and preservatives.

Effects of deficiency: Nausea; diarrhea, muscle cramps, dehydration, hypotension.

Effects of excess: Edema if inadequate excretion or excessive parenteral fluids.

Sulfur Amino Acids

Function and metabolism: Constituent of cellular protein; cocarboxylase; melanin; mucopolysaccharides, vitreous humor, synovial fluid, connective tissues, cartilage, heparin, insulin; metabolism of nerve tissue; detoxification mechanisms; SH group in coenzyme A, cystathionine, and glutathione. Only sources utilized are cystine and methionine; inorganic forms unavailable to body; excreted as inorganic sulfate or ethereal sulfate via urine and bile.

Daily requirements (mg/24 hr): 0–6 mo (6 kg) 52; 7–12 mo (9 kg) 32; 1–3 yr (13 kg) 25; 4–8 yr (22 kg) 21.

Sources: Protein foods contain about 1%.

Effects of deficiency: Not known; growth failure from protein deficiency may be due in part to deficiency of sulfur-containing amino acids.

Effects of excess: Not harmful, excreted in urine as sulfates.

Zinc

Function and metabolism: Constituent of several enzymes; carbonic anhydrase (in erythrocytes) essential for CO_2 exchange; carboxypeptidase of intestine for hydrolysis of protein; dehydrogenase of liver; supplements of zinc is useful in diarrhea.

Found in liver and organs, muscles, bones, red and white blood cells; higher tissue concentration in young subjects; excreted chiefly from intestine, competes with copper.

Daily requirements (mg/24 hr): 0–6 mo (6 kg) 2; 7–12 mo (9 kg) 3; 1–3 yr (13 kg) 3; 4–8 yr (22 kg) 5.

Sources: Meat, grain, nuts, cheese.

Effects of deficiency: Dwarfism, iron-deficiency anemia, hepatosplenomegaly, hyperpigmentation and hypogonadism, acrodermatitis enteropathica, depression of immunocompetence, poor wound healing.

Functional zinc depletion syndrome includes: Hepatosplenomegaly, dermatitis, anemia, stunted growth, impaired immune function.

Effects of excess: Gastrointestinal upsets (from galvanized iron cooking utensils); copper deficiency; decreased high-density lipoprotein.

Greenbaum LA. Micronutrient mineral deficiencies. In: Kliegman RM, Behrman RE, Jenson HB, Stanton BF (eds). *Nelson Textbook of Pediatrics.* 18th edn. Vol. 1. Philadelphia: Saunders, 2007; 265–6.

Needlman RD. Nutritional requirements. In: Behrman RE, Kliegman RM, Jenson HB (eds). *Nelson Textbook of Pediatrics.* 17th edn. Philadelphia: Saunders, 2004; 153–7.

Prasad AS. Zinc deficiency. BMJ 2003; 326: 409–10.

3.9 FLUOROSIS

The disease fluorosis is caused by an element known as fluorine, the 13th most abundant element available in the earth crust. Being included in the list of trace element for human consumption, to a certain extent (as per WHO; 0.6 ppm) fluoride ingestion is useful for bone and teeth development, but excessive ingestion causes a disease known as fluorosis. While the WHO standards permit only 1.5 mg/L as a safe limit of fluoride in drinking water for human consumption. People in several districts in Rajasthan are consuming water with fluoride concentrations of up to 44 mg/L. Main sources of fluoride for human are water, food, air, medicaments.

Extent of problem: The countries identified for the problem of fluorosis: India, Pakistan, Bangladesh, China, Argentina, United States of America, Morocco, Middle East countries, Japan, South African Countries, New Zealand, Thailand, etc. In India, the problem has reached alarming proportions affecting at least 17 states of India: Andhra Pradesh, Bihar, Delhi, Gujarat, Haryana, Jammu & Kashmir, Karnataka, Kerala, Rajasthan, Madhya Pradesh, Maharashtra, Odisha, Punjab, Tamil Nadu, Uttar Pradesh, and West Bengal.

Pathogenesis: Ingested fluoride is rapidly absorbed through gastrointestinal tract and lungs. The peaks are reached after 30 min in blood. The rapid excretion takes place through renal system over a period of 4 to 6 hr. In children less than three years of age only about 50% of total absorbed amount is excreted, but in adults and children over 3 yrs about 90% is excreted. Approximately 90% of the fluoride retained in the body is deposited in the skeleton and teeth. The biological half-life of bound fluoride is several years. Fluoride also passes through the placenta and also appears in low concentrations in saliva, sweat, and milk.

Clinical manifestations: The clinical presentation of fluoride intoxication may be of two types: acute fluoride intoxication, and chronic fluoride ingestion.

1. *Acute fluoride intoxication:* The acute effects of the ingestion of massive doses of fluoride are first those of an irritant poison, and later become apparent in enzyme systems such as those engaged in metabolism, energetic, and cellular respiration and in endocrine functions. However, no system of the body can be considered exempt. Thus, in cases of acute poisoning, early involvement of the alimentary, cardiovascular, respiratory and central nervous systems, with corresponding symptoms, is a characteristic feature and such cases commonly have a fatal outcome in two to three days. After ingestion of fluorine compounds in high doses, there is diffuse abdominal pain, diarrhea and vomiting. There is excessive salivation, with thirst, perspiration and painful spasms in the limbs. The

acute lethal dose of fluoride for man is probably about 5 g as NaF.

2. *Chronic fluoride ingestion:* Fluorosis may cause dental fluorosis, musculoskeletal fluorosis, systemic manifestations and final stages it causes premature aging.

Diagnosis: The diagnosis of fluorosis needs the following criteria:

1. High fluoride contents of the drinking water.
2. Endemicity of the fluorosis in the area.
3. Clinical manifestations of fluorosis in the population: Dental, clinical, skeletal fluorosis.
4. *Clinical examination:* Examination of teeth and three simple diagnostic tests:
   a. The individual is made to bend and touch the toes without bending the knees. If there is pain or stiffness in the backbone, hip and joints, this exercise will not be possible.
   b. The individual is made to touch the chest with the chin. If there is pain or stiffness in the neck, this exercise will not be possible.
   c. The individual is made to stretch the arms sideways, fold the arm and try to touch the back of the head. If there is pain or stiffness in the shoulder joint and backbone, this exercise will not be possible.
5. Biochemical evaluation.
6. Radiological evaluation (osteosclerosis; periosteal bone formation; calcification of interosseous membrane, ligaments, capsules, muscular attachments, and tendons; exostoses, osteophytosis).
7. Histopathological evaluations, e.g. bone biopsy, muscle biopsy, etc.

Differential diagnosis: Dental fluorosis should be distinguished from dental caries or decay/cavity formation; periodontal disease or pyorrhea, whereas skeletal fluorosis should be distinguished from rheumatoid and ankylosing spondylitis, renal osteodystrophies, rickets, and congenital malformations. Non-skeletal fluorosis should be differentiated from poliomyelitis.

Treatment and prevention: Three approaches are suggested: Health education, treatment and preventive measures.

1. Health education is needed for creating disease awareness, sources of the fluoride and in implementing the need based preventive measures in the affected community.
2. Treatment. Vitamins C and D, and, salts of calcium, magnesium or aluminum are prescribed in an attempt to reverse these effects.
3. Prevention by:
   a. Providing defluoridated water for drinking purpose.
   b. Changing the dietary habits. The main aim should be to restrict use of fluoride rich food, avoiding use of fluoride rich cosmetics and use of food rich in calcium, vitamin C and proteins.
   c. Water harvesting (alternative water source).

Agrawal KC, Gupta SK and Gupta AB. Development of New Low Cost Defluoridation Technology (Krass). Water Science and Technology, UK1999 Sept; 40(2): 167–73.

Gopalan C, Ramasastri BV, Balasubramanian SC. Nutritive value of Indian foods. National Institute of Nutrition, Indian Council of Medical Research, Hyderabad 1993.

Gupta SK, Gambhir S, Mithal A, Das BK. Skeletal scintigraphic findings in endemic skeletal fluorosis. Nucl-Med-Commun 1993 May; 14(5): 384–90.

Gupta SK, Gupta RC, Seth AK and Gupta A. Reversal of fluorosis in children. Acta Pediatrica Japonica 1996:38:513–9.

3.10 LATHYRISM

Lathyrism is a paralyzing disease and in humans it is referred to as neurolathyrism because it affects the nervous system. In India, neurolathyrism is prevalent in some parts of the country, where lathyrus is eaten, e.g., Madhya Pradesh, Uttar Pradesh, Bihar, Odisha, Maharashtra, West Bengal, Rajasthan, Assam, and Gujarat; it has also been reported to occur in Spain and Algeria.

Lathyrus sativus is commonly known as "Khesari dhal." The seeds of lathyrus have a characteristic triangular shape and grey color; when dehusked the pulse looks similar to red gram dhal or Bengal gram dhal (pulse). It has been reported that diets containing over 30% of this dhal (pulse) if taken over a period of 2–6 mo will result in neurolathyrism. The toxin present in lathyrus seeds is Beta oxalyl amino alanine (BOAA), which has been isolated in crystalline form and is water soluble. The toxin of the pulse is removed by soaking it in hot water and rejecting the soaked water.

Clinical manifestations: The disease affects mainly individuals between the age of 15 and 45 yrs and manifest in five stages:

i. *Latent stage:* The patient is apparently healthy, but walks with difficulty. The physical findings of spastic paralysis (upper motor neuron) can be elicited. At this stage, if pulse is withdrawn from the diet, it will result in complete remission of the disease.

ii. *No-stick stage:* The patient walks with short jerky steps without the aid of a sick. A large number of patients are found at this stage.

iii. *One-stick stage:* The patient walks with a crossed gait with a tendency to walk on toes, due to muscular stiffness.

iv. *Two-stick stage:* The symptoms are more severe. Due to excessive bending of knees and crossed legs, the patient needs two crutches for support.

v. *Crawler stage:* Finally, the erect posture become impossible as the knee joints cannot support the weight of the body. There is also atrophy of the thigh and leg muscles. The patient is reduced to crawling by throwing the weight on his hands.

Treatment: Although the condition is believed to be irreversible, in certain instances the damages could be repaired by daily administration of 500–1,000 mg of ascorbic acid or so.

Prevention: Ascorbic acid in the lathyrogenic diet may prevent damage. Use of pulse after removal of toxins, because the toxins are water soluble and can be removed by soaking the pulse in hot water for two hours, draining the soaked water, washing again with clean water and dried in sun or parboiling or soaking in lime water overnight followed by boiling.

Control of lathyrism: Banning the crop: The Prevention of Food Adulteration Act (PFA) in India has banned lathyrus in all forms–whole, split or flour. Educating the public regarding the dangers of consuming this pulse is also important.

Park K. Nutrition and Health. In: Park's Textbook of Preventive and Social Medicine. 19th edn. Jabalpur: M/s Banarsidas Bhanot, 2005; 480–533.

The Prevention of Food Adulteration Act & Rules. Sale of Kesari gram prohibited. New Delhi: Confederation of Indian Industry, 2002; 118–9.

3.11 EPIDEMIC DROPSY

Epidemic dropsy is a form of edema due to intoxication with *Argemone mexicana* (Mexican prickly poppy). In Northern India, epidemic dropsy occurs as a food adulterant disease where use of mustard oil as cooking medium is common. When mustard oil is adulterated deliberately (as in most cases) or accidental contamination with argemone oil, proteinuria (specifically loss of albumin) occurs, with a resultant edema as would occur in nephrotic syndrome. Other symptoms are bilateral pitting edema of extremities, headache, nausea, loose bowels, erythema and breathlessness. In severe cases fatalities are reported due to congestive heart failure. The toxic effects of argemone oil have been attributed to the presence of benzophenanthridine alkaloids, sanguinarine and dihydrosanguinarine. It has been reported that the sanguinarine alkaloid content in argemone oil varies from 0.44 to 0.50%.

Besides India, widespread epidemics have been reported from Mauritius, Fiji Islands, Northwest Cape districts of South Africa, Madagascar and Nepal. Apart from South.

The earliest reference to argemone oil poisoning was made by Lyon (1889), who reported four cases of poisoning in Calcutta in 1877 from the use of this oil in food. Since then, epidemic dropsy has been reported from various states of India, mainly due to consumption of food cooked in argemone oil mixed mustard oil or occasionally by body massage with contaminated oil.

Mechanism of toxicity: It has been suggested that the impairment of hepatic phase I and phase II enzymes by argemone oil may decrease the rate of metabolism of the alkaloid, which in turn may be responsible for the slow elimination of the compound/metabolite through urine and feces. The retention of sanguinarine in the gastrointestinal tract, liver, lung, kidney, heart, and serum even after 96 hrs of exposure indicates these as the likely target sites of argemone oil toxicity. The inhibition of Na^+–K^+–ATPase activity of heart by sanguinarine is due to interaction with the cardiac glycoside receptor site of the enzyme, which may be responsible for producing degenerative changes in cardiac muscle fibers in the auricular wall of rats fed argemone oil and could be related to tachycardia and cardiac failure in epidemic dropsy patients.

The other facet of argemone oil toxicity, *in vitro* studies have shown that the toxicity of argemone oil is due to the production of reactive oxygen species (ROS) and which in turn may cause enhancement in lipid peroxidation (LPO) in various hepatic subcellular fractions including microsomes and mitochondria of rats. Recent studies in the blood of dropsy patients has revealed that there is extensive ROS production in the argemone oil intoxication leading to depletion of total antioxidants in the body and especially lipid soluble antioxidants such as vitamins E and A (tocopherol and retinol) are highly depleted in dropsy patients. There is an extensive damage to the anti-oxidant defense system (anti-oxidant enzymes and anti-oxidants) of the blood.

Babu CK, Khanna SK, Das M. Adulteration of mustard cooking oil with argemone oil: do Indian food regulatory policies and antioxidant therapy both need revisitation? Antioxid Redox Signal 2007 Apr; 9(4): 515–25.

Das M, Khanna SK. Epidemic dropsy. Natl Med J India 1998; 11(5): 207–8.

Sharma BD, Malhotra S, Bhatia V, Rathee M. Epidemic dropsy in India. Postgrad Med J 1999; 75: 657–61.

3.12 PROBIOTICS

Probiotics have been defined as living micro-organisms, which upon ingestion in certain numbers, exert health benefits beyond general nutrition. The most commonly used probiotics are latic acid bacteria such as lactobacilli and bifidobacteriae, but other non-pathogenic bacterial strains, including Streptococcus,

Escherichia coli and non-bacterial organisms such as nonpathogenic yeast *Saccharomyces boulardii* also have been used. Probiotics are either available in the form of fermented dairy foods such as yoghurt and other dairy products, fruit juices and other drinks, or as powdered supplements containing freezed bacteria and also medicinal probiotics that are sold as specific medical indications. Diseases for which probiotics have been suggested are listed in Box 3.3.

Sources of probiotics: Probiotics can be broadly divided in to two broad groups:
a. Probiotics as functional food, and
b. Medicinal probiotics

Probiotics as functional food: A food can be said to be functional if it contains a component (which may or may not be a nutrient) that affects one or a limited number of functions in the body in a targeted way, leading to positive effects that may justify functional or even health claims. The live microbial agents for the purpose of disease prevention and treatment (functional food) include intestinal microflora and probiotics. It is in the form of natural food and formula food. The natural food includes breast milk, animal milk (contains probiotics but in lesser amount than breastmilk), and yoghurt. Yoghurt deserves its reputation as a healthful food. It is a great source of protein and calcium. When made with non- or low-fat milk, it is low in fat. If it contains live starter cultures, it can aid digestion. *Lactobacillus casei* and *Bifidobacterium bifidum* which are present in yoghurt/curd and milk products that are partially fermented. Some manufacturers add other cultures during processing to enhance the health-promoting potential of yoghurt. The most commonly added cultures include *Lactobacillus acidophilus*, *L. casei*, *L. reuteri* and *Bifidobacterium bifidum*. These "probiotic" bacteria pass through the stomach to the gastrointestinal tract. The claim most substantiated is yoghurt's beneficial effect on digestion in some individuals. People who are lactose intolerant have a hard time digesting milk products because they lack the enzyme that breaks down the main carbohydrate in milk. Yoghurt is a unique dairy food because the starter cultures actually produce that enzyme during fermentation. Thus, the milk sugar in yoghurt is more easily digested, even for lactose-intolerant individuals. Many people who commonly experience gas, bloating or discomfort from dairy foods can digest yoghurt more easily.

The formula food includes infant formula and follow-up formula containing probity's *Bifidobacterium lactis* 10'000'000 cfu/g and *Streptococcus thermophilus* 5'000'000 cfu/g dosage) are marketed in some countries.

Medicinal probiotics: Medicinal probiotics contain either lactobacilli or lactobacilli and *bifidobacterium* or *saccharomyces boulardii* (yeast). Lactobacilli are also available in combination with vitamin B complex and vitamin C, zinc, and antibiotics.

Mathur GP, Mathur Sarla. Probiotics. In: Mathur GP, Mathur Sarla (eds). Current Trends in Pediatrics. Vol 2. Delhi: Academa Publishers, 2006; 126–32.

Mishra L (ed). Drug Today. Vol 1 and Vol 2. Delhi: Lorina Publications (India) Inc., 2005 (Oct–Dec); 222–45, 495, 505,734–68.

Probiotics in childhood. Annales Nestlé 2003;61(2):1–88.

3.13 PREBIOTICS

A prebiotic is defined as "a nondigestible food ingredient that beneficially affects the host by selectively stimulating the growth and/or activity of one or a limited number of bacteria in the colon" especially, but not exclusively, lactobacilli and bifidobacteria. Prebiotics are digestion resistant carbohydrate foods. They work in the colon. Prebiotics are oligosaccharides, chains of sugar units linked together. Inulin is a long-chain oligosaccharide (from 2–60 sugars) and fructo-oligosaccharides (FOS) are short-chain oligosaccharides (from 2 to 7 sugars). In general inulin has a larger degree of polymerization compared to oligofructoses. Galacto-oligosaccharides and lactulose also fulfill the criteria for a prebiotic. There is need for continuous supply of prebiotics to provide nutrition to friendly live bacteria.

Fiber intakes for infants and children: Currently, there is a lack of scientific data available to define appropriate fiber intakes for infants and children < 2 yrs of age. The current American Academy of pediatrics recommendation for fiber intake in healthy children

---

Box 3.3: Diseases for which probiotics have been suggested

- Intestinal infections
  - Acute viral gastroenteritis
  - Acute bacterial gastroenteritis
  - Antibiotic associated diarrhea
  - Travelers' diarrhea
- Inflammatory bowel diseases
- Irritable bowel syndrome
- Lactose intolerance
- Upper respiratory infections
- Invasive neonatal infections
- Enhancement of immune system
- Prevention and treatment of allergic diseases
- Dental caries
- Reduction of serum cholesterol
- Prevention of cancer and tumor growth

>2 yrs of age is to consume the amount in gram equal to or greater than their age (in years) plus 5 g/day. Therefore, at 3 yrs of age, the fiber intake would be eight (3+5) g/day and incrementally increase to 25 g/day by age of 20 yrs. This level of fiber intake is within a range thought to provide known health benefits without compromising either mineral balance or energy intake in children >3 yrs of age.

Sources of prebiotics: Prebiotics occur naturally both in plants and milk. Various types of prebiotics are also produced industrially. Prebiotics is available from i) vegetable source: asparagus, banana (used as ripe fruit, or as vegetable unripe banana), beans, cereal (e.g. wheat, rice, maize), chicory, garlic and honey; ii) milk source: Breastmilk for infants, bovine milk, curd-thick, soft substance formed when milk turns sour; also used to make cheese, Yoghurt-fermented liquor made from milk; iii) products manufactured for infants: Infant formula, cereal based weaning foods;. Drug: Lactulose.

Breastmilk contains oligosaccharides (prebiotics) and bifidus (probiotics), and therefore, the ideal and best food for infants and children for first two years; for first six months exclusive breastfeeding, and after six months food items containing prebiotics in addition to breastfeeding.

Oligosaccharides in infant formulae, follow-on-formulae and cereal based weaning foods is derived from vegetable source.

Various types of prebiotics produced industrially are oligosaccharides including inulins and their derivatives, the fructo-oligosaccharides and galacto-oligosaccharides.

Galacto-oligosaccharides (GOS) are present naturally in human and cow's milk and are also produced from lactose by galactosidase.

Lactulose is a laxative with bifidogenic edge. It improves osmotic effect on stool in colon; increases gut motility and overcome constipation. It avoids watery stool and dehydration. It treats constipation physiologically, enhances microflora; stimulates growth of bifidobacteria—the gut friendly bacteria. Bifidobacteria ferment carbohydrate to acetic acid and lactic acid and acidification of stool promotes NH_4^+ elimination. It is safe in children, pregnancy, and elderly.

Mechanism of action: A prebiotic resists host digestion and absorption in the stomach and the small intestine and reaches the large bowel unmodified, where it is fermented by the microflora of colonizing the gastrointestinal system. Once in the large bowel, it selectively stimulates the growth or activity of one or a limited number of potentially beneficial bacteria, particularly bifidobacteria and lactobacilli, while decreasing the number of facultative anaerobic strains such as *Escherichia coli* and clostridia. in the large bowel, the breakdown of the prebiotic molecules by bacterial enzymes, such as β-fructosidase and β-galactosidase, results in the production of lactate and short-chain fatty acids (SCFA), acetate, propionate and butyrate, as end products of fermentation. These molecules decrease the intraluminal pH, directly inhibiting the growth and activities of harmful microorganisms, and contributing to stimulation of the growth of bifidobacteria, which compete with the enteropathogens for nutrients and epithelial adhesion sites. The short-chain fatty acids produced by fermentation are absorbed across the large-bowel wall and provide nutrition for the colonocyte and a source of energy for the body. In this way as much as 70% of the energy in the carbohydrate is salvaged by this mechanism.

Benefits of prebiotics: Published clinical trials have evaluated prebiotic substances in dietetic products for term and preterm infants, respectively. A study was conducted on 1300 children between 12 and 36 mo of age in New Delhi (2nd World Congress) for a period of one year revealed that the milk fortified with the probiotic and prebiotic (oligosaccharides) offered significant protection from dysentery (22%), nondiarrheal diseases (16%), sickness with high temperature (32%), ear infection (7%) and less likely to need antibiotics (6%) compared with the milk powder without the prebiotic and probiotic. A clinically meaningful reduction in iron deficiency anemia of 35% was also observed in the group of children drinking milk fortified with prebiotic and probiotic compared to children drinking the control milk, despite both groups were receiving iron in the milks. According to the researchers, milk with prebiotic and probiotic bacteria, can prevent major, often fatal, childhood diseases such as diarrhea and pneumonia, and have a significant impact of growth.

Moro et al have tested a synergistic mixture of neutral galacto-oligosaccharides (GOS derived from lactose) and long-chain fructo-oligosaccharides (FOS derived from chicory). After 28 days of feeding, the term infants fed formula supplemented with the GOS/FOS mixture, at concentration of 0.4 g/100 ml or 0.8 g/100 ml, respectively, exhibited a dose-dependent stimulating effect on the growth of bifidobacteria and lactobacilli in the intestine. This combination resulted also in an increase of stool frequency and a reduction of stool consistency, closer to reference breastfed infants.

Marini et al (2003) have reported that prolonged administration of probiotics in preterm babies induces a rise of specific IgA and IgM antibodies against probiotic. This fact explains why presence of living germs in stools almost disappeared in spite of continuous administration. However, some positive influences were observed: decreased ratio of aerobic/anaerobic and increased ratio of gram+/gram– germs. Prebiotic administration induces after 28 days a significant increase of fecal bifidobacteria and frequency and consistency of stools were more similar to those observed in subjects fed with human milk.

Other nutritional effects: Dietary fibers generally may have unwanted side effects, such as a negative influence on vitamin or mineral absorption, allergic reactions, and an undesirable influence on the gut flora and their metabolism. No such negative effects have been found for inulin and oligofructose. On the contrary, recent research suggests that the effects on mineral absorption and gut flora might well be positive. It was seen that addition of inulin to infant formula caused a 27% increase in availability of calcium and did not alter the availability of calcium and of zinc and iron.

Combined prebiotic and probiotic: Symbiotic is a term that is being used increasingly to denote a synergistic relationship between viable beneficial bacteria and their selective substrate. The symbiotic concept combines both the probiotic and prebiotic approaches. According to this approach, a food or food supplement will include both the live cells of beneficial bacteria and a selective substrate. The idea is that beneficial

bacteria cells that survive their transit through the stomach can grow quickly and competitively because of the presence of the selective substrate and establish their predominance.

Prebiotics Use as Food and Medicine

Natural food: We are already eating prebiotics in our food, without realizing how important they are in maintaining the colonic friendly bacteria (probiotics).

Infant formulae and cereal based weaning foods: Some infant formulae, follow-on-formulae and cereal based weaning foods with added prebiotics are already marketed in many countries.

Medicine: Lactulose is a laxative with bifidogenic edge. It treats constipation physiologically, enhances microflora; stimulates growth of bifidobacteria—the gut-friendly bacteria. Lactulose can therefore, can be safely used in medical conditions where indicated.

Gibson GR, Roberfroid MB. Dietary modulation of the human colonic microbiota: introducing the concept of prebiotics. J Nutr 1995;124:1401–12.

Ghisolfi J. Dietary fibre and prebiotics in infant formulas. Proc Nutr Soc 2003;62:183–5.

Marini A, Negretti F, Boehm G, Li-Destri M, Clerici-Bagozzi D, Mosca F, Agosti M. Pro- and prebiotics administration in preterm infants: colonization and influence on faecal flora. Acta Paediatrica 2003; 92 (Suppl. 441): S80–81.

Mathur GP, Mathur Sarla. Prebiotics. In: Mathur GP, Mathur Sarla (eds). Current Trends in Pediatrics. Vol 3. Delhi: Academa Publishers, 2007; 446–56.

4 Pathophysiology of Body Fluids and Fluid Therapy

4.1 COMPOSITION OF BODY FLUIDS

Total body water: Water is the most important constituent of the human body. The other components of the body include protein, carbohydrate, fat, vitamins and minerals. Total body water (TBW) as a percentage of body weight varies with age and sex. The fetus has a very high TBW, which gradually decreases to about 75% of birth weight for a term infant. Premature infants have a higher TBW content than term infants. During the first year of life, TBW decreases to about 60% of body weight and remains at this level until puberty. At puberty, the fat contents of girls increases more than boys, who acquire more muscle mass than girls. Because fat has very low water content and muscle has higher water content, by the end of puberty, TBW in boys remains at 60%, but TBW in girls decreases to 50% of body weight. In overweight children high fat content causes a decrease in TBW as a percentage of body weight. During dehydration the TBW decreases and remains in a smaller percentage of body weight.

Fluid compartments: TBW is divided between two main compartments: intracellular fluid (ICF) and extracellular fluid (ECF). In the fetus and newborn, the ECF volume is larger than the ICF volume. The postnatal diuresis causes an immediate decrease in the ECF volume. This is followed by continuous expansion of the ICF volume, which results from cellular growth. By 1 yr of age the ratio of the ICF to the ECF volume approaches adult levels. The ECF volume is about 20–25% of body weight and the ICF volume is about 30–40% of body weight, close to twice the ECF volume.

With puberty, the increased muscle mass of boys causes them to have a higher ICF volume than girls. There is no significant difference in the ECF volume between postpubertal girls and boys.

The ECF volume is divided into two compartments: Interstitial fluid 15% and plasma water 5% of body weight. The blood volume, given to a hematocrit of 40%, is usually close to 8% of body weight, although it is higher in newborns and young infants. In premature newborns it is around 10% of body weight. The volume of plasma water can be altered by a variety of pathologic conditions, such as dehydration, anemia, polycythemia, heart failure, abnormal plasma osmolality, and hypoalbuminemia. The interstitial fluid can increase in diseases associated with edema such as heart failure, liver failure, nephrotic syndrome, kwashiorkor and other causes of hypoalbuminemia. An increase in interstitial fluid occurs when patients develop ascites and pleural effusions.

There is normally a delicate equilibrium between the intravascular fluid and the interstitial fluid. The balance between hydrostatic and oncotic forces regulates the intravascular volume, which is critical for proper tissue perfusion. The intravascular fluid has a higher concentration of albumin than the interstitial fluid, and the consequent oncotic force draws water into the intravascular space. The maintenance of this gradient depends on the limited permeability of albumin across the capillaries. The hydrostatic pressure of the intravascular space, which is due to the pumping action of the heart, drives fluid out of the intravascular space. These forces favor movement into the interstitial space at the arterial ends of the capillaries. The decreased hydrostatic forces and increased oncotic forces, which result from the dilutional increase in albumin concentration, cause movement of fluid into the venous end of the capillaries. Overall, there is usually a net movement of fluid out of the intravascular space, but this fluid is returned via the lymphatics to the circulation. An imbalance in these forces may cause expansion of the interstitial volume at the expanse of the intravascular volume. In children with hypoalbuminemia, the decreased oncotic pressure of the intravascular fluid contributes the development of *edema*. Loss of fluid from the intravascular space may compromise the intravascular volume, placing the child at risk for inadequate blood flow to vital organs. In case of children with *heart failure*, there is an increase in venous hydrostatic pressure from expansion of the intravascular volume, which is caused by impaired pumping by the heart, and the increase in venous pressure causes fluid to move from the intravascular space to the interstitial space. Expansion of the intravascular volume and increased intravascular pressure also cause the edema that occurs in children with *acute glomerulonephritis*.

Electrolyte composition. The composition of the solutes in the ICF and ECF (plasma) is listed in Table 4.1. Sodium and chloride are the dominant cations and anions respectively in the ECF and their concentrations are much lower in ICF. Potassium is the most abundant cation in the ICF, and its concentration within the cells is approximately 30 times higher than in the ECF. Calcium (Ca^+) and magnesium (Mg^+) is present in the plasma and magnesium (Mg^+) is present in the cells. Proteins ($Prot^-$), organic anions, phosphates ($Phos^-$), bicarbonate (HCO_3^-), Chlorides (Cl^-) are the most plentiful anions in the ICF. The dissimilarity between the anions in the ICF and the ECF is largely determined by the presence of intracellular molecules that do not

cross the cell membrane, the barrier separating the ECF and the ICF. In contrast, the difference between the distribution of cations—sodium and potassium is due to the activity of the Na^+ and K^+-ATPase, which uses cellular energy to extrude sodium from cells and move potassium into cells. The chemical gradient between the intracellular potassium concentration and extracellular potassium concentration creates the electrical gradient across the cell membrane. Specifically, the concentration dependent movement of potassium out of the cell makes the intracellular space negative relative to the extracellular space.

Osmolarity: The ICF and ECF are in osmotic equilibrium because the cell membrane is freely permeable to water. If the osmolarity in one compartment changes, then water movement leads to a rapid equalization of osmolarity. This can lead to significant shifts of water between the ICF and ECF. The osmolarity of the ECF can be determined, and this equals the ICF osmolality. The plasma osmolarity is normally 285–295 mOsm/kg.

4.2 ACID–BASE BALANCE

Close regulation of pH is necessary for cellular enzymes and other metabolic processes that function optimally at a normal pH. A normal pH is 7.35–7.45 (Table 4.2). Chronic mild derangements in acid–base status may interfere with normal growth and development, whereas acute severe changes in pH can be fatal. Control of acid–base balance depends on kidneys, lungs, and intracellular and extracellular buffers. Buffers are divided into the bicarbonate and non-carbonate buffers. The non-carbonate buffers include proteins, phosphate, and bone. Protein buffers consist of extracellular proteins, mostly albumin and intracellular proteins, including hemoglobin. Clinically, we measure the extracellular pH, but it is the intracellular pH that affects the cell function. Acidemia is a pH below normal (<7.35) and alkalemia is a pH above normal (>7.45).

Metabolic acidosis: Diarrhea is the most common cause of a metabolic acidosis; it causes a loss of bicarbonate from the body. Three basic mechanisms are involved in the causation of metabolic acidosis:
1. Loss of bicarbonate from the body
2. Impaired ability to excrete acid by the kidney, and

Table 4.1: Concentration of the major cations and anions in the intracellular space and the plasma

Plasma		Intracellular	
Cations		*Cations*	
Na^+	140 mEq/L	K^+	140 mEq/L
K^+ 4 mEq/L		Na^+	13 mEq/L
Ca^+ 2.5 mEq/L			
Mg^+ 1.1 mEq/L		Mg^+	1.1 mEq/L
Anions		*Anions*	
Cl^-	104 mEq/L	$Phos^-$	107 mEq/L
HCO_3^-	24 mEq/L	$Prot^-$	40 mEq/L
$Prot^-$	14 mEq/L	HCO_3^-	10 mEq/L
Other	6 mEq/L		
$Phos^-$	2 mEq/L	Cl^-	3 mEq/L

Table 4.2: Normal values of an arterial blood gas

pH	7.35–7.45
(HCO_3^-)	20–28 mEq/L
PCO_2	35–45 mmHg

3. Addition of acid to the body (exogenous or endogenous).

The plasma anion gap is useful for evaluating patients with a metabolic acidosis. It divides patients into two diagnostic groups: normal anion gap or increased anion gap. A normal anion gap is 8–16. The following formula determines the anion gap:

$$\text{Anion gap} = [Na^+] - [Cl^-] - [HCO_3^-]$$

Metabolic alkalosis: Metabolic alkalosis in children is most commonly secondary to emesis or diuretic use. Kidneys normally respond promptly to a metabolic alkalosis by increasing base excretion. Two processes are usually present to produce a metabolic alkalosis. The first process is the generation of the metabolic alkalosis. This requires addition of base to the body. The second process is the maintenance of the metabolic alkalosis. This requires impairment in the kidney's ability to excrete base.

Respiratory acidosis: Respiratory acidosis is characterized by an inappropriate increase in the blood carbon dioxide (PCO_2). Carbon dioxide, which is a byproduct of metabolism, is removed from the body by the lungs. During a respiratory acidosis, there is a decrease in the effectiveness of carbon dioxide removal by lungs.

Respiratory alkalosis: A respiratory alkalosis is an inappropriate reduction in the carbon dioxide concentration. This is usually secondary to hyperventilation, initially causing removal of carbon dioxide surpass production.

4.3 MAINTENANCE AND REPLACEMENT THERAPY

Parenteral or oral fluid therapy is employed to maintain or restore the normal volume and composition of body fluids. Fluid therapy consists of three categories: maintenance, deficit, and replacement therapies. Maintenance intravenous fluids are used in a child who cannot be fed enterally. Along with maintenance fluids, children may require concurrent replacement fluids if they have excessive losses that may occur with drainage from a nasogastric (NG) tube or high urine output due to nephrogenic diabetes insipidus. In addition, if dehydration is present, the patient needs to receive deficit therapy. A child awaiting surgery may only need maintenance fluid, whereas a child with diarrheal dehydration needs maintenance and deficit therapy and may also require replacement fluids if the diarrhea continues.

Maintenance Therapy

Maintenance fluids are generally composed of a solution of water, electrolytes and glucose. Patients loose water, sodium, and potassium in their urine and stool; water is also lost from the skin and lungs. Maintenance fluids replace these losses and therefore avoid the development of dehydration and deficiencies of sodium and potassium. But a patient on maintenance intravenous fluids is receiving inadequate calories and will actually loose 0.5 to 1% of weight each day.

Maintenance of water: Water is an essential component of maintenance fluid therapy. Table 4.3 provides a system for calculating maintenance water based on the patient's weight. This system emphasizes the higher water needs of smaller patients. But the calculations based on weight do overestimate the water needs of over weight patients. However, there is an upper limit of 2–2.5 L/24 hrs in adult sized patients. Intravenous fluids are written as an hourly rate and therefore it is always helpful to use the formulas mentioned in Box 4.1 to quickly calculate the rate of maintenance fluids.

Maintenance of electrolytes: The electrolytes—sodium, potassium and chlorides are given in maintenance fluids to replace losses from urine and stool. Maintenance requirements for sodium and potassium are shown in Box 4.2. Adequate chloride is provided as long as at least half of the sodium and potassium are given as chloride salts.

Glucose: Maintenance fluids usually contain 5% dextrose (D5), which provides 17 calories per 100 ml and close to 20% of the daily caloric needs. This is

Table 4.3: Body weight method for calculating maintenance fluid volume	
Body weight	*Fluid per day*
0–10 kg	100 ml/kg
10–20 kg	1,000 ml + 50 ml/kg for each kg >10 kg
> 20 kg	1,500 ml + 20 ml/kg for each kg >10 kg*

*The maximum total fluid per day is normally 2,400 ml

Box 4.1: Hourly maintenance of water rate

0–10 kg: 4 ml/kg/hr
10–20 kg: 40 ml/hr + 2 ml/kg/hr × (wt 10 kg)
>20 kg: 60 ml/hr + 1 ml/kg/hr × (wt 20 kg)*

*The maximum fluid rate is normally 100 ml/hr

Box 4.2: Maintenance of electrolytes

Sodium: 2–3 mEq/kg/24 hr
Potassium: 1–2 mEq/kg/24 hr

enough to prevent ketone production and helps minimize protein degradation, but a child will loose weight on this regimen. This is the principal reason to start on parenteral nutrition after a few days of maintenance fluids if enteral feedings are still not possible. Maintenance fluids are also lacking in protein, fat, vitamins, and minerals.

Intravenous solutions: In designing fluid management, it is important to know the components of the commonly available solutions (Table 4.4). Normal saline (NS) and Ringer lactate are isotonic solutions; they have approximately the same tonicity as plasma. Isotonic fluids are generally used for the acute correction of intravascular volume depletion (deficit therapy). Half NS and 1/4 NS are the usual choices for maintenance fluid therapy in children. These solutions are available with 5% dextrose. In addition, these solutions are available with 20 mEq/L of potassium chloride, 10 mEq/L of potassium chloride, or no potassium.

A normal plasma osmolality is 285–295 mOsm/kg. Infusing the intravenous solution peripherally with a much lower osmolality can cause water to move into red blood cells, causing hemolysis. Thus, intravenous fluids are generally designed to have an osmolality that is either close to 285 or greater (moderately higher osmolality fluids do not cause problems). Thus, ¼ NS (osmolality = 77) should not be administered peripherally, but D5 ¼ NS (osmolality = 355) or D5 ½ NS + 20 mEq/L KCl (osmolality = 472) can be administered.

Selection of maintenance fluids: After calculation of water needs and electrolyte needs, children typically receive either D5 ¼ NS + 20 mEq/L KCl or D5 ½ NS + 20 mEq/L KCl. Children weighing less than about 20–25 kg do best with the solution containing ¼ NS because of their high water needs per kilogram, whereas larger children and adults may receive the solution with ½ NS. These solutions work well in children who have normal homeostatic mechanisms for adjusting urinary excretion of water, sodium, and potassium. In children with complicated pathophysiologic derangements (for example renal impairment), it may be necessary to empirically adjust the electrolyte composition and rate of maintenance fluids based on electrolyte measurements and assessing of fluid balance.

Replacement Therapy

Replacement fluid therapy is designed to replace ongoing abnormal fluid and electrolyte losses (Box 4.3). Because the constituents of these losses often are quite different than the composition of maintenance fluids, simply increasing the volume of maintenance fluids in an attempt to compensate for these losses may be hazardous. Measuring the electrolyte content of these losses and replacing them mEq for mEq and ml for ml may be preferable. Third space losses are due to a shift of fluid from the intravascular space into the interstitial space. Third space losses can be massive and lead to intravascular volume depletion, despite the patient's weight gain and edema. For the patient under severe physiologic stress or undergoing extensive surgery (e.g. abdominal surgery), calculate third space losses and adjust in the

---

Box 4.3: Various sites of ongoing abnormal electrolytes and fluid losses

GI losses: stool (diarrhea); gastric content (emesis, gastric aspiration)
Urine losses: oliguria/anuria (renal failure, syndrome of inappropriate antidiuretic hormone); polyuria (nephrogenic diabetes insipidus)
Surgical drains and chest tubes
Third space losses (despite weight gain and edema)

Table 4.4: Composition of intravenous solutions

Fluid	[Na⁺]	[Cl⁻]	[K⁺]	[Ca²⁺]	[Lactate⁻]
Normal saline (0.9% NaCl)	154	154	–	–	–
½ Normal saline (0.9% NaCl)	–	77	77	–	–
¼ Normal saline (0.9% NaCl)	38.5	38.5	–	–	–
Ringer lactate	130	109	4	3	28

Ringer lactate each 100 ml contains:
Lactic acid 0.24 ml (sodium lactate 0.32 g)
Sodium chloride 0.6 g
Potassium chloride 0.04 g
Calcium chloride 0.027 g
Constituents approximately mmol/L: Sodium 131; Potassium 5; Calcium 2; Bicarbonate as Lactate 29; Chloride 111.
500 ml bottle

amount of replacement fluid for third space losses based on continuing assessment of the patient's intravascular volume status. Third space losses are isotonic and require replacement with an isotonic fluid such as normal saline or Ringer lactate.

4.4 DEFICIT THERAPY

Deficit is described as losses per kg of body weight, and deficit therapy is designed to replace abnormal losses of fluid and electrolytes, usually as a result of illness. Dehydration, frequently the result of diarrhea, is a common problem in children. Most cases can be managed with oral rehydration (*see* Fig. in CD).

Clinical manifestations: The first step is to asses the degree of dehydration. Table 4.5 summarizes the clinical features that are present with varying degrees of dehydration. The history usually points to the etiology of dehydration and may predict whether the patient will have a normal sodium concentration (isotonic dehydration), hypotonic dehydration, or hypertonic dehydration (Table 4.6). The neonate with dehydration due to poor intake of breast milk often has hypernatremic dehydration. Hypernatremic dehydration is likely in any child with losses of hypotonic fluid and poor water intake such as may occur with diarrhea and poor oral intake due to anorexia or emesis. In contrast, hyponatremic dehydration occurs in the child with diarrhea who is taking large quantities of low salt fluid such as water or diluted formula. Pinching and gently twisting the skin of the abdominal or thoracic wall detects tenting of the skin. Tented skin remains in a pinched position rather than springing quickly back to normal. It is difficult to properly assess tenting of the skin in premature infants or severely malnourished children. Tachycardia is due to activation of the sympathetic nervous system due to intravascular volume depletion; diaphoresis may also be present. Tachypnea in children with dehydration may be present secondary to metabolic acidosis from stool losses of bicarbonate, or due to lactic acidosis from poor tissue perfusion.

Laboratory findings: The serum sodium, potassium, and creatinine concentration, blood urea nitrogen (BUN) and urinalysis are useful investigations for evaluating a child with dehydration. Metabolic acidosis may be due to stool bicarbonate losses in children with diarrhea, secondary renal insufficiency, or lactic acidosis from decreased tissue perfusion. In contrast, emesis and nasogastric losses usually cause a metabolic alkalosis. Hypokalemia is as a result of diarrheal potassium losses, gastric potassium losses,

Table 4.5: Clinical evaluation of severity of dehydration			
Signs and symptoms	*Mild dehydration*	*Moderate dehydration*	*Severe dehydration*
Body weight loss (%)	3–5%	6–9%	10% or more
General appearance and condition:			
Infants and young children	Alert, restless	Thirsty, restless or lethargic, irritable to touch	Lethargic or comatose; limp. cold, sweaty, cyanotic; poor peripheral perfusion
Older children and adults	Thirsty, alert, restless	Thirsty, alert, postural hypotension	Usually conscious; apprehensive; cold, sweaty, cyanotic; wrinkled skin of fingers and toes; muscle cramps
Radial pulse	Normal rate and strength	Rapid and weak	Rapid, feeble, sometimes not palpable
Blood pressure	Normal	Normal or low; orthostatic hypotension	Low, may be unrecordable
Respiration	Normal	Deep, may be rapid	Deep and rapid
Anterior fontanel	Normal	Sunken	Very sunken
Eyes	Normal	Sunken	Grossly sunken
Tears	Present	Absent or reduced	Absent
Mucous membranes	Moist	Dry	Very dry
Skin elasticity (over abdominal wall)	Pinch, retracts immediately	Pinch, retracts slowly	Pinch, retracts very slowly
Urine flow	Normal	Reduced amount and dark	Anuria/severe oliguria
Capillary refill	Normal	±2 sec	>3 sec
Estimated fluid deficit (ml/kg)	30–50	60–90	100 or more

Table 4.6: Dehydration and serum sodium concentration

Type of dehydration	Electrolyte status	Occurrence in population*
Isotonic or isonatremic	Serum Na 130–150 mEq/L	70–80%
Hypotonic or hyponatremic	Serum Na <130 mEq/L	10–15%
Hypertonic or hypernatremic	Serum Na >150 mEq/L	10–15%

*Approximate estimate

urinary potassium losses, and metabolic alkalosis. In contrast, metabolic acidosis and renal insufficiency may lead to hyperkalemia.

Urine specific gravity is usually elevated in cases of significant dehydration but returns to normal after rehydration. A specific gravity less than 1,020 indicates mild or no dehydration or indicates a urinary concentrating defect, as in chronic renal diseases or primary or secondary diabetes insipidus. Urinalysis may show hyaline and granular casts, a few white cells and red cells, and 30–100 mg of proteinuria with dehydration, which are not usually associated with significant renal pathology, and they remit with rehydration.

Hemoconcentration as a result of dehydration causes an increase in the hematocrit, hemoglobin and serum proteins, which normalize with rehydration. A normal hemoglobin concentration during acute dehydration may mask an underlying anemia. A decreased albumin in a dehydrated patient suggests malnutrition, nephrotic syndrome, liver disease, or acute or chronic protein loosing enteropathy.

Calculation of deficits: The child with dehydration looses water, sodium, and potassium. Most patients have isotonic dehydration, and therefore, have normal serum sodium values. The guidelines in Box 4.4. are used in calculating the deficits in isotonic dehydration due to gastroenteritis.

Approach to dehydration: The child with dehydration requires immediate intervention and requires restoration of the intravascular volume with an isotonic solution such as normal saline (NS), or Ringer lactate (Box 4.5). The child is given a fluid bolus, usually 20 ml/kg, over about 20 minutes. A child with mild dehydration does not usually require a fluid bolus. In contrast, the child with severe dehydration may require multiple fluid boluses, and may need to receive the boluses at a faster rate.

Blood, 5% albumin, and plasma are occasionally used for fluid boluses. Blood transfusion is indicated in the child with severe anemia or blood loss. The child with hypoalbuminemia may benefit from 5% albumin. Plasma is useful in children with a coagulopathy.

The initial rehydration is complete when the child has an adequate intravascular volume. The child will have some general clinical improvement, including a lower heart rate, a normalization of the blood pressure, improved perfusion, and a more alert affect.

When there is adequate intravascular volume, plan the fluid therapy for the next 24 hr, which is mentioned in Box 4.5. In isotonic dehydration, the entire fluid deficit is corrected over 24 hr. The child receives normal maintenance fluids and the fluid deficit. The total amount of water and electrolytes are added together and then an appropriate fluid is selected. For the patient with isotonic dehydration D5½ normal saline with 20 mEq/L potassium chloride is usually an appropriate fluid. For a child weighing less than 10–20 kg with only mild dehydration, a reduction of sodium concentration is usually reasonable (¼ NS) because the majority of the administered fluid is maintenance fluid. Children with mild dehydration do not require intravenous therapy unless enteral

---

Box 4.4: Calculation of deficit water and electrolytes

Water deficit
Percent dehydration × weight
Sodium deficit
Weight deficit × 80 mEq/L
Potassium deficit
Weight deficit × 30 mEq/L

Box 4.5: Fluid management of dehydration

Restore intravascular volume
Normal saline: 20 mL/kg over 20 min
(Repeat until intravascular volume restored)
Calculate 24 hr water needs
Calculate maintenance water
Calculate deficit water
Calculate 24 hr electrolyte needs
Calculate maintenance sodium and potassium
Calculate deficit sodium and potassium
Select an appropriate fluid (based on total water and electrolyte needs)
Administer half the calculated fluid during the first 8 hr, first subtracting any boluses from this amount
Administer the remainder over the next 16 hr
Replace the ongoing losses as they occur

therapy is not possible. Potassium is not usually included in the intravenous fluids until the patient voids. Half of the total fluid is given over the first 8 hr; previous boluses are subtracted from this volume. The remainder is given over the next 16 hr. It is important to consider ongoing fluid losses of the patient. For example, the child with copious diarrhea must receive an additional replacement solution; otherwise the rehydration will not be complete.

Monitoring and adjusting therapy: It is important to monitor the patient during treatment and to modify therapy based on the clinical situation. The general approach to monitoring therapy is outlined in Box 4.6. The patient's vital signs are useful indicators of intravascular volume status. The child with a decreased blood pressure and increased heart rate will benefit from a fluid bolus. The central venous pressure is an excellent indicator of fluid status (depletion or overload) in the critically ill child.

The patient's intake and output are important. The child, who, after 8 hr of therapy, has more output than input due to continuing diarrhea, needs to be placed on a replacement solution. The presence of a good urine output indicates that rehydration has been successful. This is supported by a decreased urine specific gravity. It may be appropriate in such patients to decrease the intravenous fluid rate. The presence of dehydration on physical examination suggests the need for continued rehydration, whereas when signs of overhydration, such as edema or pulmonary congestion appear it is desirable to discontinue hydration. A daily weight measurement is important for management of the dehydrated child, a gain in weight suggests successful therapy. At least daily electrolyte measurements are appropriate for any child who is receiving intravenous rehydration, as these children are at risk for disorders of sodium, potassium, and acid–base.

Hyponatremic dehydration: The pathogenesis of hyponatremic dehydration is usually due to a combination of sodium and water loss and water retention to compensate for the volume depletion. The patient has a pathologic increase in fluid loss, and this fluid contains sodium. The risk of hyponatremia is further increased if the volume depletion is due to loss of fluid with a higher sodium concentration, as may occur with renal salt wasting, third space losses, or diarrhea with high sodium content as occurs in cases of cholera.

The initial goal in treating hyponatremia is correction of intravascular volume depletion with isotonic fluid (NS or Ringer lactate). Most patients with hyponatremic dehydration do well with the same basic strategy that is outlined in Box 4.5. As with isotonic dehydration half the fluid can be administered over the first 8 hr, and potassium is not given until the patient voids. Despite the increased sodium deficit in these patients compared with isotonic dehydration, D5½ normal saline with 20 mEq/L potassium chloride is usually an appropriate fluid.

The patient's sodium concentration is monitored to ensure appropriate correction. Patients with ongoing losses require an appropriate solution. Patients with neurologic symptoms (e.g. seizures) from hyponatremia need to receive an acute infusion of hypertonic (3%) saline to rapidly increase the serum sodium concentration.

Hypernatremic dehydration: Hypernatremic dehydration is the most dangerous form of dehydration due to complication of hypernatremia and of therapy. Hypernatremia can cause serious neurologic damage including hemorrhages and thrombosis, which is secondary to movement of water from the brain cells into the hypertonic extracellular fluid, causing brain cell shrinkage and tearing blood vessels within the brain. Children with hypertonic dehydration are often lethargic, but irritable when touched. Hypernatremia may cause fever, hypertonicity, and hyperreflexia. More severe neurologic symptoms may develop if cerebral bleeding occurs. If cerebral edema develops during correction of hypernatremia, symptoms can range from seizures to brain herniation and death. During the development of hypernatremia there is generation of idiogenic osmoles to increase the osmolality within the cells of brain, providing protection against brain cell shrinkage caused by movement of water out of cells into the hypertonic extracellular fluid. However, these idiogenic osmoles dissipate slowly during correction of hypernatremia. With overly rapid lowering of the extracellular osmolality during correction of hypernatremia, there may be an osmotic gradient created that causes water movement from the extracellular space into the cells of the brain, producing cerebral edema. To minimize

---

Box 4.6: Monitoring therapy

Vitals
Pulse
Blood pressure
Intake and output
Fluid balance
Urine output and specific gravity
Physical examination
Weight
Clinical signs of depletion or overload
Electrolytes

the risk of cerebral edema, the serum sodium concentration should not decrease by >12 mEq/L every 24 hr. Severe hypernatremic dehydration may need to be corrected over 2–4 days (Box 4.7). The initial management requires restoration of intravascular volume with normal saline. Ringer lactate should not be used because it may decrease serum sodium rapidly especially if multiple fluid boluses are necessary.

Seizures are the most common manifestation of cerebral edema, which results from an overly rapid decrease of the serum sodium concentration during correction of hypernatremic dehydration. Acutely, increasing the serum sodium concentration via an infusion of 3% sodium chloride can reverse the cerebral edema. Each ml/kg of 3% sodium chloride increases the serum sodium concentration by approximately 1 mEq/L. An infusion of 4–6 ml/kg often results in resolution of symptoms.

In patients with severe hypernatremia, oral fluids must be used cautiously. Less hyponatremic fluid, such as an oral rehydration solution, may be more appropriate initially. If oral intake is allowed, amount of water intake must be taken into account of and adjustment in the intravenous fluid is usually appropriate. Monitoring of the serum sodium concentration is essential.

Box 4.7: Treatment of hypernatremic dehydration

Restore intravascular volume

Normal saline: 20 mL/kg over 20 minutes
(Repeat until intravascular volume restored)

Determine the time for correction based on the initial sodium concentration

[Na]: 145–157 mEq/L: 24 hr
[Na]: 158–170 mEq/L: 48 hr
[Na]: 171–183 mEq/L: 72 hr
[Na]: 184–196 mEq/L: 84 hr

Administer fluid at a constant rate over the time for correction

Typical fluids: D5¼ NS or D5½ NS (both with 20 mEq/L KCl unless contraindicated)
Typical rate: 1.25–1.5 times maintenance

Follow serum sodium concentration

Adjust fluid based on clinical status and serum sodium concentration
Signs of volume depletion: Administer NS (20 mL/kg)
Sodium decreases too rapidly
    Increase sodium concentration of intravenous fluid, or
    Decrease rate of intravenous fluid
Sodium decrease too slowly
    Decrease sodium concentration of intravenous fluid, or
    Increase rate of intravenous fluid

Replace ongoing losses as they occur

4.5 ORAL REHYDRATION THERAPY (ORS + ZINC)

Oral rehydration is a simple, safe, and effective way to treat most children with mild to moderate dehydration. Oral solutions rely on the coupled transport of sodium and glucose in the intestine. New WHO ORS formula is as effective as the old WHO ORS formula with the added advantage of reducing the stool output and no chance of having the danger of hypernatremia. This is done by reducing the osmolality of the ORS to avoid possible adverse effects of hypertonicity on net fluid absorption. The osmolality is reduced by decreasing the concentration of salt and glucose in the solution. WHO and UNICEF now recommend the use and manufacture of the new formula instead of previously recommended ORS solution (*see* Chapter 16) along with zic sulfate tablet.

4.6 PERIOPERATIVE FLUIDS THERAPY

Preoperatively, preparing a patient having no pre-existing deficit or in whom the deficit has been repaired consists mainly of supporting adequate carbohydrate for sustenance and protein sparing and the usual maintenance requirements of water and electrolytes. Young infants who are not vomiting should receive carbohydrate and electrolyte mixtures by mouth until 3 hr before the operation. Such fluids are readily absorbed from the gastrointestinal tract. In the case of newborn infant, deficits of water and electrolytes from vomiting or from stasis caused by intestinal obstruction should be replaced before the surgery. In cases of intestinal obstruction, conjugated bilirubin may be deglucuronidated by intestinal enzymes; enterohepatic circulation of unconjugated bilirubin can then lead to high serum levels and kernicterus. Hypoprothrombinemia should be prevented by administering 1 mg of vitamin K.

During surgery, blood, plasma, saline, or other volume expanders may be given, if blood loss, tissue trauma, third space losses, or excessive evaporative loss occurs. The most common error in administering parenteral fluid during and after surgery is excessive administration, particularly of dextrose in water, rather than use of isotonic solutions. Under most circumstances, little to no potassium need be administered during this time, because extensive tissue trauma or anorexia may result in the release of large amounts of intracellular potassium, with the potential of causing hyperkalemia. If shock occurs, acute renal failure may ensue, impairing the ability to eliminate through the renal route large amounts of released potassium.

Postoperatively, fluid intake should be limited for 24 hr. Thereafter, the usual maintenance therapy is gradually resumed. The water intake should not exceed 85 ml/100 kcal metabolized, because of antidiuretics resulting from trauma, circulatory readjustment, general anesthesia, or narcotic pain relief, unless renal ability to concentrate the urine is limited, as in patients with sickle cell disease, chronic pyelonephritis, or obstructive uropathy. If the intake of water is not limited, whether given parenterally or orally water intoxication may occur associated with severe hyponatremia and even fatal cerebral edema. Postoperatively some children have elevated blood antidiuretic hormone (ADH) levels due to syndrome of inappropriate ADH (SIADH) or to an appropriate response to fluid restriction and resultant volume contraction. If decreasing urine output after surgery is the result of SIADH, the patient is euvolemic and has a normal circulatory status, stable to slightly increased weight, and an elevated urinary excretion. If a child has oliguria related to third space losses and true depletion of intravascular volume, there is decreased sodium excretion associated with clinical signs of hypovolemia, such as weight loss, tachycardia, changes in skin turgor and peripheral perfusion, and hypotension; isotonic solutions are indicated.

Greenbaum LA. Pathophysiology of Body Fluids and Fluid Therapy. In: Behrman RE, Kliegman RM, Jenson HB (eds). *Nelson Textbook of Pediatrics*. 17th edn. Philadelphia: Saunders, 2004; 191–252.

Rice HE, Caty MG, Glick PL: Fluid therapy for the pediatric surgical patient. Pediatr Clin North Am 1998 Aug;45(4):719–27.

5 ◆ Child Psychiatry

5.1 HISTORY TAKING AND EXAMINATION

History

i. *Reason for referral:* The problems as seen from various points of view, i.e. parents, teachers, referring doctor, and child. Expectations about the referral.

ii. *Detailed description of present problem:* Onset, course, consequences including effect on family, help given to date.

iii. **Systematic questioning on recent behavior and emotional state**
  • General health; eating, sleeping, elimination, physical complaints, fits or faints.
  • Interests, activities, hobbies.
  • Social relationships with siblings, peers, adults, opposite sex; reactions to new people or situations.
  • *Emotions:* Happy, miserable, fearful, worried at home or at school.
  • Rituals, tics, or mannerisms.
  • Antisocial behavior.
  • Attention and persistence, activity levels, co-ordination.
  • Schooling.

iv. *Family structure and history*
  • Draw a family tree indicating the patient by an arrow. Note also consanguinity and whether left-handed.

  • *Sibs:* Dates of birth, weights. Also note any miscarriages of mother's pregnancies.
  • Family occurrence of developmental disorders, and illness; causes of death.
  • Personality, education, and occupation of each family member and relationships with patient.
  • Home circumstances, finances and character of the neighborhood.

v. *Family life and relationships*
  • Parental relationship—how do the parents get on? What do they enjoy doing together? Father's involvement with child care and household tasks.
  • Parent–child interaction—things done with child. Going out together and playing together. Help with homework.
  • Child's participation in family activities—child's help with washing up, errands and shopping.
  • Pattern of family relationships—mother or father's child? Who does the child confide in? More like father or mother?
  • Discipline—amount of freedom or restriction, methods of punishment. Who reprimands?

vi. *Personal history*
  • Pregnancy was it wanted? Complications, duration.
  • *Delivery:* Route, complications, birth weight (compare with sibs).

- Neonatal problems: Breathing, feeding, jaundice, seizures.
- Early development (compare details of referrals and treatment) immunizations, illnesses or disabilities, seizures or behavioral problems.
- Separations from parents.
- Schools attended, progress.

vii. *Temperamental or personality attributes*
- Meeting new people, e.g. adults, children, approach to strangers.
- New situations—places, foods, toys.
- Emotional expression—how vigorous in expression of feelings? How happy or miserable before present problem?
- Affections and relationships: How are feelings shown? Affectionate? Confiding? Quality of relationships?
- Regularity of functions—sleeping, bowels, appetite.
- Sensitivity—response to the injury of another person or an animal. Reaction when something wrong.

Examination

It may be possible with older children to follow something like the same procedure used to examine an adult's mental state but, particularly in young children, formal examination of the mental state may be impossible. Every opportunity should be taken to observe the child's behavior and this should be recorded systematically and objectively. Avoid global clinical impressions. Do not forget to obtain the child's view of the situation including his likes, dislikes, and hopes for the future.

Mental State

General Behavior

- Dress, appearance.
- Parent–child interaction and separation.
- Emotional responsiveness and relationship with the doctor.
- Restless, disinhibited, assertive, or aggressive.

Mood

- Signs of tension and sadness including facial expression, tearfulness, and apprehension.
- Preoccupation with fear, worries, depressing thoughts.
- Apathetic, withdrawn, shy.

Talk (form)

- Spontaneity, flow.
- Defects of articulation or sentence structure.
- Coherence.

Attention and Persistence

- Degree and duration of interest in topics, activities, or objects.
- Whether easily distracted.
- Unexplained interruptions of attention.

Activity Levels

- General Activity.
- Fidgeting.

Intellectual Function

- Rough assessment of reading level, spelling, arithmetic, writing, general knowledge.
- Write name and address, draw a man, copy triangle, diamond, cross, and circle (according to age).
- If possible, testing by *clinical or educational psychologist* should be arranged including assessment of basic intellectual ability, educational attainments, and specific learning problems.

(A *school report* about progress and general behavior should always be obtained or, for younger children, an account from nursery school or playgroup.)

Physical State

General

- Physique, sexual maturity.
- Height, weight, head circumference (use percentile charts).
- Congenital abnormalities, e.g. asymmetry or other physical abnormality.

Neurological

- Head: size and shape of skull.
- Vision and hearing. Other cranial nerves.
- Preferred hand, eye, foot.
- Posture, involuntary movements.
- Co-ordination of fingers and limbs.
- Limb tone, power, reflexes.
- Constructional skills.
- Right-left differentiation.
- Speech and language.

Personality and Mental State of the Parents

Note in Particular

- Attention for child.
- Excessive indulgence or anxiety.
- Degree, type and consistency of discipline and control of child.
- Negligence.
- Lack of self-confidence in parental ability, fear if the child.

• Understanding of previous diagnosis and management.

(Home visits by *social workers* are a valuable way of collecting this type of information).

Assessment

The different psychological measures in use with children and the mentally retarded are given in Table 5.1.

Achenbach TM, Conaughty SH. *Empirically based Assessment of Child and*
Adolescent Psychopathology. SAGE Publications, Newbury Parkm, 1987.

Barker P. *Basic Child Psychiatry*. Blackwell, Oxford, 1994.

5.2 PSYCHIATRIC DISORDERS

In india, the children below 15 yr of age constitute about 42% of the population but the health resources devoted to them are meager (not even 1–2%).

Table 5.1: Some psychological methods in use with children		
Test category	*Range*	*Test description*
1. **Developmental scales** Gasell infant scale Catell infant scale	8 wk–3.5 yr	Mostly motor development in the first year with some social and language assessment
Bayley infant scale Denver developmental	8 wk–2.5 yr	Motor and social
Screening test	2 mo–6 yr	Screening
Yale revised developmental scale	1 month–6 yr	Gross motor, fine motor, adaptive personal and social language
2. Social maturity behavior Vineland adaptive Behavior scales—survey	0–adult	Interview with parents or teachers on communication skills, daily living, socialization and leisure time
form (parental) Vineland adaptive behavior Scales—survey form—classroom (revised teacher)	3–12.5 yr	
3. Motor skills Bruninks-Oseretsky test of motor Proficiency.	4.5–14.5 yr	Eight subtests, gross and fine motor balance
4. Perceptual and Perceptuomotor	4–12 yr	Perceptuomotor tests
Bender visual-motor Gestalt test	All ages	Also used to rule out organicity
Draw a person Benton Visual retention test	8 yr adult	
5. Speech and language Peabody picture vocabulary	2.5 yr adult	Screening
Test of early language development	3–8 yr	
6. Intelligence Stanford Binet	2–24 yr	Verbal reasoning, abstract visual, reasoning, qualitative reasoning, short-term memory composite score. Verbal
Wechsler intelligence scale for children—revised (WISC-R)	6–17 yr	
Wechsler preschool and primary scale for intelligence (WPPSI)	4–6.5 yr	performance and full scale IQ
Kaufman assessment battery for children	2.5–12.5 yr	Sequential processing, simultaneous process, achievement, processing
Peabody individual achievement test.	5–18 yr	Composite score Word identification, spelling, maths, reading comprehension.
7. Personality	3 yr adult	Projection tests.
Rorschach test	2.5 yr adult	
Children appreciation test (CAT)	7 yr adult	
Thematic appreciation test	7–13 yr	
Junior eysenck personality inventory (EPI)		Objective test (an adaptation of adult EPI)

It is estimated that about 1–2% children in India have some underlying emotional or behavioral problems. There are about 15 million mentally retarded persons. About 4 to 6% of total children are in employment (which deprives them of their potentialities, literacy and full development).

The important common psychiatric disorders seen in children may be classified as:

1. **Developmental disorders**
   a. Mental retardation
   b. Autistic disorder and pervasive developmental disorder
   c. Specific developmental disorder
2. **Developmental disorders**
   a. Anxiety neurosis
   b. Phobic neurosis
   c. Hysteria
   d. Obsessive compulsive disorder
   e. Depressive disorder
3. **Problems of movements**
   a. Head banging
   b. Breath holding spells
   c. Temper tantrums
   d. Hyperkinetic syndrome
   e. Tic disorder (Gilles de la Tourette syndrome)
4. **Problems of habit**
   a. Thumb sucking
   b. Nail-biting
   c. Pica
   d. Trichotillomania (hair-plucking)
5. **Problems of toilet training**
   a. Enuresis
   b. Encopresis
6. **Problem of speech**
   a. Stammering (stuttering)
   b. Selective (elective) mutism
7. **Problems at school**
   a. School phobia
   b. Impaired school performance
8. **Sleep disorders**
   a. Nightmare
   b. Night terror
   c. Somnambulism
   d. Excessive/inadequate sleep
9. **Eating disorders**
   a. Anorexia nervosa
   b. Bulimia nervosa
   c. Obesity
   d. Pica
   e. Rumination disorder
   f. Failure to thrive
10. **Suicide and deliberate self-harm**
11. **Children under peculiar circumstances**
    a. Battered child syndrome (child abuse)
    b. Sibling rivalry
    c. Adopted child
12. **Psychiatric aspects of**
    a. Physical handicaps
    b. Medical disorders
13. a. Drug addiction
    b. Antisocial behavior
14. **Disorders of adolescence**
15. **Prevention of childhood and adolescent psychiatric disorders**

American Psychiatric Association. *Diagnostic and Statistical Manual of Mental Disorders*. 4th edn. (DSM-IV). Washington DC, APA, 1994.

Sartorius N, Graham P. Child mental health: experience of eight countries. *WHO Chronicle* 1984; 38: 208–11.

World Health Organization. *International Classification of Mental and Beahavioural Disorders*. Geneva, WHO, 1992.

5.3 DEVELOPMENTAL DISORDERS

Mental Retardation

Mental retardation is not a disease but a condition in which the intellectual faculties are never manifested or have never been developed sufficiently to enable the retarded person to acquire such an amount of knowledge as persons of his own age and placed in similar circumstances with himself are capable of receiving. Mental retardation is defined as:

i. Significantly subaverage general intellectual functioning (i.e. 2 standard deviation below the mean). IQ below 70.
ii. Significant deficit or impairment in adaptive functioning (i.e. person's ability to meet the responsibilities of social personal, interpersonal and occupational areas of life according to his age and sociocultural and educational background.
iii. Which manifests during the period of development (i.e. before 18 yr of age) (*see* Fig. in CD).

Epidemiology: There are about 15 million mentally retarded in india (2–3% children of general population). The highest incidence in school age children with peak at ages 10 to 12. It is twice as common in boys and girls. There are four types of mental retardation (depending on IQ and adaptive behavior).

i. *Mild mental retardation:* (IQ 50 to 70). This constitutes about 85% of total mentally retarded. Usually their appearance is unremarkable and any motor or sensory deficits are slight. Most people in this group develop more or less normal language abilities and social behavior during the preschool yr and their mental retardation may not be detected until the start of schooling. In adult life, most of them can live independently in ordinary surroundings, though they may need help when under some usual stress. They can achieve academic level up to 6–8th standard and usually belong to low socioeconomic class.

ii. *Moderate mental retardation:* (IQ 35 to 49). This accounts for about 7% of the mentally retarded. Communicates; some independence in self-care; housekeeping with supervision; job skills learned with much repetition; uses public transport with some supervision.

iii. *Severe mental retardation:* (IQ 20 to 34). Needs continuous support and supervision; may communicate wants and needs.

iv. *Profound mental retardation:* (IQ below 20). Less than 1% mentally retarded, only few of them learn to care for themselves completely. Some eventually achieve some simple speech and social behavior.

Disorders Frequent Among Mentally Retarded

A. *Physical Disorders*

i. **Sensory disorders** (about 20%)
Defects in vision or hearing

ii. **Motor disorders**
- Spasticity
- Ataxia
- Athetosis
- Epilepsy (common among severely retarded)

B. *Psychiatric Disorders (All Varieties)*

i. **Schizophrenia:** Characterized by poverty of thinking, less elaborate delusions, simple and repetitive hallucinations; also called "*Pfropf Schizoiphrenie*", treatment is same as of patient with normal intelligence; diagnosed only if there is deterioration in intellectual or social functioning. Difficult to diagnose if IQ below 45.

ii. **Mood disorder**
- *Depressive disorder:* Diagnosed on appearance of sadness, retardation or agitation, suicide attempts may be seen.
- *Mania:* Diagnosed mainly on overactivity and behavioral signs suggestive of elevation of mood.

iii. **Neurosis:** Common in less severely retarded especially while facing changes in the routine of their lives. Clinical picture is often missed. Treated by increased adjustment to environment.

iv. **Personality disorder:** Common in mentally retarded.

v. **Organic psychiatric disorders:** Dementia is usually diagnosed after age 18 yr or when there is definite decline in intellectual capacity and adaptive behavior.
- There is particular association between Alzheimer's disease and Down's syndrome.

- The underlying cause may lead to organic psychoses, e.g. delirium.

vi. *Autism and overactivity syndromes*

vii. *Behavior disorders*
- Mannerisms, head banging and rocking are common among severely retarded (seen in about 40% of children and 20% of adults).
- Repeated self injurious behavior.
- Hyperkinetic syndrome.
- Others, e.g. temper tantrums, self-stimulation, pica, undue dependency, legal problems (rarely).

viii. *Sexual problems*
- Masturbation in public is the most frequent problem.
- Severely mentally retarded are not likely to become good parents.
- All types of mental retardation are not inherited.

Effects of Mental Retardation on the Family

Parents show:
- Distress, feelings or rejection.
- Depression, guilt, shame or anger.
- Rejection of child.
- Overindulgence.
- Social problems.
- Marital disharmony (in some).
- Burden of care for their child.
- Dissatisfaction about medical and social services (even when they are normal).

Predisposing factors: Important predisposing factors are low socioeconomic strata, low birth weight (of child), advanced maternal age and consanguinity.

Differential Diagnosis

- Delayed maturation (specific developmental disorders).
- Blindness or other sensory defects.
- Childhood psychosis (childhood onset schizophrenia).
- Childhood autism.
- Severe neuroses.
- Systemic disorders with physical handicap.
- Deprived children with insufficient stimulation.
- Epilepsy.
- States due to the side effects of drugs (e.g. antipsychotics, anticonvulsants, etc).

Management: No satisfactory treatment is available till today. No drugs are available to increase the level of intelligence. Most of the mentally retarded children brought for treatment can only be benefited only to a limited extent. Management of mentally retarded patients is directed at the following levels:

i. *Primary prevention*
   a. *Health promotion:* It is directed at

- Good antenatal care and encouraging deliveries in hospitals under proper supervision and care.
- Improving the socioeconomic status of the country.
- Education of the public to help in early detection of mental retardation and also, to remove various misconceptions about its causes and treatment.
- Facilitating research to identify the causes, and to invent new methods of treatment.

b. *Specific protection*
- Good prenatal, natal and postnatal care to the pregnant mothers at risk.
- Genetic counseling to at risk patients, e.g. in phenylketonuria.
- Avoiding childbirths in late age of the mother (e.g. to prevent Down syndrome).
- Avoiding consanguinal marriages in case the hereditary factor is operative.
- Avoiding marriages of mentally retarded (especially to mentally retarded) where strong inheritable factors are operating, e.g. tuberous sclerosis.
- Vaccination of girls with rubella vaccine to prevent teratogenicity in fetus due to rubella.
- Avoid giving pertussis vaccine to children with history of convulsions or neurological abnormalities.

ii. *Secondary prevention (early diagnosis and treatment)*
- Early detection and treatment of the preventable disorders (metabolic, endocrinal and nutritional disorders), e.g. cretinism (thyroxine is given), phenylketonuria (restrict phenylalanine in diet), maple syrup disease (diet with low branched chain amino acids).
- Amniocentesis and medical termination of pregnancy on medical grounds.
- Early detection of correctable disorders, e.g. nutritional deficiencies (replacement), infections (antibiotics), hydrocephalus and skull configuration disorders (surgery) or situations (understimulation) and their treatment.
- Early detection of physical handicaps (sensory and motor) and psychological handicaps (e.g. epilepsy, behavioral disorders) and early intervention.
- Prevent them against abuse, e.g. (physical or sexual abuse) by legal or by medical measures (e.g. tubectomy of severely retarded girls).

iii. *Tertiary prevention*
a. *Disability limitation*
- Treatment of physical and psychological problems (by drugs, behavior modification).

- Institutionalization of severe mentally retarded or those with psychological problems.
- Education (if educable) and training to avoid handicaps.
- Physiotherapy to treat the associated deficits.

b. *Rehabilitation:* This is the cornerstone of management of the mentally retarded children. It depends on the patient's level of intelligence and his aptitude. These patients need warmth, love, appreciation and discipline. Rehabilitation is aimed at physical (appliances for handicaps), social (social skills training) and occupational areas (e.g. by teaching and training the patients to make them self sufficient). Day care centres and schools, integrated schools, vocational training centres, sheltered farms and workshops are useful.

Counseling to parents: Parents should be explained about the causation, and prognosis of mental retardation (to alley their misconceptions, fear and unwarranted expectations of miraculous cure).
- To educate mothers and families in-caring for the mentally handicapped (e.g. training mentally retarded girls in household activities).
- Special supervision for the physically handicapped or those severely and profoundly mentally retarded.
- Treatment of psychological problems in parents (e.g. depression in mother resulting in understimulation of a child resulting in retardation).

Hospitalization: It is estimated that about 4/1000 children are severely mentally retarded and about one-fourth to one-third of these need hospitalization.

Indications

a. *Behavioral difficulties* due to
- Attention deficit disorder with hyperkinesis.
- Destructive, assaultive or self-mutilative behavior.
- Psychoses.
- Organic psychoses.

b. *Social factors*
- Overcrowding.
- Incompetent parents.
- Mentally retarded or psychotic parent.
- Single parenthood.
- No one to look after.

American psychiatric association. *Diagnostic and Statistical Manual of Mental Disorders.* 4th edn (DSM-IV). Washington DC, APA, 1994.

Holmes LB, Moser HW, Halldorsan S, Mark SC, Matzilevich B. *Mental Retardation.* An Atlas of Diseases with Associated Physical Abnormalities. London, MacMillan, 1972.

Master RS. Multidisciplinary rehabilitation of the mentally retarded. *Indian J Psychiatry* 1984;26:88–92.

Master RS. Mental Retardation. In: Bhatia MS, Dhar NK (eds). *Textbook of Child and Adolescent Psychiatry.* CBS Publishers and Distributors, New Delhi, 1996; 531–9.

World Health Organization. *International Classification of Mental and Beahavioural Disorders.* Geneva, WHO, 1992.

Shapiro BK, Batshaw ML. Mental retardation (intellectual Disability). In: Kliegman RM, Behrman RE, Jenson HB, Stanton BF (eds). *Nelson Textbook of Pediatrics.* 18th edn. Vol. 1. Philadelphia: Saunders, 2007; 191–7.

Autistic Disorder and Pervasive Developmental Disorders

They are a diverse group of conditions characterized by massive deficits across many areas of functioning, leading to a pervasive disruption of developmental processes which are not merely slow or limited, but is "atypical" or deviant. These disorders are mainly classified as:

i. Infantile autism
ii. Childhood onset schizophrenia

a. *Autistic disorder:* The condition was described by Leo Kanner (1943) as "autistic disturbances of affective contact".

Epidemiology: By definition the onset is in infancy or childhood. The prevalence of the disorder is 4 to 5 per 10,000 in children under 16 yr of age. The male-to-female ratio is 2 to 5 : 1.

Etiology: The higher concordance in monozygotic than dizygotic twins (36% versus 0%) suggests a genetic factor. There is an elevated incidence of early developmental problems such as postnatal neurological infections (meningitis, encephalitis), congenital rubella and cytomegalovirus, phenylketonuria and rarely perinatal asphyxia. The other inborn errors of metabolism associated with autism are tuberous sclerosis and neurofibromatosis. About 2 to 5% appear to have Fragile X chromosome syndrome. Seizure disorder appears in 35 to 50% by age 20. Low IQ is associated with a higher incidence of seizures, social impairment, self-mutilatory and bizarre behavior and a poorer prognosis. Neurological abnormalities are present in about one-quarter of cases ("Soft signs"). Kanner had described the parents of autistic children as intellectual, obsessive, socially reserved, cold and emotionally detached (so-called *"refrigerator parents"*) but this has not been substantiated subsequently. Altered catecholamines (especially dopaminergic) function has been implicated as a component of behavioral impairments in autism.

Clinical features: The characteristic features are:

i. *Autism* (inability to make warm emotional relationships with people). This is manifested as:

 • Autistic aloofness.

 • Unresponsiveness to parent's affectionate behavior by smiling or cuddling.
 • Gaze avoidance or lack of eye-to-eye contact.
 • Dislike being touched or kissed.
 • Behave towards people and inanimate objects in a similar eye.
 • Lack of attachment to parents and no separation anxiety.
 • No or impaired imitation.
 • No or abnormal seeking of comfort at times of distress (seeks comfort in a stereotyped way, e.g. says 'cheese, cheese' whenever hurt).
 • Gross impairment in ability to make peer friendships.
 • Marked lack of awareness of the existence or feelings of others.
 • Anger or fear without apparent reason and absence of fear in presence of danger.

ii. *Communication:* There is marked qualitative impairment in verbal (language) or nonverbal communication and in imaginative activity. It is manifested as:

 • No mode of communication such as communicative babbling, facial expression, gesture, mime, etc.
 • Marked abnormal nonverbal communication as in the use of eye-to-eye contact, facial expression, body posture or gestures to initiate social interaction.
 • Absence of imaginative activity such as play acting of adult roles, fantasy characters or animals; lack of interest in imaginative stories.
 • Marked abnormalities in the production of speech (volume, pitch, stress, rhythm, rate, etc.).
 • Marked abnormalities in the form or content of speech including stereotyped or repetitive use of speech, use of "you" when 'I' is meant; idiosyncratic use of phrases.
 • Marked impairment in the ability to initiate or sustain a conversation with others, despite adequate speech.

iii. *Activities:* Marked restricted repertoire of activities and interests.

 • Stereotyped body movements, e.g. hand flicking, or twisting, spinning, head banging, etc.
 • Persistent preoccupation with parts of objects (e.g. spinning wheels of toy cars) or attachment to unusual objects (e.g. insists on carrying a piece of ring).
 • Marked distress over changes in trivial aspects of environment, e.g. when a vase is moved from usual position.
 • Unreasonable insistence on following routines in precise details.

• Markedly restricted range of interests and a preoccupation with one narrow interest (e.g. lining up of objects).

iv. *Other features*

• Mental retardation (more than half of autistic children have moderate to profound retardation whereas about 25% have mild mental retardation).

• *Idiot savant syndrome:* In spite of a pervasive or abnormal development as in schizophrenia.

• Kanner's *"autistic triad":* Kanner said that autistic aloofness, speech and language disorder and obsessive desire for sameness constitute a triad characteristic of infantile autism.

Prognosis: About 10 to 20% autistic children begin to improve between 4 and 6 yr of age and eventually attend an ordinary school and obtain work. 10 to 20% can live at home but need to attend a special school or training center and cannot work. 60% improve little and unable to lead an independent life, most needing long-term residential care. Those who improve may continue to show language problems, emotional coldness and odd behavior.

Differential Diagnosis (Tables 5.2 and 5.3)

i. *Childhood schizophrenia:* An infantile autism in contrast to childhood schizophrenia there is little or no period of normal development, retardation and epilepsy are common, have symptoms suggestive of negative symptoms of schizophrenia and there are no hallucinations or delusions (Table 5.3).

ii. *Reactive attachment disorder of infancy (RADI).* This disorder is characterized by a failure to establish normal attachment to a caregiver or an indiscriminate sociability and is the result of psychosocial deprivation or abuse, but these children have potential for normal imaginative play and normal responses to the environment, lacks motor abnormalities and are not mentally retarded.

iii. *Elective mutism:* There is absence of speech in some but not necessarily all environments. This may be acute (following identified stressor) or chronic (following social or familial factors). These children communicate via gesture, nodding or short mono-syllabic utterances.

iv. *Others:* The other disorders need to be differential are Tourette's disorder, habit disorder, obsessive compulsive disorder, attention deficit disorder, specific developmental (language) disorder, acquired aphasia with convulsions, schizoid personality, heating or neurodegenerative diseases and mental retardation.

Management: There is no 'specific' treatment. The main modes of treatment used are:

i. *Behavior modification*

• Positive reinforcement to teach self-care skills.

• Speech therapy (also sign language teaching).

• Structured classroom training (to learn new material and maintain the acquired learning; "special schooling").

• Development of regular routine with minimum or no changes.

• Behavioral techniques to encourage social and interpersonal interactions.

This treatment is often carried out at home by the patients (instructed and supervised by a clinical psychologist).

ii. *Counseling and supportive therapy* for parents. Family based therapies are used.

iii. *Medication:* Various drugs have been tried in the treatment of infantile autism.

a. *Antipsychotics:* Haloperidol is helpful in decreasing hyperactivity and other disruptive (temper tantrums, etc.) behavior.

b. *Dopamine agonists* CNS stimulants (amphetamines or methylphenidate) improve hyperactivity and other behavioral problems but children may develop irritability, tics, stereotypies or aggressive behavior. Levodopa is useful in autistic cases (hypoactive children, but stereotypes and interference with learning are side effects).

c. *Fenfluramine* structurally similar to amphetamine, is a serotonin releasing agent known to reduce blood serotonin levels. It may cause reduced motor symptoms, enhanced social relatedness, improved attention and sleep patterns and increased IQ.

d. *Naloxone and naltrexone* are pure opiate receptor antagonists. Naltrexone is a potent, oral long acting agent. It decreases self-injurious behavior, aggressiveness, hyperactivity, impulsivity, withdrawal and stereotypies.

e. *Others,* e.g. antiepileptic drugs (carbamazepine, phenytoin) to control seizures and aggressive behavior.

Comments: According to ICD-10 and DSM-IV, childhood autism manifests before the age of three yr (not 2.5 yr as was included in previous classifications). The other type is atypical autism.

b. *Atypical autism:* It is a type of pervasive developmental disorder that differs from autism in terms of either age of onset or failing to fulfill diagnostic criteria (i.e. disturbance in reciprocal social interactions, communication and restrictive stereotyped behavior). Atypical is seen in profoundly retarded individuals whose very low level of functioning provides little scope for exhibition of the specific deviant behavior required for the diagnosis of autism. It also occurs in individuals with a severe specific developmental disorder of receptive language. They are also known as mental retardation with autistic features; atypical childhood psychosis.

c. *Rett syndrome:* A condition, so far reported only in girls, for which the cause is not known, but which has been differentiated on the basis of a characteristic onset, course and patterns of symptomatology.

- Typically apparently normal or near-normal early development is followed by partial or complete loss of acquired hand skills and of speech together with deceleration in head growth, usually with an onset between 7 and 24 mo of age.
- Loss of purposive hand movements, hand wringing stereotypes and hyperventilation.
- Arrest of social and play development in the first two or three years but social interest tends to be maintained.
- Truncal ataxia and apraxia with scoliosis or kyphoscoliosis, in middle childhood.
- Sometimes choreoathetoid movements.
- Severe mental handicap and fits (during early or middle childhood generally before the age of 8 years).
- Deliberate self-injury and complex stereotyped preoccupation are rare.

For comparison between autistic disorder, rett syndrome and Asperger syndrome (Table 5.2).

d. *Childhood disintegrative disorder:* A type of pervasive developmental disorder (other than Rett syndrome) that is defined by the presence of a definitely normal development prior to the onset of this disorder and by a definite phase of loss of previously acquired skills over the course of a few months, that extends across at least several areas of development; together with the onset of characteristic abnormalities of social, communicative and behavioral functioning. Often there is prodromal period of vague illness; the child becomes restive, irritable, anxious and over-reactive. This is then followed by an impoverishment and then a loss of speech and language accompanied by behavioral disintegration. In some cases loss of skill is persistently progressive but a limited improvement may be seen. The prognosis is usually very poor with most individual left with severe mental retardation.

Table 5.2: Comparison between autistic disorder, Rett syndrome and Asperger syndrome

	Autistic disorder	Rett syndrome	Asperger syndrome
1. Incidence per 10,000	4–5	0.5–1	1
2. Age of onset	<36 mo	5–48 mo	>36 mo
3. Sex	M	F	M
Deficits			
1. Cognitive	50% MR	MR, severe to profound	–
2. Eye gaze	+	?	+
3. Language	+	+	–
4. Motor	–	+++	
5. Stereotypies	++	++	+
6. Social	+	+	+
7. Prognosis	High IQ: Fair low IQ poor	Worse	Less symptoms in adulthood

There is uncertainty on the extent to which condition is different from autism. In some cases there is associated encephalopathy but the diagnosis should be made on the behavioral features.

It resembles dementing conditions of adult life but it differs in 3 key respects; a lack of evidence of any identifiable organic disease or damage; loss of skills followed by a degree of recovery; and impairment in socialization and communicative rather than intellectual decline.

The other terms used are *Heller's syndrome,* disintegrative psychosis, symbiotic psychosis; dementia infantilis. It needs differentiation from pervasive developmental disorder, schizophrenia, Rett syndrome, elective mutism and epilepsy with acquired aphasia.

e. *Asperger syndrome:* A disorder of uncertain classification, characterized by the same type of qualitative impairment of reciprocal social interaction that typifies autism together with a restricted stereotyped repetitive repertoire of interests and activities. It differs from autism primarily in the fact that there is *no general delay or retardation in language or in cognitive development.* Most individuals are of normal general intelligence but are clumsy. This occurs primarily in boys (boys : girls = 8 : 1). The abnormalities tend to persist into adolescence and adult life and the characteristics are not affected by environmental influences. Psychotic episodes occasionally occur in early adult life.

The other names are—autistic psychopathy and schizoid disorder of childhood. It needs differentiation from pervasive developmental disorder, schizotypal disorder, simple schizophrenia, attachment disorder of childhood, anarchistic personality disorder and obsessive compulsive disorder.

f. ***Childhood onset schizophrenia:*** The differences of childhood onset schizophrenia from pervasive developmental disorder are given in Table 5.3.

Schizophrenia is almost unknown before seven years of age and seldom begins before late adolescence. Schizophrenia in childhood can be differentiated clearly from other childhood psychosis on the basis of its symptoms (while rare as seen in adults). Before its onset, four-fifth of the affected children are odd, timid and sensitive. In nearly half the cases, there is a history of delayed speech development. E.M. Creak's (1963) nine points of childhood schizophrenia are:

i. Gross and sustained impairment of emotional relationships with people.

ii. Apparent unawareness of his own identity to a degree inappropriate to his age.

iii. Pathological preoccupation with particular objects or certain characteristics of them without regard to their accepted functions.

iv. Sustained resistance to change in the environment and a striving to maintain or restore sameness.

v. Abnormal perceptual experience (in the absence of discernible organic abnormality).

vi. Acute, excessive and seemingly illogical anxiety as a frequent phenomenon.

vii. Speech either lost or never acquired or showing failure to develop beyond a level appropriate to an earlier age.

viii. Distortion in mobility patterns.

ix. A background of serious retardation in which islets of normal, near normal or exceptional intellectual function or skill may appear.

Specific Developmental Disorders

i. ***Developmental arithmetic disorder:*** Difficulty with arithmetic is probably the second most common specific learning disorder that cannot be explained in terms of generally low IQ. Little is known about it. It is believed to be quite common.

The clinical features are:

• Arithmetic skills as measured by a standardized individually administered test are markedly below the expected level, given the person's schooling and intellectual capacity (as measured by IQ tests, e.g. Wechsler's scales— WISC, WAIS).

Table 5.3: Comparison of pervasive development disorder and childhood onset schizophrenia

Characteristic	Pervasive developmental disorders (PDD)	Childhood onset schizophrenia
i. Age of onset	—	8 yr or older
ii. Sex ratio	Before 3 yr.	1 : 1
iii. Incidence	4 : 1	4 5/1,000
iv. Family history	Autism—4–5 in 10,000, other PDD: 2–16/10,000 Slightly increased incidence of schizophrenia Increased incidence of autism, cognitive and language disorders and mental retardation	Marked increased incidence
v. Socioeconomic class	Evenly distributed	More in lower classes
vi. Prenatal and perinatal complications	Possible increased incidence	Possible increased incidence
vii. Previous development	Impaired in first yr of childhood Uneven pattern of abilities	Deterioration from normal function
viii. Intelligence	70–80% retarded (Severe to mild)	18% (borderline to mild)
ix. Clinical features	Gaze avoidance, abnormal preoccu-pations, disinterest in people, poor supervised play, stereotypies, echolalia, overactivity	Hallucinations, disorder of thought content, blunted affect, incongruous ideation and affect
x. Prevalence of Seizures	Approximately 25%	Low
xi. Types of seizures	Grand mal	Temporal lobe
xii. Course	Autism continues, worsens or improves but no remissions. Resembles negative type of schizophrenia	Chronic course or remissions

- It significantly interferes with academic achievement or activities of daily living requiring arithmetic skills.
- Not due to a defect in visual or hearing acuity or a neurological disorder.

Although it causes a less severe handicap in everyday life than reading difficulties. It can lead to secondary emotional difficulties while the child is at school.

Etiology: Factors that produce slow academic development include neurological, genetic, psychological, socioeconomic conditions, learning experiences. Arithmetical ability correlates with IQ and classroom training. Approximately 6% of the population is affected and low socioeconomic conditions show overrepresentation.

Management involves special education, with initial evaluation and subsequent monitoring of need for psychiatric and neurological intervention. It is likely that this disorder may be quietly present in many adults who make accommodations in their lives and work to manage the residue of dysfunctions that there were evident during school years.

ii. *Developmental expressive writing disorder:* Difficulties in spelling, grammar, sentence and paragraph formation and punctuation are characteristic.

Symptoms include slow writing speed and low volume output, illegibility, letter reversals, word finding and syntax errors, erasures, rewritings, spacing errors and punctuation and spelling problems. Low productivity, refusal to complete work or submit assignments and chronic underachievement may be suggestive of development output failure.

These deficits may result from underlying problems with graphemotor (hand and pencil control), fine motor and visuomotor function, attention, memory, concept formation and organization as well as expressive language function. It results from neurocortical characteristics as modified by environmental experiences.

Prevalence is not determined, but there appears to be the standard 3–4 : 1 male predominance seen in most learning disorders.

Genuine remedial therapy is possible with educational interventional typically consisting of alternative writing formats and skill buildings. The recent availability of commercial word processors may contribute to remediation of same cases.

iii. *Developmental reading disorder:* Common 'dyslexia' is characterized by a slow acquisition of reading skills. Slow reading speed, impaired comprehension, word omissions and distortions and letter reversals are outside to the expected performance levels based on age and IQ. This disorder is seen in the presence of normal intelligence, appropriate education, motivation and emotional control.

Etiology: For reading acquisition to develop in a numerous neurological and psychiatric functions must be intact, e.g. eye control, spatial orientation, verbal sequencing, grasping the structural sense of a sentence and abstraction and categorization cortical integration, attention, motivation and effort.

Difficulty in reading may result due to disturbance in any of the above functions, mental retardation, brain damage, psychiatric and inadequate schooling. The neuropathological studies have shown widespread neuronal ectopias, dysplasia and micropolygyria.

Characteristics: These individuals show difficulty in the "paired-associate task" of translating verbal symbols (letters) into auditory based words. There is also, left-right disorientation, impairment in sound discrimination, perceptual-motor skills (i.e. letter reversals (b, d), word transposition (saw, was), omissions (truck, tuck), and substitution (truck, trick), spelling problems (severe and long lasting), verbal language deficits, seizures or symptoms of left hemisphere injury, attentional difficulties, conduct disorder, etc. and many have mental expressive writing disorder, developmental articulation disorder, developmental coordination disorder and poor handwriting.

Epidemiology: Prevalence about 3 to 10% in general population with male female ratio 3–4 : 1. Increased prevalence is in low socioeconomic classes, large family size and social disadvantage.

Assessment and management: Assessment is carried out by an educational or clinical psychologist. Treatment is given by remedial teachers. Early Educational intervention is essential. Self-esteem may need to be bolstered to help the child (or adult) tolerate the remedial efforts. Treatment is directed at reading disorder and the possibly associated specific developmental disorders, conduct disorder and hyperkinetic disorder. Parental involvement is also important.

Prognosis: This varies with the severity of the condition. About a quarter of those with a mid-childhood achieve normal reading skills by adolescence. Those with substantial difficulties in adolescence retain them.

iv. *Developmental coordination disorder (specific motor retardation):* Some children have delayed motor development, which results in clumsiness in schoolwork or play apraxia. Now the term clumsiness is used. About 5% of children have significant impairments of gross or fine motor functions which are manifested in running, throwing a ball, buttoning, holding a pencil, or general awkwardness and clumsiness. Common concomitants include attention deficit disorder with hyperkinesis and common complications include scapegoating, impaired self-esteem and sports avoidance.

These children are sometimes referred to a psychiatrist because of a secondary emotional disorder. An explanation of the nature of the problem should be given to the child, the family and the teachers. Special training can be tried though without great hope of success. It may be necessary to exempt the child from organized games or other school activities involving motor-coordination.

v. *Developmental speech and language disorders:* Half of the children use words with meaning by 12.5 mo and 97% do so by 21 mo. Half form words into simple sentences by 23 mo. Vocabulary and complexity of language development rapidly during the preschool years. However, when they start school, 1% of children are seriously retarded in speech and 5% have difficulty in making themselves understood by strangers. There may be developmental articulation disorder, expressive or receptive language disorder. Children with developmental speech and language disorder have marked delay in acquiring normal speech, in the absence of any of the primary causes. Many speak freely and appear to understand speech, but their own speech is hard to understand because the words are ill formed. They have greater difficulty with longer words and tend to omit the end of words. Consonants are usually more difficult than vowels.

Speech therapy is the usual treatment and is beneficial in many patients.

vi. *Mixed disorder of scholastic skills:* This is an ill-defined inadequately conceptualized (but necessary) residual category of disorders (in ICD-10), in which both arithmetical and reading or spelling skills are significantly impaired, but in which the impairment is not solely explicable in terms of general mental retardation or of inadequate schooling.

It needs differentiation from specific developmental disorders (of reading or spelling or arithmetical skills).

American Psychiatric Association. *Diagnostic and Statistical Manual of Mental Disorders.* 4th edn (DSM-IV). Washington DC, APA, 1994.

Bhatia MS. Essentials of Psychiatry. New Delhi, CBS Publishers & Distributors, 2004.

Larner J. Children with Learning Disabilities. Houghton, Niffin,1971.

Treffert DA. Epidemiology of Infantile autism. *Arch Gen Psychiatry* 1970; 22:431–438.

Verghese A, Beigh A. Psychiatric disturbances in children–An epidemiological study. *Indian J Med Res* 1974; 62:1538–44.

World Health Organization. *International Classification of Mental and Behavioral Disorders.* Geneva, WHO, 1992.

5.4 DEPRESSION

Depression is a common illness and is among the ten major illness causing disability.

Prevalence: Though large epidemiological studies are not available for India, but a few studies reported prevalence in different populations. Prevalence has been reported to be 0.5 to 1.5%.

Diagnosis: According to DSM-IV, marked loss of interest in almost all activities, apathy and either loss of weight or failure to gain expected weight are major symptoms of childhood depression. Tantrums, frustration, lack of cooperation, withdrawal from family and friends, impaired school performance are other presentations of childhood depression.

Management

Pharmacological: In recently published guidelines, selective serotonin reuptake inhibitors (SSRIs) were placed as the first line therapy for the management of adolescent depression, followed by norepinephrine-serotonin reuptake inhibitors. Another SSRIs, sertraline is associated with faster improvement in children. Duloxetine, which is recommended for the depressive with prominent somatic symptoms in adults, is also found to be efficacious in a girl child with severe pain and dissociative symptoms. Venlafaxine is found to be effective in depressed adolescents but not in children with depression.

Psychotherapy: Improvement is better in younger adolescents, who were less chronically depressed, less hopeless with less suicidal ideation, had lesser melancholic features and had greater expectations from the treatment. Combination of fluoxetine and cognitive behaviour therapy (CBT) is more effective with mild to moderate depression, especially when depression is associated with cognitive distortions. There are two evidence-based psychotherapies for the management of depression—interpersonal therapy and cognitive therapy.

Adolescent under cognitive therapy improve with the treatment. Some of them may develop worsening of depression in the initial phase of treatment, termed as depression spike; others start to improve from the beginning. It is more efficacious in the treatment of recurrent major depressive disorder and in subjects with good coping skills.

Yoga for the treatment of depression: Yoga is helpful in improvement of not only the depression, but also its accessory symptoms. Sahaj yoga has been found to remit depression as well as executive functioning, manipulation of information, attention span and visuomotor speed in depressed patients.

Sudarshan kriya yoga is thought to produce chemicals in mind that travel from nervous system to immune cells and thus improving overall state of body and mind. Sudarshan kriya yoga involves essentially rhythmic hyperventilation at different rates of breathing with the sounds of So-hum A thirty minute everyday session of Sudarshan kriya yoga can improve stress, anxiety, post-traumatic stress disorder (PTSD), depression, stress-related medical illnesses and substance abuse. It also enhances well-being, mood, attention, mental focus, and stress tolerance.

Curry J, Rohde P, Simons A, Silva S, Vitiello B, Kratochvil C, Reinecke M, Feeny N, Wells K, Pathak S, Weller E, Rosenberg D, Kennard B, Robins M, Ginsburg G, March J; TADS Team. Predictors and moderators of acute outcome in the Treatment for Adolescents with Depression Study (TADS). *J Am Acad Child Adolesc Psychiatry* 2006; 45:1427–39.

Malhotra S, Nitin G, Gagandeep S. Retrospective study of affective disorders in children attending a child psychiatry clinic. *Indian J Med Res* 1999;109:71–75.

Srinath S, Girimaji SC, Gururaj G, Seshadri S, Subbakrishna DK, Bhola P, et al. Epidemiological study of child and adolescent psychiatric disorders in urban and rural areas of Bangalore, India. *Indian J Med Res* 2005; 122: 67–79.

Hughes CW, Emslie GJ, Crismon ML, Posner K, Birmaher B, Ryan N, Jensen P, Curry J, Vitiello B, Lopez M, Shon SP, Pliszka SR, Trivedi MH; Texas Consensus Conference Panel on Medication Treatment of Childhood Major Depressive Disorder. Texas Children's Medication Algorithm Project: update from Texas Consensus Conference Panel on Medication Treatment of Childhood Major Depressive Disorder. *J Am Acad Child Adolesc Psychiatry* 2007;46:667–686.

Sharma VK, Das S, Mondal S, Goswami U, Gandhi A. Effect of Sahaj Yoga on neuro-cognitive functions in patients suffering from major depression. *Indian J Physiol Pharmacol* 2006;50:375–83.

5.5 ANXIETY DISORDERS

Anxiety disorders are probably one of the most common categories of childhood mental disorders. In the DSM-IV classification (APA 1994), two sections of the manual include anxiety disorders. The general category of 'Anxiety Disorders' include panic disorders, agoraphobia, social phobia, specific phobia, obsessive compulsive disorder, post-traumatic stress disorder, acute stress disorder, generalized anxiety disorder, anxiety disorder due to a general medical condition, substance-induced anxiety disorder and anxiety disorders not otherwise specified. If the criteria for the diagnosis for these disorders are fulfilled, then many of these disorders may be diagnosed in children. Another section includes 'Separation Anxiety Disorders' of childhood and adolescence.' The over anxious disorder of childhood has been included in generalized anxiety disorder.

Epidemiology: Recent epidemiological work has demonstrated that anxiety disorders are the most common psychiatric problems encountered in childhood (Table 5.4).

Etiology: Controlled family studies of anxiety disorder patients confirms a familial pattern in these disorders. A higher number of environmental stressors have been documented in children with anxiety disorders.

Differential diagnosis: The differential diagnosis (i) separation anxiety disorder, (ii) overanxious disorder and (iii) avoidant disorder is listed in Table 5.4.

Obsessive Compulsive Disorder

Obsessive compulsive disorder is identical in adults and children. Many adults who come for treatment give a history of onset in childhood. The average age of onset in a large study was 12.8 yr. Boys seem to be more affected than girls. The onset is usually gradual but may be sudden.

Clinical features: Obsessions consist of repeated, unwelcome and unpleasant thoughts over which the person has no control and which may be quite persistent. These are followed by ritual actions, the performance of which in some way helps in "undoing" the thoughts and provides a temporary relief. These actions are known as compulsions.

When the symptoms are mild and mixed with other anxiety features then the prognosis is better. In its full-fledged form obsessive compulsive neurosis is as difficult to treat in the child as in the adult.

The *differential diagnosis* should consider impending psychosis and psychotic features and the presence of other abnormal thought should be ruled out by psychological tests and psychiatric evaluation.

Treatment: Behavior modification in the form of systematic desensitization and relaxation therapy may help. Cognitive behavior therapy (CBT) is useful. Antidepressants have been used with some success and SSRIs, e.g. fluoxetine, fluvoxamine or clomipramine seems to be the antidepressant of choice.

Phobias

Mild fears are quite frequent in children. If these fears are associated with one of the anxiety

	Table 5.4: Differential diagnosis of anxiety disorders		
	I. Separation anxiety disorder	*II. Overanxious disorder*	*III. Avoidant disorder*
Definition	Excess anxiety (panic) on separation from major attachment figures home or familiar surroundings	Excessive worrying and fearful behavior that is not focused on a specific situation or object and that is not due to a recent psychosocial stressor,	Extreme social inhibition of sufficient severity to interfere with peer relationships
Epidemiology	Before 3 yr, normal. Less than 2% in general population. About 5% among child guidance clinic attendance. Equally common in both sexes	Apparently common disorder. More common in boys, especially in rural areas	Apparently rare especially after 4 yr of age. Always begins in childhood. More common in girls
Etiology	There is a specific development stage between 12 and 35 mo, in which normal separation anxiety may become constelled, through fixation and regression. It result when excessive and unrealistic symptoms impede growth and creativity. More common among family members (a communicative or inherited disorder)	Unconscious conflict may play a role. Depressive setting in the family. More common among family members (A communication or inheritable disorder)	Children who have been victims of abuse, neglect or from minority groups or conditions of social and geographic isolation
Clinical features	Excessive anxiety concerning separation as manifested by : unrealistic and persistent worry about possible harm to attachment figure; persistent reluctance or refusal to go to school, sleep or being alone; complaints of physical symptom nightmares or excessive distress duration of at least 2 wk and onest before age 18	Excessive or unrealistic anxiety or worry of at least 6 mo duration characterized by: excessive or unrealistic worry about future events, or appropriation of past behavior or competence; somatic complaints, marked self-consciousness, excessive need for reassurance, marked feelings of tensions; does not meet the criteria of generalized anxiety disorder	Excessive shrinking from contact with unfamiliar person for a period of at least 6 mo Interfere with social functioning in peer relationships. Warm and satisfying relationship with family members. Age at least 2 yr
Differential diagnosis	Pervasive developmental disorder or schizophrenia. Overanxious and avoidance disorder. Major depression. Conduct disorder	Separation anxiety disorder Attention deficit disorder Others: Major depression, obsessive compulsive disorder, Pervasive developmental disorder or schizophrenia	Avoidant personality disorder Adjustment disorder Overanxious disorder
Prognosis	Spontaneous remission Young and acute cases and with empathic parents have good prognosis	Spontaneous remission common. Some cases may continue into adulthood	Spontaneous remission Favorable response to treatment
Treatment	Anti-depressants (SSRIs, e.g. fluoxetine). Behavior (cognitive behavior therapy or CBT) and individual psychosocial therapy	CBT and/or SSRIs anxiolytics, e.g. Benzodiazepines	Combined therapy

Table 5.5: Clinical features of childhood hysteria

Motor symptoms	Seizures, paralysis, weakness, abnormal movements, disturbed gait (astasia abasia)
Sensory symptoms	Pain, paresthesia, hypoesthesia, anesthesia, hyperesthesia, deafness, blindness, anosmia, loss of taste
Dissociative phenomenon	Amnesia, fugues, multiple personality, somnambulism
Others	Mutism, unconsciousness, somatic symptoms, possession states, headache, hyperventilation, suicidal attempts, etc.

syndromes then they are treated as part of the respective disorder. If the fear is isolated, specific, persistent and a well defined stimulus and if the child shows deficits in normal functioning because of the fear, then the diagnosis of phobia may be made.

Phobias are more common in girls than in boys. Simple phobias have a prevalence rate of 2.4% in children.

Depending on the type of phobia the age of onset will vary—social phobias seem to have a later onset than animal phobias while situational phobias, e.g. fear of dark, fear of storms, etc. have a variable onset.

Treatment: Supportive psychotherapy and behavior modification are the most effective methods of treatment. Psychotherapy includes parental counseling, suggestions for environmental manipulation and reduction of generalized anxiety level. Desensitization has been useful. It may be difficult to get a child to train in relaxation procedures but he can be exposed to a graded series of exposures to the object of fear by being able to talk about it, see pictures of it and to gradually see the object and become involved with it. Flooding can also be tried if the child has enough confidence in the therapist. Minor tranquilizers can be given for short intervals while the intervention procedures are being undertaken.

American Psychiatric Association. *Diagnostic and Statistical Manual of Mental Disorders* 4th edn Washington DC : American Psychiatric Press,1994.

Rapoport JL, Inoff-Germain G. Treatment of obsessive compulsive disorder in children and adolescents. *J Child Psychol Psychiatry* 2000; 41:419–31.

Stafford B, Boris NW, Daton R. Anxiety disorders. In: Kliegman RM, Behrman RE, Jenson HB, Stanton BF (eds). *Nelson Textbook of Pediatrics.* 18th edn. Vol. 1. Philadelphia: Saunders, 2007; 117–120.

5.6 CHILDHOOD HYSTERIA

Hysteria, the "(uterus) of Greeks; the Sacred Disease" described by Hippocrates (400 BC) was considered to be due to the diabolical possession in the middle ages. Sigmund Freud in 1902 declared that the symptoms of hysterical patients are based on highly significant but forgotten events usually of sexual nature from their past which were suppressed and got converted into somatic symptoms. In simple non-Freudian terms, the dynamism—conversion is an unconscious expression in physical symptoms of emotional conflicts.

Epidemiology: The incidence of hysteria in all age-groups ranged from 6.5 to 10.6% in various studies probably because of variations in the diagnostic criteria used by different workers. The age of onset reported by most of the workers is usually in adolescence or early adulthood.

Clinical features: The clinical features are listed in Table 5.5.

Differential diagnosis: Differentiation of common hysterical manifestations, i.e. malingering and pseudo-seizure are given in Tables 5.6 and 5.7, respectively.

Treatment: Children with hysteria and their parents make reluctant psychiatric patients; they are usually seen by many other medical specialists before the referral to psychiatry which is almost universally made by pediatricians, often in the face of initial parental opposition and even hostility. This is partly explained by the fact that the symptoms frequently start in the context of some, usually minor physical illness or of an accident. Sexual abuse or sexual stressors need to be excluded in children with hysteria, especially pseudoseizures.

First step in the treatment of hysteria is *symptom removal*. This can be achieved by suggestion, assurance and only sometimes use of narcosuggestion.

Symptom removal should always be followed by *individual psychotherapy* for the child and casework for the parents to uncover the psychopathology.

Cognitive behavior therapy (CBT) is used to modify patients at attitudes and interpretations of the symptoms. Regular physiotherapy and strong suggestions of improvement are must in cases of hysterical paralysis to prevent muscle wasting or contractures in rare instances. Useful goals of treatment should be to alleviate the associated psychiatric problems and prevent iatrogenic damages because of excessive inappropriate use of drugs. Doctors shopping should be discouraged.

Prognosis: The prognosis of hysteria in children appears to be good. Most patients appear to be free

Table 5.6: Differences between conversion hysteria and malingering

	Conversion hysteria	Malingering
Nature of symptoms	Nonanatomic, nonphysiological, dysfunction rather than pain	Anatomic or nonanatomic dysfunction or pain
Emotional response to symptoms	Relative indifference	Exaggerated concern
Onset	Sudden in response to conflict	Gradual planned
Volitional or nonvolitional etiology	Nonvolitional	Volitional
Presumed motivation	Resolution of psychological or situational conflict	Compensation or prosecution
Pre-existing physical pathology	Absent/present	Absent
Suggestibility	High	Low
Cognitive state	Dissociation memory or attention deficit	Intact
Response to treatment	Sudden, dramatic for short-term	None

Table 5.7: Differences between pseudoseizure and true seizure

Pseudoseizure	True seizure
I. History	
a. Pattern	
No neurophysiological pattern	Same pattern
b. Precipitant	
Obvious emotional precipitant and occurrence in presence of others	May be there but less obvious and presence of others not associated
c. Occurrence in sleep	
Not there	May occur
d. Treatment	
Intractable dispute adequate medication	Often responds
e. Other features	
History of sexual or other abuse	History of incontinence or self injury
II. Observations	
a. Onset	
Gradual	Abrupt
b. Duration	
Time variable but longer (10–15 minutes)	Short duration up to 1–2 minutes
c. Consciousness	
Usually preserved with bilateral motor activity. May be fluctuating but some response to pain	Lost and unresponsive to pain
d. Aura	
Aura unusual except for symptoms of hyperventilation	Aura usual
e. Moaning	
Swoon or faint, may moan, cry, scream or weep	Monotonous epileptic cry
f. Movements	
• Nonsynchronous out of phase movements (may be mild, jerfy, side-to-side head movements, pelvic thrusting, limping, motionless, unresponsive)·	Generalized tonic clonic movements starting with fast small amplitude movements to slower larger movements
• Opisthotonic posturing or rigidity for extended periods	Briefer rigidity, supplementary movements (e.g. arms in abduction)
g. During sleep	
Uncommon during physiologic sleep	May occur
h. Injury	
Self-protection before fall, seldom self injury	Frequent self injury, bite tongue , hit head, hurt limb

(Contd.)

Table 5.7: Differences between pseudoseizure and true seizure (*Contd.*)

Pseudoseizure	*True seizure*
i. Reflexes No pathological reflexes	Babinski reflex and papillary constriction after seizure
j. Postictal confusion Little and patient unconcerned	Postictal confusion or transient paralysis
k. Amnesia Better memory for event; nonorganic amnesia	Amnesia
l. In presence of significant others Usually occur	Unconcerned
m. Independent witness Absent	Present
n. Induction by suggestion Readily induced or stopped	Not
o. Induction by sleep, photic stimuli, sleep deprivation, hyperventilation Not readily	Often precipitated
p. Others Avoidance behavior, arm drop, eye opening, genotropic eye movement	Seeking help, tiredness, look blank, pupillary reflexes
III. Testing	
a. pH immediately after attack Normal	May change
b. Creatinine kinase after attack Normal	Rises (significant if positive)
c. Prolactin after attack Normal	Rises (significant if positive)
d. EEG	
• No epileptic form discharge, maintenance of alpha rhythm with only discontinuous muscle activity record during attack and absence of slowing with immediate reappearance of previous occurred alpha rhythm	Epileptic changes in majority (VEEG preferred) a. Takes time to recovery (VEEG useful)
• EEG may be abnormal in 10–53% and prompt clinical and EEG recovery from a generalized convulsive episode.	
e. Provocative methods Psychiatric interview, suggestion, placebo medication or hypnosis	Hyperventilation, photic stimuli or sleep deprivation

of symptoms and showing good psychosocial adjustment within one to eleven years of treatment, with no reports of physical symptoms substitution.

Bhatia MS, Choudhary S. Hysteria—a chamaleon or a fossil? *Indian J Med Sci* 1998;52:227–30.

Mathew C, John JK. The changing trend of hysteria over the decade. *Indian J Psychiatry* 1995;37:12–17.

Freud S. *Collected Papers*. Vol. 1. New York: Churchill Livingstone, 1954.

Nandi DN, Banerjee G, Nandi S, Nandi P. Is hysteria on the wane? A community survey in West Bengal, India. *Br J Psyhiatry* 1992; 160: 87–91.

5.7 ADJUSTMENT DISORDERS AND IMPULSE DISORDERS

Adjustment Disorders

The important diagnostic feature of these disorders is a *maladaptive reaction* to an identifiable psychosocial stressor, that occurs *within three mo after* the onset of the stressor.

Epidemiology: Prevalence is 0.1 to 10% depending on the sample studied. It is twice common in women as compared to men.

Clinical picture: Adjustment disorder with depressed mood/anxious mood/mixed emotional features/disturbance of conduct/mixed disturbance of emotions and conduct/work (or academic) inhibition/withdrawal/physical complaints.

Etiology: These factors include the intensity or severity of the stress (or life events), the quality of the support and vulnerability of the individual.

Differential diagnosis: Conditions not attributable to a mental disorder, personality disorders or psychological factors affecting physical condition.

Management: These are several different approaches, usually referred to as crisis interventions, in the treatment of adjustment disorders. Crisis intervention involves identifying the traumatic events and determining the significance of these events to the individual. Group therapy, family or marital therapy may also be used, if indicated.

Disorders of Impulse

The *essential features* of disorders of impulse control are:

i. *Failure to resist,* an impulse, drive or temptation to perform same act that is harmful to the individual or others.

ii. *An increasing sense of tension:* Before committing the act.

iii. *An experience of either pleasure, gratification or release:* At the time of committing the act.

a. *Kleptomania:* The diagnostic feature is a recurrent failure to resist impulses to steal objects that are for immediate use or their monetary value; the objects taken are either given away, returned surreptitiously or kept and hidden.

Epidemiology

Little is known about the epidemiology of kleptomania. The age at onset may be as early as childhood.

Clinical Picture

The individual experiences an increasing sense of tension before committing the act and intense gratification while committing it. The diagnosis is not made if the stealing is due to conduct disorder or antisocial personality disorder.

The individual often displays signs of depression, anxiety and guilt.

Etiology

Kleptomania is believed to be dominated by the Oedipus complex, which is certainly far from accident. There is also an association of stealing with psycho-

social stress. To punish others by punishing themselves; hysterical secondary gain; or in the newly poor, to keep up appearances.

Differential Diagnosis

Ordinary stealing, malingering, conduct disorder, antisocial personality disorder or mania, schizophrenia, organic mental disorders.

Management

The only treatment reasonably well documented in the literature is psychoanalysis. There are reports of treating kleptomaniacs with systematic desensitization and a covert punishing contingency respectively.

b. *Pyromania*

- Deliberate and purposeful fire-setting on more than one occasion.
- Increased tension or affective arousal immediately before setting the fire.
- Fascination with, interest in, curiosity about or attraction to fire.
- Intense pleasure, gratification or relief when setting fires or witnessing.
- Fire setting is not done for monetary gain, as an expression of sociopolitical ideology, to conceal criminal activity, to express anger or vengeance, to improve one's living circumstances, or in response to a delusion or hallucination.

Pyromania has been described as '"*motivationless arson*".

Epidemiology

Onset is usually in childhood. The disorder is diagnosed far more commonly in males than females.

Clinical Picture

Individuals are recognized as regular *"watchers"* at fires in their neighbourhoods, frequently set off false alarms and show interest in fire-fighting paraphernalia.

Etiology

A symbolic solution to his conflict between instinct and reality. *Sigmund freud* considered fire setting as a masturbatory equivalent with homosexual features.

Differential Diagnosis

i. Young children's experimentation and fascination.
ii. Conduct disorder, antisocial personality disorder.
iii. Schizophrenia.
iv. Organic mental disorder.

Management

Psychoanalysis has been reported as a successful treatment in some cases.

Most behavioral researchers have used aversive therapy to treat fire setters, although some have used positive reinforcement with threats of punishment, stimulus satiation and operant structured fantasies with positive reinforcement.

American Psychiatric Association. *Diagnostic and Statistical Manual of Mental Disorders.* 4th edn. (DSM-IV). Washington DC: APA, 1994.

Bhatia MS. *Essentials of Psychiatry.* New Delhi: CBS Publishers and Distributors, 2004.

Sadock BJ, Sadock VA (eds). *Kaplan and Sadock's Synopsis of Psychiatry.* 9th edn. Baltimore: Lippincott-Williams & Wilkins, 2003.

World Health Organization. *International Classification of Mental and Beahavioural Disorders.* Geneva, WHO, 1992.

5.8 EATING DISORDERS

Anorexia Nervosa

Anorexia nervosa (AN) is a disorder characterized by a preoccupation with body weight and food: behavior directed towards losing weight; peculiar patterns of handling food, weight loss; intense fear of gaining weight, disturbance of body image and in women, amenorrhea.

Epidemiology: Indian studies are lacking but other studies have found a prevalence of 113.1 per 100,000 (203.9 for female and 16.9 for male residents) in Rochester. Its lifetime prevalence was estimated to be 5.2% in females while 0% in men.

Clinical features: The term "anorexia nervosa" is a *misnomer* as the patient with this disorder may neither show "anorexia" (i.e. decreased appetite) nor be "nervous". These patients suffer from a range of abnormalities including behavior, cognition, perception, emotions and physical functioning.

The DSM-IV TR criteria for anorexia nervosa are

a. Refusal to maintain body weight at or above a minimally normal weight for age and height (e.g. weight loss leading to maintenance of body weight less than 85% of expected; or failure to make expected weight gain during period of growth, leading to body weight less than 85% of that expected)
b. Intense fear of gaining weight or becoming fat, even though underweight.
c. Disturbance in the way in which one's body weight or shape is experienced, undue influence of body weight or shape on self-evaluation, or denial of seriousness of current low body weight.
d. In postmenarchal females, amenorrhoea, i.e. the absence of at least three consecutive menstrual cycles.

Comorbidity and complications: It is frequently comorbid with anxiety and mood disorders and also, anxious personality disorder, psychosis and mental retardation.

Differential diagnosis: Table 5.8.

Management: The immediate aim of treatment is to restore the patient's nutritional state to normal
a. *Behavioral therapy:* Most behavior therapy programmes follow an operant conditioning, with positive reinforcement, negative reinforcement or response prevention technique is applied.
b. *Drug treatment:* Antidepressants (newer and classical) are also frequently been used in the treatment. Lithium is *contraindicated* in patients who vomit or abuse laxatives.
c. *Family therapy:* Parental conflicts in one-third to one-half of anorectic families require appropriate attention.
d. *Individual psychotherapy:* Individual psychotherapy should focus on making the patients aware of their behavior and the effect it has on maintaining their illness.
e. *Electroconvulsive therapy:* ECT is preferred as a life saving measure, when a patient is grossly emaciated and often dehydrated, and adamantly refuses to eat or drink, or persistently vomits back everything she ingests. ECT is given to lift depression and improve the patient's emotional state.

Bulimia Nervosa

Bulimia nervosa (BN) was first recognized in 1970 as a disorder and the first case was published by Russel.

Epidemiology: British study found that incidence of 6.6 per lac population.

Etiology: The etiology of bulimia nervosa is uncertain. There are a few predisposing factors that are known, e.g. being female, adolescence, personal or family history of obesity, presence of mood disorder and genetic factors. It also appears that strong esthetic ideas for thinness, profession that requires keeping the body in perfect shape, large capacity stomach and lesser secretion of cholecystokinin from intestine (that leads to satiety) and personality types particularly the affective-perfectionist cluster.

Clinical features: The DSM-IV TR criteria for bulimia nervosa are:

a. Recurrent episodes of binge eating. An episode of binge eating is characterized by both of the following:
   1. Eating in discrete period of time (e.g. within any 2-hr period) an amount of food that is definitely larger than most people would eat during a similar period of time and circumstances.

Table 5.8: Differential diagnosis of eating disorders

Feature	Obesity	Anorexia nervosa	Bulimia	Pica	Rumination
Age Group	20–50	12–20	15–30	1.5 to 6 children	3–12 mo or young (yr)
Sex ratio	More in females	91–96% females	5–10 times in females	Young children—equal: Older—more in girls	Equal
Prevalence (%)	30–60% of American adults	Not known (rare) 0.2 to 11 per lac	1.8–13	10–32	Not known
Social class	Lower	Upper and middle	Upper and middle	Lower	Lower
Etiology	Not known (? Metabolic signal theory? Genetic factors or brain damage? Developmental or emotional determinants;? Endocrine disorders or drugs)	Not known (? Phobic avoidance response? Personality or familial predisposition? Norepinephrine and/or dopamine depletion? Endocrine disturbance	Not known ? HPA axis defect ? Positive reinforcement? Variant of psychomotor epilepsy?	Not known (? Disturbed Parent–child interaction? Zinc or iron deficiency? Cultural practice)	Lower (ANS dysfunction? Disturbed parent–child interaction?
Core symptom	Overweight (40 to 100% of average weight)	Fear of becoming obese	Binge eating with fear or becoming obese	Eating of non-edible substance (commonly dirt)	Repeated regurgitation of food
Complications	CVS problems (hypertension, hyperlipidemia) GIP problems (Gall stones, hernias), Metabolic problems Diabetes mellitus, (Gout). Malignancy (Colorectal, prostate in males, ovarian uterine, cervical, breast in females	Starvation, hypotension, hypothermia, circulatory collapse	Physical: Hypokalemia dehydration, parotitis, caries, etc. Physiological" depression, impulsivity, adjustment problems	Physical: Lead poisoning Intestinal obstruction, hypocalcemia Psychological: Mental retardation	Physical: Dehydration, malnutrition. Physiological: Maternal neglect, developmental delays
Diagnostic criteria	Stunkard Brownell	DSM-IV, ICD-10	DSM-IV, Russell	DSM-IV	DSM-IV
Differential diagnosis	Fluid retention, due to cardiac, hepatic or renal disease	Depression, somatization disorder, Bulimia Schizophrenia Medical illness	Anorexia nervosa Schizophrenia Neurological disorders	Cultural practice Mental retardation, zince or iron deficiency	Congenital, anomalies like pyloric stenosis hiatus hernia
Main treatment	Behavior therapy (BT)	BT	BT	BT	BT
Associated treatment	Diet, exercise Drugs or surgery	Family therapy	Individual or groups therapy Drugs like antidepressants, etc.	Environmental manipulation. Treatment of zinc or iron deficiency.	Surgery

2. A sense of lack of control over eating during the episode (e.g. a feeling that one can not stop eating or control what or how much one is eating)

b. Recurrent inappropriate compensatory behavior in order to prevent weight gain, such as self-induced vomiting; misuse of laxatives, diuretics, enemas, or medications; fasting or; excessive exercise.

c. The binge eating and inappropriate compensatory behaviors both occur, on average, at least twice a wk for 3 mo.

d. Self-evaluation is unduly influenced by body shape and weight.

e. The disturbance does not occur exclusively during episodes of anorexia nervosa.

Medical complications and co-morbidity, Table 5.8.

Differential diagnosis, Table 5.8.

Treatment: Goals of treatment are to terminate abnormal behaviors as early as possible and completely.

The treatment begins with the estimation of medical status of the patient. Since medical complications can be life-threatening, they must be dealt first. In such cases opinion of physician must be taken and according to need patient must be hospitalized.

Cognitive behavior therapy (CBT) is the treatment of choice for core symptoms. It focuses on the distorted ideas about shape, size of the body, rigid rules regarding food consumption, pressure to diet and triggers of episodes. It is highly structured and usual duration is 3–6 mo.

SSRI are also commonly used for the treatment and commonly Fluoxetine in doses up to 60 mg/day used. Sibutramine has also been tried in binge eating disorder and it is well tolerated.

Efficacy of transcranial magnetic stimulation has also been described in bulimia.

Other Eating Disorders

Food avoidance emotional disorder (FAED): Described by Higgs et al in 1989, it has not been given due attention, it deserved. This condition is described in children and adolescents who have a disorder of emotions in which food avoidance play a prominent part but there is a failure to meet diagnostic criteria of anorexia nervosa. Other symptoms of emotional disorder are present such as depression, obsessional behavior or school attendance difficulties. Whether FAED is an independent disorder or intermediate between anorexia nervosa and emotional disorder of childhood, or a partial syndrome of anorexia nervosa, with less severe symptoms, is exactly not known.

Selective eating: This term is applied to those children and adolescents who have for many years had a very restricted range of foods. Typically they eat three or four different foods, usually carbohydrate based, such as biscuits, potatoes and bread. Initially they present as food fads, but unlike other faddy children, their range of foods does not increase. Often they present to the pediatrician or psychiatrist between the ages of about 8 to 12, because of parental concern about their child's health. These children are within normal range of weight and height but their social functioning is disturbed due to their concerns about eating. These children do not show any benefit from treatment aimed at increasing their range of foods, but with the guidance of parents, their social problems can be removed.

Pervasive refusal syndrome: Lask et al described this condition in girls between ages of 8 and 14 and is manifested by a profound and pervasive refusal to eat, drink, walk, talk or indulge in any form of self-care. Initially these children present with features fairly typical of anorexia nervosa, but food avoidance is gradually becomes generalized, with a marked fear response. There is no separate category for these children, but the intense and frightened avoidance behavior suggests the possibility of post-traumatic stress disorder. Some of these cases might be victims of physical and sexual violence, and had been silenced by repeated threats. This syndrome further leads to avoidance of participation and problems in self-care and communication.

Bryant-Waugh R, Lasj B. Annotation: Eating disorders in children. *J Child Psychol Psychiat* 1995; 36:191–206.

Higgs J, Goodyer I, Birch J. Anorexia nervosa and food avoidance emotional disorder. *Arch Dis Child* 1989; 64: 346–51.

Lask B, Britten C, Kroll L, Magagna J, Tranter M. Pervasive refusal in children. *Arch Dis Child* 1991;66:866–9.

Lucas AR, Beard CM, O'Fallon WM, Kurland LT. Anorexia nervosa in Rochester, Minnesota: a 45-year study. *Mayo Clin Proc* 1988; 63(5): 433–42.

Taraldsen KW, Eriksen L, Gotestam KG. Prevalence of eating disorders among Norwegian women and men in a psychiatric outpatient unit. *Int J Eat Disord* Sep 1996; 20(2):185–90.

5.9 SLEEP PROBLEMS

Proper sleep is considered one that is adequate in duration, is good quality and refreshing. Quality of sleep also varies and is dependent upon the corporal and environmental factors. Since quality of sleep differs from person to person and is dependent upon one's expectations regarding sleep, hence 'refreshing' sleep is the surrogate marker. Refreshing means that one is able to work in best of his capacity after leaving the bed provided he is not having any other problem. In essence, one must seek the advice from the physician when he is not able to get the refreshing sleep.

Prevalence: Majority of adolescents are sleeping one hour less than required duration in the respective age and it is culminating in their school performance. Western data show that at a given time around 15% persons in a given community suffer from insomnia.

Etiology: Environmental factors, e.g. extremes of temperature, poor sleeping place, overcrowded room, mosquitoes, noisy surroundings, poor ventilation, bright lighting may cause non refreshing sleep. Medical disorders, e.g. pain anywhere in the body, difficulty breathing in lying down situation, certain brain tumors, e.g. psychiatric disorders, e.g. primary insomnia, depression, stress, anxiety, e.g. frequently changing work shifts or time zones, strange surroundings, e.g. substance dependence, e.g. sleeping pills, alcohol, cannabis, and cocaine, may cause or contribute to the illness.

Perpetuating factors include cognitive and behavioral factors. Negative conditioning with the sleeping environment is an important issue. Insomnia sufferers in absence of proper guidance and quick relief adopt some antagonistic behaviors, e.g. changing sleep schedule, sleeping pills, heavy intake of caffeine during waking period, performing activities in the bed for which it is not meant, e.g. reading books, watching television, lying wake up in the bed waiting for the sleep.

Management: The evaluation starts with the information regarding your complaints and includes complete physical examination, systemic examination, psychiatric evaluation and sometimes laboratory investigations. We will not go into details of all these. Sleep promoting behaviors are also called, good sleep hygiene and they are helpful not only therapy of the insomnia but also its prevention. These are mentioned in Table 5.9.

Stimulus control therapy: In this therapy, patient is asked to follow simple instructions as follows:

a. Use the bed for sleeping only
b. Leave the bed when not able to sleep
c. Indulge in relaxing exercises while out of bed, and
d. Lastly, when feels sleepy, go to bed. This therapy has proven very effective when instituted in the right candidates and does not include any kind of pill-popping.

Sleep-restriction therapy: This therapy increases the internal sleep pressure and thus helps in achieving the normal sleep wake cycle. For example, if you spend 8 hr in bed and sleep for five hours only, your time in bed is reduced to 5 hr only. When you are able to sleep for approximately 90% of your time in bed (determined by sleep diaries), time in bed is increased gradually.

Cognitive behavior therapy: In coordination with the patient, these beliefs are identified and then challenged gradually. This therapy can be combined with any of the above mentioned methods to achieve total control over the situation.

Pharmacological management: Newer hypnotic drugs, e.g. zolpidem, eszopiclone, zopiclone, are preferred drugs (as they cause no hangover or withdrawal, produce low dependence, and there are few drug interactions.

Barker P. *Basic Child Psychiatry*. Oxford: Blackwell, 1994.

Sadock BJ, Sadock VA (eds.). *Kaplan and Sadock's Synopsis of Psychiatry*. 9th edn. Baltimore: Lippincott-Williams Wilkins, 2003.

Singhal PK, Bhatia MS. *Problems of Behaviour in children*. Delhi: CBS Publishers & Distributors, 1994; 15–37.

5.10 DISORDERS OF MOVEMENTS

The disorders of movements are listed in Box 5.1. Characteristics of different problems of movements are documented in Table 5.10.

Gilles de la Tourette's disorder: A type of tic disorder characterized by both multiple motor and one or more vocal tics which occur many times a day (usually in

Table 5.9: Helpful guidelines for proper sleep	
Do's	*Don'ts*
Maintain a regular sleep-wake schedule	Do not take caffeinated beverages/coffee/tea before four hr of bed
Should take adequate amount of food before going to bed	Do not indulge in heavy exercise before going to bed
Indulge in physical exercises during the day	Avoid daytime naps
Take balanced diet	Surrounding environment should not be crowded, very cold or hot, noisy, etc.
Go to bed only when sleepy	Avoid alcohol close to bedtime
Always leave the bed at the same time in the morning	Avoid doing your work in the bed
	Should not be hungry or do not eat too much in the dinner
	Do not watch TV while in bed

<table>
<tr><td>

Box 5.1: Disorders of movements

Head banging
Breath holding spells
Temper tantrums
Attention deficit hyperkinetic disorder
Tic disorders

</td></tr>
</table>

bouts) nearly everyday or intermittently throughout a period of 1 yr. The onset is usually before age 21 yr and it is not during CNS stimulant drug abuse or neurological disease, e.g. Huntington's chorea and post viral encephalitis. The anatomic location number, frequency, complexity and severity change over time.

Bhatia MS, Malik SC. Attention Deficit Hyperactivity Disorder among pediatric outpatients. *J Child Psychol Psychiatry* 1991;32:297–306.

Bhatia MS, Choudhary S, Sidana A. Attention Deficit Hyperactivity Disorder among pediatric outpatients. *Indian Pediatr* 1999;36:583–7.

Cantwell DP. *Genetic Studies of Hyperactive Children*. In: Fieve R R, Rosenthal D, Brill H (eds). Genetic Research in Psychiatry. Baltimore, John Hopkins University Press, 1975.

Comings DE, Coming BG. Tourette syndrome: Clinical and psychological aspects of 250 cases. *Am J Human Gen* 1985;37: 435–50.

5.11 PROBLEMS OF HABIT

The common habit disorders are:
a. Thumb sucking
b. Nail biting
c. Pica
d. Trichotillomania (hair-plucking).

The characteristics of these disorder are listed in Table 5.11.

Bhatia MS, Singhal PK, Nigam VR, Malik SC. Nail Biting-An Analysis of 160 children. *Indian Med Gaztte* 1989;5:188–91.

Bhatia MS, Singhal PK, Rastogi V, Dhar NK and Nigam VR. Clinical profile of trichotillomania. *J Indian Med Assoc* 1991; 89:137–8.

Singhal PK, Bhatia MS. *Problems of Behaviour in children*. Delhi, CBS Publishers & Distributors, 1994;15–37.

Singhal PK, Bhatia MS, Dhar NK, Nigam VR. Habit disorders-prevalence and etiology. *Indian Pediatr* 1987; 24: 475–479.

Singhal PK, Bhatia MS, Nigam VR and Bhatia N. Thumb Sucking: An Analysis of 150 cases. *Indian Pediatr* 1988; 25: 647–53.

5.12 PROBLEMS OF TOILET TRAINING

Enuresis (Bed-wetting)

Enuresis (bed-wetting) a common symptom of childhood and adolescence, has been a problem in most cultures for centuries. Enuresis refers to the wetting of one's clothes or one's bed, past the age of *five years*. If the child has never attained bladder control, it is called *primary enuresis* and if the child has once attained the bladder control for about one year and then gets this disease, it is known as *Secondary Enuresis*. Bed-wetting is repetitive, inappropriate, involuntary passage of urine.

Epidemiology: It is found in all countries and races, in all socioeconomic groups, in both sexes, afflicts those who are of normal and subnormal intelligence.

It is estimated that 3–7% of children (3% girls, 7% boys) wet at the age of five while in adults, the prevalence varies from 0.5 to 3.8%. 80% of enuretics wet only during night while 15% during day and night and rest during day only. More common in males and in winter, enuresis is often familial and seen more in children coming from joint families.

Etiology: The psychological, social and biological components appear to contribute to the problem in varying proportions. The causes can be classified as:

i. *Genetic:* Enuresis is more common in children who have family history of this problem in parents or siblings. It is also more prevalent in mentally retarded children.

ii. *Psychological:*
   • Separation from parents.
   • Disturbed family (marital disharmony, etc.).
   • Death or illness of a parent.
   • School phobia.
   • Birth of a sibling.
   • Excessive anxiety or depression.
   • Anger, punishment or rejection from caretakers.

iii. *Physiological*
   • Delayed or lax or coercive toilet training

iv. *Organic*
   • Metabolic causes like diabetes mellitus.
   • Worms infestation.
   • Urinary obstruction (e.g. posterior urethral valves) and infection (common in females).
   • Epilepsy and sleep disorders.
   • Deformities like spina bifida, weak bladder musculature, etc.

This problem is commonly associated with other psychological conditions like sleep-walking, sleep talking, night terrors (fearful dreams), encopresis (involuntary passage of feces), thumb sucking, etc.

Complications and impairment: The degree of impairment is primarily a function of the individual's self esteem, the degree of social ostracism by peers and anger, punishment and rejection from caretakers. Enuretic children are more prone to urinary infection (pyelonephritis).

	Head banging	Breath holding spells	Temper tantrums	Hyperkinetic syndrome	Tic disorder
Epidemiology	Incidence— 20–30% (more in younger children) Common group 11–14 mo More common in boys, first born	Relatively uncommon. Common in 1–5 yr of age. (Begins usually before 18 mo of age). Common in girls, and those from lower social class and unclear families	20–25 in 2–12 yr. Common up to first five yr. Peak age 3–5 yr. More common in boys, first born and of joint families. More common in boys, first born and of joint families.	1–5% of all children Usually starts before age of 3 yr 6–10 times more in boys Common in children of lower socioeconomic strata	12–20% children. Peak 5–7 yr. Boys: girls: 3 : 1 Facial tics commonest followed by neck, eye, leg tics
Etiology	Exact unknown tension relieving device, to gain pleasure to neutralize pain of teething Mean to gratify or seek attention Result of discomfort or frustration *Precipitants:* fear, loss of joy, teething period, institutionalization, separation from parent	*Multifactorial parental factors* over solicitatious, strict, separation, or marital discord, etc. *Child personality.* Generally active, energetic, obstinate, using attention seeking devices. *Others:* Fear, punishment, social deprivation *Precipitants:*Anger, frustration fall, pain, fear, birth of a sibling, iron deficiency	*Parental factors* overprotection, overindulgence inconsistency *Child personality* Active, determined, energetic, when in period of resistance, imitativeness, fear of insecurity. *Others:* Sibling jealousy, physical illness, psychosocial problems in family, postnatal trauma	*Multifactorial Genetic:* about 1/3 have family history. *CNS:* maturational lag, CNS damage, (fever, trauma) *Biochemical* Altered homeostasis in epinephrine metabolism; imbalance related to dopamine *Emotional:* Disturbed or inadequate family neglect, overprotection	*Multifactorial Genetic:* 10–15% have family history *CNS:* Defect in striopallidal connections *Biochemical:* Increased dopaminergic activity in corpus striatum *Emotional:* Ambitious over-expecting parents strictness, overprotection, neglect
Clinical features	Rocking, head banging, crying, obstinancy, refusal of feeds	Violent crying, followed by arrest of respiration, usually lead to pallor (pallid type) and also cyanosis (cyanotic type)	*Precipitants:* Not meeting demands, interruption of play, threat of abandonment, meeting a stranger, criticism imitation	Inattentiveness, distractibility, impulsivity, hyperactivity, impairment in visuospatial tasks	*Precipitants:* Tension, anger frustration Infections (sinusitis, conjunctivitis in facial tics, encephalitis)
Complications	Head injury, meeting accidents, social embarrassment to parents	Seizures, brain damage, unconsciousness	Screening, hammering, stamping feet, thrashing arms, kicking, thrusting on the floor, strikes people, throws	Learning difficulties (school failure), conduct disorders tantrums,	Grimacing writing grunting, sighing, blinking, writhing hands, wrinkling or scra-

(Contd.)

Table 5.10: Characteristics of different problems of movements (*Contd.*)

	Head banging	*Breath holding spells*	*Temper tantrums*	*Hyperkinetic syndrome*	*Tic disorder*
			things, abuses Breaking things, injuries, head injury	accidents, drug abuses	tching nose, thigh rubbing. Personality, social, physical and learning problems.
Differential diagnosis	Mental retardation, conduct disorder epilepsy, organic lesions, tantrums, hyperkinetic syndrome	Epilepsy, respiratory, or heart problems, tetany	Hyperkinetic syndrome, mental retardation, epilepsy	Mental retardation, conduct disorder, epilepsy	Focal epilepsy, hyperkinetic syndrome
Management	Ceases spontaneously replacement of rhythmic movement with a rhythmic auditory stimulus such as metronome. Helmet for protection Sedative tranquilizers in some cases. Changes in parental attitudes	Ceases spontaneously Tapping on the back to break apnea, avoid injuries. Removal of precipitants Change in parental attitudes. Iron therapy in iron deficient cases	Ceases with age Remove underlying insecurity, overprotection, or faulty parental attitude. Cut down opportunities for resistance ignore	Ceases in most cases with age Drugs—CNS stimulants (amphetamine, methylphenidate, pemoline), neuroleptics, antidepressants. Behavior and situational manipulation Avoid chocolate, synthetic drinks, tea, coffee, food additives, etc.	Drugs—haloperidol, pimozide clonidine, nifedipine Behavior modification—self training, relaxation techniques, biofeedback. Treat situational difficulties or any physical problems

Table 5.11: Characteristics of important habit disorders

	Thumb (finger) sucking	*Nail biting*	*Pica*	*Trichotillomania*
Definition	Habit of putting thumb into the mouth most of the time. (Usually diagnosed after 3 yr of age)	Habit of biting (or eating) nails most of the time. (Usually diagnosed after 3 yr of age)	Eating of non-edible substances (e.g. mud, plaster, cloth, paper, pencils). Usually diagnosed after the age of 18 mo	The irresistible urge to pull (pluck) one's hair
Epidemiology	Earliest and commonest form of habit disorders (peak age 4–7 mo) 15–20% in 3–12 yr (prevalence decreases with age). More common in boys especially those of upper (middle and upper) socioeconomic class	7–12% of children in 3–12 yr. Peak age 5–7 yr, 13–15 yr. More common in females. Found in all socioeconomic classes and prevalence falls with age	25–30% in 1–2 yr of children. Peak age 20–26 mo. More common in males Prevalence falls with age. More common in lower socioeconomic classes	Relatively uncommon in 0.05–0.1%. Exact details not known. More common in females (especially with long hair). Found in all socioeconomic classes

(Contd.)

Table 5.11: Characteristics of important habit disorders (*Contd.*)

	Thumb (finger) sucking	Nail biting	Pica	Trichotillomania
Etiology	*Devolment* A gratifying action especially under unpleasant and unsatisfying feeding situation *Psychological* A model of infantile sexual manifestation (freud) correlate with adulthood desire for perverse kissing, smoking and drinking	*Development* Common in the biting, teething stage as gratifying oral habit *Psychological* Unconscious and displaced form of masturbatory activity	*Cultural acceptance* In pregnant mother, and as a cure of many GIT problems, mud eating is common and may be seen in young children *Organic* Mental retardation, iron deficiency, lead poisoning, etc.	*Psychological* Parent child conflict *Organic* Mental retardation
Precipitants	Neglect, strictness of parents, over-protection, loneliness, rivalry, boredom, etc.	Parental neglect, strictness, stress (of exam), excessive fear	Neglect, parental disharmony, strictness, sibling rivalry, separation from present	Pica, inadequate emotional satisfaction, loneliness, boredom, stress of exam, parental discord, separation, anxiety
Complications	Teething problems, respiratory and GIT infections	Worm infestation, cholera, enteric, respiratory infections	Lead poisoning, worm infestation, cholera, typhoid, constipation	Alopecia, trichobezoar (hair ball in stomach), intestinal obstruction
Treatment	Most children grow out of his habit by age 5 or 6 yr or by removal of precipitants. Behavior modification (promise of a reward, wearing gloves)	Identification and removal of causes of tensions. Distraction (by preoccupation with toys and children) Behavior modification	Identify and remove precipitants. Change in parental attitudes Oral substitutions in child	Identify and remove the cause. Distraction and avoid wearing cap and hairy toys

Very often the individual feels ashamed or embarrassed and may wish to avoid situations that might lead to embarrassment, such as camp or overnight visits to relatives and friends.

Management: The various modes of treatment available are:

i. *Parental counseling:* To avoid psychological factors leading to this problem like separation from parents, parental neglect, marital disharmony, excessive punishment to children, criticism in front of others, etc. The toilet-training should be given properly and should be started by the age of two years. In mentally retarded children, the toilet training can be delayed to five years of age.

ii. *Behavior modification methods:* Mowrer and Mowrer devised an apparatus (available also in India) in 1938, consisting of an *alarm buzzer* which could be set off by the discharge of urine onto a detector circuit and child wakes up from sleep to pass urine at a proper place. Good results have been reported in as much as 70–85% children with this device.

iii. *Drugs:* The drugs like Oxybutynin (2.5 to 5 mg 2 to 4 times/d), desmopressin, imipramine (25–50 mg, avoided in children below 6 yr), etc. can be given during bed time.

iv. *Situational manipulation:* These include waking the child during course of the night, restricting fluids (water, milk, etc.) atleast 1–2 hr before sleep and avoiding certain kinds of spices or nutrients (lemon juice, tea, sweets, etc.).

The other methods like penile ligatures, rubber bags inserted into the vagina, pelvic elevation, burning the sacrum, etc. should be avoided because they lead to many fatal complications.

Encopresis (Soiling)

Encopresis has been a common clinical problem in children. It involves repeated, involuntary evacuation of feces into clothing without gross organic cause after the age of four years, with or without constipation. The other terms which are commonly used to describe this condition are "soiling", 'bowel accidents', 'incontinentia alvi', 'psychogenic megacolon', etc.

Epidemiology: The prevalence of encopresis among children is 4 to 8 percent. It is three to four times more common among boys than girls. World Health Organization (WHO) has put the maximum age of normal bowel control as four years. Encopresis is more common in children of age group 4 to 8 yr. Encopresis is more common in the first child, where there is family history and in children belonging to lower classes, socially and emotionally incompetent or disorganized families.

Types: Encopresis can be *continuous type* (never trained, an aggressive, overactive, shameless, child from a lax, dirty, lower socioeconomic class family; also called primary infantile encopresis), *discontinuous type* (once toilet trained but soils later in response to stress, a neurotic, inhibited, ashamed child from a rigid, compulsive, higher class family; also called primary reactive encopresis) and *retentive soilers* (also called secondary retentive type).

In a study conducted at Kalawati Saran Children's Hospital, Delhi, encopresis was found to be commonly associated with enuresis in 60–70% children. Other habit disorders like thumb sucking, nail biting, truancy, tics, refusal, temper tantrums, head rolling, sleep and speech disturbances, stomach aches are also commonly seen among soilers. Night encopresis is very rare.

Etiology: Several researchers have noted a high rate of language disorder and characteristic findings of maturational lag (difficulty in controlling bodily functions, channeling aggressive impulses or problems in the use of verbal and symbolic behaviour) in children who have family history of encopresis. Children may become encopretic in presence of fever, dyspepsia, anal fissure, diarrhoea, abuse of laxatives, calcium and potassium deficiency, after operation, spinal cord injury, colonic atony, worms manifestation, tuberculosis, spasticity of anal sphincter, chronic obstipation, etc. Unpleasant or coercive toilet training, an unsatisfactory relationship to the familial environment, separation from the mother, birth of a sibling, start of school, poor peer relationship, tense or step mothers, negativism and possibly, a maturational lag, all combine to produce this syndrome.

Clinical features: In primary encopretics, the frequency of soiling varies from once to several times daily, whereas the secondary soilers have episodes of two to three times weekly. Nocturnal encopresis is very rare and during the day, it occurs at school, on the way home from school, or at home and in proximity of the mother. Most encopretics are tense, easily frightened children, very prone to anxiety reactions and with poor self-esteem, body image, marked passivity, difficulty in self-assertion and excessive hostility. Encopretic children are usually pale, poorly coordinated with a sickly, asthenic look. Withdrawn and stubborn, they spend little time with peers. Characteristically, the encopretic child refuses to use a pot or toilet or postpones such use. Usually, the consistency of the feces is normal but when retention of feces is present, a foul smelling fluid can be discharged.

A five-year-old girl, Meena, unwanted even before birth, whose domineering, obsessively clean mother nagged her to go to the toilet, refused to give her foods eaten by the rest of the family, demanded unnatural quiet, and would scold and strike the child at any resistance or disobedience, mother trained her at the age of two years; obedience and cleanliness were demanded with threats of sending her to an institution. Though constipation was present for many years, encopresis was precipitated by starting schools, an event equated by the child with desertion by the mother and placement in an institution.

Management

i. *General measures:* Toilet training should be started at an appropriate age (between two and three years of age) and coercive toilet training should be avoided. The violent maternal response to toilet accidents by these children can also paralyse learning.

The use of enemas, large doses of laxatives are undesirable. The measures like anal strapping, putting foreign bodies into the rectum should be discouraged because it can lead to fatal complications.

ii. *Specific measures:* Any contributory organic factors should be ruled out. The key pediatric approach is to advise the parents to ignore the incontinence and so to reduce pressure on the child, to avoid unnecessary discussion with the child, and to stop record keeping and tallying. Around 10 percent children improve within a few wk.

The psychotherapy (with child and parents) and eventual interpretation of conflicts relieves the psychological stress.

Telling parents about proper age and correct method of toilet training and about diet and mild laxatives is useful.

Behavior modification through the introduction, rearrangement or withdrawal of reinforcement contingencies is very effective. Examples of such reinforcers are social, maternal, token and activity. Reinforcers have been hugs, praise, attention, goodies to eat, pennies, books, coupons, toys and freedom of movement. By careful temporal patterning of toilet after meals, during situations correlated with high incidence of soiling, the desired behavior occurs and can be reinforced. The various drugs like imipramine (25–75 mg daily), tincture belladona (one to two tea spoons daily), etc. have been used with good results.

Bhatia MS, Dhar NK, Rai S, Malik SC. Enuresis: an analysis of 82 cases. *Indian J Med Sci* 1990;12:337–42.

Bhatia MS, Singhal PK, Dhar NK, Bohra N, Malik SC, Mullick DN. Family and the pattern of childhood psychiatric problems. *Indian Practitioner* 1990;43:893–900.

Bhatia MS, Singhal PK, Dhar NK, Rai S, Nigam VR, Malik SC. Encopresis: A review of 40 cases. *Indian Practitioner* 1990; 42:971–5.

Singhal PK, Bhatia MS. Drugs in childhood psychiatric disorders. *Indian Pediatr* 1994;28:537–49.

Singhal PK, Bhatia MS. *Problems of Behaviour in children.* Delhi, CBS Publishers & Distributors, 1994;15–37.

6 Social Issues and Special Health Needs

6.1 ADOPTION

Adoption is a social, emotional, and legal process that provides a new family for children when the birth family is unable or unwilling to parent. Over the past several years, there have been significant increases in the number of children adopted from the foster care system. International adoptions have increased substantially in the recent years. Infant is a gift from God but there are a number of incidents of infants being thrown into garbage dump, hidden at such places where they can be bitten or chewed by all sorts of animals, insects, reptiles, etc. or may even die due to unbearable atmospheric conditions. Restoring to such type of horrifying abandonment of a newly born is indeed uncalled for especially when surrendering of the child can be done with a recognized/licensed adoption agency. By doing so, you are sure that your child will survive and you can take him/her back in your households, if you so desire. The recognized adoption agencies provide useful counseling to the person(s) who is bent upon surrendering their child. Even counseling is kept confidential. There are instances when the parent(s)/guardian(s) change their idea of surrendering after counseling. So never abandon a baby, but if you must, do it in a secure place of a recognized/licensed adoption agency, a list of which is available www.adoptionindia.nic.in. Remember you have the right to reclaim the baby within 60 days of surrender at the recognized/licensed adoption agency. There is a Central Adoption Resource Authority (CARA) (An autonomous body of the Ministry of Women and Child Development, Govt. of India, Delhi).

Adoption is the legal act of permanently placing a child with a parent or parents other than the birth (or "biological") mother or father. An adoption order has the effect of severing the parental responsibilities and rights of the birth parents and transferring those responsibilities and rights onto the adoptive parent(s). After the finalization of an adoption, there is no legal difference between adopted children and those born to the parents (Table 6.1).

Adoption from India: India has a long history of adoption to the United States. Because of economic conditions, many children are relinquished to orphanages by parents who are unable to provide for them. Children's Hope International (CHI) works with several well-run and respected orphanages. The children are cared for by dedicated and loving staff members.

India has established a governmental body that regulates adoptions. Only agencies approved by India's central government may place children, and only agencies enlisted by India's central government may receive children for their applicant families. Our office in Oregon has such a license from the government of India.

Families must travel to bring their children to the United States. Escorts will be allowed under extenuating circumstances. The prepared documents

Table 6.1: Do's/Don'ts for prospective adoptive parents (PAPs) in India

Do's	*Dont'ts*
• Adopt only from a recognised placement agency or LAPA or shishu greh (for the list, please visit the Website: http://www.adoptionindia.nic.in)	• Do not adopt from nursing homes or hospitals directly as it is illegal and will render you liable to legal action
• Obtain a copy of the receipt of your registration from the adoption agency	• Do not adopt from un-recognized agency or unrelated persons
• Pay adoption fee as prescribed under guidelines and obtain fee receipt (for details: www.adoptionindia.nic.in)	• Do not succumb to the demand for donation and any amount more than the prescribed adoption fees
• The consent of children above 6 years should be taken for the adoption	• Take informed decision based on facts made available to you
• Ask for doing home study report (within 2 months from Registration)	
• The child study report with PER should be signed by both adoptive parents	

are sent over, a court hearing is done in which guardianship of the child is granted to the adoptive parents, and the child can then travel home.

Important information: Once you have said yes to a particular child, your case will go to the Central Adoption Resource Agency (CARA) and then on to court. The child's picture, videos (when available) and medical information is forwarded to CHI and then on to you during the CARA approval and court process (approximately 6–9 mo). Once court approval is granted, traveling families will leave in about 5–6 wks to pick up their child. Both boys and girls are available for adoption. Most of the children have medium to dark skin, lovely big brown eyes, and Caucasian features. Little or nothing is known about the children's backgrounds. At the present time, it takes about 12 mo after all documents are submitted before there is a referral to families. You will receive your child approximately 6–9 mo later. (It can take longer if unforeseen circumstances occur such as strikes, holidays, vacations, and litigation.) You will travel to pick up your child, spending about a wk to 10 days in India. You will be assisted while in India to complete any required adoption processes. Legal custody of your child will be retained by the agency until the final adoption is completed in the US. This is required by law to ensure that the child will remain the legal responsibility of the agency. If the adoption is disrupted, the adoptive parent will be responsible for airfare for the child and an escort to travel to the child's new family. Post-placement supervisory visits by a licensed social worker are required prior to the finalization of the adoption. All children must be adopted in the US. Final adoption must be completed within 2 years. The adoptive parents are financially responsible for all adoption costs.

Box 6.1: Recommended screening tests for newly arriving adoptees

Infectious disease screening
Hepatitis B and C virus
HIV virus
Mantoux test
Treponema pallidum
Stool for ova, cyst and parasites
Other screening tests
Complete blood cell count
Thyroxine and thyroid stimulating hormone
Determination of lead levels
Determination of aspartate aminotransferase, alanine aminotransferase, bilirubin, and alkaline phosphatase
Urinalysis
Visual and hearing screening
Developmental testing
Other screening tests to consider depending on clinical findings and age of the child
Newborn screening including hemoglobin electrophoresis, glucose-6-phosphate dehydrogenase deficiency
Stool cultures for bacterial pathogens
Detection of *Helicobacter pylori* antibody or ^{13}C-urea breath test

Role of pediatricians: Pediatricians can help prospective adoptive parents evaluate the health and developmental history of a child and available background information from birth families in order to assess actual and potential problems or risks that children may have (Box 6.1). Adoption agencies obtain from birth mother and birth fathers information about their own health and genetic histories and the histories of their children so that this information can be shared with adoptive families. Assistance in evaluating the child's current status and future health risks should be provided.

Pediatricians also can promote positive adjustment of the child and family by providing guidance and support at all stages of the adoption. After the child is settled in the new home, pediatricians should encourage adoptive parents to seek a comprehensive assessment of the child's health and development. Most adopted children and families adjust well and lead healthy, productive lives.

Central Adoption Resource Authority (CARA), Ministry of Women & Child Development, West Block 8, Wing 2, 2nd Floor, R.K. Puram, New Delhi-110066 (India).

Central Adoption Resource Authority (CARA). (An autonomous body of the Ministry of Women and Child Development, Govt. of India, Delhi.Website: www.adoption-india.nic.in; Email: cara@bol.net.in.)

Simms MD, Freundlich M. Adoption. In: Kliegman RM, Behrman RE, Jenson HB, Stanton BF (eds). Nelson Textbook of Pediatrics. 18th edn. Vol 1. Philadelphia: Saunders, 2007; 163–4.

6.2 FOSTER CARE SERVICES

The objective of the Foster Care Services is to provide near home atmosphere of a foster family, to children who become destitute at a very early age. Home is the best place for the satisfaction of the physical, mental and emotional needs of the children, in the circumstances when the family is not in a position to provide care and security to the child it is advisable that he should be placed in an environment which is similar to the home. This is more important for child below 6 years, if an adoption of a destitute child cannot be readily arranged it would be desirable to place him with a foster family rather than in an institution. Children who enter foster care have high rates of medical, developmental, and mental health problems. Most children suffer from behavioral and adjustment problems.

Successful foster home placement requires provision of a fair amount of allowances for foster parents and a well developed machinery of case work, investigation and supervision. The process of matching of the family with the child according to his personality make-up is a difficult task. It needs to be handled only by a trained social worker having skills in the proper placement of children with families. Care is needed to ensure proper facilities of adjustments and development for the child frequent replacements on account of maladjustment can prove disastrous to the machinery and social growth of the child. The foster care placement, therefore, requires to be planned carefully on the basis of proper understanding of the child as well as the family.

The tradition and the custom of family life in India encourage adoption of children primarily within the same caste and/or religion. In the programme of Foster Care Services, efforts are made to find parents who have similar social atmosphere in their homes as that of the child. The matching of family with the requirement of the child is basic to Foster Care Services. In addition, the case worker who maintains the systematic follow-up with the families ensures that the child is properly taken care of and is provided with the facilities of development. If any difficulties are experienced by the child, the family is helped to correct the situation immediately by the case worker. Normally the foster care placement is to be confined to children below the age of 6 years. This is for two reasons. Families accept children at this tender age primarily with the motive of helping them. The relationship develops easily between the child at the tender age and the members of the foster family. The second reason is that the grown-up is likely to be exploited by some parents using his services for assistance in the home. This requires to be avoided under all circumstances. But if circumstances warrant the benefits of the scheme might be extended to children even up to the age of 12 years in exceptional cases, in the case of children of the age group 6–12 such penalties could be made available to them for further period. The Committee that is formed for selecting the foster parents should approve the list of parents in advance. Through an advertisement, the names of the families are cleared. The case worker makes visits to these families and ensures the proper atmosphere before placing any child with them. The list should be revised from time to time after proper scrutiny.

The Foster Care Services will be promoted with the help of voluntary child and family welfare organizations which have established high standard of services for children. The programme will be entrusted to them after ensuring the existence of adequate facilities for its promotion. Services of one Foster Care Organizer and one clerk-cum-cashier will be provided to the organization for dealing with 50 cases of children placed under Foster Care. In the initial stage a very sizeable number of families will have to be investigated to find out their suitability for placing children with them. As a practice, out of 5 families investigated, one family is selected for the placement of children.

The benefits of the foster care programme in India is available to beneficiaries in the metropolitan cities of Delhi, Mumbai, Kolkata and Chennai and also State/Union Territory capitals and other towns with a population of not less than two lakhs, if good voluntary organizations come forward for implementation of the programme.

In United States foster care home is a temporary home for children. Children in foster care home have clearly defined permanency goals (return home, placement with relatives, adoption) for 2 yr from the time they entered foster care and that there be periodic court reviews of children placements and progress toward their permanency goals. Adoption is viewed as an important option for children in foster care. A permanency plan must be made for a child in the foster care no longer than 12 mo from the child's entry into care and a petition to terminate parental rights must be filed to free the child for adoption when a child has been in foster care for 15 of the most recent 22 mo (with some exceptions).

Scheme for the Foster Care Services Grant in Aid from Delhi state and Government of India.

Simms MD, Freundlich M. Foster Care. In: Kliegman RM, Behrman RE, Jenson HB, Stanton BF (eds). *Nelson Textbook of Pediatrics*. 18th edn. Philadelphia: Saunders, 2007; 164–6.

6.3 CHILD CARE

Child care is defined as care provided by individual outside the nuclear family or in a setting separate from the child's home and is inclusive of such services as baby sitting, day care, preschool, early childhood program and remedial education programs, nursery school. Child care is used for children of all ages.

Due to profound social and demographic changes, an increase number of children receiving a portion of their care from someone other than their parents. For working parents' child care services is the necessity.

The effect of child care on children's development depends on a number of interrelated factors, including the quality and quantity of the child care experience, as well as characteristics of the child and family. Despite the substantial time spent by children in child care settings, the predominant influences on children's adjustment and development are the parents and the home environment. Children in whom more time is spent in non-maternal care during preschool years may be associated with more aggressive, assertive, and defiant behaviors. Pediatricians can help parents informed regarding the advantages and disadvantages of various child care options and information about child care in the community.

Child Day Care Services

With increased opportunities for employment for women and the need to supplement household income more and more women are entering the job market. With the breaking up of joint family system and the increased phenomenon of nuclear families, working women need support in terms of quality, substitute, and care for their young children while they are at work. Crèche and Day care Services are not only required by working mothers but also women belonging to poor families, who require support and relief from child care as they struggle to cope with burden of activities, within and outside the home. Effective day care for young children is essential and a cost effective investment as it provides support to both the mothers and young children. Hence, there is an urgent need for improved quality and reach of child day care services for working women among all socio-economic groups in both in the organized and unorganized sectors.

The need for child care services has been emphasized in the National Policy for Children, 1994, National Policy for Education, 1986 and National Policy for Empowerment of Women, 2001 and the National Plan of Action for Children, 2005. Rajiv Gandhi National Crèche Scheme for the Children of Working Mothers government of India is providing assistance for developing comprehensive day care services for the babies (0–6 years) of working and other deserving women provided the monthly income of both the parents does not exceed Rs. 12000/- for eight hours, i.e. from 9.00 A.M. to 5.00 P.M.

The present scheme will provide assistance to NGOs for running crèches for babies (0–6 years) and would provide assistance to ensure sleeping facilities, health care, supplementary nutrition, immunization, etc. for running a crèche for 25 babies for eight hours i.e. from 9.00 A.M. to 5.00 P.M. The government assistance can only be on a limited scale.

Monitoring of the crèches being run under the scheme will be conducted through independent agencies, to be identified in each state, which will submit reports direct to the central government.

The component of training has been added to the scheme to orient the crèche workers as well as the implementing agencies to provide better services and to build up child-friendly environment in the centre. A short-term training will be provided to every crèche worker and helper.

Physical infrastructure and service delivery: A crèche centre must have a minimum space of 6–8 sq. ft. per child to ensure that they can play, rest, and learn without any hindrance. The centre should be clean, well lighted with adequate ventilation. A fan should also be installed in the centre where electricity supply is available. The centre must have clean toilet and sanitation facility that caters to the needs of small children.

There should be adequate safe play area outside the centre also. Within the centre, there should be sleeping facilities for children, i.e. mattresses, cradles, cots, pillows and basic infrastructure to meet the requirement of the children. Essential play material and teaching and learning material must be available to meet the needs of pre-school children.

Implementing agencies and the crèche workers must ensure linkages with the local primary health centre or sub-primary health centre in the area. They should also have a tie-up with the nearby anganwadi centres and its workers for health care inputs like immunization, polio drops, basic health monitoring.

Food and other essentials: The centre must at all times be equipped with a basic First Aid Kit containing pediatric medicines for common ailments like fever, vomiting, cough and cold, dehydration, common stomach ailments, minor injuries, ointments, band-aids, cotton wool, disinfectants. The centre must have adequate cooking facility. The centre must have a safe and regular drinking water source. If necessary, chlorination or boiling of drinking water must be done. Food provided to the children must have adequate nutritional value and there should be variety in the food that is given to the children everyday. Weekly visits by doctors should be carried out for treatment and checkup.

Users charges: Rs. 20/- per child per month may be collected from children from below poverty line (BPL) families and Rs. 60/- per child per month from other families. This will ensure of participation with the community and also increase the centres' resources which can be utilized as rent or for better facilities at the crèche. It should be ensured that 50% of the children coming to these crèche are from BPL families.

Dworkin PH. Child Care. In: Behrman RE, Kliegman RM, Jenson HB (eds). Nelson Textbook of Pediatrics. 17th edn. Philadelphia: Saunders, 2004; 115–6.

Rajiv Gandhi National Crèche Scheme for the Children of Working Mothers government of India. Department of Women & Child Development, Ministry of Human Resource Development, New Delhi.

6.4 IMPACT OF VIOLENCE ON CHILDREN

Violence is a public health epidemic, affecting victim, witness, and perpetrator. The source of first exposure of violence for children is often domestic violence. Family violence is most likely to be perpetrated by those between ages 18 and 30 years—the child-rearing years. Most of the children are injured when they intervene to protect their mother from her husband. Another source of witnessed violence is community violence. The most important source of exposure to violence for children is television (TV).

Bullying and School Violence

Bullying: Bullying is the assertion of power through aggression targeting to a weaker victim through social, emotional, or physical means. Bullying is a common occurrence for school children and occurs in all countries, affecting children 12–18 yr more commonly. Boys are twice as likely as girls to be bullies, more than three times as likely to be bully-victims, and twice as likely to be victims. Involvement in bullying is associated with poorer psychosocial adjustment; bullies, victims, and bully-victims report greater health problems and poorer emotional and social adjustment. Victims tend to be either physically weak and emotionally vulnerable or provocative, with attention or conduct problems.

Bullying occurs most frequently at school when there is minimal supervision during breaks, recess, and lunch at playgrounds, in hallways and en route to and from school. The Internet is also another venue for the behavior and takes place through mass emailing, chat rooms, and message boards. Bullying can be direct, involving physical aggression such as hitting, stealing, and threatening with a weapon or verbal aggression such as name calling, public humiliation, and intimidation, or it can be indirect, involving relational aggression such as spreading rumors, social rejection, exclusion from peer groups, and ignoring. Childhood bullies have a fourfold increase in criminal behavior by their mid twenties and are at higher risk of dropping out of school. The bully-victim has problems with poor relationships and high rates of depression, loneliness, alcohol use, and weapon carrying.

School violence: Bullying may be an important precursor to more serious school violence. School violence and weapon carrying occurs worldwide. There is more school violence in areas with higher crime rates and more street gangs. These risks take away students' ability to learn in a safe environment and leave many children with traumatic stress and grief reactions.

Symptoms of bullying: Signs of a child being bullied include physical complaints such as insomnia, stomachaches, headaches, and new onset enuresis. Psychologic symptoms such as depression, loneliness, anxiety, and suicidal ideation may occur. Behavioral changes such as irritability, poor concentration, school avoidance and substance abuse are common. School problems such as academic failure, social problems, and lack of friends can also occur. The physical, psychologic, behavioral, and school symptoms of bullying may overlap with other conditions such as medical illness, obesity or physical deformities, and students in special education, learning problems, and psychologic disorders.

Treatment and prevention of bullying and school violence: Management of bullying involves interventions with parents, victims, bullies, and the school. School violence prevention programs should include: i. Problem solving, basic interpersonal skill building, and nonviolent conflict resolution found to be effective; ii. Parents and community organizations with the school can reduce violence by increasing rewards for academic achievements and; iii. Addressing access to firearms, the sensitivity of youth's fragile self-esteem, and the gap between youth and adults are important in creating a safe school climate.

Effects of War on Children

The impact of war is devastating, and its effects can last for decades after hostilities have ceased. Many more children are physically harmed than killed. Children bear the psychological scars of war resulting from exposure to violent events, loss of primary caregivers, and forced removal from their homes. During periods of war, children are more susceptible to exploitation in the forms of forced conscription as soldiers, sexual exploitation and slavery. After cessation of hostilities children are still at risk for life-endangering injuries from landmines and unexploded ordnance.

Protection of children from the effects of war: War and Terror violate the human rights of children. Several international treaties and conventions have been ratified beginning with 4th Geneva Convention (1949). The United Nations Convention on the Rights of the Child (1990) delineated specific human rights inherent to every child (defined as any individual younger than the age of 18 yr). The Rome Statute of the International Criminal Court that was enacted in the year 2002 declared that the conscription or enlistment of children younger than the age of 15 yr is a prosecutable war crime. These treaties better serve in heightening awareness regarding the protected status of children in wartime, and perhaps deter high ranking leaders who fear being held accountable for war crimes. Several organizations either nongovern-mental or under the auspices of the United Nations are involved in mitigating the effects of war on children. These organizations, which include the International Red Cross, UNICEF, United Nations Refugee Agency, World Health Organization and Medicins Sans Frontiéres (Doctors Without Borders) have had a significant impact on reducing violence-related casualties in war-torn regions.

Role of pediatricians and allied health professionals: Health providers need to be prepared to treat childhood casualties resulting from military or terrorist activity as well as caring for children suffering from the aftermath of war or related violence. Pediatricians need to be cognizant of the effects that war and terror can have on parents and children. They can be instrumental in educating parents to be more aware of inappropriate responses by children to war and violence. When necessary, pediatricians can serve their families by referring them to appropriate support services.

Augustyn M, Zuckerman B. Impact of violence on children. In: Kliegman RM, Behrman RE, Jenson HB, Stanton BF (eds). *Nelson Textbook of Pediatrics*. 18th edn. Philadelphia: Saunders, 2007; 166–7.

Krug EG, Dahlberg LL, Mercy JA, et al (eds). World Report on Violence and Health. Geneva: World Health Organization, 2002.

Vanderbilt D, Augustyn M. Bullying and school violence. In: Kliegman RM, Behrman RE, Jenson HB, Stanton BF (eds). Nelson Textbook of Pediatrics. 18th edn. Philadelphia: Saunders, 2007;168–9.

Wexler ID, Kerem E. Effects of war on children. In: Kliegman RM, Behrman RE, Jenson HB, Stanton BF (eds). *Nelson Textbook of Pediatrics*. 18th edn. Philadelphia: Saunders, 2007; 169–71.

6.5 CHILD LABOR

Every year on June 12, World Day Against Child Labour reminds us that "child labour is a social evil. It jeopardizes children's health, education, human rights and future". The ban imposed by the labor ministry on Tuesday (August 1, 2006), under the Child Labor (prohibition and regulation) Act, 1986 will come into effect from October 31 (Box 6.2). For any assistance in the rescue and rehabilitation of child labor, contact state labor department or toll free help line 1098 (child line) or local police.

Child labor ban would not work. The National Human Rights Commission (NHRC) of India has said that a complete withdrawal of children from work is not a practical solution to the problem of child labor. Therefore, we have to look at it from a holistic angle. Children should be allowed to study and work at the same time. They can be made to learn while they earn. They must also be given enough time to play. So their hours of work must be reduced as they need time to study.

Ministry of Labor & Employment, Government of India, visit website at http://labour.nic.in for more details.

Box 6.2: What the constitution of India says

Article 21A casts a duty on the state to provide free and compulsory education to all children of the age of six and 14 years in such manner as the state, may, by law, determine.

Article 24 of the constitution says: "No child below the age of 14 years shall be employed to work in any factory or mine or engaged in any other hazardous employment."

Article 39 (f) of the constitution says: "The state shall, in particular direct its policies towards securing that children are given opportunities and facilities to develop in a healthy manner and in conditions of freedom and dignity and that childhood and youth are protected against exploitation and against moral and material abandonment."

Child Labor: (Prohibition and regulation) Act, 1986 prohibits he employment of children below the age of 14 in factories, mines, ad in other forms of hazardous employment."

Under the child labor (P&R) Act, 15 occupations and 57 processes are prohibited for employment of children below 14 years. Some of these prohibited occupations/processes are *Bidi* making, domestic servants, dhaba/tea-shop/hotel work, building and construction, carpet weaving, stone grinding, mechanized fishing, state stone mining, cinder picking, etc.

Penalty against anyone employing a child in the prohibited category is a fine up to Rs 20.000/- and/or imprisonment up to one year.

Under national child labor project (NCLP) scheme, children withdrawn from hazardous work are put into special schools, where they are provided with bridging education (pre-vocational skills, stipend, mid-day meal, health care facilities, etc.).

6.6 ABUSE AND NEGLECT OF CHILDREN

The abuse and neglect (maltreatment) of children are pervasive problems worldwide, with short- and long-term physical and mental health and social consequences. Abuse is defined as acts of commission and neglect as acts of omission. The US government defines child abuse as "any recent act or failure to act on the part of a parent or caretaker, which results in death, serious physical or emotional harm, sexual abuse or exploitation, or an act or failure to act which presents an imminent risk of serious harm."

Physical abuse includes beating, shaking, burning, and biting, and fractures, abusive head trauma, and abdominal trauma. Corporal punishment is widely accepted in many countries. The World Health Organization (WHO) reported in 2006 that 106 countries do not prohibit the use of corporal punishment in schools, 147 do not prohibit it within alternative care settings, and only 16 prohibit its use in home.

Sexual abuse has been defined as "the involvement of dependent, developmentally immature children and adolescents in sexual activities which they do not fully comprehend, to which they are unable to give consent, or they violate the social taboos of family roles." Sexual abuse includes exposure to sexually explicit materials, oral-genital contact, genital-to-genital contact, genital fondling, and genital to anal contact. Any touching of private areas by parents or caregivers in context other than necessary care is inappropriate. Sexual abuse may also be defined as any sexual behavior or action toward a child that is unwanted. Some legal definitions distinguish sexual abuse from sexual assault; the former being committed by a caregiver or household member, and the latter being committed by someone with a noncustodial relationship or no relationship with the child, *see* Section 13.11.

Neglect refers to omissions in care, resulting in actual or potential harm. Omissions may include health care, education, supervision, protection from hazards in the environment, physical needs (e.g. clothing, food), and/or emotional support.

Psychological abuse includes verbal abuse and humiliation and acts that scare or terrorize the child.

Incidence and prevalence: Child abuse and neglect are not rare and occur worldwide. WHO has estimated that 40 million children under the age of 15 yr suffer from abuse and neglect; over 1 million children have been trafficked. More than 80% children suffer physical punishment in their homes, with over 30% experiencing severe physical punishment.

Etiology: Child maltreatment seldom has a single cause. Rather risk factors usually exist at 4 levels.

1. At the individual level, a child's disability or a parent's depression or substance abuse predispose a child to maltreatment.
2. At the familial level, intimate partner (or domestic) violence presents risk for children.
3. Influential community factors include stressors, such as dangerous neighborhoods or a lack of recreational facilities. Professional inaction may contribute to neglect, such as when the treatment plan is not clearly communicated.
4. Broad societal factors such as poverty and its associated burdens, also contribute to maltreatment.

WHO estimates the rate of homicide of children is approximately twofold higher in lower income compared to high-income countries. However, children in all social classes can be maltreated.

In contrast, protective factors such as family supports, or a mother's concern for her child, may buffer risk factors and protect children from maltreatment. Identifying and building on protective factors can be vital to intervening. Child maltreatment results from a complex interplay among risk and protective factors.

Outcomes of child maltreatment: Child maltreatment often has significant short- and long-term medical, mental health, and social sequelae. Physically abused children are at risk for behavioral and functional problems, including conduct disorders, aggressive behavior, decreased congestive functioning and poor academic performances. Neglect is similarly associated with many potential problems. Even if a maltreated child appears to be functioning well, health care professionals and parents need to know that there may be the possibility of problems in adulthood. Maltreated children are at risk for becoming abusive parents.

Prevention of child abuse and neglect: Parent and child education regarding medical conditions helps to ensure implementation of the treatment plan and to prevent neglect. Screening for major psychosocial risk factors for maltreatment (depression, substance abuse, intimate partner violence, major stress) and helping address identified problems, often via referrals, may help prevent maltreatment. Child health care professionals should recognize their limitations in providing referral to other community resources when indicated. Finally, the problems support child maltreatment, such as poverty, parental stress, substance abuse and limited child-rearing resources require policies and programs that enhance families' abilities to care for their children adequately. Child care professionals can help advocate for such policies and programs.

American academy of Pediatrics Committee on Child Abuse and Neglect: Shaken baby syndrome: rotational cranial injuries-technical report. Pediatrics 2001;108:206–10.

Dubowitz H, Lane WG. Abused and neglected children. In: Kliegman RM, Stanton BF, St.Geme JW, NF Schor NF, Behrman RE. *Nelson Textbook of Pediatrics.* 19th edn. New Delhi: Elsevier, 2011;135–46.

WHO. Report on the consultation on child abuse prevention. Geneva: World Health Organization, 2002.

World Health organization. Injuries and violence prevention: child abuse and neglect. Email http://www.who.int/health_topics/child_abuse/en.

6.7 FAILURE TO THRIVE

Failure to thrive (FTT) is usually refers to growth below the 5th percentile or a change in growth that has changed two major growth percentiles (i.e. from above the 75th percentile to below the 25th) in a short time. Children with FTT can be arbitrarily divided in to two categories: organic FTT (*see* Chapter 3, page 64) and nonorganic FTT (NOFTT) or psychosocial FTT. Organic and nonorganic etiologic factors may also occur together, for example in children who are victims of abuse and neglect or temperamentally difficult premature infants.

Nonorganic Failure to Thrive

Nonorganic Failure to Thrive (NOFTT) or psycho-social FTT occurs when a child, usually an infant, is not fed adequate calories. The mother may neglect proper feeding because she is involved with external demands and the care of others; is preoccupied with inner problems or depressed; is ignorant about appropriate feeding; is abusing substances; does not like or understand the infant; is having multiple and continuing crises, frequently compounded by the physical absence of the father; is poor (poverty may also prevent a caregiver not getting adequate food for a child); is retarded and emotionally disturbed (may not have the capacity to provide proper care).

Treatment

Children with NOFTT should be hospitalized and given unlimited feedings of a diet appropriate for age for a minimum of 1 wk; this diet usually approaches 150 kcal/kg (ideal weight)/24 hr. Infants with NOFTT usually gain more than 2 oz every 24 hr for 1 wk (approximately 1 lb per week), or have a gain that is significantly greater than that achieved during a similar period at home. These infants have a ravenous appetite. A nursing plan should include careful charting of intake, weight, and observations of the mother's feeding style and the amount of time she spent with the child. For older infants and young children with psychological FTT meal times should be 20–30 min, solid foods should be offered before liquids, environmental disturbances should be minimized, and children should eat with other people and not be forced fed. High-caloric foods, such as whole milk, butter, cheese, and dried fruits, should be emphasized. The rule of 3s is quite helpful—3 meals, 3 snacks, and 3 choices. Infants who are difficult to feed because of neurologic or mechanical problems may gain weight as a result of the intensive efforts by the hospital staff.

Prognosis: After hospital management, approximately 75% of infants recover. Weight loss and understature from malnutrition are reversible, but normal head circumference and brain growth may not be achieved if the infant has suffered from NOFTT more than

6 mo of age. More than half of these children with psychosocial FTT have social and emotional problems. Ongoing assessment and monitoring of cognitive and emotional development, with appropriate intervention, is necessary for all children.

Munchausen Syndrome by Proxy (MSBP)

The term Munchausen syndrome was usually to describe situations in which adults falsified their own symptoms. In MSBP, a parent, invariably the mother simulates or causes disease in a child. The parent may (i) fabricate a medical history; (ii) cause symptoms by repeatedly exposing the child to a toxin, medication, infectious agent, or physical trauma, including smothering; or (iii) alter laboratory samples or temperature measurements. Depending on the parent's sophistication and secrecy, a variety of convincing, novel, and exotic diseases may be simulated or created. The parent may deny any involvement, and in instances of intentional poisoning, smothering, or trauma, may continue the action while the child is hospitalized. MSBP is inflicted on children who are either unable or unwilling to identify the true offense or offender. The abusing caregiver gains attention from the relationships formed with health care providers or her own family as the result of the problems created.

Clinical manifestations: The child's symptoms, their pattern, or the response to treatment may not be compatible with a recognized disease. The mother may have a history of Munchausen syndrome (MS) and seem relatively unconcerned about the severity of the child's illness. Apnea and seizures are two common manifestations of MSBP. The observations may be falsified or may be created by partial suffocation. The clinical pattern is variable. It includes forced ingestion of medications such as ipecac to cause chronic vomiting or laxatives to cause diarrhea, or injection of insulin with consequent seizures. The skin, which is more easily accessible to the perpetrator, may be burned, dyed, tattooed, lacerated or punctured to simulate acute or chronic skin conditions. Infectious or toxic agents may be administered in any available orifice. Provision of intravenous lines during hospitalization may provide an opportunity for injection of infectious agents from feces, toxins, and pharmacologic agents. Urine and blood samples may be contaminated with foreign blood or stool. Older children may become convinced that they have an illness.

Diagnosis: In establishing the diagnosis parents of children hospitalized for evaluation should be videotaped. All laboratory information should be critically reviewed.

Treatment: After all laboratory information is collected and the diagnosis is established, the offending parent should be confronted by a non accusatory physician and staff who offer help. Any approach may be met with resistance, denial, and threats.

Prognosis: The consequences of MSBP include persistence of abuse, emotional problems, chronic disability, and death. Other siblings may be or may have been, at risk; there is a association of this syndrome with unexplained infant deaths.

Bauchner H. Failure to thrive. In: Kliegman RM, Behrman RE, Jenson HB, Stanton BF (eds). *Nelson Textbook of Pediatrics.* 18th edn. Vol. 1. Philadelphia: Saunders, 2007; 184–7.

Johnson CF. Abuse and Neglect of Children. In: Kliegman RM, Behrman RE, Jenson HB, Stanton BF (eds). *Nelson Textbook of Pediatrics.* 18th edn. Vol. 1. Philadelphia: Saunders, 2007; 171–84.

Rosenberg DA. Munchausen Syndrome by Proxy: Medical diagnostic criteria. Child Abuse Negl 2003;27:421–30.

6.8 DEVELOPMENTAL DISABILITIES

India has a large number of children with developmental disabilities, the prevalence of which is on the rise. Efforts should be undertaken at all levels to promote growth and maximize opportunities for development, socialization and strengthening of bonds between the child, family, and community. Developmental disabilities represent a large proportion of childhood illnesses and disorders. A disability is any restriction or inability to perform any activity in the manner or within the range considered normal for a human being, which has resulted from impairment (any loss or abnormality of psychological, physiological or anatomical structure or function). According to the Federal Disability Act, USA (1978), a developmental disability has been defined as a 'severe chronic disability that is attributed to mental or physical impairment, is manifested before the person attains the age of 22 years, is likely to continue indefinitely; results in substantial functional limitation in three or more areas of major life specified as self-care, language, learning, motility, self-direction, capacity for independent living and economic self sufficiency and that reflects the persons need for life-long and individually planned services'.

Causes of developmental disabilities: According to UNICEF statistics, at least one in ten children is born with or acquires a physical, mental or sensory impairment. What is critical to understand is that as much as 50% of these can be prevented or postponed. Acquired causes are listed in Table 6.2. The common congenital causes include structural anomalies, genetic disorders, inborn errors of metabolism and various dysmorphology syndromes. In quite a large proportion of children the cause may be unidentified. Brief descriptions of the developmental disabilities have been provided in Table 6.3.

Classification systems: Taking into consideration the heterogeneity of the entities which are included in childhood disabilities it is not surprising that formulation of an optimal classification system is extremely challenging. Definitions of these terms have been provided in Table 6.4.

Early detection of disabilities: Timely identification of impairment can reduce the impact on the functional level of the individual and prevent it from becoming a disability.

Table 6.2: Causes of acquired developmental disabilities

Timing of insult	Causes
Prenatal	• Maternal nutritional status • Maternal infections • Maternal illnesses • Antenatal exposure to teratogens • Maternal metabolic state • Pregnancy related complications
Perinatal	• Complications in labor • Prematurity (with its morbidities) • Neonatal morbidities
Postnatal	• Hypoxic-ischemic events • Traumatic (accidental or battered baby syndrome) • Infectious • Nutritional • Toxins and drugs

Table 6.3: Definitions/descriptions of individual developmental disabilities

Terms	Description
Locomotor disabilities	Cerebral palsy or any disability due to bones, joints or muscles which lead to substantial restriction of the movement of the limbs (i.e. neuromuscular disorders, orthopedic disorders, post-traumatic).
Cerebral palsy	A group of disorders of the development of movement and posture, causing limitation in activity, that is attributable to non-progressive disturbances occurring in the fetal or infant brain.
Neuromuscular disorders	A group of disorders which may involve any of the following: Anterior horn cells, peripheral nerve, neuromuscular junction or the muscle.
Mental retardation	Below average intellectual functioning with an intelligence quotient (IQ) below 70–75 (measured by standardized tests) and significant limitations in two or more adaptive skill areas
Global developmental delay	A significant delay in two or more developmental domains, i.e. gross motor, fine motor, cognition, speech and language, personal/social and activities of daily living.
Hearing impairment	Full or partial decrease in the ability to detect or understand sounds
Blindness	A corrected visual acuity of the better eye of less than 3/60
Severe visual impairment	A corrected visual acuity of the better eye of less than 6/60 but equal to or better than 3/60
Learning disorders	A heterogeneous group of neurobehavioral disorders manifested by significant, unexpected, specific and persistent difficulties in the acquisition and use of efficient reading (dyslexia), writing (dysgraphia) and mathematical abilities (dyscalculia) despite conventional instruction, intact senses, normal intelligence, proper motivation and adequate social-cultural opportunity.
Speech and language disorders	A heterogeneous group of communication disorders manifested by significant unexpected, specific and persistent difficulties in the acquisition and use of speech and language disabilities.
Attention deficit hyperactivity disorder (ADHD)	A persistent (for at least 6 months) pattern of inattention and/or hyperactivity-impulsivity that is more frequently displayed and more severe than is typically observed in an individual at a comparable level of development. The behavior should be present in two or more settings and should cause significant impairment in social, academic or occupational functioning.
Pervasive developmental disorder (PDD)	A group of behavioral and neurodevelopmental disorders which are characterized by a severe and pervasive impairment in several areas of development.
Epilepsy	A condition characterized by recurrent (two or more) epileptic seizures, unprovoked by any immediate identified cause.

Table 6.4: Definitions of terms used in classification systems: ICIDH*, ICF**

System of classification	Definitions/descriptions	
ICIDH*	**Impairment**	Any loss or abnormality of psychological, physiological or anatomical structure or function
	Disability	Any restriction or lack (resulting from an impairment) of ability to perform an activity in the manner or within the range considered normal for a human being
	Handicap	A disadvantage for a given individual, resulting from impairment or a disability, that limits or prevents the fulfillment of a role that is normal (depending on age, sex, and social and cultural factors) for that individual
ICF**	**Functioning**	All body functions, activities and participation
	Body functions	Physiological and psychological functions of the body systems
	Body structures	The anatomical parts of the body such as organs, limbs and their components
	Activity	The execution of a task or action by an individual
	Participation	The involvement in a life situation
	Disability	An umbrella term for impairments, activity limitations and participation restrictions
	Impairments	Problems in body function or structure such as a significant deviation or loss
	Activity limitations	Difficulties an individual may have in executing activities.
	Participation restrictions	Problems an individual may experience in involvement in life situations
	Environmental factors	The physical, social and attitudinal environment in which people live and conduct their lives

*ICIDH: International classification of impairments, disabilities and handicaps.
**ICF: International classification of functioning, disability and health.

Assessment of disabilities: The next step in management is the evaluation and subsequent formulation of an individualized intervention program. This needs to be developed by a multidisciplinary team which should comprise the following (as per individual requirement): a child development specialist/developmental pediatrician, pediatric neurologist, ENT specialist, audiologist, ophthalmologist/optometrist, child developmental psychologist, speech pathologist, occupational and physical therapist, special educator and social worker. In ideal circumstances they should be under the same roof, so that the child and his parents do not have to run from pillar to post to get optimum intervention. An assessment should include nature of disability (congenital or acquired; single or multiple; progressive or static; any specific cure available); and associated co-morbidities. Also enquire whether the child is receiving education (if IQ permits) and the family is aware of any special benefits to which he may be entitled (i.e. certificates, concessions, income tax rebates).

Management: The conditions resulting in childhood disability are extremely heterogeneous and the specific needs and management of such a diverse group vary widely. However, it is important to remember that as a group, children with disabilities do have common needs. These include the need for basic health maintenance and health promotion measures (basic medical care, nutrition, and immunizations), coordination of services with communication between health and education fields, psychological and family support, technical assistance, and funding resources. Rehabilitation is the process aimed at enabling persons with disabilities to reach and maintain their optimal physical, sensory, intellectual, psychiatric or social functional levels. An ideal intervention program needs to involve the following components (as required on an individualized basis):

i. *Motor skills:* Occupational therapy, oral motor therapy, motor planning intervention and physical therapy.

ii. *Cognitive:* Special education, classroom modification, organizing skills, study skills, tutoring and remediation.

iii. *Sensory:* Sensory integration and sensory modulation.

iv. *Language and communication:* Speech and language therapy, listening and auditory processing programs, language enhancement and oral motor therapy.

v. *Overall social/relational approach:* One on one communication skills and play therapy.

vi. *Behavioral approach* applied behavioral analysis, discrete trial learning and behavioral modification and intervention programs.

vii. *Provision of aids:* Visual aids, hearing aids, loco-motor aids, special technologies, etc.

viii. *Genetic counseling* including prenatal diagnosis (if available).

ix. *Medical:* Treatment of associated medical and psychiatric co-morbidities.

x. *Nutritional counseling:* Improving eating patterns and providing optimum diets.

xi. *Family support:* Social worker, family support groups, guidance regarding various resources and benefits.

Working off this framework, health maintenance and promotion measures should be then further individualized to suit the child and family's specific needs. It is very important to emphasize and strengthen the family's role as the central determinant of child health and development. The advantages are multiple. It enhances development and minimizes the potential for delay, minimizes the need for special education and related services and also minimizes the likelihood of institutional or other restrictive care outcomes.

Prevention: Developmental disabilities need to be addressed at each level (primary, secondary, or tertiary) to reduce the expression, duration or impact of disabilities. At the primary level the goal is to reduce risk factors. Strategies should focus at the underlying cause. For environmental causes these include: increasing immunization; improving nutritional status especially adolescent girls; increasing the use of family planning services; providing good quality antenatal, obstetric and neonatal care; creating awareness of basic child safety measures; improving basic health services; providing education about medical care seeking attitudes; and providing education about factors influencing human reproduction (age at marriage and childbearing, child spacing, family size). For genetic disorders measures comprise genetic counseling and prenatal diagnosis and certain pre-conceptual interventions when possible, i.e. folic acid administration for reducing incidence of neural tube defects. At a secondary prevention level, the goal is to reduce the extent of manifested disability and shorten its duration. This can be achieved by infant stimulation and remediation programs which focus on family involvement. At the tertiary level, the aim is to prevent or reduce the complications of disability (physical and behavioral) that may subsequently lead to a need for

institutionalization. At this level, there may be a need for family counseling and other intensive supports.

Legislation and disability rights: It is the responsibility of the physician to make parents aware of their rights and benefits as caregivers of a child with disabilities. Legislative initiatives on disability gained momentum in India after the United Nations Economic and the Social Commission for Asia and Pacific (UNESCAP) convened a meeting to launch the Asian and Pacific Decade of Disabled Persons, 1993–2002. The meeting adopted the 'Proclamation on the Full Participation and Equality of People with Disabilities in the Asian and Pacific Region', to which India is a signatory and for which India enacted the following act:

1. The Persons with Disabilities (Equal Opportunities, Protection of Rights and Full Participation) Act, (PDA) 1995.
2. National Trust for welfare of Persons with Autism, Cerebral Palsy, Mental Retardation and Multiple Disabilities Act.

Chakrabarty S, Dutt D. Rapid Assessment of Childhood Disabilities Through Key Informant Approach. Indian Pediatr 2004; 41:1064–6.

Developmental disabilities assistance and bill of rights act, 42 USCA, Section 6000 seq, West Supp 1993.

Gulati S, Wasir V. Prevention of developmental disabilities. Indian J Pediatr 2005; 72:975–8.

World Health Organization (WHO). International Classification of Impairments.

Disabilities and Handicaps. Geneva, Switzerland: World Health Organization, 1981.

World Health Organization (WHO). International Classification of Functioning, disability and Health. Geneva, Switzerland: World Health Organization, 2003.

6.9 CHILDREN AT SPECIAL RISK

The majority of children at special risk need a nurturing environment but their futures get compromised by actions or policies arising from their families, schools, communities, and nation. The main task is to improve the environment of these children so that most can achieve their full potential. The causes of their problems are many, but similar in majority of children whether it is the problem of homeless children, runaways, children in foster care, or other disadvantaged groups. From a preventive point of view, the most effective approach involves alleviation of poverty, poor housing, and lack of jobs. From a treatment point of view, optimal care of these children requires specially organized programs, multidiscipline teams and special financing.

Children in poverty: Many factors associated with poverty are responsible for the illnesses seen in these children include crowding, poor hygiene and health care, poor diet, environmental pollution, poor education, and stress.

Children of migrant farm workers and construction workers: The medial problems of children of migrant farm workers and construction workers (construction of houses and roads and bridges) are similar to those of children of homeless families: increased frequency of infections (including human deficiency virus [HIV] and AIDS), trauma, poor nutrition, poor dental care, low immunization rates, exposures to toxic chemicals, anemia, and developmental delays.

Children of immigrants: Refugee children who escape from war or political violence (usually from border countries) and whose families have been subjected to extreme stress are a subset of immigrant children. They have a particularly high incidence of mental and behavioral problems and traumatic stress disorder.

Homeless children: Homeless children have an increased frequency of illness, including intestinal infections, anemia, neurologic disorders, mental illness, and dental problems, as well as increased frequency of trauma and substance abuse. They have higher school failure rates, and the likelihood of their being victims of abuse and neglect is much higher. There is increased frequency of psychosocial problems such as developmental delays, severe depression, or learning disorders in these children.

Runaway and thrown-away children: Runaway and thrown-away children and youths have no secure and safe place to stay. Teenagers make up most of both groups. The usual definition of a runaway is a youth younger than 18 yr who is gone for at least one night from his or her home without parental permission. Most runaways leave home only once, stay overnight with friends, and have no contact with the police or other agencies. This group is no different from their 'healthy' peers in psychological status. A smaller number become multiple or permanent "runners" and are significantly different from the one-time runners. Thrown-aways include children directly told to leave the household, children who have been away from home and are not allowed to return, abandoned or deserted children, and children who runaway but whose caretakers makes no effort to recover them or does not care if they return. The causes include environmental problems (family dysfunction, abuse, poverty), personal problems of the young person (poor impulse control, psychopathology, substance abuse, or school failure). Thrown-aways experienced more violence and conflicts within their families.

Behrman RE. Children at special risk. In: Behrman RE, Kliegman RM, Jenson HB (eds). Nelson Textbook of Pediatrics. 17th edn. Philadelphia: Saunders 2004; 148–52.

Khurana S, Sharma N, Jena S, et al. Mental health status of runaway adolescents. Indian J Pediatr 2004; 71(5):405–9.

6.10 PEDIATRIC PALLIATIVE CARE

In 1990 the World Health Organization defined palliative care as "The active total care of patients whose disease is not responsive to curative treatment. Control of pain, of other symptoms, and of psychological, social and spiritual problems is paramount. The goal of palliative care is achievement of the best quality of life for patients and their families." Palliative care is provided in hospitals and in the home whenever is possible and desired. Pediatric palliative care has:

1. Smaller number of dying children.
2. A broad spectrum of illnesses, including many rare diseases that often require involvement of a number of disciplines.
3. Unpredictable illness with significant prognostic uncertainty. It is often difficult to predict accurately the progression of illness for many life-threatening illnesses.
4. More uncertainty about whether treatments are supportive/palliative versus those that primarily cure or prolong life. It is not always possible with emerging technologies such as noninvasive respiratory ventilation whether a specific treatment is palliative or life prolonging.

Advances in pediatric medicine have resulted in an increase in the number of children who live longer, often with significant dependence on new (and expensive) technologies.

Care planning: Although it may not be possible to accurately determine how long a child may live, there is often a delay between the time when a terminal prognosis is first recognized by physicians and when the prognosis is first understood by parents. The best time is when the physician recognizes a significant possibility of patient mortality to initiate discussions concerning resuscitation, symptom control, and end-of-life care planning. Home care of the dying child requires 24 hr per day acceptability to experts in pediatric palliative care, a team approach, and an identified coordinator who serves as a link between hospitals, the community, and specialists, and can arrange for hospital admissions and respite care, as needed. Good end-of-life care can be effectively carried out in a hospital setting but only when institutions are flexible enough to modify protocols that may present unnecessary obstacles to the care of dying patients, especially in tertiary care hospitals (the neonatal and pediatric intensive care units [ICUs]) where most children die.

Communication Issues and Anticipatory Guidance

The Child: Children may ask questions about death, such as "What's happening to me? Am I dying?" This requires careful explanation keeping in mind that the child may ask more questions.

Sibling: Brothers and sisters are at a special risk both during the course of illness and after their death. Parents should involve siblings with their sick brother and sister and should be encouraged to maintain the routines of daily living. Siblings who are most involved with their sick brothers or sisters before death usually adjust better both at the time of and after the death.

Parents: Parents may blame themselves for their child's illness even when logic dictates that they had nothing to do with what is happening to their child. They think that "if they had taken him early to the doctor" or spent considerable energy and resources looking for "miracle cures." The physician should be sensitive to these possible and other parental concerns, which they may not like to disclose. Physicians should provide support to parents at these times by engaging in active listening. In communication with the child and family, the physician should avoid giving estimates of survival length, even when these are explicitly asked for. A more appropriate approach may be to tell ranges of time in general terms ("weeks to months," "months to years").

Decision-making: During the course of child's life-limiting illness, a series of difficult decisions need to be made in relation to truth-telling and disclosure, location of care, medications with risks and benefits (e.g. steroids), double beneficent use of analgesics, withholding and or withdrawing life-prolonging technologies, experimental treatments in research protocols, and the use of alternative therapies. Decision-making should remain focused on the goals of therapy rather than on specific limitations of the care; e.g. "This is what we can offer", instead of "This what we can no longer do". Once the goals of therapy are agreed upon, the physician may draft a letter that outlines the end-of-life care plan for the child, including suggestions for medications and the telephone numbers of caregivers who know the patient best. Such a letter, given to the patients, with copies to involved caregivers and institutions, can be a useful aid in communication, especially at times of crisis. Conflicts in decision-making can occur within families, within health care teams, between the child and family, and between the family and professional caregivers. Although frequently encountered, differences in opinion are often manageable, because the main goals of care to provide comfort and quality of life are agreed upon.

Management: Dying children have a multitude of symptoms in addition of pain, for significant periods before their death. Pain control is of paramount importance in reducing the suffering of the child, family, and care givers, but many dying children do not have their pain successfully treated (see Chapter 7, page 166). Guidelines for treatment of pain and other symptoms are summarized as follows:
1. Maintaining comfort is the priority.
2. Anticipate and plan symptoms before they occur.
3. Utilize a stepwise approach to pain management.
4. Choose the least invasive route for medications—by mouth whenever possible.
5. Prescribe regular medications for constant pain.
6. *Consider opioids:* Begin with weak opioids (e.g. codeine). Replace with strong opioids (e.g. morphine) for unresponsive or persisting pain.
7. *Consider use of adjuvant drugs*
   - Antidepressants and anticonvulsants—neuropathic pain
   - Neuroleptics—nausea, agitation
   - Sedatives and hypnotics—anxiety or muscle spasm
   - Steroid—resistant pain
8. Consider anesthetic blocks for regional pain. Use topical local anesthetics when possible.
9. Always include cognitive (guided imagery, distraction), physical (TENS, physiotherapy, message), and behavioral (biofeedback, behavior modification) techniques (TENS—transcutaneous electrical nerve stimulation).

Respiratory symptoms such as dyspnea (the subjective sensation of shortness of breath) are common because many children with chronic illness have difficulty swallowing and handling their airway secretions. Excessive airway secretions and salivation owing to poor swallowing are accumulated and may cause noisy respiration, sometimes referred to as death rattle. Use of an anticholinergic drug such as hyoscine, may be helpful in decreasing secretions. Dyspnea can be relieved with the use of regularly scheduled plus as-needed doses of opioids. Oxygen may be helpful in certain cases to relieve hypoxemia related headaches. However, giving oxygen to a child with cyanosis who is otherwise quiet and relaxed has no impact on patient distress. Pneumonia is a frequent complication in dying patient.

Neurologic symptoms include seizures that are often part of the antecedent illness but may increase in frequency and severity towards the end of life. Anticonvulsants should be administered and parents should be taught to use rectal diazepam at home.

Increased irritability occurs in some neuro-degenerative disorders and children have prolonged crying. Judicious use of sedatives in the daytime (e.g. benzodiazepines) combined with hypnotics at night (e.g. chloral hydrate) may achieve a balance that can improve the quality of life for both child and caregivers.

Feeding and hydration issues raise ethical questions that include the use of nasogastric and gastrostomy feedings for the child who cannot take by mouth. These questions should be considered in the light of risks and benefits of artificial feeding and functional level and prognosis. At times it may be appropriate to initiate a trial of tube feedings with the understanding that they may be discontinued at the later stage of illness. Hydration by administering intravenous fluids to a dying patient is associated with deleterious effects in the form of increased secretions, need for frequent urination, and exacerbation of dyspnea and therefore, sensation of thirst may be alleviated by keeping the mouth moist and clean.

Nausea demands prompt treatment after a search for common causes (drug effects, constipation, primary disease, metabolic disturbance). Drugs such as metoclopramide, phenothiazines, ondansetron, and steroids may be used depending on the cause and desires secondary effect. Vomiting may accompany may occur with nausea and without nausea in the presence of intestinal obstruction. Constipation is common in neurologic disorder. Children with minimal solid intake may be comfortable with bowel movements as infrequent as weekly. Children with regular opioids should routinely be placed on laxative agents (senna derivatives, lactulose). Diarrhea may be particularly difficult for the child and family and may be treated with loperamide and opioids. Paradoxical diarrhea, a result of overflow resulting from constipation, may also be considered.

Hematologic issues include consideration of transfusions for anemia and thrombocytopenia. Most children in the palliative phase may be managed by intermittent red cells and platelets for bleeding that interferes with the quality of life.

Skin care issues include the prevention of problems such as bedsores by the early use of foam, mattresses and careful attention to positioning. Pruritus may be secondary to systemic disorders or drug therapy. Treatment includes avoiding excessive use of soap, using moisturizers, trimming fingernails, wearing loose-fitting clothings and use of topical or systemic steroids, oral histamines and other specific therapies may also be indicated (e.g. cholestyramine in biliary disease).

When discussing possible therapies or inter-ventions, it is important to raise the issue of complementary or alternative medicine therapy. Most of these are unproven, but some are inexpensive therapies and provide relief to individual patients. Other therapies may be expensive, painful, intrusive, and even dangerous. The physician can offer advice on the safety of different therapies and may help avoid expensive and dangerous interventions.

The terminal phase: As the death approaches the major tasks of the physician to help prepare the child and family for expected problems and issues and continued to stay involved in care. If the child is at home, regular phone calls should be made to help manage new symptoms as they occur (e.g. terminal airway secretions, seizures, irritability, myoclonus, vomiting). In an intensive care setting, where technology can put distance between the child and parent, the physician should discontinue the use of unneeded equipment. While in ICU, even children on ventilation can be placed in their parent's arms.

The physician should discuss the option of an autopsy and organ donation; answering questions that parents may be reluctant to ask ("Will the face be disturbed?"). Parents might also be reminded that they may have questions later that can be answered by autopsy ("Will present and future siblings and grand children be affected?"). The parents can also be offered genetic counseling when appropriate.

The pediatrician: Most pediatricians have little formal palliative care education and limited clinical experience in how to care for a dying child. Like many aspects of medical practice, palliative medicine requires that physicians evolve their own knowledge, skills, and attitudes about healing and their role in caring even when death is the unavoidable outcome for their patients.

American Academy of Pediatrics: Palliative care for children. Pediatrics 2000;106(2):351–7.

Goldman A (ed). Care of the Dying Child. 2nd Printing. Oxford: Oxford University Press, 1998.

Liben S. Pediatric Palliative Care. In: Kliegman RM, Behrman RE, Jenson HB, Stanton BF (eds). *Nelson Textbook of Pediatrics*. 18th edn. Vol 1. Philadelphia: Saunders, 2007; 200–6.

6.11 SEPARATION AND LOSS

All children experience involuntary separation from loved ones, think about death, and encounter death in everyday events. The initial reaction of young children to separation may involve crying, either of a tantrum like, protesting type or of a sadder type. After a few hours or a day or so of separation, children may become appear subdued, withdrawn, and quiet, or irritable, fussy, moody, and resistant to authority. Disturbance of appetite may occur, and there may be special difficulty at bedtime such as reluctance to go to bed and problems in getting to sleep, with resurgence of old fears, and in younger children, perhaps such regressive behavior as bed-wetting. Children may repeatedly ask where the absent parent is and when he or she will return home. The child may go to the window or door or out into the neighborhood looking for an absent parent; a few may even leave home or their places of temporary placement to search for their parents.

A child's response to union may surprise or alarm a parent. A parent who joyfully returns to the family finds the child after a brief interaction of affection may move away from the parent and seem indifferent to his or her return. Immediately after the reunion or after a few days, some children particularly younger ones may become more clinging and dependent than they were before separation, while continuing any regressive behavior that had occurred during separation. Parents should not try to ameliorate a child's behavior by threatening to leave.

Experiences of loss such as divorce or placement in foster care can give rise to the same type of reactions listed earlier but they are more intense and possibly more lasting. School-aged children may respond with evident depression, seem indifferent or be markedly angry. Other children appear to deny or avoid the issue, behaviorally or verbally.

In response to separation or divorce of parents, older children and adolescents commonly show more intense anger. Almost all children will cling to their parents with the belief that they will reunite after divorce.

When the family moves, this effect on children and families, but if changes in the family structure as divorce or death precipitate moves, children face the stresses created by both the precipitating events and moving itself. Children who move loose their old friends, the comfort to the familiar house, and their ties to schools and community. Frequent moves during the school years are likely to have adverse consequences on social and academic performance.

Migrant children and families not only need to adjust to a new community, school, and house but also need to adjust to a new culture and in many cases, to a new language. Children have faster language acquisition, they may even function as translators for the adults in their families.

Parents should prepare children well in advance of any move and allow them to express any unhappy feelings or misgivings. Parents should assist the entry of their children into the new community, and exchanges of letters, phone/mobile/internet with old friends and visits, whenever is possible should be encouraged.

Dalton R. Separation and Loss. In: Behrman RE, Kliegman RM, Jenson HB (eds). *Nelson Textbook of Pediatrics*. 17th edn. Philadelphia: Saunders, 2004;116–7.

7 ◆ Acutely Ill Child

7.1 EVALUATION OF THE SICK CHILD

There are many reasons for a sick child to visit the clinic/hospital, but most are due to acute intercurrent infections, and often the child is febrile. The acutely ill child with a serious illness is identified by careful observation, history taking, physical examination, age and body temperature, and the relevant screening laboratory tests. Six observation items and their scales (Acute Illness Observation Scales) that have identified serious illness in febrile children are shown in Table 7.1. The chance of serious illness is 1–2% if the total score is 10 or less; if the score is more than 10, the risk of serious illness increases by at least 10 fold.

Check six observation items and their scales that describe your child's appearance and observation. A normal finding is scored as 1; a moderate impairment as 3; and severe impairment as 5. The best possible score is 6 items × 1 = 6; the worst score is 6 items × 5 = 30. *Vital signs* (pulse, blood pressure, temperature, respiratory rate) are quite valuable in assessing the ill child. If the child appears ill or the history or physical examination suggests a serious illness, definitive laboratory tests appropriate for those findings are indicated. A follow-up examination often yields a diagnosis in a child as an outpatient in whom no specific diagnosis has been established. For the child in whom a diagnosis has already been established and who does not require hospitalization, follow-up in the outpatient department (OPD)/clinic visit should be used to monitor the course of the illness and to further educate and support the parents.

McCarthy PL. Evaluation of the sick child in the Office and Clinic. In: Kliegman RM, Behrman RE, Jenson HB, Stanton BF (eds). *Nelson Textbook of Pediatrics.* 18th edn. Vol. 1. Philadelphia: Saunders, 2007; 363–6.

7.2 INJURY CONTROL

Injuries are the most common cause of death during childhood and adolescence beyond first few months of life, and are preventable. The reduction of morbidity and mortality from injuries can be accomplished not only through *primary* prevention (averting the event or injury in the first place) but also through *secondary* and *tertiary* prevention. The latter two approaches include appropriate emergency medical services for injured children and specialized pediatric rehabilitation services that attempt to return children to their prior level of functioning. This broadened scope of prevention is covered in *injury control.* Various types of injuries include motor vehicle injuries (occupants, teenage drivers); bicycle injuries; pedestrian injuries; fire and burn related injuries; poisoning; drowning; firearm injuries; suffocation; homicide; suicide; work related injuries

Principles of injury control: Children at high injury risk are likely to be relatively poorly supervised, have disorganized or stressed families, and live in

Table 7.1: Acute illness observational scales for use in clinical evaluation of the well and sick child

Observation item	Normal	Moderate impairment	Severe impairment
1. **Quality of cry**	Strong with normal tone OR Content and not strong	Whimpering OR Sobbing	Weak OR Moaning OR High pitched
2. **Reaction to parent stimulation** (Effect on crying when held, patted on back, jiggled on lap or carried)	Cries briefly, then stops OR Content and not crying	Cries off and on	Continual cry OR Hardly responds
3. **State variation** (Going from awake to asleep or asleep to awake)	If awake stays awake OR If asleep and stimulated, then wakes up quickly	Eyes close briefly, then awakens OR Awakens with prolonged stimulation	Will not rouse OR Falls to sleep
4. **Color**	Pink	Pale hands, feet OR Acrocyanosis (blue hands and feet)	Pale OR Blue OR Ashen (Gray) OR Mottled
5. **Hydration** (Moisture in skin, eyes, mouth)	Skin normal and eyes, mouth moist	Skin, eyes normal and mouth slightly dry	Skin doughy OR tented and eyes may be sunken and dries eyes and mouth
6. **Response to social overtures** (Being held, kissed, hugged, touched, talked to, comforted)	Smiles OR Alerts (2 months or less)	Brief smile OR Alerts briefly (2 months or less)	No smile, face anxious OR Dull, expressionless OR No alerting (2 months or less)

Source: McCarthy PL, Sharpe MR, Spiesel SZ, et al. Observation scale to identify serious illness in febrile children. Pediatrics 1982;70:802.

hazardous environments. Efforts to control injuries include *education or persuasion, changes in product design, and modification of the social and physical environment.* Persuading individuals, particularly parents, to change their behaviors is important in injury control efforts. Speaking with parents specifically about using car seat restraints and bicycle helmets, installing smoke detectors, and checking the tap water temperature is likely to be more useful rather than advising them about supervising the child closely, being careful, and 'childproofing' the home. The information should be presented in the form of anticipatory guidance. Important topics to discuss at each developmental stage are shown in Box 7.1. The most successful injury prevention strategies are listed in Table 7.2. These *passive* interventions protect all individuals in the population, regardless of cooperation or level of skill, and are likely to be more successful than *active* measures that require repeated behavior change by the parent or child. Prevention campaigns combining two or more of theses approaches have been particularly effective in reducing injuries. Government has to play an important role especially making legislation.

American Academy of Pediatrics Committee on Injury Prevention and Poison Prevention. *Injury prevention and control for children and youth.* 3rd edn. Elk Grove Village, IL, American academy of Pediatrics, 1977.

Rivara FP, Grossman D. Injury control. In: Kliegman RM, Behrman RE, Jenson HB, Stanton BF (eds). *Nelson Textbook of Pediatrics.* 18th edn. Vol. 1. Philadelphia: Saunders, 2007; 366–75.

> **Box 7.1:** Injury prevention topics for anticipatory guidance by the pediatrician

Newborn
Car seats
Tap water temperature
Smoke detectors

Infant
Car seats
Tap water temperature
Bath safety

Toddler and prescooler
Car seats
Pedestrian skills training
Water safety
Childproof caps on medicines and household poisons

Primary school child
Pedestrian skills training
Water skills training
Seat belts
Bicycle helmets
Removal of firearms from home

Middle school child
Seat belts
Removal of firearms from home
Pedestrian skills

High school and older adolescents
Seat belts
Alcohol use, especially while driving, boating, and
    swimming
Occupational injuries
Removal of firearms from home

7.3 EMERGENCY MEDICAL SERVICES FOR CHILDREN

Most children who require emergency medical care come to physicians' offices, clinics, community emergency departments (EDs) and not to specialized pediatric EDs. This requires a community-based approach to emergency care of the child. Emergency medical services for children (EMS-C) is a concept that embodies a continuum of care and encompasses prevention, prehospital care and transport, ED and inpatient care, and necessary follow-up, including rehabilitation.

Pediatric critical care: Children having acute neurologic deterioration, respiratory distress, cardiovascular compromise, or life-threatening traumatic injuries constitute the most common admissions to a pediatric intensive care unit (PICU). Unlike pediatric patients who require general care, these patients usually have a disease process that affects more than one organ system, commonly referred to as multiple system organ failure (MSOF) or dysfunction (MSOD).

Patients are admitted to a PICU because they require a very high level of monitoring of vital signs and other body functions not available in other parts of the hospital. These patients may need mechanical ventilation, invasive intravascular monitoring, and frequent attention by both the nursing and the medical staffs (Table 7.3).

Interfacility transfer of the critically ill infant and child: Specialized transport programs (interfacility transport) bring patients from community facilities to the recognized pediatric intensive care unit (PICU). The members of the transport team must have the cognitive and technical skills required for the needs of pediatric patients and should be supervised by an attending physician (medical control physician [MCP]). *Ground ambulance* is used for the majority of transports. *Helicopters* enable a more rapid response, but are expensive; the greatest hazards are poor weather and landing in poorly visualized or nondesignated landing areas. Helicopters are most useful for transports within a 150–300 kilometer radius and for going directly to the site of an injury (e.g. to pick up a trauma victim). All vehicles must have the capability of radio or telephone contact with the MCP or the base station. In addition, each vehicle must be able to provide to on-board oxygen, electrical power, and suction and must have space for adequate supplies and equipment, and pharmacy packs.

Dowd MD, Rivara FP. Emergency Medical Services for Children. In: Kliegman RM, Behrman RE, Jenson HB, Stanton BF (eds). *Nelson Textbook of Pediatrics.* 18th edn. Vol. 1. Philadelphia: Saunders, 2007; 376–80.
Frankel LR. Interfacility Transfer of Critically Ill Infant and Child. In: Kliegman RM, Behrman RE, Jenson HB, Stanton BF (eds). *Nelson Textbook of Pediatrics.* 18th edn. Vol. 1. Philadelphia: Saunders, 2007; 380–2.

Table 7.2: Injury control interventions

Product modification	Environmental modification	Education
Child-resistant caps	Cabinet locks	Anticipatory guidance
Airbags	Roadway design	Public service announcements
Fire-safety	Smoke detectors	School safety programs

Table 7.3: Criteria for PICU and PIICU admission and discharge

Admission criteria	Discharge criteria
PICU	**PICU**
Patients who need invasive monitoring: Arterial and central venous catheters, pulmonary arterial lines, ICP catheters	Patient may be discharged from the PICU once the disease process has reversed itself and care can be provided in a less intense environment
Patients with evidence of:	
Respiratory impairment or failure	Patient no longer requires invasive monitoring
Cardiovascular compromise: shock, hypotension, hypertensive crisis	Patient can protect his/her airway (cough and gag reflexes)
Acute neurologic deterioration, coma, status epilepticus, increased ICP. Acute renal failure requiring dialysis or CVVH	Patient is hemodynamically stable
Bleeding disorders that necessitates massive transfusions	
PIICU	**PIICU**
Patients who do not require respiratory assistance for acute respiratory failure but may require continuous noninvasive monitoring of vital signs, BP, SaO_2, TcO_2, $TcCO_2$	Patient may be discharged from the PIICU when it is determined that care can be provided in general care areas
Patients who require chronic respiratory support via tracheotomies or noninvasive ventilation	
Patients who are in early cardiovascular failure and require monitoring of vital signs (noninvasive monitoring)	
Patients with acute neurologic injury but with a patent airway that they can protect themselves	
Patients with MSOD who do not need a PICU, but nursing care is not available elsewhere (e.g. trauma victims, DKA)	

BP: blood pressure; CVVH: Continuous venovenous hemofiltration; DKA: Diabetic ketoacidosis; ICP: Intracranial pressure; MSOD: Multiple system organ dysfunction; PICU: Pediatric intensive care unit; PIICU: Pediatric intermediate intensive care unit; SaO_2: Arterial oxygen saturation; TcO_2: Transcutaneous oxygen; $TcCO_2$: Transcutaneous carbon dioxide.

7.4 EFFECTIVE COMMUNICATION WITH FAMILIES IN THE PICU

There is sadness, fright, and anger in families of the child admitted in a pediatric intensive care unit (PICU). Families may wish to review their child's medical chart. This should be arranged at a time convenient when both the family and treating physician can be present together. Such a review may provide an opportunity to answer questions and explain unfamiliar terminology, which can provide further family reassurance. The goal should be to speak to the family with simple honesty and compassion about the child's condition and prognosis, unless certain circumstances would make such a frank discussion problematic (e.g. psychiatric or other serious illness in a parent).

Informed consent: The goal of informed consent is to provide patients or parents or other adults who are responsible for representing the interests of a child with a full understanding of their choices and the benefits and risks of each potential course of action. Caregivers should make efforts to ensure that proper communication occurs despite language barriers or differences in educational or cultural backgrounds.

Uncooperative or hostile families: The vast majority of families, despite the stress and anxiety provoked by their child's serious illness, want to work with the medical staff toward the goal of improving their child's health. However, the frustrations, sadness, and anger associated with the illness of a child can lead some families to become suspicious, aggressive, and occasionally violent. If there is a threat intimidation or violence against the medical staff, hospital security and the administration should be alerted that a serious conflict has occurred. In such instances, visitation privileges may be limited, allowed only when a security guard is present, and carried out in the company of an appropriate chaperone. But the focus should be to care for the child.

Communication regarding end-of-life decisions: When a child's condition irreversibly deteriorates and death is a likely event, health care staff must discuss the possibility of limiting or terminating support. If the possibility of tissue or organ donation exists, then discussion regarding limitation of support must be tailored to that purpose. Even death is the tragic outcome of a child's hospitalization; the PICU staff can be a source of strength and compassion and may help families to know that in his or her final days a child will be treated with respect, and genuine concern. In addition, to this, the need to recognize and respond to the family's shock and pain is equally important.

Mathers LH, Frankel LR. Effective communication with families in the PICU. In: Behrman RE, Kliegman RM, Jenson HB (eds). *Nelson Textbook of Pediatrics*. 17th edn. Philadelphia: Saunders, 2004; 270–2.

Young Seideman R, Watson MA, et al. Parent stress and coping in NICU, and PICU. *J Pediatr Nurs* 1977;2:69–77.

7.5 PEDIATRIC EMERGENCIES AND RESUSCITATION

Pediatric emergencies are of various types: respiratory, cardiac, endocrine, traumatic, and infectious. Most pediatrics arrests are respiratory and not cardiac. The most common life-threatening illnesses in children are those involving respiratory, cardiac, or neurologic failure. Pediatric patients suffering from acute failure of the liver, kidneys, or adrenals are also at risk.

Detecting and assessing physiologic instability: A simple and consistent approach is necessary for rapid and efficient evaluation of a pediatric patient who may be in serious distress. First determine alertness of the patient, including response to stimuli, spontaneous vocalization or movement, and muscle tone. In basic life support, this is assessed by asking "Are you all right?" This is followed by assessment of the vital signs (heart rate, blood pressure, respiratory rate, and temperature) and other basic indicators of the physiologic state (Table 7.4). To help define poor perfusion, the lower limit of systolic BP should be less than 60 mm Hg for neonates; less than 70 mm Hg from 1 mo to 1 yr; less than 70 mm Hg + 2 × age from 1 to 10 yr; less than 90 mm Hg if older than 10 yr.

Adequate cardiac output is reflected in good *perfusion* of the skin (central and distal extremities). Skin perfusion may be assessed by the temperature of the skin or by capillary refill time (the time required for color to return to the skin after pressure blanching that part of skin is released). Normally capillary refill time is 2 seconds or less; however, low environmental temperature may cause peripheral vasoconstriction and lengthening of capillary refill. Pulse oximetry is meant to measure hemoglobin oxygen saturation and for that there is need to have adequate perfusion for reliable measurement; the presence of a strong signal indicates good peripheral perfusion.

The normal temperature range for humans is constant throughout life (36°–37°C; 96.8°–98.6°F), less than 99°F (37.2°C). Normal body temperature also varies in a regular pattern each day (> 37°C; > 98.6°F). This circadian temperature rhythm, or *diurnal variation*, results in lower body temperatures in the early morning and temperatures approximately 1°C higher in the late afternoon or early evening. Premature infants and small term infants may have difficulty maintaining their appropriate *core temperature* if they are left uncovered in a cool environment. Infants may not be able to generate an elevated temperature in response to infection. Temperatures in excess of 41°C (> 41°C) is known as hyperpyrexia. Temperature is less than normal (< 36°C) and when the body core temperature falls below 35°C, the syndrome of hypothermia occurs. In healthy individuals 18–40 yr of age, the mean oral temperature is 36.8° ± 0.4°C (98.2° ± 0.7°F), with low levels at 6 AM and higher levels at 4–6 PM. *An* **AM** *temperature of* > 37°C (> 98.9°F) *or a* **PM** *temperature of* > 37.7°C (> 99.9°F) *would define a*

Table 7.4: Vital signs at various ages			
Age	*Heart rate (beats/min)*	*Blood pressure (mm Hg)*	*Respiratory rate (breaths/min)*
Premature	120–170*	55–75/35–45†	40–70#
0–3 mo	100–150*	65–85/45–55	35–55
3–6 mo	90–120	70–90/50–65	30–45
6–12 mo	80–120	80–100/55–65	25–40
1–3 yr	70–110	90–105/55–70	20–30
3–6 yr	65–110	95–110/60–75	20–25
6–12 yr	60–95	100–120/60–75	14–22
12 yr	55–85	110–135/65–85	12–18

*In sleep, infant heart rates may drop significantly lower, but if perfusion is maintained, no intervention is required.
†A blood pressure cuff should cover approximately two-thirds of the arm; too small a cuff yields spuriously high blood pressure readings, and too large a cuff yields spuriously low blood pressure readings
#Many premature infants require mechanical ventilatory support, making their spontaneous respiratory rate less relevant

fever. The normal daily temperature variation is typically 0.5°C (0.9°F).

Assessing metabolic status: Two important acute destabilizing metabolic disorders are acidosis and hypoglycemia. Hypoglycemia produces weakness and lethargy and can lead to seizures and coma. Emergency resuscitation should usually include intravenous administration of glucose (250–500 mg/kg, infused over 1–2 min).

Central nervous system function assessment: The integrity of the CNS is assessed by the history and physical examination to determine the possibility of trauma, toxic and/or drug ingestions, seizures, ischemia, and signs of any expanding intracranial lesion (hemorrhage, tumor, abscess, vascular malformations). Tables 7.5 and 7.6 show important scoring or staging criteria used to assess neurologic status. These scores should be used serially over time to detect disease improvement or progression. Glasgow Coma Scale (GCS) used in patients with altered level consciousness, especially those who have sustained a traumatic head injury. Patients with a GCS score of 8 or less may require aggressive management, including mechanical ventilation and intracranial pressure monitoring.

Resuscitation

The main objective in pediatric resuscitation is to maintain adequate oxygenation and perfusion of blood throughout the body while steps are taken to stabilize a child and establish long-term homeostasis. An orderly sequence of events should be instituted, beginning with the ABCs: **A** = airway, **B** = breathing and **C** = circulation. Children with a respiratory arrest,

Table 7.5: Glasgow Coma Scale (GCS)

Eye opening (total points 4)

Spontaneous	4
To voice	3
To pain	2
None	1

Verbal response (total points 5)

Older children		*Infants and young children*	
Oriented	5	Appropriate words; smiles, fixes, and follows	5
Confused	4	Consolable crying	4
Inappropriate	3	Persistently irritable	3
Incomprehensible	2	Restless, agitated	2
None	1	None	1

Motor response (total points 6)

Obeys	6
Localizes pain	5
Withdraws	4
Flexion	3
Extension	2
None	1

Source: Adapted and modified from Teasdale G, Jennett B. Assessment of coma and impaired consciousness: A practical scale. *Lancet* 1974; 2: 81

Table 7.6: Clinical staging of encephalopathy

Clinical stage 1	*Clinical stage 2*	*Clinical stage 3*	*Clinical stage 4*	*Clinical stage 5*
Lethargic	Combative	Comatose	Comatose	Comatose
Follows commands	Inconsistent following of commands	Occasional respond to commands	Responds only to pain	No response to pain
Pupils reactive	Pupils sluggish	Eyes may deviate	Weak papillary response	No papillary response
Breathing normal	May hyperventilate	Irregular breathing	Very irregular breathing	Requires mechanical ventilation
Normal muscle tone	Reflexes inconsistent	Decorticate posturing	Decerebrate posturing	Absent tendon reflexes—flaccid

a short duration of CPR, and a pulse present at the time of apnea have the best chance of survival.

Respiratory support: If *no obstruction by a foreign body* is found and if a child has no spontaneous respirations, steps should be immediately taken to breathe for the child. A common cause of airway obstruction in an unresponsive child is the tongue occluding the airway. Assessment includes opening the airway (head tilt/chin lift or jaw thrust if the cervical spine is unstable) and looking for the rise and fall of the chest as well as a foreign body, listening at the nose and mouth for breathing, and feeling air existing the child's airways (Figs 7.1 and 7.2). This should be done in less than 10 seconds. If *a foreign body is seen*, it should be removed; perform a tongue/jaw lift if a foreign body is suspected

but not initially visualized. If the patient resumes adequate spontaneous ventilation, the patient's body is turned on its side to the recovery position with the head to the side (if in the field).

Rescue breathing should be done by *mouth-to-mouth or mouth-to-nose breathing*, or bag-mask respirations (Figs 7.3 and 7.4). Successful rescue breathing will provide good chest rise and relief of deep cyanosis. Exhaled air is 16–17% oxygen, which corresponds to

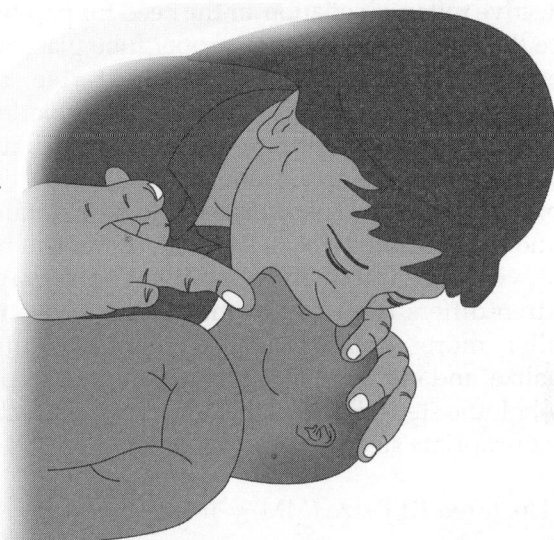

Fig. 7.3: Rescue breathing in an infant: The rescuer's mouth covers the infant's nose and mouth, creating a seal. One hand performs head tilt while the other hand lifts the infant's jaw. Avoid head tilt if the infant has sustained head or neck trauma.

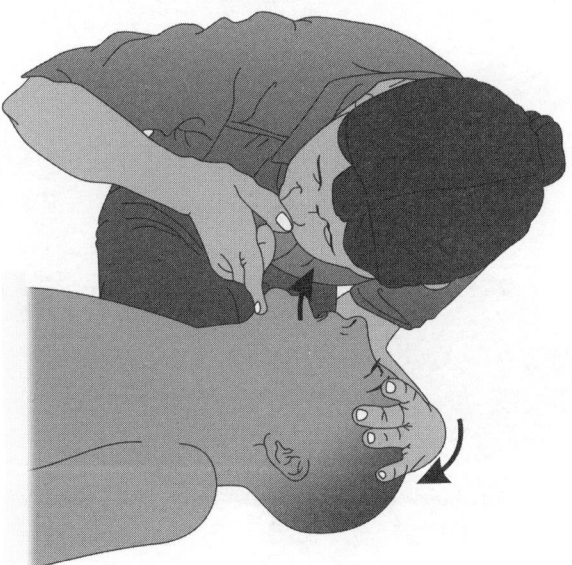

Fig. 7.1: Opening the airway with the head-tilt/chin-lift maneuver: One hand is used to tilt the head, extending the neck. The index finger of the rescuer's other hand fits the mandible outward by lifting the chin. Head-tilt should not be performed if a cervical spine injury is suspected.

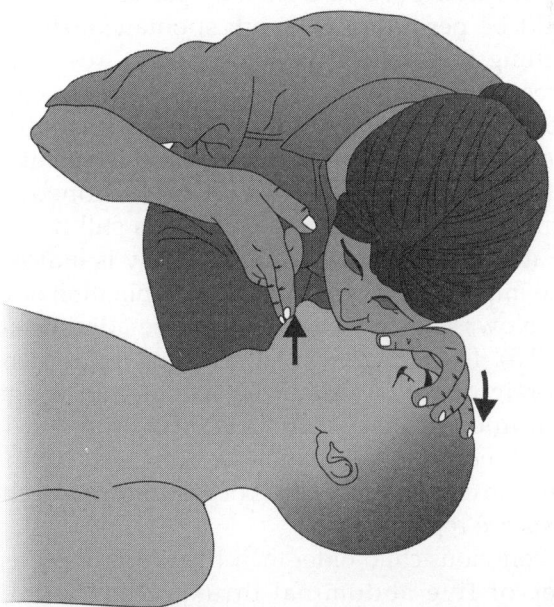

Fig. 7.4: Rescue breathing in a child: The rescuer's mouth covers the mouth of the child, creating a mouth-to-mouth seal. One hand maintains head tilt; the thumb and forefinger of the same hand are used to pinch the child's nose.

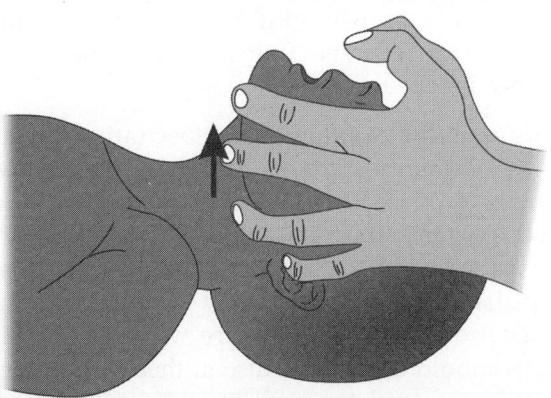

Fig. 7.2: Jaw thrust: Combined jaw thrust-spine stabilization maneuver for the pediatric trauma victim.

an alveolar oxygen pressure of 80 mm Hg in the patient. If these measures do not facilitate adequate air entry, recheck that the airway is patent and the seal is tight; if so endotracheal intubation is indicated. Indicators for endotracheal intubation include apnea, loss of CNS control of respirations, airway obstruction unrelieved by airway opening maneuvers, increased work of breathing that may lead to fatigue, the need for positive end-expiratory pressure (PEEP) or a high peak inspiratory pressure (PIP), poor airway protective reflexes, sedation, or the need for paralysis. Once the patient is intubated, proper tube placement is assessed by breath sounds, chest rise, and instantaneous analysis of exhaled carbon dioxide by a calorimetric device placed within the respiratory tubing near the endotracheal tube (ETT). The respiratory rate parameters that should be maintained are indicated in Table 7.4. In the field, competent bag-mask ventilation may be preferable. The airway in children differs from that of the adult because it is smaller, more anteriorly placed, more difficult to visualize, and more prone to mucosal injuries leading to subglottic stenosis. A simple formula for selecting the appropriate size ETT is as follows:

$$\text{Uncuffed ETT size (MM)} = 16 + \frac{\text{Age in year}}{4}$$

Foreign body aspiration always should be suspected if respiratory distress has had a sudden onset or if the chest does not rise when ventilation is first attempted in an unconscious, apneic infant or child. A conscious child suspected of a foreign body partial obstruction should be permitted to cough spontaneously until coughing is not effective (or aphonic), respiratory distress and stridor increase, or the child becomes unconscious. The airway is then opened with the head-tilt/chin-lift maneuver, and ventilation is attempted. If unsuccessful, the airway is repositioned and ventilation again attempted. If there is still no chest rise, attempts to remove a foreign body is indicated. In the infant younger than 1 yr, a combination of five back blows and five chest thrusts are administered (Fig. 7.5). The foreign body is removed if it is seen. If no foreign body is visualized, ventilation is again attempted. If this is unsuccessful, the head is repositioned and ventilation is attempted again. If there is no chest rise, the series of back blows and chest thrusts are repeated.

A conscious child older than 1 yr is administered a series of five abdominal thrusts (the Heimlich maneuver) with the child standing or sitting (Fig. 7.6). If unconscious, this is done with the child lying down (Fig. 7.7). After the abdominal thrusts, the airway is examined for a foreign body, which should be

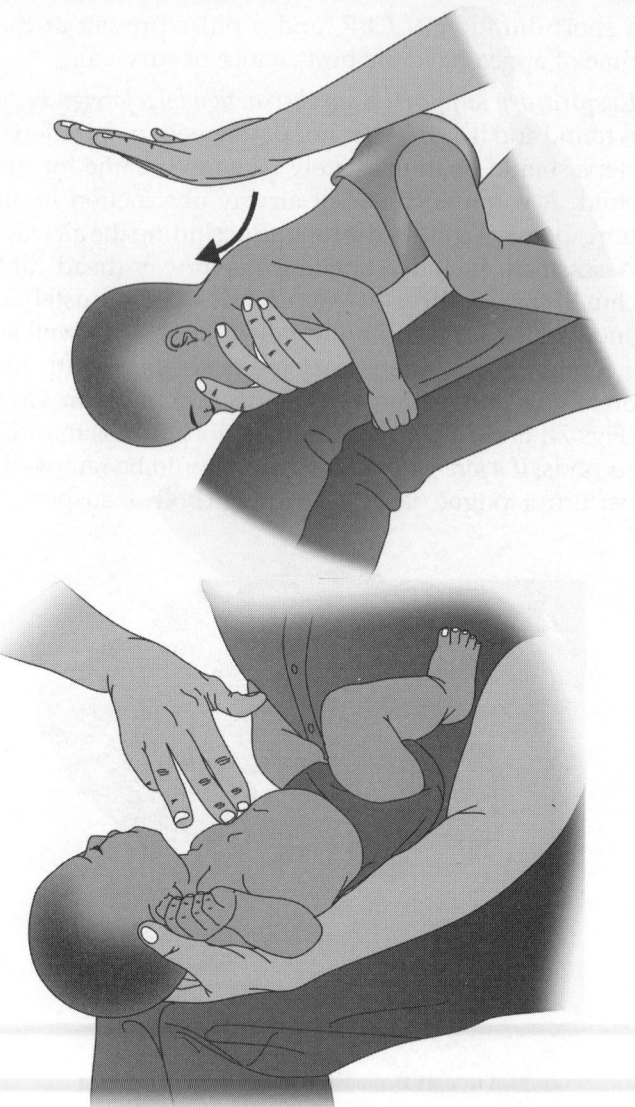

Fig. 7.5: Back blows (top) **and chest thrusts** (bottom) to relieve foreign body airway obstruction in the infant.

removed if visualized. If no foreign body is seen the head is repositioned and ventilation attempted. If unsuccessful, repositioning of head and attempted ventilation are repeated. If unsuccessful, the Heimlich sequence is repeated.

Cardiovascular support: As resuscitation proceeds and ventilation is started, support of the *circulation* should be provided to sustain adequate blood flow to deliver oxygen to the tissues (Figs 7.8 and 7.9). Circulation is assessed by lay rescuers without checking for the pulse, it actually delays cardiopulmonary resuscitation; while health care workers or trained parents should check for pulse. If there is no pulse or the pulse is less than 60 beats/min with poor perfusion, chest compressions must be given. Chest compressions are given without interrupting

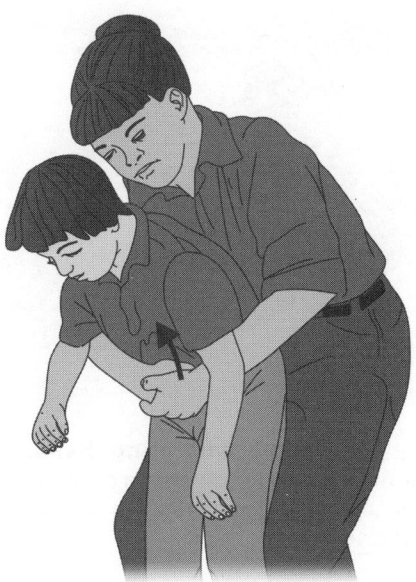

Fig. 7.6: Abdominal thrusts with victim standing or sitting (conscious).

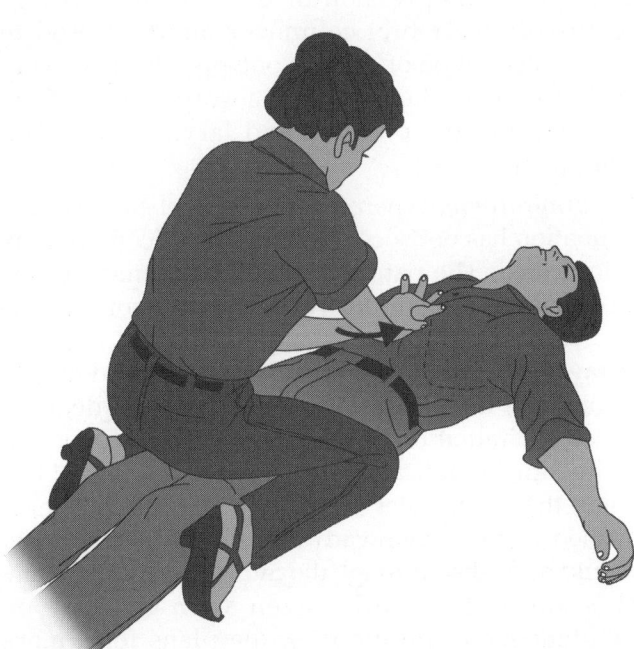

Fig. 7.7: Abdominal thrusts with victim lying (conscious or unconscious).

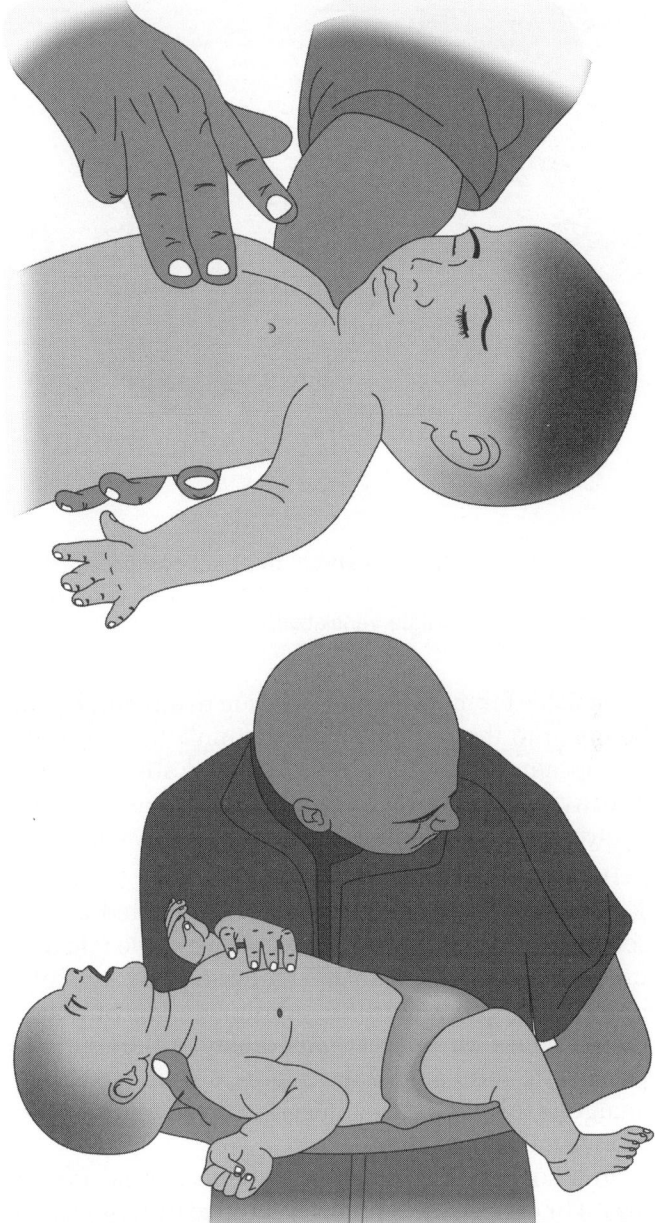

Fig. 7.8. Cardiac compressions: The infant is supine on palm of the rescuer's hand for performing CPR (top); CPR is performed while carrying the infant or small child. Note that the head is kept level with the torso (bottom).

ventilations. The effectiveness of chest compressions is determined by the presence of a palpable pulse. The rate of chest compressions varies with age and size (Table 7.7). Chest compressions in small infants and newborns may be performed by placing two thumbs on the midsternum with the hands encircling the thorax, or by two fingers over the midsternum and compressing, or by holding the child in the supine posture on one's lap. When feasible, a cardiac resuscitation board should be placed under the child's back to maximize efficiency of compressions. The

resuscitation effort should pause periodically to make an assessment of the possible return of spontaneous heart rate, pulse and respirations. If the resuscitative efforts do not succeed in re-establishing respiration and heartbeat, the medical team must decide whether continued efforts are warranted or if the resuscitation should be stopped. If resuscitation is to continue and spontaneous heart rate and respirations have not returned, then the patient should be intubated, vascular access established, and administration of resuscitative drugs initiated. If appropriate equipment

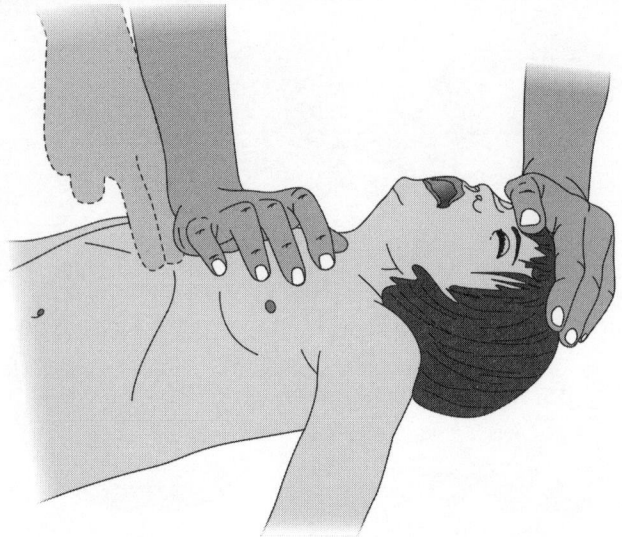

Fig. 7.9: Locating hand position for chest compression in a child. Note that the rescuer's other hand is used to maintain head position to facilitate ventilation.

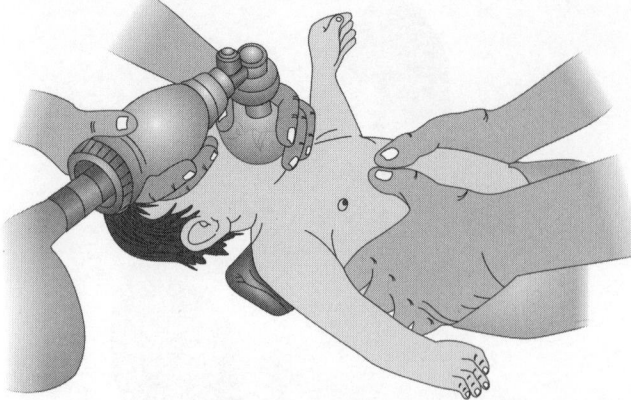

Fig. 7.10. Two thumb-encircling hands for chest compression: One rescuer to perform chest compressions in an infant and another rescuer to resuscitate the infant with bag and mask (2 rescuers).

is available for monitoring ECG drug treatment should be given to the particular dysrhythmia (amiodarone or lidocaine for ventricular tachycardia; adenosine for supraventricular tachycardia; cardioversion for ventricular fibrillation—usually used in older children).

Intubation and mechanical ventilation: Children 1 month of age or older should be pretreated with a sedative, an analgesic, and possibly a muscle relaxant unless the situation is an emergency (apnea, asystole, unresponsiveness) and the administration of drugs would cause an unacceptable delay; although it is possible to intubate awake infants without sedation, analgesia, or paralysis, analgesia is recommended to reduce metabolic stress.

In a controlled intubation, patients should fast at least 4 hr or have their stomach emptied by nasogastric tube. The history and physical examination should be reviewed for any allergies or evidence of unusual airway anatomy or risk of malignant hyperthermia, and informed consent should be obtained. Equipment necessary for intubation and bag-mask ventilation and an emergency cricothyrotomy tray should be available.

Because the stomach generally cannot be emptied before rapid sequence intubation (RSI) the **Sellick maneuver** (compression of the cricoids cartilage against the vertebral column) should be used to prevent aspiration of gastric contents, which are very likely to occur when the laryngoscope and ETT are inserted into the pharynx and larynx (*orotracheal intubation*).

Cricothyrotomy: When the airway is obstructed and intubation has not succeeded, needle cricothyrotomy is indicated. The patient should be supine with the face looking directly upward. The midpoint of the cricothyroid membrane is palpated, and a 14-gauge intravenous catheter with stylet is advanced slowly through it, inclined interiorly at about 45 degrees. Quick aspiration of air through a syringe connected to the catheter indicates entry into the trachea. At this point, the metal stylet is removed and the catheter is pushed further downward into the trachea. Oxygen should be flushed through the catheter at 10–15 L/min. This supports a child, even with little or no spontaneous respirations, while plans for a more secure airway are made. *Surgical cricothyrotomy* is rarely necessary in children. It involves making a transverse incision in the cricothyroid membrane and

	Neonate	1–8 year	>8 year
Table 7.7: Chest compressions: ventilation relationships			
Compression rate	120	At least 100	100
Compression to ventilation ratio*	3 : 1	5 : 1	15 : 2[†]
Pulse check[‡]	Umbilical artery	Brachial	Carotid

*Ventilation should be given without interrupting chest compression; it is synchronous.
[†]Once intubated go to 5 : 1.
[‡]For lay rescuers no pulse check is necessary; it actually delays cardiopulmonary resuscitation. Lay rescuers should check for signs of circulation; cyanosis, breathing, coughing, and movement.

advancing a large catheter through the incision downward into the lower trachea. The risk of bleeding, upper airway obstruction, and pneumothorax are significantly greater.

Interosseous line placement: Interosseous cannulation should be performed in those patients for whom intravenous access is difficult or unattainable, even in older children and in an arrest situation within 1 min if venous access is not available.

Administration of drugs through endotracheal tube (ETT): Administration of certain drugs is also possible through the ETT include lidocaine, atropine, naloxone and epinephrine.

Drug therapy and defibrillation: If ventilation and chest compressions do not restore the circulation and spontaneous respirations, medications may be needed. If there is ECG evidence of a potentially perfusing rhythm but no pulse is palpated, one should consider the causes of pulseless electrical activity (electrical mechanical dissociation). These include hypothermia, hypoxia, hypovolemia, hyperkalemia, tension pneumothorax, pericardial tamponade, toxins, and pulmonary thromboembolism. If there is bradycardia, asystole, ventricular tachycardia, or ventricular fibrillation, the patient requires drug therapy and when indicated, defibrillation. Epinephrine should initially be used in the standard dose (0.01 mg/kg, which is 0.1 ml/kg of 1:10,000 solution). If the first dose is ineffective, it may be repeated every 3 min or increased to 0.1–0.2 mg/kg dose. Vasopressin may also be effective as a one-time dose (40 U in adults) after epinephrine (not recommended in children younger than 8 yr of age). Atropine may be effective for pulseless electrical activity, bradycardia, or asystole. Amiodarone is indicated in patients with ventricular fibrillation or pulseless ventricular tachycardia that is shock refractory; lidocaine and procainamide are second choice alternate drugs. *Torsades de pointes* may respond to intravenous administration of 25 mg/kg magnesium sulfate. Intravenous or intraosseous fluids should be normal saline or Ringer lactate without glucose to support circulation and to avoid hyperglycemia, which is a poor prognostic factor during an arrest.

Arterial access: The *radial artery* is commonly used for cannulation. The other arteries used for cannulation are ulnar, brachial, femoral, posterior tibial, and dorsalis pedis. Arterial catheters require special care for insertion and subsequent management because the blood flow to tissue can be compromised and considerable hemorrhage can occur if a catheter is dislodged. The adequacy of perfusion distal to the catheter must be monitored (e.g. warmth, capillary filling, edema). Catheters usually need to be heparinized (0.5–1 U/ml) to minimize clotting.

Thoracentesis and chest tube placement: *Thoracentesis* is the placement of a needle or catheter (chest tube) into the pleural space to evacuate fluid, blood, or air. Most insertions are performed in an intercostal space between the 4th and 9th ribs, along the midclavicular line in the anterior chest wall (in adolescents and adults), or in the plane of the midaxillary line. After the chest tube is inserted, it should be secured firmly to the chest wall and connected to a source of suction (e.g. Pleurovac) at a pressure of 15–20 cm H_2O. A radiograph should be obtained to verify chest tube placement and evacuation of the pleural space.

Pericardiocentesis: When fluid, blood or gas accumulates in the pericardial sac, a danger is that the heart will be compressed and will not be able to fill and empty with normal volumes of blood, leading to diminution in cardiac output.

Postresuscitation care: When *resuscitation is successful*, continuous PICU care is usually needed to attend to the potential post ischemic multiple organ dysfunction syndrome and continued need for cardiac inotropic support. Most patients do not require hyperventilation. Hyperglycemia and hyperthermia should be avoided. Continuous observation for immediate neurologic deterioration and long-term permanent neurodevelopment sequelae are imperative.

When *resuscitation fails and the patient dies* attention is focused on comforting the grieving family. Finally, someone on the team must be mindful of the legal and procedural duties involved in a death, such as contact with the organ/tissue transplant bank, completion of the death certificate, and arrangements for disposition of the remains of the deceased, depending on local regulations, family wishes, and customs.

Eisenberg MS, Mengert TJ. Cardiac resuscitation. *N Engl J Med* 2001; 344:1304–13.

Emergency Cardiac Care Committee and Subcommittee, American Heart Association. Pediatric basic life support, part 5. *JAMA* 1992; 268:2251.

Mathers LH, Frankel LR. Pediatric emergencies and resuscitation. In: Kliegman RM, Behrman RE, Jenson HB, Stanton BF (eds). *Nelson Textbook of Pediatrics*. 18th edn, Vol. 1. Philadelphia: Saunders, 2007; 387–405.

Parfitt A. Resuscitation guidelines. *Lancet* 2006; 367:282–4.

7.6 MECHANICAL VENTILATION

Positive pressure ventilators are used to provide mechanical ventilation in adult, pediatric and neonatal ICUs. During positive pressure mechanical ventilation, the flow of gas during inspiration and exhalation is driven by the airway pressure gradient between the airway opening and the alveoli. Pressure may be administered at the airway opening by a tight-fitting mask connected to a ventilator-mask CPAP (continuous positive airway pressure); to a compressible bag attached to a gas source—bag-mask ventilation; or to both—mask BiPAP (bilevel positive airway pressure). In a PICU, the ventilatory support is frequently provided through an endotracheal tube (ETT) or occasionally with a tracheostomy cannula. The ETT adapter, which attaches to the ventilator tubing, is considered the airway opening. During inspiration, the airway opening pressure is greater than alveolar pressure, thereby driving gas into the lungs and inflating them. Exhalation is usually passive and occurs because, at the end of inspiration, alveolar pressure becomes greater than airway pressure.

Use of Mechanical Ventilators

Pressures: Peak inspiratory pressure (PIP) occurs during maximal inspiration. *Positive end-expiratory pressure* (PEEP) helps maintain the end-expiratory resting lung volume. The maximum pressure ingredient is the difference between PIP and PEEP. The mean airway pressure is a measure of the average pressure to which the lungs are exposed during the respiratory cycle. Mean airway pressure can be increased by increasing PEEP, PIP, the ratio of inspiratory time to expiratory time (I : E ratio), or the inspiratory flow.

Components of the ventilator breath: Each complete ventilator breath has an allotted time for inspiration (I time) before the ventilator must cycle into exhalation time (E time). The sum of the I time and E time equals the allotted time per breath. The ventilator delivers a set number of breaths per minute, the *ventilator frequency*. The frequency determines the length of each breath. For example, a frequency of 20 would result in 3 sec/breath. Most ventilators allow setting either the I time or the I : E ratio. For example, if an I time of 1 sec is ordered and the breath is 3 sec, the I:E ratio will be 1 sec:2 sec. If an I : E ratio of 1 : 3 is ordered, then the I time would be 0.75 sec, and the E time would be 2.25 sec.

The change in lung volume during the inspiratory period is defined as the *tidal volume* (V_T). It is the volume above the *functional residual capacity* (FRC), that is, the volume above the end-expiratory lung volume. By convention the gas flows is in units of L/min and the I time is in seconds; in pediatrics the V_T is usually expressed in milliliters. From the alveolar gas equation, to adjust $PaCO_2$, either the V_T or the ventilator frequency is changed.

Alveolar ventilation = (tidal volume – dead space) × frequency

---

Box 7.2: Comparison of pressure-controlled and volume-controlled ventilation

Pressure-controlled ventilation

Constant pressure delivered

Variable volume delivered; reduced risk of barotraumas

Changes in patient's compliance or resistance may lead to alterations in delivered volumes as pressure remains constant

Changes in tidal pressures may result in changes in minute ventilation

Volume-controlled ventilation

Constant volume (V_T) delivered; less risk of hypoventilation or hyperventilation

Variable pressure (PIP) delivered

Changes in patient's compliance or resistance leads to potential for dangerously high inflating volume delivered and therefore closure monitoring is required of tidal volume and carbon dioxide, and pressure alarms.

V_T: Tidal volume; PIP: Peak inspiratory pressure

Pressure-controlled vs. volume-controlled ventilation: These are the two primary forms of positive pressure ventilators (Box 7.2). Pressure-controlled ventilators allow a clinician to set the PIP and PEEP. Whereas in volume-controlled ventilation, the V_T is present as a product of setting flow and I time. The airway pressure rises throughout inspiration and reaches its peak when the entire V_T has been delivered. Thus, PIP is not set but rather is determined by both the V_T and the pulmonary mechanics of the patient.

Ventilator-patient interactions: When children are not attempting to breathe spontaneously, the ventilator completely controls the respiratory pattern. But for children who can attempt to breathe, the degree to which a ventilator is able to synchronize with the patient's own respiratory efforts may have significant clinical effects.

Synchronized intermittent mandatory ventilation (SIMV): SIMV allows better response by the ventilator to the patient. During SIMV, the ventilator allows the child to trigger a breath by spontaneously attempting to inspire. If the patient takes too long to initiate a spontaneous breath, then inspiration is time triggered by the ventilator: a mandatory breath. Many ventilators allow both pressure support and SIMV.

Monitoring and alarms: In pressure-controlled ventilation, the V_T is monitored. In volume-controlled ventilation, the airway pressure is monitored; safety precautions include pop-off limits to the peak airway pressure. An oxygen analyzer allows monitoring of FiO_2 (fraction of inspired oxygen, e.g. breathing oxygen at room air with a concentration of 21%—a FiO_2 of 0.21%).

Alarms can be set for a wide array of events. The common alarms are for high or low airway pressure, absence of flow (apnea), loss of electrical power, high or low exhaled V_T, and high or low minute volume. When alarms occur, they must then be evaluated to determine if there is a malfunction of the ventilator or a change in the patient. Frequent physical examination is the fastest means of diagnosing a variety of ventilator problems, such as patient-ventilator dyssynchrony (in patients receiving less sedation or having anxiety when their lung disease is improving), ETT obstruction, barotraumas, pneumothorax, and accidental extubation.

Approach to mechanical ventilation: Respiratory diseases result in decreased lung compliance or increased airway resistance or both. Ventilator strategies are designed to ameliorate physiologic derangements and resulting ventilation-perfusion mismatch.

Diseases of decreased compliance include various diseases that affect the lung parenchyma, such as acute respiratory distress syndrome (ARDS), atelectasis, pneumonia, pulmonary edema, and pulmonary hemorrhage. Fractional residual capacity (FRC) is reduced in all these diseases as terminal spaces are flooded or collapsed, owing to the presence of abnormal fluid with in the alveoli or atelactasis from the decreased amount of surfactant lining the alveoli. Intrapulmonary shunt is increased when blood flows to poorly ventilated lung units. Decreased compliance requires a higher pressure gradient to achieve a given V_T. With volume-controlled ventilation, the PIP will be higher than it would for a patient with normal lungs. If the ventilator is pressure-controlled, then a given PIP may result in a V_T that will be lower than that of a patient with normal lungs. These diseases of decreased compliance also may respond to higher ventilator rates as the lungs empty and fill more quickly. If decreased compliance is not compensated then hypercarbia develops.

Diseases of increased resistance include various diseases that decrease the caliber of the airway lumen by edema, spasm, or obstructing material. Because airways decrease in caliber during exhalation, increased resistance affects expiratory flow more than inspiratory flow. Diseases in which airway resistance

	Normal lungs	*Decreased compliance*	*Increased resistance*
Tidal volume (V_T)	8–12 ml/kg (set of volume-controlled and derived if pressure-controlled ventilation)	10–12 ml/kg (may need to useless if the inflating pressures are too high, i.e. risk of volutrauma)	10–12 ml/kg (may need to use less volume if the inflating pressures required are too high, i.e. barotrauma)
Rate (breaths/min)	Physiologic norm for age or lower (depending on the V_T used, e.g. infant rate = 30; toddler rate = 20; adolescent rate = 16)	May require higher rates to maintain adequate minute ventilation	Often requires lower rates to allow adequate emptying time
Peak inspiratory pressure—PIP (cm H_2O)	Initial PIP = 20–25 cm H_2O, monitor for adequate chest expansion and V_T	May require higher PIP to obtain acceptable V_T	May require higher PIP to obtain acceptable V_T
Positive end-expiratory pressure (PEEP)	2–4 cm H_2O to prevent atelectasis	Frequently requires higher PEEP to achieve oxygenation and improved compliance (e.g. 6–10 cm H_2O) Anticipate decreased venous return and cardiac output	May need to maintain low PIP to avoid exacerbation of gas trapping and overinflation
Oxygen concentration (FiO_2)	May not need supplemental oxygen; however, one usually begins with FiO_2 of 1.0 and may the quickly wean to an $FiO_2 \leq 0.5$	Begin with an FiO_2 of 1.0 Attempt to wean to ≤ 0.6 by adjusting mean airway pressures/PEEP	Begin with an FiO_2 of 1.0, wean to maintain adequate oxygenation and avoid oxygen toxicity
Inspiratory time (I time)	Normal for age I : E = 1 : 2, 1 : 3	Generous I time to allow recruitment of collapsed lung segments (e.g. 1 : 1.2)	Ensure adequate I time and E time, especially E time, to avoid gas trapping (e.g. I : E of 1 : 3 or 1 : 4)

Table 7.8: Guidelines for initiating mechanical ventilation

is increased include asthma, bronchiolitis, bronchopulmonary dysplasia, smoke inhalation, and cystic fibrosis. Diseases of increased resistance are often accompanied by both increased intrapulmonary shunt and dead space ventilation.

Mechanical ventilation is initiated to provide support for lungs that function normally or for diseases of decreased compliance, or of increased resistance (Table 7.8).

Complications: There are many pulmonary and systemic complications of mechanical ventilation. Lung injury may result from positive pressure (barotrauma), oxygen toxicity, or excessive volume changes in the lung-volutrauma. Volutrauma may be manifested acutely as pulmonary air leak, such as pneumothoraces, pneumomediastinum, pulmonary interstitial emphysema, and bronchopleural fistula and may also be a cause of chronic repetitive lung injury.

Positive pressure ventilation also may have effects on the cardiovascular system, which may be beneficial or detrimental, depending on the overall cardiovascular status of the child. In general, high mean airway pressures require close observation and may necessitate support with fluids and inotropic drugs.

An ETT may become obstructed owing to mucus, purulent material, or blood from trauma to the airway or from the child biting on the tube and are immediately life-threatening complications. An ETT also may cause injury to the tracheal mucosa resulting in subglottic stenosis, which may resolve with time or may require surgical intervention. Prolonged intubation and mechanical ventilation may predispose the child to nosocomial infections, often by bacteria with resistance to numerous antibiotics. Nosocomial infection, sepsis, and other organ system failures are the leading cause of death of patients with respiratory failure.

Other approaches: Other approaches to the care of the critically ill child with acute respiratory failure include high-frequency modes of ventilation (HFV), the application of permissive hypercapnia and the use of prone positioning. All three modes of HFV (oscillatory, jet, and flow interruption) utilize very small tidal volume (< 1 ml/kg), very rapid rates (150–1,000 breaths/min), and lower mean airway pressures to provide a gentler form of mechanical ventilation. Permissive hypercapnea [allowing the patient's $Paco_2$ to rise into the 60–70 mm Hg range as long as the patient is adequately oxygenated (SaO_2 > 92%)] and the patient is able to tolerate the degree of acidosis. This is used to limit the amount of barotraumas and volutrauma to the patient. Positioning the patient in the prone position has been shown to improve oxygenation and reduce ventilator-induced lung injury in patients with severe lung injury.

Long-term Mechanical Ventilation

Children younger than 10 yr of age with life-threatening or life-shortening medical conditions commonly require long-term ventilator assistance. Patients are often maintained on long-term ventilation until they recover from the initial pulmonary insult, or indefinitely, for progressively neuromuscular disease. These patients can be also managed in home.

Chronic respiratory failure is pulmonary insufficiency for a protracted period, usually 28 days, but this time limit is an approximation and varies with the specific clinical situation.

Patients in an ICU in whom extubation is unsuccessful because of muscle weakness are candidates for long-term support. These patients may require more than 4–6 wk for the acute pulmonary process to completely resolve and to regain respiratory muscle strength; they also need some rehabilitation. Patients who have progressive neuromuscular disease and signs and symptoms of muscle fatigue should be considered for this treatment. Patients who have any central nervous system insult and cannot appropriately protect their airway should be considered for a tracheostomy, but may also need mechanical ventilation due to hypoventilation or apnea.

Curley MA. Prone positioning of patients with acute respiratory distress syndrome: A systemic review. *Am J Crit Care* 1999; 8: 397–405.

Frankel LR, Kache S. Mechanical ventilation. In: Kliegman RM, Behrman RE, Jenson HB, Stanton BF (eds). *Nelson Textbook of Pediatrics*. 18th edn Vol. 1. Philadelphia: Saunders, 2007; 424–31.

Matthews BD, Noviski N. Management of oxygenation in pediatric acute hypoxemic respiratory failure. *Pediatr Pulmonol* 2001; 32: 459–470.

7.7 DROWNING AND NEAR-DROWNING

The definitions of drowning and near-drowning are somewhat arbitrary, but are still widely used. Death within 24 hr of a submersion is termed *drowning*, which may be immediate or may follow resuscitation. Survival after more than 24 hr is termed *near-drowning*, regardless of whether the victim later dies or recovers. After submersion in the liquid medium, suffocation and asphyxia may occur, with or without pulmonary aspiration. Drowning is death by suffocation from being submerged in water. If a person has been rescued from a near-drowning situation, first aid and medical attention is critical.

Most drownings occur within a short distance of safety. Immediate action and first aid can prevent death. A person who is drowning usually cannot shout for help. Be alert for signs of drowning. Suspect an accident if you see someone in the water fully clothed. Watch for uneven swimming motions, which indicate a swimmer is getting tired. Often the body sinks, and only the head shows above the water. Children can drown in only a few inches of water. It may be possible to revive a drowning victim even after a prolonged period of submersion, especially if the person was in very cold water. As a cause globally, drowning ranked 11th for children younger than 5-yr-old and 4th for children aged 5–14 yr.

Pathophysiology: Young children can only struggle for 10–20 sec before a final submersion event occurs. Once submission occurs, all organs and tissues are at risk for hypoxia. In a short period, hypoxia can lead to cardiac arrest and ischemia. The combination of *hypoxia and ischemia* is a common injury mechanism associated with submission events. *Pulmonary aspiration* can further exacerbate hypoxia and subsequent respiratory failure. The majority of submersion victims do not aspirate large enough volumes of fluid to result in significant *electrolyte disturbances*. Massive seawater ingestion or aspiration can lead to hypernatremia and fluid shifts because of its high sodium concentration and osmolarity, whereas massive fresh water ingestion or aspiration can cause hyponatremia and hemodilution. In both the situations, free water overload may be seen with excess antidiuretic hormone (SIADH), which can accompany pulmonary or brain injury. Excess free water can also increase cerebral edema and intracranial pressure (ICP).

Hypothermia (core temperature of less than 35°C) is common after submersion. Children are at increased risk of developing hypothermia owing to their relatively high body surface area to mass ratio, decreased subcutaneous fat, and limited thermogenic capacity. Hypothermia can develop as a result of prolonged surface contact with cold water, after swallowing or aspirating of large quantities of very cold fluid and further drops in body temperature occurs after the child is removed from the water due to cold air, wet clothes, hypoxia, and hospital transport. Compensatory mechanisms will usually attempt to restore normothermia at body temperatures above 32°C; below this temperature thermoregulation fails and spontaneous rewarming will not occur. Moderate hypothermia (core temperature 32–35°C) increases oxygen consumption owing to shivering thermogenesis and increased sympathetic tone. Below 32°C (severe hypothermia), shivering ceases and the

cellular metabolic rate decreases approximately 7% per °C in the absence of active thermogenesis. With moderate to severe hypothermia progressive bradycardia, impaired myocardial contractibility, and loss of vasomotor tone contribute to inadequate perfusion, hypotension and shock. Deep coma with fixed and dilated pupils and absent reflexes at very low body temperatures (< 25–29°C) may give the false appearance of death. Hypothermia in non-icy water near-drowning is most commonly an unfavorable prognostic sign. *Rewarming shock* may be observed

---

Box 7.3: Causes of drowning

Leaving small children unattended around bathtubs and pools
Drinking alcohol while boating or swimming
Inability to swim or panic while swimming
Falling through thin ice
Blows to the head or seizures while in the water
Attempted suicide

Box 7.4: Treatment should adhere to the following sequence of priorities

1. Remove the victim from the water as soon as possible and stabilize the patient's head and neck if trauma is suspected.
2. Immediately follow the ABCs of cardiopulmonary resuscitation—even in the water if this does not endanger the rescuer.
3. If the patient is unconscious, protect the airway as needed with endotracheal intubation.
4. Establish venous excess as soon as possible.
5. Provide supplemental oxygen and ventilatory support until each is no longer needed. This can be judged from analysis of arterial blood for oxygen tension, carbon dioxide tension, and pH.
6. Monitor cardiac rhythm with the electrocardiogram as soon as possible.
7. Monitor body temperature and restore as soon as possible.
8. If the patient has persistent respiratory insufficiency, provide intensive pulmonary support with continuous positive airway pressure (CPAP) and mechanical ventilation therapy as necessary.
9. If the patient has cardiovascular instability, evaluate cardiac output and effective circulatory volume by invasive monitoring, and serum electrolyte concentrations. Intravenous fluid replacement should be provided as necessary.
10. Evaluate and treat renal function and cerebral status as indicated.

Note: Glucocorticoid therapy, prophylactic antibiotic therapy, and monitoring of intracranial pressure are no longer recommended.

after rescue. The causes of drowning are listed in Box 7.3.

Clinical manifestations and treatment: The clinical course and outcome are primarily determined by the circumstances of the incident, the duration of submersion, the speed of the rescue, and the effectiveness of resuscitative efforts (Box 7.4). Two groups may be identified based on responsiveness at the scene: (i) children who require minimal amounts of resuscitation at the scene commonly have good prognosis and experience a low incidence of complications. They should be transferred to the ED for further evaluation, (ii) victims in cardiac arrest require aggressive or prolonged resuscitation and have a high risk of multiorgan system complications, major neurologic morbidity or death. Grief, guilt, and anger are frequent. Friends and family may blame the parents for the event. Counseling should be considered for all drowning victims and their families.

Prognosis: The great majority of near-drowning victims either have good outcomes (intact or mild neurologic injury) or bad outcomes (persistent vegetative state or death), with very few exhibiting intermediate neurologic injury. Neurologic examination and progression during the 24–72 hr are presently the best prognosticators of long-term CNS outcome. Children, who regain consciousness within 72 hr, even after prolonged resuscitation, are unlikely to suffer serious neurologic sequelae.

Prevention: Parents must be made aware that anybody of water, no matter how innocuous, poses a drowning risk, especially to children 1 yr of age and younger. Parents should be told about the risks of common household fixtures such as bathtubs, buckets, toilets and washing machines.

Kallas HJ. Drowning and Submersion Injury. In: Kliegman RM, Behrman RE, Jenson HB, Stanton BF (eds). *Nelson Textbook of Pediatrics*. 18th edn, Vol. 1. Philadelphia: Saunders, 2007; 438–49.

Mathur GP, Kushwaha KP, Mathur Sarla. Drowning and Near-Drowning. In: Mathur GP, Mathur Sarla (eds). *Current Trends in Pediatrics*. Vol 1. Delhi: Academa Publishers, 2005; 393–7.

Summerton C, Shetty P, Sandle LN, et al. Drowning/Near-Drowning. In: Haslett C, Chilvers ER, Boon NA, Colledge NR, Hunter JAA (eds). *Davidson's Principles and Practice of Medicine*. 19th edn. Edinburgh: Churchill Livingstone, 2002; 333–4.

7.8 SEASICKNESS

Seasickness is a benign condition experienced after spending time on a ship, boat, submarine, craft or any vessel in water. It is a type of *motion sickness* and not a distinct entity in itself. The people who are particularly vulnerable to the condition can feel seasick even if there is a little movement of the ship in completely calm sea. Despite engineering advances and the sophisticated and comfortable modern ships, motion sickness remains a problem for contemporary sea-goers. Surveys have shown that up to 100% of ship passengers become seasick under very rough sea conditions.

Clinical manifestations: All persons with normal vestibular function are susceptible to varying degree of seasickness. The susceptibility may differ in different background and force levels of the body motion. About one-third of the population is highly susceptible to sea sickness, a third experience it in fairly rough conditions, and another third become sick only in extreme conditions. There is increased susceptibility for sea sickness in certain clinical groups. They are; (i) children aged 3 to 12 years, (ii) people who have migraine headaches, and (iii) women, particularly during menstruation and pregnancy. Individuals with total loss of vestibular function are immune to motion sickness and those with half-sided loss are less susceptible than normal people. Severity of symptoms is directly proportional to the turbulence of sea state. A rough sea will cause increasingly severe symptoms. Seasickness can produce following signs and symptoms:

- Nausea
- Epigastric symptoms (epigastric discomfort, nausea, vomiting)
- Skin signs (pallor, cold sweating, dry mouth)
- Central nervous system features (headache, dizziness, drowsiness/lethargy, eye strain, apathy)
- Generally feeling unwell (excessive production of saliva, headache, nausea, dizziness, hyperventilating, heavy sweating, weakness)
- Losing color in the face or turning red

The development of symptoms follows an orderly sequence that varies with the intensity of the stimulus and the susceptibility of the individual. The initial symptom is usually discomfort around the upper abdomen ("stomach awareness"), which is followed by nausea and increasing malaise. Concurrently, the face or area around the mouth becomes pale, and the individual starts to sweat. With rapid worsening of symptoms ("avalanche syndrome") there can be increased salivation, feelings of body warmth, a lightness of the head, and often depression and apathy. This is followed by vomiting.

Additional symptoms are frequent but more variable. These include belching and flatulence, hyperventilation, sighing and yawning, headache, tightness around the forehead or a "buzzing" sensation, drowsiness, lethargy and somnolence, and panic or confusion. The lethargy, fatigue, and drowsiness can persist after the stimulus stops and nausea lessens.

Over time, there is a tendency to adapt ("to get one's sea legs"). For most individuals this occurs by 2 to 3 days, although about 5% are said not to adapt and to remain symptomatic if the stimulus persists.

In some individuals the distressing symptoms of sea sickness are usually relieved when the individual comes back to the shore. This is not always true. Rarely, there are people who suffer symptoms for a few days even after the trip is over. This is called "mal de embarquement" syndrome or, more properly, the "mal de debarquement" syndrome. ("Mal de embarquement" is embarkment or departure sickness while "mal de debarquement" is disembarkment or arrival sickness.)

Complications: In severe motion sickness with multiple bouts of vomiting, alkalosis may develop because of hydrogen ion loss and lead to increased renal excretion of potassium bicarbonate resulting in potassium deficiency which can cause muscle weakness, constipation, and cardiac arrhythmias. Sodium loss can lead to hypotension. Levels of antidiuretic hormone release also become elevated.

Prevention of seasickness: To prevent the symptoms of seasickness the following can be tried to the ease symptom:

1. *The night before the voyage*
   • Eat and drink moderately.
   • Take an advance dose of medicine, if there is a previous history of seasickness or motion sickness

2. *The morning of the voyage*
   • Eat only a light breakfast, avoiding rich or fatty foods.
   • Take a small quantity of beverages like tea or coffee.
   • Take a second dose of drug.

3. *On the boat/ship*
   • Take a position with a good outside view, low and near the center of the boat if possible.
   • Avoid smells of exhaust, fuel, the galley (kitchen), and the toilet.
   • Avoid reading or work requiring close-up focus.
   • Move around and get fresh air.
   • Avoid alcohol and tobacco.

4. *If you start feeling sick*
   • Acknowledge the situation and tell the captain or crew.
   • Avoid going below or into enclosed spaces

   If the individual feels he is going to vomit
   • Vomit over the side, on the downwind side, or in the head. Be considerate to others on the boat.

   • Many people feel much better after vomiting.

5. *If your companions are seasick*
   • Protect them from injury or falling overboard.
   • Encourage them to drink water or solution such as oral rehydration solution (ORS).

6. *Traditional remedies:* A number of natural remedies have been tried such the chewing or sucking of ginger was known to the ancient Chinese sea farers. In the Indian naval ships there is tradition of serving spicy dish called *rasum*; it is known to suppress seasickness.

The use of popular accupressure bands (sea bands), which are worn around the wrist to apply pressure to the P6 point, also showed no benefit for combating motion sickness.

Psychological therapies have also been investigated. Biofeedback does little to reduce symptoms or to increase tolerance to motion. Cognitive behavioral training can help to build some tolerance to provocative motion stimuli and to reduce the need for antimotion medications, but the process is quite time-consuming and thus impractical for most people.

Wearing of prism glasses has been shown to decrease the seasickness. The prism glasses are thought to decrease discrepancy between visual and vestibular cues and thus to reduce the negative effects of vertigo.

Anti-motion sickness treatment should aim at minimizing symptoms and preventing complications. Symptoms can be controlled by a variety of drugs and other non-pharmacologic therapies. Complications can be prevented primarily by ensuring adequate hydration.

Pharmacologic treatment: Two classes of drugs are known to be effective against motion sickness; these are central cholinergic blockers and drugs that enhance dopamine-norepinephrine activity. These drugs act on various sites such as the vestibular receptors and nuclei, the cerebellum, the reticular area, and the vomiting center. All antimotion medications are also effective antiemetic agents.

Cholinergic blockers include scopolamine, atropine, dimenhydrinate, cyclizine, meclizine, and promethazine. The effective sympathomimetics include d-amphetamine, methamphetamine, premoline, phenmetrazine, phenemine, and methylphenidate. Drugs taken orally must be taken in a sufficient dosage at least an hour in advance to be effective; otherwise, they must be administered intramuscularly in most cases if motion sickness symptoms have already surfaced.

Scopolamine is the single most effective antimotion sickness drug, consistently providing more protection than any other single medication in clinical trials. Although some drowsiness may be a welcome side effect for travelers who are not operating a vehicle or equipment, this and other performance side effects of scopolamine can be eliminated by adding 5 to 10 mg of the sympathomimetic medication d-amphetamine (Dexedrine). The drowsiness produced by scopolamine and the excitement produced by d-amphetamine effectively cancel each other. This combination also produces the fastest rate of habituation in motion sickness, but also leads to increased dry mouth symptoms.

Evans RW, Marcus D, Furman JM. Motion sickness and migraine. *Headache* 2007; 47(4): 607–10.

Kohl RL, Sandoz GR, Reschke MF, et al. Facilitation of adaptation and acute tolerance to stressful sensory input by doxepin and scopolamine plus amphetamine. *J Clin Pharmacol* 1993;33:1092–1103.

Kozarsky PE. Prevention of common travel ailments. *Infect Dis Clin North Am* 1998;12:305–24.

Parrott AC. Transdermal scopolamine: a review of its effects upon motion sickness, psychological performance, and physiological functioning. *Aviat Space Environ Med* 1989;60:1–9.

Stewart JJ, Wood MJ, Wood CD, et al. Effects of ginger on motion sickness susceptibility and gastric function. *Pharmacol* 1991;42:111–20.

Wood CD. Pharmacological countermeasures against motion sickness. In: Crampton GH (ed). *Motion and Space Sickness*. Boca Raton: CRC Press, 1990;344.

Wood CD. Antimotion sickness and antiemetic drugs. *Drugs* 1979;17:471–9.

7.9 BURN INJURIES

A burn can be caused by heat (flames, hot grease, or boiling water), the sun (solar radiation), chemicals or electricity. Burn injury can be accidental, suicidal, or homicidal. Approximately half of the burn injury occurs at home and the usual victims are the lady of the house and the children surrounding her. The articles used in cooking are very inflammable (*Angethi* in which coal or small pieces of dry wood is burnt; kerosene stove) and a little bit of carelessness causes the accident. In *urban areas*, the leakage of cooking gas in closed, small kitchen is producing the utmost burn cases. Accidents occur with crackers, firework and lightening too.

Burn injury: The burn injuries are caused by thermal, electrical, chemical or solar radiation.

Thermal: Fire burn (dry burn) caused by open fire or contact with the hot object is less common than scald burn. Anoxia and not the actual burn is a major cause of morbidity and mortality in house fires. Scald burns accounts for 85% of total injuries and are most prevalent in children younger than 4 yr of age. It is caused by hot liquid like boiling water, milk, tea, hot sugar syrup or hot soup and curry and oil, but usually the burn injury is not as deep in scald as with dry fire, because the hot liquid is bound to loose some heat while coming in contact with the body. Kitchen and bathroom are the usual place of occurrence.

Electrical: It is mostly accidental. Usually the carelessness of the people causes this type of burn. They work at some place and leave the live wire open, and it causes the accident. In this mostly small children are the sufferers. Some time the children put the plug or wire in the mouth and chew them. In rural areas high voltage live wires snap and fall on the agriculture lands and it causes electric burn of very severe type, which mostly leads to amputation. Some time, workers of electric appliances get burnt too by their carelessness.

Chemical: It is caused by strong alkali and acid contact with the body. Mostly it is accidental when the students are doing practical work in a laboratory or somebody is working in a workshop and factory. Sometime it is homicidal too, when somebody throws acid on another, then usually face is attacked and it causes burn of eyes and nose too. Usually it is very deep burns with very bad scarring.

Solar radiation burn: Burns caused by solar radiation may be painful and may also produce blister.

Inhalational injury: Inhalation airway injury may occur from (i) direct heat (greater problems with steam burns), (ii) acute asphyxia, (iii) carbon monoxide poisoning, and (iv) toxic fumes, including cyanides from combustible plastics. Sulfur and nitrogen oxides and alkalis formed during the combustion of synthetic fabrics produce corrosive chemicals that may erode mucosa and cause significant sloughing. Inhalation injury and burn injury are synergistic, and the combined effect can increase morbidity and mortality.

Classification of burn: Burn is classified into three grades according to the depth of skin involved in the injury (Table 7.9). Skin is a multi-layered organ of body. In *superficial burn* there is partial thickness burn of skin, only the epidermis and part of dermis is burnt, and there is enough layers of skin left for spontaneous healing to take place. The healing takes place within three weeks time. In *deep burn* all the layers of skin is burnt and healing takes place only by skin grafting or, if left as such, by fibrosis. It is difficult to differentiate the type of burn just immediately after the injury whether it is deep or superficial. Only time is the factor which makes the decision. So before excising the tissue one should wait for some time so that the difference is confirmed.

Clinical manifestations: The history usually reveals a common pattern: scald burn to the side of face, neck,

	First degree	Second degree partial thickness	Third degree full thickness
Surface appearance	Dry, no blisters; minimal or no edema	Moist blebs, blisters	Dry, leathery eschar
Color	Erythematous	Mottled pink and white with good capillary refill	Mixed white, waxy, khaki. Mahogany, soot stained
Pain	Very painful	Very painful	No pain, insensitive
Histologic depth	Epidermal layer only	Epidermis, papillary and reticular layers of dermis; may include domes of subcutaneous layers	Skin and may include fat, subcutaneous tissue, fascia, muscle, tendon and bone
Healing time	2–5 days with no scarring	Superficial: 5–21 days with no grafting; deep partial 21–35 days with no infection, if infected converts to full thickness	Large areas require grafting; small areas may heal from the edges after weeks

Table 7.9: Classification of degree of burn

and arms if liquid is pulled from a table, open hearth or stove; a pant leg area burn if clothing ignites; slash areas from cooking; and palm of hand contact with a hot object. In young children burns of hands and feet, single area deep burns on the trunk, buttocks, or back, and small-area full thickness-burns (cigarette-burn) should raise the suspicion of child abuse. Scald burn tends to cause a superficial burn, whereas electrical, chemicals and direct flame cause deep burn. Very hot agent for momentary contact cause less severe type of burn than the less hot substance for a longer duration. Inner side of arm and thigh sustain more burn than the outer side of arm and thigh and the skin of palm and sole, because the skin is more delicate in that part. Similarly women and children get more severe burn due to their tender skin than the men.

An area, which looks superficial burn, may turn into deep due to thrombosis of the blood vessels. Red, erythematous area is in favor of superficial burn. Deep burn area is a white, depressed patch. There is no pain or very dull pain in deep burn. A person is sick with pain in superficial burn. The more is the TBSA (total burn surface area), the more is the percentage of deep burn. The contact of hot object causes radiation of burn in concentric, circular wave to travel away from the point of contact. It involves the blood supply directly and makes the center of the area avascular. So more is the area involved, more is the avascular area in center, producing deep burn.

Estimation of total burn surface area (TBSA): The area from the wrist crease to finger crease (the palm) in the child equals 1% of the child's body surface area. In small burns under 10% of TBSA, the "rule of palm" may be used, especially in outpatient settings.

In the case of children because of variable growth rate of the head and extremities throughout childhood TBSA should be calculated with the chart shown in

Table 7.10: Chart to determine developmentally related percent body burn surface area

	Newborn	3 year	6 year	12 year
Head	18%	15%	12%	6%
Trunk	40%	40%	40%	38%
Arms	16%	16%	16%	18%
Legs	26%	29%	32%	38%

Courtesy: Shrines Hospital for Crippled Children, Burn Institute, Boston Unit

Table 7.10. The "Rule of Nine" and "Rule of Five " are rapid and easy way of calculating TBSA (Tables 7.11 and 7.12). In an adult burn of head and neck and one upper extremity, each comprises 9%, trunk 36%, each lower extremity comprises 18% area of the body and remaining 1% area consist of the genitalia. The "Rule of Nine" used in adults may be used only in children older than age 14 yr or as a very rough estimate to institute therapy before transfer to a burn center.

Table 7.11: Rapid estimation of surface area by "Rule of Nine"

Front	Back
Head 9%	Head 9%
Upper limb, Rt 9%	Upper limb, Rt 9%
Upper limb, Lt 9%	Upper limb, Lt 9%
Trunk 18%	Trunk, Rt side 18%
	Trunk, Lt side 18%
Lower limb, Rt 18%	Lower limb, Rt 18%
Lower limb, Lt 18%	Lower limb, Lt 18%

Treatment

Treatment will include first aid measures, emergency care, and care involving large areas of the body (Box 7.5) and outpatient treatment of minor burns.

Table 7.12: Rapid estimation of surface area of "Rule of Five"

	Infants	Child*	Adult**
Head	20%	15%	5%
Upper limb, Rt side	10%	10%	10%
Upper limb, Lt side	10%	10%	10%
Trunk, front	20%	20%	20%
Trunk, back	20%	20%	20%
Lower limb, Rt side	10%	15%	10%
Lower limb, Lt side	10%	15%	10%
Total	**100%**	**105%**	**95%**

*5% may be subtracted from the trunk in the case of child.
**5% may be added to the anterior of both feet in the case of adult.

First aid measures: These measures include the following:

1. Extinguish flames by rolling on the ground; cover the child with blanket, coat, or any clothing material.
2. After determining that the airway is patent, remove smoldering clothing or clothing saturated with hot liquid and remove or cut away jewelry, particularly rings and bracelets to prevent constriction and vascular compromise during the edema phase in the first 24–72 hr post term.
3. In the case of chemical injury, brush off any remaining material if powered or solid; then use copious irrigation or wash the affected area with water (especially someone has thrown acid).
4. Cover the burned area with clean, dry sheeting and apply cold (not iced) wet compresses to small injuries, but significant large burn surface area injury (TBSA > 15–20%) decreases body temperature

Box 7.5: Acute treatment of burns

Fist aid measures
Fluid resuscitation
Nutritional care
Pain control
Tetanus prophylaxis
Prevention of infection—early excision and grafting
H₂ blockers—ranitidine
Ileus and associated vomiting; intragastric tube can be used to decompress the stomach.
Control of bacterial wound flora
Indwelling catheter to collect the urine passed to assess the kidney function
Respiratory complication due to inhalation of burn fumes
Treatment of associated injuries
Head end should be elevated so that the edema of the face and head may be reduced rapidly and there will be less difficulty in breathing.
Dressings to close wound

control, therefore, the use of cold compress dressings are contraindicated.

5. If the burn is caused by hot tar, use mineral oil to remove the tar.
6. Do not go near the victim with electrical burns unless you are sure the power source has been turned off.
7. Protect the burn caused by solar radiation by staying out of the sun. If you must go in the sun, wear a sunscreen and apply caladryl (containing calamine 8%) on the affected area and reapply it frequently. Be sure to cover up any existing sunburn if you are going to be outside again.
8. Tetanus prophylaxis consist of tetanus toxoid and Tetanus immune globulin (TIG) (250 U IM, and 500 U for highly tetanus-prone wounds)

Emergency care: Life support measures include:

1. Rapid review of the cardiovascular and respiratory status
2. Maintenance of adequate airway and providing humidified oxygen by mask or endotracheal intubation
3. Intravenous fluid resuscitation in children with burns greater than 15% of body surface area
4. Evaluation of associated injuries (spine, bones, and thoracic or intra-abdominal organs)
5. No oral fluids to children with burns greater than 15% of body surface area because they may develop ileus; insertion of a nasogastric tube may be required to prevent aspiration
6. Foley catheter to be inserted to monitor urine output, and
7. All wounds to be wrapped with sterile towels.

Debridement of eschar: Usually within three weeks the superficial burn wounds heal and what is left, is covered with slough produced by burning or by a caustic, which is known as 'eschar'. It has to be removed. A natural process of putrefaction takes place under the dead tissue and it helps in the removal of the eschar; the rest is removed surgically. After the removal of the eschar the raw area is prepared for skin grafting.

Nutritional care: Children with a 40% TBSA require approximately 50% above predicted basal energy expenditure for their age. Usually from third day onward solid food is added. Calories are provided at one and one half times the basal metabolic rate, 3–4 g/kg of protein per day. Multivitamins, particularly the B vitamin group, vitamin C, vitamin A, and zinc, are also necessary. For the adequate treatment of burn, blood transfusion has a great role. Hemoglobin level is kept at 70–75%. It helps in the healing process of the burn wound and take-up of the skin graft when applied.

Outpatient treatment of minor burns: Patients with burn involving small area of the body can be treated in the outpatient department (OPD). The part is thoroughly washed with normal saline or Savlon (chlorhexidine gluconate 0.3% and cetrimide 0.6%) solution. Approximately one half of the patients, need treatment for pain only.

Pain relief and psychological adjustment: Children having burn injury show frequent and wide fluctuations in pain intensity. Opiate analgesia in an adequate dose and timed to cover dressing changes is essential to comfort management. Anxiolytic medication (lorazepam) added to the analgesic is helpful in anxious patients.

Reconstruction and rehabilitation: To ensure maximum cosmetic and functional outcome, occupational and physical therapy must begin on the day of admission, continue throughout the hospitalization and for some patients continue after discharge.

Prognosis: As soon as a patient of major burn injury is admitted anxious relatives and patients are to know the prognosis regarding the survival of the patient, duration of stay in the hospital, operated or not, and scar formation. However, it is difficult to answer all the questions of anxious parents and patients just after admission, but there are following a few guidelines will help the doctor to discuss with patient and relatives:

1. Always overestimate the percentage of burn.
2. Extremes of ages tolerate the burn injuries poorly.
3. Men are more tough against burn injury.
4. Obesity is an ardent enemy of the burn injury.
5. A burn patient requires 1 to 1.5 hospital day/% of TBSA.
6. Any burn wound needing graft will need twice as long hospitalization as extensive (>30%) burn.

Box 7.6: Preventive measures to reduce the incidence of burns

- Not to wear synthetic clothes during cooking.
- Do not cover head and face while cooking. Tight fitting cotton dress should be advocated.
- Persons during cooking should be less distracted.
- Involvement of non-governmental organizations (NGOs) and government agencies to educate the masses through media (radio, television and news papers), street show, work-shop and seminars.
- Inclusion of a chapter in the school books and teachers can educate the students in detail about the measures to be taken to save them from burn injury.

Prevention: To prevent burn incidence, drastic change in life style, particularly in rural and slum areas is needed (Box 7.6).

Antoon AY, Donovan MK. Burn Injuries. In: Behrman RE, Kliegman RM, Jenson HB (eds). *Nelson Textbook of Pediatrics.* 17th edn. Philadelphia: Saunders, 2004;330–7.

Monafo W. Initial management of burns. *N Engl J Med* 1996; 335:1581–6.

Sheridan RL, Hinson M, et al. Long-term outcomes of children surviving massive burns. *JAMA* 2000;283:69–73.

Sinha Mala. Burn. In: Mathur GP, Mathur Sarla (eds). *Current Trends in Pediatrics.* Vol 2. Delhi: Academa Publishers, 2006;323–32.

7.10 HEAT INJURIES

1. *Heat cramps:* Heat cramps are the most common heat injury. These painful muscle cramps occur most commonly in the legs affecting the calf and hamstring muscles following vigorous exercise in hot weather. There is no elevation of core temperature. The mechanism is considered to be extracellular sodium depletion following electrolyte loss as a result of persistent sweating with replacement of water but no salt. The syndrome is also encountered in athletes undertaking heavy physical work in hot conditions. Symptoms usually respond rapidly with salt replacement (oral rehydration with ORS) and with gentle stretching.

2. *Heat syncope* is fainting after prolonged exercise attributed to poor vasomotor tone and depleted intravascular volume, and it responds to fluids, cooling, and supine positioning.

3. *Heat edema* is mild edema of the hands and feet during initial exposure to heat; it resolves with acclimatization.

4. *Heat tetany* is carpopedal tingling or spasms caused by heat-related hyperventilation. It responds to moving to a cooler environment and decreasing respiratory rate (or rebreathing by breathing into a bag).

5. *Heat exhaustion:* Heat exhaustion occurs when there is an elevation in core (rectal) temperature between 37°C (98.6°F) and 40°C (104°F) and is usually seen when an individual is undertaking vigorous physical work in a hot environment. A high work rate, extreme ambient temperature or impairing evaporative heat loss due to high humidity or inappropriate clothing may all combine to overcome thermoregulatory control. The diagnosis is based on the finding of an elevated core temperature associated with hyperventilation and symptoms of tiredness or fatigue, muscular weakness, dizziness and collapse. *Blood examination* may show evidence of dehydration with mild

elevation of the blood urea, sodium concentration and hematocrit. *Treatment* consists of removal of the patient from the heat, active cooling using cool sponging, and fluid replacement. This may be achieved by using oral rehydration salt based on WHO formula and water or intravenous isotonic saline. Frequent monitoring of blood electrolytes is important, especially in those patients receiving intravenous replacement.

6. *Heat stroke:* Heat stroke occur when the core body temperature rises above 40°C (104°F) and is a severe and life-threatening condition provoked by a failure of heat regulatory mechanisms. The symptoms of heat exhaustion progress to include headache, nausea, and vomiting. Neurological manifestations include a coarse muscle tremor and confusion, which may progress to loss of consciousness. The patient's skin feels very hot and sweating is often absent due to failure of thermoregulatory mechanisms. The condition may progress from heat exhaustion or present acutely in a patient who has become progressively dehydrated without symptoms. Coincidental illness, age and drug therapy, particularly phenothiazines, diuretics may be important contributory factors.

Complications include hypovolemic shock, lactic acidosis, disseminated intravascular coagulation, rhabdomyolysis, hepatic and renal failure, and cerebral edema. *Investigations* include coagulation studies, muscle enzymes, hematology and biochemistry depending on the complications take place. *Treatment* is immediate whole-body cooling via cold water immersion. Airway, breathing, circulation, core temperature, and CNS status should be monitored constantly. Rapid cooling should be ceased when core temperature is ~38.3°–38.9°C/101°–102°F. IV fluid at a rate of 800 ml/m^2 in the 1st hr with normal saline or lactated Ringer solution improves intravascular volume and the body's ability to dissipate heat. Physician clearance is required for athletes before return to exercise.

Prevention: Dehydration is common to all heat illness; therefore measures to prevent dehydration may also prevent heat illnesses. Thirst is not an adequate indicator of hydration status because it is initiated at 2–3% dehydration. Athletes are advised to be well hydrated before exercise and should drink every 20 min during exercise (150 ml for those weighing 40 kg, 300 ml, and 300–350 ml for those > 60 kg).

Bytomsky JR, Squire DL. Heat illness in children. *Curr Sports Med Rep* 2003;2:320–4.

Landry GL. Heat injuries. In: Kliegman RM, Behrman RE, Jenson HB, Stanton BF (eds). *Nelson Textbook of Pediatrics.* 18th edn. Vol. 2. Philadelphia: Saunders, 2007; p-2864.

Summerton C, Shetty P, Sandle LN, et al. Hyperthermia and heat illness. In: Haslett C, Chilvers ER, Boon NA, Colledge NR, Hunter JAA (eds). *Davidson's Principles and Practice of Medicine.* 19th edn. Edinburgh: Churchill Livingstone, 2002; 330–1.

7.11 COLD INJURIES

Frostnip: With frostnip there is firm, cold white areas on the face, ears, or extemities initially, then blistering and peeling may occur over the next 24–72 hr. Treatment consists of warming the area with an unaffected hand or warm object before numbness supervenes.

Immersion foot (trench foot): This occurs in cold weather when the feet remain in damp or wet, poorly ventilated boots. The feet become cold, numb, pale, edematous and clammy. Tissue maceration and infection may occur along with prolonged autonomic disturbances such as increased sweating, pain, and hypersensitivity to temperature changes, which may persist for years. Treatment consists of using well-fitting insulated, waterproof, nonconstricting footwear, keeping the affected area dry, and well ventilated, preventing or treating infection and supportive measures for control of autonomic symptoms.

Frostbite: With frostbite, initial stinging or aching of the skin progresses to cold, hard, white anesthetic and numb areas. On rewarming, the area becomes blotchy, itchy, and often red, swollen and painful. Treatment consists of warming the damaged area, analgesia, and maintenance of good nutrition. Oxygen is of help only at high altitudes. Meticulous local care, prevention of infection, and keeping the warm area dry, open, and sterile provide optimal results. With treatment there is complete recovery or if early relief is not obtained, extensive tissue damage, even gangrene may occur.

Hypothermia: Hypothermia may occur in winter sports, drowning and near drowning and high altitude illness. The decrease in rectal temperature to less than 34°C (93°F) is diagnostic of hypothermia. As the core temperature of the body falls, an insidious onset of extreme lethargy, fatigue, incoordination, clumsiness, irritability, hallucinations, and finally bradycardia occur. Treatment at the scene aims at prevention of further heat loss and early transportation to adequate shelter. If no pulse is detected at the initial review, cardiopulmonary resuscitation is indicated. During transfer, jarring and sudden motion should be avoided, because these may cause ventricular arrhythmia. If the patient is conscious, mild muscle activity should be encouraged and a warm drink offered. If the patient is unconscious, external warming should be initially undertaken using blankets and a sleeping bag. On arrival at a treating center, inhalation of warm, moist air or oxygen, heating pads, or thermal blankets should be used while a warming bath of 45–48°C (113–118°F) is prepared. Monitoring of serum chemistry values and electrocardiogram are necessary until the core temperature rises above 35°C (95.0°F) and can be stabilized. Control of fluid, pH, blood pressure, and oxygen all are necessary in the early phases of the warming period and resuscitation. If pulse or breathing absent start, start CPR; defibrillate VF/pulseless VT up to a maximum of 3 shocks. Infuse warm normal saline (43°C; 109.4°F) in patients with marked abnormalities; warming measures such as gastric or colonic irrigation with warm saline or peritoneal dialysis may be considered, but the effectiveness of these measures to treat hypothermia is not known. In accidental deep hypothermia (core temperature 28°C; 82.4°F) with circulatory arrest, rewarming with cardiopulmonary bypass may be life-saving for previously healthy individuals.

Prevention is of extreme importance for those who participate in winter sports. They should wear layers of warm clothing, gloves, socks within insulated boots and a warm head covering. Ample food and fluid need to be provided during exercise. Application of petrolatum (Vaseline) to nose and ears give certain protection against frost bite.

Chilblain (pernio): In chilblain (pernio) erythematous, vesicular or ulcerative lesions are most often found at the ears, tips of fingers, and toes and on exposed areas of the legs. They are often itchy and may be painful and result in swelling and scabbing. The lesions last for 1–2 wk but may persist longer. Treatment consists of avoiding prolonged chilling and protecting potentially susceptible areas with a cap, gloves, and stockings; prazosin and phenoxybenzamine may be helpful in improving circulation if this is a recurrent problem. Local corticosteroid preparation is useful if there is itching.

Cold-induced fat necrosis (panniculitis): This cold injury occurs on exposure to cold air, snow, or ice and is manifested in exposed surfaces, rarely in covered surfaces as red (or, less often purple to blue) macular, papular, or nodular lesions. The lesions may last 10 days to 3 wk. Treatment is with nonsteroidal anti-inflammatory agents.

Antoon AY, Donovan MK. Cold Injuries. In: Kliegman RM, Behrman RE, Jenson HB, Stanton BF (eds). *Nelson Textbook of Pediatrics.* 18th edn. Vol. 1. Philadelphia: Saunders, 2007; 458–60.

Shepherd RJ. Metabolic adaptations to exercise in the cold: An update. *Sports Med* 1993;16:266–89.

7.12 HIGH ALTITUDE ILLNESS

High altitude related illnesses are common and should be recognized promptly to avoid unnecessary morbidity and mortality. Altitude related illnesses usually occur above altitudes of 3000 meters (although the effects may be felt by 2500 m). High altitude related medical problems cause significant avoidable morbidity and mortality. Many high altitude places are remotely located and away from medical help. It is imperative for persons travelling to such places to be able to recognize symptoms of common problems and manage them accordingly. Eye problems are often unrecognized and can cause problems. The basic problems of high altitude trips relate to: (i) remoteness of location, (ii) high altitude effects on the human body. Remote locations make access to medical help difficult if not impossible. The speed of evacuation of injured or ill trekkers or climbers is often dictated by the availability of porters, pack animals or helicopters. The last option is dependent on the weather, availability of aircraft and whether the victim possesses a valid insurance certificate.

Pathophysiology: Tissue hypoxia caused by a reduced ambient partial pressure of oxygen is the basis for pathophysiological changes in altitude related illness. Altitude related illnesses are a spectrum of disorders from the common and relatively mild acute mountain sickness (AMS) to the life threatening forms such as high altitude pulmonary edema (HAPE) and high altitude cerebral edema (HACE). The partial pressure of ambient air falls with increasing altitude due to the reduced mass of the atmospheric air above. Below 2500 meters the reduction in oxygen saturation is small and few symptoms occur other than some exertional breathlessness. Above 2500 meters a number of altitude syndromes may occur. Sudden ascents to altitudes above 6000 meters as experienced by aviators, balloonists, and astronauts, may result in decompression illness. Decompression illness varies in severity from a mild rash or musculoskeletal pain to life-threatening circulatory collapse. The majority of patients develop symptoms within 4 hr. Rapid ascents to altitude above 7000 meters may result in loss of consciousness. Despite this most altitude illness occurs in travelers or mountaineers.

Common high altitude medical problems: Three types of altitude syndromes may occur: Acute mountain sickness (AMS); high-altitude pulmonary edema (HAPE); high altitude cerebral edema (HACE). Acute mountain sickness (AMS) is common and preventable with sensible altitude gain. If it occurs, AMS is usually mild and self-limiting if it is recognized and managed properly. Severe and potentially fatal manifestations such as high altitude pulmonary edema (HAPE) and high altitude cerebral edema (HACE) must be diagnosed and managed without delay.

1. *Acute mountain sickness (AMS):* AMS is a syndrome characterized by headache along with fatigue, anorexia, nausea and vomiting, difficulty in sleeping and dizziness. Ataxia and peripheral edema may be present. Symptoms appear 6–24 hr of an ascent to altitudes > 2500–3000 m and vary in severity from trivial to completely incapacitating.

Occasionally, symptoms may not appear till a day after ascent. If no further altitude gain is made, these symptoms usually resolve within 24–72h. The rate at which different individuals acclimatize is extremely variable and has little bearing on sea level fitness. The barometric pressure decreases in an exponential manner as altitude is gained. The pressure at 5800 m (e.g. Everest Base Camp) is approximately half that at sea level so that the PO_2 of moist inspired gas is 70 mm Hg, compared with approximately 150 mmHg at sea level and at the summit of Mt Everest (8848 m), the inspired PO_2 is only 43 mm Hg. Clearly then, the basis of pathophysiological changes is tissue hypoxia. The greater the hypoxic stress (i.e. the faster the rate of ascent), the less time the body has to adapt to it, the greater the severity of the illness.

Treatment of AMS: One should treat the person as for AMS even if one is doubtful regarding the diagnosis; stop further ascent, treat headache with simple analgesics such as paracetamol, rest and rehydrate. Symptoms usually resolve after 12–48 hr at a stable altitude but may recur with further ascent. Persistent symptoms may respond to acetazolamide. Steroids may be helpful, but descend is the best option. Descend if there is no improvement or if symptoms worsen. Immediate descent/evacuation if there are symptoms and signs of HAPE or HACE, with concomitant initiation of pharmacological therapy. Note that the use of hyperbaric chamber should not delay descent/evacuation unless movement in adverse weather conditions imposes an even greater risk of morbidity to both patient and rescuers. [Treatment of AMS **Mild:** Rest (no further altitude gains); symptomatic treatment, e.g. paracetamol for headache; **Severe:** DESCENT; Oxygen; Acetazolamide 250 mg 8 hr, PO; Dexamethasone 4 mg 6 hr, PO or IM/IV; Hyperbaric chamber].

Prevention of AMS: The usual recommendation is modest altitude gains of not more than 300 m per day above 3000 m and to spend 2 nights in the same place every 1000 m. This rule of thumb has been widely quoted, and most trekkers appear to acclimatize reasonably with this rate of ascent, although a minority does not acclimatize well. Recently, a suggestion has been made to spend a night or two at intermediate altitudes below 3000 m before ascending further. Drug prophylaxis using acetazolamide is well-established. However, this is not a substitute for gradual ascent. It is usually recommended only for those who have shown to be susceptible to AMS, or who have to make large altitude gains over a short period, e.g. military or rescue personnel, or tourists flying into high altitude destinations such as Leh, Ladakh (3514 m) or Lhasa (3658 m). The current dose recommendations made by the Himalayan Rescue Association (Phone: 262746 Thamel Mall Building, Jyatha Thamel, Kathmandu, Nepal) is 125 mg BD. This dose is as effective as the previously recommended dose of 250 mg BD whilst reducing the unpleasant side effects of tingling of hands and feet and diuresis. Since acetazolamide is a diuretic, the trekker or climber is well advised to make efforts to drink enough liquids to remain well hydrated, as dehydration appears to hamper acclimatization as well. Gradual ascent without excessive exertion allows the normal processes of acclimatization to occur and reduces the risk of altitude illness. Acclimatization results in an increase in ventilation over a few days, associated with a respiratory alkalosis and renal compensation, and a slower rise in hemoglobin. These changes promote the availability of oxygen to tissues. An ascent (300 meter/day above 3000 meters) may permit acclimatization, but is too slow for travelers' plans.

Acetazolamide (children and adults: 8–30 mg/kg/24 hr PO divided q 6–8 hr (max: 1 g/24 hr) taken in a dose of 250 mg 8 hourly commencing 24–48 hr before ascent reduces the incidence and severity of symptoms of acute mountain sickness (AMS), and also of HAPE, and HACE, but may produce some minor side effects of peripheral paresthesia. Nifedipine provides protection against HAPE, but no effect on AMS symptoms.

2. *High-altitude pulmonary edema (HAPE):* HAPE is a serious and potentially fatal condition. It appears to occur in susceptible subjects, youth, rapidity of ascent, the presence of mountain sickness and heavy exertion. Following of recent ascent, symptoms of dry cough, breathlessness, and extreme fatigue develop. Later, the cough is productive containing blood in sputum. It is associated with crepitations in lungs, profound hypoxemia, pulmonary hypertension, and radiological evidence of diffuse alveolar edema.

HAPE can occur within 24–48 hr after ascent to 3000 m in susceptible people, the risk of increasing with greater sudden altitude gains. It is usually preceded by symptoms of AMS. It is associated with raised pulmonary artery (PA) pressures, and high protein lung lavage fluid. It is made worse by physical exertion, and relieved by nifedipine, oxygen and rest. Typically, the person experiences diminishing effort tolerance leading to breathless at rest. A cough, initially dry will become wet and productive. Auscultation of the lungs reveals crackles. With poor gas exchange, the patient becomes increasingly cyanosed. HAPE is a medical emergency. The mainstay of treatment is immediate descent of at least a 1000 m or to below where the person was last asymptomatic. Deaths have occurred when diagnosis or descent was delayed.

Treatment consists of reversal of hypoxia with descent where possible and administration of oxygen, reduction of pulmonary arterial pressure with nifedipine. Nifedipine 10 mg stat (sublingual) followed by 10–20 mg SR 6 hr should be started. Oxygen if available improves symptoms. As exertion and cold increase PA pressure, the person should be assisted or carried and kept warm. Hyperbaric bags or portable altitude chambers (PAC) may be used if there is no means of safely evacuating the person but should never delay descent. If the HAPE victim is treated in a PAC, he should be maintained in a position of slight (30°) head up tilt to reduce orthopnea. If HACE is also present, dexamethasone should also be given. The use of acetazolamide in this instance may worsen the tachypnea.

[Treatment of HAPE: 1. DESCENT; 2. Nifedipine 10 mg SL stat, 10–20 mg SR 6hr; 3. Oxygen; 4. Hyperbaric bag].

3. *High altitude cerebral edema (HACE):* It is a rare and potentially fatal condition associated with recent ascent, usually follows AMS. It is most likely seen above altitudes of 3500 meters. The clinical manifestations include hallucinations or behavioral change, confusion, visual loss and later loss of consciousness. Ataxia is usually present, papilledema and retinal hemorrhages are common, and focal neurological signs may be found. The diffuse cerebral edema appears to be related to the rapid increase in cerebral blood flow and capillary permeability.

HACE is a severe cerebral manifestation of altitude illness. Like HAPE, it can be rapidly fatal. Whilst persons with AMS have very mild neurological symptoms, very few actually develop full blown HACE. However, HACE is often associated with HAPE. It appears that vasogenic edema in response to hypoxia is a culprit but certain biochemical mediators may play a role in altering the blood–brain barrier (BBB). The "tight fit" hypothesis proposes that individual anatomical differences in the craniospinal axis determines tolerance to mild brain swelling and the apparent random nature of HACE.

HACE should be suspected when a person complains of severe headache, becomes confused, ataxic or irrational. They may become lethargic and sleepy and if left alone in their tents "to sleep it off", may be found comatose or dead the next day.

Treat as for HACE, even in doubt and descend immediately. Dexamethasone 8 mg stat (PO/IM) and 4 mg 6 hr should be started, oxygen administered if available. A PAC may be used if immediate descent is impossible. [Treatment of HACE 1. DESCENT; 2. Dexamethasone 8 mg stat, 4 mg 6 hr; 3. Oxygen; 4. Hyperbaric bag.]

Eye problems at altitude: Eye problems at altitude are often overlooked. Briefly, they consist of snow blindness (this is not confined to high altitude), problems of myopes having had radial keratotomy (RK) and high altitude retinopathy.

The amount of ultraviolet A (UV A) and ultraviolet B (UV B) radiation to the eye is greater at altitude than at sea level. This effect is often compounded by rays bouncing of bright snow resulting in snow blindness. The best way to prevent this is the use of proper high altitude sunglasses that filter out all UV A/UV B, up to 70–100% infra red (IR) and are much darker than ordinary sunglasses used at sea level. Treatment includes padding the eyes, steroid and lubricant eye drops, a cycloplegic and simple analgesic for pain. Symptoms usually subside in a day or two. Local anesthetic eye drops are not usually recommended. It is now well documented that patients who have had RK for correction of myopia experience refractive changes at altitude. These changes range from minor irritations to severe disability. Retinopathy in the form of retinal hemorrhage often goes unnoticed, unless they are large enough to impair vision or occur near the macula. Asymptomatic hemorrhages have been found inpatients with HACE and AMS. Suggested etiology includes raised intracranial pressure, cerebral blood flow and decreased intraocular pressure. This coupled with extreme physical exertion and valsalva maneuvers during mountain climbing may lead to hemorrhages.

Portable hyperbaric chambers (PACs): Portable hyperbaric chambers which can simulate a descent of approximately several hundred to 1000 m have been shown to be useful in the management of altitude illnesses. They can best be described as single person chambers constructed from lightweight materials and closed with a zipper producing an airtight seal. There are usually transparent panels though which the patient can be monitored. After the patient is placed inside, the bag is inflated with a foot pump to a preset working pressure. Continuous pumping is necessary to maintain fresh airflow into the bag and prevent carbon dioxide buildup. The minimum treatment time in the bags is an hour, after which the patient may be reassessed. Further time in the bag may be required if the patient is still symptomatic. After emergence from the bag, symptoms may recur and it is wise to descend to lower altitude. It cannot be overemphasized that the hyperbaric bag is not substitute for descent. Unfortunately, the provision of such a device by trekking agencies have lulled some groups into a false sense of security and the use of it by persons unfamiliar with the bag has led in certain instances to avoidable morbidity and mortality.

Management: Descent is the most important treatment for all forms of mountain illness. Portable pressurized bags (Gamow bags) provide a means of temporarily increasing the patient's ambient pressure and are used to relieve symptoms where immediate descent is impossible. The medications commonly used include analgesic, acetazolamide, nifedipine, and steroids.

Analgesics: Treat headache with simple analgesics such as paracetamol in the doses of 10–15 mg/dose 4–6 times a day.

Acetazolamide (Diamox): It is a carbonic anhydrase inhibitor and is a sulpha drug and should be avoided by those with sensitivity to sulpha drugs. It produces a mild metabolic acidosis and stimulates respiration, leading to an increase in alveolar PO_2 and improves sleep quality at altitude. Persistent symptoms may respond to acetazolamide. Acetazolamide (children and adults: 8–30 mg/kg/24 hr PO divided q 6–8 hr (max: 1 g/24 hr) taken in a dose of 250 mg 8 hourly commencing 24–48 hr before ascent reduces the incidence and severity of symptoms of acute mountain sickness (AMS), and also of HAPE, and HACE, but may produce some minor side effects of peripheral paresthesia. Drug prophylaxis using acetazolamide is well-established.

Nifedipine (Calcigard): It is a calcium channel antagonist. The reduction of pulmonary arterial pressure occurs with nifedipine. As exertion and cold increase PA pressure, the person should be assisted or carried and kept warm. 10 mg stat (sublingual) followed by 10–20 mg SR 6 hr should be started (infants and children: 0.25–0.5 mg/kg per dose per oral; Adolescents and Adults: 10 mg/dose (maximum 120–180 mg/24 hr).

Dexamethasone). It is given in severe cases of AMS and HACE.

Prevention: The key messages to high altitude travelers include:
a. Slow ascent to allow acclimatization
b. Descent is the best treatment for any altitude illness
c. Acetazolamide is useful in reducing the symptoms of acute mountain sickness; and
d. Susceptible subjects tend to have similar symptoms on subsequent ascents.

Basnyat B, Suede D, Sleggs J, et al. High-altitude illness. *N Engl J Med* 2001;245:107–14.

Hackett PH, Oelz O. The Lake Louise Consensus on the definition and quantification of altitude illness. In: Sutton JR, Coates G, Houston CS (eds). *Hypoxia and Mountain Medicine.* Burlington: Queens City Printers, 1992;327–30.

Mathur GP, Mathur Sarla, Vaidya Kamala, et al. High Altitude Illness. In: Mathur GP, Mathur Sarla (eds). *Current Trends in Pediatrics.* Vol 1. Delhi: Academa Publishers, 2005;452–9.

Oelz O, Maggiorini M, Ritter M, et al. Nifedipine for high altitude pulmonary oedema. *Lancet* 1989;2:1241–44.

Subedi N. Disoriented and ataxic pilgrims: an epidemiological study of acute mountain sickness and high altitude cerebral edema at a sacred lake at 4300 m in the Nepal Himalayas. *Wilderness and Environmental Med* 2000;11:89–93.

Summerton C, Shetty P, Sandle LN, et al. High altitude illness. In: Haslett C, Chilvers ER, Boon NA, Colledge NR, Hunter JAA (eds). *Davidson's Principles and Practice of Medicine.* 19th edn. Edinburgh: Churchill Livingstone, 2002; 334–5.

Sutton JR, Houston CS, Mansell AL, et al. Effect of acetazolamide on hypoxemia during sleep at high altitude. *N Engl J Med* 1979;301:1329–31.

Wiedman M, Tabin GC. High-altitude retinopathy and altitude illness. *Ophthalmology* 1999; 106:1924–1936; discussion 1927.

Zafren K. Gamow bag for high altitude cerebral edema. [Letter]. *Lancet* 1998;352:325.

7.13 WITHDRAWAL OF WITHHOLDING OF LIFE SUPPORT, BRAIN DEATH, AND ORGAN PROCUREMENT

The goal of treatment of children with life-threatening illness is their survival with minimal residual injury or cure. When a physician realizes that further treatment is futile in not preventing death and perhaps harmful to a patient, the family should be compassionately informed.

Withholding or withdrawing of life support: Two basically different groups of patients die in a PICU: (i) previously healthy children who have recently experienced a catastrophic event (motor vehicle, near drowning, or a serious infection); and (ii) children with a serious chronic illness that has become terminal (major congenital malformations, cystic fibrosis, severe inborn errors of metabolism). For these latter children and their families it may be possible to provide appropriate terminal care in a more comfortable setting such as home. The management of a dying patient should include consideration of resuscitation measures, comfort care, and symptom management such as pain, nausea, anxiety, and dyspnea.

Some children may have a very limited quality of continuing life, although not fulfilling the criteria of death, such as children with the *persistent vegetative state* (PVS). This is a state of perpetual unconsciousness in which there may be neurologic responsiveness to some external stimuli. In these children brainstem continues to function and therefore legally they are not brain dead and thus are not dead. PVS exists when

Table 7.13: Diagnosis of brain death	
Brain death criteria	*Evaluated by*
Prerequisites	
1. A recognized cause of coma, sufficient to explain the irreversible cessation of all brain function	History, clinical examination, laboratory, technical investigation
2. Potentially reversible causes of coma must be excluded:	
a. Sedatives and neuromuscular blocking drugs	
b. Hypothermia	

c. Metabolic and endocrine disturbances
     Severe electrolyte disturbances
     Severe hypo- or hyperglycemia	

d. Uncontrolled hypotension	
e. Surgically remedial intracranial conditions	
f. Any other sign that suggests a potentially reversible cause of coma	
Clinical evaluation	
1. Absence of higher brain function	Lack of consciousness, voluntary movement or responsiveness except for spinal reflexes (stimuli applied to anybody region may not elicit motor response within cranial nerve distribution); preferably test in a cranial (trigeminal) dermatome rather than a spinal dermatome, no decorticate or decerebrate posturing, no convulsions
2. Absence of brainstem function:	
a. Absence of sympathetic and parasympathetic regulation of the pupils	Pupils in midposition or dilated showing neither direct nor indirect reaction to light
b. Disruption of the pathways controlling eye movement in the brainstem	Absence of spontaneous eye movement, absence of reaction to injection of iced water into the ear (vestibulo-ocular reflex), absence of doll's eye phenomenon (oculocephalic reflexes)
c. Disruption of afferent trigeminal and efferent facial nerve pathways	Absence of blink response to (careful) corneal stimulation
d. Disruption of the afferent and efferent pathways of cranial nerves IX and X in the medulla oblongata	Absence of gag response to stimulation of posterior pharynx, absence of cough on suctioning of the trachea
e. Absence of vagal efferent activity	No significant increase of heart rate on administration of intravenous atropine or on pressure applied to the eyeballs (oculocardiac reflex)
f. Disruption of respiratory control centers of the medulla oblongata	No respiratory movement (as assessed by observation ± capnography) at a $PaCO_2$ above a set limit during a standardized apnea testing
Confirmatory tests	
1. Confirmation of absence of higher brain function	Electrocerebral silence on EEG during at least 30 min
2. Confirmation of complete infarction of the brain	Four vessel contrast angiography or radionuclide imaging brainstem by confirmation of absence of blood flow
Observation	
Confirmation of irreversibility	Observation during a set time; ± request formal physical examination and confirmatory tests

Source: Lutz-Dettinger N, de Jaeger A, Kerremans I. Care of the potential pediatric organ donor. *Pediatr Clin North Am* 2001; 48: 715–49

there has been lack of neurologic recovery for at least 6 mo with preservation of only the autonomic nervous system, resulting in the maintenance of vital signs (heart rate, blood pressure, respirations and temperature). Such patients may require nursing care, including feeding (usually via gastrostomy), bathing, assistance with bladder and bowel function, skin care to prevent pressure ulcers (bed sores), airway access via a tracheotomy, and passive range of motion exercises to minimize joint contractures. Patients in PVS are susceptible to infections and death usually occurs from pneumonia, urinary tract infection or complications of a skin lesion. These children may be cared for at home or in long-term care nursing facilities. After months or years of caring for a child in PVS, a family may decide to limit various treatment modalities after careful consideration of the risks and benefits of further interventions for the child.

Withdrawal of support represents cessation of medical treatment and support already being provided to patients. This should be the standard in brain dead children. It must be made very clear to a family that as life support is withdrawn from a child who is not brain dead but is dependent on the treatment, the outcome is most likely to be death.

There are children with *"locked-in-syndrome"* which is characterized by absent outward signs of responsiveness owing to paralysis, muscular dysfunction, or acute neurologic insult, but consciousness persists. This syndrome can occur with injuries to the lower brainstem, sparing the neocortex, and should be suspected and ruled out before withdrawal of

support is considered, which will lead to death of the patient.

Brain death: Death is defined as irreversible cessation of circulatory and respiratory functions or irreversible cessation of all functions of the brain, including the brainstem. Brain death criteria are listed in Table 7.13. Guidelines for assessing brain death in children of different ages are presented in Box 7.7. Brain death is equivalent to cardiovascular death, and child should be considered legally dead at the time brain death criteria is fulfilled. This determination is crucial to the process of organ procurement that requires harvesting heart, lung, liver, or bowel from a donor whose heart is beating. When the diagnosis of brain death has been made and the family wishes to pursue organ donation then the consent is obtained, and organ procurement is carried out.

Frankel LR, Mathers LH. Withdrawal or Withdrawing of Life Support, Brain Death, and Organ Procurement. In: Behrman RE, Kliegman RM, Jenson HB (eds). *Nelson Textbook of Pediatrics.* 17th edn. Philadelphia: Saunders, 2004;340–2.

Lutz-Dettinger N, de Jaeger A, Kerremans I. Care of the potential pediatric organ donor. *Pediatr Clin North Am* 2001; 48:715–49.

Task Force for Determination of Brain Death in Children: Guidelines for the determination of brain death in children. *Pediatrics* 1987;80:298–300.

7.14 PEDIATRIC PAIN MANAGEMENT IN CHILDREN

The International Association for Study of Pain defines pain as 'an unpleasant sensory and emotional pain experience associated with actual or potential tissue damage or described in terms of such damage'. Pain should be managed using a broad range of demonstrated tools that include pharmacologic, regional anesthesia, behavioral and alternative therapies. Acute and chronic pain can be best handled when they are approached in a multidisciplinary fashion, because pharmacologic techniques and nonpharmacologic approaches complement one another.

Pharmacological Treatment of Pain

A. *Non-steroidal Anti-inflammatory Drugs*

1. *Acetaminophen (paracetamol):* It is mainly an antipyretic and a weak analgesic indicated for mild pain or as an adjunct for treatment of moderated or severe pain. It is safe to use in neonates because it is primarily metabolized in the liver. As neonates have immature hepatic function, they are less likely to produce toxic metabolites. Oral doses of 10–15 mg/kg, although antipyretic are not analgesic until doses of 20–35 mg/kg are used. Rectal doses of 40–

Box 7.7: Age specific criteria for brain death*

Children 1 week to 2 mo of age: fulfillment of the clinical criteria described in Table 7.13 in two separate examinations at least 48 hr apart, or one clinical examination followed by an isoelectric EEG at least 48 hr later.

Children 2 mo–1 yr of age: fulfillment of the clinical criteria described in Table 7.13 in two separate examinations at least 24 hr apart, or one clinical examination followed by an isoelectric EEG or negative results of a cerebral blood flow study at least 24 hr later.

Children > 1 yr of age: fulfillment of the clinical criteria described in Table 7.13 in two separate examinations at least 12 hr apart.

EEG: Electroencephalogram

*Criteria for brain death in infants in infants younger than 1 wk of age have not been determined but should be at least as stringent as for those 1 wk–2 mo of age. It is often very difficult to diagnose brain death in premature infants; the wait period should be at least 72 hr (wait period for the adults is 6 hr). Once brain death is determined, that is the medical time of death.

45 mg/kg are needed to achieve effective plasma concentrations.

2. *COX 2 inhibitors:* None of these have received approval for use in children, though use of diclofenac and ketorolac has been reported. Ketorolac is the only parenteral NSAID available.

B. Opioids

Opioids are an integral part of providing analgesia.

1. *Morphine and fentanyl:* Premature and term newborns show reduced clearance of morphine and prolonged elimination half-life. Till 3 to 6 months doses up to 1/4 to 1/2 are used. After that morphine pharmacokinetics resembles that in older children and adults.

   Fentanyl also has a diminished clearance in premature infants and newborns. But in infants older than 3 months, clearance is actually double that in older children. It should be used with caution in infants with increased intra-abdominal pressure, as fentanyl clearance is dependant on hepatic blood flow. Fentanyl infusions are widely used with a loading dose of 1–4 mcg/kg followed by infusions of 2–4 mcg/kg per hour. Nausea, vomiting, pruritus, urinary retention, dysphoria, constipation and somnolence are side effects which need to be treated promptly. If a child is having significant pain at current infusion rate, a bolus dose of approximately 50% of the standard dose for age should be administered followed by a rate increase of 10–20%.

2. *Codeine:* It is a commonly prescribed oral opioid analgesic that is often used for mild to moderate pain. However, nausea, vomiting, constipation and hepatic metabolism (which depends upon cytochrome P450 2D6 isozyme and is absent or diminished in 5–10% of certain ethnic population causing markedly diminished analgesic response) has led many to switch to other drugs.

3. *Tramadol:* It is a synthetic analog of codeine. Dose is 1–2 mg/kg per dose every 6 hr. It should be used with caution with tricyclic antidepressants.

4. *Hydromorphone, methadone, oxycodone:* Hydromorphone is 5 times more potent than morphine with less pruritus and less respiratory depression. Methadone is used in weaning opioid tolerant patients. Oxycodone is available as liquid, tablets and in various fixed combinations.

C. Other Drugs

1. *Clonidine:* This drug is used as an analgesic regiment for postoperative and cancer pain. Dose is 3–5 mcg/kg oral and has been used orally, caudal, transdermal or neuraxial.

2. *Ketamine:* It has been used as an adjunct.

3. *Tricyclic antidepressants:* Provide analgesia in a variety of chronic pain conditions including neuropathic pain. Because of anticholinergic side effects these should be slowly titrated to an effective dose.

4. *Anticonvulsants:* These have been used for chronic pain management. Commonly used drugs are phenytoin, carbamazepine, sodium valproate and gabapentin (Table 7.14).

Acute Pain Management

Cutaneous anesthesia can be utilized for venepuncture, circumcision, lumbar puncture, bone marrow aspiration, laceration repair, etc. and can be done with application of local anesthetic creams like EMLA. EMLA (Eutectic Mixture of Local Anesthetic) is a mixture of 2.5% lidocaine and 2.5% prilocaine. This is applied to skin for 60 minutes with an occlusive dressing which leads to effective cutaneous anesthesia.

Patient controlled analgesia (PCA): The rationale for PCA analgesia is that the usual doses of as needed medication can lead to episodes or cycles of pain, followed by rescue dosing that causes excessive sedation and other opioid side effects. More frequent, smaller doses of opioids, which can be self-administered by patient lead to better analgesic titration with fewer side effects. The child's control over his or her own analgesia has considerable psychological benefits. Parent and nurse controlled analgesia is another way to use PCA technology, when the patient is incapable of delivering doses, due to either immaturity, developmental delay or medical

Table 7.14: Tricyclic and anticonvulsant drugs for relief of pain		
Drug	*Dose*	*Comments*
Amitriptyline	Initial: 0.2 mg/kg per day Target: 0.5–1 mg/kg per day	Once each night; 1–2 hrs before bed
Carbamazepine	Initial; 5–10 mg/kg per day Target: 15–30 mg/kg per day	Divide into 2–3 doses
Gabapentin	Initial: 5 mg/kg per day Target: 15–30 mg/kg per day	Divide into 3 doses
Sodium valproate	Initial: 10 mg/kg per day	Divide into 3 doses

Table 7.15: Morphine and fentanyl for relief of pain			
Drug	PCA dose	PCA hr max (mg/kg)	Basal rate (mg/kg/hr)
Morphine	0.01 to 0.03	0.1	0.01 to 0.03
Fentanyl	0.5 to 2 mcg/kg per dose	3.5–5 mcg/kg/hr	1–2 mcg/kg

condition. It is important to initiate PCA in the recovery room or the emergency department to avoid potential long delay (Table 7.15).

Continuous intravenous opioids: Continuous infusion of opioids is a means of managing postoperative pain in infant's and young children unable to use a PCA device. Morphine dosages of 0.02 to 0.03 mg/kg per hr can provide consistent levels of analgesia with minimal respiratory depression.

Epidural analgesia—Pulmonary function maybe enhanced with effective epidural analgesia after upper abdominal surgery and thoracic procedures. Also postoperative ventilation could be avoided by combining general anesthesia with epidural analgesia. Single shot caudal analgesia with bupivacaine is very safe, can last as long as 6-8 hr, and has been effectively used for outpatient procedures. The epidural space can be approached at any level: Caudal, lumbar or thoracic. Air should be avoided in children in injecting in epidural space to avoid the risk of air embolus, if a patent foramen ovale, a VSD or ASD. Epidural catheters should be inserted below the first or second lumbar vertebra as they are below the termination of spinal cord. To minimize the side effects of epidural analgesia a combination of local anesthetic and opioids is used to permit using a lower dose of each agent. Morphine and fentanyl are frequently combined with 0.0625 to 0.1% bupivacaine. In general, fentanyl can be reloaded every 4 hr, whereas redosing of morphine depends on amount initially administered and the elapsed time.

When the catheter tip is close to dermatome of surgery, fentanyl is the opioid of choice, when the tip is farther from the site of operation, such as a lumbar catheter in a patient with thoracotomy, more water soluble opioid such as morphine are chosen. The morphine load is usually 30–35 mcg/kg and fentanyl is 0.5 to 2 mcg/kg. Infusion rates of bupivacaine must be kept below 0.2 mg/kg per hr in neonate and infant under 4–6 mo of age and below 0.4–0.75 mcg/kg per hr in child over 2 yrs of age to avoid toxicity and cardiovascular instability. Contraindications to placement of epidural catheter include intrinsic coagulopathy or use of anticoagulant, sepsis and infection in the skin at the site of insertion.

Chronic Pain Management

Chronic pain has become a significant problem in the pediatric population. Signs of sympathetic nervous system arousal rarely accompany chronic pain in contrast to acute pain. Formerly, chronic pain was defined as having pain for longer than 6 mo, but it is now recognized that chronic pain can be evident much earlier. Chronic pain can be differentiated from acute pain in that acute pain signals a specific nociceptive event and is self limited. Chronic pain may start as an acute event but continues beyond the normal time expected for recovery. To evaluate and treat chronic childhood pain effectively and efficiently a multidisciplinary approach is most successful. The evaluation of a patient with chronic pain should begin with a complete history. Factors to investigate include the time frame for painful condition, the description of pain, how it affects patient's activities, alternative forms of pain therapies taken by the patient, social history, recent stressors (death, parental separation), how family perceives the pain. The psychologist should interview both the family and the child separately. Physician then examines the child. Common chronic pain problems include the following:

1. ***Headache:*** As many as 20% children younger than 5 years have headache. At puberty migraine headaches become common with an incidence of 10 to 27%. Tension type headache is also common. A detailed neurological evaluation including a MRI to rule out brain tumors, vascular anomalies and other structural abnormalities should be carried out. Eye and sinus conditions should be looked into. Viral illnesses, temporomandibular joint dysfunction can also result in recurrent bitemporal headaches. Treatment is aimed at preventive and abortive therapy including NSAIDs acetaminophen, ergotamines, beta blockers, SSRI, TCA. Chronic headache treatment should include cognitive behavioral therapy which may include biofeedback relaxation techniques, cognitive reframing and a variety of standard psychotherapeutic intervention.

2. ***Chronic abdominal pain:*** Only 10% of children with recurrent abdominal pain have recognizable organic illness accounting for the pain complaints. Organic causes include lactose intolerance, ulcerative colitis, and infection and Crohn's disease. Even if organic causes are excluded, there is some evidence that

these patients may have some forms of irritable bowel syndrome with associated visceral hyperalgesia. A multidisciplinary approach is taken, incorporating medications (NSAIDS, amitriptyline, tramadol, SSRI, COX 2 inhibitors), behavioral approaches to manage stress and anxiety, sleep hygiene, biofeedback training and encouragement of return to normal activities.

3. *Myofascial pain/ fibromyalgia:* It is characterized by widespread pain, multiple tender points on physical examination, fatigue, sleep difficulties, abdominal pain, headaches and mood disturbance and is estimated to occur in 1–6% of the juvenile population. Current management includes improving sleep hygiene, regular physical activity, cognitive behavioral strategies and low dose TCAs to improve both pain and sleep disturbances. Acupuncture can also be tried.

4. *Complex regional pain syndrome* (CRPS type I formerly known as reflex sympathetic dystrophy RSD): CRPS refers to a syndrome of persistent neuropathic pain associated with nondermatomal autonomic dysfunction. It is often seen after minor injury and patients have findings that include temperature and color changes, edema, cyanosis and eventual trophic changes of the skin and osteoporotic changes, if left untreated. The current IASP diagnostic criteria include (i) at least 2 neuropathic pain descriptors (burning, dysesthesias, paresthesia, and hyperalgesia to cold, and (ii) at least 2 physical signs of autonomic dysfunction (cyanosis, mottling, hyperhidrosis, 3°C lower temperature in affected limb, edema).

   The cause of pain is not completely understood but is thought to be related to abnormal discharges in sympathetic afferent nerves along with nociceptive effects produced by incidental trauma. Conservative treatment includes physical therapy, TENS, TCAs, cognitive behavioral therapies and relaxation therapies. Sympathetic blockade, intensive physical therapy cognitive behavioral therapy neuromodulating drug therapy, psychotherapy, intensive family psychotherapy have all been tried.

5. *Sickle cell anemia:* It is an inherited hemoglobinopathy that results in recurrent acute and chronic pain due to red cell sickling and obstruction of the microvasculature with subsequent embolism and inflammation. Painful vaso-occlusive episodes occur in the hands and feet, extremity long bones, chest and abdomen leading to frequent hospitalizations for intensive pain management with intravenous opioids. The superimposition of unpredictable acute pain crises on top of chronic pain compounds the chronic pain assessment of these patients. It is imperative to complete a thorough evaluation of all the biologic and psychological aspects of the individual and his or her family and support system. Emotional support, possible chronic transfusions, hydroxyurea and selective administration of NSAIDs or TCAs with liberal use of short and long acting opioids can help the patient who has sickle cell crises. As most have used opioids for pain control, they may have a high tolerance to opioid analgesics. Regional anesthesia maybe a good choice to help manage a sickle cell crisis in lower extremity or pelvis. It may also be quite beneficial in the management of acute chest syndrome. Epidural anesthesia with local anesthetics administered alone or in combination with fentanyl has been shown to effectively treat sickle cell vaso-occlusive crisis unresponsive to conventional methods with fewer side effects such as sedation or respiratory depression.

6. *Cancer* in children may have pain that can be classified into four broad categories: Cancer related pain (bone pain, neuropathic pain, somatic pain terminal care); treatment related pain from chemotherapy, radiation, infection and phantom limb pain; procedure related pain; pain unrelated to cancer (pre-existing pain such as headache, trauma or other medical problems such as appendicitis. For almost 15 years, cancer pain treatment has been guided by WHO analgesic ladder. Mild pain can be treated with nonopioids first, with it kept in mind that these agents have a ceiling effect and side effects that include inhibition of platelet function, gastritis and decreased renal blood flow. Moderate pain can be treated with an oral opioid plus nonopioids. Severe pain can be managed with potent intravenous opioids. A more appropriate conceptualization of the ladder demands selecting the analgesic agent that seems best matched to the severity of the patient's pain. In addition, some pain in cancer can be opioid resistant such as spinal cord or nerve root compression. In this case, the prompt addition of adjuvant analgesics such as TCAs or gabapentin is indicated. Unless the individual has unusual intermittent pain episodes, a regimen of around the clock with long acting opioids should be chosen with a short acting immediate release available for breakthrough pain. Under rare circumstances, the terminally ill children with cancer may benefit from invasive neuraxial therapy delivered via an implanted intraspinal or epidural catheter. Management of side effects of opioids is important. Constipation can be treated with stool softeners, laxatives, and small doses of stimulants, antihistaminics, and antiemetics.

Alternative Forms of Pain Management

Alternative forms of pain management include cognitive behavioral interventions, TENS, and acupuncture.

1. *Cognitive behavioral interventions:* Children are highly responsive to pain reducing strategies that involve their imagination and sense of play. Children younger than 6 years can be distracted by blowing bubbles, playing with pop up toys or looking through a kaleidoscope. Older children engage well in external or abstract interventions such as guided imagery, counting creating techniques. A potential physiologic explanation of the effectiveness of hypnosis in reducing pain is that hypnosis inhibits transmission of pain signals from peripheral fibers at the level of the dorsal horn. Alternatively, hypnosis may work by causing amnesia of the event surrounding the hypnotic trance. Progressive muscle relaxation is designed to help children recognize and reduce tension associated with pain, decrease anxiety and decrease discomfort. Learning to decrease body tension is an acquired skill and relaxation training requires initial instruction and then frequent practice to be successful. An occupational therapist or a psychologist often teaches these skills. Biofeedback uses alpha electroencephalography, muscle electromyography, skin temperature and temporal pulse feedback to modify the level of tension in the body.

2. *Transcutaneous electrical nerve stimulation (TENS):* TENS can be an additive technique for pain management. A TENS unit generates a nonpainful stimulus at peripheral nerves and appears to facilitate the closing of the gate for transmission of pain.

3. *Acupuncture:* Acupuncture is among the most commonly used forms of complementary medicine for various pain problems. It may provide analgesia through a mechanism similar to TENS. Stimulation of small pain fibers may inhibit spinal transmission of other pain signals. It has been found that acupuncture significantly reduced pediatric pain associated with headaches, limb pain, chest pain and abdominal pain when used in a multimodal approach to pain.

Anand KJS, Craig KD: New perspectives on the definition of pain. *Pain* 1996;67:3–6; discussion 209–211, 1996.

Bieri D, Reeve RA, Champion GD, et al. The Faces Pain Scale for the self-assessment of the severity of pain experienced by children: Development, initial validation and preliminary investigation for ratio scale properties. *Pain* 1990;41:139–50.

Breau LM, Finley GA, mcGrath PJ, et al. Validation of the Non-communicating Children's Pain Checklist—Postoperative Version. *Anesthesiology* 2004;96:528–35.

Grazzi LD, Amico D, Leone M, et al. Pharmacological and behavioral treatment of pediatric migraine and tension type headache. *Ital J Neurol Sci* 1998;19:59–64.

Merskey H, Bogduk N (eds). Classification of chronic pain, IASP Task Force on Taxonomy. Seattle: IASP Press, 1994.

Rusy LM, Weisman SJ. Complementary therapies for acute pediatric pain management. *Pediatr Clin North Am* 2000;47:589–99.

Wiffen P, Collins S, McQuay H, et al. Anticonvulsants drugs for acute and chronic pain. *Cochrane Database Syst Rev* CD 001133, 2000.

7.15 SHOCK

Shock is an acute syndrome characterized by inadequate circulatory provision of oxygen, so that the metabolism demands of vital organs and tissues are not met. Shock is clinically divided into five types (Table 7.16). There is significant overlap in these categories, especially in septic and distributive shock. Hypovolemia (hemorrhage, diarrhea-dehydration) and septic shock are the most common causes of shock in children. Refractory shock is present if despite 1 hr of appropriate therapy shock persists.

Pathophysiology of Shock

It is common for more than one of these processes to occur simultaneously:

1. *Extracorporeal fluid loss:* Hypovolemic shock may be due to the direct blood loss through hemorrhage or abnormal loss of body fluids (diarrhea, vomiting, burns, diabetes insipidus, nephrosis, adrenal insufficiency).

2. *Lowering plasma oncotic forces:* Hypovolemic shock may also result from hypoproteinemia (nephrotic syndrome, malnutrition, hepatic dysfunction, acute severe burns or as a progressive complication of increased capillary permeability)

3. *Abnormal vasodilation:* Distributive shock (neurogenic, anaphylaxis, or septic shock) occurs when intravascular fluid shifts into the extracellular space owing to increase in the rate of blood flow, and blood volume, or hydrostatic pressure in the vascular compartment (sympathetic blockade, local substances affecting permeability, acidosis, drug effects, and spinal cord transection).

4. *Increased vascular permeability:* Sepsis may change the vascular permeability in the absence of any change in capillary hydrostatic pressure (endotoxins from sepsis, excess histamine release in anaphylaxis).

5. *Cardiac dysfunction:* Peripheral hypoperfusion may result from any condition that affects the heart's ability to pump blood efficiently (ischemia, acidosis, drugs, constrictive pericarditis, pancreatitis, and sepsis).

Table 7.16: Clinical classification of shock

Type of shock	Characteristics	Causes
1. Hypovolemic	Reduced fluid volume reduces cardiac output; metabolic acidosis can result from low intravascular volume and poor tissue perfusion; serious electrolyte abnormalities may occur	Diarrhea Vomiting Hemorrhage Extensive burns Diabetes insipidus Adrenal insufficiency
2. Septic	Infectious organisms release toxins that affect fluid distribution, cardiac output, and so on	Bacterial Viral Fungal (all are more likely in immunocompromised state)
3. Cardiogenic	Primary pump failure produces inadequate tissue perfusion; results in metabolic acidosis which further impairs cardiac function	Ischemic insult Cardiomyopathy Congenital heart disease
4. Distributive	Neurologic disturbances, may cause uneven distribution of fluids, leading to acidosis Overdose of drugs can alter fluid distribution	Neurogenic (disturbance of vasomotor tone) Anaphylaxis Toxins Allergic reactions
5. Obstructive	Poor cardiac output, cyanosis, hypotension, narrow pulse pressure	Tension Pnumothorax Pericardial tamponade

Clinical manifestations: The clinical manifestations of shock are presented in Table 7.17.

Treatment

Initial management: In most patients with early shock, a fluid bolus of 20 ml/kg of normal saline or lactated Ringer solution should be given rapidly (5–10 min). If it is not possible to insert an intravenous catheter into a peripheral vein within 90 seconds or within three attempts, an intraosseous needle should be inserted to administer fluids. After this infusion, the patient reassessed to determine if more fluid is required or other forms of therapy should be initiated (e.g., antibiotics, vasoactive agents or other types of fluids). Children in severe hypovolemic shock may require and tolerate fluid boluses totaling 60–80 mL/kg within

Table 7.17: Clinical manifestations of shock

Type of shock	Clinical manifestations
Hypovolemic	Changes in mental status, tachypnea, tachycardia, hypotension, cool extremities, and oliguria
Septic	Compensated or "warm shock" with warm extremities [from peripheral vasodilation secondary to systemic vascular resistance (SVR)], bounding pulses and tachycardia (from high stroke volume and widened pulse pressure), tachypnea, adequate urination, and mild metabolic acidosis
Cardiogenic	Cool extremities, delayed (> 2–3 sec.) capillary filling time, hypotension, tachypnea, increasing obtundation, and decreased urination (all caused by peripheral vasoconstriction and decreased cardiac output)
Late (regardless of its etiology)	Uncompensated or "cool shock" due to high vascular resistance; delayed capillary refill, mottled, cyanotic, cool extremities; tachycardia, hypotension; tachypnea; oliguria/anuria; ileus; agitated/confused, stuporous, coma
Hemorrhagic shock encephalopathy syndrome (HSES)	Encephalopathy, fever, shock, watery diarrhea, severe disseminated intravascular coagulation (DIC), and renal and hepatic dysfunction; may develop seizures and other neurologic findings as a result of cerebral edema; usually seen in children younger than 3-year-old; very high mortality rate

the first 1–2 hr of presentation. However, the risk of fluid overload must be continually reassessed. If the child's hypovolemia is from loss of blood or protein rich fluid, replacement with fresh frozen plasma, albumin, whole blood, or packed red blood may be appropriate. The overall goal is to restore oxygen delivery to vital tissues. This can be accomplished by improving oxygen-carrying capacity (maintain normal hematocrit at 35–40%), improving oxygen saturation (95–99%).

Cardiovascular management: Septic, cardiogenic, distributive, and rarely, hypovolemic shock may require various drugs to stimulate heart rate (*chronotropic*), cardiac contractility (*inotropic*), and enhance peripheral vascular resistance (*blood pressure*). These drugs should be infused through a central venous catheter in intensive care unit. These drugs increase oxygen consumption and the risk of dysrhythmias. If after appropriate fluid resuscitation, the patient continues to demonstrate poor perfusion and shock, vasoactive agents are needed.

Dopamine (1–5 mg/kg/min) is the most frequently used initial drug and is preferred for cardiogenic shock.

Epinephrine (0.05–3 mg/kg/min) is more effective in increasing perivascular tone and has a greater effect on the heart and poses a greater risk of dysrhythmias.

Dobutamine (1–20 mg/kg/min) provides afterload reduction in cardiogenic shock.

Norepinephrine (0.05–1.5 mg/kg/min) and *phenylephrine* (0.5–2 g/kg/min) are particularly effective in counteracting low systemic vascular resistance. Various inotropic drugs are also given in combination, including low-dose *dopamine with epinephrine*, *dobutamine with norepinephrine*, or *dopamine with dobutamine*. Intravenous *vasopressin* is used to treat shock that is unresponsive to catecholamines. Some patients with septic shock and in all patients who are on or who were recently weaned from steroids, intravenous *hydrocortisone* in stress doses should be started. Afterload reduction is seldom indicated in early shock but may be useful in the recovery phase of cardiogenic shock.

Amrinone (load with 1.5–5 mg/kg bolus over 20 min, followed by 5–10 mg/kg/min) and more often *milrinone* have demonstrated beneficial effects in the advanced treatment of cardiogenic shock, intravenous *methylene blue* and *angiotensin II* (40 times more potent as a vasoconstricting agent as norepinephrine) have been used in patients with unresponsive shock.

Butt W. Septic shock. *Pediatr Clin North Am* 2001;48:601–26.

Frankel LR, Kache S. Shock. In: Kliegman RM, Behrman RE, Jenson HB, Stanton BF (eds). *Nelson Textbook of Pediatrics.* 18th edn. Vol. 1. Philadelphia: Saunders, 2007; 413–21.

8 The Fetus and Newborn Infant

8.1 THE NEWBORN

The neonatal period is an extremely important period for an infant, because of infant's transition from intrauterine to extrauterine life requiring many biochemical and physiologic changes. Many newborn infants have special problems related to poor adaptation because of asphyxia, premature birth, life-threatening congenital anomalies, or the adverse effects of delivery.

Definitions Based on World Health Organization (WHO)

Gestation (Independent of birth weight)

1. Preterm = less than 37 completed weeks of gestation (258 days)
2. Full term = between 37 wk and 42 completed wk of gestation (259–293 days)
3. Post-term or postmature = more than 42 completed weeks (294 days)

Dates are taken from the first day of the last menstrual period. Conception is presumed to be approximately 2 wk after this date.

Ultrasound dates are based on conception and have to be altered to fit the dates estimated from the last menstrual period.

Birth Weight (Independent of gestation)

1. Low birth weight = less than 2500 g
2. Very low birth weight = less than 1500 g
3. Extremely low birth weight (very, very low birth weight) = less than 1000 g
4. Inappropriately or incredibly low birth weight = less than 750 g

Size for Gestation

1. Small for gestation (SGA) = less than 10th percentile in weight expected for gestation (small for dates)
2. Appropriate for gestation (AGA) = between 10th and 90th percentiles of weight expected for gestation
3. Large for gestation (LGA) = more than 90th percentile in weight expected for gestation

NB. The expected weight in percentiles will vary with the population. The term immature, premature and dysmature should no longer be used.

In Utero

1. Less than 1 wk = fertilized egg to the formation of the blastocyst
2. 1–12 wk = embryo
3. 24 wk or more = current period of 'legal' validity

Abortion is the expulsion of the dead fetus prior to 24 wk's gestation (168 days).

A dead fetus expelled after this time is *still birth*.

Note that a *live born baby* is a baby of any gestation that has signs of life (e.g. only a heart beat) at delivery. Many miscarriages before 20 wk of gestation will show signs of life.

The Neonate

1. Perinatal period—the period from 24 wk gestation or the time of the live birth if less than 24 wk of gestation to 7 days of postnatal age.
2. Early neonatal period = the first 7 days of life of a live born infant of any gestation
3. Late neonatal period = 8–28 days after birth
4. Neonatal period = first 28 days of life of a live born infant of any gestation
5. Infancy= the first year of life

Mortality Rate

1. Still birth rate = number of still birth per 100 total births.
2. Perinatal mortality rate (PMR) = number of still stillbirths + early (up to 7 days) neonatal deaths per 1000 total births
3. Neonatal mortality rate (NMR) = number of deaths in the first 28 days per 1000 live births
4. Infant mortality rate (IMR) = number of deaths in the first 365 days per 1000 live births

8.2 EXAMINATION OF NEWBORN

History

The *neonatal history* should:
1. Identify disabling diseases that are amenable to prompt preventive action or treatment (respiratory distress syndrome)
2. Anticipate conditions that may be of later importance (gonococcal conjunctivitis), and
3. Screening inborn errors of metabolism that may explain pathologic conditions regardless of their immediate or future significance.

The *perinatal history* should include demographic and social data (socioeconomic status, age, race); past medical illnesses in the mother and family, including previous siblings (cardiopulmonary disorders, infectious diseases, genetic disorders, anemia, jaundice, diabetes mellitus); previous maternal reproductive problems (stillbirth, prematurity, blood group sensitization); infant feeding practices (breastfed or not, reasons not breastfed); events occurring in the present pregnancy (vaginal bleeding, medications, acute illness, duration of rupture of membranes); and a description of the labor (duration, fetal presentation, fetal distress, fever) and delivery (cesarean section, anesthesia or sedation, use of forceps, Apgar score, need for resuscitation).

Physical Examination

Examination of a newborn requires patience, gentleness, and procedural flexibility. If the infant is quiet and relaxed at the beginning of the examination, palpation of the abdomen or auscultation of the heart should be performed first before other more disturbing manipulations are attempted. The *initial examination* should be performed as soon as possible after delivery to detect abnormalities and to establish a baseline for subsequent examination. In newborn infants temperature, heart rate, respiratory rate, color, type of respiration, tone, activity, and level of consciousness should be monitored every 30 min after birth for 2 hr or until stabilized. For high-risk deliveries, this examination should take place in the delivery room, and focus on congenital anomalies and patho-physiologic problems that may interfere with normal cardiopulmonary and metabolic adaptation to extrauterine life. After a stable delivery room course, a *2nd and more detailed examination* should be performed within 24 hr of birth. With a healthy infant, the mother should be present during this examination; even minor, insignificant anatomic variations should be explained. No infant should be discharged from the hospital without a final examination because certain abnormalities, particularly heart murmurs, often appear and disappear in the immediate neonatal period; in addition, evidence of disease that has just been acquired may be noted. The pulse (normal, 120–160 beats/min), respiratory rate (normal, 30–60 breaths/min), temperature, weight, length, head circumference, and dimensions of any visible or palpable structural abnormality should be recorded (*see* Section 2.4; page-16). Blood pressure is determined if a neonate appears ill or has a heart murmur.

General appearance: Physical activity may be absent during the relaxation of normal sleep, or it may be decreased by the effects of illness or drugs; an infant may be either lying with the extremities motionless (to conserve energy for the effort of difficult breathing), or be vigorously crying with accompanying activity of the arms and legs. Both active and passive muscle tone and any unusual posture should be recorded. Coarse, tremulous movements with ankle or jaw myoclonus are more common and less significant in newborn infants than at any other age. Such movements tend to occur when an infant is active, where as convulsive twitching occurs in a quiet state. Edema of the eyelids commonly results from irritation caused by the administration of silver nitrate. Generalized edema may occur with prematurity, hypoproteinemia secondary to severe erythroblastosis fetalis, nonimmune hydrops, congenital nephrosis, Hurler's syndrome, or unknown cause. Localized edema suggests a congenital malformation of the lymphatic system; when confined to one or more extremities of a female infant; it may be the initial sign of Turner syndrome.

Skin: Note harmless cyanosis (*acrocyanosis*) of the hands and feet, especially when they stop crying and are cool, mottling may be associated with serious illness or related to a transient fluctuation in skin temperature, *harlequin color change* (a division of the body from the forehead to the pubis in to red and pale halves a transient and harmless condition), *cyanosis*, and *pallor*. The *ruddy red appearance* of plethora is seen with polycythemia. The vernix and common transitory macular capillary hemangiomas of the eyelids and neck are present. Slate-blue, well demarcated areas of pigmentation known as *mongolian spots* are seen over the buttocks, back, and sometimes other parts of the body, tend to disappear within the 1st yr. The vernix, skin, and especially the cord may be stained brownish yellow if the amniotic fluid has been colored by the passage of meconium during or before birth.

The skin of premature infants is thin and tends to be deep red; in extremely premature infants, the skin appears almost gelatinous and bleeds and bruises easily. Fine soft immature hair, *lanugo*, frequently covers the scalp and brow and may also cover the face of premature infants. *Tufts of hair* over the lumbosacral spine suggest an underlying abnormality such as occulta spina bifida, a sinus tract or a tumor. The nails are rudimentary in very premature infants, but they may protrude beyond the finger tips in infants born past term. Post-term infants may have a peeling, parchment-like skin, a severe degree of which suggests ichthyosis congenita.

In many neonates, small, white, occasionally vesiculopustular papules on an erythematous base develop 1–3 days after birth, this benign rash is known *as erythema toxicum*. The erythema toxicum rash persists for as long as 1 wk, contains eosinophils, and is usually distributed on the face, trunk and extremities. *Pustular melanosis*, a benign lesion predominantly seen in black neonates, contains neutrophils and is present at birth as a vesiculopustular eruption around the chin, neck, back, extremities, and palms or soles; it lasts 2–3 days.

Skull: Head circumference of newborn infants should be measured and charted. The skull may be molded, particularly if the infant is the first-born and if the head is engaged for a considerable time. The parietal bones tend to override the occipital and frontal bones. The head of an infant born by cesarean section or from a breech presentation is rounded in shape. The suture lines and the size and fullness of the anterior and posterior fontanels should be determined digitally by palpation (*see* Box 24.1).

Face: The general appearance should be noted with regard to dysmorphic features, such as epicanthal folds, widely or narrowly spaced eyes, microphthalmos, asymmetry, long philtrum, and low-set ears that are often associated with congenital syndromes. Symmetric facial palsy suggests absence or hypoplasia of the 7th cranial nerve nucleus (*Möbius syndrome*).

Eyes: The eyes often open spontaneously if the infant is held up and tipped gently forward and backward. This maneuver, a result of labyrinthine and neck reflexes should be used for inspecting the eyes than is forcing the lids apart. Conjunctival and retinal hemorrhages may be present but are usually benign. The iris should be examined for colobomas and heterochromia. A cornea larger than 1 cm in diameter in a term infant (with photophobia and tearing) suggests congenital glaucoma and prompt intervention by an ophthalmologist is required. The presence of bilateral red reflexes suggests the absence of cataracts and intraocular pathology. Leukokoria (white pupillary reflex) suggests cataracts, tumor, choreoretinitis, retinopathy of prematurity, or a persistent hyperplastic primary vitreous and an ophthalmologist should be consulted.

Ears: Deformities of the pinnae are occasionally seen. Unilateral or bilateral preauricular skin tags occur frequently. The tympanic membrane can be seen by otoscope through the short, straight external auditory canal and normally appears dull gray.

Nose: The nose may be slightly obstructed by mucus accumulated in the narrow nostrils. Unilateral or bilateral choanal atresia results in respiratory distress.

Mouth: Natal (present at birth) or neonatal (eruption after birth) teeth in the lower incisor position or aberrantly placed rarely present in normal mouth; these teeth are shed before the deciduous ones erupt. The soft and hard palate should be inspected and palpated for a complete or submucosal cleft and the contour noted if the arch is excessively high or the uvula bifid. On the hard palate on either side of the raphe there may be temporary accumulations of epithelial cells called *Epstein pearls*. Neonates do not have active salivation. The tongue appears relatively larger; the frenulum may be short, but rarely is shortness (*tongue-tied or ankyloglossia*) a reason for cutting it.

Neck: The neck appears relatively short. Abnormalities include goiter, cystic hygroma, branchial cleft rests, teratoma, hemangioma, and lesions of the sterno-cleidomastoid muscle that are presumably traumatic or due to a fixed positioning *in utero* that produces either a hematoma or fibrosis, respectively. Congenital torticollis causes the head to turn toward and the face to turn away from the affected side. Redundant skin or webbing in a female infant suggests intrauterine lymphedema and Turner syndrome. Both clavicles should be palpated for fractures.

Chest: Breast hypertrophy is common and milk may be present but should not be expressed. Look for supernumerary nipples, inverted nipples, or widely spaced nipples with a shield-shaped chest; the latter suggests Turner syndrome.

Lungs: Observe breathing and note variations in rate and rhythm and fluctuations in relation to infant's physical activity, state of wakefulness, or the presence of crying. Under these circumstances, the rate for normal term infants is 30–40/min; in premature infants the rate is higher and fluctuates more widely.

Heart: The location of the heart should be determined to detect dextrocardia. Transitory murmurs heard are usually due to a closing ductus arteriosus. The pulse may vary normally from 90/min in relaxed sleep to 180/min during activity.

Abdomen: The liver is usually palpable, sometimes as much as 2 cm below the rib margin. The abdominal wall is normally weak especially in premature infants and diastasis recti and umbilical hernias may occur.

Genitals: The genitals and mammary glands normally respond to transplacentally acquired maternal hormones to produce enlargement and secretion of the breasts in both sexes and prominence of the female genitals, often with nonpurulent discharge. These are transitory manifestations and no intervention is required. The testes should be in the scrotum or palpable in the inguinal canals of term infants. The prepuce of a newborn infant is normally tight and adherent. Urine is usually passed during or immediately after birth; a period without voiding may normally follow. Most void by 12 hr, and about 95% of preterm and term infants void within 24 hr.

Anus: Some passage of meconium usually occurs within the 1st 12 hr after birth and 99% term infants and 95% of premature infants pass meconium within 48 hr of birth. Imperforate anus is not always visible and may be detected by gentle insertion of little finger or a rectal tube.

Extremities: The extremities should be examined in spontaneous or stimulated activity to detect a fracture or nerve injury associated with delivery. The effects of fetal posture should be noted so that their cause and usual transitory nature can be explained to the mother. Such explanations are particularly important after breech presentations. The hands and feet should be examined for polydactyly, syndactyly, club foot, developmental dysplasia of hip and abnormal dermatographic patterns, such as simian crease. The hip joints of all infants should be examined with specific maneuvers to rule out congenital dislocation (Ortolani test, Barlow test) (*see* Chapter 31).

Ortolani test: The examiner grasps the child's thigh between the thumb and index finger, and with the 4th and 5th fingers, lifts the greater trochanter while simultaneously abducting the hip. When the test is positive, the femoral head will slip into the socket with a delicate "clunk" that is palpable but usually not audible. It should be a gentle, nonforced maneuver.

A hip click is the high-pitched sensation (or sound) felt at the very end of abduction during testing for DDH with Ortolani and Barlow maneuvers. Classically a hip click is differentiate from a hip "clunk," which is heard and felt as the hip goes in and out of joint. Hip clicks usually originate in the ligamentum teres or occasionally in the fascia lata or psoas tendon and do not indicate a significant hip abnormality.

Barlow test: the Barlow provocative maneuver assesses the potential for dislocation of a nondisplaced hip. The test is performed with the patient's knees and hips flexed. The examiner holds the patient's limbs gently, with the thigh in adduction and then applies a posteriorly directed force in an effort to dislocate the femoral head. In a positive test, the hip will be felt to slide out of the acetabulum. As the examiner relaxes the proximal push, the hip can be felt to slip back into the acetabulum. This test is positive in a dislocatable hip. The Ortalani test is the reverse of Barlow test: the examiner attempts to reduce a dislocated hip.

Neurological Assessment

State: Normal babies show different states of alertness. Babies who are continually in one state may be abnormal. Inability to rouse a baby from sleep is pathological.

Posture, spontaneous movement and tone: Normal muscle offers a resistance to stretch felt by the examiner as tone. Tone increases with gestational age and is high in term babies. Term babies lie with their limbs flexed and adducted in supine position unlike preterm babies who adopt an extended posture. Tone can alter in relation to feeds and sleep state, and repeated examination is required to confirm physical signs.

A term newborn makes smooth, spontaneous symmetrical limb movements which stop when the baby's attention is diverted. Finger movements are elegant and varied, involving the thumb which can be abducted away from the palm at term. In general, the movements of the newborn have writhing quality which changes to fidgety after 1 month of age. A persistently adducted thumb (cortical thumb) is abnormal, and brain damaged babies often have fisted hands and a paucity of fine finger movements and jitteriness.

The normal term newborn is in a state of hypertonicity, with brisk reflexes tending to clonus. This 'transient spasticity' gradually relaxes over the first 8–10 mo in a caudocephalad direction. The high tone can lead to the clinical sign of jittering. Jittering is high frequency, generalized symmetrical tremor of the limbs which is stilled by flexion or by inducing the baby to suck on a finger. Jittering is common in the first 2 or 3 days in term babies but if it is excessive or persistent it deserves investigation. Repetitive chewing movements or tongue thrusting are not part of jitteriness and imply seizures. Jitteriness is stimulus-sensitive whereas seizures are not. In seizure the movement has a fast and slow component whereas in jittering the tremor is symmetrical. Jittering is never accompanied by physiological changes due to the autonomic nervous system such as tachycardia, hypertension or apnea.

Limb tone and power: Failure to move part or whole of a limb may be due to pain or paralysis. Limb tone is influenced by the tonic neck reflex in newborns, which means it is important to have the head in midline before beginning to elicit passive movements. These involve gentle flexion of the upper and lower limbs, then rapid extension and observation of recoil. These include the popliteal angle, the foot dorsiflexion angle and clusters of abnormal signs have been shown to be sensitive indicator of later outcome.

Trunk and neck tone and power: Normal term babies have sufficient power in their neck muscles to lift their heads slightly when prone or supine. Preterm babies can manage to turn their heads from side to side but have much less power with complete head lag when pulled to sit. In order to judge tone in the neck and trunk, babies should be pulled to sit by holding them at the shoulders and then allowed to fall back again to the couch. If the head is unsupported it will gradually fall forwards or backwards. Normal term babies will be able to raise their heads to the vertical again from either direction. There is balance between the neck flexors and extensors during pull-to-sit and back-to-lying maneuvers at term so that the head in line with the body in both phases. Immature babies usually have better control in back-to-lying. To assess truncal tone, lay the child on its back and try to push his bottom towards his head using his thighs. With the baby lying on his side, hold the lumbar region and pull both legs backwards with the other hand grasping the ankles. Trunk flexion should always exceed extension. Arching of the trunk is abnormal; backwards arching of the whole back and neck is called opisthotonos.

Tendon and Babinski reflexes: Knee and biceps jerks can be obtained. Reflexes at term are very brisk, because of the high tone and a few beats of clonus at the ankle is usual. Very brisk reflexes and clonus are not reliable indicators of an upper motor neuron lesion until about 6 mo of age. A crossed adductor response to the knee jerk is also usual in the first few months of life, whereas the sign is abnormal later on. The plantar response of Babinski is always extensor in babies and often results in a withdrawal response.

Sensory testing: Babies respond to pin prick stimuli with gross body movement or grimacing and even the preterm babies feel pain. The classical withdrawal response of flexion of the lower limbs and extension of the opposite leg in response to pricking of the sole of the foot requires motor integrity also and habituates easily.

Special Senses

Eyes and vision: Pupil reactions to light are present after 31 wk gestation. Visual fixation of a suitable target is present from 32 wk gestation and by 34 wk babies track briefly. By term, babies can reliably fix and track an object held 20–30 cm away from the face, and persistent failure to follow a suitable object should give rise to concern. Blinking in response to a bright light is a subcortical response. Opticokinetic nystagmus is present from 36 wk.

Hearing: Babies from 28 wk gestation onwards can be shown to respond to noise, usually by turning the head or increased body movements.

Smell: Babies including preterm babies can detect smells. Babies of all gestations have been found to respond to odors such as peppermint, or breast pads-soaked in their own mother's breast milk.

Occipitofrontal head circumference and fontanels: Neurological examination is not complete without measuring and charting the occipitofrontal circumference and noting the presence and tension of the fontanels.

Primitive reflexes: Primitive reflexes appear and disappear in sequence during specific periods of development (Table 8.1). Their absence or presence beyond a given time frame signifies dysfunction of CNS. Persistence of primitive reflexes can inhibit normal movement in children with cerebral palsy.

Rooting, sucking and swallowing: Stroking the upper lip or around the mouth of a baby results in the baby searching for the nipple and opening the mouth. This reflex tests the sensation in the distribution of the Vth cranial nerve and the motor pathways of the cranial nerves V, VII, and XII. Swallowing also involves cranial nerves IX and X. The sensory input for the sucking reflex comes from the hard palate, not the tongue or cheek. Sucking begins during the 11th wk of intrauterine life. Coordination between sucking and swallowing exists from 28 wk's of gestation but the strength to sustain it and to synchronize the process breathing is only adequate after 32–34 wk' gestation (*see* Chapter 3, page-48).

Moro reflex: The head of the infant in supine position is supported over the palm of one hand and another is placed below over the crib. The *Moro reflex* is obtained by placing the infant in a semi-upright position. The head is momentarily allowed to fall backward, with immediate resupport by the examiner's hand. The child symmetrically abducts and extends the arms, flexes the thumbs, followed by flexion and adduction of the upper extremities or embrace equivalent. An asymmetric response may signify a fractured clavicle, brachial plexus injury or a hemiparesis. Absence of the Moro reflex in a term newborn signifies dysfunction of the CNS. Persistence beyond 6 mo is always abnormal.

Palmar grasp response is elicited by placing a finger or object in the open palm of each hand. Normal infants grasp the object, and with attempted removal, the grasp is reinforced, that is often strong enough to lift the baby from the crib.

Plantar response is elicited by stroking the ball of the foot results in curling of the toes in a similar manner to the palmar response.

Tonic neck reflex is produced by manually turning the head to one side while supine. Extension of the arms occurs on that side of the body corresponding to the direction of the face, while flexion develops in the contralateral extremities (fencing posture). This is known as asymmetrical tonic neck reflex. An obligatory tonic neck response, by which the infant remains "locked" in the fencer's position, is always abnormal and implies a CNS disorder. The reflex appears by 35 wk gestation, is very prominent by about 1 month of age and disappears by about 7 mo. Symmetric tonic neck reflex helps the baby to push up on his arms later: when the head is extended on the neck, tone increases in the upper limbs and when it is flexed tone reduces.

Crossed extension (adduction) reflex: One leg is held in extension and the sole of the foot is rubbed. The other leg is first withdraws and then extends with fanning of the toes. The third and final component of the fully developed reflex brings the other foot towards the side that was stimulated. Eliciting the knee jerk often produces this reflex in the neonatal period, which should not persist after 8 mo of age.

Parachute reflex is demonstrated by suspending the child by the trunk and by suddenly producing forward flexion as if the child were to fall. The child spontaneously extends the upper extremities as a protective mechanism. The parachute reflex appears before the onset of walking.

Placing and stepping reflex: By stimulating the dorsum of the foot, usually by bringing it into contact with the edge of the couch, a mature baby can be induced to 'sit' over the edge. The baby's toes fan out and he lifts his foot up and then places it on the surface. Babies will extend their legs on to a flat surface and support their weight when held under the arms. With the feet in contact with a solid surface and the body tilted forwards the baby will 'walk'.

Glabellar tap reflex: Tapping of nasion is followed by blink response. The response normally disappears after 3 to 4 taps due to habituation.

Table 8.1: Timing of selected primitive reflexes			
Reflex	*Onset*	*Fully developed*	*Duration*
Palmar grasp	28 wk	32 wk	2–3 mo
Rooting	32 wk	36 wk	Less prominent after 1 mo
Moro	28–32 wk	37 wk	5–6 mo
Tonic neck	35 wk	1 mo	6–7 mo
Parachute	7–8 mo	10–11 mo	Remains throughout life

8.3 ROUTINE DELIVERY ROOM CARE

Note the time, date and sex of delivered baby. Tie the umbilical cord 2.5 cm above the umbilicus, cut and clamp with the umbilical clamp. Note whether one or two umbilical arteries. Receive the baby in the tray and dry the baby with warm cloth. *Low risk infants* may initially be placed head downward after delivery to clear the mouth, pharynx, and nose of fluid, mucus, blood, and amniotic debris by gravity; gentle suction with a bulb syringe or soft rubber catheter should be used if there is a significant amount of fluid. Wiping the palate and pharynx with gauze should not be done because it may lead to abrasions and the development of thrush, pterygoid ulcers (Bednar aphthae), or rarely tooth bud infection with maxillary osteomyelitis and retrobulbar abscess formation. The stomachs of infants delivered by cesarean section may contain more fluid than those of infants delivered vaginally. The stomachs may need to be emptied by gastric tube if a significant amount of fluid is suspected to prevent aspiration of gastric contents. Naso- or orogastric tube placement is a potentially noxious stimulus that may predispose to future poor experiences with pain. If not necessary, tube placement should be avoided. Most healthy infants who appear to be in satisfactory condition may be given directly to their mothers for immediate bonding and nursing without undergoing oropharyngeal or gastric suctioning. If respiratory distress is considered, infants should be placed under a warmer with the head dependent. Take weight, length and head circumference of the baby. Palpate anterior and posterior fontenale.

All newborn infants should be assessed immediately after birth by *Apgar score* to identify those requiring resuscitation and to predict survival in the neonatal period (Table 8.2). The 1 min Apgar score may signal the need for immediate resuscitation, and the 5–, 10–, 15–, and 20– min scores may indicate the probability of successfully resuscitating an infant. A low score may be due to a number of factors, including the drugs given to the mother during labor and immaturity (Table 8.3). The Apgar score was not designed to predict neurologic outcome; the score is normal in most patients in whom cerebral palsy subsequently develops and the incidence of cerebral palsy is low in infants with Apgar scores of 0–3 at 5 min (but higher than in infants with Apgar scores of 7–10). The Apgar score and umbilical artery blood pH predict neonatal death. Apgar score of 0–3 at 5 min is a better predictor of neonatal death than an umbilical artery pH of 7.0 or less. The presence of both variables increases the relative risk of neonatal mortality in term and preterm infants. Infants who fail to initiate respiration should receive prompt resuscitation and close observation. Regardless of the etiology, a low Apgar score because of fetal asphyxia, immaturity, central nervous system depression, airway obstruction identifies an infant needing immediate resuscitation.

Table 8.2: Apgar evaluation of newborn infants			
Sign	*0*	*1*	*2*
Heart rate	Absent	Below 100	Over 100
Respiratory effort	Absent	Slow, irregular	Good, crying
Muscle tone	Limp	Some flexion of extremities	Active motion
Response to catheter in nostril (tested after oropharynx is clear)	No response	Grimace	Cough or sneeze
Color		Blue, pale	Body pink, extremities blue	Completely pink

Sixty second after complete birth (disregarding the cord and placenta), the five objective signs above are evaluated and each is given a score of 0, 1, or 2. A total score of 10 indicates an infant in the best possible condition. An infant with a score of 0–3 requires immediate resuscitation.

Source: Modified from Apgar V. *Res Anesth Analg* 1953;32: 260.

Table 8.3: Factors affecting the Apgar score	
False positive (no fetal acidosis or hypoxia; low Apgar)	*False negative* (acidosis; normal Apgar)
Immaturity; analgesics, narcotics, sedatives; magnesium sulphate; acute cerebral trauma; precipitous delivery; congenital myopathy; congenital neuropathy; spinal cord trauma; cerebral nervous system anomaly; lung anomaly (diaphragmatic hernia); airway obstruction (choanal atresia); congenital pneumonia and sepsis; previous episodes of fetal asphyxia (recovered); hemorrhage-hypoxemia	Maternal acidosis; some fetal catecholamine levels; some full-term infants

Maintenance of body heat: Relative to body weight, the body surface area of a newborn infant is approximately three times that of an adult, and in low birth weight infants, the insulating layer of subcutaneous fat is thinner. The estimated rate of heat loss in a newborn is approximately four times that of an adult. Under the usual delivery room conditions (20–25°C), an infant's skin temperature falls approximately 0.3°C/min and deep body temperature decreases approximately 0.1°C/min during the period immediately after delivery; these rates generally result in a cumulative loss of 2–3°C in deep body temperature (corresponding a heat loss of approximately 200 kcal/kg). The heat loss occurs by convection of heat energy to cooler surrounding air, by conduction of heat to the cooler materials on which the infant is lying, by heat radiation from the infant to other nearby cooler solid objects, and by evaporation from moist skin and lungs.

Metabolic acidosis, hypoxemia, hypoglycemia, and increased renal excretion of water and solutes may develop in term infants exposed to cold after birth. Heat production is augmented by increasing the metabolic rate and oxygen consumption in part by releasing nor-epinephrine which results in nonshivering thermogenesis through oxidation of fat, particularly brown fat. Hypoglycemic or hypoxic infants cannot increase their oxygen consumption when exposed to a cold environment and their central temperature decreases. On the 1st day after birth naked newborn can tolerate a limited range of temperature between 32 and 36°C. The temperature requirement of naked newborns ranges between 28–36°C through neonatal period and 24–32°C if clothed. Therefore, to reduce heat loss, it is desirable that infants are dried and either wrapped in blankets or placed under a warmer. *Skin-to-skin contact* with the mother (the kangaroo method; Boxes 8.2 and 8.3) is the optimal method to maintain temperature in the stable newborn. A radiant heat source should be used to warm the baby during resuscitation, because it is difficult to carry out resuscitative measures on a covered infant, or one enclosed in an incubator.

It is important to maintain temperature within normal range because the newborns are prone to develop hypothermia after birth due to change in environmental temperature and various factors. Series of measures should be taken at birth and during the 1st days of life to ensure that the newborn baby does not become either too cold (hypothermia) or too hot (hyperthermia) and maintains a normal body temperature of 36.5–37.5°C (97.7–99.5°F).

Antiseptic skin and cord care: Blood from the skin should be removed after birth as this may reduce the risk of infection with blood borne agents. The first bath is given with warm water and nonmedicated soap after a healthy infant's temperature has stabilized (an axillary temperature > 97.5°F). Umbilical care include one application of topical antibiotics, such as bacitracin followed by twice daily alcohol swabbing (until the cord falls off) reduces colonization, exudates and foul odor of the umbilicus. Keeping the cord dry promotes earlier detachment of the umbilical stump. Nursery personnel should use chlorhexidine or iodophor-containing antiseptic soap for routine handwashing before caring each infant. Rigid enforcing hand-to-elbow washing for 2 min in the initial wash and 15–30 sec in the second wash is essential for staff and visitors entering the nursery. Equally thorough washes between handling infants are also required.

Other measures
1. An intramuscular injection of 1 mg of water-soluble vitamin K_1 (phytonadione) is recommended for all infants immediately after birth to prevent hemorrhagic disease of the newborn.
2. Eyes of all infants must be protected against gonococcal infection by instilling 1% silver nitrate drops, which is the best therapy; erythromycin (0.5%) and tetracycline (1%) sterile ointments are alternative measures that add coverage for chlamydia. This procedure may be delayed during the initial short-alert period after birth to promote bonding, but once applied; drops should not be rinsed out.
3. Detection of any *congenital abnormality* if present should be noted and discussed with the parents.
4. Neonatal screening is available for various genetic, metabolic, hematologic, and endocrine diseases. Laboratory tests performed on infant heel puncture blood samples include those for hypothyroidism, phenylketonuria, galactosemia, maple syrup urine disease, homocystinuria, biotinidase deficiency, adrenal hyperplasia, hemoglobinopathy, cystic fibrosis, tyrosinemia, and other organic acid defects or aminoacidopathies. Screening program must include not only high-quality laboratory tests but also follow-up of infants with abnormal test results; education, counseling, and psychologic support for families; and prompt referral of the neonates for accurate diagnosis and therapy.
5. Hearing impairment, that affects speech and language development, may be severe in 2/1,000 and overall affects 5/1,000 births. Screening of infants is recommended to ensure early detection of hearing loss and appropriate, timely intervention.

Nursery Care

Non-high-risk healthy infants may be placed in the mother's room or taken to the newborn nursery if the hospital does not have rooming-in facility.

The bassinet, preferably of clear plastic to allow for easy visibility and care, should be cleaned frequently. All professional care should be given in the bassinet, including the physical examination, clothing changes, temperature taking, skin cleansing, and other procedures. The clothing and bedding should be minimal. The nursery temperature should be kept at approximately 24°C (75°F). The *infant's temperature* should be taken by axillary measurement. In case the temperature is required, the interval between the temperatures need be shorter than 4 hr during the 1st 2–3 days and 8 hr thereafter. Axillary temperatures of

36.4–37.0°C (97.0–98.5°F) are within normal limits. *Weighing* should be taken at birth and daily thereafter. Healthy infants should be *placed supine* to reduce the risk of sudden infant death syndrome (SIDS).

Vernix is spontaneously shed within 2–3 days, much of it adhering to the clothing, which should be completely changed daily. The diaper should be checked before and after feeding and when baby cries; it should be changed when wet or soiled. Meconium or feces should be cleansed from the buttocks with sterile cotton moistened with sterile water. The foreskin of a male infant should not be retracted. Circumcision is an elective procedure.

Vaccination: BCG is given at birth or before baby is discharged from the hospital (*see* Table 15.5). In some hospitals first dose of OPV and hepatitis B vaccine (HBV) are also given along with BCG. The BCG site should be checked for 'take' response after 4 wk. Persistent and recurrent ulceration at the site of vaccination or regional adenitis responds to oral administration of erythromycin in a dose of 30 mg/kg/day for 14 days or INH 10 mg/kg/day for 3 mo.

Discharge: Early discharge (< 48 hr) or very early discharge (< 24 hr) may increase the risk of rehospitalization for hyperbilirubinemia, sepsis, failure to thrive, dehydration, and missed congenital anomalies. Early discharge requires follow-up at home (visiting nurse) or in the hospital within 48 hr.

Parent–infant Bonding

Normal infant development depends partly on a series of affectionate responses exchanged between a mother and her newborn infant that binds them together psychologically and physiologically. It is initiated before birth with the planning and confirmation of pregnancy and with the growing acceptance of the fetus as an individual. After delivery and during the ensuing weeks sensory (visual, auditory, olfactory) and physical contact between the mother and baby triggers various mutually rewarding and pleasurable interactions such as the mother touching the infant's extremities and face with her fingertips and encompassing and gently massaging the infant's trunk with her hands. Touching an infant's cheek eliciting responsive turning towards the mother's face or towards the breast with nuzzling and licking the nipple, a powerful stimulus for prolacting secretion. An infant's initial quiet, alert state provides the opportunity for eye-to-eye contact, which is particularly important in stimulating the loving and possessive feelings of the parents for their babies. Delayed or abnormal maternal-infant bonding is seen after prematurity, infant or maternal illness, birth defects or family stress, but this may adversely affect the infant development and maternal caring ability. Hospital routines should be designed to encourage parent-infant contact. This maternal-infant bonding is further facilitated and reinforced by the emotional support of a loving family.

Hospital Practices

Many hospital practices contribute to difficulties in breastfeeding by enforcing 4 hr feeding schedules, limiting nursing time, using only one breast at feeding, washing nipples with substances other than water, delaying the 1st feeding, providing formula supplements, and using heavy intrapartum sedation.

In order to encourage and promote exclusive breastfeeding to enhance child survival, the Baby-Friendly Hospital Initiative (BFHI) was launched jointly by WHO and UNICEF in March, 1992. BFHI is a global effort with hospitals to provide support to the mother before, during, and after delivery so that she has a joyful breastfeeding experience. These hospitals must fully practice "ten steps to successful breastfeeding" given in a joint WHO/UNICEF document (Box 8.1). Hospital practices that encourage successful breastfeeding include immediate post-partum mother–infant contact with suckling, rooming-in, demand feeding, inclusion of fathers in prenatal breastfeeding education, and support from experienced women. Nursing at least 5 minutes at each breast is reasonable and allows a baby to obtain most of the available breast contents and provides effective stimulation for increasing the milk supply. Nursing episodes then can be extended according to the comfort and desire of the mother and infant. A confident and relaxed mother, supported by an encouraging home and hospital environment, is likely to nurse well.

The concept of supporting mothers to breastfeed is important. But promotion of breastfeeding alone is not enough to make a hospital baby-friendly. This should also include practices which will make hospital safe for newborns and their mothers such as:

i. Safe delivery practices
ii. Proper care of the umbilical cord
iii. Warming and temperature regulation after birth; and
iv. Early diagnosis and management of conditions such as absence of spontaneous breathing, aspiration, sepsis, hypoglycemia, hypocalcemia, etc.

Kangaroo-mother Care

Kangaroo-mother care is a nonconventional method of caring for low birth weight and preterm newborns

Box 8.1: Ten steps to successful breastfeeding

Every facility providing maternity services and care for newborn infants should

1. Have a written breastfeeding policy that is routinely communicated to all health care staff
2. Train all health care staff in skills necessary to implement this policy
3. Inform all pregnant women about the benefits and management of breastfeeding
4. Help mothers initiate breastfeeding within half-hour of birth
5. Show mothers how to breastfeed, and how to maintain lactation, even if they should be separated from their infants
6. Give newborn infants no food or drink other than breast milk, unless medically indicated
7. Practice rooming in-allow mothers and infants to remain together 24 hr a day
8. Encourage breastfeeding on demand
9. Give no artificial teats or pacifier like dummies or soothers to breastfeeding infants
10. Foster the establishment of breastfeeding support groups and refer mother to them on discharge from the hospital or clinic

after initial stabilization. Kangaroo-mother care (KMC), adapted from kangaroos, and involves placing the newborn infant in close skin-to-skin contact with the mother. It is an effective way to meet baby's needs for warmth following birth and in the immediate postnatal period. The key features are listed in Box 8.2. For providing kangaroo-mother care steps to be followed are discussed in Box 8.3. The kangaroo method may be tiring for the mother and restrict her freedom of movement. A lot of support is therefore required from relatives and health workers to help mother to accept and practice this method correctly. Another man or woman can also provide skin-to-skin contact.

Breastfeeding

See Section 3.2, page-50.

Box 8.2: Key features of kangaroo-mother care

1. Early, continuous, prolonged skin-to-skin contact between the mother and the baby
2. Assists in maintaining the temperature of infant
3. Facilitates breastfeeding (particularly exclusive breastfeeding)
4. Help to increase the duration of breastfeeding
5. Improves mother–infant bonding and increases the mother's confidence, ability and involvement in the care of her newborn
6. Early discharge from the hospital

Box 8.3: Steps to be followed for providing kangaroo-mother care

1. Dress the newborn with cap, socks, kurta and napkin
2. Place the newborn in a prone and upright (or diagonal) position between the mother's breasts, and covered with a mother's clothes and a cloth/blanket/shawl, for most of the day and night
3. Let the baby suckle at breasts as often as he/she wants, but at least every 2 hourly
4. Mother should sleep propped up so that the baby stays upright
5. Make sure that baby stays warm at all times
6. If environmental temperature is low, dress the baby with extra clothing and cover his head
7. When mother wants to go to toilet, bathe or rest†, ask the father or another family member to 'kangaroo' the baby or wrap infant in several layers of warm clothing, covered with blankets and keep in a warm place
8. Take neonate for regular check ups for vaccination and weight record.

†Another man or woman can also provide skin-to-skin contact

Drugs and Breastfeeding

Maternal medications may affect the production and safety of breast milk (Table 8.4). Most commonly used medications are safe. But the safety of any drug to be used while a woman is breastfeeding, must be confirmed before a new drug is initiated and/or breastfeeding is continued. Maternal sedatives may result in sedation of the infant.

Medical contraindications to breastfeeding include infections with HIV (in developing countries after discussing with the parents, breastfeeding to be discontinued), human T cell leukemia virus type 1 and 2, cytomegalovirus (preterm infants), active tuberculosis (until appropriately treated ≥ 2 wk and not considered contagious), and hepatitis B virus (until an infant receives hepatitis B immune globulin and vaccine).

Hosalkar HS, Horn D, Friedman JE, Dormans JP. The Hip. In: Kliegman RM, Behrman RE, Jenson HB, Stanton BF (eds). *Nelson Textbook of Pediatrics.* 18th edn. Vol 1. Philadelphia: Saunders, 2007;2800–11.

IAP-NNF National Task force: Temperature Regulation. *IAF-NNF Guidelines 2006 on level II Neonatal Care* 2006;15–36.

Kasser JR. Orthopedic problems. In: Cloherty JP, Eichenwald EC, Stark AR (eds). *Manual of Neonatal Care.* 6th edn. New Delhi: Wolters Kluwer (India) Pvt. Ltd., 2008; 536–9.

Melentosh N, Stenson B. The Newborn. In: Melntosh N, Helms PJ, Smyth RL (eds). *Forfar & Arneil's Textbook of Pediatrics.* 6th edn. Edinburgh: Churchill Livingstone, 2003;177–403.

Philipp BL, Merewood A. The baby-friendly way: The breastfeeding start. *Pediatr Clin N Am* 2004;51:761–83.

Stoll BJ. The newborn infant. In: Kliegman RM, Behrman RE, Jenson HB, Stanton BF (eds). *Nelson Textbook of Pediatrics.* 18th edn. Vol 1. Philadelphia: Saunders, 2007;671–83.

Table 8.4: Drugs and breastfeeding
Contraindications: Amphetamine; antineoplastic agents; bromocriptine; chloramphenicol; clozapine; cocaine; cyclophosphamide; diethylstilbestrol; doxorubicin; ergots; gold salts; heroin; immunosuppressants; iodides; lithium; methimazole; methamphetamine; phencyclidine (PCP); radiopharmaceuticals; thiouracil
Avoid or give with caution: Alcohol; amiodarone; anthraquinones (laxative); aspirin (salicylates); atropine; β-adrenergic blocking agents; birth control pills; bromides; calciferol; cascara; ciprofloxacin; danthron; dihydrotachysterol; domperidone; estrogens; metoclopramide; metronidazole; meperidine; phenobarbital*; primidone; psychotropic drugs; reserpine; sulfasalazine
Probably safe: Acetaminophen; acyclovir; aldomet; anesthetics; antibiotics (not chloramphenicol); antiepileptics; antihistamines*; antithyroid (not methimazole); bishydroxycoumarin; chlorpromazine*; codeine*; cyclosporine; dipo-provera; digoxin; diuretics; fluoxetine; furosemide; haloperidol*; hydralazine; indomethacin, other nonsteroidal anti-inflammatory drugs; low molecular weight heparin; metformin; methadone*; morphine; muscle relaxants; phenytoin; proxetine; prednisolone; propranolol; propylthiouracil; sedatives*; sertaline; theophylline; vitamins; warfarin

*Watch for sedation

Wong CM, Laing IA. History taking and physical examination. In: Melntosh N, Helms PJ, Smyth RL (eds). *Forfar & Arneil's Textbook of Pediatrics*. 6th edn. Edinburgh: Churchill Livingstone, 2003;21–47.

8.4 RESUSCITATION OF NEWBORN

The neonatal period is an extremely important period for an infant, because of infant's transition from intrauterine to extrauterine life requiring many biochemical and physiologic changes. Of the nearly 100 million babies born annually worldwide nearly 90% successfully make a transition from the maternal-fluid filled environment to an air-filled environment. 10% of newborns require some assistance to begin breathing at birth and only 1% requires intensive resuscitative efforts. Birth asphyxia contributes to nearly 1/5th of all neonatal deaths. The way in which an asphyxiated infant is managed in the first few minutes of life can have consequences over an entire lifetime, directly affecting the quality of the individual's life. In addition to resuscitation of asphyxiated infants, resuscitation is needed in very low birth weight infants, infants with meconium aspiration, birth trauma, multiple births, hydrops fetalis, congenital defects, and other problems.

Although the need for resuscitation of the newborn infant often can be predicted, such circumstances may arise suddenly without any prior warning. Therefore, it is essential that the knowledge and skills required for resuscitation—be learned by all providers of neonatal care—neonatal advanced life support (NALS). With adequate anticipation, it is possible to optimize the delivery setting with appropriately prepared equipment and trained personnel who are capable of functioning as a team during neonatal resuscitation.

All newborns are assessed at birth for their resuscitatory needs. Resuscitation is done as per requirement of the individual baby. Quick assessment for further need of resuscitation is done at the end of each step of resuscitation. Most newborn infants require only the initial steps, but for those who require further intervention, the most crucial action is establishment of adequate ventilation. Only a very small percentage will need chest compressions and medications.

Delivery Room Emergencies

Most neonates complete the transition to extrauterine life without difficulty; however, in a small percentage of neonates' resuscitation after birth is required. The most common delivery room emergency for neonates is secondary to failure to initiate and maintain effective respirations. Less frequently, but of major importance are shock, severe anemia, plethora, convulsions and management of life-threatening congenital malformations.

Common congenital anomalies are choanal atresia, cleft lip and cleft palate, Pierré-Robin syndrome, diaphragmatic hernia, tracheoesophageal fistula, intestinal obstruction (volvulus, duodenal atresia, ileal atresia), anorectal anomalies, abdominal wall defects (gasrroschisis, omphalocele), renal agenesis, Potter syndrome, neural tube defects (anencephalus, meningocele, myelomeningocele) and congenital cyanotic heart disease.

Respiratory distress and failure: Disorders of respiration in newborn infants are either central indicating central nervous system (CNS) failure due to depression or failure of the respiratory center, or peripheral respiratory difficulty indicating interference with the alveolar exchange of oxygen and carbon dioxide. Cyanosis occurs in both groups. Most common respiratory problems encountered in the delivery room are those due to airway obstruction and depression of the CNS (maternal medications, asphyxia) with an absence of adequate respiratory effort. Pulmonary causes of respiratory difficulty are discussed in Section 8.9, page-216.

Failure to initiate or sustain respiration: Failure to initiate or sustain respiration effort usually originates in the CNS due to asphyxia or peripherally due to neuromuscular disorders. The lungs in these infants may be noncompliant, and standard efforts to begin respirations may be inadequate to initiate sufficient ventilation.

Cleft lip and cleft palate: In Pierré-Robin syndrome, cleft palate is associated with micrognathia and large tongue, with a tendency for glossoptosis. Feeding is difficult in cases of cleft palate. For the first few days, gavage feeding or spoon-feeding may be done. Bottle-feeding may be tried with a soft nipple with rubber flange which close the cleft and help the baby in sucking. If this is not successful, palatal prosthesis may be used. These babies are prone to develop otitis media and should be treated as and when required (*see* Section 27.4, page-826).

Narcosis results from administration of morphine, meperidine, fentanyl, barbiturates, or tranquilizers to the mother shortly before delivery or from maternal anesthesia given during the 2nd stage of labor. Prenatal or perinatal hypoxia, if sufficiently severe produces brainstem depression and secondary apnea that is unresponsive to sensory stimulation. Treatment includes external cardiac massage, correction of acidosis, and circulatory support with drugs in addition to ventilation in the severely asphyxiated infant, provided that the basic cause of the hypoxia can be eliminated within a reasonable time.

Meconium: Meconium staining of the amniotic fluid may be an indication of fetal stress.

Shock: Circulatory insufficiency may be present at birth as a result of severe asphyxia or hemorrhage, during gestation, labor, or delivery. Shock from overwhelming infection may also be present after birth. Supportive treatment with type O Rh-negative blood or normal saline is indicated for hemorrhage or hypovolemia, respectively.

Pneumothorax: Infants may develop pneumothorax in the delivery room resulting in respiratory distress and hypoxia. Approximately 1–2% of infants develop a pneumothorax after birth. A 23-gauge butterfly needle or angiocath attached to a stopcock and syringe should be inserted perpendicular to the chest wall above the rib in the 4th intercostal space at the level of the nipple. The air is evacuated. The catheter is then inserted with constant negative pressure and the air is then evacuated.

Airway obstruction: Fetal and then neonatal airway obstruction presents an emergency in the delivery room. The ex-utero intrapartum procedure (*EXIT procedure*) allows time to secure the airway in infants known to have airway obstruction due to laryngeal atresia or stenosis, teratomas, hydromas, and oral tumors before the infants are separated from the placenta. Uteroplacental gas exchange is maintained throughout the procedure. High risk perinatal care has led to more frequent prenatal diagnosis of many disorders known to cause critical airway obstruction.

Abdominal wall defects: See Section 8.17, page-247.

Injury during delivery (birth trauma): See Section 8.8, page-215.

Neonatal Advanced Life Support (NALS)

NALS in short is discussed below:
- Prevent heat loss
  - Place on warmer
  - Dry thoroughly
  - Remove wet towel
  - Open airway
  - Place the baby
  - Suction mouth first and then nose (suction trachea—if meconium stained fluid)
- Initiate breathing
  - Tactile stimulation of sole
- Evaluate infant (Apgar score) (not necessary in diagnosing respiratory distress—respiratory effort; response to catheter)
  - Breathing
  - Heart rate
  - Color

Evaluate respiration—Spontaneous → HR—above 100 → Evaluate color → Pink or Acrocyanosis → Observe and Monitor

Evaluate respiration—Spontaneous → HR—above 100 → Evaluate color-Blue → Provide oxygen

Evaluate respiration—Spontaneous → HR—below 100—PPV 15–30 sec → Drug Depressed → Give Narcan → HR

Evaluate respiration—None → HR—below 60 – continue ventilation and chest compression—Initiate medication if: HR—below 80 after 30 sec; PPV with 100% oxygen and chest compression

Evaluate respiration—None → HR—60–100–HR not increasing—continue ventilation-chest compressions-Initiate medication if: HR—below 80 after 30 sec; PPV with 100% oxygen and chest compression

Evaluate respiration—None → HR—60–100—HR increasing—continue ventilation

Evaluate respiration—None → HR 60–100—Watch for spontaneous respirations—then discontinue ventilation

Physiology of Asphyxia—Apnea

Apnea: When infants become asphyxiated (either *in utero* or following delivery), they undergo a well defined sequence of events.

i. *Primary apnea:* When a fetus or infant is deprived of oxygen, an initial period of rapid breathing occurs. If the asphyxia continues, the respiratory cease, the heart rate begins to fall, and the infant enters a period of apnea known as primary apnea. Exposure to oxygen and stimulation during the period of primary apnea in most instances will induce respirations.

ii. *Secondary apnea:* If the asphyxia continues, the infant develops deep gasping respirations, the heart rate continues to decrease, and the blood pressure begins to fall.

The respirations become weaker and weaker until the infant takes a last gasp and enters a period of apnea called secondary apnea. During secondary apnea the heart rate, blood pressure and oxygen in the blood (PaO_2) continue to fall farther and farther. The infant now is unresponsive to stimulation and artificial ventilation with oxygen (positive-pressure ventilation) must be initiated at once. The longer an infant is in secondary apnea, the greater is the chance that brain damage will occur.

Primary vs. secondary apnea: As a result of fetal hypoxia, the infant may go through primary apnea and into secondary apnea while *in utero*. Thus, an infant may be born in either primary or secondary apnea. In a clinical setting, primary and secondary apnea is virtually indistinguishable from one another. In both instances the infant is not breathing, and the heart may be below 100 per minute. A newborn infant in primary apnea will reestablish a breathing pattern (although irregular and possibly ineffective) without intervention. An infant in the secondary apnea will not resume breathing of his or of her own accord. Positive pressure ventilation (PPV) will be required to establish respirations.

Assume secondary apnea: As one cannot distinguish primary and secondary apnea, we must assume that we are dealing with secondary apnea, and resuscitation should begin immediately.

Being Prepared for Resuscitation

In order to provide prompt and effective intervention two major factors must be given proper attention. These two factors are: Anticipating the need for resuscitation, and adequate preparation, both of equipment and personnel.

Anticipation: Asphyxiation in a newborn at birth may sometimes come as a surprise. Some infants, in spite of being at risk for asphyxia, will do well following delivery and will require no resuscitative assistance.

Antepartum/Intrapartum history: Delivery of a depressed or asphyxiated infant can be anticipated in many cases on the basis of information found in both the antepartum and the intrapartum histories. Antepartum factors are mentioned in Box 8.4. In the intrapartum history, any of the factors listed in Box 8.5 should alert you to the possibility that the infant may be asphyxiated.

Adequate preparation: The minimum preparation for any delivery should include as follows:

A *radiant warmer*, heated and ready for use.

All *resuscitation equipment* immediately available and in working order. A complete list of neonatal resuscitation equipment is listed in Box 8.6.

Box 8.4: Antepartum factors

Maternal diabetes mellitus
Pregnancy-induced hypertension
Chronic hypertension
Previous Rh sensitization
Previous stillbirth
Bleeding in 2nd or 3rd trimester
Maternal infection
Polyhydramnios
Oligohydramnios
Post-term gestation
Multiple gestation
Size-date pregnancy
Drug therapy (reserpine; lithium carbonate, magnesium, adrenergic blocking drugs)
Maternal drug abuse

Box 8.5: Intrapartum factors

Elective or emergency cesarean section
Abnormal presentation
Premature labor
Rupture of membranes more than 24 hr prior to delivery
Foul-smelling amniotic fluid
Precipitous labor
Prolonged labor (greater than 24 hr)
Prolonged second stage of labor (greater than 2 hr)
Non-reassuring fetal heart rate patterns
Use of general anesthesia
Uterine tetany
Narcotics administered to mother within 4 hr of delivery
Meconium-stained amniotic fluid
Prolapsed cord
Abruptio placenta
Placenta previa

Staff: Two trained individuals capable of working together to perform all aspects of resuscitation.

In the event of a multiple gestation, a full complement of equipment, as well as staff, must be available for each anticipated infant.

Personnel for "normal" deliveries: At every delivery, there should be at least one person (physician, nurse, respiratory therapist, etc.), who has the skills required to perform a complete resuscitation. He or she must be skilled in ventilation with bag and mask, endotracheal intubation, chest compressions, and the use of medications. Another person attending the delivery of a neonate should be able to assist with resuscitation.

When *asphyxia is anticipated.* Two people possessing the skills already described must be available, who will be managing the infant only. With multiple births, such a team is needed for each infant.

The TABC of Resuscitation

The components of TABC resuscitation for neonates are mentioned as follows:

T—Provide *warmth*

A—Establish an open *airway*:
- Position the infant.
- Suction the mouth (first) and then nose and some instances the trachea.
- If necessary, insert an endotracheal tube to assure an open airway.

B—Initiate *breathing*:
- Use tactile stimulation to initiate respirations.
- Employ positive-pressure ventilation when necessary using either:
  – Bag and mask or
  – Bag and endotracheal tube.

C—Maintain *circulation*:
- Stimulate and maintain the circulation of blood with:
  – Chest compressions, and
  – Medications.

Principles of a Successful Resuscitation

The following three principles, if followed, will increase the likelihood of a successful resuscitation.

1. Personnel adequately trained in neonatal resuscitation should be physically present at every delivery. Each person should know what his or her responsibilities are?
2. Personnel in the delivery must be able to do it efficiently and effectively.
3. Personnel involved in resuscitating an infant must work together as a coordinated team.

Consequences of Delayed or Inefficient Resuscitative Efforts

The consequences of delayed or inefficient resuscitative efforts are increased likelihood of brain damage and making the resuscitation more difficult.

The brain must have a constant supply of oxygen in order to function properly. The longer the brain remains without oxygen, the greater are the chances of irreparable damage of the brain cells. In addition to that damage to other organs such as kidneys, lungs, heart, and bowel can result of oxygen lack.

Preventing Heat Loss

To avoid the metabolic problems brought on by cold stress, the first step in the management of the newborn infant is to prevent the loss of body heat ("T" of TABC). Heat loss is prevented by placing the infant under a radiant heat source (on heated radiant warmer) and quickly drying him or her of amniotic fluid. Infants who suffer heat loss have an increased metabolic rate and require more oxygen-factors that can create serious problems for infants who already suffer from asphyxia. An *overhead radiant warmer* provides a suitable thermal environment that minimizes radiant and convective heat loss. It is important to preheat the radiant warmer so that the infant is placed on a warm mattress. A *radiant warmer* allows access to and full visualization of the infant. Blankets and clothings should not be used to cover the infant since they prevent the radiant heat waves from reaching the skin.

As soon as an infant is placed on the radiant warmer, the body and head should be quickly dried to remove amniotic fluid (*drying the infant*) and to prevent evaporative heat loss. It is preferred to dry the infant with a prewarmed towel. Remove the wet towel, otherwise evaporative heat loss will continue. The act of drying has a second benefit: it provides gentle stimulation, which may initiate or help maintain respirations.

Opening the Airway

Once the infant is placed under a preheated radiant warmer and dried the next step is to assure the "A" of TABC—the establishment of an open airway. This is accomplished by *positioning* the infant correctly and *suctioning* the infant's mouth and then nose (if necessary, the trachea).

Positioning (position the infant): The neonate should be placed on his or her back or side in a slight Trendelenburg position with the neck slightly extended. Care should be taken to prevent the hyperextension or underextension of the neck since in either position the air entry is decreased. To help

Box 8.6: Neonatal resuscitation supplies and equipment

Suction equipment

Bulb syringe

DeLee mucus trap with #10 Fe, catheter or mechanical suction

Suction catheters #5 or #6, #8, #10 Fr.

#8 Fr, feeding tube and 20 cc syringe

Bag-and-mask equipment

Infant resuscitation bag with a pressure-release valve or pressure gauge the bag must be capable of delivering 90–100% oxygen.

Face masks newborn and premature sizes (cushioned rim masks preferred).

Oral airways newborn and premature sizes.

Oxygen with flowmeter and tubing.

Intubation equipment

Laryngoscope with straight blades No. 0 (premature) and No. 1 (newborn)

Extra bulbs and batteries for laryngoscope

Endotracheal tubes sizes 2.5, 3.0, 3.5, 4.0 mm

Stylet

Scissors

Gloves

Medications

Epinephrine 1: 10,000 3cc or 10 cc ampules

Naloxane hydrochloride (neonatal NARCAN) 0.02 mg/cc–2 cc ampules

Volume expander—one or more:

   Albumin 5% solution

   Normal saline

   Ringer lactate

Sodium bicarbonate 4.2% (5 mEq/10 cc) 10 cc ampules

Dextrose 10% 250 cc

Sterile water 30 cc

Normal saline 30 cc

Miscellaneous

Infant resuscitation manikin

Intubation head (5 only)

Radiant warmer

Stethoscope

Cardiotachimeter with ECG oscilloscope (desirable)

Adhesive tape ½ or ¾ inch width

Syringes—1 cc, 3 cc, 5 cc, 10 cc, 20 cc, 50 cc.

Needles—25, 21, 18

Alcohol sponges

Umbilical artery catheterization tray

Umbilical tape

Umbilical catheters 3 ½, 5 Fr.

3-way stopcocks

#5 Fr. feeding tube

maintain the correct position, rolled towel or blanket is placed under the shoulders raising them 3/4 to 1 inch of the mattress. This shoulder roll may be particularly useful if the infant has a large occiput resulting from molding, edema, or prematurity. In this position resuscitation with bag and mask can be carried out. If the infant has copious secretions coming from the mouth turn the head to the side. This will allow secretions to collect in the mouth, where they can be easily removed, rather than in the posterior pharynx.

Suctioning: As soon as the infant is positioned, *the mouth (first) and then nose should be suctioned.* The mouth is suctioned first in order to make sure that there is nothing for the infant to aspirate if he or she should gasp when the nose is suctioned. The very act of suctioning provides a degree of *tactile stimulation.* In some cases, this all provides the stimulation that is needed to initiate respirations in the infant. If the material in the mouth and nose is not removed before the infant establishes respirations, it can be aspirated into the trachea and lungs. When this occurs, the respiratory consequences can be serious. Suction can be carried out by using a bulb syringe, DeLee suction catheter or a mechanical suction to remove material. Stimulation of the posterior pharynx during the first few minutes after birth can produce a vagal response causing severe bradycardia and/or apnea while suction is carried out. In healthy infants, gentle suctioning with a bulb syringe is usually adequate to remove secretions. When using a mechanical suction apparatus, the suction pressure should be set so that when the suction tubing is occluded, the negative pressure does not exceed 100 mm Hg.

Meconium in Amniotic Fluid

It is extremely important to observe whether meconium is present in the amniotic fluid. When meconium is present in the amniotic fluid, there is a chance that the meconium will be aspirated into the infant's mouth and potentially into the trachea and lungs. Appropriate steps should be taken depending upon whether the meconium is thin, watery or thick as mentioned below:

Thin, watery: Small amounts of meconium passed by the fetus well before delivery may merely discolor the amniotic fluid, with *no particles* of meconium visible. Such fluid is often described as thin or watery meconium-stained fluid. Special management of these infants is not necessary.

Thick, particulate: In those infants in whom the amniotic fluid contains thick meconium-amniotic fluid like "pea soup" in appearance or contains particles of meconium suctioning must take place when the head is delivered, and when the infant has been placed on a warmer to clear the airway of meconium. Soon as the baby's head is delivered (prior to delivery of shoulders) the mouth, oropharynx, and hypopharynx should be thoroughly suctioned, using a 10 Fr. DeLee suction catheter or other flexible suction catheter. After delivery of the infant, the trachea should be intubated and any residual meconium removed from the lower airway. Suction can be applied to the endotracheal tube by use of an adapter and a regulated wall suction device. Reintubation followed by suctioning should be repeated until returns are free of meconium.

Providing Tactile Stimulation

Both drying and suctioning in the infant produces stimulation, which for many infants is enough to induce respiration. If the infant does not immediately breathe, additional tactile stimulation should be provided in an attempt to initiate respirations. The two safe and appropriate methods of stimulating breathing are: slapping or flickering the soles of the feet, and rubbing the infant's back which will usually stimulate breathing in an infant in primary apnea. This should not be done more than twice. Gentle rubbing of the trunk, extremities, or head also produces tactile stimulation. If the infant remains apneic, tactile stimulation should be abandoned, and bag-and-mask ventilation should be started immediately. Some harmful actions used in the past to provide tactile stimulation to apneic neonates that can harm the baby should never be used (Table 8.5).

Practice Performing all the Steps

It is extremely important to practice performing all the steps on a manikin, quickly with in 20 sec (Box 8.7). Repeat the above steps several times until you can perform them smoothly. Can you carry out within 20 sec? How would you alter the steps if the amniotic fluid contained thick meconium?

Evaluating the Infant

Positioning, suctioning, and stimulating are necessary in every infant at birth and are carried out to clear the airway and to initiate respirations. The next steps in the resuscitation process will depend on your evaluation of the infant. You should evaluate the infant on the basis of three vital signs: 1 Respiratory effort, 2. Heart rate, 3. Color.

Box 8.7: Practice performing all the steps on a manikin or doll, quickly with in 20 seconds

Place on radiant warming table (or table top for practice)
Wipe fluid from body and head
    Remove towel
    Quickly position
    On back
    Slight Trendelenburg
    Neck slightly extended
    Roll under shoulders (optional)
Suction mouth and then
Suction nose
Provide tactile stimulation
    Slap/flick feet, or
    Rub back

Steps in the evaluation
- Observe and evaluate the infant's respirations. If normal go on to the next sign. If not, begin positive-pressure ventilation.
- Check the baby's heart rate. If above 100 beats/min go on. If not, initiate positive-pressure ventilation.
- If an infant is breathing and the heart rate is above 100, evaluate the infant's color; if central cyanosis is present, administer oxygen.

Respiratory effort: The first vital sign to be evaluated is the infant's respiratory effort. Adequate oxygenation of the infant primarily depends upon adequate respirations. The rate and depth of respirations should increase in the first few seconds after the first slap or flick of the foot or rub of the back may provide the necessary stimulation. Time should not be taken to stimulate the baby more than twice. After stimulating the baby observe whether the infant shows respiratory effort.

Breathing: If there is chest movement, then check the heart rate.

Apneic: Infants who show no respiratory response to stimulation should be given positive-pressure ventilation (PPV) using bag and mask.

Heart rate: As soon as respiratory effort is evaluated (and appropriate action taken, if needed) monitor the baby's heart rate. Respirations may be present but may

---

Table 8.5: Harmful actions and potential consequences	
Harmful actions	*Potential consequences*
Slapping the back	Bruises
Squeezing the rib cage	Fractures; pneumothorax
Forcing thighs on to abdomen	Rupture of liver or spleen; hemorrhage
Dilating anal sphincter	Tearing of anal sphincter
Using hot or cold compresses or baths	Hypothermia, hyperthermia, burns
Blowing cold oxygen or air onto face or body	Hypothermia

not be adequate to sustain a heart rate above 100 beats per minute. If the heart rate is above 100, and the infant has spontaneous respirations, evaluate the next sign- color. Anytime the heart rate is below 100, positive pressure ventilation (PPV) is indicated, even though the infant may have spontaneous respirations.

Color: When the infant's respirations and heart rate improve significantly, the skin should also begin to turn pink. This improvement in color is due to increased oxygen entering the blood. The infant may still be cyanotic (central cyanosis) even if the heart rate is above 100/minute, and the respirations are adequate. In this case, there is enough oxygen crossing the lungs and entering the bloodstream to sustain the heart rate, but there is not enough to fully oxygenate the infant.

If central cyanosis is present in an infant with spontaneous respirations and an adequate heart rate, free flow oxygen should be given. Oxygen is not necessary for infants who have blue extremities only (peripheral cyanosis)—a condition that is present in most infants the first few minutes after birth. Peripheral cyanosis is caused by a combination of cool delivery room and initially sluggish circulation. It is not due to oxygen lack.

Use of Free-flow Oxygen

At birth most infants have some degree of cyanosis. As respirations are established, oxygenation improves so that by 60–90 seconds, most infants are beginning to become pink, although peripheral cyanosis may still be present. Persistent cyanosis can also be due to a congenital defect that interferes with pulmonary function (e.g. diaphragmatic hernia) or congenital heart disease. To relieve cyanosis in infants with normal respirations and a heart rate above 100 beats/minute, positive pressure ventilation is not indicated. Instead, free-flow oxygen should be given to improve the color.

Principles in managing free-flow oxygen

i. Initially
ii. Once the infant becomes pink; iii. And if cyanosis persists.

Initially: A newborn infant who has central cyanosis after respirations are established and a heart rate above 100, should initially receive a high concentration of oxygen, at least 80%.

When pink: Once the infant becomes pink, the oxygen should be gradually withdrawn, until the infant remains pink while breathing room air, as clinically appropriate.

When cyanosis persists: Infants who become cyanotic as the oxygen withdrawn should continue to receive just enough oxygen to remain pink and no more.

Free-flow oxygen: Free-flow oxygen refers to blowing oxygen over the infant's nose so that the infant breathes oxygen-enriched air. For a brief period, this can be accomplished by holding the end of an oxygen tube close to the nose or by holding an oxygen mask over the mouth and nose.

Actual concentration of oxygen: Wall or portable oxygen source sends 100% oxygen through the tubing, it mixes with room air. The concentration of oxygen that reaches to the infant's nose is determined by the amount of 100% oxygen coming from the tube (stated in liter flow per minute) and the amount of room air it must pass through to reach the infant. Room air contains 21% oxygen. Thus, when 100% oxygen is mixed with room air, the concentration of oxygen reaching the infant is less than 100% (Table 8.6).

Caution: Remember that you are to provide just enough oxygen for the infant to become pink. After the acute resuscitation, once you have established the infant on oxygen, immediately move him or her into an area where assessment of oxygen concentration (FiO$_2$) can be based on blood gas (PaO$_2$) values.

Equipment

1. Resuscitation bags
   - Anesthetic bag
   - Self-inflating bag
2. Pressure gauge, if one is used
3. Oxygen reservoir, if necessary

Self-inflating resuscitation bag: The self-inflating bag is designed so that it inflates automatically as you release your grip on the bag. It does not require a compressed gas source in order to fill.

Table 8.6: Oxygen concentration chart 100% oxygen at 5 liter per minute		
O$_2$ concentration	*Tubing*	*Mask*
Approx 80%	½ inch from nares	Mask held firmly on face
Approx 60%	1 inch from nares	Mask held firmly on face
Approx 40%	½ inch from nares	Mask held loosely on face

Note: To prevent heat loss and drying of the respiratory mucosa, oxygen given neonates should be heated and humidified. However, during emergency dry oxygen can be given briefly to stabilize the infant's condition. If oxygen is to be continued for more than a few minutes, it should be heated and humidified.

Parts: There are four parts of the self-inflating bag: Air inlet, oxygen inlet, patient outlet, valve assembly.

Air inlet: As the bag re-expand following compression, air is drawn into the bag through a one-way valve that may be located at either end of the bag, depending on its design. This valve is called the air inlet.

Oxygen inlet: Every self-inflating bag has an oxygen inlet, which is usually located near the air inlet. The oxygen inlet is a small nipple or projection to which oxygen tubing can be attached when oxygen is needed. In the self-inflating bag, an oxygen tube does not need to be attached in order for the bag to function. It does need to be attached if the infant is to be resuscitated with an oxygen-enriched air mixture rather than with room air.

Patient outlet: The patient outlet is where air exists from the bag to the infant and is where the mask and ET tube attach.

Resuscitation mask: Anatomically shaped masks are shaped to fit the contours of the face. It is easier to obtain a seal with this type of mask. For a mask to be of a correct size, the rim must cover the tip of the chin, the mouth and the nose, but not the eyes.

Fingertip control: If the mask has been properly applied and seal is tight, you will be able to squeeze the resuscitation bag with just your *fingertips*. Avoid compressing the bag with the palm of your hand. Grasping the bag with your palm can result in poor control of ventilation as well as excessive pressures and an excessive volume of air being delivered to the infant. As the volume of the infant's lungs is only a fraction of the volume of the bag (20–30 ml air—lungs of an infant and 240 mL air in the bag), one should never has to squeeze a bag empty to inflate the lungs of an infant.

Indications: Positive-pressure ventilation should be initiated as soon as it is indicated. To delay ventilating an infant in whom it is indicated will only prolong the resuscitative efforts and place the infant at a risk for further damage.

Preceding events: Immediately after birth the infant should be:
1. Placed under a radiant warmer
2. Wiped dry

3. Properly positioned
4. Suctioned, and
5. Provided with tactile stimulation. It is only after the infant has reached this point that a decision regarding positive-pressure ventilation should be made.

Two indications for ventilation: After tactile stimulation has occurred, the use of bag-and-mask ventilation should be initiated in any infant who is apneic or whose respirations are at any time insufficient to maintain a heart rate above 100 beats/minute. Thus, *positive-pressure ventilation* should begin when:
a. Infant is apneic, or
b. Heart rate is 100 beats/minute or below.

Exception to using a mask: A bag and mask are adequate for ventilating most infants. However, infants suspected of having a diaphragmatic hernia should be ventilated via an endotracheal tube rather than mask.

Heart-rate decisions: Heart rate decisions are summarized in Table 8.7.

Improvement

It is indicated by three signs
1. Increasing heart rate
2. Spontaneous respirations
3. Improving color.

Signs of improvement: As the heart rate keeps increasing toward normal, you should continue ventilating the baby at the rate of 40 breaths per minute. Monitor the rise of the chest to prevent over- or under-inflation of the lungs.

Heart rate: When the heart rate stabilizes above 100 beats/minute, stop ventilating but continue to provide a high-oxygen environment and observe whether the baby can sustain spontaneous respirations.

Respirations: If the infant is breathing spontaneously and the heart rate is reached an acceptable level, you may provide tactile respiration by rubbing the infant's back until the rate and depth of respirations are normal. Continue to monitor the infant to determine whether or not the improved signs stabilize.

Color: With improvement, the infant should become pink. If there is central cyanosis, provide free-flow

Table 8.7: Decisions based on heart rate		
Below 60	*60–100*	*Above 100*
Continue ventilation	HR not increasing	Watch for spontaneous respirations
Chest compressions	Chest compressions—if HR is below 80	Then, discontinue ventilation

oxygen and withdraw the free-flow oxygen slowly, once the color improves.

Deterioration

Initial Actions: If with continued assisted ventilation, the infant's condition continues to deteriorate or fails to improve, check adequacy of ventilation and start chest compressions if the heart rate is less than 80 beats/minute.

Chest compressions: Provide chest compressions if despite assisted ventilation, the heart rate remains below 80 beats/minute, chest compressions should be initiated.

Additional procedures: If the infant's condition continues to deteriorate or fails to improve despite assisted ventilation and chest compressions, the infant may require:
  i. Medications, and/or
  ii. Endotracheal intubation.

Administer medications: Discussed in Table 8.10.

Consider intubation: A bag and mask is usually effective for neonatal ventilation. However, if ventilation with bag and mask is ineffective, the infant should be intubated. In addition, when the need for prolonged ventilation is anticipated, it is often easier to continue the ventilation if the infant is intubated. Thus, there are two main reasons for switching to ventilation via an endotracheal tube:
  i. *For effectiveness:* If bag-and-mask ventilation is not providing effective ventilation
  ii. *For convenience:* If ventilation is to be continued for a prolonged period of time.

Use of a resuscitation bag and mask: Procedure
Situation: An infant has just born, provided with thermal management, positioned, suctioned, and given tactile stimulation. The infant is apneic, but no problem has been detected in the lungs. Establish ventilation in this infant using a bag and mask.

Ventilates for 15–30 seconds:
• Rate—40 times/minute
• Pressure—15–20 cm H_2O for normal lungs

Check heart rate with stethoscope for 6 seconds
Result (Table 8.8).

Overview of Chest Compressions

The purpose of chest compression is to assure that the infant maintains a minimal, life-sustaining *circulation*.

Why perform circulation? The heart circulates blood throughout the body, furnishing the tissues and vital organs with oxygen. When an infant has suffered hypoxia, the heart not only slows in rate but also decreases its effectiveness in terms of myocardial contractility. As a result of bradycardia and less powerful contractions, there is a diminished flow of blood, and thus oxygen, to the vital tissues of the body. The decreased supply of oxygen to these tissues can lead to irreparable damage to essential organs such as the brain, heart, kidneys, and bowel.

What is needed then is a means of assuring that life-sustaining circulation is maintained. Chest compression (CC) is the procedure that does this. *Chest compressions must always be accompanied by ventilation with 100% oxygen.* Ventilation must be performed to assure that the blood being circulated during chest compressions is oxygenated.

What is chest compression? Chest compression, sometimes referred to as external cardiac massage, consists of rhythmic compensations of the sternum that:
• Compresses the heart against the spine,
• Increase the intrathoracic pressure, and
• Circulate blood to the vital organs of the body.

The heart lies in the chest, between the sternum and the spine. Compressing the sternum compresses the heart and increases the pressure in the chest, causing blood to be pumped into the arteries. When pressure on the sternum is released, blood enters the heart from the veins.

Indications for Chest Compressions

An adequate heart rate is necessary in order for blood to be circulated throughout the body. Most of the time, ventilation alone with100% oxygen will be

Table 8.8: Ventilation on the basis of heart rate with stethoscope for 6 seconds

A	B	C	D
Below 60	60–100, not increasing	60–100, increasing	Above 100
Continue ventilation	Continue ventilation	Continue ventilation	
Initiate chest compressions	Initiate chest compressions if HR below 80		
No spontaneous respirations		With spontaneous respirations	
Continue ventilation		Discontinue ventilation	
Indicate monitoring		Provide tactile stimulation	
		Indicate monitoring	

sufficient to raise the infant's heart rate to an adequate level. If, despite being ventilated with 100% oxygen, an infant fails to achieve an adequate heart rate, chest compressions must be performed.

Initial period of PPV: In a newborn, bradycardia usually results from a lack of proper oxygenation. In most infants with bradycardia, the heart rate begins to improve as soon as adequate ventilation with 100% oxygen is established. Therefore, the decision to begin chest compressions should be based on the heart rate obtained after 15–30 seconds of PPV with 100% oxygen—not on a heart rate obtained at the time of delivery.

When to begin: Current recommendations include two indications for initiating chest compressions if after 15–30 seconds of PPV with 100% oxygen the heart rate is:

- Below 60, or
- Between 60 and 80 beats/minute and not increasing.

When to stop: Once the heart rate is 80 beats/minute or greater, chest compressions should be discontinued.

Summary: The steps leading to initiating and discontinuing chest compressions are:

1. Ventilate infant with 100% oxygen for 15–30 seconds.
2. Evaluate heart rate
3. Initiate chest compressions if: HR less than 60, or between 60 and 80 and not increasing.
4. Evaluate heart rate: (i) Below 80 continue chest compressions; (ii) 80 or above discontinue chest compressions.

Positioning for Chest Compressions

When the decision to initiate chest compressions is made, the infant is already positioned for positive-pressure ventilation and is being ventilated with 100% oxygen. The person performing chest compressions must gain access to the chest and place his or her hands appropriately. It is important that the two people position themselves in such a way that each one can do an effective job without interfering with others.

Two different techniques used in performing chest compressions. These techniques are:

  i. Thumb technique.
  ii. Two-finger technique.

Thumb technique: With the thumb technique, the two thumbs are used to depress the sternum, with the hands encircling the torso and the fingers supporting the back.

Two-finger technique: With the two-finger technique, the tips of the middle finger and either the index finger or ring finger of one hand are used to compress the sternum. The other hand is used to support the infant's back if firm surface is not available.

These two techniques have several things in common:

- Position of the infant
- Firm support for the back
- Neck slightly extended
- Compressions
- Same location, depth, and rate.

It is advantageous to learn these two methods of performing chest compressions, as each method has advantages and disadvantages.

Location of compressions: When chest compressions are performed on a neonate, pressure is applied to the lower third of the sternum. Care must be used to avoid applying pressure to the xiphoid. To locate the area, imagine a line drawn between the nipples. The lower third of the sternum is just below this line.

Using the thumbs for compressing the sternum: This is accomplished by encircling the torso with both hands and placing the thumbs on the sternum and the fingers under the infant. The thumbs can be placed side by side or, on a small infant, one over the other. The thumbs will be used to compress the sternum, while your fingers provide the support needed for the back. Care must be taken not to squeeze the chest (ribs) with your whole hand during compression. If the chest is squeezed, the infant may suffer fractured ribs or a pneumothorax. The thumb technique has some restrictions. It cannot be used effectively if the infant is large or your hands are small. It also makes access to the umbilical cord more difficult when medications become necessary. However, the thumb technique is less tiresome than the two-finger technique if chest compressions are required for a prolonged period of time.

Using two-finger technique for compressing the sternum: Your other hand can be used to support the infant's back, so that the heart can be more effectively compressed between the sternum and spine (if the infant is positioned on a firm surface, this may not be necessary). With the second hand supporting the back, you can feel the pressure and the depth of the compressions. This technique is more tiring than the thumb technique if chest compressions are required for a prolonged period of time. However, the two-finger method can be used regardless of the size of the infant or the size of your hands. An additional advantage of this technique is that it leaves the umbilicus free, in case medications need to be administered via the umbilical route.

Position of the infant: The infant who is being ventilated and whose chest is being compressed must be properly positioned for both procedures. The infant's neck must be slightly extended to provide an open airway for ventilation.

Thumb method: Use your fingers to support the infant's back, and use both thumbs to compress the sternum.

Two-finger method: Use the tip of two fingers of one hand to compress the sternum, and use your other hand or a firm surface to support the infant's back.

Position of resuscitators: In addition to positioning the infant properly, the persons providing ventilation and chest compressions must position themselves so that each can do an effective job without restricting the other.

Indications for Endotracheal Intubation

When positive pressure ventilation (PPV) is required on a newborn, it can usually be effectively delivered with a resuscitation bag and mask. A major advantage of the bag and mask is that the ventilation can be initiated immediately, without the delay necessitated by the insertion of an endotracheal tube. There are four situations in which endotracheal intubation are necessary. These are when:

- Prolonged positive-pressure ventilation is required.
- Bag-and-mask ventilation is ineffective.
- Tracheal suctioning is required.
- Diaphragmatic hernia is suspected.

Prolonged PPV required: A bag and mask can be used to ventilate the neonate effectively over a period of time. However, when prolonged assisted ventilation is anticipated, it is easier if the infant is intubated.

Bag-and-mask ineffective: If a bag-and-mask ventilation is ineffective, as evidenced by inadequate chest expansion, the infant should be intubated.

Tracheal suctioning: Intubation is required in order to suction the trachea of an infant born with thick or particulate meconium in the amniotic fluid. Tracheal suctioning is also indicated in infants suspected of having aspirated formula or other foreign material.

Diaphragmatic hernia suspected: If a diaphragmatic hernia is suspected, ventilation should be performed using an ET tube rather than a mask. This prevents air from entering the bowel and compromising lung expansion.

Supplies and Equipment

The supplies and equipment necessary to perform endotracheal intubation should be kept together on either a resuscitation cart or intubation tray. Each delivery room, nursery, and emergency room should have a completed set of the items listed below.

The supplies and equipment essential for intubating a neonate include:

- Laryngoscope with an extra set of batteries and extra bulb.
- *Blades*
  Size 1 (full term infant)
  Size 0 (preterm infant)
  (Straight rather than curved blades are preferred for optimal visualization)
- Endotracheal tubes with an internal diameter (ID) of 2.5 mm, 3.0 mm, 3.5 mm. and 4.0 mm.
- Wire stylet
- Suctioning device, DeLee mucus trap with 10 Fr catheter, suction setup with 10 Fr suction catheter
- Shoulder roll
- Roll of ½- or ¾- adhesive tape
- Scissors
- Resuscitation bag and mask capable of providing a high concentration of oxygen
- Oxygen tubing (this must be available to oxygenate the infant, should the need arise, during the procedure. Once the tube is inserted, the bag alone is needed to check the tube placement and for ventilation).

Preventing contamination: Intubation is best performed as a clean procedure: the laryngoscope blades, endotracheal tubes, and stylet should be sterile and protected from contamination. The laryngoscope handle should be thoroughly cleaned following each use.

Endotracheal tubes: Sterile disposable tubes of nonirritating material should be used. They should be of uniform diameter throughout the length of the tube—not tapered near the tip. One disadvantage of the tapered tube is that during intubation, your view of the tracheal opening is easily obstructed by the wide part of the tube.

Vocal cord guide: The endotracheal tubes manufactured for neonates have a black line near the tip of the tube, which is called "vocal cord guide". Such tubes should be inserted so that the vocal cord guide is placed at the level of the vocal cords. This usually positions the tip of the tube above the bifurcation of the trachea. As you know that the length of the trachea in a premature infant is less than that of full term infant 3 cm vs. 5–6 cm. Therefore, the smaller the tube, the closer is the vocal cord guide is to the tip of the tube. In 2.5 mm tubes, it is 2.2 cm from the tip, whereas in a 4.0 mm tube it is positioned 2.8 cm from the tip.

Centimeter markings: Endotracheal tubes made for neonates come with centimeter markings along the tube, identifying the distance from the tip of the tube. When the tube is first inserted, take note of the centimeter marking that appears at the upper lip. This can serve to alert you if the tube's position has changed.

Inserting the laryngoscope and visualizing the glottis: As soon as the infant is properly positioned, the laryngoscope should be inserted, and the glottis (the opening of the trachea) visualized. This is the most difficult and critical part of the procedure. Once there is a clear view of the glottis, inserting an ET tube is accomplished relatively easily.

Preparing for insertion: Stand at the head of the infant. Turn on the laryngoscope light and hold the laryngoscope in your left hand between your thumb and the first three fingers with the blade pointing away from you.

Note: The laryngoscope is designed to be held in the left hand by both right and left handed individuals. If held in the right hand, the closed, curved part of the blade may block your view of the glottis, as well as make insertion of the ET tube impossible. Stabilize the infant's head with your right hand.

Introducing blade: The goal in inserting the laryngoscope blade is to slide it over the tongue with the tip of the blade resting in the vallecula (the area between the base of the tongue and the glottis) (Table 8.9).

Exception: In general, the blade should be placed in the vallecula. However, in extremely premature infants the vallecula may be too small, in which case it may be necessary to use the blade to gently lift the epiglottis. To properly visualize the blade, introduce the blade into the infant's mouth between the tongue and palate. Gently advance the tip to just beyond the base of the tongue.

Visualizing glottis: Once the blade is inserted to the desired distance, lift it slightly, it will lift the tongue out of the way to expose the pharyngeal area. When lifting the blade, raise the entire blade by pulling up in the direction the handle is pointing. *Do not just lift the tip of the blade by using the rocking motion and pulling the handle towards you.* The latter will not produce the view of the glottis you desire and will put excessive

pressure on the alveolar ridge and possibly harm future tooth formation.

Assess landmarks: With the blade properly inserted and slightly elevated, the pharyngeal area is exposed. The next step is to look for landmarks. It is important to identify where the tip of the blade is. This will enable you to take immediate corrective action (if necessary) in an attempt to visualize the glottis.

Correct blade position: If the tip is correctly positioned in the vallecula, you should see the epiglottis at the top with the glottic opening below.

Incorrect blade position: An incorrectly positioned blade is either inserted too far, not far enough, or too far to the right or left. The landmarks that signal each of these positions are given here, along with the appropriate corrective action.

If these corrective measures fail to bring the epiglottis and glottis into view, withdraw the laryngoscope, ventilate the infant with a bag and mask, and begin again.

Stop after 20 seconds: To minimize hypoxia, intubations attempts should be limited to 20 seconds. The infant should be stabilized between attempts by ventilating with a bag and mask.

External tracheal pressure: In some infants, particularly very small ones, pressure on the neck over the trachea will help lower the trachea, maximizing the view of the glottis. This is accomplished by using the fourth or fifth finger of the left hand, or asking an assistant to apply the pressure.

Suction: When inserting the laryngoscope blade, if you encounter secretions blocking the airway, suction the area with an appropriate DeLee mucus trap or a suction catheter. Suctioning secretions prior to inserting the blade is essential for visualizing the glottis and preventing aspiration, should the infant gasp.

Summary: As stated earlier, the most difficult part of the procedure is obtaining an unobstructed view of the glottis. This involves the following steps:
1. Insert blade to just beyond base of tongue.

Table 8.9: Blade position and corrective action		
Position	*Landmarks*	*Corrective action*
Not inserted far enough	You see the tongue surrounding the blade	Advance the blade farther
Inserted too far	You see the wall of the esophagus surrounding the blade	Withdraw the blade slowly until the epiglottis and glottis come into view
Inserted off to the side	In the posterior pharynx, you see part of the trachea to the side of the blade	Gently move the blade back to the midline, then advance or retreat according to the landmarks seen

2. Lift the blade and identify landmarks (ideally, as you lift the blade, the glottis and epiglottis will come into view).
3. If landmarks are not seen:
   Determine blade placement:
   • On tongue?
   • In esophagus?
   • To the side?
   • Take corrective action, and reassess landmarks.
   • Use external tracheal pressure if necessary to lower the trachea.
   • Use suction to clear airway.

If 20 seconds have passed, stop and ventilate with a bag and mask.

Use of medicines: Use of medications, indications and effects is shown in Table 8.10.

Routes of drug administration: The routes of drug administration include:
• Umbilical vein
• Peripheral veins
• Intratracheal/instillation.

Umbilical vein: The umbilical vein is the preferred route for administering drugs in the delivery room because it can be easily located and cannulated. A 3.5 or 5.0 Fr umbilical catheter with a single end hole and radiopaque marker should be used. The catheter should be inserted in to the vein of the umbilical stump until the tip of the catheter is just below the skin level, but the free flow of the blood is present. If the catheter is inserted farther, there is risk of infusing solutions into the liver and possibly causing damage. The umbilical venous catheter should be removed once resuscitation procedure is over. If vascular access is desired for continuing care, an umbilical artery or a peripheral vein should be used.

Peripheral vein: Veins in the scalp and extremities can be used for administering drugs or solutions, but are difficult to access especially during resuscitation.

Endotracheal instillation: Some drugs may be injected directly into the bronchial tree via the endotracheal tube (IT). Immediately after the drug is injected, the infant should be given positive pressure ventilation to distribute the drug deep into the bronchial tree. Because some of the drugs may adhere to the endotracheal tube, many prefer to insert a 5-Fr, feeding tube through the endotracheal tube. The drug is then injected via a feeding tube, which is then flushed with enough normal saline to clear the drug from the feeding tube (0.5 ml for a 15-inch 5 Fr tube). The feeding tube is then removed and positive-pressure ventilation provided to distribute the drug into the bronchial tree.

Cloherty JP, Eichenwald EC, Stark AR. Manual of Neonatal Care. 6th edn. Philadelphhia: Lippincott Williams & Wilkins, 2008;1–762.

Chaudhri S, Kadam S. Oxygen Therapy in Neonates. In: Mathur GP, Mathur Sarla (eds). *Current Trends in Pediatrics.* Vol 1. Delhi: Academa Publishers, 2005;52–56.

		Table 8.10: Medications II: Indications and effects		
Medication	*Indication*	*Effects*	*Response*	*Follow-up if no response*
Epinephrine	HR zero or below 80/minute, after 3 sec of PPV and CC	Inotropic, chronotropic, peripheral vasoconstrictor	HR 100 or above after 30 sec	If HR is below 100: Repeat epinephrine every 5 min Consider volume expander/sodium bicarbonate.
Volume expanders	Acute bleeding with signs of hypovolemia	Increased intravascular volume, better tissue perfusion, less acidosis	Better pulses, high BP, improved pallor expander	If hypovolemia pesists: Repeat volume Consider sodium bicarbonate/dopamine
Sodium bicarbonate	Documented metabolic acidosis, Apgar score—3 or less at 5 min	Correction of pH, volume expansion	HR 100 or more after 30 sec	If HR is below 100: Consider epinephrine, volume expander, dopamine
Naloxone	Severe respiratory depression with history of narcotic administration 4 hr before delivery	Narcotic antagonist	Spontaneous respiration	If poor response, consider repeat dose.
Dopamine	Persisting hypotension	Better cardiac output, higher BP	Improved BP	

Chaudhri S, Kadam S. Assisted Ventilation in Neonates. In: Mathur GP, Mathur Sarla (eds). *Current Trends in Pediatrics.* Vol 1. Delhi: Academa Publishers, 2005;63–76.

Kattwinkel J (ed). *Textbook of neonatal resuscitation.* 4th edn. American Heart Association: American Academy of Pediatrics, 2000.

Malik GK. Neonatal Resuscitation—Current Concepts. In: Mathur GP, Mathur Sarla (eds). *Current Trends in Pediatrics.* Vol 1. Delhi: Academa Publishers, 2005;421–31.

Perlman JM, Risserr R. Cardiopulmonary resuscitation in the delivery room: Associated clinical events. *Arch Pediatr Adolesc Med* 1995; 149:20–25.

Saugstad OD. Practical aspects of resuscitating asphyxiated newborn infants. *Eur J Peditr* 1998;157 (suppl 1): S11–15.

Shah NK, Mathur NB. Neonatal resuscitation. *IAP-NNF Guidelines 2006 on Level II Neonatal Care.* Delhi: UNICEF, 2006; 1–13.

Stoll BJ. The newborn infant. In: Kliegman RM, Behrman RE, Jenson HB, Stanton BF (eds). *Nelson Textbook of Pediatrics.* 18th edn. Vol 1. Philadelphia: Saunders, 2007; 675–83.

Stoll BJ, Adams-Chapman I. Delivery room emergencies. In: Kliegman RM, Behrman RE, Jenson HB, Stanton BF (eds). *Nelson Textbook of Pediatrics.* 18th edn. Vol 1. Philadelphia: Saunders, 2007; 723–8.

Wolkoff LI, Davis IM. Delivery room resuscitation of the newborn. *Clin Perinatol* 1999;26:641–58.

8.5 HIGH RISK PREGNANCY

Pregnancy is a physiological event in the life of a woman. Under certain various circumstances, a pregnancy may be detrimental to the health of either the mother or the fetus. Such a pregnancy is termed as high risk.

Identification of High Risk Factors

Women with established medical condition or with a history of medical complication in a prior pregnancy are encouraged to seek preconceptional counselling. The counselling covers the following points:

1. High risk groups are identified (Box 8.8)
2. The potential effect that risk factors can have on pregnancy
3. The effect of pregnancy on the identified risk factors
4. Potential maternal or fetal disability
5. The specialized investigations required for monitoring maternal and fetal well-being
6. Establishment of management regimen using the safest medications in the lowest possible doses for a pre-existing medical condition prior to and during the critical first trimester of pregnancy, that is, during organogenesis.

Role of scoring system: Identification of a high risk may be achieved by a scoring system. Each system incorporates a list of condition known to be poor prognostic indicators in pregnancy. Most of these systems give different numerical values to the high

---

Box 8.8: Recognised high risk groups

Maternal: Hypertension; renal disease; respiratory disease; cardiac disease; hemoglobinopathy; psychiatric conditions; infections (e.g. varicella); drug misuse; extremes of age; obesity

Perinatal: "Bad obstetric history"; recurrent pregnancy loss; Prematurity (including rupture of membranes and labour); rhesus disease; diabetes mellitus; monozygotic multiple pregnancy; fetal anomaly; assisted conception.

Complications developing (during pregnancy): Placenta previa; fetal growth restriction

Critical emergencies: Fulminating pre-eclampsia/eclampsia; massive obstetric hemorrhage; coagulopathy; amniotic fluid embolism; severe sepsis; other 'life-threatening' conditions.

---

risk factor. Advantage of such systems is that it helps to identify and document the high risk factor–documentation is of value in medicolegal case. They have limited role in predicting outcome as it is influenced by medical intervention.

Role of ultrasonography: Ultrasound has developed from a separate formal investigation to a "hands on bedside service". There has been an expansion of its role from an anomaly scan to a modality for assessing fetal well-being. A timely anomaly scan would help to identify high risk pregnancy and should be offered to every pregnancy. Ultrasound for assessment of fetal well being is now being recommended as a part of routine examination of fetus. When compared with clinical abdominal examination, it has helped to identify the at-risk fetus in a low risk population—a growth restricted fetus, which have a perinatal mortality 4–10 times higher than normally grown fetuses.

Antepartum Fetal Surveillance in High Risk Pregnancies

The widespread use of antepartum fetal surveillance is primarily based on circumstantial evidence because there have been no definitive randomised clinical trials. According to American College of Obstetrics and Gynaecologist (1999), the main goal of antepartum fetal surveillance is to prevent fetal death. Tests to assess antepartum fetal surveillance include:

1. Daily fetal movement count
2. Non-stress test
3. Contraction stress test
4. Biophysical profile
5. Umbilical artery Doppler velocimetry

Fetal movements: Passive fetal movements commence as early as 7 wk and become more sophisticated and coordinated by the end of pregnancy. The decrease or cessation of fetal movements has an ominous implication and may be associated with fetal distress or death. Thus, fetal movement counting has been proposed as a method for evaluating fetal health. The objective is to recognise a decrease in movement and to follow that recognition with further testing to confirm or rule out the existence of fetal distress. The main drawback to this test is maternal non-compliance.

Non-stress test (NST): It is the most commonly used test for antepartum evaluation of fetal well-being. The principle underlying this test is that fetal movements are associated with fetal heart rate accelerations. This is indicative of a normal interaction between the parasympathetic and sympathetic system of fetus suggestive of fetal well-being. A reactive test is defined as presence of two or more fetal heart rate (FHR) accelerations during a period of 20 minutes, each acceleration of 15 or more beats per minute and lasting for 15 or more seconds usually occurring simultaneously with episodes of fetal activity.

Drawbacks to this test are
- High frequency of false-positive results (50% for morbidity and 80% for mortality), and an extremely low false negative rate (3.2 per 1000).
- The possibility that a truly abnormal result reflects an advanced rather than an early stage of fetal distress.
- Interpretation relies on one variable (i.e. presence of accelerations of fetal heart rate associated with fetal movements) and it ignores other important variables like fetal heart rate variability and presence or absence of decelerations.
- Absence of accelerations in a 20-minute period may correspond to fetal sleep requiring an extended NST of 40 minutes or vibro-acoustic stimulation of the fetus.

Contraction stress test (CST): It is one of the best available tests for primary fetal surveillance of high risk pregnancies. It is based on the evidence that uterine contraction result in a decrease in the uteroplacental blood flow resulting in a hypoxic stress for the fetus. A healthy fetus is able to tolerate this stress but a fetus with chronic or acute problem will not be able to tolerate such a decrease in oxygen supply and will demonstrate this by decelerations of fetal heart rate. The end point of CST is presence or absence of late deceleration of the FHR following uterine contractions induced by intravenous oxytocin or nipple stimulation. Such late deceleration could be due to uteroplacental insufficiency. It has a false-negative rate of 0.4 per 1000 and false-positive rate with respect

to fetal morbidity 50%. Drawback is that on an average the test requires 90 minutes to complete.

Biophysical profile (BPP): It was devised by Manning and colleagues (1980). It entails the observation by ultrasound of fetal breathing movements, fetal body movements, fetal tone, amniotic fluid volume, and fetal heart reactivity. These factors are dependent on the integrity of the fetal central nervous system and are affected in situations of fetal compromise. It has a negative predictive value of 98.5% (similar to NST 98%) but the positive predictive value of an abnormal BPP (50.8%) better than non-reactive NST.

Drawbacks of BPP test are
- That each criterion is assigned a score of either zero or two points, despite the possibility that each of these variables may have different importance in assessing fetal situation. A normal BPP corresponds to a score of 8 or greater but this value must include a normal amniotic fluid volume.
- Decreased body movements and fetal tone are found only when the fetal compromise is severe and by the time of discovery, the value of intervention is suboptimal.
- Difficulty in evaluating fetal tone.

Modified BPP
Vintzileos et al (1987) proposed modification of BPP. *It includes:* Non-stress test with vibro-acoustic stimulation and estimation of amniotic fluid volume. It combines observation of an index of acute fetal hypoxia and a second index indicative of chronic fetal problems.

Umbilical artery Doppler velocimetry: It is a non-invasive technique to assess blood flow by characterising downstream impedance. The umbilical artery systolic/diastolic echo (S/D), the commonly used index, is considered abnormal if it is elevated above the 95th percentile for gestational age or if the diastolic flow is either absent or reversed. Absent or reversed diastolic flow is associated with fetal growth restriction and may suggest fetal compromise. Williams and colleagues (2000) in their study of 1240 high risk women found that nonstress test and Doppler velocimetry are equivalent in their ability to predict pregnancy outcome. American College of Obstetricians and Gynaecologists (1999, 2000), concluded no benefit for umbilical artery velocimetry for conditions other than suspected fetal growth restriction. No benefit has been demonstrated for other conditions such as post-term pregnancy, diabetes mellitus, systemic lupus erythematosus or anti-phospholipid antibody syndrome.

Recommendations for antenatal assessment of fetal well-being: According to American College of

Obstetricians and Gynaecologists (1999), there is no overall agreement regarding the best test to evaluate fetal well-being. The three commonly used testing systems—contraction stress test, non-stress test, and biophysical profile—have different end points that are considered depending on the clinical situation.

Most authorities recommend that testing should begin by 32 to 34 wk of pregnancies in high risk pregnancies. Pregnancy with severe complications might require testing as early as 26–28 wk. The frequency for repeating tests has been arbitrarily set at 7 days, but more frequent testing is often done depending on the clinical situation.

An important and unanswered question is whether antepartum fetal surveillance identifies fetal asphyxia early enough to prevent fetal brain damage. Studies by Todd and co-workers (1992) attempted to correlate cognitive development in infants up to 2 yr following either abnormal Doppler velocimetry or non-stress test. Abnormal non-stress test were associated with marginally poorer cognitive outcomes, but not those associated with abnormal Doppler velocimetry, thus these investigators concluded that by the time fetal compromise is diagnosed with antenatal testing, fetal damage has already been sustained.

Intrapartum fetal surveillance of high risk pregnancy: Management of high risk pregnancies should be undertaken in a tertiary care centre with a neonatal intensive care unit. During labor, these patients require very stringent monitoring of fetal heart rate, where available, continuous electronic fetal heart rate monitoring is preferable. At risk fetuses do not tolerate labor well and the incidence of cesarean section is very high. The neonate should be received by a neonato-logist competent in handling suspected complications.

Fetal Outcomes of High Risk Pregnancy

Outcome of high risk pregnancy is normal or else premature/small for gestational age infant. Thus, the two most common fetal problems associated with high risk pregnancies are prematurity and fetal growth restriction.

1. Prematurity

Preterm births can be prevented in less than half of the mothers who present in labor before 37 wk. The goals of management are listed in Box 8.9.

Corticosteroid therapy: It is presently the only treatment shown to improve fetal survival when given to a woman in preterm labor between 24 and 34 wk of gestation. Studies have shown decreased incidence of intraventricular hemorrhage, respiratory distress and mortality even when treatment lasts less than 24 hr,

---

Box 8.9: Goals of management

1. Early identification of risk factors
   Previous preterm delivery
   Decidual hemorrhage (abruptio placenta)
   Uterine over distension (multiple pregnancies, polyhydramnios)
   Cervical incompetence (trauma, uterocervical malformations, hormonal change—maternal and fetal stress)
   Uteroplacental insufficiency—hypertension, diabetes mellitus, drug abuse, smoking, alcohol
   Maternal infections—STD, vaginitis, UTI
2. Timely diagnosis of preterm labor
3. Identification the etiology
4. Evaluate fetal well-being
5. Provide proper pharmacological treatment to reduce the incidence of respiratory distress syndrome
6. Corticosteroid therapy
7. Tocolytic therapy
8. Antibiotic therapy
   STD: Sexually transmitted diseases; UTI: Urinary tract infection

---

although the optimal benefits begin after 24 hrs. Recommended drug is betamethasone in a dosage of 12 mg given intramuscularly every 24 hrs—2 doses or dexamethasone in a dose of 6 mg every 6 hr for 24 hrs. Dexamethasone is not preferred as it causes ventriculomalacia in infants.

Antibiotic therapy: Infections account for about 30–40% of spontaneous preterm labour and preterm birth. These infections affecting an immunocompromised host like the fetus may cause tissue damage and long term sequelae such as bronchopulmonary dysplasia, cerebral palsy, and bacterial infections. They are major cause of morbidity and mortality in a preterm infant. Prophylactic antibiotics do not have a role in prolonging labour but decrease prenatal morbidity in established infections. The ORACLE study has established role of erythromycin in prolonging labor and decreasing the incidence of respiratory distress in fetuses of women with premature rupture of membranes. In the West, Group B streptococcal infection is very common in the neonate of patients with preterm labor. There is a role of ampicillin therapy in established infection to decrease mortality or morbidity in the neonate.

2. Fetal Growth Restriction (FGR)

Fetal growth restriction is associated with substantial perinatal morbidity and mortality affecting 5–10% births. It is defined as fetal weight or abdominal circumference deviate below 10th percentile of the gestational age, which constitute the threshold. It is associated with fetal demise, birth asphyxia, meconium aspiration, neonatal hypoglycemia and hypothermia, prevalence of abnormal neurological development. Post-natal growth and development of the growth restricted fetus depends on the cause of restriction, nutrition in infancy, and social environment.

Management

Once a growth restricted fetus is diagnosed the American College of Obstetricians and Gynaecologists (2000) does not opine for diagnosing anomalies or to determine poor psychological condition. Instead the timing of delivery is crucial.

Growth restricted fetus near term

- Prompt delivery is the best outcome
- In the presence of severe oligohydramnios, most fetuses are delivered if gestational age has reached 34 wk
- In the presence of reassuring fetal heart patterns, vaginal delivery may be attempted. Unfortunately such fetuses tolerate labor less well and cesarean section rate is higher.

Growth restriction remote from term

In a growth restricted fetus diagnosed prior to 34 wk, if amniotic fluid volume and antepartum surveillance are normal, observation is recommended. A sonographic search for fetal anomalies is recommended. Antepartum surveillance is continued if growth and fetal evaluation is normal and pregnancy is allowed to continue till fetal lung maturity is achieved. No specific treatment is available which will ameliorate the condition. Nutrient supplementation, plasma volume expansion, oxygen therapy, antihypertensive drugs, heparin, aspirin have not shown to be effective (American College of Obstetricians and Gynaecologists, 2000).

American College of Obstetricians and Gynecologists. Antepartum fetal surveillance. *Practice Bulletin No. 9, 1999* (October).

American College of Obstetricians and Gynecologists. Intrauterine growth restriction. *Practice Bulletin No. 12,* January 2000a (January).

American College of Obstetricians and Gynecologists. Intrauterine growth restriction. *Practice Bulletin* No. 12, January 2000 (January).

Arias F. Identification and antepartum surveillance of the high-risk patient. In: Arias F (ed). *Practical Guide to High Risk Pregnancy and Delivery*, 2nd edn. Bangalore: Harcourt Asia Pvt. Ltd; 2000:3–21.

Gyetvai K, Hannah ME, Hodnett ED, et al. Tocolysis for preterm labour: a systematic overview. *Obstet Gynecol* 1999; 94:869–77.

Kleigman RM. Intrauterine growth retardation. In: Fanuroft AA, Martin RJ (eds). *Neonatal-perinatal Medicine*, 6th edn, New York: Mosby, 1997;203.

Manning FA, Platt LD, Sipos L. Antepartum fetal evaluation: Development of fetal biophysical profile. *Am J Obstet Gynecol* 1980;136:787–95.

Manning FA, Lange IR, Morrison I, et al. Fetal biophysical profile score and non-stress test: A comparative trial. *Obstet Gynecol* 1984;64:326–31.

National Institute of Health Consensus. Development Conference: Statement of Repeat Course of Antenatal Corticosteroid. Bethesda, MD. August 17–18, 2000. http://consensus.nih.gov

Todd AL, Tridinger BJ, Cole MJ, et al. Antenatal tests of fetal welfare and development at age 2 yr. *Am J Obstet Gynecol* 1992;167:66–71.

Vintzileos AM, Gaffney SE, Salinger LM, et al. The relationship among the fetal biophysical profile, umbilical cord pH and Apgar score. *Am J Obstet Gynecol* 1987;157:627–31.

Williams KP, Farquharson DF, Bebbington M, et al. A randomised controlled clinical trial comparing non-stress test in a high risk population (Abstract 315). *Am J Obstet Gynecol* 2000;182:S109.

8.6 HIGH RISK INFANTS

Neonates at risk should be identified as early as possible to decrease neonatal morbidity and mortality. Neonate at risk include: Birth weight < 2,500 or > 4,000 g; birth before 37 wk or after 42 wk of gestation; SGA, LGA, growth status; tachypnea, cyanosis; congenital malformation; pallor, plethora, petechiae. Examination of fresh placenta, cord, and membranes may help the physician to think newborn infants at high risk and may confirm a diagnosis in a sick infant. Fetal blood loss may be indicated by placental pallor and retroplacental hematoma. Placental edema and secondary possible immunoglobulin G deficiency in newborns may be associated with fetofetal transfusion syndrome, hydrops fetalis, congenital nephrosis, or hepatic disease. Amnion nodosum (granules on the amnion) and oligohydramnios are associated with pulmonary hypoplasia and renal agenesis, whereas small whitish nodules on the cord suggest a candidal infection. Short cords and noncoiled cords occur with chromosome anomalies and omphalocele. True umbilical cord knots are seen in about 1% of births and are associated with prematurity, abruptio placentae, polyhydramnios, and intrauterine growth restriction (IUGR). Meconium staining suggests *in utero* stress. Opacity of the fetal placental surface suggests infection. Single umbilical arteries are associated with an increased incidence of congenital renal abnormalities and syndromes. See also Box 8.7 for recognised high risk groups.

Many prematurely born infants are small for gestational age (SGA), have significant perinatal asphyxia, are breech, or are born with life-threatening congenital anomalies. The highest risk of neonatal mortality occurs in infants whose weigh < 1,000 g at birth and whose gestation is < 28 wk. The lowest risk of neonatal mortality occurs in infants with a birthweight of 3,000–4,000 g and a gestational age of 38–42 wk. Neonatal mortality rates rise sharply for infants weighing over 4,000 g at birth and for those whose gestational period is 42 wk or longer. Neonatal mortality mostly occurs within the 1st hr and days after birth, but with increasing postnatal survival mortality decreases.

Multiple Gestation Pregnancies

The reported incidence of spontaneous twinning is highest among blacks and East Indians, followed by Northern European whites, and it is lowest in the Asian races. Triplets are estimated to occur in 1 in 86^2 pregnancies and quadruplets in 1 in 86^3 pregnancies in the United States.

Etiology: The occurrence of monovular twins appears to be independent of genetic influence. Polyovular pregnancies are more frequent beyond the 2nd pregnancy, in older women, and in families with a history of polyovular twins. Twin-prone women have higher levels of gonadotropin. Polyovular pregnancies occur in many women treated for infertility.

Conjoined twins (Siamese twins-incidence, 1/50,000) probably result from relatively late monovular separation, as does the presence of two separate embryos in one amniotic sac. The site of connections varies: thoraco-omphalopagus (28%), thoracopagus (18%), omphalopagus (10%), craniopagus (6%), and incomplete duplication (10%). Difficult to separate conjoined twins have occasionally survived to adulthood. Most conjoined twins are female.

Superfecundation, or fertilization of an ovum by an insemination that takes place after one ovum has already been fertilized, and *superfetation,* or fertilization and subsequent development of an ovum when a fetus is already present in the uterus, results in differences in size and appearance of certain twins at birth.

The diagnosis of pregnancy with twins is suggested by a uterine size that is greater than that expected for gestational age, auscultation of two fetal hearts, and elevated maternal serum α-fetoprotein or human chorionic gonadotropin levels, and it is confirmed by ultrasound.

Monozygotic vs dizygotic twins: Identifying twins as monozygotic or dizygotic (monovular or polyovular) is important because studying monozygotic twins is useful in determining the relative influence of heredity and environment on human development and disease.

Examination of the placenta: If the placentas are separate, they are always dichorionic (present in 75%), but the twins are not always dizygotic because initiation of monovular twinning at the 1st cell division or during the morula stage may result in two amnions, two chorions, and even two placentas. One-third of monzygotic twins are dichorionic and diamnionic. An apparently single placenta may be present with either monovular or polyovular twins; yet inspection of a polyovular placenta usually reveals that each twin has a separate chorion. Separate or fused dichorionic placentas may be disproportionate in size. The fetus attached to the smaller placenta or the smaller portion of the placenta is usually smaller than its twin or malformed. *Monochorionic twins* may be presumed to be monovular. They are usually diamnionic, and almost invariably, the placenta is single.

Problems of twin gestation include polyhydramnios, hyperemesis gravidarum, pre-eclampsia, premature rupture of membranes, vasa previa, velamentous insertion of the umbilical cord, abnormal presentations (breech), and premature labor. *Placental vascular anastomoses* occur with high frequency only in monochorionic twins; the vascular anastomoses may be artery-to-artery, vein-to-vein, or artery-to-vein. A combination of artery-to-artery and vein-to-vein anastomoses is associated with the condition of lethal acardiac fetus. In the *fetal transfusion syndrome,* an artery from one twin acutely or chronically delivered blood that is drained into the vein of the other. The latter becomes plethoric and large, and the former is anemic and small. Maternal hydramnios in a twin pregnancy suggests fetal transfusion syndrome.

Postnatal identification: The physical criteria used to determine whether twins are monovular are listed in Box 8.10.

Prognosis: Most twins are born prematurely, and maternal complications of pregnancy are more common than with single pregnancies. Because most twins are premature by weight, their overall mortality is higher than that of single births. The perinatal mortality of twins is about four times that of singletons. The mortality for multiple gestations with four or more fetuses is excessively high for each fetus. Because of this poor prognosis, selective fetal reduction (with transabdominal intrathoracic fetal injection of KCL) to two to three fetuses has been offered as a treatment option. Monozygotic twins have an increased risk of one twin dying *in utero.* The surviving twin has a greater risk for cerebral palsy and other neurodevelopmental sequelae.

Treatment: Prenatal diagnosis enables the obstetricians and pediatricians to anticipate the birth of infants who

Box 8.10: Physical criteria to determine monovular twins

1. Both must be of the same sex;
2. Their features, including ears and teeth, must be obviously alike (but they need not resemble each other more than the lateral halves of one individual);
3. Their hair must be identical in color, texture, natural curl, and distribution;
4. Their eyes must be of the same color and shade;
5. Their skin must be of the same texture and color (nevi may be differently distributed);
6. Their hands and feet must be of the same conformation and of similar size; and
7. Their anthropometric values must show close agreement.

are at high risk because of twinning. Close observation is needed during labor and in the immediate neonatal period so that prompt treatment of asphyxia or fetal transfusion syndrome can be initiated. Immediate blood transfusion in a severely anemic "donor twin" or to perform a partial exchange transfusion of a "recipient twin" should be based on clinical judgment.

Prematurity and Intrauterine Growth Restriction

Low Birth Weight (LBW)

Live-born infants delivered before 37 wk from the 1st day of the last menstrual period are termed premature by the World Health Organization (WHO). Ideally, definitions of LBW for individual populations should be based on data that are as genetically and environmentally homogeneous as possible. Therefore, in India and various other developing countries, *infants with birth weight less than 2,500 g are considered low birth weight (LBW)*. LBW is due to prematurity, poor intrauterine growth restriction (IUGR) or both. Prematurity and IUGR are associated with increased neonatal morbidity and mortality.

Very low birth weight (VLBW) infants are those with a weight less than 1,500 g and extremely low birth weight (ELBW) infants are those with weight less than 1,000 g. The VLBW rate is an accurate predictor of the infant mortality rate (IMR). Very low birth weight contributes significantly to neonatal mortality. VLBW infants account for over 50% of neonatal deaths and 50% of handicapped infants; their survival is directly related to birth weight, with approximately 20% of those between 500 and 600 g and over 90% of those between 1,250 and 1,500 g surviving. Perinatal care has improved the rate of survival of VLBW infants. The survival of VLBW infants is dependant on quality of care in (equipment and personnel) intensive neonatal units. Establishment of these units is very effective in reducing mortality among VLBW babies.

When compared with term infants, VLBW neonates have higher incidence of rehospitalization during the 1st yr of life for sequelae of prematurity, infections, neurologic complications and psychological disorders.

Factors Related to Premature Birth and Low Birth Weight

It is difficult to separate completely the factors associated with prematurity from those associated with IUGR. There is a strong positive correlation between both preterm birth and IUGR and low socioeconomic status. Families of low socioeconomic status have higher rates of maternal undernutrition, anemia, and illness; inadequate prenatal care; drug misuse; obstetric complications; and maternal histories of reproductive insufficiency (abortions, stillbirths, premature or LBW infants). Other associated factors such as single-parent families, teenage pregnancies, short interpregnancy interval, and mothers who have borne more than four previous children are also encountered more frequently. Systematic differences in fetal growth have also been described in association with maternal size, birth order, sibling weight, social class, maternal smoking, and other factors. The etiology of preterm birth is multifactorial and involves a complex interaction between fetal, placental, uterine, and maternal factors (Table 8.11).

Intrauterine Growth Restriction (IUGR)

IUGR is associated with medical conditions that interfere with the circulation and efficiency of the placenta, with the development or growth of the fetus, or with the general health and nutrition of the mother

Table 8.11: Causes of preterm birth	
Fetal	Fetal distress
	Multiple gestation
	Erythroblastosis
	Nonimmune hydrops
Placental	Placental dysfunction
	Placenta previa
	Abruptio placentae
Uterine	Bicornuate uterus
	Incompetent cervix (premature dilatation)
Maternal	Pre-eclampsia
	Chronic medical illness infection (*Listeria monocytogenes*, group B streptococcus, urinary tract infection, bacterial vaginitis, choreoamnionitis)
	Drug abuse (cocaine)
Other	Premature rupture of membranes
	Polyhydramnios
	Iatrogenic
	Trauma

(Table 8.12). IUGR is similar to malnutrition and may be present in both term and preterm infants. Neonates affected by IUGR are usually undernourished and have loose skin folds on the face and on the gluteal region, absence of subcutaneous fat and peeling of skin. Many factors are common to both born preterm and LBW infants with IUGR. IUGR is associated with decreased insulin production or insulin [or insulin-like growth factor (IGF)] action at the receptor level. Infants with IGF-1 receptor defects, pancreatic hypoplasia, or transient neonatal diabetes have IUGR. Genetic mutations affecting the glucose-sensing mechanisms of the pancreatic islet cells that result in decreased insulin release (loss of function of the glucose-sensing glucokinase gene) give rise to IUGR. IUGR may be a normal fetal response to nutritional or oxygen deprivation, and the ongoing risk is of malnutrition or hypoxia. Similarly some preterm births need early delivery because of a potentially disadvantageous intrauterine environment. Problems of infants with IUGR are noted in Table 8.13. Other problems include pulmonary hemorrhage and those common in gestational age-related risk of prematurity if born at less than 37 wk.

The most widely used definition of IUGR is a fetus whose estimated weight is below the 10th percentile for its gestational age and whose abdominal circumference is below the 25th percentile. At term, the cutoff birth weight for IUGR is 2,500 g (5 lb, 8 oz). Growth percentiles for fetal weight versus gestational age are shown in Fig. 8.1. Approximately 70 percent of fetuses with a birth weight below the 10th percentile for gestational age are constitutionally small. In the remaining 30 percent, the cause of IUGR is pathologic.

Classification of IUGR: IUGR is classified as reduced growth that is symmetric or asymmetric.
1. *Symmetric IUGR:* In symmetric IUGR the head circumference, length, and weight are equally

affected. Symmetric IUGR often has an earlier onset and is associated with diseases that seriously affect fetal cell number, such as conditions with chromosomal disorders, genetic, malformation, teratogenic, infections or severe maternal hypertensive etiologies. The baby is proportionately

Table 8.12: Causes of intrauterine growth restriction (IUGR)

Fetal	Chromosomal disorders (autosomal trisomies)
	Chronic fetal infections (cytomegalic inclusion disease, congenital rubella, syphilis)
	Congenital anomalies syndrome complexes
	Multiple gestation
	Irradiation
	Pancreatic hypoplasia
	Insulin deficiency
	Insulin like growth factor type 1 deficiency
Placental	Decreased placental weight or cellularity or both
	Decrease in surface area
	Villous placentitis (bacteria, viral, parasitic)
	Infarction
	Placental separation
	Tumor (choreoangioma, hydatidiform mole)
	Twin transfusion syndrome
Maternal	Toxemia
	Hypertension or renal disease or both
	Hypoxemia (high altitude, cyanotic cardiac or pulmonary disease)
	Malnutrition (micro or macronutrient deficiencies)
	Chronic illness
	Sickle cell anemia
	Drugs (narcotics, alcohol, cigarettes, cocaine, antimetabolites

Table 8.13: Problems of IUGR (SGA) infants

Problem	Pathogenesis
Intrauterine fetal demise	Hypoxia, acidosis, infection, lethal anomaly
Perinatal asphyxia	Decreased uteroplacental perfusion during labor ± chronic fetal hypoxia—acidosis, meconium aspiration syndrome
Hypoglycemia	Decreased tissue glycogen stores, decreased gluconeogenesis, hyperinsulinism, increased glucose needs of hypoxia, hypothermia, large brain
Polycythemia—hyperviscosity	Fetal hypoxia with increased erythropoietin production
Reduced oxygen consumption/hypothermia	Hypoxia, hypoglycemia, starvation effect, poor subcutaneous fat stores
Dysmorphology	Syndrome anomaly, chromosomal genetic disorders, oligohydramnios induced deformation, TORCH infection

IUGR: Intrauterine growth restriction; SGA: Small for gestational age; TORCH: Toxoplasmosis, other agents, rubella, cytomegalovirus, hepatitis simplex

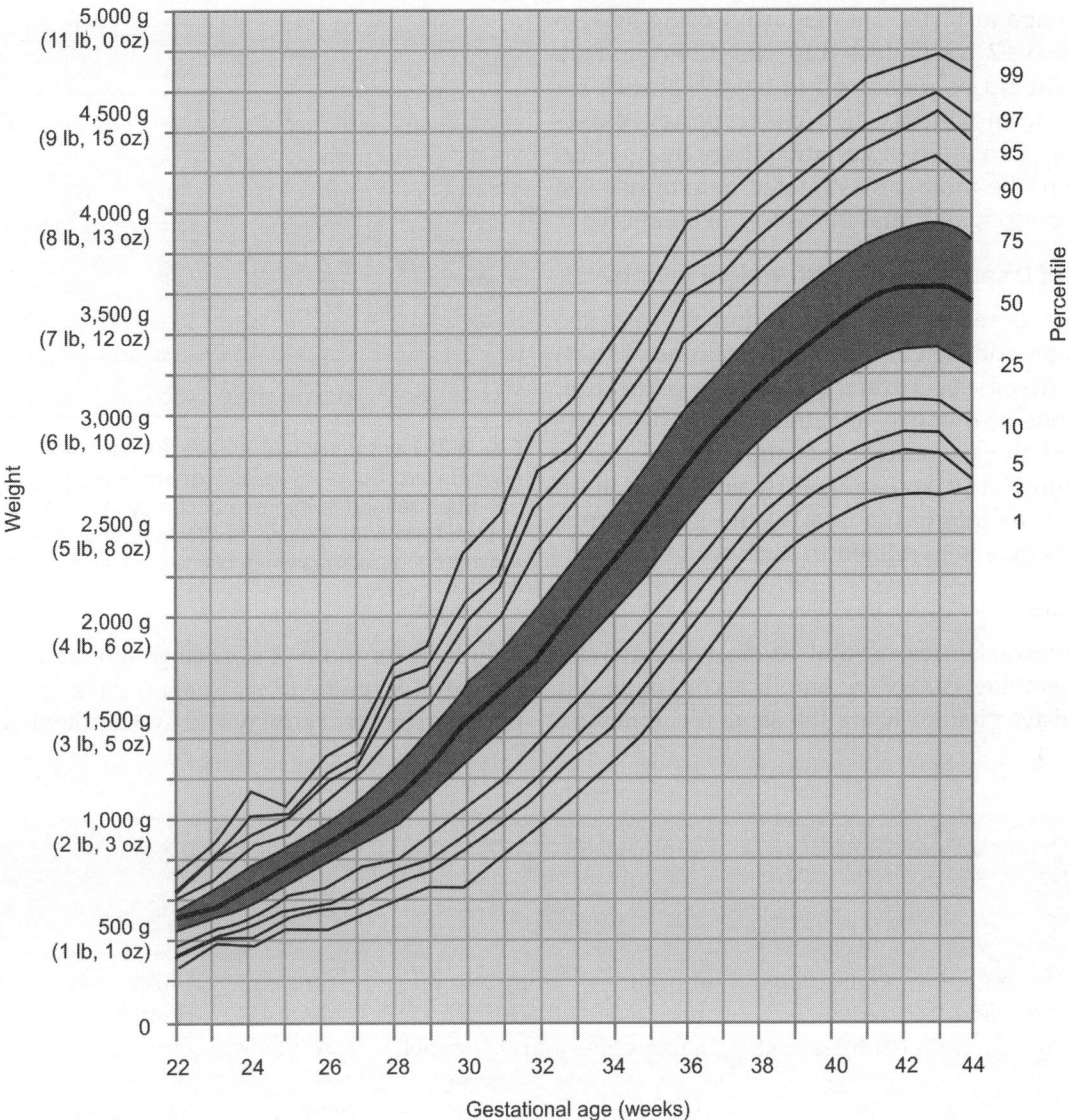

Fig. 8.1: Fetal weight percentiles throughout gestation.

smaller in all parameters, i.e. head circumference, weight and the length.

2. *Asymmetric IUGR:* In asymmetric IUGR there is relative sparing of head growth. Asymmetric IUGR is often of late onset, demonstrates preservation of Doppler waveform velocity to the carotid vessels and is associated with poor maternal nutrition or with late onset or exacerbation of maternal vascular disease (pre-eclampsia, chronic hypertension). The baby appears marasmic with loose folds of skin, a shrunken scaphoid abdomen, large anterior fontanel and an umbilical cord that is twice as thick as in a normal baby. The head appears large and the trunk is under-grown. Their potential for growth is preserved.

Ponderal index (PI) is used for defining newborn babies with intrauterine growth restriction (IUGR). Ponderal index is an index of body mass and is calculated by [birth weight (g) ÷ crown-heel length $(cm)^3$ × 100]. This parameter is usually less than 2 in asymmetrically growth retarded baby and 2 or more in a baby who has either normal growth or has symmetrical growth restriction (length is measured by infantometer in centimetre).

Assessment of Gestational Age at Birth

When compared with a premature infant of appropriate weight, an infant with IUGR has a reduced birth weight, and may appear to have a disproportionately larger head relative to body size; infants in both groups lack subcutaneous fat. Neurological maturity (nerve conduction velocity), in the absence of asphyxia, correlates with gestational age despite reduced fetal weight. Physical signs may be useful in estimating gestational age at birth. The Ballard scoring system is accurate to ±2 wk (Tables 8.14 and 8.15; Fig. 8.2). An infant should be presumed to be at high risk for mortality or morbidity if a discrepancy exists between the estimation of gestational age by physical examination, the mother's estimated date of her last menstrual period, and fetal ultrasonic evaluation.

Spectrum of Disease in Low Birth Weight Infants

Immaturity increases the severity but reduces the distinctiveness of the clinical manifestations of most neonatal diseases. Immature organ function, complications of therapy, and the specific disorders that caused the premature of labor contribute to neonatal morbidity and mortality associated with premature, LBW infants (Table 8.16). In VLBW infants, morbidity is inversely related to birth weight.

Nursery Care

At birth, the measures needed to clear the airway, initiative breathing, care of the umbilical cord and eyes, and administer vitamin K are the same for immature

	-1	0	1	2	3	4	5
Posture							
Square window (wrist)	< 90°	90°	60°	45°	30°	0°	
Arm recoil		180°	140–180°	110–140°	90–110°	<90°	
Popliteal angle	180°	160°	140°	120°	100°	90°	< 90°
Scarf sign							
Heel to ear							

Fig. 8.2: Neuromuscular criteria for maturity. The expanded New Ballard Score includes extremely premature infants and has been refined to improve accuracy in more mature infants. *Source:* Ballard JL, Khoury JC, Wedig K, et al. New Ballard Score, expanded to include extremely premature infants. *J Pediatr* 1991;119: 417–23.

infants as for those of normal weight and maturity (*see* Chapter 8, page-183). Special care is required to maintain a patent airway and avoid potential aspiration

Table 8.14: Physical criteria for maturity. The expanded New Ballard Score includes extremely premature infants and has been refined to improve accuracy in more mature infants

Physical maturity	1	0	1	2	3	4	5
Skin	Sticky, friable, transparent	Gelatinous, red, translucent	Smooth, pink, visible veins	Superficial peeling and/or rash, a few veins	Cracking, pale areas, rare veins	Parchment, deep cracking, no veins	Lethargy, cracked, wrinkled
Lanugo Breast	None Impercep-tible	Sparse Rarely perceptible	Abundant Flat areola—no bud	Thinning Stripped areola, 1–2 mm bud	Bald areas Raised areola, 3–4 mm bud	Mostly bald Full areola, 5–10 mm bud	
Eye/Ear	Lids fused loosely (–1), tightly (–2)	Lids open, pinna flat, stays folded	Slightly curve pinna; soft; slow recoil	Well-curved pinna; soft but ready recoil	Formed and firm, instant recoil	Thick cartilage, ear stiff	
Genitals, male	Scrotum flat and smooth	Scrotum empty, faint rugae	Testes in upper canal, rare rugae	Testes descending, a few rugae	Testes down, good rugae	Testes pendulous, deep rugae	
Genitals, female	Clitoris prominent, labia flat	Prominent clitoris, small labia minora	Prominent clitoris, enlarging minora	Majora and minora equally prominent	Majora large, minora small	Majora cover clitoris and minora	
Plantar surface	Heal-toe 40–50 mm –1< 40 mm^2	< 50 mm, no crease	Faint red marks	Anterior transverse crease only	Creases on anterior 2/3	Creases over the entire sole	

Source: Ballard JL, Khoury JC, Wedig K, et al. New Ballard Score, expanded to include extremely premature infants. *J Pediatr* 1991;119:417–23.

Table 8.15: Maturity rating. The physical and neurologic scores are added to calculate gestational age

Maturity score	Rating weeks	Maturity score	Rating weeks
–10	20	25	34
–5	22	30	36
0	24	35	38
5	26	40	40
10	28	45	42
15	30	50	44
20	32		

Source: Ballard JL, Khoury JC, Wedig K, et al. New Ballard Score, expanded to include extremely premature infants. *J Pediatr* 1991;119:417–23

Table 8.16: Neonatal problems associated with premature infants

Respiratory	Respiratory distress syndrome (hyaline membrane disease—a common problem)
	Bronchopulmonary dysplasia
	Pneumothorax, pneumomediastinum, interstitial emphysema
	Congenital pneumonia
	Pulmonary hypoplasia
	Pulmonary hemorrhage
	Apnea#
Cardiovascular	Patent ductus arteriosus#
	Hypotension
	Hypertension
	Bradycardia (with apnea)#
	Congenital malformations
Hematologic	Anemia (early or late onset)
	Subcutaneous, organ (liver, cranial, adrenal) hemorrhage#
	Disseminated intravascular coagulopathy
	vitamin K deficiency
	Hydrops—immune or nonimmune
Gastrointestinal	Poor gastrointestinal function—poor motility#
	Necrotizing enterocolitis
	Hyperbilirubinemia—direct or indirect#
	Congenital anomalies producing polyhyramnios
	Spontaneous gastrointestinal isolated perforation
Metabolic-Endocrine	Hypocalcemia#
	Hypoglycemia#
	Hyperglycemia#
	Late metabolic acidosis
	Hypothermia#
	Euthyroid but low thyroxine status
Central nervous system	Intraventricular hemorrhage#
	Periventricular leukomalacia
	Hypoxic ischemic encephalopathy
	Seizures
	Retinopathy of prematurity
	Deafness
	Hypotonia#
	Congenital malformations
	Kernicterus (bilirubin encephalopathy)
	Drug (narcotic) withdrawal
Renal	Hyponatremia#
	Hypernatremia#
	Hyperkalemia#
	Renal tubular acidosis
	renal glycosuria
	Edema
Other	Infections#

Common *Source:* Ballard JL, Khoury JC, Wedig K, et al. New Ballard Score, expanded to include extremely premature infants. *J Pediatr* 1991;119:417–23.

of gastric contents, thermal control and monitoring of the heart rate and respiration, oxygen therapy, feeding, and safeguards against infection. Routine procedures that disturb these infants may result in hypoxia. There is need of regular and active participation by the parents in the infant's care in the nursery, where instruction to the mother in at-home care of her infant and regarding the growth and development should also be given.

Thermal control: LBW and sick infants should be cared at or near their *neutral thermal environment.* Incubators or radiant warmers can be used to maintain body temperature. Body heat is conserved through provision of a warm environment and standard conditions of humidity 40–60%. The optimal environmental temperature for minimal heat loss and oxygen consumption of for an unclothed infant is one that maintains the infant's core temperature at 36.5–37.0°C. It depends on an infant's size and maturity; the smaller and more immature the infant, the higher the environmental temperature required. An additional heat shield or head cap and body clothing may be required to keep an extremely LBW (ELBW) preterm infant warm. Infant warmth can be maintained by heating the air to a desired temperature or by servo-controlling the infant's body temperature at a desired set point. Continuous monitoring of the infant's temperature is required so that the environmental temperature can be adjusted to maintain optimal body temperature. Kangaroo mother care is a safe alternative (*see* Boxes 8.2 and 8.3).

Maintaining a relative *humidity* of 40–60% aids in stabilizing body temperature by reducing heat loss at lower environmental temperatures; by preventing drying and irritation of the lining of respiratory passages, especially during the administration of oxygen and after or during endotracheal intubation (usually 100% humidity); and by thinning viscid secretions and reducing insensible water loss from the lungs. An infant should be weaned and then removed from the incubator or radiant warmer only when the gradual change to atmosphere of the nursery does not result in a significant change in the infant's temperature, color, activity, or vital signs.

Oxygen administration: Oxygen is administered to reduce the risk of injury from hypoxia and circulatory insufficiency, but must be balanced against the risk of hyperoxia to the eyes (retinopathy of prematurity) and oxygen injury to the lungs. Oxygen should be administered via a head hood, nasal cannula, continuous positive airway pressure apparatus, or endotracheal tube to maintain stable and safe inspired oxygen concentrations. The concentration of inspired oxygen must be adjusted in accordance with the oxygen tension of arterial blood (PaO_2) or noninvasive methods such as continuous pulse oximetry or transcutaneous oxygen measurements.

Fluid requirements: The fluid requirements vary according to gestational age, environmental conditions, and disease states. Very premature preterm infants (< 1,000 g) may loose as much as 2–3 ml/kg/hr, partly because of immature skin, lack of subcutaneous tissue and a large exposed area. Insensible water loss is increased under radiant warmer, during phototherapy, and in febrile infants. It is diminished when infants are clothed, are covered by a inner heat shield, breathe humidified air, or are of advanced postnatal age. Larger premature infants (2,000–2,500 g) nursed in an incubator may have an insensible water loss of approximately 0.6–0.7 ml/kg/hr. Adequate fluid intake is essential for excretion of the urinary solute load (urea, electrolytes, phosphate). Renal solute loads may vary between 7.5 and 30 mOsm/kg.

Water intake in term infants is usually begun at 60–70 ml/kg on day 1 and increased to 100–120 ml/kg by days 2–3. Smaller, more premature infants may need to start with 70–80 ml/kg on day 1 and advance gradually to 150 ml/kg/day. Daily weights, urine, and serum urea nitrogen and sodium levels should be monitored to determine water balance and fluid needs. Fluid overload may lead to edema, heart failure, patent ductus arteriosus, and bronchopulmonary dysplasia.

Total parenteral nutrition (TPN): Total parenteral nutrition is needed in infants before complete enteral feeding has been established or when enteral feeding is impossible for prolonged periods. Total intravenous alimentation may provide sufficient fluid, calories, amino acids, electrolytes, and vitamins to sustain the growth of LBW infants. TPN has been life-saving technique for VLBW infants and those having intractable diarrheal syndromes or extensive bowel resection. Infusions may be administered through a percutaneously or less often surgically placed indwelling central venous catheter or through a peripheral vein. The umbilical vein may also be used for a short time. The purpose of parenteral alimentation is to deliver sufficient calories from glucose, protein, and lipids to promote optimal growth. The infusate should contain 2.5–3 g/dL of synthetic amino acids, 10–15 g/dL of glucose, fat emulsions such as 20% Intralipid (2.2 kcal/mL) may be administered and *appropriate quantities of electrolytes, trace minerals, and vitamins.* If a peripheral vein is used, the glucose concentration should be kept below 12.5 g/dl; in central vein glucose concentrations as high as 25 g/dl may be used (rarely). Intralipid may be initiated at 0.5 g/kg/24 hr and advanced to 3 g/kg/24 hr, if triglyceride levels remain normal. The contents of each day's infusate should be determined after assessing the infant's clinical and biochemical status. Slow and continuous infusion is advisable.

After a caloric intake of > 100 kcal/kg/24 hr is established by total parenteral intravenous nutrition, LBW infants can be expected to gain about 15 g/kg/24 hr, with a positive nitrogen balance of 150–200 mg/kg/24 hr in the absence of episodes of sepsis, surgical procedures, or other severe stress. This goal can be achieved by peripheral vein infusion of 2.5–3.5 g/kg/24 hr of an amino acid mixture, 10 g/dl of glucose, and 2–3 g/kg/24 hr of intralipid.

Complications of intravenous alimentation are related to both the catheter and metabolism of the infusate. Sepsis is a problem of central vein infusions, caused commonly by coagulase-negative staphylococci. It can be minimized by meticulous catheter care, and aseptic preparation of the infusate; a vancomycin-heparin solution also reduces the risk of line sepsis. Treatment includes appropriate antibiotics and if an infection persists, the line must be removed. Thrombosis, exravasation of fluid, and accidental dislodgment of catheters have also occur. Phlebitis, cutaneous sloughing, superficial infection and sepsis (rarely) may occur. Metabolic complications of parenteral nutrition include hyperglycemia from the high glucose concentration of the infusate, which may lead to osmotic diuresis and dehydration; azotemia; nephrocalcinosis; hypoglycemia from sudden accidental cessation of the infusate; hyperlipidemia and possibly hypoxemia from intravenous lipid infusions; and hyperammonemia, which may be due to high levels of certain amino acids. Metabolic bone disease and/or cholestatic jaundice and liver disease may develop in infants who require long-term parenteral nutrition and receive no enteral nutrition.

Feeding: In feeding LBW infant it is important to avoid fatigue and aspiration of food by regurgitation or by the feeding process. Oral feeding (nipple) should not be initiated or should be discontinued in infants with respiratory distress, hypoxia, circulatory insufficiency, excessive secretions, gagging, sepsis, central nervous system depression, severe immaturity, or signs of severe illness. These high-risk infants require parenteral nutrition or gavage feeding to supply calories, fluids and electrolytes. Oral administration should be considered when in addition to a strong sucking effort, coordination of swallowing, epiglottal, and uvular closure of the larynx and nasal passages, and normal esophageal motility, a synchronized process is present in preterm infants at 34 wk of gestation or more (that is usually absent before 34 wk of gestation). Preterm infants at 34 wk of gestation or more can often be fed by bottle or at the breast. Breast-feeding is less likely to succeed until the infant matures. Bottle-feeding of expressed breast milk may be a temporary alternative. In bottlefeeding, effort may be reduced by use of special small, soft nipples with large holes. Smaller or less vigorous infants should be fed by gavage. A soft plastic tube with No. 5 Fr external and appropriately 0.05 cm internal diameters and with a rounded atraumatic tip and two holes on alternate sides is preferable. The tube is passed through the nose until approximately 2.5 cm (1 inch) of the lower end is in the stomach. The free end of the tube has an adapter into which the tip of a syringe is fitted, and a measured amount of fluid is given by pump or gravity. Such tubes may be left in place for 3–7 days before being replaced by a similar tube through the alternate nostril. Infants occasionally have enough local irritation from an indwelling tube that they may gag or secretions may gather around it in the nasopharynx. In such cases, a catheter may be passed through the mouth and removed at the end of each feeding.

The LBW infant may be fed with intermittent bolus feeding or continuous feeding. In an infant with feeding intolerance, nasojejunal feeding may be successful. Intestinal perforation is a risk with nasojejunal feeding. Gastrostomy feeding is not usually indicated in premature infants except as an adjunct to surgical management of specific gastro-intestinal conditions or in permanently neurologically injured patients unable to suck and swallow normally. A change to breastfeeding or bottle-feeding may be instituted gradually as soon as an infant shows general vigor adequate for oral feeding without fatigue.

Initiation of feeding: The optimal time to introduce enteral feeding to a sick LBW is controversial. *Trophic feeding* is the practice of feeding very small amounts of enteral nourishment to VLBW preterm infants to stimulate development of the immature gastrointestinal tract. The benefits of trophic feeding include enhanced gut motility, improved growth, decreased need for parenteral nutrition, fewer episodes of sepsis, and shortened hospital stays. Once the infant is stable, small-volume feedings are given in addition to intravenous fluids/nutrition. Feeding is gradually advanced and parenteral nutrition decreased. This approach may reduce the incidence of necrotizing enterocolitis. Early feeding of breast milk or formula tends to reduce the risk of hypoglycemia, dehydration, and hyper-bilirubinemia without the additional risk of aspiration, provided that the presence of respiratory distress or other disorders does not present. In an infant who is well, having no distress and making sucking movements, oral feeding may be attempted, although most infants weighing < 1,500 g require tube feeding because they are unable to coordinate breathing, sucking, and swallowing. Intestinal readiness for feeding may be determined by active bowel sounds, passage of meconium, and absence of abdominal distension, bilious gastric aspirates, or emesis.

For infants under 1,000 g, the initial feedings are half-or full-strength breast milk or preterm formula at 10 ml/kg/24 hr as a continuous nasogastric drip (or given by intermittent gavage every 2–3 hr). If the initial feeding is tolerated, the volume is increased by 10–15 ml/kg/24 hr. The daily milk volume increment should not exceed 20–30 ml/kg/24 hr. Once a volume of 150 ml/kg/24 hr has been achieved, the caloric content may be increased to 24 or 27 kcal/oz. Intravenous fluids are needed until feedings provide approximately 120 ml/kg/24 hr. The feeding protocol for premature infants weighing over 1,500 g is initiated at a volume of 20–25 ml/kg/24 hr of breast milk or preterm formula given as a bolus every 3 hr. Increments in total daily formula volume should not exceed 20 ml/kg/24 hr. The expected weight increments for premature infants of various birth weights are shown in Fig. 8.3.

Regurgitation, vomiting, abdominal distension or gastric residuals from previous feedings should arouse suspicion of sepsis, necrotizing enterocolitis, or intestinal obstruction. A change in the feeding schedule is indicated and increase subsequent feedings slowly or to change to intravenous alimentation and consider for more serious problems. Weight gain may not be achieved for 10–12 days, and a daily intake of 130–150 ml/kg or more may be necessary for some infants. In vigorous infants whose feeding schedule is advanced successfully in calories or volume, weight gain may appear within a few days.

When tube feeding is used, the contents of the stomach should be aspirated before each feeding. If only air or small amounts of mucus are obtained, the feeding should be continued as planned. If all or a substantial part of the previous feeding is aspirated, the amount of the feeding should be reduced and proceed more gradually with subsequent increases in feeding amounts.

The digestive enzyme systems of infants older than 28 wk gestation are mature and adequate digestion and absorption of protein and carbohydrate occur. Fat is less well absorbed, primarily because of inadequate amounts of bile salts; unsaturated fats and the fat of human milk are absorbed better than those of cow's milk. The weight gain of infants weighing under 2,000 g at birth should be adequate when human milk or "humanized" milk premature formula (40% casein

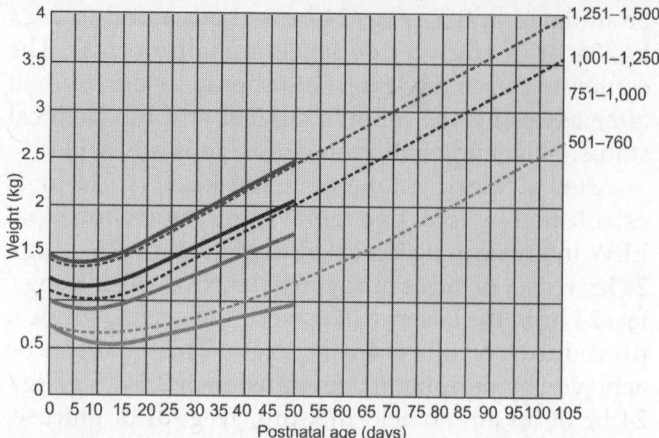

Fig. 8.3: Average daily weight (kg) vs postnatal age (days) for infants with birth weight ranges of 501–750 g, 751–1,000 g, 1,001–1,250 g, and 1,251–1,500 g (*dotted lines*), plotted with the curves of Dancis and colleagues for infants with birth weights of 750 g, 1,000 g, 1,250 g, 1,500 g (*solid lines*). *Source:* Wright K, Dawson JP, Fallis D, et al. New postnatal growth grids for very low birth weight infants. *Pediatrics* 1993;91:922–6.

and 60% whey) with a protein intake of 2.25–2.75 g/kg/24 hr is fed. These two alternatives should provide all amino acids essential for premature infants including tyrosine, cystine, and histidine. Higher protein intake may be well tolerated and is generally safe, especially in older rapidly growing infants. Protein intake as high as 4–5 g/kg/24 hr may be hazardous. High-protein formulas may cause abnormal plasma aminograms, elevations in blood urea nitrogen, ammonia, and sodium concentrations; metabolic acidosis (cow's milk formulas); and untoward effects on neurologic development.

Breast milk from the infant's mother is the preferred milk for all infants, including VLBW infants. In addition to nutritional advantages, the benefits of breast milk include protection against a wide range of infections (through both specific and nonspecific anti-infective factors in breast milk and beneficial effects on intestinal flora), a decreased risk of necrotizing enterocolitis in preterm infants, a lower risk of sudden infant death syndrome, and lower risk of childhood/adolescent obesity and improved neurodevelopmental outcome. Once a premature infant takes 120 ml/kg/24 hr, breast milk fortifiers are added to supplement breast milk with protein, calcium and phosphorus. If breast milk is unavailable, special preterm formulas should be used. An approximately 34–36 wk gestation, infants who are not receiving breast milk should be switched to a term formula (unless metabolic bone disease is present) because hypercalcemia may develop as a result of the preterm formula's higher calcium and vitamin D levels.

Although formula in amounts necessary for adequate growth probably contains adequate quantities of all vitamins, the volume of milk sufficient to satisfy these requirements may not be ingested by the LBW infant for several weeks. Therefore, LBW infants should be given supplemental vitamins. Because requirements for these infants have not been precisely established, the recommended daily allowances for term infants should be given. Furthermore, these infants may have a special need for certain vitamins such as vitamin C needed partly for intermediary metabolism of phenylalanine and tyrosine; decreased vitamin D and other fat soluble vitamins and calcium due to decreased fat absorption with increased fecal fat loss (VLBW infants are prone to develop osteopenia, but their total intake of vitamin D should not exceed 1,500 IU/24 hr); folic acid, essential for the formation of DNA and production of new cells; vitamin E functions as an antioxidant; vitamin K deficiency results in hemorrhagic disease of the newborn.

In LBW infants, physiologic anemia as a result of postnatal suppression of erythropoiesis is exacerbated by smaller fetal iron stores and greater expansion of blood volume from the more rapid growth than that of term infants and the anemia develops earlier. Fetal or neonatal blood loss accentuates this problem. Iron stores, even in VLBW neonates, are usually adequate until an infant's birth weight has doubled; iron supplementation (2 mg/kg/24 hr) should then be started. If erythropoietin is used, iron supplementation is also required.

Premature infants may have from 1 to 6 daily stools of semisolid consistency. It is a matter of concern if there is sudden increase in the number of stool, change to a watery consistency or appearance of occult or gross blood. Premature infants should not vomit or regurgitate. They should be satisfied and relaxed after a feeding but may normally show the activity of hunger shortly before the next feeding.

Management of inadequate weight gain: Inadequate weight gain is a common and pertinent problem in LBW infants. Management consists of the following steps:

1. Counseling and adequate support for breastfeeding positioning/attachment, managing sore/flat nipple, etc.
2. Explain the frequency and timing of both breastfeeding and spoon feeds and importance of demand feeding and night-feeding.
3. Giving expressed breast milk (EBM) by spoon after breastfeeding also helps in preterm infants who tire out easily while sucking from the breast.

4. Proper demonstration of the correct method of expression of milk and spoon feeding.
5. Initiate fortification of breast milk when indicated.

Prevention of infection: Premature infants have an increased susceptibility to infection. Preventive measures include strict compliance with hand washing and universal precautions, limiting nurse-to-patient ratio and avoiding crowding, minimizing the risk of catheter contamination, meticulous skin care, encouraging early appropriate advancement of enteral feeding, education and feedback to staff, and surveillance of nosocomial infection rates in the nursery. Universal precautions require gloves to be worn with all patient contact. No one with an active infection should be permitted in nursery. Preventing transmission of infection from infant to infant is difficult because neither term nor premature newborn infants have clear clinical evidence of an infection.

Early and frequent participation by parents in the nursery care of their infant does not significantly increase the risk of infection when preventive precautions are maintained. Routine immunizations should be given on the regular schedule at standard doses (*see* Section 15.1, page-428).

Immaturity of drug metabolism: Renal clearance of almost all substances excreted in the urine is diminished in newborn infants, but more so in premature ones. The glomerular filtration rate increases with increasing gestational age, therefore, drug dosing recommendations vary with age. Intervals between doses should be extended when administering drugs excreted chiefly by the kidneys. Drugs detoxified in the liver or requiring chemical conjugation before renal excretion should also be given with caution and in doses smaller than usual. When possible, blood levels should be determined for potentially toxic drugs, especially if renal or hepatic dysfunction is present. Decisions about the choice, dose and route of administration of antibacterial agents should be considered keeping in mind the dangers of:

1. Development of infections with organisms resistant to antibacterial agents
2. Inhibition of the intestinal bacteria that manufacture significant amounts of essential vitamins (vitamin K and thiamine), and
3. Harmful interference in important metabolic processes. Many drugs apparently safe for adults on the basis of toxicity studies may be harmful to newborn infants, especially premature ones.

Prognosis: Infants born weighing 1,501–2,500 g have a 95% or greater chance of survival, but those weighing less have significantly high mortality. The post-discharge mortality rate of LBW infants is higher than that of term infants during the 1st 2 yr of life, mostly due to infection (respiratory syncytial virus). In addition, premature infants have an increased incidence of failure to thrive, sudden infant death syndrome, child abuse, and inadequate maternal-infant bonding. Congenital anomalies are present in approximately 3–7% LBW infants.

In the absence of congenital abnormalities, central nervous system injury, VLBW, or marked IUGR, the physical growth of LBW infants tends to approximate that of term infants by the 2nd yr; it occurs earlier in premature infants with larger birth size. VLBW infants may not catch up, especially if they have severe chronic sequelae, insufficient nutritional intake, or an inadequate caretaking environment (Table 8.17). Many surviving LBW infants have hypotonia before 8 mo corrected age, which improves by the time they are 8 months to 1 yr old. Infants with IUGR (SGA) who grow poorly and do not demonstrate catch-up growth may benefit from recombinant human growth hormone therapy beginning at age 4 yr. The greater the immaturity and the lower the birth weight, the greater the likelihood of intellectual and neurologic deficit; as many as 50% of 500–750 g infants have a significant neurodevelopmental impairment (blindness, deafness, mental retardation, cerebral palsy). Small head circumference at birth may be similarly related to a poor neurobehavioral prognosis. Factors associated with a risk for poor academic performance include birth weight below 750 g, severe IVH, periventricular leukomalacia, bronchopulmonary dysplasia, cerebral atrophy, post-hemorrhagic hydrocephalus, IUGR, low socioeconomic status, and possibly, low thyroxine levels. Adolescents who were VLBW report satisfactory health, are mostly integrated in regular classes despite neurosensory disabilities (hearing, vision, cerebral palsy, cognition).

Premature and IUGR infants are also at risk for significant metabolic conditions (obesity, type II diabetes mellitus) and cardiovascular disorders (ischemic heart disease, hypertension) as adults. This fetal origins hypothesis of adult morbidities may be due to insulin resistance, which may be evident in early childhood.

Predicting neonatal mortality: Birth weight and gestational age have been used as strong indicators for the risk of neonatal death. Survival at 22 wk of gestation is poor, particularly in those infants requiring aggressive resuscitation in the delivery room. Clinical judgment (based on birth weight, illness severity, low Apgar score, bronchopulmonary dysplasia, IUGR, therapeutic requirements) provide reasonable information regarding the risk of mortality.

Discharge from the hospital: Before discharge from the hospital, a **premature infant** should be taking all nutrition by nipple, either breast or bottle. Some medically fragile infants may be discharged home on gavage feedings after the parents have received appropriate nursing and education. Growth should be occurring at steadily increments of approximately 10–30 g/24 hr. Temperature should be stabilized in an open crib. Infants should have had no recent episodes of apnea or bradycardia, and parenteral drug administration should have been discontinued or converted to oral dosing. Stable patients recovering from bronchopulmonary dysplasia may be discharged on a regimen of oxygen given by nasal cannula as long as follow-up is arranged with frequent pulse oximetry monitoring and outpatient visits. All infants with birth weight under 1,500 g and those between 1,500 and 2,000 g with an unstable course requiring oxygen should have an eye examination to screen for retinopathy of prematurity. All LBW infants should

Table 8.17: Sequelae of low birth weight	
Immediate	*Late*
Hypoxia, ischemia	Mental retardation, spastic diplegia, microcephaly, seizures, poor school performance
Intraventricular hemorrhage	Mental retardation, spasticity, seizures, hydrocephalus
Sensorineural injury	Hearing, visual impairment, retinopathy of immaturity, strabismus, myopia
Respiratory failure	Bronchopulmonary dysplasia, cor pulmonale, bronchospasm, malnutrition, subglottic stenosis, iatrogenic cleft palate, recurrent pneumonia
Necrotizing enterocolitis	Short bowel syndrome, malabsorption, malnutrition, infectious diarrhea
Cholestatic liver disease	Cirrhosis, hepatic failure, hepatic carcinoma, malnutrition
Nutrient deficiency	Osteopenia, fracture, anemia, vitamin E, growth failure
Social stress	Child abuse or neglect, failure to thrive, divorce
Other	Sudden infant death syndrome, infections, inguinal hernia, cutaneous scars (chest tube, patent ductus arteriosus ligation, intravenous infiltration), gastroesophageal reflux, hypertension, craniosynostosis, cholelithiasis nephrocalcinosis, cutaneous hemangiomas

have hearing test prior to discharge. Those who had indwelling umbilical arterial catheters should have their blood pressure examined for renal vascular hypertension. The hemoglobin level or hematocrit should be checked to evaluate for possible anemia. If all major medical problems have resolved and the home setting is adequate, premature infants may then be discharged when their weight approaches 1,800–2,100 g; close follow-up plus easy access to health care providers is essential for early discharge protocols. In case the medical or social environment is not ideal, high-risk neonates who have been transported to neonatal intensive care units and whose major illness has resolved may be returned to their hospital of birth for an additional period of hospitalization. Standard vaccinations with full doses should commence after discharge or, if in the hospital, with vaccines that do not contain live viruses.

Home care: The mother should receive instruction on how to care for the baby after discharge from the hospital. Ideally, at least one visit to her home for evaluating domestic arrangements and advising about any needed improvements.

Post-term Infants

Post-term infants are those born after 42 wk of gestation, as calculated from the mother's last menstrual period, regardless of weight at birth. Approximately 25% of all pregnancies end on or after the 287th day of gestation, 12% on or after the 294th day, and 5% on or after the 301st day. The cause of post-term birth or postmaturity is unknown. Large size of the infant correlates poorly with late delivery but does correlate with large size of either parent, multigravidity, or a prediabetic or diabetic state in the mother.

Clinical manifestations: Post-term infants may be clinically indistinguishable from term infants, but some infants are designated as postmature because their appearance and behavior suggest that they are 1–3 wk of age. These post-term infants, postmature characteristic findings are listed in Box 8.11. If placental insufficiency occurs, the amniotic fluid and fetus may be meconium stained, and abnormal fetal heart rates may be observed; the infant may have growth retardation. Although this syndrome is frequently confused with postmaturity, only about 20% of infants with placental insufficiency syndrome are post-term. The majority of these affected are term and preterm infants particularly those SGA who are infants of toxemic mothers, older primigravidas, and women with chronic hypertension. The placentas are often small or poorly attached. This syndrome results from degenerative changes in the placenta that progressively reduces oxygen and nourishment to the fetus.

Infants born post-term in association with presumed placental insufficiency may have physical signs, including desquamation, long nails, abundant hair, pale skin, alert faces, and loose skin especially around the thighs and buttocks, give them the appearance of having recently lost weight; meconium-stained nails, skin, vernix, umbilical cord, and placental membranes may also be noted.

Prognosis: When delivery is delayed 3 wk or more beyond term, mortality is significantly increased. Mortality can be lowered markedly through improved obstetric management.

Treatment: Obstetric monitoring, including nonstress testing, biophysical profile, or Doppler velocimetry, usually provides a rational basis for choosing a course of nonintervention, induction of labor or cesarean section. Induction of labor or cesarean may be indicated in older primigravidas who go more than 2–4 wk beyond term, particularly if fetal distress is present. Newborns having any medical problem should be treated.

Large for Gestational Age

The mortality rates increases after 4,000 g birth weight. These oversized infants are usually born at term, but preterm infants with weights high for gestational age also have a significantly higher mortality than do infants of the same size born at term. Maternal diabetes mellitus and obesity are the predisposing factors. Infants large for gestational age, regardless of their gestational age have higher incidence of birth injuries and congenital anomalies (Table 8.18).

Infant Transport

High risk neonates should be transported to neonatal intensive care units (NICU) in hospitals at which they are not born. Ideally, high-risk mothers should be transported to and their babies delivered at centers where these specialized units are located. Neonate

---

Box 8.11: Characteristic findings of post-term, postmature infants

Increased birth weight (often)
Absence of lanugo
Decreased or absent vernix caseosa
Long nails
Abundant scalp hair
White parchment-like or desquamating skin
Increased alertness

should be transported after securing an airway, providing oxygen, assisting with infant ventilation, providing antimicrobial therapy, maintaining the circulation, providing a warmed environment, and placing intravenous or arterial lines or chest tubes should all be initiated, if indicated, before transport. Infant and maternal records, laboratory reports, and a tube of clotted maternal blood should also be provided. Before departing, the mother should be reassured and allowed to see her stabilized infant, if practical; the father should follow the transport vehicle to the unit. The transport officer or nurse should also call ahead to inform the receiving unit about the nature of the patient's illness.

The transport vehicle should be equipped with appropriate medicines, fluids, oxygen cylinders, catheters, chest tubes, endotracheal tubes, laryngoscopes, and an infant warming device. It should be well illuminated and have ample room for emergency procedures and monitoring equipment. With efficient transport and proper nursing and medical staff at the referring hospitals, the mortality of "outborn" neonates should not be more than those born within the tertiary care center.

Baker P, Tower C. Fetal growth, intrauterine growth restriction and small-for-gestational-age babies. In: Rennie JM (ed). *Roberton's Textbook of Neonatology*. 4th edn. London: Elsevier, Churchill Livingstone, 2005;167–76.

Bland RD. The Newborn Infant. In: Rudolph C D, Rudolph A (eds). *Rudolph's Textbook of Pediatrics*. 21st edn. New York: McGraw Hill, 2003;55–222.

Garite TJ, Clark R, Thorp JA. Intrauterine growth restriction increases morbidity and mortality among premature neonates. *Am J Obstet Gynecol* 2004;191:481–87.

Gilbert WM, Danielsen B. Pregnancy outcomes associated with intrauterine growth restriction. *Am J Obstet Gynecol* 2003; 188:1596–601.

Jain N, Jain VM. Feeding and Nutrition, Fluids Electrolyte Management. In: Jain N, Jain VM (eds). *The Neonate*. New Delhi: Aditya Medical Publishers, 2003; 63–77.

Mathur NB, Krishnamurthy Sriram. Very Low Birth Weight and Extremely Low Birth Weight Infants. In: Mathur GP, Mathur Sarla (eds). *Current Trends in Pediatrics*. Vol 3. Delhi: Academa Publishers, 2007;20–29.

Shah NK, Mathur NB. Neonatal resuscitation. *IAP-NNF Guidelines 2006 on Level II Neonatal Care*. Delhi: UNICEF, 2006; 1–13.

Stoll BJ, Adams-Chapman I. The high-risk infant. In: Kliegman RM, Behrman RE, Jenson HB, Stanton BF (eds). *Nelson Textbook of Pediatrics*. 18th edn. Vol 1. Philadelphia: Saunders, 2007;683–711.

Tucker J, McGuire W. Epidemiology of preterm birth *Br Med J* 2004;329:675–78.

Walther F, Ramaekers L. The ponderal index is a measure of nutritional status at birth and its relation to some aspects of neonatal morbidity. *J Perinatal Medicine* 1982;10:42–47.

8.7 HYPOXIC-ISCHEMIC ENCEPHALOPATHY

Hypoxic-ischemic encephalopathy (HIE) is an important cause of mortality in neonatal period and those survive suffer from permanent neurodevelopmental abnormalities (cerebral palsy, mental retardation). The greatest risk of adverse outcome is seen in infants with fetal acidosis (pH < 7.0), a 5 min Apgar score of 0–3, hypoxic-ischemic encephalopathy (altered tone, depressed level of consciousness, seizures), and other multi-organ system signs.

Etiology: Most neonatal encephalopathic or seizure disorders, in the absence of major congenital malformations or syndromes, are due to perinatal events rather than prenatal events. *Fetal hypoxia* may be caused by various disorders in the mother, including:

1. Inadequate oxygenation of maternal blood from hypoventilation during anesthesia, cyanotic heart disease, respiratory failure, or carbon monoxide poisoning.
2. Low maternal blood pressure, from acute blood loss, spinal anesthesia, or compression of the vena cava and aorta from the gravid uterus.
3. Inadequate relaxation of the uterus to permit placental filling as a result of uterine tetany caused by the administration of excessive oxytocin.
4. Premature separation of the placenta.

Table 8.18: Birth injuries and congenital anomalies in large for gestational age infants

Birth injuries	Congenital anomalies#
Cervical injuries	Congenital heart disease
Brachial plexus injuries	Intellectual and developmental retardation
Phrenic nerve damage with paralysis of the diaphragm	
Fractured clavicles	
Cephalhematomas	
Subdural hematomas	
Ecchymoses of the head and face	

Statistically more common than in infants of appropriate weight for gestational age.

5. Impedance to the circulation of blood through the umbilical cord as a result of compression or knotting of the cord, and
6. Placental insufficiency from toxemia and postmaturity.

After birth, hypoxia may be caused by:
1. Failure of oxygenation as a result of severe forms of cyanotic congenital heart disease or severe pulmonary disease.
2. Anemia severe enough to lower the oxygen content of the blood (severe hemorrhage, hemolytic disease), and
3. Shock severe enough to interfere with the transport of oxygen to vital organs from overwhelming sepsis, massive blood loss, and intracranial or adrenal hemorrhage.

Clinical manifestations: Intrauterine growth restriction (IUGR) with increased vascular resistance may be the first indication of fetal hypoxia. *During labor* the fetal heart rate slows, and beat-to-beat variability declines. Continuous heart rate recording may reveal a variable or late (type II) deceleration pattern, and fetal scalp blood analysis may show a pH < 7.20. The acidosis usually has both metabolic and respiratory components. In infants near term, these signs should lead to the administration of high concentrations of oxygen to the mother and immediate delivery to avoid fetal death or CNS damage.

At delivery the presence of yellow, meconium-stained amniotic fluid indicates that fetal distress has occurred. At birth, these infants are frequently depressed and fail to breathe spontaneously. During the ensuing hours they may remain hypotonic, or change from hypotonic to hypertonic, or their tone appear normal.

After delivery hypoxia is due to respiratory failure and circulatory insufficiency. The severity of neonatal encephalopathy depends on the duration and timing of injury. Symptoms develop over a series of days (Table 8.19). During the initial hours after an insult, infants have depressed level of consciousness, periodic breathing with apnea, bradycardia, and hypotonia, but may pass to stage 3. It is, therefore, important to perform serial neurological examination.

Diagnosis: No specific test excludes or confirms a diagnosis of HIE. The diagnosis is based on the history and physical examination. Choice of tests (serum electrolytes, renal function studies [serum creatinine, creatinine clearance, and BUN] and echocardiography depends on the evolution of symptoms). Test results should be interpreted in conjunction with clinical history and the findings of physical examination.

Ultrasound provides a quick assessment of brain lesions, although its utility in evaluation of hypoxic injury in the term infants is limited; it is the preferred modality in evaluation of the preterm infant. CT scans are helpful in identification of local hemorrhagic, diffuse cortical injury, and damage to the basal ganglia, but it has limited ability to identify cortical injury within the 1st few days of life. Diffusion-weighed MRI is the preferred imaging modality because of its increased sensitivity and specificity early in the process and its ability to outline the topography of the lesion.

Amplitude integrated EEG (aEEG) determines which infants are at highest risk for significant brain injury. Continuous aEEG monitoring detects sub-clinical seizures during the subacute phase.

In infants with HIE, a hearing test is preferable because of an increased incidence of deafness among HIE infants requiring assisted ventilation and retinal

Signs	Stage 1	Stage 2	Stage 3
Table 8.19: Sarnat and Sarnat stages of hypoxic-ischemic encephalopathy (HIE) in term infants			
Level of consciousness	Hyperalert	Lethargic	Stuporous, coma
Muscle tone	Normal	Hypotonic	Flaccid
Posture	Normal	Flexion	Decerebrate
Tendon reflexes/clonus	Hyperactive	Hyperactive	Absent
Myoclonus	Present	Present	Absent
Moro reflex	Strong	Weak	Absent
Pupils	Mydriasis	Miosis	Unequal, poor light reflex
Seizures	None	Common	Decerebration
Electroencephalographic	Normal	Low voltage, changing to seizure activity	Burst suppression to isoelectric
Duration	< 24 hr if progressive; otherwise, may remain normal	24 hr to 14 days	Days to weeks
Outcome	Good	Variable	Death, severe deficits

and ophthalmic examination may be valuable, particularly as part of an evaluation for developmental abnormalities of the brain.

Treatment: Systemic or selective cerebral hypothermia for acute management of HIE may be neuroprotective. The optimal level of hypothermia for maximal neuroprotection is not known. Extreme hypothermia may cause significant systemic side effects.

Up to 48–72 hr of cooling may be needed to prevent secondary neuronal loss. The greater the severity of the initial injury, the longer the duration of hypothermia needed for optimal neuroprotection. Cooling must be begun early, within 1 hr of injury, if possible; however, favorable outcome may be possible if cooling is begun up to 6 hr after injury. Selective cerebral hypothermia, cools the head, is not effective in infants with the most severe aEEG findings, but is effective in those with less severe aEEG changes. Some investigators believe that total body cooling may be superior to selective head cooling. Hypothermia may cause significant side effects, including coagulation defects, leukocyte malfunctions, pulmonary hypertension, and worsening of metabolic acidosis.

Seizures should be treated early and be well controlled, since even asymptomatic seizures (i.e. seen only on EEG) may continue to injure the brain. Seizures should be treated with phenobarbital (the drug of choice), which is given with an intravenous loading dose (20 mg/kg); additional doses of 5–10 mg/kg (up to 40–50 mg/kg total) may be needed. Phenytoin (20 mg/kg loading dose) or lorazepam (0.1 mg/kg) may be needed for refractory seizures. This may need continuous electroencephalographic monitoring. Phenobarbital levels should be monitored 24 hr after the loading dose and maintenance therapy (5 mg/kg/hr) are begun. Therapeutic phenobarbital levels are 20–40 μg/ml. Seizures in asphyxiated newborns may also be due to hypocalcemia, hypoglycemia, or infection and should be appropriately treated.

Maintain adequate ventilation, perfusion, and metabolic status; most infants with HIE need ventilatory support during the first week. Prevent hypoxia, hypercapnia, and hypocapnia; the latter is due to inadvertent hyperventilation, which may lead to severe hypoperfusion of the brain. Maintain the blood gases and acid–base status in the physiological ranges including partial pressure of arterial oxygen (PaO$_2$), 80–100 mm Hg; partial pressure of arterial carbon dioxide (PaCO$_2$), 35–40 mm Hg; and pH, 7.35–7.45.

Maintain the mean BP above 35 mm Hg (for term infants). Dopamine or dobutamine can be used to maintain adequate cardiac output.

Fluid, electrolyte, and nutritional status should be monitored and corrected and adequate calories and proteins provided.

Avoid hypoglycemia or hyperglycemia, as both are known to cause brain injury. In the first 2 days of life, restrict intravenous fluids to two-thirds of the daily requirement for gestational age and nursing environment. When infants begin to improve, urinary output increases, and fluid administration must be adjusted.

In most cases (particularly in moderately severe and severe HIE), the infant is restricted to nothing by mouth (NPO) during the first 3 days of life or until the general level of alertness and consciousness improves. Begin trophic feeding with expressed breast milk or dilute formula about 5 ml every 3–4 hr. Monitor abdominal girth and the composition of stools and for signs of gastric retention; any of these may be an early indicator of necrotizing enterocolitis, for which infants with perinatal asphyxia are at high risk. Individualize increments in feeding volume and composition.

Close physical therapy and developmental evaluation are needed before discharge. Severely disabled children may need to be monitored in multispecialty clinics and by a developmental neurologist.

Prognosis: Accurate prediction of the severity of long-term complications is difficult, although the following pointers may be used:
1. Lack of spontaneous respiratory effort within 20–30 minutes of birth is associated with almost uniform mortality.
2. The presence of seizures is an ominous sign, particularly if seizures occur frequently and are difficult to control.
3. Abnormal clinical neurological findings such as hypotonia, rigidity, weakness persisting beyond the first 7–10 days of life usually indicate poor prognosis.
4. Persistent feeding difficulties also suggest significant CNS damage.
5. Poor head growth during the postnatal period and the first year of life predicts higher frequency of neurologic deficits.

Adams-Chapman I, Stoll BJ. Nervous system disorders. In: Kliegman RM, Behrman RE, Jenson HB, Stanton BF (eds). *Nelson Textbook of Pediatrics.* 18th edn. Vol 1. Philadelphia: Saunders, 2007;713–722.

Rennie JM. Assessment of the neonatal nervous system. In: Rennie JM. *Roberton's Textbook of Neonatology.* 4th edn. London: Elsevier, Churchill Livingstone, 2005:1093–105.

Sarnat HB, Sarnat MS: Neonatal encephalopathy following fetal distress: A clinical and electroencephalographic study. *Archives of Neurology* 1976;33:696–705.

Sarnat HB, Sarnat MS. Neonatal encephalopathy following fetal distress: A clinical and electroencephalographic study. *Arch Neurol* 1976;33:695–705. Copyright 1976 American Medical Association.

8.8 BIRTH TRAUMA

The birth process is a blend of compression, contractions, torques, and traction. When fetal size, presentation, or neurologic immaturity complicates this event, such intrapartum forces may lead to tissue damage, edema, hemorrhages, or fractures in the neonate. The use of obstetric instrumentation may further amplify the effects of such forces or may induce injury alone. Under certain conditions, delivery by cesarean delivery can be an acceptable alternative, but it does not guarantee an injury-free birth. Factors predisposing to birth injury are listed in Box 8.12.

Caput succedaneum is a serosanguineous, subcutaneous, extraperiosteal fluid collection with poorly defined margins; it is caused by the pressure of the presenting part against the dilating cervix. Caput succedaneum extends across the midline and over suture lines and is associated with head molding. Caput succedaneum does not usually cause complications and usually resolves over the first few days. Analogous swelling, discoloration, and distortion of the face are seen in face presentation. Management consists of observation only.

Cephalohematoma is a subperiosteal collection of blood secondary to rupture of blood vessels between the skull and the periosteum; suture lines delineate its extent. Most commonly parietal, cephalohematoma may occasionally be observed over the occipital bone. Resolution occurs within 2 wk–3 mo, depending on their size, occasionally with residual calcification. They may begin to calcify by the end of the 2nd wk. A few remain for yr as bony protuberances and are detectable by X-ray as widening of the diploic space.

Subgaleal hematoma is bleeding in the potential space between the skull periosteum and the scalp galea aponeurosis. Ninety percent of cases result from vacuum applied to the head at delivery. Subgaleal

hematoma has a high frequency of occurrence of associated head trauma, such as intracranial hemorrhage or skull fracture.

Sternocleidomastoid (SCM) injury is also referred to as congenital or muscular torticollis. Torticollis can arise during delivery as the muscle is hyperextended and ruptured, with development of a hematoma and subsequent fibrosis and shortening. Torticollis may be present at birth with a palpable 1 to 2 cm mass in the SCM region and head tilt to the side of the lesion. More often it is noted at 1 to 4 wk of age. Facial asymmetry may be present on the side of the lesion. Prompt treatment may lessen or correct the torticollis.

Intracranial hemorrhage (IVH) in the newborn may result from trauma or asphyxia and, rarely from a primary hemorrhagic disturbance or congenital vascular anomaly. IVH falls into four grades. The higher the grade, the more severe is the bleeding. Grades I and II involve a small amount of bleeding and do not usually cause long-term problems. Grades III and IV involve more severe bleeding, which presses on or leaks into brain tissue. Blood clots can form and block the flow of cerebrospinal fluid, leading to increased fluid in the brain (hydrocephalus).

Spine and spinal cord injury incurred during delivery results from excessive traction or rotation. Traction is more important in breech deliveries and torsion is more significant in vertex deliveries. The lower cervical and upper thoracic region for breech delivery and the upper and midcervical region (most commonly at the level of the 4th cervical vertebra) for vertex delivery are the major sites of injury. There is stillbirth or neonatal death with failure to establish adequate respiratory function. Treatment of the survivors is supportive; patients often remain permanently disabled.

Peripheral nerve injuries include brachial plexus injury, phrenic nerve paralysis, facial nerve palsy, and laryngeal nerve injury. Brachial plexus injuries occur frequently with shoulder dystocia or breech delivery. In *Erb-Duchenne paralysis*, the injury occurs in the 5th and 6th cervical nerves. The characteristic position consists of adduction and internal rotation of the arm with pronation of forearm. The infant cannot abduct the arm from shoulder, rotate the arm externally, and supine the forearm; the Moro reflex is absent on the affected side. The outer aspect of the arm may have some sensory impairment. Power in the forearm and hand grasp is preserved unless the lower part of the plexus is also injured; the presence of the grasp reflex is a favorable prognostic sign. If there is injury to the phrenic nerve, alteration in diaphragmatic excursion may be observed fluoroscopically. In *Klumpke paralysis*, injury to the 7th and 8th cervical

Box 8.12: Factors predisposing to birth injury

Prima gravida
Cephalopelvic disproportion, small maternal stature, maternal pelvic anomalies
Prolonged or rapid labor
Deep transverse arrest of descent of presenting part of the fetus
Oligohydramnios
Abnormal presentation (breech)
Use of midcavity forceps or vacuum extraction
Versions and extractions
Very low birth weight infant or extreme prematurity
Fetal macrosomia
Large fetal head
Fetal anomalies

nerves and the 1st thoracic nerve produces a paralyzed hand (weakness of the intrinsic muscles of the hand; grasp reflex is absent) and ipsilateral ptosis and miosis (*Horner syndrome*) if the sympathetic fibres of the 1st thoracic root are also injured. **Treatment** consists of partial immobilization and appropriate positioning to prevent the development of contractures. If the paralysis persists without improvement for 3–6 mo, neuroplasty, neurolysis, end-to-end anastomosis, and nerve grafting should be considered.

Phrenic nerve paralysis: Phrenic nerve injury (3rd, 4th, 5th cervical nerves) with diaphragmatic paralysis must be considered when cyanosis and irregular and labored respirations develop.

Facial nerve palsy: Facial palsy is usually a peripheral paralysis that results from pressure over the facial nerve *in utero*, from efforts during labor, or from forceps use during delivery. The prognosis depends on whether the nerve was injured by pressure or whether the nerve fibers are torn. Improvement occurs within a few weeks when facial nerve was injured by pressure.

Laryngeal nerve injury: Disturbance of laryngeal nerve function may affect swallowing and breathing. Laryngeal nerve injury appears to result from an intrauterine posture in which the head is rotated and flexed laterally.

Skeletal injuries: Fractures are most often observed following breech delivery and/or shoulder dystocia in macrosomia infants. The clavicle is the most frequently fractured bone in the neonate during birth. Loss of spontaneous arm or leg movement is an early sign of long bone fracture, followed by swelling and pain on passive movement. Separation of humeral or femoral epiphysis occurs through the hypertrophied layer of cartilage cells in the epiphysis.

Intra-abdominal injuries: Hemorrhage is the most serious acute complication, and the liver is the most commonly damaged internal organ. Intra-abdominal injuries are liver hematoma, splenic hematoma, adrenal hemorrhage, and renal hemorrhage.

Soft tissue injuries include petechiae and ecchymoses, lacerations and abrasions (may be secondary to scalp electrodes and fetal scalp sampling or injury during birth), and subcutaneous fat necrosis.

Abdulhayoglu E. Birth Trauma. In: Cloherty JP, Eichenwald EC, Stark AR (eds). *Manual of Neonatal Care.* 6th edn. Philadelphia: Lippincott Williams & Wilkins, 2008;228–36.

Adams-Chapman I, Stoll BJ. Nervous system disorders. In: Kliegman RM, Behrman RE, Jenson HB, Stanton BF (eds). *Nelson Textbook of Pediatrics.* 18th edn. Vol 1. Philadelphia: Saunders, 2007;713–22.

Rennie JM. Assessment of the neonatal nervous system. In: Rennie JM. *Roberton's Textbook of Neonatology.* 4th edn. London: Elsevier Churchill Livigstone, 2005:1093–105.

Schullinger JN: Birth trauma. *Pediatr Clin North Am* 1993; 40(6): 1351–58.

Uhing MR. Management of birth injuries. *Clin Perinatal* 2005; 32:19–38.

Volpe JJ: Injuries of extracranial, cranial, intracranial, spinal cord, and peripheral nervous system structures. In: *Neurology of the Newborn.* 3rd edn. Philadelphia: WB Saunders Company, 1995;769–92.

8.9 RESPIRATORY SYSTEM DISORDERS

Hyaline Membrane Disease (HMD) or Respiratory Distress Syndrome (RDS)

HMD almost always occurs in preterm babies often less than 34 wk of gestation. It is the commonest cause of respiratory distress in a preterm neonate. The overall incidence is 10–15% but can be as high as 80% in neonates < 28 wk. In addition to prematurity, asphyxia, acidosis, maternal diabetes and cesarean section can increase the risk of developing HMD.

Etiopathogenesis: In HMD the basic abnormality is surfactant deficiency. Surfactant is a lipoprotein containing phospholipids like phosphatidylcholine (lecithin) and phosphatidylglycerol and proteins. Surfactant is produced by type II alveolar cells and helps to reduce surface tension in the alveoli. In the absence of surfactant, surface tension increases and alveoli collapse during expiration. During inspiration more negative pressure is needed to keep alveoli patent. There is inadequate oxygenation and increased work of breathing. Hypoxemia and acidosis result in pulmonary vasoconstriction and right to left shunting across the foramen ovale. This worsens the hypoxia and the neonate eventually goes into respiratory failure. Ischemic damage to the alveoli causes transudation of proteins into the alveoli.

Clinical manifestations: Respiratory distress usually occurs within the first 6 hr of life. Clinical features include tachypnea, retractions, grunting, cyanosis, and decreased air entry. Diagnosis can be confirmed by chest X-ray. Radiological features of HMD include reticulogranular pattern, ground glass opacity, low lung volume, air bronchogram, and a whiteout lung in severe disease.

Prenatal diagnosis can be made by determining the L/S (Lecithin/Sphingomyelin) ratio in the amniotic fluid. L/S ratio > 2.0 indicates adequate lung maturity. A simple bedside test, **shake-test** can be done on the amniotic fluid or gastric aspirate to determine lung maturity. The gastric or amniotic fluid is mixed with absolute alcohol and shaken for 15 seconds and allowed to settle. Copious bubbles are formed in the presence of adequate surfactant indicating extent of lung maturity.

Management: The basic defect requiring treatment is inadequate pulmonary exchange or oxygen and carbon dioxide; metabolic acidosis and circulatory insufficiency are secondary manifestations.

Oxygen therapy: Warm, humidified oxygen is given with a head box preferably with a FiO_2 meter and pulse oximeter monitoring to determine the amount of oxygen required. Soft nasal cannulae may also be used to give oxygen. Small changes in FiO_2 (fraction of inspired oxygen) are made and monitored on the pulse oximeter. At saturation of 90–95%, the PaO_2 (arterial partial pressure of oxygen) may be between 60 to 98 mm Hg and above 95% saturation, PaO_2 is well above 100 mm Hg. Clearing of airway, ensuring adequate breathing and circulation are the first line of management. A baby in obvious respiratory distress needs to be on continuous pulse oximeter monitoring to decide when intubation and ventilation is required.

Surfactant replacement therapy: Surfactant is the drug of choice in a baby with HMD. This may be given either prophylactically at birth if the baby is less than 28 wk of gestation or within the first two hours of onset of symptoms in older babies. Prophylactic surfactant is given in the labor room after the baby has been stabilized. Rescue therapy is most effective if given within the first two hours of birth. Surfactant is given in a dose of 100 mg/kg through the endotracheal tube in small aliquots with intermittent bagging to prevent desaturation during administration and it should be followed by ventilatory support.

Respiratory support: Respiratory support is given in the form of continuous positive airway pressure (CPAP) or intermittent mandatory ventilation (IMV). Short nasal or longer nasopharyngeal prongs are preferred to endotracheal CPAP as latter markedly increases the work of breathing and tires the infant. CPAP should be started early in a preterm with HMD. Indications for starting CPAP are a Downes' or Silverman score of > 6 at birth or a FiO_2 requirement of > 0.4 to maintain an acceptable saturation on pulse oximeter. CPAP is a gentler form of non-invasive ventilatory support as compared to IMV. CPAP is said to have failed when the FiO_2 requirement is >0.6 or the pressure required to maintain oxygenation exceeds 7–8 cm of H_2O.

Intermittent mandatory ventilation (IMV): Time cycled pressure limited ventilation is the modality of choice for ventilation of a neonate in respiratory failure. Respiratory failure is defined a $PaCO_2$ > 60 mm or PaO_2 < 50 mm Hg or saturation < 85% in 100% O_2 with or without a pH of < 7.25. If patient-triggered ventilation is used it is given as synchronized intermittent mandatory ventilation (SIMV) or assist control mode ventilation (ACMV). For best outcomes this should be given to babies in impending respiratory failure or failed CPAP rather than in complete respiratory failure

Supportive Therapy

a. *Fluid and electrolyte management:* Electrolyte balance, fluids, calcium and glucose homeostasis are all equally important. Fluids are usually started at a minimum of 60 ml/kg/day of 10% dextrose or three fourth of daily maintenance which ever is more. This will ensure a glucose infusion rate of about 4 mg/kg/min which is the minimum required for adequate glucose homeostasis. Excess fluid administration may cause pulmonary edema and increases the risk for a symptomatic PDA. By the second day usually add sodium (2–3 mEq/kg/day), potassium (1 mEq/kg/day), and calcium in the dose of 4–8 mL/kg/day of calcium gluconate to the fluids.

b. *Nutritional support* is essential in the care of infants with respiratory insufficiency. Parenteral nutrition should be initiated as soon after birth as possible to prevent catabolism and to promote postnatal growth and healing. Enteral nutrition should be initiated as soon as the patient is likely to tolerate it in order to further optimize nutrient uptake and to decrease the risk of infection from long-standing indwelling intravenous catheters.

c. *Maintenance of adequate hemoglobin:* Any neonate with respiratory distress should have a hematocrit above 40%. Packed cell transfusion should be given to maintain hematocrit above 40%.

d. *Antibiotics:* Since pneumonia can duplicate the signs of RDS; preterm babies with respiratory distress should be started on broad spectrum antibiotics after obtaining blood cultures and complete blood counts.

e. *Closure of patent ductus arteriosus (PDA):* PDA in premature babies can prolong the course of HMD. Therapeutic closure of PDA with indomethacin (0.1–0.2 mg/kg every 12–24 hours—3 doses) is indicated in cases of a symptomatic PDA in any premature infant, or may be considered for any asymptomatic but persistent PDA by Doppler evaluation in an extremely premature infant. Prophylactic therapy with indomethacin (0.1 mg/kg every 24 hr—3 doses) started within 12 hr after birth to prevent PDA is frequently used in extremely premature infants (28 wk gestation). Contraindications to indomethacin therapy include thrombocytopenia (< 50,000/mm^3), bleeding disorders, oliguria (1 ml/kg/hr), necrotizing enterocolitis, isolated intestinal perforation, and an elevated plasma creatinine level (> 1.8 mg/dL). Early closure also decreases the incidence of bronchopulmonary dysplasia (BPD).

Prognosis: With good intensive care in a neonatal intensive care unit (NICU), the outcome of neonates with respiratory distress has improved remarkably in the past decade with a survival rate of > 60% in babies weighing > 1,000 g.

Transient Tachypnea of Newborn (TTN)

Transient tachypnea of the newborn is a benign, self-limiting disease occurring usually in term neonates. It is due to delayed clearance of lung fluid. These babies have tachypnea with minimal or no respiratory distress. Respiratory rate is commonly 60–80/min but sometimes 100/min. Chest X-ray may show prominent perihilar markings, vascular markings and prominent interlobar fissure. Oxygen treatment is often adequate and ventilatory support is not required. Tachypnea usually resolves in 2–3 days. Prognosis is good.

Meconium Aspiration

Meconium staining of amniotic fluid occurs in 10–15% of pregnancies. Neonates born to mother with thick or thin meconium stained liquor can aspirate the meconium into the lungs and develop respiratory distress. This is known as meconium aspiration syndrome (MAS). Aspiration of meconium can occur *in utero*, during birth or immediately after birth. Thick meconium can cause chemical pneumonitis. Thick meconium aspiration can block the large and small airway causing areas of atelectasis and emphysema which can progress to develop air leak syndromes like pneumothorax.

Clinical manifestations and course: MAS usually occur in post mature and small for date babies. Respiratory distress usually develops in the first 24 hr of life; if untreated distress can progress to respiratory failure. Complications include pneumothorax, other air leak syndromes (pneumo-pericardium, pneumomediastinum) and persistent pulmonary hypertension. Chest X-ray shows hyperinflation and patchy infiltration.

Management: IV fluids and oxygen are needed for mild distress and ventilatory support for severe disease. Potential therapies include surfactant replacement. Steroids have no definite role. Assisted ventilation should be provided early when respiratory failure is impending. Infants with MAS are ventilated with high flow rates, reduced positive end-expiratory pressure (PEEP), and short inspiratory time to reduce

trapping. Hyperventilation is used to wash out CO_2 and produce alkalosis when persistent pulmonary hypertension of the newborn (PPHN) sets in. ECMO (extracorporeal membrane oxygenation) and iNO (inhaled nitric oxide) are the other modalities.

Prevention: All babies born to mother with meconium stained liquor should have oropharyngeal suction before delivery of shoulder. Immediately after delivery endotracheal suction should be done in non-vigorous babies. This is done to prevent postnatal aspiration of meconium into the lungs.

Prognosis: The mortality rate of meconium-stained infants is considerably higher than that of non-stained infants.

Aspiration of Foreign Material (Fetal Aspiration Syndrome, Aspiration Pneumonia)

During prolonged labor and difficult deliveries, infants often initiate vigorous respiratory movements *in utero* because of interference with the supply of oxygen through the placenta. Under such circumstances, the infant may aspirate amniotic fluid containing vernix caseosa, epithelial cells, meconium, blood, or material from the birth canal, which may block the smallest airways and interfere with alveolar exchange of oxygen and carbon dioxide. Pathogenic bacteria may accompany the aspirated material, and pneumonia may ensue. Roentgenographic findings will show coarsely granular pattern with irregular aeration.

Postnatal pulmonary aspiration may also occur in newborn infants as a result of tracheoesophageal fistula, esophageal and duodenal obstruction, gastroesophageal reflux, improper feeding practices, and administration of depressant medicines.

To avoid aspiration of gastric contents, the stomach should be aspirated using a soft catheter just before surgery or other major procedures that require anesthesia or conscious sedation. In case the aspiration is sudden and overwhelming, immediate laryngoscopy and suctioning under direct visualization may prevent the aspirated material from reaching the lungs. The treatment of aspiration pneumonia includes respiratory support and systemic antibiotics. Gradual improvement generally occurs over 3–4 days.

Pneumonia

Pneumonia may be caused by infections acquired transplacentally, during birth process, and postnatally. Premature rupture of membranes, i.e. more than 24 hrs, unclean vaginal examinations, foul smelling liquor, febrile maternal illness, fetal hypoxia and prolonged labor are possible risk factors. Viral infections transmitted by transplacental route include enteroviruses, adenoviruses, influenza viruses, rubella virus, varicella-zoster virus, herpes simplex virus, cytomegalovirus and HIV. Transplacental bacterial infections caused by *L. monocytogenes, M. tuberculosis,* or *T. pallidum* are less common than viral infections. Neonatal pneumonia is most commonly acquired during birth process. Group B Streptococcus is the most common pathogen; other pathogens (e.g. gram-negative enteric bacteria) are less common. Most common viral agents acquired during birth process are herpes simplex virus and cytomegalovirus. *C. trachomatis* is also acquired during delivery and usually presents at 2–8 wk of age with persistent cough and absence of fever and wheezing. History of conjunctival infection may or may not exist.

Inadequate hand washing and exposure to respiratory equipment or humidified incubators may contribute to infection, especially with *S. aureus* and gram-negative enterobacteria.

Other causes of postnatal infections include respiratory syncytial virus, parainfluenza viruses, influenza viruses, herpes simplex virus, cyto-megalovirus, and fungi (*C. albicans*). Infants with pneumonia present with respiratory distress. Chest radiography shows interstitial or alveolar infiltrates or consolidation. With suspected bacterial pneumonia in newborn, blood and spinal fluid cultures should be performed and treatment should begin immediately while awaiting culture results.

Pulmonary Air Leaks

It refers to the group of disorders in which air escapes through ruptured alveoli into any of several potential spaces. Air leak can occur spontaneously, secondary to pulmonary disease, or as a complication of mechanical ventilation. Extra-alveolar air may compress air spaces, resulting in decreased lung compliance and respiratory insufficiency. Prompt recognition and evacuation can be life-saving. Pneumothorax occurs spontaneously in as many as 1% of live births, and complicates 5–10% cases of RDS and 20% cases of MAS. Other locations of air leaks are pneumomediastinum, pneumopericardium, pneumo-peritoneum, and pulmonary interstitial emphysema (PIE). PIE is a unique form of air leak in which air from ruptured alveoli dissects into perivascular spaces, causing hyperinflation of non-gas-exchanging areas of the lungs.

Pulmonary Hemorrhage

About 5–10% of neonatal autopsies show evidences of pulmonary hemorrhage. Predisposing factors in neonatal period include perinatal asphyxia, septicemia with DIC, and mechanical ventilation, especially in those with respiratory distress syndrome. Accom-panying respiratory distress is bloody fluid, which oozes from nose, mouth, or endotracheal tube. Treatment includes blood replacement, PEEP (positive end-expiratory pressure), suctioning to clear the airway, intratracheal administration of epinephrine, and in some cases HFV (high-frequency ventilation). Mechanical ventilation with high PEEP helps to decrease the leakage of blood in alveoli and prevent collapse. Depending on the severity of bleeding, chest radiography may show spectrum of findings ranging from patchy infiltrates to opacification of lungs.

Bronchopulmonary Dysplasia (BPD)

Diagnosis is suspected when a preterm neonate continues to have respiratory distress and remains oxygen or ventilator dependent for long time. Criteria for diagnosis are oxygen requirement beyond 36 wk post-conceptional age or beyond 28 days of life. BPD occurs because of barotrauma, volutrauma and oxygen toxicity. This causes damage to the alveolar cells. Inflammatory mediators are released and there is increased permeability causing leakage of water and protein. In late stage, there is fibrosis and cellular hyperplasia. Severe lung damage leads to respiratory failure. These babies continue to require prolonged ventilation and oxygen therapy. Diuretics may improve respiratory function in infants with BPD but care should be taken to maintain electrolyte homeostasis. Corticosteroids may help in weaning ventilator settings. Long or multiple courses are associated with worse neuro-developmental outcome (especially cerebral palsy) in premature infants and should be avoided. Systemic vs. inhaled steroids dosing is under investigation. Bronchodilators such as salbutamol may improve respiratory mechanics in infants with established chronic lung disease; however, excessive dosing can lead to tachyarrhythmias.

Apnea

Apnea may be defined as cessation of respiration for 20 seconds with or without bradycardia and cyanosis or bradycardia. Apnea is a common problem in preterm neonates. It could be central, obstructive or mixed. Apnea of prematurity occurs in preterm neonates between the 2nd and 5th days of life and is because of the immaturity of the developing brain. Central apnea can also occur because of pathological cause like sepsis, metabolic problem (hypoglycemia, hypocalcemia), temperature instability, respiratory distress, anemia and polycythemia. Obstructive apnea can occur because of block to the airway by secretion, improper positioning, etc. Treatment is supportive and correction of underlying cause. Drugs used include aminophylline, caffeine and doxapram. In unresponsive case, continuous positive airway pressure may be required. Prognosis is good in apnea of prematurity. In other cases it depends on the underlying cause.

Upper Airway Obstruction

The newborn may be born with stridor or may develop it later. It may be constant or intermittent and with or without respiratory difficulty. Feeding difficulty and choking may be associated with stridor due to any cause such as choanal atresia, micrognathia/retrognathia/Pierre Robin sequence, laryngomalacia, laryngeal atresia, laryngeal webs, subglottic stenosis, esophageal atresia, extrinsic airway compression (vascular rings and slings, teratomas and cystic hygromas, hemangiomas), trauma (vocal cord paralysis caused by birth or surgical trauma, bilateral paralysis can cause severe respiratory distress).

Persistent pulmonary hypertension of the newborn (persistent fetal circulation, *see* Section 19.1.

Bhutani VK. Differential diagnosis of neonatal respiratory disorders. In:Spitzer AR (ed). *Intensive care of fetus and neonate.* Mosby year book 1996;494–505.

Dudell GG, Stoll BJ. Respiratory tract disorders. In: Kliegman RM, Behrman RE, Jenson HB, Stanton BF (eds). *Nelson Textbook of Pediatrics.* 18th edn. Vol 1. Philadelphia: Saunders, 2007;728–53.

Greenough A, Robertson MRC. Acute respiratory disease in the newborn. In: Rennie JM (ed). *Textbook of Neonatology.* 4th edn. China: Churchill Livingstone, 2005;512–7.

Singh M, Deorari AK. Pneumonia in the newborn. *Indian J Pediatr* 1995;62:293–306.

8.10 GASTROINTESTINAL DISORDERS

Neonatal Necrotizing Enterocolitis (NEC)

NEC is the most common life-threatening emergency of the gastrointestinal tract in the newborn period. The incidence of NEC is 1–5% of infants in neonatal intensive care unit (NICU).

Pathology and pathogenesis: The cause of NEC remains unclear but is most likely multifactorial. Many factors may contribute to the development of a necrotic segment of intestine, gas accumulation in the submucosa of the bowel wall (pneumatosis intestinalis), and progression of the necrosis to perforation, peritonitis, sepsis and death. The distal part of the ileum and the proximal segment of the colon are involved most frequently; in fatal cases, the gangrene may extend from the stomach to the rectum. The triad of intestinal ischemia (injury), enteral nutrition (metabolic substrate), and pathogenic organisms has been linked to NEC. Coagulation necrosis is the characteristic histologic finding of intestinal specimens. Various bacterial and viral agents, including *Escherichia coli*, *Klebsiella*, *Clostridium perfringens*, *Staphylococcus epidermidis*, and rotavirus, have been recovered from cultures, but in most cases no pathogen is identified. The greatest risk factor for NEC is prematurity, rarely occurs in term infants. NEC rarely occurs before the initiation of enteral feeding and is less common in infants fed human milk. Aggressive enteral feeding may predispose to the development of NEC.

Clinical manifestations: The clinical features of NEC can be divided into systemic and abdominal signs. Most infants have a combination of both. *Systemic signs* include respiratory distress, apnea, and/or brady-cardia, lethargy, temperature instability, irritability, poor feeding, hypotension (shock), decreased peripheral perfusion, acidosis, oliguria, and bleeding diathesis. *Abdominal (enteric) signs* include bloody stools, abdominal distension or tenderness, gastric aspirates (feeding residuals), vomiting (of bile, blood, or both), ileus (decreased or absent bowel sounds), abdominal wall erythema or induration, persistent localized abdominal mass, or ascites.

The course of the disease varies among infants. Most frequently, it will appear as fulminant, rapidly progressive presentation of signs consistent with intestinal necrosis and sepsis, or as a slow, paroxysmal presentation of abdominal distension, ileus, and possible infection.

Diagnosis: Early diagnosis of NEC is the most important factor in determining outcome. A very high index of suspicion in treating preterm at-risk infants is crucial. The finding of pneumatosis intestinalis (air in the bowel wall) confirms the clinical suspicion of NEC and is diagnostic. Portal venous gas is a sign of severe disease, and pneumoperitoneum indicates a perforation. Hepatic ultrasonography may detect portal venous gas despite normal abdominal roent-genograms. Triad of thrombocytopenia, persistent metabolic acidosis, and severe refractory hypo-natremia confirms the diagnosis. Serial measurements of C-reactive protein (CRP) may also be helpful in the diagnosis and assessment of response to therapy of severe NEC. Analysis of stool for blood and carbohydrate has been used to detect infants with NEC. Although grossly bloody stools may be an indication of NEC, occult hematochezia does not correlate well with NEC. Carbohydrate malabsorption as reflected in a positive stool Clinitest result can be a frequent and early indicator of NEC. Bell staging criteria with the Walsh and Kleigman modification contributes uniformity of diagnosis and treatment based on severity of illness (Table 8.20).

Differential diagnosis: The differential diagnosis of NEC includes specific infections (systemic or intestinal), gastrointestinal obstructions, volvulus and isolated intestinal perforations. Idiopathic focal intestinal perforation can occur spontaneously or after the early use of postnatal steroids and indomethacin. Pneumoperitoneum develops in such patients, but they are usually less ill than those with NEC.

Treatment: Rapid initiation of therapy is required for suspected as well as proven NEC cases. The therapy is directed at supportive care and preventing further injury with cessation of feeding, nasogastric decompression, and administration of intravenous fluids. Careful attention to respiratory status, coagulation profile, and acid–base and electrolyte balance are important in managing these cases (Table 8.20). Once blood is drawn for culture, systemic antibiotics (with broad coverage based on the antibiotic sensitivity patterns of the gram-positive, gram-negative, and anaerobic organisms in the neonatal ICU) should be started immediately. If present, umbilical catheters should be removed while maintaining good intravenous access. Ventilation should be assisted in the presence of apnea or if abdominal distension is contributing to hypoxia and hypercapnia. Intravascular volume replacement with crystalloid or blood products, cardiovascular support with volume and/or inotropes, and correction of hematologic, metabolic, and electrolyte abnormalities are essential to stabilize the infant.

The patient's course should be monitored closely by performing frequent physical assessments; sequential anteroposterior and cross-table lateral or lateral decubitus abdominal X-rays to detect intestinal

Table 8.20: Management of necrotizing enterocolitis		
Bell staging criteria	*Diagnosis*	*Management#*
Stage I (suspect)	Clinical signs and symptoms Nondiagnostic radiograph	NPO with IV fluids Nasogastric drainage CBC KUB q 6–8 hr × 48 hr Blood culture Stool heme test and Clinitest Ampicillin and gentamicin × 48 hr
Stage II (definite)	Clinical signs and symptoms Pneumatosis intestinalis on radiograph Mildly ill Moderately ill with systemic toxicity	NPO with parenteral nutrition (by CVL once sepsis is ruled out) Nasogastric drainage CBC KUB (AP and lateral) q 6–8 hr × 48–72 hr, then pm Blood culture Stool heme test and Clinitest Ampicillin, gentamicin, and clindamycin × 14 days Surgical consultation
Stage III (advanced)	Clinical signs and symptoms Critically ill Pneumatosis intestinalis or pneumoperitoneum on radiograph Impending IP Proven IP	NPO with parenteral nutrition (by CVL once sepsis is ruled out) Nasogastric drainage CBC KUB (AP and lateral) q 6–8 hr × 48–72 hr, then pm Stool heme test and Clinitest Ampicillin, gentamicin, and clindamycin × 14 days Surgical consultation, with intervention, if indicated. Resection with enterostomy or primary anastomosis in selected cases (usually < 1,000 g and unstable) bedside drainage under local anesthesia

AP : Anteroposterior; CBC : Complete blood count; CVL : Central venous line; IP : Isolated intestinal perforation; KUB : Kidney, ureter, bladder X-ray; NPO : Nothing by mouth.
Usual attention to respiratory, cardiovascular and hematologic resuscitation presumed.

perforation, and serial determination of hematologic, electrolyte, and acid–base status.

Indications for surgery include evidence of perforation on abdominal roentgenograms (pneumoperitoneum) or positive abdominal paracentesis (stool or organism on Gram stain from peritoneal fluid). Ideally, surgery should be performed after intestinal necrosis develops, but before perforation and peritonitis occurs. Peritoneal drainage may be helpful for patients who are too unstable to undergo surgery (Section 8.10).

Prognosis: Medical management fails in about 20–40% of patients with pneumatosis intestinalis at diagnosis; of these, 10–30% die. Early postoperative complications include wound infection, dehiscence, and stomal problems (prolapse, necrosis). Late complications include **intestinal strictures** that develop at the site of the necrotizing lesion in about 10% of surgically or medically managed patients. Resection of the obstructing stricture is curative. After massive intestinal resection, complications from postoperative NEC include short bowel syndrome (malabsorption, growth failure, malnutrition), complications related to central venous catheters (sepsis, thrombosis), and cholestatic jaundice. There is increased risk for adverse growth and neurodevelopmental outcome in those premature infants with NEC who require surgical intervention or who have concomitant bacteremia.

Prevention: Exclusively breastfed newborn infants have a reduced risk of NEC. Early initiation of aggressive feeding may increase the risk of NEC in VLBW infants, whereas a gut stimulation protocol of minimal enteral feeds followed by judicious volume advancement may decrease the risk. Prebiotic preparations have also decreased the incidence of NEC.

Eichenwald EC. Necrotizing Enterocolitis. In: Cloherty JP, Eichenwald EC, Stark AR (eds). *Manual of Neonatal Care*. 6th edn. Philadelphia: Lippincott Williams & Wilkins, 2008;608–15.

Jaundice and Hyperbilirubinemia in the Newborn

Jaundice is observed approximately in 60% term infants and in 80% of preterm infants during the first week of life. Jaundice may be present at birth or may appear at anytime during the neonatal period, depending on the cause. The neonatal production rate of bilirubin is 6–8 mg/kg/24 hr in contrast to 3–4 mg/kg/24 hr in adults. Bilirubin is of two types: unconjugated and conjugated. Unconjugated bilirubin (designated *indirect* acting by nature of the van den Bergh reaction) is an end product of heme-protein catabolism from a series of enzymatic reactions by hemeoxygenase and biliverdin reductase and non-enzymatic reducing agents in the reticuloendothelial cells. Unconjugated bilirubin by the enzyme uridine diphosphoglucuronic acid (UDP)-glucuronyl transferse that has undergone conjugation in the liver cell microsome form conjugated bilirubin [water-soluble glucuronide of bilirubin (direct reacting)].

The bilirubin may have a physiologic role as an antioxidant. The unconjugated bilirubin is neurotoxic for infants at certain concentrations and under various conditions. Conjugated form is not neurotoxic but it indicates a potentially serious hepatic disorders or systemic illnesses.

Etiology: Unconjugated hyperbilirubinemia may be caused or increased by any factor that:
1. Increases the load of bilirubin to be metabolized by the liver (hemolytic anemia, polycythemia, shortened red cell life as a result of immaturity or transfused cells, increased extrahepatic circulation, infection)
2. Damages or reduces the activity of the transferase enzyme or other isolated enzymes (genetic deficiency, hypoxia, infection, or thyroid deficiency
3. Competes for or blocks the transferase enzyme (drugs, and other substances requiring glucuronic acid conjugation); or
4. Leads to an absence or decreased amounts of the enzyme or to reduction of bilirubin uptake by liver cells (genetic defect or prematurity).

Toxic effects of elevated serum levels of unconjugated bilirubin are increased by factors that reduce the retention of bilirubin in the circulation (hypoproteinemia, displacement of bilirubin from its binding sites on albumin by competitive binding of drugs such as sulfisoxazole and moxalactam, Chuen-Lin herbal tea, acidosis, and increased free fatty acid concentration secondary to hypoglycemia, starvation, or hypothermia). Neurotoxic effects are directly related to the permeability of the blood–brain barrier and nerve cell membranes, and also to neuronal susceptibility to injury, all of which are adversely influenced by asphyxia, prematurity, hyperosmolality, and infection. Early and frequent feeding decreases, whereas breastfeeding and dehydration increase serum levels of bilirubin. Delay in passage of meconium, which contains 1 mg bilirubin/dl, may contribute to jaundice by enterohepatic circulation after deconjugation by intestinal glucunidase. Drugs such as oxytocin and chemicals used in the nursery such as phenolic detergents may also produce unconjugated hyperbilirubinemia.

Clinical manifestations and laboratory evaluation: Jaundice may be present at birth or may appear at anytime during the neonatal period, depending on etiology (Table 8.21). Jaundice usually becomes apparent in a cephalocaudal progression starting on the face and progressing to the abdomen and then feet, as serum levels increase. Dermal pressure may reveal the anatomic progression of jaundice (face, ~ 5 mg/dL; mid-abdomen, ~15 mg/dL; soles, ~ 25 mg/dL), but this clinical examination cannot be depended on to estimate serum levels. Jaundice to the mid-abdomen, signs or symptoms, high-risk factors that suggest nonphysiologic jaundice, or hemolysis must be evaluated further (Tables 8.21 and 8.22). Transcutaneous of bilirubin (TcB) measurement that correlates with serum levels may be used to screen infants, but determination of serum bilirubin level is indicated in patients with elevated age-specific transcutaneous measurement, progressing jaundice, or risk for either hemolysis or sepsis. Jaundice from deposition of indirect bilirubin in the skin tends to appear bright yellow or orange, whereas jaundice of the obstructive type (direct bilirubin) has a greenish or muddy yellow cast. Signs of kernicterus rarely appear on the 1st day; affected infants may present with lethargy and poor feeding and, without

Table 8.21: Causes of jaundice in the neonatal period (based on first appearance of jaundice)

At birth or appears with in the first 24 hr
Erythroblastosis fetalis
Concealed hemorrhage
Sepsis
Congenital infections, including syphilis, cytomegalovirus, rubella, and toxoplasmosis
Intrauterine blood transfusions for erythroblastosis fetalis

2nd or 3rd day
Physiologic
Familial nonhemolytic icterus (Crigler-Najjar syndrome)
Early-onset breastfeeding jaundice

After 3rd day and within the 1st week of life
Bacterial sepsis
Urinary tract infections
Other infections (syphilis, cytomegalovirus, toxoplasmosis, enterovirus)
Extensive ecchymosis or hematoma especially in premature infants#
Polycythemia

After the 1st week of life
Breast milk jaundice
Septicemia
Congenital atresia or paucity of bile ducts
Hepatitis
Galactosemia
Hypothyroidism
Cystic fibrosis (CF)
Congenital hemolytic anemia (spherocytosis, pyruvate kinase and other glycolytic enzyme deficiencies, hereditary nonspherocytic anemia)
Drug induced hemolytic anemia (as in congenital deficiencies of enzymes glucose-6-phosphate dehydrogenase [G6PD], glutathione synthetase, reductase, or peroxidase)

Persistent jaundice during the 1st month of life
Inspissated bile syndrome (which may follow hemolytic disease of the newborn)
Hyperalimentation-associated cholestasis
Hepatitis
Cytomegalic inclusion disease
Syphilis
Toxoplasmosis
Familial non-hemolytic icterus
Congenital atresia of the bile ducts
Galactosemia
Rarely, physiologic jaundice may be prolonged for several weeks, as in infants with hypothyroidism or pyloric stenosis

#Jaundice may occur during the first day or later.

treatment, can progress to acute bilirubin encephalopathy. Jaundice and hyperbilirubinemia is discussed under four headings:
1. Physiologic jaundice (icterus neonatorum)
2. Pathological hyperbilirubinemia
3. Jaundice associated with breastfed infants, and
4. Kernicterus

Differential diagnosis: The causes of jaundice in the neonatal period are mentioned in Table 8.21. Jaundice consisting of either indirect or direct bilirubin that is present at birth or appears within the 1st 24 hr of life requires immediate attention. Hemolysis is suggested by a rapid rise in serum bilirubin > 5 mg/dl/hr, anemia, pallor, reticulocytosis, hepatosplenomegaly, and a positive family history. In infants who have received intrauterine transfusions for erythroblastosis fetalis may have jaundice due to usually high proportion of direct-reacting bilirubin.

Full-term, low risk, asymptomatic infants may be evaluated by monitoring total serum bilirubin (TSB) levels. A complete diagnostic evaluation (determination of direct and indirect bilirubin fractions, hemoglobin, reticulocyte count, blood type, Coombs test, and peripheral blood smear) should be performed in patients with significant hyperbilirubinemia and those with symptoms or signs, regardless of gestation or time of appearance of jaundice (Table 8.22).

1. *Physiologic jaundice (Icterus neonatorum):* Under normal circumstances, the level of indirect-reacting bilirubin in umbilical cord serum is 1–3 mg/dl and rise at a rate of < 5 mg/dl/24 hr; thus, jaundice becomes visible on the 2nd–3rd day, usually peaking between the 2nd and 4th days at 5–6 mg/dl and decreasing to below 2 mg/dl between the 5th and 7th days of life. Jaundice associated with these changes is designated *physiologic* and results from increased bilirubin production from the breakdown of fetal red blood cells combined with transient limitation in the conjugation of bilirubin by the immature neonatal liver. In premature infants the rise in serum bilirubin tends to be the same or somewhat slower but of longer duration than in term infants. Peak levels of 8–12 mg/dl are not usually reached until the 4th–7th day, and jaundice is infrequently observed after the 10th day, corresponding to the maturation of mechanisms for bilirubin metabolism and excretion.

The diagnosis of physiologic jaundice in term or preterm infants can be established only by precluding known causes of jaundice on the basis of the history, clinical findings and laboratory data (Table 8.23). In general, a search to determine the cause of jaundice should be made if
1. It appears in the 1st 24–36 hr of life
2. Serum bilirubin is rising at a rate faster than 5 mg/dl/24 hr
3. Serum bilirubin is > 12 mg/dL in full-term infants (especially in the absence of risk factors) or 10–14 mg/dl in preterm infants
4. Jaundice persists after 10–14 days of life, or
5. Direct-reacting bilirubin is > 2 mg/dL at any time.

Other factors suggesting a nonphysiologic cause of jaundice are family history of hemolytic disease, pallor, hepatomegaly, splenomegaly, failure of phototherapy to lower bilirubin, vomiting, lethargy, poor feeding,

Table 8.22: Laboratory evaluation of the jaundiced infant of 35 or more weeks gestation

Indications	*Assessments*
Jaundice in first 24 hr	Measure TcB and/or TSB
Jaundice appear excessive for infant's age	Measure TcB and/or TSB
Infant receiving phototherapy or TSB rising rapidly (i.e. crossing percentiles (Fig. 8.30) and unexplained by history and physical examination	Blood type and Coombs' test, if not obtained with cord blood
	Complete blood count and smear
	Measure direct or conjugated bilirubin
	It is an option to perform reticulocyte count, G6PD, and ETCO, if available
	Repeat TSB in 4–24 hr depending on infant's age and TSB level
TSB concentration approaching exchange levels or not responding to phototherapy	Perform reticulocyte count, G6PD, albumin, ETCO, if available
Elevated direct (or conjugated) bilirubin level	Do urinalysis or urine culture. Evaluate for sepsis if indicated by history and physical examination
Jaundice present at or beyond age 3 wk or sick infant	Total and direct (or conjugated) bilirubin level, if direct bilirubin is elevated, evaluate for causes of cholestasis. Check results of newborn thyroid and galactosemia screen and evaluate infant for signs or symptoms of hypothyroidism

ETCO : End tidal carbon monoxide; G6PD : Glucose-6-phosphate dehydrogenase; TcB : Transcutaneous bilirubin
Source: AAP subcommittee on hyperbilirubinemia: Management of hyperbilirubinemia in the newborn infant 35 or more weeks of gestation. *Pediatrics* 2004;114:297–316.

excessive weight loss, apnea, bradycardia, abnormal vital signs including hypothermia), light-colored stools, dark urine positive for bilirubin, and signs of kernicterus.

2. *Pathological hyperbilirubinemia:* Jaundice and its underlying hyperbilirubinemia are considered pathologic if their time of appearance, duration, or pattern of serially determined serum bilirubin concentrations varies significantly from that of physiological jaundice, or if the course is compatible with physiologic jaundice but other reasons exist to suspect that the infant is at special risk for neurotoxicity. Many of these infants have associated risk factors such as Asian race, prematurity, breastfeeding, weight loss or probably a deficiency or inactivity of bilirubin glucuronyl transferase (Gilbert syndrome). The greatest risk associated with indirect hyperbilirubinemia is the development bilirubin-induced neurologic dysfunction, which typically occurs with high indirect bilirubin levels and the development of kernicterus (bilirubin encephalo-pathy).

Neonatal hepatitis: The term neonatal hepatitis implies intrahepatic cholestasis. *Idiopathic neonatal hepatitis* can occur in either a sporadic or a familial form is a disease of unknown cause (*see* Section 17.2, p-482).

Table 8.23: Diagnostic features of the various types of neonatal jaundice

Diagnosis	Nature of van den Bergh reaction	Jaundice Appears	Disappears	Peak bilirubin concentration mg/dl	Age in days	Bilirubin rate of accumulation mg/dl/day	Remarks
"Physiologic	Indirect	2–3 days	4–5 days	10–12	2–3	< 5	Usually relates to degree
Jaundice" Full-term Premature	Indirect	3–4 days	7–9 days	15	6–8	< 5	of maturity
Hyperbilirubinemia due to metabolic factors Full-term Premature	Indirect Indirect	2–3 days 3–4 days	Variable Variable	> 12 > 15	1st week 1st week	< 5 < 5	Metabolic factors: hypoxia, respiratory distress, lack of carbohydrate Hormonal influences: Cretinism, hormones, Gilbert syndrome Genetic factors: Crigler-Najjar syndrome, Gilbert syndrome Drugs: vitamin K, novobiocin
Hemolytic states and hematoma	Indirect	May appear in 1st 24 hr	Variable	Unlimited	Variable	Usually > 5	Erythroblastosis: Rh, ABO, Kell congenital hemolytic states: Spherocytic, nonspherocytic, Infantile pyknocytosis Drugs: Vitamin K enclosed hemorrhage, hematoma
Mixed hemolytic and hepatotoxic factors	Indirect and direct	May appear in 1st 24 hr	Variable	Unlimited	Variable	Usually > 5	Infection: Bacterial sepsis, pyelonephritis, hepatitis, toxoplasmosis, cytomegalic inclusion disease, rubella, syphilis Drugs: Vitamin K
Hepatocellular damage	Indirect and direct	Usually 2–3 days, may appear by 2nd week	Variable	Unlimited	Variable	Variable, can be > 5	Biliary atresia, paucity of biliary ducts, familial cholestasis, galactosemia, hepatitis, infection

Source: Brown AK. Neonatal jaundice. *Pediatr Clin North Am* 1962; 9: 575-603.

Aagenaes syndrome (see Section 17.2, page-482).

Zellweger (cerebrohepatorenal) syndrome (*see* Section 17.2, page-482).

Neonatal iron storage disease (NISD; neonatal hemochromatosis) (NISD) (*see* Section 17.3, page-485).

Congenital atresia of the bile ducts: Jaundice persisting more than 2 wk or associated with acholic stools and dark urine suggests biliary atresia. All such infants should have an immediate diagnostic evaluation, including determination of direct bilirubin.

Inspissated bile syndrome is a rare occurrence of persistent icterus in association with significant elevations in direct and indirect bilirubin in infants with hemolytic disease. Jaundice clears spontaneously within a few weeks and months.

3. *Jaundice associated with breastfed infants:* Two varieties of jaundice are observed in breastfed infants-breast milk jaundice and breastfeeding jaundice.

Breast milk jaundice: In about 2% breastfed term infants significant elevation in unconjugated bilirubin (breastmilk jaundice) develops after the 7th day of life, reaching maximum concentrations as high as 10–30 mg/dl during the 2nd and 3rd week. If breast-feeding is continued, the bilirubin gradually decreases but may persist for 3–10 wk at lower levels. If breastfeeding is discontinued, the serum bilirubin falls rapidly, usually reaching normal levels with in a few days. With resumption of breastfeeding, bilirubin levels seldom return to previously high levels. Phototherapy may be of benefit. Although uncommon, kernicterus can occur in patients with breastmilk jaundice. The etiology of breastmilk jaundice is not clear, but may be attributed to the presence of glucuronidase in some breastmilk.

Breastfeeding jaundice: Breastmilk jaundice should be distinguished from an early-onset accentuated unconjugated hyperbilirubinemia known as breast-feeding jaundice, which occurs in the first week of life in breastfed infants who normally have higher bilirubin levels than formula-fed infants. Hyperbili-rubinemia (>12 mg/dl) develops in 13% of breast-fed infants in the 1st wk of life and may be due to decreased milk intake with dehydration and/or reduced caloric intake. Those infants who are given glucose water to breastfed infants are associated with higher bilirubin levels, in part because of reduced intake of the higher caloric density of breast milk. Frequent breastfeeding (> 10/24 hr), rooming-in with night feeding, discouraging 5% dextrose or water supplementation, and ongoing lactation support may reduce the incidence of early breastfeeding jaundice.

4. *Kernicterus*, or bilirubin encephalopathy, is a neurologic syndrome resulting from the deposition of unconjugated (indirect) bilirubin in the basal ganglia and brainstem nuclei. The clinical features of kernicterus are listed in Table 8.24.

Treatment: Kernicterus is a medical emergency. Regardless of the cause, the goal of therapy is to prevent indirect-reacting bilirubin related neuro-toxicity. The treatment of bilirubin hyperbilirubinemia is phototherapy, exchange transfusion and drugs. Phototherapy and if unsuccessful, exchange transfusion remain the primary treatment modalities to be used to keep the maximal total serum bilirubin below the pathologic levels (Fig. 8.4; Table 8.25). The risk of injury to the central nervous system from bilirubin must be balanced against the potential risk of treatment. Because phototherapy may require 6–12 hr to have a measurable effect, it must be started at bilirubin levels below those indicated for exchange transfusion. When identified, underlying medical causes of elevated bilirubin and physiologic factors that contribute to neuronal susceptibility should be treated (antibiotics for septicemia and correction of acidosis).

Phototherapy: Clinical jaundice and indirect hyperbilirubinemia are reduced on exposure to a high intensity of light in the visible spectrum. Bilirubin absorbs light maximally in the blue range from 420 to 470 nm. Broad spectrum white, blue, and special narrow spectrum (super) blue lights have been

Table 8.24: Clinical features of kernicterus

Acute form

Phase 1 (1st 1–2 days): Poor sucking, stupor, hypotonia, seizures

Phase 2 (middle of 1st week): Hypertonia of extensor muscles, opisthotonos*, retrocollis*, fever

Phase 3 (after the 1st week): Hypertonia

Chronic form

First year: hypotonia, active deep tendon reflexes, obligatory tonic neck reflexes, delayed motor skills

After 1st year: Movement disorders (choreoathetosis, ballismus, tremor), upward gaze, sensorineural hearing loss

*Retrocollis (backward arching of the neck, in which the head is drawn backward); and backward arching of the back-Opisthotonos

Source: Dennery PA, Seidman DS, Stevenson DK. Neonatal hyperbilirubinemia. *N Engl J Med* 2001;344:581–90.

effective in reducing bilirubin levels. Bilirubin in the skin absorbs light energy causing photochemical reactions. One major product from phototherapy is a result of a reversible photo-isomerization reaction converting the toxic native unconjugated 4Z, 15Z-bilirubin into the unconjugated configurational isomer 4Z, 15E-bilirubin. The latter can then be excreted in bile without conjugation. The other major product from phototherapy is lumirubin, which is an irreversible structural isomer converted from native bilirubin and can be excreted by the kidneys in the unconjugational state.

The therapeutic effect of phototherapy depends on the light energy emitted in the effective range of wavelengths, the distance between the lights and the infant, and the surface area of exposed skin, as well as the rate of hemolysis and *in vivo* metabolism and excretion of bilirubin. The phototherapy units vary considerably in spectral output and the intensity of radiance emitted; therefore, the wattage can be accurately measured only at the patient's skin surface. The nude infant may be exposed under a portable or fixed light source at a distance of about 35–45 cm from the skin. Before initiating phototherapy, the infant's eyes should be closed and adequately covered to prevent light exposure and conceal damage. Eyes should be covered properly to avoid pressure injury to the closed eyes, corneal excoriation if the eyes can be opened under the binding and nasal occlusion. The infant should be shielded from bulb-breakage. Dark skin does not reduce the efficacy of phototherapy. Maximal intensive phototherapy should be used when indirect bilirubin levels approach those noted in Fig. 8.4 and Table 8.25. Such therapy includes "special blue" fluorescent tubes, placing the lamps within 15–20 cm of the infant, and placing a fiberoptic phototherapy blanket under the infant's back to increase the exposed surface area.

The use of phototherapy has decreased the need for exchange transfusion in term and preterm infants with hemolytic and non-hemolytic jaundice.

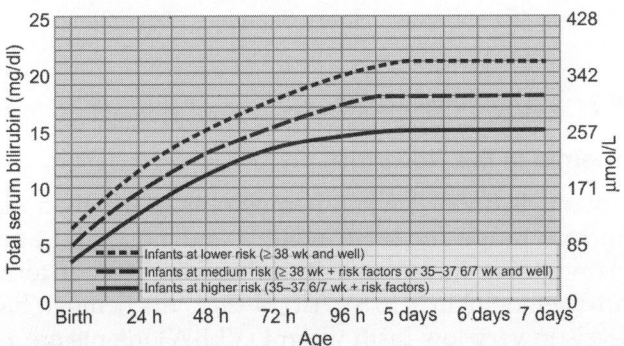

Fig. 8.4: Guidelines for phototherapy in hospitalized infants of 35 or more weeks gestation

Phototherapy should not be used as a substitute, when indications for exchange transfusion are present. However, phototherapy may reduce the need for repeated exchange transfusions in infants with hemolysis. Conventional phototherapy is applied continuously, and the infant is turned frequently for maximal skin surface area exposure. It should be discontinued as soon as the indirect bilirubin concentration has reduced to levels considered safe with respect to the infant's age and condition. Serum bilirubin levels and hematocrit should be monitored every 4–8 hr in infants with hemolytic disease or those with bilirubin levels near toxic range for the individual infant. Others, particularly older infants may be monitored less frequently. Serum bilirubin monitoring should continue for at least 24 hr after cessation of phototherapy in patients with hemolytic disease because unexpected rise in bilirubin may occur and require further treatment. Skin color should not be relied on for evaluating the effectiveness of phototherapy, because the skin of babies exposed to light may appear to be almost without jaundice in the presence of marked hyperbilirubinemia. It is reported that addition of intravenous fluid may be beneficial in dehydrated patients or those with high bilirubin levels nearing exchange transfusion.

Complications associated with phototherapy include loose stools, erythematous macular rash, purpuric rash associated with transient porphyrinemia, overheating, dehydration (increased insensible water loss, diarrhea), hypothermia from exposure and a benign condition called *bronze baby syndrome*. Phototherapy is contraindicated in the presence of porphyria. Body temperature should be monitored. Irradiance should be measured directly and details of the exposure recorded (type and age of the bulbs, duration of exposure, distance from the light source to the infant). In infants with hemolytic disease, care must be taken to monitor for the development of anemia. Anemia may develop despite lowering of bilirubin levels, which may require transfusion.

The term *bronze baby syndrome* refers to dark, grayish-brown skin discoloration in infants undergoing phototherapy. Infants with this syndrome have had significant elevation of direct-reacting bilirubin and other evidence of obstructive liver disease. The discoloration may be due to photo-induced modification of porphyrins, which are often present during cholestatic jaundice and may last for many months. Phototherapy can continue in bronze baby syndrome if required.

Phenobabitone: Phenobarbitone/Phenobarbital (in a dose of 3 to 8 mg/kg/24 hr q 12–24 hr), induces microsomal enzymes, increases bilirubin conjugation and excretion, and increases bile flow.

Intravenous immunoglobulin: The administration of intravenous immunoglobulin is an adjunctive treatment for hyperbilirubinemia due to isoimmune hemolytic disease. It is advised to use when serum bilirubin is approaching exchange levels despite maximal interventions including phototherapy. Intravenous immunoglobulin (0.5–1.0 g/kg/dose; repeat in 12 hr) has been shown to reduce the need for exchange transfusion in both ABO and Rh hemolytic disease, presumably by reducing hemolysis.

Exchange transfusion: Double volume exchange transfusion is performed if intensive phototherapy has failed to reduce bilirubin levels to a safer range and if the risk of kernicterus exceeds the risk of the procedure. Potential complications from exchange transfusion include metabolic acidosis, electrolyte abnormalities, hypoglycemia, hypocalcemia, thrombocytopenia, volume overload, arrhythmias, NEC, infection, graft versus host disease, and death. The treatment is repeated if necessary to keep indirect bilirubin levels in a safe range (Fig. 8.5, Table 8.25).

Prevention: Prevention of neonatal hyperbilirubinemia is the best way to minimize the risk of bilirubin neurotoxicity. The following guidelines may help in prevention of neonatal hyperbilirubinemia and thus, kernicterus: (i) evaluate all cases of jaundice appearing in the first 24 hrs, (ii) interpret all bilirubin levels according to infant's age in hours, (iii) allow early discharge (< 48 hrs) only if a healthy status is confirmed and appropriate follow up is assured, (iv) promote and support successful exclusive breast-feeding, and (v) provide parents with written and oral information about neonatal jaundice.

Prognosis: The spectrum of neurological disability from kernicterus can range from mild to severe. Overt neurologic signs have a grave prognosis. Many infants die; the survivors may appear to recover and for 2–3 mo show a few abnormalities. Mildly affected infants only have mild to moderate neuromuscular incoordination, partial deafness, or "minimal brain dysfunction," occur singly or in combination, that may not be apparent until the child enters school. Mental retardation, deafness and spastic quadriplegia are common. Infants at risk should be subjected to screening hearing tests.

American Academy of Pediatrics Subcommittee on Hyperbilirubinemia. Management of hyperbilirubinemia in the newborn infant 35 or more weeks of gestation. *Pediatrics* 2004; 114: 247–316.

Eichenwald EC. Necrotizing enterocolitis. *Manual of Neonatal Care.* 6th edn. Philadelphia: Lippincott Williams & Wilkins, 2008;608–15.

Gartner LM, Herschel M. Jaundice and Breastfeeding. In: Schanler RJ (ed.). The Pediatric Clinics of North America (Breast-feeding 2001, Part II: The Management of Breastfeeding). Philadelphia: WB Saunders Co., 2001;48(2):389–99.

Gottstein R, Cooke RWI. Systemic review of intravenous immunoglobulin. *Arch Dis Child Fetal Neonatal Ed* 2003;88:F6–10.

Huang MJ, Kua KE, Teng HC, et al. Risk factors for severe hyperbilirubinemia in neonates. *Pediatr Res* 2004;56:682–9.

La Torre A, Targioni G, Rubaltelli FF. Beta-glucuronidase and hyperbilirubinemia in breastfed babies. *Biol Neonate* 1999; 75:82–84.

Malik GK. Kernicterus. In: Mathur GP, Mathur Sarla (eds). *Current Trends in Pediatrics.* Vol 3. Delhi: Academa Publishers, 2007;130–7.

Martin CR, Cloherty JP. Neonatal Hyperbilirubinemia. In: Cloherty JP, Eichenwald EC, Stark AR (eds). *Manual of Neonatal Care.* 6th edn. Philadelphia: Lippincott Williams & Wilkins, 2008;181–212.

Mathur GP, Dadhich JP, Mathur Sarla, et al. Jaundice in the Neonatal Period. In: Mathur GP, Mathur Sarla (eds). *Current Trends in Pediatrics.* Vol 1. Delhi: Academa Publishers, 2005; 130–8.

Piazza AJ, Stoll BJ. Digestive system disorders. In: Kliegman RM, Behrman RE, Jenson HB, Stanton BF (eds). *Nelson Textbook of Pediatrics.* 18th edn. Vol 1. Philadelphia: Saunders, 2007; 753–66.

Volpe JJ (ed). Bilirubin and brain injury. In: *Neurology of the Newborn.* 4th edn. Philadelphia: Saunders, 2001; 521–46.

8.11 BLOOD DISORDERS

Anemia in the Newborn

Anemia is defined when hemoglobin is less than the normal range for birth weight and postnatal age. Hemoglobin increases with advancing age: at term cord hemoglobin is 16.8 g/dl (14–20 g/dl); hemoglobin levels in very low birth weight (VLBW) infants are 1–2 g/dl below those at term. A "physiologic" decrease in hemoglobin content is noticed at 8–12 wk in term

Table 8.25: Suggested maximal indirect serum bilirubin concentration (mg/dl) in preterm infants		
Birth weight (g)	*Uncomplicated*	*Complicated**
< 1000	12–13	10–12
1,000–1,250	12–14	10–12
1,251–1,499	14–16	12–14
1,500–1,999	16–20	15–17
2,000–2,500	20–22	18–20

Phototherapy is usually started at 50-70% of the maximal indirect level, if values greatly exceed this level, if phototherapy is unsuccessful in reducing the maximal bilirubin level, or if signs of kernicterus are evident, exchange transfusion is advised

*Complications include perinatal asphyxia, acidosis, hypoxia, hypothermia, hypoalbuminemia, meningitis, intraventricular hemorrhage, hemolysis, hypoglycemia, or signs of kernicterus

infants (hemoglobin, 11 g/dl) and at about 6 wk in premature infants (7–10 g/dl). Anemia at birth is manifested as pallor, heart failure, or shock.

Etiology: Anemia may be due to acute or chronic fetal blood loss, hemolysis, or underproduction of erythrocytes. The causes of anemia are listed in Table 8.26.

Transplacental hemorrhage with bleeding from the fetal into the maternal circulation occurs in 5–15% of pregnancies. Unless anemia is severe, clinically apparent anemia does not occur.

Acute blood loss is accompanied by severe distress at birth, initially with a normal hemoglobin level, no hepatosplenomegaly and early onset of shock. In contrast, *chronic blood loss in utero*, produces marked pallor, less distress, a low hemoglobin level with microcytic indices, and, if severe, heart failure.

Anemia of prematurity occurs in low birth weight infants 1–3 mo after birth, is associated with hemoglobin levels below 7–10 g/ml, and is clinically manifested as pallor, poor weight gain, decreased activity, tachypnea, tachycardia, and feeding problems. The causes that contribute to anemia of prematurity is shown in Table 8.26. The oxygen available to neonatal tissue is lower than that in adults, but a neonate's erythropoietin response is attenuated for the degree of anemia and, as a result, hemoglobin and reticulocyte levels are low. In VLBW infants, delayed clamping of the umbilical cord with infant held below the level of the placenta may enhance placental-infant transfusion and reduce postnatal transfusion needs. But any needed resuscitation should not be delayed for this maneuver; this may also lead to hyperviscosity.

Table 8.26: Causes of anemia
Specific causes of anemia
Hemolytic disease of the newborn
Tearing or cutting of the umbilical cord during delivery
Abnormal cord insertion
Communicating placental vessels
Placenta pervia or abruption
Nuchal cord incision in to the placenta
Internal hemorrhage (liver, spleen, intracranial)
Alpha-thalassemia
Congenital parvovirus infection or other hypoplastic anemias
Twin-twin transfusion in monozygotic twins with arteriovenous placental connections
Anemia appearing in the first few days after birth#
Hemolytic disease of the newborn
Hemorrhagic disease of the newborn
Bleeding from an improperly tied or clamped umbilical cord
Large cephalhematoma
Intracranial hemorrhage
Subcapsular bleeding from rupture of the liver, spleen, adrenals, or kidneys
Delayed anemia appearing later in the neonatal period
Hemolytic disease of the newborn, with or without exchange transfusion or phototherapy
Congenital hemolytic anemia (spherocytosis) occasionally appears during the 1st mo of life
Hereditary nonspherocytic hemolytic anemia secondary to deficiency of G6PD deficiency and pyruvate kinase
Bleeding from hemangiomas of the upper gastrointestinal tract or from ulcers caused by aberrant gastric mucosa in a Meckel diverticulum or duplication
Repeated blood sampling of infants requiring frequent monitoring of blood gas and chemistry parameters among hospitalized infants
Total parenteral nutrition due to deficiency of minerals such as copper
Anemia of prematurity
Repeated phlebotomy for blood tests
Shortened RBC survival
Rapid growth
Physiologic effects of the transition from fetal (low PaO_2 and hemoglobin saturation) to neonatal life (high PaO_2 and hemoglobin saturation)

G6PD deficiency-glucose-6-phosphate dehydrogenase deficiency
#Rapid decreases in hemoglobin or Hct values during the first few days of life may be the initial clue to these conditions.

Treatment may involve intravenous fluids followed by a blood transfusion or an exchange blood transfusion. Transfusion protocol is documented in Table 8.27. The treatment by blood transfusion depends on the severity of symptoms, the hemoglobin level, and the presence of co-morbid diseases (bronchopulmonary dysplasia, cyanotic congenital heart disease, respiratory distress syndrome) that interfere with oxygen delivery. The need for treatment with blood should be balanced against the risks of transfusion, including hemolytic transfusion reactions, exposure to blood product preservatives, and other potential toxins, volume overload, possible increased risk of retinopathy of prematurity and necrotizing enterocolitis, graft vs host reaction, and transfusion-acquired infection (cytomegalovirus, HIV, parvovirus, hepatitis B and C). The risk of CMV infection can be almost eliminated by the use of leukoreduced blood. In the infant under 1,500 g, CMV antibody-negative leukoreduced blood should be used.

Asymptomatic full-term infants with a hemoglobin level of 10 g/dl may be monitored, whereas symptomatic neonates born after abruptio placentae or with severe hemolytic disease of the newborn warrant immediate transfusion. No transfusion is needed to replace blood removed for testing or for mild asymptomatic anemia. Asymptomatic neonates with reticulocytopenia and hemoglobin levels of 7 g/dL or lower may require transfusion. Packed RBC transfusion (10–20 ml/kg) is given at a rate of 2–3 mL/kg/hr to raise the hemoglobin concentration; 2 mL/kg raises the hemoglobin level 0.5–1 g/dl. Hemorrhage should be treated with whole blood, if available; alternatively fluid resuscitation is initiated and followed by packed RBC transfusion.

Recombinant human erythropoietin (r-HuEPO), supplemented with oral iron and vitamin E has been used to prevent or treat chronic anemia associated with prematurity, bronchopulmonary dysplasia and the hyporegenerative anemia of erythroblastosis fetalis. But does not have a major impact on transfusion requirements; therefore, routine use of erythropoietin in VLBW infants is not recommended.

Hemolytic Disease of the Newborn (Erythroblastosis Fetalis)

Erythroblastosis fetalis is caused by the transplacental passage of maternal antibody active against paternal RBC antigens of infant and is characterized by an increased rate of RBC destruction. The disease is primarily with D antigen of the Rh group and with incompatibility of ABO factors. There are more than 60 different RBC antigens capable of eliciting an antibody response. Rarely,

hemolytic disease may be caused by C or E antigens or by other RBC antigens such as C^w, C^x, D^u, K (Kell), M, Duffy, S, P, MNS, Xg, Lutheran, Diego, and Kidd.

Hemolytic Disease of the Newborn Caused by Rh Incompatibility

The Rh antigenic determinants are genetically transmitted from each parent, determine the Rh type, and direct the production of a number of blood group factors (C, c, D, d, E, and e). Each factor can elicit a specific antibody response under suitable conditions; 90% are due to D antigen and remainder to C or E.

Pathogenesis: Isoimmune hemolytic disease from D antigen occurs in two ways: (i) When Rh-positive blood is infused into a Rh-negative woman through error, or (ii) when small quantities usually more than 1 ml of Rh-positive fetal blood containing D antigen inherited from an Rh-positive father enter the maternal circulation during pregnancy, with spontaneous or induced abortion, or at delivery, antibody formation against D antigen may be induced in the unsensitized Rh-negative recipient mother. Once sensitization has taken place, considerably smaller doses of antigen can stimulate an increase in antibody titer. Initially, a rise in IgM antibody occurs, which is later replaced by IgG antibody; the latter readily crosses the placenta and causes hemolytic manifestations.

Hemolytic disease rarely occurs during a first pregnancy because transfusion of Rh-positive fetal

Table 8.27: Transfusion protocol	
Hct/Hb	*Transfusion volume*
Hct ≤ 35/Hb ≤ 11	15 ml/kg RBCs* over period of 2–4 hr
Hct ≤ 30/Hb ≤ 10	15 ml/kg RBCs over period of 2–4 hr
Hct ≤ 25/Hb ≤ 8	20 ml/kg RBCs over period of 2–4 hr (divide into 2–10 ml/kg volumes if fluid sensitive)
Hct ≤ 20/Hb ≤ 7	20 ml/kg PRBCs over period of 2–4 hr (2–10 ml/kg volumes)

*RBCs should be irradiated before transfusion.
CPAP: continuous positive airway pressure; FiO$_2$: Fractional inspired oxygen; Hct : Hematocrit; Hb : Hemoglobin; HR: Heart rate; MAP: Mean airway pressure; PRBC: Packed red blood cells; RR: Respiratory rate
Source: Ohls RK, Ehrenkranz RA, Wright LL, et al. Effects of early erythropoietin therapy on the transfusion requirements below 1250 g birth weight: A multicentric randomized control trial. *Pediatrics* 2001;108:934–42.

blood into an Rh-negative mother occurs near the time of delivery, too late for the mother to become sensitized and transmit antibody to her infant before delivery. The facts that 55% of Rh-positive fathers are heterozygous (D/d) and may have Rh-negative offspring and that fetal to maternal transfusion occurs in only 50% of pregnancies reduces the chance of sensitization, as does small family size, in which the opportunities for its recurrence are reduced. Finally, the capacity of Rh-negative women to form antibodies is variable, some producing low titers even after adequate antigenic challenge. Thus, the overall incidence of isoimmunization of Rh-negative mothers at risk is low, with antibody to D detected in less than 10%, and even after five or more pregnancies, only about 5% ever have babies with hemolytic disease.

When the mother and fetus are also incompatible with respect to group A or B, the mother is partially protected against sensitization by rapid removal of Rh-positive cells from her circulation by her pre-existing anti-A or anti-B, which are IgM antibodies and do not cross the placenta. Once a mother has been sensitized, her infant is likely to have hemolytic disease. The severity of Rh illness worsens with successive pregnancies.

Clinical manifestations: Hemolytic disease in affected infants born to sensitized mothers occurs with varying severity. In mild hemolysis (15% of cases) the diagnosis is based on laboratory evidence to severe anemia. Whereas in severe anemia there is compensatory hyperplasia of erythropoietic tissue leading to hepatosplenomegaly, signs of cardiac decompensation (cardiomegaly, respiratory distress), massive anasarca and circulatory collapse. This clinical picture of excessive abnormal fluid in two or more fetal compartments (skin, pleura, pericardium, placenta, peritoneum, amniotic fluid), termed *hydrops fetalis*, frequently results in death *in utero* or shortly after birth. With the use of anti-D gamma globulin to prevent Rh sensitization, nonimmune (non-hemolytic) conditions have become frequent causes of hydrops.

Jaundice may be absent at birth because of placental clearance of lipid soluble unconjugated bilirubin, but in severe cases, bilirubin pigments stain the amniotic fluid, cord, and vernix caseosa yellow. Jaundice is generally evident on the 1st day of life because the infant's bilirubin-conjugating and excretory systems are unable to cope with the load resulting from massive hemolysis. Indirect-reacting bilirubin therefore, accumulates postnatally and may rapidly reach extremely high levels and present a significant risk of bilirubin encephalopathy. Hypoglycemia occurs frequently in infants with severe isoimmune hemolytic disease and may be related to hyperinsulinism and hypertrophy of the pancreatic islet cells in these infants.

Infants born after intrauterine transfusion for prenatally diagnosed erythroblastosis may be severely affected because the indications for transfusion are evidence of already severe disease *in utero* (hydrops, fetal anemia). Such infants usually have very high cord levels of bilirubin, which reflects the severity of the hemolysis and its effects on hepatic function. Infants treated with intra-umbilical vein transfusions *in utero* may also have a benign postnatal course if the anemia and hydrops resolve before birth. Anemia from continuing hemolysis may be masked by the previous intrauterine transfusion, and the clinical manifestations of erythroblastosis may be superimposed on various degrees of immaturity resulting from spontaneous or induced premature delivery.

Laboratory findings: Before treatment, the direct Coombs' test is usually positive and anemia is generally present. The cord blood hemoglobin content varies and is usually proportional to the severity of the disease; with hydrops fetalis it may be as low as 3–4 g/dl. Despite hemolysis, the hemoglobin level may be within the normal range because of compensatory bone marrow and extramedullary hematopoiesis. The blood smear shows polychromasia and a marked increase in nucleated RBCs. The reticulocyte count is increased. The white blood cell count is usually normal but may be elevated; thrombocytopenia may develop in severe cases. Cord bilirubin is generally between 3 and 5 mg/dl; direct reacting (conjugated) bilirubin may also be elevated, especially if there was an intrauterine transfusion. Indirect-reacting bilirubin rises rapidly to high levels in the 1st 6 hr of life.

After intrauterine transfusions, cord blood may show a normal hemoglobin concentration, negative direct Coombs' test, predominantly type O Rh-negative adult RBCs, and a relatively normal smear.

Diagnosis: The diagnosis of erythroblastosis fetalis is based on demonstration of blood group incompatibility and corresponding antibody bound to the infant's RBCs.

Antenatal diagnosis: In Rh-negative women, a history of previous transfusions, abortion, or pregnancy should suggest the possibility of sensitization. Expectant parents' blood types should be tested for potential incompatibility, and the maternal titer of IgG antibodies to D antigen should be assayed at 12–16, 28–32, and 36 wk. Fetal Rh status may be determined by isolating fetal cells or fetal DNA (plasma) from the maternal circulation. The presence of elevated antibody titers at the beginning of pregnancy, a rapid rise in titer or a titer of 1 : 64 or greater suggests significant hemolytic disease, although the exact titer correlates poorly with the severity of disease. The severity of fetal disease should be monitored by Doppler ultrasonography of the middle cerebral artery and then percutaneous umbilical blood sampling (PUBS) if indicated. Real-time ultrasonography is used to detect the progression of disease, with hydrops defined as skin or scalp edema, pleural or pericardial effusions, and ascites. Early ultrasonographic signs of hydrops include organomegaly (liver, spleen, heart), the double-bowel wall sign (bowel edema), and placental thickening. Hydrops is present when fetal hemoglobin is < 5 g/dl, frequent when < 7 g/dl and variable between 7 and 9 g/dl.

Amniocentesis and cordocentesis are invasive procedures with risks to the fetus and mother, therefore, noninvasive measurements to detect fetal anemia should be performed. In fetuses without hydrops, moderate to severe anemia can be detected noninvasively by demonstration in an increase in the peak velocity of systolic blood flow in the middle cerebral artery by Doppler ultrasound.

If Doppler and real-time ultrasonography suggest an affected fetus, PUBS is performed to determine fetal hemoglobin levels and to transfuse packed RBCs in those with serious fetal anemia (Hct of 25–30%).

Postnatal diagnosis: Immediately after the birth of an infant to an Rh-negative woman, blood from the umbilical cord or from the infant should be examined for ABO blood group, Rh type, Hct and hemoglobin, and reaction of the direct Coombs' test. If the Coombs' test is positive, a baseline serum bilirubin level should be measured and RBC panel should be used to identify RBC antibodies present in the mother's serum; both tests being performed not only to establish the diagnosis but also to ensure selection of the most compatible blood for exchange transfusion should it be necessary. The direct Coombs' test is strongly positive in clinically affected infants and may remain so for a few days up to several months.

Treatment: The two main objectives of treatment are to (i) prevent intrauterine or extrauterine death from severe anemia and hypoxia, and (ii) avoid neurotoxicity from hyperbilirubinemia.

Treatment of an unborn infant: Intravascular (umbilical vein) transfusion of packed RBCs is the treatment of choice for fetal anemia, replacing intrauterine transfusion into the fetal peritoneal cavity. Hydrops or fetal anemia (Hct < 30%) is an indication for umbilical vein transfusion in infants with pulmonary immaturity. Intravascular fetal transfusion is facilitated by maternal and hence fetal sedation with

diazepam and by fetal paralysis with pancuronium. Packed RBCs are given by slow-push infusion after cross-matching with the mother's serum. The cells should be obtained from a CMV-negative donor and irradiated to kill lymphocytes to avoid graft vs. host disease (leukoreduction alone without irradiation does not prevent graft vs. host disease). Transfusions should achieve a post-transfusion Hct of 45–55% and can be repeated every 3–5 wk. Indications for delivery include pulmonary maturity, fetal distress, complications of PUBS, or 35–37 wk of gestation. The survival rate for intrauterine transfusions is 89%; the complication rate is 3%. Complications include rupture of the membranes and preterm delivery, infection, fetal distress requiring emergency cesarean section, and perinatal death.

Treatment of a liveborn infant: The birth should be attended by a physician skilled in neonatal resuscitation. Fresh, low titer, group O, leukoreduced and irradiated Rh-negative blood cross-matched against maternal serum should be immediately available. If clinical signs of severe hemolytic anemia (pallor, hepatosplenomegaly, edema, petechiae, and ascites) are evident at birth, immediate resuscitation and supportive therapy, temperature stabilization, and monitoring before proceeding with exchange transfusion may save some severely affected infants. Such therapy should also include correction of acidosis with 1–2 mEq/kg of sodium bicarbonate; a small transfusion of compatible packed RBCs to correct anemia; volume expansion for hypotension, especially in those with hydrops; and provision of assisted ventilation for respiratory failure.

Exchange transfusion: When an infant's clinical condition at birth does not require an immediate full or partial exchange transfusion the decision to perform one should be based on a judgment that the infant has high risk of rapid development of a dangerous degree of anemia or hyperbilirubinemia. Cord hemoglobin of 10 g/dl or less and bilirubin of 5 mg/dl or more suggest severe hemolysis, but inconsistently predict the need for exchange transfusion. Some physicians consider previous kernicterus or severe erythroblastosis in a sibling, reticulocyte counts > 15% and prematurity may be the additional factors supporting a decision for early exchange transfusion. Intrauterine, intravascular transfusions have decreased the need for exchange transfusion.

The hemoglobin concentration, Hct, and serum bilirubin level should be measured at 4–6 hr intervals initially, with extension to longer intervals if and as the rate of change diminishes. The decision to perform an exchange transfusion is based on the likelihood that the trend of bilirubin levels plotted against hours of in Fig. 8.5 and Table 8.27. Term infants with levels of

20 mg/dl or higher have an increased risk of kernicterus. Ordinary transfusions of compatible Rh-negative, leukoreduced, and irradiated RBCs may be necessary to correct anemia at any stage of the disease up to 6–8 wk of age, when the infants own blood-forming mechanism may be expected to take over. Weekly determinations of hemoglobin or Hct should be done until a spontaneous rise has been demonstrated.

Type of blood: Blood withdrawn < 72 hr before is preferred. Heparin or citrate-phosphate-dextrose-adenine (CPDA) solution is used as an anticoagulant. In an emergency, frozen RBC reconstituted in saline or plasma is used. ABO compatible, blood is used for erythroblastosis fetalis and O group Rh compatible blood is used for ABO incompatibility.

Quantity: 170 ml/kg (double the normal volume of 85 ml/kg) blood is used for one exchange transfusion. This ensues that 87% of blood volume is removed and exchanged by the donor blood.

Procedure: The most commonly used technique is the push pull method in the umbilical vein (other peripheral vein or peripheral artery may be used). For this, a single syringe and a special 4-way stopcock (two three way stopcocks can be connected to make on four way system) are required. The size of the aliquots during each push or pull should be 20 ml; smaller aliquotes (5–10 ml) may be indicated for sick and premature infants. A double volume exchange transfusion (2 × 85 ml/kg) should take 45 min to 1 hr and probably longer in sick infants (Table 8.27).

Complication: These occur frequently and include bacterial sepsis, thrombocytopenia, especially after repeated exchanges, portal vein thrombosis, inspissated bile syndrome, umbilical or portal vein perforation, arrhythmia, cardiac arrest, hypocalcemia, hypoglycemia, hypomagnesemia, metabolic acidosis, alkalosis, HIV, hepatitis B and C infection, and graft vs. host disease.

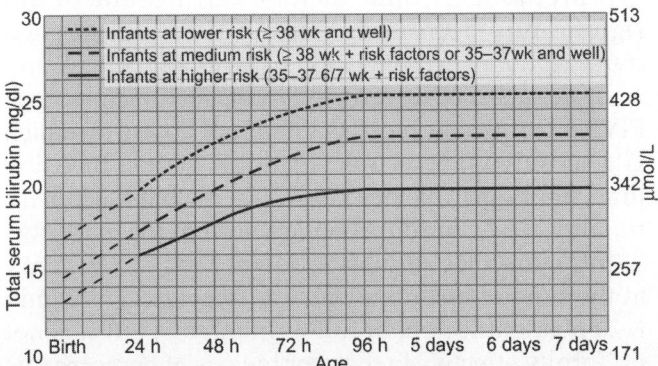

Fig. 8.5: Guidelines for exchange transfusion in infants 35 or more weeks gestation

Prevention of Rh sensitization: The risk of initial sensitization of Rh-negative mother has been reduced to less than 1% by the intramuscular injection of 300 µg human anti-D immunoglobulin within 72 hr of delivery of an Rh-positive infant, ectopic pregnancy, abdominal trauma in pregnancy, amniocentesis, chorionic villus biopsy, or abortion. This quantity is sufficient to eliminate ~ 10 ml of potentially antigenic fetal cells from the maternal circulation. Large fetal-to-maternal transfers of blood may require proportionately more human anti-D immunoglobulin. Human anti-D immunoglobulin administered at 28–32 wk and again at birth (40 wk) is more effective than a single dose. The use of this technique, combined with improved methods of detecting maternal sensitization and measuring the extent of fetal-to-maternal transfusion, plus the use of fewer obstetric procedures that increase the risk of such fetal-to-maternal bleeding (version, manual separation of the placenta), should further reduce the incidence of erythroblastosis fetalis.

Hemolytic Disease of the Newborn Caused by Blood Group A and B Incompatibility

ABO incompatibility is the most common cause of hemolytic disease of the newborn, but is a milder disease than Rh incompatibility. Maternal antibody may be formed against B cells, if the mother is type A or against A cells if the mother is type B. Usually, the mother is type O and the infant is type A or B. Although ABO incompatibility occurs in 25–30% of pregnancies, hemolytic disease develops only 10% of such offspring, and the infants are generally type A_1, which is more antigenic than A_2. Low antigenicity of the ABO factors in the fetus and the newborn infant may account for the low incidence of severe ABO hemolytic disease relative to the incidence of incompatibility between the blood groups of the mother and child. Approximately 15% of live births are at risk, but manifestations of disease develop in only 0.3–2.2%.

Clinical manifestations: Most cases are mild, with jaundice being the only clinical manifestation. Jaundice usually appears during the 1st 24 hr. The infant is not generally affected at birth; pallor is not present, and hydrops fetalis is extremely rare. The liver and spleen are not greatly enlarged. Rarely, infant may become severe, and symptoms and signs of kernicterus develop rapidly.

Diagnosis: A presumptive diagnosis is based on the presence of ABO incompatibility, a weakly to moderately positive direct Coombs test, and spherocytes in the blood smear. The hemoglobin level is usually normal but may be as low as 10–12 g/dl. Hyperbilirubinemia is present, and in 10–20% of affected infants, the unconjugated serum bilirubin level may reach 20 mg/dl or more unless phototherapy is administered. Reticulocytes may be increased to 10–15%, with extensive polychromasia and increased numbers of nucleated RBCs.

Treatment: Phototherapy may be effective in lowering serum bilirubin levels. In rare severe cases, treatment is directed at correcting dangerous degrees of anemia or hyperbilirubinemia by exchange transfusions with type O blood of the same Rh type as the infant (Section 8.11). Some infants with ABO hemolytic disease may require transfusion of packed RBCs at several weeks of age because of slowly progressive anemia. Hemoglobin/Hct should be monitored in newborns with ABO hemolytic disease after discharge.

Plethora in the Newborn Infant (Polycythemia)

Plethora, a deep red-purple appearance associated with a high Hct, is often due to polycythemia, defined as a central Hct of 65% or higher. Peripheral (heelstick) Hct values are higher than central values. The incidence of neonatal polycythemia is increased in high altitudes; in postmature, and in small for gestational age; during the 1st day of life (peak, 2–3 hr); in the recipient infant of a twin-twin transfusion; after delayed clamping of the umbilical cord; in infants of diabetic mothers; in trisomy 13, 18, or 21; in adrenogenital syndrome, in neonatal Graves' disease, in hypothyroidism; in infants of hypertensive mothers or those on propranolol; and in Beckwith-Wiedeman syndrome. Infants of diabetic or hypertensive mothers and those with growth restriction may have been exposed to chronic fetal hypoxia, which stimulates erythropoietin production and increases RBC production.

Clinical manifestations include irritability, lethargy, tachypnea, respiratory distress, cyanosis, feeding disturbances, hyperbilirubinemia, hypoglycemia and thrombocytopenia. Severe complications include seizures, stroke, pulmonary hypertension, necrotizing enterocolitis, renal vein thrombosis, and renal failure. Many affected infants are asymptomatic. Hyperviscosity is present in most infants with central Hct values of 65% or higher and accounts for the symptoms of polycythemia.

Treatment of symptomatic polycythemic newborn is partial exchange transfusion (with normal saline). Partial exchange will lower the Hct and viscosity and improve acute symptoms. The volume to be exchanged is calculated from the following formula:

Volume of exchange (ml) = Blood volume × (Observed – Desired hematocrit)/Observed hematocrit

Reported adverse outcomes include speech deficits, abnormal fine motor control, reduced IQ, school problems, and other neurologic abnormalities. The underlying etiology (chronic intrauterine hypoxia) and hyperviscosity contribute to adverse outcomes. Most asymptomatic infants develop normally.

Hemorrhage in the Newborn Infant

Hemorrhagic disease of the newborn: A moderate decrease in factors II, VII, IX, and X normally occurs in all newborn infants by 48–72 hr after birth, with a gradual return to birth levels by 7–10 days of age. This transient deficiency of vitamin K-dependent factors is probably due to lack of free vitamin K from the mother and absence of the bacterial intestinal flora normally responsible for the synthesis of vitamin K. Rarely, in term infants and more frequently in premature infants accentuation and prolongation of this deficiency between the 2nd and 7th days of life result in spontaneous and prolonged bleeding. Breast-milk is a poor source of vitamin K, and hemorrhagic complications are more frequent in breastfed than in formulafed infants. Classic form of hemorrhagic disease of the newborn, which is responsive to and prevented by vitamin K therapy, must be distinguished from disseminated intravascular coagulopathy and from congenital deficiencies of one or more of the other factors that are unresponsive to vitamin K. Early-onset life-threatening vitamin K deficiency-induced bleeding (onset from birth to 24 hr) also occurs if the mother has been treated with drugs that interfere with vitamin K function. Late onset (> 2 wk) is often associated with malabsorption as noted in neonatal hepatitis or biliary atresia. The common sites of bleeding are gastrointestinal, nasal, subgaleal, intracranial, or postcircumcision. Prodromal or warning signs (mild bleeding) may occur before serious intracranial hemorrhage. The prothrombin time (PT), blood coagulation time and partial thromboplastin time are prolonged, and level of prothrombin (II) and factors VII, IX, and X are significantly decreased. Vitamin K facilitates post-transcriptional carboxylation of factors II, VII, IX and X. In the absence of carboxylation, such factors form PIVKA (protein induced in vitamin K absence), which is a sensitive marker for vitamin K status. Bleeding time, fibrinogen, factors V and VIII, platelets, capillary fragility, and clot retraction are normal for maturity.

Intramuscular administration of 1 mg of vitamin K at the time of birth prevents the decrease in vitamin K-dependent factors in full-term infants, but it is not uniformly effective in the prophylaxis of hemorrhagic disease of the newborn in premature infants. The disease is treated with a slow intravenous infusion of

1–5 mg of vitamin K_1, with improvement in coagulation defects and cessation of bleeding noted within a few hours. Serious bleeding particularly in premature infants or those with liver disease may require a transfusion of fresh frozen plasma or whole blood. The mortality rate is low in treated patients.

Infants born to mothers receiving anticonvulsive medications (phenobarbital and phenytoin) develop a severe form of deficiency of vitamin K-dependent coagulation factors. They may have severe bleeding with onset within the 1st 24 hr of life; the bleeding is usually corrected by vitamin K_1. A PT should be obtained on cord blood and the infant given 1–2 mg of vitamin K_1 intravenously. If the PT is greatly prolonged and fails to improve, 10 ml/kg of fresh frozen plasma should be administered.

Disseminated intravascular coagulopathy in newborn infants results in consumption of coagulation factors and bleeding. Affected infants are premature may be associated with asphyxia, hypoxia, acidosis, shock, hemangiomas, or infection. Treatment is directed at correcting the primary clinical problem, such as infection, and interrupting consumption and replacing clotting factors.

Infants with central nervous system or other bleeding posing an immediate threat to life should receive fresh frozen plasma, vitamin K_1 and blood if needed as soon as possible after blood has been drawn for coagulation studies (including blood platelet count).

In the swallowed blood syndrome blood or bloody stools are passed, usually on the 2nd or 3rd day of life, may be confused with hemorrhage from the gastrointestinal tract. The blood may be swallowed during delivery or from a fissure in the mother's nipple. Differentiation from gastrointestinal hemorrhage is based on the fact that the infant's blood contains mostly fetal hemoglobin, which is alkali-resistant, whereas swallowed blood from a maternal source contains adult hemoglobin, which is promptly changed to alkaline hematin after the addition of alkali. Apt devised the following test for differentiation of fetal hemoglobin present in infant's blood from adult hemoglobin:

1. Rinse a blood-stained diaper or some grossly bloody (red) stool with a suitable amount of water to obtain a distinctly pink supernatant hemoglobin solution.
2. Centrifuge the mixture and decant the supernatant solution.
3. To five parts of the supernatant fluid add one part of 0.25 N (1%) sodium hydroxide. Within 1–2 min a color reaction takes place: A yellow-brown color indicates that the blood is maternal in origin; a persistent pink indicates that it is from the infant.

A control test with known adult or infant blood, or both, is advisable.

Widespread subcutaneous ecchymoses in premature infants at or immediately after birth result from fragile superficial blood vessels rather than a coagulation defect; vitamin K_1 administration to the mother during labor has no effect. Infant born with petechiae or generalized bluish suffusion limited to the face, head, and neck, probably as a result of venous obstruction by a nuchal cord or sudden increases in intrathoracic pressure during delivery usually disappear in 2–3 wk time.

Neonatal thrombocytopenia (*see* Section 20.8, page-659).

Bizzarto MJ, Colson E, Ehrenkranz RA. Differential diagnosis and management of anemia in the newborn. *Pediatr Clin Norh Am* 2004;51:1087–107.

Christou HA, Shannon K, Rowitch DH. Anemia. In: Cloherty JP, Eichenwald EC, Stark AR (eds). *Manual of Neonatal Care*. 6th edn. Philadelphia: Lippincott Williams & Wilkins, 2008;436–44.

Goorin AM. Polycytemia. In: Cloherty JP, Eichenwald EC, Stark AR (eds). *Manual of Neonatal Care*. 6th edn. Philadelphia: Lippincott Williams & Wilkins, 2008;450–5.

Goorin AM, Cloherty JP. Throbocytopenia. In: Cloherty JP, Eichenwald EC, Stark AR (eds). *Manual of Neonatal Care*. 6th edn. Philadelphia: Lippincott Williams & Wilkins, 2008; 455–462.

Greer FR. Are breastfed infants vitamin K deficient? *Adv Exp Med Biol* 2001;501:391–5.

Moise Jr KJ. Diagnosing hemolytic disease of the fetus-time to put the needles away. *N Engl J Med* 2006;355:192–4.

Stoll BJ. Blood disorders. In: Kliegman RM, Behrman RE, Jenson HB, Stanton BF (eds). *Nelson Textbook of Pediatrics*. 18th edn. Vol 1. Philadelphia: Saunders, 2007;766–75.

8.12 GENITOURINARY PROBLEMS IN NEONATES

Urinary tract anomalies (hydronephrosis, dysplasia, cystic and solitary kidney) are frequently identified by prenatal ultrasonography. After birth, anomalies, needs to be confirmed and followed. Follow-up of urinary anomalies diagnosed *in utero* requires renal ultrasonography after birth.

Renal vein thrombosis (RVT) see Section 21.2, page-636.

Acute renal failure (ARF) is a frequent clinical condition in NICU. Acute renal failure should be suspected in neonates with oliguria (urine output less than 0.5 ml/kg/hr), raised blood urea (> 50 mg%) and creatinine level more than 1.0 mg%. It can be of 3 types:

1. Pre-renal (75– 80%)
2. Intrinsic renal (10–15%)
3. Post renal (5%). Persistence of insult can convert pre-renal or post-renal failure to intrinsic renal failure.

Anomalies of external genitalia include phimosis, undescended testis (cryptorchidism), hypospadias and ambiguous external genitalia.

Bhutani VK. Neonatal Acute Renal Failure. *J Neonatal* 2001; 15(1):16–22.

Davis ID, Avner ED. Conditions particularly associated with hematuria. In: Kliegman RM, Behrman RE, Jenson HB, Stanton BF (eds). *Nelson Textbook of Pediatrics.* 18th edn. Vol 1. Philadelphia: Saunders, 2007; 2183–4.

Stoll BJ. Genitourinary system. In: Kliegman RM, Behrman RE, Jenson HB, Stanton BF (eds). *Nelson Textbook of Pediatrics.* 18th edn. Vol 1. Philadelphia: Saunders, 2007;p-775.

8.13 UMBILICUS

Umbilical cord: The **navel** known clinically, as the **umbilicus** is the depression in the center of the surface of the abdomen indicating the point of attachment of the umbilical cord to the embryo. It is the site through which vessels provide nutrients to the fetus from the mother during development. The skin around the waist at the level of the umbilicus is supported by the tenth thoracic spinal nerve (T10 dermatome). The umbilicus itself lies at the level between L3/L4 vertebrae.

The cord contains two umbilical arteries, one umbilical vein, rudimentary allantois, remnant of the omphalomesenteric duct and a gelatinous substance called Wharton's jelly. The sheath of the umbilical cord is derived from the amnion. The muscular umbilical arteries contract readily, but the vein does not. The vein retains a fairly large lumen after birth. The normal cord at term is 55 cm long. The fetal blood is oxygenated in the placenta not in the lungs and the fetal circulation depends on the three short-circuiting arrangements, all of which cease to function at the time of birth: the ductus venosus, the foramen ovale and the ductus arteriosus.

Common problems of umbilical cord: The common problems of umbilical cord are short cord, long cord, delayed separation, single umbilical artery, patency of the omphalomesenteric duct, persistent urachus, and umbilical infection. Abnormally *short cords* are associated with antepartum abnormalities including fetal hypotonia, oligohydramnios, and uterine constraint. It is also associated with increased risk for complications of labor and delivery for both mother and infant. Length more than 70 cm is defined as *long cord.* It has the risk for true knots, wrapping around fetal parts (neck or arm) or prolapse. Long straight untwisted cords are associated with fetal distress, anomalies and intrauterine fetal demise. The separation of the cord after more than one month (*delayed separation*) has been associated with

overwhelming bacterial infection and neutrophilic chemotactic defects. A *single umbilical artery* is present in about 5–10 per 1,000 births. The frequency is about 35–70/1,000 in twin birth. Approximately 30% of infants with a single umbilical artery have congenital abnormalities, usually more than one. Many such infants are still born or die shortly after birth. Trisomy 18 is one of the more frequent anomalies. It is important that at every delivery the cut cord and the maternal and fetal surfaces of the placenta be inspected and the number of arteries present is recorded. Many recommend renal ultrasonography. *Patency of the omphalomesenteric (vitelline) duct* may be associated with intestinal obstruction, intestinal fistula with fecal or bilious draining, prolapse of the bowel, a polyp (cyst), or a Meckel diverticulum. Therapy is surgical excision of the anomaly. *Persistent urachus* (urachal cyst, sinus, patent urachus, or diverticulum) is due to failure of closure of the allantoic duct and is associated with bladder outlet obstruction. Patency is suspected if a clear, light yellow, urine-like fluid is being discharged from the umbilicus. Symptoms include drainage, a mass or cyst, abdominal pain, local erythema, or infection. Urachal anomalies should be investigated by ultrasonography and a cystogram. Therapy is surgical excision of the anomaly and correction of any bladder outlet obstruction if present. Modern perinatal practices, rigorous asepsis, proper handwashing and cord care has reduced the incidence of *umbilical infection* (omphalitis) to less than 1%. The risk factors are home deliveries, low birth weight, use of umbilical catheters and septic delivery. Omphalitis may remain localized or may spread to the abdominal wall, the peritoneum, the umbilical or portal vessels, or the liver. Portal vein phlebitis may develop and result in the later onset of extrahepatic portal hypertension. Infants with abdominal wall cellulitis or those with necrotizing fasciitis have a high incidence of associated bacteremia. Treatment includes prompt antibiotic therapy (effective against *Staphylococcus aureus* and *Escherichia coli*) and, if abscess formation has occurred, surgical incision and drainage. Necrotizing fasciitis is often polymicrobial and has a high mortality.

Umbilical hernia: See Section 16.15, page-471.

Umbilical granuloma: The umbilical cord usually dries and separates within 6–8 days after birth. The raw surface becomes covered by a thin layer of skin; scar tissue forms, and the wound is usually healed within 12–15 days. Mild infection or incomplete epithelization may result in a moist granulation tissue at the base of the cord. The tissue is soft, 3–10 mm in size, vascular and granular, and dull red or pink, and it may have a seropurulent secretion. *Treatment* is cauterization with silver nitrate, repeated at intervals of several days until the base is dry. Umbilical granuloma must be differentiated from umbilical polyp, a rare anomaly resulting from persistence of all or part of the omphalomesenteric duct or the urachus. The tissue of the polyp is firm and resistant, is bright red and has a mucoid secretion. If the polyp is communicating with the ileum or urinary bladder, small amounts of fecal matter or urine may be discharged intermittently. Histologically, the polyp consists of intestinal or urinary tract mucosa. Treatment is surgical excision of the entire omphalomesenteric or urachal remnant.

Tumors of the umbilicus are rare and include angioma, enteroteratoma, dermoid cyst, myxosarcoma, and cysts of urachal or omphalomesenteric duct remnants.

Hemorrhage from the umbilical cord may be due to trauma, inadequate ligation of the cord, hemorrhagic disease of the newborn or other coagulopathies (especially factor XIII deficiency), septicemia, local infection or failure of normal thrombus formation. The infant should be observed frequently during the first few days of life so that if hemorrhage does occur, it will be detected promptly.

Amch EA, Nmadu PT. Major complications of omphalitis in neonates and infants. *Pediatr Surg Int* 2002; 18: 413–416.

Mason WH, Andrews R, Ross LA, et al: Omphalitis in the newborn infants. *Pediatrics Infect Dis J* 1989; 8: 521–525.

Pomeranz A. Anomalies, abnormalities, and care of the umbilicus. *Pediatr Clin North Am* 2004; 51: 819–827.

Stoll BJ. The umbilicus. In: Kliegman RM, Behrman RE, Jenson HB, Stanton BF (eds). *Nelson Textbook of Pediatrics.* 18th edn. Vol 1. Philadelphia: Saunders, 2007; 775–777.

8.14 METABOLIC PROBLEMS

Hyperthermia in the newborn (transitory fever of the newborn, dehydration fever): Elevations of temperature (38–39°C or 100–103°F) are occasionally noted on the 2nd–3rd day of life in infants who are otherwise normal. This problem is particularly noted in breastfed infants whose intake of fluid has been low or in infants who are overdressed or are exposed to high environmental temperatures, either in an incubator, in a bassinette near a radiator, or in the sun.

The infant may loose weight, urinary output and the frequency of voiding diminish, and fontanel may be depressed and diminished intake of fluids. But the apparent vigor and activity shows that the infant is not "sick" from an infection. The rise in temperature may be associated with an increase in serum levels of protein and sodium and increase in hematocrit. The possibility of local or systemic infection should be excluded. Administration of oral or parenteral fluids or lowering the environmental temperature brings down prompt reduction of the fever and alleviation of symptoms. Additional nursing (breastfeeding) or formula should be given along with oral fluids and not simply water because of the risk of hyponatremia.

Severe form of neonatal hyperthermia: A more severe form of neonatal hyperthermia occurs in both newborn and older infants when they are warmly dressed for outdoor low temperatures that actually do not exist in their immediate indoor environment. The diminished sweating capacity of newborn infants is a contributing factor. Body temperature may become as high as 41–44°C (106–111°F). The skin is hot and dry, infant usually appears flushed and apathetic and tachypnea and irritability may be noted. This stage may be followed by stupor, grayish pallor, coma, and convulsions. Hypernatremia may contribute to the convulsions. Mortality and morbidity rates (brain damage) are high. Hyperthermia is associated with sudden infant death and with hemorrhagic shock and encephalopathy syndrome. The condition is prevented by dressing infants in clothing suitable for the temperature of the immediate environment. In newborn infants, exposure of the body to usual room temperature or immersion in tepid water brings the temperature back to normal levels. Older infants may require cooling for a longer time. Fluid and electrolyte disturbances should be treated.

Neonatal cold injury: It usually occurs in abandoned infants or those in inadequately heated homes during damp cold spells when outside temperature is in the freezing range. The initial features are apathy, refusal of food, oliguria, and coldness to touch. The body temperature is usually between 29.5 and 35°C (85–95°F). Immobility, edema and redness of extremities, especially hands and feet and face, rhinitis, and hemorrhagic manifestations are observed. Hypoglycemia and acidosis occur. Treatment consists of warming and correcting hypotension and metabolic disturbances, particularly hypoglycemia. Prevention consists of providing adequate heat. The mortality rate is about 10%; about 10% of survivors have evidence of brain damage.

Edema may be generalized or localized. *Generalized edema* occurs in association with hydrops fetalis and in the offspring of diabetic mothers. In premature infants edema is due to their decreased ability to excrete water or sodium. Infants with respiratory distress syndrome may become edematous without heart failure. Edema may be associated with heart failure. A sudden large increase in intake of electrolytes, particularly with feeding of concentrated cow's milk formulas may result in edema due to a lag in renal excretion of electrolytes and water. High-protein formulas may also cause edema as a result of the excessive renal solute load, particularly in premature infants. Idiopathic hypoproteinemia with edema lasting weeks or months is rarely observed in term infants; the disturbance is benign. Generalized edema with hypoproteinemia may be seen in the neonatal period with congenital nephrosis and rarely with Hurler syndrome, or after feeding hypoallergic formulas in infants with cystic fibrosis of pancreas.

Localized edema: Edema of the face and scalp may be caused by pressure from the umbilical cord around the neck, and transient localized swelling of the hands or feet may similarly be due to intrauterine pressure. Persistent edema of one or more extremities may represent congenital lymphedema (Milroy disease) or, in females, Turner syndrome.

Sclerema neonatorum: It is an uncommon disorder of adipose tissue that present abruptly in preterm, gravely ill infants as diffuse, yellowish-white woody induration of the skin. Affected skin becomes stony in consistency, cold and nonpitting. The face assumes a mask-like expression, and joint mobility may be compromised because of inflexibility of the skin. Histopathologic findings consist of an increase in the size of fat cells and an increase in the width of the fibrous connective tissue septa. Sclerema neonatorum is almost always associated with serious illness, such as sepsis, congenital heart disease, multiple congenital anomalies, or hypothermia. The outcome depends on the response of the underlying disorder to treatment.

Hypoglycemia: See Section 8.15, page-240.

Hypocalcemia (Tetany): Congenital rickets occurs when there is severe maternal vitamin D deficiency during pregnancy. Maternal risk factors include poor dietary intake of vitamin D, lack of adequate sun exposure, and closely spaced pregnancies. These newborns may have symptomatic hypocalcemia, intrauterine growth restriction (IUGR), and decreased bone ossification, along with classic rachitic changes. Subtler maternal vitamin D deficiency may have an adverse effect on neonatal bone density and birth weight and cause a defect in dental enamel, and predispose infants to neonatal hypocalcemic tetany. The treatment of congenital rickets includes vitamin D supplementation and adequate intake of calcium and phosphorus. Use of prenatal vitamins containing vitamin D prevents this entity.

Metabolic bone disease: It is a common complication in very low birth weight preterm infants. Progressive osteopenia with demineralized bones and occasionally pathologic fractures may develop. The major cause is inadequate intake of calcium and also poor intake of phosphorus and vitamin D. The contributing factors include prolonged parenteral nutrition, vitamin D and calcium malabsorption, intake of unsupplemented human milk, immobilization, and urinary calcium losses from chronic diuretic use. Serum alkaline phosphatase level is used to monitor metabolic bone disease. Fortified human milk and formulas designed for preterm infants provide improved intake of calcium, phosphorus, and vitamin D. Treatment of fractures requires immobilization and administration of calcium and, if needed phosphorus (for hypophosphatemia) and vitamin D (not more than 1,000 IU/day unless severe cholestasis or vitamin D resistance is present).

Hypomagnesemia occurs when serum magnesium levels fall below 1.5 mg/dl (0.62 mmol/L), although clinical signs do not develop until serum magnesium levels fall below 1.2 mg/dl. Hypomagnesemia may occur in newborn infants:

1. In association with inefficient stores of skeletal magnesium secondary to deficient placental transfer, decreased intestinal absorption, neonatal hypoparathyroidism, hyperphosphatemia, renal loss (primary or secondary to drugs, e.g. amphotericin B)
2. Due to a defect in magnesium and calcium homeostasis
3. In iatrogenic deficiency caused by loss incurred during exchange transfusion or insufficient replacement during total intravenous alimentation
4. During exchange transfusion with citrated blood
5. In infants of diabetic mothers; and
6. Rarely hypomagnesemia of unknown cause usually in association with hypocalcemia. The clinical manifestations of hypomagnesemia are indistinguishable from those of hypocalcaemia and tetany and may actually contribute to the accompanying hypocalcemia. Immediate treatment consists of intramuscular injection of magnesium sulfate (newborn infants: 25–50 mg/kg/dose q 8 hr for 3–4 doses). The accompanying hypocalcemia usually corrects itself as the hypomagnesemia resolves. Same daily dose can be given for oral maintenance therapy. Four to 5 times higher doses may be required in malabsorption states. In most cases, the metabolic defect is transient and treatment can be discontinued after 1–2 wk. A few patients may have permanent form of the disease that requires continuous oral therapy to prevent recurrence of hypomagnesemia. No residual damage to the central nervous system occurs after prompt treatment.

Hypermagnesemia may occur in newborn infants of mothers treated with magnesium sulfate during labor and in those associated with failure to pass meconium (**meconium plug syndrome**). The upper limit of normal magnesium is 2.8 mg/dl (1.15 mmol/l, but serious symptoms rarely occur at levels below 5 mg/dl (2.1 mmol/l). At high serum levels, the central nervous system is depressed and infants have profound respiratory depression requiring mechanical ventilation. Lower levels may result in hypoventilation, lethargy, flaccidity, hyporeflexia, and poor sucking. In most cases no specific therapy other than supportive care and maintenance of respiratory support is required. Intravenous calcium and diuresis will reduce magnesium levels. In rare cases, exchange transfusion has been used for rapid removal of magnesium ion from the blood.

Substance abuse and neonatal abstinence (Withdrawal): Substance abuse during pregnancy is a serious problem for both the mother and her newborn. Pregnancy in women who use illegal drugs or alcohol is by definition, high risk. Prenatal care is usually inadequate, and these women have a higher incidence of sexually transmitted infections, including syphilis, HIV, and hepatitis. In addition, the risk of premature labor, intrauterine growth restriction, premature rupture of membranes, and perinatal morbidity and mortality is higher. Physiologic addiction to narcotics occurs in most infants born to actively addicted mothers because opiates cross the placenta. Withdrawal may be manifested even before birth by increased activity of fetus when the mother feels a need for the drug or withdrawal symptoms develop. Heroin and methadone are the drugs frequently associated with withdrawal syndromes, but such syndromes may also occur with alcohol, nicotine, phenobarbital, pentazocine, codeine, propoxyphene, hydroxyzine, amphetamines, neuroleptics, antidepressants, and benzodiazepines.

Fetal alcohol syndrome (FAS): High levels of alcohol ingestion during pregnancy can be damaging to embryonic and fetal development. Both moderate and high levels of alcohol intake during early pregnancy may result in alterations in growth and morphogenesis of the fetus; the greater the uptake, the more severe the signs. Additional maternal risk factors associated with FAS are advanced maternal age, low socio-economic status, poor psychologic indicators, and binge drinking.

Characteristics of fetal alcohol syndrome (FAS) include:
1. Prenatal onset and persistence of growth deficiency for length, weight, and head circumference
2. Facial abnormalities, including short palpebral fissures, epicanthal folds, maxillary hypoplasia, micrognathia, smooth philtrum, and a thin, smooth upper lip
3. Cardiac defects, primarily septal defects
4. Minor joint and limb abnormalities, including some restriction of movement and altered palmar crease patterns, and
5. Delayed development and mental deficiency varying from borderline to severe. FAS is a common identifiable cause of mental retardation. The severity of dysmorphogenesis may range from severely affected infants with full manifestations of fetal alcohol syndrome to those mildly affected with only a few manifestations. Alcohol may impair placental transfer of essential amino acids and zinc, both necessary for protein synthesis, which may account for the intrauterine growth restriction.

There is no specific therapy. These infants may remain hypotonic and tremulous despite sedation, and the prognosis is poor. Counseling with regard to recurrence is important. Prevention is best achieved by eliminating alcohol intake after conception.

Greenbaum LA. Rickets and hypervitaminosis D. In: Kliegman RM, Behrman RE, Jenson HB, Stanton BF (eds). *Nelson Textbook of Pediatrics.* 18th edn. Vol 2. Philadelphia: Saunders, 2007;253–62.

Johnson K, Gerada C, Greenough A. Treatment of neonatal abstinence syndrome. *Arch Dis Child Fetal Neonatal Ed* 2003; 88:F2-5.

Morelli JG. Diseases of subcutaneous tissue. In: Kliegman RM, Behrman RE, Jenson HB, Stanton BF (eds). *Nelson Textbook of Pediatrics.* 18th edn. Vol 2. Philadelphia: Saunders, 2007; 2721–4.

Stoll BJ. Metabolic disturbances. In: Kliegman RM, Behrman RE, Jenson HB, Stanton BF (eds). *Nelson Textbook of Pediatrics.* 18th edn. Vol 1. Philadelphia: Saunders, 2007;775–82.

8.15 ENDOCRINE SYSTEM

Pituitary dwarfism is not usually diagnosed at birth, although panhypopituitary male infants may have neonatal hypoglycemia, hyperbilirubinemia, and micropenis.

Congenital hypothyroidism: See Section 23.3, page-688.

Transient hypothyroxinemia of prematurity is most common in ill very low birth weight (VLBW) infants. These infants are probably chemically euthyroid, as suggested by normal levels of serum thyrotropin and other tests of the pituitary-hypothalamic axis. They may be manifested as tetany of the newborn.

Transient hyperthyroidism may occur at birth in infants of mothers with hyperthyroidism or in infants whose mothers have been receiving thyroid medication.

Adrenal glands disturbances may become apparent and require life-saving treatment during the neonatal period. *Acute adrenal hemorrhage* and failure may occur after breech or other traumatic deliveries or in association with overwhelming infection. Congenital adrenal hyperplasia is suggested by vomiting, diarrhea, dehydration, hyperkalemia, hyponatremia, shock, ambiguous genitals and hypertension. Because the condition is genetically determined, newborn siblings of patients with the salt-loosing variety of adrenocortical hyperplasia should also be closely observed for manifestations of adrenal insufficiency. Congenitally hypoplastic adrenal glands may also give rise to adrenal insufficiency during the first few weeks of life.

Gonadal dysgenesis should be suspected in female infants with webbing of the neck, lymphangiectatic edema, hypoplasia of the nipples, cutix laxa, low hairline at the nape of the neck, low-set ears, high-arced palate, deformities of the nails, cubitus valgus, and other anomalies.

Transient diabetes mellitus: See Section 23.7, page-722.
Syndrome of transient diabetes mellitus in the newborn: See section 23.7, page-722.

Infants of Diabetic Mother

Women with diabetes in pregnancy (Type 1, Type 2, and gestational diabetes) are at increased risk for adverse pregnancy outcomes. Gestational diabetes is when carbohydrate intolerance occurs only during pregnancy and affects about 2% of pregnant women. Therefore, adequate glycemic control before and during pregnancy is essential for improving outcome. Diabetic mothers have a high incidence of polyhydramnios, pre-eclampsia, pyelonephritis, preterm labor and chronic hypertension. The fetal mortality rate is higher at all gestational ages, especially after 32 wk, and is greater than that of non-diabetic mothers. Fetal loss is associated with poorly controlled maternal diabetes (**especially ketoacidosis**) and congenital anomalies. Most infants born to diabetic mothers are large for gestational age. If the diabetes is complicated by vascular disease, infants may be growth restricted, especially those born after 37 wk of gestation. The neonatal mortality rate is more than 5 times that of infants of non-diabetic mothers. Mortality is higher at all gestational ages and in every birth weight for gestational age category.

Pathophysiology: Maternal hyperglycemia causes fetal hyperglycemia, and the fetal pancreatic response leads to fetal hyperinsulinemia; fetal hyperinsulinemia and hyperglycemia then cause increased hepatic glucose uptake and glycogen synthesis, accelerated lipogenesis and augmented protein synthesis. This results in hypertrophy and hyperplasia of the pancreatic islets with a disproportionate increase in the number of beta cells; increased weight of the placenta and infant organs except for the brain; myocardial hypertrophy; increased amounts of cytoplasm in liver cells; and extrapulmonary hematopoiesis. Hyperinsulinism and hyperglycemia produce fetal acidosis, which may result in an increased rate of stillbirth.

Separation of the placenta at birth suddenly interrupts glucose infusion into the neonate without a proportional effect on the hyperinsulinism, resulting in hypoglycemia and attenuated lipolysis during the first hours after birth. Hyperinsulinemia has been documented in infants of gestational diabetic mothers and in those of insulin-dependent diabetic mothers without insulin antibodies.

Although hyperinsulinism is probably the main cause of hypoglycemia, the diminished epinephrine and glucagon responses that occur may be the contributory factors. Chronic fetal hypoxia, indicated by elevated amniotic fluid erythropoietin levels, is associated with increased fetal and neonatal morbidity. Birth trauma is a common sequela of fetal macrosomia.

Clinical manifestations: Infants of diabetic and gestational diabetic-mothers often have resemblance to each other. They are:

1. Large and plump as a result of increased body fat and enlarged viscera, with puffy and plethoric facies, resembling patients, who are receiving corticosteroids; or
2. Normal or low birth weight particularly if they are delivered before term or if there is associated maternal vascular disease.

Hypoglycemia develops in about 25–50% of infants of diabetic mothers and 15–25% of infants of mothers with gestational diabetes, but only few infants become symptomatic. The infants tend to be jumpy, tremulous, and hyperexcitable during the 1st 3 days of life, although hypotonia, lethargy, and poor sucking may also occur. They may have any of the diverse manifestations of hypoglycemia. Early appearance of these signs is more likely to be related to hypoglycemia and later appearance related to hypocalcemia; these abnormalities may also occur together. Hypomagnesemia may be associated with the hypocalcemia. Perinatal asphyxia or hyperbilirubinemia may produce similar signs. These manifestations may also occur in the absence of hypoglycemia, hypocalcemia, or asphyxia.

Tachypnea develops in many infants of diabetic mothers during the 1st 2 days of life and may be manifestation of hypoglycemia, hypothermia, polycythemia, cardiac failure, transient tachypnea, or cerebral edema from birth trauma or asphyxia.

Infants of diabetic mothers have a higher incidence of **respiratory distress syndrome (RDS)** than do infants of nondiabetic mothers born of comparable gestational age; the greater incidence is due to an antagonistic effect of insulin on stimulation of surfactant synthesis by cortisol.

Cardiomegaly is common (30%) and **heart failure** occurs in 5–10% of infants of diabetic mothers. **Congenital heart disease** is more common in infants of diabetic mothers and **asymmetric septal hypertrophy** may occur and become manifested similar to transient idiopathic hypertrophic subaortic stenosis.

Neurologic development and ossification centers tend to be immature and correlate with the brain size (which is not increased) and gestational age rather than with total body weight.

These infants have increased incidence of **hyperbilirubinemia, polycythemia, and renal vein thrombosis** (suspect in the presence of a flank mass, hematuria and thrombocytopenia).

The incidence of **congenital anomalies** is increased threefold in infants of diabetic mothers; cardiac malformation (VSD, ASD, coarctation of aorta, transposition of great vessels, truncus arteriosus, double outlet right ventricle, tricuspid atresia) and lumbosacral agenesis are most common. Additional anomalies include neural tube defects, renal abnormalities (hydronephrosis, renal agenesis and dysplasia, double ureter), gastrointestinal (duodenal or anorectal atresia, small left colon syndrome characterized by abdominal distension), situs inversus, and holoprosencephaly.

Treatment: It should be initiated before birth by frequent prenatal evaluation of all pregnant women with overt or gestational diabetes, by evaluation of fetal maturity, by biophysical profile, by Doppler velocimetry, and by planning delivery of these infants in hospitals where expert obstetric and pediatric care is continuously available. Periconception glucose control reduces the risk of anomalies, and glucose control during labor reduces the incidence of neonatal hypoglycemia. It is important that all infants born from diabetic mothers should initially receive intensive observation and care. Asymptomatic infants should have a blood glucose determination within 1 hr of birth and then every hour for the next 6–8 hr. If the infant is clinically well and normoglycemic, oral or gavage feedings with breastmilk or formula should be started as soon as possible and continued at 3 hr intervals for 24–48 hr. If the infant is unable to tolerate oral feeding, the feeding should be discontinued and glucose given by intravenous infusion at a rate of 4–8 mg/kg/ minute. Even in asymptomatic infants hypoglycemia should be treated with intravenous infusions of glucose sufficient to keep the blood levels well above this level. Avoid use of bolus injections of hypertonic glucose, because they may cause further hyperinsulinemias and potentially produce rebound hypoglycemia. The treatment of hypocalcemia and hypomagnesemia, hyaline membrane disease and polycythemia is discussed in separate chapters.

Women with Type 1 diabetes who have tight glucose control during pregnancy (average daily glucose levels < 95 mg/dl) deliver infants with birth weights and anthropometric features that are similar to those of infants of nondiabetic mothers. Treatment of gestational diabetes also reduces complications. The treatment includes dietary advice, glucose monitoring, and insulin therapy as needed decrease the rate of serious perinatal outcomes (shoulder dystocia, bone fracture, nerve palsy or death).

Prognosis: The incidence of diabetes in infants from diabetic mothers is increased. Oversized infants may be predisposed to childhood obesity that may extend into adult life. Both premature and full term infants are at risk of impaired intellectual function that has symptomatic hypoglycemia.

Langer O, Yogev Y, Most O, et al. Gestational diabetes: The consequences of not treating. *Am J Obstet Gynecol* 2005;192:989–97.

Nold JL, Georgieff MK. Infants of diabetic mothers. *Pediatr Clin North Am* 2004;51:619–37.

Stoll BJ. The endocrine system. In: Kliegman RM, Behrman RE, Jenson HB, Stanton BF (eds). *Nelson Textbook of Pediatrics.* 18th edn. Vol 1. Philadelphia: Saunders, 2007;782–86.

8.16 INFECTIONS OF THE NEONATAL INFANT

Infections frequently affect newborn and are the important cause of neonatal and infant morbidity and mortality. As many as 2% of fetuses are infected *in utero*, and up to 10% of infants have infections in 1st month of life. The outcome depends mainly the timing of infection during gestation:

1. First trimester infection may alter embryogenesis, with resulting congenital malformations (congenital rubella)
2. Third trimester infection often results in active infection at the time of delivery (toxoplasmosis, syphilis); and
3. Infections that occur late in gestation may lead to a delay in clinical manifestations until some time after birth (syphilis).

The modes of transmission are: (i) *intrauterine infection*; (ii) *ascending bacterial infection*; (iii) *late-onset postnatal infections:* Transmitted by direct contact with hospital staff, the mother, or other family members or from breastmilk (HIV, CMV), or from inanimate sources such as contaminated equipment.

Congenital pneumonia may be caused by CMV, rubella virus, and *T. pallidum* and less commonly, by the other agents producing transplacental infection. The microorganisms responsible for nosocomial pneumonia include bacteria (staphylococcal species, gram-negative enteric aerobes, and occasionally, *Pseudomonas*); fungi (candida); respiratory viruses (acquired from respiratory syncytial virus, para-influenza virus, influenza viruses, and adenovirus).

Neonatal meningitis is caused by GBS, *E. coli*, *L. monocytogenes*. *S. pneumoniae*, other streptococci, non-typable *Haemophilus influenzae*, coagulase positive and negative staphylococci, *Klebsiella*, *Enterobacter*, *Pseudomonas*, and *T. pallidum*. *Mycobacterium tuberculosis* may also produce meningitis.

Clinical manifestations: The clinical manifestations of transplacental infections are:

 i. Intrauterine growth restriction
 ii. Congenital anatomic defects (cataracts, heart defects, hydrocephalus, intracranial calcification, limb hypoplasia, microcephaly, microphthalmos)
 iii. Neonatal organ involvement (anemia, carditis, encephalitis, hepatitis, hepatosplenomegaly, hydrops, lymphadenopathy, osteitis, petechiae, purpura, pneumonitis, retinitis, rhinitis, skin lesions, thrombocytopenia)
 iv. Late sequelae (convulsions, deafness, dental/skeletal, endocrinopathies, eye pathology, hepatitis, mental retardation, nephrotic syndrome).

Bacterial sepsis: Neonates with bacterial sepsis may have either nonspecific signs and symptoms or focal signs of infection including temperature instability, hypotension, poor perfusion with pallor and mottled skin, metabolic acidosis, tachycardia or bradycardia, apnea, respiratory distress, grunting, cyanosis, irritability, lethargy, seizures, feeding intolerance, abdominal distension, jaundice, petechiae, purpura, bleeding, cutaneous manifestations (impetigo, cellulitis, mastitis, omphalitis, subcutaneous abscesses and ecthyma gangrenosum), pneumonia and neonatal tetanus. The initial manifestation may involve only limited symptomatology and only one system such as apnea alone or tachypnea with retractions or tachycardia, or it may be an acute catastrophic manifestation with multiorgan dysfunction. Respiratory distress syndrome secondary to surfactant deficiency can coexist with bacterial pneumonia.

Diagnosis

The maternal history may provide important information about maternal exposure to infection (including sexually transmitted infections from pregnant mothers and their partners), maternal immunity (natural or acquired), maternal colonization, and obstetric risk factors (prematurity, prolonged ruptured membranes, maternal chorioamnionitis).

Suspected intrauterine infection: The acronym *TORCH* refers to toxoplasmosis, other agents (syphilis, etc), rubella, CMV, and HSV. CMV and HSV require culture or polymerase chain reaction (PCR) methods; whereas syphilis, toxoplasmosis, and rubella are diagnosed by specific serologic methods.

Suspected bacterial or fungal infections: Bacterial or fungal infection is diagnosed by isolating the etiologic agent from a normally sterile body site (blood, CSF, urine, joint fluid). Obtaining 2 blood culture specimens by venepuncture from different sites avoids confusion caused by skin contamination and increases the likelihood of bacterial detection. Documentation of a positive blood culture is the first diagnostic criterion that must be met with sepsis.

When the clinical findings suggest an acute infection and the site of infection is unclear, additional studies should be performed, including blood cultures, lumbar puncture, urine examination, and a chest X-ray. Urine should be collected by catheterization or suprapubic aspiration. Demonstration of bacteria and inflammatory cells in Gram-stained gastric aspirates on the 1st day of life may reflect maternal amnionitis, which is a risk factor for early-onset infection. Stains of endotracheal secretions in infants with early-onset pneumonia may demonstrate intracellular bacteria and cultures may reveal either pathogens or upper respiratory tract flora. Examination of the placenta can be helpful in the diagnosis of both chronic and acute intrauterine infections. In an asymptomatic term infant whose mother has chorioamnionitis, two blood cultures should be performed and presumptive treatment initiated. The diagnosis of pneumonia in a neonate is usually presumptive; microbiologic proof of infection is generally lacking because lung tissue is not easily cultured. Blood culture results are usually negative, and sufficient pleural fluid for culture is rarely present.

The diagnosis of meningitis is confirmed by examination of CSF and identification of a bacterium, virus, or fungus by culture, antigen, or the use of PCR. Gram stain of CSF yields a positive result in most patients with bacterial meningitis. The leukocyte count is usually elevated, with a predominance of neutrophils (> 70–90%); the number is often > 1,000 and may be < 100 in infants with neutropenia or early in the disease. Contamination of CSF by bacteria after traumatic lumbar puncture may occur rarely. Culture-negative meningitis may be seen with antibiotic pretreatment, a brain abscess, or infection with *Mycobacterium hominis*, *U. urealyticum*, *Bacteroides fragilis*, enterovirus, or HSV. Head ultrasonography or, more often, CT with contrast enhancement may be helpful in diagnosing ventriculitis and brain abscess.

Sepsis screen: Indirect markers of neonatal infection constitute a useful sepsis screen for clinically doubtful cases. Sepsis screen is considered positive if two of these parameters are positive. The diagnosis of sepsis can be reasonably excluded if two screens 12–24 hr apart are negative.

1. White blood count (WBC < 5,000 cells per mm^3)
2. Absolute neutrophil count (ANC < 2,000 cells per mm^3)
3. Immature to total neutrophil ratio (I : T ratio of >0.3); and
4. C-reactive protein (CRP) concentration above 1 mg/dl.

Treatment

Treatment of suspected bacterial infection is determined by the pattern of disease and the organisms that are common for the age of the infant and the flora of the nursery. Once appropriate culture have been obtained, intravenous or, less often, intramuscular antibiotic therapy should be instituted immediately. Initial empirical treatment of early-onset bacterial infections should consist of ampicillin and an aminoglycoside (usually gentamicin). Nosocomial infections acquired in a NICU are more likely to be caused by staphylococci, various *Enterobacteriaceae*, *Pseudomonas* species, or *Candida* species. Thus, an antistaphylococcal drug (methicillin or nafcillin for *S. aureus* or, more often, vancomycin for coagulase-negative staphylococci or methicillin-resistant *S. aureus*) should be substituted for ampicillin. Third-generation cephalosporins such as cefotaxime are valuable additions for treating documented neonatal sepsis and meningitis. Therapy for most bloodstream infections should be continued for a total of 7–10 days or for at least 5–7 days after a clinical response has occurred. A blood culture taken 24–48 hr after initiation of therapy should yield negative results. If the blood culture remains positive, the possibility of an infected indwelling catheter, endocarditis, an infected thrombus, an occult abscess, subtherapeutic antibiotic levels, or resistant organisms should be considered. A change in antibiotics, longer duration of therapy, or removal of the catheter may be indicated.

Treatment of newborn infants with early-onset sepsis, whose mothers received antibiotics during labor, be continued until it is shown that *no infection* has occurred (the infant remains asymptomatic for 24–72 hr) or clinical and laboratory evidence of recovery is apparent. It is also important to consider that the organism causing infection to the newborn infant may be resistant to the antibiotic given to the mother, which may influence the choice of antibiotic use in the infant.

For pneumonia developing in the 1st 7–10 days of life, a combination of ampicillin and an aminoglycoside or cefotaxime is appropriate. Nosocomial pneumonia, generally manifested after this time, can be treated empirically with methicillin or vancomycin and an aminoglycoside or a 3rd generation cephalosporin.

Presumptive antimicrobial therapy for bacterial meningitis should include ampicillin in meningitic doses and cefotaxime or gentamicin unless staphylococci are likely which an indication for vancomycin. Meningitis caused by GBS usually responds within 24–48 hr and should be treated for 14–21 days. Treatment of gram-negative meningitis should be continued for 21 days or for at least 14 days after sterilization of the CSF, whichever is longer. Metronidazole is the treatment of choice for infection caused by *B. fragilis*. Prolonged antibiotic administration, with or without drainage for treatment and diagnosis, is indicated for neonatal cerebral abscesses. CT scans are recommended for patients with suspected ventriculitis, hydrocephalus, or cerebral abscess and for those with an unexpectedly complicated course (prolonged coma, focal neurologic deficits, persistent or recurrent fever). Neonatal herpes meningoencephalitis should be treated with acyclovir, and empirical therapy should be considered in symptomatic infants with a CSF mononuclear pleocytosis. Treatment of Candida infection is discussed in Section 14.11. It is important to remember that nonbacterial infectious agents can produce the syndrome of neonatal sepsis.

Disseminated intravascular coagulation (DIC) may complicate neonatal septicemia. Platelet counts, hemoglobin, and clotting studies should be monitored. DIC is treated by management of the underlying infection, but if bleeding occurs, DIC may require fresh frozen plasma, platelet transfusions, or whole blood.

Careful attention to respiratory and cardiovascular status is mandatory. Adequate oxygenation of tissues should be maintained; ventilator support is frequently necessary for respiratory failure caused by sepsis, pneumonia, pulmonary hypertension or ARDS. Refractory hypoxia and shock may require extra-corporeal membrane oxygenation, which has reduced mortality rates in full-term infants with respiratory failure. Shock and metabolic acidosis if present should be managed with fluid and inotropic agents. Corticosteroids should be administered only for adrenal insufficiency. Fluids, electrolytes, and glucose levels should be monitored and correction of hypovolemia, hyponatremia, hypocalcemia, and hypoglycemia should be done. if hyperbilirubinemia is present, it should be treated with phototherapy and/or exchange transfusion because the risk of kernicterus increases in the presence of sepsis and meningitis. Seizures should be treated with anticonvulsants. Infants who cannot sustain enteral feeding should be given parenteral nutrition.

Prevention

A number of intrauterine infections are preventable through maternal immunization, including hepatitis B, rubella, and VZV. Toxoplasmosis is preventable with appropriate diet and avoidance of exposure to cat feces. Malaria during pregnancy can be minimized with chemoprophylaxis. Congenital syphilis is prevented by early diagnosis and appropriate early treatment of infected pregnant women. Neonatal tetanus can be prevented by maternal tetanus immunization and proper care of the umbilical cord. Treatment of suspected maternal chorioamnionitis with antibiotics during labor, along with rapid delivery of the infant, reduces the risk of early-onset neonatal sepsis. Vertical transmission of GBS (Group B streptococcus) is significantly reduced by selective intrapartum chemoprophylaxis. Neonatal infection with *Chlamydia* can be prevented by identification and treatment of infected pregnant women. Mother-to-child transmission is reduced by maternal anti-retroviral therapy during pregnancy, labor, and delivery, cesarean section delivery prior to rupture of membranes and antiretroviral treatment of the infant after birth.

Prevention of nosocomial infection: Most nosocomial infections in the NICU are bloodstream infections associated with an intravenous catheter. The skin is an important mechanical barrier to infection. VLBW infants are born with an ineffective epidermal barrier that results in increased transepidermal water loss and an increased risk for infection. Hence, reduce traumatic injury to this immature skin, including reduction in the number of heelsticks. Handwashing is the most important and effective means of reducing nosocomial infections. Ongoing education of staff regarding practices that are likely to reduce nosocomial infections and active surveillance of infection rates are important components of nosocomial infection control.

Adams-Chapman I, Stoll BJ. Systemic inflammatory response syndrome. *Semin Pediatr Infect Dis* 2001;12:5–16.

Adams-Chapman I, Stoll BJ. Prevention of nosocomial infections in the neonatal intensive care unit. *Curr Opin Pediatr* 2002;14:157–64.

Stoll BJ. Infections of the Neonatal Infant. In: Kliegman RM, Behrman RE, Jenson HB, Stanton BF (eds). *Nelson Textbook of Pediatrics*. 18th edn. Vol 1. Philadelphia: Saunders, 2007;794–811.

Vergnano S, Sharland M, Kasembe P, et al. Neonatal sepsis: An international perspective. *Arch Dis Child Fetal Neonatal Ed* 2005;90:F220–4.

8.17 NEONATAL SURGICAL EMERGENCIES

Neonates requiring emergency surgical intervention are an integral part of pediatric surgical practice. The neonatal surgical emergencies are listed in Box 8.13.

1. *Bilious vomiting* in a neonate is always abnormal. An initial bilious aspirate on insertion of nasogastric tube of more than 15 ml is highly suggestive. The common conditions presenting as bilious vomiting are duodenal atresia and stenosis, malrotation, intestinal atresias, meconium ileus, necrotizing enterocolitis, Hirschsprung's disease and entero-colitis.

Duodenal atresia and stenosis: The site of obstruction is usually beyond the ampulla of Vater (post ampullary) but may also be preampullary or may involve other parts of the duodenum. Antenatal diagnosis may be suspected on account of polyhydramnios, which is seen in one half of cases. The dilated stomach and proximal duodenum may be visualized on antenatal ultrasonography . The neonate presents usually with persistent bile stained vomiting usually within the first few hours of life. Bilious aspirate of more that 20 ml of gastric or bilious fluid suggests intestinal obstruction and a plain abdominal roentgenogram usually demonstrates a dilated stomach and the proximal duodenum (double-bubble appearance). Presence of intestinal gas beyond duodenum indicates an incomplete obstruction like stenosis or malrotation. Treatment consists of initial period of gastric decompression and fluid and electrolyte management. A diamond shaped side-to-side duodenoduodeno-stomy is the procedure of choice for the bypass of atresias, annular pancreas and some cases of stenosis.

Malrotation and volvulus: See Section 16.13, page-466.

Small bowel obstruction: See Section 16.13, page-468.

Meconium ileus is a neonatal intraluminal intestinal obstruction caused by inspissated meconium blocking the distal ileum. Cystic fibrosis is the predominant cause of meconium ileus and about 15% of patients with cystic fibrosis develop meconium ileus. Meconium ileus is classified into two types: (i) Simple meconium ileus: The distal small bowel (10–30 cm of distal ileum) is relatively small, measuring less than 2 cm in diameter and contains concretions of gray, inspissated meconium with the consistency of thick

Box 8.13: Neonatal surgical emergencies

Bilious vomiting
Non-bilious vomiting
Respiratory distress
Anorectal malformation
Abdominal wall defects
Congenital neurosurgical

glue or putty. (ii) Complicated meconium ileus: Usually occurs during the prenatal period associated to volvulus, atresias, gangrene, perforation or peritonitis. Newborn infant presents with intestinal obstruction, often on the first day of life with abdominal distention and bilious vomiting. Non-operative management is the initial procedure of choice in uncomplicated meconium ileus. It consists of giving gastrograffin enema, which draws water into the bowel lumen and tend to loosen the meconium pellets. Repeat contrast enema or saline enema with acetyl cystine may be done in refractory cases. Surgical therapy is indicated in complicated meconium ileus and in patients' refractory to medical management.

Neonatal necrotizing enterocolitis: See Chapter 8.

Hirschsprung's disease and enterocolitis: Hirschsprung's disease (HD) is due to the failure of ganglion cells (from neural crest) to reach the distal most portion of the alimentary tract. This non-innervated bowel then acts as a functional obstruction leading to constipation, acute intestinal obstruction and enterocolitis. It is believed that the classical HD may have an autosomal recessive inheritance with low penetration, whereas the longer segment variant has an autosomal dominant with incomplete penetration.

The basic pathophysiology in HD is a lack of propagation of propulsive waves and an abnormal or absent relaxation of internal anal sphincter due to aganglionosis. Most children with HD present with intestinal obstruction or severe constipation during the neonatal period. The child also does not pass meconium within the first 24 hr and develops severe abdominal distension. Older children usually present with constipation or repeated episodes of enterocolitis. Enterocolitis presents with diarrhea, with increasing abdominal distention and pain. More severe forms can lead to life-threatening megacolon with fever, bile stained vomiting, explosive diarrhea, abdominal distension, and shock. It may lead to perforation and eventual sepsis.

The *plain radiograph of the abdomen* usually demonstrates air-fluid levels in the dilated colon with an absence/paucity of gas in the rectum. Occasionally, a plain radiograph may demonstrate the presence of free gas in the cavity suggesting a perforation of the

proximal colon. A *barium enema* is often performed in these cases, and is especially useful to confirm the length of aganglionosis and the level of the transition zone. Recently, the *intestinal transit times* are being studied to identify the eventual transition zone and to distinguish neuronal dysplasias from HD. *Anorectal manometry* has also been utilized for the diagnosis of ultra short/short segment HD and to assess anal function after surgery. Manometry shows an absence of rectal inhibitory response on rectal distention and the presence of multisegmental rhythmical contractions, which are pathognomonic of HD. *Rectal biopsy* is the gold standard for the diagnosis of HD. Various methods of biopsy include full-thickness, submucosal biopsy, and the suction rectal biopsy. Full thickness biopsy has been in vogue since the 60s. This method is beset with complications such as bleeding, scarring, and requires general anesthesia. Submucosal biopsy was also introduced the same time, but has since been refined into the rectal suction biopsy. The absence of ganglion cells in both the submucosal and the intermuscular plexus is the hallmark of the disease. There is also an associated marked increase in the submucosal nerve fibers.

Treatment: Once the diagnosis has been reached, the treatment consists of one of the varieties of pull-through procedures where, the aganglionic bowel is removed and the normally ganglionated bowel is brought very close to the anal verge.

2. *Non-bilious vomiting:* The commonest surgical condition presenting with non-bilious vomiting in a neonate is hypertrophic pyloric stenosis. Gastric antral webs, pyloric atresia and gastric volvulus are other causes, but these are exceedingly rare.

Hypertrophic pyloric stenosis (HPS): Pyloric stenosis is an abnormality of the pyloric musculature (hypertrophy) causing gastric outlet obstruction in the neonatal period. The infant usually presents with nonbilious, projectile vomiting which usually start from the first few days of life. The emesis usually occurs shortly after feeding and the infant is constantly hungry. Examination reveals epigastric distention with visible peristaltic waves. Palpation of a firm, mobile, ~ 2 cm in length, olive shaped, hard, best palpated from the left side, and located above and to the right of the umbilicus in the midepigastrium beneath the liver edge. Ultrasonography of abdomen is the most sensitive test to diagnose HPS in the absence of a palpable olive mass; the criteria for diagnosis include pyloric thickness > 4 mm or an overall pyloric length > 14 mm. Contrast upper gastrointestinal study demonstrate an elongated pyloric channel, a bulge of the hypertrophic pyloric muscle into the antrum (shoulder sign), and parallel streaks of barium seen in the narrowed channel producing a "double tract sign". The treatment consists of correction of hypochloremic alkalosis and dehydration. Intravenous fluid therapy is begun with 0.45–0.9% saline, in 5–10% dextrose, with the addition of potassium chloride in concentration of 30–50 mEq/L. Fluid therapy should be continued until the infant is rehydrated and the serum bicarbonate concentration is < 30 mEq/L, which indicates that the alkalosis has been corrected. This is followed by a Ramsteadt pyloromyotomy. Feeds can be resumed within 8–10 hr after surgery.

3. Respiratory distress: Congenital diaphragmatic hernia, esophageal atresia and congenital cystic and solid lesions of the lung may commonly present with respiratory distress in a newborn.

Congenital diaphragmatic hernia: See Chapter 16.

Esophageal atresia and tracheoesophageal fistula: Esophageal atresia (EA) is the most frequent congenital anomaly of the esophagus, affecting ~1/4,000 neonates. Of these, >90% have an associated tracheoesophageal fistula (TEF). There are five most commonly encountered forms of esophageal atresia and tracheoesophageal fistula (TEF). In the most common form of EA, the upper esophagus ends in a blind pouch and the TEF is connected to the distal esophagus. The types of EA and TEF and their relative frequencies are shown in Fig. 8.6.

These children present in the neonatal period with frothing and bubbling at the mouth and nose. There will be excessive salivation and choking, coughing and cyanosis with feedings (3Cs). The mother often had a history of polyhydramnios and an antenatal ultrasonography may demonstrate a small or absent stomach bubble, which is suggestive of an atresia. Inability to pass a stiff No. 10 nasogastric tube into the stomach confirms the diagnosis. The infant with an isolated TEF in the absence of EA (H-type fistula) may come to medical attention later in life with chronic respiratory problems, including refractory bronchospasm and recurrent pneumonias. The chest radiograph will often confirm that the nasogastric tube is coiled up in the cervical region. The presence of air in the stomach points to the presence of a fistula to the distal pouch, whereas a gasless, scaphoid abdomen is evidence of a pure atresia. A contrast study of the upper esophagus may demonstrate the blind upper pouch, but is rarely used because of the risk of aspiration pneumonitis. Recently, direct sagittal computerized tomography has been used to evaluate patients with EA and is useful in assessing the interpouch distance and associated aortic arch and cardiac anomalies. Fifty percent of

infants are nonsyndromic without other anomalies while the rest have associated anomalies. Associated anomalies include musculoskeletal, cardiovascular, gastrointestinal and genitourinary anomalies. They may occur individually or as part of an association of abnormalities known as VATER (vertebral and vascular, anal, tracheal, esophageal, radial, and renal) or the VACTERAL (vertebral, anal, cardiac, tracheal, esophageal, renal and limb) association. Tracheomalacia and disordered esophageal motility is seen very commonly. Radiographs of the chest and the abdomen, echocardiography and ultrasonography of the abdomen are often used to diagnose these associated anomalies. The management includes correction of dehydration, acid–base disturbances, respiratory distress and decompression of the upper esophageal pouch. Prone positioning minimizes movement of gastric secretions into a distal fistula, and esophageal suctioning minimizes aspiration from a blind pouch. Chest physiotherapy and antibiotics may be indicated in case of associated pneumonitis. Surgical ligation of the TEF and primary end-to-end anastomosis of the esophagus are performed when feasible.

Congenital lobar emphysema (CLE): CLE is a postnatal overdistention of one or more lobes of a histologically normal lung and is believed to be due to a cartilaginous deficiency in the tracheobronchial tree. This causes bronchomalacia producing a check valve type of obstruction leading to severe air trapping within the affected lobe. The affected portion of the lung is dilated, which compresses the normal lobes and often causes mediastinal shift away from the affected side. The left upper lobe is most commonly involved followed by the right middle and upper lobes. Lower lobar involvement is unusual. Neonates with CLE often have a dramatic presentation with severe respiratory distress. Radiographs of the chest demonstrate lobar hyperinflation, flat diaphragm and mediastinal shift. The compressed normal lobes are often visible on the radiographs as peripheral opacities. Associated cardiac anomalies (VSD and PDA) are

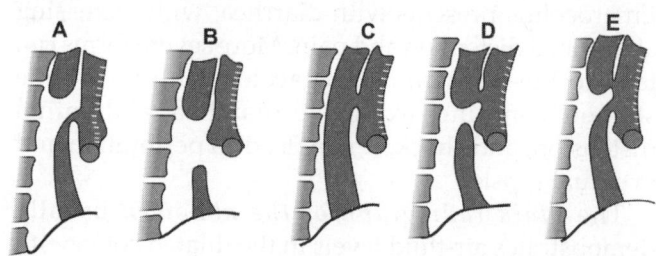

Fig. 8.6: Five major anatomical types of esophageal anomalies shown in order of frequency (A 87%; B 8%; C 4%; D < 1%; E < 1%)

frequent. Symptomatic neonates with congenital variant of lobar emphysema require a lobectomy.

Congenital cystic adenomastoid malformation (CCAM): CCAM is a developmental hamartomatous abnormality of the lung with adenomastoid proliferation of cysts resembling bronchioles and is believed to result from focal arrest in fetal lung development before the seventh week of gestation secondary to a variety of pulmonary insults. CAM differs from normal lung tissue because of a combination of increased cell proliferation and decreased apoptosis. A well-defined intrapulmonary bronchial system is lacking, and normally formed bronchi supplying the mass are absent. Radiographic pattern appears as an expansible soft-tissue mass containing multiple air-filled cystic masses of varying size and shifting of the mediastinum, which are separated from each other by wisps of pulmonary tissue.

Bronchogenic cyst: Bronchogenic cysts (BC) are benign congenital lesions of the respiratory tract that have the potential to develop complications creating a dilemma in diagnosis and treatment. BC are commonly located in the mediastinum (2/3) or lung parenchyma (1/3) arising from anomalous budding along the primitive tracheobronchial tube (foregut duplication errors). Other atypical locations are cervical, subcutaneous, paravertebral, etc. They commonly present with symptoms caused by infection of the cyst or by compression of adjacent structures. The most common presentation is as respiratory distress or dysphagia. Complete surgical resection is the treatment of choice.

Pulmonary sequestration: Pulmonary sequestration is an uncommon usually cystic mass of nonfunctioning primitive tissue that does not communicate with the tracheobronchial tree. In addition, it receives its blood supply from an anomalous systemic artery rather than the pulmonary circulation. Multiple feeding vessels may be present in 15–20% of cases. The 2 forms of pulmonary sequestration include intrapulmonary (IS), which is surrounded by normal lung tissue, and extrapulmonary (ES), which has its own pleural investment. Management consists of resection to alleviate symptoms and avoid complications.

4. *Anorectal malformations:* See Chapter 16.

5. *Abdominal wall defects: Omphalocele and Gastroschisis:* The three most common abdominal wall defects in newborns are umbilical hernia, gastroschisis and omphalocele. An **omphalocele** is a central defect of the umbilical ring, through which bowel and other abdominal viscera herniated (Table 8.28). The contents are covered by a membrane composed of an inner layer of peritoneum, an outer layer of amnion and the Wharton's jelly in the middle. Primary closure with correction of the malrotation should be attempted whenever possible. If this is not possible, then a plastic mesh/silastic chimney is fashioned around the defect to cover the intestinal contents and the contents slowly reduced over 5–14 days.

Gastroschisis consists of a defect in the abdominal wall lateral to the intact umbilical cord with herniation of the viscera through the small defect (Table 8.28). Treatment of gastroschisis is identical to omphalocele, except that intestinal atresias need to be repaired along with the primary closure.

Table 8.28: Differential features of omphalocele and gastroschisis	
Omphalocele	*Gastroschisis*
Usually midline defects	Paraumbilical defects
Cord insertion on the herniated mass	Usually on the right side of the cord insertion
Hernia contains intestines, liver or both fluid	Herniated small bowel loop floating free in amniotic
Covered by a membrane (peritoneum and amnion)	Not covered by any membrane
Associated with chromosomal anomaly 40–60%	Not associated with chromosomal anomaly
Prognosis often poor	Prognosis good

Alexander F, Johanningman J, Markin LW. Staged repair improves outcome of high-risk premature infants with esophageal atresia and tracheoesophageal fistula. *J Pediatr Surg* 1993;28:151–4.

Aziz D, Chait P, Kreichman F, et al. Image-guided percutaneous gastrostomy in neonates with esophageal atresia. *J Pediatr Surg* 2004 Nov; 39(11):1648–50.

Finder JD, Michelson PH. Congenital disorders of the lung. In: Kliegman RM, Behrman RE, Jenson HB, Stanton BF (eds). *Nelson Textbook of Pediatrics.* 18th edn. Vol 2. Philadelphia: Saunders, 2007;1783–87.

Orenstein S, Peters J, Khan S, Youssef N, Hussain SZ. Congenital anomalies: Esophageal atresia and tracheoesophageal fistula. In: Kliegman RM, Behrman RE, Jenson HB, Stanton BF (eds). *Nelson Textbook of Pediatrics.* 18th edn. Vol 2. Philadelphia: Saunders, 2007; 1543–44.

Robert W. Intestinal atresia, stenosis, and malrotation. In: Kliegman RM, Behrman RE, Jenson HB, Stanton BF (eds). *Nelson Textbook of Pediatrics.* 18th edn. Vol 2. Philadelphia: Saunders, 2007; 1558–62.

Samujh Ram, Sinha Arvind. Neonatal surgical emergencies. In: Mathur GP, Mathur Sarla (eds). *Current Trends in Pediatrics.* Vol 2. Delhi: Academa Publishers, 2006;312–22.

Wyllie R. Motility disorders and Hirschsprung's disease. In: Kliegman RM, Behrman RE, Jenson HB, Stanton BF (eds). *Nelson Textbook of Pediatrics.* 18th edn. Vol 2. Philadelphia: Saunders, 2007;1564–68.

9 Human Genetics

9.1 HUMAN GENOME

Human genome has approximately 25,000 genes, which are the individual units of heredity of all traits. Reproductive or germ line cells contain one copy (N) of this genetic complement and are haploid, whereas somatic (non-germ line) cells contain two complete copies (2N) and are diploid. Humans (including all different racial and ethnic groups) are 99.9% identical at the functional gene level, implying that there is no genetic basis for precise racial categorization. Nevertheless, various genes and genetic markers are specific for different races.

The genes are organized into long segments of deoxyribonucleic acid (DNA), which, during cell division, are compacted into intricate structures with proteins to form chromosomes. Each somatic cell has 46 chromosomes [22 pairs of autosomes, or non-sex chromosomes, and 1 pair of sex chromosomes (XY in a male and XX in a female)]. Germ cells (eggs, sperm) contain 22 autosomes and 1 sex chromosome, for a total of 23. At fertilization, the full diploid chromosome complement of 46 is again present in the embryo.

The DNA molecule has three building blocks: a pentose sugar (deoxyribose), a phosphate group, and four types of bases, either purines [adenine (A) and guanine (G)] or pyrimidines [thymine (T) and cytosine (C)]. These four bases form the alphabet of the genetic code. The basic subunit of DNA is the *nucleotide*, composed of one deoxyribose, one phosphate group, and one base. The structure of the DNA molecule is that of a double helix and is a twisted ladder, with the two sides of the ladder formed by the sugar and phosphate components, and the rungs of the ladder composed of the bases. Each "rung" contains one purine and one pyrimidine, binding with one another in a predictable way: "A" with "T" and "C" with "G". Different long sequences of the nucleotide bases code for different proteins. Only 10% of the total DNA of the cell is functioning working material during the metabolically active portion of the cell cycle. Some of the "inactive" genetic material may be important in the regulation of gene expression or in chromosome structure and function.

Most of the genetic material is contained in the cell's nucleus. The mitochondria (the cell's energy-producing organelles) contain their own genome. The *mitochondrial chromosome* consists of a double-stranded circular piece of DNA, which contains 16,568 base pairs (bp) of DNA and is completely sequenced. The proteins that comprised the mitochondria may either be produced in the mitochondria (from information contained in the mitochondrial genome) or produced from information contained in the nuclear genome and transported into the organelle. All mitochondria are maternally derived (because sperm usually do not carry mitochondria in the fertilized eggs). The different mitochondria within a single cell with a variety of genomes reflect the maternal lines from which they descended.

Structure and function of genes: The basic purpose of genes is the production of structural proteins and enzymes. This occurs through a series of events, termed *transcription*, *processing*, and *translation*. DNA transmits its information by unwinding into single-stranded DNA, with one strand or the other or both, acting as a template to be copied. If this occurs during cell replication, each of the DNA strands is copied, forming two new double-stranded daughter DNA molecules during a process termed *replication*. If this process occurs during the metabolically active portion of the cell cycle, only one strand is copied, forming a strand of messenger RNA (mRNA) during *transcription*. The complete DNA sequence of each gene is transcribed into mRNA, including the information used to encode amino acids (*exons*) and noncoding sequences between exons (*introns*). The resultant mRNA differs from DNA in the substitution of the sugar ribose for deoxyribose and the pyrimidine uracil (U) for thymine (T). This primary transcript of mRNA is processed before leaving the nucleus, by a mechanism in which the noncoding introns are removed from the molecule and the remaining sections are spliced together to form the functional mRNA, which then migrates to the cytoplasm for translation. During *translation*, the mRNA directs the production of proteins on the ribosome by forming base pairs between three of its nucleotides, called *codons*, and the three complementary nucleotides on a transfer RNA molecule (tRNA), termed *anticodons*. As the ribosome moves along the RNA sequence codon by codon, an enzyme joins together the adjacent amino acids associated with the tRNA molecules by forming covalent peptide bonds. The structure of polypeptide chains and, ultimately, proteins is determined by the mRNA sequence.

Mutations and their consequences: Medical genetics is concerned with the study of human genetic variation. The basis of that variation is mutation or change in the DNA sequence. Mutations can and do occur in every cell of the body. When they occur in somatic cells, there is risk of cancer development; when they occur in germ line, there is a risk that an offspring may inherit a structural or functional disability. Many mutations are benign or silent; others explain variation in the severity of a genetic disease (polymorphisms), whereas others produce serious consequences. The male mutation rate is approximately twice that of the female mutation rate.

Genotype-phenotype correlations in genetic disease: *Genotype* is defined as the genetic constitution of an individual and refers to which particular alternative version (*allele*) of a gene is present at a specific location (*locus*) on a chromosome. *Phenotype* is defined as the observed structural, biochemical and physiologic characteristics of an individual, determined by the genotype, and refer to the observed structural and functional effects of a mutant allele at a specific locus. Many mutations result in predictable phenotypes. Therefore, identification of a specific mutation in an individual can often be used to predict clinical outcomes and plan appropriate treatment strategies.

Genotype-phenotype correlations are observed in cystic fibrosis (CF), long QT syndrome, and fibrillin-1 gene associated with Marfan syndrome.

9.2 ETHICAL ISSUES IN GENETIC TESTING

Genetic disorders can present at any age, some of the most severe diseases begin in childhood. The majority of chronic diseases in children has an obvious genetic component or is influenced by genetic susceptibility. Major categories of genetic disorders in children include single gene, chromosomal, and multifactorial conditions.

Genetic testing is often performed to diagnose children with malformation syndromes, mental retardation, or other disabilities wherein there is a clear benefit to the child. In other cases, the decision whether to test a child is more difficult.

The American College of Medical Genetics and the American Society of Human Genetics have suggested that the following points be fully discussed with families considering genetic testing for their children.

1. A mature minor and the parents should receive education and counseling about the genetic testing being considered and consent should be obtained by the physician before testing is done. Adolescents who are 14–15 yr of age or older are usually considered mature minors, and assent/consent should be sought from them. If a child between the ages of 7 and 14 yr is to be tested, "assent" of the child should be obtained. Assent is the child's affirmative agreement to agree with the decision of the parents.

2. The primary justification for undergoing testing should be timely medical benefit. If the test will not provide medical benefit in terms of prevention or treatment, its necessity should be questioned.

3. If medical benefit is not apparent, one must consider whether substantial psychosocial benefits to the older child or adolescent can justify testing.

4. Genetic testing should be deferred until after age 18 yr if the benefits of testing will not become apparent until adulthood.

5. In the case of a competent adolescent, if the balance of benefits and harms is unknown, the physician should follow the decision of the adolescent regarding testing, even if it conflicts with the wishes of the parents.

6. The pediatrician should evaluate whether testing is in the best interest of the child, and, if the potential harms of testing overweigh the potential benefits, the physician should dissuade the parents from testing.

9.3 PATTERNS OF INHERITANCE

Genetic versus familial disorders: A *genetic disorder* is one caused completely or partially by altered genetic material; some genetic disorders occur in multiple family members, others occur sporadically in single individuals in a family with no instances of recurrence. A *familial disorder* is one that is more common in relatives of an affected individual than in the general population; some familial disorders are genetic, and others are caused by environmental exposures (lead poisoning). Recognition of pattern of inheritance assists in clinical diagnosis and also provides essential information for counseling family members about recurrence risks in future pregnancies.

Pedigree: A *pedigree* is a diagram of a family history and illustrates relationships among family members; it shows which family members are affected with specific medical conditions. Information for a three-generation pedigree should be obtained from a family being evaluated for a genetic disorder. The patient through whom the family is ascertained is called *proband*. Individuals who share half of their genetic material with the proband are *first-degree relatives* (brothers, sisters, children, parents); those who share one-fourth of their genetic material are *second degree relatives* (grandparents, grandchildren, aunts, uncles, nieces, nephews). *Third* and *fourth degree relatives* share one-eighth and one-sixteenth of their genetic material, respectively with the proband.

Patterns of Genetic Inheritance

Six patterns of genetic inheritance are reported in human beings. Autosomal genes are one of the 22 pairs of non-sex chromosomes. X-linked disorders are associated with altered genes on the X chromosome. X-linked genes behave like autosomal genes. Because of X-inactivation (a random process occurring early in female embryogenesis), only one chromosome is active in each cell. Therefore, a female who is heterozygous for a mutant X-linked allele will produce 50% of the normal amount of gene product, similar to a heterozygote for an autosomal recessive condition. Because a male inherits only one X-chromosome, he is hemizygous for all of the genes present at all loci along the chromosome and all of the genes are expressed. If a male inherits an altered X-linked gene, he will express the condition, because the Y-chromosome contains no normal allele to compensate for the mutated gene.

1. *Autosomal dominant inheritance:* The examples of autosomal dominant disorders are mentioned in Box 9.1.

Box 9.1: Examples of autosomal dominant disorders

Achondroplasia	Neurofibromatosis 1
Ehlers-Danlos syndrome	Noonan's syndrome
Familial hypercholesterolemia	Osteogenesis imperfecta
Huntington's disease	Otosclerosis
Marfan's syndrome	Polyposis coli
Myotonic dystrophy	Tuberous sclerosis

2. *Autosomal recessive inheritance:* Examples of autosomal recessive disorders are listed in Box 9.2.

Box 9.2: Examples of autosomal recessive disorders

Congenital adrenal hyperplasia	Oculocutaneous albinism
Cystic fibrosis	Phenylketonuria
Familial dysautonomia	Sickle cell disease
Fanconi anemia	Tay-Sachs disease
Galactosemia	Thalassemia
Gaucher's disease	Werdnig-Hoffmann disease
Hurler syndrome (MPS I)	

3. *X-linked recessive inheritance:* The examples of X-linked recessive disorders are mentioned in Box 9.3.

Box 9.3: Examples of X-linked recessive disorders

Color blindness (red-green)
Duchenne and Becker muscular dystrophies
Fragile X syndrome
Glucose-6-phosphatase deficiency (G6PD)
Hemophilia A and B
Hunter syndrome (mucopolysaccharidosis II)

4. *X-linked dominant inheritance:* The examples of X-linked dominant disorders are hypophosphatemic rickets (vitamin D-resistant rickets), incontinentia pigmenti.

5. *Multifactorial inheritance:* The examples of multifactorial inheritance are listed in Box 9.4.

Box 9.4: Examples of multifactorial inheritance

Congenital anomalies	Disorders of adult life
Neural tube defects	Diabetes mellitus
Cleft lip	Hypertension
Cleft lip with cleft palate	Stroke
Isolated cleft palate	Coronary artery disease
Club feet	Schizophrenia
Cardiac septal defects (VSD, ASD)	

6. *Nontraditional patterns of inheritance:* Certain diseases display an atypical mode of inheritance because they result from mutations in mitochondrial DNA (mtDNA) (*see* Section 9.6). The examples of non-traditional patterns of inheritance are listed in Box 9.5.

Boright AP, Kere J, Scherer SW. The genetics of childhood disease and development: A series of review articles. *Pediatr Res* 2003;53:4–9.

Descartes M, Carroll AJ. Cytogenetics. In: Kliegman RM, Behrman RE, Jenson HB, Stanton BF (eds). *Nelson Textbook of Pediatrics.* 18th edn. Philadelphia: Saunders, 2007;502–17.

Korf BR. The human genome. In: Kliegman RM, Behrman RE, Jenson HB, Stanton BF (eds). *Nelson Textbook of Pediatrics.* 18th edn. Philadelphia: Saunders, 2007;487–92.

Hoyme HE. The molecular basis of genetic disorders. In: Behrman RE, Kliegman RM, Jenson HB (eds). *Nelson Textbook of Pediatrics.* 17th edn. Philadelphia: Saunders, 2004;367–71.

Hoyme HE. Molecular diagnosis of genetic diseases. In: Behrman RE, Kliegman RM, Jenson HB (eds). *Nelson Textbook of Pediatrics.* 17th edn. Philadelphia: Saunders, 2004;371–376.

Hoyme HE. Patterns of inharitance. In: Behrman RE, Kliegman RM, Jenson HB (eds). *Nelson Textbook of Pediatrics.* 17th edn. Philadelphia: Saunders, 2004;376–82.

9.4 CHROMOSOMAL CLINICAL ABNORMALITIES

Human Chromosome

The chromosomes are made up of DNA and other protein complexes and contain most of the genetic information that is passed from one generation to the next generation. There are two types of cell division: mitosis and meiosis. *Mitosis* is the type of cell division that occurs in most cells of the body. It is during mitosis, specifically the prophase stage of mitosis that chromosomes are visible and easy to identify for karyotyping. In mitosis, two genetically identical daughter cells are produced from a single parent cell after passing through four stages: prophase, metaphase, anaphase, and telophase. *Meiosis* is the form of cell division that occurs to produce germ cells or gametes (sperm and egg). A diploid cell (with two sets or 46 chromosomes) divides to form haploid cells (with one set or 23 chromosomes).

Chromosomes are arranged by size in pairs (Fig. 9.1). Chromosome 1 is the largest and the smallest is chromosome 21 and then the sex chromosomes X and Y. The X chromosome is a large submetacentric chromosome, and the Y chromosome is a small acrocentric chromosome. The position of the centromere in regard to the chromosome arms is another distinguishing feature of each chromosome. The short arm of the chromosome is referred to as p (for petite)

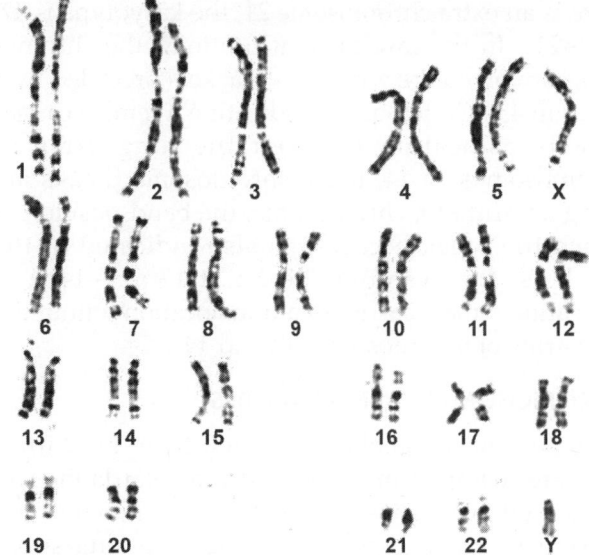

Fig. 9.1: Karyotype of normal male with chromosomes in late prophase

and the long arm as q (for the next letter in the alphabet) (Fig. 9.2).

A karyotype is the designation for the visual display of chromosomes and is obtained after the chromosomes are arrested during cell division in prophase and is photographed and arranged according to size. The visual display can be produced by the computer. A description of a karyotype consists of three parts: (i) the number of chromosomes, (ii) the sex chromosome constitution, and (iii) any abnormality found. Centromere position determining the three types of chromosomes seen in the normal human karyotype are metacentric, submetacentric and acrocentric. The normal karyotype is 46, XX for females, and 46, XY for males. If an abnormality is found, it is noted after the sex chromosome constitution. For example, in the case of a female with cri-du-chat syndrome in which a piece of the short arm of the chromosome 5 is missing, karyotype would be 46, XX, 5p–. In a male with Down syndrome in which

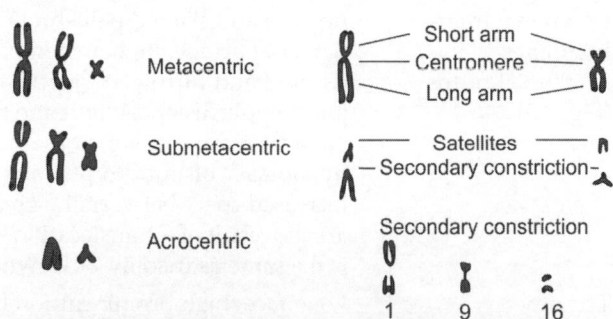

Fig. 9.2: Centromere position, demonstrating the three types of chromosomes seen in the normal human karyotype- metacentric, submetacentric, and acrocentric

there is an extra chromosome 21, the karyotype is 47, XY, +21. In the case of translocations, the chromosomes involved are written in brackets preceded by a "t" as in 45, XX, t(13q14q), indicating a female carrier of a translocation between the long arms of chromosomes 13 14. If the chromosome breaks are along an arm of a chromosome, the band position at which the break occurred is also indicated in the brackets, for example, 45, XY, t(13q2.1–14q1.3) indicating a male carrier of a translocation within the long arms of chromosomes 13 and 14.

CHROMOSOMAL ABNORMALITIES

Chromosomal anomalies occur in 0.4% of live births. They are an important cause of mental retardation and congenital anomalies. Chromosomal anomalies are present in much higher frequencies among spontaneous abortions and stillbirths. The phenotypic anomalies that result from chromosomal aberrations are mainly due to imbalance of genetic information. Identification of these chromosomal aberrations is important for counseling families about prognosis and reproductive risks in future pregnancies. Chromosomal anomalies include abnormalities of *chromosome number* and *structure*.

Abnormalities of Chromosome Number

Aneuploidy and polyploidy: When the human cell has 23 chromosomes, it is referred as a haploid cell (the number of chromosomes in an ova or sperm). Any number of chromosomes that is an exact multiple of the haploid number (e.g. 46, 69, 92 in humans) is referred to as euploid. Euploid cells with more than the normal diploid number of 46 chromosomes are called polyploid cells. Polyploid conceptions are usually not viable, but they may be present in mosaic (more than one cell line) forms, which allow survival. Cells with three sets of chromosomes are called triploid and are frequently seen in abortus material and occasionally in viable humans, usually in mosaic form. Cells deviating from the multiples of the haploid number are called aneuploid (and not euploid), indicating a missing or extra chromosome.

Trisomies: These are the most common abnormalities of chromosome number (aneuploidy). They occur when there are three representatives of a particular chromosome instead of the usual two. Trisomies are usually the result of meiotic nondisjunction (failure of a chromosome pair to separate). Trisomy may be present in all cells or may occur in mosaic form. The most frequent trisomy is trisomy 21 (Down syndrome). Trisomies of chromosome 18, 13, and 8 are also relatively common (Table 9.1) (*see* Figs 9.1 and 9.2 in CD).

Monosomies: Monosomies occur when only one representative of a chromosome is present. They may be complete or partial. Complete monosomies may be the result of nondisjunction or anaphase lag. In

Table 9.1: Chromosomal trisomies and their clinical manifestations	
Syndrome	Clinical manifestations
Trisomy 13, Patau syndrome **Incidence** 1/10,000 births	Cleft lip often midline, flexed fingers with polydactyly, ocular hypotelorism, bulbous nose, low-set malformed ears; small abnormal skull; cerebral malformation, especially holoprosencephaly, microphthalmia; cardiac malformations; scalp defects; hypoplastic or absent ribs; visceral and genital anomalies
Trisomy 18, Edwards' syndrome **Incidence** 1/6,000 births	Low birth weight, closed fists with index finger overlapping the 3rd digit and the 5th digit overlapping the 4th, narrow hips with limited abduction, short sternum, rocker-bottom feet, microcephaly, prominent occiput, micrognathia, cardiac and renal malformations, and mental retardation; 95% of cases are lethal in the 1st yr
Trisomy 21, Down syndrome **Incidence** 1/600–800 births (Fig. 9.3)	Hypotonia, short stature, moderate-to-severe mental retardation, brachycephaly, flat face, upward and slanted palpebral fissures and epicanthic folds, speckled irises (Brushfield spots), flat nasal bridge, high arched palate, open mouth with a tendency of tongue protrusion, a fissured and furrowed tongue, macroglossia, small ears with an over-folded helix, decreased inter-nipple distance, short and broad hands, dermal patterns of palm (single flexion transverse palmar crease [simian crease], axial triradius in distal position, ulnar loops on all 10 digits), hypoplasia of middle phalanx of 5th finger (clinodactyly), hyperextensible finger joints, increased space between the great toe and the second toe, 4% of patients with Down syndrome are the result of a translocation—t(14q21q), t(15q21q), and t(13q21q)—in which the phenotype is the same as trisomy 21 Down syndrome
Trisomy 8, Mosaicism **Incidence** 1/20,000 births	Long face, high prominent forehead, wide upturned nose, thick everted lower lip, microretrognathia, low-set ears, high arched, sometimes cleft palate, osteoarticular anomalies are common; moderate mental retardation

nondisjunction during cell division, the two chromosomes in a replicating pair fail to separate; one cell ends up with only one copy (monosomic) and the other with three copies (trisomic) of the specific chromosome. In anaphase lag, the chromosome fails to move into the new daughter cell and is lost. All complete autosomal monosomies appear to be lethal early in development and only survive in mosaic forms. Partial monosomies are usually the offspring of a translocation carrier.

Abnormalities of Chromosome Structure

Deletions: Deletions occur when a piece of a chromosome is missing. Deletions may be located at the chromosome ends or in interstitial segments of the chromosome and are usually associated with mental retardation and malformations. Small telomeric deletions may be relatively common in nonspecific mental retardation with minor anomalies. The most common deletions are 4p–, 5p–, 9p–, 13q–, 18p–, 18q– and 21q– (Table 9.2).

Microdeletions are defined as small chromosome deletions that are detectable only in high-quality (pro) metaphase preparations (Table 9.3).

Translocations: Translocations involve the transfer of chromosomal material from one chromosome to another. Translocations may be Robertsonian or reciprocal. They occur with a frequency of 1/500 liveborn human infants. They may be inherited from a parent or appear *de novo*, with no affected family members. *Robertsonian translocations* involve two acrocentric chromosomes that fuse near the centromeric region with subsequent loss of the nonfunctional, very truncated short arms. The translocation chromosome is made up of the long arms of two fused

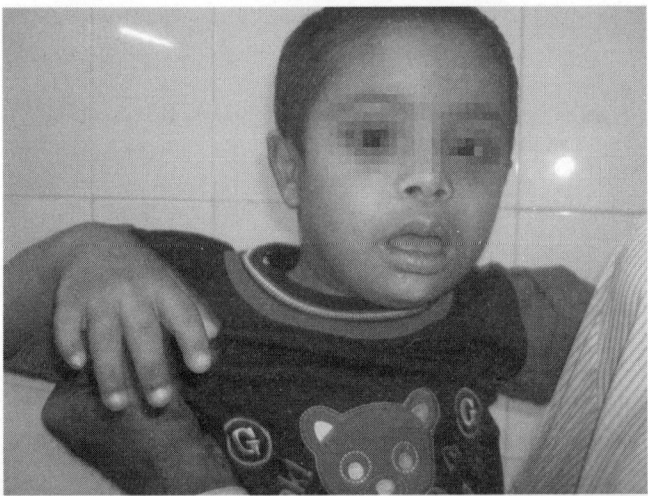

Fig. 9.3: A nine-year-old male Down syndrome child (trisomy 21) with open mouth and tongue protrusion; moderate mental retardation with an IQ approximately 50.

chromosomes; hence the resulting count is only 45 chromosomes. Although carriers of a Robertsonian translocation are usually phenotypically normal, they are at increased for miscarriages and abnormal offspring. *Reciprocal translocations* are the result of breaks in nonhomologous chromosomes with reciprocal exchange of the broken segments. Carriers of a reciprocal translocation are usually phenotypically normal but also have an increased risk of having chromosomally abnormal offspring and miscarriages.

Inversions: Inversions require the chromosome to break at two points. The broken piece is then inverted and joined into the same chromosome. Inversions have a frequency of 1/100 liveborns and may be pericentric and paracentric.

Ring chromosomes: Ring chromosomes are rare, but they have been found for all human chromosomes. The formation of a ring involves a deletion at each end of the chromosome. The "sticky" ends then join to form the ring. The phenotype of a ring chromosome ranges from mental retardation and multiple congenital anomalies to normal or near normal depending on the amount of chromosomal material that is lost.

Duplications: A duplication is the presence of extra genetic material from the same chromosome. Duplications may result from the abnormal segregation in carriers of translocations or inversions.

Insertions: Insertions occur when a piece of chromosome breaks at two points and is incorporated into a break in another part of a chromosome. This requires three breakpoints and may occur between two chromosomes or within one.

Telomere/subtelomere deletions: Because chromosomes "cross over" during meiosis, small deletions and duplications of the regions toward the ends of the chromosomes occur relatively frequently. Subtelomeric rearrangements are reported in 5–10% children with unexplained moderate to severe mental retardation without very obvious dysmorphic seizures. Submicroscopic subtelomeric deletions (smaller than 2–3 mb) are the second most common cause of mental retardation after trisomy 21.

Sex Chromosome Anomalies

There are three common sex chromosome anomalies: Turner's syndrome, Klinefelter's syndrome, and Fragile X syndrome.

Turner's Syndrome

Turner's syndrome (45, XO) occurs in about in 1/1,500–2,500—liveborn females (*see* Fig. 9.3 in CD).

Table 9.2: Common deletions and their clinical manifestations	
Deletion	*Clinical manifestations*
4p–	Wolf-Hirschhorn syndrome: Typical "Greek helmet" facies with ocular hypertelorism, prominent glabella, and frontal bossing; microcephaly, dolichocephaly, hypoplasia of the eye socket, ptosis, strabismus, nystagmus, bilateral epicanthic folds, cleft lip and palate, beaked nose with prominent bridge, hypospadias, cardiac malformations and mental retardation
5p–	Cri-du-chat syndrome: hypotonia, short stature, characteristic cry, microcephaly with protruding metopic suture, moon-like face, hypertelorism, bilateral epicanthic folds, high arched palate, wide and flat nasal bridge, and mental retardation
9p–	Craniofacial dysmorphology with trigonocephaly, slanted palpebral fissures, discrete exophthalmos, arched eyebrows, flat and wide nasal bridge, short neck with pterygium colli, genital anomalies, long fingers and toes, cardiac malformations, and mental retardation
13q–	Low birth weight, failure to thrive; facial features include microcephaly, flat wide nasal bridge, hypertelorism, ptosis, micrognathia; ocular manifestations; hands have hypoplastic or absent thumbs and syndactyly, and mental retardation
18p–	Approximately 15% of patients are severely affected with cephalic and ocular manifestations, cleft lip and palate, and varying degrees of mental retardation; most (80%) have only minor malformations and mild mental retardation
18q–	Hypotonia with "frog-like" position with the legs flexed, externally rotated, and in hyperabduction; characteristic face with depressed midface and apparent protrusion of the mandible, deep-set eyes, short upper lip, everted lower lip ("carp-like" mouth); very prominent antihelix of the ears; mental retardation and belligerent personality.
21q–	Hypertonia, microcephaly, downward-slanting palpebral fissures, high palate, prominent nasal bridge, large low-set ears, micrognathia, mental retardation; may have skeletal malformations

Table 9.3: Microdeletions and their clinical manifestations	
Syndrome	*Clinical manifestations*
Williams **Deletion 7q11.23**	Round face with full cheeks and lips, stellate pattern in iris, strabismus, supraventricular stenosis and other cardiac malformations, a very friendly personality and varying degrees of mental retardation
Langer-Giedion or tricho-rhino-phalangeal, type II **Deletion 8q24.1–**	Sparse hair, multiple cone-shaped epiphyses, multiple cartilaginous exostoses, bulbous nasal tip, upturned nares, prominent philtrum, large protruding ears, and mild mental retardation
WAGR **Deletion 11p13–**	Hypernephroma (Wilms' tumor), aniridia, male genital hypoplasia of varying degrees, gonadoblastoma, long face, upward slanting palpebral fissures, ptosis, beaked nose, low-set poorly formed auricles, and mental retardation
Prader-Willi **Deletion 15q11–13** (pat)	Severe hypotonia at birth, obesity, short stature, small hands and feet, hypogonadism and mental retardation
Angelman **Deletion 15q11–13** (mat)	Hypotonia, fair hair, midface hypoplasia, prognathism, seizures, jerky ataxic movements, uncontrollable bouts of laughter, and severe mental retardation
Rubinstein-Taybi **Deletion 16p13–**	Microcephaly, ptosis, beaked nose with low-lying philtrum, broad thumbs and large toes, and mental retardation
Smith-Magenis **Deletion 17p11.2**	Brachycephaly, midfacial hypoplasia, prognathism, myopia, cleft palate, short stature, behavioral problems and mental retardation
Miller-Dieker **Deletion 17p13.3–**	Microcephaly, lissencephaly, pachygyria, narrow forehead, hypoplastic male external genitals, growth retardation, seizures, and profound mental retardation
Alagille syndrome **Deletion 20p12–**	Bile duct paucity with cholestasis, heart defects, particularly pulmonary artery stenosis, ocular abnormalities (posterior embryotoxin), skeletal defects such as butter fly vertebrae, long nose with broad midnose
Velocardiofacial DiGeorge syndrome **Deletion 22q11.2**	Hypoplasia or agenesis of the thymus and parathyroid glands, hypoplasia of auricle and external auditory canal, conotruncal cardiac anomalies, cleft palate, short stature, behavioral problems

Clinical manifestations: Turner's syndrome is recognizable at birth. The characteristic features are listed in Box 9.6. Short stature is the cardinal finding in all girls. Sexual maturation fails to occur at the expected age. The most common skeletal abnormalities are shortening of the 4th metacarpal (a short fourth metacarpal is best seen when making a fist) and metatarsal bones, epiphyseal dysgenesis in the joints of the knees and elbows, scoliosis, and in older patients, inadequate osseous mineralization. Associated defects are common and include congenital heart disease (bicuspid aortic valve, coarctation of aorta, aortic stenosis, mitral valve prolapse, and anomalous pulmonary venous drainage), renal malformations, type 2 diabetes, thyroid disease, inflammatory bowel disease (e.g. Crohn's disease, ulcerative colitis), recurrent bilateral otitis media, and sensorineural hearing defects.

Box 9.6: Features of Turner's syndrome

Recognized at birth in females:

Lymphedema over the dorsal surface of the hands and feet

Loose skin folds at the neck of the nape

Low birth weight and decreased length

Short stature

Webbing of the neck

Low posterior hair line

Small mandible

Prominent ears

Epicanthal folds

High arched palate

Broad chest with widely spaced nipples

Cubitus valgus

Shortening of the 4th metacarpal

Hyperconvex finger nails

Failure of sexual maturation at the expected age

CVS— bicuspid aortic valves, coarctation of aorta

Renal—horseshoe kidney

Laboratory findings: Chromosomal analysis must be considered in all short girls. Ultrasonography of the heart, kidneys, and ovaries is indicated after the diagnosis is established. Plasma levels of follicle-stimulating hormone (FSH) are markedly elevated. Thyroid antiperoxidase antibodies should be checked periodically and if positive, levels of thyroxine and thyroid-stimulating hormone should be obtained. Radiographs will show skeletal abnormalities. Echocardiography should be performed to exclude congenital cardiac defects.

Treatment: The treatment with recombinant human growth hormone (hGH) increases height velocity and ultimate stature in most but not in all children. Many girls achieve heights of greater than 150 cm with early initiation of treatment. Replacement therapy with estrogens is indicated. Premarin, a conjugated estrogen, 0.3–0.625 mg, or estrace 0.5 mg (micronized estradiol), given daily for 3–6 months is usually effective in inducing puberty. The estrogen then is cycled (taken on day 1–23), and provera, a progestin, is added (taken on days 10–23) in a dose of 5–10 mg daily. In the reminder of the calendar month, during no treatment is given, withdrawal bleeding usually occurs.

Psychosocial support for these girls is an integral component of treatment. Successful pregnancies have been carried to term using ovum donation and its *in vitro* fertilization.

Klinefelter's Syndrome (XXY syndrome)

It is a relatively common (1:500–1000 live male births) abnormality associated with tall stature, mild mental retardation, gynecomastia, and decreased upper body: lower body segment ratio. They usually have azoospermia, testes are invariably small, although androgen production by Leydig cells, and are infertile. These individuals have a male karyotype with an extra X chromosome, 47, XXY, and the phenotype is male. The 47, XXY complement is the most common chromosomal pattern in persons with Klinefelter's syndrome (80%); some have mosaic patterns. Even with as many as four X chromosomes, the Y chromosome determines a male phenotype.

Klinefelter's syndrome is caused by the presence of an additional X chromosome in a male. About 50–60% of cases are due to maternal nondisjunction (75% meiosis I errors). In cases, in which these maternal meiosis I errors are identified, maternal age is increased. The remaining cases are due to paternal nondisjunction. The most common karyotype is 47, XXY (about 80–90% of all cases). Mosaicism (46, XY/ 47,XXY) is observed in about 10% of cases. Other variant karyotypes, including 48,XXYY, 48,XXXY, 49,XXXYY, and 49,XXXXY, are rare. The best time to reveal the condition to an affected male is probably mid-to-late adolescence when he is old enough to understand his condition.

Clinical manifestations: The diagnosis is rarely made before puberty. The patients tend to be tall, slim and underweight and to have relatively long legs, but body habitus can vary markedly. The features of Klinefelter's syndrome are tall stature, poor school performance, decreased testicular volume and azoospermia, decreased body hair, decreased sexual function, gynecomastia, increased gonadotropins, and decreased testosterone. The testes tend to be small for age, but this sign may become apparent only after puberty, when normal testicular growth fails to occur. The phallus tends to be smaller than average and cryptorchidism or hypospadias may occur in a few patients.

Pubertal development is delayed. Some degree of androgen deficiency is usually detected, although some children may undergo normal virilization. About 80% adults have gynecomastia; they have sparser facial hair, most shaving less often daily. The height of patients tends to be increased. There is an increased incidence of pulmonary disease, varicose veins, and cancer of the breast. Mediastinal germ cells tumors have been reported; some of these tumors produce hCG and cause precocious puberty in young boys. They may be associated with leukemia, lymphoma, and other hematologic neoplasia. The highest cancer risk (relative risk 2.7) occurs in the 15–30 yr age group. In adults with XY/XXY mosaicism, the features of Klinefelter's syndrome are decreased in severity and frequency. Children with mosaicism have a better prognosis for virilization, fertility, and psychosocial adjustment. When the number of X chromosomes exceeds two, the clinical manifestations, including mental retardation and impairment of virilization, are more severe. The most common testicular lesions are spermatogenic arrest and Sertoli cell predominance. The sperm have a high incidence of sex chromosomal aneuploidy. Azoospermia and infertility are usual. Antisperm antibodies have been detected in one quarter of tested specimens. In nonmosaic tested patients, most testicular sperm (94%) have a normal pattern of sex chromosome segregation.

Laboratory findings: The chromosomes should be examined in all patients suspected of having Klinefelter's syndrome. Echocardiography is performed to detect mitral valve prolapse. Radiographs are performed to detect lower bone mineral density, radioulnar synostosis, and taurodontism. Klinefelter's syndrome can be detected prenatally by amniocentesis and cytogenetic analysis of amniotic fluid.

Treatment: The long acting testosterone preparation (enanthate ester) may be used in patients 11–12 yr of age, in a starting dose of 25–50 mg injected intramuscularly every 3–4 wk, 50 mg increment every 6–9 mo until a maintenance dose for adults (200–250 mg every 3–4 wk) is achieved. At that time, testosterone patches or testosterone gel may be substituted for the injections. There is increase in prostate volume and prostate-specific antigen levels. Fertility is possible by an intracytoplasmic sperm injection technique. A multidisciplinary team approach will help speech impairments, academic difficulties, and other psychosocial and behavioral problems.

Prognosis: XXY babies differ little from other children. The recurrence risk is not increased above that of the general population. Although boys with 47,XXY may have limited academic success, some can complete graduate education and have a normal level of functioning. Lifespan is presumably normal. Hypogonadism, low libido, and psychosocial problems can be helped by testosterone treatment. Gynecomastia can be corrected by mastectomy.

47, XYY Male

The frequency of XYY males has been estimated to be 1/1,000. In most, the extra Y is generated by non-disjunction at meiosis II after normal chiasmate meiosis I. Children are at an increased risk of learning disabilities, cognitive skill impairments, and difficulties in psychosocial adaptation. The XYY adult has a few phenotypic manifestations. He tends to be tall and to have severe nodulocystic acne. Genital abnormalities, prolonged PR intervals on electro-cardiography, radioulnar synostosis, renal agenesis and cystic dysplasia of the kidney, hematologic malignancies have been reported. The most common reason for a 47, XYY male to be karyotyped is developmental delay or behavioral problems, or both. Stable, supportive, and compassionate family environments promote improved adaptation of these children and adolescents.

Fragile X Syndrome

Fragile sites are defined as regions of chromosomes that show a tendency of separation, breakage, or attenuation under particular growth conditions. Numerous fragile sites have been identified. The fragile site located on the distal long arm of chromosome X at Xq27.3 is associated with the *fragile X syndrome*, which is the most common heritable form of mental retardation in males. This fragile site (FRAXA) becomes visible in chromosome studies only when it is induced under special culture techniques. The diagnosis of fragile X is made by DNA studies, which demonstrates an expanded segment of DNA from the Xq27.3 region. The length of the expanded segment reflects the number of nucleotide triplet repeats. There are two other fragile sites on the X chromosome (FRAXE and FRAXF) also associated with mental retardation and allelic expansion. The clinical manifestations of fragile X syndrome in affected males are mental retardation, autistic behavior, macroorchidism, large size, characteristic facial features, including long face, prominent jaw, and large prominent ears; stereotyped behavior and speech. Females affected with fragile X show varying degrees of mental retardation, but it is less frequent cause of mental retardation in girls.

Other Chromosomal Abnormalities

Chromosome instability syndrome: Chromosomal instability syndrome, formerly known as chromosomal breakage syndrome are characterized by an increased risk of malignancy and specific phenotypes There are a number of recessive disorders that are associated with breakage or rearrangement of chromosomes or both. The chromosome instability syndromes are Fanconi anemia, ataxia-telangiectasia, Nijmegen syndrome, Bloom syndrome, Werner syndrome, Roberts' syndrome, and ICF (immunodeficiency, centromere instability, and facial anomalies) syndrome.

Mosaicism is the term used to describe an individual who has two or more different cell lines derived from a single zygote (fertilized egg). At least 2% of all conceptions are mosaic for chromosomal anomalies at or before 10 wk of pregnancy. *Germline mosaicism* refers to the presence of mosaicism in the germ cells found in the gonad. This type of mosaicism may be suspected in cases in which there is more than one affected offspring with the same genetic abnormality (usually inherited as a chromosomal or autosomal dominant disorder) with phenotypically normal parents. If germ line mosaicism is present, there is an increased risk for recurrence of an affected child.

Pallister-Killian syndrome: This syndrome is characterized by coarse facies, pigmentary skin anomalies, localized alopecia, diaphragmatic hernias, cardiovascular anomalies, supernumerary nipples, and profound mental retardation. The disorder is due to mosaicism for isochromosome 12p.

Hypomelanosis of Ito: This disorder is characterized by unilateral or bilateral macular hypopigmented whorls, streaks, and patches. Abnormalities of the eyes, musculoskeletal system, and central nervous system may also be present. Patients have two genetically distinct cell lines. The mosaic chromosome anomalies involve both autosomes and sex chromosomes and have been demonstrated in about 50% of cases.

Acquired cytogenetic abnormalities: Chromosomal changes are seen in most cancers. It is thought that the chromosomal change affects cancer-promoting and cancer-suppressing genes. Loss, gain, and translocations of chromosomes are seen in cancerous tissue, which appear to alter the function of cancer related genes. The particular rearrangements may be useful in predicting prognosis and suggesting the most efficacious therapy.

Uniparental disomy (UPD) is the term used when both chromosomes of a pair of chromosomes in a person with a normal number of chromosomes have been inherited from only one parent. Uniparental disomy most likely arises because a pregnancy starts off as a trisomy. Uniparental isodisomy means that the two chromosomes are identical, whereas uniparental heterodisomy means that the two chromosomes are different members of a pair, both of which were inherited from one person. Three types of phenotypic effects are seen in UPD:

1. Those related to imprinted genes, that is, the absence of a gene that is expressed only when inherited from a parent of a specific gender
2. Those related to autosomal recessive disorders, and
3. Those related to a vestigial aneuploid producing mosaicism.

Maternal uniparental disomy involving chromosomes 2, 7, 14, and 15 and paternal uniparental disomy involving chromosomes 6, 11, 15, and 20 are associated with phenotypic abnormalities of growth and behavior. UPD maternal 7 is associated with a phenotype similar to Russell-Silver syndrome with intrauterine growth restriction. UPD for chromosome 15 is seen in some cases of Prader-Willi syndrome and Angelman syndrome.

Imprinting: Genomic imprinting refers to observation that phenotypic expression depends on the parent of origin for certain genes and chromosome segments. Imprinting in humans is noted by phenotypic differences seen in cases of Prader-Willi syndrome and Angelman syndrome, which are associated with deletion and uniparental disomy of the same region of chromosome 15. Thus, in cases of Prader-Willi syndrome, the deletion when it occurs, is always of the paternally derived chromosome 15, in contrast, when there is a deleted chromosome 15 in Angelman syndrome, the deleted chromosome is always maternal in origin, and the UPD is always parental, that is, there is lack of maternal information.

Cunniff C. American Academy of Pediatrics Committee on Genetics: Prenatal screening and diagnosis for pediatricians. *Pediatrics* 2004;114:889–94.

Hall JG. Chromosomal clinical abnormalities. In: Behrman RE, Kliegman RM, Jenson HB (eds). *Nelson Textbook of Pediatrics.* 17th edn. Philadelphia: Saunders, 2004;382–91.

Jacquemont S, Hagerman PJ, Lechey MA. Fragile-X syndrome and Fragile-X associated tremor-ataxia syndrome: two faces of FMRI. Lancet Neurol 2007;6:45–55.

Lanfranco F, Kamischke A, Zitzmann M, et al. Klinefelter's syndrome. *Lancet* 2004;364:273–83.

Mathur Sarla, Prasad Piyush, Mathur GP. Down Syndrome. In: Mathur GP, Mathur Sarla (eds). *Current Trends in Pediatrics.* Vol 3. Delhi: Academa Publishers, 2007;292–300.

Rapport R. Disorders of the gonads. In: Behrman RE, Kliegman RM, Jenson HB (eds). *Nelson Textbook of Pediatrics.* 17th edn. Philadelphia: Saunders, 2004;1921–46.

Ranke MB, Saenger P. Turner's syndrome. *Lancet* 2001;358: 309–14.

Roizen NJ, Patterson D. Down syndrome. *Lancet* 2003; 361:1281–88.

Sybert VP, McCauley E. Turner's syndrome. *N Engl J Med* 2004;351:1227–38.

9.5 MANAGEMENT OF GENETIC DISORDERS

Gene therapy is defined as the introduction of nucleic acids into a tissue to prevent, inhibit, or revert a pathologic process. Diseases considered for genetic therapy include *Single gene defects:*

1. Severe combined immunodeficiency
2. α_1-antitrypsin deficiency
3. Cystic fibrosis
4. Hemophilia A and B
5. Gaucher's disease
6. β-hemoglobinopathies
7. Hypercholesterolemia, familial
8. Phenylketonuria

Complex traits

9. Cancer
10. HIV-1

As safety and success become demonstrable, gene therapy is likely to impact disease prevention. At present, there is only one accepted therapeutic benefit in treated patients with X-linked severe combined immunodeficiency (SCID). There are a few genetic disorders which are amenable to curative therapies. But all individuals/families should be provided information about the disorder, genetic counseling, specific medical therapies, and surgical management. Surgical management is available for many conditions that are associated with congenital anomalies or predisposition to tumors. Specific medical therapies for genetic disorders can be classified into physiologic, pharmacologic, and replacement therapies.

Physiologic therapies are used in the treatment of inborn errors of metabolism. The underlying defect itself is not altered by treatment. These include dietary management, such as avoidance of phenylalanine for children with phenylketonuria; coenzyme supplementation for some patients with methylmalonicacidemia; provision of substrates to excrete ammonia for those with urea cycle disorders; bisphosphonate treatment for those with osteogenesis imperfecta to reduce bone fractures; and avoidance of cigarette smoking for individuals with α_1-antitrypsin deficiency. Physiologic treatments are most effective when begun early in life before irreversible damage has occurred.

Pharmacologic therapies directly target a defective cellular pathway that is altered by an abnormal or a missing gene product. In cases of chronic myeloid leukemia (CML) and several other malignancies development of imatinib; this is a small molecule that blocks ATP binding in the fusion protein. Many physiologic therapies use pharmaceuticals (e.g. to remove ammonia in those with urea cycle disorders).

Replacement therapies include replacement of a missing metabolite, an enzyme, an organ, or a specific gene. **Enzyme replacement** therapy is useful for the treatment of cystic fibrosis to manage intestinal malabsorption by pancreatic enzymes. Enzyme replacement therapies are available for Gaucher's and Fabry's diseases, some mucopolysaccharidoses, and Pompe disease. **Organ transplantation** is an effective approach for replacing a defective gene. Aside from transplantation to replace damaged tissues, transplantation of liver or bone marrow is also used mainly in cases of inborn errors of metabolism, and hematologic or immunologic disorders.

Balicki D, Beutler E. Gene therapy of human disease. *Medicine* 2002;81:69–86.

Kay MA. Gene therapy. In: Behrman RE, Kliegman RM, Jenson HB (eds). *Nelson Textbook of Pediatrics.* 17th edn. Philadelphia: Saunders, 2004;391–95.

Korf BR. Integration of genetics into pediatric practice. In: Kliegman RM, Behrman RE, Jenson HB, Stanton BF (eds). *Nelson Textbook of Pediatrics.* 18th edn. Vol. 1. Philadelphia: Saunders, 2007;522–25.

9.6 GENETIC COUNSELING

Genetic counseling has an integral role in the management of genetic disorders. Counseling should be nondirective, psychoeducational and involves good communication with latest information, confidentiality, and truthfulness. Pediatricians are the primary physicians for the diagnosis, and management of children and high risk couples with genetic disorders. Also besides treating the patients, physicians should make the parents or couple aware of the genetic disorder, risk of recurrence, prognosis and prenatal diagnosis.

Definition and aims of genetic counseling: The American Society of Human Genetics (ASHG) defined genetic counseling as a communication process that deals with the human problems associated with the occurrence or the risk of recurrence of a genetic disorder in a family. The process involves an attempt by one or more appropriately trained persons to help the individual or family to understand, choose, and adjust (Table 9.4).

While genetic counseling is a comprehensive activity, the particular focus will depend upon the family situation. A pregnant couple at high genetic risk may need to make urgent decisions concerning prenatal diagnosis; parents of a newly diagnosed child with a rare genetic disorder may be desperate for further prognostic information, while still coming to terms with the diagnosis; a young adult at risk of a late onset degenerative disorder may be well informed about the condition, but require ongoing discussions about whether to go ahead with a presymptomatic test; and a teenage girl, whose brother has been affected with an X-linked disorder, may be apprehensive to learn about the implication for her future children. Being able to establish the individual's and the family's particular agenda, to present information in a clear manner, and to address psychosocial issues are all crucial skills required in genetic counseling.

Indications of genetic counseling: Based on indications (Box 9.7) genetic counseling can be grouped into three subspecialities: reproductive genetic counseling, pediatric/adult genetic counseling, and genetic counseling for common disease.

Reproductive genetic counseling: It offers options to patients related to testing (prenatal or carrier) and childbearing. The majority of clients are not adapting to a genetic condition or birth defect in their family but rather considering of how to avoid having an affected child. The focus of the counseling is often on consultant decision making including accepting the consequences of the choice(s) as it is the consultant and his family who has to live with the decision. *The goal of reproductive counseling is to promote the* consultant's *self-determination in exercising choices* because of the uncertainty associated with the chances for most birth defects to occur and lack of preventive options currently available.

Pediatric/adult genetic counseling: In majority of this kind of counseling, there is a proband and consultand or counselee (person who needs counseling) seeks to understand the diagnosis, prognosis and recurrence risks. Genetic counseling thus focuses on under-

---

Box 9.7: Indications of genetic counseling

History of a previous child or family history of unexplained mental retardation/dysmorphism/multiple malformations

History of a previous child or family history of degenerative brain disease-regression of mile stones

Acutely sick neonate or infant, failure to thrive, recurrent vomiting, acidosis, convulsions

Neuromuscular disorders

Childhood deafness

Down syndrome and other chromosomal disorders

Relatives of a person with chromosomal translocation

Exposure to teratogens

Unexplained still birth(s) with or without congenital malformation

Skeletal dysplasia (proportionate/disproportionate short stature)

Ambiguous genitalia, primary amenorrhea, infertility

Familial cancers and cancer prone disease

Single gene disorder like thalassemia, spinal muscular atrophy, hemophilia or family pedigree suggestive of a typical pattern of inheritance (AR, AD, X-linked)

Multifactorial/polygenic—hypertension, diabetes, obesity, psychotic disorders

Consanguineous marriage

Advanced maternal age

Positive maternal serum screen

Patient or family member with a known mendelian disorder

Previous child with a chromosomal disorder

Abnormal ultrasonographic (USG) findings

Recurrent pregnancy loss/still births

---

standing, accepting and adapting to a genetic diagnosis or risk (uncertainty) and their impact on the individual and family.

Genetic counseling for common disease: Here, genetic counseling addresses risk for more common diseases (cancer, Alzheimer, Parkinson, coronary artery disease

---

Table 9.4: Aims of genetic counseling to help the individual or family to understand, choose, and adjust		
Understand	*Choose*	*Adjust*
The diagnosis, prognosis and available management The genetic basis and chance of recurrence The options available (including genetic testing) for dealing with the risk of recurrence	The course of action appropriate to their personal and family situation and their ethical and religious standards and act in accordance with the decision	To the psychosocial impact of the genetic condition in the family

etc.) and increasingly include offers of predictive genetic testing. The goal includes specific aims, which are listed in Box 9.8.

Box 9.8: Specific aims of genetic counseling

To promote health enhancing behaviors

To enhance accurate and useful risk perceptions

To facilitate adaptation to genetic risk

To prevent disease

Genetic counseling case management: It is a multistep process and involves clinical expertise similar to any other medical speciality listed in Box 9.9.

Steps in evaluation of a child with genetic disorder: The steps taken in evaluating a child is listed in Box 9.10.

1. History and Pedigree Analysis

- Draw at least 3 generation pedigree using standard set of symbols (Tables 9.5 and 9.6)
- Male lines are placed on left
- All the members of same generation are placed on same horizontal levels
- Define generations with Roman and Arabic numerals are used to indicate each individual within a generation
- Write name and age of each member of pedigree
- History suggestive of maternal infections or antenatal drug exposure

---

Box 9.9: Genetic counseling case management

Information gathering—by

History with particular emphasis on pedigree construction and analysis

Detailed clinical examination

Diagnosis

Investigations of the patient and/or family members

Information giving—about

Nature and course of disorder

Recurrence risk

Possible treatment

Availability of further or future testing

Prenatal diagnosis if possible

Decision making

Referral to other specialists, health agencies, support groups

Follow up—for

Continuing clinical assessment especially if no diagnosis

Psychological support

Box 9.10: Steps taken in evaluating a child

History with particular emphasis on pedigree construction and analysis

Clinical examination

Diagnosis

Management with strong emphasis on genetic counseling regarding recurrence risk and prenatal diagnosis if possible.

- Developmental milestones
- Identify consanguineous marriages, miscarriages, infertility, congenital malformations, and similarly affected individuals in a family
- Identify pattern of inheritance depending upon the detailed history.

2. Clinical Examination

- Complete anthropometric measurements along with percentile depending upon the suspected disorder
- Head to toe examination for facial dysmorphism, any skin abnormalities, any malformation or deformities
- Any dysmorphic facial features with relevant facial measurements
- Presence of any minor or major malformation or neurocutaneous stigmata
- Complete general and systemic examination
- Clinical photograph of the patient
- Examination of parents

3. Diagnosis

A. Clinical

i. *Syndromic diagnosis* is based on identification of known syndromes based on the clinical phenotype. There are excellent texts available for understanding this interesting field of clinical genetics. In addition there are computer databases available for syndrome search such as London Dysmorphology Database and Pictures of Standard Syndromes and Undiagnosed Malformations (POSSUM). Referring to the books giving detailed descriptions of syndromes and diagnostic approaches is also of great help.

ii. *Chromosomal* (to be confirmed by cytogenetic analysis): Important indicators of a chromosomal abnormality are failure to thrive, presence of dysmorphism, confirmation or exclusion of the diagnosis of known chromosomal syndromes, for example Down syndrome, unexplained mental retardation with or without dysmorphism, multiple malformation syndrome, X-linked

Table 9.5: Common pedigree symbols, definitions and abbreviations

Instructions

Key should contain all information relevant to interpretation of pedigree (e.g. define shading)

For clinical (non-published) pedigrees include

a. Family names/initials, when appropriate

b. Name and title of person recording pedigree

c. Historian (person relaying family history information)

d. Date of intake/update.

Recommended order of information placed below symbol (below to lower right, if necessary)

a. Age/date of birth or age at death

b. Evaluation

c. Pedigree number (e.g. I-1, I-2, I-3)

	Male	*Female*	*Sex unknown*	*Comments*
Individual	b. 1925	30 y	4 mo	Assign gender by phenotype. Square represents male; circle represents a female; a diamond represents whose sex in not known. Age/date of birth can be given at the bottom right hand corner
Affected individual				Fillings can be shading, hatches, dots, lines, etc.
Multiple traits in an individual				For 2 conditions the symbols are partitioned correspondingly, each quadrant with different fillings/patterns representing different features.
Multiple individuals; number known	6	6	6	Number of the siblings is written inside the symbols; affected individuals should not be grouped
Multiple individuals; number unknown	n	n	n	"n" is used in the place of "?"
Deceased individual	d. 35y	d. 4 mo		If known, write "d" with age at death below symbol
Stillbirth (SB)	SB 28 wk	SB 30 wk	SB 34 wk	Birth of a dead child with gestational age noted
Pregnancy (P)	P	P / LMP. 7/1/94 Or 20 wk	P	Gestational age and karyotype (if known) below symbol. Light shading can be used for affected and defined in key/legend
Proband	P	P	P	First affected family member coming to medical attention
Consultand				Individual(s) seeking genetic counseling/testing

(Contd.)

Table 9.5: Common pedigree symbols, definitions and abbreviations (Contd...)

Male	Female	Sex unknown	Comments
	▯ (square divided vertically)	⊘ (circle divided vertically)	Presymptomatic carriers who may manifest disease later
	▣ (square with dot)	⊙ (circle with dot)	Carrier of autosomal or X-linked recessive trait who will not become affected
□—○			Two parents are joined by a horizontal line
□═○			Consanguineous mating are indicated by a double line
□—○ (with offspring)			Two parents joined by a horizontal line from which falls an inverted T to which their offspring are attached by short vertical lines
□—○ (single child)			A single child is attached by a long vertical line directly to the parents' horizontal mating line
□—○ (with twins)			Twins attach at the same spot along the inverted T if nonidentical; if identical they branch from a short vertical line and connected by a line

recessive syndrome manifesting in a female, two or more than two monogenic disorders in a patient, pregnancy at a risk of aneuploidy because of previous chromosomally abnormal child, maternal serum screening, advanced maternal age, or abnormality detected on fetal ultrasound scanning,

Table 9.6: Pedigree symbols and abbreviations for pregnancies not carried to term

Instructions

Symbols are smaller than standard ones and individual's line is shorter. (Even if sex is known, triangles are preferred to a small square/circle; symbol may be mistaken for symbols given in the previous table, especially in hand drawn pedigrees)

If gender and gestational age known, write below symbol in that order

	Male	Female	Sex unknown	Comments
Spontaneous abortion (SAB)	△ male	△ female	△ ECT	If ectopic pregnancy, write ECT below symbol
Affected SAB	▲ male	▲ female	▲ 16 wk	If gestational age known, write below symbol. Key/legend used to define shading
Termination of pregnancy (TOP)	◿ male	◿ female	◿	Other abbreviations (e.g. TAB, VTOP, Ab) not used for sake of consistency
Affected TOP	◢ male	◢ female	◢	Key/legend used to define shading

Table 9.7: Empiric risk of recurrence of isolated malformation

Malformation	Frequency per 1000 births	Recurrence for normal parents of one affected child
Anencephaly/spina bifida	4–5	5%
Cardiac malformation	6–8	3–4%
Cleft lip and cleft palate	2	4–5%
Cleft palate alone	0.5	2–6%
Pyloric stenosis	2–3	3%
Talipes equinovarus	3–4	2–8%
Dislocation of hip	3–4	3–4%
Hirschsprung's disease	0.1	6%

abnormalities of sexual differentiation and development, infertility, recurrent miscarriages or still births.

iii. *Single gene disorder* (thalassemia, neurometabolic disorder, etc)

B. *Laboratory*

a. *Cytogenetic* (Conventional/HRB) and/or FISH if a specific micro-deletion syndrome is suspected. 2 ml blood in heparin with asepsis is required and should be sent to lab within 24 hr.

b. *Molecular studies* for a specific suspected single gene disorders like—DNA diagnostic test are extremely important for prenatal diagnosis and carrier detection. Presently DNA diagnosis for thalassemia, hemoglobinopathies, hemophilia, Duchenne muscular dystrophy, fragile-X mental retardation, cystic fibrosis, megalencephalic leukodystrophy and spinal muscular atrophy are available in India. For providing prenatal diagnosis, the DNA diagnosis of the affected child in the family needs to be done beforehand. Sample for molecular tests should be saved in EDTA vials. Unless the type of mutations in the proband or carrier parents is identified, prenatal diagnosis is not feasible. It results in unambiguous results, diagnosis before appearance of clinical features, carrier status. Almost any tissue can be used. It is limited by high cost, genetic heterogeneity, and ethnic difference of disease prevalence.

c. *Enzyme studies* for lysosomal storage disorders like Gaucher's disease, mucopolysaccharidosis.

4. Management

Management with strong emphasis on genetic counseling regarding recurrence risk and prenatal diagnosis if possible.

4.1. *Nondirectiveness in genetic counseling:* The main principle of genetic counseling is nondirectiveness which is the art of presenting facts without influencing decision. It promotes the autonomy or self determination and personal control of the client. To maintain the sense of psychological well being amongst the clients, genetic counseling has also been defined as a dynamic psychoeducational process centered on genetic information. With a therapeutic relationship established between providers and clients, clients are helped to personalize technical and probabilistic genetic information, to promote self determination and to enhance their ability to adapt over time. The goal is to facilitate client's ability to use genetic information in a personally meaningful way that minimizes psychological distress and increases personal control. It promotes understanding, decision making, personal control, adaptation to stress inducing events and reduces psychological distress. As it is evident genetic counseling is a complex process and ideally requires (i) a correct diagnosis, (ii) a trained counselor with good knowledge of genetics and excellent communication skills, and (iii) psychosocial support to the family in coping up with the disorder and making decision with nondirective counseling. In addition to medical specialists, trained persons with various backgrounds like nursing, social work education and psychology can function as genetic counselors.

4.2. *Psychosocial issues:* The psychosocial impact of a genetic diagnosis for affected individuals and their families cannot be over emphasized. The diagnosis of any significant medical condition in a child or adult may have psychological, financial and social implications, but if the condition has a genetic basis a number of additional issues arise. These include guilt and blame, the impact on future reproductive decisions and the genetic implications to the extended family in addition to bereavement and long-term support and follow-up.

Guilt and blame: Feelings of guilt arise in relation to a genetic diagnosis in the family in many different situations. Parents very often express guilt at having transmitted a genetic disorder to their children, even when they had no previous knowledge of the risk. On the other hand, parents may also feel guilty for having taken the decision to terminate an affected pregnancy. Healthy members of a family may feel guilty that they have been more fortunate than their affected relatives and at-risk individuals may feel guilty about imposing a burden onto their partner and partner's family. Although in most situations the person expressing guilt will have played no objective causal role, it is important to allow him or her to express these concerns and for the counselor to reinforce that this is a normal human reaction to the predicament. Blame can sometimes occur in families where only one member of a couple carries the genetic risk ("It wasn't *our* side"), but again this is less likely to occur when the genetic situation has been explained and is understood.

Reproductive decision making: Couples aware of an increased genetic risk to their offspring must decide whether this knowledge will affect their plans for a family. Some couples may be faced with a perplexing range of options including different methods of prenatal diagnosis and the use of assisted reproductive technologies. For others the only available option will be to choose between taking the risk of having an affected child and remaining childless. Couples may need to reconsider these choices on repeated occasions during their reproductive years. Decision making may be more difficult in particular circumstances, including marital disagreement, religious or cultural conflict, and situations where the prognosis for an affected child is uncertain. For many genetic disorders with variable severity, although prenatal diagnosis can be offered, the clinical prognosis for the fetus cannot be predicted. When considering reproductive decisions, it can also be difficult for a couple to reconcile their love for an affected child or family member, with a desire to prevent the birth of a further affected child.

Impact on the extended family: The implications of a genetic diagnosis usually reverberate well beyond the affected individual and his or her nuclear family. For example, the parents of a boy just diagnosed with Duchenne muscular dystrophy will not only be coming to terms with his anticipated physical deterioration, but may have concerns that a younger son could be affected and that daughters could be carriers. They also face the need to discuss the possible family implications with the mother's sisters and female cousins who may already be having their own children.

Bereavement: Bereavement issues arise frequently in genetic counseling sessions. These may pertain to losses that have occurred recently or in the past. A genetic disorder may lead to reproductive loss or death of a close family member. The grief experienced after termination of pregnancy following diagnosis of abnormality is like that of other bereavement reactions and may be made more intense by parents' feelings of guilt. After the birth of a baby with congenital malformations, parents mourn the loss of the imagined healthy child in addition to their sadness about their child's disabilities, and this chronic sorrow may be ongoing throughout the affected child's life.

Long-term support and follow-up: Many families will require ongoing information and support following the initial genetic counseling session, whether coping with an actual diagnosis or the continued risk of a genetic disorder. Follow-up sessions may be needed to reinforce the informations (usually forgotten or wrongly remembered), to answer new queries, to provide latest information and to provide psychological support to the family during the process of coping up, till the acceptance and adjustments take place.

4.3. Counseling around genetic testing: Genetic counseling is an integral part of the genetic testing process and is required because of the potential impact of a test result on an individual and family, as well as to ensure informed choice about undergoing genetic testing. The extent of the counseling and the issues to be addressed will depend upon the type of test being offered, which may be diagnostic, presymptomatic, carrier or prenatal testing. Common pedigree symbols, definitions and abbreviations are mentioned in Table 9.5. Pedigree symbols and abbreviations for pregnancies not carried to term are shown in Table 9.6. Some relevant points regarding counseling of common pediatric genetic problems with different pattern of inheritance are given below:

1. Single gene disorders

Mendelian diseases are defined as disorders, which are the result of a single mutant gene leading to a large effect on the phenotype and are classified as follows:

- *Autosomal:* If the causative genes are present on the any of the autosomes (chromosome 1 to chromosome 22)
- *X-linked:* If they are present on the X chromosome
- *Dominant:* Those conditions which are expressed in heterozygous state
- *Recessive:* Those conditions which are expressed in homozygous state.

Males are hemizygous for the genes on X and Y chromosomes because they have only a single copy of each gene. This categorizes the mendelian disorders based on the transmission pattern as:

1. Autosomal dominant
2. Autosomal recessive
3. X-linked dominant
4. X-linked recessive
5. Y-linked inheritance

Autosomal Dominant Inheritance

- Vertical transmission is a characteristic feature
- An affected person usually has at least one affected parent
- Both sexes are affected in equal numbers
- Both sexes transmit the trait with equal probability
- Marriage between affected and normal individual results in offspring each with 50% chance of being affected (Fig. 9.4).

Autosomal Recessive Inheritance

- Characteristic pedigree pattern is horizontal because the affected individuals tend to be limited to a single sibling and not found in multiple generations
- Males and females are affected with equal probability
- Affected people are usually born to unaffected parents
- Parents of affected people are usually asymptomatic carriers

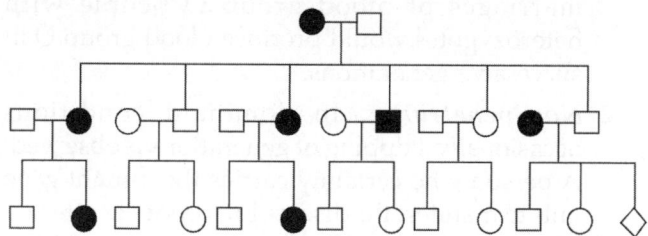

Fig. 9.4: Autosomal dominant pedigree

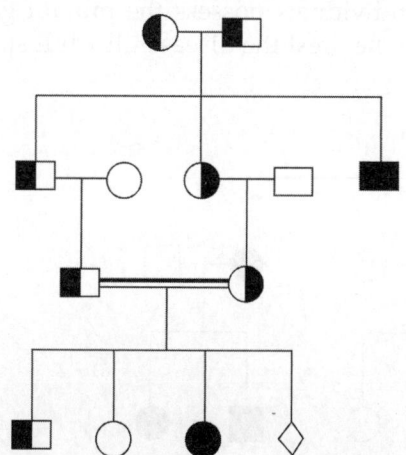

Fig. 9.5: Autosomal recessive pedigree

- There is an increased incidence of parental consanguinity
- When both the parents are carriers there is a 25% chance of each fetus being affected (Fig. 9.5).

X-linked Recessive Inheritance

- Usually only males are affected.
- Affected males are usually born to unaffected parents; mother is normally an asymptomatic carrier and may have affected male relatives.
- There is no male to male transmission in the pedigree.
- Usual mating is between a carrier woman and a normal male resulting in each son having a 50% chance of inheriting the mutant gene and being affected; each daughter having 50% chance of being a carrier of the mutant gene but clinically normal. In a second type of mating (as in hemophilia) between an affected man and a homozygous normal woman, all the sons are normal and all the daughters are obligate carriers. Lack of male to male transmission is a characteristic feature of X-linked inheritance.
- Females may be affected in certain situations such as, if the father is affected and the mother is a carrier, resulting in homozygosity for a X-linked recessive disorder; occasionally as a result of non-random inactivation of the normal X chromosome, so that the active X-chromosome is the one bearing the mutant gene; if a woman is hemizygous for the X-chromosome, as in Turner's syndrome; rare translocation between an autosome and X-chromosome might result in a female expressing an X-linked disease (Fig. 9.6).

X-linked Dominant Inheritance

- Although uncommon, these disorders manifest in the heterozygous female as well as in the male,

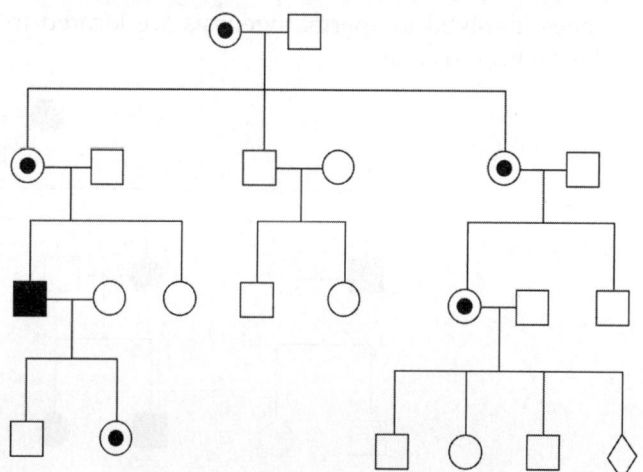

Fig. 9.6: X-linked recessive pedigree

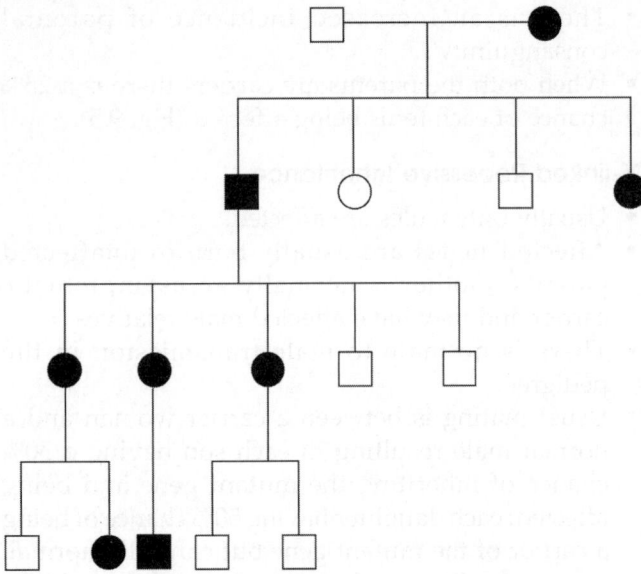

Fig. 9.7: X-linked dominant pedigree

carrying the mutant allele in his single X-chromosome.

- Resembles an AD trait because both sons and daughters of an affected female have a 1 in 2 (50%) chance of being affected.
- Important difference from an AD disease being that an affected male transmits the disorder to all his daughters but to none of his sons.
- Characteristically, such families have an excess of affected females and direct male to male transmission cannot occur.
- Vitamin D-resistant rickets is an example of X-linked dominant disorder (Fig. 9.7).

Y-linked Inheritance

- Only males are affected.
- Affected male transmits Y-linked traits to all his sons but none to his daughters.
- Hairy ears, H-Y histocompatibility antigen and genes involved in spermatogenesis are located in the Y-chromosome.

2. *Mitochondrial inheritance:* Mitochondrial genome is small; but contributes significantly to human genetic diseases. The mutation rate of mitochondrial DNA is high when compared to the nuclear DNA. Genes present on the mitochondria exhibit mitochondrial inheritance and cells may contain a mixture of mutant and normal mitochondria, referred to as heteroplasmy.

Mitochondrial inheritance is usually observed in diseases associated with the mitochondria because all the mitochondria in a zygote are derived from the ovum and the sperm does not contribute the same. So the mitochondrial diseases affect both sexes but are passed through affected mothers only. Essentially, all the offsprings of an affected mother inherit the disease (Fig. 9.8). Examples include MELAS (*m*yopathy, *e*ncephalopathy, *l*actic *a*cidosis, and *s*troke-like episodes), MERRF (*m*yoclonic *e*pilepsy associated with *r*agged *r*ed *f*ibers), and Kearns-Sayre syndrome (ophthalmoplegia, pigmentary retinopathy, and cardiomyopathy)

3. *Deviations in inheritance patterns (non-traditional/non-mendelian inheritance).*

   1. *Pseudodominant pedigree patterns.* If a recessive character is common in the population, then there is a high chance that the pedigree pattern resembles dominant inheritance, e.g. repeated marriages of blood group O people with heterozygotes would produce blood group O in successive generations.

   2. *Non-penetrance.* In dominant conditions occasionally skipping of generations is observed. A person who certainly carries the mutant gene fails to manifest the disease but produces affected offspring. This is described as non-penetrance, which is a major pitfall in genetic counseling.

   3. *Delayed onset* (age related penetrance) is observed in certain genetic conditions. Though the individuals possess the mutant genes they don't manifest the disease till adult stage.

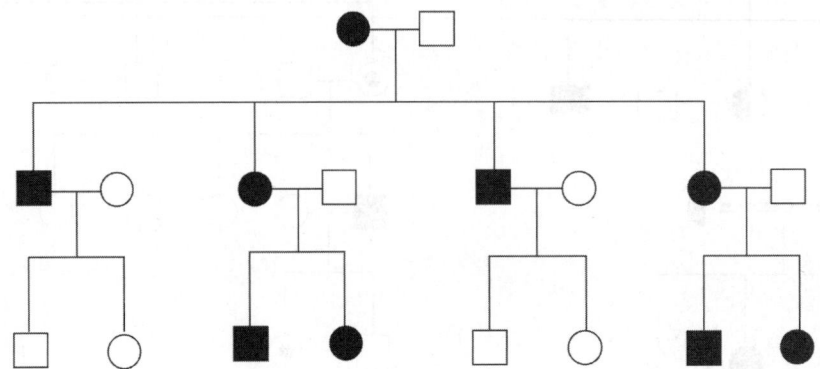

Fig. 9.8: Pedigree showing a classical mitochondrial inheritance

4. *Variable expression* is associated with non-penetrance and observed in dominant conditions. Different family members show different features of the syndrome.

5. *Anticipation* is defined as a condition in which the disease becomes more severe in successive generations. This is observed in some variable dominant conditions. For example, fragile X, myotonic dystrophy, Huntington's disease, etc.

6. *Genomic imprinting.* Certain autosomal dominant characters are transmitted by parents of either sex, but they manifest only when inherited from a parent of one particular sex. This parental sex effect is called **genomic imprinting.** Examples are Prader-Willi inherited from the paternal mutant allele on chromosome 15 and Angelman syndrome inherited when the same mutant allele is inherited from the maternal chromosome.

7. In some **X-linked dominant conditions** absence of the normal allele is lethal before birth. Thus, affected males are not born and we only see affected females who pass on the defective X chromosome to half their daughters but none of their sons. There may be a history of miscarriages.

8. New mutations often complicate pedigree interpretation and could be due to *germ line mosaicism.* When a couple with no relevant family history have a child with severe abnormalities deciding the mode of inheritance and recurrence risks can be very difficult: the problem might be autosomal recessive, autosomal dominant with a fresh mutation, X-linked recessive if the child is male, or non-genetic.

 Majority of genetic diseases exhibit **genetic heterogeneity** where different gene mutations lead to identical phenotype.

4.4. *Multifactorial disorders.* Counseling and risk of recurrence in these disorders is based on empiric risk figures available in literature. Table 9.7 shows risk of recurrence of some common malformations.

4.5. *Chromosomal disorders.* Majority of chromosomal disorders have associated mental retardation, e.g. Down syndrome (trisomy 21), Edwards' syndrome (trisomy 18), Patau syndrome (trisomy 13). In all *de novo* numerical and structural chromosomal abnormalities have a low risk of recurrence (< 1%). Risk is higher if either of the parents is carrying a balanced translocation. Extended family studies will be required if a parent has a balanced structural rearrangement. Counseling depends on the specific type of chromosomal abnormality detected.

4.6. *Points to remember*

1. Hereditary diseases may manifest at the time of birth or several years later in life.

2. All congenital defects observed at the time of birth are not necessarily inherited. Some of these may be due to teratogenic effect of drugs, infections or irradiation during the first trimester of pregnancy.

3. All familial diseases are not necessarily inherited disorders. Children share not only genes, but also the environment.

4. Different genetic disorders may result in similar clinical picture. Thus, several clinical syndromes, which were once considered as a single entity, are now known to be caused by several different genes. This is called genetic heterogeneity. It is, therefore, necessary to make a precise diagnosis of the genetic disorder, to provide accurate genetic counseling.

5. A degree of clinical variability exists in the presentation of certain genetic disorders. This variable expression of the mutant gene is attributed to the degree of penetration of the gene. Thus, one member of the family may show all the features of a genetic disease, while his or her siblings may show only mild forms of the disorders with one or the other sign.

6. Difficulty in genetic counseling may arise if the socially accepted father is not the real biologic father.

7. Genetic counselor should interpret the anticipated risk of recurrence of the inherited disorder in the future siblings in a meaningful manner, so that the family can arrive at a rational decision. The counselor has a particularly important responsibility in reassuring the parents that the risk of recurrence is low in case of disorders with multifactorial inheritance. In sporadic mutations and most of chromosomal disorders, there is only a small or no risk of recurrence.

8. While conveying information to the parents the physician should be extremely cautions. He should take special care not to infuse a sense of guilt in the parents. In case of X-linked disorders, it will be desirable to temper the blame on the mother, lest she is castigated by her husband or in-laws (Indian scenario).

Biesecker BB. Goals of Genetic Counseling. *Clinical Genet* 2001;60:323–30.

Buyse ML. Birth Defect Encyclopedia. Oxford: Blackwell Scientific Publication, 1990.

Fraser FC. Genetic Counseling. *Am J Human Genet* 1974;26:636–61.

Gardner RJM, Day TC, Sutherland GR. Chromosomal Abnormality and Genetic Counseling. 3rd edn. New York: Oxford University Press, 2003.

Hall JG. Genetic counseling. In: Behrman RE, Kliegman RM, Jenson HB (eds). *Nelson Textbook of Pediatrics.* 17th edn. Philadelphia: Saunders, 2004;395–96.

Harper PS. Practical Genetic Counselling. 5th edn. New York:A Oxford University Press, 2004.

Jones KL, Smith WS. Smith's Recognizable Patterns of Human Malformation. 6th edn. Philadelphia: WB Saunders, 2005.

10 Disorders of the Immunologic System

10.1 EVALUATION OF IMMUNODEFICIENCY DISORDERS

Immunodeficiency diseases (ID) are a group of disorders involving defects in one or more components of the immune system, and are characterized by an increased incidence of infections, autoimmunity, and malignancies. Immunodeficiency disorders can be primary or secondary, the latter being far more common. Primary immune deficiency diseases arise because of defects of the adaptive or innate immune system. Table 10.1 outlines important causes of secondary immunodeficiency. Pediatricians should maintain a high index of suspicion of defects of immune system because early diagnosis and treatment improves quality of life of patients. In case of detection of primary immunodeficiency, life saving procedures and genetic counseling can be done.

Healthy young children may experience up to 6 upper respiratory tract infections per year and even 10 or more if exposed to day care, school going sibs or smoking. These infections should clear promptly and in the case of bacterial infections, should respond rapidly to antibiotics. Evaluation of immune system should be initiated in children with clinical manifestations of a specific immune disorder or recurrent infections which are severe, complicated, in multiple locations, resistant to treatment, caused by unusual organisms. Table 10.2 summarizes the common organisms involved with specific defects.

History

A. *History Suggestive of Immunodeficiency Disease*

• *Severe eczema and petechiae:* Wiskott-Aldrich syndrome
• Delayed separation of umbilical stump of more than 8 wks or poor wound healing suggests leukocyte adhesion defect
• Post-vaccination disseminated BCG or paralytic polio in T cell or B cell disorders
• Hypocalcemic tetany of the neonate in DiGeorge anomaly

Table 10.1: Common causes of secondary immunodeficiency	
Infections	Human immunodeficiency virus infection (HIV), Epstein-Barr virus (EBV), *Mycobacterium tuberculosis*, measles, cryptococcus, severe sepsis and severe malnutrition
Collagen vascular disorders	Systemic lupus erythematosus, rheumatoid arthritis
Lymphoreticular malignancies	Lymphoma, leukemia
Medications	Glucocorticoids, cyclophosphamide, azathioprine, phenytoin
Loss of lymphocytes or antibodies	Severe burns, nephrotic syndrome, protein losing enteropathy
Bone marrow transplantation	
Metabolic	Diabetes mellitus, severe liver disease, uremia

Table 10.2: Pathogens associated with various immunodeficiencies	
T cells	*Pneumocystis carinii,* mycobacteria, *Cryptococcus neoformans,* herpes viruses
B cells	*Streptococcus pneumoniae, Haemophilus influenzae, Giardia lamblia,* enteroviruses, staphylococci, *Campylobacter* spp
Complement	*Neisseria* spp
Phagocytes	Staphylococci, *Aspergillus* spp, *Burkholderia cepacia*

- Graft-versus-host disease caused by maternal engraftment or non-irradiated blood transfusion in T cell defects
- Arthritis which does not fit in the defined categories of juvenile idiopathic arthritis (JIA) in agammaglobulinemia (but also in acquired immunodeficiency syndrome)
- Autoimmunity of B cell-related disorders: Early complement component deficiencies
- Generalized molluscum contagiosum or extensive warts: T cell disorders.

B. *Family History Suggestive of Immunodeficiency Disease*

- Unexplained death in infancy or recurrent infection history in maternal male relatives may be a clue to *X-linked immunodeficiency* where the mother is a carrier of the condition.
- A history of autoimmunity in family members may be positive for the patient with common variable immunodeficiency or IgA deficiency.
- It is important to remember that a negative family history does not exclude PID which can also be due to new mutations.

Examination

A thorough physical examination is very important in the diagnostic process.
- *General appearance* especially features of chronic illness such as pallor, wasting, clubbing and especially listlessness for which there is no other obvious explanation.
- *Detailed weight and height measurement*
- *Dysmorphic* features of DiGeorge anomaly with micrognathia, hypertelorism, anti-mongoloid slant of eyes and low-set and posteriorly rotated ears or those of trisomy 21 may be apparent.
- *Skin and mucosal membranes:* Gingivostomatitis and dental erosions are characteristic of patients with phagocytic defect, such as leukocyte adhesion deficiency. Recurrent oral ulcers are characteristic of patients with cyclic neutropenia. Extensive mucous membrane candidiasis suggests T cell defect.

- Examination of pharynx and nasal cavity for signs of sinusitis, including posterior pharyngeal cobble stoning, postnasal discharge or purulent nasal discharge. Evidence of scarred or perforated tympanic membranes with purulent discharge may be present.
- Absence of lymphoid tissue including tonsillar tissue in the presence of chronic infections may alert to X-linked agammaglobulinemia with inability to form immunoglobulins due to absence of B cells.
- *Systemic examination* frequently reveals rales on auscultation of the chest (bronchiectasis), hepatosplenomegaly due to chronic immune activation or hepatomegaly with or without jaundice as part of T cell disorders and intrahepatic chronic infections. Detailed neurological examination should be evaluated particularly in the presence of telangiectasia—although ataxia and immunodeficiency can also occur without the hallmark ocular findings.

Laboratory Evaluation

History and physical examination are helpful but must be supplemented by immune function testing. Prenatal testing is available for many disorders and is indicated if there is a family history of immunodeficiency and the mutation has been identified in family members.

Initial testing: If the findings on the history and physical examination are suggestive of primary immunodeficiency, appropriate laboratory tests should be ordered. If a specific secondary immunodeficiency disorder is suspected clinically, testing should focus on that disorder (e.g. diabetes, HIV infection, cystic fibrosis, primary ciliary dyskinesia, bronchiectasis.

Initial screening tests should include:
a. CBC with manual differential
b. Quantitative Ig measurements
c. Antibody titers
d. Skin testing for delayed hypersensitivity (Mantoux test) and chest X-ray, and
e. HIV serology.

If results are normal, immunodeficiency (especially Ig deficiency) can be excluded. If results are abnormal, further tests in specialized laboratories are needed to identify specific deficiencies. If chronic infections are objectively documented, initial and specific tests may be done simultaneously.

Important Issues in Primary Care

1. Prompt recognition of infection and aggressive treatment to avoid life-threatening complications and improve prognosis and quality of life.
   i. Initiation of early empiric coverage for suspected pathogens, obtaining appropriate cultures, and ongoing communication with the consulting immunologist are important measures.
   ii. Prophylactic antibiotics (trimethoprim-sulfamethoxazole) for children with significant T cell defects because of the risk for *Pneumocystis carinii* pneumonia.
   iii. Children with B cell immunodeficiencies who continue to experience recurrent infections despite adequate intravenous immunoglobulin replacement treatment also should be considered for concomitant antimicrobial therapy to avoid complications, such as chronic lung disease and bronchiectasis.
2. For routine childhood immunizations, live attenuated vaccines, such as OPV, varicella and BCG should not be given to children with suspected or diagnosed antibody or T cell immunodeficiency because vaccine-induced infection is a risk in these patients. IPV instead of live-attenuated OPV should be given to household members to prevent transmission of the virus that can occur by shedding of the attenuated virus in the stool. MMR, varicella and BCG can be given to family members.
3. If blood transfusion is needed, only irradiated, leukocyte-poor, and virus-free (i.e. CMV) products should be used in patients with T cell defects to avoid graft-versus-host reaction and CMV infection.
4. In some patients, varicella-zoster immunoglobulin may be indicated following varicella exposure.
5. Recurrent infections may predispose children to poor weight gain and growth; therefore, monitoring of the height and weight should be performed frequently and appropriate nutritional interventions initiated early if problems arise.

Specific Treatment Options

1. *Bone marrow transplantation:* Treatment of choice for most forms of significant cellular immunodeficiency (e.g. SCID, Wiskott-Aldrich syndrome, hyper IgM syndrome). For it to succeed, the procedure should be done in early infancy.
2. *Immunoglobulin replacement:* Definitive treatment for well-documented and symptomatic antibody-deficiency disorders (ADDs), frequent and severe infections or in infants, the development of failure to thrive, are initial indications for considering immunoglobulin replacement therapy, which would be instituted after a diagnosis of hypogammaglobulinemia or specific antibody deficiency has been confirmed. Children with X-linked agammaglobulinemia and common variable immunodeficiency need to be administered 3–4 weekly injections of IV immunoglobulin (IVIG). A minimum starting dosage is 200 mg/kg/mo which can be titrated upward as necessary.
3. *Enzyme replacement:* For C1 esterase inhibitor deficiency, prophylactic danazol therapy results in significant improvement, but injections of C1 esterase inhibitor may be required whenever there is laryngeal involvement and consequential airway compromise.
4. *Stem cell transplantation:* Candidate diseases for treatment with allogeneic stem cell transplantation (SCT) include: i) Severe combined immunodeficiency disorder (SCID); ii) Chediak-Higashi syndrome; iii) Wiskott-Aldrich syndrome; iv) leukocyte adhesion deficiency (LAD); v) combined immunodeficiency; vi) chronic granulomatous disease (CGD).
5. *Gene therapy:* Retroviral vector gene therapy has been successful in a few patients with X-linked and adenosine deaminase (ADA)-deficient SCID, but this treatment is not widely used because some patients with X-linked SCID developed leukemia.

Buckley RH. Evaluation of the immune system. In: Behrman RE, Kliegman RM, Jenson HB (eds). *Nelson Textbook of Pediatrics.* 18th edn. Philadelphia, PA: WB Saunders Co; 2007:867–73.

Candotti F. The potential for therapy of immune disorders with gene therapy. *Pediatr Clin North Am* 2000;47:1389–407.

Horwitz ME. Stem cell transplantation for inherited immunodeficiency disorders. *Pediatr Clin North Am* 2000;47:1371–87.

Tangsinmankong N, Bahna SL, Good RA. The immunologic workup of the child suspected of immunodeficiency. *Ann Allergy Asthma Immunol* 2001;87:362–70.

Woroniecka M, Ballow M. Office evaluation of children with recurrent infection. *Pediatr Clin North Am* 2000;47:1211–24.

10.2 THE T, B, NK CELL SYSTEMS

Defense against infectious agents is secured through a combination of anatomic physical barriers including the skin, mucous membranes, mucous blanket, and ciliated epithelial cells, as well as of the various components of the immune system. The immune system also helps to protect against malignancy and autoimmunity.

The immune system integrates two fundamental response mechanisms—innate (natural) and acquired (adaptive). 1. Innate (natural) immunity responds to infection regardless of previous exposure to the agent and includes polymorphonuclear leukocytes, dendritic and mononuclear phagocytic cells, various receptors that recognize common pathogenic antigens (Toll-like receptors) and the complement system. 2. Acquired (adaptive) immunity includes T lymphocytes, B lymphocytes, and natural killer (NK) cells.

Buckley RH. The T, B, NK cell systems. In: Kliegman RM, Behrman RE, Jenson HB, Stanton BF (eds). *Nelson Textbook of Pediatrics.* 18th edn. Vol 1. Philadelphia: Saunders, 2007;873–95.

10.3 THE PHAGOCYTIC SYSTEM

Neutrophils and mononuclear phagocytes share primary functions including the unusual ability to ingest large particles. Neutrophils are of only one type, but there are many varieties of mononuclear phagocytes, including the tissue macrophages, and their circulating precursors, monocytes, and remain for only 6 hr in the circulation.

The pluripotential stem cells give rise to more mature stem cells, including cells that are committed to either lymphoid or myeloid development. Lymphoid stem cells give rise to T and B cell precursors and their mature progeny.

Granulocytes survive for only 6–12 hr in the circulation, and therefore, daily production of 2×10^4 granulocytes/μl of blood is required to maintain a level of circulating granulocytes of 5×10^3/μl. In contrast, *lymphocytes* can exhibit lifetimes measured in months or years and require daily renewal of lymphocytes progenitors at rates substantially lower than the other hematopoietic progenitors. Proliferation of myeloid cells consisting of approximately five divisions takes place only during the 1st three stages of neutrophil development (myeloblast, promyelocyte, myelocyte). After the myelocyte stage, the cells terminally differentiate into metamyelocytes, bands, and neutrophils. Neutrophil maturation is associated with changes in the nucleus and with production of azurophilic primary nucleus, and a deficiency of granules. Promyelocytes acquire peroxidase-positive azurophilic granules, and myelocytes acquire specific granules. Chromatin condensation, loss of nucleoli, and the shape changes of the nucleus result in the morphometric characteristic of the segmental neutrophil.

Monocytes, Macrophages, and Dendritic Cells

Mononuclear phagocytes (monocytes, macrophages) have a central and essential role in innate host defense against infection, in tissue repair and remodeling, and in the antigen-specific adaptive immune response. No human has been identified as having congenital absence of this cell line, probably because macrophages are required to remove primitive tissues during fetal development as new tissues develop to replace them. Monocytes and tissue macrophages in their various forms constitute the molecular phagocyte system. Monocytes, the circular precursors of tissue macrophages, develop more rapidly in the bone marrow and remain longer in the circulation than do neutrophils. The 1st recognizable monocyte precursor is the monoblast, followed by the promonocyte, a somewhat larger cell with cytoplasmic granules and an indented nucleus containing finely divided chromatin, and finally, the fully developed monocyte. A mature monocyte is larger than a neutrophil and has cytoplasm filled with granules containing hydrolytic enzymes. The transition from monoblast to mature circulating monocyte requires about 6 days. Migration of monocytes into the different tissues appears to occur randomly in the absence of localized inflammation. Once in the tissues, monocytes undergo transformation into tissue macrophages with morphologic and sometimes functional properties that are characteristic for the tissue in which they reside. All macrophages have at least three major functions in common: presentation of antigens to lymphocytes, phagocytosis, and immunomodulation through release of a variety of potent hormone-like factors termed cytokines. At sites of inflammation, monocytes and macrophages can fuse to form multinucleated giant cells, the terminal stage of development in the mononuclear phagocyte line. Numerous functions are upregulated when the macrophage is activated in response to infection. Ingestion and killing of such intracellular pathogens as *Mycobacterium tuberculosis, Listeria, Leishmania, Toxoplasma,* and some fungi, but macrophages also clear from the bloodstream and eliminate such exracellular pathogens as *Streptococcus pneumoniae.*

Myeloid dendritic cells (DCs): Cells with dendritic (branched) extensions originate from myeloid progenitors in the bone marrow and function as highly efficient antigen-presenting cells. They phagocytose, though less well than macrophages. DCs are of four types:

i. Langerhans' cells in the epithelial surfaces of skin and mucosa

ii. Dermal or interstitial DCs in subepithelial skin and interstitial of solid organs

iii. Monocyte-derived DCs, which can leave the circulation and enter a site of pathogen invasion; and

iv. Plasmacytoid DCs, the principal source of IFN-α and IFN-β in response to viral infection.

Abnormalities of Monocyte-Macrophage or Dendritic Cell Function

1. Mononuclear phagocytes, as well as neutrophils, from patients with chronic granulomatous disease exhibit a profound defect of phagocyte killing. The inability of affected macrophages to kill ingested organisms leads to abscess formation and characteristic granulomas at sites of macrophage accumulation beneath the skin and in the liver, lungs, spleen, and lymph nodes.

2. The monocyte-macrophage system is prominently involved in several lipid storage diseases, the sphingolipidoses.

3. The cytokine interleukin 12 (IL-12) is a powerful inducer of IFN-γ production by T cells, and natural killer cells. Individuals with inherited deficiency in macrophage receptors for IFN-γ or lymphocyte receptors for IL-12, or in IL-12 itself, suffer a severe, profound, and selective susceptibility to infection by nontuberculous mycobacteria such as *Mycobacterium avium* complex, or bacillus Calmette-Guérin (BCG). About half of these patients have had disseminated *Salmonella* infection. These abnormalities are now grouped under the term leukocyte mycobactericidal defects.

4. Mixed mononuclear cells from newborns produce less IFN-γ and IL-12 than adult cells do, and macrophages cultured from cord blood are not activated normally by IFN-γ. This combination of deficiencies would be expected to blunt the newborn's response to infection by viruses, fungi, and certain bacteria as *Listeria*.

5. There are two disorders in which macrophage activation is pathologically excessive. *Familial hemophagocytic lymphohistiocytosis* is characterized by uncontrolled activation of T cells and macrophages, with resultant fever, hepatosplenomegaly, lymphadenopathy, pancytopenia, marked elevation of serum proinflammatory cytokines, and macrophage hemophagocytosis. Up to 5% of children with systemic onset juvenile rheumatoid arthritis develop an acute severe complication termed *macrophage activation syndrome*, with persistent fever (rather than typical febrile spikes), hepatosplenomegaly, pancytopenia, macrophage hemophagocytosis, and coagulopathy, which can progress to disseminated intravascular coagulation and death if not recognized.

Eosinophils

Eosinophils are nondividing fully differentiated cells with a diameter of ~ 8 μm and a bilobed nucleus. They differentiate from stem cell precursors in the bone marrow under the control of T cell-derived interleukin 3 (IL-3), granulocyte-macrophage colony-stimulating factor (GM-CSF), and especially IL-5. Blood eosinophil numbers do not always reflect the extent of eosinophil involvement in disease-affected tissues. The absolute eosinophil count, calculated as the white blood cell (WBC) count/μl × percent of eosinophils, is usually < 450 cells/μl in the blood and varies diurnally, being more abundant in the early morning and diminishing as endogenous glucocorticoid levels rise.

Eosinopenia occurs after corticosteroid administration and with some bacterial and viral infections.

Eosinophilia: The absolute eosinophilia count is used to quantitate eosinophilia. Many diseases are associated with moderately severe (1,500–5,000 cells/μl) or severe (> 5,000 cells/μl) eosinophilia. Patients with sustained blood eosinophilia may develop organ damage, especially cardiac damage as found in the idiopathic hypereosinophilic syndrome, and should be monitored for evidence of cardiac disease. Many cases of moderately severe eosinophilia often have no clear etiology. Eosinophilia is associated with:

a. *Allergic diseases:* Drug fever, atopic dermatitis, eczema, pemphigus, urticaria, and toxic epidermal necrolysis.

b. *Infectious diseases:* Helminthic parasites infection (due to visceral larva migrans caused by *Toxocara*); fungal diseases (allergic bronchopulmonary aspergillosis and coccidioidomycosis).

c. *Hypereosinophilic syndrome:* Idiopathic hyper-eosinophilic syndrome is characterized by sustained overproduction of eosinophils.

d. *Miscellaneous diseases:* Eosinophilia is observed in patients with primary immunodeficiency syndromes, especially hyper-IgE syndrome and Wiskott-Aldrich syndrome, syndromes of thrombocytopenia with absent radii, familial reticuloendotheliosis, Hodgkin's disease, ulcerative colitis, Crohn's disease, and chronic hepatitis.

Leukopenia

Marked developmental changes in normal values for the total white blood cell (WBC) count occur during childhood. The mean WBC count at birth is high, followed by a rapid fall beginning at 12 hr until the end of 1st week. Thereafter, the values are stable until 1yr of age. A slow, steady WBC count occurs throughout childhood until reaching the adult value during adolescence. Leukopenia in adolescents and adults is defined as a total WBC count < 4,000 cells/μl. Evaluation of patients with leukopenia, or lymphopenia begins with a history, physical examination, family history, and screening laboratory tests.

Neutropenia

Neutropenia is an absolute neutrophil count (ANC) calculated as the WBC count/µl × % of neutophils and bands, more than two standard deviations below the normal mean. Normal neutrophil counts must be stratified for age and race. For whites, the lower limit of normal for neutrophil count is 1,500/µl, for blacks, the lower limit of normal is 1,200/µl. The relatively lower limit in blacks probably reflects a relative decrease in neutrophils in the storage compartment of the bone marrow. There are various causes of neutropenia.

a. *Infectious causes: Transient neutropenia* often accompanies viral infections, usually occurs during 1st 1–2 days of illness and may persist for 3–8 days. *Bacterial sepsis* is a particularly serious cause of neutropenia and all neonates are particularly vulnerable to developing neutropenia because of a deficient pool of reserve neutrophils and bands in the bone marrow. *Chronic neutropenia* often accompanies infection with HIV as a finding associated with AIDS. The neutropenia associated with AIDS probably arises from a combination of impaired neutrophil production and the accelerated destruction of neutrophils mediated by antineutrophil antibodies.

b. *Drug induced neutropenia:* Drug-induced neutropenia has several underlying mechanisms (immune-mediated, toxic, idiosyncratic, hypersensitivity reactions) and should be differentiated from the severe neutropenia that occurs after large doses of cytoreductive cancer drugs or radiotherapy. Drugs, such as penicillin, propylthiouracil, phenothiazines, chloramphenicol, phenytoin, and phenobarbital causes neutropenia.

c. *Bone marrow replacement:* Various acquired disorders may lead to neutropenia accompanied by anemia, and thrombocytopenia. The causes are:
   1. Hematologic malignancies (most important cause) including leukemia and lymphoma, and metastatic solid tumors such as neuroblastoma, rhabdomyosarcoma, and Ewing's sarcoma that infiltrate the bone marrow, resulting in suppression of myelopoiesis
   2. Myelodysplastic disorders or preleukemic syndromes characterized by peripheral cytopenias and macrocytic blood cells associated with impaired production of myeloid precursors, and
   3. Aplastic anemia arising from acquisition of damaged stem cells.

d. *Reticuloendothelial sequestration:* Splenic enlargement resulting from intrinsic splenic disease, portal hypertension, or other causes of splenic hyperplasia can lead to neutropenia.

e. *Immune neutropenia:* Immune neutropenias are associated with the presence of circulating anti-neutrophil antibodies, which may mediate neutrophil destruction by complement-mediated lysis or splenic phagocytosis of opsonized neutrophils. In other conditions such as systemic lupus erythematosus and autoimmune lymphoproliferative disease, accelerated apoptosis of myeloid precursors or neutrophils themselves may underlie the pathogenesis of the neutropenia.

f. *Alloimmune neonatal neutropenia (ANN):* ANN occurs after transplacental transfer of maternal alloantibodies directed against antigens on the infant's neutrophils, analogous to Rh hemolytic disease.

g. *Alloimmune neonatal neutropenia (ANN):* ANN occurs after transplacental transfer of maternal alloantibodies directed against antigens on the infant's neutrophils, analogous to Rh hemolytic disease. The pathogenesis of ANN usually involves phagocytosis of antibody-coated neutophils by splenic macrophages. Symptomatic infants may present with delayed separation of the umbilical cord, mild skin infections, fever, and pneumonia within the 1st 2 wk of life. By 7 wk of age, the neutrophil count usually returns to normal, reflecting the duration of maternal antibodies in the infant's circulation.

h. *Autoimmune neutropenia:* Autoimmune neutropenia is analogous to autoimmune hemolytic anemia and thrombocytopenia. Autoimmune neutropenia frequently occurs in children with congenital and acquired forms of immune deficiencies, including dysgammaglobulinemia, immune-mediated thyroiditis, autoimmune hemolytic anemia, and thrombocytopenia.

i. *Autoimmune neutropenia of infancy (ANI):* Patients having ANI have severe neutropenia on presentation with an ANC usually < 500/µl, but the total WBC count is always within normal limits. Monocytosis or eosinophilia may occur. The age at diagnosis is usually between 5 and 15 mo, with a female : male ratio of 6 : 4. None of the affected children has evidence of other autoimmune diseases. Children with ANI present with minor infections such as otitis media, gingivitis, respiratory tract infections, gastroenteritis and cellulitis.

j. *Neonatal autoimmune neutropenia:* Mothers with autoimmune disease may give birth to infants who develop transient neutropenia. It persists in most cases for a few weeks to a few months. Neonates almost always remain asymptomatic.

k. *Cyclic neutropenia:* Cyclic neutropenia, a congenital granulopoietic disorder is inherited in an autosomal dominant manner in some patients. It is characterized by regular, periodic oscillation in the number of peripheral neutrophils from normal to neutropenic values with a mean oscillatory period of 21± 3 days. During the neutropenic phase, most patients suffer from oral ulcers, fever, stomatitis, or pharyngitis, occasionally associated with lymph node enlargement. Serious infections occur occasionally, include pneumonia, chronic periodontitis, and recurrent ulcerations of the oral, vaginal, and rectal mucosa, and sepsis notably with *Clostridium perfringens*.

l. *Severe congenital neutropenia*: Severe congenital neutropenia, or Kostmann disease, is characterized by an arrest in myeloid maturation at the promyelocyte stage of the bone marrow, resulting in an ANC of < 200/μl. The disorder occurs sporadically or as an autosomal dominant or recessive disorder. Patients typically show monocytosis, eosinophilia, and anemia and suffer from recurrent, severe pyogenic infections, especially of the skin, mouth, and rectum.

m. *Shwachman-Diamond syndrome:* Shwachman-Diamond syndrome is an autosomal recessive disorder characterized by pancreatic insufficiency and abnormally low WBC counts (neutropenia) with the ANC periodically < 1,000/μl associated with hypoplastic myelopoiesis. The initial symptoms are usually diarrhea and failure to thrive because of malabsorption, which develops in almost all infants by 4 mo of age.

n. *Cartilage-hair hypoplasia:* Cartilage-hair hypoplasia is a multisystem autosomal recessive disorder and is common among the Finnish and Amish. The major symptoms include abnormalities of the spine, hyperextensible fingers, and very fine, thin hair, eyebrows, and eyelashes. Cartilage-hair hypoplasia is associated with decreased cell-mediated immunity, neutropenia, macrocytic anemia, and increased rates of malignancy. Stem cell transplantation has been used which restores cellular immunity and corrects the neutropenia.

o. *Glycogen storage disease type 1b:* Recurrent infections with neutropenia are a distinctive feature of glycogen storage disease (GSD) type 1b.

p. *Severe chronic neutropenia:* Acquired idiopathic chronic symptomatic neutropenia is characterized by onset of neutropenia after 2 yr of age and more frequently among adults. Patients with an ANC persistently < 500/μl are afflicted with recurrent pyogenic infections involving the skin, mucous membranes, lungs, and lymph nodes. Bone marrow examination reveals variable patterns of myeloid formation with arrest generally occurring between the myelocyte and band forms.

q. *Chronic benign neutropenia:* Chronic benign neutropenia of childhood represents a group of disorders characterized by mild to moderate neutropenia that does not lead to an increased risk of pyogenic infections. Spontaneous remissions are also reported.

Lymphopenia

Lymphocytes account for about 30% of the circulating WBCs in a newborn. The proportion of lymphocytes then increases rapidly within the 1st mo, reaching an average of 60% by 2 yr of age. The normal lymphocyte count in children < 2 yr of age is 3,000–9,500/μl and in adults is 1,000–4,800/μl. At 6 yr of age, the lower limit of the normal is 1,500/μl. Almost 65% of blood T lymphocytes are CD4 (helper) T lymphocytes. Most patients with lymphocytopenia have a reduction in the absolute number of T lymphocytes, particularly in the number of CD4 T lymphocytes. The average number of CD4 T lymphocytes in adult blood is 1,000/μL (range 300–1,300/μl), and the average number of CD8 (suppressor) T lymphocytes is 600/μl (range 100–900/μl), with the normal CD4 : CD8 ratio of 1.8:2.0.

Lymphocytopenia is detected in recurrent viral, fungal, and parasitic infections. Inherited causes of lymphocytopenia include inherited immunodeficiency disorders, Wiskott-Aldrich syndrome, adenosine deaminase deficiency and purine nucleoside phosphorylase deficiency. Acquired lymphocytopenia is the result of depletion of blood lymphocytes. AIDS is the most common infectious disease associated with lymphocytopenia, which results from destruction of CD4 T cells infected with HIV 1 or HIV 2. Other viral and bacterial diseases may be associated with lymphocytopenia. Iatrogenic lymphocytopenia is usually caused by cytotoxic chemotherapy, radiation therapy, and long-term administration of anti-lymphocyte globulin. Long-term treatment of psoriasis with psoralen and ultraviolet irradiation may destroy T lymphocytes. Corticosteroids can cause lymphopenia through increased cell destruction. Systemic autoimmune diseases such as systemic lupus erythematosus are associated with lymphocytopenia. Other conditions such as protein loosing enteropathy and aberrant or surgical drainage of the thoracic duct are associated with lymphocyte depletion, leading to lymphocytopenia.

Leukocytosis

Leukocytosis is an elevation in the total leukocyte, or white blood cell (WBC), count that is two standard deviations above the mean count for a particular age. A WBC count exceeding 50,000/µl is termed a leukemoid reaction because of the similarity to features of leukemia. Leukemoid reactions are usually neutrophilic and are most frequently associated with septicemia and severe bacterial infections including shigellosis, salmonellosis, and meningococcemia. Infection in children with leukocyte adhesion deficiency results in WBC counts approaching or exceeding 1, 00,000/µl. A significant proportion of > 5% of immature to mature neutrophil cells is termed a *shift-to-the-left* and indicates rapid release of cells from the bone marrow. This may result in increased circulating neutrophilic cells, or metamyelocytes and myelocytes, which are not usually found in the peripheral circulation. Higher degrees of shift to the left with more immature neutrophil precursors indicate serious bacterial infections, trauma, burns, surgery, and acute hemolysis or hemorrhage.

Neutrophilia: Neutrophilia is an increase in the total number of blood neutrophils, which for older children and adults is > 8,000/µl. During the 1st day of life, the upper limit of the normal neutrophil count ranges from 7,000 to 12,000/µl. In the 1st month of life, the neutrophil count ranges from 1,800 to 5,400/µl, and by 1 yr of age, the range is 1,500–8,500/µl. Myelocytes are not released to the blood except under extreme circumstances.

i. *Acute acquired neutrophilia:* Neutrophilia is usually an acquired disorder and is a common finding with inflammation, infection, injury, surgery, sickle cell disease, chronic hemolytic anemia, heatstroke, burns, diabetic ketoacidosis, stress and drugs (epinephrine, corticosteroids, and recombinant growth factors such as rhG-CSF and rhGM-CSF).

ii. *Chronic acquired neutrophilia:* Chronic neutrophilia is usually associated with continued stimulation of neutrophil production resulting from persistent inflammatory reactions or chronic infections such as tuberculosis, vasculitis, postsplenectomy states, Hodgkin's disease, chronic myelogenous leukemia, chronic blood loss, prolonged administration of corticosteroids, and exogenously administered hematopoietic growth factors such as rhG-CSF.

iii. *Lifelong neutrophilia:* Congenital asplenia, leukocyte adhesion deficiency, familial myeloproliferative disease, Down syndrome, and Rac-2 mutation are associated with lifelong neutrophilia.

Monocytosis: The average absolute blood monocyte count varies with age. Most commonly, monocytosis occurs in patients recovering from myelosuppressive chemotherapy and indicates the return of the neutrophil count to normal. Monocytosis is often a sign of an acute bacterial, viral, protozoal, or rickettsial infection, chronic neutropenia, and postsplenectomy states.

Lymphocytosis: The common causes of lymphocytosis are acute viral illnesses (infectious mononucleosis, cytomegalovirus, and viral hepatitis), chronic bacterial infections (tuberculosis, brucellosis, and pertussis), and endocrine disorders (thyrotoxicosis and Addison disease). Persistent or profound lymphocytosis suggests acute lymphocytic leukemia.

Basophilia: Basophilia occurs when the basophil count exceeds 100–120 cells/µl. Basophil is a nonspecific sign of a wide variety of disorders and is usually of limited diagnostic importance. Basophilia is most often present in hypersensitivity reactions.

Borregaard N, Boxler LA. Disorders of neutrophil function. In: Beutler E, Kipps TJ, et al (eds). *Williams Hematology*. 7th edn. New York: McGraw-Hill, 2006.

Boxer LA. Neutrophils. In: Kliegman RM, Behrman RE, Jenson HB, Stanton BF (eds). *Nelson Textbook of Pediatrics*. 18th edn. Vol 1. Philadelphia: Saunders, 2007;895–9.

Boxer LA. Eosinophils. In: Kliegman RM, Behrman RE, Jenson HB, Stanton BF (eds). *Nelson Textbook of Pediatrics*. 18th edn. Vol 1. Philadelphia: Saunders, 2007;902–3.

Boxer LA. Leukopenia. In: Kliegman RM, Behrman RE, Jenson HB, Stanton BF (eds). *Nelson Textbook of Pediatrics*. 18th edn. Vol 1. Philadelphia: Saunders, 2007;909–15.

Boxer LA. Leukocytosis. In: Kliegman RM, Behrman RE, Jenson HB, Stanton BF (eds). *Nelson Textbook of Pediatrics*. 18th edn. Vol 1. Philadelphia: Saunders, 2007;915–17.

Dale DC, Bolyard AA, Aprikyan A. Cyclic neutropenia. *Semin Hematol* 2002;39:89–94.

Johnston RB, (Jr). Monocytes, macrophages, and dendritic cells. In: Kliegman RM, Behrman RE, Jenson HB, Stanton BF (eds). *Nelson Textbook of Pediatrics*. 18th edn. Vol 1. Philadelphia: Saunders, 2007;899–902.

10.4 THE COMPLEMENT SYSTEM

The complement system is an essential component of innate immunity. Complement is a system of interacting proteins. Complement was originally defined as the nonspecific, heat-labile complementary principle required with specific antibody to lyse bacteria. The 1st four components were number in the order of their discovery and are termed the classical pathway, but the components fix to the immune complex are in a different order, C1423. Complement emerges as a logical, exquisitely balanced, and highly influential system that is fundamental to the clinical expression of host defense and inflammation.

Neutralization of virus by antibody can be enhanced with C1 and C4 and further enhanced by the additional fixation of C3b through the classical or alternative pathway. Complement may therefore is particularly important in the early phases of a viral infection when antibody is limited. Antibody and the full complement sequence can also eliminate infectivity of at least some viruses by the production of typical complement "holes" as seen by electron microscopy.

Activation of the entire complement sequence can result in lysis of virus-infected cells, tumor cells and most types of microorganisms. Bactericidal activity of complement has not appeared to be important to host defense, except for the occurrence of *Neisseria* infections in patients lacking later-acting components of complement.

A defect of complement function should be considered in any patient with recurrent angioedema, autoimmune disease, chronic nephritis, or partial lipodystrophy or with recurrent pyogenic infections, or a second episode of bacteremia at any age.

Most patients with primary C1q deficiency have systemic lupus erythematosus (SLE), an SLE-like syndrome without typical SLE serology, a chronic rash that has shown an underlying vasculitis on biopsy, or membranoproliferative glomerulonephritis (MPGN). Some C1q-deficient children have serious infections, including septicemia and meningitis. Partial deficiency of C1q has occurred in patients with severe combined immunodeficiency disease or hypogammaglobu-linemia, apparently secondary to the deficiency of IgG, which normally binds reversibly to C1q and prevents its rapid catabolism. Patients with C2 deficiency often have repeated life-threatening septicemic illnesses, most commonly due to pneumococci.

Newborn infants have mild to moderate deficiencies of all plasma components of the complement system. Complement activity is even lower in preterm infants.

Patients with severe chronic cirrhosis of the liver, hepatic failure, malnutrition, or anorexia nervosa may also have significant depletion of components and functional activity of complement. Immune complexes initiated by microorganisms or their by-products can induce complement consumption.

Burns can induce massive activation of the complement system, especially the alternative pathway, within a few hours after injury. In patients with erythropoietic protoporphyria or porphyria cutanea tarda, exposure of the skin to light of certain wavelengths activates complement, generating chemotactic activity. Phototoxicity is associated histologically with lysis of capillary endothelial cells, mast cell degranulation, and the appearance of neutrophils in the dermis.

Treatment: No specific therapy is available at present for genetic deficiencies of the complement system except hereditary angioedema.

Davis AE III. The pathophysiology of hereditary angioedema. *Clin Immunol* 2005;114:3–9.

Johnston RB, (Jr). The complement system. In: Kliegman RM, Behrman RE, Jenson HB, Stanton BF (eds). *Nelson Textbook of Pediatrics.* 18th edn. Vol 1. Philadelphia: Saunders, 2007; 918–24.

10.5 HEMATOPOIETIC STEM CELL TRANSPLANTATION

Hematopoietic stem cells are used to cure malignant and non-malignant disorders. *Autologous* (from the same individual) transplantation is employed as a rescue strategy after delivering otherwise lethal doses of radiotherapy and chemotherapy. *Allogeneic* transplantation is used to treat children with genetic diseases of blood cells, such as thalassemia and primary immunodeficiency diseases and hematologic malignancies, such as leukemia and lymphoma.

Protocols for allogeneic HSCT consist of two parts: the preparative regimen and transplantation itself. During the preparative conditioning regimen, chemotherapy, often associated with irradiation, is administered to destroy the patient's hematopoietic system and to suppress the immune system, especially T cells, so that graft rejection is prevented. In patients with malignancies, the preparative regimen also serves to reduce the tumor burden. The patient then receives an intravenous infusion of hematopoietic cells from the donor.

The immunology of HSCT is distinct from that of other types of transplant because, in addition to stem cells, the graft contains mature blood cells of donor origin, including T cells, natural killer (NK) cells, and dendritic cells. These cells repopulate the recipient's lympho-hematopoietic system and give rise to a new immune system, which helps eliminate residual leukemia cells that survive the conditioning regimen. The effect is known as the graft *versus leukemia (GVL) effect.* The donor immune system exerts its GVL effect through T cell-mediated alloreactions directed against recipient histocompatibility antigens displayed on recipient leukemia cells. Because histocompatibility antigens are also displayed on tissues, T cell-mediated alloreactions may ensue. The *optimal donor* for any patient undergoing HSCT is an HLA-identical sibling. Because polymorphic HLA genes are closely linked and usually constitute a single genetic locus, any pair of siblings has a 25% chance of being HLA identical. This allows approximately one-third of patients to receive their transplant from an HLA-identical sibling.

Autologous Hematopoietic Stem Cell Transplantation

Autologous transplantation, using the patient's own stored marrow, is associated with a very low risk of life-threatening transplant-related complications, although the main cause of failure is disease recurrence. Autologous HSCT is employed primarily to prevent relapse in patients with AML who achieve complete remission after induction therapy, and also for selected children with relapsed lymphomas and selected solid tumors (Box 10.1).

HSCT from Alternative Sources and Donors

Two-thirds of patients do not have an HLA-identical sibling for hematopoietic stem cell transplantation (HSCT). Alternative sources of hematopoietic stem cells are used and include matched unrelated donors (MCDs), unrelated umbilical cord blood (UCB), and haploidentical relatives with one HLA mismatched.

Unrelated donor transplants: Outcomes from a fully matched or a single allelic disparate unrelated volunteer donor are now similar to those of HSCT from an HLA-identical sibling, as indicated by results of unrelated donor transplantation in children with acute lymphoblastic leukemia (ALL) in the second complete remission, juvenile myelomonocytic leukemia, or thalassemia.

The outcome of unrelated donor transplants is poorer for patients with other disorders such as Fanconi anemia, mainly because of a high incidence of transplant-related complications.

Umbilical cord blood transplants: UCB transplantation is an option for children who require allogeneic HSCT. Despite the low incidence of acute and chronic GVHD, the risk of recurrence of leukemia is not increased after UCB transplantation. The long-term results of UCB transplants are similar to those after transplantation from other sources of hematopoietic stem cells. Results are particularly promising with acute myeloid leukemia transplanted with cord blood cells from an unrelated donor and in children with hemoglobinopathies given a related UCB transplantation.

Box 10.1: Indications to autologous hematopoietic stem cell transplantation for pediatric diseases

Acute myeloid leukemia in 1st and 2nd complete remission

Acute lymphoblastic leukemia after an isolated extra-medullary relapse

Relapsed Hodgkin's or non-Hodgkin's lymphoma

Stage IV neuroblastoma

Stage IV rhabdomyoblastoma

High-risk relapsed or resistant brain tumors

Stage IV Ewing's sarcoma

Life-threatening autoimmune diseases resistant to conventional treatments

---

Haploidentical transplants: Haploidentical transplantation offers an immediate source of hematopoietic stem cells to almost all leukemia patients who fail to find a matched donor, whether related or unrelated, or a suitable cord blood unit. Nearly all of these children have at least one haploidentical, three loci mismatched family member who is promptly available as donor. A few patients who reject the haploidentical transplant have the advantage of another immediately available donor within the family circle.

Donor vs recipient NK cell alloreactivity: Donor vs recipient natural killer (NK) cell alloreactivity is a biologic phenomenon that is unique to the mismatched transplant. Transplantation from NK-alloreactive haploidentical donors controls acute myeloid leukemia (AML) relapse and improve engraftment without causing GVHD.

Graft-Versus-Host Disease (GVHD) and Rejection

The major cause of mortality and morbidity after allogeneic hematopoietic stem cell transplantation (HSCT) is GVHD, which is caused by engraftment of immunocompetent donor lymphocytes in an immunologically compromised host with histocompatibility differences between the graft and the host that result in donor T cell activation against host major histocompatibility complex (MHC) antigen. GVHD is classified as acute GVHD, which occurs within 3 mo of transplantation and chronic GVHD, which, though related, is a different disease.

Acute GVHD: Acute GVHD usually develops from 2–5 wk post-transplantation. The primary manifestations are an erythematous maculopapular rash, persistent anorexia, vomiting and/or diarrhea, and liver disease with increased serum levels of bilirubin, alanine aminotransferase, aspartate aminotransferase, and alkaline phosphatase. Diagnosis may require skin, liver, or endoscopic biopsy for confirmation. Endothelial damage and lymphocytic infiltrates are seen in all affected organs. The epidermis and hair follicles of the skin are damaged, the hepatic small bile ducts show segmental disruption, and there is destruction of the crypts and mucosal ulceration of the gastrointestinal tract. Grade I acute GVHD (skin rash alone) has a favorable prognosis and often no treatment is required. Grade II GVHD is a moderately severe multiorgan disease requiring therapy, Grade III GVHD is a severe multiorgan disease, and Grade IV GVHD is a life-threatening, often fatal condition. The standard prophylaxis of GVHD is the post-transplant administration of immunosuppressive drugs such as cyclosporin or tacrolimus or combinations of either with methotrexate or prednisolone, anti-T cell antibodies, mycophenolate mofetil, and other immunosuppressive agents. An alternative approach is the attempt to remove T lymphocytes from the graft (T cell depletion). Any form of GVHD prophylaxis in itself may impair post-transplant immunologic reconstitution, increasing the risk of infection-related deaths. Despite prophylaxis, significant acute GVHD develops in ~30% of recipients of HSCT from matched siblings and about 60% of HSCT recipients from unrelated donors. The risk of acute GVHD is increased in older donor and recipient ages, in patients given an unmanipulated allograft, in patients with the diagnosis of malignant disease, and GVHD prophylaxis with only one drug. Acute GVHD is usually treated with glucocorticoids, antithymocyte globulin, extracorporeal photopheresis, or monoclonal antibodies targeting molecules expressed on T cells, cytokines during the inflammatory cascade, which underlies the physiopathology of GVHD.

Chronic GVHD: Chronic GVHD develops or persists > 3 mo of post-transplantation and is the most frequent late complication of allogeneic HSCT with an incidence of ~25% in pediatric patients. Chronic GVHD is the major cause of nonrelapse mortality and morbidity in long-term HSCT survivors. Chronic GVHD is a disorder of immune regulation characterized by autoantibody production, increased collagen deposition and fibrosis, and clinical symptoms similar to those seen in patients with autoimmune diseases. The ongoing immune reactivity results in clinical features resembling a systemic autoimmune disease with lichenoid and sclerodermatous skin lesions, malar rash, sicca syndrome, arthritis, joint contractures, obliterative bronchiolitis, and bile duct degeneration with cholestasis.

Patients with chronic GVHD involving only the skin and liver have a favorable course. Extensive multi-organ disease may be associated with recurrent infections associated with prolonged immuno-suppressive regimens to control GVHD, and a high mortality rate. Morbidity and mortality are highest in patients with a progressive onset of chronic GVHD that follows acute GVHD, intermediate in those with a quiescent onset after resolution of acute GVHD, and lowest in patients with de novo onset in the absence of acute GVHD. Prednisolone or cyclosporin is the standard treatment, although other agents, including thalidomide and extracorporeal photopheresis, have been employed with variable success. Patients with chronic GVHD are particularly susceptible to infections, and should receive appropriate antibiotic prophylaxis, including trimethoprim-sulfamethoxazole. Chronic GVHD resolves in most patients without recurrence of disease, but may require 1–3 yr of immunosuppressive therapy.

Graft failure: Graft failure is a serious complication exposing patients to a high risk of fatal infection. *Primary graft failure* is defined as failure to achieve a neutrophil count of $0.2 \times 10^9/L$ by 21 days post-transplant. *Secondary graft failure* is loss of peripheral blood counts following initial transient engraftment of donor cells. Causes of graft failure after autologous and allogeneic transplantation include transplant of an inadequate stem cell dose, and viral infections such as with cytomegalovirus (CMV) or human herpesvirus type 6 (HHV6), which are often associated with activation of recipient macrophages. Graft failure after allogeneic transplantation is mainly caused by immunologically mediated rejection of the graft by residual recipient-type T cells that survive the conditioning regimen. *Diagnosis* of graft failure resulting from immunologic mechanisms is based on examination of peripheral blood and marrow aspirate and biopsy, along with molecular analysis of chimerism status. Persistence of lymphocytes of host origin in allogeneic transplant recipients with graft failure indicates immunologic rejection. *Treatment* of graft failure usually requires removing all potentially myelotoxic agents from the treatment regimen and administration of a short trial of hematopoietic growth factors, such as G-CSF. Graft failure due to relapse is managed by either donor lymphocytic infusions (DLI) or cytoreductive chemotherapy followed by DLI and/or a second myeloablative regimen and transplant. When caused by rejection, it is treated with a second myeloablative regimen and transplant. Standard preparative regimens are generally poorly tolerated if started within 100 days of a 1st transplant because of cumulative toxicities. Regimens containing anti-CD3 antibodies along with high-dose corticosteroids have been successful in achieving engraftment in > 50% of patients.

Infectious Complications of HSCT

Hematopoietic stem cell transplantation (HSCT) recipients experience a transient but profound state of immune deficiency. Immediately after transplantation, because neutrophils are absent, patients are particularly susceptible to bacterial and fungal infections. Despite prophylactic use of antibiotics or antifungal treatment during the conditioning regimen, most patients develop fever and signs of infection in the early post-transplant period. The common pathogens include enteric bacteria, and fungi such as *Candida* and *Aspergillus*. An indwelling central venous line in all children given HSCT, is a significant risk factor for bacterial (particularly staphylococcal species) and fungal (particularly *Candida*) infections. HSCT recipients remain at increased risk of developing severe infections even after the neutrophil count has normalized because T cell number and function remain below normal for months after transplantation. Aspergillus (causing invasive aspergillosis), cytomegalovirus (CMV) and Epstein-Barr virus (EBV) remain the most common and potentially severe infections encountered in HSCT recipients.

Late Effects of HSCT

Many children given hematopoietic stem cell transplantation (HSCT) become long term survivors. Besides chronic graft-vs-host disease (GVHD), long-term complications include impaired growth, neuroendocrine dysfunction, delayed puberty, infertility, second malignancies, cataracts and other ocular complications, leukoencephalopathy, and cardiac and pulmonary dysfunction. Children given HSCT before puberty may develop *growth impairment*, precluding achievement of the genetic target for adult height, and is frequent in patients given total body irradiation (TBI) as part of the preparative regimen. The use of craniospinal radiotherapy before transplantation plays a synergistic detrimental role with TBI in favoring growth impairment. Growth impairment of patients given TBI is mainly due to direct damage of cartilage plates and the effect of TBI on the hypothalamic-pituitary axis, which leads to an inappropriately low production of growth hormone (GH). GH deficiency is susceptible to at least partial correction through administration of hormonal replacement therapy. Annual growth evaluation should be performed in all children after HSCT.

The use of TBI during preparative regimen that involves the thyroid gland in the irradiation field may result in *hypothyroidism*. Children < 7 yr at the time of allograft are at greater risk of developing hypothyroidism. Therapy with thyroxine is very effective for overt hypothyroidism, but treatment of compensated hypothyroidism is more controversial, although there is evidence that hormonal replacement therapy may reduce the risk of thyroid carcinoma through a suppression of thyroid-stimulating hormone (TSH). Despite treatment of hypothyroidism, the incidence of thyroid carcinoma is not negligible.

Gonadal hormones are essential for normal pubertal growth as well as for development of secondary sexual characteristics. A significant proportion of patients receiving TBI-containing regimens show *delayed development of secondary sexual characteristics*, resulting from primary ovarian or testicular failure. Laboratory evaluation of these patients reveals elevated follicle-stimulating hormone (FSH) and luteinizing hormone (LH) levels with depressed estradiol and testosterone. Supplementation of gonadal hormones is useful for primary gonadal failure and is administered with growth hormone to promote pubertal growth.

The overall risk of developing a *secondary form of cancer* is significantly higher after HSCT than in general population. Several types of secondary tumors have been identified; most frequently are brain tumors, epithelial cancers, and thyroid carcinoma. Young age, male gender, use of TBI during the preparative regimen, chronic GVHD, and an intrinsic genetic predisposition to develop cancer (Fanconi anemia) have been reported to be risk factors for development of secondary malignancies after HSCT.

Cataracts mainly occur in children given a radiotherapy-based on preparative regimen, which is particularly high if TBI is delivered as a single fraction (800–1,000 cGy) and is markedly reduced (~10–20% patients) if given as fractionated TBI. Corticosteroids, frequently employed for treating GVHD, have also been demonstrated to promote development of cataracts. A dry eye syndrome, or keratoconjunctivitis sicca, may also affect HSCT recipients. It is often related to chronic GVHD and postradiotherapy fibrosis of lacrimal gland, and is treated with artificial tears and lubricants.

Blume KG, Forman SJ, Appelbaum FR (eds). *Hematopoietic Cell Transplantation*. 3 rd edn. Blackwell, 2004.

Damodar Sharat. Pediatric Aplastic Anemia—Bone Marrow Transplantation. In: Mathur GP, Mathur Sarla (eds). *Current Trends in Pediatrics*. Vol 3. Delhi: Academa Publishers, 2007; 28–38.

Ferrara JLM, Cooke KR, Deeg J (eds). *Graft-vs-Host Disease*. 3rd edn. Marcel Dekker, 2004.

Steward CG, Jarish A. Haemopoietic stem cell transplantation for genetic disorders. *Arch Dis Child* 2005;90:1259–63.

Velardi A, Locatelli F. Hematopoietic stem cell transplantation. In: Kliegman RM, Behrman RE, Jenson HB, Stanton BF (eds). *Nelson Textbook of Pediatrics*. 18th edn. Vol 1. Philadelphia: Saunders, 2007;924–34.

11 Allergic Disorders

11.1 ALLERGY

The term allergy was first coined in 1906 by von Pirquet, who used it to refer to patients who expressed an "altered state of reactivity" to common environmental allergens. Atopy is derived from the Greek *atopos,* meaning "out of place" and often used to describe patients with IgE-mediated diseases. The increase in allergic disease prevalence is attributed to environmental factors. Children spend the majority of their time in indoor environments, including the home. Examination of indoor environments suggests that house dust mite, cat, dog, and cockroach allergens are the most common significant triggers of allergic disease in these settings; exposures to allergens from other pets, pests, fungi, and respiratory irritants such as cigarette smoke can also be a problem. Control of these environmental measures is necessary in the management of allergic disorders. Allergic diseases arise from the acute or chronic exposure of a sensitized individual to a specific allergen by inhalation, ingestion, contact, or injection. Symptoms most often involve the nose, eyes, lungs, skin, or gastrointestinal tract either individually or in combination. The basic principles of the treatment of allergic disease include the avoidance of exposure to allergens and irritants that trigger symptoms and the pharmacological management of symptoms caused by inadvertent allergen exposures and allergen immunotherapy in selected patients. Pharmacologic therapy include adrenergic agents (salbutamol, albuterol, salmeterol and formoterol); anticholinergic agents (ipratropium bromide); antihistamines; chromones (cromolyn sodium and nedocromil sodium); glucocorticoids; leukotriene-modifying agents; theophylline; monoclonal anti-IgE antibodies (anti-IgE). Histamine exerts its effects through binding with one of its three receptors, referred to as H_1-, H_2-, or H_3-receptors. First generation antihistamines include antazoline, pyrilamine, tripelennamine, carminoxamine, clemastine, diphenhydramine, brompheneramine, chlorpheneramine, triprolidine, cyclizine, hydroxizine, meclizine,

Table 11.1: Classification of antihistamines (H_1-antagonists)

Cetirizine: 0.2 mg/kg once a day PO. Non sedating, long acting

Clemastine: 1–3 yr: 0.25–0.5 mg BD, 3–6 yr: 0.5 mg BD

Chlorpheniramine maleate: Children 0.35 mg/kg/day q 4–6 hr. *Adverse events:* hypotension, sedation, urinary retention, oculogyric spasms

Cyproheptadine hydrochloride: 0.25 mg/kg/day q 8 hr PO. *Adverse events:* Same as in chlorpheniramine

Diphenhydramine hydrochloride: 5 mg/kg/day q 6 hr (max 300 mg/24 hr) PO.

Fexofenadine: 30 mg bid for children < 12 yr and 60 mg bid or 120 mg OD > 12 yr children

Hydroxizine hydrochloride: 2 mg/kg/day q 6 hr PO; 0.5–1 mg/kg/dose q 4–6 hr IM

Loratadine: > 3 yr up to 30 mg/kg 5 mg/day PO; 12 yr 10 mg once a day PO

Methdilazine hydrochloride: > 3 yr 4 mg q 6–12 hr PO
Pheniramine maleate (Avil): 0.5 mg/kg/day 8 hourly PO, IM, IV. *Adverse events:* same as in chlorpheniramine
Promethazine (Phenargan): 0.1 mg/kg/day q 6–8 hr or 0.5 mg/kg/dose PO HS

azatadine, cyproheptadine, methdilazine, promethazine. Second generation antihistaminies include acrivastine, cetirizine, fexofenadine, loratadine (Table 11.1). First generation antihistamines are associated with sedative effects and cognitive impairment, but second generation antihistamines are nonsedating or much less so than first generation antihistamines.

Atkins D, Leung DYM. Principles of treatment of allergic diseases. In: Kliegman RM, Behrman RE, Jenson HB, Stanton BF (eds). Nelson Textbook of Pediatrics. 18th edn. Vol. 1. Philadelphia: Saunders, 2007;942–49.

Leung DYM. Allergy and the immunologic basis of atopic disease. In: Kliegman RM, Behrman RE, Jenson HB, Stanton BF (eds). *Nelson Textbook of Pediatrics*. 18th edn. Vol. 1. Philadelphia: Saunders, 2007;935–8.

11.2 ALLERGIC RHINITIS

Two perquisites for the expression of allergic rhinitis (AR) are sensitivity to an allergen and its presence in the environment. AR is currently classified as *seasonal or perennial*. Inhalant allergens are the main cause of AR. *Seasonal* (intermittent) *AR (SAR)* follows a well defined course of cyclical exacerbation, while *perennial* (persistent) *AR (PAR)* causes year round symptoms. Approximately 20% are strictly seasonal, 40% perennial, and 40% mixed (perennial with seasonal exacerbations).

Clinical manifestations: AR is an inflammatory disorder of the nasal mucosa characterized by nasal congestion, rhinorrhea, and itching and often accompanied by sneezing and conjunctival irritation. Nasal itching brings on grimacing, twitching, and picking at the nose that may result in epistaxis. Children with AR often perform the *allergic salute*, an upward rubbing of the nose with an open palm or extended index finger. This maneuver relieves itching and briefly unblocks the airway. It also gives rise to the nasal crease, a horizontal skin crease over the bridge of the nose. Patients may have headaches, wheezing, and coughing, and may loose their sense of smell and taste. Nasal congestion is usually more severe at night, causing mouth-breathing and snoring, which interferes with sleep and arousing irritability.

Signs of physical examination include: Abnormalities of facial development; dental malocclusion; *allergic gape*, which is continuous open mouth breathing; chapped lips; *allergic shiners*, which are dark circles under the eyes; and the nasal crease. Conjunctival edema, itching, tearing, and hyperemia are frequent findings. Nasal examination may reveal clear nasal secretions; edematous, boggy, and bluish mucous membranes with little or no erythema, and swollen turbinates that may block the nasal airway. Thick, purulent nasal secretions indicate the presence of infection. Sinusitis, conjunctivitis, otitis media, serous otitis, and eczema are often associated in children with AR. AR is frequently associated with co-morbid conditions: chronic sinusitis is a common complication of AR, with an inflammatory process that is characterized by marked eosinophilia, mucosal thickening, and nasal polyposis. Allergens, possibly fungal, may be the inciting agent. The sinusitis of *triad asthma* (asthma, sinusitis with nasal polyposis, and aspirin sensitivity) often shows poor response to therapy. AR is a risk factor for asthma and often precedes it.

Diagnosis: The diagnosis of AR is based on recurrent symptoms of sneezing, rhinorrhea, nasal itching, and congestion that occur most often in the absence of an upper respiratory tract infection or structural abnormalities. The diagnosis is supported by laboratory findings of elevated IgE, specific IgE antibodies, blood eosinophilia, and positive allergy skin tests. Evaluation of AR includes a thorough history including details of the patient's environment and diet; family history of allergic conditions such as AR, eczema, and asthma; risk factors include family history of atopy and IgE > 100 IU/ml before 6 yr of age; physical examination and laboratory investigations.

Differential diagnosis: SAR differs from PAR by the time of occurrence and skin test results. Allergic rhinitis is seasonal, perennial or perennial with seasonal exacerbation. Nonallergic rhinitides cause sporadic symptoms that may resemble PAR. Nonallergic inflammation rhinitis with eosinophils (NARES) imitates AR in presentation and response to treatment but the patients do not have elevated IgE antibodies.

Treatment: The removal and avoidance of offending allergen is advised. The only effective measure for avoiding animal allergens in the home is the removal of the pet. Sealing the mattress, pillows, and covers in allergen-proof encasings reduces the exposure to mite allergens. Bed linens and blankets should be washed every week in hot water (> 103°F). Avoidance of pollens and outdoor molds can be accomplished by staying in a controlled environment. Air-conditioning allows for keeping windows and doors closed lowering the pollen exposure.

Oral antihistamines (Table 11.1) are administered as needed in patients with mild, intermittent symptoms of sneezing and rhinorrhea. Four oral antihistaminics are approved for children: cetirizine and desloratadine for > 6 mo of age, loratadine for > 2 yr of age, and fexofenadine for > 6 yr of age. Azelastine is a topically active antihistamine that is available as a nasal spray for children > 5 yr of age. The anticholinergic nasal spray ipratropium bromide may be used for serous rhinorrhea. Intranasal decongestants should be used for < 3–5 days, not to be repeated > 1 cycle a month. Sodium cromoglycate is effective but requires frequent administration.

Patients with more persistent, severe symptoms require intranasal corticosteroids which are the most effective therapy for AR. These agents reduce all symptoms of AR caused by eosinophilic inflammation, but not of rhinitis associated with neutrophils or free of inflammation. Mometasone, fluticasone, and budesonide offer greater topical activity with lower systemic exposure and a better safety profile. Mometasone is approved for children > 2 yr of age, fluticasone for > 4 yr of age, and budesonide for > 6 yr of age. More severely affected patients may benefit from combination treatment with antihistamines, intranasal corticosteroids, and other medications such as ipratropium bromide, azelastine, cromolyn sodium, oxymetazoline, and phenylephrine.

Specific allergen immunotherapy should be considered for children in whom IgE-mediated allergic manifestations cannot be adequately controlled by symptomatic treatment, especially in the presence of co-morbid conditions. Allergen immunotherapy interferes with IgE production and allergen-induced symptoms and is effective in the treatment of AR.

Prognosis: Treatment with antihistamines and intranasal corticosteroids significantly improves health-related quality of life measures in patients of all ages, as long as they continue to take their medication.

Milgrom H, Leung DYM. Allergic rhinitis. In: Kliegman RM, Behrman RE, Jenson HB, Stanton BF (eds). *Nelson Textbook of Pediatrics.* 18th edn. Vol. 1. Philadelphia: Saunders, 2007; 949–52.

Plaut M, Valentine MD. Allergic rhinitis. *N Engl J Med* 2005; 353:1934–44.

Sly RM. Epidemiology of allergic rhinitis. *Clin Rev Allergy Immunol* 2002;22:67–103.

11.3 CHILDHOOD ASTHMA

Asthma is a chronic inflammatory condition of the lung airways resulting in episodic airflow obstruction. A combination of environmental and genetic factors in early life shape how the immune system develops and responds to ubiquitous environmental exposures.

Genetics: More than 22 loci on 15 autosomal chromosomes have been linked to asthma. Asthma has been consistently linked with loci containing pro-allergic, proinflammatory genes [the interleukin (IL)-4 gene cluster on chromosome 5].

Environment: Recurrent wheezing episodes in early childhood are associated with common respiratory viruses, including respiratory syncytial virus, rhinovirus, influenza virus, parainfluenza virus, adenovirus, and human metapneumovirus. Injurious viral infections of the airways manifesting as pneumonia or bronchiolitis requiring hospitalization are risk factors for persistent asthma in childhood. Indoor and home allergen exposures in sensitized individuals can initiate airways inflammation and hypersensitivity to other irritant exposures, and are strongly linked to disease severity and persistence. Environmental tobacco smoke (ETS) and air pollutants (ozone, sulfur dioxide) aggravate airways inflammation and increase asthma severity. Cold dry air and strong odors can trigger bronchoconstriction when airways are irritated, but do not worsen airways inflammation or airways hyper-responsiveness (AHR).

Persistent asthma: Approximately 80% of all asthmatics report disease onset prior to 6 yr of age. Of all young children who experience recurrent wheezing, only a minority will suffer from persistent asthma in later childhood. Early childhood risk factors for persistent asthma have been identified and are listed in Box 11.1.

A modified Asthma Predictive Index (Table 11.2) optimizes risk factor assessments of young children to predict the risk for persistent asthma in later childhood. Allergy in young children is a major risk factor for the persistence of childhood asthma. Through a statistically optimized model for pre-school age children with frequent wheezing in the past year, one major criterion or two minor criteria provide a high specificity (97%) and positive predictive value

Box 11.1: Early childhood risk factors for persistent asthma

Parental asthma

Allergy

   Atopic dermatitis

   Allergic rhinitis

   Food allergy

   Inhalant allergen sensitization

Severe lower respiratory tract infection

   Pneumonia

   Bronchiolitis requiring hospitalization

Wheezing apart from cold

Male gender

Low birth weight

Environmental tobacco smoke exposure

Table 11.2: Asthma predictive index for children	
Major criteria	*Minor criteria*
Parent asthma	Allergic rhinitis
Eczema	Wheezing apart from cold
Inhalant allergen sensitization	Eosinophils ≥ 4%
	Food allergen sensitization

Source: Modified from Castro-Rodriguez JA, Holberg CH, Wright AL, et al. A clinical index to define risk of asthma in young children with recurrent wheezing. *Am J Respir Crit Care* 2000;162:1403–06; and Guilbert TW, Morgan WJ, Zeirger RS, et al. Atopic characteristics of children with recurrent wheezing at high risk for the development of childhood asthma. *J Allergy Clin Immunol* 2004;114:1282–87

(77%) for persistent asthma in later childhood (Tucson Children's Respiratory study, Tucson AZ).

Types of childhood asthma: There are two main types of childhood asthma: (i) *recurrent wheezing* in early childhood, primarily triggered by common viral infections of the respiratory tract; and (ii) *chronic asthma* associated with allergy that persists into later childhood and often adulthood. A 3rd type of childhood asthma typically emerges in females who develop obesity and early onset puberty (by 11 yr of age). *Triad asthma*—asthma associated with hyperplastic sinusitis/nasal polyposis and hypersensitivity to aspirin and nonsteroidal anti-inflammatory medications (ibuprofen), rarely has its onset in childhood. The most common persistent form of childhood asthma is that associated with allergy.

Pathogenesis: Airflow obstruction in asthma is the result of numerous pathological processes. In the small airways, airflow is regulated by smooth muscles encircling the airways lumens; bronchoconstriction of these bronchiolar muscular bands restricts or blocks airflow. A cellular inflammatory infiltrate and exudates contains eosinophils and also other inflammatory cell types (neutrophils, monocytes, lymphocytes, mast cells, and basophils), can fill and obstruct the airways and induce epithelial damage and desquamation into the airways lumen. Helper T lymphocytes and other immune cells that produce pro-allergic, proinflammatory cytokines (IL-4, IL-5, IL-13) and chemokines mediate this inflammatory process. Pathogenic immune responses and inflammation may also result from a breach in normal immune regulatory processes [regulatory T lymphocytes that produce IL-10 and transforming growth factor (TGF)-β] that dampen effector immunity and inflammation when they are no longer needed. Airways inflammation is linked to airways hyper-responsiveness (AHR) or hypersensitivity of airways smooth muscle to

Box 11.2: Asthma triggers
Common viral infections of the respiratory tract
Aeroallergens in sensitized asthmatics
   Animal dander
   Indoor allergens
   Dust mites
   Cockroaches
   Molds
   Seasonal aeroallergens
   Pollens (trees, grasses, weeds)
   Seasonal molds
Environmental tobacco smoke
Air pollutants
   Ozone
   Sulfur dioxide
   Particulate matter
   Wood- or coal-burning smoke
   Endotoxin, mycotoxins
   Dust
Strong or noxious odors or fumes
   Perfumes, hairsprays
   Cleaning agents
Occupational exposures
   Farm and barn exposures
   Formaldehydes, cedar, paint fumes
Cold air, dry air
Exercise
Crying, laughter, hyperventilation
Co-morbid conditions
   Rhinitis
   Sinusitis
   Gastroesophageal reflux

numerous provocative exposures that act as asthma triggers (Box 11.2).

Clinical manifestations and diagnosis: Intermittent dry coughing and/or respiratory wheezing are the most common chronic symptoms of asthma. Older children and adults also complain of shortness of breath and chest tightness; younger children more commonly report intermittent, nonfocal chest pain. Respiratory symptoms can be worse at night, especially during prolonged exacerbations triggered by respiratory infections or inhalant allergens. Daytime symptoms often linked with physical activities or play. A history of symptomatic improvement with asthma medications (bronchodilators) supports the diagnosis of asthma. Lack of improvement with broncodilator and corticosteroid therapy is inconsistent with underlying asthma.

Asthma symptoms can be triggered by numerous events or exposures (Box 11.2). Exposures induce always inflammation include infections [respiratory viral infections (mentioned in etiology), *Mycoplasma pneumoniae, Chlamydia pneumoniae*] and inhaled allergens. Numerous occupational exposures incite asthma in some adults. Similarly, some children might be chronically exposed airways toxicants in their home or school environments, leading to "occupational" type asthma in children. An environmental history is essential for optimal asthma diagnosis and management. The presence of risk factors (Box 11.1) supports the diagnosis of asthma. During routine clinic visits, children with asthma commonly present without abnormal signs, which stresses the importance of the medical history in diagnosing asthma. Some may exhibit a dry, persistent cough. The chest examination is often normal. Deeper breaths can some time elicit otherwise undetectable wheezing. In clinic, quick resolution (within 10 min) or convincing improvement in symptoms and signs of asthma with administration of a short-acting inhaled beta-agonist is supportive of the diagnosis of asthma.

During asthma exacerbations, expiratory wheezing and a prolonged expiratory phase is appreciated by auscultation. Decreased breath sounds in some of the lung fields, commonly the right lower posterior lobe, are consistent with regional hypoventilation owing to airways obstruction. Crackles can sometimes be heard, resulting from excess mucus production and inflammatory exudates in the airways. In severe exacerbations, the greater extent of airways obstruction causes labored breathing and respiratory distress manifested as expiratory wheezing, increased prolongation of expiration, poor air entry, suprasternal and intercostals retractions, nasal flaring, and accessory respiratory muscle use. In extreme condition, the airflow may be so limited that wheezing cannot be heard.

Differential diagnosis: Many childhood respiratory conditions can present with symptoms and signs similar to asthma (*see* Chapters 18 and 29). Besides asthma other common causes of chronic, intermittent coughing include rhinosinusitis and gastroesophageal reflux (GER). In some localities, hypersensitivity pneumonitis (e.g. farming communities, homes of bird owners), pulmonary parasitic infestations (e.g. rural

---

Box 11.3: Lung function abnormalities in asthma

Spirometry

Airflow limitation

  Low FEV_1 (relative to percentage of predicted norms)

  FEV_1/FVC ratio < 0.8

Bronchodilator response (to inhaled β_2-agonist)

  Improvement in $FEV_1 \geq 12\%$*

Exercise challenge

  Worsening in $FEV_1 \geq 15\%$*

Peak flow morning-to-afternoon variation $\geq 20\%$*

*Main criteria consistent with asthma

FEV_1: forced expiratory volume in 1 sec; FVC: forced vital capacity

---

areas of developing countries), or tuberculosis may be common causes of chronic coughing and/or wheezing.

Laboratory findings: Lung function tests can help to confirm the diagnosis of asthma and determine disease severity.

Pulmonary function testing: Forced expiratory air flow measures are helpful in children with asthma. *Spirometry* is helpful as an objective measure of airflow limitation (Box 11.3). Valid spirometric measures are dependent on a patient's ability to perform properly a full, forceful, and prolonged expiratory maneuver, usually feasible in children > 6 yr of age (with some younger exceptions). Reproducible spirometric efforts are an indicator of test validity; if, on 3 attempts, the FEV_1 (forced expiratory volume in 1 sec) is within 5%, then the *highest* FEV_1 effort of the 3 is used. This standard utilization of the highest of 3 reproducible efforts is indicative of the effort-dependence of reliable spirometric testing. In asthma, airways blockage results in reduced airflow with forced exhalation and smaller partial-expiratory lung volumes. The comparative values of spirometric volume-time curves in a non-asthmatic and asthmatic child are mentioned in Table 11.3 (*see* Figs 11.1 to 11.3 in CD).

Peak expiratory flow (PEF) monitoring is performed by a peak flow meter. It is a simple and inexpensive home-use tool to measure airflow. Poor perceivers of airflow obstruction due to asthma can benefit by monitoring PEFs daily to assess objectively airflow as an indicator of asthma control or problems that would

---

Table 11.3: Comparative values of spirometric volume-time curves in a non-asthmatic and asthmatic child	
Child 1. A non-asthmatic child	*Child 2. An asthmatic child*
FEV_1 = 3.4 (100% of predicted)	FEV_1 = 2.1 (62% of predicted)
FVC = 3.8 (100% of predicted)	FVC = 3.8 (97% of predicted)
FEV_1/FVC = 0.86	FEV_1/FVC = 0.57

be more sensitive than their symptom perception. PEFs vary in their ability to detect airflow obstruction; in some patients, PEFs decline only when flow obstruction is severe. Therefore, PEF monitoring should be started by measuring morning and evening PEFs (best of 3 attempts) for several weeks for patients to practice the technique, to determine a "personal best," and to correlate PEF values with symptoms (and ideally spirometry). PEF variation $\geq 20\%$ is consistent with asthma (Box 11.3).

PEFs performed and recorded twice daily in the morning and evening daily over 1 mo in an asthmatic child. This child's "personal best" PEF is 220 L/min; therefore green zone (> 80–100% of best) is 175–220 L/min; yellow zone (50–80%) is 110–175 L/min; and red zone (< 50%) is less than 110 L/min. This child's (A) evening PEFs are almost always in the green zone, whereas his morning PEFs are often in the yellow or red zone. This illustrates the typical diurnal morning-to-evening variation of inadequately controlled asthma. Another child (B) PEFs performed twice daily, in the morning and evening, over 1 mo is an asthmatic child who developed a viral respiratory tract infection. This child's PEF values are initially in the green zone. A viral respiratory tract infection led to asthma worsening, with a decline in PEF to the yellow zone that continued to worsen until PEFs were in the red zone. At that point, a 4-day prednisolone course was administered, followed by improvement in PEF back to green zone.

Measuring of fractional exhaled nitric oxide (FENO), a marker of airway inflammation in asthma, can help titrate medications and confirm the diagnosis of asthma.

Radiology: Chest radiographs [posteroanterior (PA) and lateral views] in children with asthma often appear to be normal except subtle and nonspecific findings of hyperventilation (flattening of the diaphragm) and peribronchial thickening. Chest radiographs can identify asthma masqueraders (aspiration pneumonitis, hyperlucent lung fields in bronchiolitis obliterans), and complications during asthma exacerbations (atelectasis, pneumomediastinum, pneumothorax). Some lung abnormalities can be better appreciated with high-resolution, thin-section chest CT scans. Bronchiectasis is clearly seen on CT scan.

Treatment: The goals of childhood asthma management for children are mentioned in Box 11.4. There are four components of optimal asthma management (Box 11.5).

Regular assessment and monitoring: Asthma management should include regular clinic visits every 2–4 wk until good asthma control is achieved. Two to four regular annual asthma check-ups are recomm-

---

Box 11.4: Goals of childhood asthma management

Maintain normal activity
   Regular school or daycare attendance
   Full participation in physical exercise, athletics, and other recreational activities
Prevent sleep disturbance
Prevent chronic asthma symptoms
Keep asthma exacerbations from becoming severe
Maintain normal lung function
Experience little to no adverse effects of treatment

Box 11.5: Four components of optimal asthma treatment

1. Regular assessment and monitoring
Asthma check-ups
   Every 2–4 wk until good control is achieved
   2–4 per yr to maintain good control
Lung function monitoring
2. Control of factors contributing to asthma severity
Eliminate or reduce problematic environmental exposures
Treat co-morbid conditions: rhinitis, sinusitis, gastro-esophageal reflux
3. Asthma pharmacotherapy
Long-term control versus quick-relief medications
Classification of asthma severity from anti-inflammatory pharmacotherapy
Step-up, step-down approach
Asthma exacerbation management
4. Patient education
Provide a two-part care plan
   Daily management
   Action plan for asthma exacerbations

---

ended to maintain good asthma control. During these visits, asthma control can be assessed by asking about:
1. The frequency of asthma symptoms during the day and night, and with physical exercise
2. The frequency of "rescue" short-acting α-agonist medication use
3. The number and severity of asthma exacerbations since the last visit; and
4. Participation in school, sports, and other preferred activities.

Spirometry is recommended annually and more often if asthma is inadequately controlled. PEF monitoring (Box 11.3) at home can be especially helpful when assessing asthmatic children with poor symptom perception, other causes of chronic coughing in addition to asthma, moderate-to-severe asthma, or a history of severe asthma exacerbations.

Control of factors contributing to asthma severity: Controllable factors that can significantly worsen asthma generally grouped as (i) external exposure and (ii) co-morbid conditions (Box 11.6).

Eliminate or reduce problematic environmental exposures: Eliminating or minimizing environmental exposures (Box 11.6), can reduce the asthma symptoms, disease severity, and the amount of medication needed to achieve good asthma control. Common viral infections of the respiratory tract are difficult to avoid. Annual influenza vaccination is recommended for all asthmatic children (except for those with egg allergy).

Treat co-morbid conditions: Rhinitis, sinusitis, and gastroesophageal reflux (GER) commonly accompany asthma and can worsen disease severity (Box 11.6). These conditions are also common causes of chronic coughing. Effective management of these co-morbid conditions can often improve asthma symptoms and disease severity, so that less medication is needed to achieve good asthma control.

Asthma pharmacotherapy: The National Asthma Education and Prevention Program (NAEPP) guidelines classify asthma in four disease severity groups (mild intermittent, mild persistent, moderate persistent, and severe persistent asthma). The classification of asthma severity is based on the following four parameters:
1. Frequency of daytime or

Box 11.6: Control of factors contributing to asthma severity

Eliminate or reduce problematic environmental exposures

Environmental tobacco smoke elimination or reduction in home and automobiles

Allergen exposure elimination or reduction in sensitized asthmatics
  Animal danders
  Pets (dogs, cats, rodents, birds)
  Pests (mice, rats)
  Dust mites
  Cockroaches
  Molds
Other airway irritants
  Wood- or coal-burning smoke
  Strong chemical odors and perfumes (e.g. house-hold cleaners)
  Dusts
Treat co-morbid conditions
Rhinitis
Sinusitis
Gastroesophageal reflux
Get annual influenza vaccination (unless egg-allergic)

---

2. Night-time symptoms
3. Degree of airflow obstruction by spirometry and/or
4. PEF (peak expiratory flow) variability (Tables 11.4 to 11.6).

In case of younger children (<5 yr of age), management is primarily based on symptoms since young children cannot perform the maneuvers required for conventional lung function measurements. The objective of this approach is to identify and treat all "persistent" asthma with anti-inflammatory controller medication. Inhaled corticosteroids (ICSs) therapy is recommended as preferred therapy for all levels of asthma severity except for the mild intermittent category. Leukotriene pathway modifiers or sustained-release theophylline (only for patients > 5 yr of age) are considered alternative controllers for mild persistent asthmatics. Combination therapy of a low-to-medium dose ICS with a long-acting β-agonist (LABA) or a leukotriene modifier or theophylline is a mainstay therapy for moderate persistent asthma in older children and adults. While the use of medium-dose ICS alone is an alternative therapy for older children and adults with moderate persistent severity, for infants and young children, it is considered a preferred treatment for moderate persistent asthma. Severe persistent asthmatics should receive high-dose ICSs, a long-acting bronchodilator, and routine oral corticosteroids if needed. Daily controller therapy is not recommended for mild intermittent asthma. Short-acting β-agonists (SABAs) are the recommended quick-reliever medications for all asthma severity levels. They are to be used as needed for acute symptoms.

"Step-Up, Step-Down" Approach. The NAEPP guidelines online a stepwise approach to asthma therapy that emphasizes initiating higher-level controller therapy at the outset to establish prompt control, with measures to "step-down" therapy once good asthma control is achieved (Tables 11.5 and 11.6).

Inhalation medications: Various inhalation medications are delivered as an aerosolized form in a metered-dose inhaler (MDI), as a dry powder inhaler (DPI) formulation, or in a suspension or solution form delivered via a nebulizer (Table 11.6). Mouth rinsing is recommended after inhaled corticosteroid (ICS) use to rinse out ICS deposited on the oral mucosa and reduce the swallowed ICS and the risk of thrush. Nebulizers have been the mainstay of aerosol treatment for infants and young children (*see* Fig. 11.4 in CD).

The most commonly encountered adverse effects from inhaled corticosteroids (ICSs) are local: oral candidiasis (thrush) and dysphonia (hoarse voice).

Table 11.4: Stepwise approach for managing asthma severity classification and management*						
Asthma severity	Days with symptoms	Nights with symptoms	Lung function	Long-term-control medication	Quick-relief medication	Education
Step 1: *Mild intermittent*	< 3 per wk	< 3 per mo	FEV_1 or PEF $\geq 80\%$ Predicted; PEF variability < 20%	No daily medication is needed	**Short-acting β-agonist** as needed and before exercise; Use ≥ 3 times per wk may indicate need to initiate long-term-control therapy	Asthma facts, MDI and spacer technique
Step 2: *Mild persistent*	< 3 per wk	3–4 per mo	FEV_1 or PEF $\geq 80\%$ Predicted; PEF variability 20–30%	**Anti-inflammatory:** Either low dose **inhaled glucocorticoid, cromolyn, nedocromil, or leukotriene modifier.** Sustained release theophylline is an alternative	**Short-acting β-agonist** as needed and before exercise; daily use or increasing use may indicate need for additional long-term-control therapy	Step 1 actions plus: Self-monitoring, group education, review and update self-management plan
Step 3: *Moderate persistent*	Daily symptoms, daily use of short-acting β-agonists	> 1 time per wk	FEV_1 or PEF > 60% and $\leq 80\%$ Predicted; PEF variability > 30%	**Anti-inflammatory: inhaled glucocorticoid**	**Short-acting β-agonist** as needed and before exercise; daily use or increasing use may indicate need for additional long-term-control therapy	Step 1 actions plus: Self-monitoring, group education, review and update self-management plan
Step 4: *Severe persistent*	Continual symptoms, limited physical activity, frequent exacerbations	Frequent	FEV_1 or PEF $\leq 60\%$ Predicted; PEF variability > 30%	**Anti-inflammatory: inhaled glucocorticoid**	**Short-acting β-agonist** as needed and before exercise; daily use or increasing use may indicate need for additional long-term-control therapy	Step 2 and 3 actions plus: Referral for individual education/counseling

*Based on clinical features before treatment; classifications is determined by the patient's most severe feature; bold prints indicates preferred medication; asthma patients with "persistent" disease of any severity should be treated with a "long-term-control" anti-inflammatory medication.

Source: Modified from the National Asthma Education and Prevention Program: Expert Panel Report II: Guidelines for the Diagnosis and Management of Asthma. Bethesda, MD, National Institutes of Health, National Heart, Lung, and Blood Institute, 1997. From Liu AH, Spahn JD, Leung DYM. Childhood asthma. In: Behrman RE, Kliegman RM, Jenson HB (eds). *Nelson Textbook of Pediatrics.* 17th edn. Philadelphia: Saunders, 2004;760–74.

Table 11.5: Asthma medications by category

Category	Examples of medications

Quick-relief medications ("relievers")	Short-acting inhaled β-agonists (SABAs):
	  Albuterol/Salbutamol
	    Levalbuterol
	    Terbutaline
	    Pirbuterol
	    Metaproterenol
	Inhaled anticholinergics:
	  Ipratropium
	  Atropine
	Short-course systemic glucocorticoids:
	  Prednisone
	  Prednisolone
	  Methylprednisolone
	  Methylprednisolone sodium succinate

Long-term-control medications ("controllers")	Nonsteroidal anti-inflammatory agents:
	  Cromolyn
	  Nedocromil
	Inhaled corticosteroids
	  Beclomethasone
	  Flunisolide
	  Budesonide
	  Fluticasone
	  Triamcenalone
	  Mometasone
	Sustained-release theophylline
	Long-acting inhaled β-agonists:
	  Salmeterol
	  Formoterol
	Leukotriene modifiers
	  Montelukast
	  Zafirlukast
	  Zileuton
	Oral corticosteroids
	  Prednisolone/Prednisone
	  Methylprednisolone

Thrush results from propellant-induced mucosal irritation and local immunosuppression. Dysphonia occurs from vocal cord myopathy. These effects are dose-dependent and are most common in individuals on high-dose ICS and/or oral corticosteroid therapy. The incidence of these local effects can be greatly minimized by using a spacer with MDI ICS because spacers reduce oropharyngeal deposition of the drug and propellant (*see* Figs 11.5 to 11.8 in CD).

Combination pharmacotherapy: Most children will have their asthma well controlled on a single controller medication. In children who continue to be symptomatic on low to moderate doses of inhaled glucocorticoid therapy: a superior outcome when a long-acting β-agonist or leukotriene pathway modifier is added to the original dose of inhaled glucocorticoids rather than doubling the dose of inhaled glucocorticoid. Thus, lung function and asthma control can be optimized without increasing the potential for systemic effects from inhaled glucocorticoids.

Adherence: Asthma is a chronic condition that is often best managed with daily controller medication. Adherence with a daily regimen is commonly suboptimal; ICSs are underused most of the time. Individuals who require an oral corticosteroid course due to an asthma exacerbation had used their ICS the least. Adherence is poorer when prescribed frequency of medication administration is greater (3–4 times/24 hr). Controller formulations for twice- and even once-daily dosing can improve patient adherence. Misconceptions about controller medication efficacy and safety often underlie poor adherence and can be addressed by asking about such concerns at each visit.

Table 11.6: Inhaled glucocorticoids daily dosage guidelines*			
Glucocorticoid	*Low dose*	*Medium dose*	*High dose*
Beclomethasone			
42, 84 µg/puff	84–336 µg/puff	336–672 µg/puff	> 672 µg/puff
(40 µg/puff HFA-propellant)	(2–8 puffs of 42 µg/puff or 1–4 puffs of 84 µg/puff)	(8–16 puffs of 42 µg/puff or 4–8 puffs of 84 µg/puff)	(> 16 puffs of 42 µg/puff or > 8 puffs of 84 µg/puff)
Budesonide			
Turbuhaler	200–400 µg/	400–800 µg/	> 800 µg/ (> 4 inhalations)
(DPI) 200 µg/inhalation	(1–2 inhalations)	(2–4 inhalations)	2000 µg
Respules (Nebulizer)	500 µg OD	1000 µg OD	
250–500 µg/vial			
Flinisodide			
250 µg/puff (MDI)	500–750 µg (2–3 puffs)	500–750 µg (2–3 puffs)	500–750 µg (2–3 puffs)
Fluticasone			
44, 110, 220 µg/puff (MDI)	88–176 µg	176–440 µg	> 440 µg
	(2–4 puffs of 44 µg/puff)	(4–10 puffs of 44 µg/puff or 2–4 puffs of 110 µg/puff or 1–2 puffs of 220 µg/puff)	(> 4 puffs of 110 µg/puff > 2 puffs of 220 µg/puff)
Triamcinolone			
100 µg/puff (MDI with spacer)	400–800 µg (4–8 puffs)	800–1200 µg (8–12 puffs)	> 1200 µg (> 12 puffs)

*Estimated comparative daily doses for children ≤ 12 yr of age
Source: Modified from the National Asthma Education and Prevention Program: Expert Panel: Guidelines for the Diagnosis and Management of Asthma. Update on Asthma Selected Topics 2002. Bethesda, MD, National Institutes of Health, National Heart, Lung, and Blood Institute, 2002

Systemic corticosteroids: With ICS therapy large majority of children with asthma can maintain good disease control without oral corticosteroids. Oral corticosteroid therapy is used primarily to treat asthma exacerbations and in rare patients with severe disease who remain symptomatic despite optimal use of other asthma medications (Table 11.5). In these severe asthmatics, every attempt should be made to exclude any co-morbid conditions and to keep the oral corticosteroid dose at ≤ 20 mg (no maintenance oral corticosteroids). Doses exceeding this amount are associated with numerous adverse effects (Box 11.7). To determine the need for continued oral cortico-steroid therapy, a taper of the oral corticosteroid dose (over weeks to several months) should be considered, with close monitoring of the patient's symptoms and lung function. When administered orally, prednisone, prednisolone, and methylprednisolone are rapidly and nearly completely absorbed, with peak plasma concentrations occurring within 1–2 hr. Prednisone is an inactive pro-drug that requires biotransformation via first-pass hepatic metabolism to prednisolone, its active form. Corticosteroids are metabolized in the liver into inactive compounds, with the rate of metabolism influenced by drug interactions and disease states. Anticonvulsants (phenytoin, pheno-barbital, carbamazepine) increase the metabolism of prednisolone, methylprednisolone, and dexametha-sone, with methylprednisolone most significantly affected. Rifampin also enhances the clearance of corticosteroids and can result in diminished thera-peutic effect. Other medications (ketoconazole, oral contraceptives) can significantly delay corticosteroid metabolism. Macrolide antibiotics (erythromycin, clarithromycin, toleandomycin) delay the clearance of only methylprednisolone.

Long-acting inhaled β-agonists (LABA): They are considered to be daily controller medications, not intended for use as "rescue" medication for acute asthma symptoms or exacerbations, nor as mono-therapy for persistent asthma (Table 11.5). Salmeterol has a prolonged onset of action, with maximal bronchodilation about 1 hr after administration, whereas formoterol has an onset of action within 5–10 min. Both medications have a prolonged duration of effect of at least 12 hr. They are used for patients with nocturnal asthma, during the day to prevent exercise-induced bronchospasm, and as an "add-on" agent in patients who are suboptimally controlled on ICS therapy alone.

Leukotriene modifying agents: Leukotrienes are potent pro-inflammatory mediators that can induce bronchospasm, mucus secretions, and airways edema. There are two classes of leukotriene modifiers: inhibitors of leukotriene synthesis and leukotriene receptor antagonists (LTRA). Zileuton, the only leukotriene synthesis inhibitor, is not approved for use

> **Box 11.7:** Adverse effects associated with chronic systemic glucocorticoid use
>
> **Metabolic/endocrinologic effects**
> Hypokalemia
> Hyperglycemia
> Hyperlipidemia
> Adrenal suppression
> Growth suppression
> Delayed sexual maturation (delayed puberty)
> Weight gain
> Cushingoid habitus (central obesity with wasting of extremities)
> Diabetes mellitus
> **Musculoskeletal effects**
> Osteoporosis/vertebral compression fractures
> Aseptic necrosis of bone (hips, shoulders, knees)
> Myopathy (acute and chronic form)
> **Dermatologic effects**
> Dermal thinning and striae
> Increased skin fragility
> Acne
> Hirsutism
> **Ophthalmologic effects**
> Cataracts
> Glaucoma
> **Immunologic effects**
> Diminished IgG levels
> Loss of delayed type of hypersensitivity
> Potential for increased risk of opportunistic infection, reactivation of latent tuberculosis, or severe varicella infection
> **Hematologic effects**
> Lymphopenia
> Neutrophilia
> **Cardiovascular effects**
> Hypertension
> Atherosclerosis
> **Psychologic/neurologic effects**
> Mood swings
> Steroid withdrawal syndrome
> Pseudomotor cerebri
> Psychosis

in children < 12 yr of age. LTRAs have bronchodilator and targeted anti-inflammatory properties and reduce exercise-, aspirin-, and allergen-induced bronchoconstriction. They are recommended as an alternative treatment for mild persistent asthma and as an "add-on" medication to ICS for moderate persistent asthma. Two LTRAs (Montelukast and Zafirlukast) approved for use in children, improve asthma symptoms, decrease need for rescue β-agonist use, and improve lung function. Montelukast, used in children ≥ 1 yr of age, is administered once daily. Zafirlukast, used in children ≥ 5 yr of age, is administered twice daily. LTRAs are not thought to have significant adverse effects.

Nonsteroidal anti-inflammatory agents: Cromolyn and nedocromil are nonsteroidal anti-inflammatory agents that can inhibit allergen-induced asthmatic responses and reduce exercise-induced bronchospasm. Both drugs are considered alternative anti-inflammatory drugs for children with mild persistent asthma. These medications though devoid of adverse effects, but must be administered frequently (2–4 times/day) and are not nearly as effective daily controller medications as ICSs and leukotriene modifying agents. Because they inhibit exercise induced bronchospasm, they can be used in place of SABAs especially in children who develop untoward adverse effects with β-agonist therapy (tremor, and elevated heart rate).

Theophylline has bronchodilator effects. When used chronically theophylline can reduce asthma symptoms and the need for rescue short-acting inhaled β-agonist (SABA) use. It is still considered an alternative monotherapy controller agent for older children and adults with mild persistent asthma, but is not considered a first-line agent for small children in whom there is significant variability in the absorption and metabolism of different theophylline preparations, necessitating frequent monitoring (blood levels) and adjustments. Theophylline overdosage and elevated theophylline levels have been associated with headaches, vomiting, cardiac arrhythmias, seizures, and death.

Anti-IgE (Omalizumab): Omalizumab is a humanized monoclonal antibody. It binds IgE, thereby preventing its binding to the high affinity IgE receptor and blocking IgE-mediated allergic responses and inflammation. It is FDA-approved for patients > 12 yr old with moderate to severe asthma, having hypersensitivity to perennial aeroallergens, and inadequate disease control with inhaled and/or oral corticosteroids. It is given every 2–4 wk subcutaneously based on body weight and serum IgE levels. It is generally well tolerated, but local injection site reactions can occur.

Quick reliever medications: Quick-relief "rescue" medications are listed in Table 11.5.

Short-acting inhaled β-agonist (SABA) is given for their rapid onset of action, effectiveness, and 4–6 hr duration of action. SABAs are the first drugs of choice for acute asthma symptoms (rescue medication) and for preventing exercise-induced bronchospasm. β-agonists bronchodilate by inducing airway smooth muscle relaxation, reducing vascular permeability, reducing airways edema, and improving mucociliary clearance. Overuse of β-agonists is associated with an increased risk of death or near-death episodes from asthma. This is an important major concern for some patients with asthma who rely on the frequent use of SABAs for their asthma, rather than using controller medications in a preventive manner. It is, therefore, important to monitor the frequency of SABA use, in that use of at least 1 MDI/month or at least 3 MDIs/year (200 inhalations/MDI) indicates inadequate asthma control and need for improving other aspects of asthma therapy and management.

Anticholinergic agents: As bronchodilators, the anticholinergic agents (ipratropium bromide) are much less potent than the β-agonists. When used in combination with albuterol/salbutamol, ipratropium can improve lung function and reduce the rate of hospitalization in children who present to the emergency department with acute asthma. Ipratropium is the anticholinergic formulation of choice for children because it has few central nervous system adverse effects. It is available in both MDI and nebulizer formulations. It is approved for children > 12 yr of age.

Asthma exacerbations and their management: Asthma exacerbations (asthma asthmaticus) are acute or subacute episodes of progressively worsening symptoms or airflow obstruction. Often, asthma exacerbations worsen during sleep (between midnight and 8 AM) when airways inflammation and hyper-responsiveness are at their peak. SABAs, which are first-line therapy for asthma symptoms and exacerbations, increase pulmonary blood flow through obstructed, unoxygenated areas of the lungs with increasing doses and frequency. When airways obstruction is not resolved with SABA use, ventilation-perfusion mismatching can cause significant hypoxemia, which can perpetuate bronchoconstriction and further worsen the condition. Severe, progressive asthma exacerbations need to be managed in a medical setting, with administration of supplemental oxygen as first-line therapy and close monitoring for potential worsening. Complications that can occur during severe exacerbations include atelectasis and air leaks in the chest (pneumomediastinum, pneumothorax). A severe exacerbation of asthma that does not improve with standard therapy is termed status asthmaticus. Immediate management of asthma exacerbations involves a rapid evaluation of the severity of obstruction and assessment of the risk for further

clinical deterioration. Most of the patients will improve with frequent bronchodilator treatments and a systemic corticosteroid course. However, the optimal management of a child with an asthma exacerbation should include a more comprehensive assessment of the events leading up to the exacerbation and underlying disease severity. Actually, the frequency and severity of asthma exacerbations helps to define the severity of a patient's asthma. Severe asthma exacerbations, resulting in respiratory distress, hypoxia, hospitalization, and/or respiratory failure are the best predictors of future life-threatening exacerbations or a fatal asthma episode. When extreme, respiratory failure occurs due to fatigue mechanical ventilation will be required for several days. In contrast, some children experience abrupt-onset exacerbations that may result from extreme AHR (airway hypersensitiveness) and physiological susceptibility to airways closure, are initially associated with very high arterial PCO_2 levels and they require only brief periods of supportive ventilation.

Home management of asthma exacerbations: All children with asthma should have a written action plan to guide their recognition and management of exacerbations, along with necessary medications and tools to manage them. The NAEPP guidelines recommend immediate treatment with "rescue" medication (inhaled SABA, up to 3 treatments in 1 hr). A good response is characterized by resolution of symptoms within 1 hr, no further symptoms over the next 4 hr and improvement in PEF (peak expiratory flow) to at least 80% of personal best. The child's physician should be contacted for follow-up, especially if bronchodilators are required repeatedly over the next 24–48 hr. If the child has an incomplete response to initial treatment with rescue medication (persistent symptoms and/or a PEF < 80% of personal best), a short course of oral corticosteroid therapy [predni-solone 1–2 mg/kg/day (not to exceed 60 mg/day) for 4 days] in addition to inhaled β-agonist therapy should be instituted. The physician should also be contacted for further instructions. Immediate medical attention should be sought for severe exacerbations, persistent signs of respiratory distress, lack of expected response or sustained improvement after initial treatment, further deterioration, or high-risk factors for asthma morbidity or mortality (previous history of severe exacerbations). For patients with severe asthma and/or a history of life-threatening episodes, especially if abrupt-onset in nature, providing an injectable form of epinephrine and possibly portable oxygen at home should be considered. Use of either of these extreme measures for home management would be an indication to call for emergency support services.

Emergency department management of asthma exacerbations: In the emergency department, the primary goals of asthma management include correction of hypoxemia, rapid improvement of airflow obstruction, and prevention of progression or recurrence of symptoms. Indications for a severe exacerbations include breathlessness, dyspnea, retractions, accessory muscle use, tachypnea or labored breathing, cyanosis, mental status changes, a silent chest with poor air exchange, and severe airflow limitation (PEF or FEV1 < 50% of personal best or predicted values). Initial treatment includes supplemental oxygen, inhaled β-agonist every 20 min for 1 hr, and if necessary, systemic corticosteroids given either orally or intravenously. Inhaled ipratropium may be added to the β-agonist treatment if no significant response is seen with the 1st inhaled β-agonist therapy. An intramuscular injection of epinephrine or other β-agonist may be administered in severe cases. Oxygen should be administered and continued for at least 20 min after the last injection to compensate for possible ventilation-perfusion abnormalities caused by SABAs.

Close monitoring of clinical status, hydration, and oxygenation are essential elements of immediate management. The patient may be discharged to home if there is sustained improvement in symptoms, normal physical findings, PEF > 70% of predicted or personal best, an oxygen saturation > 92% on room air for 4 hr. Discharge medications include administration of an inhaled β-agonist up to every 3–4 hr plus a 3–7 day course of an oral corticosteroid. The addition of ICS (inhaled corticosteroids) to a course of oral corticosteroid in the emergency department setting reduces the risk of exacerbation recurrence over the subsequent month.

Hospital management of asthma exacerbations: Patients with moderate to severe exacerbations who do not adequately improve within 1–2 hr of intensive treatment, overnight observation and/or admission to the hospital is likely to be needed. Admission to an intensive care unit is included for patients with severe respiratory distress, poor response to therapy, and concern for potential respiratory failure and arrest. Supplemental oxygen, frequently or continuously administered inhaled bronchodilator, and systemic corticosteroid therapy are the conventional interventions for children admitted to the hospital for status asthmaticus. Supplemental oxygen is administered because many children hospitalized with acute asthma will have or develop hypoxemia, especially at night with increasing SABA administration. SABAs can be delivered frequently (every 20 min to 1 hr) or continuously (at 5–15 mg/hr). When administered

continuously, significant systemic absorption of β-agonist occurs, and as a result continuous nebulization can obviate the need for intravenous β-agonist therapy. Adverse effects of frequently administered β-agonist therapy include tremor, irritability, tachycardia, and hypokalemia. Patients requiring frequent or continuous nebulized β-agonist therapy should have ongoing cardiac monitoring. Frequent β-agonist therapy can cause ventilation-perfusion mismatch and precipitate hypoxemia, therefore, oximetry is indicated. Inhaled ipratropium bromide is often added to albuterol or salbutamol every 6 hr if patients do not show a remarkable improvement. In addition to its potential to provide a synergistic effect with a β-agonist agent in relieving severe bronchospasm, it may be beneficial in patients with mucous hypersecretion or on β-blockers.

Short-course systemic corticosteroids therapy is recommended for use in moderate to severe asthma exacerbations to hasten recovery and prevent recurrence of symptoms. Oral corticosteroid therapy can often be used, although children with sustained respiratory distress and unable to tolerate oral preparations or liquids are candidate for intravenous corticosteroid therapy.

Patients with persistent severe dyspnea and high-flow oxygen requirements require additional evaluations such as arterial blood gas, complete blood cell counts, serum electrolytes, and chest radiograph to monitor for respiratory insufficiency, co-morbidities, infection, and/or dehydration. Hydration status monitoring is particularly in infants and young children whose increased respiratory rate (insensible losses) and decreased oral intake put them at increased risk for dehydration. Further complicating this situation is the association of increased antidiuretic hormone (ADH) secretion with status asthmaticus. Administration of fluids at or slightly below maintenance fluid requirements is recommended.

Some asthmatic children remain critically ill and at risk for respiratory failure, intubation, and mechanical ventilation. Complications (air leaks) related to asthma exacerbations increase with intubation and assisted ventilation. Every effort should be made to relieve bronchospasm and prevent respiratory failure. Methylxanthines (2.5 g, intravenously over 20 min), and magnesium sulfate (25–75 mg/kg, maximum dose 2.5 g, intravenously over 20 min), and inhaled heliox have demonstrated some benefit as adjunctive therapies in severe status asthmaticus patients. Administration of either methylxanthine or magnesium sulfate requires monitoring of serum levels and cardiovascular status. Parenteral (subcutaneous, intramuscular, or intravenous) epinephrine or terbutaline sulfate may be effective in patients with life-threatening obstruction who are not responding to high doses of inhaled β-agonists, since inhaled medication may not reach the lower airway.

A severe asthma exacerbation in children rarely results in respiratory failure and intubation and mechanical ventilation is necessary. Mechanical ventilation aims to achieve adequate oxygenation while tolerating mild to moderate hypercapnia (PCO_2 50–70 mm Hg) to minimize barotraumas. Volume-cycled ventilators, using short inspiratory and long expiratory times, 10–15 mL/kg tidal volume, 8–15 beats/min, peak pressures < 60 cm H_2O and without positive end-expiratory pressure are starting mechanical ventilation parameters that can achieve these goals.

In children, management of severe exacerbations in medical centers is usually successful, even when extreme measures are required. Consequently, asthma deaths in children rarely occur in medical centers; most occur at home or in community settings.

Special Management Circumstances

Management of infants and young children: Recurrent wheezing episodes in pre-school-age children are very common as much as 1/3 of this population. Of them, most will improve and even become asymptomatic during the prepubescent school-age years, while others will have lifelong persistent asthma. All require management of their recurrent wheezing problems (Table 11.4). The updated NAEPP guidelines recommend a modified Asthma Predictive Index (Table 11.2) to identify pre-school-age children who are likely to have persistent asthma. These at-risk children may be candidates for conventional asthma management; including daily controller therapy and early intervention with exacerbations (Table 11.4). Nebulized budesonide and montelukast are more effective than cromolyn. For young children with a history of moderate to severe exacerbations, nebulized budesonide used as a controller medication could prevent subsequent exacerbations. There are 2 aerosol therapy delivery systems for inhaled medications for this age group: the nebulizer and the MDI with spacer/holding chamber and face mask.

Home management of asthma exacerbations: The goals of asthma management during pregnancy should include prevention of exacerbations and control of chronic symptoms by using medications that cause minimal risk to the mother and fetus because most drugs cross the placenta. It is safer for pregnant asthmatic women to be treated with controller medications than it is to have uncontrolled symptoms and severe exacerbations. Albuterol/Salbutamol is the preferred SABA for use during pregnancy. Budesonide is currently the preferred ICS (inhaled corticosteroid) for pregnant women. Nonpharmacotherapeutic approaches to improve asthma control such as avoidance of environmental tobacco smoke (beginning prenatally), prolonged breastfeeding (up to 2 yr of age), an active lifestyle, and a healthy diet should be emphasized. A multidisciplinary approach with monthly evaluation (including pulmonary function test when not contraindicated) and ongoing consultation with the obstetrician and asthma specialist is recommended. Frequent fetal and maternal surveillance is especially important for adolescents with suboptimal asthma control, those with moderate to severe asthma, and those with recent exacerbation.

Management of asthma during surgery: Patients with asthma are at-risk from disease-related complications from surgery such as bronchoconstriction and asthma exacerbations, atelectasis, impaired coughing, respiratory infection, and latex exposure that may induce asthma complications in patients with latex allergy. All patients with asthma should be evaluated before surgery, and those who are inadequately controlled should be given time for intensified treatment in order to improve asthma stability before surgery if possible. A systemic corticosteroid course may be indicated for patients who are having symptoms and/or FEV1 or PEF < 80% of the patient's personal best. In addition, patients who have received more than 2 wk of systemic corticosteroid and/or moderate-to-high dose ICS therapy may be at risk of intraoperative adrenal insufficiency. For these patients, anesthetic should be alerted to provide "stress" replacement doses of systemic corticosteroid for the surgical procedure and possibly the postoperative period if needed.

Patient education: With education, the child and family become essential partners in the asthma management process (Table 11.7). In initial patient visits, a basic understanding of the pathogenesis of asthma can help children and their parents to understand the importance of recommendations aimed at reducing airways inflammation. The expectations of good asthma control resulting from optimal asthma management should be specified. In addition to addressing concerns about potential adverse effects of asthma pharmacotherapy, and especially their risks relative to their benefits, are essential in achieving long-term adherence with asthma pharmacotherapy and environmental control measures.

Table 11.7: Specific educational element in the clinical care of children

Specify goals of asthma management	Normal activity——*see* Box 11.5
Explain basic facts about asthma	Contrast normal vs asthmatic airways
	Long-term control and quick-relief-medications
Address concerns about potential adverse effects of asthma pharmacotherapy	This will help parents to continue medications
Teach, demonstrate, and have patient show proper technique	Inhaled medication use (spacer use with MDI)
	Peak flow measures
Investigate and manage factors that contribute to asthma severity	Environmental exposures
	Co-morbid conditions
Written two-part asthma management plan	Daily management
	Action plan for asthma exacerbations
Regular follow-up visit	Twice yearly (more often if not well controlled)
	Monitor lung function annually

Children with asthma and their families benefit from a written asthma management plan with 2 main components: (i) a daily "routine" management plan describing regular asthma medication use and other measures to keep asthma under good control; and (ii) an action plan for asthma exacerbations, describing action to take when asthma worsens, including what medications to take and when to contact the regular physician and/or for urgent/emergent medical care. Regular follow-up visits can help to maintain optimal asthma control.

Prognosis: Recurrent coughing and wheezing occurs in approximately 35% of pre-school-age children. Of these, 1/3 continues to have persistent asthma into later childhood, while 2/0 improve on their own. Asthma severity by the ages of 7–10 yr of age is predictive of asthma persistence in adulthood. Children with moderate to severe asthma and with lower lung function measures are likely to have persistent asthma as adults. Children with milder asthma and normal lung function are likely to improve over time, with some becoming periodic (disease-free mo to yr); however, complete remission for 5 yr in childhood is uncommon.

Prevention: Anti-inflammatory interventions, the cornerstone of asthma control in young children with recurrent wheezing fail to cure. Several nonpharmaco-therapeutic measures such as avoidance of environmental tobacco smoke (beginning prenatally), prolonged breastfeeding (up to 2 yr of age), an active lifestyle, and a healthy diet-might reduce the likelihood of asthma development. Immunizations are currently not considered to increase the likelihood of developing asthma. Therefore, all standard immuniza-tions are recommended for children with asthma, including varicella and influenza vaccines.

Anderson HR. Prevalence of asthma. Br Med J 2005;350: 1037–38.

Biscardi S, Lorrot M, Marc E, et al. Mycoplasma pneumonia and asthma in children. Clin Infect Dis 2004;38:1341–46.

Guglani Lokesh, Kabra SK. Acute Exacerbation of a Child with Asthma. In: Mathur GP, Mathur Sarla (eds). Current Trends in Pediatrics. Vol 1. Delhi: Academa Publishers, 2005; 158–73.

Liu AH, Covar RASpahn JD, LeungDYM. Childhood asthma. In: Kliegman RM, Behrman RE, Jenson HB, Stanton BF (eds). *Nelson Textbook of Pediatrics*. 18th edn. Vol. 1. Philadelphia: Saunders, 2007; 963–70.

Lipworth BJ. Phosphodiesterase-4 inhibitors for asthma and chronic obstructive pulmonary disease. Lancet 2005;365:167–75.

National Asthma Education and Prevention Program: NAEPP guidelines for the diagnosis and management of asthma-update on selected topics, 2002, Washington, DC, NIH, 2002 (NIH publication no. 02–5075).

Struck RC, Bloomberg GR. Omalizumab for asthma. N Engl J Med 2006;354:2689–95.

Vonk JM, Postma DS, Boezen HM, et al. Childhood factors associated with asthma remission after 30 yr follow-up. Thorax 2004;59:925–9.

11.4 ATOPIC DERMATITIS (ATOPIC ECZEMA)

Atopic dermatitis (AD) is an eczematous eruption that is extremely pruritic, recurrent, flexural and symmetric. It occurs in atopic persons, who have personal or a family history of allergic rhinitis, asthma or hay fever, and have increased ability to form IgE to common environmental allergens.

Precipitating factors: There are several possible precipitating factors responsible for allergic dermatitis such as:

1. Inhalant allergens [house dust mite (*Dermato-phagoides pteronyssinus*), grass pollens, and animal dander]

2. Food allergy and intolerance (eggs, milk, peanuts, soya beans, tree nuts, fish and wheat)
3. Irritants (woolen material, shiny nylon materials and some acrylics, soap in excess and bubble baths excessively, perfumed and "medicated" products applied)
4. Microbial products (exotoxins secreted by *staphylococcus aureus*, lipophillic yeast, *P. ovale* and superficial dermatophyte *Trichophyton rubrum*); and
5. Psychological issues (child feels physically unattractive, often lacks confidence and has poor self image).

Diagnostic criteria: There are no laboratory tests available to confirm the diagnosis of AD. The diagnostic criteria of atopic dermatitis (AD) include pruritus; facial and extensor involvement in infant and children; flexural lichenification in adults; chronic or relapsing dermatitis; personal or family history of atopic disease. Additional features identified in patients are scaling of the scalp and peri-auricular fissures.

Clinical Manifestations

AD typically begins during infancy. Approximately 50% of patients develop this illness by the first year of life and an additional 30% between the age of 1 and 5 yr. Nearly 80% of patients with AD eventually develop allergic rhinitis or asthma later in childhood.

1. *Infantile phase (birth to less than 2 yr):* Infants are rarely born with AD, but they typically develop the first sign of inflammation during the third month of life. The lesions most frequently start on the face, but may occur anywhere on the skin surface. Most commonly, during winter months, child develops red, dry, scaly areas confined to the cheeks but sparing perioral and paranasal areas. Chin is often involved. Habitual lip licking by an atopic child results in oozing, crusting and scaling on the lips and perioral skin. When the child begins to crawl, the exposed surfaces, especially the extensor surface of the knees is most involved. The lesions consist of erythema and discrete or confluent edematous papules. The papules are intensely itchy, and may become exudative and crusted as a result of repeated scratching. At this stage the infant is uncomfortable, has disturbed sleep and becomes restless. Secondary infection and lymphadenopathy are common.
2. *Childhood phase (2 to 12 yr):* The most common presentation is the inflammation in flexural areas (i.e. ante-cubital fossa, neck, wrist and ankles) (*see* Fig. 11.9 in CD). These areas of repeated flexion and extension perspire with exertion. The act of perspiring stimulates burning and intense itching and initiates the itch-scratch cycle. Tight clothing further aggravates the problem. The eruption consists of papules that may coalesce to form plaques, which eventually become lichenified. The exudative lesions typical of the infant phase are not as common. However, when vigorously scratched, they may become bright red and scaly with erosions. Exacerbating factors like heat, cold, low humidity and emotional stress may lead to the extension of inflammation beyond the confines of crease areas. Most patients achieve remission by the age of 30, but in few others the disease becomes a lifelong chronic disease.

3. *Adult phase (12 yr to adults):* Localized flexural inflammation with lichenification is the most common presentation. Hand dermatitis, periocular and genitofemoral eczema are probably more common in patients with AD. The disease is chronic with periods of exacerbation and remission often related to the seasons.

Complications

1. *Infections:* Viral (herpes simplex and vaccinia virus) bacterial (*S. aureus*) and fungal (*Trichophyton rubrum* and *Pitytosporum ovale*) skin infections.
2. Hand dermatitis especially in those patients involved in wet work occupations.
3. *Exfoliative dermatitis/erythroderma:* Generalized scaling, erythema, systemic toxicity and fever. It may be due to staphylococcal or herpes simplex superinfection, inappropriate irritant therapy or withdrawal of systemic steroids.
4. *Ocular problems:* Eyelid dermatitis, chronic blepharitis, atopic keratoconjunctivitis, keratoconus and cataract.

Associated problems include dry skin and xerosis, ichthyosis vulgaris, keratosis pilaris, hyperlinear palmar crease, pityriasis alba, atopic pleats (Dennie-Morgan folds), cataracts and keratoconus.

Differential diagnosis: Atopic dermatitis (AD) should be differentiated from scabies, infantile seborrhoeic dermatitis, severe combined immunodeficiency, Wiskott-Aldrich syndrome, contact allergic dermatitis.

Management

General measures:
a. Explanation and counseling are a vital part of the successful management of childhood eczema.
b. Precipitating factors should be avoided as far as possible for successful treatment.

Specific measures: First line agents include moisturizers and emollients, topical steroids, antihistaminics (like promethazine given at bedtime is useful as effective antipruritic agent), antimicrobials (see Section 30.11, page 906). Second line agents include:

a. Topical (Pimecrolimus cream 1%; Tacrolimus ointment (0.03% and 0.15)
b. Systemic (steroids, cyclosporin)
c. Phototherapy
d. UV irradiation [both UVA (60–400) and UVB or combination of the two]
e. Desensitization. However, the compliance should be checked and antibiotic resistant infection should be excluded.

Antibiotics: Infection of the skin by staphylococcal organisms may exacerbate the eczema and should be promptly treated with penicillin or macrolide group of antibiotics. In patients with recurrent flares of atopic dermatitis, the use of long-term antibiotics therapy may suppress the formations of the superantigen.

Holden CA, Parish WE. Atopic Dermatitis. In: Champion RH, Burton JL, Burns DA, Breathnach SM (eds). *Rooks Textbook of Dermatology.* 6th edn, Vol 1. Oxford: Blackwell publications, 1998; 681–708.

Khanna N. Eczematous Dermatitis. In: Khanna N (Ed). Illustrated synopsis of Dermatology and Sexually Transmitted Disease. 1st edn. Delhi: Peepee Publishers, 2005; 64–82.

Leung DYM, Tharp M, Beguniewicz M. Atopic Dermatitis. In: Freedberg IM, Eisen AZ, Wolfe K et al (eds). Fitzpatrick's Dermatology in General Medicine. 5th edn, Vol 1. New York: McGraw-Hill, 1999; 1464–79.

Singal Archana, Mehta Shilpa. Eczema in Pediatric Age Group. In: Mathur GP, Mathur Sarla (eds). Current Trends in Pediatrics. Vol 2. Delhi: Academa Publishers, 2006;296–306.

11.5 URTICARIA AND ANGIOEDEMA

Urticaria (hives) and angioedema affect 20% of individuals at some point in their lives. Episodes of urticaria that continue for < 6 wk are considered acute, and those that persist for > 6 wk are designated chronic. Urticaria is transient, pruritic, erythematous, raised wheals, with flat tops and edema that may become tense and painful. Individual lesions usually last 20 min to 3 hr, and rarely more than 24 hr. The lesions often disappear and reappear. Angioedema involves the deeper subcutaneous tissues such as the eyelids, lips, tongue, genitals, and dorsum of the hands or feet. Acute urticaria and angioedema are often caused by an allergic IgE mediated reaction (Table 11.8).

Physical Urticaria

Physically induced urticaria and angioedema are induced by environmental factors such as a change in temperature or by direct stimulation of the skin with pressure, stroking, vibration, or light.

Cold urticaria: Cold urticaria is characterized by the rapid onset of localized pruritus, erythema, and urticaria/angioedema after exposure to a cold stimulus. Cold urticaria has also been reported after viral infections.

Cholinergic urticaria: It is characterized by the onset of small punctuate wheals surrounded by a prominent erythematous flare associated with exercise, hot showers, and sweating. When the patient cools down, the rash usually subsides in 30–60 minutes.

Urticaria factitia: The ability to write on skin, termed dermatographism (also called dermographism or urticaria factitia), can occur as an isolated disorder or accompany chronic urticaria or other physical urticaria such as cholinergic and cold urticaria.

Pressure induced urticaria and angioedema: Pressure induced urticaria or angioedema symptoms usually occur 4–6 hr after pressure has been applied. Symptoms occur at sites of tight clothing; foot swelling is common after walking; and buttock swelling may be present after sitting for a few hours.

Solar urticaria: Solar urticaria is a rare disorder in which urticaria develops within 1–3 min of sun exposure. The pruritus occurs first in about 30 sec, followed by edema confined to the light-exposed area

Table 11.8: Etiology of acute urticaria	
Foods	Egg, milk, wheat, peanuts, tree nuts, soy, shellfish, fish, strawberries (direct mast cell degranulation)
Medications	Suspect all medications, even over-the-counter or homeopathic
Insect stings	Hymenoptera (honey bee, yellow jacket, hornets, wasp, fine ants), biting insects (papular urticaria)
Infections	Bacterial (streptococcal pharyngitis, *Mycoplasma*, sinusitis); viral (hepatitis, mononucleosis [EBV], coxsackievirus A and B); parasitic (*Ascaris, Ancylostoma, Echinococcus, Fasciola, Filaria, Schistosoma, Strongyloides, Toxocara, Trichinella*); fungal (dermatophytes, *Candida*)
Contact allergy	Latex, pollen, animal saliva, nettle plants, caterpillars
Transfusion reactions	Blood, blood products, or IV immunoglobulin administration
Idiopathic	-

EBV, Epstein-Barr virus

and surrounded by a prominent erythematous zone. The lesions usually disappear within 1–3 hr after sun exposure is avoided. When large areas of the body are exposed, systemic symptoms may occur, including hypotension and wheezing. Erythropoietic protoporphyria can be confused with solar urticaria because of the development of itching and burning of exposed skin immediately after sun exposure. In erythropoietic protoporphyria, fluorescence of UV-irradiated red blood cells can be demonstrated.

Aquagenic urticaria: Patients with aquagenic urticaria develop small wheals after contact with water, regardless of its temperature. These patients can be distinguished from patients with cold urticaria or cholinergic urticaria.

Chronic Idiopathic Urticaria and Angioedema

This is a common disorder of unknown origin that is often associated with normal routine laboratory studies and no evidence of systemic disease. Chronic urticaria does not appear to be an allergic reaction. It differs from allergen-induced skin reactions or from physically induced urticaria in that histologic studies reveal a cellular infiltrate predominantly about small venules. Skin examination reveals infiltrative urticarial lesions with palpably elevated borders, sometimes varying greatly in size and/or shape but generally being rounded. Biopsy of the typical lesion reveals non-necrotizing, perivascular, mononuclear cellular infiltration. The incidence of elevated thyroid antibodies in patients with chronic urticaria is 12% compared with 3–6% in the general population. 35 to 40% of patients with chronic urticaria have a positive autologous skin test; if serum from the patient is intradermally injected into their skin, a significant wheal and flare reaction develops.

Treatment: Acute urticaria is a self-limited illness. Cetirizine, hydroxyzine, diphenhydramine, loratadine, and fexofenadine are effective and commonly used antihistamines. Epinephrine 1:1, 000, 0.01 ml/kg (maximum: 0.3 ml) usually provides rapid relief of acute, severe urticaria/angioedema. A short-course of corticosteroids should only be given for very severe episodes of urticaria and angioedema.

Most forms of physical urticaria respond to avoidance of triggering stimuli in combination with oral antihistamines; delayed pressure urticaria often requires oral corticosteroids and for cold-induced urticaria cyproheptadine in divided doses is the drug of choice.

Treatment of dermatographism (urticaria factitia) consists of local skin care and antihistamines in order to decrease pruritus. A combination of antihistamines, sunscreens, and avoidance of sunlight are helpful for most patients.

Chronic urticaria only rarely responds favorably to dietary manipulation. Removal of urticarial aggravators, such as salicylates, alcohol, or β-blockers, should be considered. A combined use of H1- and H$_2$-type antihistamines are sometimes helpful to control chronic urticaria when H1-type antihistamines alone, even at higher than standard doses do not work. If urticaria persists after maximal H1- and H2-receptor blockade has been achieved, alternate-day therapy with corticosteroids is the most effective treatment. Prednisolone (or prednisone) 20 mg orally as a single morning dose on alternate days is used, with the dosage decreased by 2.5–5.0 mg every 1–3 wk depending on the clinical response; the objective is the slow reduction of the use of this drug. Antileukotriene agents in combination with antihistamines may also be helpful. Treatment of autoimmune chronic urticaria refractory to medical therapy includes intravenous immunoglobulin, plasmapheresis, or both.

Boguniewicz M. Chronic urticaria in children. Allergy Asthma Proc 2005;26:13–17.

Dibbern DA Jr, Dreskin SC. Urticaria and angioedema: An overview. Immunol Allergy Clin North Am 2004;24:141–62.

Lasley MV, Kennedy MS, Altman LC. Urticaria and angioedema. In: Altman LC, Backer JW, Williams PV (eds). Allergy in Primary Care. Philadelphia: WB Saunders, 2000; 232 and 234.

Leung DYM, Dreskin. Urticaria (Hives) and angioedema. In: Kliegman RM, Behrman RE, Jenson HB, Stanton BF (eds). *Nelson Textbook of Pediatrics*. 18th edn. Vol. 1. Philadelphia: Saunders, 2007;979–82.

Sheikh J. Advances in the treatment of chronic urticaria. Immunol Allergy Clin North Am 2004;24:317–34.

11.6 INSECT ALLERGY

The allergic responses to stinging or biting insects vary from localized cutaneous reactions to systemic anaphylaxis. Most reactions to biting and stinging insects such as those induced by mosquitoes, flies and fleas are limited to a primary lesion isolated to the area of the bite and do not represent an allergic response. Systemic allergic responses to insects are attributed to IgE antibody-mediated responses, which are caused almost entirely by stings from venomous insects of the order Hymenoptera. Members of this order include rapids (honeybee, bumblebee), vespids (yellow jacket, wasp, hornet), and formicids (fire and harvester ants).

Clinical manifestations: Insect bites are usually urticarial but may be papular or vesicular. Papular urticaria affecting the lower extremities in children is caused by multiple bites. Clinical reactions to stinging venomous insects are categorized as local, large local, generalized cutaneous, systemic, toxic, and delayed/late. Simple local reactions involve limited swelling and pain, and generally last < 24 hr. Large local reactions develop over hours and days, involve swelling of extensive areas (> 10 cm) that are continuous with the sting site, and may last for days. Generalized cutaneous reactions typically progress within minutes and include cutaneous symptoms of urticaria, angioedema, and pruritus beyond the site of the sting. Systemic reactions are identical to anaphylaxis from other triggers and may include symptoms of generalized urticaria, laryngeal edema, bronchospasm, and hypotension. Stings from a large number of insects at once may result in toxic reactions of fever, malaise, emesis, and nausea owing to the chemical properties of the venom in large doses. Serum sickness, nephrotic syndrome, vasculitis, neuritis, or encephalopathy may occur in delayed/late reactions to stinging insects.

Inhalant allergy caused by insects' results in clinical disease similar to that induced by other inhalant allergens such as pollens. Depending on individual sensitivity and exposure, reactions may result in seasonal or perennial rhinitis, conjunctivitis, and asthma.

Treatment: For local cutaneous reactions caused by insect bites and stings, treatment with cold compresses, topical medications to relieve itching, and occasionally the use of a systemic antihistamine and oral analgesic are needed. Stingers should be removed promptly by scrapping, with caution not to squeeze the venom sac because this could inject more venom. Anaphylactic reactions after a Hymenoptera sting are treated in an identical fashion to anaphylaxis from any cause (*see* anaphylaxis).

Prevention: It is essential to avoid stings and bites. To reduce the risk of stings, sensitized individuals should avoid attractants such as perfumes and bright-colored clothing outdoors, wear gloves when gardening, and wear long pants and shoes with socks when walking in the grass or through fields. Nests should be removed if they are close to the home. Individuals who have had generalized cutaneous or systemic reactions to hymenoptera stings should have immediate access to self-injectable epinephrine. Individuals at risk for anaphylaxis from an insect sting should also wear an identification bracelet indicating their allergy.

Bircher AJ. Systemic immediate allergic reactions to arthropod stings and bites. Dermatology 2005;210:119–27.

Sicherer SH, Leung DYM. Insect allergy. In: Kliegman RM, Behrman RE, Jenson HB, Stanton BF (eds). *Nelson Textbook of Pediatrics.* 18th edn. Vol. 1. Philadelphia: Saunders, 2007;975–77.

11.7 ANAPHYLAXIS

Anaphylaxis is a clinical condition characterized by cutaneous (urticaria, angioedema, flushing), respiratory (bronchospasm, laryngeal edema), cardiovascular (hypotension, dysrhythmias, myocardial ischemia), and gastrointestinal symptoms (nausea, colicky abdominal pain, vomiting, diarrhea) as a result of sudden release of potent biologically active mediators from mast cells and basophils.

Etiology: Anaphylaxis in children is different for hospital and community settings. Anaphylaxis occurring in the hospital is primarily the result of allergic reactions to medications and latex, whereas food allergy (most common pea nut allergy) is the most common cause of anaphylaxis occurring outside the hospital (Table 11.9). Patients with latex allergy also may experience food allergic reactions from homologous proteins in fruits such as bananas, kiwi, avocado, chestnuts, and passion fruit.

Pathogenesis: The anaphylaxis is the result of activation of mast cells and basophils via cell-bound allergen-specific IgE molecules. In IgE mediated reaction, patients must first be exposed to the responsible allergen to generate allergen-specific antibodies. The initial exposure to a child may be from passage of food proteins in maternal breastmilk.

Clinical manifestations: The onset of symptoms are acute but vary some what depending on the cause of the reaction; reactions from ingested allergens (foods, medications) are delayed in onset (minutes to 2 hr) compared with injected allergen (insect sting, medications). The initial symptoms are pruritus about the mouth and face, a sensation of warmth, weakness and apprehension. They may develop flushing, urticaria and angioedema, oral pruritus, tightness in the throat, dry staccato cough and hoarseness, periocular pruritus, nasal congestion, sneezing, dyspnea, deep cough and wheezing. Nausea, abdominal cramping, and vomiting are common with ingested allergens. In women low back pain will occur due to uterine contractions. Faintness and loss of consciousness occurs in severe cases. Some degree of obstructive laryngeal edema also occurs in severe reactions. The acute onset of severe bronchospasm in a previously well asthmatic even in the absence of cutaneous symptoms should suggest the diagnosis of anaphylaxis.

Diagnosis: The diagnosis of anaphylaxis is usually apparent owing to the acute and characteristic combination of cutaneous and respiratory manifestations, especially when accompanied by hypotension.

Table 11.9: Common causes of anaphylaxis in children	
Food	Peanuts, tree nuts (walnut, hazelnut, cashew, pistachio, Brazil nut), milk, eggs, fish, shellfish (shrimp, crab, lobster, clam, scallop, oyster), seeds (sesame, cotton seed, pine nuts, psyllium), fruits (apple, banana, kiwi, peaches, oranges, melon), grains (wheat)
Drugs	Penicillins, cephalosporins, sulfonamides, nonsteroidal anti-inflammatory agents, opiates, muscle relaxants, vancomycin, dextrin, thiamine, vitamin B_{12}, insulin, thiopental, local anesthetics
Hymenoptera venom	Honeybee, yellow jacket, wasp, hornet, fire ant
Latex	
Allergen immunotherapy	
Exercise	Food specific exercise, postprandial (non-food-specific) exercise
Vaccinations	Tetanus, measles, mumps, influenza
Miscellaneous	Radiocontrast media, gammaglobulin, cold temperature, chemotherapeutic agents (asparaginase, cyclosporin, methotrexate, vincristine, 5-fluorouracil), blood products, inhalants (dust and storage mites, grass pollen)
Idiopathic	

Differential diagnosis: Sudden collapse in the absence of cutaneous symptoms, consider the possibility of other conditions such as vasovagal collapse, seizure disorder, aspiration, myocardial infarction or pulmonary embolism. Laryngeal edema, especially with abdominal pain, suggests hereditary angioedema.

Treatment: Anaphylactic reaction is an emergency and should be treated aggressively with intramuscular epinephrine, intramuscular or intravenous H_1 and H_2 antihistamine antagonists, oxygen, intravenous fluids, inhaled β-agonists, and corticosteroids. Patients may experience a biphasic reaction, which occurs when anaphylactic symptoms recur after apparent resolution. The mechanism of this phenomenon is not known. It is seen if the therapy is initiated late and symptoms at presentation are more severe. It is not affected by the administration of corticosteroids during the initial therapy. More than 90% of biphasic responses occur within 4 hr, so patients should be observed for at least 4 hr before being discharged from the emergency department.

A. Patient Emergency Management (dependent on severity of symptoms)

Epinephrine: (adrenaline) 0.01 mg/kg up to 0.3 mg (0.15 mg); IM 8–25 kg (0.3 mg); IM > 25 kg in a case of anaphylaxis, bronchospasm, cardiac arrest

Cetirizine (liquid) (5 mg/5 ml): 0.25 mg/kg up to 10 mg PO

Alternative: Diphenhydramine (Benadryl: 12.5 mg/5 ml) 1.25 mg/kg up to 50 mg PO

Transport to an Emergency Facility

B. Emergency Personnel Management (dependent on severity of symptoms)

i. Supplemental oxygen and airway management
ii. *Epinephrine* (adrenaline) 0.01 mg/kg up to 0.3 mg (0.15 mg); IM 8–25 kg (0.3 mg); IM > 25 kg; 0.01 ml/kg/dose of 1: 1,000 solution up to 0.3 ml IM; 0.01 ml/kg/dose of 1: 10,000 slow IV push in case of anaphylaxis, bronchospasm, cardiac arrest
iii. *Volume expanders:* **Crystalloids** (normal saline or Ringer lactate) 30 ml/kg in first hour, rate titrated against BP response

Cetirizine: (liquid) (5 mg/5 ml) 0.25 mg/kg up to 10 mg PO

Alternative: **Diphenhydramine:** (Benadryl: 12.5 mg/5 ml) 1.25 mg/kg up to 50 mg IM

Alternative: **Nebulized albuterol:** α-agonist (0.83 mg/ml (3 ml) via mask with O_2

Corticosteroids: **Methylprednisolone:** Solution (IV), Depo (IM)

Prednisolone: 1 mg/kg up to 75 mg PO

Ranitidine: (25 mg/mL) 1 mg/kg up to 50 mg IV should be administered slowly

Alternative: **Cimetidine** (25 mg/mL) 4 mg/kg up to 200 mg IV should be administered slowly

C. Post-emergency management

Cetirizine (5–10 mg qid) or loratidine (5–10 mg qid) for 10 days

Prednisolone (1 mg/kg up to 75 kg) daily PO for 3 days

Preventive treatment: Follow-up evaluation to determine/confirm etiology.

Immunotherapy for insect sting allergy; prescription for epinephrine and antihistamine

Provide written plan outlining patient emergency management.

Patient education

a. Instruction on avoidance of causative agent
b. Information on recognizing early signs of anaphylaxis
c. Stress on early treatment of allergic symptoms to avoid systemic anaphylaxis

Prevention: Patients experiencing anaphylactic reactions to food should avoid their use. Patients with egg allergy should be tested before receiving the influenza or yellow fever vaccines, which contain egg protein. Children experiencing systemic anaphylactic reactions to an insect sting should be treated with immunotherapy. Children with food-associated exercise-induced anaphylaxis must not exercise within 2–3 hr of ingesting the triggering food. Patient who had previous reactions to medications and food must inform the doctor, so that they are not prescribed (advised). Reactions to medications are less by using oral medications in preference to injected forms. Hypoosmolar radiocontrast dyes can be used in cases where previous reactions are suspected. In children undergoing multiple surgeries powder-free, low allergen gloves and materials should be used. Any child with food allergy and history of asthma, peanut or tree nut allergy should be given an EpiPen (epinephrine), liquid cetirizine (or alternatively, diphenhydramine), and a written emergency plan in case of accidental ingestion.

Dibs SD, Baker MD. Anaphylaxis in children: A 5-yr experience. *Pediatrics* 2000;106:762–66.

Lee JM, Greenes DS. Biphasic anaphylactic reactions in pediatrics. *Pediatrics* 2000;106:762–66.

Sampson HA. Anaphylaxis and emergency treatment. *Pediatrics* 2003;111:1601–08.

Sampson HA, Leung DYM. Anaphylaxis. In: Kliegman RM, Behrman RE, Jenson HB, Stanton BF (eds). *Nelson Textbook of Pediatrics*. 18th edn. Vol. 1. Philadelphia: Saunders, 2007; 983–85.

11.8 SERUM SICKNESS

Serum sickness is a systemic, immune complex-mediated hypersensitivity vasculitis due to the therapeutic administration of foreign serum proteins. Serum sickness is a classic example of a Gell and Coombs' type III hypersensitivity reaction caused by antigen-antibody complexes.

Clinical manifestations: The symptoms of serum sickness generally begin 7–12 days after injection of the foreign material, but may appear as late as 3 wk afterward. The onset of symptoms may be accelerated if there has been earlier exposure or previous allergic reaction to the same antigen. A few days before the onset of generalized symptoms, the site of injection may become edematous and erythematous. Symptoms usually include fever, malaise, and rashes. Urticaria and the morbilliform rashes are the predominant types of skin eruptions, and pruritus is common.

Diagnosis: Circulating immune complexes are usually detectable, with peak levels at 10–12 days. Serum complement levels (C3 and C4) are generally decreased and reach a nadir at about day 10. C3a anaphylatoxin may be increased. ESR is usually elevated and thrombocytopenia is often present. Mild proteinuria, hemoglobinuria and microscopic hematuria may be seen. In serum sickness caused by horse serum proteins, antibodies of the IgG, IgA, IgM, and IgE classes may be found detected against various horse serum proteins. Direct immunofluorescence studies of skin lesions often reveal immune deposits of IgM, IgA, IgE, or C3.

Treatment: It is primarily supportive with antihistamines and analgesics. When the symptoms are severe, systemic corticosteroids can be used initially in high doses and then rapidly reduced as the patient improves.

Prevention: Seek alternative therapies, if available such as non-equine-derived formulations, partially digested antibodies of animal origin and engineered (humanized) antibodies. In these therapies serum sickness-like disease appears low. When only equine antitoxin/antivenom is available, skin tests should be performed before administration of serum. The positive results of allergy skin test indicate an increased likelihood and a negative test indicating a small, but not absent, risk of anaphylaxis.

Sicherer SH, Leung DYM. Serum sickness. In: Kliegman RM, Behrman RE, Jenson HB, Stanton BF (eds). *Nelson Textbook of Pediatrics*. 18th edn. Vol. 1. Philadelphia: Saunders, 2007; 985–6.

11.9 OCULAR ALLERGIES

The eye is the common target of allergic disorders because of its marked vascularity and direct contact with allergens in the environment. The conjunctiva is the most immunologically active tissue of the external eye. Ocular allergies can occur as isolated target organ disease or more commonly in conjunction with nasal allergies.

Clinical Manifestations

Allergic conjunctivitis is the most common hypersensitivity response of the eye. It is caused by direct exposure of the mucosal surfaces of the eye to environmental allergens.

Patients complain of variable ocular itching, rather than pain, with increased tearing.

Clinical signs include bilateral injected conjunctivae with vascular congestion that may progress to chemosis, or conjunctival swelling, and a watery discharge. Allergic conjunctivitis occurs in a seasonal or, less commonly, perennial form.

Vernal keratoconjunctivitis: Vernal keratoconjunctivitis is a severe bilateral chronic inflammatory process of the upper tarsal conjunctival surface that occurs in a limbal or palpebral form. It may threaten eyesight if there is corneal involvement. It occurs most frequently in children with seasonal allergies, asthma, or atopic dermatitis. Vernal keratoconjunctivitis affects boys twice as often as girls, and is more common in persons of Asian and African origin. It affects primarily children in temperate areas, with exacerbations in the spring and summer. Symptoms include severe ocular itching exacerbated by exposure to irritants, light, or perspiration, severe photophobia, foreignbody sensation, and lacrimation. Giant papillae occur predominantly on the upper tarsal plate, described as cobblestoning. Other signs include a stringy or thick ropy discharge, cobblestone papillae, transient yellow-white points in the limbus (Trantas dots) and conjunctiva (Horner points), corneal "shield" ulcers, and Dennie lines (Dennie-Morgan folds), which are prominent symmetric skinfolds that extend in an arc from the inner canthus beneath and parallel to the lower lid margin. Children with vernal keratoconjunctivitis have longer eyelashes.

Atopic keratoconjunctivitis: Atopic keratoconjunctivitis is a chronic inflammatory ocular disorder most commonly involving the lower tarsal conjunctiva. It may threaten eyesight if there is corneal involvement. Almost all patients have atopic dermatitis, and a significant number have asthma; rarely present before late adolescence. Secondary staphylococcal blepharitis is common.

Giant papillary conjunctivitis: Giant papillary conjunctivitis has been linked to chronic exposure to foreign bodies such as contact lenses, both hard and soft, ocular prostheses, and sutures.

Contact allergy: Contact allergy involves the eyelids but can also involve the conjunctivae. It is commonly associated with topical medications, contact lens solutions, and preservatives.

Diagnosis: Nonallergic conjunctivitis can be viral, bacterial, or chlamydial in origin. It is typically unilateral but can be bilateral with symptoms initially developing in one eye. Symptoms include stinging or burning rather than itching, and often a foreign body sensation. Ocular discharge can be watery, mucoid, or purulent. Ocular allergy should be distinguished from nasolacrimal duct obstruction, foreign body, blepharoconjunctivitis, dry eye, uveitis, and trauma.

Treatment: Primary treatment of ocular allergies includes avoidance of allergens, cold compresses, and lubrication. Secondary treatment regimens include the use of oral or topical antihistamines and, if necessary, topical decongestants, mast cell stabilizers, and anti-inflammatory agents. Combined use of an antihistamine and a vasoconstrictive agent is more effective than use of either agent alone.

Azelastine hydrochloride (antihistamine) 0.05%: children ≥ 3 yr: bid; Emedastine difumarate (antihistamine) 0.05%: children ≥ 3 yr: qid; Pheniramine maleate (antihistamine/vasoconstrictor) 0.03%: children > 6 yr: 1–2 qid avoid prolonged use (> 3–4 days 0; Cromolyn sodium (antihistamine/mast cell stabilizer) 4%: children > 4 yr: 1–2 q 4–6 hr; Olopatadine hydrochloride (antihistamine/mast cell stabilizer) 0.1%: children ≥ 3 yr: bid (8 hr apart).

Tertiary treatment of ocular allergy includes topical or, rarely, oral corticosteroids. Local administration of topical corticosteroids may be associated with increased intracranial pressure, viral infections, and cataract formation.

Allergen immunotherapy can be very effective in seasonal and perennial allergic conjunctivitis, especially when associated with rhinitis, and the need for oral or topical medications to control allergy symptoms can decrease.

Boguniewicz M, Leung DYM. Ocular allergies. In: Kliegman RM, Behrman RE, Jenson HB, Stanton BF (eds). *Nelson Textbook of Pediatrics.* 18th edn. Vol. 1. Philadelphia: Saunders, 2007; 978–79.

Leibowitz HM. The red eye. *N Engl J Med* 2004;351:2203–17.
Stahl JL, Barney NP. Ocular allergic disease. *Curr Opin Allergy Clin Immunol* 2004;4:455–9.

11.10 ADVERSE REACTIONS TO FOODS

Adverse reactions to foods consist of any untoward reaction following the ingestion of a food or food additive and are classically divided into *food intolerance*, which are adverse physiologic responses, and *food hypersensitivities*, which include adverse immunologic responses and allergies. From a clinical and diagnostic point of view, it is most useful to subdivide food hypersensitivity disorders by the predominant target organ and immune mechanism.

Gastrointestinal manifestations: Gastrointestinal food allergies are often the first form of allergy to affect infants and young children and typically present as irritability, vomiting or 'spitting-up," diarrhea, and poor weight gain. Symptoms are most commonly provoked by cow's milk or soy protein-based formulas but also occur from food proteins passed in maternal breast milk. A similar enterocolitis syndrome occurs in older infants and children from rice, oat, wheat, egg, peanut, nuts, and chicken, turkey, or fish sensitivity. Hypotension occurs in about 15% of cases after allergen ingestion. *Gastrointestinal anaphylaxis* generally presents as acute abdominal pain and vomiting that accompany IgE-mediated allergic symptoms in other target organs.

Skin manifestations: Cutaneous food allergies are also common in infants and young children, such as atopic dermatitis (*see* page 294) and acute urticaria and angioedema (*see* page 297).

Respiratory manifestations: Respiratory food allergies are uncommon as isolated symptoms. *Food-induced rhinoconjunctivitis* symptoms typically accompany allergic symptoms on other target organs, such as skin, and consist of typical allergic rhinitis symptoms (periocular pruritus and tearing, nasal congestion and pruritus, sneezing, rhinorrhea. Wheezing occurs in about 25% of IgE-mediated food allergic reactions, but only about 10% of asthmatic patients have food-induced respiratory symptoms.

Cardiovascular manifestations: In addition to the rapid onset of cutaneous, respiratory, and gastrointes-tinal symptoms, patients may develop **cardiovascular symptoms**, including hypotension, cardiovascular collapse and cardiac dysrhythmias, presumably caused by massive mast cell-mediator release.

Anaphylaxis: Food allergic reactions are the single most common cause of anaphylaxis seen in hospital emergency departments. *Food-associated exercise-induced anaphylaxis* is occurring more frequently among teenage athletes, especially females.

Diagnosis: A detailed medical history is necessary to differentiate whether a patient's symptomatology represents an adverse reaction, whether the adverse food reaction is an intolerance or hypersensitivity reaction. Prick skin tests and radioallergosorbent tests are useful for demonstrating IgE sensitization. A negative skin test virtually excludes an IgE-mediated form of food allergy. Serum food-specific IgE levels ≥ 15 KUa/L for milk (≥ 5 KUa/L for children ≥ 1 yr), ≥ 7 KUa/L for egg (≥ 2 KUa/L for children < 3 yr), and ≥ 14 KUa/L for peanut are associated with a > 95% likelihood of clinical reactivity to these foods.

Treatment: Appropriate identification and elimination of foods responsible for food hypersensitivity reactions are the only correct treatment. Complete elimination

of common foods (milk, egg, soy, wheat, rice, chicken, fish, peanut, nuts) is very difficult because of their widespread use in a variety of processed food. The Food Allergy and Anaphylaxis Network (www. foodallergy.org) provides information to help parents deal with both the practical and emotional issues regarding these diets. Children with asthma and IgE-mediated food allergy, peanut or nut allergy, or history of a previous severe reaction should be given self-injectable epinephrine and a written emergency plan in case of accidental ingestion (*see* page 299). Since many food allergies are outgrown, children should be reevaluated periodically. Anti-IgE immunoglobulin therapy may be more definitive means of treating food allergies or raise the threshold for adverse reactions.

Prevention: For prevention of food allergies, recommendations include promotion of breastfeeding (excluding breastfeeding for first 6 mo and to continue breastfeeding for 2 yr) with maternal exclusion of peanut or nut products from the mother's diet and delay in introducing major allergenic foods: cow's milk until 1 yr of age; egg until 18–24 mo of age; and peanut, tree nuts, and seafood until 3 yr of age. Skin preparations containing peanut oil should be avoided.

Bischoff SC, Crowe S. Gastrointestinal food allergy: New insights into pathophysiology and clinical perspectives. *Gastrointestinal* 2005;128:1089–113.

Fleischer DM, Conover-Walker LK, Christie L, et al. Peanut allergy: Recurrence and its management. *J Allergy Clin Immunol* 2004;114:1195–201.

Sampson HA, Leung DYM. Adverse reactions to food. In: Kliegman RM, Behrman RE, Jenson HB, Stanton BF (eds). *Nelson Textbook of Pediatrics.* 18th edn. Vol. 1. Philadelphia: Saunders, 2007; 986–90.

11.11 ADVERSE DRUG REACTIONS (ADR)

Definitions: The World Health Organization (WHO) definition of adverse drug reactions (ADR), which has been in use for about 30 yr, is a response to a drug that is noxious and unintended and occurs at doses normally used in man for the prophylaxis, diagnosis or therapy of disease, or for modification of physiological function'. But, this definition seems to be restrictive because it considers only incidents in which the use of a drug is appropriate, whereas many adverse events are due to errors in drug administration and non-compliance. Such conservative definitions help to avoid over estimation of the ADR rates in children. When immunologic mechanisms have been shown, these reactions should be classified as *drug allergy*.

The terms, ADR and adverse drug event (ADE) are often used interchangeably. But, this is not always correct. ADE relate to any undesirable event experienced by a patient whilst taking a medicine, regardless of whether the drug is suspected of being related to the event. ADR is a subset of adverse events including those that are suspected of being related to the drug. ADE is defined as 'an injury resulting from medical intervention related to a drug'. These events include non-preventable ones such as unpredictable drug rashes, expected ones such as complications of chemotherapy, and incidents caused by errors in prescribing, dispensing or administering drugs.

Types/classification: ADR in children may be broadly divided into two types, type A and type B. Type A reactions are the more common (80%) and may be predicted from the known properties of the drug. These are dose-dependent and predictable based on the pharmacology of the drug. The more dangerous are Type B reactions. Typically, these are unrelated to the known pharmacology of the drug and are not dose-dependent. These are idiosyncratic and may depend heavily on host factors. Some have an immunological basis and not much is known about the underlying mechanisms. Type B reactions account for 20% of ADRs and carry a high mortality rate.

Clinically, ADR may be classified into three basic categories: (i) **pharmacologic reactions** which are an extension of the drug's desired effect, (ii) **hypersensitivity** reactions and (iii) **idiosyncratic reactions,** which are unrelated to dose or serum drug concentration. Idiosyncratic reactions can affect any organ system and include IgE-mediated reactions such as anaphylaxis, teratogenicity and carcinogenicity, as well as reactive metabolite syndromes such as hypersensitivity-syndrome reactions, serum sickness like reactions, and drug-induced lupus. These ADRs are not dose-related and may be related to an unusual biotransformation of the drug to a reactive intermediate. This intermediate, then may act as a hapten or may injure cells directly. Vervloet (1998) has classified ADR based on the susceptibility; drug overdosage, side effects and interactions that occur in any child versus drug intolerance, allergy and idiosyncrasy that occur in susceptible children. This classification is given in Table 11.10. ADR may also be classified as predictable or unpredictable. Predictable ADRs may either be avoidable or modifiable, such as toxicity, drug interactions and secondary effects. Unpredictable and unavoidable ADR include idiosyncratic or allergic reactions as well as drug intolerance.

Mechanisms of ARD in children: The mechanisms for ADRs include the following: pharmacologic/dose-related, drug interactions, idiosyncratic and immunologic drug interactions. Immunologic processes can lead to ADRs through classic anaphylaxis—Type I IgE mediated penicillin allergy or through any other type of immune response: Type II (IgG mediated cytotoxicity/hemolytic anaemia due to alpha-methyldopa and Type III IgG mediated serum sickness due to penicillins or Type IV cell-mediated hypersensitivity due to topical agents.

Risk factors for ADR: Risk factors for ADRs in children include multiple drug exposure, complex multisystem illness, inappropriate medication prescribing or monitoring, prior history of ADRs, genetic predisposition, younger age, prolonged hospital stay and parent or prescriber related increase in administered dosage. The developmental

Table 11.10: Types of adverse drug reactions in children according to susceptibility	
Reactions that may occur in any child	*Reactions that occur only in susceptible children*
Drug overdose Toxic reactions linked to excess dose or impaired excretion, or to both	**Drug intolerance** A low threshold to the normal pharmacological action of a drug
Drug side effect Undesirable pharmacological effect at recommended doses	**Drug idiosyncrasy** A genetically determined, qualitatively abnormal reaction to a drug related to a metabolic or enzyme deficiency
Drug interaction Action of a drug on the effectiveness or toxicity of another drug	**Drug allergy** An immunologically mediated reaction, characterised by specificity, transferability by antibodies or lymphocytes, and recurrence on re-exposure
	Pseudoallergic reaction A reaction with the same clinical manifestations as an allergic reaction (e.g., as a result of histamine release) but lacking immunological specificity

Source: Vervloet D, Durham S. ABC of allergies: Adverse reactions to drugs *BMJ* 1998;316:1511–4

processes in children may be susceptible to certain agents and a number of drugs used in pediatric disease can produce specific ADR, unique to children.

ADR in neonates: The neonate is potentially at significant risk for ADR because of underdeveloped mechanisms and systems for handling drugs. The 'Gray Baby Syndrome' with chloramphenicol is a classic example. This is because infants in neonatal intensive care units are often critically ill with multiple organ system dysfunctions, on multiple drugs and they may present with an ADR as a result of exposure as a fetus. Neonates are also exposed to many drugs before birth because of transplacental transfer of drugs. The lack of information on drug action in neonates and altered disposition, metabolism and renal excretion of drugs could be another reason for the less reported ADR in neonates.

Detection of ADR and monitoring: Most hospitals identify ADR and ADEs using spontaneous reporting, but this approach lacks sensitivity. *Chart review* is an excellent method for detecting errors in drug ordering and has a proven track record in the research arena. But this method is personnel intensive, costly, and only marginally effective at detecting errors in drug administration and monitoring. *Computer-based approaches to ADR identification* appear promising, but they have not been directly compared with chart review and they are not widely used. Implementation of a computer monitoring system that automatically generates laboratory signals may help to identify ADRs in children and to reduce morbidity and hospital stay, as well as costs. The detection rate of ADRs would almost be doubled by a computerized monitoring system that analyzes laboratory data. Patient safety indicators based on discharge coding have been proposed to identify children at risk for an ADE.

Reporting: ADR reporting systems may serve as the first-line surveillance method to identify ADRs of newly approved drugs as well as serious and unknown adverse reactions related to drugs that have been longer on the market in large patient populations. *Post-marketing surveillance* is essential for getting insight into the ADRs among children and their determinants may prevent unnecessary damage by drugs in future use. Simplifying the reporting process can encourage physicians and nurses to document ADRs themselves or to solicit follow-up reporting of ADRs by pharmacists.

Management: Methods reported to reduce the occurrence of ADR in children include improving the documentation of patient allergy/drug reaction histories, educating staff about proper medication administration, improving techniques for patient monitoring, and pursuing further investigation through formal drug utilization evaluations. The management of severe ADRs may well entail multiple changes in therapy and the use of corticosteroids as a 'blanket measure' to reduce inflammation and immuno-logical responses. It has also been recommended that treatment decision-making should be shared with the patients/parents and that efforts should be made to improve the communication process between doctors and the family.

Edwards IE, Aronson JK. Averse drug reactions: definitions, diagnosis and management. *Lancet* 2000;356:1255–1259.

Jha AK, Kuperman GJ, Teich JM, et al. Identifying adverse drug events: Development of a Computer-based Monitor and comparison with Chart Review and Stimulated Voluntary Report. *J American Medical Informatics Association* 1998;(5)3:305–14.

Knowles SR, Uetrecht J, Shear NH. Idiosyncratic drug reactions: The reactive metabolite syndromes *Lancet* 2000;356:1587–91.

Kramer MS, Hutchinson TA, Kenneth M, et al. Adverse drug reactions in general pediatric outpatients. *J Pediatr* 1985;06:305–10.

Lazarou J, Pomeranz B, Corey P. Incidence of adverse drug reactions in hospitalized patients. *JAMA* 1998; 279:1200–05.

McKnight A. Adverse drug reactions in neonates. J Clin Pharmacol 1994;34:128–35.

Rheumatic Diseases of Childhood

12.1 JUVENILE RHEUMATOID ARTHRITIS

Juvenile rheumatoid arthritis (JRA) is a common rheumatic disease of children and a major cause of chronic disability. The American college of Rheumatology (ACR) has defined it as arthritis of one or more joints, with age of onset < 16 years, and persisting for at least 6 wk with exclusion of other specific disease such as juvenile ankylosing spondylitis, juvenile psoriatic arthritis or arthritis associated with inflammatory disease. The estimated prevalence rates varies in the range of 0.4–1.3 per 1000 children. A new nomenclature, juvenile idiopathic arthritis (JIA), is increasingly used and is replacing the term JRA.

Etiopathogenesis: JRA is an autoimmune disease with major histocompatibility complex (MHC) associated with genetic predisposition. α-HLA class I antigen A2 is associated with early onset oligoarthritis in girls and HLA B27 with late onset oligoarthritis in boys. Specific HLA class II antigens are also associated with certain pattern of JRA. Polyarthritis is associated with HLA-DR4, particularly the DRB1*0401 and 0404 alleles. Oligoarthritis is associated with HLA alleles at the DR8, particularly DRB1*0801, and DR5, particularly DRB1*1104.

Both humoral and cell-mediated immunity are involved in the pathogenesis of JRA. T cell from the synovial fluid or membrane has increased expression of activation markers. CD8 suppressor T-lymphocyte deficiency or altered function may permit over-production of auto-antibodies. Abnormal expression of inflammatory cytokines IL-6, IL-1 and TNF-α may be present in systemic onset JRA, whereas IL-2α is elevated in polyarticular or oligoarticular JRA. B cell abnormalities include increase in immunoglobulin level, antibodies to specific virus and auto-antibodies.

Complement activation and consumption also play a role in the perpetuation of inflammatory reaction in JRA. Several environmental trigger include infection (parvovirus B19, rubella, Epstein-Barr virus), *Mycobacterium tuberculosis, Mycoplasma pneumonia*) are linked to the onset of JRA.

Classification: The ACR classifies JRA into 3 distinct subtypes: Pauciarticular JRA, Polyarticular JRA, and systemic JRA (Table 12.1). The ACR criteria for the classification of JRA are the simplest and most widely used.

Clinical manifestations: Initial symptoms may be subtle or acute, and often include morning stiffness, easy fatigability, particularly after school in the early afternoon, joint pain later in the day, and objective joint swelling. The involved joints are often warm, resist full range of motion, painful on motion, limping may be observed in involvement lower extremity and weight loss.

Oligoarthritis (Pauciarticular JRA) is defined as arthritis that involves ≤ 4 joints in the first 6 months of disease. Chronic involvement can result in atrophy of extensor

	Polyarthritis	Oligoarthritis Type I	Type II	Systemic
Table 12.1: ACR classification of JRA				
Frequency of case	30%		60%	10%
No. of joints involved	> 5		< 4	Variable
Pattern of joint involvement	Large as well as small joints	Large joint	Large joint usually lower limb, asymmetrical	
Age of onset childhood peak 1–3 year	Throughout peak 1–2 year	Early childhood >8 year	Older children childhood. No peak	Throughout
Sex ratio (F : M)	3 : 1	5:1	Commonly in boys	1 : 1
Systemic involvement	Moderate	Absent	Absent	Prominent
Occurrence of uveitis	5%	20% may occur	Rare, acute uveitis	Rare
Frequency of seropositivity				
• **Rheumatoid factor**	10%	Rare	Rare	Rare
• **Antinuclear antibodies**	40–50%	75–85%	Rare	10%
• **HLA B27**	Absent	Absent	Present	Rare
Outcome	Guarded to moderately good	Excellent except for eyesight		Moderate to poor

muscles in the thigh, tight hamstring ligaments, and knee flexion contractures. Leg length discrepancies occur in the involved limb with asymmetric arthritis. Isolated involvement of upper extremity large joints is not characteristic of this type of onset.

Polyarthritis (polyarticular JRA) is generally involves ≥ 5 joints involves characterized by involvement of both large and small joints of both upper and lower extremities. Severe limitations in motion are usually accompanied by muscle weakness and decreased physical function. Low grade fever can accompany the arthritis. Rheumatoid nodules on the extensor surfaces of the elbows and over the Achilles tendons, while unusual, are associated with a more severe course. Presence of rheumatoid factor (RF) differentiates the two forms of polyarticular disease of JRA. Children are also at risk for developing chronic iridocyclitis or uveitis especially those who are ANA positive. Specific articular complications are cervical spine involvement leading to atlantoaxial subluxation and temporo-mandibular joint involvement leading to micrognathia.

Systemic-onset JRA is characterized by arthritis and prominent visceral involvement that includes hepatosplenomegaly, lymphadenopathy, muscle tenderness, pericarditis, pleuritis, myocarditis, or pericardial effusion. Typical rash, fever and arthritis are characteristic of systemic-onset JRA, independent of the number of joints involved. Each febrile episode is accompanied by a characteristic faint, erythematous,

macular rash; these evanescent salmon-colored lesions with a linear distribution commonly over the trunk and proximal extremities. *The Koebner phenomenon* is cutaneous hypersensitivity to superficial trauma resulting in a localized recurrence of the rash, and is suggestive of systemic-onset disease. Heat, such as warm bath, also evokes a reappearance of the rash.

Laboratory investigation reveals hematologic abnormalities often reflect the degree of systemic or articular inflammation, with elevated white blood cell and platelet counts and decreased hemoglobin concentration and mean corpuscular volume. Elevated antinuclear antibody (ANA) titers are present in at least 40–85% of children with oligoarticular or polyarticular JRA, but are unusual in children with systemic-onset disease. Rheumatoid factor (RF) is present in less than 10% of children with JRA. Synovial fluid aspiration for microscopy and culture is indicated if septic arthritis is suspected. X-ray of the affected joints in the early stages only reveals periarticular soft tissue swelling, increased joint space and juxta-articular osteoporosis. It is only in the later stage that joint space narrowing, marginal erosions, subluxation and ankylosis are observed.

Differential diagnosis: Arthritis can be the presenting manifestation for any of the rheumatic diseases of childhood, including systemic lupus erythematosus (SLE), juvenile dermatomyositis, sarcoidosis and the vesiculating syndromes (*see* Figs 12.1 to 12.3 in CD).

Management: The objective of the management of the JRA is to control inflammation and the disease process so that these children retain maximum functional capacity, normal physical growth, minimize impact of the chronic disease on the family, educate the child and family and finally rehabilitate the child.

Non-steroidal anti-inflammatory drugs (NSAIDs): NSAIDs are analgesics, antipyretics, and anti-inflammatory. Naproxen is effective in management of joint inflammation in a dose of 15–20 mg/kg/day in two divided doses. Other NSAIDs include ibuprofen (35–45 mg/kg/day), piroxicam (0.3 mg/kg/day), tolmetin, indomethacin (1–2 mg/kg/day) and diclofenac (2–3 mg/kg/day).

Disease modifying antirheumatic drugs (DMARDs): DMARDs are stated if the child does not improve with a 'reasonable' trial of NSAID. In the past a number of drugs (e.g. hydroxychloroquine, d-penicillamine and gold salts) were believed to have significant DMARDs activity. However, they are no longer used as first line drugs. Most children with polyarticular disease or with systemic-onset disease require additional anti-inflammatory therapy. The DMARDs include methotrexate, leflunomide and sulfasalazine. *Methotrexate* remains the remission-inducing agent of first choice for seropositive polyarticular JRA. *Sulphasalazine (SSZ)* has been effective in children with oligoarthritis, spondylitis or seronegative spondyloarthropathies at doses 30–50 mg/kg/day.

Corticosteroid: Corticosteroid therapy is recommended for management of overwhelming inflammatory or systemic illness, for bridge therapy early in disease in lower doses for the child who has not yet responded to conventional therapy. Intra-articular corticosteroid injection is used to treat oligoarthritis. The dosage regimen for triamcinolone hexacetonide is 1 mg/kg for large joint and 0.5 mg/kg for small joints. Local steroids are also indicated in uveitis.

Other drugs: TNF inhibitors (infliximab, etanercept), Cox-2 inhibitors (celecoxib, and rofecoxib) or anti-IL–6R (Tocilizumab) have not been adequately studied in pediatric patients, and the role of these agents, (except for etanercept) in children with JRA remains to be determined. Cytotoxic drug such as azathioprine, cyclosporin, and cyclophosphamide, are reserved for resistant cases.

Autologous hemopoietic stem cell transplantation (AHSCT) has been described as a possible treatment for severe autoimmune disease refractory to conventional treatment.

Physiotherapy: All children with arthritis should be referred to a physiotherapist for an effective rehabilitation program. Good physiotherapy is essential so that contracture can be prevented deformities can be minimized. Occupational therapy is required for continuing the activities of daily living.

Complications

Systemic-onset JRA includes endarteritis, pericarditis, hemolytic anemia, disseminated intravascular coagulopathy, and macrophage activation syndrome (MAS). The acute development of a profound anemia associated with thrombocytopenia or leukopenia with a high, spiking fever, lymphadenopathy, and hepatosplenomegaly occurs with the MAS, a rare and occasionally fatal complication of systemic JRA. This diagnosis is suggested by clinical criteria and confirmed by bone marrow biopsy demonstrating hemophagocytosis.

Pauciarticular JRA is associated with knee flexion contractures, uveitis, and leg length discrepancy.

Polyarticular JRA is associated with skeletal abnormalities: Swan-neck or Boutonniere deformities, joint subluxation, and cervical spine involvement.

Prognosis: The course of JRA in an individual child is unpredictable. Children with oligoarthritis, particularly girls with onset of arthritis at an age of < 6 yr, are at risk to develop chronic uveitis. The child with polyarticular disease often has a more prolonged course of active inflammation of the joints. The child with systemic-onset disease is often the most difficult to control in terms of both articular inflammation and systemic manifestations. Marked systemic disease is usually present only during the 1st few years after onset and tends to regress over time. Prognosis is dependent on the number of joints involved, duration of active inflammation, and the severity of the arthritis.

Adams A, Lehman TJ. Update on the pathogenesis and treatment of systemic onset juvenile rheumatoid arthritis. *Curr Opin Rheumatol* 2005;17(5):612–16.

Ilowite NT. Current treatment of juvenile rheumatoid arthritis. *Pediatrics* 2002;109(1):109–15.

Petty RE, Southwood TR, Manners P, et al. International League of Associations for Rheumatology classification of juvenile idiopathic arthritis: second revision, Edmonton, 2001. *J Rheumatol* 2004;31(2):390–92.

Ravelli A, Martini A. Early predictors of outcome in juvenile idiopathic arthritis. *Clin Exp Rheumatol* 2003;21(5 Suppl 31):S89–93.

Schwartz MM, Simpson P, Kerr KL, et al. Juvenile rheumatoid arthritis in African Americans. *J Rheumatol* 1997; 24(9):1826–29.

12.2 ANKYLOSING SPONDYLITIS AND OTHER SPONDYLOARTHROPATHIES

Juvenile ankylosing spondylitis (JAS), psoriatic arthritis, arthritis accompanying inflammatory bowel diseases, and chronic reactive arthritis following enteric or genitourinary tract infections are referred to as spondyloarthropathies. These arthritic conditions can cause disease and inflammation in the spine, other joints, eyes, skin, mouth, and various organs. The spondyloarthropathies are linked by common genetics (*HLA B27*) and a common pathology (enthesitis). Genes possibly associated with ankylosing spondylitis include *ANKH* and *HLA DRB1*. The cause of ankylosing spondylitis is unknown, but a combination of genetic and environmental factors works in concert to produce clinical disease. JAS (juvenile ankylosing spondylitis) occurs most frequently in older boys, adolescents, and young adults. Psoriatic arthritis is common in young girls. The arthropathies of inflammatory bowel diseases (IBDs) and reactive arthritis are much less common in childhood. **Spondyloarthropathies are characterized by inflammation of joints of the axial skeleton as well as the limbs, by the presence of enthesitis, and by the absence of rheumatoid factor. Symptoms include back pain, peripheral enthesitis, arthropathy, and constitutional manifestations. Morning stiffness is characteristic, and fatigue is common. Fever and weight loss may occur during periods of active disease.**

Enthesitis is characterized by chronic inflammation, and calcification of ligaments and fusion of joints. Tenosynovitis and periostitis may occur. Chronic reactive arthritis may follow enteric infection with Salmonella, *Shigella*, *Yersinia enterocolitica*, *Campylobacter jejuni*, or *Giardia intestinalis*. The cause of the other spondyloarthropathies is considered as molecular mimicry.

Laboratory findings: Laboratory evidence of systemic inflammation is often present with elevated ESR, mild leukocytosis and thrombocytosis. The serum IgA level may be elevated. Rheumatoid factor is absent in all children with spondyloarthropathies. HLA B27 is present in > 90% of children with JAS. Radiographic changes include periarticular osteoporosis, loss of sharp cortical margins in areas of enthesitis, and erosions of the sacroiliac joints. The inflammatory lesions at vertebral enthuses may result in sclerosis of the superior and inferior margins of the vertebral bodies, called shiny corners (Romanus lesion). MRI or CT scanning of the sacroiliac and peripheral joints may reveal evidence of early sacroiliitis, erosions, and enthesitis that are not apparent on standard radiographs. The characteristic of advanced ankylosing spondylitis in adults is bamboo spine caused by calcification of ligaments but very rare in childhood.

Treatment: The goal of treatment for JAS is to reduce pain and stiffness, prevent deformities, and help the child maintain as normal and active a lifestyle as possible. Nonsteroidal anti-inflammatory drugs, such as naproxen (15–20 mg/kg/day), may be sufficient. It may be necessary to add sulfasalazine (up to 50 mg/kg/day; maximum: 3 g/day). In patients not responsive to these medications, oral or subcutaneous methotrexate may be considered. The TNF-blocking medications (etanercept or infliximab) have been shown to be extremely effective for treating ankylosing spondylitis in adults. Surgery is useful to correct spinal deformities or to repair damaged peripheral joints. Exercise to maintain range of motion in the back, thorax, and affected joints should be instituted early in the disease course.

Complications: Acute iridocyclitis or anterior uveitis occurs in about 25% of patients with JAS. Chronic iridocyclitis occurs in approximately 15% of children with psoriatic arthritis. Aortic valve insufficiency is a rare but important complication of ankylosing spondylitis. Atlantoaxial subluxation has also been reported.

Prognosis: JAS is often have long periods of active disease followed by long periods of inactivity. Poor physical function at onset and early hip involvement are predictors of severe chronic disease. Psoriatic arthritis tends to be a chronic unremitting disease. Reactive arthritis may be brief (several weeks or months), but may become chronic and progress to ankylosing spondylitis. In children with inflammatory bowel disease, the peripheral arthritis is usually controlled when the gastrointestinal inflammation is controlled; if the arthritis is associated with HLA B27, the course tends to be more chronic.

Braun J, Sieper J. Ankylosing spondylitis. *Lancet* 2007; 369(9570):1379–90.

Dincer U, Cakar E, Kiralp MZ, Dursun H. Diagnosis delay in patients with ankylosing spondylitis: possible reasons and proposals for new diagnostic criteria. *Clin Rheumatol* 2008;27(4):457–62.

Reveille JD, Arnett FC. Spondyloarthritis: update on pathogenesis and management. *Am J Med* 2005;118(6):592–603.

Tse SM, Laxer RM. Juvenile spondyloarthropathy. *Curr Opin Rheumatol* 2003;15(4):374–9.

van der Linden S, van der Heijde D. Ankylosing spondylitis. Clinical features. *Rheum Dis Clin North Am* 1998;24(4):663–76.

12.3 REACTIVE ARTHRITIS

Reactive arthritis is a joint inflammation developing after or during an infection elsewhere in the body, but the organism cannot be isolated from the joint. Reactive arthritis has been associated with gastrointestinal infections with *Shigella*, *Salmonella*, and *Campylobacter* species as well as with genitourinary infections (especially with *Chlamydia trachomatis*).

Reactive arthritis usually develops 2–4 wk after a genitourinary or gastrointestinal infection. Inflammation of joints, axial skeleton, skin, mucous membranes, gastrointestinal tract, and eyes may occur. Urinary tract inflammation commonly involves the urethra. About 10% of people with reactive arthritis, especially those with prolonged disease will develop cardiac manifestations including aortic regurgitation and pericarditis. *Reiter triad* includes urethritis, conjunctivitis, and arthritis may occur. The likelihood of developing reactive arthritis is increased 50-fold in patients who are HLA B27 positive.

Laboratory findings: ESR and CRP (C-reactive protein) are elevated at the onset of the disease and later may become normal in the chronic stage of the disease. There may be mild leukocytosis and anemia in the early phase. The rheumatoid factor is usually negative. Gram staining and bacterial culture of the synovial fluid should be performed to differentiate from septic arthritis.

Treatment: The main goal of treatment is to identify and eradicate the underlying infectious source with the appropriate antibiotics if still present. NSAID, corticosteroids and immunosuppressant may be needed for patients with severe reactive symptoms that do not respond to any other treatment. Sulfasalazine may be beneficial in some patients. Methotrexate can be used in patients who present with rheumatoid-like disease.

Barth WF, Segal K. Reactive arthritis (Reiter's syndrome). *Am Fam Physician* 1999;60(2):499–503, 507.

Keat A. Reiter's syndrome and reactive arthritis in perspective. *N Eng J Med* 1983;309:1606–15.

Kvien T, Glennas A, Melby K, et al. Reactive arthritis: Incidence, triggering agents and clinical presentation. *J Rheumatol* 1994;21:115.

Wu IB, Schwartz RA. Reiter's syndrome: The classic triad and more. *J Am Acad Dermatol* 2008;59(1):113–21.

12.4 SYSTEMIC LUPUS ERYTHEMATOSUS

Etiology: The cause and disease mechanisms of lupus remain unknown. Many factors, including genetic predisposition, hormones, and environment, potentially trigger immune dysregulation. The hallmark of lupus is autoantibody production against many self antigens, particularly antinuclear antibodies (ANAs) to DNA and other nuclear antigens, such as ribosomes, small nuclear (anti-Sm) and cytoplasmic (anti-Ro, anti-La) ribonuclear proteins, platelets, coagulation factors, immunoglobulins, erythrocytes, and leukocytes.

Epidemiology: The incidence of lupus is not known but varies by location and ethnicity. Prevalence rates of 4–250/100,000 have been reported, with increased prevalence among Asians, Native Americans, Hispanics, and African-Americans. Disease onset before 8 yr of age is unusual, although lupus has been diagnosed even in the 1st yr of life. Female preponderance varies from 4 : 1 before puberty to 8:1 afterwards.

Pathogenesis: Lupus is characterized by production of autoantibodies and polyclonal activation of B lymphocytes that results in elevated immunoglobulin levels, which also contribute to elevated autoantibody levels. Possible causes include nonspecific responses to antigenic stimuli such as viral agents, or following loss of either B cell immune tolerance to self antigens or suppressor T cell function. Fibrinoid deposits resulting from changes in collagen fibers and ground substance are found in blood vessel walls of affected organs. The parenchyma may contain *hematoxylin bodies*, most likely representing degenerated cell nuclei. Rheumatoid nodules and granulomas are sometimes also found in affected tissues.

Clinical manifestations: Children most frequently present with fever, fatigue, hematologic abnormalities, arthralgia or arthritis, rash, and renal disease. Symptoms may be intermittent or persistent (Table 12.2) (*see* Figs 12.1 to 12.7 in CD).

Diagnosis: The diagnosis of lupus is confirmed by the combination of clinical and laboratory manifestations revealing multi-system disease. The presence of 4 of 11 criteria serially or simultaneously strongly suggests the diagnosis (Table 12.2). Patients suspected to have lupus demonstrating fewer than 4 criteria should receive appropriate medical attention. In 1997, revised criteria replaced the LE prep with anticardiolipin antibodies or a positive test for lupus anticoagulant. A positive ANA test is not required for diagnosis; absence of ANA in lupus is very rare. Hypocomplementemia is not diagnostic and extremely low levels or absence of total hemolytic complement suggests the possibility of complement component deficiency. Renal biopsy is useful to confirm the diagnosis of lupus nephritis and to guide treatment.

Differential diagnosis: The lupus must be considered in the differential diagnosis of many problems, ranging from fevers of unknown origin to arthralgias, anemia, and nephritis. Lupus should be considered in patients with multiorgan symptoms, especially if there are hematologic or urinalysis abnormalities. *Drug-induced lupus* is a lupus-like disease that is precipitated by exposure to certain drugs, notably many anticonvulsants, sulfonamides, and antiarrhythmic agents. The typical symptoms of fever, rash, and pleuropericardial disease typically abate with discontinuation of the

Table 12.2: 1997 revised classification criteria for systemic lupus erythematosus

Criterion*	Definition
1. Malar rash	Fixed erythema, flat or raised, over the malar eminences, tending to spare the nasolabial folds
2. Discoid rash	Erythematous raised patches with adherent keratotic scaling and follicular plugging; atrophic scarring may occur in older lesions
3. Photosensitivity	Rash as a result of unusual reaction to sunlight (elicited by patient history or physician observation)
4. Oral ulcers	Oral and nasopharyngeal ulceration, usually painless observed by physician
5. Arthritis	Non-erosive arthritis involving two or more peripheral joints characterized by tenderness, swelling, or effusion
6. Serositis	Pleuritis: Convincing history of pleuritic pain or rub heard by a physician or evidence of pleural effusion or pericarditis documented by ECG or rub or evidence of pericardial effusion
7. Renal disorder	Persistent proteinuria > 0.5 g/day or > 3 plus (+++), if quantitation not performed or Cellular casts: may be red blood cell, hemoglobin, granular, tubular, or mixed
8. Neurologic disorder	Seizures: In the absence of offending drugs or known metabolic derangements (e.g. uremia, ketoacidosis, or electrolyte imbalance) or psychosis: In the absence of offending drugs or known metabolic derangements (e.g. uremia, ketoacidosis, or electrolyte imbalance)
9. Hematologic disorder	Hemolytic anemia with reticulocytosis or leukopenia: $< 4000/mm^3$ total on two or more occasions or lymphopenia: $< 1500/mm^3$ on two or more occasions or thrombocytopenia $< 100,000/mm^3$
10. Immunologic disorder	Anti-DNA antibody to native DNA in abnormal titer or Anti-Smith: presence of antibody to Smith nuclear antigen or positive finding of anti-phospholipid antibodies based on (i) an abnormal serum level of IgG or IgM anticardiolipin antibodies; (ii) a positive test result lupus anticoagulant using a standard method; or (iii) a false-positive serologic test for syphilis known to be positive for at least 6 mo and confirmed by *Treponema pallidum* immobilization or fluorescent treponemal antibody absorption test (FTA-ABS), standard methods should be used in testing for the presence of antiphospholipid
11. Antinuclear antibody	An abnormal titer of antinuclear antibody by immunofluorescence or an equivalent assay at any time and in the absence of drugs known to be associated with "drug-induced lupus syndrome"

*This proposed classification is based on 11 criteria. For the purpose of identifying patients in clinical studies, a person shall be said to have SLE, if any 4 or more of the 11 criteria are present seriously or simultaneously during any interval of observation. (Source: Tan EM, Cohen AS, Fries JF, et al. The 1982 revised criteria for the classification of systemic lupus erythematosus. *Arthritis Rheum* 1982;25:1271–7.)

An approved modification deletes the positive LE cell preparation from the immunologic disorder criteria and substitutes the presence of a biologic false-positive test for syphilis. (From Hochberg MC. Updating the American College of Rheumatology revised criteria for the classification of systemic lupus erythematosus. *Arthritis Rheum* 1997; 40:1725. Reprinted with permission of Wiley-Liss, Inc., a subsidiary of John Wiley & Sons, Inc.)

drug. The serum complement usually remains normal and complications, including renal disease, are rare.

Laboratory findings: Elevated ANA titers are often present in children with active lupus. Elevated ANA is an excellent screening tool, although ANA can be found without any disease or can be associated with rheumatic and other conditions. Conditions associated with antinuclear antibodies (ANAs) include systemic lupus erythematosus; juvenile arthritis; drug-induced lupus; juvenile dermatomyositis; vasculitis syndromes; infectious mononucleosis; chronic active hepatitis; hyperextensibility. Levels of anti-double-stranded DNA, which are more specific for lupus, often reflect the degree of serologic disease activity. Serum levels of total hemolytic complement (CH_{50}), C3, and C4 are decreased in active disease. Anti-Smith antibody, found specifically in patients with lupus, does not measure disease activity. Many autoantibodies can be found (Table 12.3). Hypergammaglobulinemia is common but nonspecific. The *lupus anticoagulant*, found in 2/3 of patients is associated with antiphospholipid antibodies. It reacts with cardiolipin used in the serologic test for syphilis and may result in a false-positive test, and also reacts with the phospholipid reagent used in the partial thromboplastin time (PTT), causing an elevated result. It is associated with increased incidence of deep venous thrombosis and neurologic disease including stroke and psychosis.

Table 12.3: Autoantibodies often found in systemic lupus erythematosus

Antibody	Manifestation
Coombs' antibodies	Hemolytic anemia
Antiphospholipid antibodies	Antiphospholipid antibody syndrome
Lupus anticoagulant	Coagulopathy (thrombosis)
Antithyroid antibodies	Hypothyroidism
Antiribosomal P antibody	Lupus cerebritis

Treatment: The goal of management of SLE patients is to prevent disease flares, and hence delay/prevent morbidity and mortality. Lupus is a lifelong illness, and patients require monitoring indefinitely. Deaths early in the course of disease are usually due to infections and active disease, and those that occur later in the disease course are often due to atherosclerotic vascular and renal complications. Timely and aggressive therapy, is therefore crucial. The first 3 years of disease may be most critical, requiring close monitoring of patients and good control of disease activity. The severity of the disease decreases 5 years after the onset.

Patients and parents must learn to cope with and monitor their own disease. In order to minimize exacerbation of a flare, it is prudent that patients can recognize triggers. Common triggers are prolonged sunlight or fluorescent light exposure, smoking, stress. Computer screens can also be a source of ultraviolet rays. Dietary modification may also be necessary. Animal studies have shown dietary fat restriction and low zinc intake is beneficial. Fish oil supplementation with a low saturated fat diet has also been shown to be helpful.

The treatment regimen depends on the affected target organs and disease severity. Sun exposure should be minimized and include use of a sunscreen. Patients are treated to promote clinical well-being, using serologic markers of disease activity as guidelines, including serum complement levels. *Nonsteroidal anti-inflammatory agents*, used to treat arthralgia and arthritis, are used with caution because patients with lupus are more susceptible to hepatotoxicity. *Hydroxychloroquine* is often used to treat mild manifestations including skin lesions, fatigue, arthritis, and arthralgia; may also reduce the risk of thromboembolic disease and lowers lipid levels.

Patients with thrombosis and antiphospholipid antibodies or a lupus anticoagulant should receive anticoagulant medication at least until lupus is in remission. Low molecular weight *heparin* is the anticoagulant of choice; warfarin can also be used.

Corticosteroids control symptoms and autoantibody production in lupus. Treatment with corticosteroids has improved kidney disease and the rate of survival. All patients should have PPD, when possible, before corticosteroids are initiated. Patients with systemic disease are often started on 1–2 mg/kg/24 hr of oral prednisolone (or prednisone) in divided daily doses. When complement levels increase to within the normal range, the dose is carefully tapered to the lowest effective dose. Alternate-day high-dose corticosteroids once disease is controlled to prevent the adverse effects of daily corticosteroid administration may be used instead of daily lowest effective dose. Severely ill patients may require pulse intravenous corticosteroid therapy (30 mg/kg/dose, maximum 1 g/day, given over 60 min, for 3 days). Intermittent high-dose intravenous therapy in combination with low-dose daily oral corticosteroids may be used as an alternative regimen. Adverse effects of corticosteroids include hypertension, gastritis, cataracts, osteopenia, and cushingoid body habitus. *Methotrexate, cyclosporin*, and *mycophenolate mofetil* are used as steroid-sparing agents.

Patients with severe disease may require *cytotoxic* therapy. *Cyclophosphamide* is used to treat vasculitis, pulmonary hemorrhage, and central nervous system involvement. Pulse intravenous cyclophosphamide has maintained renal function and prevented progression in patient with lupus nephritis, particularly diffuse proliferative glomerulonephritis. *Azathioprine* has been used to prevent renal disease progression. Adverse effects of cytotoxic therapy include secondary infections, gonadal dysfunction, and possibly increased risk of later malignancies. Prepubertal children, compared with those who have entered puberty, may be at less risk for subsequent gonadal dysfunction from cytotoxic agents. Other potential therapies include autologous stem cell and allogeneic bone marrow transplantation.

Renal biopsy for staging can help determine whether an immunosuppressive agent such as cyclophosphamide needs to be added to a corticosteroid regimen. Biopsy findings according to the World Health Organization classification, which was modified in 2004, correlate with the morbidity and mortality, classified in to six classes. The six classes include: Class I minimal mesangial change without proteinuria or hematuria; Class II mesangial proliferation; Class III focal proliferative glomerulonephritis; Class IV diffuse segmental or global proliferative glomerulonephritis; Class V meningoproliferative glomerulonephritis; and Class VI advanced sclerosing nephritis and demonstrates diffuse, chronic damage suggesting progression to renal failure. Both Class I and class II are associated with excellent prognosis. Intravenous pulse cyclophosphamide can decrease the risk of Class IV renal disease.

Complications: The major causes of death in patients with lupus currently include infection, nephritis, central nervous system disease, pulmonary hemorrhage, and myocardial infarction. Lupus nephritis occurs in most children show evidence of progression within 2 yr after onset of symptoms. Persistent leukopenia, anemia or thrombocytopenia may develop.

Prognosis: Untreated lupus may be followed by spontaneous remission, years of smoldering disease, or rapid death. Early diagnosis and treatment to the particular problems of each individual patient significantly improves the course of the disease. The 5 yr survival rate is > 90%. A few patients die of complications of the disease in late adulthood.

Neonatal Lupus

Lupus in newborns results from maternal transfer of IgG autoantibodies, usually anti-Ro/SSA or anti-La/SSB, between the 12th and 16th wk of gestation. Only a small percentage of offspring of mothers with autoantibodies to Ro and/or La develop disease. Symptoms usually derive from a single organ, although multiple organ involvement may occur and include congenital heart block, cutaneous lesions, hepatitis, thrombocytopenia, neutropenia, and pulmonary and neurologic disease. Cutaneous lesions occur after ultraviolet exposure at about 6 wk of life and last 3–4 mo. The rash most frequently occurs on the face and scalp. Treatment is supportive. Most manifestations resolve, although congenital heart block is permanent and often requires cardiac pacing, either after birth or, when detected and severe, antenatally. Corticosteroid treatment of the pregnant mother after heart block is detected early *in utero* and postnatal steroids may be effective. Cardiomyopathy is a rare serious sequela.

Antiphospholipid Antibody (APLA) Syndrome or Antiphospholipid Syndrome (APS) or Hughes Syndrome

The APLA syndrome is an autoimmune hyper-coagulable state caused by antiphospholipid antibodies present mostly in young women. People with this disorder may be otherwise healthy or they also may suffer from an underlying disease most frequently SLE. The term 'primary antiphospholipid syndrome' is used when APLA occurs in the absence of any other related disease. In rare cases, APLA leads to rapid organ failure due to generalized thrombosis, this is termed 'catastrophic antiphospholipid

syndrome' (CAPS) and is associated with a high risk of death. It is a common cause of hypercoagulable states in children and can manifest with arterial and venous thrombosis, livedo reticularis and thrombocytopenia. This presentation may result in fatality. Laboratory diagnosis is based on the detection of anticardiolipin antibodies (IgM and IgG) and the lupus anticoagulant. There is no cure, but medication can be effective in reducing risk of blood clots. It often requires treatment with anticoagulant medication such as heparin to reduce the risk of further episodes of thrombosis and improve the progress of pregnancy.

Ahluwalia J, Singh S, Garewal G. Antiphospholipid antibodies in children with systemic lupus erythematosus: a prospective study from Northern India. *Rheumatoid Int* 2005; 25:530–3.

Ali US, Dalvi RB, Merchant RH, Mehta KP, et al. Systemic lupus erythematosus in Indian children. .*Indian Pediatr* 1989; 26(9):868–73.

Asherson RA, Cervara P, de Groot PG, et al. Catastrophic antiphospholipid syndrome: international consensus statement on classification criteria and treatment guidelines. *Lupus* 2003; 12(7):530–4.

Bongu A, Chang E, Ramsey-Goldman R. Can morbidity and mortality of SLE be improved? *Best Pract Res Clin Rheumatol* 2002;16:313–32.

Gitelman MK, Reiff Andreas, Silverman ED. Systemic Lupus Erythematosus in Childhood. *Rheumatic Disease Clinics of North America* 2002;28:561–77.

Grossman JM, Kalunian KC. Definition, classification, activity and damage indices. In: Wallace D, Hahn BH (eds). *Dubois' Lupus Erythematosus*. 7th edn. Philadelphia, PA: Lippincott, Williams & Wilkins, 2007;16–31.

Iqng IC, Icornich IIIC, Dcrnstcln DII. The clinical spectrum of systemic lupus erythematosus. Proceedings of the conference of rheumatic diseases of childhood. *Arthritis Rheum*.1977; 20(supple2):287–94.

Klein-Gitelman MS, Miller ML. Systemic Lupus erythematosus. In: Kliegman RM, Behrman RE, Jenson HB, Stanton BF (eds). *Nelson Textbook of Pediatrics*. 18th edn. Vol. 1. Philadelphia: Saunders, 2007;1015–19.

Kumar A. Indian guidelines of management of SLE. *J Indian Rheumatol Assoc* 2002;10:80–96.

Petty RE, Cassidy JT. Systemic lupus erythematosus. In: Petty RE, Cassidy JT (eds). *Textbook of Pediatric Rheumatology*. 4th edn. Philadelphia: WB Saunders, 2001;396–449.

Vaidya S, Samant RS, Nadkar MY, et al. Systemic lupus erythematosus—a review of 220 patients. *J Indian Rheumatol Assoc* 1997;5:14–18.

12.5 JUVENILE DERMATOMYOSITIS

Juvenile dermatomyositis (JDM) is characterized by proximal symmetrical muscle weakness, skin rash and vasculitis. The average age at the disease onset is 6.9 yr, with > 25% of children < 4 yr of age. The characteristic cutaneous features include heliotrope rash and Gottron papules. Heliotrope or "lilac" rash is a periorbital violaceous erythema may cross the bridge of the nose, in a mask-like distribution and involve the ears. Gottron's sign is an erythematous, scaly eruption occurring in symmetric fashion over the metacarpophalangeal and interphalangeal joints. Shawl (or V-) sign is a diffuse, flat, erythematous lesion over the chest and shoulders or in a "V" over the anterior neck and chest, worsened with ultraviolet light. Erythroderma is a flat, erythematous lesion located in the malar region and the forehead. Children with an initial myopathic form, with rash may develop myositis and calcinosis later.

Muscle involvement manifests as proximal muscle weakness, detected by difficulty in climbing stairs, walking, rising from a sitting position or combing their hair. Neck flexor weakness is an especially sensitive indicator of muscle weakness. The child usually keeps the limbs in a flexed position, which promotes development of flexion contractures and soft tissue calcification.

Viruses (coxsackievirus, parvovirus, HIV), *Toxoplasma* and *Borrelia* species, and drugs like penicillamine; quinidine agents may trigger the diseases.

Laboratory findings: Elevated serum levels of creatinine kinase, aspartate aminotransferase, serum glutamic-oxaloacetic transaminase, alanine aminotransferase, and lactic dehydrogenase are present. ESR is usually normal, the rheumatoid factor is negative and a positive antinuclear antibody (ANA). Electromyography shows changes suggestive of myopathy. Muscle biopsy shows a mixed B and T cell perivascular inflammatory infiltrate and perifascicular atrophy.

Treatment: Use of intravenous bolus of parenteral steroid (methyl prednisolone 30 mg/kg/day) followed by oral prednisolone (1–2 mg/kg/day) therapy is the method of treatment. If the skin rash is very prominent, hydroxychloroquine is used along with topical steroids and lubricants. Unresponsive children are treated with methotrexate (15–20 mg/m^2/wk), cyclosporin or cyclophosphamide. IV gammaglobulin (1–2 gm/kg) used in resistant cases. The prognosis for survival is improved following use of corticosteroids.

Ansell BM. Juvenile dermatomyositis. *Rheum Dis Clin North Am* 1991;17:931–42.

Feldman BM, Rider LG, Reed AM, et al. Juvenile dermatomyositis and other idiopathic inflammatory myopathies of childhood. *Lancet* 2008;371:2201–12.

Singh S, Kumar L, Ravi Shankar K. Juvenile dermatomyositis in North India. *Indian Pediatr* 1997;34:193–8.

12.6 SCLERODERMA AND RAYNAUD PHENOMENON

Scleroderma affects the skin to cause widespread signs of inflammation that can lead to skin tightness or hardening and affect the fingers, feet, face, and neck. Skin pigmentary changes include a salt-and-pepper appearance, with areas of hyperpigmentation alternating with hypopigmentation, or an overall appearance of tanned skin that persists long after sun exposure. Loss of subcutaneous tissue in the face can result in a small oral stoma. Scarring of the esophagus with difficulty swallowing or localized central chest pain may occur. Calcinosis may develop on the fingers and extremities, usually the extensor side of the forearms and the prepatellar areas. *Raynaud phenomenon* results from arterial spasm which is induced by exposure to cold and mostly affects finger tips, toes, ears, tips of the nose. The typical sequence of color change is blanching (pallor), cyanosis (blue) and then hyperanemia (erythema) may occur. Pain and paresthesias are often present. Abnormalities of nail fold capillaries are seen as capillary dropouts and dilated loops. *CREST syndrome* refers to manifestation of calcinosis, Raynaud's phenomenon, esophageal dysmotility, sclerodactyly and telangiectasia.

Laboratory findings: Investigation shows presence of antinuclear antibodies and anticentromere antibody. Anti-Scl-70 antibody (antitopoisomerase I antibody) is seen in diffuse scleroderma patient.

Treatment: There is no direct cure for scleroderma. Penicillamine increases soluble collagen and is the preferred drug for the treatment of skin thickening (Dose: start with 125–250 mg OD then to 250 mg BD). Additional treatment includes physical and occupational therapy to improve flexion contractures and maintain muscle strength, and spring-loading splints in selected patients. Raynaud phenomenon can be treated with calcium channel blockers (sustained release, nifedipine 30–60 mg, PO, QD; amlodipine besylate); angiotensin-converting enzyme inhibitors (captopril, enalapril), and topical vasodilators (nitroglycerin paste) may be useful in preventing or ameliorating fingertip ulcerations. Vascular compromise threatening to lead to gangrene and autoamputation of the distal digits may respond to parenteral administration of prostaglandin E$_1$ (alprostadil). Local measures keeping the hands warm with leather gloves during cold exposure are extremely important.

Miller M L. Scleroderma and Raynaud phenomenon. In: Kliegman RM, Behrman RE, Jenson HB, Stanton BF (eds). *Nelson Textbook of Pediatrics*. 18th edn. Vol. 1. Philadelphia: Saunders, 2007;1024–27.

Sapadin AN, Fleischmajer R. Treatment of scleroderma. *Arch Dermatol* 2002;138 (1):99–105.

Tripathi KD (Ed). Antirheumatoid and antigout drugs. In: *Essential Medical Pharmacology*. 6th edn. New Delhi: Jaypee Brothers Medical Publishers (P) Ltd, 2008;202–10.

Zulian F. Systemic sclerosis and localized scleroderma in childhood. *Rheum Dis Clin North Am* 2008;34(1):239–55.

12.7 BEHÇET DISEASE

Behçet disease (BD) is a small blood vessel vasculitis of unknown origin. The disease is uncommon in children with most cases reported from the Eastern Mediterranean. International criteria for the diagnosis of BD are: Recurrent oral ulceration that recurs at least 3 times within 12 months plus 2 of the following: * Recurrent genital ulceration, *Eye lesions like anterior uveitis, posterior uveitis, or retinal vasculitis, *Skin lesions like erythema nodosum, pseudofolliculitis, and papulopustular lesions or acneiform nodules,* Positive pathology test. **Positive cutaneous pathology test manifesting as an erythematous sterile pustule or papules surrounded by erythema develops 24–48 hrs. after needle prick.** Less common manifestations of the disease include gastrointestinal involvement, central nervous system abnormalities. Occlusion of major veins and arteries and aneurysms often causes bleeding, infarction, organ failure. There is an increased risk for thrombophlebitis and large vessel thrombosis including the superior or inferior vena cava and hepatic veins (*Budd- Chiari syndrome*). Myocarditis, pericarditis, myositis, nephritis may occur rarely.

Laboratory tests: Finding of HLA B51 supports the diagnosis. The ESR, CRP value, and other acute phase reactants may be elevated during the active stage.

Treatment: Corticosteroids oral or topical represent the initial therapy. Other drugs, including colchicine, chlorambucil, azathioprine, cyclosporin, thalidomide and tacrolimus, have been used. Anti-tumor necrosis factor-α (TNF-α) therapy or interferon-α-2a is used in severe or intractable cases.

Kastner DL. Intermittent and periodic arthritic syndromes. In: Koopman WJ (Ed). Arthritis and allied conditions. *A Textbook of Rheumatology*. 13th edn. Vol. 1. Baltimore: Williams & Wilkins, 1997;1279–306.

Kaklamani VG, Variopoulos G, Kaklamanis PG. Behçet's disease. *Semin Arthritis Rheum* 1998;27:197–217.

Sakane T. New perspective on Behçet's disease. Int Rev Immunol 1997;14:89–96.

12.8 SJÖGREN SYNDROME

Sjögren syndrome (SS) is an autoimmune disease characterized by progressive lymphocytic and plasma cell infiltration of the salivary and lacrimal glands. It is uncommon in pediatric age group. SS consists of the triad of xerostomia, keratoconjunctivitis sicca (KSS) and abnormalities of the salivary gland. Primary SS is the gland inflammation that is not associated with another connective tissue disease whereas secondary SS is associated with a connective tissue disease, such as rheumatoid arthritis, systemic lupus erythematosus or scleroderma. The common symptoms are photophobia, burning and itching eyes, blurred vision, decreased sense of taste, dental caries, dysphagia, fissured tongue, and angular cheilitis. At the onset of the disease, recurrent parotid gland enlargement and parotitis is the common manifestation.

Laboratory findings: Investigation shows elevated ESR with normal CRP levels and positive antinuclear antibody (ANA), hypergammaglobulinemia, and presence of IgM rheumatoid factor (RF) levels.

Treatment: Symptomatic treatment includes the use of artificial saliva, sugarless chewing gum, oral lozenges, artificial tears, and fluids. Corticosteroids, NSAID, and hydroxychloroquine are commonly used drugs. Immunosuppressive agents such as cyclosporin and cyclophosphamide are reserved for severe functional disorders and life-threatening complications.

Anaya JM, Ogawa N, Talal N. Sjögren's syndrome in childhood. *J Rheumatol* 1995;22(6):1152–8.

Fox RI. Sjögren's syndrome. *Lancet* 2005;366(9482):321–31.

Gedalia A. Sjögren syndrome. In: Kliegman RM, Behrman RE, Jenson HB, Stanton BF (eds). *Nelson Textbook of Pediatrics*. 18th edn. Vol. 1. Philadelphia: Saunders, 2007;1028–9.

Singer NG, Tomanova-Soltys I, Lowe R. Sjögren's syndrome in childhood. *Curr Rheumatol Rep* 2008;10(2):147–55.

12.9 AMYLOIDOSIS

Amyloidosis is a group of diseases characterized by deposition of insoluble fibrous amyloid protein in various body tissues. Symptoms result from abnormal functioning of the organs like heart, kidneys, liver, bowels, skin, nerves, joints, and lungs which are affected. Symptoms are vague and can include fatigue, shortness of breath, weight loss, lack of appetite, numbness, tingling, weakness, enlarged tongue, and swelling. Amyloidosis affecting the kidney leads to "nephrotic syndrome," characterized by proteinuria and edema. Involvement of the gastrointestinal system manifests as chronic diarrhea, GI bleeding and malabsorption. Anemia, hepatomegaly and spleno-megaly may be present. *Diagnosis* is made by detecting the amyloid protein of involved tissue in a biopsy specimen with a special Congo red dye. The best sites to biopsy are the abdominal fat pad and rectal mucosa. Other sites have poor sensitivity for the diagnosis include the salivary glands, skin, tongue, gingiva, stomach, and bone marrow. *Treatment* is directed at maintaining the function of affected organs and management of the underlying infectious and inflammatory disease. Autologous stem cell transplantation is another possible treatment.

Georgiades CS, Neyman EG, Barish MA, et al. **Amyloidosis: Review and CT Manifestations.** *Radiographics* 2004;24:405–16.

Husby G. Amyloidosis and rheumatoid arthritis. *Clin Exp Rheumatol* 1985;3:173–80.

Nakamura T. Clinical strategies for amyloid. A amyloidosis secondary to rheumatoid arthritis. *Mod Rheumatol* 2008;18:109–18.

Pepys MB. Amyloidosis. *Annu Rev Med* 2006;57:223–41.

Westermark P, Benson MD, Buxbaum JN, et al. A primer of amyloid nomenclature. *Amyloid* 2007;14:179–83.

12.10 SARCOIDOSIS

Sarcoidosis, a term derived from Greek meaning a "flesh-like condition" is a chronic multi-systemic granulomatous disease that primarily affects the lungs and lymphatic systems of the body. It is less common in children than in adults. Lung is the most frequently affected organ in the children and presents with coughing, shortness of breath, chest pain, dyspnea on exertion, and hemoptysis. Parenchymal lung disease may lead to airway obstruction and bronchiectasis, airway hyperactivity. Chest radiography is used in staging the disease. Stage I disease shows bilateral hilar lymphadenopathy (BHL). Stage II disease shows BHL plus pulmonary infiltrates. Stage III disease shows pulmonary infiltrates without BHL. Stage IV disease shows pulmonary fibrosis. Extrathoracic lymphadeno-pathy, eye changes consisting of uveitis or iritis, skin lesions, and hepatic and bone marrow involvement occur frequently. Neurologic involvement is rare in childhood but may present with seizures, cranial nerve involvement, mass lesions, and hypothalamic dysfunction. Definitive *diagnosis* requires demonstra-tion of the non-caseating granulomatous lesions in a biopsy of tissue, usually taken from the most readily available affected organ. CT of the thorax may demonstrate lymphadenopathy or granulomatous infiltration. The **Kveim test** takes 4–6 wk after injection for histologically examining noncaseating granuloma formation. Bronchoalveolar lavage fluid reveals excessive lymphocytes with an increased CD4+/CD8+ ratio of 2 : 1 to 13 : 1. *Treatment* of choice for patients with pulmonary disease, inflammatory ocular lesion, neurologic involvement, and hypercalcemia is oral corticosteroids. The dose of prednisone is 1 mg/kg/day for 8–12 wk until manifestations improve, with a gradual taper over 6–12 month to the minimal effective dose that controls symptoms. Methotrexate used in severe cases that are unresponsive to corticosteroid therapy. The overall prognosis is good, but half of

patients have some degree of permanent organ dysfunction.

Lannuzzi MC, Rybicki BA, Teirstein AS. Sarcoidosis. *N Engl J Med* 2007;357:2153–65.

Leigh MW. Sarcoidosis. In: Kliegman RM, Behrman RE, Jenson HB, Stanton BF (eds). *Nelson Textbook of Pediatrics.* 18th edn. Vol. 1. Philadelphia: Saunders, 2007;1035–6.

Shetty AK, Gedalia A: Sarcoidosis in children. *Curr Probl Pediatr* 2000;30:149–76.

12.11 KAWASAKI DISEASE

Kawasaki disease (KD), formerly known as muco-cutaneous lymph node syndrome is an acute febrile illness with inflammation of medium-sized blood vessels throughout the body. It is a self-limited acute vasculitic syndrome of unknown etiology, first described by Tomisaku Kawasaki in 1967. Multiple theories exist, including an infectious disease caused by bacteria or bacterial superantigens (*Streptococcus pyogenes*) or virus infectious etiology, genetic disposition and an immunological abnormality. The illness occurs > 80% of cases are seen in young children below < 5 years. It is more common in males than in females (M : F 1.5 : 1).

Diagnostic criteria: For *classic KD*, the diagnostic criteria require the presence of fever for at least 5 days and at least four of five of the other characteristic clinical features of illness. In *atypical or incomplete KD*, the patient has persistent fever but with fewer than four other features of the illness. The diagnostic criteria for classic KD are as follows:

A. Fever persisting at least 5 days

B. Presence of at least 4 principal features:
- *Changes in extremities:* Erythema, edema, and desquamation. Desquamation of the fingers and toes begins in the periungual region, may involve the palms and soles, and is usually observed 1–2 wk after the onset of fever.
- Polymorphous rash (not vesicular) is usually generalized but may be limited to the groin or lower extremities.
- Bilateral bulbar conjunctival injection without exudates.
- *Changes in lips and oral cavity:* Erythema, lips cracking, strawberry tongue, diffuse injection of oral and pharyngeal mucosae
- Cervical lymphadenopathy (> 1.5 cm diameter), usually unilateral

C. Illness not explained by any other known disease process.

The above clinical feature evolves sequentially over a period of a few days and all need not be present at one particular point of time. Other clinical features of the disease may include extreme irritability especially prominent in infants, aseptic meningitis, urethritis, orchitis, arthritis/arthralgia, abdominal pain, vomiting, diarrhea, sterile pyuria, hepatitis, and gallbladder distension. Cardiac involvement occurs in the form of myocarditis, pericarditis, pericardial effusion or decreased ventricular function. Coronary artery aneurysms develop in up to 25% of untreated patients in the 2nd–3rd wk of illness.

Clinical manifestations: KD is generally divided into three clinical phases.

1. **The acute febrile phase**, which usually lasts 1–2 wk, is characterized by fever and the other acute signs of illness. The hands and feet develop the erythema and edema. The tongue and oral mucosa become red and cracked. The cardiac manifestation is myocarditis and pericarditis.
2. **The subacute phase** begins when fever and other acute signs have abated, but irritability, anorexia, and conjunctival injection may persist. This phase should end by the 4th wk. This phase is associated with desquamation, thrombocytosis and the development of coronary aneurysms. Children are at greatest risk of sudden death during this phase.
3. **The convalescent phase** begins when all clinical signs of illness have disappeared and continues until the erythrocyte sedimentation rate (ESR) and C-reactive protein (CRP) return to normal, ~ 6–8 wk after the onset of illness. The significant clinical finding that persists through this phase is the presence of coronary artery aneurysms.

Diagnosis: The diagnosis of KD is based on the presence of characteristic clinical signs. There is no specific laboratory test that definitely diagnoses KD. Laboratory tests reveal leukocytosis with neutrophilia and immature forms; elevated ESR, CRP, and other acute phase reactants; normocytic normochromic anemia; platelet count normal in the 1st wk of illness and rapidly increases by the 2nd–3rd wk of illness, sometimes exceeding $1,000,000/mm^3$; abnormal plasma lipids; hypoalbuminemia; tests for antinuclear antibody and rheumatoid factor negative; sterile pyuria; mild elevations of the hepatic transaminases; cerebrospinal fluid pleocytosis present; and elevated serum transaminases and serum gamma-glutamyl transpeptidase.

Two-dimensional echocardiography, is the most useful test to monitor potential development of coronary artery abnormalities.

Differential diagnosis: The differential diagnosis of Kawasaki disease includes measles, adenovirus infection, scarlet fever, toxic shock syndrome, drug hypersensitivity reactions including Stevens-Johnson syndrome, leptospirosis, and juvenile rheumatoid arthritis.

Complication: Complication of KD is development and rupture of coronary artery aneurysms. These aneurysms may also cause heart problems in later life. Other complications include dehydration and limited mobility from joint inflammation.

Treatment: Treatment should be started within the first 10 days of the onset of illness and include intravenous (IV) immunoglobulin and high-dose oral aspirin. Acute stage: IV immunoglobulin 2 g/kg over 10–12 hr with aspirin 80–100 mg/kg/day divided every 6 hr orally until 14th illness day. Convalescent stage: Aspirin 3–5 mg/kg once daily orally until 6–8 wk after illness onset. Long-term therapy for those with coronary abnormalities: Aspirin 3–5 mg/kg once daily orally ± clopidogrel 1 mg/kg/day (max 75 mg/day). Patients with larger or numerous aneurysms may require the addition of clopidogrel, warfarin, or low molecular weight heparin therapy.

Prognosis: Recovery is complete and without apparent long-term effects for patients who do not develop coronary disease. The prognosis for patients with coronary abnormalities depends on the severity of coronary disease. Recurrent acute illness occurs rarely.

Newburger JW, Takahashi M, Gerber MA, et al. Diagnosis, treatment, and long-term management of Kawasaki disease: A statement for health professionals from the Committee on Rheumatic Fever, Endocarditis, and Kawasaki Disease, Council on Cardiovascular Disease in the Young, American Heart Association. *Pediatrics* 2004;114:1708–33.

Pinna GS, Kafetzis DA, Tselkas OI, et al. Kawasaki disease: an overview. *Curr Opin Infect Dis* 2008;21(3):263–70.

Rowley AH, Shulman ST. Kawasaki syndrome. *Pediatr Clin North Am* 1999; 46(2):313–29.

12.12 VASCULITIS SYNDROMES

1. *Henoch-Schönlein Purpura*: Henoch-Schönlein purpura (HSP), also known as anaphylactoid or allergic purpura, is a small vessel vasculitis. HSP is an inflammatory disorder of unknown cause characterized by immunoglobulin A (IgA), C3, and immune complex deposition in arterioles, capillaries, and venules. It represents a diffuse vasculitis secondary to hypersensitivity. Infectious agents like staphylococcal infections, various viruses like parvovirus B19, *Mycoplasma pneumonia*, enteric organisms as well as drugs, foods, vaccination and insect bites may act as triggering factors for HSP. It was first described by Schönlein in 1837 and then by Henoch in 1874. It is most frequent in children between 2 and 8 years and has a 2 : 1 male preponderance. The criteria for the diagnosis of childhood HSP are given in Table 12.4.

Clinical manifestations: The disease onset may be acute, with the appearance of several manifestations simultaneously, or insidious, with sequential occurrence of symptoms over a period of weeks or months. Low grade fever and fatigue are present in more than half of the affected children.

Rash: A palpable rash (non-thrombocytopenic) of erythematous papules typically appear on the lower extremities and buttocks, but may also involve the upper extremities, face and trunk, and are accentuated in areas of pressure. In the first a few days of illness, the skin rashes may be urticarial or macular and can be difficult to diagnose but all skin lesions eventually become petechial, purpuric, or ecchymotic.

Abdominal pain: Gastrointestinal involvement occurs in approximately two-thirds of the cases of HSP, is usually manifested by abdominal pain, and symptoms precede the rash in 14 to 36% of patients. Vomiting, diarrhea, periumbilical pain mimicking appendicitis, and bloody stools are the main abdominal symptoms. Severe cases may complicate to intussusception, hemorrhage and shock.

Arthritis: About 80% of people with HSP have pain and swelling in their joints, usually in the knees and ankles, less frequently in the elbows and wrists.

Renal disease: Renal manifestations are observed in 20 to 50% of cases and are generally hematuria that most often is macroscopic but may be microscopic and either transient, persistent, or recurrent. Usually, there is associated proteinuria, and the frequency of the nephrotic syndrome is also extremely variable. Deterioration of GFR may occur, and azotemia or end-stage renal failure may occur in 10% of patients. Renal histopathology may include minimal change to severe glomerulonephritis that is indistinguishable from IgA nephropathy.

Other systemic manifestations are myocardial infarction, pulmonary hemorrhage and pleural effusion. Severe neurological manifestations occur secondary to cerebral vasculitis and/or hemorrhage, hypertension presents with headache, seizures, and behavior changes. Peripheral nervous system lesions may appear as mononeuropathies. Other unusual involvements include optic neuritis, parotiditis, scrotal swelling and testicular torsion.

Diagnosis: The diagnosis of HSP depends on clinical findings and history. There may be a non-specific increase in total serum IgA level. The complete blood count may reveal a normal or elevated white blood cell count and possible eosinophilia. Erythrocyte sedimentation rate may be elevated. C-reactive protein mildly elevated and electrolytes may be affected secondary to gastrointestinal involvement. Urinalysis may show hematuria. Microscopic hematuria is often present at the beginning of HSP but usually resolves in the first month to two months after onset of the HSP. A normal platelet count differentiates HSP from thrombocytopenic purpura. Abdominal ultrasonography is used to diagnose intussusceptions. Renal biopsy is required only in children with persistent or severe renal abnormalities. Skin biopsy shows a leukocytoclastic vasculitis with deposition of IgA and C3 on direct immunofluorescence.

Differential diagnosis: The differential diagnosis of HSP includes bacterial endocarditis, rheumatoid arthritis, rheumatic fever, idiopathic thrombocytopenic purpura, systemic lupus erythematosus, drug reactions, pancreatitis, meningitis, encephalitis, and septicemia.

Treatment: There is no specific treatment for HSP. The main goals of treatment are to relieve symptoms such as joint pain, abdominal pain, or swelling. The treatment includes bed rest, supportive care and maintenance of adequate hydration. Nonsteroidal anti-inflammatory drugs (NSAIDs) may help joint pain. Corticosteroids are used in patients with severe abdominal pain and not recommended for treatment of rash, joint pain or renal disease alone. Prednisolone (1–1.5 mg/kg/day) for 2 wk and then tapered over 2 more weeks has been shown to improve gastrointestinal symptoms. Other treatment regimens have included azathioprine, cyclophosphamide, cyclosporin, dipyridamole, plasmapheresis, IV immunoglobulin G.

Prognosis: HSP is generally a benign disease with an excellent prognosis. In the absence of renal disease and central nervous system involvement, the prognosis is excellent and majority of the children have no permanent sequelae. The illness lasts four to six weeks in most patients. Long-term follow-up is necessary for patients with renal disease.

2. *Takayasu arteritis:* Takayasu arteritis (or nonspecific aortoarteritis or pulseless disease), is a chronic vasculitic disease of the aorta, the proximal portions of its major branches, and the pulmonary artery. It leads to progressive wall fibrosis and lumen

Table 12.4: Classification criteria for Henoch-Schönlein purpura

Palpable purpura in the presence of at least one of the following four features:
- Diffuse abdominal pain
- Any biopsy showing predominant IgA deposition
- Arthritis or Arthralgia
- Renal involvement (any hematuria and/or proteinuria)

stenosis or rarely aneurysm formation. It is most common in women (90%) of Asian descent between the ages of 15 and 45 years, but also occurs in children and infants. The etiology of TA is unknown, but an association with tuberculosis has been reported. The acute, active phase of the illness lasts for weeks to months, and may have a remitting and relapsing course. Constitutional symptoms like fever, anorexia, loss of weight, night sweats, arthralgia, skin rash, myalgia, cough, hemoptysis, pleuritis, episcleritis, headache, neurologic deficits may occur. During early part of this phase, the peripheral pulses and blood pressure may be normal. In late chronic phase, extremity claudication, bruits over the cervical, supraclavicular and abdominal regions, absent pulses, systolic blood pressure difference greater than 10 mmHg between arms may be present. Skin vasculitis resembling erythema nodosum or ulcerating nodular lesions may be seen. In India, TA is believed to be the commonest cause of renovascular hypertension. *Complications* may include retinopathy, stroke, seizures, congestive heart failure, secondary hypertension, aortic regurgitation, and aneurysm formation.

Diagnosis: Angiography shows narrowing or blockage of the entire aorta, its primary branches, or large arteries in the arms or legs. ESR is significantly elevated. Microcytic hypochromic anemia with leukocytosis is present. In 1/3 of cases polyclonal hypergammaglobulinemia is present. TA must be differentiated from acute rheumatic fever and juvenile rheumatoid arthritis.

Treatment: In the initial phase, prednisolone 1–2 mg/kg/day for approximately 1 month followed by slow tapering over several months as symptoms subside. Cytotoxic agents like azathioprine, methotrexate, and cyclophosphamide are used for patients with steroid resistance or relapsing Takayasu arteritis. Mycophenolate mofetil has been used in patients unresponsive to other immunosuppressor agents. Surgical treatment is needed when complications of stenosis or occlusion or less frequently aneurysm develop. In addition, balloon dilatation or stenting is often necessary. Angioplasty may be needed to prevent development of chronic hypertension and decreased perfusion. More than 50% cases achieve remission.

3. *Polyarteritis nodosa:* Polyarteritis nodosa (PAN) is also called Kussmaul disease or Kussmaul-Maier disease represents the classic form of focal segmental necrotizing vasculitis and is associated with aneurysmal nodules along the wall of the small- and medium-sized arteries. Most commonly involve organs are the skin, joints, peripheral nerves, gastrointestinal tract (GIT),

and renal system. Skin manifestation includes vascular purpura, subcutaneous nodules, livedo reticularis, distal gangrene, and ischemic atrophy. Renal involvement manifests as hematuria, proteinuria, hypertension, nephrotic syndrome, or rapidly progressive glomerulonephritis. Arthromyalgias, arthritis, and myositis are common. Central nervous system involvement may cause motor deficits, strokes, brain hemorrhages, psychosis, weakness, sensory changes and diffuse encephalopathy. Cardiac involvement characterized by myocarditis result in myocardial ischemia and heart failure. Less frequent findings include orchitis, retinal arteritis, and GIT disease (bleeding, ulceration). PAN has been described in all age groups and rarely found in children. Boys and girls appear to be equally affected, with a mean age of 9 yr of age. The cause is unknown, although the occurrence of PAN after drug exposure and infection due to hepatitis B virus or *Streptococcus* species has implicated immune complexes. Other infection which is responsible for the disease includes infectious mononucleosis, tuberculosis, Parvovirus B19 and cytomegalovirus.

Laboratory findings: Increased platelet activating factor levels and increased factor VIII-related antigen (von Willebrand factor antigen) are present. Hepatitis B surface antigen should be tested in all patients independent of liver function tests. Antinuclear antibody (ANA) in low titer, cryoglobulins, and diminished serum complement (i.e. C3, C4) may be observed. Other laboratory abnormalities depend on specific organ involvement.

Treatment: Corticosteroid and immunosuppressive drug have increased the survival rate. If hepatitis B is identified with PAN, specific antiviral therapy should be added. Plasma exchange is useful as a second-line treatment in PAN to conventional therapy. The course of PAN varies from mild disease with a few complications to a severe, overwhelming, multiorgan disease leading to death.

4. *Wegener granulomatosis:* Wegener granulomatosis (WG) is a necrotizing granulomatous vasculitis of small size vessels characterized by the upper and lower respiratory tracts involvement and glomerulonephritis. Pulmonary manifestation includes infiltrate, nodules, hemoptysis and dyspnea. Nasal (Saddle nose) deformity and subglottic stenosis are common in children. Other clinical manifestations include ocular findings (conjunctivitis, keratitis, scleritis and proptosis); cutaneous lesions (palpable purpura, papules, subcutaneous nodules, and ulcerations); arthritis, pericarditis, and cranial or peripheral neuropathies. The disease is rare in children, but it may present as early as 2 wk of age. There is a female predominance of 3 : 1. The etiology is unknown.

Diagnosis is established by the detection of the granulomatous inflammation on biopsy of the upper airway, lung, kidney or skin. cyclase-antineutrophil cytoplasmic antibody with PR3 specificity is most specific for WG. Antibodies to antineutrophil cytoplasmic antibody (ANCA) are absent in other granulomatous disease such as sarcoidosis and tuberculosis. Churg-Strauss syndrome is a vasculitis that can cause chronic sinus lesions; a history of asthma, circulating eosinophilia, and an eosinophilic cutaneous vasculitis distinguish this syndrome from WG.

Treatment consists of corticosteroids, cyclophosphamide and methotrexate.

Bahl VK, Seth S. Takayasu arteritis Revisited. *Indian Heart J* 2002;54:147–51.

Gardener-Medwin JM, Dolezalova P, Cummins C, et al. Incidence of Henoch-Schönlein purpura, Kawasaki disease, and rare vasculitides in children of different ethnic origins. *Lancet* 2002;(19) 360:1197–202.

Guillevin L, Lhote F. Treatment of polyarteritis nodosa and microscopic polyangiitis. *Arthritis Rheum* 1998;41(12):2100–05.

Hellmich B, Lamprecht P, Gross WL. Advances in the therapy of Wegener's granulomatosis. *Curr Opin Rheumatol* 2006;18(1):25–32.

Miller ML, Pachman LM. Vasculitis syndromes. In: Kliegman RM, Behrman RE, Jenson HB, Stanton BF (eds). *Nelson Textbook of Pediatrics*. 18th edn. Vol. 1. Philadelphia: Saunders, 2007;1042–49.

Rai A, Nast C, Adler S. Henoch-Schönlein Purpura Nephritis. *J Am Soc Nephrol* 1999;10:2637–44.

Sharma BK, Sagar S, Singh AP, Suri S. Takayasu Arteritis in India. *Heart Vessels Suppl* 1992;7:37–43.

Silvia Maffei, Michela Di Renzo, Giovanni Bova, *Alberto Auteri, Anna Laura Pasqui*. Takayasu's arteritis: a review of the literature. *Intern Emerg Med* 2006;1 (2):105–12.

Wung PK, Stone JH. Therapeutics of Wegener's granulomatosis. *Nat Clin Pract Rheumatol* 2006;2(4):192–200.

13 ◆ Special Health Problems during Adolescence

13.1 HEALTH PROBLEMS IN ADOLESCENCE

Adolescence has been described as the transition period in life when an individual is no longer a child, but not yet an adult. A complex myriad of physiological as well psychological changes take place as a child evolves into an adult. This period of adolescence is marked by visible changes of growth and puberty and invisible changes such as maturation of all organs, neuroendocrinal changes as well as psychological maturation. It is a period of sexual and reproductive maturity. The individual capacity for abstract and critical thinking also develops. The World Health Organization refers to people aged 10–19 yr as adolescents. The term 'young people' refers to those between 10 and 24 years. The United Nations definition of youth is those between the ages of 15 and 24 years.

The major problems of adolescent health in a developing country are:
a. Nutritional disorders
b. Infections and immunization, and
c. Social and mental health problems related to lifestyle of the society in transition.

A. *Nutritional disorders:* The rapid growth and increase in physical activity creates special nutritional needs which are higher during adolescence than at any other time in life. Failure to consume adequate diet at this time can potentially retard physical growth, intellectual capacity and delay sexual maturation. The nutrition of female adolescent is of special importance given the far reaching effects of maternal undernutrition. Overweight is more prevalent in affluent class, the major factors being lack of daily exercise, excess of junk-food and television (TV) / computer watching in excess. Iron requirements peak during adolescence due to rapid growth with sharp increase in lean body mass, blood volume and red cell mass. Inability to meet this increased demand can lead to iron deficiency and iron deficiency anemia. Iodine deficiency is a community disease that affects virtually all sections of community. Foci of endemic goiter are prevalent far and wide throughout India.

B. *Infections and immunization:* In developing countries the immunization of infants is a priority and concerted efforts are made to increase the immunization coverage. However, this should not undermine continued need for appropriate vaccination as the child grows into adolescence.

C. *Health problems related to lifestyle:* **Substance abuse** is an alarming problem with its deep seated relationship with adolescence. The abuse of alcohol, tobacco, marijuana and opium is a continuum starting from incidental use to regular use followed by abuse and dependency. The *sexual behavior of adolescents* is largely influenced by sociocultural factors. The risk taking and experimentation may include experimenting with sex in societies where dating and having sex is considered a part of growing up. The main reproductive health risks facing adolescents are early pregnancy, unsafe abortion, sexually transmitted diseases such as AIDS, sexual abuse and exploitation including harmful traditional practices such as female genital mutilation. *Teenage pregnancy* during the period of rapid growth can pose a threat to their nutritional and health status as well as that of their offspring. *Injury and violence* is an important cause of death and disability in adolescence. Accidental injuries in this age group can be: (a) related to vehicles; (b) falls; (c) drowning; (d) burns and electric shock; and (e) injury in school/sport ground or workplace. Suicide is another form of intentional injury. In India, there has been an alarming increase in suicides and suicidal attempts in the last few years.

Clustering of problem behavior: It has been seen that problem behavior cluster together. Teenagers who engage in one risk taking behavior are often involved in other risky practice. Those who smoke are more likely to use illicit drugs, drink alcohol, do poorly at school and to be involved in antisocial behavior and traffic accidents. This may be due to underlying behavior/emotional dysfunction of the adolescent or as a result of maladjusted family, which requires attention and appropriate therapy.

Aneja S. Health Problems in Adolescence. In: Mathur GP, Mathur Sarla (eds). *Current Trends in Pediatrics.* Vol 1. Delhi: Academa Publishers, 2005;442–51.

Health Information of India. Central Bureau of Health Intelligence. Director General of Health Services, New Delhi, Government of India, 1968.

Kushwaha KP, Rai AK, Rathi AK, et al. Pregnancies in adolescents–Fetal, neonatal and maternal outcome. *Indian Pediatr* 1993;30:501–5.

Pandav CS, Lochupillai N, Karmarker MG, Ramchandran K, Gopinath PG, Bath LM. Endemic goiter in Delhi. *Indian J Med Res* 1980;72:81–88.

Pathak P, Singh P, Kapil U, et al. Prevalence of iron, vitamin A, and iodine deficiencies amongst adolescent pregnant mothers. *Indian J Pediatr* 2003;70:299–301.

13.2 DELIVERY OF HEALTH CARE TO ADOLESCENTS

The leading causes of death and disability among adolescents are preventable. It is the responsibility of the society to prevent morbidity and mortality and to promote optimal health and development of adolescents by adequately addressing their health needs. The World Health Organization in collaboration with United Nations International Children's Emergency Fund and United Nations Population Fund has developed a common agenda for action for healthy development in the 2nd decade of life by advocating for youths for opportunities to:

1. Acquire accurate health information about their health needs
2. To build the life skills needed to avoid risk-taking behavior

3. Obtain counseling, especially during crisis situation
4. Have access to health services (including reproductive health services) and
5. Live in a safe and supportive environment.

Enhancement of health status: The health status of adolescents may be enhanced by preventive measures and anticipatory guidance. Prevention of infectious diseases will include immunization and counseling. Prevention of sexually transmitted infections and pregnancy should be addressed in sexually adolescents. Prevention of harmful illicit drugs and alcohol and the potential for related injuries, of automotive accidents and interpersonal conflicts ending violently, the leading killer of accidents, and of smoking, the leading killer of adults should also be discussed. Also provide him or her support in successfully negotiating through school, job, and personal and family relations.

Adolescent Medicine: State of the Art Reviews: The office visit. *Adolesc Med* 2003;14:263–72.

American Medical Association: *Guidelines for Adolescent Preventive Services, Recommendations Monograph.* 3rd edn. Chicago: American medical Association, 1996.

Jenkins RR. Delivery of health care to adolescents. In: Kliegman RM, Behrman RE, Jenson HB, Stanton BF (eds). *Nelson Textbook of Pediatrics.* 18th edn. Vol. 1. Philadelphia: Saunders, 2007;816–20.

World Health Organization: *Overview of Child and Adolescent Health and Development,* available at: www.who.int/child-adolescent-health/OVERVIEW/AHD/adh_over.htm (accessed November 20, 2005).

13.3 IMMUNIZATION IN ADOLESCENCE

See Section 15.2, page 433.

13.4 DEPRESSION

See Section 5.4, page 106.

13.5 CHILD AND ADOLESCENT SUICIDE

Suicide is one of the common causes of death among children and adolescents. The suicide rates in this group have been increasing in the past two decades. The physical, psychological, emotional and social changes that take place in the day to day life of children and adolescents, increases the stress level in them. They suffer a feeling of loss of their childhood and undergo a difficult period of adjustment to their new adult identity. Achievement-oriented, highly competitive society puts pressure on the children and adolescents to succeed, often focusing them to set unrealistically high personal expectations. There is increased pressure to stay in school, where success is narrowly defined and difficult to achieve. In an affluent society which emphasizes immediate rewards, children are not taught to handle frustration. Suicidal behavior is the end result of a complex interaction of physical, social and familial factors. Recent stressful events can activate suicidal behaviors particularly in impulsive youth. There are far more suicidal attempts and gestures than actual completed suicides. Suicide also affects the health of the community. Family and friends of the children and adolescents who commit suicide may feel shock, anger, guilt and depressed. Children who survive a suicidal attempt continue to be at risk for completed suicide, violent death and poor psychological outcomes.

Definition of Terms

The definition of terms is listed in Table 13.1.

Epidemiology: Suicide is the second leading cause of death among children and adolescents. Worldwide there is a rise in child and adolescent suicide rates both in the developed and developing countries. In the United States suicide is the third leading cause of death for individuals between 15 and 24 yr old and sixth leading cause from 5 to 14 yr old.

Methods of suicide: The common methods of suicide used by child and adolescent are poisoning. The common poisons include pesticides employed. Over the counter medication is also used for suicide and attempted suicide in urban settings. Drug over-dose with medication, commonly available over-the-counter (e.g. benzodiazepines, antidepressants, pain-killers, etc.) is also common. The other methods of suicide commonly employed by older people are used by children and adolescents, although much less frequently. Drowning, hanging, burning oneself (self immolation), jumping from tall structures and electrocution are rarer options. While poisoning is common in both sexes, girls and young women also employ drowning and burning while boys tend to choose hanging as options.

Protective factors: The protective factors that help children and adolescents to cope with life stressors which will aid in the prevention of suicidal attempts are family cohesion, religiosity, positive self esteem, optimism, good coping, problem solving skills, close relationships and social support.

Aaron R, Joseph A, Abraham S, et al. Suicide in young people in rural south India. *Lancet* 2004; 363(9415):1117–8.

Manoranjitham S, Abraham S, Jacob KS. Towards a national strategy to reduce suicide in India. *The Medical Journal of India* 2005;18(3):118–22.

Manoranjitham S, Helen C, Saravanan B. Perception about suicide: a qualitative study from south India. *The Medical Journal of India* 2007; 20(4):176–79.

Sharma BR, Gupta M, Sharma AK, et al. Suicides in Northern India: Comparison of trends and review of literature. *J Forensic and Legal Medicine* 2007;14(6):318–26.

13.6 VIOLENT BEHAVIOR

Violence is a leading worldwide public health problem. The World Health Organization (WHO) defines *violence* as "The intentional use of physical force or power, threatened or actual, against oneself, another person, or against a group or community that either results in or has a high likelihood of resulting in injury, death, psychological harm, maldevelopment or deprivation."

Clinical manifestations: There are clinical entities directly associated with violent behavior in adolescents such as: mental retardation, learning disabilities, attention deficit/hyperactivity disorder, mood disturbance, anxiety, and disruptive behavior disorders.

Diagnosis: An adolescent at risk, or with a history of, violent behavior or victimization should be assessed. The FISTS mnemonic provides guidance for structuring the assessment (Box 13.1).

Treatment: In the case of acute injury secondary to violent assault the treat plan should include the stabilization of the injury, evaluation and treatment of the injury, evaluation of the assault circumstances, psychologic evaluation of the functioning of the victim, rehabilitation of the injury, and outpatient follow-up of the behavioral and physical sequelae, and management of sexual assault victims.

Table 13.1: Definition of terms	
Term	*Definition*
Suicide	The process of purposefully ending one's own life
Suicidal behaviors/self injurious behaviors/ Deliberate self harm	Deliberately hurting self without the intention to end one's own life
Attempted suicide	An act that was intended to cause death but was unsuccessful
Suicidal ideation	Formal suicidal thoughts and plan without the suicidal act or attempt

---

Box 13.1: FISTS mnemonic to assess an adolescent's risk of violence

F: **Fighting** (How many fights were you in last year? What was the last?)

I: **Injuries** (Have you ever been injured? Have ever injured someone else?)

S: **Sex** (Have your partner hit you? Have you hit your Partner? Have you ever been forced to have sex?)

T: **Threats** (Has someone with a weapon threatened you? What happened? Has anything changed to make you feel safer?)

S: **Self-defense** (What do you do if someone tries to pick a fight? Have you carried a weapon on self-defense?)

Prevention: A multifactorial approach to prevention has been suggested by the WHO, includes: individual approaches, relationship approaches, community approaches, and socialistic approaches. *Individual approaches* concentrate on changing attitudes and behaviors to avoid aggressive and violent behavior for all children and youths who have already displayed some violent tendencies. *Relationship approaches* focus more on victims, families, and peer relationships. *Community-based approaches* raise public awareness in an effort to stimulate action by community members to reduce violence and protect vulnerable community members. *Societal approaches* include broader advocacy and legislative actions, as well as societal and cultural environmental changes.

American Academy of Pediatrics, Committee on Adolescence: Care of the adolescent sexual assault victim. *Pediatrics* 2001;107:1476–9.

Hennes HMA, Calhoun AD (eds). Violence among children and adolescents. *Pediatr Clin North Am* 1998;45:269–80.

Zwi A, Grove N, Kelly P, et al. Child health in armed conflict; time to rethink. *Lancet* 2006;367:1886–8.

13.7 EPILEPSY IN ADOLESCENCE

Epilepsy in adolescence is a significant neurologic burden to an individual. Many people with epilepsy experience their first seizure before the age of 20. Eight epilepsy syndromes with onset in adolescence are discussed in detail.

1. *Epilepsy with grand mal on awakening:* Epilepsy with grand mal on awakening (GMA) is a syndrome of IGE characterized by generalized tonic-clonic (GTC) seizures occurring predominantly or exclusively shortly after awakening (without respect to the time of day) or in the evening with relaxation. The age at onset is broader than the other idiopathic generalized epilepsies (IGEs), but a clear peak occurs around puberty.

2. *Juvenile absence epilepsy (JAE)* is an infrequent IGE with onset in adolescence. There probably exists an overlap between JAE and juvenile myoclonic epilepsy (JME). The absence seizure frequency is less than in childhood absence epilepsy (CAE), with absences occurring sporadically. The majority of patients also have generalized tonic-clonic (GTC) seizures.

3. *Juvenile myoclonic epilepsy* (Janz syndrome): *See* Section 24.8, page 751.

4. *Mesial temporal lobe epilepsy:* Mesial temporal lobe epilepsy (MTLE) is associated with hippocampal sclerosis is the most common form of human epilepsy and represents a discrete syndrome that can be recognized in adolescence. Diagnosis of medically refractory MTLE before or during adolescence is important, because the seizures and their consequences can be eliminated by surgical therapy (anteromesial temporal lobectomy) in 80–90% of patients, and early surgical intervention provides the greatest opportunity for complete psychosocial rehabilitation.

5. *Psychogenic non-epileptic seizures:* Psychogenic non-epileptic seizures (PNES) occur typically between 10 and 18 yr of age and are more frequently seen in females. Significant rise in serum prolactin is seen in epileptic seizures whereas there is no change in PNES.

6. *Photosensitive epilepsy:* Photosensitive epilepsy usually presents between the ages of 7 and 19 yr and may account for 10% of all new cases of epilepsy in this age group. There is a 3 : 2 female preponderance and greatest expression in adolescence. The commonest seizure types are generalized tonic-clonic, absence and myoclonic seizures.

7. *Progressive myoclonic epilepsies:* Progressive myoclonic epilepsies (PMEs) are rare, accounting for only 1% of all epilepsy cases in childhood and adolescence. A PME syndrome is characterized by the association of:

   a. A myoclonus syndrome involving massive myoclonus and asymmetric myoclonus

   b. Generalized tonic clonic seizures

   c. mental deterioration resulting in dementia, and

   d. A neurologic syndrome with cerebellar manifestations.

8. *Reading epilepsy:* During reading, the EEG usually shows focal epileptiform activity in the left frontotemporal region or synchronous activity over both hemispheres. Bickford et al (1975) described two groups of patients with seizures precipitated by reading.

Group I had the following features

1. Seizures occur only with reading
2. Onset with clicking sensation in the jaw or jaw movement, followed by generalized seizure activity if reading is not stopped
3. Paroxysmal discharges of bilaterally synchronous 3–6 Hz activity, which is maximum posteriorly
4. Normal resting EEG, and
5. No evidence of brain pathology.

Group II had the following features

1. Seizures sometimes precipitated with stimuli other than reading (photic stimulation, visual patterns, writing, calculation, recall)
2. Jaw clicking does not occur, and
3. Sometimes evidence for brain damage. Reading epilepsy usually begins in the second decade of life and may settle subsequently as the patient learns personal tricks to avoid the onset of facial jerks. Seizures may be controlled by clonazepam or sodium valproate.

Special Issues Related to Adolescent Girls

Catamenial epilepsy: Some adolescent girls experience a marked increase in seizure frequency around the time of menses. This is thought to reflect either the effects of estrogen and progesterone on neuronal excitability or changes in epileptic drug levels due to altered protein binding. Acetazolamide (250–500 mg/day) may be effective as adjunctive therapy in some cases when started 7–10 days prior to the onset of menses and continued until bleeding stops. Some patients may benefit from increases in antiepileptic drug dosages during this time or from control of menstrual cycle through the use of oral contraceptives. Natural progestins may be of benefit to a subset of women.

Pregnancy: Most adolescent girls with epilepsy who become pregnant will have uncomplicated gestation and deliver a normal baby. Seizure frequency remains unchanged in 50% of women, increase in 30%, and decrease in 20%. The incidence of fetal abnormalities in children born to mother with epilepsy is more (5–6%), compared to 2–3% in healthy women. Part of the higher incidence is due to teratogenic effects of antiepileptic drugs, and the risk increases with the number of antiepileptic drugs used (e.g. 10% risk of malformations with 3 drugs). It is known that fetal abnormalities occur with first-line drugs (i.e. phenytoin, valproic acid, carbamazepine). However, little is currently known about the safety of newer drugs.

It is important to put the patient where possible on monotherapy at the lowest effective dose, especially during the first trimester. Patients should also take folic acid tablet (1–5 mg/day), since the antifolate effects of anticonvulsants are thought to play role in the development of neural tube defects, although the benefits of this treatment remain unproved in this setting. Enzyme inducing drugs such as phenytoin, phenobarbital, and primidone cause a transient and reversible deficiency of vitamin K-dependent clotting factors in approximately 50% newborn infants. Although neonatal hemorrhage is uncommon, the mother should be treated with oral vitamin K (20 mg daily) in the last 2 wk of pregnancy, and the infant should receive vitamin K (1 mg IM) at birth.

Contraception: Women who are taking oral contraceptives should not be prescribed antiepileptic drugs such as carbamazepine, phenytoin, phenobarbital, and topiramate as they can significantly antagonize the effects of oral contraceptives via enzyme induction and other mechanisms. Patients should be advised to consider alternative forms of contraception.

Breastfeeding: Antiepileptic drugs are excreted into breast milk to a variable degree. The ratio of drug concentration in breast milk relative to serum is 80% for ethosuximide, 40–60% for phenobarbital, 50% for carbamazepine, 15% for phenytoin, and 5% for valproic acid. In view of the benefit of breastfeeding and lack of evidence of long-term harm to infant, mother should be encouraged to breastfeed. This should be reconsidered if there is any evidence of drug effect on infant such as lethargy or poor feeding with the antiepileptic drug she is taking.

Preparing for Adulthood

With support teenager can learn that epilepsy does not have to rule their life. Provided they are sensible, there is no reason why young people with epilepsy should not take part in sports, traveling, going to discos and having boyfriends or girlfriends. As a parent it can be hard to acknowledge that children have adult desires. However, at some stage parent will need to discuss sex and relationships. Boys and girls need to know that epilepsy would not stop them enjoying sex. Girls should be aware that medication can affect absorption of the contraceptive pill and may need to talk this over with the doctor. And both sexes need to know that there is absolutely no reason why they cannot have a partner or children.

There is no reason an adolescent should not enjoy every aspect of student life. Like all students, adolescents with epilepsy will need to decide for themselves where they stand on matters such as alcohol, smoking, street drugs and how they conduct their social life. In making such choices, they will, of course, need to take into account how these are likely to affect their epilepsy. If they encounter particular problems linked to epilepsy, they can discuss them with their parents, a personal tutor or student counselor.

Bickford et al. Reading epilepsy: Clinical and electro-encephalographic studies of a new syndrome. *Trans Am Neurol Assoc* 1975;81:100.

Conry JA. Progressive myoclonic epilepsy. J Child Neurol 2002;17:80S–84.

Janz D. Juvenile myoclonic epilepsy. Cleve Clin J Med 1989; 56 (suppl): S23–S33.

Johnston MV. Seizures in childhood. In: Kliegman RM, Behrman RE, Jenson HB, Stanton BF (eds). *Nelson Textbook of Pediatrics*. 18th edn. Vol 2. Philadelphia: Saunders, 2007; 2457–75.

Mathur GP, Mathur S. Myoclonus. In: Mathur GP, Mathur S (eds). *Movement disorders in children and adolescents*. 1st edn. New Delhi: Jaypee Brothers Medical Publishers (P) Ltd., 2003; 48–61.

Mathur GP, Kushwaha KP, Mathur Sarla, et al. Epilepsy in Adolescence. In: Mathur GP, Mathur Sarla (eds). *Current Trends in Pediatrics*. Vol 2. Delhi: Academa Publishers, 2006;149–159.

Pack AM, Morrell MJ. Treatment of women with epilepsy. *Semin Neurol* 2002;22:289.

Wheless JW, Kim HL. Adolescent seizures and epilepsy syndromes. Epilepsia 2002;43 (suppl):S33–S52.

Wolf P. Juvenile absence epilepsy. In: Roger J, Bureau M, Dravet C, et al (eds). *Epileptic syndromes in infancy, childhood and adolescence*. 2nd edn. London: John Libbey, 1992;307–12.

Wolf P. Epilepsy with grand mal on awakening. In: Roger J, Bureau M, Dravet C, et al (eds). *Epileptic syndromes in infancy, childhood and adolescence*. 2nd edn. London: John Libbey, 1992; 329–41.

13.8 EATING DISORDERS

See Section 5.8, page 113.

13.9 SUBSTANCE ABUSE

According to World Health Organization (WHO) substance abuse refers to the harmful or hazardous use of psychoactive substances, including alcohol and illicit drugs. Repeated and prolonged or heavy use of such substances can lead to dependence, which is characterized by continued use of the substance despite physical and mental problems, difficulty in controlling use, strong desire to take the substance, neglect of other activities and interests, increased tolerance, and sometimes a withdrawal syndrome if use is ceased or reduced. Withdrawal can range from mild anxiety to seizures and hallucinations. Drug overdose may also cause death. Behaviors such as rebelliousness, poor school performance, delinquency, criminal activity, and personality traits such as low self-esteem are frequently associated with or predate

the onset of drug use. Some of the most commonly abused drugs include alcohol, tobacco, amphetamines, barbiturates, benzodiazepines, cocaine, heroin, and opium alkaloids. An estimated 4.7% of the global population aged 15 to 64, or 185 million people, consume illicit drugs annually.

Screening for substance abuse disorders: The annual health maintenance examination provides an opportunity for identifying adolescents with substance use or abuse issues. Mnemonics specifically designed for adolescents are in use (CRAFFT) (Box 13.2).

Prevention: The Center for Substance Abuse Prevention has identified 6 program characteristics that have produced statistically significant reduction in 30-day substance use for adolescents:

1. Life skills focus-promoting attitudinal and behavioral life skills
2. Emphasis on building connectedness-emphasizing connectedness to positive peers and adults
3. Coherent Program Design and Implementation-linking activities to articulated and coherent preventive theory
4. Introspective orientation-encouraging youth to examine their own attitudes and behaviors and their contextual impact
5. Intensive contact—4 or more contact hours per week; and
6. After school setting as compared to classroom delivery. Programs that delivered at least 5 of the 6 characteristics demonstrated strong prevention benefits through an 18 month follow-up period.

Approaches to managing drug abuse: Finding effective treatment for and prevention of substance abuse has been difficult. Studies have made it clear that drug education and prevention aimed at children and adolescents offers the best chance to curb abuse nationally. There are two strategies:

Box 13.2: CRAFFT mnemonic tool

Have you ever ridden in a Car driven by someone (including yourself) who was high or had been using alcohol or drugs?

Do you ever use alcohol or drugs to relax feel better about yourself or fit in?

Do you use alcohol or drugs while you are by yourself (alone)?

Do you ever forget things you did while using alcohol or drugs?

Do your family or friends ever tell you that you should cut down on your drinking or drug use?

Have you evergotten into trouble while you went using alcohol or drugs?

1. *Harm reduction:* The harm-reduction strategies, which focus on reducing the societal costs of drug abuse and other drug use. Techniques include education to avoid overdose, needle exchange programs to reduce the spread of blood-borne diseases, and opiate substitution therapy to reduce crime related to the procurement of drugs. This pragmatic approach is known as the harm reduction paradigm. Harm reduction also addresses special populations, such as drug-using parents, pregnant drug users and users with psychiatric comorbidity.

2. *Abstinence-based:* Abstinence-based approaches set as a goal complete abstinence from all addictive substances, including both licit and illicit, prescribed and unprescribed. While the harm-reduction approach has been demonstrated to work well with opiates, the abstinence-based approach is the medical community standard of care for sedative (including alcohol) dependence.

Medical treatment: Beyond the sociological issues, many drugs of abuse can lead to addiction, chemical dependency, or adverse health effects, such as lung cancer or emphysema from cigarette smoking. Medical treatment therefore centers on two aspects:

1. Breaking the addiction
2. Treating the health problems.

Most countries have health facilities that specialize in the treatment of drug abuse, although access may be limited to larger population centers and the social taboos regarding drug use may make those who need the medical treatment reluctant to take advantage of it. Important features of successful long-term management include continuing medical education after detoxification. Patients may require acute and long-term maintenance treatment and relapse prevention, and the provision of developmentally appropriate psychosocial support system.

Anglin TM. Evaluation by interview and questionnare. In: Schydlower M (ed). *Substance abuse: A Guide for Health Professionals.* 2nd edn. Elk Grove Village. IL: American Academy of Pediatrics, 2002;69.

Bonomo Y, Proimos J. Substance misuse: Alcohol, tobacco, inhalants, and other drugs. *Br Med J* 2005;330:777–80.

George A, Verghese C, Sankaranaryanan R, Nair MK. Use of tobacco and alcoholic beverages by children and teenagers in a low income coastal community in South India. *J Cancer Educ* 1994;9:111–3.

Jenkins RR, Adger H. Substance abuse. In: Kliegman RM, Behrman RE, Jenson HB, Stanton BF (eds). *Nelson Textbook of Pediatrics.* 18th edn. Vol. 1. Philadelphia: Saunders, 2007; 824–34.

Kapoor SK, Anand K, Kumar G. Prevalence of tobacco use among school and college going adolescents of Haryana. *Indian J Pediatr* 1995;62:461–6.

Kushwaha KP, Singh YD, Rathi AK, et al. Prevalence and abuse of psychoactive drugs in children and adolescents. *Indian J Pediatr* 1992;59:261–8.

Rimsza ME, Moses KS. Substance abuse on the college campus. *Pediatr Clinic North Am* 2005;52:307–19.

Sunday SR, Folan P. Smoking in adolescence: What a clinician can do to help. *Med Clin North Am* 2004;88:1495–515.

13.10 SEXUALLY TRANSMITTED DISEASES

See Section 30.8, page 884.

13.11 RAPE IN CHILDREN AND ADOLESCENTS

Sexual violence is defined as, "any sexual act, attempt to obtain a sexual act, unwanted sexual comments or advances, or trafficking of women for sex, using coercion, threats or harm or physical force, by any person regardless of the relationship to the victim, in any setting, including but not limited to home and work". The sexual violence in children and adolescence encompasses:

- Attempted/accomplished sexual coercion.
- Sexual assault with any object, instrument or sexual organ.
- Sexual harassment including sexual humiliation.
- Forced marriage or cohabitation including child marriage.
- Forced prostitution and trafficking.
- Forced abortion.
- Denial of right to use contraception or protection from diseases.
- Female genital mutilation and social virginity inspections.
- Child sexual abuse.
- Sexual violence in war situations.

Although the incidents of sexual exploitation of children and adolescents can be traced in history since time immemorial, its prevalence has increased exponentially during last century in spite of enactments of numerous laws all over the world. Rape is amongst the commonest sexual violence even in the present day so-called modern civilized society. The term rape, though, literally means taking away anything by force, has different meaning in different countries. From legal and clinical perspectives, *rape* is defined as "forced sexual intercourse" that occurs because of physical force or psychologic coercion. Rape involves vaginal, anal, or oral penetration by the offender. This definition also includes incidents in which penetration is with a foreign object, such as a bottle, or situations in which the victim is unable to give consent because of intoxication or developmental disability. The terms *acquaintance rape* and *date rape* are applied to those situations in which the assailant and victim know each other.

In India, legally rape has restricted meaning and is defined under Section 375 of Indian Penal Code as, "unlawful sexual intercourse by a man with a woman," under following condition:

- With his own wife under the age of 15 years, or
- With any other women under the age of 16 yr with or without her consent, or
- With any other woman above the age of 16 years, against her will or without consent, or
- With her consent, when the consent has been obtained by putting her or any person in whom she is interested, in fear of death or hurt, or
- With her consent, when the man knows that he is not her husband that her consent is given because she believes that he is another man to whom she is or believes to be lawfully married, or
- With her consent, when at the time of giving the consent, by the reason of unsoundness of mind or intoxication or the administration of any stupefying or unwholesome substance, she is unable to understand the nature and consequences of that to which she gives consent.

As per state amendment to this law, in state of Manipur the ages of valid consent to sexual intercourse by unmarried and married females has been reduced to 14 and 13 yr respectively.

In countries like India only vaginal intercourse is taken as rape and anal and/or oral intercourse is not included under rape, while in other countries like UK varieties of other sexual activities, if they are performed against will and without consent are taken as rape. Also, in India male children and adolescents cannot be raped. The same is not true for some other countries, where the crime applies equally to both the sexes. Since, we are discussing this topic in Indian context, we shall concise ourselves regarding rape to the definition as provided in Indian law. As per Indian law, even partial penetration of the penis within the labia majora or the vulva or pudenda with or without emission of semen or even an attempt at penetration is sufficient to construed crime of rape.

Epidemiology: The rape, being a sexual crime is still associated with social stigma and hence incidence is grossly under reported especially from children and adolescent age group. With this caveat, however 2 rape cases are reported every hour and overall number of cases reported from India exceeds 16000 per year. An increasing trend in cases of rape has been observed during 2006–2008. A mixed trend in the incidence of rape has been observed during 2008–2010 (Table 13.2).

Table 13.2: Incidence of child rape in India 2008–2010

Year	Number
2008	5446
2009	5368
2010	5484

From: Crime in India, 2010. National Crime Records Bureau. Ministry of Home Affairs, Govt. of India, New Delhi, September, 2011

Role of pediatricians: With the increase in the prevalence of child and adolescent rape their evaluation is increasingly becoming a part of general pediatric practice. Since, pediatricians usually have trusted relationship with patients and their families; they are often able to gain information about sexual assault that may not be readily available to others.

A raped child may be encountered in a variety of circumstances:

1. Routine physical examination or for care of a medical illness, behavioral condition or physical findings that would include rape as differential diagnosis.
2. They have been or thought to have been raped and brought by parent/social worker or law enforcing agencies for evaluation, evidence collection and crisis management.

Managing a rape victim-child and adolescent: The task of managing a rape victim is challenging and requires experience. However, it can be made simple by dividing into compartments—psychological, physical and medicolegal. In adherence to other medical case, the raped child should be managed by:

a. History taking
b. General and physical examination
c. Investigations and collection of evidences
d. Opinion
e. Treatment.

History taking: While interviewing the child, it is important to:

- Ensure privacy, safety and adequate time to develop confidence in the child.
- Acknowledge the child's courage and encourage speaking.
- Accept the child's story in non-judgmental way (it is the role of police to investigate veracity of story).
- Start interview with non-related, general, non-leading questions.
- Avoid showing strong emotions such as shock or disbelief and maintain, "tell me more", or "what happened next" approach.
- While interviewing young child and adolescent line drawings, dolls or other aids can be used.

- Focus on whether the symptoms are explained by sexual abuse and/a physical abuse to the genital area, or to other medical conditions.
- Children who are sexually abused generally are coerced into secrecy and a high level of suspicion may be required to recognize the problem.
- Gently try to obtain history about the incident's time, place, person, relative position in relation to accused, urination, change of clothes (especially under garments) and about menstrual cycle.
- Interview the child in her own language.

General and physical examination: It should always be kept in mind that the examination of the raped child should not result in additional emotional trauma. It should be explained beforehand to the child as well as to her guardian. No unauthorized person should be present at the place of examination. However, some workers advocate the presence of chaperone (a supportive adult not suspected to involve in the assault) during examination. In the state of Haryana and Punjab, the examination of a rape victim can be performed only by a female doctor as per the direction of Punjab and Haryana High Court. In other states also, it is always advisable to have a female attendant/lady medical practitioner at the time of examination, whenever this examination is performed by a male doctor. Section 53(2) of the criminal procedure code of India also states that when a female is to be medically examined, such examination must be performed only by (or under the supervision) of a lady medical practitioner.

As per the draft guidelines of National Human Rights Commission, the Investigating Officer shall ensure that medical examination of the victim of sexual assault and the accused is done preferably within 24 hr in accordance with Cr. PC Sec. 164 A. Instruction be issued that the Chief Medical Officer ensures the examination of victim immediately on receiving request from Inquiry officer (IO). The gynecologist, while examining the victim should ensure recording the history of incident.

The child should have a thorough pediatric examination including behavioral and emotional status. Special attention should be paid to the growth parameters and sexual development of the child. In some cases where the child is uncooperative, sincere efforts should be made to perform the examination because of the likelihood of trauma, infection and/or the need of forensic sample collections. Consideration should be given to using sedation with careful monitoring. Instruments that magnify and illuminate the genital and rectal area like colposcope can be used as they offer better visualization and simultaneous documentation and are also fitted with still and radio

camera. The photography and video-films taken during examination can latter be reviewed by experts (if needed), thereby avoiding repeated examinations of the children, and also become an important piece of evidence in the court of law.

During examination after complete general examination special attention should be paid to the areas involved in sexual activity like mouth, breasts, genital, perianal region, buttocks, anal area and upper thighs. It is preferable to document the findings of the examination diagrammatically or by photography. During genital examination, look at the inner aspect of thighs, labia majora and minora, clitoris, urethra, periurethral tissue, hymen, hymenal opening, fossa navicularis and posterior fourchette. Speculum or digital examination of vagina should not be performed on the prepubertal child. Note for the presence or absence of:

a. Signs of injury like bruise, abrasion, laceration, etc.
b. Pathological lesions like warts, inflammation, etc.
c. Discharge likes blood, semen, pus, etc.
d. Foreign bodies like tampons, cotton pads, hairs, etc.
e. Hymenal injury/deficit.
f. Laxity of anal sphincter.
g. Congenital lesions.

Investigation and collection of evidence: It is always better to inform all such cases of rape to the nearest police station for further necessary action and also preferably involve a forensic expert for further management of the case. In all such cases following evidences from the child should be collected and preserved:

a. Clothing (if they are the same worn at the time of assault).
b. Head hair combing/brushing.
c. Pubic hair combing/brushing.
d. Vaginal, anal and oral swabbing.
e. Finger nails clippings.
f. Debris like blood, semen and saliva from skin.
g. Blood and urine sample.

The child should also be investigated for:
a. Dental and radiological assessment for age;
b. Sexually transmitted diseases including HIV; and
c. Pregnancy.

Opinion: Never give an opinion as "Rape". Since, rape is neither a medical illness/disease nor a diagnosis. Rape is a legal entity (a crime). Opinion should always be expressed in terms of whether evidence of sexual activity (recent or past) present or not. To arrive at such a conclusion the medical practitioners should consider the following aspects of the case in totality:
a. History of the case;
b. Condition of clothing (in recent case);

c. Psychological assessment;

d. Abrasion/bruising of inner thigh/genitalia;

e. Scarring/tears of labia minora;

f. Scarring/tear or distortion of the hymen;

g. Scarring/injury of fossa navicularis and/or posterior fourchette;

h. Anal injuries/scarring;

i. Positive test for semen/pregnancy; and

j. Positive test for sexually transmitted disease.

Treatment: The need of treatment varies with:

a. Age and symptoms of child;

b. Reporting time after assault; and

c. Nature of physical and psychological trauma.

Role of psychiatrist/counselor is very important in most of the cases. At times a surgeon/gynecologist may be needed for surgical/gynecological intervention such as in case of severe lacerations of vagina/rectum. In case of adolescent rape, emergency contraception must be kept in mind, if the rape was unprotected or the victim is not sure or intoxicated/unconscious at the time of assault. The first dose of regimen should be given as soon as possible and 2nd dose should be repeated after 12 hr. The emergency contraception can be offered up to 3 and possibly up to 5 days after the assault.

Similarly, possibility of chemoprophylaxis and vaccination against STDs, hepatitis B and C depending upon the assessment of case should be kept in mind and proper follow ups at regular intervals should be advised. Although, it is not easy to get victims back for follow up in these cases.

Legal and ethical issues: All pediatricians in the US are required under the laws of each state to report suspected as well as known cases of child sexual abuse. So, whenever there is a case with strong suspicion of child/adolescent rape (especially under 16 yr of age), the victim/guardian should be persuaded to report the matter to the police themselves. However, if they are reluctant, the matter may be brought to the notice of police by the treating doctor.

In addition, there are professional liability risks for pediatricians who fail to diagnose abuse or who misdiagnose other conditions as abuse. Thus, one must keep this thing in mind while labeling any case as a case of child abuse.

Because of the high probability of court involvement in cases of child and adolescent rape, the documentation of examination with proper maintenance of chain of custody of all the evidences preserved is needed. So that when the doctor is required to testify in the court of law, is better prepared and will feel more comfortable if his records are complete and accurate.

Recommendations: (As per American Academy of Pediatrics, committee on Adolescence)

1. Pediatricians should be knowledgeable about the epidemiology of sexual assault in children.

2. Pediatricians should be knowledgeable about the current reporting requirements for sexual assault in their communities.

3. Pediatricians should be knowledgeable about sexual assault and rape evaluation services available in their communities and when to refer a child for a forensic examination.

4. Pediatricians should screen children for a history of sexual assault and potential sequelae.

5. Pediatricians should be prepared to offer psychologic support or referral for counseling and should be aware of the services in the community that provide management, examination, and Counseling for the child and adolescent patient who has been sexually assaulted.

6. Pediatricians should provide preventive counseling to their child and adolescent patients regarding avoidance of high-risk situations that could lead to sexual assault.

American Professional Society on the Abuse of Children. Use of Anatomical dolls in child sexual Abuse Assessments. Chicago, IL: American Professional society on the Abuse of Children, 1995.

American Academy of Pediatrics, Section on Child Abuse and Neglect. *A guide to references and Resources in child abuse and neglect.* 2nd edn. Elk Grove Village II: American Academy of Pediatrics, 1997.

American Academy of Pediatrics, committee on Adolescence. Care of the Adolescent Sexual Assault Victim. Pediatrics 2001;107:1476–9.

Crime in India, 2010. National Crime Records Bureau. Ministry of Home Affairs, Govt. of India, New Delhi, September, 2011.

Indian Penal Code, 1860.

Verma SK. Rape, Sexual abuse and Hymen: A review. *Asian J Obst & Gynae Practices* 1999;3(3):40–44.

Verma SK, Agarwal BBL. Medical aspects of rape victims: Indian perspective. International *J Med Toxicol Legal Med* 1999; 1(2):23–26.

Verma SK, Agarwal BBL. Medicolegal issues concerning adolescent girls. In: Agarwal M, Suneja A (eds). *Paediatric and Adolescent Gynaecology.* New Delhi: Jaypee Brothers Med Pub (P) Ltd., 2003;368–79.

Verma SK. Rape in Children and Adolescents. In: Mathur GP, Mathur Sarla (eds). *Current Trends in Pediatrics.* Vol 1. Delhi: Academa Publishers, 2005;221–6.

Vij K. *Textbook of Forensic Medicine and Toxicology.* 2nd edn. New Delhi: BI Churchill Livingstone, 2002.

13.12 ROAD TRAFFIC ACCIDENTS IN CHILDREN

Trauma evaluation and management: Road traffic injuries are the tenth leading cause of death among all ages, accounting for 2.2% of the global mortality. It is important to stress that management of the traumatized child is a multidisciplinary process. Evaluation and resuscitation of the polytraumatized child begins with the ABCs (airway, breathing, and circulations) of trauma. It is presumed that cervical spine pathology exists unless ruled out clinically and radiographically. The relatively large head of a child forces the cervical spine into flexion if the child is laid on an adult backboard. This cervical flexion can be avoided with a backboard with a cutoff for the head or by elevating the torso by placing a roll under the shoulders. One should keep these precautions in mind before proceeding with airway management. After opening the airway with jaw thrust or lift, clear the nostrils, mouth and oropharynx of any obvious foreign material (food, mucus, blood, vomit, etc.). If required, use of endotracheal intubation may help in procuring a secure airway.

Once an adequate airway has been obtained, breathing and circulation should be assessed. The child should be auscultated to assess lung fields. Assessment of blood volume status in a child can be deceptive, owing to their large physiologic reserves. Although children often maintain normal blood pressure despite significant volume loss, hypovolemia often manifests as tachycardia. Life-threatening hemorrhage in children is usually the result of solid visceral injury, as children are less likely than adults to sustain massive blood loss from pelvic or extremity trauma.

Fluid resuscitation begins with a crystalloid bolus equal to one-fourth of the circulating blood volume (20 ml/kg). If tachycardia or other signs of hypovolemia persist after two crystalloid boluses, consideration should be given to transfusion of packed red blood cells. Urine output is monitored preferably by passing a Foley's catheter in child's bladder.

Following resuscitation, a quick assessment of details of accident, medical allergies, medications and significant past medical history is inquired into. It is essential to understand that initial assessment may not be complete and reassessment at frequent intervals may be necessary. Continuous reassessment will help identify the 'missed injuries' that are noted in up to 12% of poly-traumatized patients. Secondary assessment begins as soon as primary assessment is completed. The secondary survey includes calculation of the Glasgow Coma Scale (GCS) score and radiographs of chest (AP), cervical spine (lateral) and pelvis (AP). The GCS should be noted on arrival in the trauma centre and should be repeated 1 hr after the child arrives at the hospital. The Glasgow Coma Scale is adopted with some modifications in paediatric group who are preverbal or in the early verbal stages of development. Children's best verbal response is graded as follows (smiles, orients to sound, follow objects, interacts-5; consolable when crying, interacts inappropriately-4; inconsistently consolable, moans inconsolably, irritable-3; restless-2, no response-1). The criteria for eye opening and motor response are applicable similar to adult group.

Additional studies (CT head, abdomen, radiographs of extremities and spine), MRI of spine, ultrasonography of abdomen should be performed as indicated. Continuous monitoring of airway, breathing and circulation must continue during the investigations. Deterioration of vital signs or GCS score may warrant emergency consultation with a neurosurgeon or a trauma surgeon.

Orthopedic management of the injured child: In a child with multiple closed fractures, splinting is needed at the time of the initial resuscitation. Definitive treatment should proceed expeditiously once the child's condition has been stabilized. In specific situations, surgical management and operative fixation of fractures may result in decreased morbidity and better functional results.

Rehabilitation: Formal physical therapy and rehabilitation are not generally necessary for the majority of injured children. However, in a multiply injured child, long-term rehabilitation may be needed. Ideally the rehabilitation should be initiated in treatment centre itself because children with severe head, spinal, and musculoskeletal injuries are most often in need of prolonged rehabilitation. Use of orthoses and prostheses requires special care in children because child continues to grow and frequent modifications are necessary. Another aspect of rehabilitation in an injured child is psychologic rehabilitation. Children may also require help with education to catch up with their peers.

Road Traffic Accidents Preventive Measures

1. Seat belts decrease death and severe injury for motor vehicle occupants. A baby up to 9 months of age is to be strapped in on the back seat in a carry cot; a toddler between 9 months to 5 yr of age is to be seated in a bucket seat with harness in the rear. A child greater than 5 yr to 12 yr can be seated in an ordinary harness in the rear.

2. Children less than 8 are not fit to cycle in traffic alone and are only really fully competent by age of around 13. Helmets reduce head and facial injuries in cycle and motorcycle users.

3. Some interventions limit vehicle speed through various traffic calming measures, such as by placing

speed breakers or rumble and reduction in average speeds.

4. School and community based traffic safety education in classroom settings/or simulated traffic environment and via theoretical performance in community settings can help a young child to interact in real traffic conditions comfortably.

Gururaja G, Thomas AA, Reddi MN. Under reporting of road traffic injuries in Bangalore: implications for road safety policies and programmes. In: *Proceedings of the 5th World Conference on injury prevention and control.* Delhi: Macmillan India Ltd., 2000;54–55.

Thompson DC, Rivara FP, Thompson R. Helmets for preventing head and facial injuries in bicyclists. *Cochrane Database Syst Rev* 2000;(2):CD001855.

14 Infectious Diseases

14.1 FEVER

Fever is defined as a controlled increase in body temperature over the normal values for an individual. Fever is regulated in the same manner as normal temperature is maintained in a cool environment, the difference being that the body's thermostat has been reset at a higher temperature. Body temperature is regulated by *thermosensitive neurons* located in the preoptic or anterior hypothalamus that respond to changes in blood temperature as well as to direct neural connections with cold and warm receptors located in skin and muscle. Thermoregulatory responses include redirecting blood to or from cutaneous vascular beds, increased or decreased sweating, extracellular fluid volume regulation (via arginine vasopressin) and behavioral responses, such as seeking a warmer or cooler environmental temperature. Normal body temperature also varies in a regular pattern each day. This circadian temperature rhythm, or diurnal variation, results in lower body temperatures in the early morning and temperatures approximately 1°C higher in the late afternoon or early evening. Temperature can be recorded from oral cavity, and axilla, groin, rectum, and ear.

Pathogenesis: Regardless of the cause of fever, the thermostat is reset in response to "*endogenous pyrogens*" including the cytokines interleukin 1 (IL-1) and IL-6, tumor necrosis factor-α (TNF-α), and interferon-β (IFN-β) and IFN-γ. Stimulated leukocytes and other cells produce lipids that also serve as endogenous pyrogens. The most important lipid mediator is prostaglandin E_2 (PGE_2).

Microbes, microbial toxins, or other products of microbes are the most common *exogenous pyrogens* which are substances that come from outside of the body, stimulate macrophages and other cells to produce endogenous pyrogens, and result in fever. Some substances produced within the body are not pyrogens but are capable of stimulating endogenous pyrogens, such as antigen-antibody complexes in the presence of complement, complement components, lymphocyte products, bile acids and androgenic steroid metabolites. *Endotoxin* is one of the few substances that can directly affect thermoregulation in the hypothalamus as well as stimulate endogenous pyrogen release. In humans, increased temperatures are associated with decreased microbial reproduction and an increased inflammatory response. Thus, fever is an adaptive response and should be treated only in selected circumstances. However, heat production associated with fever increases oxygen consumption, carbon dioxide production, and cardiac output, and may exacerbate cardiac insufficiency in patients with heart disease, or chronic anemia (e.g. sickle cell disease), pulmonary insufficiency in those with chronic lung disease, and metabolic instability in children with diabetes mellitus or inborn errors of metabolism. Furthermore, children between the ages of 6 mo and 5 yr are at increased risk for benign febrile seizures, whereas those with idiopathic epilepsy may have an increased frequency of seizures associated with a febrile illness. The causes of fever are listed in Box 14.1. Factitious fever, or self induced fever, may be due to intentional manipulation of the thermometer or injection of pyrogenic material.

Clinical manifestations: Fever per se is not often helpful in determining a specific diagnosis. In general, a single isolated fever spike is not associated with an infectious disease, but can be attributed to the infusion of blood products, some drugs, some procedures or manipulation of a catheter on a colonized or infected body surface. Similarly, temperatures > 41°C are most often associated with a noninfectious cause. Causes of very high temperatures (> 41°C) include *central fever* (resulting from central nervous system dysfunction involving the hypothalamus), malignant hyperthermia, malignant neuroleptic syndrome, drug fever, or heatstroke. Temperatures that are lower than normal (< 36°C) can be associated with overwhelming sepsis but are more commonly related to cold exposure,

---

Box 14.1: Causes of fever

1. Infection
2. Vaccines
3. Biologic agents (granulocyte-macrophage colony stimulating factor, interferon, interleukins)
4. Tissue injury (infarction, pulmonary emboli, trauma, intramuscular injections, burns)
5. Malignancy (leukemia, lymphoma, hepatoma, metastatic disease)
6. Drugs (cocaine, amphotericin B, drug fever)
7. Immunologic-rheumatologic disorders (systemic lups erythematosus, rheumatoid arthritis)
8. Inflammatory diseases (e.g. inflammatory bowel disease)
9. Granulomatous diseases (sarcoidosis)
10. Endocrine disorders (thyrotoxicosis, pheochromo-cytoma)
11. Metabolic disorders (gout, uremia, Fabry disease, type 1 hyperlipidemia)
12. Genetic disorder (familial Mediterranean fever)
13. Unknown or poorly understood entities
14. Factitious fever

Table 14.1: Temperature ranges in celsius and fahrenheit

Celsius		Fahrenheit
Normal	36.6–37.2	98–99
Febrile	< 36.6	< 98
Hyperpyrexia	>41.6	>107
Hypothermia	<35	<95

hypothyroidism, or overuse of antipyretics (Table 14.1).

Intermittent fever is an exaggerated circadian rhythm that includes a period of normal temperatures on most days; extremely wide fluctuations may be termed *septic or hectic fever. Sustained fever* is persistent and does not vary by more than 0.5°C/24 hr. *Remittent fever* is persistent and varies by more than 0.5°C/24 hr. *Relapsing fever* is characterized by febrile periods that occurs on the 1st and 3rd days (malaria caused by *Plasmodium vivax*), and quartan fever occurs on the 1st and 4th days (malaria caused by *Plasmodium malariae*). *Biphasic fever* indicates a single illness with 2 distinct periods (*camelback fever pattern*) in various illnesses such as poliomyelitis a classic example, leptospirosis, dengue fever, yellow fever, Colorado tick fever, spirillary rat-bite fever (*Spirillum minus*), and the African hemorrhagic fevers (Marburg, Ebola, and Lassa fever). *Periodic fever is* used to describe fever syndromes with a regular periodicity (cyclic neutropenia, and *p*eriodic fever, *a*phthous stomatitis, *p*haryngitis, and *a*denopathy [PFAPA]) or more broadly to include disorders characterized by recurrent episodes of fever that do not follow a strictly periodic pattern (familial Mediterranean fever, hyper IgD syndrome).

The relationship between a patient's pulse rate and temperature can provide useful information. *Relative tachycardia*, when the pulse rate is elevated out of proportion to the temperature, is usually due to noninfectious diseases or infectious diseases in which a toxin is responsible for the clinical manifestations. *Relative bradycardia (temperature-pulse dissociation)*, when the pulse rate remains low in the presence of fever, suggests typhoid fever, brucellosis, leptospirosis, or drug fever. Bradycardia in the presence of fever also may be a result of a conduction defect resulting from cardiac involvement with acute rheumatic fever, Lyme disease, viral myocarditis or infective endocarditis.

Treatment: Fever with temperature less than 39°C in healthy children generally do not require treatment. Other than providing symptomatic relief, antipyretic therapy does not change the course of infectious diseases. Antipyretic therapy is beneficial in high-risk patients who have chronic cardiopulmonary diseases,

metabolic disorders, or neurologic diseases and in those who are at risk for febrile seizures. Hyperpyrexia (> 41°C) indicates greater risk for severe infection, hypothalamic disorders, or central nervous system hemorrhage, and should always be treated with antipyretics. High fever during pregnancy may be teratogenic. Acetaminophen, aspirin, ibuprofen are inhibitors of hypothalamic cyclo-oxygenase, thus inhibiting PGE_2 synthesis. These drugs all are equally effective antipyretic agents. Because aspirin has been associated with Reye syndrome in children and adolescents, it is not recommended for the treatment of fever. Acetaminophen (paracetamol), 10–15 mg/kg orally every 4 hr, is not associated with significant adverse effects; however, prolonged use may produce renal injury, and massive overdose may produce hepatic failure. Ibuprofen, 5–10 mg/kg orally every 6–8 hr, is also effective and may cause dyspepsia, gastrointestinal bleeding, reduced renal blood flow, and rarely, aseptic meningitis, hepatic toxicity, or aplastic anemia. Serious injury from ibuprofen overdose is unusual. Alternating acetaminophen and ibuprofen Q 4–6 hr or giving both drugs at the same time are also effective. Tepid sponge bathing in warm water is another recommended method of reducing hyperpyrexia due to infection or hyperthermia resulting from external causes (heatstroke). The decline of body temperature after antipyretic therapy does not distinguish serious bacterial from less serious viral diseases.

Cunna BA. The clinical significance of fever patterns. *Infect Dis Clin North Am* 1996;10:33–44.

Powell KR. Fever. In: Kliegman RM, Behrman RE, Jenson HB, Stanton BF (eds). *Nelson Textbook of Pediatrics*. 18th edn. Vol. 1. Philadelphia: Saunders, 2007;1084–7.

Saper CB, Breder CD. The neurologic basis of fever. *N Engl J Med* 1994;330:1880–6.

Fever: Without a Focus

Fever is a common manifestation of infectious diseases but is not predictive of severity. There are high-risk groups on the basis of age, associated diseases, or immunodeficiency status, require more extensive evaluation, and in certain situations, prompt antimicrobial therapy before a pathogen is identified.

Fever without localizing signs: Fever without localizing signs and symptoms, usually of acute onset and present for < 1 wk is seen in children < 36 mo of age.

Infants < 3 mo of age: An infectious agent, usually viral, is identified in 70% of infants < 3 mo of age with fever (rectal temperatures approximately of ≥ 38°C); the remainder are presumed to have self-limited but undiagnosed viral infections. However, fever in an infant < 3 mo of age should always suggest the possibility of serious bacterial disease. These infections include sepsis, meningitis, urinary tract infections, enteritis, osteomyelitis, and suppurative arthritis. Pyelonephritis is more common in uncircumcised infant boys, neonates and infants with urinary tract anomalies, and young girls. Other potential bacterial diseases in this age group include otitis media, pneumonia, omphalitis, mastitis, and other skin and soft tissue infections. Bacteremia is present in 5% of febrile infants < 3 mo of age.

The approach to febrile patients < 3 mo of age includes a detailed history and physical examination. Ill-appearing (toxic) febrile infants < 3 mo of age require prompt hospitalization and immediate parenteral antimicrobial therapy after cultures of blood, urine, and cerebrospinal fluid (CSF) are obtained. Ceftriaxone (50 mg/kg/dose every 24 hr with normal CSF findings, or 80 mg/kg/dose every 24 hr with CSF pleocytosis) or cefotaxime (50 mg/kg/dose every 6 hr) plus ampicillin (50 mg/kg/dose every 6 hr) to cover for *L. monocytogenes* and enterococcus, is an effective initial antimicrobial regimen for ill-appearing infants without focal findings. This regimen is effective against the usual bacterial pathogens causing sepsis, urinary tract infections, and enteritis in young infants. However, if meningitis is suspected, because of CSF abnormalities, vancomycin (15 mg/kg/dose every 6 hr) should be included to cover for possible penicillin-resistant *S. pneumoniae*, in addition to the ceftriaxone/cefotaxime and ampicillin, until the results of culture and susceptibility tests are known.

Occult bacteremia in children 3 mo to 3 yr of age: Approximately 30% of febrile children 3 mo to 3 yr of age have no localizing signs of infection. Occult bacteremia (bacteremia without an apparent focus of infection) can occur due to *S. pneumoniae*, *N. meningitidis*, and *Salmonella*. Risk factors indicating increased probability of occult bacteremia include temperature ≥ 39°C, WBC count ≥ 15,000/µl, or an elevated absolute neutrophil count, band count, erythrocyte sedimentation rate, or C-reactive protein. Occult bacteremia may resolve spontaneously without sequelae, may persist, or may lead to localized infections such as pneumonia, meningitis, cellulitis, pericarditis, osteomyelitis, or suppurative arthritis without therapy.

Treatment of toxic-febrile children 3–36 mo of age who do not have focal signs of infection includes hospitalization and prompt institution of antimicrobial therapy after specimens of blood, urine, and CSF are obtained for culture. For non-toxic appearing infants with a rectal temperature of ≥ 39°C, there are two options:

1. Obtain a blood culture and give empirical antimicrobial therapy (ceftriaxone, a single dose of 50 mg/kg, not to exceed 1 g), or
2. If the WBC count is ≥ 15,000/µl, obtain a blood culture and begin empirical antimicrobial therapy.

Fever with petechiae: Irrespective of age, fever with petechiae in an ill-appearing patient with or without localizing signs indicates high risk for life-threatening bacterial infections such as bacteremia, sepsis, and meningitis, and Rocky Mountain spotted fever. Management includes prompt hospitalization, culture of blood and CSF, and administration of appropriate parenteral antimicrobial agents. Well-appearing patients with fever and petechiae can be evaluated with a complete blood count and platelet count as well as a blood culture. If no further petechiae develop or if they are secondary to emesis or coughing and the patient remain well, the patient can be managed as an outpatient with or without antibiotics depending on the most likely cause of the petechiae.

Fever in patients with sickle cell disease: The incidence of infection is greatest among children < 5 yr of age. The increased risk of infection is due in part to functional asplenia and a defect in the properdin (alternate complement) pathway. Fever without localizing signs of infection is caused by *S. pnumoniae* (sepsis, pneumonia, and meningitis), *H. influenzae* type b (meningitis), *S. aureus* (osteomyelitis), *Salmonella* (osteomyelitis), and *E. coli* (pyelonephritis). The managements of patients requires culture of blood and if indicated, CSF, stool, and bone, and administration of antimicrobial agents. Children who appears seriously ill have temperatures of ≥ 40°C, have a WBC count of < 5,000/µl or > 30,000/µl, or who have pulmonary infiltrates or complications of sickle cell disease or severe pain should be hospitalized. Other febrile infants can be given intramuscular ceftriaxone after taking appropriate specimens for culture and cared for as outpatients. Prevention of pneumococcal sepsis is possible by giving long-term penicillin therapy continued until adolescence (oral penicillin V, 125 mg twice daily for children < 5 yr of age and 250 mg twice daily for children ≥5 yr of age).

Hyperpyrexia: Hyperpyrexia (temperatures > 41°C) is uncommon should be carefully evaluated as for all children with fever.

Fever of unknown origin: The term *fever of unknown origin* (FUO) is best reserved for children with a fever documented by a health care provider and for which the cause could not be identified after 3 wk of evaluation as an outpatient or after 1 wk of evaluation in hospital. Patients with fever not meeting these criteria, and specifically those admitted to the hospital with neither an apparent site of infection nor a noninfectious diagnosis may be considered to have *fever without localizing signs*. But over a relatively short period these children will develop additional clinical manifestations which will confirm the infectious nature of illness.

The principal causes of PUO in children, using these rigorous criteria, are infectious and rheumatologic (connective tissue or autoimmune) diseases (Box 14.2). The other three causes associated with fever are neoplastic disorders, drug fever, and factitious fever. In neoplastic disorders most children with malignancies do not have fever alone. Drug fever is usually sustained and not associated with other symptoms. Discontinuation of the drug is associated with resolution of the fever, generally within 72 hr, although certain drugs such as iodides are excreted for a prolonged period with fever that may persist for as long as one month after drug withdrawal. If factitious fever (inoculation of pyrogenic material or manipulation of the thermometer by the patient or parent) is suspected, the presence and pattern of fever should be documented in the hospital. PUO lasting more than 6 mo is uncommon in children and suggests granulomatous or autoimmune disease. Repeat interval evaluation, including history, physical examination, and roentgenographic studies is required.

Diagnosis: The evaluation of PUO requires a detailed history, physical examination (including ophthalmoscopic and otoscopic and rectal examination), laboratory and radiographic tests as indicated by the history or abnormalities found on examination. A complete blood cell count with a differential WBC count and a urinalysis should be part of the initial laboratory evaluation. Biopsy is occasionally helpful in establishing a diagnosis of PUO. Bronchoscopy, laparoscopy, mediastinoscopy, and gastrointestinal endoscopy may provide direct visualization and biopsy material when organ-specific manifestations are present.

Treatment: Fever and infection in children are not synonymous, antimicrobial agents should not be used as antipyretics, and empirical trials of medication should generally be avoided. An exception may be the use of antituberculous treatment in critically ill children with suspected disseminated tuberculosis. Serious cases will need hospitalization for investigation and treatment.

Prognosis: The prognosis in children with PUO is better than adults. The outcome in a child is dependent on the primary disease process, which is usually an atypical presentation of a common childhood illness. In many cases, no diagnosis can be established and fever bates spontaneously. In as many as 25% of cases in which fever persists, the cause of the fever remains unclear, even after thorough evaluation.

Bonsu BK, Harper MB. Fever interval before diagnosis, prior antibiotic treatment, and clinical outcome in young children with bacterial meningitis. *Clin Infect Dis* 2001;32:566–71.

Powell KR. Fever. In: Kliegman RM, Behrman RE, Jenson HB, Stanton BF (eds). *Nelson Textbook of Pediatrics.* 18th edn. Vol. 1. Philadelphia: Saunders, 2007;1087–93.

Roberts KB. Young, febrile infants. A 30 yr odyssey ends where it started. *JAMA* 2004;291:1261–2.

Infection Associated with Medical Devices

Many factors are important in the pathogenesis of device-related infection, including the susceptibility of the host, the composition of the device, the ability of the micro-organisms to adhere to the device itself or to the biofilm that quickly forms on it, and environmental factors that include the insertion technique and maintenance of the device.

1. *Intravascular access devices:* Intravascular access devices range from short stainless steel needles to multilumen implantable synthetic plastic catheters that are expected to remain in use for years.
2. *Cerebrospinal fluid shunts:* The cerebrospinal fluid (CSF) shunt is required for the treatment of children with hydrocephalus.
3. *Peritoneal dialysis catheters:* During the 1st year of peritoneal dialysis for end-stage renal disease, majority of children will have one or more episodes of peritonitis.
4. *Urethral catheters:* Urinary catheters are frequent cause of nosocomial infection.

Box 14.2: Principal causes of pyrexia of unknown origin (PUO)	
Systemic infectious diseases	Salmonellosis, tuberculosis, rickettsial diseases, syphilis, Lyme disease, cat scratch disease, atypical prolonged presentation of common viral diseases, infectious mononucleosis, cytomegalovirus (CMV) infection, viral hepatitis, coccidioidomycosis, histoplasmosis, malaria, kala-azar, toxoplasmosis, tularemia, brucellosis, leptospirosis, rat-bite fever, and AIDS
Rheumatologic (connective tissue or autoimmune) diseases	Juvenile rheumatoid arthritis (JRA), systemic lupus erythematosus, inflammatory bowel disease, rheumatic disease, Kawasaki disease

5. *Orthopedic prostheses:* Infection most often follows introduction of microorganisms at surgery or via hematogenous spread.

Flynn PM, Barrett FF. Infection Associated with Medical Devices. In: Kliegman RM, Behrman RE, Jenson HB, Stanton BF (eds). *Nelson Textbook of Pediatrics.* 18th edn. Vol. 1. Philadelphia: Saunders, 2007;1108–10.

Subba Rao SD, Mary J, Radhika L, et al. Infections related to Vascular Catheters in a Pediatric Intensive Care Unit. *Indian Pediatr* 2005;42:667–72 .

Subba Rao SD, Joseph MP. Catheter related problems in children. In: Mathur GP, Mathur Sarla (eds). *Current Trends in Pediatrics.* Vol 3. Delhi: Academa Publishers, 2007;70–78.

14.2 BACTERIAL INFECTIONS

Diphtheria

Etiology: Corynebacteria are aerobic, nonencapsulated, non-spore forming, mostly nonmotile, pleomorphic, gram-positive bacilli. *Corynebacterium diphtheriae* is by far the most commonly isolated agent of diphtheria. Four *C. diphtheriae* biotypes (mitis, intermedius, belfanti, and gravis) are capable of causing diphtheria and are differentiated by colonial morphology, hemolysis, and fermentation reactions.

Epidemiology: C. diphtheriae is an exclusive inhabitant of human mucous membranes and skin. Spread is primarily by airborne respiratory droplets, direct contact with respiratory secretions of symptomatic individuals, or exudates from infected skin lesions. Organisms can remains viable in dust or on fomites for up to 6 months.

Pathogenesis: Within the 1st few days of respiratory tract infection (usually in the pharynx), a dense necrotic coagulum of organisms, epithelial cells, fibrin, leukocytes and erythrocytes forms, advances and becomes a gray-brown, leather-like adherent pseudomembrane. Removal is difficult and reveals a bleeding edematous submucosa. Paralysis of the palate and hypopharynx is an early local effect of diphtheritic toxin. Toxin absorption can lead to systemic manifestations: kidney tubule necrosis, thrombocytopenia, cardiomyopathy, and/or demyelation of nerves.

Clinical manifestations: The manifestations of C. diphtheriae depend on the anatomic site of infection, the immune status of the host, and the production and systemic distribution of toxin.

Respiratory tract diphtheria: The primary focus of infection is the tonsils or pharynx, with the nose and larynx are the next two most common sites. After an incubation period of 2–4 days, local signs and symptoms develop. Infection of the anterior nares, which is more common among infants, causes serosanguineous, purulent, erosive rhinitis with membrane formation. Shallow ulceration of the external nares and upper lip is characteristic. In tonsillar and pharyngeal diphtheria, sore throat is the early symptom and fever, dysphagia, hoarseness, malaise or headache occurs in some cases. Mild pharyngeal injection is followed by unilateral or bilateral tonsillar membrane formation, which can extend to involve the uvula (which may cause toxin-mediated paralysis), soft palate, posterior oropharynx, hypopharynx, or glottic areas. Underlying soft tissue edema and enlarged lymph nodes can cause a bull-neck appearance.

The characteristic adherent pseudomembrane (gray-brown, leather-like and difficult to remove and reveals a bleeding edematous submucosa), extension beyond the faucial area, dysphagia, and relative lack of fever help differentiate diphtheria from exudative pharyngitis caused by *Streptococcus pyogenes* or Epstein-Barr virus. Infection of the larynx, trachea, and bronchi can be primary or a secondary extension from the pharyngeal infection; hoarseness, stridor, dyspnea, and croupy cough will show involvement. Differentiation from bacterial epiglottis, severe viral laryngotracheobronchitis, and staphylococcal or streptococcal tracheitis depends on visualization of the adherent pseudomembrane at the time of laryngoscopy and intubation. Patients with laryngeal diphtheria are at a greater risk for suffocation because of local soft tissue edema and airway obstruction by the diphtheritic membrane.

Infection at other sites: Cutaneous diphtheria is characterized by a superficial, ecthymic, nonhealing ulcer with a gray-brown membrane. *C. diphtheriae* occasionally causes infections of other sites, such as the ear (otitis externa), the eye (purulent and ulcerative conjunctivitis), and the genital tract (purulent and ulcerative vulvovaginitis). The clinical setting, ulceration, membrane formation, and submucosal bleeding help differentiate diphtheria from other bacterial or viral causes.

Diagnosis: Specimens for culture should be obtained from the nose and throat and any other muco-cutaneous lesions. A portion of membrane should be removed and submitted with underlying exudates. Culture isolates of coryneform organisms should be identified to the species level, and toxigenicity and antimicrobial susceptibility tests should be performed for *C. diphtheriae* isolates.

Complications: The complications include respiratory tract obstruction, toxic cardiomyopathy and toxic neuropathy.

1. *Respiratory tract obstruction* by pseudomembranes may require bronchoscopy or intubation and mechanical ventilation.

2. *Toxic cardiomyopathy* occurs in 10–25% of patients with respiratory diphtheria and is responsible for 50–60% of deaths. The 1st evidence of cardiac toxicity characteristically occurs during the 2nd and 3rd wk of illness as the pharyngeal disease improves, but can appear acutely as early as the 1st wk, a poor prognostic sign, or insidiously as late as 6th wk of illness. Tachycardia out of proportion to fever is common and may be evidence of cardiac toxicity or autonomic nervous system dysfunction. The other findings include a prolonged PR interval and the ST-T wave changes on electrographic tracing, dilated and hypertrophic cardiomyopathy detected by echocardiogram. Single or progressive cardiac dysrhythmias can occur including 1st, 2nd, and 3rd degree heart block. Heart failure may appear insidiously or acutely. Elevation of the serum aspartate aminotransferase concentration closely parallels the severity of myonecrosis. Recovery from the myocarditis is often slow but usually complete. Corticosteroids do not diminish the complications and are not recommended.

3. *Toxic neuropathy:* Neurologic complications occur acutely or 2–3 wk after the onset of oropharyngeal inflammation. Hypesthesia and local paralysis of the soft palate is the common finding. Weakness of the posterior pharyngeal, laryngeal, and facial nerves may follow, causing a nasal quality in the voice, difficulty in swallowing, and risk for aspiration. Cranial neuropathy characteristically occurs in the 5th wk, leading to occulomotor and ciliary paralysis, which can cause strabismus, blurred vision, or difficulty with accommodation. Symmetric polyneuropathy occurs 10 days to 3 mo after oropharyngeal infection and causes principally motor deficits with diminished tendon reflexes. Distal muscle weakness in the extremities that progresses proximally is more commonly described than proximal muscle weakness with distal progression. Clinical and cerebrospinal fluid findings are indistinguishable from those of Guillain-Barré syndrome. Paralysis of the diaphragm may ensue. Complete neurologic recovery occurs but is often slow and rarely 2–3 wk after onset of illness. Vasomotor dysfunction can cause hypotension or cardiac failure. Corticosteroids are not recommended as they do not diminish the complications.

Treatment: Specific antitoxin is the main therapy and should be administered on the basis of clinical diagnosis. Because it neutralizes only free toxin, antitoxin efficacy diminishes with elapsed time after the onset of mucocutaneous symptoms. Antitoxin [diphtheria antitoxin (Haffkine) 10,000 IU in 10 ml and 5 mL] is administered as a single empirical dose of 20,000–120,000 U based on the degree of toxicity, site and size of the membrane, and duration of illness. Antitoxin is probably of no value for local manifestations of cutaneous diphtheria, but its use is prudent because toxic sequelae can occur. Antitoxin is not recommended for asymptomatic carriers.

The role of antibiotic therapy is to halt toxin production, treat localized infection, and prevent transmission of the organisms to contacts. Erythromycin or penicillin is recommended; erythromycin is marginally superior to penicillin for eradication of nasopharyngeal carriage. Appropriate therapy is erythromycin (40–50 mg/kg/day divided every 6 hr PO; maximum 2 g/day), aqueous crystalline penicillin G (100,000–150,000/day divided every 6 hr IV), or procaine penicillin (25,000–50,000 U/kg/day divided every 12 hr IM). Therapy is given for 14 days. Some patients with cutaneous diphtheria have been treated for 7–10 days. At least two successive negative cultures from the nose and throat (or skin) obtained 24 hr apart after completion of therapy confirm eradication of the organism. Treatment with erythromycin is repeated if either culture yields *C. diphtheriae.*

Supportive care: Bed rest is essential during the acute phase of disease, usually for ≥ 2 wk until the risk for symptomatic cardiac damage has passed, with a return to physical activity guided by the degree of toxicity and cardiac involvement.

Prognosis: Mechanical obstruction from laryngeal diphtheria or bull-neck diphtheria and the complications of myocarditis account for most diphtheria-related deaths.

Prevention: Asymptomatic case contacts: All household contacts and those who have had intimate respiratory or habitual physical contact with a patient are closely monitored for illness through the 7 day incubation period. Antimicrobial prophylaxis is presumed effective and is administered regardless of immunization status using erythromycin (40–50 mg/kg/day divided qid PO for 7 days; maximum 2 g/day) or a single injection of benzathine penicillin G (600,000 U IM for < 30 kg, 1,200,000 U IM for ≥ 30 kg). Diphtheria toxoid vaccine, in age-appropriate form, is given to immunized individuals who have not received a booster dose within 5 yr. When an *asymptomatic carrier* is identified, antimicrobial prophylaxis is given for 7 days and an age-appropriate preparation of diphtheria toxoid is administered immediately if a booster has not been given within 1 yr, *see* Chapter 15 and vaccines in Chapter 40.

Buescher ES. Diphtheria (*Corynebacterium diphtheriae*). In: Kliegman RM, Behrman RE, Jenson HB, Stanton BF (eds). *Nelson Textbook of Pediatrics*. 18th edn. Vol. 1. Philadelphia: Saunders, 2007;1153–57.

Hadfield TL, McEvoy P, Polotshy Y, et al. The pathology of diphtheria. *J Infect Dis* 2000;181(Suppl 1): S116–20.

Pertussis

Etiology: *Bordetella pertussis* and *B. parapertussis* are gram-negative, non-motile, pleomorphic, coccobacilli, responsible for causing pertussis. It was first isolated by Bordet in 1906. Only *B. pertussis* expresses pertussis toxin (PT), the major virulence protein. During epidemics, *B. pertussis* has been observed to be the sole causative agent. *B. parapertussis* has been occasionally isolated in sporadic cases.

Epidemiology: Pertussis continues to be endemic worldwide, with an estimated 50 million cases occurring annually, 90% of which are in developing countries. Children in 0–5 yr age group, especially infants, are most vulnerable. Immunity against pertussis begins to wane 3–5 yr after vaccination and is undetectable after 12 years, therefore an injection of *Tdap* vaccine should be given before 12 yr (at 10 yr). Pertussis is transmitted by respiratory droplets. It is extremely contagious, with attack rates as high as 100% in susceptible individuals.

Clinical manifestations: Classically pertussis is a 6 wk disease divided into catarrhal, paroxysmal and convalescent stages. The *catarrhal stage* begins insidiously after an incubation period ranging from 3–12 days. It is accompanied by low grade fever, sneezing, lacrimation and conjunctival congestion. This is the most infectious stage with patients remaining communicable even after 2–3 wks of onset of cough. As initial symptoms wane, coughing marks the onset of the *paroxysmal stage*. After the most insignificant startle from a light, sound, and sucking, or stretching, a well appearing young infant begins to choke, gasp, with flail extremities, face becomes reddened. Cough (expiratory grunt) may not be prominent. Whoop (forceful inspiratory gasp) infrequently occurs in infants < 3 mo of age who are exhausted or lack muscular strength to create sudden negative intrathoracic pressure. A playful toddler with similarly insignificant provocation suddenly expresses an anxious aura and may clutch a parent or an adult before beginning bursts of uninterrupted coughs, chin and chest held forward, tongue protruding maximally, eyes bulging and watering, face purple, until coughing ceases and a loud whoop follows as inspired air traversers the still partially closed airway. Cyanosis can follow a coughing paroxysm, or apnea can occur without a cough. Adults describe a sudden feeling of strangulation followed by uninterrupted coughs, feeling of suffocation, bursting headache, diminished awareness, and then a gasping breath, usually without a whoop. Post-tussive exhaustion occurs in every case. The number and severity of paroxysms progress over days to a week (more rapidly in young infants) and remain in this condition for days to weeks. At the peak of the paroxysmal stage, patients may have more than one episode hourly. As the paroxysmal stage fades into the *convalescent stage*, the number, severity, and duration of episodes diminish.

Diagnosis: Pertussis should be suspected in any individual who has pure or predominant complaint of cough, especially if the following findings are absent: fever, malaise or myalgia, exanthema, or enanthem, sore throat, hoarseness, tachycardia, wheezes, and crackles. Post-tussive emesis is common in pertussis at all ages and is a diagnostic clue in adolescents and adults. Leukocytosis (15,000–100,000 cell/mm^3) due to absolute lymphocytosis is characteristic finding in the catarrhal stage. Isolation of *B. pertussis* in culture remains the gold standard for diagnosis. Direct fluorescent antibody (DFA), culture and polymerase chain reaction (PCR) are all positive in unimmunized children during the catarrhal and paroxysmal stage of disease.

Differential diagnosis: Adenoviral infections are usually distinguishable by associated features, such as fever, sore throat, and conjunctivitis. Mycoplasma causes protracted episodic coughing, but patients have history of fever, headache and frequent finding of crackles on auscultation of the chest.

Complications: The principal complications of pertussis are apnea, secondary infections (such as otitis media and pneumonia, bronchiectasis), physical sequelae of forceful coughing (such as conjunctival and scleral hemorrhages, petechiae on the upper body, epistaxis, hemorrhage in the central nervous system and retina, pneumothorax and subcutaneous emphysema, umbilical and inguinal hernias, and laceration of the lingual frenulum) and following post-tussive vomiting (dehydration, post-tussive alkalosis, and malnutrition). Rectal prolapse occurs in malnourished children with pertussis. Seizures are usually a result of hypoxemia.

Treatment: For patients aged 1 month or older, macrolide antibiotics have been shown to be effective in treating pertussis, such as: erythromycin (40–50 mg/kg/day in 4 divided doses for 14 days) or clarithromycin (15 mg/kg/day in 2 divided doses for 7 days) or azithromycin (10 mg/kg/day PO in a single dose on day 1 followed by 5 mg/kg/day PO for days 2–5). Trimethoprim-sulphamethoxazole (TMP 8 mg/

kg/day, SMZ 40 mg/kg/day in 2 divided doses for 14 days) combination can be used alternatively. The same drugs and dosage can be administered as prophylaxis to *household contacts of index case*. If the age of the contact is < 7 years, vaccination with *DTPw* (DTP whole cell vaccine) or *DTPa* (DTP acellular vaccine) should be completed. In children ≥ 9 yrs of age, *Tdap* vaccine should be given, if it has not been previously given. For prevention, see Chapter 15 and Chapter 40 (vaccination).

American Academy of Pediatrics. Pertussis. In: Pickering LK ed. *Red Book: 2006 Report of the Committee of Infectious Disease.* 2006; 498–520.

Long SS. Pertussis *(Bordetella Pertussis and Bordetella Parapertussis).* In: Kliegman RM, Behrman RE, Jenson HB, Stanton BF (eds). *Nelson Textbook of Pediatrics.* 18th edn. Vol. 1. Philadelphia: Saunders, 2007; 1178–1182.

Enteric Fever (Typhoid Fever)

Etiology: Typhoid fever is caused by *Salmonella enterica* serovar Typhi (*S. typhi*), a gram-negative bacterium. A very similar but often less severe disease is caused by *S. paratyphi* A and rarely by *S. paratyphi* B (Schotmulleri) and *S. paratyphi* C (Hirschfeldii). The ratio of disease caused by *S. typhi* to that caused by *S. paratyphi* is about 10:1.

Epidemiology: Humans are the only natural reservoir of *Salmonella typhi*. Persons with typhoid fever carry the bacteria in their bloodstream and intestinal tract. In addition, a small number of persons, called carriers, recover from typhoid fever but continue to carry the bacteria. Both patients and carriers shed *S. typhi* in their feces.

Pathogenesis: One can get typhoid fever after eating food or drinking beverages handled by patient or a carrier, or due to improper sanitation, when sewage contaminated with *S. typhi* bacteria gets into the drinking water. Once *S. typhi* bacteria are eaten or drunk, they multiply and spread into the bloodstream causing fever and other signs and symptoms. Pathology occurs in the Payer's patches. Initially *S.* Typhi proliferates in the small intestine from where systemic dissemination occurs, to the liver, spleen, and mesenteric glands.

Clinical manifestations: The incubation period of typhoid fever is usually 7–14 days, but is also dependent on the infecting dose (range 3–30 days). Typhoid fever usually presents with high-grade fever with a wide variety of associated features such as generalized myalgia, anorexia, abdominal pain, and hepatosplenomegaly. In children, diarrhea may be present in the earlier stages of illness and may be followed by constipation. The fever may rise

gradually, but the classic step-ladder rise of fever is relatively rare. In about 25% of cases, a macular or maculopapular rash (rose spots) may be seen around the 7th–10th day of illness, and lesions may appear in crops of 10–15 at the lower chest and abdomen and lasts for 2–3 days. Multidrug resistant *S. typhi* infection is a more severe clinical illness with higher rates of toxicity, complications, and case fatality rates. If no complications occur, the symptoms and physical findings gradually resolve within 2–4 wk, with malnutrition in a number of affected children. Paratyphoid fever classically regarded as milder illness may also be severe, with significant morbidity and complications.

Complications: The complications include altered liver function (hepatitis, jaundice, and cholecystitis), intestinal hemorrhage (< 1%) and perforation (0.5–1%), toxic myocarditis, neurologic (delirium, psychosis, increased intracranial pressure, acute cerebellar ataxia, chorea, deafness, and Guillain-Barré syndrome), bone marrow necrosis, disseminated intravascular coagulation (DIC), hemolytic uremic syndrome, pyelonephritis, nephrotic syndrome, meningitis, endocarditis, parotitis, orchitis, and suppurative lymphadenitis.

Individuals who excrete *S. typhi* for ≥3 mo after infection are regarded as *chronic carriers*; in general rates of chronic carriage are lower in children than adults. The propensity to become a carrier follows the epidemiology of gall bladder disease, increasing with age and antibiotic resistance of the prevalent strains.

Diagnosis: A positive culture from blood, stool, urine, or bone marrow is diagnostic of typhoid fever. Results of blood cultures are positive in 40–60% of the patients in early course of disease, and stool and urine cultures become positive after the 1st wk. However, the sensitivity of blood cultures in diagnosing typhoid fever is limited as widespread antibiotic prescribing may render bacteriologic confirmation difficult. The organism can be cultured from the bone marrow in as many as 96% of patients even if the patient has started antibiotics. Blood leukocyte counts are frequently low in relation to the fever and toxicity; in younger children leukocytosis is a common finding.

The Widal test measures antibodies against O and H antigens of *S. typhi* but lacks sensitivity and specificity in endemic areas. Because many false-positive and false-negative results occur, diagnosis of typhoid fever by Widal test alone is prone to error. Two specimens of serum are required at an interval of 7–10 days and a four-fold rise in the titres of H (flagellar) or O (somatic) agglutinins indicates a strong likelihood of the disease. Previous immunisations may leave residual titres of H agglutinins for years, thus only a rise in O agglutinins is relevant. However, the Widal test can be performed on a single serum; elevated titres of O and H agglutinins (e.g. > 1 : 160) in unvaccinated subjects is strongly suggestive of *S. typhi* infection if the person comes from a non- endemic area or if a child less than 10 yrold in an endemic area. A 60 minutes dot enzyme immunoassay for the rapid detection of *Salmonella typhi* specific IgM and IgG antibodies test is reported to be 95% sensitive.

Differential diagnosis: The early stages of enteric fever may be confused with acute gastroenteritis, bronchitis, or bronchopneumonia. Subsequently, the differential diagnosis includes malaria, sepsis, tuberculosis, brucellosis, leptospirosis, rickettsial diseases, dengue fever, acute hepatitis, and infectious mononucleosis.

Treatment: Treatment should not be delayed for confirmatory tests since prompt treatment drastically reduces the risk of complications and fatalities. Patients with persistent vomiting, severe diarrhea, and abdominal distension may require hospitalization and parenteral antibiotic therapy. Adequate rest, hydration, and soft, easily digestible diet should be continued unless the patient has abdominal distension or ileus. Antipyretic therapy (paracetamol 10–15 mg/ kg every 4–6 hr PO) should be provided as required. Most antibiotic regimens are associated with a 5–20% recurrence risk. Antibiotic therapy minimizes complications. Traditional therapy with chloram-phenicol, trimethoprim-sulfamethoxazole or amoxicillin is associated with relapse, whereas quinolones and 3rd degree cephalosporins (cefixime, ceftriaxone) are associated with higher cure rates. There is also emergence of multidrug resistant strains of *S. typhi*. Persons given antibiotics usually begin to feel better within 3 to 5 days, but the antibiotics are continued until a week after the fever subsides. Most complications tend to occur in the relapses and not in the primary typhoid fever. Dexamethasone (3 mg/kg for the initial dose, followed by 1 mg/kg every 6 hr for 48 hr) has been recommended among severely ill patients with shock, obtundation, stupor or coma, this must be done carefully and signs of abdominal complications may be masked.

- Uncomplicated typhoid fever (fully sensitive) give amoxicillin 75–100 mg/kg/day for 14 days, or ofloxacin 15 mg/kg/day for 5–7 days#, or chloramphenicol 50–75 mg/kg/day for 14–21 days.
- Uncomplicated typhoid fever (multidrug resistant) give ofloxacin 15 mg/kg/day for 5–7 days, or cefixime 15–20 mg/kg/day for 7–14 days, or azithromycin 8–10 mg/kg/day for 7 days.

- Uncomplicated typhoid fever (quinolone resistant) give azithromycin 8–10 mg/kg/day for 7 days, or ceftriaxone 75 mg/kg/day for 10–14 days, or cefixime 20 mg/kg/day for 7–14 days.
- Severe typhoid fever (fully sensitive) give ampicillin 100 mg/kg/day for 14 days, or ceftriaxone 60–75 mg/kg/day for 10–14 days, or ofloxacin 15 mg/ kg/day for 5–7 days#, or ciprofloxacin 15 mg/kg/ day for 5–7 days#.
- Child with relapse treat with the same drug as used for primary therapy but for at appropriate dose and duration. If the isolate is nalidixic acid sensitive and fluoroquinolones were not used for primary therapy, they should be used.
- Chronic carrier individuals give 1.5 g ampicillin with 0.5 g of probenecid 4 times a day for a period of 6 wk.

Surgery is usually indicated in cases of intestinal perforation (*see* Chapter 16). Simple closure of the perforation with drainage of the peritoneum is preferred for small perforations. Small-bowel resection is indicated for patients with multiple perforations. If antibiotic treatment fails to eradicate the hepatobiliary carriage, cholecystectomy is preferred although it is not always successful in eradicating the carrier state because of persisting hepatic infection.

Prognosis: The prognosis depends on early diagnosis and administration of appropriate antibiotic therapy. Infants and children with malnutrition and those infected with multi-drug resistant isolates are at higher risk for adverse outcomes.

Prevention: The three basic actions can protect from typhoid fever:
1. Avoid risky and raw foods and contaminated drinks
2. Keep good personal and social hygiene; and
3. Get vaccinated against typhoid fever (*see* Chapters 15 and 40).

Bhutta ZA. Salmonella. In: Kliegman RM, Behrman RE, Jenson HB, Stanton BF (eds). *Nelson Textbook of Pediatrics*. 18th edn. Vol. 1. Philadelphia: Saunders, 2007; 1182–91.

Bhutta ZA. Current concepts in the diagnosis and treatment of typhoid fever. *Br Med J* 2006;333:78–82.

Parry CM, Hien TT, Dougan G, et al: Typhoid fever. *N Engl J Med* 2003;347:1770–82.

Cholera

Etiopathogenesis: *Vibrio cholerae*, a comma-shaped gram-negative, aerobic, non-spore-forming bacillus is responsible for causing the epidemic diarrheal disease—cholerae. The antigenic structure of *V. cholerae* consists of a flagellar 'H' antigen and a somatic 'O' antigen. Presently *V. cholerae* O1 El Tor is the

#A 3 days course is also effective particularly for epidemic containment.

predominant strain responsible for the epidemics. Other strains of *V. cholera* apart from O1 and O139 can cause mild diarrhea but do not develop into epidemics. After colonization *V. cholerae* O1 and O139 produce an enterotoxin that promotes the secretion of fluids and electrolytes into the lumen of the small intestine. Humans are the only known vertebrate reservoirs of *V. cholerae*. Cholera exists in sporadic, endemic, epidemic, and pandemic forms. Transmission is usually by fecal-oral spread with contaminated water as the main vehicle but contaminated food and utensils and houseflies may also play important roles.

Clinical manifestations: The incubation period between ingestion of the organism and onset of manifestations is 18 hr to 5 days. Cholera is characterized by an acute onset of copious watery diarrhea and vomiting without abdominal cramps or fever. The stools are colorless with small flecks of mucus ('rice-water') and having a fishy odor. At first, children may be restless or extremely thirsty. Other signs of dehydration may rapidly manifest. Some individuals have mild diarrhea, indistinguishable from other diarrheal diseases.

Diagnosis: Dark-field microscopy involves examining a wet mount of stool sample for "darting" organisms, which is a characteristic feature of *V. cholerae*. The diagnosis is confirmed by isolation of the organism in stool cultures. Molecular diagnostic tests, such as PCR, are now being developed for both clinical and environmental monitoring of *V. cholerae* O1 and O139.

Treatment: Fluid and electrolyte replacement either by oral rehydration or intravenous fluid therapy is the main treatment. Oral rehydration is indicated in patients with no or some dehydration and who are able to accept fluids orally with WHO-ORS (osmolarity 245 mOsm/L). Treat severe dehydration with IV fluids as mentioned in Chapter 16.

Antimicrobial agents in children < 9 yr of age, trimethoprim-sulfamethoxazole (8–10 mg/kg/day trimethoprim and 40 mg/kg/day sulfamethoxazole, PO, divided bid), or erythromycin (40 mg/kg/day, maximum 2 g/day PO), or furazolidone (5–8 mg/kg/ day, maximum 400 mg, PO) is prescribed. For children > 9 yr of age, tetracycline (50 mg/kg/day divided PO qid for 3 days; maximum 2 g/day) or doxycycline (5 mg/kg PO as a single dose, maximum 200 mg/day) is given.

Prevention: Provision for safe water supply and environmental sanitation are effective preventive measures at community level. Travelers to endemic areas should be especially careful about, what they eat and drink. During an epidemic various measures include early identification of cases through surveillance and case-finding, establishment of treatment centres, notification to health authorities and health-education, and proper disposal of human waste (*see* Chapters 15 and 40).

Deen JL. Cholera (*Vibrio cholerae*). In: Kliegman RM, Behrman RE, Jenson HB, Stanton BF (eds). *Nelson Textbook of Pediatrics.* 18th edn. Vol. 1. Philadelphia: Saunders, 2007; 1196–99.

Sharma NC, Mandal PK, Dhillon R, et al. Changing profile of *Vibrio cholerae* O1, O139 in Delhi and its periphery (2003–2005). *Indian J Med Res* 2007;125:633–4.

Brucellosis

Etiopathogenesis: Human brucellosis is caused by organisms of the genus *Brucella*. *Brucella abortus* (cattle), *B. melitensis* (goat/sheep), *B. suis* (swine), and *B. canis* (dog) are the most common organisms responsible for human disease. These organisms are small, aerobic, non-spore-forming, nonmotile, gram-negative coccobacillary bacteria.

Human brucellosis is a major public health problem worldwide. Brucellosis is an occupational risk among adults working with livestock. Brucellosis in children is food-borne and is associated with consumption of unpasteurized milk products. It is also a potential agent of bioterrorism (*see* Chapter 35).

Clinical manifestations: Brucellosis is a systemic illness, symptoms usually nonspecific appear 2–4 wk after inoculation. The classic triad of fever, arthralgia/arthritis, and hepatosplenomegaly can be demonstrated in most patients. Joints frequently involved include sacroiliac joints, hips, knees, and ankles. Infection of the nervous system occurs in about 1% of cases. Neonatal and congenital infections have been transmitted transplacentally, from breastmilk, and through blood transfusions.

Diagnosis: Routine laboratory examinations of blood reveal thrombocytopenia, neutropenia, anemia, or pancytopenia. A history of exposure to animals or ingestion of unpasteurised dairy products may be more helpful. A definitive diagnosis is established by recovering the organisms in the blood, bone marrow, or other tissues. Isolation of the organism may require as long as 4 wk from a blood culture sample. The serum agglutination test (SAT) is used and detects antibodies against *B. abortus*, *B. melitensis*, and *B. suis*. In most patients with acute infections the titers of ≥ 1:160 are diagnostic. The enzyme immunoassay appears to be the most sensitive method for detecting *Brucella* antibodies.

Differential diagnosis: Brucellosis may be confused with other infections such as typhoid fever, cat scratch disease, *Mycobacterium tuberculosis*, atypical mycobacteria, rickettsiae, and Yersinia.

Treatment: The onset of initial antimicrobial therapy may precipitate a Jerisch-Herxheimer-like reaction, presumably due to a large antigen load. It is rarely severe and does not require corticosteroid therapy.

- *Age ≥ 8 yr:* Doxycyline 2–4 mg/kg/day; maximum 200 mg/day PO 4–6 wk + Rifampin 15–20 mg/kg/day; maximum 600–900 mg/day PO 4–6 wk.
- *Age < 8 yr:* Trimethoprim-sulfamethoxazole, TMP (10 mg/kg/day; max 400 mg/day) and SMZ (50 mg/kg/day; max 2.4 g/day) PO 4–6 wk.
- *Meningitis, osteomyelitis, endocarditis:* Doxycyline 2–4 mg/kg/day; 200 mg/day PO 4–6 mo + Gentamicin 3–5 mg/kg/day IV 1–2 wk + Rifampin 15–20 mg/kg/day; maximum 600–900 mg/day PO 4–6 mo.

Prevention: Brucellosis can be prevented by effective eradication of organism from cattle, goats, and swine herds as well as from other animals. Pasteurization of milk and dairy products for human consumption is an important aspect of prevention.

Pappas G, Akritidis N, Bosilkovski M, et al. Brucellosis. *N Engl J Med* 2005;352:2325–36.

Schutze GE, Jacobs RF. Brucella. In: Kliegman RM, Behrman RE, Jenson HB, Stanton BF (eds). *Nelson Textbook of Pediatrics.* 18th edn. Vol. 1. Philadelphia: Saunders, 2007;1214–16.

Cat Scratch Disease

Etiopathogenesis: Cat scratch disease (CSD) is caused by *Bartonella hensalae*. Transmission between cats is arthropod borne by the cat flea, *Ctenocephalides felis*. Distribution is worldwide. Cat scratches appear to be more common among children. Boys are affected more often than girls.

Clinical manifestations: After an incubation period of 7–12 days (range 3–30 days), 1 or more 3–5 mm red papules develop at the site of cutaneous inoculation, often reflecting a linear cat scratch. Lymphadenopathy generally is evident within a period of 1–4 wk. Chronic regional lymphadenitis is the hallmark, affecting the 1st or 2nd set of nodes draining the entry site in order of frequency include the axillary, cervical, submandibular, preauricular, epitrochlear, femoral and inguinal glands. Fever and transient rashes are reported in a few cases. More severe, disseminated illness includes high fever, hepatosplenomegaly, granulomatous osteolytic lesions, neuroretinitis, and encephalitis. The most common atypical presentation is *Parinaud oculoglandular syndrome*, which is unilateral conjunctivitis followed by preauricular lymphadenopathy, due to direct eye inoculation as a result of rubbing with the hands after cat contact.

Various complications include facial nerve paralysis, myelitis, radiculitis, compression neuropathy, cerebellar ataxia, retinopathy and hematologic manifestations (hemolytic anemia, purpura and eosinophilia).

Diagnosis: Diagnosis can be suspected on clinical grounds with the history of exposure to cat. If tissue specimens are obtained, bacilli may be visualized with Warthin Starry and Brown-Hopp tissue Gram stains. *Bartonella* DNA can be identified by PCR on tissue specimens. White blood cell count may be normal or mildly elevated. Hepatic transaminases may be elevated in systemic disease. Ultrasonography or CT may reveal many granulomatous nodules in the liver and spleen, appearing as hypodense round irregular lesions.

Differential diagnosis: The differential diagnosis of CSD includes pyogenic lymphadenitis, primarily from staphylococcal or streptococcal infections, atypical mycobacterium infections, tularemia, brucellosis, sporotrichosis, and malignancy. Epstein-Barr virus, cytomegalovirus, or *Toxoplasma gondii* infections usually cause more generalized lymphadenopathy.

Treatment: Oral azithromycin (500 mg on day 1, then 250 mg on days 2–5; for smaller children 10 mg/kg/24 hr on day 1 and 5 mg/kg/24 hr on days 2–5) has shown to decrease in initial lymph node volume in 50% of patients during the 1st 30 days but after 30 days there is no difference in lymph node volume. Children with hepatosplenic CSD appear to respond well to rifampin (dose 20 mg/kg for 14 days), either alone or in combination with trimethoprim-sulfamethoxazole.

Stechenberg BW. Cat-scratch disease. In: Kliegman RM, Behrman RE, Jenson HB, Stanton BF (eds). *Nelson Textbook of Pediatrics.* 18th edn. Vol. 1. Philadelphia: Saunders, 2007;1219–23.

Botulism

Etiopathogenesis: Botulism is caused by the neurotoxin produced by *Clostridium botulinum*, a gram-positive, spore-forming, obligate anaerobe whose natural habitat worldwide is soil, dust, and marine sediments. It is also found in fresh and cooked agricultural products. Botulinum toxin is carried by the blood stream to peripheral cholinergic synapses, where it binds irreversibly, blocking acetylcholine release and causing impaired neuromuscular and automatic transmission. *Inhalational botulism* occurs when aerosolized botulinum toxin is inhaled. A bioterrorist attack could result in large or small outbreaks of inhalational or food-borne botulism (*see* Chapter 35).

Clinical manifestations: Botulinum toxin is distributed hematogenously. Because relative blood flow and density of innervation are greatest in the bulbar musculature, all forms of botulism manifest neurologically as a symmetric, descending, flaccid paralysis beginning with the cranial nerve musculature. It is not possible to have botulism without having multiple bulbar palsies. In infants such symptoms as poor feeding, weak suck, feeble cry, drooling, and even obstructive apnea are of bulbar in origin. Loss of head control is a prominent sign. Food-borne botulism begins with gastrointestinal symptoms of nausea and vomiting, or diarrhea in about 1/3 of cases. Constipation may occur once flaccid paralysis becomes evident. Illness usually begins 12–36 hr (range 2 hr to 8 days) after ingestion of the contaminated food. The incubation period in wound botulism is 4–14 days. Fever may be present in wound botulism but is absent in food-borne botulism unless a secondary infection (pneumonia) is present.

Diagnosis: The classic triad of botulism is the acute onset of a symmetric flaccid descending paralysis with clear sensorium, no fever, and paresthesias. The diagnosis of botulism is established by demonstrating the presence of botulinum toxin in serum or of *C. botulinum* toxin or organism in wound material, enema fluid, or feces. An epidemiologic diagnosis of food-borne botulism can be established when *C. botulinum* organisms and toxin are found in food eaten by patients.

Differential diagnosis: The botulism is to be differentiated from Guillain-Barré syndrome, myasthenia gravis, spinal muscular atrophy, and central nervous system diseases.

Treatment: Human botulism immune globulin (BIG-IV) is for the treatment of infant botulism caused by botulinum toxin. Treatment with BIG-IV consists of a single intravenous infusion of 50 mg/kg that should be given as soon as possible after infant botulism is suspected. Older patients with suspected food, wound, or inhalational botulism may be treated with 1 vial of equine botulinum antitoxin. Antibiotics should be used for the treatment of secondary infections, and in the absence of antitoxin therapy, a nonclostridiocidal antibiotic such as trimethoprim-sulfamethoxazole is preferred. Wound botulism requires aggressive treatment with antibiotics and antitoxin in a manner analogous to tetanus. In the absence of complications (pneumonia, urinary tract infection or otitis media), there is full and complete recovery in infants.

General management: Correct positioning is important to protect airway and improve respiratory mechanics. About half of patients with infant botulism require endotracheal intubation, which is best done prophylactically. Feeding should be done by a nasogastric or nasojejunal tube until sufficient oropharyngeal strength and coordination enable feeding by breast or bottle. Honey is an unsafe food for any child younger than 1 yr of age.

Arnon SS. Botulism (*Clostridium botulinum*). In: Kliegman RM, Behrman RE, Jenson HB, Stanton BF (eds). *Nelson Textbook of Pediatrics.* 18th edn. Vol. 1. Philadelphia: Saunders, 2007; 1224–7.

Fox CK, Keet CA, Strober JB. Recent advances in infant botulism. *Pediatr Neurol* 2005;32:149–54.

Sobel J. Botulism. *Clin Infect Dis* 2005;41:1167–73.

Tetanus

Etiopathogenesis: Tetanus is caused by the neurotoxin produced by *Clostridium tetani*, a motile, gram-positive, spore-forming obligate anaerobe whose natural habitat world-wide is soil, dust, and the alimentary tract of various animals. *C. tetani* causes illness through the effect of a single toxin, tetanospasmin, more commonly referred as tetanus toxin. Most cases of tetanus are associated with a traumatic injury, contaminated suture material, after intramuscular injection of medicines, animal bites, abscesses (including dental abscess), ear and other body piercing, chronic skin ulceration, burns, compound fractures, frostbite, gangrene, intestinal surgery, ritual scarification, infected insect bites and circumcision. Tetanus toxin blocks the normal inhibition of antagonistic muscles on which voluntary coordinated movement depends; in consequence, affected muscles sustain maximal contraction and cannot relax. The autonomic nervous system is also rendered unstable in tetanus. The human lethal dose of tetanus toxin is estimated to be 10^{-5} mg/kg.

Clinical manifestations: Tetanus may be either generalized or localized. The incubation period is 2–14 days, but it may be as long as months after the injury. In *generalized tetanus*, the presenting symptom in about half of cases is *trismus* (masseter muscle spasm, or lockjaw). Headache, restlessness, and irritability are early symptoms, often followed by stiffness, difficulty chewing, dysphagia, and neck muscle spasm. The so-called *sardonic smiles of tetanus* (*risus sardonicus*) results from intractable spasms of facial and buccal muscles induced by sight, sound or touch (*see* Fig. 14.1 in CD). When paralysis extends to abdominal, lumbar, hip and thigh muscles, the patient may assume an arched posture of extreme hyperextension of the body, or *opisthotonos*, with the head and the heels bent backward and the body bowed forward with only the back of the head and the heels touching the supporting surface (typical board-like rigidity of tetanus). Laryngeal and respiratory muscle spasm can lead to airway obstruction and asphyxiation. Because tetanus toxin does not affect cortical function or sensory nerves, the patient remains conscious, in extreme pain, and in fearful anticipation of the next tetanic seizure. These seizures are characterized by sudden, severe tonic contractions of the muscles, with the fist clenching, flexion, and adduction of the arms and hyperextension of the legs. Without treatment, the seizures range from a few seconds to a few minutes in length with intervening respite periods, but as the illness progresses, the spasms become sustained and exhausting. The smallest disturbance by sight, sound, or touch may trigger a tetanic spasm. Dysuria and urinary retention result from bladder sphincter spasm; forced defecation may occur. Fever occasionally as high as 40°C, is common because of the substantial energy consumed by spastic muscles. Autonomic effects include tachycardia, dysrhythmias, labile hypertension, diaphoresis, and cutaneous vasoconstriction. The tetanic paralysis is usually more severe in the 1st wk after onset, stabilizes in the 2nd wk, and ameliorates gradually over the ensuing 1–4 wk.

Neonatal tetanus (tetanus neonatorum), manifests in the form of generalized tetanus within 3–12 days of birth as progressive difficulty (sucking and swallowing), associated hunger, and crying. Paralysis or diminished movement, stiffness and rigidity to the touch, and spasms with or without opisthotonos, are characteristic features. The umbilical stump may contain remnants of dirt, dung, clotted blood, or serum, or it may appear relatively benign.

Localized tetanus results in painful spasms of the muscles adjacent to the wound site and may precede generalized tetanus. *Cephalic tetanus* is a rare form of localized tetanus involving the bulbar musculature that occurs with wounds, chronic otitis media, and foreign bodies in the head, nostrils, or face. Cephalic tetanus is characterized by retracted eyelids, deviated gaze, trismus, risus sardonicus, and spastic paralysis of the tongue and pharyngeal musculature.

Diagnosis: The typical findings in an unimmunized patient or newborn who was injured within the preceding 2 wk (and/or mother), who presents with trismus, other rigid muscles, and a clear sensorium. Peripheral leukocytosis may be observed from a secondary bacterial infection of the wound or may be stress induced from the sustained tetanic spasms. The cerebrospinal fluid is normal, although the intense muscle contractions may raise intracranial pressure.

Differential diagnosis: Both rabies and tetanus may follow an animal bite, but rabies may be distinguished from tetanus by hydrophobia, marked dysphagia, predominantly clonic seizures, and pleocytosis. Strychnine poisoning may result in tonic muscle spasms and generalized seizure activity but it seldom produces trismus and generalized relaxation usually occurs between spasms. Hypocalcemia may produce tetany that is characterized by laryngeal and carpopedal spasms, but trismus is absent. Epileptic seizures, narcotic withdrawal, or other drug reactions may suggest tetanus.

Treatment: Surgical wound excision and debridement are often needed to remove the foreign body or devitalized tissue that created anaerobic growth conditions; surgery should be performed promptly after administration of human tetanus immunoglobulin (TIG) and antibiotics. Excision of the umbilical stump in neonatal tetanus is not recommended. Infiltration of TIG into the wound is now considered unnecessary.

TIG should be given as soon as possible in order to neutralize toxin that diffuses from the wound into the circulation before the toxin can bind at distant muscle groups. A single intramuscular injection of 500 U of TIG is sufficient to neutralize systemic tetanus toxin, but total doses as high as 3,000–6,000 U are also recommended.

Penicillin G (1, 00,000 U/kg/day divided every 4–6 hr IV for 10–14 days) is the antibiotic of choice because of its clostridiocidal action and its diffusibility to injured tissue. Metronidazole (500 mg every 8 hr IV for adults) appears to be equally effective. Erythromycin and tetracycline (for persons > 8 yr of age) are alternatives for penicillin-allergic patients.

All patients with generalized tetanus need muscle relaxants. Diazepam provides both relaxation and seizure control. The initial dose of 0.1–0.2 mL/kg every 3–6 hr given intravenously is subsequently titrated to control the tetanic spasms, after which it is sustained for 2–6 wk before its tapered withdrawal. Magnesium sulfate, other benzodiazepines (midazolam), chlorpromazine, dantroline, baclofen, neuromuscular agents (vecuronium and pancuronium), and morphine are also used.

Supportive care: Because tetanic spasms may be triggered by minor stimuli, the patient should be sedated and protected from all unnecessary sounds, sights, and touch; and all therapeutic and other manipulations must be carefully scheduled and coordinated. Early tracheostomy should be considered in severe cases not managed by pharmacologically induced flaccid paralysis. Cardio-respiratory monitoring, frequent suctioning, and maintenance of substantial fluid, electrolyte, and caloric needs are essential. Nursing attention to mouth, skin, bladder, and bowel function is needed to avoid ulceration, infection, and obstipation.

Complications: Various complications reported include aspiration of secretions and pneumonia, pneumothorax and mediastinal emphysema, seizures may result in laceration of tongue or mouth, venous thrombosis, pulmonary embolism, gastric ulceration with or without hemorrhage, paralytic ileus, decubitus ulceration, cardiac arrhythmias, and renal failure.

Prognosis: Most fatalities occur within the 1st wk of illness. Reported case fatality rates for generalized tetanus are 5–35%, and for neonatal tetanus extend from < 10% with intensive care treatment to > 75% without it. Cephalic tetanus has a poor prognosis because of breathing and feeding difficulties.

Prevention: A serum antibody titer of ≥ 0.01 U/ml is considered protective. Tetanus is an entirely preventive disease (*see* Chapters 15 and 40).

Arnon SS. Tetanus (*Clostridium tetani*). In: Kliegman RM, Behrman RE, Jenson HB, Stanton BF (eds). *Nelson Textbook of Pediatrics*. 18th edn. Vol. 1. Philadelphia: Saunders, 2007; 1228–30.

Brook I. Tetanus in children. *Pediatr Emerg Care* 2004;20:48–51.

Pseudomembranous Colitis

Etiopathogenesis: C. difficile is an obiquitous, spore-bearing, gram-positive anaerobic bacillus. Administration of antibiotics that impair growth of normal flora but not *C. difficile* is the most common risk factor, but any process that disrupts the normal bowel flora (weaning, chemotherapy) or bowel motility (bowel stasis, bowel surgery) predisposes to *C. difficile*-associated diarrhea.

Clinical manifestations: Illness varies from a mild self-limited diarrhea without pseudomembranous, to explosive watery diarrhea with occult blood, to the classic picture of pseudomembranous colitis with bloody diarrhea accompanied by fever, cramps, abdominal pain, nausea, and vomiting.

Diagnosis: The diagnosis is confirmed by detecting *C. difficile* or its toxin in the stool. Findings of sigmoidoscopy or colonoscopy include pseudomembranous nodules and plaques characteristic of toxin-related colitis.

Treatment: If possible discontinue current antibiotics, which is sufficient in most cases in combination with appropriate fluid and electrolyte replacement. If symptoms persist, antibiotics cannot be discontinued, or illness is severe, then oral metronidazole (20–40 mg/kg/day divided every 6–8 hr PO) should be given for 7–10 days. Appropriate use of antibiotics can prevent pseudomembranous colitis.

Fisher MC. Pseudomembranous Colitis (*Clostridium difficile*).In: Kliegman RM, Behrman RE, Jenson HB, Stanton BF (eds). *Nelson Textbook of Pediatrics*. 18th edn. Vol. 1. Philadelphia: Saunders, 2007;1230–31.

Mylonakis E, Ryan ET, Calderwood SB. *Clostridium difficile*-associated diarrhea. A review. *Arch Intern Med* 2002;161:525–33.

14.3 CHILDHOOD TUBERCULOSIS

Introduction: Tuberculosis is prevalent throughout the world. The World Health Organization (WHO) estimates that > 8 million new cases of tuberculosis occur and approximately 3 million people die of the disease worldwide each year. Almost 1.3 million cases and 450,000 deaths occur in children each year. More than 1/3 of the world's population is infected with *Mycobacterium tuberculosis*. Infection rates are highest in Africa, Asia, and Latin America. Currently, 95% of tuberculosis cases occur in developing countries where HIV/AIDS epidemics have had the greatest impact, and where resources are often unavailable for proper identification and treatment of these diseases.

The incidence of drug-resistant tuberculosis has increased throughout the world. In some countries, drug resistance rates range from 20 to 50%. The major reasons for the development of drug resistance are poor patient adherence to treatment and provision of inadequate regimens by the physician or national tuberculosis program.

Etiology: M. tuberculosis is the single most important cause of tuberculous disease in humans. The tubercle bacilli are non-spore-forming, nonmotile, pleomorphic, weakly gram-positive curved rods 2–4 μm long. They are obligate aerobes that grow in Loewenstein-Jensen culture media. A hallmark of all mycobacteria is acid fastness. There are 5 closely related mycobacteria in the *M. tuberculosis* complex: *M. tuberculosis, M. bovis, M. africanum, M. microi,* and *M. canetti.*

Transmission: Transmission of *M. tuberculosis* is person to person, usually by airborne mucus droplet nuclei, particles 1–5 μm in diameter that contains *M. tuberculosis*. A tuberculous patient discharges tubercle bacilli in his sputum or nasopharyngeal secretions during bouts of coughing or sneezing. The infected sputum spit carelessly by open cases of tuberculosis dries up and tubercle bacilli are resuspended in dust and spread in the air. This may be a source of infection through breathing in the overcrowded area. Most adults no longer transmit the organism within several days to 2 wk after beginning adequate chemotherapy, but some patients remain infectious for many weeks. Young children with tuberculosis rarely infect other children or adults. However, children and adolescents with adult-type cavity or endobronchial pulmonary tuberculosis can transmit the organism. A primary lesion, a tuberculous chancre, results when *M. tuberculosis* or *M. bovis* gains access to the skin or mucous membranes through trauma.

Human infection with *M. bovis* is rare in developed countries as a result of the pasteurization of milk and effective tuberculosis control programs for cattle. Milk can carry bovine tuberculosis if the milk is not boiled before use. When infection with *M. bovis* happens, the primary infection will be in the intestine or tonsils.

Pathogenesis: The lung is the portal of entry of tubercle bacilli in > 98% of cases. The primary focus, the draining lymphatics and the inflamed regional lymph nodes are collectively called as the **"primary complex"**. The inhaled tubercle bacilli multiply initially within the pulmonary alveoli and alveolar ducts. Most of the bacilli are killed, but some survive within nonactivated macrophages, which carry them through lymphatic vessels to the regional lymph nodes. When the primary infection in the lungs, the hilar lymph nodes usually are involved, although an upper lobe focus may drain into paratracheal nodes. The tissue reaction in the lung parenchyma and lymph nodes intensifies over the next 2–12 wk as the organisms grow in number and tissue hypersensitivity develops. The parenchymal portion of the primary complex often heals completely by fibrosis or calcification after undergoing caseous necrosis and encapsulation. Occasionally this portion continues to enlarge, resulting in focal pneumonitis and pleuritis. If caseation is intense, the center of the lesion liquefies and empties into the associated bronchus, leaving a residual cavity.

The foci of infection in the regional lymph nodes develop some fibrosis and encapsulation, but healing is usually is less complete than in the parenchymal lesion. Viable *M. tuberculosis* can persist for decades in these foci. In most cases of initial tuberculosis infection the lymph nodes remain normal in size, but if hilar and paratracheal lymph nodes enlarge significantly as part of the host inflammatory reaction they may encroach on a regional bronchus. Partial obstruction of the bronchus caused by external compression may cause hyperinflation in the distal lung segment, whereas complete obstruction results in atelectasis. Inflamed caseous nodes can attach to the bronchial wall and erode through it, causing endobronchial tuberculosis or a fistula tract and causes complete obstruction of the bronchus.

During the development of the primary complex (Ghon complex), which is the combination of a parenchymal pulmonary lesion and a corresponding lymph node site, tubercle bacilli are carried to most tissues of the body (reticuloendothelial system, lung apices, brain, kidneys, and bones) through the blood and lymphatic vessels. Disseminated tuberculosis occurs if the number of circulating bacilli is large and the host cellular immune response is inadequate. In most cases the number of bacilli is small, leading to clinically inapparent metastatic foci in many organs. These remote foci usually become encapsulated, but

they may be the origin of both extrapulmonary tuberculosis and reactivation tuberculosis.

The time between initial infection and clinically apparent disease is variable. In disseminated and meningeal tuberculosis it is within 2–6 mo of acquisition, in significant lymph node or endobronchial tuberculosis within 3–9 mo, and in renal lesions it may become evident decades after infection. The risk for dissemination of *M. tuberculosis* is very high in HIV-infected persons. Reinfection also can occur in persons with advanced HIV or AIDS.

Pregnancy and the newborn: Pulmonary and particularly extrapulmonary tuberculosis other than lymphadenitis in a pregnant woman is associated with increased risk for prematurity, fetal growth retardation, low birth weight, and perinatal mortality. Congenital tuberculosis is rare because most common result of female genital tract tuberculosis is infertility. Congenital transmission of infection usually occurs from a lesion in the placenta through the umbilical vein. Primary infection in the mother just before or during pregnancy is more likely to cause congenital infection than is reactivation of a previous infection. The tubercle bacilli first reach the fetal liver, where a primary focus with peripheral lymph node involvement may occur. Organisms pass through the liver into the main fetal circulation and infect many organs. The bacilli in the lung usually remain dormant until after birth, when oxygenation and pulmonary circulation increase significantly. Congenital tuberculosis may also be caused by aspiration or ingestion of infected amniotic fluid. However, the most common route of infection for the neonate is postnatal airborne transmission from an adult with infectious pulmonary tuberculosis.

Immunity: Conditions that adversely affect cell-mediated immunity predispose to progression from tuberculosis infection to disease. Cell-mediated immunity develops 2–12 wk after infection, along with tissue hypersensitivity. After bacilli enter macrophages, lymphocytes that recognize mycobacterial antigens proliferate and secrete lymphokines and other mediators that attract other lymphocytes and macrophages to the area. Certain lymphokines activate macrophages, causing them to develop high concentrations of lytic enzymes that enhance their mycobactericidal capacity. A discrete subset of regulator helper and suppressor lymphocytes modulates the immune response. Development of specific cellular immunity prevents progression of the initial infection in most individuals.

The pathologic events in the initial tuberculosis infection depend on the balance among the mycobacterial antigen load; cell-mediated immunity, which enhances intracellular killing; and tissue hypersensitivity, which promotes extracellular killing. When the antigen load is small and the degree of tissue sensitivity is high, granuloma formation results from the organization of lymphocytes, macrophages, and fibroblasts. When both antigen load and the degree of sensitivity are high, granuloma formation is less organized. Tissue necrosis is incomplete, resulting in formation of caseous material. When the degree of tissue sensitivity is low, as is often the case in infants or immunocompromised individuals, the reaction is diffuse and the infection is not well contained, leading to dissemination and local tissue destruction. Tumor necrosis factor and other cytokines released by specific lymphocytes promote cellular destruction and tissue damage in susceptible individuals.

Latent tuberculosis infection (LTBI) occurs after inhalation of infective droplet nuclei containing *M. tuberculosis*. A positive tuberculin skin test and the absence of clinical and radiographic manifestations are the characteristic features of this stage. The word *tuberculosis* refers to disease, which occurs when signs and symptoms or radiographic changes become apparent. Untreated infants with *LTBI* have up to a 40% likelihood of developing tuberculosis, with the risk of progression decreasing gradually through childhood to adult lifetime rates of 5–10%. The greatest risk for progression occurs in the 1st 2 yr after infection.

Clinical manifestations and diagnosis: The majority of children with tuberculous infection develop no signs or symptoms at any time. Occasionally, infection is marked by low grade fever and mild cough, and rarely by high fever, cough, malaise, and flu-like symptoms that resolve within one week.

Primary pulmonary disease: The primary complex includes the parenchymal pulmonary focus and the regional lymph nodes. About 70% of lung foci are subpleural, and localized pleurisy is common. All lobar segments of lung are at equal risk for initial infection. In primary pulmonary tuberculosis there is relatively large size of the regional lymphadenitis compared with the relatively small size of the initial lung focus. As delayed-type hypersensitivity (DTH) develops, the hilar lymph nodes continue to enlarge in some children, especially infants, compressing the regional bronchus and causing obstruction. The usual sequence is hilar lymphadenopathy, focal hyperinfla-tion, and then atelectasis. The radiographic shadows have been called collapse-consolidation or segmental tuberculosis. In some cases, inflamed caseous nodes attach to the endobronchial wall and erode through it, causing endobronchial tuberculosis or a fistula tract.

The caseous material causes complete obstruction of the bronchus, resulting in extensive infiltrate and collapse. Enlargement of the subcarinal lymph nodes can cause compression of the esophagus and, rarely, a bronchoesophageal fistula. Most cases of tuberculous bronchial obstruction in children resolve fully with appropriate treatment, but in a few cases calcification of primary focus or regional lymph nodes. The appearance of the calcification implies that the lesion has been present for at least 6–12 mo. Healing of the segment can be complicated by scarring or contraction associated rarely with cylindrical bronchiectasis.

Children may have lobar pneumonia without impressive hilar lymphadenopathy. If the primary infection is progressively destructive, liquefaction of the lung parenchyma can lead to formation of a thin-walled primary tuberculosis cavity. Bullous tuberculous lesions can occur in the lungs rarely and if they rupture pneumothorax occur. Erosion of a parenchymal focus of tuberculosis into a blood or lymphatic vessel may result in dissemination of the bacilli and a military pattern, with small nodules evenly distributed on the chest radiograph.

The symptoms and physical signs of primary pulmonary tuberculosis in children are minimal considering the degree of radiographic changes often seen. Nonproductive cough and mild dyspnea are the most common symptoms. Fever, night sweats, and failure to thrive occur less often. Some infants and young children with bronchial obstruction have localized wheezing or decreased breath sounds that may be accompanied by tachypnea or, rarely, respiratory distress. These pulmonary symptoms and signs are occasionally alleviated by antibiotics, suggesting bacterial superinfection.

The most important diagnostic finding of pulmonary tuberculosis is isolation of *M. tuberculosis*. Sputum specimens for culture should be collected from adolescents and older children who are able to expectorate. Induce sputum with a jet nebulizer and chest percussion followed by nasopharyngeal suctioning is effective in children as young as one month. Sputum induction provides samples for both culture and smear staining, whereas gastric aspirates are usually cultured. The culture specimen in young children is the early morning gastric acid obtained before the child has arisen and peristalsis has emptied the stomach of the pooled secretions that have been swallowed over night. Even under optical conditions, though, 3 consecutive morning gastric aspirates yield the organisms in < 50% cases. Negative culture never excludes the diagnosis of tuberculosis in a child. The presence of a positive tuberculin skin test, an abnormal chest radiograph consistent with tuberculosis, and history of exposure to an adult with infectious tuberculosis is adequate proof that the disease is present. Drug susceptibility test results of the isolate from the adult source can be used to determine the best therapeutic regimen for the child. Cultures should be obtained from the child whenever the source case is unknown or the source case has possible drug resistant tuberculosis.

Progressive primary pulmonary disease: The disease in a child occurs when the primary focus enlarges steadily and develops a large caseous center. Liquefaction may cause formation of a primary cavity associated with large numbers of tubercle bacilli. The enlarging focus may slough necrotic debris into the adjacent bronchus, causing further intrapulmonary dissemination. Significant signs or symptoms are frequent in locally progressive disease in children. High fever, severe cough with sputum production, weight loss, and night sweats are common. Physical findings include diminished breath sounds, rales, and dullness or egophony over the cavity. The prognosis with appropriate treatment is excellent, but the recovery is slow.

Reactivation tuberculosis: Pulmonary tuberculosis in adults is usually endogenous reactivation of a site of tuberculosis infection established previously in the body. This form of tuberculosis may occur in adolescence. This form of tuberculosis may be highly contagious if there is significant sputum production and cough. The most frequent pulmonary sites are the original parenchymal focus, lymph nodes, or the apical seedings (Simon foci) established during the hematogenous phase of the early infection. Older children and adolescents with reactivation tuberculosis have fever, anorexia, malaise, weight loss, night sweats, productive cough, hemoptysis, and chest pain. Physical findings usually are minor or absent. The most common radiographic findings are extensive infiltrates or thick-walled cavities in the upper lobes. The prognosis for full recovery is excellent when patients are given appropriate therapy.

Pleural effusion: Tuberculous pleural effusions, focal or general, originate in the discharge of bacilli into the pleural space from a subpleural pulmonary focus or caseated lymph node. Asymptomatic local pleural effusion is frequent in primary pulmonary tuberculosis. Large and clinically significant effusions occur months or years after the primary infection. Effusions are usually unilateral but can be bilateral. Clinical onset of tuberculous pleurisy is often sudden, characterized by low or high fever, shortness of breath, and chest pain on deep inspiration. Physical findings include dullness on percussion and diminished breath sounds. Radiologic abnormality is characteristic of pleural effusion. The tuberculin test is positive in only 70–80% of cases. Examination of pleural fluid and the pleural membrane is important to establish the diagnosis of tuberculous pleurisy. The pleural fluid is usually yellow, specific gravity 1.012–1.025, protein level 2–4 g/dl, glucose concentration in the low-normal range (20–40 mg/dl), and several hundred to several thousand white blood cells per cubic millimeter with an early predominance of polymorphonuclear cells followed by a high percentage of lymphocytes. Acid-fast smears of the pleural fluid are rarely positive. Cultures of the fluid are positive in only < 30% of cases. Biopsy of the pleural membrane is more likely to yield a positive acid-fast stain or culture, and granuloma formation usually can be demonstrated.

Pericardial disease: Pericarditis occurs in 0.5–4% of tuberculosis cases in children and usually arises from direct invasion or lymphatic drainage from subcarinal lymph nodes. The presenting symptoms are non-specific, including low-grade fever, malaise, and weight loss. Chest pain is unusual in children. A pericardial friction rub or distant heart sounds with pulsus paradoxus may be present. The pericardial fluid is typically serofibrinous or hemorrhagic. Acid-fast smear of the fluid rarely reveals the organism, but cultures are positive in 30–70% of cases. The culture yield from pericardial biopsy may be higher, and the presence of granulomas often suggests the diagnosis. Partial or complete pericardiectomy may be required when constrictive pericarditis develops.

Lymphohematogenous (disseminated) disease: Tubercle bacilli are disseminated to distant sites, including liver, spleen, lymph nodes, skin, and lung apices, in all cases of tuberculosis infection. The clinical picture produced by lymphohematogenous dissemination depends on the quantity of organisms released from the primary focus and the adequacy of the host immune response. Lymphohematogenous spread is usually asymptomatic. Rare patients experience protracted hematogenous tuberculosis caused by the intermittent release of tubercle bacilli as a caseous focus erodes through the wall of a blood vessel in the lung. Multiple organ involvement is common, leading to hepatomegaly, splenomegaly, lymphadenitis in superficial or deep nodes, and papulonecrotic tuberculids appearing on the skin. Bones and joints or kidneys also may become involved. Meningitis occurs late in the course of disease.

The most clinically significant form of disseminated tuberculosis is *miliary disease*, which occurs when massive numbers of tubercle bacilli are released into the bloodstream, causing disease in 2 or more organs.

Military tuberculosis occurs within 2–6 mo of initial infection. The disease is most common in infants and young children, it is also found in adolescents and older adults, resulting from the breakdown of a previously healed primary pulmonary lesion. Lesions are often larger and more numerous in the lungs, spleen, liver, and bone marrow than other tissues.

The onset of military tuberculosis is sometimes explosive, and the patient may become gravely ill. More often, the onset is insidious, with early systemic signs, including anorexia, weight loss, and low grade fever. Generalized lymphadenopathy and hepato-splenomegaly develop within several weeks in about 50% of cases. The fever may then become higher and more sustained. Within several weeks, the lungs may become filled with tubercles, and dyspnea, cough, rales, or wheezing occurs. The lesions of military tuberculosis are usually smaller than 2–3 mm in diameter when first visible on chest radiograph. The smaller lesions coalesce to form larger lesions and sometimes extensive infiltrates. As the pulmonary disease progresses, an alveolar-air block syndrome may result in frank respiratory distress, hypoxia, and pneumothorax, or pneumomediastinum. Chronic or recurrent headache in a patient with military tuberculosis usually indicates the presence of meningitis, whereas the onset of abdominal pain or tenderness is a sign of tuberculous peritonitis. Cutaneous lesions include papulonecrotic tuberculids, nodules, or purpura. Choroid tubercles occur in 13–87% of patients (see Fig. 14.2 in CD).

Diagnosis of disseminated tuberculosis is difficult and a high index of suspicion by the physician is required. The most important clue is usually history of recent exposure to an adult with infectious tuberculosis. Choroid tubercles are highly specific for the diagnosis of tuberculosis. Tuberculin skin test is nonreactive in up to 40% of patients with disseminated tuberculosis. Early sputum or gastric cultures have a low sensitivity. Biopsy of the liver or bone marrow with appropriate bacteriologic and histologic examinations more often yields an early diagnosis. Chest radiograph shows military tubercles.

The resolution of military tuberculosis is slow; fever usually declines within 2–3 wk of starting chemo-therapy, but the chest radiographic abnormalities may not resolve for many months. Corticosteroids hasten symptomatic relief, especially when air block, peritonitis, or meningitis is present. The prognosis is excellent if the diagnosis is made early and adequate treatment is given.

Upper respiratory tract disease: Children with laryngeal tuberculosis have a croupy cough, sore throat, hoarseness, and dysphagia. Most children with laryngeal tuberculosis have extensive upper lobe pulmonary disease (diagnosed by X-ray chest). Tuberculosis of the middle ear results from aspiration of infected pulmonary secretions into the middle ear or from hematogenous dissemination in older children. The clinical features include painless unilateral otorrhea, tinnitus, decreased hearing, facial paralysis, perforated tympanic membrane, and preauricular or anterior cervical lymph nodes enlargement. Diagnosis is difficult because stains and cultures of ear fluid are frequently negative, and histology of the affected tissue often shows a nonspecific acute and chronic inflammation without granuloma formation.

Lymph node disease: Tuberculosis of the superficial lymph nodes, often referred to as *scrofula*, is the most common form extrapulmonary tuberculosis in children. Scrofula can be caused by drinking unpasteurized cow's milk laden with *M. bovis*, but most current cases occur within 6–9 mo of initial infection by *M. tuberculosis*, although some cases appear years later. The tonsillar, anterior cervical, submandibular, and supraclavicular nodes become involved secondary to extension of a primary lesion of the upper lung fields or abdomen. Infected nodes in the inguinal, epitrochlear, or axillary regions result from regional lymphadenitis associated with tuberculosis of the skin or skeletal system. The nodes usually enlarge gradually, and are firm but not hard, discrete, and nontender. The nodes often feel fixed to underlying or overlying tissue. As infection progresses, multiple nodes are infected, resulting in a mass of matted nodes. Disease is most often *unilateral*, but bilateral involvement may occur because of the crossover drainage patterns of lymphatic vessels in the chest and lower neck. Systemic signs and symptoms other than a low-grade fever are usually absent. The tuberculin skin test is usually positive, but chest radiograph is normal in 70% of cases. The onset of illness is occasionally more acute, with rapid enlargement of lymph nodes, high fever, tenderness, and flatulence. Lymph node tuberculosis more often progresses to caseation and necrosis. The capsule of the node breaks down, resulting in the spread of infection to adjacent nodes. Rupture of the node usually results in a draining sinus tract that may require surgical removal.

A definitive diagnosis of tuberculous adenitis usually requires histologic or bacteriologic confirmation, which is best accomplished by fine needle aspiration for culture, stain, and histology. If fine-needle aspiration is not successful in establishing a diagnosis, excisional biopsy of the involved node is indicated. Culture of lymph node tissue yields the organism in only about 50% of cases. Tuberculous adenitis should be differentiated from infection due to nontuberculous mycobacteria (NTM) (see in the CD), cat scratch disease (*Bartonella henselae*), tularemia, brucellosis, toxoplasmosis, tumor, branchial cleft cyst, cystic hygroma, and pyogenic infection. In NTM infections, granulomas are noncaseating, ill-defined, and irregular or serpiginous.

Tuberculous lymphadenitis responds well to antimicrobial therapy, although the lymph nodes do not return to normal size for months or even years. Surgical removal is not always necessary, and must be combined with antituberculous medication because the lymph node disease is only a part of a systemic infection.

Central nervous system disease: Tuberculosis of the central nervous system (CNS) occurs in two forms: Tuberculous meningitis and tuberculoma. Tuberculous meningitis is the most serious complication in children and is fatal without prompt and appropriate treatment. The clinical progression of tuberculous meningitis may be rapid or gradual. More commonly the signs and symptoms progress slowly over several weeks and can be divided into 3 stages. The *1st stage*, which typically lasts 1–2 wk, is characterized by nonspecific symptoms such as fever, headache, irritability, drowsiness, and malaise. Focal neurologic signs are absent. The *2nd stage* usually begins more abruptly. The most common features are lethargy, nuchal rigidity, seizures, positive Kernig or Brudzinski signs, hypertonia, vomiting, cranial nerve palsies, and other focal neurologic signs. The accelerating clinical illness usually correlates with the development of hydrocephalus, increased intracranial pressure, and vasculitis. Some children have no evidence of meningeal irritation but may have signs of encephalitis, such as disorientation, movement disorders, or speech impairment. The *3rd stage* is marked by coma, hemiplegia or paraplegia, hypertension, decerebrate posturing, deterioration of vital signs, and eventually death. The prognosis of tuberculous meningitis correlates most closely with the clinical stage of illness at the time treatment is initiated. The majority of patients in the 1st stage have an excellent outcome, whereas most patients in the 3rd stage who survive have permanent disabilities, including blindness, deafness, paraplegia, diabetes insipidus, or mental retardation. The prognosis for young infants is generally worse than for older children. It is imperative that antituberculosis treatment be considered for any child who develops basilar meningitis and hydrocephalus, cranial nerve palsies, or stroke with no other apparent etiology.

The diagnosis of tuberculous meningitis in early stage of disease requires a high degree of suspicion on the part of clinician. Identifying an adult in contact with the child who has infectious tuberculosis is helpful in arriving to the correct diagnosis. The tuberculin skin test is negative in up to 50% of cases, and 20–50% of children have a normal chest radiograph. The most important laboratory test for the diagnosis of tuberculous meningitis is examination and culture of CSF. The CSF examination will show 10–500 cells/mm^3, polymorphonuclear leukocytes may be present initially, but lymphocytes predominate in the majority of cases; glucose < 40 mg/dl but rarely < 20 mg/dL, and protein level may be markedly high (400–5,000 mg/dL) secondary to hydrocephalus and spinal block. Although the lumbar CSF is grossly abnormal, ventricular CSF may have normal findings because this fluid is obtained from a site proximal to the inflammation and obstruction. During early stage 1, the CSF may resemble that of viral aseptic meningitis. When 5–10 ml of lumbar CSF can be obtained (small amounts of CSF are unlikely to demonstrate), the acid-fast stain of the CSF sediment is positive in up to 30% of cases and the culture is positive in 50–70% of cases. Cultures of other fluids, such as gastric aspirates or urine, may help confirm the diagnosis. Radiographic studies may aid in the diagnosis of tuberculous meningitis. CT or MRI of the brain of the patients with tuberculous meningitis may demonstrate basilar enhancement and communicating hydrocephalus with signs of cerebral edema or early focal ischemia and in some small children one or several tuberculomas in the cerebral cortex or thalamic regions (*see* Fig. 14.3 in CD).

Another manifestation of CNS tuberculosis is the *tuberculoma*, a tumor-like mass resulting from aggregation of caseous tubercles that usually presents clinically as a brain tumor. Tuberculomas account for up to 40% of brain tumors in some areas of the world. In adults tuberculomas are most often supratentorial, but in children they are often infratentorial, located at the base of the brain near the cerebellum. Lesions are most often singular but may be multiple. The most common symptoms are headache, fever, and convulsions. The tuberculin skin test is usually positive, but the chest radiograph is usually normal. Corticosteroids are usually administered during the 1st few weeks of treatment or in the immediate postoperative period to decrease cerebral edema. On CT or MRI of the brain, tuberculomas usually appear as discrete lesions with a significant amount of surrounding edema. Contrast medium enhancement may result in a ring-like lesion.

Bones and joint diseases: Bones and joint infection complicating tuberculosis is most likely to involve the vertebrae. The classic manifestation of tuberculous spondylitis is progression to Pott disease (Pott's spine), in which destruction of vertebral bodies leads to gibbus deformity and kyphosis.

Abdominal and gastrointestinal disease: Tuberculosis of the oral cavity or pharynx is quite unusual. The most common lesion is a painless ulcer on the mucosa, palate, or tonsil with enlargement of the regional lymph nodes. Tuberculosis of the parotid gland or esophagus can rarely occur. These forms of tuberculosis are usually associated with extensive pulmonary disease and swallowing of infectious respiratory secretions

Generalized peritonitis may arise from subclinical or miliary hematogenous dissemination. Localized peritonitis is caused by direct extension from an abdominal lymph node, intestinal focus, or genitourinary tuberculosis. Rarely, the lymph nodes, omentum, and peritoneum become matted and can be palpated as a *"doughy"* irregular nontender mass. Abdominal pain or tenderness, ascites, anorexia, and low-grade fever are typical manifestations. The tuberculin test is usually positive. The diagnosis can be confirmed by paracentesis with appropriate stains and cultures, but this procedure must be performed carefully to avoid entering a bowel that is intertwined with the matted omentum.

Tuberculous enteritis is caused by hematogenous dissemination or by swallowing tubercle bacilli discharged from the patient's own lungs. The jejunum and ileum near Peyer's patches and the appendix are the most common sites of involvement. The typical findings are shallow ulcers that cause pain, diarrhea, or constipation, and weight loss and low grade fever. Mesenteric adenitis usually complicates the infection. The enlarged nodes may cause intestinal obstruction or erode through the omentum to cause generalized peritonitis. The disease should be suspected in any child with chronic gastrointestinal complaints and a positive tuberculin skin test. Biopsy, acid-fast stain, and culture of the lesions are usually necessary to confirm the diagnosis.

Tuberculosis of skin and subcutaneous tissue: Tuberculosis can affect the skin both at the stage of primary infection and during the time when bacilli are spreading in the blood stream. All forms of cutaneous disease are caused by *M. tuberculosis*, *M. bovis*, and occasionally by the bacille Calmette-Guérin (BCG), an attenuated vaccine form of *M. bovis.*

A primary lesion, a tuberculous chancre, results when *M. tuberculosis* or *M. bovis* gains access to the skin or mucous membranes through trauma. The face, lower extremities, and genitals are commonly affected. The initial lesion develops 2–4 wk after introduction of the organism into the damaged tissue. A red-brown papule gradually enlarges to form a shallow, firm, sharply demarcated ulcer. Satellite abscesses may be present. Some lesions acquire a crust resembling impetigo, and others become heaped up and verrucous at the margins. The primary lesion occurs in 30% of cases as a painless ulcer on the conjunctiva, gingiva, or palate and occasionally as a painless acute paronychia. Painless regional adenopathy appears ~3–8 wk after inoculation and may be accompanied by lymphangitis, lymphadenitis, or perforation of the skin surface, forming *scrofuloderma. Erythema nodosum* develops in ~10% of cases. Untreated lesions heal with scarring within ~12 mo but may reactivate, may form lupus vulgaris, or rarely, may progress to the acute military form. *M. tuberculosis* or *M. bovis* can be cultured from the skin lesion and local lymph nodes, but acid-fast staining of histologic sections, often does not reveal the organism. The differential diagnosis includes a syphilitic chancre; deep fungal or atypical mycobacterial infection; leprosy; tularemia; cat scratch disease, leishmaniasis; and papular acne rosacea.

Direct cutaneous inoculation of the tuberculous bacillus into a previously infected individual with a moderate to high degree of immunity initially produces a small papule with surrounding inflammation. *Tuberculosis verrucosa cutis* (warty tuberculosis) forms when the papule becomes hyperkeratotic and warty, and several adjacent papules coalesce or a single papule expands peripherally to form a brownish-red to violaceous, exudative, crusted verrucous plaque. Irregular extension of the margins of the plaque produces a serpiginous border. Lesion in children is most commonly present on the lower extremities after trauma and contact with infected material such as sputum or soil. Regional lymph nodes are involved only rarely. Spontaneous healing with atrophic scarring occurs slowly. Healing with antituberculous therapy is also gradual.

Lupus vulgaris is a rare, chronic, progressive form of cutaneous tuberculosis that develops in individuals with a moderate to high degree of tuberculin sensitivity induced by previous infection. Lupus vulgaris develops as a result of direct extension from underlying joints or lymph nodes; through lymphatic or hematogenous spread, or, rarely, by cutaneous inoculation with BCG vaccine. Lupus vulgaris is also preceded by scrofluoderma. 90% cases of lupus vulgaris are present on the head and neck, most commonly on the nose or cheek. Involvement of the trunk is uncommon. A typical solitary lesion consists of a soft, brownish-red papule. Expansion of the papule peripherally, or occasionally the coalescence of several papules, forms an irregular lesion of variable size and form. One or several lesions may develop, including nodules or plaques that are flat and serpiginous, hypertrophic and verrucous, or edematous in appearance. Spontaneous healing occurs centrally, and lesions reappear within the area of atrophy. Chronicity is characteristic, and persistence and progression of plaques over many years is common. Vegetative masses and ulceration involving the nasal, buccal, or conjunctival mucosa; the palate; the gingival; or the oropharynx may cause extensive deformities. Squamous cell carcinoma, with a relatively high metastatic potential, may develop, usually after several years of the disease. The differential diagnosis includes sarcoidosis, atypical mycobacterial infection, actinomycosis, leishmaniasis, tertiary syphilis, and leprosy. Small lesions can be excised. Antituberculous drug therapy usually halts further spread and induces involution.

Scrofuloderma results from enlargement, cold abscess formation, and breakdown of a lymph node, most frequently in a cervical chain, with extension to the overlying skin. Linear or serpiginous ulcers and dissecting fistulas and subcutaneous tracts studded with soft nodules may develop. As spontaneous healing may take years, cord-like keloid scars are formed. Lupus vulgaris may also develop. Scrofuloderma of a cervical lymph node often originates in the larynx and was linked in the past to ingestion of milk containing *M. bovis*. Lesions may also originate from an underlying infected joint, tendon, bone or epididymis. Constitutional symptoms are typically absent. The differential diagnosis includes syphilitic gumma, deep fungal infections, and actinomycosis. Antituberculous therapy is effective.

Orofacial tuberculosis presents on the mucous membranes and periorificial skin after autoinoculation of mycobacteria from sites of progressive infection. Lesions are painful, yellowish or red nodules that form punched-out ulcers with inflammation, and edema of the surrounding mucosa. It is a sign of advanced internal disease and carries a poor prognosis. Treatment consists of identification of the source of infection and initiation of antituberculous therapy.

Military tuberculosis (hematogenous primary tuberculosis) rarely presents cutaneously and occurs most commonly in infants and in individuals who are immunosuppressed after chemotherapy or infection with measles or HIV. The eruption consists of crops of symmetrically distributed, minute, erythematous to purpuric macules, papules, or vesicles. The lesions may ulcerate, drain, crust, and form sinus tracts or may form subcutaneous gummas, particularly in malnourished children with impaired immunity. Constitutional signs and symptoms are common. A leukemoid reaction or aplastic anemia may develop.

Tubercle bacilli are identified in an active lesion. A fulminant course should be anticipated, and antituberculous treatment should be immediately started.

Single or multiple metastatic tuberculous abscesses (**tuberculous gummas**) may develop on the extremities and trunk by hematogenous spread from a primary focus of infection during a period of decreased immunity, especially in malnourished and immuno-suppressed children. The fluctuant, nontender, erythematous subcutaneous nodules may ulcerate and form fistulas.

Vaccination with BCG characteristically produces a papule ~2 wk after vaccination. The papule expands in size, typically ulcerates within 2–4 mo, and heales slowly with scarring. In ~ 1–2 per million vaccinations, a complication caused specifically by the BCG organism occurs, including regional lymphadenitis, lupus vulgaris, scrofuloderma, and subcutaneous abscess formation.

Tuberculids: The lesions appear in an individual who usually has moderate to strong tuberculin reactivity, has a history of previous tuberculosis of other organs, and usually shows a therapeutic response to antituberculous treatment. Most patients are in good health with no clear focus of disease at the time of the eruption. The most common tuberculid is the papulonecrotic tuberculid. Recurrent crops symmetrically distributed asymptomatic, firm, sterile, dusky-red papules appear on the extensor aspects of the limbs, the dorsum of the hands and feet, and the buttocks. The papules may undergo central ulceration and eventually heal, leaving sharply delineated, circular, depressed scars. The duration of the eruption is variable, but it usually disappears promptly after treatment of the primary infection. Tuberculids are skin reactions that exhibit tuberculoid features histologically but do not contain detectable mycobacteria. Lichen scrofulosorum, another form of tuberculid, is characterized by asymptomatic, grouped, pinhead-sized, often follicular pink or red papules that form discoid plaques, mainly on the trunk. Healing occurs without scarring.

Genitourinary disease: Renal tuberculosis is rare in children because incubation period is several years or longer. Tubercle bacilli usually reach the kidney during lymphohematogenous dissemination. The organisms often can be recovered from the urine in cases of military tuberculosis and in some patients with pulmonary tuberculosis in the absence of renal parenchymal disease. In true renal tuberculosis, small caseous foci develop in the renal parenchyma and release *M. tuberculosis* into the tubules. A large mass develops near the renal cortex that discharges bacteria through a fistula into the renal pelvis. Infection then spreads locally to the ureters, prostate, or epididymis. Renal tuberculosis in early stages is marked only by sterile pyuria and microscopic hematuria. Dysuria, flank or abdominal pain, and gross hematuria develop as the disease progresses. Superinfection by other bacteria, which often causes more acute symptoms, occurs more frequently but may also delay recognition of the underlying tuberculosis. Hydronephrosis or ureteral strictures may complicate the disease. Renal tuberculosis is most often unilateral. The tuberculin skin test is negative in up to 20% of patients. Urine cultures for *M. tuberculosis* are positive in 80–90% of cases, and acid-fast stains of large volumes of urine sediment are positive in 50–70% of cases. An intravenous pyelogram or CT scan often reveals mass lesions, dilatation of the proximal ureters, multiple small filling defects, and hydronephrosis if ureteral stricture is present.

Tuberculosis of the genital tract usually originates from lymphohematogenous spread, although it can be caused by direct spread from the intestinal tract or bone, although it can be caused by direct spread from the intestinal tract or bone. It is uncommon in both males and females before puberty. Adolescent girls may develop genital tract tuberculosis during the primary infection. The fallopian tubes are most often involved (90–100% of cases) followed by the endometrium (50%), ovaries (25%), and cervix (5%). The most common symptoms are lower abdominal pain and dysmenorrhea or amenorrhea. Systemic manifestations are usually absent and the chest radiograph is normal in most of the cases. The tuberculin skin test is usually positive. Genital tuberculosis in adolescent males causes epididymitis or orchitis. The condition usually manifests as a unilateral nodular painless swelling of the scrotum. Involvement of glans penis is extremely rare. Genital abnormalities and a positive tuberculin skin test in an adolescent male or female is suggestive of genital tract tuberculosis.

Disease in HIV-infected children: Tuberculosis disease in HIV-infected children is higher than in non-HIV infected and is often more severe, progressive, and likely to occur in extrapulmonary sites. Fever and weight loss are the most common complaints. Rates of drug-resistant tuberculosis tend to be higher in HIV-infected adults, and probably, are also higher in HIV-infected children. The mortality rate of HIV-infected children with tuberculosis is high, especially as the CD4 lymphocyte numbers decrease. Therefore, HIV-infected children with potential exposures and/or recent infection should be promptly evaluated and treated for tuberculosis. All children with tuberculosis disease should be tested for HIV co-infection, because of the potential benefits of early diagnosis and treatment of HIV infection, and because the presence of HIV may necessitate a longer duration of treatment. Establishing the diagnosis of tuberculosis in an HIV-infected child may be difficult because tuberculin skin test is usually negative, culture confirmation is difficult, and the clinical features of tuberculosis are similar to many other HIV-related infection and conditions. X-ray chest findings are similar to those in children with normal immune systems, but lobar disease and lung cavitation are more common.

Perinatal disease: Symptoms of congenital tuberculosis may be present at birth but more commonly begin by the 2nd or 3rd wk of life. The most common signs and symptoms are respiratory distress, fever, hepatic or splenic enlargement, poor feeding, lethargy or irritability, lymphadenopathy, abdominal distension, failure to thrive, ear drainage, and skin lesions. Many infants have an abnormal chest radiograph, most often a military pattern. Some infants with no pulmonary findings early in the course of the disease later develop profound radiographic and clinical abnormalities. Generalized lymphadenopathy and meningitis occur in 30–50% of patients. The clinical presentation of tuberculosis in newborns is similar to that caused by bacterial sepsis and other congenital infections such as syphilis, toxoplasmosis, and cytomegalovirus. The diagnosis should be suspected in an infant with signs and symptoms of bacterial or congenital infection whose response to antibiotic and supportive therapy is poor and diagnosis of other infections could not be made. The most important clue for rapid diagnosis of congenital tuberculosis is a maternal or family history of tuberculosis. Frequently the mother's disease is discovered only after the neonate's diagnosis is suspected. The infant's tuberculin skin test is negative initially but may become positive in 1–3 mo. A positive acid-fast stain of an early morning gastric aspirate from a newborn usually indicates tuberculosis. Direct acid-fast stains on middle-ear discharge, bone marrow, tracheal aspirate or biopsy tissue of the liver can be useful in making diagnosis of tuberculosis. The CSF should be examined and cultured, although the yield for isolating *M. tuberculosis* is low. The mortality rate of congenital tuberculosis is high because of delayed diagnosis but a complete recovery occurs if the diagnosis is made promptly and adequate anti-tuberculous therapy is started.

Diagnosis: Diagnosis of tuberculosis is more difficult in children than adults because sputum usually is not available and in only less than 20% are AFB positive in smear of sputum and gastric aspirate as compared to 75% in adults. Unlike adults children often have primary disease with radiological findings and may be asymptomatic. Diagnosis of childhood tuberculosis is based on triad of clinical features, history of contact and investigations.

A. *Clinical features:* Take history of immunization, measles, pertussis and HIV. Clinical manifestations already mentioned.

B. *History of contact:* Child in contact with an individual who has positive sputum for AFB on smear examination or negative sputum smear but culture +ve or clinical evidence of an active pulmonary tuberculosis but prior AFB smear were not obtained or has laryngeal tuberculosis or extrapulmonary tuberculosis are more likely to become infected.

C. *Investigations*

a. *Tuberculin skin test:* Detects delayed hypersensitivity to antigen (protein of tubercle bacilli) of *Mycobacterium tuberculosis*. Infected persons responds usually with positive test after 6–10 wk of infection.

The *Mantoux (Mx) tuberculin skin text* is the intradermal injection of 0.1 ml containing 5 tuberculin units (TU) of purified protein derivative (PPD) stabilized with Tween 80. T cells sensitized by prior infection are recruited to the skin where they release lymphokines that induce induration through local vasodilatation, edema, fibrin deposition, and recruitment of other inflammatory cells to the area. 5 TU of PPD 0.1 ml is injected intradermally in the volar aspect of left arm, and a wheal of 8 mm should be raised. Read 48–72 hrs after administration. Induration area (not erythema) with transverse diameter of more then 10 mm constitutes positive reaction. If Mantoux text is negative BCG test may be performed.

False negative results: Faulty technique, loss of potency, improper concentration, bacterial contamination or inadequate dose. Host factors interfering with delayed hypersensitivity reactions include extremes of age (infants < 6 mo), overwhelming tubercular illness (miliary tuberculosis, TBM), coincidental viral infections (measles, influenza, etc.), immunosuppressive therapy, malnutritional states, neoplastic diseases (especially Hodgkin, non-Hodgkin lymphomas), chronic renal failure (less commonly).

BCG test: Reconstituted BCG vaccine 0.1 ml given intradermal above insertion of deltoid of left arm by raising a wheal of 5 mm. Accelerated response with nodule formation of more then 5 mm size after 72 hrs is considered as positive test.

b. *Complete blood counts and ESR.* Lympocytosis and raised ESR are only supportive tests.

c. *X-ray chest.* Posteroanterior (PA) and lateral chest X-ray is suggestive for tuberculosis disease when it shows: 1. enlarged hilar, mediastinal or subcarinal lymph nodes, 2. lung parenchymal changes, 3. segmental hyperinflation, 4. atelectasis, 5. alveolar consolidation, 6. pleural effusion, 7. focal mass, and 8. unchanged radiological finding after 2 wk of antibacterial therapy.

d. *Sputum and gastric aspirate* for smear and culture for AFB. Early morning gastric aspirate of empty stomach is used for AFB smear and culture as children < 7 yr are unable to bring out sputum voluntarily. Smear and culture may also be done in samples of cerebrospinal fluid, pleural fluid, ascitic fluid and bronchial aspirate whenever indicated.

e. *Histopathology.* Fine needle aspiration cytology (FNAC) or biopsy may be required in specific circumstances when lymph nodes are enlarged.

f. *Bronchoscopy* is useful in the diagnosis of tuberculosis and excluding other causes of pulmonary abnormality particularly in immuno-compromised/HIV-infected children.

g. *CT scan/MRI.* In selected cases only helpful to demonstrate endobronchial disease, subcarinal lymph nodes, pericardial invasion, early cavitation and bronchiectasis resulting from pulmonary tuberculosis and various lesions of CNS tuberculosis.

h. *ELISA* to detect IgG, IgM and IgA antibodies is of no utility in the diagnosis of childhood tuberculosis. The positive IgG indicates old or chronic infection; the positive IgM indicates current infection, and the positive IgA indicates active disease.

i. *Polymerase chain reaction.* Sensitivity and specificity of PCR for CSF and pleural fluid is high and that for gastric aspirate is low. PCR is expensive and false-positive reaction can occur.

Treatment

Drugs used in treatment of tuberculosis: Antitubercular drugs are divided into first line and second line drugs. Majority of the patients can be successfully treated with the first line drugs. Second line drugs are used in drug resistant cases and in situation where first line drugs cannot be used due to toxicity or some other constraints (Tables 14.2 and 14.3). The *second line*

Table 14.2: Antitubercular drugs	
First-line drugs	*Second-line drugs*
Isoniazid (H)	Cycloserine (Cs)
Rifampicin (R)	Ethionamide (Eto)
Ethambutol (E)	Capreomycin
Pyrazinamide (Z)	Kanamycin (Km)
Streptomycin (S)	

drugs include: fluoroquinolones, kanamycin, amikacin, capreomycin, cycloserine, ethionamide, prothionamide, PAS.

Antituberculous regimen: Newly diagnosed patients of pulmonary tuberculosis and extrapulmonary tuberculosis are nowadays treated with short-course chemotherapy regimen. It consists of two phases:

Intensive phase: The object is to eliminate bacterial load and prevent emergence of resistance, at least 3 drugs (bactericidal) should be used.

Continuation phase: At least two bactericidal drugs are used to continue and complete the therapy.

IAP recommendations: Indian Academy of Pediatrics classifies treatment of tuberculosis into 5 groups (Table 14.4).

Directly Observed Treatment Short-Course (DOTS)

DOTS is the recommended strategy for treatment of tuberculosis and all pediatric tuberculosis patients should be registered under Revised National Tuberculosis Control Program (RNTCP). Intermittent short-course chemotherapy given under direct observation as advocated in the RNTCP (Table 14.5) should be used in children. Administration of DOTS to a child at the center means the incumbent will have dependability upon either parent and could be miss the school due to clash with center timing. However, this regime is worth considering when compliance is poor.

Use of corticosteroids: Corticosteroids may be used in patients with CNS involvement (tuberculous meningitis, evidence of cerebral edema, focal neurological deficits); miliary tuberculosis; tuberculosis of serous layers, and endobronchial tuberculosis. Prednisolone is used in the doses of 1–2 mg/kg/day. The dose is gradually reduced when there is clinical improvement and discontinued usually after 8–12 weeks.

Drugs Resistance in Children

It may be primary (already resistant to a particular drug) or secondary (resistance develops during treatment). Multidrug Resistant (MDR) tuberculosis is resistant to at least isoniazid and rifampicin with or without other drugs. Diagnosis of MDR tuberculosis can be made by culture and sensitivity tests.

Treatment: In known drug resistant cases the initial regimen should include at least 3 drugs to which the isolate is susceptible and preferably those, which have never been taken by the patient before. Drugs for MDR tuberculosis are listed in Box 14.3. Surgery should actively be considered for all MDR tuberculosis cases.

Treatment Regimens for MDR Tuberculosis

a. *Where drug resistance is suspected:* No bacteriologic proof is available: 2 SHRZE/1 HRZE/6 HRE
b. *Proven drug resistance*
   i. *INH resistant:* a. HIV-negative—12 RZE; b. HIV-positive—18 RZE or 12 mo after culture negative.
   ii. *Rifampicin resistant:* a. HIV-negative —18–24 HZE; b. HIV-positive—18–24 HZE or 12 months after culture negative.

Table 14.3: Recommended doses of drugs for children		
Drug/route of administration	*Daily regimen*	*Intermittent regimen*
Isoniazid (H) Oral	5–10 mg/kg/day (max dose 300 mg)	10–15 mg/kg (max dose 600 mg)
Rifampicin (R) Oral	10 mg/kg/day (max dose 600 mg)	15 mg/kg/day (max dose 900 mg)
Pyrazinamide (Z) Oral	25 mg/kg/day	30 mg/kg/day
Ethambutol (E) Oral	15 mg/kg/day	15 mg/kg/day (30 mg/kg/day)
Streptomycin (S) Intramuscular (IM)	20 mg/kg/day (max dose 1 g)	30 mg/kg/day (max dose 1 g)
Prednisolone Oral	1–2 mg/kg/day	

Group	Clinical presentation	Description of therapy
	Table 14.4: Treatment regimens for tuberculosis: IAP Recommendations	
1	a. Asymptomatic, Mx +ve aged < 3 yrs b. Asymptomatic, Mx +ve aged < 5 yrs with grade III or IV malnutrition c. Children < 3 yrs with history contact d. Children < 5 yrs with history of contact with grade III or IV malnutrition e. Recent converter, no signs but Mx +ve	6 HR
2	a. Primary complex b. Symptomatic, Mx +ve < 3 yrs without localization c. Symptomatic, Mx +ve < 5 yrs with grade III or IV malnutrition without localization d. Isolated lymphadenitis e. Pleural effusion	2 HRZ + 4 HR
3	a. Progressive pulmonary disease b. Tubercular lymphadenitis involving multiple nodes. Extend continuation phase by 3 month in event of non-resolution	2 HRZE + 4 HR
4	a. Miliary tuberculosis b. Disseminated tuberculosis c. Cavitary tuberculosis d. Tubercular bronchopneumonia e. Bone and joint tuberculosis f. Abdominal, pericardial and genitourinary tuberculosis	2 HRZE + 7 HR
5	CNS tuberculosis, i.e. tuberculoma or tubercular meningitis	2 HRZE + 10 HRE

Mx test: Mantoux test
Note: In immunocompromised/seropositive HIV-continuation phase is extended 3 mo. In children less then 5 yrs or who are not evaluated visually, streptomycin can be used in place of ethambutol

Numerical denotes number of months for which the drug is to be given, e.g. 6 HR means giving 6 mo isoniazid and rifampicin.

Category of patients	Type of patients	Intensive	Continuation phase
	Table 14.5: RNTCP treatment regimens		
Category I	a. New sputum smear +ve tuberculosis b. Seriously ill sputum smear –ve pulmonary. tuberculosis c. Seriously ill extrapulmonary. tuberculosis	2 H3R3Z3E3	4 H3R3
Category II	a. Sputum smear +ve relapse b. Sputum smear +ve treatment c. Sputum smear +ve patients after default	2 S3H3R3Z3E3 1 H3R3Z3E3	5 H3R3E3
Category III	a. Sputum smear –ve and extrapulmonary tuberculosis not seriously ill	2 S3H33R3Z3E3	4 H3R3

iii. *Multi-drug resistant:* a. HIV–negative—3 sensitive drug 2 yrs after culture negative; b. HIV-positive–same as above

Treatment of Special Cases

1. ***Interrupted or incomplete treatment of a child with active tuberculosis and drug susceptible:*** Interrupted or incomplete treatment is defined as the "interruption or non-completion of ATT for at least 1/3 of the intended regimen" (e.g. two or more consecutive months or intermittent interruption totaling two months of six months regimen or interruption of three months or more of nine months regimen).

Deciding to restart treatment: Following points should be considered when a child returns after a lapse in treatment:

a. If child has a lapse in therapy early (e.g. during the first three months);

Box 14.3: Drugs used for MDR-tuberculosis cases

Amino glycosides	*Cycloserine*
Kanamycin	
Amikacin	*Newer drugs*
Capreomycin	Imipenem
	Interferon
Thionamides	Rifamycin
Ethionamide	Rifabutin
Prothionamide	Rifapentine
	Interleukin-2
Pyrazinamide	Immunotherapy
	M. vaccae vaccine
Quinolones	
Ofloxacin	

b. Has extensive disease, especially military, neurotuberculosis or cavitary;
c. Is immunocompromised, especially with HIV;
d. Has incompletely treated tuberculosis, stopped treatment more then six months previously.

Length of retreatment
1. If one or more criteria above are met, the length of retreatment should correspond to that indicated by the original protocol.
2. If one or more criteria above are met, treatment should be rearmed so as to complete that original protocol. (For example, if treatment lapsed for two months) after 3 mo of intended six months regimens, the patients should receive treatment for an additional 3 mo (mo 6, 7, 8) so as to complete six months of total treatment.

2. *Treatment failure:* Individual with active tuberculosis is originally drug susceptible. Treatment failure is defined by one or more of the following:
 i. Mantoux or BCG positivity
 ii. Clinical deterioration
 iii. Worsening of chest X-ray findings
 iv. A positive culture any time after three months of ATT. Or reversion from –ve culture after three months of treatment to a +ve culture during anti-tuberculosis treatment.

In these cases:
a. For pulmonary tuberculosis—three consecutive, daily sputum/gastric aspirate sample should be sent for AFB smear, culture and susceptibility testing from the child and contact if possible.
b. For extrapulmonary tuberculosis—renewed attempts should be made to obtain appropriate specimen for AFB smear, culture and susceptibility testing.

Treatment
a. If the individual is clinically stable they may be maintained on the current tuberculosis regimens, until susceptibility results are available to guide the choice of medications.
b. If the child is clinically deteriorating, treat as MDR TB.

3. *Relapse: Definition:* Reappearance of signs and symptoms of tuberculosis disease within 2 yrs of cure after completion of specialized therapy. Relapses are rare in children.
 Suggested drug regimen: Treat as suspected drug resistance in the absence of bacteriological proof.

Clinical evaluation during treatment of tuberculosis: A child receiving antituberculosis treatment should receive, at a minimum, a monthly medical assessment by the treating doctors. Monitor: a. Symptoms and signs of tuberculosis; b. Side-effecters to anti tuberculosis medications; c. Weight of the child: Increase in weight while being treated for tuberculosis may be a sign of clinical improvement. Doses of medications should be adjusted according to the individual's weight. The commonly encountered adverse reactions to antitubercular drugs are listed in Table 14.6.

Laboratory tests during ATT: Complete blood count and platelets, SGPT/SGOT/alkaline phosphate. Other laboratory tests should be ordered based on elicited side effects.

An expectorated or induced sputum examination for AFB should be ordered monthly, at a minimum.
Evaluation at the end of treatment: At the end of treatment for pulmonary tuberculosis, one sputum culture and chest X-ray should be done.
 i. If child was immunocompetent and has tuberculosis susceptible to all first line anti-tuberculosis medication—farther evaluation is not necessary. they should be instructed to return for reevaluation if they experience prolonged cough/loss of appetite/weight loss/ fever/night sweats/chest pain, etc.
 ii. Post-treatment evaluation should be done every six months for two years after completion of a full course of anti-tubercular treatment on the following: a. seropositive-HIV; b. children treated for MDR tuberculosis.

Chemoprophylaxis regimens: Protocols applies to
 i. A symptomatic child < 5 yr or 5 yr with tuberculin skin test +ve with grade III and IV PEM
 ii. A symptomatic recent converter with normal X-ray
 iii. Child < or 5 yr. With history of contact with active infections tuberculosis (sputum +ve) with grades III and IV malnutrition.

A combination of isoniazid and rifampicin should be used for above mentioned cases for at least six months.

Table 14.6: Commonly encountered adverse reactions to anti-tubercular drug

Adverse reactions	Anti-tubercular drugs
1. Hepatitis	Isoniazid, Rifampicin, PZA
2. Gastritis	Rifampicin, rarely PZA
3. Peripheral neuritis/ paresthesias of hands/feet	Isoniazid (INH)
4. Gout-like symptoms/signs	Pyrazinamide
5. Renal (hematuria, azotemia) rifampicin, amino glycosides	
6. Leukopenia, thrombo-cytopenia	Isoniazid, rifampicin, PZA, ethambutol
7. Loss of vision/color blindness	Ethambutol

Chemoprophylaxis options in children with MDR tuberculosis contact

a. *Children who are immunocompetent:* Consider at least two drugs for preventive treatment with anti-tubercular medications. This is especially important to consider for recent tuberculin test convertors. Duration of chemoprophylaxis is minimum of nine months of continuous therapy.

b. *Children who are severely immunocompromised* or seropositive HIV or at risk of HIV infection should be placed on at least two drugs preventive treatment for 12 months.

Management of neonate with mother suspected or active case of tuberculosis

i. *If mother is infectious* use face mask while handling baby and chemoprophylaxis (short-term chemotherapy) till mother becomes sputum –ve for AFB (3 sputum smears negative). After 15 days gap BCG is administered—if accelerated response (BCG test +ve), do X-ray chest-if findings are also present in X-ray chest: Extend chemotherapy for 6 months in total (preferably with HR). If no accelerated response, discontinue chemoprophylaxis.

ii. *If asymptomatic* therapy with RH × 3 months. Do Mx test—if negative, discontinue therapy and give BCG. *If* + ve, continue therapy for 6 months.

iii. *Symptomatic:* +ve chest X-ray finding: Give anti-tuberculosis therapy.

Prevention: The highest priority of any tuberculosis control program should be case finding and treatment, which interrupts transmission of infection between close contacts. All children and adults with symptoms suggestive of tuberculosis disease and those in close contact with an adult suspected of having infectious pulmonary tuberculosis should be tuberculin skin tested and examined as soon as possible. On an average, 30–50% of household contacts to infectious cases will be tuberculin skin test positive and 1% of contacts already have overt disease. Children, particularly young infants, should receive high priority during contact investigations because their risk for infection is high and they are more likely to rapidly develop severe forms of tuberculosis. Public awareness is essential for getting their active cooperation.

Bacille calmette-guérin vaccination: The vaccine against tuberculosis is BCG, named for the 2 French investigators responsible for its development. The BCG vaccine contains attenuated *M. bovis* (the only widely used live bacterial vaccine). See vaccine in Chapter 40.

Amdekar YK. DOTS Program in Children and Adolescents. In: Mathur GP, Mathur Sarla (eds). *Current Trends in Pediatrics.* Vol 2. Delhi: Academa Publishers, 2006;216–19.

American Thoracic Society, Centres for Disease Control and Prevention, Infectious Disease Society of America: Treatment of tuberculosis. *Am J Respir Crit Care Med* 2003;167:603–62.

Central TB Division (CTD), DGHS, MOHF, Govt. of India. TB India 2003: RNTCP status report Delhi CTD; 2003.

Indian Academy of Pediatrics, treatment of childhood tuberculosis consensus statement of IAP working group. *Indian Pediatr* 1997;34:1093–6.

Khatri GR, Frieden TR. Rapid DOTS expansion in India. *Bull World Health Organ* 2002;80(6):457–63.

Powell DA. Nontuberculous mycobacteria. In: Kliegman RM, Behrman RE, Jenson HB, Stanton BF (eds). *Nelson Textbook of Pediatrics.* 18th edn. Vol. 1. Philadelphia: Saunders, 2007; 1259–63.

Starke JR, Munoz FM. Tuberculosis (*Mycobacterium tuberculosis*). In: Kliegman RM, Behrman RE, Jenson HB, Stanton BF (eds). *Nelson Textbook of Pediatrics.* 18th edn. Vol. 1. Philadelphia: Saunders, 2007;1259–64.

Statement Management. Pediatric Tuberculosis under the revise National Tuberculosis Central Program (NTCP). *Indian Pediatr* 2004;41:910–5.

Tripathi VN, Tiwari Bhavana. Tuberculosis in Children. In: Mathur GP, Mathur Sarla (eds). *Current Trends in Pediatrics.* Vol 2. Delhi: Academa Publishers, 2006;208–15.

Udani PM. Tuberculosis in children. *J International Med* 1994; Supplement 6:41–51.

WHO. Treatment of Tuberculosis, Guidelines for National Program. Geneva; WHO; 2003 (WHO/CDS/TB 2003–313).

14.4 LEPTOSPIROSIS

Etiopathogenesis: Leptospirosis is a worldwide zoonosis caused by spirochetes of the genus Leptospira in both tropical and subtropical countries. This is further divided into the pathogenic variants (*Leptospira interrogans)* and the nonpathogenic variants (*Leptospira biflexa).* The rat is the principal source of infection to man, although other domestic mammals can also be infected. Transmission is via infected urine (direct contact or contact with contaminated water and soil) and rarely animal bite or person to person transmission. Although leptospirosis is most common among adult males due to occupational (handlers and farmers) and recreational exposures, outbreaks have been reported in which more than 40% of patients were children.

Clinical manifestations: Clinically letospirosis can be classified as anicteric (90% of cases) and icteric leptospirosis or Weil disease (10% of cases). The septicemic phase of anicteric leptospirosis is an acute febrile illness with nonspecific symptoms like fever, myalgia, arthralgia, headache, lethargy, emesis, abdominal pain and cough. On examination conjunctival hyperemia, myositis, abdominal tenderness and generalized lymphadenopathy may be present. In the immune phase there is recurrence of fever; aseptic meningitis and uveitis may also be seen. Although less common, the presentation of Weil disease is more severe with a higher mortality rate. The septicemic phase of icteric is similar to that seen in anicteric leptospirosis. However, the immune phase manifests mainly as hepatic dysfunction/failure and renal failure. Occasionally pulmonary hemorrhage and myocarditis may occur.

Diagnosis: The diagnosis is mainly clinical. Serological tests include genus specific and serogroup specific microscopic agglutination tests and ELISA. A 4-fold or greater increase in titer in paired sera confirms the diagnosis. Agglutinins usually appear by the 12th day of illness and reach a maximum titer by the 3rd wk.

Treatment: Empiric therapy should be started in a patient with compatible symptoms and a plausible history of exposure, because drugs may be more effective in decreasing the severity of symptoms and reducing the duration of illness when the treatment is started before the 7th day of illness. The drug of choice is parenteral penicillin G (6–8 million units/m²/day in divided every 4 hr IV for 7 days). Tetracycline (10–20 mg/kg/day divided every 6 hr PO or IV for 7 days) in children 9 yr of age or older can be used in penicillin sensitive individuals. Oral amoxicillin is an alternative therapy for children < 9 yr of age.

Prevention: Simple measures like rodent control, use of protective clothing and immunization of livestock and family pets are helpful. Although animal vaccines do prevent symptomatic disease, infection and transmission may still occur. Prophylactic doxycycline (200 mg PO weekly) can be used in travelers to endemic areas for a short period.

Azimi P. Leptospira. In: Kliegman RM, Behrman RE, Jenson HB, Stanton BF (eds). *Nelson Textbook of Pediatrics.* 18th edn. Vol. 1. Philadelphia: Saunders, 2007;1270–1.

14.5 LYME DISEASE

Etiopathogenesis: Lyme disease is a vector-borne disease that occurs worldwide. It is caused by the spirochete *Borrelia burgdorferi*, which is transmitted by an infected tick of Ixodes species (Ixodes scapularies in the USA and Ixodes pacificus is on the Pacific Coast). The risk of transmission of *B. burgdorferi* from an infected tick to a human depends on the length of exposure. It takes hours for the tick to attach fully, and it requires as much as 48–72 hr for transmission of *B. burgdorferi* to occur.

Clinical manifestations: The illness has two phases; early and late. The early disease occurs usually 7–14 days after a tick bite and can be further classified as early localized and early disseminated. The early localized disease is characterized by rash known as erythema migrans (EM), a confluent erythematous macule that develops a central clearing, can occur anywhere on the body and gradually expands. A flu like illness with fever, chills, myalgias, arthrologies, headache, and malaise may be present. The early disseminated disease develops 3–10 wk after inoculation. During this phase multiple secondary EM lesions develop which differ from the primary lesions by being smaller, oval, evanescent and non-expansile. In addition to flu like symptoms aseptic meningitis, cranioneuropathies (seventh nerve) and carditis with complete heart block may occur.

The late disease develops weeks to months after inoculation. Untreated patients may present in the later stages without apparently having any symptoms of the early phase. Migratory arthritis is the hallmark of this stage with involvement of the large joints (knees in 90% of cases). The symptoms last for several weeks in a single joint. After resolution it recurs in another joint. Some individuals with arthritis may have persistent symptoms even after clearance of the infection, possibly due to autoimmunity. Another late manifestation is tertiary neuroborreliosis that affects the CNS and is rarely seen in children.

Diagnosis: In the early localized stage diagnosis is mainly based on the presence of erythema migrans (EM), as only a third of patients have a positive serological result. For patients with suspected Lyme disease in whom an EM rash is absent, serial titers can be used for confirmation eventually. Although isolation of the organism from a symptomatic patient is considered diagnostic, the organism is difficult to culture.

Treatment: All stages of Lyme disease require antibiotics. Those older than 8 yr are given 100 mg doxycycline bid for 14–21 days. Patients younger than

8 yr or those who cannot be given the above drug are administered amoxicillin or cefuroxime for the same duration. In early disseminated disease with carditis or meningitis, therapy is ceftriaxone or penicillin for 14–28 days and 28 days for those with late disease. The prognosis for Lyme disease is generally excellent when patients are treated early with appropriate antibiotic regimens, although some patients develop a Jarisch-Herxheimer reaction.

Prevention: Appropriate clothing should be worn in areas of likely tick exposure. Tick should be only removed vertically with a tweezer, never by twisting.

Shapiro ED. Lyme Disease (*Borrelia burgdorferi*). In: Kliegman RM, Behrman RE, Jenson HB, Stanton BF (eds). *Nelson Textbook of Pediatrics.* 18th edn. Vol. 1. Philadelphia: Saunders, 2007;1274–8.

14.6 RICKETTSIAL INFECTIONS

Rocky mountain spotted fever (RMSF) is caused by *Rickettsia rickettsia*. Ticks are the natural hosts, reservoirs, and vectors of *R. rickettsia*.

Clinical manifestations: The highest incidence of RMSF is seen in children < 10 yr of age. Boys are affected more than girls. The incubation period in children varies from 2 to 14 days, with a median of 7 days. History of removal of an attached tick, exposure in an endemic area, playing or hiking in wooded areas, typical season, similar illness in close contacts and close contact with a dog (especially a dog who has been sick) are all important clues to suspect rickettsial infection. The illness initially is nonspecific, with headache, fever, anorexia, myalgias, calf muscle pain and tenderness and gastrointestinal symptoms (nausea, vomiting, diarrhea, and abdominal pain). Skin rash is usually present after 2–4 days of illness. The typical clinical triad of headache, fever and rash is observed in < 50% of cases. Rash are initially discrete, pale, rose-red blanching macules or maculopapules appearing on the extremities, including the ankles, wrists, and lower legs. The rash then spreads rapidly to involve the entire body, including the soles and palms. After several days the rash becomes petechial or hemorrhagic, sometimes with palpable purpura. In severe disease, the petechiae may enlarge into ecchymoses, which can become necrotic. Severe vascular obstruction secondary to the rickettsial vasculitis and thrombosis can result in gangrene of the digits, earlobes, scrotum, nose, or an entire limb. Central nervous system infection often produces meningismus and changes in sensorium. CSF is usually normal, but in some cases there is mononuclear pleocytosis and elevated protein. In addition, patients may manifest ataxia, seizures, coma, or auditory deficits. Pulmonary disease is more commonly seen in adults than in children. Other findings reported include periorbital edema, dorsal hand and feet edema, hepatosplenomegaly, conjunctival suffusion, myocarditis, acute renal failure, and vascular collapse. Persons with glucose-6-phosphate dehydrogenase (G6PD) deficiency are at increased risk for fulminant RMSF.

Diagnosis: Delays in diagnosis and therapy are significant factors associated with death or severe illness. Since no reliable diagnostic test is available to confirm RMSF in its acute stage, the initial diagnosis and decision to initiate treatment of RMSF must be based on clinically suspicious illness with compatible epidemiologic and laboratory features. Laboratory abnormalities are nonspecific, include normal or low white blood cell count, but leukocytosis develops as the illnesses progresses, a left-shifted leukocyte differential, anemia, thrombocytopenia, hyponatremia and elevated serum aminotransferase activities. If a rash is present, a vasculotropic rickettsial infection can be diagnosed as early as day 3 of illness by immuno-histologic demonstration of specific rickettsial antigen in the endothelium in skin biopsy samples of petechial lesions. Diagnostic serologic criteria include a 4-fold increase in antibody titer, usually by indirect fluorescent antibody (IFA) assay in acute and convalescent sera (2–4 wk apart) or a single elevated IFA titer ≥ 64 in convalescent serum. A case is considered probable if a single titer of ≥ 128 is found. Serious complications include noncardiogenic pulmonary edema from pulmonary microvascular leakage, cerebral edema from meningoencephalitis, and multiorgan damage. Learning disabilities and behavioral problems are the most common sequelae among children who have survived severe disease.

Differential diagnosis: Other rickettsial infections are easily confused with RMSF, especially murine typhus. RMSF can mimic meningococcemia, measles, and enteroviral exanthemas. Negative blood cultures may aid in reaching a correct diagnosis. Other diseases sometimes included in the differential diagnosis are typhoid fever, secondary syphilis, lyme disease, leptospirosis, rat-bite fever, scarlet fever, toxic shock syndrome, rheumatic fever, rubella, parvovirus infection, Kawasaki disease, idiopathic thrombocyto-penic purpura, thrombotic thrombocytopenic purpura, Henoch-Schönlein purpura, hemolytic uremic syndrome, aseptic meningitis, acute gastrointestinal illness, acute abdomen, hepatitis, infectious mono-nucleosis, hemophagocytic syndromes, dengue fever, and drug reactions.

Treatment: The treatment of choice is doxycycline (2.2 mg/kg/dose bid PO or IV; maximum dose 200 mg/day). Alternative treatments include tetracycline (25–50 mg/kg/day divided every 6 hr PO; maximum dose 2 g/day), or chloramphenicol (50–100 mg/kg/day divided every 6 hr IV, maximum 3 g/day). Chloramphenicol should be reserved for patients with doxycycline allergy and for pregnant women. If used should be monitored to maintain serum concentrations of 10–30 µg/ml. Therapy should be continued for a minimum of 5–7 days and until the patent has been afebrile for at least 3 days to avoid relapse. Doxycycline as a single 200 mg oral dose (4.4 mg/kg if < 45 kg) is also reported an effective therapy.

Prevention: Prevention of RMSF is best accomplished by eliminating the tick infestations of dogs, avoiding wooded or grassy areas where ticks reside, using insect repellents containing DEET, wearing protective clothing, and carefully inspecting children who have been playing in the woods or fields. Recovery from infection yields lifelong solid immunity. Prompt and complete removal of attached ticks helps diminish the risk for transmission. Ticks should not be squeezed or crushed because their fluid may be infectious. Tick disposal should be accomplished by soaking the tick in alcohol or flushing it down the toilet, followed by good hand washing.

Mediterranean spotted fever (MSF) or Boutonneuse fever is caused by *Rickettsia conorii*. Transmission occurs after the bite of the brown dog tick, *R. sanguineus* or other tick species. The peak incidence is seen during July and August in the Mediterranean basin, but in other regions it occurs during warm seasons when ticks are active. Typically symptoms include fever, headache, myalgias, and a maculopapular rash that appears 3–5 days after onset of symptoms. In about 70% patients, a painless **eschar** at the initial site of tick attachment and regional lymphadenopathy are present. Persons with glucose-6-phosphate dehydrogenase (G6PD) deficiency, alcoholic liver disease or diabetes mellitus are at increased risk for fulminant infection. The disease is milder in children. The complications of MSF are similar to those of RMSF. The complications of MSF are similar to those of RMSF. The case fatality rate is approximately 2%. Severe infections have been noted in patients with underlying medical conditions, including G6PD deficiency and diabetes mellitus. Laboratory diagnosis of MSF is the same as that for RMSF and may be accomplished by immunohistologic demonstration of rickettsiae on skin biopsy. The differential diagnosis is similar to that of RMSF, with the inclusion of conditions associated with single

eschars such as anthrax, bacterial ecthyma, spider bite, rat-bite fever (caused by *Spirillum minus*), and other rickettsioses. Treatment and prevention is same as mentioned in RMSF. Intensive care may be required for hemodynamic management of severely affected individuals.

Rickettsialpox is caused by *Rickettsia akari*, which is transmitted by the mouse mite *Allodermanyssus sanguineus*. The mouse host for this mite is widely distributed in the USA, Europe, and Asia. Initially there is typical macular or maculopapular rash, distributed over the trunk, head, and extremities, which may become vesicular in some cases. At presentation, most patients have fever, headache and chills. There is a painless papular or ulcerative lesion or eschar at the initial site of inoculation in up to 90% of cases, which may be associated with regional, often tender lymphadenopathy. The infection resolves, even without therapy. Doxycycline will hasten resolution but is often withheld in children < 9 yr of age in view of mildness of illness. However, some experts limit treatment to a brief course (2 days) of doxycycline to young children with more significant illness. Complications and fatalities are rare.

Sexton DJ, Kaye KS. Rocky mountain spotted fever. *Med Clin North Am* 2002;86:351–60.

Siberry GK, Dumler JS. Spotted fever group Rickettsioses. In: Kliegman RM, Behrman RE, Jenson HB, Stanton BF (eds). *Nelson Textbook of Pediatrics.* 18th edn. Vol. 1. Philadelphia: Saunders, 2007;1289–94.

Scrub typhus or Tsutsugamushi fever is caused by *Orientia tsutsugamushi*. *O. tsutsugamushi* is transmitted via the bite of the larval stage (chigger) of a trombiculid mite (*Leptotrombidium*), which serves as both vector and reservoir. The disease is prevalent in many parts of the Eastern hemisphere. Most patients present with fever for 9–11 days (range 1–30 days) before seeking medical care. Regional and generalized lymphadenopathy, hepatomegaly, splenomegaly, and gastrointestinal symptoms, including abdominal pain, vomiting, and diarrhea are reported. A single painless eschar with an erythematous rim at the site of the chigger bite and a maculopapular rash may be present. Serious complications include pneumonitis, meningoencephalitis, acute renal failure, myocarditis, or a septic shock-like syndrome in some cases. Thrombocytopenia and leukocytosis may occur. Serologic tests such as indirect fluorescent antibody (IFA) or immunoperoxidase assays confirm the diagnosis of *O. tsutsugamushi*. Differential diagnosis includes fever of unknown origin, enteric fever, typhoid fever, dengue hemorrhagic fever, other rickettsioses, tularemia, anthrax, dengue, leptospirosis, malaria, and infectious mononucleosis.

Treatment and prevention is similar to that recommended for RMSF.

Dumler JS, Siberry GK. Scrub Typhus (*Orientia tsutsugamushi*). In: Kliegman RM, Behrman RE, Jenson HB, Stanton BF (eds). *Nelson Textbook of Pediatrics*. 18th edn. Vol. 1. Philadelphia: Saunders, 2007;1295–6.

Murine typhus is caused by *Rickettsia typhi*, a rickettsia transmitted from infected fleas to rats, other rodents, or opossums and back to fleas. *R. typhi* normally cycles between rodents or midsize animals such as opossums and their fleas. Human acquisition of murine typhus occurs when rickettsiae infected flea feces contaminate flea bite wounds. The incubation period varies from 1 to 2 wk. Fever of undetermined origin the most frequent presentation. Other clinical presentation includes rash, myalgias, vomiting, cough, headache, diarrhea or abdominal pain, lymphadenopathy and hepatomegaly. In a few patients neurologic involvement is reported. Macules, maculopapules or petechial rash (in a few children) distributed on the trunk and extremities is reported. The rash can involve both the soles and palms. Confirmation of the diagnosis is usually made by comparing acute and convalescent phase antibody titers obtained with the indirect fluorescent antibody assay. Treatment is similar to that recommended for RMSF. Control of murine typhus includes elimination of the flea reservoir and control of flea hosts.

Epidemic typhus is caused by *Rickettsia prowazekii* and its recrudescent form, Brill-Zinsser disease. Human body lice (*Pediculus humanus* subspecies *corporis*) become infected by feeding on rickettsemic persons. The ingested rickettsiae infect the midgut epithelial cells of the lice and are passed into the feces, which in turn are introduced in to a susceptible human host through abrasion or perforations in the skin, through the conjunctivae, or rarely through inhalation of dried infected louse excreta present in clothing, bedding, or furniture. The incubation period is usually < 14 days. The typical clinical manifestations include fever, severe headache, abdominal tenderness, and rash in most patients. The rash is initially pink or erythematous and blanches appear predominantly on the trunk. *Brill-Zinsser disease* is an unusual form of typhus that becomes recrudescent months to yr after primary infection. Thrombocytopenia and leukocytosis may occur. Treatment is similar to that recommended for RMSF. Antibiotic therapy and delousing measures used to prevent the disease.

Dumler JS, Siberry GK. Typhus group rickettsioses. In: Kliegman RM, Behrman RE, Jenson HB, Stanton BF (eds). *Nelson Textbook of Pediatrics*. 18th edn. Vol. 1. Philadelphia: Saunders, 2007;1296–98.

Q fever is caused by *Coxiella burnetii*. The disease is reported worldwide, except in New Zealand. Two forms of Q fever (acute and chronic) occur. *Acute Q fever* is most frequent and develops about 3 wk (range 14–39 days) after exposure to the causative agent, usually presenting in children as fever only or as an influenza-like illness with interstitial pneumonitis.

Chronic Q fever usually involves the native heart valves, prosthetic valves, or other cardiovascular prostheses and osteomyelitis. Q fever should be considered in children with fever of unknown origin. The diagnosis Q fever is confirmed serologically by testing acute and convalescent sera (2–4 wk apart), which show a 4-fold increase in indirect fluorescent antibody titers to phase I and phase II *C. burnetii* antigens. Predominant, elevated, or increasing titers of phase II antibody are characteristic of acute Q fever and the appearance and persistence of elevated titers of phase I and phase II antibody are indicative of chronic Q fever. Treatment of acute Q fever should be started within 3 days of onset of symptoms with doxycycline (2.2 mg/kg/dose bid PO or IV, maximum 200 mg/day). Chloramphenicol should be reserved for patients with doxycycline allergy and for pregnant women. During pregnancy, Q fever is best treated with trimethoprim-sulfamethoxazole. For chronic Q fever, especially endocarditis, therapy for 18–36 mo is mandatory with the bacteriostatic drugs doxycycline or tetracycline in combination with hydroxychloroquine or with bactericidal drugs such as rifampicin, ofloxacin, or pefloxacin. For patients with heart failure, valve replacement may be warranted and should be accompanied by an effective antibiotic regimen to avoid reinfection of the prosthetic valves. Recognition of the disease in livestock or other domestic animals should alert communities to the risk for human infection. Milk from infected herds must be pasteurized at temperatures sufficient to destroy *C. burnetii*.

Dumler JS, Siberry GK. Q fever (*Coxiella burnetii*). In: Kliegman RM, Behrman RE, Jenson HB, Stanton BF (eds). *Nelson Textbook of Pediatrics*. 18th edn. Vol. 1. Philadelphia: Saunders, 2007;1301–03.
Maltezou HC, Raoult D. Q fever in children. *Lancet Infect Dis* 2002;2:686–91.

14.7 FUNGAL INFECTIONS

Candidiasis is responsible for neonatal and congenital infection and infections in immunocompetent and immunocompromised children and adolescents.

1. *Neonatal infections:* The various presentations of *Candida* infections in the newborn can be separated into the following categories:

i. *Mucocutaneous candidiasis*, which includes oropharyngeal involvement (thrush) or diaper dermatitis

ii. *Systemic candidiasis:* Common presenting symptoms are respiratory distress, apnea, and thrombocytopenia and localized signs of candidal infection at one or more of the following sites:

   a. *Skin and mucous membranes* (oral thrush, diaper rash) (*see* Fig. 14.4 in CD)

   b. *Central nervous system:* Meningitis.

   c. *Eyes: Candida* endophthalmitis.

   d. *Heart: Candida* endocarditis. Right-sided intra-cardiac fungal masses can manifest with heart failure or even with pulmonary fungal embolism.

   e. *Kidneys: Candida* is the most frequent cause of urinary tract infection.

   f. *Bones and joints:* Warmth and swelling of the extremities in combination with radiographic evidence of osteolysis or arthritis.

iii. *Catheter-related infections without multi-organ involvement:* Catheter-related *Candida* infection refers to candidemia that resolves rapidly after catheter removal and initiation of therapy.

iv. *Invasive focal infection* includes meningitis, urinary tract infections, peritonitis, endophthalmitis, osteomyelitis, and septic arthritis.

2. *Congenital candidiasis:* Two forms have been described.

   i. *Congenital cutaneous candidiasis* is associated with extensive skin rash presents within 12 hr of birth. A macular erythema that may evolve from a pustular, papular or vesicular phase finally results in extensive desquamation.

   ii. *Congenital systemic candidiasis:* Presenting signs are pneumonia (most common), meningitis, candiduria and/or candidemia. Treatment includes removal of vascular catheters associated with transient fungemia or disseminated infection should, followed by treatment with intravenous antifungal therapy for 2–3 wk. Amphotericin B is the gold standard neonatal antifungal therapy (0.5–1.0 mg/kg/day IV) for systemic candidiasis and is active against both yeast and mycelial forms. The total recommended dose is 20–30 mg/kg.

3. *Infections in immunocompetent children and adolescents* include:

   i. *Oral thrush* (*see* Chapter 30)

   ii. *Diaper dermatitis (syn. diaper rash)* (*see* Chapter 30)

   iii. *Ungual and periungual infections* (*see* Chapter 30)

   iv. *Vulvovaginitis:* The principal symptoms of *Candida* vulvovaginitis are vulvar and/or vaginal pruritus and a thick vaginal discharge. Other possible symptoms are vulvar pain and dyspareunia. Fungal cultures are performed if microscopic studies are negative and the index of suspicion for *Candida* vulvovaginitis continues to be high. Vaginal creams or troches of nystatin, clotrimazole, econazole, terconazole or miconazole are effective in treating candidal vulvovaginitis. Oral therapy with a single dose of fluconazole has been found to be as effective as topical clotrimazole. Persistent vulvovaginal candidiasis can be treated with fluconazole.

4. *Infections in immunocompromised children and adolescents:* In HIV-infected children, malignancy/organ transplant patients, and children with indwelling catheters infections range from superficial mucocutaneous infection like oral thrush to severe sepsis and shock. Intravenous amphotericin B/liposomal amphotericin B is the treatment of choice alone or with the addition of fluconazole. Fluconazole prophylaxis in bone marrow transplant recipients decreases incidence of candidemia.

Bendel CM. Nosocomial neonatal candidiasis. *Pediatr Infect Dis J* 2005;24:831–2.

Patterson TF. Advances and challenges in management of invasive mycoses. *Lancet* 2005;166;1013–25.

Weisse ME, Aronoff SC, *Candida* In: Kliegman RM, Behrman RE, Jenson HB, Stanton BF (eds). *Nelson Textbook of Pediatrics.* 18th edn. Vol. 1. Philadelphia: Saunders, 2007;1307–10.

Cryptococcus neoformans is one of the presenting manifestations of AIDS. Primary infection occurs through inhalation of fungal spores from soil contaminated with pigeon fecal droppings. Pneumonia is the most common form of crypttococcosis. If the host immune status is compromised, dissemination follows with involvement of the brain, meninges, skin, eyes, skeletal system and the prostate.

Diagnosis is based on recovery of the fungus by culture from the clinical specimen or demonstration of fungus in infected tissue or detection of cryptococcal antigen in serum and CSF in titers of > 1 : 4.

Treatment depends on the sites of involvement and the host immune status. Pneumonia is treated with oral fluconazole (200–400 mg/day) or itraconazole (200–400 mg/day) for 3–12 mo depending on the clinical response. Disseminated disease/relapse is treated with amphotericin B (0.7–1 mg/kg/day) plus flucytosine (100 mg/kg/day) for 2 wk.; it may be extended till 10 wk. This is followed by therapy with oral fluconazole or itraconazole for 6–12 months. The treatment may be continued lifelong in immuno-compromised children. Surgical intervention may be required in patients with hydrocephalus and skeletal infections. Individuals at high risk should avoid exposures such as bird droppings. Effective antiretroviral therapy for persons with HIV infection reduces the risk of cryptococcal disease.

Flood RG, Aronoff SC. *Cryptococcus neoformans*. In: Kliegman RM, Behrman RE, Jenson HB, Stanton BF (eds). *Nelson Textbook of Pediatrics*. 18th edn. Vol. 1. Philadelphia: Saunders, 2007; 1310–2.

Jaiswani SP, Hemwani N, Sharma N, et al. Prevalence of fungal meningitis among HIV positive and negative subjects. *Indian J Med Sci* 2002;56:325–9.

Malassezia

See Chapter 30, Tinea Versicolor.

Aspergillosis in children most commonly is caused by *A. fumigates*. Aspergillus-associated diseases may be immunoglobulin E (IgE) mediated (hypersensitivity syndromes), saprophytic (noninvasive), or invasive.

Hypersensitivity syndromes include asthma, extrinsic alveolar alveolitis, and allergic bronchopulmonary aspergillosis (ABPA). The episodes of hypersensitivity syndromes can be treated with oral prednisolone 0.5 mg/kg/day daily for 7 days, followed by 0.5 mg/kg every alternate day until symptoms abate and serum IgE returns to pre-illness levels. Corticosteroid therapy usually lasts for 6 wk. If asthma symptoms recur as steroid treatment is withdrawn inhaled steroids and/or bronchodilators are indicated.

Saprophytic (noninvasive) syndromes include otomycosis, primary cutaneous aspergillosis, sinusitis, and pulmonary aspergilloma. Colonization and fungal proliferation occur in the cavity of the lung by spores of *Aspergillus* in patients with pre-existing chronic pulmonary disease, e.g. tuberculous cavities, bronchiectasis, congenital pulmonary cysts, healed abscess cavities. This results in formation of amorphous mycelial mass ('fungus ball'). This lesion is known as *aspergilloma*. The treatment of otomycosis includes proper cleaning of the affected part and application of topical antifungal agents such as nystatin, tolnaftate, or dilutes acetic acid and topical corticosteroids. Oral itraconazole is also beneficial. Early recognition of primary cutaneous aspergillosis and therapy with amphotericin B is essential to prevent systemic disease.

Invasive disease is characterized by propensity of the hyphal elements of *Aspergillus* to infiltrate blood vessels leading to infarction and necrosis of the tissue/organ supplied by them. Systemic anti-fungal therapy with amphotericin B or voriconazole and surgical debridement (if indicated), are cornerstone of treatment.

Denning DW. Invasive aspergillosis. *Clin Infect Dis* 1998; 26:781–803.

Gefter W B. The spectrum of pulmonary aspergillosis. *J Thoracic Imaging* 1992;7:56–74.

Tynan M, Aronoff SC. Aspergillus. In: Kliegman RM, Behrman RE, Jenson HB, Stanton BF (eds). *Nelson Textbook of Pediatrics*. 18th edn. Vol. 1. Philadelphia: Saunders, 2007; 1313–16.

Histoplasmosis is caused by an intra-cellular, dimorphic fungus, *Histoplasma capsulatum*.

The endemic areas are located in the United States, Latin America, Brazil, and India. Infection is usually acquired by inhalation of microconidia (fungal spores). There are 3 forms of histoplasmosis:

1. *Acute pulmonary histoplasmosis* (45%) is characterized by prolonged illness with fever, cough, chest pain (*bronchopneumonia*), headache, myalgia, and fatigue.
2. *Chronic pulmonary histoplasmosis* is an opportunistic infection in adult patients with centrilobular emphysema.
3. *Progressive disseminated histoplasmosis* (5%) presents with fever, weight loss, lymphadenopathy, interstitial pneumonia, hepatosplenomegaly. Other sites of involvement include bone (osteolytic lesions), bone marrow (anemia, thrombocytopenia), oral cavity (ulceration), brain and meninges (meningoencephalitis), retina (chorioretinitis), skin (cutaneous nodules), heart (endocarditis), adrenal glands (Addison's disease). In HIV positive patients, histoplasmosis usually presents as a disseminated infection and is categorised as an AIDS defining illness in such patients.

Diagnosis is based on recovery of *H. capsulatum* by culture or detection of *Histoplasma* associated antigen by radio-immunoassay in urine, blood, bronchoalveolar lavage sample, and CSF. Complement fixation test detecting specific antibody titres ≥ 1 : 32 is diagnostic and indicates recent infection.

Treatment is not indicated asymptomatic cases. Oral itraconazole or fluconazole should be considered in patients with acute pulmonary infections (bronchopneumonia). Advanced pulmonary lesions with respiratory distress warrant use of IV amphotericin B (0.7 mg/kg/day) or amphotericin B lipid complex (3 mg/kg/day) until improvement and continued therapy with oral itraconazole for 12 weeks. Lifelong prophylaxis with oral itraconazole (2–5 mg/kg/day) is indicated in HIV-infected cases.

McCoy ACS, Aronoff SC. Histoplasmosis (*Histoplasma capsulatum*). In: Kliegman RM, Behrman RE, Jenson HB, Stanton BF (eds). *Nelson Textbook of Pediatrics*. 18th edn. Vol. 1. Philadelphia: Saunders, 2007;1316–8.

Singhi MK, Gupta L, Kacchawa D, et al. Disseminated primary cutaneous histoplasmosis successfully treated with itraconazole. *Indian J Dermatol Venereol Leprol* 2003; 69:405–407.

Subhramanium S, Abraham OC, et al. Disseminated histoplasmosis. *J Assoc Physicians India* 2005;53:185–9.

Blastomycosis is caused by a dimorphic fungus *Blastomyces dermatitidis*. It has been reported in Canada, India, Africa, and Central and South America.

Infection is acquired via inhalation of the conidia. Incubation period averages 4–6 weeks. The clinical presentation is highly variable and ranges from asymptomatic to acute, chronic, or disseminated disease. *Pneumonia* is the most common form of symptomatic blastomycosis. *Extrapulmonary or disseminated disease* occur any organ, but the common sites includes skin and neurologic involvement.

Diagnosis can be made by growth of the fungus in a culture. *Treatment* is not required in asymptomatic patients. Amphotericin B remains the antifungal agent of choice. Surgical debridement may be required in for removal of devitalized bone and for pulmonary lesions not responding to medical therapy.

Chakrabarti A, Chatterjee SS, Shivprakash MR. Overview of opportunistic fungal infections in India: *Jpn J Med. Mycol* 2008;49:165–72.

Fleece DM, Aronoff SC, Blastomycosis (*Blastomyces dermatitidis*). In: Kliegman RM, Behrman RE, Jenson HB, Stanton BF (eds). *Nelson Textbook of Pediatrics.* 18th edn. Vol. 1. Philadelphia: Saunders, 2007;1318–9.

Savio J, Muralidharan S, Macaden RS, et al. Blastomycosis in a South Indian patient after visiting an endemic area in USA. *Med Mycol* 2006;44:523–9.

Coccidioidomycosis is an infection caused by the soil-inhabiting, dimorphic fungus *Coccidioides immitis.* These fungi are endemic to certain regions of North, Central and South America. Coccidioidomycosis has been rarely seen in India. Progression in symptoms may rarely occur in an otherwise healthy individual, but it more often occurs in patients with the following underlying risk factors: HIV, AIDS, thymectomy, lymphoma, taking immunosuppressive medications (transplant patients) and first year of organ transplant, chemotherapy for solid tumors, corticosteroids (> 20 mg prednisone), antitumor necrosis factor therapy, diabetes mellitus, pregnancy (highest in third trimester), and preexisting cardiopulmonary conditions.

Sixty percent patients (*asymptomatic*) have subclinical disease that never comes to medical attention, and the infection resolves spontaneously. Common sites of symptomatic infection include lungs, meninges, skin, soft tissue, bones, and joints. *Acute pneumonia* occurs in 30–40% cases approximately 1–3 wk following inhalation of arthrospores. *Diagnosis* requires isolation of the organism in culture, via histologic specimens, or with serologic testing. Bone scanning is a sensitive test for identifying sites of dissemination (e.g. skull, hands, feet, spine, and tibia). *Treatment* is not required in asymptomatic cases. Amphotericin B, fluconazole, itraconazole, ketoconazole are the antifungal agents, currently recommended as first-line agents for the treatment of rapidly progressing or disseminated coccidioidal infection only.

Chakrabarti A, et al. Overview of opportunistic fungal infections in India. Jpn J Med. Mycol 2008;49:165–72.

Pappagianis D. Coccidioidomycosis (Coccidioides). In: Kliegman RM, Behrman RE, Jenson HB, Stanton BF (eds). *Nelson Textbook of Pediatrics.* 18th edn. Vol. 1. Philadelphia: Saunders, 2007;1319–22.

Paracoccidioidomycosis is caused by a dimorphic fungus, *paracoccidioides brasiliensis.* Paracoccidioidomycosis is endemic to South and Central America. Pulmonary infection is the most common manifestation secondary to inhalation of conidia or mycelial fragments; however, following dissemination, paracoccidioidomycosis frequently involves the mucous membranes, skin, and lymph nodes. Patients with AIDS are more likely to develop hematogenous dissemination and multiple organ involvement.

Diagnosis is based on demonstration of the fungus by direct wet mount of sputum, exudates or pus with potassium hydroxide (KOH) and consist of a demonstration of large, multiple budding yeasts (blastoconidia). Immunodiffusion/Western Blotting tests are used to detect circulating *P. brasiliensis* antibodies.

Treatment of choice is itraconazole (50–400 mg/day) orally for 6 mo. Fluconazole, ketoconazole and amphotericin B are other alternatives.

Mccoy ACS, Aronoff SC. *Paracoccidioides brasiliensis.* In: Kliegman RM, Behrman RE, Jenson HB, Stanton BF (eds). *Nelson Textbook of Pediatrics.* 18th edn. Vol. 1. Philadelphia: Saunders, 2007;1322–3.

Sporotrichosis is caused by *Sporothrix schenckii* that thrives on dead and decaying organic matter. The fungus is found in the environment in the mycelial (mold) form and in tissues as yeast. It has a worldwide distribution but, preponderance of cases has been reported from North and South America, South Africa, Japan, and India. Lymphocutaneous sporotrichosis accounts for > 75% of reported cases. Extracutaneous sporotrichosis is rare in children and most cases are in adults affecting commonly skeletal infection. Pulmonary sporotrichosis usually presents as a chronic pneumonitis similar to the presentation of pulmonary tuberculosis (*see* Figs 14.5 and 14.6 in CD).

Diagnosis requires isolation of the fungus form the site of infection by culture. In case of disseminated disease, demonstration of serum antibody against *S. Schenckii*-related antigens is diagnostic.

Treatment for simple cutaneous forms is a saturated solution of potassium iodide in a dose of 5–10 drops 3 times a day in milk, juice or water. Itraconazole (5 mg/kg PO daily for 6–12 wks) is the drug of choice for infections outside the central nervous system. Terbinafine can also be used as an alternative drug. Amphotericin B is used to treat more severe forms of sporotrichosis (pulmonary, osteoarticular, meningeal, disseminated).

Fleece DM, Aronoff SC, **Sporotrichosis (Sporothrix Schenckii)**. In: Kliegman RM, Behrman RE, Jenson HB, Stanton BF (eds). *Nelson Textbook of Pediatrics*. 18th edn. Vol. 1. Philadelphia: Saunders, 2007;1323–4.

Ghosh A, Chakrabarti A, Sharma VK, Singh K,Singh A. Sporotrichosis in Himachal Pradesh (North India). *Trans Royal Soc Trop Med Hyg* 1999; 93:41–45.

Randhawa HS, Chand R, Mussa AY, et al. Sporotrichosis in India: first case in a Delhi resident and an update. *Indian J Med Microbiol* 2003;21(1):12–16.

Zygomycosis is cased by *Rhizopus arrhizus* (*Rhizopus oryzae*), followed by *Rhizopus rhizopodiformis*. These organisms rarely cause disease in immunocompetent hosts, but they have emerged as the third most common cause of invasive fungal infection in immuno-compromised patients, during the past decade. The primary route of infection is inhalation of spores from the environment. These organisms have a particular predilection for invading major blood vessels, with ensuing ischemia, necrosis, and infarction of adjacent tissues. Cutaneous or percutaneous routes of infection may lead to cutaneous and subcutaneous zygomycosis. Ingestion of contaminated food or drinks has been associated with gastrointestinal diseases. The five major clinical forms include rhinocerebral zygo-mycosis, pulmonary zygomycosis, cutaneous zygomycosis, gastrointestinal zygomycosis and disseminated zygomycosis. **Diagnosis** is confirmed on direct morphologic examination. **Treatment** includes correction of the underlying predisposing factors. Hyperglycemia and ketoacidosis should be corrected, neutropenia should be adequately managed. Steroids or deferoxamine should be discontinued. Ampho-tericin B desoxycholate (1–1.5 mg/kg/day to a total dose of 70 mg/kg or 3–4 g over several weeks) or amphotericin B lipid complex (3–5 mg/kg/day) are the current mainstay of therapy for all forms of zygomycosis. Early and aggressive surgical debridement of all infected tissue should be carried out.

Chakraborti A et al. Ten years' experience in zygomycosis at a tertiary care centre in India. *J Infect* 2001 (May); 42(4): 261–6.

Chakrabarti A *et al*; Overview of opportunistic fungal infections in India. *Jpn J Med. Mycol* 2008; 49: 165–172.

Diwakar A, Dewan RK, Chowdhary A, et al. Zygomycosis—a case report and overview of the disease in India. *Mycoses* 2007;50 (4):247–754.

Tynan M, Aronoff SC. Zygomycosis (Mucormycosis). In: Kliegman RM, Behrman RE, Jenson HB, Stanton BF (eds). *Nelson Textbook of Pediatrics*. 18th edn. Vol. 1. Philadelphia: Saunders, 2007;1324–5.

Pneumocystis jiroveci (formerly *Pneumocystis carinii*) is a common extracellular parasite found in the lungs of mammals worldwide responsible for causing life-threatening pneumonia in immunocompromised patients. *P. carinii* is commonly found in the lungs of normal immune-competent individuals. The mortality rate is high in immunosuppressed patients who require mechanical ventilation (*see* Fig. 14.7 in CD).

Diagnosis requires demonstration of *P. carinii* in the lung in the presence of clinical signs and symptoms of the infection.

Treatment of choice in cases of *P. carinii* pneumonia is trimethoprim-sulfamethoxazole (15–20 mg TMP and 75–100 mg SMZ/kg/day divided qid) administered IV or orally if there is mild disease and no malabsorption or diarrhea. The duration of treatment is 3 wk for patients with HIV–AIDS and 2 wk for other patients. Other drugs used in the treatment include pentamidine isethionate and atovaquone.

Prophylaxis of choice is trimethoprim-sulfamethoxazole [5 mg TMP and 25 mg SMZ/kg/day once (or divided into two doses) daily PO] given for 3 consecutive days each week, or, alternatively, each day. Alternatively, dapsone, atovaquone, and aerosolized pentamidine can be used. The prophylaxis must be continued as long as the patient remains immunocompromised.

Gigliotti F, Wright TW. *Pneumocystis carinii (Pneumocystis jiroveci)*. In: Kliegman RM, Behrman RE, Jenson HB, Stanton BF (eds). *Nelson Textbook of Pediatrics*. 18th edn. Vol. 1. Philadelphia: Saunders, 2007;1325–27.

Mishra M, Thakar YS, Akulwar SL, et al. Detection of *Pneumocystis carinii* is induced sputum samples of HIV positive patients. *Indian J Med Microbiol* 2006;24:149–50.

14.8 VIRAL INFECTIONS

Measles

Etiopathogenesis: Measles is caused by an RNA virus belonging to the Paramyxovirus family. High incidence is seen in children aged 1 to 5 yrs. One attack confers solid immunity. It spreads person to person through respiratory route (inhalation). Measles virus can be transmitted from 3 days before the rash up to 4–6 days the onset of the rash. As the virus resides in the mucus lining in the nose and throat of the infected person, droplets carrying viruses spread in the air during coughing and sneezing which subsequently inhaled by a susceptible person during breathing. Further, the viruses also enter into susceptible persons when they put their fingers in their mouth or nose after handling an infected surface or person. The virus remains active and contagious on infected surfaces for up to two hours. The incubation period is 8–12 days (around 10 days).

Clinical manifestations: After an incubation period of 8–12 days, the prodromal phase begins typically with a mild to moderate fever, accompanied by rash, cough, running nose, and red-watery eyes (conjunctivitis). The enanthem, Koplik spots is the pathognomonic sign of measles and appear 1 to 4 days prior to the onset of rash. They first appear as discrete red lesions with bluish white spots in the center on the inner aspects of the cheeks at the level of the premolars. They may spread to involve the lips, hard palate, and gingiva. They may occur in conjunctival folds and in the vaginal mucosa.

Symptoms increase in intensity for 2–4 days until the 1st day of the rash. The rash begins around the forehead (around the hairline), behind the ears, on the upper neck as a red macular eruption. It then spreads downward to the chest and back, and finally to the feet covering full-body, from face to the extremities, reaching the palms and soles in up to 50% of cases. The exanthema frequently becomes confluent on the face and upper trunk [Body temperature often increased as high as ±40°C (104 or 105°F)]. After about a week, the rash begins fading in the same sequence that it appeared, often leaving a fine desquamation of skin and brownish discoloration, this fades over the next 10 days. Of the major symptoms of measles, the cough lasts the longest, often up to 10 days. In more severe cases, generalized lymphadenopathy may be present with cervical and occipital lymph nodes especially prominent.

Diagnosis: The diagnosis of measles is based on clinical findings like characteristic rash, Koplik spots and a history of at least three days fever and epidemiologic findings. Laboratory findings in the acute phase include reduction in the total white blood cell count, with lymphocytes decreased more than neutrophils. Confirmatory diagnosis of measles can be made by detecting specific IgM antibodies and isolation of virus. IgM antibody appears 1–2 days after the onset of the rash and remains detectable for about 1 mo. Serologic confirmation may also be made by demonstration of a 4-fold rise in IgG antibodies in acute and convalescent specimens taken 2–4 wk later.

Differential diagnosis: Rashes similar to measles should be differentiated from other infections, including Rubella, erythema subitum (in infants), erythema infectiosum (in older children), adenoviruses, enteroviruses, Epstein-Barr virus, *Mycoplasma pneumoniae*, group A streptococcus, and Kawasaki syndrome.

Complications: Approximately 20% of reported measles affected individuals experience one or more complications like respiratory infections, diarrhea, vomiting, conjunctivitis, myocarditis, seizures, encephalitis and sub-acute sclerosing panencephalitis (SSPE). Measles during pregnancy can also cause miscarriage, premature birth, or low-birth-weight baby.

Complications are more common among children under 5 yr and adults over 20 yr of age. Respiratory infections include acute otitis media, croup, tracheitis, bronchitis, bronchiolitis, pneumonia [caused by bacterial pathogens such as *S. pneumoniae, H. influenzae* and *S. aureus*, and giant cell pneumonia (caused directly by the viral infection)]. All most all patients (90%) recover from encephalitis but there may be complications (deafness, seizures and mental disorders). Measles is also associated with malnutrition particularly the vitamin A deficiency.

Measles infection is known to suppress skin test responsiveness to purified tuberculin antigen. There may be an increased rate of activation of pulmonary tuberculosis in individuals infected with *Mycobacterium tuberculosis.*

A severe form of measles rarely seen is *hemorrhagic or "black measles".* It is presented with hemorrhagic skin eruption and is often fatal. Keratitis, appearing as multiple punctuates epithelial foci, resolves with recovery from the infection. Thrombocytopenia sometimes has occurred following measles.

Very rarely (7 in 1,000,000 cases) the patients may develop a serious complication known as *sub-acute sclerosing pan-encephalitis (SSPE),* which begins insidiously 7–13 yr after primary measles infection—a progressive and usually fatal disease characterized by behavioral changes followed by loss of motor control and coordination. There are jerky movements known as myoclonic seizures. The *diagnosis of SSPE* can be established through documentation of a compatible clinical course and at least one of the following supportive findings:
1. Measles antibody detected in CSF
2. EEG showing suppression-burst episodes in the myoclonic phase, or
3. Typical histologic findings and/or isolation of virus or viral antigen in brain tissue obtained by biopsy or postmortem examination. CSF analysis reveals normal cells but elevated IgG and IgM antibody titers in dilutions of > 1 : 8. Management of SSPE is primarily supportive and similar to care provided to patients with other neurodegenerative diseases.

Treatment: Management of measles is supportive. Children with measles need full rest to help them recover. The symptoms usually last for about two weeks. Patients with measles should be closely monitored for any symptoms of complications such as croup, and infections like bronchitis, bronchiolitis, pneumonia, conjunctivitis, otitis media, myocarditis and encephalitis. Antipyretics are used to control fever. For patients with respiratory tract involvement, airway humidification and supplemental oxygen may be of benefit. Respiratory failure due to croup or pneumonia may require ventilatory support. Oral rehydration therapy is effective in most cases, but severe dehydration may require intravenous therapy. Secondary bacterial infections, if any, should be treated accordingly. In case of encephalitis and SSPE, care should be provided accordingly. It is usually safe for a child to return to school only 7 to 10 days after the fever and rash disappear or after consulting a doctor.

Vitamin A therapy should be administered in children [in a single dose of 200,000 IU orally for children ≥1 yr of age (100,000 IU for children 6 mo to 1 yr of age)], because of increased mortality in children with vitamin A deficiency associated with measles.

Prevention: Exposure of susceptible individuals to measles patients should be avoided, because patients shed measles virus from 7 days after exposure to 4-6 days after the onset of rash. Immunocompromised patients with measles will shed for the duration of the illness, and isolation should be maintained throughout (*see* Chapters 15 and 40).

Postexposure prophylaxis: Susceptible individuals exposed to measles may be protected from infection either by vaccine administration or immunization with immunoglobulin. The vaccine is effective in prevention or modification of measles if given within 72 hr of exposure. Immune globulin may be given up to 6 days following exposure to prevent or modify infection. Immunocompetent children should receive 0.25 ml/kg intramuscularly and immunocompromised children should receive 0.5 ml/kg. Immune globulin is indicated for susceptible household contacts of measles patients, especially infants < 6 mo of age, pregnant women, and immunocompromised persons.

Rubella

Etiopathogenesis: Rubella is caused by Rubella virus (a single-stranded RNA virus). It is also known as German measles (German term likely comes from the Latin term *"germanus"* meaning "similar") or three-day measles. It is distributed worldwide. Humans are the only known reservoir of Rubella virus. Modes of infections include inhalation, direct contact with the respiratory secretions of infected persons and congenital (transplacental). The virus multiplies in the cells of the respiratory tract, extends to local lymph nodes, and then spread to target organs via blood circulation (viremia). Subsequent replication in selected target organs such as the spleen and lymph nodes, leads to a secondary viremia with wide dissemination of the virus. During this period (approximately 7 days after infection and 7 to 10 days before the onset of rash), the virus can be detected in the blood and respiratory secretions. Virus shedding from the respiratory tract may continue for up to 28 days following the onset of rash. It primarily affects the lymph nodes and skin. The most important factor for severe congenital defects is the stage of gestation at the time of infection. Maternal infection during the first 8 wk of gestation results in the most severe and wide spread defects. The risk for congenital defects has been estimated at 90% for maternal infection before 11 wk of gestation. Defects occurring after 16 wk of gestation are uncommon. Infection acquired congenitally may cause severe complications including abortion, stillbirth and other congenital abnormalities like low-birth weight, intrauterine growth restriction (IUGR), deafness, vision impairment and cardiac impairment. Outbreaks occur during spring and early summer.

Clinical manifestations: Incubation period of rubella is 14 to 21 days. Infection may begin with mild fever (1 or 2 days), malaise and swollen and tender lymph nodes (lymphadenopathy), usually suboccipital, postauricular, and anterior cervical lymph nodes are most prominent. Macular rash is the first sign of illness. Rash first appears on the face and neck, and it spreads to the trunk and limbs. The rash fades from the face as it extends to the rest of the body so that the whole body may not be involved at any one time. About the time of onset of the rash, examination of the throat may reveal tiny, rose-colored lesions (*Forchheimer spots*) or petechial hemorrhages on the soft palate. The rubella rash is similar to other viral rashes. The pink or light red spots may merge to form evenly colored patches. The rash lasts for up to three days, and it usually resolves without desquamation. Other symptoms of rubella, which are more common in teens, may include headache, loss of appetite, mild conjunctivitis, a stuffy or runny nose, swollen lymph nodes in different parts of the body, and pain and swelling in the joints (arthralgia). When rubella occurs in a pregnant woman, it may cause congenital rubella syndrome (CRS).

Diagnosis: Rubella may be apparent from the clinical findings, i.e. typical rash accompanied by lymphadenopathy. But, it is usually confirmed by the detection of specific antibodies (serology) or virus culture. IgM antibodies are detectable in the first few days of illness and are considered diagnostic.

Differential diagnosis: It is frequently confused with other viral exanthematous diseases such as measles, adenoviruses, parvovirus B19, Epstein-Barr virus, enteroviruses and *Mycoplasma pneumoniae.*

Complications: Complications following postnatal infection with rubella are infrequent and include thrombocytopenia, arthritis, myocarditis, encephalitis, progressive rubella panencephalitis (PRP), Guillain-Barré syndrome, and peripheral neuritis. PRP is an extremely rare complication of either acquired rubella or congenital rubella syndrome. It has an onset or course similar to those of the SSPE associated with measles. The clinical findings and course are indistinguishable from SSPE and other "slow virus" neurodegenerative syndromes. Death occurs 2–5 yr after onset. In addition to PRP, these include diabetes mellitus (20%), thyroid dysfunction (5%), and glaucoma and visual abnormalities associated with the retinopathy.

Congenital rubella syndrome (CRS): Nerve deafness is the single most common finding among infants with CRS. Pathological findings of congenital rubella syndrome are listed in Table 14.7.

Table 14.7: Pathological findings of congenital rubella syndrome

System	Pathologic findings
Cardiovascular	PDA; pulmonary artery stenosis; VSD; myocarditis
CNS	Chronic meningitis; parenchymal necrosis; vasculitis with calcification
Eye	Microphthalmia; cataract; iridocyclitis; ciliary body necrosis; glaucoma; retinopathy
Ear	Cochlear hemorrhage
Lung	Chronic nononuclear interstitial pneumonitis
Liver	Hepatic giant cell transformation; fibrosis; lobular disarray; bile stasis
Kidney	Interstitial nephritis
Adrenal glands	Cortical cytomegaly
Bone	Malformed osteoid; poor mineralization of osteoid; thinning cartilage
Spleen, lymph nodes	Extramedullary hematopoiesis
Thymus	Histiocytic reaction; absence of germinal centres
Skin	Erythropoiesis in dermis

CNS: Central nervous system; PDA: Patent ductus arteriosus; VSD: Ventricular septal defect

Treatment: There is no specific treatment available for either acquired rubella or CRS. Children who have rubella usually recover within one week, but adults may take longer. Intravenous immunoglobulin or corticosteroids can be considered for severe, nonremitting thrombocytopenia. Management of children with CRS is more complex and requires pediatric, cardiac, audiologic, ophthalmologic, and neurologic evaluation and follow-up. Hearing screening is of special importance since early intervention may improve outcomes.

Prognosis: The prognosis of rubella in childhood is the infection usually confers permanent immunity, although reinfection may occur. The incidence of reinfection on exposure to wild virus in among those with a history of previous rubella infection is less than among those with a history of previous rubella vaccination. Long-term outcomes of CRS are less favorable and somewhat variable.

Prevention: Patients with postnatal infection should be isolated from susceptible individuals for 7 days after onset of the rash. Children with CRS may excrete the virus in respiratory secretions up to 1 yr of age and should be maintained in contact precautions until then unless repeated cultures of urine and pharyngeal secretions are negative.

Exposure of susceptible pregnant women poses a potential risk to the fetus. For pregnant women exposed to rubella, a blood specimen is obtained as soon as possible for rubella IgG specific antibody testing. If the rubella antibody test result is positive, the mother is likely immune. A negative 1st specimen and a positive test result in either the 2nd or 3rd specimen indicate the mother has seroconverted, suggesting recent infection. Counseling should be provided about the risks and benefits of termination of pregnancy. The routine use of immune globulin for susceptible pregnant women exposed to rubella is not recommended and is only considered if termination of pregnancy is not an option based on maternal preferences. In such circumstances, immune serum globulin 0.55 ml/kg IM may be given with the understanding that prophylaxis may reduce the risk for clinically apparent infection but does not guarantee prevention of fetal infection (*see* Chapters 15 and 40). Vaccine should not be administered during pregnancy. If pregnancy occurs within 28 days of immunization, the patient should be counseled on the theoretical risks to the fetus.

Varicella-Zoster Virus

Etiopathogenesis: Varicella-zoster virus (VZV) is a neurotropic human herpesvirus with similarities to herpes simplex virus, which is also α-herpesvirus. These viruses are enveloped with double-stranded DNA genomes that encode more than 70 proteins, including proteins that are targets of cellular and humoral immunity. VZV is transferred through direct contact with the broken chickenpox blisters and through inhalation. The infectious period lasts from about three days before the rash appears until all the blisters have formed scabs. The incubation period of chickenpox is 10 to 21 days. VZV after entering into the host replicates in the nasopharynx. In seronegative individuals, virus spread to skin through blood (viremia) resulting in primary infection manifested as varicella (chickenpox) and establishment of a lifelong latent infection of sensory ganglion neurons. Reactivation of the latent infection causes herpes zoster.

Clinical manifestations: The illness usually begins 14–16 days after exposure, although the incubation period can range from 10 to 21 days. Prodromal symptoms may be present, particularly in older children and adults. Fever, malaise, anorexia, headache, and occasionally mild abdominal pain may occur 24–48 hr before the rash appears. Temperature elevation is usually from 100 to 102°F but may be as high as 106°F. Fever and other systemic symptoms persist during the 1st 2–4 days after the onset of the rash. Varicella lesions often appear first on the scalp, face, or trunk. The initial exanthema consists of intensely pruritic erythematous macules.

The lesions (blisters) start as a 2 to 4 mm red papule which develops with an irregular outline (rose petal). A thin-walled, clear vesicle develops on top of the area of redness resembling "dew drop on a rose petal" which is characteristic for chickenpox. Clouding of the fluid and umbilication of the lesions begin in 24–48 hr and subsequently the vesicle is broken leaving a crust. The fluid is highly contagious and remains so until the lesion crusts are subsided. The crust usually falls off after 7 days, sometimes leaving a crater-like scar. However, new lesions appear every few days for several days (about a week) and lesions of different stages of maturation are found next to each other. Varicella (chickenpox) is most frequently confused with smallpox though smallpox is now eradicated. However, chickenpox also has a much greater concentration of lesions on the trunk than on the face and extremities seen in smallpox. Furthermore, varicella lesions are much more superficial and are almost never found on the palms or soles. Ulcerative lesions involving the mucosa of oropharynx and vagina are also common, many children have vesicular lesions on the eyelids and conjunctivae, but corneal involvement and serious ocular disease is rare. The average number of varicella lesions is about 300, but healthy children may have fewer than 10 to more than 1,500 lesions. The disease is more severe in older children and adults. The exanthema may be much more extensive in children with skin disorders, such as eczema or recent sunburn. Hypopigmentation or hyperpigmentation of lesion sites persists for days to weeks in some children, but severe scarring is unusual unless the lesions were secondarily infected. The differential diagnosis of varicella includes vesicular rashes, caused by other infectious agents, such as herpes simplex virus, enterovirus, rickettsial pox, or *S. aureus*; drug reactions; contact dermatitis; and insect bites. Because of concerns about *smallpox as a potential bioterrorism threat*, both smallpox and smallpox vaccine rashes must be considered again in the differential diagnosis of severe chickenpox.

Varicella in vaccinated individuals ("Breakthrough varicella"): Varicella vaccine is > 95% effective in preventing severe varicella and in about 80% (range 70–100%) effective in preventing all disease after exposure to wild-type VZV. Exposure to VZV, as may occur in a household or an outbreak setting in a school or daycare center, 1 of every 5 vaccinated children may develop breakthrough varicella. Breakthrough disease is varicella that occurs in a person vaccinated > 42 days before rash onset and is caused by wild-type VZV. The rash in breakthrough disease is frequently atypical, predominantly maculopapular, vesicles are seen less commonly, and the illness is mild with < 50 lesions and little or no fever. Children with breakthrough disease should be considered potentially infectious and excluded from school until lesions have been crusted or, if there are no vesicles present until no new lesions are occurring.

Progressive varicella: Progressive varicella, with visceral organ involvement, coagulopathy, severe hemorrhage, and continued vascular lesion development, is a dreaded complication of primary VZV infection. Unusual clinical findings of varicella, including lesions that develop a unique hyperkeratotic appearance and continued new lesion formation for weeks or months, have been described in children with HIV infection. Immunization of HIV-infected children who have a CD4 count greater than 15% as well as children with leukemia and solid organ tumors who are stable on maintenance chemotherapy has reduced this problem.

Neonatal chickenpox: Newborns whose mothers develop varicella in the period from 5 days prior to delivery to 2 days afterward are at high risk for severe varicella. The infant acquires the infection transplacentally as a result of maternal viremia, which may occur up to 48 hr prior to the maternal rash. The infant's rash may occur toward the end of the 1st wk to the early part of the 2nd wk of life. Every premature infant born at < 28 wk of gestation to a mother with active chickenpox at delivery should receive varicella-zoster immune globulin (VariZIG). Because perinatally acquired varicella may be life threatening, the infant should be treated with acyclovir (10 mg/kg every 8 hr IV) when lesions develop. Infants with community acquired chickenpox who develop severe varicella, especially those who develop a complication such as pneumonia, hepatitis, or encephalitis, should also receive treatment with intravenous acyclovir (10 mg/kg every 8 hr IV).

Congenital varicella syndrome: When pregnant women contract chickenpox early in pregnancy as many as 25% of fetuses may become infected. But up to 2% of fetuses whose mothers had varicella in the 1st 20 wk of pregnancy may demonstrate a VZV embryopathy. Fetuses infected at 6–12 wk of gestation appear to have maximal interruption with limb development; fetuses infected at 16–20 wk may have eye and brain involvement. In addition, viral damage to the sympathetic fibers in the cervical and lumbosacral cord may lead to divergent effects such as Horner syndrome and dysfunction of the urethral or anal sphincters. The characteristic cutaneous lesion has been called a cicatrix, a zigzag scarring, in a dermatomal distribution, often associated with atrophy of the affected limb. This may result in one or more shortened extremities. The remainder of the torso may be entirely normal in appearance. Alternatively, there may be neither skin nor limb abnormalities, but the infant may show cataracts or even extensive aplasia of the entire brain. The diagnosis of VZV fetopathy is based mainly on the history of chickenpox combined with the stigmata seen in the fetus. Viral DNA may be detected in tissue samples by polymerase chain reaction (PCR). Since the damage caused by fetal VZV infection does not progress in the postpartum period, antiviral treatment of infants with congenital VZV syndromes is not indicated.

Herpes zoster: Herpes zoster manifests as vesicular lesions clustered within 1 or less commonly 2 adjacent dermatomes. In children, the rash is mild, with new lesions appearing for a few days; symptoms of acute neuritis is minimal; and complete resolution usually occurs within 1–2 wk. In contrast to adults, postherpetic neuralgia is very unusual in children. Immunocompromised children may have more severe herpes zoster, which is similar to that in adults, including postherpetic neuralgia. The risk for herpes zoster in healthy vaccinated children may be lower than in children who had wild-type varicella disease.

Diagnosis: Leukopenia occurs during the 1st 72 hr; it is followed by a relative or absolute lymphocytosis.

Patients with neurologic complications of varicella or uncomplicated herpes zoster have a mild lymphocytic pleocytosis and a slight to moderate increase in protein in the CSF; the glucose concentration is usually normal. VZV can be identified quickly by direct fluorescence assay of cells from cutaneous lesions, and by PCR amplification testing and helps to distinguish from the smallpox virus infection. VZV IgG antibody tests can also determine the immune status of individuals whose clinical history of varicella is unknown or equivocal.

Treatment: Only a symptomatic treatment, with a little sodium bicarbonate in baths or antihistamine medication to ease itching, and paracetamol (acetaminophen) to reduce fever is used. It is important to maintain good hygiene and daily cleaning of skin with warm water to avoid secondary bacterial infection.

Varicella: Oral therapy with acyclovir (20 mg/kg/dose; maximum 800 mg/dose) given as 4 doses/day for 5 days should be used to treat uncomplicated varicella in nonpregnant individuals > 13 yr of age and children > 12 mo of age with chronic cutaneous or pulmonary disorders; receiving short-term, intermittent, or aerolized corticosteroids; receiving long-term salicylate therapy; and possibly 2nd cases in household contacts. Treatment should preferably be started within 24 hr of the onset of the exanthema for clinical benefit and not more than 72 hr. Intravenous therapy is indicated for severe disease and for varicella in immunocompromised patients (even after 72 hr duration of rash). Any patient who has signs of disseminated VZV, including pneumonia, severe hepatitis, thrombocytopenia, or encephalitis, should receive immediate treatment. Acyclovir (500 mg/m² every 8 hr IV) therapy initiated within 72 hr of development of initial symptoms will decrease progressive varicella and visceral dissemination in high-risk patients. Treatment is continued for 7 days or until no new lesions have appeared for 48 hr.

Herpes zoster: In children, oral acyclovir (20 mg/kg/dose, maximum 800 mg/dose) may be given to shorten the duration of the illness. Immunocompromised children are at high risk for developing disseminated disease, should receive acyclovir (500 mg/m² or 10 mg/kg every 8 hr IV). Oral acyclovir, famciclovir or valacyclovir can be used for treatment of immunocompromised patients with uncomplicated herpes zoster and there is low risk for visceral dissemination.

Complications: The complications of VZV infection occur with varicella or with reactivation of infection, more common in immunocompromised patients. Complications of varicella includes mild hepatitis, mild thrombocytopenia (occurs in 1–2% of children), purpura, hemorrhagic vesicles, hematuria, cerebellar ataxia (occurs in 1 in every 4,000 cases), encephalitis, pneumonia, nephritis, nephrotic syndrome, hemolytic-uremic syndrome, arthritis, myocarditis, pericarditis, pancreatitis, orchitis, and secondary bacterial infections of the skin usually caused by group A streptococci and *S. aureus*.

Prognosis: Lowest case fatality occurs among children with varicella 1–9 yr of age, compared with these age groups, infants have a 4 times greater risk of dying and adults have a 25 times greater high risk of dying. The most common complications for mortality are pneumonia, CNS complications, secondary infections, and hemorrhagic conditions.

Prevention: (*See* Chapters 15 and 40). Varicella vaccine is contraindicated in children with cell-mediated immune deficiencies, although the vaccine may be administered with acute lymphoblastic leukemia, who are in remission and HIV infected children with a CD4 count greater than 15%. Both these groups should receive 2 doses of vaccine, 3 months apart. Vaccine virus establishes latent infection, but the risk for developing subsequent herpes zoster is lower after vaccine than after natural VZV infection among immunocompromised children.

Postexposure prophylaxis: Vaccine given to normal children within 3–5 days after exposure (as soon as possible is preferred) is effective in preventing or modifying varicella, especially in a household setting where exposure is very likely to result in infection. Varicella vaccine is now recommended for postexposure use, for outbreak control. High-titer anti-VZV immune globulin as postexposure prophylaxis is recommended for immunocompromised children, pregnant women, and newborns exposed to maternal varicella.

Roseola (Human Herpesviruses 6 and 7)

Etiopathogenesis: HHV6 and HHV7 belong to the β-herpesvirus subfamily of herpesviruses. Two distinct types of HHV-6 (types A and B) exist. Type B causes more than 99% of HHV-6 associated roseola cases. Primary HHV-6 infection occurs early in life. Most (> 90%) of newborn infants are HHV-6 positive, reflecting transplacental transfer of maternal antibodies. Primary infection with HHV-7 generally occurs slightly later than HHV-6 infection. Roseola occurs through out the year. The incubation period averages 10 days, with a range of 5–15 days. Most adults excrete HHV-6 and HHV-7 in saliva and may serve as primary sources for virus transmission to children.

Clinical Manifestations

Roseola infantum: It is also known as "exanthem subitum" (meaning sudden rash). Roseola is a mild febrile, exanthematous illness occurring exclusively during infancy. Typically the disease affects children between six months and three years of age, with a peak at 6–15 mo of age. Transplacental antibodies likely protect most infants until 6 mo of age. The rashes appear in a dramatic manner right after the fever. The initial signs and symptoms of roseola include a sudden high fever (102–104°F) that lasts for 3 to 5 days, and then typically resolves rather abruptly ("crisis"). Occasionally, the fever may gradually diminish over 24–36 hr ("lysis"). As the fever subsides, the rash appears as discrete, small (2–5 mm), slightly raised pink lesions on the trunk and usually spreads to the neck, face and proximal extremities. The rash of roseola is rose colored and is fairly distinctive; not usually pruritic, and no vesicles or pustules develop. Lesions typically remain discrete but occasionally may become almost confluent. After 1–3 days, the rash fades. Some children experience evanescent rashes that resolve within a few hours. Some cases may be accompanied with mild diarrhea. In Asian countries, ulcers at the uvulopalatoglossal junction (*Nagayama spots*) are common in infants with roseola. Roseola associated with HHV-7 occurs in slightly older children with lower mean temperature, and shorter duration of fever.

HHV-6 and HHV-7 infections are also associated with nonspecific febrile illness without classic roseola, hepatitis and heterophile-negative mononucleosis are rarely associated febrile seizures in infants and pneumonitis, encephalitis and meningoencephalitis in immunocompromised patients, including patients with AIDS or organ transplants.

Diagnosis: The diagnosis of roseola can be established primarily on the basis of age, history and clinical findings. Specific diagnostic methods (serology, virus culture and PCR) for HHV-6 and HHV-7 are available. White blood cell (WBC) counts of 8,000–9,000 WBCs/mm^3 may be found during the 1st few days of fever in children with roseola, but by the time the exanthem appears, the WBC count falls to 4,000–6,000 WBCs/mm^3 with a relative lymphocytosis (70–90%). The CSF in children with HHV-6 associated febrile seizures is normal. The CSF of HHV-6 associated cases of meningoencephalitis and encephalitis have a mild pleocytosis with predominance of mononuclear cells, normal glucose, and normal to slightly elevated protein.

Differential diagnosis: Roseola rash is to be differentiated from rubella, measles, enteroviruses, and drug hypersensitivity. Development of a roseola-like illness in association with febrile seizures, meningoencephalitis, or encephalitis makes HHV-6 more likely. Hepatitis and heterophile-negative mononucleosis are rarely associated with HHV-6, and other causes for these infections should first be considered.

Treatment: There is no specific vaccine or treatment. A child with fever should be given plenty of fluids to drink, and acetaminophen or ibuprofen to reduce temperature, but do not give aspirin because of the risk of Reye syndrome. HHV-6 is inhibited by ganciclovir, cidofovir, and foscarnet (but not acyclovir); HHV-7 is inhibited by cidofovir and foscarnet. Treatment with antiviral drugs is warranted for immunocompromised children with severe disease confirmed to be associated with HHV-6 and HHV-7. No guidelines are available for prevention of HHV-6 and HHV-7 viruses.

Prognosis: The prognosis for the majority of children with roseola is excellent, with no obvious sequelae. Deaths directly attributable to HHV-6 have been reported in normal and immunocompromised patients, in whom encephalitis, hepatitis, pneumonitis, disseminated disease, or hemophagocytosis syndrome (*see* Section 34.9) developed.

Epstein-Barr Virus

Etiopathogenesis: Epstein-Barr virus (EBV), is a member of the γ-herpesviruses, causes > 90% of cases of infectious mononucleosis. Two distinct types of EBV, type 1 and type 2 (also called type A and type B) occurs; type 1 is more prevalent worldwide than type 2, although type 2, is more common in Africa than in the USA and Europe. EBV is named after Michael Epstein and Yvonne Barr, who together with Bert Achong discovered the virus in 1964. The virus occurs worldwide, and 95% of the world population becomes infected with EBV sometime during their lives. It is transmitted via penetrative sexual intercourse, and in oral secretions such as 'deep kissing.' Thus, the EBV associated disease is also called "kissing disease" and is common among teenagers. EBV is shed in oral secretions consistently for > 6 mo after acute infection and then intermittently for life. EBV is also found in male and female genital secretions and can be spread through sexual contact.

Oncogenesis: EBV was the 1st human virus to be associated with malignancy. Benign EBV-associated illnesses include infectious mononucleosis, oral-hairy leukoplakia, and lymphoid interstitial pneumonitis. Malignant EBV associated illnesses include nasopharyngeal carcinoma, Burkitt lymphoma,

Hodgkin disease, lymphoproliferative disorders, and carcinoma of salivary glands.

Clinical manifestations: The incubation period of infectious mononucleosis is 30–50 days. Illness is most often seen in adolescents and young adults with a peak incidence in the age group of 15 to 17 years. It is also seen in children. Most patients with EBV infections are asymptomatic or have mild symptoms, such as fatigue and prolonged malaise with fever and cough, abdominal pain, and chest pain; arthralgias and myalgias are less common compared with other viral diseases. This prodromal period may last 1–2 wk.

The physical examination is characterized by generalized lymphadenopathy (90% cases), spleno-megaly (50% cases), and hepatomegaly (10% cases). Lymphadenopathy occurs most commonly in the anterior and posterior cervical lymph nodes and the submandibular lymph nodes and less commonly in the axillary and inguinal lymph nodes. *Epitrochlear lymphadenopathy is particularly suggestive of infectious mononucleosis.* The sore throat is often accompanied by moderate to severe pharyngitis with marked tonsillar enlargement, occasionally with exudates. Petechiae at the junction of the hard and soft palate and rashes and edema of the eyelids are frequently seen.

Rashes are usually maculopapular resembling measles or rubella occurs in 3–15% of patients. Furthermore, EBV infected subjects are more likely to develop *"ampicillin rash"* if treated with ampicillin or amoxicillin. This vasculitic rash is probably immune mediated and resolves without specific treatment. EBV is also associated with Gianotti-Crosti syndrome, a symmetrical rash on the cheeks with multiple erythematous papules, which may coalesce into plaques, and persists for 15–50 days. The rash has the appearance of atopic dermatitis and may appear on the extremities and buttocks.

Diagnosis: The diagnosis can be made clinically from the characteristic triad of fever, pharyngitis and lymphadenopathy with skin rashes lasting for 1 to 4 weeks. Laboratory investigations show leukocytosis (usually 10,000 to 20,000 leukocytes/mm^3) with marked lymphocytosis (at least 2/3) with atypical lymphocytes (usually account for 20 to 40%). The atypical cells are mature T-lymphocytes that have been antigenically activated. Atypical lymphocytes are larger overall, with larger, eccentrically placed indented and folded nuclei with a lower nuclear to cytoplasm ratio. Other syndromes associated with atypical lymphocytosis include acquired cytomegalo-virus infection, toxoplasmosis, viral hepatitis, rubella, measles, mumps, tuberculosis, typhoid, *Mycoplasma* infection, malaria, and some drug reactions. Mild thrombocytopenia (50,000–200,000 platelets/mm^3) rarely associated purpura, and mild elevation of hepatic transaminases usually asymptomatic without jaundice also occurs in infectious mononucleosis. *Heterophile antibody test:* The transient heterophile antibodies seen in infectious mononucleosis, also known as Paul-Bunnell antibodies are IgM antibodies detected by the Paul-Bunnell-Davidson test for sheep red cell agglutination. The heterophile antibodies of infectious mononucleosis agglutinate sheep or, for greater sensitivity, horse red cells, but not guinea pig kidney cells. This adsorption property differentiates this response from the heterophile response found in patients with serum sickness, rheumatic diseases, and some normal individuals. Titers of > 1:28 or > 1:40 depending on the dilution system used, after absorption of guinea pig cells are considered positive. The false-positive rate is < 10%, usually resulting from erroneous interpretation. If the heterophile test result is negative and an EBV infection is suspected, EBV-specific testing is indicated. *EBV-specific antibody testing* is useful to confirm acute EBV infection, especially in heterophile-negative cases, or to confirm past infection and determine susceptibility to future infection.

Differential diagnosis: Infectious mononucleosis-like illnesses may be caused by primary infection with cytomegalovirus, *T. gondii*, adenovirus, viral hepatitis, HIV, or possibly rubella virus and streptococcal pharyngitis.

Treatment: There is no specific treatment for infectious mononucleosis. Therapy with high dose of acyclovir, with or without corticosteroids, decrease viral replication and oropharyngeal viral shedding, but does not reduce the severity or duration of symptoms or alter the eventual outcome. Short courses of corticosteroids [prednisolone 1 mg/kg/day (maximum 60 mg/day), for 7 days and tapered over another 7 days] should be used in patients of incipient airway obstruction, thrombocytopenia with hemorrhaging, autoimmune hemolytic anemia, seizures, and meningitis. In view of the potential hazards of immunosuppression for a virus infection with oncogenic complications, corticosteroids should not be used in uncomplicated cases of infectious mononucleosis.

Complications: The complications include subcapsular splenic hemorrhage or splenic rupture (commonly related to trauma), swelling of the tonsils and oropharyngeal lymphoid tissue, airway obstruction, headache, seizures, ataxia, meningitis, facial nerve palsy, transverse myelitis, encephalitis, Guillain-Barré syndrome, Reye syndrome, hemolytic anemia, aplastic

anemia, thrombocytopenia, neutropenia, myocarditis, interstitial pneumonia, pancreatitis, parotitis and orchitis. Perceptual distortions of sizes, shapes, and spatial relationships, known as the *Alice in Wonderland syndrome (metamorphopsia)* may be a presenting symptom.

Prognosis: The prognosis of complete recovery is excellent if no complications ensue during the acute illness. The major symptoms typically last 2–4 wk, followed by gradual recovery.

Parvovirus B19

Etiopathogenesis: Erythema infectiosum is caused by one of the parvoviruses known as PV-B19 and is a member of the genus *Erythrovirus* in the family of Parvoviridae. PV-B19 is pathogenic only to humans. Infections with parvovirus B19 are common and worldwide most prevalent in school-aged children, with 70% of cases occurring between 5 and 15 yr of age. Seasonal peaks occur in the late winter and spring, with sporadic infections throughout the year. A person infected with PV-B19 is contagious during the early part of the illness, before the appearance of rash. PV-B19 has been found in the respiratory secretions (e.g. saliva, sputum or nasal mucus) of infected persons before the onset of rash, when they experience cold. The virus is spread from person to person by inhalation. But during the viremia in addition to respiratory route, it can also be transmitted through blood and blood products. The primary target of PV-B19 infection is the erythroid cell line.

Clinical manifestations: Infected children characteristically develop the rash illness of erythema infectiosum. Parvovirus B19 infection has been associated with myocarditis in fetuses, infants, children, and a few adults. Adults, especially women, frequently develop acute polyarthropathy with or without a rash. Primary maternal infection is associated with nonimmune fetal hydrops and intrauterine fetal demise.

Erythema infectiosum (fifth disease): The most common manifestation of parvovirus B19 is erythema infectiosum, also known as fifth disease, which is a benign, self limited exanthematous illness of childhood. It was the fifth in a classification scheme of common childhood exanthems the preceding 4 exanthems were measles, scarlet fever, rubella, and Filatove-Dukes disease (an atypical scarlet fever), with roseola infantum as the sixth disease. The incubation period is 4–28 days (average 16–17 days). The prodromal phase is mild and consists of low grade fever, headache and symptoms of upper respiratory tract infection. The characteristic rash occurs in

3 stages that are not always distinguishable. This exanthem most commonly involves the malar eminences and spares the nasal bridge and perioral areas, giving a characteristic **"slapped-cheek"** appearance. The edge of the rash may be slightly raised. This stage, which often is unrecognized, corresponds with the period of viremia and the period of contagion. 1 to 4 days after the onset of facial rash, the rash spreads rapidly or concurrently over the trunk and proximal extremities as a diffuse macular erythema in the second stage. Central clearing of macular lesions occurs promptly, giving the rash a **lacy, reticulated appearance**. The rash is more prominent on the extensor surfaces, sparing the palms and soles. Affected children are afebrile and not ill appearing. Older children and adults often complain of pruritus. The exanthem may become more marked with exposure to sunlight. The rash resolves spontaneously without desquamation. The third stage is characterized by complete disappearance and re-appearance of rash for a period of 1 to 3 weeks. As the appearance of the exanthem corresponds with the development of antibody, patients with the rash are no longer contagious.

Other cutaneous manifestations: Most of these are petechial or purpuric in nature. Among these rashes is the papular-purpuric "gloves and socks" syndrome (PPGSs), which occurs in young adults and children. PPGSs is characterized by fever, pruritus, and painful edema and erythema localized to the distal extremities in a distinct "gloves and socks" distribution. The syndrome is self limited and resolves in a few weeks.

Arthropathy: Arthritis and arthralgia may occur in isolation or with other symptoms. Females are affected more than males. The joints most often affected are the hands, wrists, knees and ankles, but practically any joint may be involved. The joint symptoms are self-limited, and in the majority of patients, resolve within 2–4 wk.

Transient aplastic crisis leads to a sudden fall in serum hemoglobin in individuals with chronic hemolytic diseases, such as sickle cell disease, thalassemia, hereditary spherocytosis, and pyruvate kinase deficiency.

Immunocompromised persons: Chronic anemia is the most common manifestation, sometimes accompanied by neutropenia, thrombocytopenia, or complete marrow suppression. Chronic infections occur in patients receiving cancer chemotherapy or immuno-suppressive therapy for transplantation, and persons with congenital immunodeficiencies, AIDS, and functional defects in IgG production who are unable to generate neutralizing antibodies.

Diagnosis: The diagnosis of erythema infectiosum is usually based on clinical presentation of the typical rash-slapped cheeks appearance. Serologic tests are usually relied only for the diagnosis of B19 infection in patients with transient aplastic crisis or arthropathy. A positive B19-specific IgM antibody or a significant rise in B19-specific IgG titer is indicative of an acute or recent infection, but it is unreliable in immuno-compromised persons. In such cases, diagnosis is based on the detection of viral DNA by PCR or nucleic acid hybridization. Prenatal diagnosis of B19-induced fetal hydrops can be accomplished by detection of viral DNA in fetal blood or amniotic fluid by these methods.

Differential diagnosis: The rash of erythema infectiosum must be differentiated from rubella, measles, enteroviral infections, and drug reactions. Rash and arthritis in older children should be distinguished from juvenile rheumatoid arthritis, systemic lupus erythematosus, serum sickness, and other connective tissue disorders.

Treatment: Mostly, erythema infectiosum is a benign and self-limited disease. The symptoms such as fever, pain or itching is treated symptomatically. People with severe anemia may need hospitalization and blood transfusions. Persons with immune problems may need special medical care, including immunotherapy.

Complications: PV-B19 may cause thrombocytopenic purpura, aseptic meningitis, infection-associated hemophagocytic syndrome.

Prevention: Children with erythema infectiosum are not likely to be infectious at presentation with rash and arthropathy and isolation and exclusion from school or child care are unnecessary. Children with PV-B19-induced red cell aplasia, including the transient aplastic crisis, are infectious and should be isolated in the hospital to prevent spread to susceptible patients and staff. Isolation should continue for at least 1 wk and until after resolution of fever. Pregnant caregivers should not be assigned to these patients. No vaccine is currently available. Frequent hand-washing is recommended to decrease the chance of infections.

Cossart YE, Field AM, Cant B, et al. Parvovirus-like particles in human sera. *Lancet* 1975;1(7898):72–73.

Epstein MA, Achong BG, Barr YM. Virus particles in cultured lymphoblasts from Burkitt's lymphoma. *Lancet* 1964; 28:702–3.

Jenson HB. Epstein-Barr Virus . In: Kliegman RM, Behrman RE, Jenson HB, Stanton BF (eds). *Nelson Textbook of Pediatrics.* 18th edn. Vol. 1. Philadelphia: Saunders, 2007;1372–7.

Kids Health, Rubella (German measles), http://www.kidshealth.org/parent/infections/skin/german_measles.html.

Koch WC. Parvovirus B19. In: Kliegman RM, Behrman RE, Jenson HB, Stanton BF (eds). *Nelson Textbook of Pediatrics.* 18th edn. Vol. 1. Philadelphia: Saunders, 2007;1357–60.

Knuf M, Habermehl P, Zepp F et al. Immunogenicity and safety of two doses of tetravalent measles-mumps-rubella-varicella vaccine in healthy children. *Pediatr Infect Dis J* 2006; 25:12–18.

Kubo T, Rai SK, Sharma CM, et al. Seroepidemiological study of viral infectious diseases in Nepal. *J Inst Med (Nepal)* 1992;14:83–86.

Leach CT. Roseola (Human Herpesviruses 6 and 7). In: Kliegman RM, Behrman RE, Jenson HB, Stanton BF (eds). *Nelson Textbook of Pediatrics.* 18th edn. Vol. 1. Philadelphia: Saunders, 2007;1380–83.

Mason WH. Measles. In: Kliegman RM, Behrman RE, Jenson HB, Stanton BF (eds). *Nelson Textbook of Pediatrics.* 18th edn. Vol. 1. Philadelphia: Saunders, 2007;1331–37.

Mason WH. Rubella. In: Kliegman RM, Behrman RE, Jenson HB, Stanton BF (eds). *Nelson Textbook of Pediatrics.* 18th edn. Vol. 1. Philadelphia: Saunders, 2007;1337–41.

Myers MG, Seward JF, LaRussa PS. Varicella-Zoster Virus. In: Kliegman RM, Behrman RE, Jenson HB, Stanton BF (eds). *Nelson Textbook of Pediatrics.* 18th edn. Vol. 1. Philadelphia: Saunders, 2007;1366–72.

National Center for Infectious Diseases. Epstein-Barr virus and infectious mononucleosis. http://www.cdc.gov/ncidod/diseases/ebv.htm.

Sabella C, Goldfard J. Parvovirus B19 Infections. *Amer Family Physian* 1999;60:1455–61.

Schrör K. Aspirin and Reye syndrome: a review of the evidence. *Paediatr Drugs* 2007;9:195–204.

WHO. Progress in reducing global measles: 1999–2004. *Wkly Epidemiol Rec* 2006;81:90–94.

Herpes Simplex Virus

Etiopathogenesis: The 2 closely related herpes simplex viruses (HSVs), HSV type-1 (HSV-1) and HSV type-2 (HSV-2), cause a variety of illnesses depending on the anatomic site where the infection is initiated, the immune state of the host, and whether the symptoms reflect primary or recurrent infection. The only natural host of HSV is humans, and the mode of transmission is direct contact between mucocutaneous surfaces.

Clinical manifestations: The common clinical features of HSV infections are skin vesicles and shallow ulcers. Classical infections present with small, 2–4 mm vesicles that may be surrounded by an erythematous base. Common infections involve the skin, eye, oral cavity, and genital tract.

Acute oropharyngeal infections: Herpes gingivostomatitis affects children most often 6 mo to 5 yr. The condition is extremely painful with sudden onset, pain in the mouth, drooling, refusal to eat or drink and fever of up to 40.0–40.6°C. The gums become markedly swollen, and vesicles may develop throughout the oral cavity, including on the gums, lips, tongue, palate, tonsils, and pharynx. Vesicles may persist for a few

days before evolving into shallow erythematous ulcers that may be covered with a yellow-gray membrane. Tender submandibular, submaxillary, and cervical lymphadenopathy is common. The breath may be foul as a result of overgrowth of anaerobic oral bacteria. In older children, adolescents and college students, the initial HSV oral infection may manifest as pharyngitis and tonsillitis rather than gingivostomatitis.

Herpes labialis: Herpes labialis typically results in a single lesion. The most common site of herpes labialis is the vermilion border of the lip, although lesions sometimes occur on the nose, chin, cheek, or oral mucosa. The short-lived ulcer dries and develops a crusted scab. Complete healing without scarring occurs usually within 6–10 days.

Cutaneous infections: In the healthy child or adolescent, cutaneous HSV infections are generally the result of skin trauma with macro- or micro-abrasions and exposure to infectious secretions. This situation often occurs in play or contact sports such as wrestling (*herpes gladiatorum*) or rugby (*scrumpox*). Pain, burning, itching or tingling often precedes the herpetic eruption by a few hours to days. Lesions begin as grouped, erythematous papules that progress to vesicles, pustules, ulcers, and crusts, and then healing without scarring in 6–10 days. Cutaneous HSV infection results in multiple discrete lesions and involves a larger surface area. Regional lymph nodes are enlarged.

Herpes whitlow results from HSV infection of fingers or toes, although strictly speaking it refers to HSV infection of the paronychia. The onset of the infection is heralded by itching, pain, and erythema 2–7 days after exposure. Lesions and associated pain persist for about 10 days, followed by rapid recovery in 18–20 days. Regional lymphadenopathy is common, and lymphangitis and neuralgia may occur.

Genital herpes: Genital HSV infection may result from genital-genital transmission (usually HSV-2) or oral-genital transmission (usually HSV-1) in sexually experienced adolescents and young adults. Vesicles on mucosal surfaces are short-lived, and rupture to produce shallow, tender ulcers covered with yellowish gray exudates and surrounded by an erythematous border. Vesicles on keratinized epithelium persist for a few days before progressing to the pustular stage and then crusts are formed. Patients may develop urethritis and dysuria severe enough to cause urinary retention and bilateral, tender inguinal and pelvic lymphadenopathy. Women may have a watery vaginal discharge and men a clear mucoid urethral discharge. Local pain and systemic symptoms including fever, headache, and myalgia are common. The course of classical primary genital herpes, from onset to complete healing, is 2–3 wk. Most patients with symptomatic primary genital herpes will experience at least one recurrent infection in the following year.

Ocular infections: HSV ocular infections may involve the conjunctiva, cornea, or retina and may be primary or recurrent. Vesicular lesions may be seen on the lid margins and periorbital skin. Patients have fever. Untreated infection generally resolves in 2–3 weeks.

Central nervous system infections: HSV encephalitis is an acute necrotizing infection generally involving the frontal and/or temporal cortex and the limbic system. Beyond the neonatal period it is caused by HSV-1. HSV is also a cause of aseptic meningitis and is the most common cause of recurrent aseptic meningitis (*Mollaret meningitis*).

Infections in immunocompromised persons: Severe, life-threatening HSV infections can occur in patients with compromised immune infections, including neonates, severely malnourished, primary and secondary immunodeficiencies including AIDS, immuno-suppressive regimens, particularly for cancer and organ transplantation. Mucocutaneous infections, including mucositis and esophagitis are most common presentation.

Perinatal infections: HSV infection may be acquired *in utero*, during the birth process, or during the neonatal period. Postpartum transmission may be from the mother or another adult with nongenital (HSV-1) infection such as herpes labialis. *Infants with intrauterine infection* have skin vesicles or scarring, eye findings including chorooretinitis and keratoconjunc tivitis, and microcephaly or hydrencephaly that are present at delivery. A few infants survive without therapy, and those that do generally have severe sequelae. *Infants infected during delivery or postpartum* present with 1 of 3 patterns of disease: (i) disease localized to the skin, eyes, or mouth; (ii) encephalitis with or without *s*kin, *e*ye, or *m*outh (SEM) disease; or (iii) disseminated infection involving multiple organs, including the brain, lungs, liver, heart, adrenals, and skin.

Diagnosis: The clinical diagnosis of an HSV infection, particularly life-threatening infections and genital herpes should be confirmed by laboratory tests, preferably isolation of virus or detection of viral antigen or more often viral DNA by polymerase chain reaction (PCR). Because most HSV diagnostic tests take at least a few days, treatment should be initiated promptly in order to ensure the maximum therapeutic benefit.

Laboratory findings: Mucocutaneous infections may cause a moderate polymorphonuclear leukocytosis. In HSV meningoencephalitis there can be an increase in lymphocytosis and protein, the glucose may be normal or reduced, and red blood cells may be present. The electroencephalogram (EEG) and MRI of the brain may show temporal lobe abnormalities in HSV encephalitis beyond the neonatal period. Encephalitis in the neonatal period affects the entire brain and not limited only to the temporal lobe. Disseminated infection may cause elevated liver enzymes, thrombocytopenia, and abnormal coagulation.

Treatment: Acyclovir is used in the treatment of HSV infections. *Gingivostomatosis:* (15 mg/kg/dose 5 times a day PO for 7 days maximum 1 g/day); *Herpes labialis in adolescents:* (200–400 mg 5 times daily PO for 5 days); *Herpes gladiatorum:* (200 mg 5 times a day PO for 7–10 days); *Herpetic whitlow:* (1,600–2,000 mg/day divided in 2–3 doses PO for 10 days); *Eczema herpeticum:* (200 mg 5 times a day PO for 5 days); *HIV infections in burn patients:* (10–20 mg/kg/day divided every 8 hr IV); *Genital herpes in adolescents:* (400 mg tid PO for 7–10 days); *Genital herpes in smaller children:* (suspension can be used at a dose of 10-20 mg/kg/dose 4 times daily not to exceed the adult dose). *Herpes encephalitis in patients beyond the neonatal period:* (10 mg/kg every 8 hr given over a one hr infusion for 14–21 days). Chronic daily use of oral acyclovir (400 mg bid PO) has been used to prevent recurrences in individuals with frequent or severe recurrences. Topical trifluorothymidine, vidarabine, and idoxuridine are used in the treatment of herpes keratitis.

Infections in immunosuppressed patients: Severe mucocutaneous and disseminated HSV infections in immunocompromised patients should be treated with intravenous acyclovir (5–10 mg/kg or 250 mg/m^2 every 8 hr) until there is evidence of resolution of infection. Oral antiviral therapy, with acyclovir has been used for treatment of less severe HSV infections and for suppression of recurrences during periods of significant immunosuppression.

Perinatal infections: All patients with proven or suspected neonatal HSV infection should be begun promptly on high dose intravenous acyclovir (60 mg/kg/day divided every 8 hr IV). Treatment may be discontinued in patients in whom laboratory testing do not show HSV infection. Infants with HSV disease limited to skin, eyes, and mouth should be treated for 14 days, while those with disseminated or central nervous system disease should receive 21 days of therapy. Patients receiving high dose therapy should be monitored for neutropenia.

Prognosis: Most HSV infections are self-limiting, last from a few days to 2–3 wk and heal without scarring. Patients with genital herpes may have psychologic consequences much greater than its physiologic effects. Life-threatening conditions include neonatal herpes, herpes encephalitis, and HSV infections in immunocompromised patients, burn patients, and severely malnourished infants and children. Recurrent ocular herpes can lead to corneal scarring and blindness.

Prevention: Good hand-washing and when appropriate the use of gloves provide health care workers with protection against HSV infection at the workplace. Patients and parents should be advised good hygienic practices, including hand-washing and avoiding contact with lesions and secretions during active herpes outbreaks. Athletes with active herpes infections participating in wrestling or rugby should be excluded from practice or games until the lesions are completely healed. Genital herpes can be prevented by avoiding genital-genital and oral-genital contact. The risk for acquiring genital herpes can be reduced but not eliminated by the use of condoms. Recurrences of genital HSV infections, oral-facial (labialis) and cutaneous (gladiatorum) herpes can be prevented by the daily use of oral acyclovir.

O'Riordan DP, Golden C, Aucott SW. Herpes simplex virus infections in preterm infants. *Pediatrics* 2006;118:e1612–20.

Sprunance SL, Kriesel JD. Treatment of herpes simplex labialis. *Herpes* 2002;3:64–69.

Stanberry LR. Herpes Simplex Virus. In: Kliegman RM, Behrman RE, Jenson HB, Stanton BF (eds). *Nelson Textbook of Pediatrics.* 18th edn. Vol. 1. Philadelphia: Saunders, 2007; 1360–6.

Human Herpesvirus 8

Etiopathogenesis: HHV-8 is a member of the γ-herpesviruses. HHV-8 infection is seen in USA, Greece, Italy, Brazil, Egypt, and Central Africa. HHV-8 is shed in the saliva of most HHV-8-infected persons, and serves as a major source for intrafamilial transmission. HHV-8 is also detectable in breast milk. Homosexual males get infected with HHV-8 infection by sexual transmission. Rarely, HHV-8 has been transmitted vertically and via blood transfusion. HHV-8-associated disease in transplant recipients can be transmitted via the donor organ or can arise from reactivated recipient virus.

Clinical manifestations: Most cases of primary HHV-8 infection are subclinical or may be associated with fever and rash or mononucleosis. Immunocompromised persons may have more severe symptoms in conjunction with primary HHV-8 infection, including bone marrow failure and disseminated Kaposi sarcoma. Three malignancies occurring primarily in adults with AIDS are associated with HHV-8: Kaposi sarcoma (KS), multicentric Castleman disease, and primary effusion lymphoma.

Diagnosis: HHV-8 infection can be demonstrated by serologic testing (enzyme immunoassay, immuno-fluorescence and Western immunoblotting) or detection of HHV-8 DNA sequences by polymerase chain reaction amplification.

Treatment: Anti-retroviral therapy (ganciclovir, foscarnet, and cidofovir) has improved survival for AIDS patients with KS. Other treatment options for KS include α-interferon, cryotherapy, phototherapy, topical retinoic acid, chemotherapy, radiation therapy, and surgery.

Cannon MJ, Laney AS, Pellett PE. Human herpesvirus 8: Current issues. *Clin Infect Dis* 2003; 37:82–87.

Leach CT. Human Herpesvirus 8. In: Kliegman RM, Behrman RE, Jenson HB, Stanton BF (eds). *Nelson Textbook of Pediatrics.* 18th edn. Vol. 1. Philadelphia: Saunders, 2007; 1383–1384.

Polioviruses

Etiology: The polioviruses are non-enveloped, positive-stranded RNA viruses belonging to the Picornaviridae family, in the genus *Enterovirus*, and include 3 antigenically distinct serotypes (types 1, 2, 3).

Epidemiology: Poor sanitation and crowding are responsible for the continued transmission of poliovirus in certain developing countries in Africa and Asia, despite massive global efforts to eradicate polio, in some areas with an average of 12–13 doses of polio vaccine administered in children in the 1st 5 yr of life.

Transmission: Humans are the only known reservoir for the polioviruses, which are spread by the fecal-oral route. The polioviruses are extremely hardy and can retain infectivity for several days at room temperature. Poliovirus has been isolated from feces for > 2 wk before paralysis to several weeks after the onset of symptoms.

Pathogenesis: In the contact host, *wild-type and vaccine strains of polioviruses* gain host entry via gastrointestinal tract. The primary site of replication is in the M cells lining the mucosa of the small intestine. Regional lymph nodes are infected, and primary viremia occurs after 2–3 days. The virus seeds multiple sites, including the reticuloendothelial system, brown fat deposits and skeletal muscles. Wild-type poliovirus probably accesses the CNS along peripheral nerves. Vaccine strains of polioviruses do not replicate in the CNS, which indicates the safety of the live attenuated vaccine. Occasional *revertants* (by nucleotide substitution) of these vaccine strains develop a neurovirulent phenotype and cause *vaccine-associated paralytic poliomyelitis (VAPP)*. Reversion occurs in the small intestine and probably accesses the CNS via the peripheral nerves.

The exact mechanism of entry into the CNS is not known. Once entry is gained, the virus may traverse neural pathways, and multiple sites within the CNS are often affected. The poliovirus primarily infects motor neuron cells in the spinal cord (*the anterior horn cells*) and the medulla (*the cranial nerve nuclei*). Because of the overlap in muscle innervation by 2–3 adjacent segments of the spinal cord, clinical signs of weakness in the limbs develop when more than 50% of motor neurons are destroyed. In the medulla, less extensive lesions cause paralysis, and involvement of the reticular formation that contains the vital centres controlling respiration and circulation may have a catastrophic outcome. Involvement of the intermediate and dorsal horn and dorsal root ganglia in the spinal cord results in hyperesthesia and myalgias that are typical of acute poliomyelitis. Other neurons affected are the nuclei in the roof and vermis of the cerebellum, the substantia nigra, and occasionally the red nucleus in the pons; there may be involvement of thalamic, hypothalamic, and pallidal nuclei and the motor cortex.

Infants acquire immunity transplacentally from their mothers. Transplacental immunity disappears at a variable rate during the first 4–6 months of life. Active immunity after neural infection is probably life-long but protects against the infecting serotype only; infections from the other serotypes are possible. Poliovirus neutralizing antibodies develop within several days after exposure as a result of replication of the virus in the M cells in the intestinal tract and deep lymphatic tissues. This early production of circulating immunoglobulin G (IgG) antibodies protects against CNS invasion. Local (mucosal) immunity, conferred mainly by secretory IgA, is an important defense against subsequent reinfection of the gastrointestinal tract.

Clinical manifestations: The incubation period of poliovirus from contact to initial clinical symptoms is 8–12 days, with a range of 5–35 days. Poliovirus infections with wild type virus may follow one of several courses: (i) inapparent infection; (ii) abortive poliomyelitis; (iii) nonparalytic poliomyelitis; or (iv) paralytic poliomyelitis. Paralysis, if it occurs, appears 3–8 days after the initial symptoms. The clinical manifestations of paralytic polio caused by wild or vaccine strains are comparable, although the incidence of abortive or nonparalytic paralysis with vaccine-associated poliomyelitis is unknown.

Inapparent infection, which occurs in 90–95% of cases and causes no disease and no sequelae.

Abortive poliomyelitis: In about 5% of patients, a nonspecific influenza-like syndrome (fever, malaise, headache, vomiting) occurs 1–2 wk after infection, which is termed abortive poliomyelitis. The physical examination may be normal or may reveal nonspecific pharyngitis, abdominal or muscular tenderness, and weakness. The illness is short-lived, up to 2–3 days. Recovery is complete, and no neurologic signs or sequelae develop.

Nonparalytic poliomyelitis: In about 1% of patients infected with wild-type poliovirus, signs of abortive poliomyelitis are present, as well as stiffness of the posterior muscles of the neck, trunk, and limbs. Fleeting paralysis of the bladder and constipation are frequent. Approximately 2/3 of these children have short symptom-free interlude between the 1st phase (*minor illness*) and the 2nd phase (*CNS disease or major illness*). Nuchal and spinal rigidity are the basis for the diagnosis of nonparalytic paralysis during the 2nd phase. When open, the anterior fontanel may be tense or bulging. The superficial reflexes, the cremasteric and abdominal reflexes and the reflexes of the spinal and gluteal muscles are usually first to diminish. Changes in the deep tendon reflexes generally occur 8–24 hr after the superficial reflexes are depressed and indicate impending paresis of the extremities. Tendon reflexes are absent with paralysis. No sensory defects occur in poliomyelitis.

Paralytic poliomyelitis: Paralytic poliomyelitis develops in about 0.1% of persons infected with poliovirus causing 3 clinically recognizable syndromes:
1. Spinal paralytic poliomyelitis
2. Bulbar poliomyelitis, and (3) polioencephalitis.

Spinal paralytic poliomyelitis: Typically presents as a single phase in which prodromal symptoms and paralysis occur in a continuous fashion. The biphasic course of paralysis is rare and may occur in the 2nd phase of a biphasic illness, the first phase of which corresponds to abortive poliomyelitis. The patient then appears to recover and feels better for 2–5 days, after which severe headache, fever, severe muscle pain and sensory and motor phenomena (e.g., paresthesia, hyperesthesia, fasciculations, and spasms) occur. The distribution of paralysis is characteristically spotty. Single muscle, multiple muscles or groups of muscles may be involved. Within 1–2 days, asymmetric flaccid paralysis or paresis occurs. Involvement of one leg is most common, followed by involvement of one arm. The proximal areas of extremities are involved to a greater extent than the distal areas. To detect mild muscular weakness apply gentle resistance in opposition to the muscle group being tested. Nuchal stiffness or rigidity, muscle tenderness, initially hyperactive deep tendon reflexes (for a short period) followed by absent or diminished reflexes, and paresis or flaccid paralysis can be detected. In the spinal form there is weakness of some of the muscles of the neck, abdomen, trunk, diaphragm, thorax, or extremities. *Sensation is intact; sensory disturbances if persist, suggest a disease other than poliomyelitis.* The paralytic phase of poliomyelitis is extremely variable, some patients progress during observation from paresis to paralysis, whereas others recover, which may be slow or rapid. Paralysis occurs if more than 50% of the neurons supplying the muscles are destroyed. The extent of involvement is usually obvious within 2–3 days; only rarely does progression occur beyond this interval. Paralysis of the lower limbs is often accompanied by bowel and bladder dysfunction ranging from transient inconvenience to paralysis with constipation and urinary retention. In developing countries, where a history of intramuscular injections precedes paralytic poliomyelitis in about 50–60% of patients, patients may present initially with fever and paralysis (*provocative paralysis*). Once the temperature returns to normal, progression of paralytic manifestations stops. Little recovery from paralysis is noted in the first days or weeks, but, if it is to occur, is usually evident within 6 months. The return of strength and reflexes is slow and may continue to improve as long as 18 months after the acute disease. If there is no improvement in paralysis within the 1st several weeks or months after onset, it is indicative of permanent paralysis. Atrophy of the limb, failure of growth and deformity is common and is especially evident in the growing child (*see* Fig. 14.8 in CD).

Bulbar poliomyelitis may occur as a clinical entity without apparent involvement of the spinal cord. The disease as bulbar implies only dominance of the clinical manifestations by dysfunctions of the cranial nerves and medullary centers. The clinical findings seen with bulbar poliomyelitis with respiratory difficulty include:

  i. Nasal twang to the voice or cry caused by palatal and pharyngeal weakness
  ii. Inability to swallow smoothly, resulting in accumulation of saliva in the pharynx
  iii. Accumulated pharyngeal secretions, which may cause irregular respirations
  iv. Absence of effective coughing
  v. Nasal regurgitation of saliva and fluids as a result of palatal paralysis
  vi. Deviation of the palate, uvula or tongue
  vii. Involvement of vital centers in the medulla, which manifests as irregularities in rate, depth, and rhythm of respiration; as cardiovascular alterations, including blood pressure changes (especially increased blood pressure), alternate flushing and mottling of the skin and cardiac arrhythmias; and as rapid changes in body temperature
  viii. Paralysis of one or both vocal cords, causing hoarseness, aphonia, and ultimately asphyxia unless this is recognized by laryngoscopy and managed by immediate tracheostomy; and
  ix. The rope sign, an acute angulation between the chin and larynx caused by weakness of the hyoid muscles (the hyoid bone is pulled posteriorly, narrowing the hypopharyngeal inlet).

Bulbar disease may culminate in an ascending paralysis (Landry type), in which there is progression cephalad from initial involvement of the lower extremities. Hypertension and other autonomic disturbances are common in bulbar involvement and may persist for a week or more or may be transient. Occasionally hypertension is followed by hypotension and shock and is associated with irregular and failed respiratory effort, delirium, or coma; this kind of bulbar disease is rapidly fatal. Cranial nerve involvement is seldom permanent. Patients immobilized for long periods may develop pneumonia, and renal stones may form as a result of hypercalcemia and hypercalciuria secondary to bone resorption.

Polioencephalitis is a rare form of disease in which higher centers of the brain are severely involved. Seizures, coma, and spastic paralysis with increased reflexes may be observed. The manifestations are common to encephalitis of any cause and can only be attributed to polioviruses by specific viral diagnosis or if accompanied by flaccid paralysis.

Paralytic poliomyelitis with ventilatory insufficiency results from several components acting together resulting in hypoxia and hypercapnia. When the arms are weak, and especially when deltoid paralysis occurs, there may be impending respiratory paralysis because the phrenic nerve nuclei are in adjacent areas of the spinal cord. The clinical findings associated with involvement of the respiratory muscles include:

  i. Anxious expression;
  ii. Inability to speak without frequent pauses, resulting in short, jerky, "breathless" sentences
  iii. Increased respiratory rate
  iv. Movement of the ala nasi and of the accessory muscles of respiration
  v. Inability to cough or sniff with full depth
  vi. Paradoxical abdominal movements caused by diaphragmatic immobility due to spasm or weakness of one or both leaves; and
  vii. Relative immobility of the intercostals spaces, which may be segmental, unilateral, or bilateral. Observation of the patient's capacity for thoracic breathing while the abdominal muscles are

splinted manually indicates minor degree of paresis. Light manual splinting of the thoracic cage will help to assess the effectiveness of diaphragmatic movement.

Diagnosis: Poliomyelitis should be considered in any unimmunized or incompletely immunized child with paralytic disease. VAPP should be considered in any child with paralytic disease occurring 7–14 days after receiving the orally administered polio vaccine (OPV). VAPP can occur in any child in countries or regions, where wild-type poliovirus has been eradicated and the OPV has been administered to the child or a contact. The combination of fever, headache, neck and back pain, asymmetric flaccid paralysis without sensory loss and pleocytosis does not occur regularly in any other illness. The World Health Organization (WHO) recommends that the laboratory diagnosis of poliomyelitis be confirmed by isolation and identification of poliovirus in the stool, with specific identification of the wild-type and vaccine-type strains. In suspected cases of acute flaccid paralysis, two stool specimens should be collected 24–48 hr apart, as soon as possible after the diagnosis of poliomyelitis is suspected. Poliovirus concentrations are high in the stool in the first week after the onset of paralysis, which is the optimal time for collection of stool specimens. Polioviruses may be isolated from 80 to 90% of acutely ill patients, where as < 20% patients may yield virus within 3–4 wk after onset of paralysis. Because most children with spinal or bulbospinal poliomyelitis have constipation rectal straws may be used to obtain specimens; ideally a minimum of 8–10 g should be collected. The stool specimens should be sent to laboratories that can isolate poliovirus or to one of the WHO-certified poliomyelitis laboratories where DNA sequence analysis can be performed to distinguish between wild poliovirus and neurovirulent, revertant OPV strains. With the current WHO plan for global eradication of poliomyelitis, Americas, Europe, and Australia have been certified wild-poliomyelitis free. In these areas, poliomyelitis most often is caused by vaccine strains and it is essential to differentiate between wild-type and revertant vaccine-type strains.

The CSF is often normal during the minor illness. With CNS involvement, there is a pleocytosis of 20–3000 cells/mm^3, the cells in the CSF may be polymorphonuclear early during the course of the disease but shift to mononuclear cells soon afterward. By the second week of major illness, the CSF cell count falls to normal values. In contrast, the CSF protein is normal or only slightly elevated at the outset of CNS disease but usually rises to 50–100 mg/dl by the 2nd week of illness. In polioencephalitis, the CSF may remain normal or show minor changes. Serologic testing demonstrates seroconversion or a 4-fold or greater increase in antibody titers, when measured during the acute phase of illness and 3–6 wk later.

Differential diagnosis: Poliomyelitis should be considered in the differential diagnosis of any case of acute flaccid paralysis in children. *Poliomyelitis (Wild and VAPP):* Progression of paralysis in 24–48 hr to onset of full paralysis; proximal involvement more than distal muscles, asymmetric; reduced or absent deep tendon reflexes, residual paralysis is present; no sensory loss; pleocytosis is present in CSF.

1. *Guillain-Barré syndrome:* Onset of paralysis in hours to 10 days, acute, symmetric, ascending paralysis (1–6 days), pyramidal tract signs are present, Sensory signs and symptoms present, few cells but an elevated protein level in CSF (*see* Section 25.7).
2. *Acute transverse myelitis:* Progresses rapidly over hours to days causing an acute symmetric paralysis of the lower limbs along with anesthesia; autonomic signs of hypothermia are common in the affected limbs and there is bladder dysfunction.
3. *Intramuscular gluteal injection/traumatic neuritis:* Occurs from a few hours to a few days after the traumatic event; asymmetric, acute, and affects only one limb; reduced or absent muscle tone and deep tendon reflexes in the affected limb with pain in gluteus; sensory loss is present; CSF is normal. Conditions causing pseudoparalysis do not present with nuchal–spinal rigidity or pleocytosis. These causes, include unrecognized trauma, transient (toxic) synovitis, acute osteomyelitis, acute rheumatic fever, scurvy, and congenital syphilis (pseudoparalysis of Parrot).

Treatment: There is no antiviral treatment of poliomyelitis. The management is supportive and aimed at limiting progression of disease, prevention of ensuing skeletal deformities, and preparation of the child and family for prolonged treatment required and for permanent disability if this seems likely. All intramuscular injections and surgical procedures are contraindicated during the acute phase of the illness, especially in the 1st wk of illness, because these may result in progression of disease.

Abortive poliomyelitis: Supportive treatment with analgesics, sedatives, diet, and bed rest until the child's temperature is normal for several days is usually required. Avoidance of exertion for the ensuing 2 wk is desirable. The child should be re-evaluated for neurologic and musculoskeletal examination to detect any minor involvement.

Nonparalytic poliomyelitis: Treatment is similar to abortive form. Hot packs and gentle physical therapy may be necessary for some weeks. Such patients should be examined 2 months after apparent recovery to detect minor residual effects that might cause postural problems in later years.

Paralytic poliomyelitis: Most patients with the paralytic form require hospitalization with complete physical rest in a calm atmosphere for the first 2–3 weeks. A neutral position with the feet at a right angle to the legs, knees slightly flexed, and hips and spine straight is achieved by use of boards, sandbags, and, occasionally, light splint shells. The position should be changed every 3–6 hr. Suitable body alignment is necessary for comfort and to avoid excessive skeletal deformity. Active and passive movements are indicated as soon as the pain has disappeared. Moist hot packs may relieve muscle pain and spasm. Opiates and sedatives should only be administered if no impairment of ventilation is present or impending. Constipation is common, and fecal impaction should be prevented. If bladder paralysis occurs, bethanechol and manual compression may be tried. If catheterization, it must be performed with aseptic precaution to prevent urinary tract infection. Diet and fluids should be started unless there is vomiting.

The management of pure bulbar poliomyelitis consists of maintaining the airway and avoiding all risk of inhalation of saliva, food or vomitus. Gravity drainage of accumulated secretions is maintained by using the head-low (foot of bed is elevated 20–25 degrees) prone position with face on one side. Patients with weakness of muscles of respiration or swallowing should be nursed in a lateral or semi-prone position. Aspirations with rigid or semirigid tips are preferred for direct oral and pharyngeal aspiration, and, soft, flexible catheters may be used for nasopharyngeal aspiration. Fluid and electrolyte should be maintained by intravenous infusion. In addition to close observation for respiratory insufficiency, the blood pressure should be taken at least twice daily. Patients with pure bulbar poliomyelitis may require tracheostomy. Mechanical respirators are often needed.

Complications: Paralytic poliomyelitis may be associated with numerous complications. Acute gastric dilatation may occur abruptly during the acute or convalescent stage causing further respiratory embarrassment; immediate gastric aspiration and external application of ice bags are indicated. Melena severe enough to require transfusion may result from single or multiple superficial intestinal erosions; perforation is rare. Hypertension is common and myocarditis rarely occurs. Hypercalcemia and hypercalciuria can also occur.

Prognosis: The outcome of inapparent, abortive poliomyelitis and aseptic meningitis syndromes is uniformly good. In severe bulbar poliomyelitis the mortality rate may be as high as 60%. Maximum paralysis usually occurs 2–3 days after the onset of paralytic phase of the illness, with stabilization followed by gradual return of muscle function. The recovery phase lasts usually about 6 months, beyond which persisting paralysis is permanent. Type 1 poliovirus has the greatest propensity for natural poliomyelitis and type 3 for VAPP.

Postpolio syndrome: After an interval of 30–40 yr, as many as 30–40% of persons who survived paralytic poliomyelitis in childhood may experience muscle pain and exacerbations of existing weakness, or they may develop new weakness or paralysis. This postpolio syndrome has been reported only in persons who were infected by wild type poliovirus. Risk factors for postpolio syndrome include increasing length of time since acute poliovirus infection, presence of permanent residual impairment after recovery from acute illness and female sex.

Prevention: Immunization is discussed in Chapter 15. Vaccination is the only effective method of preventing poliomyelitis. Both the live-attenuated OPV and the inactivated polio vaccine (IPV) have established efficacy in preventing poliovirus infection and paralytic poliomyelitis. In 1988, the World Health Assembly resolved to eradicate poliomyelitis globally by 2000, and remarkable progress had been made toward reaching this target. To achieve this, the WHO used 4 basic strategies: routine immunization, National Immunization Days (NIDs), acute flaccid paralysis surveillance, and mopping up immunization. The OPV is the only vaccine recommended by the WHO for eradication (*see* Chapters 14 and 15).

Kew OM, Wright PF, Agol VI, et al. Circulating vaccine-derived polioviruses: Current state of knowledge. *Bull WHO* 2004;82:16–23.

Mathur GP, Mathur S, Gupta V, et al. Poliomyelitis with special reference to immunization status. *Indian Pediatr* 1991;28:625–7.

Mathur GP, Gahlaut IVS, Mathur Sarla, et al. Intramuscular injection as a provocative factor in paralytic poliomyelitis. *Indian Pediatr* 1994;31:529–31.

Marx A, Glass JD, Sutter RW. Differential diagnosis of acute flaccid paralysis and its role in poliomyelitis surveillance. *Epidemiol Rev* 2000;22:298–316.

Simoes EAF. Polioviruses. In: Kliegman RM, Behrman RE, Jenson HB, Stanton BF (eds). *Nelson Textbook of Pediatrics*. 18th edn. Vol. 1. Philadelphia: Saunders, 2007;1344–50.

Nonpolio Enteroviruses

Etiopathogenesis: Enteroviruses are nonenveloped, single-stranded viruses belonged to the Picornaviridae ("small RNA virus") family. The human enterovirus subgroups are polioviruses, coxsackie viruses, and echoviruses. Coxsackieviruses derive their name from Coxsackie, New York, where they were discovered. The name for ECHO viruses reflects an acronym applied to a group of viruses originally without disease associations (*enteric cytopathic human orphan viruses*). Enterovirus infections are very common and have a world wide distribution. Humans are the only known reservoir for human enteroviruses. Virus is primarily spread person to person by the fecal-oral and respiratory routes, and vertically, from mother to neonate, either prenatally or in the prepartum period. Enteroviruses can survive on environmental surfaces, permitting transmission via fomites.

Clinical manifestations: Clinical manifestations are protean, ranging from asymptomatic infection or undifferentiated febrile or respiratory illness in the majority, to, less frequently, severe diseases such as meningoencephalitis, myocarditis, and neonatal sepsis.

Herpangina: Herpangina is caused by coxsackie viruses A 1–10, 16, or 22 and less commonly coxsackie virus B 1–5, echovirus 3, 6, 9, 11, 16, 17, 22, 25, 30 and enterovirus 71.

The incubation period is usually 7 to 14 days and illness usually lasts 3 to 6 days. The illness begins abruptly. Often there is high fever (103–104°F). The mouth sores usually develop with fever or shortly afterward. The mouth blisters are surrounded by red rings and can occur in the back of the throat, on the roof of the mouth, on the tonsils, inside the cheeks, or on the tongue.

Hand, foot and mouth disease (HFMD): Coxsackie virus A16 is most frequently involved in the causation of this disease and is also caused by enterovirus 71, coxsackie A virus 5, 7, 9 and 10, and coxsackie B virus 2 and 5. HFMD is characterized by fever, mouth sores and a rash with blisters. HFMD begins with a mild fever, poor appetite, malaise and frequently with sore throat. One or two days after the fever, painful sores develop in the mouth. They begin as small red spots that blister and become ulcers usually on the tongue, gums and buccal cavity. The skin rash develops for 1 to 2 days with flat or raised red spots, some with blisters. The rash does not itch, and is usually located on the palms of the hands and soles of the feet. It may also appear on the buttocks. Hands are more commonly involved than feet. HFMD may have only the rash or mouth ulcers also.

Respiratory manifestations: Respiratory symptoms such as sore throat and coryza frequently accompany and sometimes dominate enterovirus illnesses.

Pleurodynia (Bornholm disease) is an epidemic or sporadic illness characterized by paroxysmal pain due to myositis involving chest and abdominal wall muscles. Etiologic agents most frequently are coxsackieviruses B3 and B5, as well as coxsackieviruses B1 and B2 and echoviruses 1 and 6.

Ocular manifestations: Enterovirus 70 and coxsackie virus A24 are the primary causes of epidemics of acute hemorrhagic conjunctivitis. Epidemic and sporadic uveitis in infants caused by enterovirus 11 and 19 can be associated with severe complications, including destruction of the iris, cataracts and glaucoma. Enteroviruses have been implicated in cases of chorioretinitis, uveoretinitis, optic neuritis, and unilateral acute idiopathic maculopathy.

Myocarditis and pericarditis: Coxsackie B viruses are the most common etiologic types, although coxsackie A viruses and echoviruses may be responsible for myocarditis and pericarditis in young adults and adolescents, especially in males.

Gastrointestinal and genitourinary manifestations: Gastrointestinal symptoms include emesis (especially with meningitis), diarrhea, and abdominal pain and pancreatitis. Diarrhea, hematochezia, pneumatosis intestinalis, and necrotizing enterocolitis have been reported in premature infants during nursery outbreaks. Coxsackie B viruses are 2nd only to mumps as causative agents of orchitis.

Neurologic manifestations: Enteroviruses are the most common cause of viral meningitis, particularly common in infants, especially those < 3 mo of age and disease frequently occurs as part of community epidemics. Frequently implicated serotypes include coxsackieviruses B2-5; echoviruses 4, 6, 7, 9, 11, 16, and 30; and enteroviruses 70 and 71. Other neurologic syndromes observed include cerebellar ataxia, transverse myelitis, Guillain-Barré syndrome, peripheral neuritis, optic neuritis, acute disseminated encephalomyelitis, and sudden hearing loss.

Myositis and arthritis: Although myalgia is common, direct evidence of muscle involvement, including rhabdomyolysis, muscle swelling, focal myositis, and polymyositis, has uncommonly been reported. Enteroviruses rarely cause arthritis in normal hosts.

Neonatal infections: Enterovirus infections in neonates are relatively common, with coxsackieviruses B2-5 and echoviruses 6, 9, 11, and 19. Enteroviruses may be acquired vertically before, during, or after delivery; horizontally from family members; or by transmission in hospital nurseries (sporadic or epidemic). Infection in utero may be associated with fetal demise, nonimmune hydrops fetalis, neonatal illness, and congenital anomalies and neurodevelopmental sequelae. Neonatal infection may range from asymptomatic (the majority) to benign febrile illness to severe multisystem disease (sepsis, meningo-encephalitis, myocarditis, hepatitis, coagulopathy, and pneumonitis).

Stem cell transplant recipients: Severe and/or prolonged infections have been reported in stem cell transplant recipients including progressive pneumonia, severe diarrhea, pericarditis, heart failure, and disseminated disease.

Diagnosis: Clues to enterovirus infection can be suspected on clinical grounds, especially when specific findings such as hand-foot-and-mouth disease or herpangina are present. It is best confirmed by isolating the virus from the lesions or by demonstrating a rise in specific antibody. The differential diagnosis of enterovirus infections also varies with the clinical presentation.

Treatment: Newborns, infants, and children, presenting with nonspecific febrile illnesses or meningitis frequently require diagnostic evaluations for bacterial and herpes simplex virus infection and hospitalization for presumptive treatment until tests rule out these diagnoses. There is no specific treatment available for enterovirus infections. Hence, patients should be given plenty of fluids and symptomatic treatment to provide relief from fever, aches or pain.

Prognosis: The prognosis in the vast majority of infections is excellent. Morbidity and mortality is primarily associated with myocarditis, neurologic disease, severe neonatal infections, and infections in immunocompromised hosts.

Prevention: Specific prevention for non-polio enterovirus infections is not available, but the risk of infection can be reduced by good hygienic practices. Preventive measures include frequent hand washing, especially after diaper changes.

Abzug MJ. Nonpolio Enteroviruses. In: Kliegman RM, Behrman RE, Jenson HB, Stanton BF (eds). *Nelson Textbook of Pediatrics.* 18th edn. Vol. 1. Philadelphia: Saunders, 2007; 1350–6.

Abjug MJ. Presentation, diagnosis, and management of enterovirus infections in neonates, *Paediatr Drugs* 2004;6:1–10.

National Center for Infectious Disease (Respiratory and Enteric Virus Branch). Hand, foot and mouth disease. http://www.cdc.gov/ncidod/dvrd/revb/enterovirus/hfhf.htm.

Cytomegalovirus

Etiopathogenesis: Human cytomegalovirus (CMV) is a member of the Herpesviridae family. CMV is the largest of the herpes viruses (diameter of 200 nm). CMV is widely distributed worldwide. *Transmission sources* of CMV include saliva, breast milk, cervical and vaginal secretions, urine, semen, stools, blood, and tissue or organ transplants. The spread of CMV requires very close or intimate contact, but indirect transmission is possible via contaminated fomites. The *primary infection* occurs in seronegative, susceptible host. *Recurrent infection* represents reactivation of latent infection or infection of a seropositive immune host. Disease may result from *primary* or *recurrent* CMV infection, but the former is more commonly associated with severe disease.

Clinical manifestations: The infection is subclinical in most patients. In infants and young children, primary CMV infection occasionally causes pneumonitis, hepatomegaly, hepatitis, and petechial rashes. In older children, adolescents and adults, CMV may cause mononucleosis-like syndrome characterized by headache, fever, fatigue, myalgia, hepatospleno-megaly, elevated liver enzymes, and atypical lymphocytosis. The course of CMV mononucleosis is generally mild, lasting 2–3 wk occasionally persistent fever, overt hepatitis, or a morbilliform rash may occur. Recurrent infections are asymptomatic in the immunocompetent host.

Immunocompromised persons: The risk for CMV disease is increased in immunocompromised persons, with both primary and recurrent infections. In immunocompromised persons, including transplant recipients and patients with AIDS, CMV pneumonia, retinitis, and involvement of central nervous and gastrointestinal tract are usually severe and progressive. Submucosal ulcerations can occur anywhere in the gastrointestinal tract and may lead to hemorrhage and perforation. Pancreatitis and cholecystitis may also occur.

Congenital infections: CMV is the most common cause of congenital infection, which occasionally causes the syndrome of cytomegalic inclusion disease. The characteristic signs and symptoms include intrauterine growth restriction (IUGR), prematurity, hepatospleno-megaly and jaundice, blueberry muffin-like rash, thrombocytopenia, purpura, and microcephaly and intracerebral calcifications in neonates. Other problems include choreoretinitis, sensorineural hearing loss, and mild increases in cerebrospinal fluid protein. Asymptomatic congenital CMV infection is the leading cause of sensorineural hearing loss.

Perinatal infection: Approximately 6–12% of seropositive mothers transmit CMV infection by contaminated cervical–vaginal secretions and 50% by breast milk to their infants, despite the presence of maternally derived, passively acquired antibody. These infants usually remain asymptomatic and do not exhibit sequelae. Occasionally, perinatally acquired CMV infection is associated with pneumonitis and sepsis-like syndrome. Premature and ill full-term infants may have neurologic sequelae and psychomotor retardation and the risk for hearing loss, chorioretinitis, and microcephaly.

Diagnosis: Active CMV infection is best confirmed by virus isolation from urine, saliva, bronchoalveolar washings, breast milk, cervical secretions, buffy coat, and tissues obtained by biopsy or polymerase chain reaction (PCR). The definitive method for diagnosis of congenital CMV infection is virus isolation or PCR, which should be performed at or shortly after birth. Urine and saliva are the best specimens for culture.

Treatment: The treatment is not indicated for immunocompetent persons, but is recommended for immunocompromised persons, and remains controversial for infants with symptomatic congenital infection. Ganciclovir combined with immune globulin, either standard intravenous immunoglobulin (IVIG) or hyperimmune CMV IVG has been used to treat life-threatening CMV infections in immunocompromised hosts (bone marrow, heart, and kidney transplant recipients and patients with AIDS). The two published regimens include: ganciclovir (7.5 mg/kg/day divided every 8 hr IV for 14 days) with CMV IVIG (400 mg/kg on days 1, 2, and 7 and 200/kg on day 14); and ganciclovir (7.5 mg/kg/day divided every 8 hr IV for 20 days) with IVIG (500 mg/kg every other day for 10 doses). CMV retinitis and gastrointestinal disease appear to be clinically responsive to therapy, but often recur on cessation. CMV prophylaxis with ganciclovir or acyclovir reduces the risk for morbidity in solid organ transplantation. Ganciclovir (6 mg/kg/dose every 12 hr IV) for the first 6 wk of life prevents hearing deterioration and improves or maintains normal hearing function at 6 mo of age, and may prevent the hearing deterioration that occurs after 1 yr of age.

Prognosis: Patients with CMV mononucleosis usually recover fully. CMV infection and disease may be fatal in patients with AIDS. Approximately 90% of children with symptomatic congenital infection demonstrate CNS and hearing defects in later years.

Prevention: CMV-free blood products, especially for premature newborns, and whenever possible, organs from CMV-free donors for transplantation should be used. If possible, pregnant women should have a CMV serologic test, especially if they provide care for young children who are potential CMV excreters.

Demmler GJ. Screening for congenital cytomegalovirus infection: A tapestry of controversies. *J Pediatr* 2005;146:162–4.

Stagno S. Cytomegalovirus. In: Kliegman RM, Behrman RE, Jenson HB, Stanton BF (eds). *Nelson Textbook of Pediatrics*. 18th edn. Vol. 1. Philadelphia: Saunders, 2007;1377–9.

Stagno S, Britt W. Cytomegalovirus. In: Remington JS, Klein JO (eds), *Infectious Diseases of Fetus and Newborn Infant*. 6th edn. Philadelphia: WB Saunders, 2005:739–81.

Mumps

Etiopathogenesis: Mumps virus is in the family Paramyxoviridae and the genus *Rubulavirus*. Mumps infection spreads from person to person by respiratory droplets. Virus appears in the saliva from up to 7 days before to as long as 7 days after onset of parotid swelling. The period of maximum infectiousness is 1–2 days before to 5 days after parotid swelling.

Clinical manifestations: The incubation period for mumps ranges from 12 to 25 days, but is usually 16–18 days. The typical case presents with a prodromal symptoms lasting 1–2 days consisting of fever, headache, and vomiting. Parotitis then appears and may be unilateral initially but becomes bilateral in 70% of cases. The parotid gland is tender, and parotitis may be preceded or accompanied by ear pain on the ipsilateral side. Ingestion of sour or acidic foods or liquids may enhance pain in the parotid area. As swelling progresses, the angle of the jaw is obscured and the ear lobe may be lifted upward and outward. The opening of the Stensen duct may be red and edematous. The parotid swelling peaks approximately in 3 days then gradually subsides over 7 days. Fever resolves in 3–5 days along with other systemic symptoms. A morbilliform rash is rarely seen. Submandibular salivary glands may also be involved or may be enlarged without parotid swelling. Edema over the sternum due to lymphatic obstruction may also occur.

Diagnosis: The diagnosis can be made on history of exposure to mumps infection, an appropriate incubation period, and development of typical clinical findings. Confirmation of the presence of parotiditis could be made with demonstration of an elevated amylase level. Leukopenia with a relative lymphocytosis is a common finding. A specific diagnosis of mumps should be confirmed or ruled out by virologic or serologic means. Viruses can be isolated from upper respiratory tract secretions, CSF, or urine during the acute illness. Enzyme immunoassay (EIA) for mumps IgM antibody is used to identify recent infection.

Differential diagnosis: Parotid swelling may be caused by many other infections and noninfectious conditions. Viruses that are responsible to cause parotitis include parainfluenza 1 and 3, influenza A, cytomegalovirus, Epstein-Barr virus, enteroviruses, lymphocytic choriomeningitis virus, and HIV. Purulent parotitis, usually caused by *Staphylococcus aureus*, is unilateral, extremely tender, and associated with an elevated white blood cell count, and may have purulent drainage from the Stensen duct. Submandibular or anterior cervical adenitis may also be confused with parotid swelling. Other causes of parotid swelling including obstruction of the Stensen duct, collagen vascular diseases such as Sjögren syndrome, systemic lupus erythematosus and tumor should be considered in the differential diagnosis.

Complications: The most common complications of mumps are meningitis, with or without encephalitis and gonadal involvement (orchitis and oophoritis). Uncommon complications include pancreatitis, arthritis, thyroiditis (some cases develop hypo-thyroidism), cardiac involvement (myocarditis, and mumps virus has been identified in heart tissue taken from patients with endocardial fibroelastosis), pneumonia, nephritis, conjunctivitis, optic neuritis, and thrombocytopenia.

Treatment: No specific antiviral therapy is available for mumps. Management should be aimed at reducing the pain associated with meningitis or orchitis and maintenance of adequate hydration. Antipyretics may be given for fever.

Prognosis: The outcome is always is good even when complicated by encephalitis, although fatal cases have been reported in patients with CNS involvement or myocarditis.

Prevention: Immunization is discussed in Chapters 15 and 40.

Azimi PH, Cramblett HG, Haynes RE. Mumps meningo-encephalitis in children. *JAMA* 1969;207:509–12.

Mason WH. Mumps. In: Kliegman RM, Behrman RE, Jenson HB, Stanton BF (eds). *Nelson Textbook of Pediatrics.* 18th edn. Vol. 1. Philadelphia: Saunders, 2007;1341–4.

Thompson JA. Mumps: A cause of aqueductal stenosis. *J Pediatr* 1079;94:923–4.

Influenza Viruses

Etiology: There are three types of influenza virus, A, B and C. *Influenza A viruses* are found in human, swine, equine, avian and murine population. *Influenza A viruses* possess two surface proteins, hemagglutinin (HA) (H: 1 to 15) and neuraminidase (NA) (N: 1 to 9), which are used to as for the sub-typing of viruses (e.g. H1N1, H2N2, H3N2, etc.). Wild birds serve as natural host for all influenza A virus subtypes. *Influenza B viruses* are found only in man. Although influenza type B viruses can cause epidemics, they have not been associated with pandemics. *Influenza C viruses* cause mild illness in man, and neither cause epidemics or pandemics (*see* Fig. 14.9 in CD).

Transmission: The viruses spread from person to person through aerosol particles produced during coughing and sneezing. The incubation period is short (up to five days). The viruses initially reside on the lining of the respiratory tract. The viruses begin to shed in respiratory secretions one day before the onset of

the illness and last for about three to five days. Virus is shed for longer periods of time in children receiving cancer chemotherapy and children with immuno-deficiency.

Clinical manifestations: Influenza is an acute contagious infection characterized by inflammation of the respiratory tract. The classic symptoms of influenza include symptoms of fever, malaise (a general feeling of being unwell), headache, body ache (pain in the muscles and joints), sore throat and a characteristic dry cough. The acute illness usually lasts for three to five days but recovery may be slow, and cough and tiredness may persist for few more weeks. Otitis media and pneumonia are common complications in young children.

Laboratory findings: A relative leucopenia is frequently seen. Chest radiographs show evidence of atelectasis or infiltrate in about 10% of children.

Diagnosis and differential diagnosis: Influenza is diagnosed on the basis of epidemiologic, clinical, and laboratory findings. In an epidemic, the clinical diagnosis of influenza in a young child with fever without a focus, malaise and respiratory symptoms can be made. The laboratory confirmation of influenza is made as follows: if seen early in the illness, virus can be isolated from the nasopharynx. Rapid and reliable diagnostic tests for influenza A and B use variations of polymerase chain reaction viral genome detection technology or of antigen capture such as enzyme linked immunosorbent assay. The diagnosis is confirmed serologically with acute and convalescent sera drawn around the time of the illness and tested by hemagglutination inhibition.

Treatment: Antiviral drugs zanamivir and oseltamivir are effective against both influenza A and B strains. Zanamivir is not prescribed in children 1–6 yr of age and is administered by inhalation 10 mg bid in children more than 7 yr of age. Oseltamivir is the drug of choice and is given orally in the doses of 30–75 mg bid in children (not indicated in children below 1 yr of age). Amantadine and rimantadine, can be used in influenza type A outbreaks and is given orally in the doses of 5 mg/kg/24 hr (maximum dose, 150 mg) in children between 1 and 9 yr; and in children more than 10 yr of age 100 mg bid children (not indicated in children below 1 yr of age).

Supportive care: Adequate fluid intake and rest are important components in the management of influenza. Acetaminophen or ibuprofen, but not salicylates because of the risk for Reye syndrome should be used as antipyretic to control fever. Bacterial superinfections are quite common, and in that case antibiotic therapy should be administered. Bacterial superinfection should be suspected with recrudescence of fever, prolonged fever, or deterioration of clinical status. With uncomplicated influenza, children should feel better after the first 48–72 hr.

Prognosis: Children of less than two years of age are at increased risk for influenza-related hospitalization compared with older children. Influenza associated deaths are unusual, but during an epidemic, many deaths occur.

Prevention: All children 6–59 mo of age as well as household contacts and out-of-home caregivers of children 0–23 mo of age should be administered inactivated vaccine. Because of the decreased potential for causing febrile reactions, only the split-virus vaccine is recommended for children < 12 yr of age. Two doses of vaccine (0.25 ml for 6–36 mo of age; 0.5 ml for 3–8 yr of age) at least 1 mo apart are recommended for primary immunization of children < 9 yr of age. Live-attenuated vaccines that are administered intranasally have an efficacy comparable with that of inactivated vaccine in adults can be used in ages 5 and above.

Chemoprophylaxis with the drugs (amantadine and zanamivir) is a secondary means of prevention for prophylaxis of influenza A infections. They are recommended for prophylaxis for vaccinated and unvaccinated persons and unvaccinated high-risk patients and their unvaccinated health care providers during influenza A outbreaks.

Avian Influenza Viruses (Bird Flu Viruses)

All known subtypes of influenza A virus can infect birds. Normally, avian influenza virus can not infect man. Some human cases caused by avian influenza viruses have reported in Asian countries and human to human transmission has also been confirmed. H5 infections have been documented in man, sometimes causing severe illness and death. H7 infection in humans is rare, but can occur among persons who have close contact with infected birds; symptoms may include conjunctivitis and/or upper respiratory symptoms. H9 infections in man have been confirmed (*see* Fig. 14.10 in CD).

Swine Influenza Virus (Swine Flu Virus)

Etiology: Swine flu—an infection caused by influenza A H1N1 virus that jumped from pigs to humans in Mexico. It spreads through droplets, released when a victim coughs or sneezes. H1N1's genetic code consists of 8 segments, 6 of which are related to North American swine viruses. Two come from European or Asian swine viruses. The influenza virus spreads in phases (Table 14.8).

Table 14.8: Phase by phase: The flu spreads	
Phase 1–3	Predominantly animal infection, a few human cases (bird flu is phase 3)
Phase 4	Sustained human to human infection
Phase 5	Pandemic likely, spreads to more than one continent
Phase 6	Pandemic, with worldwide infection (swine flu)

Epidemiology: Mexico was the first country affected by the swine-flu disease. With 74 countries reporting 27,737 cases of infection, including 141 deaths, the World Health Organization (WHO) on Thursday June 11, 2009 declared influenza A (H1N1), also known as swine flu, a pandemic (World's first pandemic in 41 yr). A pandemic is a disease outbreak that has widespread transmission beyond travelers, schools and immediate contacts in two countries. It is the first flu pandemic since Hong Kong flu pandemic in 1968, which killed one million people. *Swine flu* phase by phase moved to the final phase-6 stage on its six-point pandemic scale. In India, cases infected with swine flu virus A (H1N1) were detected in May 2009. Sudden spurt of swine flu cases in India have been reported in the month of December 2009.

Clinical manifestations: Symptoms include fever, lack of appetite, cough, running nose, sore throat, nausea, vomiting and/or diarrhea. Severe symptoms of rapid breathing, breathlessness, chest pain, recurrence of fever, or breathing problems need urgent medical attention.

Treatment: Oseltamivir (Tamiflu) capsule (each capsule 75 mg)—one capsule bid (150 mg/day) for 5 days is given to infected person (children over one year of age). Those exposed to the virus are given 75 mg once a day for five days. In severe cases 2 capsules BD (300 mg/day) can be given. The drug must be taken within 12–48 hr from the first appearance of the symptoms. The drug is not recommended for use during pregnancy or nursing, as the effects on the unborn child or nursing infant are unknown.

Prevention: WHO has not advised restrictions on food (eating pork) or international travel. Human to human infection occurs. It has asked all people with flu symptoms traveling through affected countries to get tested and treated. Doctors and nurses are more prone, quarantine cannot be given, so they should use mask and take Oseltamivir (Tamiflu) tablet—one tablet for 5 days. N98 mask is recommended by WHO—triple layered mask.

Arruda E, Hayden FG. Update on therapy of influenza and rhinovirus infections. *Adv Exper Med Biol* 1996;394:175–87.

Beckford-Ball J. Building awareness of the avian flu outbreak and its symptoms. *Nurs Times* 2004;100:28–29.

Brown H. WHO confirms human-to-human avian flu transmission. *Lancet* 2004;363:462.

Collins PL, McIntosh K, Chanock RM. Respiratory Syncytial Virus. In: Field's Virology (3rd Ed), Edit: Knipe DM, Howley PM, Philadelphia, USA 1995:1313–51.

Collins PL, Chanock RM, McIntosh K. Parainfluenza viruses. In: Fields Virology (3rd Ed.): Fields BN, Knipe DM, Howley PM *et al*. Lippincott Williams & Wilkins, Philadelphia, USA 1996:1205–41.

Glezen WP, Denny FW. Parainfluenza Viruses In: Evans AS, Kaslow RA (eds). *Viral Infections in Humans: epidemiology and control*. 4th edn. New York, USA: Kluwer Academic Publishers, 1997:551–67.

Rai SK, Kurokawa M, Ono K. Viruses Causing Respiratory Infections in Children. In: GP Mathur, S Mathur (eds). *Current Trends in Pediatrics*. Delhi, India: Academia Publishers, 2006: 99–110.

Wright P. Influenza viruses. In: Kliegman RM, Behrman RE, Jenson HB, Stanton BF (eds). *Nelson Textbook of Pediatrics*. 18th edn. Vol. 1. Philadelphia: Saunders, 2007;1384–87.

Human Papillomaviruses

Etiology: The papillomaviruses are small (55 nm) DNA-containing viruses that are ubiquitous in nature. More than 100 different types of HPVs have been identified. The different HPV types typically cause disease in specific anatomic sites. About 30 of the HPV types have been identified from genital tract specimens. There are no animal reservoirs for HPV; all transmission is presumably person to person.

Clinical manifestations: The clinical manifestations of HPV infection depend on the site of epithelial infection.

Skin lesions: Common warts, including palmar and plantar warts are frequently seen in children and adolescents, where they infect the hands and feet, common areas of frequent minor trauma (*see* Chapter 30, page 896); Anogenital warts (*see* Chapter 30, page 888).

Laryngeal papillomatosis contain the HPV types 6 and 11. The median age of onset of recurrent laryngeal papillomatosis is 3 yr. Children present with hoarseness, stridor, or respiratory distress. In infants there is an altered cry and sometimes stridor. Rapid growth of respiratory papillomas can occlude the upper airway, causing respiratory compromise. The lesions may recur within weeks of removal, requiring frequent surgery. The lesions do not become malignant unless treated with radiation.

Prevention: Human papillomavirus vaccine (*see* Chapter 40).

Morelli JG. Cutaneous viral infections. In: Kliegman RM, Behrman RE, Jenson HB, Stanton BF (eds). *Nelson Textbook of Pediatrics*. 18th edn. Vol. 2. Philadelphia: Saunders, 2007; 2751–4.

Moscicki AB. Human papillomaviruses. In: Kliegman RM, Behrman RE, Jenson HB, Stanton BF (eds). *Nelson Textbook of Pediatrics*. 18th edn. Vol. 1. Philadelphia: Saunders, 2007;1402–6.

Rabies

Etiology: Rabies virus is a bullet-shaped, single stranded, envelopes RNA virus from the family Rhabodviridae, genus Lassavirus. There are 7 known genotypes of Lassavirus. All 7 Lassavirus genotypes have been associated with clinical rabies in humans, although type 1 account for the majority of cases.

Epidemiology: Rabies is present on all continents except Antarctica. Rabies virus can infect any mammal that then can transmit disease to humans, but true animal reservoirs that maintain the presence of rabies virus in the population are limited to large carnivorous mammals (dogs, cats, jackals, mongooses, and raccoons, skunks, foxes, and coyotes) and insectivorous bats. Worldwide, transmission from dogs accounts for > 90% of human cases.

Transmission: Rabies virus is found in large quantities in the saliva of infected animals and transmission occurs almost exclusively through inoculation of the infected saliva through a bite or scratch from a rabid mammal. The transmission rate is increased if the victim has suffered multiple bites and if the inoculation occurs in highly innervated parts of the body such as the face and hands. Infection does not occur after exposure to intact skin to infected secretions, but virus may enter the body through intact mucous membranes. Caregivers of a hospitalized patient with rabies are advised to use full barrier precautions with patient contact.

Clinical manifestations: The incubation period for rabies (defined as the interval between virus exposure and onset of clinical disease) is usually 1–3 months but in rare cases symptoms first occur within 5 days after exposure, and occasionally the incubation period can extend to > 6 months. Rabies has 2 principal clinical forms: Encephalitic and paralytic. *Encephalitic or "furious" rabies* begins with nonspecific symptoms, including fever, sore throat, malaise, headache, nausea and vomiting and weakness. These symptoms are accompanied by paresthesias and pruritus at or near the biting site that then extend along the affected limb. Soon thereafter the patient begins to demonstrate typical symptoms of severe encephalitis with agitation, depressed mentation, and occasional seizures. Patients initially have periods of lucidity with periods of profound encephalopathy, but ultimately condition progresses to coma. The cardinal signs of rabies, hydrophobia and aerophobia are manifested by agitation and fear created by attempting to drink and fanning air in the face, which in turn produces choking and aspiration through spasms of the larynx, neck, and chest wall. The illness is progressive and death almost always occurs within 2–3 wk after onset. *Paralytic or dumb rabies* is seen much less frequently and is characterized principally by ascending motor weakness affecting both the limbs and the cranial nerves. Most patients with dumb rabies also have some element of encephalopathy.

Differential diagnosis: The differential diagnosis of rabies encephalitis includes all form of severe cerebral infections. It is important to take the history of contact with an animal belonging to one of the known reservoirs for rabies or to establish history to a rabies endemic region. Dumb rabies is most frequently confused with Guillain-Barré syndrome. Unlike rabies this latter illness usually affects the sensory peripheral nerves a well as the motor and is always associated with clear sensorium.

Diagnosis: Tests for confirming a clinically suspected case of rabies include detection of anti-rabies antibody, isolation of virus, and detection of viral protein or RNA. Rabies-specific antibody can be detected in serum or CSF samples.

Treatment and prognosis: Rabies is an almost uniformly fatal disease but is almost always preventable with appropriate postexposure prophylaxis (PEP) during the incubation period.

Prevention: Primary prevention of rabies infection includes avoiding contact with potentially rabid animals. Special efforts should be made to teach children to avoid wild animals, stray animals, and animals with unusual behavior.

Immunization of animal reservoirs: The routine rabies immunization for domestic pets has virtually eliminated infection in dogs, which are the principal transmitter of rabies to humans. Rabid bats are widely spread and this reservoir remains uncontrolled.

Postexposure prophylaxis (PEP): On the basis of the history of the exposure and local epidemiologic information, the physician must decide whether initiation of PEP is warranted. Healthy dogs, cats, or ferrets may be confined and observed for 10 days. PEP is not necessary if the animal remains healthy. If the animal develops signs of rabies during the observation period, brain should be available for examination for the presence of rabies virus. In high-risk exposures and in areas where canine rabies is endemic, rabies prophylaxis should be initiated without waiting for laboratory results. If the laboratory results prove to be negative, it may safely be concluded that the animal's saliva did not contain rabies virus, and immunization should be discontinued. If an animal escapes after an exposure, it must be considered rabid, and PEP must be initiated unless information from public health officials indicates otherwise (i.e., there

is no endemic rabies in the area). PEP may be warranted when a person present in the same space as a bat (e.g., a small child or a sleeping adult) cannot reliably rule out contact with an unrecognized bite. PEP includes local wound care and both active and passive immunization. Local wound care is essential and may decrease the risk of rabies virus infection by as much as 90%. Wound care should not be delayed, even if the initiation of immunization is postponed pending the results of the 10-day observation period. There are 3 steps in rabies PEP.

Step 1. All bite wounds and scratches should be washed thoroughly with soap and water. Other commonly used disinfectants, such as iodine containing preparations, are viricidal and should be used in addition to soap and water when available. Devitalized tissues should be debrided. Do not touch the wound with bare hand. Do not apply irritants like soil, chilies, oil, herbs, chalk, betel leaves. Tetanus prophylaxis should be given, and antibiotic treatment initiated whenever indicated.

Step 2. All previously unvaccinated persons should be passively immunized with rabies immune globulin (RIG). If RIG is not immediately available, it should be administered no later than 7 days after the first vaccine dose. After day 7, endogenous antibodies are being produced, and passive immunization may actually be counterproductive. If anatomically feasible, the entire dose of RIG (20 IU/kg) should be infused at the site of the bite; otherwise, any RIG remaining after infiltration of the bite site should be administered IM at a distant site. With multiple or large wounds, the RIG preparation may need to be diluted in order to obtain a sufficient volume for adequate infiltration of all wound sites. If the exposure involves a mucous membrane, the entire dose should be administered IM. Rabies vaccine and RIG should never be administered at the same site or with the same syringe. Human RIG preparations are much better tolerated than are the equine-derived preparations. Serious adverse effects of human RIG are uncommon. Local pain and low-grade fever may occur.

Step 3. Two purified inactivated rabies vaccines are available for rabies PEP. Five 1-mL doses of rabies vaccine should be given IM in the deltoid area on days 0, 3, 7, 14, and 28. The anterolateral aspect of the thigh is also acceptable in children. Injection in to the gluteal area has been associated with a blunted antibody response, and this area should not be used. Ideally, the first dose should be given as soon as possible after exposure; failing that, it should be given without further delay. The four additional doses should be given on days 3, 7, 14, and 28. Pregnancy is not a contraindication for immunization. Glucocorticoids and other immunosuppressive medications may interfere with the development of active immunity and should not be administered during PEP unless they are essential. All persons vaccinated with the above schedule developed a serologic response within 2–4 weeks. Routine measurement of serum neutralizing antibody titers is not required, but titers should be measured 2–4 wk after immunization in immuno-compromised persons. Local reactions (pain, erythema, edema, and pruritus) and mild systemic reactions (fever, myalgias, headache, and nausea) are common; anti-inflammatory and antipyretic medications may be used, but immunization should not be discontinued. Systemic allergic reactions are uncommon, but anaphylaxis does occur rarely and can be treated with epinephrine and antihistamines. The risk of rabies development should be carefully considered before the decision is made to discontinue vaccination because of an adverse reaction.

Pre-exposure prophylaxis: Pre-exposure rabies prophylaxis should be considered for people with an occupational or recreational risk of rabies exposures, including certain travelers of rabies-endemic areas. This primary schedule consists of three doses of rabies vaccine given on days 0, 7, and 21 or 28. Serum neutralizing antibody tests help determine the need for subsequent booster doses. When a previously immunized individual is exposed to rabies, two booster doses of vaccine should be administered on days 0 and 3. Wound care remains critical. RIG should not be administered to previously vaccinated persons.

Pounder D. Avoiding rabies. *Br Med J* 2005;331:469–70.

Toltzis P. Rabies. In: Kliegman RM, Behrman RE, Jenson HB, Stanton BF (eds). *Nelson Textbook of Pediatrics.* 18th edn. Vol. 1. Philadelphia: Saunders, 2007;1423–6.

Warrell MJ, Warrell DA. Rabies and other Lascivious diseases. *Lancet* 2004;363:959–68.

Japanese Encephalitis

Etiology: Japanese encephalitis (JE) virus is a positive-sense, single-stranded RNA virus of the family Flaviviridae. JE is a mosquito-borne viral disease of humans as well as horses, swine, and other domestic animals that causes human infections. *Culex tritaeniorhynchus summarosus*, a night-biting mosquito that feeds preferentially on large domestic animals and birds but only infrequently on humans, is the principal vector of zoonotic and human JE in northern Asia. From Taiwan to India *Culex tritaeniorhynchus* and more closely related *Culex vishnui* group are vectors. Before the introduction of JE vaccine, summer outbreaks of JE occurred regularly in Japan, Korea, China, Okinawa, and Taiwan. Over the past decade, there has been a pattern of steadily enlarging recurrent seasonal outbreaks in Vietnam, Thailand, Nepal, and India. Seasonal rains are accompanied by increases in mosquito populations and increased transmission. Pigs serve as amplifying host. Children < 15 yr of age are principally affected, with nearly universal exposure by adulthood.

Clinical manifestations: After a 4–14 day incubation period, cases typically progress through 4 stages: prodromal illness (2–3 days), acute stage (3–4 days), subacute stage (7–10 days), and convalescence (4–7 wk). Onset may be characterized by abrupt onset of fever, headache, respiratory symptoms, anorexia, nausea, abdominal pain, vomiting and sensory changes and psychotic episodes. Grandmal seizures are seen in 10–24% of cases; Parkinsonian-like non-intention tremor and cogwheel rigidity are seen in a few cases. The characteristic features are rapidly changing central nervous signs (e.g. hyperreflexia followed by hyporeflexia). The sensory status of the patient may vary from confusion, disorientation, delirium or somnolence, progressing to coma. CSF usually contains a mild pleocytosis (100–1,000 cells/mm^3), initially polymorphonuclear but in a few days predominantly lymphocytic. Albuminuria is common. Fatal cases usually progress to coma, and the patient dies within 10 days.

Diagnosis: The etiologic diagnosis of JE is established by testing an acute-phase serum collected early in the illness for the presence of virus-specific immuno-globulin M (IgM) antibodies, or alternatively, demonstrating a 4-fold or greater increase in IgG antibody titers by testing paired acute and convalescent sera. The virus can also be identified by PCR.

Treatment: There is no specific treatment for JE. The treatment is intensive supportive care, including control of seizures.

Prognosis: Patient fatality rate ranges from 24–42% and are highest in children 5–9 yr of age. Sequelae include mental deterioration, severe emotional instability, personality changes, motor abnormalities and speech disturbances and are most common in patients younger than 10 yr at the onset of disease.

Prevention, see Chapters 15 and 40. Personal measures should be taken to reduce exposure to mosquito bites. This consists of avoiding evening outdoor exposure, using insect repellents, covering the body with clothing, and using bed nets or house screening. Commercial pesticides, widely used by rice farmers in Asia, are effective in reducing populations of *Culex tritaeniorhynchus*.

Halstead SB. Arboviral encephalitis outside North America. In: Kliegman RM, Behrman RE, Jenson HB, Stanton BF (eds). *Nelson Textbook of Pediatrics*. 18th edn. Vol. 1. Philadelphia: Saunders, 2007;1409–11.

Mathur A, Chaturevedi VC, Tandon HO, Agarwal AK, Mathur GP, Nag D, Prasad A. Japanese encephalitis epidemic in Uttar Pradesh, India during 1978 *Indian J Med Res* 1982; 75:161–9.

Mathur GP, Kumar R, Mathur Sarla, Singh YD, Kushwaha KP. Psychoneurological sequelae in Patients with JE Virus Encephalitis. *Indian Pediatr* 1988;25:371–3.

Mathur GP, Kushwaha KP, Mathur Sarla. Japanese Encephalitis. Gupte Suraj (ed). *Recent Advances in Pediatrics*. Vol 6. New Delhi: Jaypee Brothers, 1966;357–70.

National Institute of Communicable Diseases. Directorate General of Health Services. Ministry of Health and Family Welfare. Government of India, Delhi. 2009.

Dengue Fever and Chikungunya

1. Dengue Fever

Etiology: There are four distinct serotypes of dengue virus, but closely related, which are also prevalent in India. Dengue fever (DF) can be caused by any one of four types of dengue virus: DEN-1, DEN-2, DEN-3, and DEN-4. Recovery from infection by one provides lifelong immunity against that serotype but confers only partial and transient protection against subsequent infection by the other three.

Transmission: Dengue viruses are transmitted to humans through the bites of infective female Aedes mosquitoes. Two main species of mosquito, *Aedes aegypti* (commonest mosquito) and *Aedes albopictus* have been responsible for all cases of dengue transmitted in India. Mosquitoes generally acquire the virus while feeding on the blood of an infected person. After virus incubation for 8–10 days, an infected mosquito is capable, during probing and blood feeding, of transmitting the virus, to susceptible individuals for the rest of its life. An infected person cannot spread the infection to other persons but can be a source of dengue virus for mosquitoes for about 6 days.

Clinical manifestations: Dengue viral infection may remain *asymptomatic* or *manifest* either as uncomplicated (classic) dengue fever (DF) or dengue haemorrhagic fever (DHF) or dengue shock syndrome (DSS).

Case definition for dengue fever (DF): Symptoms of typical uncomplicated (classic) dengue (DF) usually start with (a flu-like illness) fever averages 4 to 6 days (with a range of 3 to 14 days) after bitten by an infected mosquito. The rash may appear over most of the body 3 to 4 days after the fever begins. A second rash occurs later in the disease. Dengue fever affects infants, young children and adults, but seldom causes death.

Case definition for dengue hemorrhagic fever (DHF):
1. Fever, or history of acute fever, lasting 2–7 days, occasionally biphasic
2. Hemorrhagic tendencies, evidenced by at least one of the following:
   a. Positive tourniquet test—petechiae, ecchymoses or purpura
   b. Bleeding from the mucosa, gastrointestinal tract, injection sites or other locations (bleeding from the nose, gums, or under the skin, causing purplish bruises)
   c. Hematemesis or melena)
3. Thrombocytopenia (100,000 cells per mm^3 or less)
4. Evidence of plasma leakage due to increased vascular permeability, manifested by at least one of the following:
   a. A rise in the hematocrit equal to or greater than 20% above average for age, sex and population
   b. A drop in the hematocrit following volume-replacement treatment equal to or greater than 20% of baseline
   c. Signs of plasma leakage such as pleural effusion, ascites, and hypoproteinemia)

Grading severity of dengue hemorrhagic fever (DHF): DHF is classified into four grades of severity, where grades iii and iv are considered to be DSS. The presence of thrombocytopenia with concurrent hemoconcentration differentiates grade i and ii DHF from DF (Table 14.9).

Case definition for dengue shock syndrome (DSS): All of the four criteria for DHF plus evidence of circulatory failure manifested by:
- Rapid and weak pulse, and
- Narrow pulse pressure (< 20 mmHg; or manifested by:
  - Hypotension by age, and
  - Cold, clammy skin and restlessness.

Diagnosis: The diagnosis of dengue fever is made by doing two blood tests, 2 to 3 wk apart. The tests can show whether a sample of blood contains antibodies to the virus. In epidemics, diagnosis of dengue fever can often be made by typical signs and symptoms.

Patients with a provisional diagnosis of DHF or DSS if there is:
- Virological or serological evidence of acute dengue infection, or
- History of exposure in a dengue endemic or epidemic area (during a period of epidemic transmission or significant cases of endemic transmission, it is unlikely that many such cases will have laboratory confirmation; such cases should be treated as proven cases of DHF/DSS and reported to the health authorities).

Table 14.9: Grading severity of dengue hemorrhagic fever (DHF)

Grade I. Fever accompanied by non-specific constitutional symptoms, the only hemorrhagic manifestation is a positive tourniquet test and/or easy bruising

Grade II. Spontaneous bleeding in addition to the manifestations of grade I patients, usually in the form of skin or other hemorrhages

Grade III. Circulatory failure manifested by a rapid, weak pulse and narrowing of pulse pressure or hypotension, with the presence of cold, clammy skin, and restlessness

Grade IV. Profound shock with undetectable BP or pulse

Guidance for diagnosis of DHF/DSS: The clinical observations (high fever of acute onset, hemorrhagic manifestations at least a positive tourniquet test, hepatomegaly and shock) and laboratory findings (thrombocytopenia [100,000 cells per mm^3 or less], hemoconcentration [hematocrit elevated at least 20% above average for age, sex and population]), which may help clinicians to establish an early diagnosis ideally before the onset of shock, as well as to avoid over diagnosis. The first two clinical observations, plus one of the laboratory findings (or at least a rising hematocrit), are sufficient to establish a provisional diagnosis of DHF.

Differential diagnosis: Early in the febrile phase, the differential diagnosis for DHF/DSS includes a wide spectrum of viral, bacterial and parasitic infections. Chikungunya fever may be difficult to differentiate clinically from DF and mild or early cases of DHF. By the third or fourth day, laboratory findings may establish a diagnosis before shock occurs. Shock virtually rules out a diagnosis of chikungunya fever. Marked thrombocytopenia with concurrent hemoconcentration differentiates DHF/DSS from diseases such as endotoxin shock from bacterial infection or meningococcemia.

Treatment

A. *Classic dengue fever:* There is no specific treatment for classic dengue fever, and most people will recover completely within 2 weeks. During the acute febrile phase there is some risk of convulsions. Acetaminophen (paracetamol), ibuprofen, and naproxen, are safe for relieving fever and pain for most people. Do not give aspirin. Persons with dengue fever should rest and drink plenty of fluids including oral rehydration salts (ORS).

B. *Dengue hemorrhagic fever (DHF):* DHF is treated by replacing lost fluids. Some patients need transfusions to control bleeding.

C. *Dengue shock syndrome (DSS):* Shock is a medical emergency. Fluids should be used for rapid volume expansion include the following: normal saline 0.9%, Ringer lactate, plasma or albumin (50 g/L), fresh whole blood. If shock persists, oxygen should be given and the hematocrit should be checked for evidence of decline, which may indicate internal bleeding. Fresh whole-blood transfusion (10 ml/kg, if the hematocrit is still above 35%) may be needed in such cases. A drop in hematocrit, e.g., from 50% to 40%, with no clinical improvement despite adequate fluid administration indicates a significant internal hemorrhage. IV fluids should be discontinued when the hematocrit level drops to approximately 40%, with stable vital signs. Good urine flow indicates sufficient circulation fluid. In general, IV fluid therapy is not needed for more than 48 hr after the termination of shock. A single dose of chloral hydrate (12.5–50 mg/kg), orally or rectally, is recommended (total dose not exceeding 1 g) for a restless child. Oxygen therapy should be given to all patients in shock.

Frequent recording of vital signs and determination of hematocrit are important in *evaluating the results of treatment* of patients in shock:

1. Check vital signs (pulse, BP, respiratory rate, temperature) every 30 minutes (or more often) until shock is overcome.
2. Hematocrit (or hemoglobin) every 2 hr for first 6 hr, then every 4 hr until stable.
3. A fluid balance sheet should be kept, recording the type of fluid and the rate and volume of it administration in order to evaluate its adequacy of fluid replacement. The frequency and volume of urine output should also be recorded, and a urinary catheter may be needed in cases of refractory shock.

Criteria for discharging inpatients: The criteria for discharging inpatients recovering from DHF/DSS include:

1. Absence of fever for at least 24 hr without the use of antifever therapy (cryotherapy or antipyretics)
2. Return of appetite
3. Visible clinical improvement
4. Good urine output
5. Stable hematocrit
6. Passing of an at least 2 days after recovery from shock
7. No respiratory distress from pleural effusion or ascites
8. Platelet count more than 50,000 per mm^3.

Prognosis: Most people who develop dengue fever recover completely within 2 weeks. Some, however, may go through several weeks to months of feeling tired and/or depressed.

Dengue hemorrhagic fever (DHF) is fatal in about 5 percent of cases, mostly among children and young adults.

Prevention: Both dengue and chikungunya spread through Aedes mosquitoes, which breed in clean water and bite during day time (Box 14.4). Avoid mosquito bites by use of insecticides, repellents, body covering with clothing, screening of houses, and destruction of *A. aegypti* breeding sites.

Box 14.4: Prevention tips

- Do not let water accumulate for more than a week in any container anywhere in your home or in the neighborhood.
- Make sure that all water tanks and water storage containers are covered.
- Empty and dry coolers, drums, flower vases, plant pots, bird bath etc. every week.
- Destroy old tyres, disposable cups and glasses, coconut shells, etc.
- Wear full-sleeved clothing and use mosquito repellents to prevent mosquito bites.
- In case of high fever accompanied with headache, pain behind the eyes, joint and muscular pain, skin rash and fatigue, go to your nearest hospital/health centre. Paracetamol can be taken. But, strictly avoid Aspirin.
- Dengue and chikungunya can be managed effectively with timely and proper medical care.

Issued in public interest by national vector borne disease control programme, directorate general of health services, ministry of health & family welfare, government of india, 2009.

---

2. Chikungunya Fever

Etiology: Chikungunya fever is caused by chikungunya virus (CHIKV), a member of the genus *Alphavirus,* in the family Togaviridae. CHIKV spreads by the bite of infected Aedes mosquitos (*Aedes aegypti*—India and Southeast Asia; *Aedes africanus*—Africa). Mosquitoes become infected when they feed on a person infected with CHIKV. Monkeys, and possibly other wild animals, may also serve as reservoirs of the virus. Infected mosquitoes can then spread the virus to other humans when they bite.

Clinical manifestations: CHIKV infection is characterized by fever, headache, fatigue, nausea, vomiting, muscle pain, rash, and joint pain. The incubation period (time from infection to illness) can be 2–12 days, but is usually 3–7 days. Acute chikungunya fever typically lasts a few days to a couple of weeks, but some patients have prolonged fatigue lasting several weeks. The prolonged joint pain associated with CHIKV is not typical of dengue. Co-circulation of dengue fever in many areas may mean that chikungunya fever cases are sometimes clinically misdiagnosed as dengue infections. Therefore, the incidence of chikungunya fever could be much higher than what has been previously reported. CHIKV infection (whether clinical or silent) is thought to confer lifelong immunity. No deaths, neuroinvasive cases, or hemorrhagic cases related to CHIKV infection have been conclusively documented in the scientific literature.

Treatment of chikungunya virus is symptomatic—rest, fluids including ORS, and ibuprofen, naproxen, acetaminophen (paracetamol) may relieve symptoms of fever and aching. Aspirin should be avoided.

Prevention: Preventive measures of chikungunya virus are the same as mentioned in dengue fever (Box 14.4).

Benenson AS. Dengue Fever. In: Benenson AS (Ed). *Control of communicable diseases manual. 16th* edn. Washington, DC: Am Pub Health As, 1995;34–35.

Benenson AS. Chikungunya. In: Benenson AS (Ed). *Control of communicable diseases manual. 16th* edn. Washington, DC: Am Pub Health As, 1995;128–33.

CDC's Travelers' Health website (www.cdc.gov/travel) for chikungunya virus.

Govt. of India. *Annual Report 2003–2004.* New Delhi: Ministry of Health and Family Welfare, 2004.

Halstead SB. Dengue fever and Dengue Hemorrhagic fever. In: Kliegman RM, Behrman RE, Jenson HB, Stanton BF (eds). *Nelson Textbook of Pediatrics.* 18th edn. Vol. 1. Philadelphia: Saunders, 2007;1412–5.

Mathur GP, Khare Vandana, Mathur Sarla. Dengue and Chikungunya: A major public health concern. In: Mathur GP, Mathur Sarla (eds). *Current Trends in Pediatrics.* Vol 3. Delhi: Academa Publishers, 2007;464–81.

Park K (Ed). The Dengue Syndrome. In: *Textbook of Preventive and Social Medicine.* 18th edn. Jabalpur: M/S Banarsidas Bhanot, 2007;206–9.

Park K (Ed). Chikungunya Fever. In: *Textbook of Preventive and Social Medicine.* 18th edn. Jabalpur: M/S Banarsidas Bhanot, 2007;241.

World Health Organization. Dengue hemorrhagic fever: diagnosis, treatment, prevention and control. 2nd edn. Geneva: WHO, 1997;1–84.

Yellow Fever

Etiology: Yellow fever virus circulates zoonotically as 3 genotypes: type I in Central Africa, type IIA in West Africa, and type IIB in South America. Type IIA virus is capable of urban transmission between human beings by *Aedes aegypti.*

Clinical manifestations: In its classic form, yellow fever begins with sudden onset of fever, headache, myalgia, lumbosacral pain, anorexia, nausea, and vomiting. After 2–3 days, there may be a brief period of remission, followed in 6–24 hr by reappearance of fever with vomiting, epigastric pain, jaundice, dehydration, gastrointestinal and other hemorrhages, albuminuria, hypotension, renal failure, delirium, convulsions, and coma. Death may occur after 7–10 days, with the fatality rate in severe cases approaching 50%. *Complications* of acute yellow fever include severe hemorrhage, liver failure, and acute renal failure.

Diagnosis: Specific diagnosis depends on detection virus or viral antigen in acute phase blood samples or antibody assays.

Treatment: There is no specific treatment of yellow fever. Medical care is directed in maintaining physiologic status:

1. Sponging and acetaminophen to reduce high temperature
2. Vigorous fluid replacement of losses resulting from fasting, thirsting, vomiting or plasma leakage
3. Correcting acid base balance; maintaining nutritional intake to lessen the severity of hypoglycemia; and
4. Avoiding drugs that are either metabolized by liver or toxic to the liver, kidney, or central nervous system.

Prevention: Countries that require travelers to obtain a yellow fever immunization do not issue a visa without a valid immunization certificate. Vaccination is valid for 10 yr for international travel certification, although immunization lasts at least 40 yr and probably for life.

Halstead SB. Yellow fever. In: Kliegman RM, Behrman RE, Jenson HB, Stanton BF (eds). *Nelson Textbook of Pediatrics.* 18th edn. Vol. 1. Philadelphia: Saunders, 2007;1415–6.

World Health Organization. Progress in the control of yellow fever in Africa. *Wkly Epidemiol Rec* 2005;80:50–55.

Acquired Immunodeficiency Syndrome (Human Immunodeficiency Virus)

Etiology: There are two human immunodeficiency viruses (HIV-1; HIV-2) belonging to *Lentivirus* genus of the Retroviridae family. HIV-1 genome is a single-stranded RNA of 9.2 kb in size and takes part in HIV infection. HIV-2 is a rare cause of infection in children. HIV destroys certain white blood cells called CD4+ T cells, which are critical to the normal function of the human immune system. When HIV weakens the immune system, a person is more susceptible to a variety of cancers and becoming infected with viruses, bacteria and parasites. AIDS stands for acquired immunodeficiency syndrome. A person who tests positive for HIV can be diagnosed with AIDS when a laboratory test shows that his or her immune system is severely weakened by the virus or when he or she develops at least one of about 25 different opportunistic infections-diseases that might not affect a normal person but that take advantage of damaged immune systems. The time between HIV infection and progressing to AIDS differs for each person and depends on many factors, including a person's health status and their health-related behaviors. With a healthy lifestyle, the time between HIV infection and developing AIDS-related illnesses can be 10–15 years, sometimes longer.

Epidemiology: More than 90% of HIV-infected individuals live in developing nations. Worldwide, 60% of HIV-infected individuals are women; heterosexual transmission accounts for most HIV spread. About 2.5 million people in India, between ages 15–49, are feared to be affected with HIV/AIDS, the third largest number in the world as reported on World AIDS Day (December 1, 2009).

Transmission of HIV in children: Transmission of HIV-1 occurs via sexual contact, parenteral exposure to blood, or vertical transmission from mother to child. The primary route of infection in the pediatric population is vertical transmission, accounting for almost all new cases. Baby can get infected in utero, though usually the transmission occurs at the time of birth and postpartum due to breast milk. Vertical transmission occurs due to infection of baby by maternal blood, cervicovaginal secretions or via breast milk. The baby gets infected either due to trans-placental hemorrhage or due to infection via umbilical cord or via oral and GI (gastrointestinal) mucosa while swallowing infected amniotic fluid.

Clinical manifestations: The clinical manifestations of HIV infection vary widely among infants, children, and adolescents. In most infants, physical examination at birth is normal. The clinical findings include lymphadenopathy and hepatosplenomegaly, failure to thrive, chronic or recurrent diarrhea, interstitial pneumonia, oral thrush. Symptoms found more commonly in children than adults with HIV infection include recurrent bacterial infections, chronic parotid swelling, lymphocytic interstitial pneumonitis (LIP), and early onset of progressive neurologic deterioration. The HIV classification system is used to categories the stage of the pediatric disease by using two parameters: clinical status and degree of immunologic impairment. Among the clinical categories (Table 14.10), *Category N (no signs and symptoms)* considered to be the result of HIV infection or have only one of the conditions noted in category A.

Category A (mild symptoms) includes children with at least two mild symptoms such as lymphadeno-pathy, parotitis, hepatomegaly, splenomegaly, dermatitis, and recurrent or persistent sinusitis or otitis media.

Category B (moderate symptoms) includes children with LIP, oropharyngeal thrush persisting for > 2 mo, recurrent or chronic diarrhea, persistent fever for > 2 mo, hepatitis, recurrent herpes simplex virus (HSV) stomatitis or HSV esophagitis or pneumonitis, disseminated varicella (i.e. visceral involvement, cardiomegaly or nephropathy).

Category C (severe symptoms) includes, children with 2 serious bacterial infections (sepsis, meningitis, pneumonia) in 2 yr period, esophageal or lower respiratory tract candidiasis, crypttococcosis, cryptosporidiosis (> 1 mo), encephalopathy, malignancies, disseminated mycobacterial infection, *Pneumocystis pneumonia*, cerebral toxoplasmosis (onset > 1 mo of age), and severe weight loss. Lymphocytic interstitial pneumonitis (LIP) in category B or any condition in category C is considered AIDS defining condition.

The immune classification is based on the absolute CD4 lymphocyte count or the percentage of CD4 cells (Table 14.11). Age adjustment of the absolute CD4 count is necessary because counts that are relatively high in normal infants decline steadily until 6 yr of age, when they reach adult norms. If there is a discrepancy between the CD4 count and percentage, the disease is classified into the more severe category.

Infections: Illnesses in children are recurrent bacterial infections caused primarily by encapsulated organisms such as *Streptococcus pneumoniae* and *Salmonella*. Other pathogens including, *Staphylococcus*, *Enterococcus*, *Pseudomonas aeruginosa* and *Haemophilus influenzae*, and other gram-positive and gram-negative organisms may also be seen. The most common infections are bacteremia, sepsis, and bacterial pneumonia, whereas meningitis, urinary tract infections, deep-seated abscesses, and bone/joint infection occur less frequently. Milder recurrent infections, such as otitis media, sinusitis, and skin and soft tissue infections are very common and may be chronic with atypical presentations. Oral candidiasis is the most common fungal infection seen in HIV-infected children.

Opportunistic infections seen in children with severe depression of the CD4 count include *Pneumocystis carinii (jiroveci)* pneumonia (PCP), and atypical mycobacterial infection, particularly with *Mycobacterium avium intracellulare* complex (MAC).

Viral infections, especially with the herpesvirus (HSV) group, causes problems for HIV infected children. HSV causes recurrent gingivostomatitis, which may be complicated by local and distant cutaneous dissemination and primary varicella-zoster virus (VZV) infection (chickenpox) may be prolonged and complicated by bacterial infection or visceral dissemination, including pneumonitis. Disseminated cytomegalovirus (CMV) may involve single or multiple organs (retinitis, pneumonitis, esophagitis, gastritis with pyloric obstruction, hepatitis, colitis, and encephalitis). The 1st line therapy for PCP is IV trimethoprim-sulfamethoxazole (TMP-SMZ) (15–20 mg/kg/day of TMP and 75-100 mg/kg/day of SMZ every 6 hr IV) with adjunctive corticosteroids if the PaO_2 is < 70 mmHg while breathing room air. When the patient has improved, therapy with oral TMP-SMZ should be continued for a total of 21 days while the corticosteroids are weaned. Alternative therapy for PCP includes intravenous administration of pentamidine (4 mg/kg/day). Other regimens such as TMP plus dapsone, clindamycin plus primaquine, or atovaquone are used as alternatives in adults but have not been widely used in children. Therapy for MAC should include at least 2 drugs: clarithromycin or azithromycin and ethambutol. A 3rd drug (rifabutin, rifampin, ciprofloxacin, livofloxacin or amikacin) is generally added to decrease the emergence of drug-resistant isolates. Oral nystatin suspension (2–5 ml qid) is often effective in cases of thrush infection. Clotrimazole troches are an effective alternative. In refractory cases, oral amphotericin suspension should be considered. Treatment with oral fluconazole (3–6 mg/kg/day for 7–4 days generally results in rapid improvement in symptoms.

Respiratory viruses such as respiratory syncytial virus (RSV) and adenovirus may present with prolonged symptoms and persistent viral shedding. With the increased prevalence of genital tract human papillomavirus (HPV) infection, cervical intra-epithelial neoplasia (CIN) and anal intraepithelial neoplasia (AIN) also occur with increased frequency among HIV-1-infected adult women compared with HIV-seronegative women. The relative risk for CIN is 5–10 times higher for HIV-1 seropositive women.

Table14.10: Clinical classification for children younger than 13 years				
Immunologic definitions	*N: No signs or symptoms*	*A: Mild signs or symptoms*	*B: Moderate signs or symptoms*	*C: Severe signs or symptoms*
1. No evidence of suppression	N1	A1	B1	C1
2. Evidence of moderate suppression	N2	A2	B2	C2
3. Severe suppression	N3	A3	B3	C3

Table 14.11: Pediatric HIV immunologic classification for children younger than 13 years						
Immunologic definitions	*< 12 months*		*1–5 years*		*6–12 years*	
	µl	*%*	*µl*	*%*	*µl*	*%*
1. No evidence of suppression	≥ 1500	≥ 25	≥ 1000	≥ 25	≥ 500	≥ 25
2. Evidence of moderate suppression	750–1499	15–24	500–499	15–24	200–499	15–24
3. Severe suppression	< 750	< 15	< 500	< 15	< 200	< 15

Note. To convert values in µl to systemic international units ($\times 10^9$/L, multiply by 0.001.

Central nervous system: The incidence of CNS involvement in perinatally infected children is 50–90% in developing countries but lower in developed countries, with a median onset at 19 mo of age. This may range from subtle developmental delay to progressive encephalopathy with loss or plateau of developmental milestones, cognitive deterioration, impaired brain growth resulting in acquired microcephaly and symmetric motor dysfunction. Older children may exhibit behavioral problems and learning disabilities. Neuroimaging studies demonstrate cerebral atrophy up to 85% of children, increased ventricular size, basal ganglia calcifications, and less frequently, leukomalacia. CNS lymphoma, CNS toxoplasmosis, other opportunistic infections including CMV, JC virus (progressive multifocal leukoencephalopathy), HSV and *Cryptococcus* or *Coccidioides* meningitis and cerebrovascular disorders (both hemorrhage and nonhemorrhagic strokes) can also affect the children.

Respiratory tract: Recurrent upper respiratory tract infections such as otitis media and sinusitis are very common. Although the typical pathogens (*S. pneumoniae*, *H. influenzae*, *Moraxella catarrhalis*) are most common, unusual pathogens such as *P. aeruginosa*, yeast, and anaerobes may be present in chronic infections and result in complications such as invasive sinusitis and mastoiditis. LIP is the most common chronic lower respiratory tract abnormality and is associated with a primary Epstein-Barr virus infection in children with HIV infection. PCP is the most common opportunistic infection, but other pathogens, including CMV, Aspergillus, Histoplasma, and Cryptococcus can cause pulmonary disease. Pulmonary and extrapulmonary tuberculosis has been reported with increasing frequency in HIV-infected children.

Cardiovascular system: Subclinical cardiac abnormalities in HIV infected children are common, persistent and often progressive. Electrocardiography and echocardiography are helpful in assessing cardiac function before the onset of clinical symptoms.

Gastrointestinal and hepatobiliary tract: Oral manifestations of HIV disease include erythematous or pseudomembranous candidiasis, periodontal disease (e.g. ulcerative gingivitis or periodontitis), salivary gland disease (i.e. swelling, xerostomia), and rarely ulcerations or oral hairy leukoplakia and ulcerations. Gastrointestinal tract involvement is common in HIV-infected children. A variety of pathogens can cause gastrointestinal disease, including bacteria (*Salmonella*, *Compylobacter* and MAC), protozoa (*Giardia*, *Cryptosporidium*, *Isospora*, microsporidia), viruses (CMV, HSV, rotavirus), and fungi (*Candida*). AIDS enteropathy, a syndrome of malabsorption with partial villous atrophy not associated with a specific pathogen, has been postulated to be a result of direct HIV infection of the gut. Disaccharide intolerance is common in HIV-infected children with chronic diarrhea. The most common symptoms of gastrointestinal disease are chronic or recurrent diarrhea with malabsorption, abdominal pain, dysphagia, and failure to thrive (FTT). The wasting syndrome, defined as a loss of > 10% of body weight, is not as common as FTT in pediatric patients. *Chronic liver inflammation* evidenced by fluctuating serum level of transaminases with or without cholestasis is relatively common, often without identification of an etiologic agent. Several of the anti-retroviral drugs or other drugs such as didanosine, protease inhibitors, and dapsone may also cause reversible elevation of transaminases. *Pancreatitis* with increased pancreatic enzymes with or without abdominal pain, vomiting, and fever may be the result of drug therapy (e.g. with pentamidine, didanosine, or lamivudine) or, rarely, opportunistic infections such as MAC or CMV.

Renal disease: A wide range of histologic abnormalities of HIV infection has been reported, including focal glomerulosclerosis, mesangial hyperplasia, segmental necrotizing glomerulonephritis, and minimal change disease. Nephrotic syndrome is most common manifestation of pediatric renal disease with edema. Cases resistant to steroid therapy may benefit from cyclosporin therapy.

Skin manifestations: Seborrheic dermatitis or eczema that is severe and unresponsive to treatment may be an early nonspecific sign of HIV infection. Recurrent or chronic episodes of HSV, herpes zoster, molluscum contagiosum, flat warts, anogenital warts, and candidal infections are common and may be difficult to control. Allergic drug eruptions in particular related to sulfonamides, and generally respond to withdrawal of drug or to desensitization. Epidermal hyperkeratosis with dry, scaling skin is frequently observed, and sparse hair or hair loss may be seen in the later stages of the disease.

Hematologic and malignant diseases: Anemia occurs in 20–70% of HIV-infected children, more commonly in children with AIDS. The anemia may be due to chronic infection, poor nutrition, autoimmune factors, virus-associated conditions (hemophagocytic syndrome, parvovirus B19 red cell aplasia) or the adverse effects of drugs (zidovudine). In children with low erythropoietin levels, subcutaneous recombinant erythropoietin may be used to treat the anemia.

Leukopenia occurs in 1/3 of untreated HIV infected children and neutropenia often occurs. Antineutrophil antibodies are the cause in some cases, who can be treated with intravenous immunoglobulin (IVIG). Multiple drugs used for treatment for treatment or prophylaxis for opportunistic infections such as PCP, MAC and CMV or anti-retroviral drugs (zidovudine) may also cause leucopenia and/or neutropenia. Treatment with subcutaneous granulocyte colony-stimulating factor in some cases is successful.

Thrombocytopenia has been reported in 10–20% cases, which may be immunologic (i.e. circulating immune complexes or antiplatelet antibodies), or due to drug toxicity or the cause may be unknown. Treatment with IVIG or anti-D offers temporary improvement in most cases. In ineffective cases, a 2–3 day course of high-dose steroids (30 mg/kg/day) may be tried. Anti-retroviral therapy may also reverse thrombocytopenia. Deficiency of clotting factors (factors II, VII, IX) is found in children with advanced HIV disease and is corrected by vitamin K. A few HIV infected children have anterior mediastinal multilocular thymic cysts without clinical symptoms. Spontaneous involution occurs in some cases.

Malignant diseases have been reported infrequently in HIV infected children, representing only 2% of AIDS defining illnesses. Non-Hodgkin lymphoma, primary CNS lymphoma, and leiomyosarcoma are reported in HIV infected children. EBV is associated with most lymphoma and with all leiomyosarcoma. Kaposi sarcoma, which is caused by human herpes virus 8, occurs frequently among HIV infected adults but is exceedingly uncommon among HIV-infected children.

Diagnosis: All infants born to HIV-infected mothers test antibody-positive at birth because of passive transfer of maternal-HIV antibody across the placenta during gestation. Most uninfected infants lose maternal antibody between 6 and 12 mo of age and are known as seroreverters, but a small proportion of uninfected infants continues to test HIV antibody positive for up to 18 mo of age. In any child > 18 mo of age, demonstration of IgG antibody to HIV by a repeatedly reactive enzyme immunoassay (EIA) and confirmatory test (immunoblot or immunofluorescence assay) establishes the diagnosis of HIV infection. Incorporating rapid HIV-testing during delivery or immediately after birth is critical for the care of HIV-exposed newborns whose HIV status was unknown during pregnancy. Viral diagnostic assays such as HIV DNA or RNA PCR, HIV culture, or HIV p24 antigen immune-dissociated p24 (ICD-p24), are considerably more useful in young infants, allowing a definitive diagnosis in most infected infants by 1–6 mo of age. Viral diagnostic testing should be performed within the 1st 48 hr of life. Almost 40% of HIV infected children can be identified at this time. Many of these children have a more rapid progression of their disease and deserve more aggressive therapy. In exposed children with negative serologic testing at 2 days of life, additional testing should be done at 1–2 mo of age and at 4–6 mo of age; some also favor testing at 14 days to maximize early detection of infected infants. A positive virologic assay (i.e. detection of HIV by PCR, culture, or p24 antigen) suggests HIV infection and should be confirmed by a repeat test on a 2nd specimen as soon as possible. A diagnosis of HIV infection can be made with 2 positive serologic test results obtained from different blood samples.

Perinatal use of prophylactic zidovudine to prevent vertical transmission has not affected the predictive value of viral diagnostic testing; the effect of more intensive antiviral combinations (protease inhibitors) in pregnant women on the accuracy of the infant's viral tests is unknown. HIV infection can be reasonably excluded if an infant has had at least 2 negative virologic test results with at least 1 test performed at ≥ 4 mo of age. The infection can be excluded definitely if the same parameters are met when the infant is at least 18 mo of age.

Infants born to HIV-infected mothers should be prescribed zidovudine (ZDV) prophylaxis. A complete blood count, differential leukocyte count, and platelet count should be performed at 4 wk of age to monitor ZDV toxicity. If the child is found to be HIV-infected or if the HIV-status is not clear, these tests should be continued every 1–3 mo to assess the hematologic effect of disease or its treatment (prophylactic TMP-SMZ and anti-retroviral therapy). If the child is found to be HIV infected, CD4 and CD8 lymphocyte counts should be performed at 1 and 3 mo of age and repeated every 3 mo. The frequency of test should be increased (every 4–6 wk) if the CD4 lymphocyte count or percentage declines rapidly.

Management: The currently available therapy does not eradicate the virus and cure the patient. Antiretroviral therapy can slow the progression of HIV to AIDS by decreasing the amount of virus in a person. The following 5 principles form the basis for anti-retroviral treatment:

1. Uninterrupted HIV replication causes destruction of the immune system and progression to AIDS.
2. The magnitude of the viral load predicts the rate of disease progression, and the CD4 cell count reflects the risk of opportunistic infections and HIV infection complications.
3. Combinations of highly active antiretroviral therapy **(HAART)**, which include at least 3 drugs should be the initial treatment.
4. The goal of sustainable suppression of HIV replication is best achieved by the simultaneous initiation of combinations of anti-retroviral agents to which the patient has been exposed previously and which are not cross resistant to drugs with which the patient has been treated previously.
5. Adherence to the complex drug regimens is crucial for a successful outcome.

Combination therapy: Anti-retroviral drugs are categorized by their mechanism of action, such as the ability to inhibit the HIV reverse transcriptase or protease enzymes. A. The *reverse transcriptase inhibitors* are further subdivided into: *Nucleoside (or nucleotide) reverse transcriptase inhibitors (NRTIs)* and *non-nucleoside reverse transcriptase inhibitors (NNRTIs)*. The *NRTIs* have a similar structure to the building blocks of DNA (e.g. thymidine, cytosine). When incorporated into DNA, that act like chain terminators and block further incorporation of nucleosides, which prevents viral DNA synthesis. Among the NRTIs, thymidine analogs (stavudine [d4T], zidovudine [ZDV]) are found in higher concentrations in activated or dividing cells, and nonthymidine analogs [didanosine (ddI), lamivudine (3TC)] have more activity in resting cells. Activated cells produce > 99% of the population of HIV virions, whereas resting cells account for < 1% of the population, but may serve as a reservoir of HIV. Suppression of replication in both populations is an important component of long-term viral control. *NNRTIs* (nevirapine, efavirenz) act differently than the NRTIs. They attach to the reverse transcriptase and restrict its motility, which reduces the activity of the enzyme. The *protease inhibitors* (lopinavir, nelfinavir, saquinavir) are potent agents that act farther along the viral replicative cycle. They bind to the site where the viral long polypeptides are cut to individual, mature, and functional core proteins that produce the infectious virions before they leave the cell. The 1st fusion inhibitor, enfuvirtide binds to viral gp41, which prevents fusion of the virus with the CD4+ cell and entry into the cell.

While the principal site of viral replication is lymphoid tissue, sanctuary sites such as the CNS may harbor residual virions with the potential source of local or persistent disease. Impaired penetration of drugs to these compartments could result in development of resistance. ZDV, d4T, 3TC, indinavir and nevirapine appear to achieve inhibitory concentrations in the CNS.

By targeting different points in the viral life cycle and stages of cell activation, and delivering drug to all tissue sites, maximal viral suppression is possible. Combinations of 3 drugs (thymidine analog NRTI [ZDV], a nonthymidine analog NRTI [3TC] to suppress the replication in both active and passive cells, and a protease inhibitor [lopinavir/ritonavir or nelfinavir] or an NNRTI [efavirenz]) have been shown to produce prolonged viral suppression. Less potent combinations such as triple NRTIs (abacavir, zidovudine, lamivudine), dual NRTIs, or ritonavir with stavudine may be considered in special situations when there are concerns about adherence to a complex drug regimen or when the patient and/or family prefer a simplified alternative regimen. Combination treatment increases the rate of toxicities, and complex drug-drug interactions exist among many of the anti-retroviral drugs. Most NNRTI and protease inhibitor drugs are inducers or inhibitors of the cytochrome P450 system. The protease inhibitors have serious interactions with multiple drug classes including nonsedating antihistamines and psychotropic, vasoconstrictor, antimycobacterial, cardiovascular, analgesic, and gastrointestinal (cisapride). The inhibitory effect of ritonavir (a protease inhibitor) on the cytochrome P450 system has been exploited, and small doses of the drug are added to several other protease inhibitors (lopinavir, indinavir, saquinavir) to slow their metabolism by the P450 system and to improve their pharmacokinetic profile. This provides more effective drug levels with less toxicity and, often, less frequent dosing.

Adherence: Compliance of < 80–90% results in less successful suppression of the viral load. In addition, poor adherence to prescribed medication regimens results in subtherapeutic drug concentrations and enhances development of resistance, particularly with protease inhibitors and NNRTI drugs. Intensive education on the relationship of drug adherence to viral suppression, training on drug administration, frequent follow-up visits, and commitment of the caregiver and the patient (despite the inconvenience of adverse effects, dosing schedule, unpalatable, and so on) are important for successful antiviral management.

Initiation of therapy: HIV infected children with symptoms (clinical category A, B, or C) or with evidence of immune dysfunction (immune category 2 or 3) should be treated with anti-retroviral therapy, regardless of age or viral load. Children < 1 yr of age are at high risk for disease progression, and immunologic and virologic tests to identify those likely to develop rapidly progressive disease are less predictive than in older children.

Anti-retroviral drug doses: *Newborns and premature infants,* because of the immaturity of the neonatal liver, often require an increase in the dosing interval of drugs primarily cleared through hepatic glucuronidation. *Adolescents* should have anti-retroviral dosages prescribed on the basis of sexual maturity rating (SMR) or Tanner staging of puberty. During early puberty (Tanner stages I, II, and III), pediatric dosing ranges should be used, whereas adolescents in late puberty (Tanner stages IV and V) should follow adult dosing schedules.

Changing anti-retroviral therapy: Therapy should be changed when the current regimen is judged ineffective as evidenced by increase in viral load, deterioration of the CD4 cell count, or clinical progression. Development of toxicity or intolerance to drugs is another reason to consider a change in treatment. When a change is considered, the patient and family should be reassessed for adherence problems. Ideally, when a decision is made to change the anti-retroviral therapy, all drugs should be changed. However, in many situations (previous anti-retroviral experience, intolerance, toxicity) this is not possible, and therefore at least two drugs should be changed based on the resistance mutation genotype (if available) or previous regimen used.

Monitoring anti-retroviral therapy: Virologic and immunologic surveillance (using HIV RNA copy number and CD4 lymphocyte count or percentage) and clinical assessment should be performed regularly in children taking anti-retroviral therapy. Initial virologic response should be achieved within 4 wk of initiating anti-retroviral therapy. The maximum response to therapy usually occurs within 12–16 wk. Thus, HIV RNA levels should be measured at 4 wk and 3–4 mo after therapy initiation. Once an optimal response has occurred, viral load should be measured at least every 3–6 mo. If the response is unsatisfactory,

another viral load should be performed as soon as possible to verify the results before a change in therapy is considered. Potential toxicities should be monitored closely for the 1st 8–12 wk, and if no clinical or laboratory toxicity is observed, a follow-up visit every 2–3 mo is adequate. Toxicities encountered with antiretroviral therapy (especially protease inhibitors) include hematologic complications, hypersensitivity rash, lipodystrophy (e.g. redistribution of body fat), hyperlipidemia (elevation of cholesterol and triglyceride concentrations), hyperglycemia and insulin resistance, mitochondrial toxicity leading to severe lactic acidosis, abnormal bone mineral metabolism, and hepatic toxicity including severe hepatomegaly with steatosis.

Resistance to anti-retroviral therapy: Failure to reduce the viral load to < 50 copies/ml increases the risk for developing resistance. The accumulation of resistance mutation progressively diminishes the potency of the anti-retroviral therapy. For some drugs (nevirapine, 3TC) a single mutation is associated with resistance, while for other drugs (ZDV, lopinavir) several mutations are needed before resistance develops. Two types of tests are available to assess the drug resistance. The *phenotypic assay* measures the virus susceptibility in various concentrations of the drug and the *genotypic assay* predicts the virus susceptibility from mutations identified in the HIV genome isolated from the patient. Treatment success was reported higher in patients whose antiretroviral therapy was guided by genotype or phenotype testing.

HIV and Infant feeding [breastfeeds (BF) or replacement feeds (RF)]: The biggest dilemma faced by a pediatrician in managing HIV patients is to decide whether to allow breastfeeding by HIV positive mothers. HIV is transmitted by breastmilk as proved by many studies. Firstly both the free and cell bound HIV has been isolated form human breastmilk. Free HIV can infect CD4+ cells lining the GI tract of baby. Infected maternal mononuclear cells present in breast milk can pass through mucous membranes of baby and infect the baby. Transmission to child is shown to occur from the mother infected with HIV postnatally and who breastfed the infant. Lastly, studies done have compared rate of vertical transmission in those babies who were breastfed compared to those who were exclusively top-fed and showed that there is 14% extra risk related to breastfeeding over and above other factors. HIV has been shown in high titers in colostrum as well as in breast milk for first 4 days after delivery. Some have shown it to be present for as long as 4–6 months or even beyond that after delivery. Vitamin A deficiency in mother leads to increased titers of HIV in breast milk. Other conditions like breast abscess, mastitis or sore nipple can lead to contamination of breast milk with mother's blood.

Exclusive breastfeeding will avoid problems of infection related with top feeding. It is cost effective, ideal in developing countries. It will also avoid stigma associated with not breastfeeding due to HIV. It is accepted by > 90% in developing countries. However, as discussed later mixed feeding should be avoided and the compliance to absolutely exclusive breastfeeding in general population is estimated to be only 22–35%. Hence, it is the duty of counselor and pediatrician to ensure that it is exclusive breastfeeding and not mixed feeding.

Replacement feeding may appear as a logical choice in HIV infected mothers. However, it has its own problems. Replacement feeding, especially bottle-feeding, is associated with higher infections like acute respiratory infections (ARI) and diarrhea, especially in countries with high infant mortality rate (IMR). Besides this there is problem of breast milk spillage and leakage if mother chooses to give replacement feeds. There is social stigmatization if the mother does not breast feed the baby in countries where breastfeeding is the norm.

Safe delivery practices: Vaginal delivery leads to more chances of HIV infection. The Swiss study showed that the risk of transmissions of HIV was 6% with LSCS and 20% with vaginal delivery. The chances increased to 29–31% if interventions are done during vaginal delivery like traumatic delivery or episiotomy. Hence episiotomy and other procedures should be avoided during vaginal delivery in HIV infected mothers. *Elective LSCS* done before rupture of membranes reduces the transplacental hemorrhage occurring during labor, reduces the length of exposure of the baby to cervicovaginal secretions or maternal blood, reduces the quantum of infective material, reduces swallowing of infected material by baby and reduces chances of ascending infection to baby. All this reduces HIV transmission.

Supportive care: A multidisciplinary team approach is desirable for successful management. Close attention should be paid to nutrition status, which may require nasogastric or gastric feedings or parenteral nutrition to achieve adequate caloric and protein intake. Painful oropharyngeal lesions and dental caries are frequent and may interfere with eating; oral hygiene should be encouraged. Development should be evaluated regularly with provision of necessary physical, occupational, and/or speech therapy. Effective pharmacologic and nonpharmacologic protocols for pain management should be instituted, especially during the terminal phase of the disease.

All HIV-exposed and infected children should receive standard pediatric immunizations. In general, live oral polio vaccine and live bacterial vaccines (BCG) should not be given. Varicella and measles-mumps-rubella (MMR) vaccines are recommended for children in immune categories 1 and 2, but neither varicella nor MMR vaccines should be given to severely immunocompromised children (immune category 3). Prior immunizations do not always provide protection, as evidenced by outbreaks of measles and pertussis in immunized HIV-infected children.

All infants between 6 wk and 1 yr of age who are proven to be HIV infected should receive prophylaxis regardless of the CD4 count or percentage. Infants exposed to HIV infected mothers should receive the same prophylaxis until they are proven to be noninfected. When the HIV-infected child is > 1 yr of age, prophylaxis should be given according to the CD4 lymphocyte count (1–5 yr CD4 count < 500 cells/µl or CD4 percentage < 15%; 6–12 yr CD4 count < 500 cells/µl or CD4 percentage < 15%). The best prophylactic regimen is 150/750 mg/m^2/day of TMP/SMZ given as 1–2 daily doses 3 days per week. If the patient experiences a mild allergic reaction (rash) desensitization is usually successful to allow daily TMP/SMZ prophylaxis. For severe adverse reactions to TMP/SMZ, alternate therapies include dapsone, atovaquone, or pentamidine (aerosolized or intravenous). Prophylaxis against MAC should be offered to HIV-infected children with advanced immunosuppression (i.e. CD4 lymphocyte count < 500 cells/mm^3 in children < 1 yr of age, < 75 cells/mm^3 in children 1–6 yr of age, < 50 cells/mm^3 in children > 6 yr of age). The drugs of choice are clarithromycin (7.5 mg/kg bid PO) or azithromycin (20 mg/kg once a week PO or 5 mg/kg once daily PO). Primary prophylaxis against opportunistic infections may be discontinued if patients have experienced sustained (> 6 mo duration) immune reconstitution with HAART. Even if patients have had opportunistic infections such as PCP or disseminated MAC, it may also be possible to discontinue prophylaxis if immune reconstitution has been sustained. Some experts recommend IVIG to prevent recurrent serious bacterial infections for symptomatic HIV-infected children who

i. Have suffered from at least 2 documented serious bacterial infections within 1 yr,

ii. Have laboratory documented inability to make antigen-specific antibodies, or

iii. Are hypogammaglobulinemic. The dose of IVIG is 400 mg/kg every 4 wk.

All HIV-exposed children should have skin testing (5TU PPD) for tuberculosis at 1 yr of age and be retested every 2 yr. If the child is living close contact with a person with tuberculosis, he or she should be tested more frequently. To reduce the incidence of other potential infections, parents should be counseled about:

1. The importance of good hand-washing
2. Avoiding raw or undercooked food (*Salmonella*)
3. Avoiding drinking or swimming in lake or river water or being in contact with young farm animals (*Cryptosporadium*), and
4. The risk of playing with pets (*Toxoplasma* and *Bartonella* from cats, *Salmonella* from reptiles).

Prognosis: In general the best prognostic indicators are the sustained suppression of plasma viral load and CD4 lymphocytes. High viral load (> 100,000 copies/mL) and CD4 lymphocyte percentage of < 15% are indicative of higher mortality. To define prognosis more accurately, the use of changes of both markers (CD4 lymphocyte percentage and plasma viral load) is recommended.

Prevention: Interruption of perinatal transmission from mother-to-child has been achieved by administering ZDV chemoprophylaxis (200 mg every 8 hr) to the pregnant women (started as early as 4 wk of gestation) and continued during delivery (2 mg/kg loading IV followed by 1 mg/kg/hr IV) and in the newborn for the 1st 6 wk of life (2 mg/kg every 6 hr PO). Such therapy has been documented to decrease the rate of perinatal HIV-1 transmission to < 8% in developed countries. Toxicity from ZDV therapy is minimal in both mothers and infants. The efficacy of ZDV chemoprophylaxis for reduction of perinatal transmission to the offspring of women in both the untreated, asymptomatic and immunologically intact women and with advanced disease, low CD4 counts, and prior ZDV therapy has been reported. Rates of perinatal transmission have been as low as 2% among women who received HAART and all 3 components of the ZDV regimen, even in women with advanced HIV-1 disease. Therefore, women should be treated with a HARRT regimen appropriate for their own health during pregnancy. Women whose viral load at the time of delivery is > 1,000 copies/ml should be counseled about the potential benefit of cesarean section in reducing the risk for vertical transmission. Full-term infants should be given oral ZDV at a dose of 2 mg/kg every 6 hr for 6 wk. Reduced dosages are used for preterm infants. For those who do not meet indications for or have no access to therapy, a regimen known to prevent vertical HIV-1 transmission should be offered, such as ZDV from 28 wk of pregnancy plus a single dose of nevirapine (SD NVP) during labor and 1 wk of ZDV therapy for the neonate. The recommended universal prenatal HIV-1 counseling and HIV-1 testing with consent for all pregnant women will reduce the number of new infections dramatically. For women not tested during pregnancy, the use of rapid HIV antibody testing during labor, or in the 1st day of life for the infant is a way to provide perinatal prophylaxis to at-risk infants. Combination of two drugs: Zidovudine (ZDV), nevirapine (NVP) or more has been used successfully bringing down the vertical transmission to below 2%. Most studies target the last months of gestation, labor and postpartum period of 1 wk for the mother and for 1–6 wk to the baby postnatally. The choice of ARV prophylaxis to prevent mother to child transmission (MTCT) in different situations are:

Affording mother: If the mother is affording and warrants ARV therapy, it is best to start her on combination drugs like ZDV plus 3TC plus NVP. Efavirenz should be avoided as it can lead to CNS malformations. The newborn can be given single dose NVP alone or along with 1 wk of ZDV. If the mother does not warrant ARV treatment, she should be given ZDV with or without 3TC from 28 wk and the newborn single NVP alone or with 1 wk of ZDV.

Non-affording mother: If the mother can not afford ARV treatment, she should be encouraged to take ZDV from 28 wk or as much as she can be followed by single dose of NVP at the time of delivery followed by single dose NVP with or without 1 wk ZDV to the newborn. If she can afford even this or comes late, one should offer single dose NVP to her and baby as it is quite effective and cost effective.

Late comers: If the mother comes late during labor she should be still given single dose NVP followed by same to the newborn with or without 1 wk of ZDV. If she is going to deliver within 2 hr, she should not be given NVP and in stead the newborn should be given one dose of NVP soon after birth and another dose at 72 hr of birth. If the mother has already delivered the newborn should be given single dose of NVP along with 1 wk of ZDV.

In sexually active adolescents, condoms should be an integral part of programs to reduce sexually transmitted diseases. Unprotected sex with older partners or with multiple partners and use of illicit drugs is common among HIV-infected adolescents, which increases their risks. Educational efforts are essential for older school-aged children and adolescents and should begin before the onset of sexual activity.

Prevention of mother to child transmission (PMTCT)

PMTCT involves four strategies:

a. Measures to decrease maternal HIV cases.

b. Measures to decrease viral load in HIV infected mothers, e.g. ARV therapy to mother.

c. Measures to decrease exposure of baby to maternal fluids, e.g. elective lower segment cesarean section (LSCS) or avoiding breast-feeds.

d. Measures to decrease chances of HIV in exposed babies, e.g. ZDV to baby.

Different interventions undertaken to prevent vertical transmission include:

a. Antiretroviral drugs

b. Infant feeding issues

c. Elective LSCS

d. Cleaning of birth canal during delivery

e. Vitamin A prophylaxis

f. Immunotherapy

Phases of PMTCT prevention: PMTCT prevention involves 5 phases.

Phase I: This phase involves giving information on voluntary counseling and testing, infant feeding, option of medical termination of pregnancy, family planning measures, problems of orphans, etc. to mother who is HIV positive. This will go a long way in preventing pregnancies or decrease the exposure of babies to maternal HIV.

Phase II: This phase involves giving prophylaxis to mother and child, which includes antiretroviral (ARV) drugs to mother and baby and use of safe delivery practices like elective LSCS and non-traumatic vaginal delivery.

Phase III: This phase involves issues related to replacement feeds versus breast feeds.

Phase IV(alpha) : This phase involves primary prevention of HIV in mothers and society. This includes HIV education, avoiding high-risk behaviors, treatment of sexually transmitted diseases, imparting life skills, etc.

Phase V (omega) : This phase includes care and support of already HIV infected mothers and babies, social support and economical support, etc.

Antiretroviral drugs for treating pregnant women and preventing HIV infection in infants. *Guidelines on care, treatment and support for women living with HIV/AIDS and their children in resource-constrained settings.* WHO 2004.

Kapoor A, Kapoor A, Vani SN. Prevention of Mother to Child Transmission of HIV. *Indian J Pediatr* 2004;71:247–51.

Read JS. Committee on Pediatric AIDS, Human milk, Breastfeeding and Transmission of Human immunodeficiency virus type-1 in United States. *Pediatrics* 2003;112:1196–205.

Rongkavilit C, Asmar BI. Advances in prevention of mother-to-child HIV transmission. *Indian J Pediatr* 2004;71:69–77.

Shah NK. Prevention of Mother to Child Transmission (PMTCT) of HIV. In: Mathur GP, Mathur Sarla (eds). *Current Trends in Pediatrics.* Vol 2. Delhi: Academa Publishers, 2006;5–12.

Verghese VP, Cherian AJ, Babu PG, et al. Clinical manifestations of HIV-1 infection. *Indian Pediatr* 2002;39:57–62.

Yogev R, Chadwick EG. Acquired Immunodeficiency Syndrome (Human immunodeficiency virus). In: Kliegman RM, Behrman RE, Jenson HB, Stanton BF (eds). *Nelson Textbook of Pediatrics.* 18th edn. Vol. 1. Philadelphia: Saunders, 2007; 1427–43.

14.9 PROTOZOAN DISEASES

Amebiasis

Etiopathogenesis: Entamoeba histolytica is the causative parasite for amebiasis. Amebiasis is highly endemic in India, Southeast Asia, Africa, and Latin America. Infection is established by ingestion of parasite cysts. After ingestion, the cyst resistant to gastric acidity and digestive enzymes, excysts in the small intestine to form 8 trophozoites. These large, actively motile organisms colonize the lumen of the large intestine and may invade the mucosal lining. Infection is not transmitted by trophozoites because of their rapid degeneration outside the body and especially in the low pH of normal gastric contents if swallowed.

Clinical manifestations: Clinical presentations range from asymptomatic cyst passage to amebic colitis, amebic dysentery, ameboma, and extraintestinal disease. *E. histolytica* infection is asymptomatic in about 90% of persons, but it has the potential to become invasive. Severe disease is more common in young children, pregnant women, malnourished individuals, and persons taking corticosteroids. Extraintestinal disease usually involves only the liver, but rare extraintestinal manifestations include amebic brain abscess, pleuropulmonary disease, ulcerative skin, and genitourinary lesions. The two most common forms of disease caused by *E. histolytica* are amebic colitis and amebic liver abscess.

Amebic colitis affects all age groups, but its incidence is high in children 1–5 yr of age. 4–10% of individuals infected with *E. histolytica* develop amebic colitis. Amebic colitis may occur within 2 wk of infection or be delayed for months. The onset is usually gradual with colicky abdominal pains and frequent bowel movements. Diarrhea is frequently associated with tenesmus. Stools are blood stained and contain a fair amount of mucus. Fever occurs in only 1/3 of patients.

Amebic liver abscess, a serious manifestation of disseminated infection, occurs in < 1% of infected individuals. Amebic liver abscess may occur months to years after exposure. In children, fever is present in amebic liver abscess and is frequently associated with abdominal pain, distension, and enlargement and tenderness of the liver. At the base of the right lung elevation of diaphragm and atelectasis or effusion, may also occur.

Laboratory findings: In uncomplicated amebic colitis, mild anemia may be present. In amebic liver abscess laboratory findings include slight leucocytosis, moderate anemia, high erythrocyte sedimentation rate and elevations of hepatic enzymes (particularly alkaline phosphatase) levels. Stool examination for amebae is negative in > 50% of patients with documented amebic liver abscess. Ultrasonography, CT, or MRI can localize and delineate the size of the abscess cavity. The most common finding is a single abscess in the right hepatic lobe, in half of the cases, left lobe abscess and multiple abscesses are more common than previously recognized.

Diagnosis: A diagnosis of amebic colitis is based on compatible symptoms with detection of *E. histolytica* antigens in stool by enzyme-linked immunosorbent assays (> 90% sensitivity). Microscopic examination of 3 fresh stool samples (within 30 min of passage) has a sensitivity of 90% for detecting *Entamoeba*.

Differential diagnosis: The differential diagnosis for amebic colitis includes colitis due to bacterial (*Shigella, Salmonella,* enteropathogenic *Escherichia coli, Campylobacter, Yersinia, Clostridium difficile*) and viral (cytomegalovirus) pathogens as well as noninfectious causes such as inflammatory bowel disease. Pyogenic liver abscess due to bacterial infection, hepatoma, and echinococcal cysts are to be considered in the differential diagnosis of amebic liver abscess.

Complications: The complications of amebic colitis include necrotizing colitis, ameboma, toxic megacolon, extraintestinal extension or local perforation and peritonitis. An ameboma is a nodular focus of proliferative inflammation, usually in the wall of the colon in cases of chronic amebiasis. Amebic liver abscess may be associated with rupture into the peritoneum, pleural cavity, skin, or rarely, pericardium when diagnosis and therapy are delayed.

Treatment: Invasive amebiasis is treated with a nitroimidazole such as metronidazole or tinidazole, followed by treatment with a luminal amebicide, such as diloxanide furoate or iodoquinol. Diloxanide furoate may also be used in children > 2 yr of age. Asymptomatic intestinal infection with *E. histolytica* should be treated with iodoquinol or diloxanide furoate. Tinidazole may become the preferred agent for amebiasis, as it has similar efficacy to metronidazole with shorter and simpler dosing and has less frequent adverse effects, which include

nausea, abdominal discomfort, and metallic taste that disappear after completion of therapy. For fulminant cases of amebic colitis, some experts suggest adding dehydroemetine (1 mg/kg/day subcutaneously or IM, never IV). Patients should be hospitalized for monitoring if dehydroemetine is administered, and the drug should be discontinued if tachycardia, T-wave depression, arrhythmias, or proteinuria develop. Broad spectrum antibiotic therapy may also be indicated in fulminant colitis, to treat spillage of intestinal bacteria into the peritoneum. Surgery is indicated in cases of intestinal perforation and toxic megacolon. In amebic liver abscess, image-guided aspiration of large lesions or left lobe abscesses may be necessary if rupture is imminent or if patient shows a poor clinical response 4–6 days after administration of amebicidal drugs. Chloroquine, which concentrates in the liver, may also be useful adjunct to nitromidazoles in the treatment of amebic liver abscess. Stool examination should be repeated every 2 wk until the result is negative after completion of endamoebic therapy to confirm cure. Patients with invasive disease (colitis or liver abscess) should be treated with metronidazole (35–50 mg/kg in 3 divided doses for 7–10 days) or tinidazole (colitis: 50 mg/kg/day once daily for 3 days; liver abscess: 50 mg/kg/day once daily for 3–5 days) followed by diloxanide furoate (20 mg/kg/day in e divided doses for 7 days) or iodoquinol (30–40 mg/kg/day in 3 divided doses for 20 days). Patients with asymptomatic intestinal colonization should be treated with diloxanide furoate or iodoquinol as for invasive disease.

Prognosis: Most infections evolve to either an asymptomatic carrier state or eradication. Death occurs in about 5% of persons having extraintestinal infection.

Prevention: Control of amebiasis can be achieved by exercising proper sanitary measures and avoiding fecal-oral contact.

Blessmann J, Tannich E. Treatment of asymptomatic intestinal *E. histolytica* infection. *N Engl J Med* 2002;347(17):1384.

Haque R, Houston CD, Hughes M, et al. Amebiasis. *N Engl J Med* 2003;348:1565–73.

John CC, Salata RA. Amebiasis. In: Kliegman RM, Behrman RE, Jenson HB, Stanton BF (eds). *Nelson Textbook of Pediatrics.* 18th edn. Vol. 1. Philadelphia: Saunders, 2007;1460–62.

Stanley SL, Jr. Amoebiasis. *Lancet* 2003;361:1025–34.

Primary Amebic Meningoencephalitis

Amebic meningoencephalitis has 2 distinct clinical presentations. The more common is *acute amebic meningitis* that is caused by *Naegleria* and occurs in previously healthy children and young adults. The second is *granulomatous amebic meningoencephalitis,* which is caused by *Acanthamoeba, Balamuthia, and Sappinia* is a more indolent infection that is more likely to occur in immunocompromised individuals.

Clinical manifestations: The incubation of *Naegleria* infection may be as short as 2 days or as long as 15 days. There is a sudden onset of severe headache, fever, nausea, and vomiting; signs of meningitis; and then encephalitis. Most cases end in death within 1 wk of onset of symptoms.

Granulomatous amebic meningoencephalitis may occur weeks to months after acquiring the organism. The presenting signs and symptoms include hemiparesis, personality changes, seizures, and drowsiness. Headache and fever occur sporadically, but stiff neck is seen in majority of cases. Cranial nerve palsies may be present.

Diagnosis: The CSF in *Naegleria* infection may mimic that of herpes simplex encephalitis early in the disease, and later of acute bacterial meningitis with a neutrophilic pleocytosis, elevated protein level, and low sugar level. The amebae, which may be motile, may be seen on a wet mount of the CSF. The CSF findings of granulomatous meningoencephalitis resemble those of aseptic meningitis. These amebae can be cultured.

Treatment: Naegleria infections have been successfully treated with regimens of amphotericin B, rifampin, and fluoconazole or ketoconazole; amphotericin B, rifampin, and chloramphenicol or ketoconazole; amphotericin B alone. The optimal duration of treatment is unknown. The optimal therapy for granulomatous amebic meningoencephalitis is also uncertain. Strains of *Acanthamoeba* are usually susceptible in vitro to pentamidine, ketoconazole, flucytosine, and less so to amphotericin B.

Centers for Disease Control and Prevention. Primary amebic meningoencephalitis-Georgia, 2002. MMWR 2003;52:962–4.

Weisse ME, Aronoff SC. Primary amebic meningo-encephalitis. In: Kliegman RM, Behrman RE, Jenson HB, Stanton BF (eds). *Nelson Textbook of Pediatrics.* 18th edn. Vol. 1. Philadelphia: Saunders, 2007;1458–60.

Giardiasis

Etiopathogenesis: Giardia lamblia is a flagellated protozoan that infects the duodenum and small intestine. The life cycle of *G. lamblia* is composed of 2 stages: Trophozoites and cysts. *Giardia* infects humans after ingestion of as few as 10–1000 cysts. Ingested cysts each produce 2 trophozoites in the duodenum. Trophozoites colonize the lumen of the duodenum and proximal jejunum, where they attach to the brush border of the intestinal epithelial cells and multiply by binary fission. As detached trophozoites pass down the intestinal tract, they encyst to form oval cysts. Cysts are passed in stools of infected individuals and may remain viable in water for as long as 2 mo. *Giardia* occurs worldwide. Infection is more prevalent in children than in adults. *Giardia* is endemic in areas of the world with poor levels of sanitation. *Giardia* infection usually occurs sporadically but is a frequently identified etiologic agent of outbreaks associated with drinking water. Person to person spread also occurs, particularly in areas of low hygiene standards, frequent fecal-oral contact, and crowding. Child care centers play an important role in transmission of urban giardiasis. Human milk contains glycoconjugates and secretory IgA antibodies that may provide protection to nursing infants.

Clinical manifestations: The incubation period of *Giardia* infection usually is 1–2 wk but may be longer. Children who are exposed to *G. lamblia* may experience asymptomatic excretion of organisms, acute infectious diarrhea, or chronic diarrhea with persistent gastrointestinal tract signs and symptoms, including failure to thrive and abdominal pain or cramping. Stools do not contain blood, mucus, or fecal leukocytes. Abnormal stool patterns may alternate with periods of constipation and normal bowel movement. Malabsorption of sugars, fats, and fat-soluble vitamins occurs and may be responsible for substantial weight loss.

Diagnosis: The diagnosis of giardiasis has been established by microscopy documentation of trophozoites or cysts in stool specimens, but 3 stool specimens are required to achieve a sensitivity of > 90%. Stool enzyme immunoassay (EIA) or direct fluorescent antibody tests for *Giardia* antigens are more sensitive for detecting of *Giardia* than microscopy.

Treatment: The recommended drug treatment of giardiasis is with metronidazole (15 mg/kg in 3 divided doses PO for 5–7 days) (efficacy 80–90%) or tinidazole single dose treatment (50 mg/kg once) (efficacy > 90%) or nitrozoxamide given for 3 days in two doses, with the dose depending on age (100 mg bid for 1–4 yr, 200 mg bid for 4–12 yr, 500 mg bid for > 12 yr) (efficacy 80–90%). Second line alternatives include albendazole, furazolidine, paromomycin and quinacrine.

Prevention: Infected persons and persons at risk should practice strict handwashing after any contact with feces.

Ali SA, Hill DR. *Giardia intestinalis. Curr Opin Infect Dis* 2003; 16 (5):453–60.

Homan WL, Mank TG. Human giardiasis: Genotype linked differences in clinical symptomatology. *Int J Parasitol* 2001; 31 (8):822–6.

John CC. Giardiasis and Balantidiasis. In: Kliegman RM, Behrman RE, Jenson HB, Stanton BF (eds). *Nelson Textbook of Pediatrics*. 18th edn. Vol. 1. Philadelphia: Saunders, 2007;1462–65.

Malaria

Malaria is still the world's most important parasitic disease and is responsible for the death of more people than any other communicable disease except tuberculosis. According to World Health Organization estimates, between 300 million and 500 million people are infected with malaria every year. The disease is a public health problem in more than 90 countries, which are home to some 2,400 million people, 40% the world's population.

Etiology: The causative agent of malaria is a protozoan, of the family Plasmodiidae, the genus *Plasmodium*: *P. falciparum*, *P. vivax*, *P. ovale*, or *P. malariae*. The majority of cases and almost all deaths are caused by *Plasmodium falciparum*. *Plasmodium vivax*, *Plasmodium ovale* and *Plasmodium malariae* cause less severe disease (*see* Figs 14.19 to 14.21 in CD).

Transmission: The parasite is transmitted by night-biting infected female Anopheles mosquitoes. In areas where domestically acquired malaria is rare, such cases include "runway" or "airport" malaria, in which local transmission of disease has been attributed to an infected mosquito that was transported on a long-haul flight, transmission by local mosquitoes that have acquired the infection from migrants or visitors, transfusion acquired infection and congenital infection. Congenital malaria occurs when the parasite is transmitted from the mother to the fetus via the placenta. Organ transplant is another rare mode of transmission.

Environment factors: Warm climates (temperature of 20–30°C) and abundant rain with high humidity (at least 60%) create favorable conditions for mosquitoes by increasing breeding areas and prolonging survival, thereby facilitating transmission. In India, the maximum prevalence is from July to November.

Life cycle of malaria parasite: Plasmodium species exist in the human host (asexual phase) and in the mosquito vector (sexual phase). To begin with the cycle, the female Anopheles mosquito injects sporozoites, less than 100 on each occasion, along with saliva into the circulating blood of the host and within 30 to 45 min the sporozoites enter hepatocytes thus initiating pre-erythrocytic or primary exoerythrocytic cycle. The mechanism of entry of sporozoites through the sinusoid lining into the space of Disse (or, might be through Kupffer cells on the walls of the sinusoids to reach the hepatocytes is unclear. Peptides forming part of the major surface protein on the sporozoite, the circumsporozoite protein (CSP), have been suggested to interact with receptors on the hepatocyte. Growth and division in the liver for the human malaria parasites take from approximately 6 to 15 days depending on the species. While *P. vivax* and *P. ovale* infect mainly the younger RBCs and *P. malariae* infects older cells, *P. falciparum* infects red blood cells of all ages. At the end of the pre-erythrocytic cycle, thousands of merozoites are released into the blood flowing through the sinusoids and, within 15 to 20 seconds, attach to and invade erythrocytes. Recognition and attachment are via a receptor-ligand interaction, and at least for *P. vivax* and *P. falciparum*, the host and parasite molecules involved are different. The asexual erythrocytic cycle produces more merozoites that are released with the destruction of the red blood cell after 48 or 72 hr for the human malaria parasites, depending on the species, and which then immediately invade additional erythrocytes. The asexual cycle usually continues until controlled by the immune response or chemotherapy or until the patient dies in the case of *P. falciparum*. In *P. vivax* and *P. ovale*, some of the sporozoites appear to develop for about 24 hr before becoming dormant as a hypnozoite stage; this form can remain as such for months and even years until reactivated to complete the liver cycle, releasing merozoites into the blood to precipitate a relapse infection. After invading red blood cells, eventually some merozoites differentiate into sexual forms (gametocytes) and, following ingestion by another female mosquito will mature to male and female gametes in the blood meal. After fertilization, the resulting zygote matures within 24 hr to the motile ookinete, which burrows through the midgut wall to encyst on the basal lamina, the extracellular matrix layer separating the hemocoel from the midgut. Within the developing oocysts, there are many mitotic divisions resulting in oocysts full of sporozoites. Rupture of the oocysts releases the sporozoites, which migrate through the hemocoel to the salivary glands to complete the cycle approximately 7 to 18 days after gametocyte ingestion, depending on host-parasite combination and external environmental conditions. All stages in the life cycle are thought to be haploid, apart from the diploid zygote, which immediately after fertilization undergoes a two-step meiotic division, the resulting cell containing a nucleus with four haploid genomes.

Immune response to malarial parasite: Although both non-specific as well as specific cellular and humoral immune responses are activated by malarial infection, such immune responses do not fully protect against either infection or disease. Moreover, the parasite evades the immune system because not only are the parasites in different inoculations genetically different, but during the course of each infection, the parasites from a single inoculation also undergoing clonal "antigenic variation". Therefore, to control an infection, the host must mount a new specific immune response to each new antigenic variant as it arises. Through this process, a single malarial infection can be prolonged over many months to years. Every individual in endemic area is continually exposed to malaria before they achieve some protective immunity against the diversity of malaria parasites and their antigens. However, having been achieved at such cost, effective immunity is readily lost again, perhaps within half a year to a year without reinfection.

Persons living in endemic area develop *"premunition"* that possibly protects them from serious illness but does not prevent re-infection. In premunition, parasites circulate in small numbers for long periods but do not multiply rapidly or cause severe illness. This premunition is species and strain specific and is often said to be "age dependent" (or "duration of exposure dependent"). Infants and the very young are more prone to malarial anemia, while cerebral damage due to *P. falciparum* malaria predominates in slightly older children. Yet other severe conditions, including renal, hepatic, and pulmonary failure, are most commonly seen in adults. Acquired immunity diminishes during pregnancy when women are at greatest risk of severe complication of malaria.

Newborn and young infants born to mothers residing in endemic area are protected by antibodies transferred transplacentally and through breast milk as well as due to the resistance of fetal hemoglobin (HbF) to growth of malarial parasite. Children with severe malnutrition also seem to have less incidence of severe malaria.

Genetic factors also determine the risk of acquiring malaria and having severe infection. Heterozygotes for sickle cell anemia, thalassemia, G6PD deficiency and hereditary ovalocytosis might be protected against severe falciparum malaria possibly because of defective parasite penetration into erythrocytes, its diminished growth within the red cells, rapid clearance by the reticuloendothelial system, and possibly oxidant membrane injury to erythrocytes in heterozygotes resulting in premature death of the parasite. A red cell antigen (Duffy factor) is necessary for invasion by *P. vivax* parasite and population with Duffy-negative blood type (e.g. Americans Black) are resistant to infection with *P. vivax*.

Pathophysiology: Infections caused by *P. vivax, P. ovale* and *P. malariae* are generally milder than falciparum malaria; symptoms are related to parasite burden and

cytokine release, since vaso-occlusive phenomena do not occur. The pathogenesis of malaria is best understood for *P. falciparum* infection. Disease due to *P. falciparum* is more severe and qualitatively different from disease caused by other plasmodia that infect humans. Several factors contribute to the severity of clinical disease. High parasite burdens combined with the unique ability of infected erythrocytes to adhere to host endothelium contribute to microvascular occlusion, metabolic derangement and acidosis, which lead to the manifestations of severe malaria (acute respiratory distress syndrome, renal insufficiency and cerebral malaria). In addition, a vigorous cytokine response to parasite proteins released during schizont rupture can contribute to adverse clinical outcomes. Manifestations of disease may also be related to intravascular hemolysis and parasite consumption of glucose. Host factors such as sickle cell disease and glucose-6-phosphate dehydrogenase deficiency can modify the severity of disease.

Clinical manifestations: The clinical signs and symptoms are produced by the asexual form of the parasite, which invade and destroy red cells, localize in critical organs and tissues in the body, and induce the release of many proinflammatory cytokines. Fever is the cardinal symptom of malaria. It can be intermittent with or without periodicity or continuous. Many cases have chills and rigors. Malaria should be suspected in patients residing in endemic areas and presenting with above symptoms. It should also be suspected in those patients who have recently visited an endemic area.

1. *Uncomplicated.* Disease manifestations are most classic in **non-immune individuals** and in areas where malaria transmission is seasonal. Non-immune people are at higher risk of developing severe or complicated malaria. More than 85% of travelers with malaria will experience symptoms only after they return from an endemic area. Clinically, malaria may present in different ways, but it is usually characterized by fever (which may be swinging), tachycardia, rigors, and sweating. Constitutional symptoms may include headache, body ache, fatigue and dizziness. Gastrointestinal symptoms including nausea, vomiting, abdominal pain, or diarrhea and respiratory symptoms like cough and dyspnea may accompany an attack. Fever and splenomegaly are the most frequent physical findings on examination. Less often, hepatomegaly, jaundice and abdominal tenderness are noted. The presence of rash and lymphadenopathy should suggest an additional or alternate diagnosis. The typical paroxysm resulting from lysis of parasitized RBCs has three stages. It begins with

the *cold stage* characterized by feeling of chills and rigors lasting for 1 to 2 hr. During the next few hr, the patient spikes a high fever and skin is warm and dry (*warm stage*). The last several hr are characterized by marked sweating, drop in temperature to normal or subnormal and feeling of fatigue (*wet stage*). Classically the fever has a tertian (occurring every 48 hr as in *P. vivax* or *P. ovale*) or quartan (every 72 hr as in *P. malariae*) periodicity; more commonly, the fever pattern is hectic. The classic fever pattern takes sometime to develop and often does not occur in *P. falciparum*. Lack of periodicity is common among children and does not rule out the diagnosis of malaria.

Semi-immune people such as those residing in endemic areas or those taking chemoprophylaxis may have delayed onset of illness and mild symptoms. A significant proportion (up to 80%) of semi-immune people with parasitemia may be completely asymptomatic. Fever is not a reliable indicator of malaria in endemic areas, but malaria must always be considered in the presence of fever. Headache, a feeling of cold and arthralgias are common presenting symptoms in children. Anemia, splenomegaly and hepatomegaly are commonly associated.

2. Severe malaria

Clinical manifestations: Severe manifestations can develop in *P. falciparum* infection over a span of time as short as 12–24 hr and may lead to death, if not treated promptly and adequately. Severe malaria is characterized by one or more of the following features: impaired consciousness/coma; repeated generalized convulsions; renal failure (serum creatinine > 3 mg/dl); jaundice (Serum bilirubin > 3 mg/dl); severe anemia (Hb < 5 g/dl); pulmonary edema/acute respiratory distress syndrome; hypoglycemia (plasma glucose < 40 mg/dl); metabolic acidosis; circulatory collapse/shock (Systolic BP < 80 mm Hg; < 50 mm Hg in children); abnormal bleeding and disseminated intravascular coagulation (DIC); hemoglobinuria; hyperpyrexia (temperature > 106°F or > 42°C); hyperparasitaemia (> 5% parasitized RBCs).

Foetal and maternal complications are more common in pregnancy with severe malaria; therefore, they need prompt attention.

Diagnosis of severe malaria cases negative on microscopy. Microscopic evidence may be negative for asexual parasites in patients with severe infections due to sequestration and partial treatment. Efforts should be made to confirm these cases by RDT or repeated microscopy. However, if clinical presentation indicates severe malaria and there is no alternative explanation these patients should be treated accordingly.

3. Severe and complicated malaria:
Almost invariably severe manifestations of malaria are due to *P. falciparum*. The major manifestations of severe malaria are shown in Table 14.12.

Cerebral malaria (CM): Cerebral malaria is a syndrome of diffuse encephalopathy with impairment of consciousness associated with *P. falciparum* infection (rarely with *P. vivax*) commonly seen in children 3 to 6 yr of age. Although various hypotheses have been proposed and some progress has been made using in vitro as well as in vivo models, the mechanisms of CM pathogenesis remain incompletely understood and are the subject of a continuing debate. The onset may be gradual but is generally sudden with 2 to 3 day history of fever. Alterations in consciousness range from drowsiness and/or convulsions to deep coma and brainstem abnormalities. Seizures are noted in 50–80% children. Prolonged seizures or those resistant to anticonvulsants are associated with the development of neurological sequelae or death. Findings include abnormal posturing (decerebrate, decorticate, opisthotonus), hemiplegia, absent or exaggerated deep tendon reflexes, pupillary changes, absent corneal reflexes, abnormal respiratory rhythms, and gaze abnormalities. Retinal hemorrhages have been seen in 6–36% children, while 2–12.5% shows papilledema associated with raised intracranial pressure. Parasitemia is generally high. Lumbar puncture reveals elevated pressure and cerebrospinal fluid protein with minimal or no pleocytosis and a normal glucose concentration. Case fatality rate is high (20–40%) but neurological sequelae among survivors are uncommon (10.9%) and many a times show dramatic resolution on follow-up. Sequelae have been associated with the presence of protracted seizures, deep or prolonged coma, and raised intracranial pressure. Sequelae include ataxia (common), paresis (common), hearing defects, visual field defects, aphasia, behavioral problems (restlessness, concentration problems, hallucinations, and aggression), developmental regression, recurrent convulsions (uncommon).

Anemia is a common and at times an inevitable consequence of severe malaria. A number of interacting mechanisms are believed to be responsible: removal of erythrocytes by the spleen, destruction of parasitized as well as non-parasitized RBC, dyserythropoiesis, and hemolysis associated with blackwater fever.

Renal failure and blackwater fever: This is a common complication of severe *P. falciparum* malaria that results from deposition of hemoglobin in renal tubules, decreased renal blood flow, and acute tubular necrosis.

Elevation of plasma creatinine is common but a disproportionate increase in blood urea suggests that elevated creatinine is probably caused by hypovolemia requiring aggressive repletion in intravascular volume. Blackwater fever is a rare clinical syndrome of severe intravascular hemolysis, hemoglobinuria, and renal failure usually seen in non-immune children. It is produced by a combination of complement and antibody mediated severe hemolysis leading to hemoglobinuria, oliguria and jaundice.

Hypoglycemia is commonly seen in children, pregnant women and those on quinine therapy and is associated with increased mortality and neurologic sequelae. Potential mechanisms that have been proposed including cytokine-induce suppression of gluconeogenesis, and increased glucose utilization by malarial parasite in the face increased demand due to fever and increased anaerobic glycolysis (which utilizes glucose much less efficiently to produce ATP). Quinine produces hypoglycemia by its capacity to induce hyperinsulinemia, and therefore can be prevented by administering quinine in 5% or 10% dextrose solution. Hypoglycemia should always be checked for by frequent blood glucose estimation as the symptoms of decreased level of consciousness may be confused with cerebral malaria.

Pulmonary edema may occur several days after therapy, is related to excessive intravenous fluid administration and may be rapidly fatal.

Acidosis: Lactic acidosis is one of the best markers of disease severity and mortality (Table 14.12) in malaria, and reflects increased lactate production (by anaerobic glycolysis) and its inadequate clearance by the body.

Algid malaria is a rare form *P. falciparum* malaria associate with overwhelming infection, hypotension, hypothermia, rapid thready pulse, shallow breathing and vascular collapse. Death may occur within a few hours.

Thrombocytopenia and DIC: Thrombocytopenia commonly accompanies falciparum and vivax malaria although a hemorrhagic diathesis is rare unless there is accompanying DIC. The degree of thrombocytopenia is frequently mild to moderate (> 50,000/mm^3) although it can decrease to 10,000–20,000/mm^3. It results from increased consumption of platelets during the acute infection with adequate megakaryocytes in the bone marrow. Changes in platelet aggregability also accompany thrombocytopenia.

**3. *Hyperreactive malarial syndrome (tropical splenomegaly syndrome, hyperreactive malarial splenomegaly):* ** Hyperreactive malarial syndrome (HMS) seen in patients living in endemic malaria (s)is characterized by massive splenomegaly, high concentration of total IgM and malarial antibodies of multiple immunoglobulin classes, and clinical and immunological response to antimalarial drugs. Its pathogenesis is unknown but appears to involve chronic exposure to malaria resulting in chronic stimulation of the immune system, as well as genetic factors. Any of the four species of Plasmodium may be involved. Physical examination reveals massive splenomegaly and hepatomegaly. Laboratory findings include anemia and increased reticulocyte count. Some patients have thrombocytopenia and neutropenia. Patients may have increased risk of bacterial infection. Some researchers have suggested that HMS is a premalignant condition. Treatment includes chronic chemoprophylaxis with chloroquine and/or proguanil for at least one year, and preferably lifelong.

**4. *Congenital malaria:* ** Congenital malaria is a rare entity (0.1–0.3% in semi-immune mothers and 8–10% in non-immune mothers). Newborn are protected against malaria partly by passively transferred maternal antibodies and partly because fetal hemoglobin (HbF) is resistant *P. falciparum* growth. All four types can be transmitted but *P. vivax* is more common. Clinically the baby develops poor feeding, vomiting, fever, diarrhea, irritability, anemia, thrombocytopenia, jaundice and hepatosplenomegaly. Therapy with erythrocytic schizonticidal drugs is curative. As there is no hypnozoite stage, primaquine therapy is not needed.

Relapses, recrudescence and reinfection: Recurrent infections are of three types: Relapses, recrudescence and reinfection. *Relapse* occurs because of delayed maturation of hypnozoites, the dormant liver stage parasites. *P. vivax* and *P. ovale* both give rise to hypnozoites in the liver. *P. vivax* malaria may relapse for up to 3 yr and *P. ovale* for 1–1.5 years. Only the sporozoites (introduced by the mosquitoes themselves) can penetrate the liver cells. Thus, if malaria is acquired by blood transfusion or transplacentally, no infection of the liver occurs and relapses do not occur. *P. falciparum* and *P. malariae* do not form hypnozoites, so they do not have true relapses. *Recrudescence* occurs when parasitemia caused by the surviving erythrocytic forms of the same parasite responsible for initial infection recurs after clearance or a significant reduction of initial parasitemia. This is most common with *P. falciparum* which can recrudesce for up to 1 year. *Reinfection* occurs with different parasite (than the one producing initial infection) as well as with more than one type of Plasmodium and occurs especially in areas with a high intensity of transmission. Persistent infection as a low-level parasitemia is noted with *P. malariae* that may continue to cause clinical malarial attacks even 20 yr after the original infection.

Diagnosis: All clinically suspected malaria cases should be investigated immediately by microscopy and/or Rapid Diagnostic Test (RDT). The definitive diagnosis of malaria is made by prompt microscopic examination of thick and thin blood films stained with Giemsa's or Field's stain. There is no need to wait for a fever peak before carrying out a blood film as parasites are often present throughout the red cell cycle. A negative finding on examination does not rule out malaria. Only 50% of children with malaria are smear-positive, even on repeated examination. At least 100–200 fields of a thick film should be scrutinized before a slide is reported as negative for malaria. In doubtful cases, the examination can be repeated after 4 hr. The thin blood film allows species differentiation, parasite staging as well as parasite quantification.

Polymerase chain reaction is useful for species identification and detecting low level of parasitemias, but is expensive, time consuming and requires specialized equipment which makes it suitable only for epidemiological and pharmacological studies. PCR has been especially effective at detecting sub-microscopic levels of parasitemia.

Serological tests provide confirmation of past malaria in patients and are valuable for epidemiological studies. These tests are also useful for screening donated blood and diagnosing hyperactive malarial splenomegaly. Among the tests used are the indirect fluorescent antibody test (IFAT), indirect hemagglutination antibody (IHA) test, and enzyme-linked immunosorbent assay (ELISA). All these tests produce positive results several days after malaria parasites appear in the blood and so do not help in the diagnosis of the acute infection for treatment purposes.

Rapid diagnostic tests (RDTs) are based on the detection of circulating parasite antigens. Several types of RDTs are available (http://www.wpro.who.int/sites/rdt). Some of them can only detect *P. falciparum*, while others can detect other parasite species also. The latter kits are expensive and temperature sensitive. NVBDCP (National Vector-borne Disease Control Programme) supplies RDT kits for detection of *P. falciparum* at locations where microscopy results are not obtainable within 24 hr of sample collection.

Lumbar puncture is indicated to rule out meningitis in cerebral malaria and febrile seizures with malaria.

Blood sugar: Severe *P. falciparum* malaria is often associated with hypoglycemia and low blood glucose levels are associated with higher mortality rates.

Moreover quinine administration itself can produce hypoglycemia. Hence, blood sugar should be checked not just at admission but even during the course of treatment.

Renal function test, serum electrolytes, arterial blood gas analysis, liver function test and *hemogram* may also form part of initial evaluation of complicated malaria.

Blood culture should be sent in patients who develop shock or other evidence of concomitant bacterial sepsis.

G6PD estimation may be required to differentiate blackwater fever from hemolysis due to G6PD deficiency and also prior to administration of primaquine.

Treatment

All fever cases diagnosed as malaria by RDT or microscopy should promptly be given effective treatment (Fig. 14.1; Tables 14.12 and 14.13). Table 14.12: Chloroquine (CQ) dosage schedule for *P. vivax*; Table 14.13: ACT (Artesunate + SP) dosage schedule for *P. falciparum* (Pf). Primaquine (2.5 mg base) for *P. vivax* (Pv)is given orally daily for 14 days as follows: < 1 yr (not prescribed); 1–4 yr one tablet; 5–8 yr two tablets; 9–14 yr four tablets. Do not give Primaquine to pregnant women and infants and G6PD deficiency cases. Primaquine (7.5 mg base) for *P. falciparum* (single dose on day 2) is given as follows: < 1 yr (not prescribed); 1–4 yr one tablet; 5–8 yr two tablets; 9–14 yr 4 tablets, 15 yr and above six tablets. Do not give Primaquine (PQ) to pregnant women and infants and G6PD deficiency cases.

A. *Treatment of Uncomplicated Malaria*

Treatment of P. vivax malaria: Confirmed *P. vivax* cases should be treated with chloroquine in full therapeutic doses of 25 mg/kg divided over 3 days. *P. vivax* may cause relapse in some patients (a form of *P. vivax* or *P. ovale* parasites called as hypnozytes remain dormant in the liver cells. These hypnozytes can later cause a relapse). For its prevention, primaquine should be given at a dose of 0.25 mg/kg body weight daily for 14 days under supervision. Primaquine is contraindicated in cases of G6PD deficient patients, infants and pregnant women. Primaquine can cause hemolysis in G6PD deficient patients; if such patients develop symptoms like dark colored urine, yellow conjunctiva, bluish discoloration of lips, abdominal pain, nausea, vomiting, etc. they should be advised to stop medicine immediately and should report to the doctor immediately.

Treatment of P. falciparum malaria: Artemisinin Combination Therapy (ACT) should be given to all confirmed *P. falciparum* cases found positive by microscopy or RDT. This is to be accompanied by a single dose primaquine (0.75 mg/kg body weight) on Day 2. ACT consists of an artemisinin derivative combined with a long acting antimalarial (amodiaquine, lumefantrine, mefioquine or sulfadoxine-pyrimethamine). The ACT recommended in the national programme in India is artesunate + sulfadoxine-pyrimethamine (SP). Presently, fixed dose combinations of artemether + lumefantrine, artesunate + amodiaquine and blister pack of artesunate + mefloquine are available for use in India. Oral artemisinin monotherapy is banned in India.

Treatment of malaria in pregnancy: ACT should be given for treatment of *P. falciparum* malaria in second and third trimesters of pregnancy, while quinine is recommended in the first trimester. *P. vivax* malaria can be treated with chloroquine.

Treatment of mixed infections: Mixed infections with *P. falciparum* should be treated as falciparum malaria. However, antirelapse treatment with primaquine can be given for 14 days, if indicated.

Treatment based on clinical criteria without laboratory confirmation: If RDT for only *P. falciparum* is used, negative cases showing signs and symptoms of malaria without any other obvious cause for fever should be considered as 'clinical malaria' and treated with chloroquine in full therapeutic dose of 25/kg body weight over three days. If a slide result is obtained later, the treatment should be completed according to species. Suspected malaria cases not confirmed by RDT or microscopy should be treated with chloroquine in full therapeutic dose.

General recommendations for the management of uncomplicated malaria

i. Avoid starting treatment on an empty stomach. The first dose should be given under observation.
ii. Dose should be repeated if vomiting occurs within 30 minutes.
iii. Patient should be asked to report back, if there is no improvement after 48 hr or if the situation deteriorates.
iv. Patient should also be examined for concomitant illnesses (Fig. 14.1).

B. Treatment Failure/Drug Resistance

After treatment patient is considered cured if he/she does not have fever or parasitemia till day 28. Some patients may not respond to treatment, which may be due to drug resistance, or treatment failure, especially in falciparum malaria. If patient does not respond, he/she should be given alternative treatment.

i. *Early treatment failure (EFT).* Development of danger signs or severe malaria on day 1, 2, or 3, in the presence of parasitemia; parasitemia on day 2 higher than on day 0, irrespective of axillary temperature; parasitemia on day 3 with axillary temperature $\geq$ 37.5°C; and parasitemia on day 3 $\geq$ 25% of count on day 0.
ii. *Late clinical failure (LCF).* Development of danger signs or severe malaria on days 1, 2, or 3, in the presence of parasitemia on any day between day 4 and day 28 (day 42) in patients who did not previously meet any of the criteria of early treatment failure; and presence of parasitemia on any day between day 4 and day 28 (day 42) with axillary temperature $\geq$37.5°C in patients who did not previously meet any of the criteria of early treatment failure.
iii. *Late parasitological failure (LPF).* Presence of parasitemia on any day between day 7 and day 28 with axillary temperature < 37.5°C in patients who did not previously meet any of the criteria of early treatment failure or late clinical failure is known as LPF.

Such cases of falciparum malaria should be given alternative ACT or quinine with doxycycline. Doxycycline is contraindicated in pregnancy, lactation and in children up to 8 years. Treatment failure with chloroquine in *P. vivax* malaria is rare in India.

C. Treatment of Severe Malaria

Diagnosis of severe malaria cases negative on microscopy: Microscopic evidence may be negative for asexual parasites in patients with severe infections due to sequestration and partial treatment. Efforts should be made to confirm these cases by RDT or repeated microscopy. However, if clinical presentation indicates severe malaria and there is no alternative explanation these patients should be treated accordingly.

Specific antimalarial treatment of severe malaria: Severe malaria is an emergency and treatment should be given promptly. *Parenteral artemisinin derivatives or quinine should be used irrespective of chloroquine sensitivity.*

*Artesunate 2.4 mg/kg IV or IM is given on admission (time=0), then at 12 hr and 24 hr, then once a day (dilute artesunate powder in 5% sodium bicarbonate provided in the pack).

*Quinine: 20 mg quinine salt/kg IV infusion in a 5% dextrose/dextrose saline over a period of 4 hr is given on admission, followed by maintenance dose of 10 mg/kg 8 hourly; infusion rate should not exceed

5 mg/kg/hr. Loading dose of 20 mg/kg should not be given, if the patient has already received quinine.

Never give bolus injection of quinine. If parenteral quinine therapy needs to be continued beyond 48 hr, dose should be reduced to 7 mg/kg 8 hourly.

****Artemether*** 3.2 mg/kg IM given on admission then 1.6 mg/kg/day.

***α-β Arteether** 150 mg daily IM for 3 days in adults only **(not recommended for children).**

Note:

*Once the patient can take oral therapy, further follow-up treatment should be as follows:

i. Patients receiving parenteral quinine should be treated with oral quinine 10 mg/kg three times a day to complete a course of 7 days, long with doxycycline 3 mg/kg per day for 7 days. (Doxycycline is contraindicated in pregnant women and children under 8 yr of age; instead, clindamycin 10 mg/kg 12 hourly for 7 days should be used.)

ii. Patients receiving artemisinin derivatives should get full course of ACT. However, ACT containing mefloquine should be avoided in cerebral malaria due to neuropsychiatric complications.

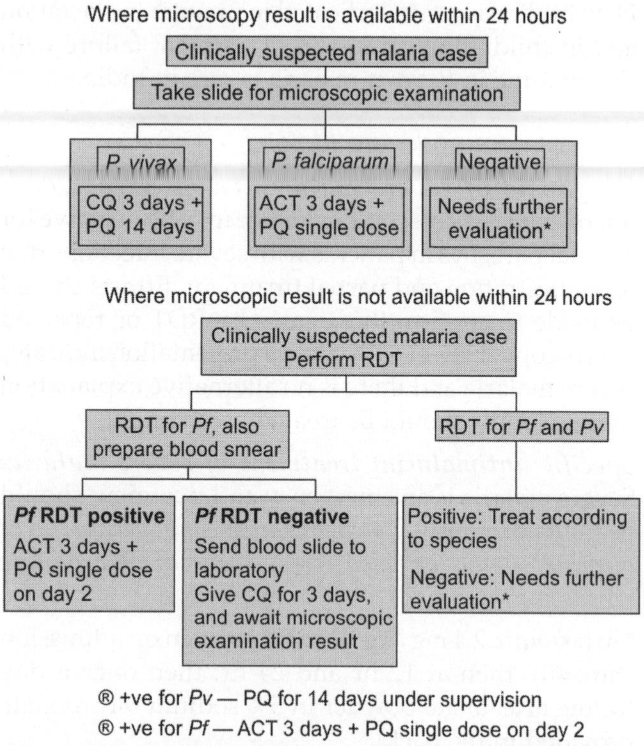

Look for other causes of fever, repeat blood slide examination after an appropriate interval. ACT: Artemesinin combination therapy; CQ: Chloroquine; PQ: Primaquine; *Pf*: *P. falciparum*; *PV*: *P. vivax*; RDT: Rapid diagnostic test

Fig.14.1: Algorithm for diagnosis and treatment of malaria

*Intravenous preparations should be preferred over intramuscular preparations. Parenteral treatment should be given for minimum of 24 hr once started.

*In first trimester of pregnancy, parenteral quinine is the drug of choice. However, if quinine is not available, artemisinin derivatives may be given to save the life of mother. In second and third trimester, parenteral artemisinin derivatives are preferred.

Severe malaria due to P. vivax: Some cases have been reported in India of severe malaria due to *P. vivax*. Severe malaria caused by *P. vivax* should be treated like severe *P. falciparum* malaria.

Requirements for management of complications: For management of severe malaria, health facilities should be equipped with the following:

i. Parenteral antimalarials, antipyretics, antibiotics, and anticonvulsants
ii. Intravenous infusion facilities
iii. Special nursing for patients in coma
iv. Blood transfusion
v. Well equipped laboratory
vi. Oxygen. If these items are not available, the patient must be referred without delay to a facility, where they are available.

Chemoprophylaxis is recommended for travelers, migrant labourers and military personnel exposed to malaria in highly endemic areas. *Short-term chemoprophylaxis* **(less than 6 weeks)** with Doxycycline (1.5 mg/kg for children more than 8 yr old and 100 mg daily in adults) should be started 2 days before travel and continued for 4 wk after leaving the malarious area. Doxycycline is contraindicated in pregnant and lactating women and children less than 8 years. Use of personal protection measures like insecticide-treated bed-nets should be encouraged for pregnant women and other vulnerable population. Mefloquine (5 mg/kg body weight (up to 250 mg) weekly should be administered two weeks before, during and four weeks after leaving the area. Mafloquine is contraindicated in cases with history of convulsions, neuropsychiatric problems and cardiac conditions.

Prevention: Reducing vector-human contact is the most effective means of individual malaria protection. Cover the body while outdoors. Wear full-length sleeves and trousers. Diethyl-m-toluamide (DEET) is an effective mosquito repellent when applied on the skin. Increased precautions are needed during the night because Anopheles species are nocturnal in habit. Sleeping under insecticide treated (permethrin 0.2 g/m^2 of material every 6 mo) mosquito nets is perhaps the most beneficial antimalarial measure available, which should be encouraged for pregnant women and other vulnerable population. Bedrooms should be sprayed with an aerosol insecticide at dusk.

Afzal K, Afzal S. Malaria in children. In: Mathur GP, Mathur Sarla (eds). *Current Trends in Pediatrics.* Vol 1. Delhi: Academa Publishers, 2005;398–420.

Drug resistance in malaria.WHO/CDS/CSR/DRS/2001.4

Guidelines for diagnosis and treatment of Malaria in India. Government of India, National vector Borne Disease Control Programme, 2010:1–14.

Hien TT, White NJ. Qinghaosu. *Lancet* 1993; 341: 603–608.

Kocar DK, Das A, Kochar SK et al. Severe *Plasmoium vivax* malaria: A report on serial cases from Bikaner in northwestern India. *Am J Trop Med Hyg* 2009;80(2):194–8.

Krause PJ. Malaria. In: Kliegman RM, Behrman RE, Jenson HB, Stanton BF (eds). *Nelson Textbook of Pediatrics.* 18th edn. Vol. 1. Philadelphia: Saunders, 2007;1477–85.

Malaria in India. Guidelines for its control. National Vector Borne Disease Control Programme. http://www.nvbdcp.gov.in/malaria-new.html

National drug policy on malaria. Ministry of Health and Family Welfare/Directorate of National Vector Borne Disease Control Programme, Govt. of India. http://www.nvbdcp.gov.in/malaria-new.html

Rapid diagnostic tests. . Website of WHO Regional Office for the Western Pacific. http://www.wpro.who.int/sites/rdt

Regional guidelines for the management of severe falciparum malaria in small hospitals. World Health Organization. Regional Office for South-East Asia (2006). New Delhi, WHO/SEARO.http://www.searo.who.int/LinkFiles/Tools_&_Guidelines_Smallhospitals.pdf

Regional guidelines for the management of severe falciparum malaria in large hospitals. World Health Organization. Regional Office for South-East Asia (2006). New Delhi, WHO/SEARO.http://www.searo.who.int/LinkFiles/Tools_&_Guidelines_Lmallhospitals.pdf

WHO Guidelines for the Treatment of Malaria, second edition. Geneva. World Health Organization (2010). http/www.who.int/malaria/publications/atoz/9789241547925/enindex.html

Leishmaniasis

Etiology: *Leishmania* organisms are members of the Trypanosomiasis family and include 2 subgenera *Leishmania* (*Leishmania*) and *Leishmania viannia*). The parasite is dimorphic, existing as a flagellate promastigote in the insect vector and as an aflagellate amastigote that resides and replicates only within mononuclear phagocytes of the vertebrate host. Within the sandfly vector the promostigote changes from a noninfective procyclic form to an infective metacyclic stage. The infective metacyclic stage is inoculated by the sandfly to the host during the blood meal, where it enters the macrophage. Once within the macrophage, the promastigote transforms to an amastigote and resides and replicates within a phagolysosome. The parasite is resistant to the acidic, hostile environment of the macrophage and eventually ruptures the cell and goes on to infect other

Table 14.12: Chloroquine dosage schedule for *P. vivax*

Age in years	Number of tablets		
	Day 1 (10 mg/kg)	Day 2 (10 mg/kg)	Day 3 (5 mg/kg)
<1	½	½	1/4
1–4	1	1	½
5–8	2	2	1
9–14	3	3	1½
15 and above	4	4	2

Table 14.13: ACT (Artesunate + SP) dosage schedule for *P. falciparum*

Age in years		Number of tablets		
		1st day	2nd day	3rd day
<1	AS	½	½	½
	SP	¼	Nil	Nil
1–4	AS	1	1	1
	SP	1	Nil	Nil
5–8	AS	2	2	2
	SP	1½	Nil	Nil
9–14	AS	3	3	3
	SP	2	Nil	Nil
15 and above	AS	4	4	4
	SP	3	Nil	Nil

AS: Artesunate 50 mg; SP: Sulfadoxine

macrophages. Infected macrophages have diminished capacity to initiate and respond to an inflammatory response, thus provided a safe heaven for the intracellular parasite. Leishmaniasis is caused by intracellular protozoan parasites of the genus *Leishmania*, which are transmitted by phlebotomine sandflies.

Clinical manifestations: The four different forms of the disease are distinct in their causes, epidemiologic features, transmission, and geographic distribution.

1. *Localized cutaneous leishmaniasis. LCL (Oriental sore)* can affect individuals of any age, but children are the primary victims in many endemic regions. It typically presents as 1 or a few popular, nodular, plaque-like, or ulcerative lesions that are usually located on exposed skin, such as the face and extremities. The lesions typically begin as a small papule at the site of the sandfly bite, which enlarges to 1–3 cm in diameter and may ulcerate over the course of several weeks to months. The shallow ulcer is usually nontender and surrounded by a sharp, indurated, erythematous margin. There is no drainage unless there is a bacterial superinfection develops. Lesions caused by *L. major* and *L. maxicana* usually heal spontaneously after 3–6 mo, leaving a depressed scar. Lesions on the ear pinna caused by *L. maxicana*, called chiclero ulcer, because they are common in chicle harvesters in Mexico and Central America, often

follows a chronic, destructive course. In general, lesions caused by *L. viannia* species tend to be larger and more chronic characterized by regional lymphadenopathy and palpable subcutaneous nodules or lymphatic cords, the so-called sporotrichoid appearance.

2. *Diffuse cutaneous leishmaniasis.* DCL is a rare form of leishmaniasis caused by *L. Mexicana* in the New World and *L. aethiopica* in the Old World. DCL manifests as large nonulcerating macules, papules, nodules, or plaques that involve large areas of the skin, particularly face and extremities. Dissemination from the initial lesion usually takes place over several years. It is thought to be an immunologic defect.

3. *Mucosal leishmaniasis. ML (espundia)* is an uncommon but serious manifestation of leishmanial infection resulting from hematogenous metastases from a cutaneous infection to the nasal or oropharyngeal mucosa. It is usually caused by parasites in the *L. viannia* complex. Approximately half of the patients with mucosal lesions have had active cutaneous lesions within the preceding 2 yr, but ML may not develop until many years after resolution of the primary lesion. Marked soft tissue, cartilage, and even bone destruction occurs late in the course of disease and may lead to visible deformity of the nose or mouth, nasal septal perforation, and tracheal narrowing with airway obstruction.

4. *Visceral leishmaniasis. VL (kala-azar)* typically affects children < 5 yr of age in the New World (*L. chagasi*) and Mediterranean region (*L. infantum*) and older children and young adults in Africa and Asia (*L. donovani*). After inoculation of the organism in to the skin by the sandfly, the child may have a completely asymptomatic infection or an oligosymptomatic illness that either resolves spontaneously or into active kala-azar. Children with *asymptomatic infection* are transiently seropositive but show no clinical evidence of disease. Children who are *oligosymptomatic* have mild constitutional symptoms (malaise, intermittent diarrhea, poor activity tolerance) and intermittent fever; most will have a mildly enlarged liver. In most of these children the illness will resolve without therapy, but in approximately 1/4 it will evolve to active kala-azar within 2–8 mo. Rarely, incubation periods of several years have been described. During the 1st few weeks to months of disease evolution the fever is intermittent, weakness and loss of energy, and the spleen begins to enlarge. Children with *classic clinical features* of kala-azar consist of high fever, marked splenomegaly, hepatomegaly, and severe cachexia typically develop approximately 6 mo after the onset of the illness, but a rapid clinical

course over 1 mo has been noted in up to 20% of patients. At the terminal stages of kala-azar there is massive hepatosplenomegaly, gross wasting, and profound pancytopenia; jaundice, edema, and ascites may be present. Severe anemia may precipitate heart failure. Bleeding episodes, especially epistaxis, are frequent. During the late stage of illness secondary bacterial infections occur. Younger age at the time of infection and underlying malnutrition are risk factors for the development of more rapid development of VL. Death occurs in > 90% of patients without specific antileishmanial treatment.

India is one of the 28 countries in world reporting leishmaniasis and HIV co-infection. The vulnerability is evident by the fact that India has almost one-half of world's VL cases; and HIV/AIDS cases are on a sharp increase. Leishmaniasis may also result from reactivation of a long-standing subclinical infection. Frequently there is an atypical clinical presentation of VL in HIV-infected individuals with prominent involvement of the gastrointestinal tract and absence of typical hepatosplenomegaly.

Few patients previously treated for VL develop diffuse skin lesions, a condition known as post-kala-azar dermal leishmaniasis (PKDL). These lesions may appear during or shortly after therapy (Africa) or upto several years later (India). The lesions of PKDL are hyperpigmented, erythematous, or nodular and commonly involve the face and torso. They may persist for several months or for many years.

The Indian term kala-azar is used for visceral leishmaniasis (VL) disease (Kala-black; Azar-sickness). Kala-azar is most often reported from Bihar, Eastern Uttar Pradesh, and Eastern Indian states. Leishmaniasis is caused by parasites of the genus Leishmania donovani, which are transmitted by female sandflies of the genus Phlebotomus (Phlebotomus agetipes). *Leishmania tropica* also has been recognized as an uncommon cause of visceral disease. Human appears to be the only reservoir of infection. Modes of transmission of infection:

i. Natural transmission of *L. donovani* from man to man by sandfly *Phlebotomus argentipes*
ii. Congenital infection of a baby *in utero*
iii. Blood transfusion
iv. Sexual intercourse
v. Accidental needle prick.

Incubation period is generally 2 to 8 mo, although it may be as long as 2 yr. The onset is insidious in most cases. All age groups including infants. Peak age is 5–9 yr; Male: female 2 : 1. Few patients previously treated for VL develop diffuse skin lesions, a condition known as post-kala-azar dermal leishmaniasis (PKDL). Treatment is done by sodium stibogluconate, amphotericin B desoxycholate, liposomal amphotericin B, aminoglycoside paromomycin (aminosidine), and miltefosine. Cure rates with sodium stibogluconate regimen of 80–100% for VL were reported in the 1990s, but lower initial cure rates have been noted recently due to clinical resistance to antimony therapy in India. Miltefosine has a cure rate of 95% in Indian patients with VL. Early recognition and treatment of cases are essential because man to man transmission is an important preventive measure.

Differential diagnosis: The differential diagnosis of LCL includes cutaneous tuberculosis, atypical mycobacterial infection, leprosy, syphilis, yaws, sporotrichosis, blastomycosis and neoplasms. Infections such as syphilis, yaws, histoplasmosis, sarcoidosis, Wegener granulomatosis, and carcinoma may have clinical features similar to those of ML. VL should be suspected in patients with prolonged fever, weakness, cachexia, marked splenomegaly, hepatomegaly, cytopenia and hypergammaglobulinemia who have had potential exposure in an endemic area. The clinical picture of VL may also be consistent with that of malaria, typhoid fever, military tuberculosis, infectious mononucleosis, schistosomiasis, brucellosis, amebic liver abscess, lymphoma, and leukemia.

Laboratory findings: Patients with cutaneous or mucosal leishmaniasis generally do not have abnormal laboratory findings unless the lesions are secondarily infected with bacteria. Laboratory findings associated with classic kala-azar include anemia (hemoglobin 5–8 mg/dl), thrombocytopenia, leulopenia (2,000–3,000 cells/µl), elevated hepatic transaminase levels, and hyperglobulinemia (> 5g/dl) that is mostly immunoglobulin G (IgG).

Diagnosis: The development of one or several slowly progressive non-tender, nodule or ulcerative lesions in a patient who had potential exposure in an endemic area should raise suspicion of LCL. Definitive diagnosis of leishmaniasis is established by the demonstration of amastigotes in tissue specimens or isolation of the organism by culture. Amastigotes can be identified in Giemsa-stained tissue sections, aspirates, or impression smears in about half the cases of LCL but only rarely in the lesions of ML. Culture of a tissue biopsy or aspirate, best performed by using Novy-McNeal-Nicolle (NNN) biphasic blood agar medium, yields a positive finding in only about 65% of cases of cutaneous leishmaniasis (CL). Identification of parasites in smears, histopathologic sections, or culture medium is more readily accomplished in DCL than in LCL. In patients with VL, smears or cultures of material from splenic, bone marrow, or lymph node aspirations are usually diagnostic (*see* Fig. 14.22 in CD). Splenic aspiration has a higher diagnostic sensitivity, but should be performed with great care because of the risk for bleeding complications. The diagnosis of species of *Leishmania* usually by isoenzyme analysis has therapeutic and prognostic significance.

Serologic tests are not useful for diagnosis of ML or LCL because they generally have low sensitivity and specificity. Serologic testing by enzyme immunoassay, indirect fluorescence assay, or direct agglutination is very useful in VL because of the very high level of antileishmanial antibodies. An enzyme-linked immunosorbent assay using a recombinant antigen (K39) has a sensitivity and specificity for VL that is close to 100%. A negative serologic test in an immunocompetent individual is against a diagnosis of VL. Serodiagnostic tests are positive in only about half of the patients who are co-infected with HIV.

Treatment: Specific antileishmanial therapy is not routinely indicated for uncomplicated LCL caused by *L. major* and *L. Mexicana*. Lesions that are extensive, severely inflamed, or located where a scar would result in disability (near a joint) or cosmetic disfigurement (face or ear), that involve the lymphatics, or that do not begin healing within 3–4 mo should be treated. Cutaneous lesions suspected or known to be caused by the members of the *Viannia* subgenus and *L. tropica* should also be treated. All patients with VL or ML should be treated.

The recommended regimen for *sodium stibogluconate* (pentavalent antimony compound) is 20 mg/kg/day intravenously or intramuscularly for 20 days (for LCL and DCL) or 28 days (for ML and VL). Repeated courses of therapy may be necessary in patients with severe cutaneous lesions, ML, or VL. An initial clinical response to therapy usually occurs in the 1st wk of therapy, but complete clinical healing (re-epithelialization and scarring for LCL and ML and regression of splenomegaly and normalization of cytopenias for VL) usually takes weeks to a few months after completion of therapy. Cure rates with this regimen of 90–100% for LCL, 50–70% for ML, and 80–100% for VL were reported in the 1990s, but lower initial cure rates have been noted recently in the regions where clinical resistance to antimony therapy is common, such as India, East Africa, and some parts of Latin America. Relapses are common in patients who do not have an effective antileishmanial cellular immune response, such as those who have DCL or are co-infected with HIV. These patients often require multiple courses of therapy or a chronic suppressive regimen. When clinical relapses occur, they are usually evident within 2 mo after completion of therapy. Adverse effects of antimony therapy are dose and duration dependent and include fatigue, arthralgias and myalgias (50%), abdominal discomfort (30%), elevated hepatic transaminase level (30–80%), elevated amylase and lipase levels (almost 100%), mild hematologic changes (slightly decreased leukocyte count, hemoglobin level and platelet count) (10–30%), and nonspecific T-wave changes on the electrocardiography (30%). Sudden death due to cardiac toxicity is usually associated with use of very high doses of pentavalent antimony and is extremely rare.

Amphotericin B desoxycholate and the amphotericin lipid formulations are very useful in the treatment of VL or ML, and in some regions replaced antimony as 1st line therapy. *Amphotericin B desoxycholate* at doses of 0.5–1.0 mg/kg every day or every other day for 14–20 doses achieved a cure rate for VL of close to 100%., but renal toxicity commonly associated with amphotericin B was common. The lipid formulations of amphotericin B are more suitable for treatment of leishmaniasis because the drugs are concentrated in the reticuloendothelial system and are less nephrotoxic. *Liposomal amphotericin B* (Ambisome, 3 mg/kg on days 1–5, and again on day 10) has been shown to be highly effective with a 90-100% cure rate for VL in immunocompetent children, some of whom were refractory to antimony therapy.

Parenteral treatment of VL with the *aminoglycoside paromomycin (aminosidine)* has efficacy (~95%) similar to that of amphotericin B in India.

Recombinant human interferon-γ has been successfully used as an adjunct to antimony therapy in the treatment of refractory cases of ML and VL. It is not effective alone and has the frequent side effects of fever and flu-like symptoms.

Miltefosine, a membrane-activating alkylphopholipid, is the 1st oral treatment for VL and has a cure rate of 95% in Indian patients with VL when administered orally at 50–100 mg/day for 28 days. Gastrointestinal adverse effects are frequent but do not require discontinuation of drug.

Treatment of LCL with oral drugs has had only modest success. Miltefosine 2.5 mg/kg/day orally for 20 days had a 91% efficacy in treating CL in Columbia (*L. panamensis*), but was significantly less effective in patients from Guatemala (*L. braziliensis*).

Fluconazole 200 mg orally once daily for 6 wk was demonstrated in adults to modestly increase the rate of healing of CL caused by *L. major* in Saudi Arabia.

Topical treatment of CL with *paromomycin plus methylbenzethonium chloride* ointment has been effective in selected cases in the both old and new world.

Prevention: Personal protective measures should include avoidance of exposures to the nocturnal sandflies and, when necessary, the use of insect repellent and permethrin-impregnated mosquito netting. Community-based residual insecticide spraying has had some success in reducing the prevalence of leishmaniasis. Early recognition and treatment of cases are essential where anthroponotic transmission, in which humans are the presumed reservoir, occurs in India, Sudan and in some urban areas of the Middle East.

Bern C, Hightower AW, Chowdhury R, et al. Risk factors for kala-azar in Bangladesh. *Emerg Infec Dis* 2005;11:655–62.

Bhattacharya SK, Jha TK, Sunder S, et al. Efficacy and tolerability of miltefosine for childhood visceral leishmaniasis in India. *Clin Infect Dis* 2004;38:217–21.

Melby PC. Leishmaniasis. In: Kliegman RM, Behrman RE, Jenson HB, Stanton BF (eds). *Nelson Textbook of Pediatrics*. 18th edn. Vol. 1. Philadelphia: Saunders, 2007; 1468–71.

Prasasd LSN. Kala-azar (Leishmaniasis) in Indian children. *Asian J Pediatr* 1977;1:31–38.

Sundar S, Mehta H, Suresh AV, et al. Amphotericin B treatment for Indian visceral leishmaniasis: Conventional versus lipid formulations. *Clin Infect Dis* 2004;38:377–83.

African Trypanosomiasis

Human trypanosomiasis, or African sleeping sickness, is a vector-borne disease caused by a parasitic trypanosome that is transmitted to humans through the bite of a tsetse fly. Symptoms usually occur within 1–4 wk of infection. The clinical syndromes of African trypanosomiasis are described as the trypanosomal chancre, hemolymphatic stage, and meningoencephalitic stage. *Trypanosomal chancre* or nodule develops in 2–3 days and within 1 wk becomes painful, hard, red nodule surrounded by an area of erythema and swelling at the site of the tsetse fly bite. Nodules are commonly seen on the lower limbs but sometimes also on the head. They subside spontaneously in about 2 wk, leaving no permanent scar. During *Hemolymphatic stage* the characteristic features occur 2–3 wk after infection includes irregular episodes of fever, headache, sweating, and generalized lymphadenopathy. *Meningoencephalitic stage* is known as *sleeping sickness*. Drowsiness and an uncontrollable urge to sleep are the major features of this stage of the disease and may become almost continuous in the terminal stages. Definitive *diagnosis* can be established during the early stages by examination of a fresh, thick blood smear, which demonstrates the motile active forms.

Treatment for the hematogenous forms is suramin (10% solution), which is administered intravenously. A test dose (10 mg for children; 100–200 mg for adults) is first administered intravenously to detect the rare idiosyncratic reactions of shock and collapse. The dose for subsequent IV injection is 20 mg/kg (maximum 1 g) administered on days 1, 3, 7, 14, and 21. Pentamidine isethionate (4 mg/kg/day IM for 10 days) is better tolerated than suramin.

Barrett MP. The rise and fall of sleeping sickness. *Lancet* 2006;367:1377–78.

Barrett MP, Burchmore RJS, Stich A, et al. The trypanosomiases. *Lancet* 2003;363:1469–80.

Bonomo RA, Salata RA. African trypanosomiasis. In: Kliegman RM, Behrman RE, Jenson HB, Stanton BF (eds). *Nelson Textbook of Pediatrics*. 18th edn. Vol. 1. Philadelphia: Saunders, 2007;1471–4.

Chagas' Disease

Etiology: Chagas' disease is caused by *Trypanosoma cruzi. (T. cruzi)* has 3 recognizable morphogenetic phases: amastigotes, trypomastigotes, and epimastigotes.

Epidemiology: Chagas' disease is found only in the Western hemisphere and is now endemic in 18 countries and in 2 ecological zones of America: Mexico and South America, particularly Brazil, Argentina, Uruguary, Chile, and Venezuela. The World Health Organization estimates that Chagas' disease affects close to 20 million people, primarily children and young adults.

Clinical manifestations: Chagas' disease occurs in acute and chronic forms. *Acute Chagas' disease* in children is usually asymptomatic or is associated with a mild febrile illness characterized by malaise, focal edema, and lymphadenopathy. Infants often demonstrate local signs of inflammation at the site of parasite entry, or chagomas (Chagoma is a local tissue reaction and the process extends to local lymph node). Approximately 50% of children come to medical attention with the *Ramoòa sign* (unilateral, painless eye swelling), conjunctivitis, and preauricular lymphadenitis. Patients complain of fatigue and headache. Fever can persist for 4–5 wk. more severe presentations can occur in children < 2 yr of age and include lymphadenopathy, hepatosplenomegaly, and meningoencephalitis. A cutaneous morbilliform eruption, anemia, lymphocytosis, hepatitis and thrombocytopenia have been described. The heart, central nervous system, peripheral nerve ganglia, and reticuloendothelial system are often heavily parasitized.

Intrauterine infection in pregnant women can cause spontaneous abortion or premature birth. In children with congenital infection, severe anemia, hepatosplenomegaly, jaundice, and convulsions can mimic congenital cytomegalovirus infection, toxoplasmosis, and erythroblastosis fetalis. *T. cruzi* can be visualized in the CSF in meningoencephalitis. Children usually undergo spontaneous remission in 8–12 wk with life-long low-grade parasitemia and development of the antibodies. The mortality rate is 5–10%, with deaths caused by acute myocarditis with resultant heart failure, or meningoencephalitis. Acute Chagas' disease must be differentiated from malaria, schistosomiasis, visceral leishmaniasis, brucellosis, typhoid fever and infectious mononucleosis.

Chronic Chagas' disease may be asymptomatic or symptomatic. The most common presentation of chronic *T. cruzi* infection is cardiomyopathy manifested by congestive heart failure, arrhythmia, and thromboembolic events. Gastrointestinal manifestations of chronic Chagas' disease occur in 8–10% of patients, clinically as megaesophagus and megacolon. Sigmoid dilatation, volvulus, and fecalomas are often found in megacolon. Megaesophagus can lead to esophagitis and cancer of the esophagus. Aspiration pneumonia and pulmonary tuberculosis are more common in patients with megaesophagus. Autonomic dysfunction and peripheral neuropathy can occur. Central nervous system involvement in Chagas' disease is uncommon. If granulomatous encephalitis occurs in the acute infection, it is usually fatal.

Immunocompromised persons: T. cruzi infections in immunocompromised persons are caused by transmission from an asymptomatic donor of blood products or activation of prior infection by immunosuppression. Organ donation to allograft recipients can result in a devastating form of the illness. Cardiac transplantation for Chagas' cardiomyopathy has resulted in reactivation despite prophylaxis and postoperative treatment with benzimidazole. HIV infection also leads to reactivation; cerebral lesions are more common. Therefore, it is necessary in immunocompromised patients at risk for reactivation for serologic testing and close monitoring.

Diagnosis: A detailed history with particular information regarding geographic origin and travel is important. Microscopic examination of a fresh preparation of a peripheral blood smear or a Giemsa-stained smear during the acute phase of illness will demonstrate motile trypanosomiasis, which is diagnostic for Chagas' disease. These are only seen in the peripheral blood in the 1st 6–12 wk of the illness. Buffy coat smears may show more parasites.

During the chronic phase of the disease, when parasites are not found in the bloodstream and clinical symptoms are not diagnostic, complement fixation is considered the most reliable immunodiagnostic method for establishing the diagnosis. Specific IgM antibodies can be detected using an enzyme-linked immunosorbent assay (ELISA) and indirect fluorescent antibody testing.

Treatment: Two drugs: nifurtimox and benzimidazoles are available for the treatment of *T. cruzi*. Neither drug is safe in pregnancy. The treatment regime with *Nifurtimox* for children 1–10 yr of age is 15–20 mg/kg/day divided qid PO for 90 days; for children 11–16 yr of age, 12.5–15 mg/kg/day divided qid PO for 90 days; and for children >16 yr of age, 8–10 mg/kg/day divided tid to qid PO for 90–120 days. The recommended treatment regimen with *Benzimidazoles* for children < 12 yr of age is 10 mg/kg/day divided bid PO for 60 days, and for those > 12 yr of age is 5–7 mg/kg/day PO for 60 days. This drug is also associated with significant toxicities, including rash, photosensitivity, peripheral neuritis, and granulocytopenia and thrombocytopenia.

A light balanced diet is recommended for megaesophagus. Surgery or dilation of the lower esophageal sphincter treats' megaesophagus; pneumatic dilaton is the superior mode of therapy. Nitrates and nifedipine have been used to reduce lower esophageal sphincter pressure in patients with megaesophagus. Treatment of megacolon is surgical and symptomatic. No vaccine or prophylactic therapy is currently available.

Barrett MP, Burchmore RJS, Stich A, et al. The trypanosomiases. *Lancet* 2003;363:1469–80.

Bonomo RA, Salata RA. American trypanosomiasis. In: Kliegman RM, Behrman RE, Jenson HB, Stanton BF (eds). *Nelson Textbook of Pediatrics*. 18th edn. Vol. 1. Philadelphia: Saunders, 2007;1474–77.

Prata A. Clinical and epidemiological aspects of Chagas' disease. *Lancet Infect Dis* 2001;1:92–100.

Toxoplasmosis

Etiopathogenesis: *Toxoplasma Gondii* is the causative protozoa for toxoplasmosis that multiplies only in living cells. *Toxoplasma* can multiply in all tissues of mammals and birds. Newly infected cats and other *Felidae* species excrete infectious *Toxoplasma* oocysts in their feces. *Toxoplasma* organisms are transmitted to cats by ingestion of infected meat containing encysted bradyzoites or by ingestion of oocysts excreted by other recently infected cats. *T. gondii* is acquired by children and adults from ingesting food that contains cysts or that is contaminated with oocysts usually from acutely infected cats. Oocysts also may be transported to food by flies and cockroaches. When the organism is ingested, bradyzoites are released from cysts or sporozoites from oocysts. The organisms enter gastrointestinal cells where they multiply, rupture cells, infect contiguous cells, enter the lymphatics, and disseminate hematogenously throughout the body. *Toxoplasma* infection is ubiquitous in animals and is one of the most common latent infections of humans throughout the world. *Toxoplasma* organisms are not transmitted from person to person except for transplacental infection from mother to fetus and, rarely, by organ transplantation or transfusion.

Clinical manifestations: The manifestations of primary infection with *T. gondii* are highly variable and influenced primarily by host immunocompetence. Immunocompetent children who acquire infection postnatally include any combination of fever, stiff neck, myalgia, arthralgia, maculopapular rash that spares the palms and soles, localized or generalized lymphadenopathy, hepatomegaly, hepatitis, reactive lymphocytosis, meningitis, brain abscess, encephalitis, pneumonia, polymyositis, pericarditis, pericardial effusion, and myocarditis. Various neurologic lesions include hydrocephalus, seizures, spinal or bulbar involvement, microcephaly, and intellectual impairment. Endocrinopathies include myxedema, persistent hypernatremia with vasopressin-sensitive diabetes insipidus without polyuria or polydipsia, sexual precocity, and partial anterior hypopituitarism.

Eyes: Almost all untreated congenitally infected infants develop choreoretinal lesions by adulthood, and about 50% will have severe visual impairment. Other ocular findings include strabismus, nystagmus, visual impairment, microphthalmia, cells and protein in the anterior chamber, large keratic precipitates, posterior synechiae, nodules on the iris, and neovascular formation on the surface of the iris, sometimes with increased intraocular pressure and glaucoma.

Ears: Sensorineural hearing loss, both mild and severe, may occur.

Immunocompromised persons: Disseminated *T. gondii* infection among older children who are immunocompromised by AIDS, malignancy, cytotoxic therapy or corticosteroids, or immunosuppressive drugs given for organ transplantation involves the CNS in 50% of cases and may also involve heart, lungs, and gastrointestinal tract.

Congenital toxoplasmosis usually occurs when a woman acquires primary infection while pregnant. There is a wide variety of manifestations of congenital infection ranging from hydrops fetalis and perinatal death to small size for gestational age, prematurity, peripheral retinal scars, persistent jaundice, mild thrombocytopenia, CSF, pleocytosis, and the characteristic triad of chorioretinitis, hydrocephalus, and cerebral calcifications.

Diagnosis: The diagnosis of acute *Toxoplasma* infection can be established by culture of *T. gondii* from blood or body fluids, identification of tachyzoites in sections or preparations of tissues and body fluids, identification of cysts in the placenta or tissues of a fetus or newborn, and characteristic lymph node histologic features. Examination of the placenta of infected newborns may reveal chronic inflammation and cysts. Tachyzoites can be seen with Wright or Giemsa stains but are best demonstrated with immunoperoxidase technique. Areas of calcification occur in the brain.

Serologic tests also are very useful for diagnosis. Polymerase chain reaction (PCR) also is useful to identify *T. gondii* DNA in CSF, amniotic fluid, infant peripheral blood, and urine to definitely establish the diagnosis.

CSF abnormalities occur in at least 1/3 of infants with congenital toxoplasmosis and a CSF protein level of > 1g/dl is characteristic of severe CNS toxoplasmosis, which is usually accompanied by hydrocephalus. CT of the brain is useful to detect calcifications, determine ventricular size, and demonstrate porencephalic cystic structures. Calcifications occur throughout the brain but more commonly occur in the caudate nucleus and basal ganglia, choroid plexus, and subependyma. MRI and contrast-enhanced CT brain scans are useful for detecting active inflammatory lesions. Ultrasonography may be useful for following ventricular size.

Treatment: Pyrimethamine plus sulfadiazine act synergistically against *Toxoplasma*, and combined therapy is indicated in many forms of toxoplasmosis. However, use of pyrimethamine is contraindicated during the 1st trimester of pregnancy. Spiramycin should be used to prevent vertical transmission of infection to the fetus of acutely infected pregnant women, and to treat congenital toxoplasmosis. Pyrimethamine inhibits the enzyme dihydrofolate reductase (DHFR), and thus synthesis of folic acid. Folinic acid, as calcium lucovorin (Recovorin tab 15 g; inj 7.5 mg/2 ml, 10 mg/5 ml) should always be administered concomitantly and for 1 wk after treatment with pyrimethamine is discontinued to prevent bone marrow suppression.

Prevention: Counseling pregnant women about the methods of preventing transmission of *T. gondii* during pregnancy can substantially reduce the acquisition of infection during gestation.

Prognosis: Early administration of specific treatment for congenitally infected infants usually cures the active manifestations of toxoplasmosis including active chorioretinitis, meningitis, encephalitis, hepatitis, splenomegaly, and thrombocytopenia.

McLeod R, Boyer K, Roizen N, et al. The child with congenital toxoplasmosis. *Curr Clin Top Infect Dis* 2000;20:189–208.

McLeod R, Remington JS. Toxoplasmosis (*Toxoplasma gondii*). In: Kliegman RM, Behrman RE, Jenson HB, Stanton BF (eds). *Nelson Textbook of Pediatrics*. 18th edn. Vol. 1. Philadelphia: Saunders, 2007;1486–95.

Mets MB, Holfels E, Boyer KM, et al. Eye manifestations of congenital toxoplasmosis. *Am J Ophthalmol* 1997;123:1–16.

Montoya JG. Laboratory diagnosis of *Toxoplasma gondii* and toxoplasmosis. *J Infect Dis* 2002;185(Suppl): S73–82.

Montoya JG, Liesenfeld O. Toxoplasmosis. *Lancet* 2004; 363: 1965–76.

14.10 HELMINTHIC DISEASES

Ascariasis

Etiopathogenesis: Ascariasis is caused by the nematode, or round worm, *Ascaris lumbricoides*. Adult worms of *A. lumbricoides* inhabit the lumen of the small intestine and have a life span of 10–24 mo. A gravid female worm produces 200,000 eggs/day. After passage in the feces, the eggs embryonate and become infective in 5–10 days under favorable environmental conditions. Transmission is primarily hand to mouth but may also involve ingestion of contaminated raw fruits and vegetables. Ascaris eggs can remain viable at 5–10°C for as long as 2 yr. Ascaris ova hatch in the small intestine after ingestion by the human host. Larvae are released, penetrate the intestinal wall, and migrate to the lungs by way of the venous circulation. The parasites then cause pulmonary ascariasis as they enter into the alveoli and migrate through the bronchi and trachea. They are subsequently swallowed and return in the intestines, where they mature into adult worms. Female ascaris begin depositing eggs in 8–10 wk.

Clinical manifestations: The most common clinical problems are due to pulmonary disease and obstruction of the intestinal or biliary tract. Larvae migrating through these tissues may cause allergic symptoms, fever, urticaria, and granulomatous disease. The pulmonary manifestations resemble Loeffler syndrome and include transient respiratory symptoms such as cough and dyspnea, pulmonary infiltrates, and blood eosinophilia. Larvae may be observed in the sputum.

Diagnosis: Microscopic examination of fecal smears can be used for diagnosis of eggs.

Treatment: The treatment options for gastrointestinal ascariasis include albendazole (400 mg PO once, for all ages), mebendazole (100 mg bid PO for 3 days or 500 mg PO once for all ages) or pyrantel pamoate (11 mg/kg PO once, maximum 1 g); piperazine citrate (150 mg/kg PO initially, followed by six doses of 65 mg/kg at 12 hr intervals PO).

Prevention: Short-term preventive measures include chemotherapy, which can be implemented in 1 of 3 ways:

1. Offering universal treatment to all individuals in an area of high endemicity
2. Offering treatment targeted to groups with high frequency of infection, such as children attending primary schools
3. Offering individual treatment based on intensity of current or past infection. Improving sanitary conditions and sewage facilities, discontinuing the practice of using human feces as fertilizer and education are the most effective long-term preventive measures.

Crompton DW. Ascaris and ascariasis. *Adv Parasitol* 2003; 48:285–375.

Dent AE, Kazura JW. Ascariasis (*Ascaris Lumbricoides*). In: Kliegman RM, Behrman RE, Jenson HB, Stanton BF (eds). *Nelson Textbook of Pediatrics*. 18th edn. Vol. 1. Philadelphia: Saunders, 2007;1495–6.

Hookworms

Etiopathogenesis: Hookworm infection is one of the most prevalent infectious diseases of humans, affecting an estimates 576 million individuals worldwide. Two major genera of hookworms, which are nematodes or round worms, infect humans—*Necator americanus* and *Ancylostoma duodenale*. The less common zoonotic species are *A. ceylanicum*, *A. caninum*, and *A. braziliensis*. Larvae infect humans either by penetrating through the skin (*Necator americanus* and *A. duodenale*) or when they are ingested (*A. duodenale*). Larvae entering the human host by skin penetration undergo extraintestinal migration through the venous circulation and lungs before they are swallowed, whereas orally ingested larvae may undergo extraintestinal migration or remain in the intestinal tract. Larvae returning to small intestine undergo two molts to become adult sexually mature male and female worms ranging in length from 5 to 13 mm. The buccal capsule of the adult hookworm is armed with cutting plates (*Necator americanus*) or teeth (*A. duodenale*) to facilitate attachment to the mucosa and submucosa of the of the small intestine. Hookworms can remain in the intestine for 1–5 yr, where they mate and produce eggs. Although approximately 2 mo is required for the larval stages of hookworms to undergo extraintestinal migration and develop into mature adults, *A. duodenale* larvae may remain developmentally arrested for many months before resuming development in the small intestine. Mature female *Necator americanus* and *A. duodenale* worms

produce > 10,000 eggs/day and about 30,000 eggs/day respectively. Eggs that are developed on soil with adequate moisture and shade develop into 1st stage larvae and hatch. Over the ensuing several days and under appropriate conditions, the larvae molt twice to the infective stage. Infective larvae migrate vertically in the soil until they either infect a new host or exhaust their lipid metabolic reserves and die.

Clinical manifestations: Clinically infected children with moderate and heavy hookworm infections suffer from intestinal blood loss resulting in iron deficiency and iron deficiency anemia and protein malnutrition, growth retardation and cognitive and intellectual deficits. Hookworm larvae elicit dermatitis, sometimes referred to as ground itch. Cough subsequently occurs when larvae migrate through the lungs to cause laryngotracheobronchitis, usually about 1 wk after the infection. Pain, anorexia, and diarrhea may be associated with intestinal hookworm infection. Some children with chronic hookworm disease acquire a yellow-green pallor known as chlorosis.

Each adult A. *duodenale* hookworm causes loss of 0.2 mL of blood/day; blood loss is less for *Necator americanus*. Hookworm disease results only when individuals with moderate and heavy infections experience sufficient blood loss to develop iron deficiency and anemia. Hypoalbuminemia and consequent edema and anasarca from the loss of intravascular oncotic pressure can also occur.

Diagnosis: Children with hookworm disease release eggs that can be detected by direct fecal examination (*see* Fig. 11.23 in CD).

Treatment: Treatment with albendazole, mebendazole or pyrantel pamoate is same as mentioned in ascariasis.

Prevention. Same as mentioned in ascariasis.

Caumes E, Danis M. From creeping eruptions to hookworm-related cutaneous larva migrans. *Lancet* 2004;4:659–60.

Hotez PJ. Hookworms (*Nector americanus and Ancylostoma duodenale*). In: Kliegman RM, Behrman RE, Jenson HB, Stanton BF (eds). *Nelson Textbook of Pediatrics*. 18th edn. Vol. 1. Philadelphia: Saunders, 2007;1496–9.

Enterobiasis

Etiopathogenesis: The cause of enterobiasis, or *pinworm* infection, is *Enterobius vermicularis*, which is a small (1 cm of length, white, threadlike nematode or roundworm that typically inhabits the cecum, appendix, and adjacent areas of the ileum and ascending colon. Gravid females migrate at night to the perianal and perineal regions where they deposit up to 15,000 eggs. Eggs embryonate within 6 hr and remain viable for 20 days. Human infection occurs by the fecal-oral route by ingestion of embryonated eggs that are carried on fingernails, clothing, bedding or house dust. After ingestion, the larvae mature to form adult worms in 36–53 days. Autoinoculation can occur in individuals who habitually put their fingers in their mouth.

Clinical manifestations: The most common complaints include itching and restless sleep secondary to nocturnal perianal or perineal pruritus. Aberrant migration to ectopic sites occasionally may lead to appendicitis, chronic salpingitis, pelvic inflammatory disease, peritonitis, hepatitis, and ulcerative lesions in the large or small bowel.

Diagnosis: A history of nocturnal perianal pruritus in children strongly suggests enterobiasis. Definitive diagnosis is established by identification of parasite eggs or worms. Digital rectal examination may also be used to obtain samples for a wet mount.

Treatment: Treatment with albendazole, mebendazole or pyrantel pamoate is same as mentioned in ascariasis. Morning bathing removes a large portion of eggs. Frequent changing of underclothes and bed sheets decreases environmental egg contamination and may decrease the risk of autoinfection.

Prevention: Household contacts can be treated at the same time as the infected individual. Repeated treatments every 3–4 mo may be required in circumstances with repeated exposure, such as with institutionalized children. Good hand hygiene is the most effective method of prevention.

Dent AE, Kazura JW. 14.12.4. Enterobiasis (*Enterobius vermicularis*). In: Kliegman RM, Behrman RE, Jenson HB, Stanton BF (eds). *Nelson Textbook of Pediatrics.* 18th edn. Vol. 1. Philadelphia: Saunders, 2007;1500–01.

Lymphatic Filariasis

Etiopathogenesis: The filarial worms *Brugia malayi* (Malayan filariasis), *Brugia timori*, and *Wuchereria bancrofti* (bancroftian filariasis) are thread-like nematodes that cause similar infections. *W. bancrofti* is transmitted in Africa, Asia, and Latin America and accounts for 90% lymphatic filariasis. *B. malayi* is restricted to the South pacific and Southeast Asia, and *B. timori* is restricted to several islands of Indonesia. Infective larvae are introduced into humans during blood feeding by the mosquito vector. Over a period of 4–6 mo the larval forms develop into adult male and female worms that reside in the afferent lymphatic vessels. Sexually mature adult female worms release large numbers of microfilariae that circulate in the bloodstream. The life cycle of the parasite is completed when mosquitoes ingest microfilariae in a blood meal, which molt to form infective larvae over a period of 10–14 days.

Clinical manifestations: The clinical manifestations of *Brugia malayi*, *Brugia timori*, and *Wuchereria bancrofti* infection are similar; manifestations of acute infection include episodic fever, lymphangitis of an extremity, lymphadenitis (especially the inguinal and axillary areas), whereas chronic filariasis (occurs mostly in adults 30 yr of age or older) is characterized by lymphatic obstruction with hydrocele and elephantiasis. Elephantiasis may involve one or more limbs, the scrotum, the breasts, or the vulva. Bacterial super-infections contribute to the morbidity of this disease.

Tropical pulmonary eosinophilia: In tropical pulmonary eosinophilia, a syndrome of filarial etiology, microfilariae are found in the lungs and lymph nodes but not in the blood stream. The presentation includes paroxysmal nocturnal cough with dyspnea, fever, weight loss, and fatigue. Crackles are found in the chest. The roentgenographic findings may occasionally be normal but increased vascular markings, discrete opacities in the middle and basal regions of the lung or diffuse miliary lesions are usually present. Recurrent episodes may result in interstitial fibrosis and chronic respiratory insufficiency in untreated individuals. Hepatospleno-megaly and generalized lymphadenopathy are often seen in children. The diagnosis is suggested by residence in a filarial endemic area, eosinophilia (> 2,000 µl), compatible clinical symptoms, increased serum IgE (> 1,000 IU/ml), and high titters of antimicrofilarial antibodies in the absence of microfilaremia. The clinical response to diethylcarba-mazine (2 mg/kg/dose tid PO for 12–21 days) is the final criterion for diagnosis; the majority of patients improve with this therapy. If symptoms recur, a second course of the anthelmintic should be administered. Patients with chronic symptoms are less likely to show improvement than those who have been ill for a short time.

Diagnosis: Demonstration of microfilaria in the blood is diagnostic; blood should be obtained between 10 o'clock at night and 2 o'clock in the morning, because microfilaria is nocturnal in most cases. Adult worms or microfilariae can be identified in tissue specimens obtained at biopsy (*see* Fig. 14.24 in CD).

Treatment: Diethylcarbamazine should be increased gradually in children, because treatment-associated complications such as pruritus, fever, generalized body pain, hypertension, and even death may occur, especially with high microbial levels. (Diethylcarba-mazine: 1 mg/kg PO as a single dose on day 1, 1 mg/kg tid PO on day 2, 1–2 mg/kg tid PO on day 3, and 6 mg/kg divided tid PO on days 4–14.) For patients with no microfilaria in the blood the full dose (6 mg/kg/

day divided tid PO) can be given beginning on day 1. Repeat doses may be necessary to further reduce the microfilaremia and kill lymph-dwelling adult parasites. *Wuchereria bancrofti* is more sensitive than *Brugia malayi* to diethylcarbamazine.

Prevention: Global programs to control and ultimately eradicate lymphatic filariasis currently recommend single annual dose of diethylcarbamazine (6 mg/kg PO once) often in combination with albendazole (400 mg PO once) for 5 years. In coendemic areas of filariasis and onchocerciasis, mass drug application with single-dose ivermectin (150 µg/kg PO once) and albendazole are used because of severe adverse reactions with diethycarbamazipine in onchocerciasis-infected individuals.

Dent AE, Kazura JW. Lymphatic filariasis (*Brugia Malayi, Brugia Timori, and Wuchereria Bancrofti*). In: Kliegman RM, Behrman RE, Jenson HB, Stanton BF (eds). *Nelson Textbook of Pediatrics*. 18th edn. Vol. 1. Philadelphia: Saunders, 2007;1502–03.

Adult Tapeworm Infections

Taeniasis

Etiopathogenesis: The beef tapeworm, *T. saginata*, and the pork tapeworm, *T. solium*, are large parasites (4–10 meters). The body of adult stage is a connected series of hundreds or thousands of flattened segments, called proglottids, whose most anterior segment, the scolex, anchors the parasite to the bowel wall. The gravid terminal segments are each packed with 50,000–100,000 eggs, and the eggs or these intact proglottids pass in the stool. These 2 tapeworms differ most significantly in that the intermediate stage of the pork tapeworm (cysticercus) can also infect humans.

When children ingest raw or undercooked infected meat, gastric acid and bile facilitate release of the immature scolex that attaches to the lumen of the small intestine. The parasite adds new segments, and after 2–3 months the terminal segments mature, become gravid, and appear in stool.

Clinical manifestations: Adult beef and pork tapeworms cause abdominal discomfort and are rare causes of intestinal obstruction, cholangitis, and appendicitis. The proglottids are seen and are also motile and sometimes produce anal pruritus.

Diagnosis: Proglottids (including gravid proglottids) are passed in stool. Eggs, by contrast, are often absent from stool. The scolex of each species is diagnostic. The scolex of *T. saginata* has only a set of four anteriorly oriented suckers, whereas *T. solium* has a double row of hooks in addition to suckers. The proglottids of *T. saginata* have more than 20 uterine branches from a central uterine structure, and those of *T. solium* have

10 or fewer. Anal pruritus may mimic symptoms of pinworm (*Enterobius vermicularis*) infection.

Treatment: Tapeworms are effectively treated with praziquantel (5–10 mg/kg PO once) An alternative treatment is niclosamide (50 mg/kg PO once for children). Praziquantel tends to cause parasite death and subsequent resorption unless purged.

Prevention: Prolonged freezing or thorough cooking kills the parasite. Because humans are the major reservoir for adult worms, health education together with improved human sanitation are important tools for preventing transmission.

Diphyllobothriasis

Diphyllobothrium latum, the fish tapeworm is the longest human tapeworm (10–20 meters). Life cycle of *D. latum* requires two intermediate hosts. Consumption of raw or undercooked fish leads to human infection with adult fish tapeworms. The life cycle of *D. latum* requires 2 intermediate hosts. The fish tapeworm is most prevalent in Europe, North America, Asia, Canada, South America and Africa. The adult worm efficiently scavenges vitamin B_{12} for its own use in the constant production of large numbers of segments and as many as 1 million eggs per day. As a result diphyllobothriasis causes megaloblastic anemia in 2–9% infections.

Infection is largely asymptomatic except those who develop B_{12} or folate deficiency. Megaloblastic anemia with leukopenia, thrombocytopenia, glossitis and signs of spinal cord posterior column degeneration (loss of vibratory sense, proprioception, and coordination) is seen in advanced nutritional deficiency due to diphyllobothriasis. The diagnosis is confirmed by the presence of characteristic eggs, ovoid and has a caplike operculum at the upper end of the egg. The treatment is with praziquantel (5–10 mg/kg PO once). Health education together with brief cooking or prolonged freezing of fish (in eliminating intermediate stage) and improved human sanitation are important tools for preventing transmission.

Hymenolepiasis

Hymenolepsis nana, the dwarf tapeworm is very common in developing countries and is a major cause of eosinophilia. Although it rarely causes overt disease, the presence of *H. nana* eggs in stool may serve as a marker for exposure to poor hygienic conditions. The intermediate stage develops in various hosts (e.g. rodents, ticks, and fleas), and the entire cycle is completed in humans. H. nana infection responds to praziquantel (25 mg/kg PO once) or niclosamide (50 mg/kg PO once for children; 2 g PO once for adults).

Dipylidiasis

Dipylidium caninum is a common tapeworm of domestic dogs and cats. Human infection requires ingestion of the parasite's intermediate host, the dog or cat flea. Infants and small children are particularly susceptible to infection. Eosinophilia, anal pruritus, vague abdominal pain and diarrhea may occur. Dipylidiasis may be confused with pinworm (*E. vermicularis*). Dipylidiasis responds to treatment with praziquantel (25 mg/kg PO once) or niclosamide (50 mg/kg PO once for children; 2 g PO once for adults). Deworming pets and flea control are the best preventive measures.

Blanton R. Adult tapeworm infections. In: Kliegman RM, Behrman RE, Jenson HB, Stanton BF (eds). *Nelson Textbook of Pediatrics.* 18th edn. Vol. 1. Philadelphia: Saunders, 2007;1512–14.

Cysticercosis

Etiopathogenesis: The pork tapeworm (*Taenia solium*), is distributed worldwide wherever pigs are raised. Intense transmission occurs in India, Indonesia, China, Korea, Central and South America and some parts of Africa. In these areas, 20–50% of cases of epilepsy may be due to cysticercosis. Infection of *Taenia solium* occurs in two ways: Consumption of undercooked pork produces intestinal infection with adult worms and infection with intermediate form by ingestion of food or water contaminated with the eggs of *Taenia solium*. Cysticercosis may therefore, develop even in individuals who do not eat pork. Individuals infected with an adult *Taenia solium* may infect themselves with the eggs by the fecal-oral route. Reverse peristalsis in the small intestine has also been implicated as a means of autoinfection. Cysticercosis is caused by infection with intermediate stage of *Taenia solium*. The intermediate stage of *Taenia solium* preferably invades the CNS, causing neurocyticercosis. In the small intestine, the egg releases an *oncosphere* that crosses the gut wall and spreads hematogenously to many tissues, primarily brain and muscles. Wherever the eggs lodge, they produce small (0.2–0.5 cm) fluid-filled bladders containing a single protoscolex, the juvenile-stage parasite.

The cystic stages of most tapeworms do not provoke strong immunologic response while they remain alive and intact. However, viable cysts can be associated with disease when the initial parasite invasion is massive or when they obstruct the flow of cerebrospinal fluid (obstructive hydrocephalus). Most cysts remain viable for 5–10 yr and then begin to degenerate, followed by a vigorous host response. Cysts resolve either by complete resorption or calcification.

Clinical manifestations: Seizures are the presenting finding in > 70% cases, although, any cognitive or neurologic abnormality from psychosis to stroke may be seen. Neurocysticercosis can be classified as parenchymal, intraventricular, meningeal, spinal or ocular on the basis of anatomic location, clinical presentation and radiologic appearance.

Parenchymal neurocysticercosis produces seizures (generalized in 80% cases) as well as focal neurologic signs. Rarely, cerebral infarction can result from obstruction of small terminal arteries or vasculitis. With extensive frontal lobe disease symptoms of intellectual deterioration with dementia or Parkinsonism may be seen. In children with massive initial infection, a fulminant encephalitis-like presentation also occurs. Intraventricular neurocysticercosis (5–10% of all cases) is associated with hydrocephalus and acute, subacute, or intermittent signs of increased intracranial pressure without localizing signs. Meningeal neurocysticercosis is associated with signs of meningeal irritation and also increased intracranial pressure. Racemose neurocysticercosis is a meningeal form of disease in which large lobulated cysts appear in the basal cisterns. Spinal neurocysticercosis presents with findings of spinal cord compression, nerve root pain, transverse myelitis, or meningitis. Ocular neurocysticercosis causes decreased visual acuity due to cysticerci floating in the vitreous, retinal detachment or iridocyclitis. Cysts can be palpated under the skin. Heavy infections in skeletal or heart muscle can result in myositis or carditis.

Diagnosis: Neurocysticercosis should be suspected in any child with onset of neurologic (seizures, hydrocephalus, unilateral visual impairment, or symptoms of encephalitis), cognitive or personality disorder. Proglottids (segments) or eggs are seen in feces only in 25% of patients. Imaging studies and serologic tests are necessary to confirm the diagnosis. In CT a solitary parenchymal cyst, with or without contrast enhancement and numerous calcifications are the most common findings. CT image of multiple cysts of neurocystecercosis are seen (*see* Fig. 14.25 in CD). Intraventricular cysts may be detected in some cases. MRI better detects intraventricular and spinal cord cysts. Serologic diagnosis using the enzyme-linked immunotransfer blot (EITB) has > 90% sensitivity and specificity; testing of CSF is not requited. Eosinophilia is frequently seen in CSF.

Differential diagnosis: Neurocysticercosis should be clinically distinguished from encephalitis, stroke, meningitis and many other conditions. On imaging studies, cysticerci can be difficult to distinguish from tuberculomas, histoplasmosis, blastomycosis, toxoplasmosis, sarcoidosis, vasculitis and tumor.

Treatment: The treatment of neurocysticercosis depends on disease presentation. But it is important to note that these patients may carry adult worms. If no anticysticercal drugs are administered, niclosamide should be used because it is not absorbed and does not provoke inflammatory response to cysticerci. Children with seizures, no hydrocephalus, and only calcified, inactive lesions on CT do not require therapy other than anticonvulsant medications. The anticonvulsant treatment should be continued for 2–3 years.

Active parenchymal lesions usually resolve spontaneously. There are two anticysticercal drugs, namely albendazole (15 mg/kg/24 hr divided bid PO for 28 days; maximum: 800 mg/24 hr) taken with a fatty meal to improve absorption and praziquantel (50–100 mg/kg/24 hr divided tid PO for thirty days). Better outcome is reported with albendazole. Antiparasitic therapy may convert quiescent parenchymal lesions to active lesions or may worsen ventricular, spinal or ocular disease, as the host responds to the dying patients with increased inflammation. Corticosteroids for 2–3 days before and during drug therapy can ameliorate worsening of symptoms that follow anticysticercal drugs. Albendazole levels are increased in the presence of corticosteroids whereas praziquantel levels are decreased as much as 50%. A ventricular shunt must be placed before medical therapy, whenever there is evidence of hydrocephalus or ventricular or spinal disease. Enucleation is frequently required in cases of ocular cysticercosis though cure using medical therapy has been reported.

Prevention: Attention to personal hygiene, proper hand washing by food handlers, and avoidance of fresh fruits and vegetables (in areas endemic for T solium) help prevent ingestion of eggs. All pork should be cooked thoroughly.

Blanton R. Cysticercosis. In: Kliegman RM, Behrman RE, Jenson HB, Stanton BF (eds). *Nelson Textbook of Pediatrics.* 18th edn. Vol. 1. Philadelphia: Saunders, 2007;1514–16.

Singh Rana Pramendra Vir. Neurocysticercosis. In: Mathur GP, Mathur Sarla (eds). *Current Trends in Pediatrics.* Vol 2. Delhi: Academa Publishers, 2006;165–77.

Echinococcosis

Etiopathogenesis: Echinococcosis (hydatid disease or hydatidosis) is the most wide spread, serious human cestode infection in the world. It is a zoonosis that is transmitted from domestic and wild members of the canine family. Two *Echinococcus* species, *E. granulosus* (cystic hydatid disease) and *E. multilocularis* (alveolar hydatid disease) are responsible for distinct clinical manifestations. Dogs, wolves, dingoes, jackals, coyotes, and foxes become infected after eating infected viscera and are the hosts of adult worms (2–7 mm). The adult worms are composed of 2–6 proglottids and have a lifespan of about 5 months. Eggs from adult worms are passed in stool and contaminate the soil and water as well as the coats of the dogs themselves.

Clinical manifestations: In the liver cysts never become symptomatic and regress spontaneously, or produce relatively nonspecific symptoms. When some cysts do take hold, increased abdominal girth, hepatomegaly, palpable mass, vomiting or abdominal pain ensues. Anaphylaxis can occur with cyst rupture or spillage spontaneously, due to trauma, or intraoperatively; protoscolex present in the cyst can form a new cyst. Jaundice due to cystic hydatid disease is rare. In the lung, cysts produce chest pain, cough or hemoptysis. Bone cysts may cause pathologic fractures, and in the genitourinary system they can produce hematuria or infertility. In alveolar hydatid disease cyst tissue continues to proliferate and may separate and metastasize distantly. The proliferating mass compromises hepatic tissue or the biliary system and causes progressive obstructive jaundice and hepatic failure. Symptoms also occur from expansion of extrahepatic foci.

Diagnosis: On physical examination, subcutaneous nodules, hepatomegaly, or a palpable abdominal mass may be found. Ultrasonography will help in the diagnosis and treatment of cystic hydatid disease of the liver, internal membranes and hydatid sand (falling echogenic cyst material), and diffuse solid tumor of alveolar disease. CT findings are similar to those of ultrasonography. CT or MRI is also important in planning a surgical intervention. Lung hydatid is usually apparent on chest X-ray (*see* Fig. 14.26 in CD).

Differential diagnosis: *Echinococcus* cyst should be differentiated from benign hepatic cysts by the absence of either internal membranes or hydatid sand. The density of bacterial hepatic abscesses is distinct from the watery cystic fluid of *E. granulosus*. Alveolar echinococcosis is confused with hepatoma and cirrhosis.

Treatment: For *E. granulosus* disease the treatment of choice is ultrasound or CT-guided *p*ercutaneous *a*spiration, *i*nstillation of hypertonic saline or another scolicidal agent, and *re*-absorption (PAIR) after 15 minutes. PAIR is appropriate for simple cysts of the liver (except larger more complicated cysts), lung cysts and renal cysts. Cysts containing bile-stained fluid should not be injected with a scolicidal agent because toxicity is increased. Spillage with PAIR is uncommon. But prophylactic albendazole therapy is recommended.

In surgery the inner cyst wall (laminate and germinal layers) is peeled from the fibrous layer and only these inner layers need to be removed.

Nonpregnant patients for *E. granulosus* cysts not amenable to PAIR or surgery, albendazole (15 mg/kg/24 hr divided bid PO for 1–6 months; maximum: 800 mg/24 hr) taken with a fatty meal to improve absorption, is the preferred drug for treatment.. A positive response occurs in 40–60% cases. Corticosteroids are not indicated unless patients have anaphylaxis or any other allergic reaction.

Medical therapy with albendazole may slow the progression of alveolar hydatidosis, but if feasible removal of infected tissue provides the best outcome.

Prognosis: Factors such as age of the cyst (< 2 years), low internal complexity of the cyst and small size respond to chemotherapy. The average mortality is 92% after 10 yr if surgical removal of alveolar hydatidosis is unsuccessful.

Prevention: Transmission can be interrupted through hand washing, avoiding contact with dogs in endemic areas, boiling or filtering water, proper disposal of animal carcasses, and proper meat inspection. Proper disposal of refuse from slaughter houses so that dogs or wild carnivores do not have access to entrails. Other useful measures include control or treatment of the feral dog population and regular praziquantel treatment of pets and working dogs in endemic areas.

Blanton R. Echinococcosis (*Echinococcus granulosus* and *Echinococcus multilocularis*). In: Kliegman RM, Behrman RE, Jenson HB, Stanton BF (eds). *Nelson Textbook of Pediatrics*. 18th edn. Vol. 1. Philadelphia: Saunders, 2007;1516–9.

Mc Manus DP, Zhang W, Li J, Bartley PB. Echinococcosis. *Lancet* 2003;362:1295–304.

15.1 IMMUNIZATION

Immunization is regarded a cost-effective and successful means of preventing infectious diseases. As a result of routine childhood immunizations, the occurrence of once common contagious diseases declined markedly both in developing and developed countries.

Vaccination is administration of any vaccine or toxoid (inactivated toxin) for prevention of disease. *Immunization* is the process of inducing immunity artificially by either vaccination (active immunization) or administration of antibody (passive immunization). Active immunization stimulates the immune system to produce antibodies and cellular immune responses that protect against the infectious agent. *Passive immunization* provides temporary protection by administrating exogenously produced antibody, such as immune globulin. Passive immunization also occurs naturally through transplacental transmission of antibodies to a fetus, which provides protection against many infectious diseases for first several months to a infant. *Vaccines* are produced from the same microorganisms or toxins that cause disease, but in either case are modified so as to be harmless to humans. Three main substances are used for the production of vaccines:

- *Live* microorganisms, e.g. weakened measles and polioviruses or tuberculosis bacteria;
- *Killed* microorganisms, e.g. pertussis microorganisms used in DPT production; and
- *Toxoids*, e.g. inactivated toxins such as tetanus toxoid and diphtheria toxoid. In addition, some vaccines are produced using genetic engineering technologies, e.g. recombinant DNA hepatitis B vaccine.

Active Immunization

Active immunization is carried out by:
1. Live-attenuated infectious agents, and
2. Inactivated or detoxified agents, their extracts, or specific recombinant products (e.g. hepatitis vaccine).

In diseases, such as poliomyelitis and typhoid fever both types of agents are used. Live-attenuated vaccines are more likely to induce an immunologic response simulating the response to natural infection. Thus, measles, rubella, and mumps vaccines are likely to confer lifelong protection with a single immunizing dose. In contrast, many inactivated or killed vaccines require booster vaccinations to provide protection. Inactivated or killed vaccines include inactivated whole organisms (e.g. whole cell pertussis and hepatitis A vaccines), detoxified exotoxins (e.g. tetanus and diphtheria toxoids), purified protein antigens (e.g. acellular pertussis and hepatitis B vaccines), polysaccharides (e.g. capsular meningococcal vaccine), capsular polysaccharides conjugated to carrier proteins (e.g. Hib and pneumococcal conjugate vaccines), and components of the organism (e.g. subunit influenza vaccine).

Immunizing agents include vaccines, toxoids, antitoxins and immune globulin derived from human or animal source (Table 15.1). Most immunizing agents contain preservatives, stabilizers, antibiotics, adjuvants, and a suspending fluid (Table 15.2).

Antibodies produced in response to vaccine constituents may be of any immunoglobulin class.

Table 15.1: Immunizing agents

Agent	Definition
Vaccine	A preparation of proteins, polysaccharides, or nucleic acids of pathogens that are derived to the immune system as single entities, as part of complex particles, or by live attenuated agents or vectors, to induce specific responses that inactivate, destroy, or suppress the antigen
Toxoid	A modified bacterial toxin that has been made nontoxic but retains the capacity to stimulate the formation of antitoxin
Immune globulin	An antibody-containing solution derived from human blood obtained by cold ethanol fractionation of large pools of plasma and used primarily for the maintenance of immunity of immunodeficient persons or for passive immunization; available in intramuscular and intravenous preparations.
Antitoxin	An antibody derived from the serum of humans of animals after stimulation with specific antigens, used to provide passive immunity

From Peter G. Immunization practices. In: Behrman RE, Kliegman RM, Jenson HB (eds). *Nelson Textbook of Pediatrics*. 17th edn. Philadelphia: Saunders, 2004;1174–84.

Table 15.2: Constituents of vaccines

Component	Use
Preservatives, stabilizers, antibiotics	Constituents (mercurials or antibiotics) can inhibit or prevent bacterial growth or stabilize the antigen. Allergic reactions to any of the additives may occur
Adjuvants	An aluminum salt is used in some vaccines to enhance the immune response (e.g. toxoids, hepatitis B)
Suspending fluid	Sterile water, saline, or more complex fluids derived from the growing media or biologic system in which the agent is produced (e.g. egg antigens, cell culture ingredients, serum proteins).

Important protective antibodies include those that inactivate soluble toxic protein products of bacteria (i.e., antitoxins), facilitate phagocytosis and intracellular digestion of bacteria (i.e. opsonins), interact with components of serum complement to damage the bacterial membrane with resultant bacteriolysis (i.e. lysins), prevent proliferation of infectious virus (i.e. neutralizing antibodies), and interact with components of the bacterial surface to prevent adhesion to mucosal surfaces (i.e. anti adhesions). Antibodies function alone or in conjunction with other components of the immune system by participating directly in the neutralization of a toxin (e.g. diphtheria); opsonization of virus (e.g. poliovirus); initiating or combining with complement and promoting phagocytosis (e.g. Pneumococcus); reacting with nonsensitized lymphocytes to stimulate phagocytosis; or sensitizing macrophages to stimulate phagocytosis.

Passive Immunity

Passive immunity is achieved by administration of preformed antibodies to reduce transient protection against an infectious agent. Passive immunity also can be induced naturally through transplacental transfer of antibodies during gestation. Maternally derived antibodies can provide protection during an infant's first months of life. Protection for some diseases may persist for as long as a year after birth. The major indications for passive immunity are to provide protection to:

1. Immunodeficient children with B-lymphocyte defects who have difficulties in making antibodies.
2. Persons exposed to infectious diseases or who are at imminent risk of exposure where there is not adequate time for them to develop an active immune response to a vaccine; and
3. Persons with an infectious disease as part of specific therapy for that disease.

Immune globulin: Immune globulin (IG) contains 15–18% protein, predominantly IgG, and is administered intramuscularly. The major indications for IG are replacement therapy for children with antibody deficient disorders, and for passive immunization for measles and hepatitis A. For replacement therapy, the usual dose of IG is 100 mg/kg or 0.66 mL/kg monthly. The usual interval between doses is 2–4 wk depending on trough IG concentrations. In practice IGIV is used for this indication and not IG. IG can be used to prevent or modify measles if administered to children within 6 days of exposure (usual dose 0.25 ml/kg for immunocompetent children, 0.5 ml/kg for immunocompromised children; maximum dose 15 ml) and to prevent or modify hepatitis A if administered to children within 14 days of exposure (usual dose 0.02 ml/kg). IG also may be administered for prophylaxis of hepatitis A for persons traveling internationally to hepatitis A-endemic areas (0.06 ml/kg), for children too young for vaccination (<1 yr of age), or in conjunction with hepatitis A vaccine when departure to the area must be undertaken <1 mo after receipt of hepatitis A vaccine. The most common adverse reaction to IG is pain and discomfort at the injection site; most serious reactions include chest pain, dyspnea, anaphylaxis, and systemic collapse, but are rare.

Immune globulin intravenous: IGIV is prepared from adult plasma donors using alcohol fractionation and is modified to allow for intravenous use. IGIV is predominantly IgG and is tested to assure minimum antibody titers to diphtheria; Hep B, measles, and polio. The major recommended indications for IVIG are replacement therapy for immunodeficiency disorders; treatment of Kawasaki disease to prevent coronary artery abnormalities and shorten the clinical course; prevention of serious bacterial infections in children with HIV; prevention of serious bacterial infections in persons with hypogammaglobulinemia in chronic B cell leukemia; immune-mediated thrombocytopenia; prophylaxis of infection following bone marrow transplantation; severe toxic shock syndrome, Guillain-Barré syndrome, and anemia caused by parvovirus B19. Reactions to IGIV range from 1 to 15%. Some of the reactions appear to be related to the rate of infusion and can be mitigated by decreasing the rate. Such reactions include fever, headache, myalgia, chills, nausea, and vomiting. More serious reactions include anaphylactoid events, thromboembolic disorders, aseptic meningitis, and renal insufficiency.

Specific immune globulin preparations: Hyper-immune globulins are specific IG preparations that are derived from donors with high titers of antibodies to specific agents and are used to provide protection against those agents.

Hyperimmune animal antisera preparations: Animal antisera preparations are derived from horses. Great care must be exercised prior to administration of such antisera because of the potential for severe allergic reactions. This includes testing for sensitivity prior to administration, desensitization, if necessary, and treatment of potential reactions, including febrile events, serum sickness, and anaphylaxis.

Monoclonal antibodies: Monoclonal antibodies are antibody preparations produced against a single antigen. The monoclonal antibody used in infectious diseases is palivizumab, which can prevent severe disease from respiratory syncytial virus (RSV) among children ≥ 24 mo of age with chronic lung disease (CD) also called bronchopulmonary dysplasia or with a

history of premature birth (< 35 wk gestation). Monoclonal antibodies also are used for preparation of transplant rejection and treatment of some types of cancer and autoimmune diseases. Serious adverse reactions to palivizumab primarily are rare cases of anaphylaxis and hypersensitivity reactions.

Basic Immunology

Whenever an immunogen is introduced in the body, since it is already attenuated, it does not produce disease but it is recognized by T& B cells and humoral and/or cellular immunity is produced. Memory cells are also stimulated by this antigen and a booster response is produced when this antigen is administered again.

Replicating and Non-replicating Antigen

Antigens which multiply in human body, there is no need for repeat administration of these antigens, e.g. Measles and BCG. And for antigens which don't multiply, there is need for recurrent administration to achieve optimum immunity, e.g. DPT. Types of antigens used in vaccines are listed in Table 15.3.

Table 15.3: Types of antigens used in various vaccines	
Live bacteria, attenuated	BCG & Ty 21a
Live virus (attenuated)	OPV, MMR, measles, varicella
Inactivated bacteria	Pertussis, Whole cell killed typhoid
Inactivated virus	IPV, rabies, HAV
Toxoid	DT, TT, Td
Capsular polysaccharides	Typhoid Vi, Hib, meningo-coccal, pneumococcal
Viral subunit	HBsAg
Bacterial subunit	Acellular pertussis

National Immunization Schedule

Table 15.4.

IAP Immunization Time Table

It should be noted that the IAP immunization time table is the 'Best individual practices' schedule for a given child and may be somewhat different from the National immunization schedule (Table 15.4). The two schedules are, however, not in conflict with each other. The fact is that the immunization needs of children in a country are quite dynamic—a vaccine which may not be considered important today may become necessary in future as more information about the epidemiology of the disease becomes available. Further in developing countries affordability of the vaccines is a critical issue and any decision on incorporation of a new vaccine in the immunization schedule has to take this fact into consideration.

Table 15.4: National immunization schedule

Age	Vaccine
Birth	BCG, OPV$_0$ (in case of institutional deliveries)
6 wk	DTP$_1$, OPV$_1$ (BCG if not given earlier)
10 wk	DTP$_2$, OPV$_2$
14 wk	DTP$_3$, OPV$_3$
9 mo	Measles
16–24 mo	DTP, OPV
5–6 yrs	DT*
10 yrs	TT**
16 yrs	TT
For pregnant women	
Early pregnancy	TT$_1$ or booster
One month after TT	TT$_2$

*A second dose of DT vaccine should be given at an interval of one month if there is no clear history or documental evidence of previous immunization with DTPw

**A second dose of TT vaccine should be given at an interval of one month if there is no clear history or documented evidence of previous immunization with DTPw, DT or TT vaccines.

Source: Government of India (1994) National Child Survival and Safe Motherhood Program, Ministry of Health and Family Welfare, New Delhi.

Vaccination that can be given after discussion with parents is listed in Table 15.5.

Indian Academy of Pediatrics (IAPs) endorses the continued use of whole cell pertussis vaccine because of its proven efficacy and safety. Acellular pertussis vaccines may undoubtedly have fewer side-effects (like fever, local reaction at injection site and irritability), but this minor advantage does not justify the inordinate cost involved in the routine use of the vaccine.

If the mother is known to be HBsAg negative, HB vaccine can be given along with DTP at 6, 10, 14 wk/6 mo. If the mother's HBsAg status is not known, it is advisable to start vaccination soon after birth to prevent perinatal transmission of the disease. The baby should be given hepatitis B immune globulin (HBIG) within 24 hr of birth along with HB vaccine, if the mother is HBsAg positive and especially HBeAg positive.

Varicella, Hepatitis A and Pneumococcal Conjugate vaccines should be offered only after one to one discussion with parents. Also refer to the individual vaccines notes for recommendations.

Combination vaccines can be used to decrease the number of pricks being given to the baby and to decrease the number of clinic visits. The manufacture's instructions should be followed strictly whenever "mixing" vaccines in the same syringe prior to injection.

At present the only typhoid vaccine available in India is the Vi polysaccharide vaccine. Revaccination may be carried out every 3–4 yr.

Under special circumstances (e.g. epidemics), measles vaccine may be given earlier than 9 mo followed by MMR at 12–15 mo.

During pregnancy, the interval between the two doses of TT should be at least one month.

Use of OPV should continue till polio is completely eradicated from India. IPV can be used additionally for individual protection. OPV must be given to children <5 yr of age at the time of each supplementary immunization activity.

Immunization in Special Circumstances

1. *Immunization in preterm infants:* In general all vaccines may be administered as per schedule according to the chronological age irrespective of birth weight or period of gestation. Very low birth weight (VLBW)/preterm infants can be given immunization after initial stabilization.

2. *Breastfeeding and vaccination:* Breastfeeding does not adversely affect immunization and is therefore, not a contraindication for any vaccine; OPV can safely be given to a breast-fed infant. Vaccines (inactivated or live vaccines) administered to a lactating woman does not affect the safety of breastfeeding infants. There is no risk of transmission of hepatitis B virus from an HBsAG carrier mother to her baby through breast milk if HB vaccination is started at birth hepatitis B vaccine is mainly useful in prevention of perinatal

Table 15.5: Vaccines given after discussion with parents

Age	Vaccine
>6 wk of age	Pneumococcal conjugate vaccine*
>15 mo of age	Varicella vaccine#
>18 mo of age	Hepatitis vaccine A+

*3 primary doses at 6, 10 and 14 wk followed by a booster dose at 15 mo

#<13 yr of age: 1 dose; >13 yr of age: 2 doses at 4–8 wk interval

+2 doses at 6–12 mo interval

transmission if given with in 48 hrs of birth along with 0.5 ml HBIG dose (10 mg). 2nd dose should be given at 1 mo and 3rd at 6 mo to 1 yr.

3. *Children receiving corticosteroids:* Children receiving oral corticosteroids in high doses (e.g., prednisolone 1–2 mg/kg/day for more than 14 days should not receive live virus vaccines until the steroid has been discontinued for at least one month. Killed vaccines are safe but may be incompletely effective in such situations. Patients on topical or inhaled steroid therapy should not be denied their age appropriate vaccines.

4. *Vaccination schedule for children not immunized in time:* Vaccination schedule for unimmunized children is documented in Table 15.6. Varicella vaccine one dose up to 13 yr of age and hepatitis A vaccine 2 doses 0 and 6 mo to be offered only after discussing with the parents.

5. *Lapsed immunization.* There is no need to restart a vaccine series regardless of the time that has elapsed between individual doses. Immunization due should be given at the next visit and the immunization schedule should be completed at the next available opportunity. However, in case of unknown or uncertain immunization status, it is appropriate to restart the schedule.

6. *Missed opportunity for immunization.* This is defined as a situation when a child visits a health care facility and is not immunized. Minor illness (e.g., fever, diarrhea, respiratory infections) and malnutrition should not be considered as contraindications to immunization. Any dose not given at a recommended age should be given at any subsequent visit when indicated and feasible.

7. *Children awaiting splenectomy.* Children with loss of splenic function are at increased risk of serious infections with encapsulated organisms. If surgical splenectomy is being planned, immunization with pneumococcal, Hib, and meningococcal vaccines should be initiated a few weeks prior to splenectomy.

8. *Vaccination of children with bleeding disorders or those receiving anticoagulants.* Needles <23G should be used for injection and the parents should be asked to apply firm pressure, without rubbing, for at least 5 minutes.

9. *Simultaneous administration of multiple vaccines.* Both killed and live vaccines can be administered simultaneously without decreasing the efficacy of the individual vaccines. However, the vaccines should be administered at different sites.

Table 15.6: Vaccination schedule for unimmunized children		
Age	*Less than 7 yr*	*More than 7 yr*
First visit	BCG*, OPV*, DPTw/DTPa, HB	Td, HB
Second visit (one mo later)	BCG*, DPTw/DTPa, HB	Td, HB
Third visit (one mo later)	Measles/MMR, typhoid	MMR, typhoid
Fourth visit (6 mo after 1st visit)	DPTw/DTPa, HB	HB
Every 3 yr	Typhoid	Typhoid

*OPV and BCG recommended up to 5 yr of age

Table 15.7: IAP recommendations for immunization of infected children with HIV		
Vaccine	*Asymptomatic HIV infection*	*Symptomatic HIV infection*
BCG	Yes (at birth)	No
DTPw/DTPa	Yes (at 6, 10, 14 wk)	Yes
OPV	Yes (at 6, 10, 14 wk)	IPV not OPV
Measles	Yes (at 6 and 9 wk)	Yes
MMR	Yes	Yes (CD 4 is >15%)
Hepatitis B	Yes (as for uninfected children)	Yes (double each dose)
Hib	Yes	Yes
Typhoid Vi	Yes	Yes
Pneumococcal	Yes	Yes
Influenza	Yes	Yes
Varicella	Yes (2 doses at 6–8 wk interval)	Yes (2 doses at 6–8 wk interval, CD 4 is >15%))
Hepatitis A	Yes	Yes

Source: Shah RC, Shah NK, Kukreja S. IAP Guide Book on Immunization. IAP Committee on immunization (2005–2006). Mumbai: Indian Academy of Pediatrics, 2007 January; 1–96.

10. *Vaccination in children with HIV infection.* Children infected by HIV are particularly vulnerable to severe, recurrent, or unusual infections by vaccine preventable pathogens. It must be emphasized that routine immunizations seem to be generally safe in such children, but the immune response following vaccination would depend upon the degree of immunodeficiency at that point of time. Consideration should be given to re-administering childhood immunizations to such children when their immune status has improved following anti-retroviral therapy. Indian Academy of Pediatrics (IAP) recommendations for immunization of infected children is listed in Table 15.7.
11. *Immunization of adolescents* (Section 15.2).
12. *Immunization for travelers* (Section 15.5).

Injection Safety Issues

Injection safety is an important issue for any immunization program. Wash or disinfect hands prior to preparing injection material. Avoid giving injections if skin is infected. Always use a sterile syringe and needle for each injection. Clean skin prior to injection with a disinfectant and wait for it to dry. Do not use cotton balls stored wet in a multi-use container. If multi-dose vials are used, always pierce the septum with a sterile needle but do not leave the needle in place in the stopper of the vial. If using an ampoule that requires a metal file to open, protect fingers with a small gauge pad when opening the ampoule. Anticipate and take measures to prevent sudden patient movement during and after injection.

All intramuscular injections in children should be given only on the anterolateral aspect of thigh at the junction of the middle and lower third. The injection in the gluteal region must be avoided as sciatic injury is a real risk.

It is important for health personnel to understand that 'sharps' must be immediately contained in a 'sharps' box. The needle must not be recapped or manually mutilated after use. To prevent reuse, the

Table 15.8: Adverse reactions following immunizations

No.	Adverse reactions	Vaccine	Symptoms	Management
1	Anaphylaxis	Any vaccine	Within minutes • Acute decompensation of circulatory system • Hypovolemic shock • Laryngospasm/edema • Acute respiratory distress	• Adrenaline • Cardiopulmonary resuscitation • IV volume expanders • Hydrocortisone • Dopamine/dobutamine
2	Hypotensive-hyporesponsive episode	DTP	• Acute paleness • Transient decreased level or loss of consciousness • Decrease or loss of muscle tone	• IV fluids • Oxygen • Sedation with Triclofos 50 mg/kg
3	Incessant cry	DTP	Within 48–72 hr of immunization • Excessive inconsolable crying	• Paracetamol (10–15 mg/kg/per dose)
4	Toxic shock syndrome	Contamination of measles vaccine with *Staphylococcus aureus*	Within 30 minutes to a few hr • Mounting fever • Vomiting • Diarrhea • Septic shock	• IV fluids • Antimicrobials Cloxacillin 50–100 mg/kg 24 hr • Steroids • Suppurative therapy
5	Lymphadenitis	BCG	Within 2 to 6 mo • Firm to soft axillary lymphadenitis 1.5 to 3 cm size	• If firm, no treatment • If soft and fluctuant aspiration/surgical excision • Anti-tuberculosis treatment (ATT) not indicated
6	Bacterial abscess	Any vaccine	After days to weeks fluctuant or firm	• Antibiotics • Antipyretics • Drainage
7	Moderate to severe local reaction	Any vaccine	Nonfluctuant swelling/redness 3–10 cm in size at the injection site	• Paracetamol
8	Seizures with fever (rare)	DTP Measles	Always generalized	• Anticonvulsants • IV fluids (if needed)

Source: Shah RC, Shah NK, Kukreja S. IAP Guide Book on Immunization. IAP Committee on immunization (2005–2006). Mumbai: Indian Academy of Pediatrics, 2007 January; 1-96.

syringe may be cut and the needle defanged using a syringe/needle destroyer. Syringes and needles should be disposed of carefully in leak-proof and puncture proof containers and needles and waste management should be given due attention. Auto-disable (AD) syringes are single-use, self-locking syringes designed in such a way that these are rendered unstable after single use.

Adverse Reactions following Immunization

Adverse reactions following immunization can be broadly classified as local and systemic (Table 15.8). Although such reactions are uncommon, every physician who is dealing with immunization should anticipate and be prepared to manage these events whenever they occur. It is mandatory for every immunization clinic to have an emergency kit for resuscitation. Local reactions are especially common after adsorbed vaccines (e.g. DTPw/DT)-no treatment other than symptomatic management is necessary. Whole cell killed typhoid vaccines are also associated with particularly significant local reactions. Ulcer formation after BCG vaccination is normal and no intervention is usually required—the ulcers may sometimes take many weeks to heal. Anaphylactic reactions have been reported following measles, MMR, Hib, and hepatitis vaccines. Such reactions may be secondary to allergy to egg (e.g. Measles, MMR, yellow fever vaccines), gelatin (e.g. MMR, varicella, yellow fever vaccines), certain antimicrobials (e.g., neomycin in MMR, varicella, and inactivated polio vaccines), or thimerosal (e.g. DPT, TT vaccines).

It is often difficult to prove a definite cause-effect relationship between a vaccine and a given complication. It is not desirable to ascribe all adverse reactions to a vaccine, which has been given in the recent past before ascertaining all facts about the case. Many adverse effects may result from inappropriate vaccination technique or storage of the product. Any suspected adverse reaction following immunization must be reported to local authority.

Surveillance for Vaccine Preventable Diseases (VPDs)

Surveillance is a French word, which means "watching with attention, suspicion and authority." Disease surveillance under the Universal Immunization Program (UIP) refers to the collection, analysis and use of data on VPD to improve action to prevent these diseases. A good surveillance system can detect program failures and impending outbreaks and can also be used to assess vaccine efficacy. Any satisfactory national immunization program should result in gradual decline of the VPDs. All cases of VPDs should

be reported to the local authority within 48–72 hr for taking prompt action at the field level.

Combination Vaccines

A combination vaccine consists of two or more separate immunogens that have been physically combined in a single preparation. Many parents opt for one single injection of combination vaccines at a given visit, rather than getting a large number of simultaneous injections. The following cautionary statements should be strictly followed when administering combination vaccines:
a. The manufacturer's recommendations should be adhered to strictly.
b. "Mixing" of vaccines in the same syringe (prior to injection) should not be done as far as possible, unless specifically recommended by the manufacturer; in the latter case the manufacturer's instructions should be followed strictly.
c. Combination vaccines should not be viewed as being more effective than vaccines given separately.

Ada G. Vaccines and vaccinations. *N Engl J Med* 2001; 395: 1042–53.

Aggarwal KC. Immunization for Reduction in Infant mortality and Maternal Mortality. In: Mathur GP, Mathur Sarla (eds). *Current Trends in Pediatrics*. Vol 1. Delhi: Academa Publishers, 2005;42–51.

American Academy of Pediatrics, Committee on Pediatric AIDS: Evaluation and Medical treatment of HIV exposed infant. *Pediatrics* 1999;909.

Essential Childhood Immunization: Govt. of NCT, Delhi publication. 2001–2002.

Murphy TV, Gargiullo PM, Marrondi MS, et al. Intussusception among infant given an oral rota virus vaccine. N Engl J Med 2001; 344: 564-572.

Orenstein WA, Pickering LK. Immunization Practices. In: Kliegman RM, Behrman RE, Jenson HB, Stanton BF (eds). *Nelson Textbook of Pediatrics*. 18th edn. Vol 2. Philadelphia: Saunders, 2007;1058–70.

Park K. Principles of epidemiology and epidemiologic methods. In: *Park's Textbook of Preventive and Social Medicine*. 19th edn. Jabalpur: M/s Banarsidas Bhanot, 2007;49–114.

Reproductive and Child Health Programme, GOI. Immunization Strengthening Project, Manage cold chain. III, 2001.

Shah RC, Shah NK, Kukreja S. IAP Guide Book on Immunization. IAP Committee on immunization (2005–2006). Mumbai: Indian Academy of Pediatrics, 2007 January; 1–96.

Standards for child and adolescent immunization practices. In: Larry K. Pickering (Ed). *Red Book 2003 report of the committee of infectious diseases*. 26th edn. American Academy of Pediatrics, 2003.

Suvedi BK. Vaccine Preventable Diseases and their Surveillance. In: Mathur GP, Mathur Sarla (eds). *Current Trends in Pediatrics*. Vol 1. Delhi: Academa Publishers, 2005;57–62.

World Health Organization. Global alliance for Vaccines and Immunizations (GAVI). WHO Fact Sheet no. 169 March 2001 (cited 14th April 2002).

World Health Organization. Vaccine Safety. Vaccine Safety Advisory Committee. Weekly Epidemiol 1999;74:337–38.

15.2 IMMUNIZATION IN ADOLESCENTS

Vaccines are not just for infants and young children contrary to the popular belief. Older children, including teens, also need to receive recommended vaccinations. Even if the child has received all recommended vaccinations in the past that's not enough. Adolescents need to be vaccinated

1. To boost the waning immunity, and for increasing the duration of effective protection from the vaccines already given earlier in life, especially in the absence of "natural" boosting from exposure to the infectious agent.
2. To accelerate disease elimination drive: Disease control initiatives frequently encompass immunizing a wide age range, including adolescents, with the aim of interrupting transmission through herd immunity or catching-up on cases missed in the past. As with the rest of the population, adolescent individuals, also benefit from the protection afforded by vaccines in the face of outbreaks or seasonal rises in infectious diseases.
3. To counter a specific risk; as for all ages, travel represents a special need for adolescent immunization, also that adolescent behavior may place them at increased risk, e.g. of hepatitis B and HIV infection through a western life style that involves drug taking or sexual experimentation with multiple partners.

Special efforts may be appropriate to immunize them with available vaccines before they enter the risk period. The adolescent risks exposure to new health threats by entering educational institutes or military training institutes. Specific measures may be needed for the same.

Vaccines required by adolescents: These 3 vaccines should be administrated beginning with child's 11–12-yr-old checkup (or as soon as possible and recommended, if child is older and has not received the vaccines).

   i. Tetanus-diphtheria-acellular-pertussis vaccine (Tdap)
  ii. Meningococcal vaccine
 iii. HBV vaccine series.

Catch up vaccination: Older children should get the following vaccinations if they did not receive all recommended doses when younger: Hepatitis B, polio, measles-mumps-rubella (MMR), varicella (chickenpox).

Additional vaccines: Some children may need additional vaccines either due to their own specific health conditions or exposure in households to other people with age-related or health-related risks. The additional vaccines for which your child should be assessed include: Pneumococcal polysaccharide vaccine, hepatitis A, influenza.

Adolescent Vaccination Schedule (as Recommended for India)

BCG: Revaccination is not required. First dose can be given in adolescence, if not given earlier.

Diphtheria as Td or Tdap if no boosters taken earlier and to control outbreaks.

Pertussis: Not being given to adolescents in India (In USA acellular vaccine Tdap is given).

Tetanus: As Td, Tdap or TT booster and also in high-risk areas and after trauma.

Polio: Used for travel to endemic areas, if immunization is not complete.

Measles should be given as a part of MMR program and in elimination campaigns.

Mumps: MMR program and also for outbreak prevention and elimination campaigns.

Rubella: MMR program and in congenital rubella syndrome (CRS) control strategy.

Hepatitis B: No boosters are recommended, primary doses recommended if not taken earlier, in high risk life style or travel to endemic area, and for institutionalized persons.

Hepatitis A: In outbreaks and travel to endemic areas.

Typhoid: Vi-capsular polysaccharide vaccine for endemic areas or travel to endemic areas and in outbreaks—every 3 yr.

Influenza: Seasonal (October to July) for high-risk adolescents.

Varicella (chickenpox): All those who have not received vaccine earlier and wish to be immunized and for immunodeficient adolescents.

Pneumococcal (unconjugated polysaccharide) for immunodeficient adolescents.

Yellow fever: In outbreaks and travel to endemic areas.

Meningococcal: In outbreak and travel to endemic areas and for military recruits and high school, etc.

Japanese encephalitis: Travel to endemic areas and in elimination campaigns.

Individual description of each vaccine (Section 15.1).

Human papillomavirus (HPV) vaccine protects cervical dysphasia and genital warts. The vaccine is also recommended for girls and women 13 through 26 yr of age who did not receive it when they were younger. HPV vaccine is given in 3 doses. First dose can be given any time after 9 yr of age (minimum age:

9 yr), second dose should ideally be 2 mo after the first dose and third dose should be 6 mo after the first dose. Boosters are not recommended. HPV vaccine may be given at the same time as other vaccines. Pregnant women should not get the vaccine. Adolescents who are breast-feeding may safely get the vaccine.

Vaccinations in special circumstances (Section 15.1)

Adolescent females of childbearing age: Those female adolescents of childbearing age who have not been immunized with tetanus toxoid (TT) in their infancy or before pregnancy, it is recommended that they receive the first dose (TT1) at first contact during pregnancy and TT2 at least 4 wk after TT1. TT3 should be given at least 6 mo after TT2. The two remaining doses should be given after subsequent intervals of one-year minimum. If pregnant women have record of prior receipt of tetanus-toxoid-containing vaccines in early childhood or school age, they may receive a booster dose during pregnancy.

Passive immunization postpartum against rhesus sensitization: One of the most effective immunological interventions post-partum is the Rh-prophylaxis in Rh-negative women who did not produce anti-Rh-D antibodies during pregnancy, and who gave birth to a Rh-positive infant. They receive anti-Rh-D 200 µg within 24–72 hr post-partum.

Post-partum rubella vaccination: The post-partum period is an appropriate time for this vaccine, because pregnancy is a relative contraindication to Rubella immunization, and the probability of pregnancy occurring within 30 days of delivery is extremely small. It has been shown to be effective. If a rubella test has been done in pregnancy and has shown the woman to be non-immune, immunization can be offered in the early puerperium to prevent congenital malformations due to rubella in subsequent pregnancies.

Immunization for travelers: Adolescent travelers should receive updated routine immunization and also destination specific vaccinations. For example, if traveling to African subcontinent they should receive yellow fever vaccine. If traveling to India from Western countries they must receive typhoid and hepatitis A vaccines.

Contraindications to adolescent immunization: There is only one permanent contraindication to adolescent immunization and that is an anaphylactic reaction to a particular vaccine or to one of its components. Temporary contraindications are: pregnancy-live vaccines, moderate to severe illness, immunodeficient states (illness or due to drugs)-live vaccines.

Children receiving daily corticosteroids for over 2 wk should not be vaccinated with live vaccines until a month after discontinuation of treatment. Killed vaccines are safe but effect cannot be guaranteed. The rule does not apply to inhaled or topical steroids.

Re-assuring about side-effects of vaccines: Vaccines are few of the safest medicines available. One must bear in mind that the potential risks associated with the diseases that these vaccines prevent are much greater than the potential risks associated with the vaccines themselves

Personal record: This record helps health care provider ensure that the adolescent is protected against vaccine-preventable diseases. The record should be carried on every visit to health care provider so that it can be reviewed each time to find out whether the "adolescent is immunized".

Bansal CP, Bhave. Adolescent immunization. *Bhave's Text book of Adolescent Medicine.* 1st edn. Delhi: Jaypee Brothers Medical Publishers 2006;109–22.

Bhave S. Overview of immunization in adolescents: Course manual for adolescent health, Part II, Indian Perspective. Delhi: Cambridge press, 2004;49–54.

Essential Childhood Immunization: Govt. of NCT, Delhi publication, 2001–2002.

Facts About Adolescent Immunization (2009). National Foundation for Infectious Disease. 4733 Bethesda Avenue, Suite 750, Bethesda, MD 2081. Retrieved from http://www.nfid.org/pdf/factsheets/adolescentqa.pdf

Standards for child and adolescent immunization practices. In: Larry K. Pickering (ed). Red Book 2003 report of the committee of infectious diseases. 26th edn. American Academy of Pediatrics, 2003.

World Health Organization. Global alliance for Vaccines and Immunizations (GAVI). WHO Fact Sheet no. 169. March 2001 (cited 14th April 2002).

World Health Organization. Vaccine Safety. Vaccine Safety Advisory Committee. *Weekly Epidemiol* 1999;74:337–8.

15.3 COLD CHAIN: STORAGE AND TRANSPORT OF VACCINE

The 'cold chain' is the system of transporting and storing vaccines within the safe temperature range of between 2° and 8°C from the place of manufacture to the point of administration. Maintenance of system requires that processes are in place to ensure that a potent vaccine reaches recipients.

Vaccine should be safe, i.e. no adverse event should follow vaccination. It should be potent to produce effective immunity otherwise once potency is lost, vaccine is no longer effective and it gives false sense of protection. Potency of vaccine is maintained by cold chain. Maintenance of temperature in prescribed limits, i.e. 2°–8°C from the site of manufacturing to site of use is called cold chain. Maintenance of prescribed temperature from site of use to site of storage is called reserve cold chain.

Vaccine vial monitor (VVM) is a time and temperature sensitive colored label that provides an indication of the cumulative heat to which the vial has been exposed. The VVM warns the end user when exposure to heat is likely to have degraded the vaccine beyond an acceptable label. It is used especially for temperature monitoring of OPV which is the most thermolabile of all vaccines. If the VVM indicates proper storage of OPV I a given center, it can be presumed that other vaccines would also be potent. VVMs increase the flexibility in handling of vaccines in the field.

Interpretation of the color change of VVM is as follows:
1. *Inner squire is lighter than outer circle:* If the expiry date has not passed, vaccine can be used.
2. *Inner square matches color of the outer circle or is darker than outer circle:* Vaccine should be discarded.

Vaccine Stability

All vaccines are sensitive biological substances that progressively lose their potency (i.e. their ability to give protection against disease). This loss of potency is much faster when the vaccine is exposed to temperatures outside the recommended storage range. Once vaccine potency has been lost, returning the vaccine to correct storage condition cannot restore it. Any loss of potency is permanent and irreversible. Thus, storage of vaccines at the correct recommended temperature conditions is vitally important in order that full vaccine potency is retained up to the moment of administration. Although all vaccines are heat-sensitive, some are far more sensitive than others. Those listed in Box 15.1 can be arranged in order of decreasing sensitivity to heat. T series of vaccine, i.e. DPT, DT, TT, hepatitis B, hepatitis A and typhoid (tyhi Vi) are least sensitive to heat, hence they should not be frozen. Vaccines listed in Box 15.2 are unstable at room temperature and must not be exposed to light.

Box 15.1: Sensitivity of vaccines arranged in order of decreasing sensitivity to heat

Live oral polio vaccine (OPV)
Measles (lyophilized
Pertussis and mumps (lyophilized)
Hepatitis B
Adsorbed diphtheria-pertussis-tetanus vaccine (DPT vaccine)
Adsorbed diphtheria-tetanus vaccine (DT, Td vaccine)
BCG (lyophilized)
Tetanus toxoid (TT)

Box 15.2: Vaccine unstable at room temperature must not be exposed to light

BCG (Bacille-Calmette-Guérin) vaccine;
Reconstituted measles-mumps-rubella (MMR) vaccine;
Oral polio vaccine (OPV).

For checking the potency of T series of vaccine shake test can be done.

Shake test: After vigorous shaking of vial, it is left for 15 minutes and presence of visible big floccule exclude usability of vaccine.

Some vaccines are also highly sensitive to being cold. Such vaccines will lose their potency entirely if frozen, although others can sustain freezing without any damage whatsoever (Box 15.3). It is therefore vitally important to know the correct storage conditions for each vaccine, and to ensure that each is kept always at the recommended conditions.

Unpacking Vaccines after Transport

Do not remove vaccines from their packaging regardless of their bulkiness. Removal from original packaging exposes vaccines to room temperature and/or lighting. Check cold chain monitors when the vaccines arrive to ensure they have not been exposed to temperatures above 8°C or below 0°C.

If cold-chain monitors (CCMs) have not been included, check that the ice packs are still partially frozen; if they are completely thawed, the vaccines have not been kept sufficiently cold and may not be effective. Do not discard any vaccines until you discuss the necessary actions with your State/Territory vaccine distribution centre, vaccine supplier, hospital pharmacy or local public health unit.

Cold Chain Equipment

The equipment used for storing and transport of vaccines at desired temperature is called cold chain equipment.
1. *Walk in freezer (WIF):* Used for bulk storage of vaccine especially OPV and measles and also used for preparation of ice packs mainly at state HQ or division level.

Box 15.3: Sensitivity of vaccines to freezing

DPT; DT; Td; TT; hepatitis B; BCG*; OPV; measles*; mumps
Note: Vaccines freeze at temperatures just below zero.

These vaccines become much more heat sensitive after they have been reconstituted with diluent.
BCG and measles vaccines must not be frozen after reconstitution
Diluents for any vaccine must never be frozen.

Tempt: –20°C

Two sizes: 16.5 M³ and 32 M³

They are provided by two identical cooling units and stand by generator set.

2. ***Walk in coolers (WIC):*** Used for bulk storage of vaccine at state/regional centre. Temperature maintenance 2° to 8°C.

Size: 16.5 M³ and 32 M³

Like WIF provided with two cooling units and standby generator set. There is provision of auto start, alarm and temperature recorder as well. They store the vaccine for 3–4 districts, i.e. 3 mo requirement with 25% extra buffer stocks.

3. Deep freezers used for storing of OPV and measles vaccine and also used for preparation of ice packs. Temperature is maintained at 18°–20°C. In case of power failure it can maintain temperature up to 24 hrs if not opened.

Sizes: 300 L and 140 L.

Chest freezer (300 L) is provided with special insulation and can store vaccines for much longer time. 140 L. Freezer can store 65,000 dosages and can make about 8–10 kg ice (i.e. 25–30 ice packs) at a time, and 35–40 ice packs (12–14 kg ice) can be frozen in one day. T series of vaccine should not be stored in them.

4. ***Ice lined refrigerators (ILRS):*** These are top opening refrigerators. It can keep safe vaccine even if there is continuous power supply for 8 hrs. in 24 hrs. Available sizes are 140 liters and 300 liters. It is named ice-lined as it is lined with water filled bottles which get frozen and keep the cold temperature for long time. In the bottom OPV, measles and MMR are stored. In the middle, BCG, DPT, TT, and hepatitis B is stored. Nowadays non-CFC deep freezer and ILR are available which do not deplete ozone layer and are environment friendly.

Electrolux ILR can act as freezer as well as ILR. Hold over time of ILR is 62 hrs at 43°C and 78 hrs at 32°C.

5. Domestic refrigerators are used for storing small quantity of vaccine at dispensary or MCH centre level and prepare frozen ice packs (Fig. 15.1). Vaccines can be placed as follows:

   1. *Freezer compartment:* OPV
   2. *Top shelf:* BCG/measles/MMR
   3. *Middle shelf:* DTP/DT/TT/typhoid/hepatitis A/Hib/hepatitis B/varicella
   4. *Lower shelf:* Diluent
   5. *Baffle tray* should be kept empty
   6. Holes so that cold air can circulate inside the boxes.

Safe vaccine storage is possible in most refrigerators if the following procedures are adhered to:
- Vaccine storage guidelines are followed;
- Door openings are kept to a minimum;
- Temperatures are checked and recorded daily;
- One person should be given responsibility for adjusting the refrigerator control (it is important that other staff are also trained to ensure continuous monitoring);
- Defrosting is done regularly and ice is not allowed to build up.

The refrigerator to be used should be dedicated to vaccine storage whenever possible. Do not store food or drink in vaccine refrigerators. Vaccines should only be stored on the middle and upper shelves in normal domestic refrigerators. If using a bar fridge, the middle shelf should be used, as vaccines stored near the evaporation plate or on the top shelf of a bar fridge can be inadvertently frozen. The lower shelves, drawers and the door of normal domestic refrigerators become to warm (above 10°C) if the refrigerator is opened frequently.

Do not crowd the vaccines by overfilling the refrigerator; allow room for the cold air to circulate within the refrigerator. Fill the lower drawers and the door with plastic bottles filled with salt water. This helps to stabilise the temperatures within the refrigerator. Allow space between the bottles for good air circulation. Add enough salt to make the water undrinkable (about 1–2 tablespoons per litre).

If a dedicated vaccine fridge is not available, store the vaccines in a (pre-cooled) Styrofoam container with lid closed and place in the middle of the refrigerator. Ensure the vaccines inside the container are monitored and place a label on the outside stating "Vaccines-Keep refrigerated".

When preparing ice packs or freezer blocks for transport, cool the thawed ice packs on the lower shelf of the refrigerator during the day before placing in the freezer. Place cooled ice packs in the freezer at the end of the day for freezing overnight. Allow a minimum of 2 days for complete freezing before using the blocks for transporting vaccines. Do not stack ice packs on top of each other in the freezer. Set them on their edge and allow space between them.

Maintaining and monitoring refrigerator temperatures: Refrigerators used for vaccines should have a minimum/maximum thermometer placed on a middle shelf and temperatures should be checked and recorded daily. The most cost effective minimum/maximum thermometer is a digital type with a probe.

If using a digital thermometer with a probe, the probe should be placed directly in contact with the vaccine vial. Do not put the probe into fluid. The recommendation of keeping the vaccine storage temp at between 2° to 8° is based on air, not fluid temperatures.

The refrigerator temperature should be read around the same time each day, preferably in the middle of the day. One person only should be responsible for adjusting the refrigerator to maintain the temperature in the recommended range of 2° to 8°C.

The door should be kept closed as much as possible. Refrigerators used for vaccine storage should have an uninterrupted power supply and door openings should be kept to a minimum.

During a power failure of 4 hr or less, the refrigerator door should be left closed. If the power fails for more than 4 hr, store vaccines in a pre-cooled, insulated container with ice packs to keep them cool (see section 'Transporting vaccines in insulated containers' for more information).

Maintenance of the vaccine refrigerator: Refrigerator breakdowns should be repaired immediately. The door seals should be in good condition so that the door closes securely. Refrigerators that are not 'frost free' should be defrosted regularly to prevent ice build-up. Ice build-up can reduce the efficiency and performance of a refrigerator.

During defrosting or cleaning of the refrigerator, move the vaccines to a second refrigerator. This temporary storage refrigerator must also be monitored to ensure the correct temperature is maintained. Alternatively the vaccines can be stored in a pre-cooled insulated container with ice packs or ice until the normal vaccine refrigerator is ready for use again.

There is more information in the section called 'Transporting vaccines in insulated containers'.

6. *Cold box:* Size 5–20 L: Lined with frozen ice packs and in between vaccines are kept. T series of vaccine should not come in contact with frozen ice packs. Hold over time 5 to 6 days. 5 L box can transport 1500 doses and 20 L box has the space for 6000 doses. It is used for transport of vaccine and in case of power failure it can store vaccine.
7. Vaccine carrier is lined by 4 fully frozen ice packs and can transport 16–20 vials in periphery. Hold over time—36 to 48 hr. Useful for peripheral use.
8. Vaccine day carrier is lined by 2 ice packs can have 6–8 vials. Hold over time 6–8 hrs.

GENERAL PRINCIPLES OF COLD CHAIN

1. Vaccines are not kept for more than 3 mo at district.
2. Vaccines are not kept more than 1 mo at PHC or MCH centre and are not stored at sub centre level at all.
3. All vaccines are stored at 2°–8°C and dial thermometer and alcohol thermometers are used for this.
4. T series of vaccines are never frozen and to check its usability shake test is used, i.e. shake it vigorously and keep it for 15 minutes and there should not be any visible floccules.
5. Principle of FIFO (first in first out) and FEFO (first expiry and first out) should be observed.
6. VVM status tells the potency of OPV vials, i.e. inner circle should be lighter or white than the outer circle then only it can be used.

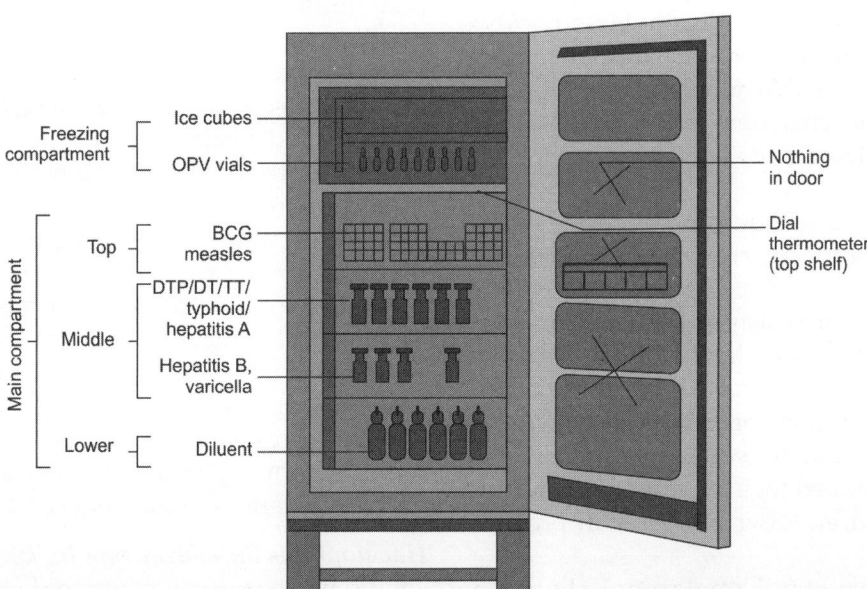

Fig.15.1: Refrigerator showing vaccines stored correctly in clinic setup. *From Shah RC, Shah NK, Kukreja S. IAP Guide Book on Immunization. IAP Committee on immunization (2005–2006). Mumbai: Indian Academy of Pediatrics, 2007 January; 1–96.*

7. Boxes should have holes while storage so that cold and air can circulate inside the boxes.
8. There should be spare cold chain equipment 10% extra so that in case of emergency, there is no interruption in cold chain.
9. There should be 25% extra voltage stabilizers for emergency use. And some mechanic should look after the wear and tear of cold chain equipment.

Aggarwal KC. Immunization for Reduction in Infant mortality and Maternal Mortality. In: Mathur GP, Mathur Sarla (eds). *Current Trends in Pediatrics.* Vol 1. Delhi: Academa Publishers, 2005;42–51.

Jacob John T, Parthsarthy A, Bhave SW. IAP Guide Book on Immunization. Committee on immunization: Indian Academy of Pediatrics, Mumbai 1996.

Reproductive and Child Health Programme, GOI. Immunization Strengthening Project, Manage cold chain. III, 2001.

Shah RC, Shah NK, Kukreja S. IAP Guide Book on Immunization. IAP Committee on immunization (2005–2006). Mumbai: Indian Academy of Pediatrics, 2007 January; 1–96.

World Health Organization. Vaccine Safety. Vaccine Safety Advisory Committee. Weekly Epidemiol 1999;74:337–8.

15.4 CHEMOPROPHYLAXIS

Chemoprophylaxis is an important method of prevention. Chemoprophylaxis implies the protection from or prevention of disease. This type of prevention is used in malaria, bacterial meningitis, diphtheria, influenza and pneumonic plague

Malaria prevention: Chemoprophylaxis is the cornerstone of malaria prevention for nonimmune children and adults who travel to malaria-endemic areas, but it is not a replacement for other protective measures because no chemoprophylaxis regimen guarantees complete protection against malaria (Section 15.5). Factors that must be considered in choosing appropriate chemoprophylaxis medications and dosing schedules include age of the child, travel itinerary (Table 15.9)

Chloroquine and mefloquine should be started 1 wk prior to departure and continued for 4 wk after last exposure.

Mefloquine resistance exists in Western Cambodia and along the Thai-Cambodia and Thai-Myanmar borders. Travelers in these areas should take doxycycline or atovaquone-proguanil.

Doxycycline should be started 1 day prior to departure and continued for 4 wk after last exposure. Do not use in children <8 yr of age or in pregnant women.

Atovaquone/proguanil (malarone) should be started 1–2 days prior to departure and continued for 7 days after last exposure.

Table 15.9: Chemoprophylaxis of malaria for children

Area	Drug	Dosage (oral)
Chloroquine-resistant area	Mefloquine	<15 kg: 4.6 mg base (5 mg salt)/kg/wk 15–19 kg: 1/4 tab/wk 20–30 kg: 1/2 tab/wk 31–45 kg: 3/4 tab/wk > 15 kg: 1 tab/wk (228 mg base)
	Doxycycline	2 mg/kg daily (max 100 mg)
	Atovaquone/proguanil (malarone)	Pediatric tabs: 62.5 mg atovaquone/25 mg proguanil Adult tabs: 250 mg atovaquone/100 mg proguanil 11–20 kg: 1 pediatric tab once daily 21–30 kg: 2 pediatric tabs once daily 31–40 kg: 3 pediatric tabs once daily >40 kg: 1 adult tab once daily
Chloroquine-sensitive area	Chloroquine phosphate	5 mg base/kg/wk (maximum 300 mg base)

Bacterial Meningitis Prevention

Chemoprophylaxis is essential to prevent contacts getting disease.

Neisseria meningitidis: Chemoprophylaxis is recommended for all close contacts of patients with meningococcal meningitis regardless of age or immunization status. Close contacts of patients should be treated with rifampin 10 mg/kg/dose every 12 hr (maximum dose of 600 mg) for 2 days as soon as possible after identification of a case of suspected meningococcal meningitis or sepsis. Close contacts include household, day care center, and nursery school contacts and health care workers who have direct exposure to oral secretions (mouth-to-mouth resuscitation, suctioning, and intubation). Exposed contacts should be treated immediately on suspicion of infection in the index patient; bacteriologic confirmation of infection should not be awaited. In addition, all contacts should be educated about the early signs of meningococcal disease and the need to seek prompt medical attention if these signs develop. Meningococcal vaccine also may be used as an adjunct with chemoprophylaxis for exposed contacts and during epidemics of meningococcal disease.

Haemophilus influenzae type b.: Rifampin prophylaxis should be given to all household contacts of patients, if any close family member younger than 48 mo has not been fully immunised or if an immunocompromised person, of any age, resides in the house-hold. A house-hold contact is one who lives in the residence of the index case or who has spent a minimum of 4 hr with the index case for at least 5 of the 7 days preceding the patient's hospitalization. Family members should receive rifampin prophylaxis immediately after the diagnosis is suspected in the index case because >50% of secondary family cases occur in the 1st wk after the index case has been hospitalized. All children should be immunized with *H. influenzae* type b conjugate vaccine beginning at 2 mo of age. The dose of the rifampin is 20 mg/kg/24 hr (maximum dose of 600 mg) given once on each day for 4 days. Rifampin color's the urine and perspiration red-orange, stains contact lenses, and reduces the serum concentrations of some drugs, including the oral contraceptives. Rifampin is contraindicated in pregnancy.

Diphtheria Prevention

Asymptomatic case contacts: All household contacts and those who have had intimate respiratory or habitual physical contact with a patient are closely monitored for illness through the 7 day incubation period. Cultures of the nose, throat, and any cutaneous lesions are performed. Antibiotic prophylaxis is administered regardless of immunization status using erythromycin (40–50 mg/kg/day divided qid PO for 7 days; maximum 2 g/day) or a single injection of benzathine penicillin G (600,000 U IM for <30 kg, 1,200,000 U IM for ≥30 kg). Diphtheria toxoid vaccine, in age-appropriate form, is given to immunized individuals who have not received a booster dose within 5 yr. Children who have not received their 4th dose should be vaccinated. Those who have received fewer than 3 doses of diphtheria toxoid or who have uncertain immunization status are immunized with an age-appropriate preparation on a primary schedule.

Asymptomatic carriers: When an asymptomatic carrier is identified, antimicrobial therapy is given for 7 days and an age-appropriate preparation of diphtheria toxoid is administered immediately if a booster has not been given within 1 yr. individuals are placed on droplet precautions (respiratory tract colonization) or contact precautions (cutaneous colonization only) until at least 2 subsequent cultures obtained 24 hr apart after cessation of therapy are negative. Repeat cultures are performed about 2 wk after completion of therapy for cases and carriers, and, if positive, an additional 10 day course of oral erythromycin should be given and follow-up cultures performed.

Influenza viral infection prevention: Amantadine and zanamivir are used for prophylaxis for vaccinated and unvaccinated high-risk patients and their unvaccinated health care providers during influenza A outbreaks in closed settings, for unvaccinated persons and health care providers during community influenza A outbreaks and during the period of peak influenza A activity, for immunodeficient persons, and for those for whom the influenza vaccine is contraindicated.

Pneumonic plague prevention: Postexposure prophylaxis should be given to close contacts of patients with pneumonic plague. Antimicrobial prophylaxis is recommended within 7 days of exposure for persons with direct close contact with a pneumonic plague patient, or those exposed to an accidental or terrorist-induced aerosol. Recommended regimens include a 7-day course of tetracycline, doxycycline, or TMP-SMZ. Contacts of cases of uncomplicated bubonic plague do not require prophylaxis.

Buescher ES. Diphtheria (Corynebacterium diphtheria). In: Kliegman RM, Behrman RE, Jenson HB, Stanton BF (eds). *Nelson Textbook of Pediatrics.* 18th edn. Vol 1. Philadelphia: Saunders, 2007;1153–57.

Murphy JR, Heresi GP. Yersinia. In: Kliegman RM, Behrman RE, Jenson HB, Stanton BF (eds). *Nelson Textbook of Pediatrics.* 18th edn. Vol 1. Philadelphia: Saunders, 2007;1202–5.

Park K. Principles of epidemiology and epidemiologic methods. In: *Park's Textbook of Preventive and Social Medicine.* 19th edn. Jabalpur: M/s Banarsidas Bhanot, 2007;49–114.

Prober CG. Central nervous system infections. In: Kliegman RM, Behrman RE, Jenson HB, Stanton BF (eds). *Nelson Textbook of Pediatrics.* 18th edn. Vol 2. Philadelphia: Saunders, 2007; 2512–24.

Wright P. Influenza viruses. In: Kliegman RM, Behrman RE, Jenson HB, Stanton BF (eds). *Nelson Textbook of Pediatrics.* 18th edn. Vol 1. Philadelphia: Saunders, 2007;1384–87.

15.5 HEALTH ADVICE FOR CHILDREN TRAVELLING INTERNATIONALLY

Infants and children under seven years of age are at higher risk of getting sick from travel to tropical and developing countries. Children have special needs, and parents of travelling children should seek advice from a health care professional at least 4 to 6 wk before travelling to obtain assessment of health risks, a schedule of vaccinations and list of medications, and instructions on dealing with disease during travel. What to bring when travelling with children is listed in Box 15.4.

Health insurance: Parents should be encouraged to determine whether their health care plan covers health care internationally. If it does, parents should ask about the need for preauthorization for medical treatment, the level of co-payment required, and whether emergency medical evacuation is covered.

Box 15.4: Items to bring when travelling with children

- Carry insect repellent in liquid form, not aerosol.
- Carry travel health kit and water-disinfectant tablets.
- Bring medication recommended by your doctor for fever, such as paracetamol.
- Take loose fitting, cotton clothes and a sun hat if you are travelling to a hot climate.
- Take well-fitting enclosed shoes for children.

Travel tips
- Air travel is not recommended for premature infants and infants younger than seven days old.
- While the plane is taking off and landing, breast-feed or bottle-feed infants. Feeding your child gets them to swallow and prevents ear pain.
- Take your child's car seat with you. It may be used on board the plane if a seat is available.

Prevention of illness: It is important to prevent the child getting ill (Box 15.5).

Box 15.5: Prevention of illness

- Use only bottled purified, or boiled and cooled water to mix formula and juices.
- Continue to breastfeed when possible.
- Consider pre-mixed liquid formula for short trips.
- Medicine to prevent traveller's diarrhea should not be given to children.

Underlying medical illness: Parents of travelling children should be asked whether the child has any current health problems or has had any problems in the past that have required medical evaluation or medication. Children with medical conditions should take with them a brief medical summary. Parents should be counseled to take a sufficient supply of prescription medications for their children and to ensure that the bottles are clearly identified. For children requiring care by specialists, an international directory for that specialty can be consulted. A directory of physicians worldwide who speak English is available from the International Association for Medical Assistance to Travelers (www.iamat.org).

A *travel health kit* consisting of prescription medications and nonprescription items such as acetaminophen, an antihistamine, oral rehydration solution packets, antibiotic ointment, bandage, insect repellent, and sunscreen is recommended for children.

Safety: Injuries and motor vehicle accidents are the major causes of serious disability, hospitalization, and loss of life during travel. The use of safety belts for children, preferably sitting in the rear seat, should be emphasized. When possible, child safety-restraint seats should be taken on the trip. Travelers to remote areas should be warned about the risks of venomous animals as snake and scorpion bites can be fatal in infants.

Infectious Disease Precautions

Infectious disease risks to traveling children can generally be divided into four categories: food-borne, insect-borne, transmitted by contact with an infected person or by needle or blood exposure, and transmitted by contact with infected animals or environments.

Food-borne infections: Ingestion of contaminated food or water is responsible for travel-associated diarrhea, the most common health complaint among international travelers. Among the bacterial and protozoan infections children can acquire from contaminated water are shigellosis, salmonellosis, *Escherichia coli* infections, cholera, giardiasis, amebiasis, and cryptosporidiosis. Viral infections, particularly rotavirus infections are also a major cause of travel-associated diarrhea in children. Boiled water, hot beverages made with boiled water, and canned or bottled carbonated beverages are generally safest. Ice should be avoided, and tap water should not be used when brushing teeth. Boiling water for at least 1 minute is the most reliable method of water disinfection. Unpeeled fruit, uncooked vegetables, unpasteurized milk, milk products such as cheese, and undercooked meat or fish may all be contaminated and should be avoided. Breast-feeding should be encouraged for young children, especially infants 6 mo of age.

Infect-borne infections: Infect-borne infections for which traveling children are at risk include malaria, yellow fever, dengue, Japanese encephalitis, and filariasis are typically caused by night-biting mosquitoes, whereas dengue is usually caused by day-biting mosquitoes. Exposure to insect bites can be avoided by restricting high-risk activities, staying indoors in a screened and protected area from dusk to dawn, wearing appropriate attire, and using insect repellents containing permethrin or N,N-diethyl-M-toluamide (DEET). Rare instances of toxic encephalopathy have been reported in young children with exposure to high concentrations of DEET, but use of repellent with no more than 40% DEET and avoidance of repeated applications minimizes the risk of this complication. Concentrations of 25–35% DEET, to be applied every 6–8 hr as needed, are recommended for children. Spraying clothing with permethrin is a safe and effective method of reducing insect bites in children. Permethrin-sprayed clothes remain effective for at least 2 wk, even with laundering. Bed nets, particularly permethrin-impregnated bed nets, also decrease the risk of insect bites.

Infections from contact with infected persons or through needle exposure: Many of the infections that may be acquired by children travelling internationally through contact with other individuals are preventable by routine childhood immunizations. Other diseases transmitted through human contact include viral respiratory and gastrointestinal infections, viral hepatitis, and sexually transmitted diseases including HIV infection. Many of these diseases are more prevalent in developing countries. Adolescent travelers should be reminded that sexual encounters and needle or blood exposure (including tattooing and body piercing) carry a significant risk of HIV and hepatitis infection. Travelers may wish to have their blood typed before departure to determine whether family members or travel companions have compatible blood types and might be able to donate blood for transfusion in an emergency situation.

Infections from infected animals or environments: Infections potentially acquired from contact with animals include rabies from stray dogs and plague from rodents, swimming or diving in contaminated water can result in serious injury and increase the risk of infections such as schistosomiasis, leptospirosis, and primary amebic meningoencephalitis.

Travel and immunizations: Make sure routine childhood immunizations are complete. Carry a written record of your child's immunizations. If you are travelling to an area with a lot of measles, measles mumps-rubella (MMR) vaccine can be given to infants between six and twelve months of age. When the vaccine is given at a young age, children still need two doses of MMR after their first birthday. The immunizations may be given to children depending on their travel destination, length of stay, and age include hepatitis A vaccine; hepatitis B vaccine; cholera vaccine; typhoid vaccine; immune globulin; yellow fever vaccine; meningococcal vaccine; Japanese encephalitis vaccine; influenza vaccine; rabies vaccine; tuberculosis. Some vaccines should not be given to infants and young children.

Traveler's diarrhea: Traveler's diarrhea, characterized by a 2-fold or greater increase in the frequency of unformed bowel movements, occurs in as many as 40% of all travelers overseas. Children <3 yr of age have a higher incidence of diarrhea, more severe symptoms, and more prolonged symptoms than adults. Traveller's diarrhea is usually acquired through ingestion of fecally contaminated food and water. Various infectious agents (bacteria, viruses, and parasites) have been associated with traveler's diarrhea; enterotoxigenic *E. coli* is still the most frequent cause. Other bacterial causes include *Shigella, Salmonella, Compylobacter, Vibrio cholerae, Vibrio parahaemolyticus, Acromonas hydrophilia,* and *Plesiomonas shigelloides.* Protozoan infections such as *Entamoeba histolytica, Giardia lamblia,* and *Compylobacter parvum,* and *Isospora* are most common in long-term travelers. Rotavirus has also been associated with traveler's diarrhea. Immunocompromised children, including children with HIV, are at increased risk for complications from bacterial causes of traveler's diarrhea, particularly Salmonella.

Treatment of Diarrhea

- Children younger than three years of age who have a lot of diarrhea should be seen by a health care professional.
- Take the child to a health care professional right away if you see any of the following signs of dehydration: Your child may be very restless or irritable, have less and darker urine than normal, and be hard to wake up. Take the child to a health care professional if the child develops bloody diarrhea, has a fever higher than 38.5°C (101.3°F), or has persistent vomiting.
- Do not give antibiotics or other medications to children to stop diarrhea unless advised by a doctor.
- Give children lots of fluids to drink. Continue breast or formula feeding throughout the illness.
- Feed children over six months of age thin porridge, rice and soups. As they recover, children can be given their usual foods when they are willing to take them.
- Give ORS by mouth if the child shows signs of mild dehydration, such as feeling thirsty and restless, but still alert.

Presumptive self-treatment is usually recommended for adults, and most experts agree that it should also be given to children. For adults ≥18 yr of age the recommended regimen is ciprofloxacin (500 mg), norfloxacin (400 mg), or ofloxacin (300 mg) orally twice daily for 3 days. For children, the drugs of choice are azithromycin (10 mg/kg/day, maximum dose of 500 mg, for 3 days) and ciprofloxacin (25–30 mg/kg/day, divided into 2 doses, maximum of 500 mg twice a day, for 3 days).

Malaria prevention: The best way to prevent malaria is to avoid being bitten by mosquitoes in the first place! If at all possible, do not take infants or young children to areas where there is malaria, particularly areas where malaria is resistant to the drug chloroquine. Breast fed babies whose mothers are taking medication to prevent malaria must also be given medication, since little of the mother's medication will be in the breast milk.

Chemoprophylaxis is the cornerstone of malaria prevention for nonimmune children and adults who travel to malaria-endemic areas (Section 15.4). If you are taking part in outdoor activities between dusk and dawn, use insect repellent (DEET) on all exposed skin. For infants less than six months of age do not use any repellants that contain DEET.

Patterns of illnesses among returning international traveler: Post-travel evaluations are part of travel medicine and continuing care. Children who will be travelling abroad for a prolonged period of time (>6 mo) should receive tuberculin skin testing before and after travel and should be tested for asymptomatic gastrointestinal parasitic infections on their return. Fever is a particularly worrisome symptom. Malaria and typhoid are the 2 important causes of fever in children returning from travel to developing countries, but numerous other illnesses acquired in these countries may cause fever (Table 15.10).

Table 15.10: Patterns of illnesses among returning international travelers

Systemic febrile illness	Malaria; typhoid fever; dengue; rickettsial infections (tick-borne spotted fever); undetermined fever source
Acute diarrhea	Giardiasis; amebiasis; *Compylobacter*; *Shigella*; *Salmonella*; *Escherichia coli*; presumed viral
Dermatologic manifestations	Insect bites; cutaneous larva migrans; abscess; superficial mycosis; animal bite; leishmaniasis; myiasis (any disease due to the larvae of flies); scabies; impetigo

Staying Healthy During Your Trip

Prevent insect bites: Many diseases, like malaria and dengue, are spread through insect bites. One of the best protections is to prevent insect bites by:
1. Using insect repellent (bug spray) with 30–50% DEET.
2. Wearing long-sleeved shirts, long pants, and a hat outdoors.
3. Remaining indoors in a screened or air-conditioned area during the peak biting period for malaria (dusk and dawn).
4. Sleeping in beds covered by nets treated with permethrin, if not sleeping in an air-conditioned or well-screened room.
5. Spraying rooms with products effective against flying insects, such as those containing pyrethroid.

Prevent animal bites and scratches
1. Prevent animal bites and scratches because animals can spread diseases like rabies or cause serious injury or illness.

2. Be sure you are up to date with tetanus vaccination.
3. Do not touch or feed any animals, including dogs and cats. Even animals that look like healthy pets can have rabies or other diseases.
4. Help children stay safe by supervising them carefully around all animals.
5. If you are bitten or scratched, wash the wound well with soap and water and go to a doctor right away.
6. After your trip, be sure to tell your doctor or state health department if you were bitten or scratched during travel.

Be careful about food and water: Diseases from food and water are the leading cause of illness in travelers. Diseases from food and water often cause vomiting and diarrhea. Make sure to bring diarrhea medicine with you so that you can treat mild cases yourself. Follow these tips for safe eating and drinking:
1. Wash your hands often with soap and water, especially before eating. If soap and water are not available, use an alcohol-based hand gel (with at least 60% alcohol).
2. Drink only bottled or boiled water, or carbonated (bubbly) drinks in cans or bottles. Avoid tap water, fountain drinks, and ice cubes. If this is not possible, learn how to make water safer to drink.
3. Do not eat food purchased from street vendors.
4. Make sure food is fully cooked.
5. Avoid dairy products, unless you know they have been pasteurized.

Avoid injuries: Car crashes are a leading cause of injury among travelers. Protect yourself from these injuries by:
1. Not drinking and driving.
2. Wearing your seat belt and using car seats or booster seats in the backseat for children.
3. Following local traffic laws.
4. Wearing helmets when you ride bikes, motorcycles, and motor bikes.
5. Not getting on an overloaded bus or mini-bus.
6. Hiring a local driver, when possible.
7. Avoiding night driving.

Prevent altitude illness and sunburn: If you visit the Himalayan Mountains, ascend gradually to allow time for your body to adjust to the high altitude, which can cause insomnia, headaches, nausea, and altitude illness. If you experience these symptoms descend to a lower altitude and seek medical attention. Untreated altitude illness can be fatal (*see* Section 7.12).

Other health tips
1. To avoid infections such as HIV and viral hepatitis do not share needles for tattoos, body piercing, or injections.

2. To reduce the risk of HIV and other sexually transmitted diseases always use latex condoms.
3. To prevent fungal and parasitic infections, keep feet clean and dry, and do not go barefoot, especially on beaches where animals may have defecated.

INFECTIONS IN INTERNATIONAL ADOPTEES

International adopted children have many health problems. Infections or infestations are common and are in part dependent on the international region, nutritional status, and prior immunizations (Table 15.11); (*see* Section 6.1). Screening tests are listed in Table 15.13. The immunization record should be checked and the child immunized against any pathogen not reported in the immunization records. Catch-up immunization should be initiated.

Relevant websites are listed in Table 15.12 to guide families planning international adoption.

Barnett ED. Immunizations and infectious disease screening for internationally adopted children. Pediatr Clin North Am 2005;52:1287–309.

Barnett ED, Chen LH. Prevention of travel-related infectious diseases in families of internationally adopted children. Pediatr Clin North Am 2005;52:1271–86.

Central Adoption Resource Authority (CARA), Ministry of Women and Child Development, West Block 8, Wing 2, 2nd Floor, RK Puram, New Delhi-110066 (India).

Central Adoption Resource Authority (CARA) (An autonomous body of the Ministry of Women and Child Development, Govt. of India, Delhi.Website: www.adoption-india.nic.in; Email: cara@bol.net.in).

Hill DR. The burden of illness in international travelers. New Engl J Med 2006;354:115–7.

John CC, Salata RA. Health advice for children traveling internationally. In: Kliegman RM, Behrman RE, Jenson HB, Stanton BF (eds). *Nelson Textbook of Pediatrics*. 18th edn. Vol 1. Philadelphia: Saunders, 2007; 1077–83.

Katz BZ. Traveling with children. Pediatr Infect Dis J 2003; 22:274–6.

Kliegman RM. Infections in international adoptees. In: Kliegman RM, Behrman RE, Jenson HB, Stanton BF (eds). Nelson Textbook of Pediatrics. 18th edn. Vol 1. Philadelphia: Saunders, 2007;1083–84.

Mackell SM. Vaccinations for the pediatric traveler. Clin Infect Dis 2003;37(11):1508–16.

Orenstein WA, Pickering LK. Immunization Practices. In: Kliegman RM, Behrman RE, Jenson HB, Stanton BF (eds). *Nelson Textbook of Pediatrics*. 18th edn. Vol 2. Philadelphia: Saunders, 2007;1058–70.

Shah RC, Shah NK, Kukreja S. IAP Guide Book on Immunization. IAP Committee on immunization (2005-2006). Mumbai: Indian Academy of Pediatrics, 2007 January; 1–96.

Simms MD, Freundlich M. Adoption. In: Kliegman RM, Behrman RE, Jenson HB, Stanton BF (eds). *Nelson Textbook of Pediatrics*. 18th edn. Vol 1. Philadelphia: Saunders, 2007; 163–4.

Table 15.11: Common infectious diseases of internationally adopted children

Disease	Comment
Tuberculosis (TB)	Latent TB in 3–20% High rates in Asia and Russia
Hepatitis B virus	Chronic carriers in 5–7% High rates in Asia, Caribbeans, Eastern Europe, Africa
Hepatitis C virus	0–2.5% incidence High rates in Eastern Europe, Middle East, Asia
HIV	<1% HIV positive High risk from Russia, Africa, Asia
Syphilis (congenital)	<2% VDRL (Venereal Disease Research Laboratory) test is positive High rates in Eastern Europe, Russia, Asia
Giardia	Very common High rates in Africa, Central and South America, Asia
Ascaris lumbricoides	Common High rtes in Asia, Africa, Central and South America
Hookworms	Unknown incidence High rates in Asia. Mediterranean, South America
Other parasitic diseases	
Dientamoeba fragilis	~2% of adoptees
Tricuris trichuria	Unknown prevalence
Enterobius vermicularis	2–30% of adoptees
Strongyloides stercoralis	Most virulent, eosinophilia present

Table 15.12: Online resources to guide families planning international adoption

Website	Comments
www.adoptionindia.nic.in; Email: cara@bol.net.in Central Adoption Resource Authority (CARA), Delhi, India	
http://travel.state.gov//family/adoption/adoption_485.html	International adoption booklet, information on US visa requirements; travel warnings
http://www.cdc.gov/nie/menus/groups.htm#intl	General health information regarding international adoption
http://www.istm.org	Travel clinic directory
http://www.cdc.gov/travel	Travel health warning and precautions; outbreaks; travel health recommendations

Table 15.13: Screening tests for infectious diseases recommended for internationally adopted children

Test	Population to be screened	Additional testing or consideration
Tuberculin skin test	All adoptees	Consider repeating in 2–3 mo or when nutrition status is improved. If negative no initial screen
Hepatitis serology Hepatitis B surface antigen (HBSAg) Hepatitis B surface antibody (HBSAb) Hepatitis B core antibody (HB core Ab)	All adoptees	Consider repeating in 6 mo
Complete blood cell count with differential, red blood cell indices, and platelet count	All adoptees	Some findings may suggest, in combination with clinical signs and symptoms, that additional evaluation is necessary as follows: Eosinophilia: parasitic infections Anemia/thrombocytopenia; malaria Thrombocytopenia: CMV Leukopenia: HIV
Syphilis serology Non-treponemal tests (RPR, VDRL, ART)	Non-treponemal test for all adoptees	
Treponemal tests (MHA-TP, FTA-ABS)	Treponemal tests if non-treponemal tests are reactive; if clinical signs and/or symptoms of syphilis are present	Children with positive test results and those diagnosed and/or treated in their birth country need additional testing
Stool examination for ova or parasites (3 specimens)	All adoptees	Repeat to those with persistent symptoms
Stool specimen for antigen for *Giardia lamblia* and *cryptosporidium parvum* (1 specimen)	All adoptees	Repeat to confirm elimination of parasites after treatment
HIV 1 and 2 ELISA (consider DNA PCR in infants)	All adoptees	Consider repeating in 6 mo if negative on initial screen
Hepatitis C	All adoptees from China, Russia, Eastern Europe and South East Asia Adoptees with risk factors for infection	Consider repeating in 6 mo if negative on initial screen

CMV: Cytomegalovirus; RPR: Rapid plasma regain; VDRL: Venereal Disease Research Laboratory (test); ART: Automated regain test; MHA-TP: Microhemagglutination test for *Treponema pallidum*; FTA-ABS: fluorescent treponemal antibody absorption; ELISA: Enzyme-linked immunosorbent assay; PCR: Polymerase chain reaction. *Source:* Barnett ED. Immunizations and infectious disease screening for internationally adopted children. *Pediatr Clin North Am* 2005;52:1287–309.

16 Gastrointestinal System

16.1 INTRODUCTION

Gastrointestinal function varies with maturity. A fetus can swallow amniotic fluid as early as 12 wk gestation, but nutritive sucking in neonates first develops at about 34 wk of gestation. The coordinated oral and pharyngeal movements necessary for swallowing solids develop within the first few months of life in term infants. Before this time, the tongue thrust is upward and outward to express the milk from the nipple instead of a backward motion, which propels solids toward the esophageal inlet. By 1 month of age, infants appear to show preferences for sweet and salty foods and interest in solid foods increases at about 4 months of age. *The current recommendation to begin solids at 6 months of age is based on nutritional concepts rather than maturation of the swallowing process.* Infants swallow air during feeding and must be stimulated to burp to prevent gaseous distension of the stomach. The functions of GIT are taking food-nutrition, digestion, absorption, and excretion.

Major Symptoms and Signs of Digestive Tract Disorders

Dysphagia: Dysphagia or difficulty in swallowing may be caused by a structural defect or motility abnormalities.

Structural defects that cause obstruction to the food bolus arise from narrowing within the esophagus, as from a stricture, web, or tumor or from extrinsic obstruction by a vascular ring. *Structural defects typically cause more problems in swallowing solids than liquids.* Nonstructural defects are caused by motility abnormalities of the oropharynx or the esophagus.

Regurgitation: Regurgitation is the effortless movement of stomach contents into the esophagus and mouth. It is not associated with distress, and infants with regurgitation are often hungry immediately after an episode. The lower esophageal sphincter prevents reflux of gastric contents in to the esophagus. Regurgitation is a result of gastroesophageal reflux through an incompetent, or in infants, immature lower esophageal structure. If regurgitation is a developmental process in an infant, it will resolve with maturity. Regurgitation should be differentiated from vomiting, which denotes an active reflex process.

Vomiting: Vomiting is a highly coordinated reflex process that may be preceded by increased salivation and begins with involuntary retching. Violent descent of the diaphragm and constriction of abdominal muscles with relaxation of the gastric cardia actively force gastric contents back up the esophagus. This process is coordinated in the medullary vomiting center, which is influenced directly by afferent innervation and indirectly by the chemoreceptor trigger zone and higher central nervous (CNS) centers. Vomiting caused by obstruction of the GIT is probably mediated by intestinal visceral afferent nerves stimulating the vomiting center. If obstruction occurs below the second part of the duodenum, vomitus is usually bile stained. With repeated vomiting in the absence of obstruction, duodenal contents are refluxed into the stomach and emesis may become bile stained. Nonobstructive lesions of the GIT can also cause vomiting, such as diseases of upper bowel, pancreas, liver, or biliary tree. CNS or metabolic derangements may lead to severe persistent emesis.

Cyclic vomiting is a syndrome with numerous episodes of vomiting (average of 12 episodes per year) interspersed with well intervals. Precipitating factors include infection, stress and excitement. Idiopathic cyclic vomiting may be a migraine equivalent (abdominal migraine), or it may result from altered intestinal motility or mutations in mitochondrial DNA.

The evaluation of a case of vomiting includes a careful history and physical examination and may include if indicated, endoscopy, contrast gastrointestinal radiography, brain MRI, and metabolic studies (lactate, organic acids, ammonia). The differential diagnosis includes gastrointestinal anomalies (malrotation, duplication cysts, and choledochal cysts), CNS disorders (neoplasm, epilepsy, and vestibular pathology), nephrolithiasis, hydronephrosis, cholelithiasis, metabolic-endocrine disorders (urea cycle, fatty acid metabolism, Addison disease, porphyria, hereditary angioedema, and familial Mediterranean fever), chronic appendicitis, and inflammatory bowel disease. Treatment includes hydration, administration of antiemetic drug and treatment of the underlying cause. Prevention may be possible with the antimigraine agent amitriptyline or cyproheptadine.

Diarrhea: See Section 16.10.

Constipation: Constipation depends on stool consistency, stool frequency, and difficulty in passing the stool. A normal child may have a soft stool only every 2nd or 3rd day without difficulty; this is not constipation. On the other hand a hard stool passed with difficulty every 3rd day should be treated as constipation. Causes of constipation are listed in Table 16.1. Functional constipation is defined by a delay or difficulty in defecation that has been present for 2 wk or longer. Functional constipation, also known as idiopathic constipation or fecal with-holding, can usually be differentiated from constipation secondary to organic causes on the basis of history and physical examination (Table 16.1).

Abdominal pain: Children greatly differ in their perception of and tolerance for abdominal pain. A child with functional abdominal pain (no identifiable organic cause) may be as uncomfortable as one with an organic cause. Causes and characteristics of pain are described in Table 16.2.

Gastrointestinal hemorrhage: Blood loss from the gastrointestinal tract is never normal and should be distinguished from swallowed blood. Maternal blood may be ingested at the time of birth or later by a nursing infant if there is bleeding near the mother's nipple. Nasal or oropharyngeal bleeding is occasionally mistaken for gastrointestinal bleeding. Red dyes in foods or drinks may turn the stool red but positive test for occult blood is absent. Bleeding can occur anywhere along the gastrointestinal tract, and identification of the site is important (Box 16.1). When bleeding originates in the abdomen, it may cause hematemesis. Red or maroon blood in stools,

Table 16.1: Causes of constipation	
1. Nonorganic (functional)—retentive **2. Organic** *Anatomic:* Anal stenosis; Imperforate anus; Anteriorly displaced anus; intestinal stricture (post-necrotising enterocolitis) *Abnormal musculature:* Prune-belly syndrome; gastroschisis; Down syndrome *Intestinal nerve or muscle abnormalities* Hirschsprung's disease; pseudo-obstruction (visceral myopathy or neuropathy); Intestinal neuronal dysplasia *Spinal cord defects:* Spina bifida; tethered cord; spinal cord trauma *Drugs:* Anticholinergics; narcotics	*Drugs:* Antidepressants; chemotherapeutic agents; pancreatic enzymes; vitamin D intoxication; lead *Metabolic disorders:* Hypokalemia; hypercalcemia; hypothyroidism; diabetes mellitus *Intestinal disorders:* Cow's milk protein intolerance; Celiac disease; cystic fibrosis Inflammatory bowel disease (stricture); tumor *Connective tissue disorders:* Systemic lupus erythematosus; scleroderma *Psychiatric diagnosis:* Anorexia nervosa

Table 16.2: Particular characteristics of pain from frequent and important causes

Cause of pain	Characteristic of pain
Peptic ulcer	Epigastric, burning or gnawing, radiates through to back, meal related, wakes the patient, relieved by antacid
Pancreatic	High epigastric, severe, felt front-to-back, immediately after eating, relieved by sitting forward
Midgut	Periumbilical, colicky, some relation to meals
Lower gut	Periumbilical or suprapubic, colicky, some relief from bowel action
Biliary	Right upper quadrant, severe, colicky (but over long time period), radiates to right shoulder, accompanied by nausea
Renal colic	Loin-to-groin, colicky, very severe, accompanied by nausea
Functional	Anywhere in the abdomen, colicky, accompanied by bloating, relieved by bowel action

Box 16.1: Differential diagnosis of gastrointestinal bleeding in childhood

Infant: *Common causes:* Bacterial enteritis; milk protein allergy; intussusception Swallowed maternal blood; anal fissure; lymphonodular hyperplasia.
Rare causes: Necrotizing enterocolitis; volvulus; Meckel diverticulum; stress ulcer, stomach; coagulation disorder (hemorrhagic disease of newborn).

Child: *Common causes:* Bacterial enteritis; anal fissure; peptic ulcer/gastritis; swallowed epistaxis; colonic polyps; intussusception; prolapse (traumatic) gastropathy; Mallory-Weiss syndrome.
Rare causes: Esophageal varices; esophagitis; Meckel diverticulum; lymphonodular hyperplasia; Henoch-Schönlein purpura; foreign body; hemangioma, arteriovenous malformation; sexual abuse; hemolytic-uremic syndrome; inflammatory bowel disease; coagulopathy.

Adolescent: *Common causes:* Bacterial enteritis; inflammatory bowel disease; peptic ulcer/gastritis; Mallory-Weiss syndrome; colonic polyps.
Rare causes: Hemorrhoids; esophagitis; esophageal varices; telangiectasia-angiodysplasia; Gay bowel disease; graft-versus-host disease.

hematochezia, signifies either a distal bleeding site or massive hemorrhage above the distal ileum. Moderate to mild bleeding from sites above the distal ileum tends to cause blackened stools of tarry consistency (malena); major hemorrhages in the duodenum or above can also cause melena. The stool is brick colored or current jelly colored in Meckel diverticulum.

16.2 ORAL CAVITY

Examine the oral cavity—tongue, lips, angle of the mouth (teeth primary, secondary, shedding of teeth, combination of all three; caries), palate, fauces, tonsils and pharynx. Disorders of teeth and surrounding structures may occur in isolation or associated with selected medical conditions (*see* Chapter 27). Various lesions include oropharyngeal infection with *Candida albicans* (thrush); aphthous ulcers; herpetic gingivostomatitis; recurrent herpes labialis; cheilitis. A **bifid uvula** may be normal or associated with a submucous cleft of the soft palate. *Ankyloglossia* or "tongue-tie" is characterized by an abnormally short lingual frenum that may hinder the tongue movement but rarely interferes with feeding or speech. *Ranula* is a cyst

associated with a major salivary gland in the sublingual area. A ranula is a large, soft, mucus-containing swelling in the floor of the mouth.

Drooling child: Drooling is the flow of saliva outside the mouth. Drooling can be caused by excessive production of saliva, inability to retain saliva within the mouth (incontinentia of saliva) or problem with swallowing (dysphagia or odynophagia). Isolated drooling in healthy infants and toddlers is normal, it may be associated with teething, upper tract infection and nasal allergies. Drooling or sialorrhea can happen in sleep. It is often the result sleeping on one side. In sleep, saliva may not reach at the back of the throat, triggering the normal swallow reflex, thus allowing for the condition. Stroke and other neurologic pathologies such as mental retardation, cerebral palsy is associated with drooling. Drooling associated with fever or trouble swallowing may be a sign of an infectious disease including retropharyngeal abscess, tonsillitis, mononucleosis, streptococcal throat infection. A sudden onset of drooling may indicate poisoning, especially pesticide.

Treatment plan depends on the etiology and incorporates several stages of care: Correction of reversible causes, behavior modification, medical treatment and surgical procedure. Treatment due to teething includes good oral hygiene and applying cold objects. Atropine sulfate tablets are used in some circumstance to reduce salivation.

Cleft lip and cleft palate: See Section 27.4.

Li BU, Misiewicz L. Cyclic vomiting syndrome: A brain-gut disorder. Gastrointestinal Clin North Am 2003;32:997–1019.

Tinanoff N. The oral cavity. In: Kliegman RM, Behrman RE, Jenson HB, Stanton BF (eds). *Nelson Textbook of Pediatrics.* 18th edn. Vol. 2. Philadelphia: Saunders, 2007;1529–41.

Wyllie R. Clinical manifestations of gastrointestinal disease. In: Kliegman RM, Behrman RE, Jenson HB, Stanton BF (eds). *Nelson Textbook of Pediatrics.* 18th edn. Vol. 2. Philadelphia: Saunders, 2007;1521–29.

16.3 ESOPHAGUS

The esophagus is a hollow muscular tube, separated from the pharynx above and the stomach below by two tonically closed sphincters. The upper esophageal sphincter (UES) at the cricopharyngeus muscle and the lower esophageal sphincter (LES) at the gastro-esophageal junction (GEJ), constrict the esophageal lumen at its proximal and distal boundaries. The muscularis propria of the upper third of the esophagus is predominantly striated, and that of the lower two-thirds is smooth muscle. Clinical conditions involving striated muscle (cricopharyngeal dysfunction, cerebral palsy) affect the upper esophagus, whereas those involving smooth muscle (achalasia, reflux esophagitis) affect the lower esophagus.

16.4 GASTROESOPHAGEAL REFLUX DISEASE (GERD)

GERD is the most common esophageal disorder in children. Gastroesophageal reflux (GER) signifies the retrograde movement of gastric contents across the lower esophageal sphincter (LES) into the esophagus. Occasional episodes of reflux are physiological. The phenomenon becomes pathologic (GERD) in children who have episodes that are more frequent or persistent, and thus produce esophagitis or esophageal symptoms, or in those who have respiratory sequelae.

Clinical manifestations: Infantile reflux manifests more often with regurgitation (especially postprandially), signs of esophagitis (irritability, arching, choking, gagging, feeding aversion), and resulting failure to thrive; symptoms resolve spontaneously in the majority in 12–24 mo. Older children, in contrast, may have regurgitation during the preschool years; complaints of abdominal and chest pain supervene in later childhood and adolescence. Some children present with neck contortions (arching, turning of

head) designated Sandifer syndrome. The respiratory clinical features are also age dependent. Respiratory symptoms in infants with GERD may manifest as obstructive apnea or as stridor or lower airway disease in which reflux complicates primary airway disease such as laryngomalacia or bronchopulmonary dysplasia. Otitis media, sinusitis, lymphoid hyperplasia, hoarseness, vocal cord nodules, and laryngeal edema may be associated with GERD. In older children with GERD airway manifestations are more frequently related to asthma or to otolaryngological disease such as laryngitis or sinusitis.

Diagnosis: A thorough history and physical examination is sufficient to reach the diagnosis of GERD initially. Other diagnoses to be considered in an infant or a child with chronic vomiting are milk and other food allergies, pyloric stenosis, intestinal obstruction (especially malrotation with intermittent volvulus), nonesophageal inflammatory diseases, infections, inborn errors of metabolism, hydronephrosis, increased intracranial pressure, rumination, and bulimia. Depending on the presentation and the differential diagnosis, diagnostic testing can then supplement the initial examination. *Contrast (usually barium) radiographic* study of the esophagus and upper gastrointestinal tract is performed in children with vomiting and dysphagia to evaluate for achalasia, esophageal strictures and stenosis, hiatal hernia, and gastric outlet or intestinal obstruction. *Endoscopy* is helpful in diagnosing erosive esophagitis and complications such as strictures, Barrett esophagitis; esophageal biopsies may diagnose histologic reflux esophagitis in the absence of erosions while simultaneously eliminating allergic and infectious causes. Endoscopy is also used therapeutically to dilate reflux-induced strictures. Radionucleotide scintigraphy using technetium may demonstrate aspiration and delayed gastric emptying when these are suspected.

Laryngotracheobronchoscopy evaluates for visible airway signs that are associated with extraesophageal GERD, such as posterior laryngeal inflammation and vocal cord nodules; it may permit diagnosis of silent aspiration (during swallowing or during reflux) by bronchoalveolar lavage with subsequent quantification of lipid-laden macrophages in airway secretions. Esophageal manometry permits evaluation for dysmotility, particularly in preparation for antireflux surgery.

Complications: The complications of GERD are: (i) esophagitis and sequelae-stricture, Barrett esophagitis, adenocarcinoma, (ii) nutritional (because of caloric deficits), (iii) respiratory (atypical) presentation (with unexplained or refractory otolaryngological and respiratory complaints), (iv) apnea and stridor and (v) dental erosions. Long-standing esophagitis predisposes to metaplastic transformation of the normal esophageal squamous epithelium into intestinal columnar epithelium, termed Barrett esophagus, a precursor of esophageal adenocarcinoma.

Management: 1. *Dietary measures* include: (i) Thickening of formula with a tablespoon of rice cereal per oz of formula results in fewer regurgitation episodes, greater caloric density (30 kcal/oz); (ii) a short trial of a hypoallergic diet can be used to exclude milk or soy protein allergy before pharmacotherapy; (iii) older children and adults should be counseled to avoid acidic or reflux-inducing foods (tomatoes, chocolate, mint) and beverages (juices, carbonated and caffeinated drinks, alcohol); and (iv) weight reduction for obese patients and elimination of smoke exposure are other important measures at all ages.

2. *Positioning measures* are particularly important for infants, who cannot control their positions independently. Seated position worsens infant reflux and should be avoided. More reflux episodes in infants in supine and side positions has been observed as compared with the prone position, but supine position reduces the risk of sudden infant death syndrome (SIDS), hence infants should always be kept in supine position during sleep. When the infant is awake and observed, prone position and upright carried position can be used to minimize reflux. Some evidence suggests a benefit to left side position and head elevation during sleep. Head elevation should utilize elevation of the head of the bed, rather than excess pillows, to avoid abdominal flexion and compression that might worsen reflux.

3. *Pharmacotherapy* is used at ameliorating the acidity of the gastric contents or at promoting their aboral movement. *Antacids* are used antireflux therapy. They provide rapid but transient relief of symptoms by acid neutralization. Long-term regular use of antacids is not recommended because of side effects of diarrhea (magnesium) and constipation (aluminum) and rarely more serious side effects of chronic use. *Histamine-2 receptor antagonists (H2RAs;* cimetidine, famotidine, nizatidine, and ranitidine) are widely used antisecretory agents that act by selective inhibition of histamine receptors on gastric parietal cells; they produce benefit in the treatment of mild-to-moderate reflux esophagitis. *Proton pump inhibitors* (PPIs; omeprazole, lansoprazole, pantoprazole, rabeprazole, and esoprazole) provide the most potent antireflux effect by blocking the hydrogen-potassium ATPase channels of the final common pathway in gastric acid secretion. PPIs are superior to H2RAs in the treatment of severe and erosive esophagitis. The dose of omeprazole is 0.7–3.3 mg/kg/day, which is higher than those used in adults on a dose per weight basis. *Prokinetic agents* include metoclopramide (dopamine-2 and 5HT-3 antagonist), bethanechol (cholinergic agonist), and erythromycin (motilin receptor agonist). Most of these increase LES pressure; some improve gastric emptying or esophageal clearance. These drugs have not shown much efficacy for GERD.

4. *Surgery*, usually *fundoplication*, is effective therapy for intractable GERD in children.

Orenstein S, Peters J, Khan S, Youssef N, Hussain SZ. Gastroesophageal Reflux Disease (GERD). In: Kliegman RM, Behrman RE, Jenson HB, Stanton BF (eds). *Nelson Textbook of Pediatrics*. 18th edn. Vol. 2. Philadelphia: Saunders, 2007;1547–50.

Orenstein S, Peters J, Khan S, Youssef N, Hussain SZ. Embryology, anatomy, and function of the esophagus. In: Kliegman RM, Behrman RE, Jenson HB, Stanton BF (eds). *Nelson Textbook of Pediatrics*. 18th edn. Vol. 2. Philadelphia: Saunders, 2007;1541–43.

16.5 STOMACH AND INTESTINES

Examination of Abdomen

The patient should be lying supine with the arms loosely by his or her sides, on a couch or mattress, the head and neck supported by enough pillows—normally one or two, for comfort. The clothing should be drawn up to just above the xiphisternum and down expose to the level of the symphysis pubis. Generalized fullness or distension may be due to (**five F**) fat, fluid, flatus, feces, or a fetus. (Note: Use F a fetus where it is relevant) (*see* Figs 16.1 and 16.2 in CD)

It is helpful when examining the patient to remember the surface anatomy of the structures related to the gastrointestinal tract and abdomen and to think of the abdomen is being divided into nine regions (Fig. 16.1). The two lateral vertical planes (also called midclavicular or mammary lines) pass through points midway between the anterior–superior iliac spines and the symphysis pubis below to cross the costal margin close to the tip of the ninth costal cartilage. The two horizontal planes, the subcostal and interiliac, pass across the abdomen to connect the lowest points on the costal margins, the inferior border of the 10th costal cartilage (above) and the tubercles of the iliac crests (below), respectively. For more general clinical descriptions, four quadrans of the abdominal cavity (right and left upper and lower quadrants) are defined by the two planes: (i) the transverse transumbilical plane, passing through the umbilicus (and the intervertebral disc between the L3 and L4 vertebrae) dividing into upper and lower halves, and (ii) the vertebral median plane passing longitudinally through the body dividing into right and left halves. The four abdominal quadrants (Fig.16.2) contain intra-abdominal organs are listed in Table 16.3.

Glynn M. Gastrointestinal system. In: Swash M, Glynn M (eds). *Hutchison's Clinical Methods*. 22nd edn. Edinburgh: Saunders Elsevier, 2007;117–46.

Moore Kl, Dalley AF, Agur AMR (eds). *Clinically Oriented Anatomy*. 6th edn. New Delhi: Wolters Kluwer India Pvt Ltd., 2010;181–325.

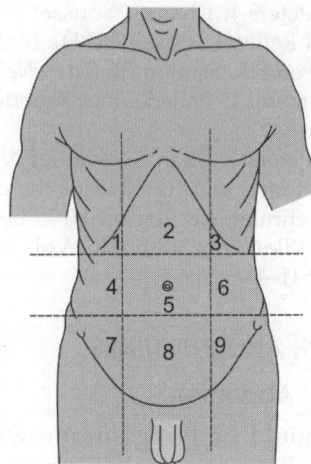

Fig.16.1: Regions of the abdomen. 1 and 3: right and left hypochondrium; 2: epigastrium; 4 and 6: right and left lumbar; 5: umbilical; 7 and 9: right and left iliac; 8: hypogastrium or suprapubic

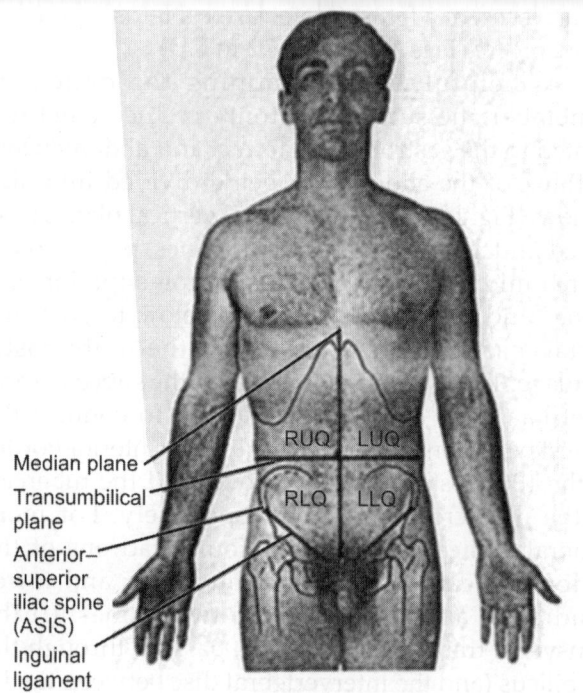

Median plane

Transumbilical plane

Anterior– superior iliac spine (ASIS)

Inguinal ligament

Fig. 16.2: Abdominal quadrants

Table 16.3: Intra-abdominal organs in four quadrants
Right upper quadrant (RUQ): Liver: right lobe; gall bladder; stomach: pylorus; duodenum parts 1–3; pancreas: head; right suprarenal gland; right kidney; right colon (hepatic) flexure; ascending colon: superior part; transverse colon: right half
Left upper quadrant (LUQ): Liver, left lobe; spleen; stomach; jejunum and proximal ileum; pancreas: body and tail; left suprarenal gland; left kidney; left colon (splenic) flexure; transverse colon: left half; descending colon: superior part
Right lower quadrant (RLQ): Cecum, appendix; most of ileum; ascending colon: inferior part; right ovary; right uterine tube; right ureter: abdominal part; right spermatic cord: abdominal part; uterus (if enlarged); urinary bladder (if very full)
Left lower quadrant (LLQ): Sigmoid colon; descending colon: inferior part; left ovary; left uterine tube; left ureter: abdominal part; left spermatic cord: abdominal part; uterus (if enlarged); urinary bladder (if very full)

16.6 FOREIGN BODIES AND BEZOARS

Foreign bodies in the stomach and intestine: Ninety five percent of all ingested objects present in the stomach pass without any difficulty through the remainder gastrointestinal tract (*see* Section 16.19). Children occasionally place objects in their rectum. Small blunt objects usually pass spontaneously, but large or sharp objects need to be retrieved. Adequate sedation is essential to relax the anal sphincter before attempted endoscopic or speculum removal. If the object is proximal to the rectum, observation for 12–24 hr usually allows the object to descend into the rectum.

Bezoars: A bezoar is an accumulation of exogenous matter in the stomach or intestine. Bezoars are classified on the basis of their composition. Trichobezoar are composed of the patient's own hair (*see* Section 30.10). Bezoars in the stomach can usually be removed endoscopically. If endoscopy is unsuccessful, surgical intervention may be needed.

Cerri RW, Liacouras CA. Evaluation and management of foreign bodies in the upper gastrointestinal tract. Pediatr Case Rev 2003;3:150–6.

Wyllie R. Foreign bodies and bezoars. In: Kliegman RM, Behrman RE, Jenson HB, Stanton BF (eds). *Nelson Textbook of Pediatrics*. 18th edn. Vol. 2. Philadelphia: Saunders, 2007;1571–2.

16.7 PEPTIC ULCER DISEASE IN CHILDREN

Peptic ulcer disease in childhood is less common. Gastric ulcers are generally located on the lesser curvature of the stomach, and 90% of duodenal ulcers are found in the duodenal bulb. Primary ulcers are most often associated with *Helicobacter pylori* infection, but up to 20% of duodenal ulcers in children are idiopathic primary peptic ulcers. Secondary peptic ulcers can result from stress due to sepsis, shock, or an intracranial lesion (Cushing ulcer) or in response to a severe burn injury (Curling ulcer); aspirin or nonsteroidal anti-inflammatory drug (NSAID) use; hypersecretory states like Zollinger-Ellison syndrome; short bowel syndrome; and systemic mastocytosis.

Clinical manifestations: School-aged children and adolescents more commonly present with epigastric pain and nausea, presentation generally seen in adults, and infants and younger children with feeding difficulty, vomiting, crying episodes, hematemesis and melena, whereas in the neonatal period gastric perforation can be the initial presentation. The classic symptom of peptic ulceration, epigastric pain alleviated by the ingestion of food, is present only in a minority of children.

Treatment: Proton pump inhibitors (omeprazole, lansoprazole) are more potent in ulcer healing. Antibiotics (amoxicillin, clarithromycin, metronidazole) in combination with a proton pump inhibitor must be used for the treatment of *H. pylori*-associated ulcers. The indications for surgery remain uncontrolled bleeding, perforation, and obstruction.

Zollinger-Ellison syndrome: This rare syndrome is characterized by refractory, severe peptic ulcer disease caused by gastric hypersecretion due to the autonomous secretion of gastrin by a neuroendocrine tumor, a gastrinoma. Clinical presentations are similar to those of peptic ulcer disease with the addition of diarrhea. The diagnosis is suspected by the presence of recurrent, multiple, or atypically located ulcers. More than 98% patients have elevated fasting gastrin levels. Zollinger-Ellison syndrome is a frequent occurrence in patients with multiple endocrine neoplasia (MEN 1) and is rarely associated with neurofibromatosis and tuberous sclerosis. Proton pump inhibitors are the drug of choice due to their long duration of action and potency.

Blanchard SS, Czinn SJ. Peptic ulcer disease in children. In: Kliegman RM, Behrman RE, Jenson HB, Stanton BF (eds). *Nelson Textbook of Pediatrics.* 18th edn. Vol. 2. Philadelphia: Saunders, 2007;1572–75.

Blecker U, Gold BD. Gastritis and peptic ulcer disease in childhood. Eur J Pediatr 1999;158:541–6.

16.8 INFLAMMATORY BOWEL DISEASE

The term inflammatory bowel disease (IBD) is used to represent two distinctive disorders of idiopathic chronic intestinal inflammation: Crohn's disease and ulcerative colitis.

Chronic ulcerative colitis: Blood in stool and diarrhea are the typical presentation of ulcerative colitis. Constipation is observed in those with proctitis. Fever, severe anemia, hypoalbuminemia, leukocytosis, and more than five bloody stools per day for 5 days, defines fulminant colitis. Chronicity is an important part of diagnosis. The clinical course of ulcerative colitis is marked by remission and relapse. The risk of colon cancer begins to increase 8–10 yr after disease and may then increase by 0.5–1% per year. Extraintestinal manifestations include pyoderma gangrenosum, sclerosing cholangitis, chronic active hepatitis, and iron deficiency and folic acid anemia. The treatment is aimed at controlling symptoms and reducing the risk of recurrence. In mild colitis sulfasalazine is used to treat ulcerative colitis and prevent recurrences in the dose of 50–75 mg/kg/24 hr (divided into two to four doses; not more than 2–3 g/24 hr). Hypersensitivity to the sulfa component of sulfasalazine occurs in 10–20% of individuals. Other less allergenic preparation of 5-aminosalicylate such as mesalamine, 50–75 mg/kg/day have been shown to treat ulcerative colitis and prevent recurrences. Hydrocortisone enemas (100 mg) are also used to treat proctitis. Children with moderate to severe pancolitis or colitis that is nonresponsive to 5-aminosalicylate therapy should be treated with oral corticosteroids (prednisolone). Children requiring frequent corticosteroids therapy should be started on immunomodulators such as azathioprine (1.5–2.5 mg/kg/day) or 6-mercaptopurine (1.5–2.5 mg/kg/day) to see a corticosteroid sparing effect. Other drugs can be used include cyclosporine and infliximab (5 mg/kg given intravenously). Probiotic agents may have a role in maintaining remission and may be as effective in preventing relapae as mesalamine. Colectomy is performed for intractable disease, complications of therapy, and fulminant disease that is unresponsive to medical management. Prompt colectomy should be performed after detection of significant dysplasia on biopsy.

Crohn's disease (regional enteritis, regional ileitis, granulomatous colitis): The initial presentation most commonly involves ileum and colon (ileocolitis) but involves the small bowel alone in ≈ 30% (70% of these patients have terminal ileitis alone) or colon alone in 10–15%. Upper gastrointestinal involvement (esophagus, stomach, and duodenum) is seen in up to 30% of children. Isolated colonic disease is common in children > 8 yr of age. Crohn's disease cannot be cured by either medical or surgical therapy. Medical treatment is same as mentioned in ulcerative colitis. The surgical approach for Crohn's disease is to remove as limited a length of bowel as possible. Crohn's disease is a chronic disorder that is associated with high morbidity but low mortality. There is risk of colon cancer in long-standing Crohn's colitis.

Hymas JS. Inflammatory bowel disease. In: Kliegman RM, Behrman RE, Jenson HB, Stanton BF (eds). *Nelson Textbook of Pediatrics*. 18th edn. Vol. 2. Philadelphia: Saunders, 2007;1575-85.

16.9 AN APPROACH TO A CHILD WITH MALABSORPTION

Malabsorption disorders/syndromes are conditions that cause insufficient assimilation of ingested nutrients due to defects in the digestion or absorption of food by the gastrointestinal system. While features like weight loss and diarrhea are common to almost all malabsorption syndromes, the specific causes are usually determined on physiological evaluation.

Laboratory diagnosis: In a child presenting with diarrhea, the initial investigations should include stool occult blood and leukocytes to exclude inflammatory disorders, stool microcopy and antibody tests for parasites such as Giardia, stool pH, and reducing substances for carbohydrate malabsorption, and quantitative stool fat examination to identify fat malabsorption. A complete blood count including peripheral smear for microcytic anemia, lymphopenia, neutropenia, and acanthocytosis (abetalipoproteinemia) is useful. If lactose intolerance, celiac disease or cystic fibrosis is suspected, more specific investigations can be planned.

Imaging Studies

Small bowel barium studies: The mucosal pattern often becomes obliterated in celiac disease. Flocculation of barium may occur in the gut lumen. Small bowel dilatation and diverticulosis are frequently seen in scleroderma. Stricture, ulceration and fistula formation may be seen in regional enteritis.

CT scan of abdomen: CT scan is especially useful to detect evidence of chronic pancreatitis, such as pancreatic calcification or atrophy. Enlarged lymph nodes are seen in Whipple disease and lymphoma.

Endoscopic retrograde cholangiopancreatogram (ERCP): This study helps to determine pancreatic/biliary tract disorders resulting in malabsorption.

Plain abdominal radiographs: Pancreatic calcification suggests chronic pancreatitis.

Upper GI endoscopy with small bowel mucosal biopsy: See Section 16.18.

Treatment

Broadly treatment aims at restoring the deficient nutrients and specific treatment of etiology.

1. *Nutritional support:* (i) **Supplementing** various **vitamins** and **minerals** like iron, calcium, magnesium, vitamins A, D, E and K. Vitamin A supplement of 5,000–10,000 IU and 400–800 IU of vitamin D per day are recommended. Vitamin K 2.5/5 mg may be given parenterally biweekly/weekly. Vitamin E supplements of 5–10 IU/kg/day. Water soluble vitamins may be given in twice the recommended daily allowances. (ii) **Protein-calorie rich diet:** This is aimed at achieving optimal nutritional status and augmenting growth and development. The main dietary goals therefore would be to provide an energy intake of 120–150% of RDA for age; protein intake of 150–200% of RDA for age; and a fat intake that provides 40% of total energy requirements. The dietary fat content should ideally provide 35–40% of the total calories; 8.5% of these should be derived from polyunsaturated fats and 10% of the calories from monounsaturated fats. (iii) **Medium chain triglycerides** can be used as substitutes for fats since they do not require micelle formation for absorption.

2. *Specific treatment:* (i) **Gluten-sensitive enteropathy/Celiac disease**. (ii) **Lactose intolerance:** A lactose free diet helps to correct the disease. (iii) **Pancreatic insufficiency, Cystic fibrosis.** (iv) **Bacterial overgrowth.** (v) Corticosteroids may be useful in regional enteritis, and Crohn's disease.

3. *Surgical correction:* Conditions requiring definitive surgical correction to cure associated malabsorption includes diverticulitis, lymphoma, stricture, and malrotation of gut.

4. *Counseling and life style modification:* This step is probably as important as specific treatment to ensure sustained efforts on part of patient to avoid treatment failure. Support groups help to build the confidence of patients and parents and motivate them to sustain treatment.

5. *Family screening:* Symptomatic family members should be screened aggressively. If tests are suggestive of disease, they must be treated too.

Gluten-Sensitive Enteropathy (Celiac Disease)

Celiac disease is an immune-mediated enteropathy caused by permanent sensitivity to gluten in genetically susceptible individuals. The prevalence of celiac disease in children between 2.5 and 15 yr in the general population ranges from 3–13/1,000 children. Celiac disease develops only after dietary exposure to the protein gluten, which is found in wheat, rye, and barley. The activity of gluten resides in the gliadin fraction, which contains certain repetitious amino acid sequences (motifs) that lead to sensitization of lamina propria lymphocytes. Celiac disease occurs at a higher frequency in children with type 1 diabetes mellitus, Down syndrome, Turner syndrome, William syndrome, thyroiditis, and selective IgA deficiency.

Clinical manifestations: The signs and symptoms include: failure to thrive, diarrhea, irritability, vomiting, anorexia, foul stools, abdominal pain, excessive appetite, rectal prolapse, wasted muscles, abdominal distension, edema, and finger clubbing.

Screening and diagnosis: Anti-tissue transglutaminase IgA antibody test is used in identifying individuals with celiac disease, which has a reported sensitivity of 96–100% and specificity of 99–100%. But it can be falsely negative with IgA deficiency, which is associated with an increased incidence of celiac disease. Measurement of serum IgA concentration is mandatory to ensure that false-negative results in IgA-deficient individuals are excluded. If celiac disease is suspected with IgA deficiency, intestinal biopsy may be required. The characteristic histologic changes include villous atrophy and loss of the normal villus to crypt ratio.

Treatment: The only treatment for celiac disease is lifelong exclusion of gluten. This requires a wheat, barley, and rye-free diet. The clinical response to a gluten-free diet usually results in improvement of appetite, mood and lessening of diarrhea within a week. Celiac disease is associated with intestinal lymphoma, and other forms of cancer, especially adenocarcinoma of the small intestine, pharynx, and esophagus.

Prognosis: Follow-up studies suggest that a gluten-free diet protects from cancer development, especially if started in the 1st years of life.

Intestinal lymphangiectasia: Obstruction of the lymphatic drainage of the intestine can be due to congenital defects in lymphatic duct formation or to secondary causes. The congenital form is often associated with lymphatic abnormalities elsewhere in the body as occurs with Turner, Noonan, and Klippel-Trénaunay-Weber syndromes. Causes of secondary lymphangiectasia include constrictive pericarditis, heart failure, retroperitoneal fibrosis, abdominal tuberculosis, and retroperitoneal malignancies. Lymph rich in proteins and lymphocytes leaks into the bowel lumen; it leads to protein-loosing enteropathy and lymphocyte depletion. Hypoalbuminemia, hypo-gammaglobulinemia, edema, lymphocytopenia, fat and fat-soluble vitamin malabsorption, and chylous ascites often occur. Intestinal lymphangiectasia can also present with ascites, peripheral edema, and a low serum albumin. The diagnosis is suggested by the typical findings along with an elevated fecal α_1-antitrypsin level. Radiologic findings of uniform, symmetric thickening of mucosal folds throughout the small intestine are characteristic. Small bowel mucosal biopsy shows dilated lacteals with distortion of villi, and no inflammatory infiltrate. Supplementing a low-fat diet with medium chain triglycerides (MCTs) oil in cooking is used in the management of older children with lymphangiectasia.

Abetalipoproteinemia: This rare autosomal recessive disorder of lipoprotein metabolism is associated with severe fat malabsorption from birth. Children fail to thrive during the 1st yr of life, have distended abdomen and their stools are pale, foul smelling and bulky. Neurological findings including absent deep tendon reflexes, loss of position sense, intention tremors occur as a result of peripheral neuropathy and involvement of the posterior columns, cerebellum, and basal ganglia. In adolescence, atypical retinitis pigmentosa develops. Diagnostic findings are acanthocytes in the peripheral blood and extremely low plasma levels of cholesterol (<50 mg/dl), triglycerides (< 20 mg/dL) and virtually absent very low density lipoproteins and low density lipoproteins (LDL). Large supplements of fat soluble vitamins A, D, E, and K should be given. Vitamin E (100–200 mg/kg/24 hr) and vitamin A (10,000 25,000 IU/day) may arrest the neurologic and retinal degeneration. Limiting long-chain fat intake can alleviate intestinal symptoms; medium chain triglycerides (MCT) can be used to supplement the fat intake.

Bacterial overgrowth: Bacteria are normally present in large numbers in the colon and have a symbiotic relationship with the host, providing nutrients and protecting the host from pathogenic organisms. Excessive numbers of bacteria in the small bowel or stomach are harmful. Bacterial overgrowth occurs in partial bowel obstruction, diverticulum, short bowel, intestinal duplications, diabetes mellitus, scleroderma, prematurity, immunodeficiency, and malnutrition. Bacterial over growth leads to steatorrhea and overproduction of D-lactate that can cause stupor, neurologic dysfunction, and shock. Diagnosis of bacterial overgrowth can be made by culturing small bowel aspirate or by lactulose hydrogen breath test. Treatment of bacterial overgrowth focuses on correction of underlying causes such as partial obstruction and oral administration of antibiotics. Initial treatment with 2–4 wk of metronidazole may provide relief for many months. Cycling of antibiotics including azithromycin, trimethoprim-sulfamethoxazole, ciprofloxacin and metronidazole is required. Other alternatives are oral non-absorbable antibiotics such as aminoglycosides. Occasionally, antifungal therapy may be needed to control fungal overgrowth of the bowel. The underlying cause of bacterial overgrowth is usually not easily reversible and may require surgery.

Tropical sprue: The etiology of tropical sprue is unclear, but an infectious etiology is suspected. The incidence appears to be decreasing, possibly due to frequent use of antibiotics for gastroenteritis in developing countries. *Clinical symptoms* include fever and malaise followed by watery diarrhea. After ≈1 wk, the acute symptoms subside and chronic malabsorption, intermittent diarrhea, anorexia result in severe malnutrition characterized by glossitis, stomatitis, cheilosis, night blindness, hyperpigmntation, muscle wasting, distended abdomen, edema, and megaloblastic anemia from folate and vitamin B_{12} deficiency. *Diagnosis* is made by bowel biopsy, which shows villous flattening, crypt hyperplasia, and a chronic inflammatory cell infiltrate of the lamina propria with adjacent lipid accumulation in the surface epithelium. Treatment includes nutritional supplementation, folate and vitamin B_{12} therapy. To prevent recurrence, 6 mo therapy with oral folic acid (5 mg) and tetracycline or sulphonamides is recommended. Relapses occur in 10–20% of patients who continue to reside in an endemic tropical region and in these patients additional courses of antibiotics may be necessary.

Short bowel syndrome: Short bowel syndrome results from congenital malformations, such as congenital short bowel syndrome, multiple atresias and gastroschisis; or small bowel resection in conditions such as necrotizing enterocolitis, volvuls with or without malrotation, volvulus with or without malrotation, long segment Hirschsprung's disease, meconium peritonitis, Crohn's disease, and trauma. At birth, the length of small bowel is between 200 and 250 cm; by adulthood, it grows to 300–800 cm. Loss of >50% of the small bowel, with or without a portion of the large intestine, can result in symptoms of generalized malabsorption disorder or in specific nutrient deficiency, depending on the region of bowel resected. The proximal 100–200 cm of jejunum is the site for carbohydrate, protein, iron, and water-soluble vitamin absorption, whereas fat absorption occurs over a larger length of the small bowel. Vitamin B_{12} and bile salts are only absorbed in the distal ileum.

After bowel resection, *treatment of short bowel syndrome* is initially directed on repletion of massive fluid and electrolyte losses as the bowel initially accommodates to absorb these losses. Nutritional support is often provided via parenteral nutrition. After the initial few weeks post resection, fluid and electrolyte losses stabilize and the focus of therapy shifts to bowel rehabilitation with the gradual reintroduction of enteral feeds containing protein hydrolysate and medium chain triglyceride. Enteral feeding will stimulate hormones and promote mucosal growth, increase pancreatobiliary flow and reduce parenteral nutrition-induced hepatotoxicity. A marked increase in stool output or evidence of carbohydrate malabsorption (stool pH<5.5 and reducing substances) contraindicates further increases in enteral feeds. Slow advancement of continuous enteral feeding rates continues until all nutrients are provided enterally. Bacterial overgrowth is common in infants with a short bowel and may delay progression of enteral feedings. Empiric treatment with metronidazole or nonabsorbable antibiotics is often useful. Long-term monitoring for deficiencies of vitamin B_{12}, folate, iron, fat soluble vitamins and trace minerals such as zinc and copper are important. Long-term complications of short bowel syndrome include those of parenteral nutrition: central catheter infection, thrombosis, hepatic cholestasis and cirrhosis, and gall stones. Renal stones can occur as a result of hyperoxaluria secondary to steatorrhea.

Enzymes Deficiencies

Carbohydrate malabsorption: Symptoms of carbohydrate malabsorption include loose watery diarrhea, flatulence, abdominal distension and pain. Disaccharidases are present on the brush border membrane of the brush border of the small border. Disaccharides deficiency can be either due to a genetic defect or secondarily due to damage to the small bowel epithelium, as occurs with infection or inflammatory disorders. Unabsorbed carbohydrates enter the large bowel and are fermented by intestinal bacteria, producing organic acids and hydrogen gas. The gas can cause discomfort and the unabsorbed carbohydrate and the organic acids cause osmotic diarrhea characterized by an acidic pH and presence of either reducing or non-reducing sugars in the stool.

Lactase deficiency: Congenital lactase deficiency is rare. Secondary lactose intolerance follows small bowel mucosal damage (celiac disease, rotavirus infection) and is usually transient, improving with mucosal healing. Lactase deficiency can be diagnosed by hydrogen breath test or by measurement of mucosal lactase concentration with small bowel biopsy. *Treatment* of lactase deficiency consists of a milk free diet. A lactose free formula (based on either soy or cow's milk) can be used in infants. Older children can ingest modest quantities of milk in which lactose is predigested by lactase. Live culture yogurt contains bacteria that produce lactase enzyme and hard cheeses (contains small amount of lactose) are generally well tolerated.

Juice drinking syndrome: Children consuming a large quantity of juice rich in fructose may present with diarrhea, abdominal distension, and slow weight gain; this can mimic carbohydrate malabsorption disorders. Restricting the amount of juice in the diet resolves the symptoms.

Sucrase-isomaltase deficiency: This is a rare autosomal recessive disorder with a complete absence of sucrase and reduced maltase digestive activity. Symptoms of sucrase-isomaltase deficiency usually begin when the infant is exposed to sucrose or a glucose polymer diet. Diarrhea, abdominal pain and poor growth are observed. Diagnosis is made with hydrogen breath test or enzyme assay of small bowel biopsy. The mainstay of treatment is lifelong dietary restriction of sucrose containing foods. Enzyme replacement with a purified yeast enzyme, sucrosidase is a highly effective adjunct to dietary restriction.

Glucose-galactose malabsorption: A rare autosomal recessive disorder, cause osmotic diarrhea. The finding of positive reducing substances in watery stools and slight glycosuria despite low blood sugar levels is highly suggestive of glucose-galactose malabsorption. The malabsorption of glucose-galactose is identified using the breath hydrogen test and by small intestinal biopsy that shows normal villous architecture and normal disaccharidase activities. Treatment consists of rigorous restriction of glucose and galactose. Fructose is the only carbohydrate that can be given safely and should be added to a carbohydrate-free formula at a concentration of 6–8%. Diarrhea immediately ceases, when infants are given such a formula. The defect is permanent, but limited amount of glucose or sucrose may be tolerated later in life.

Exocrine pancreatic insufficiency: The disorders associated with exocrine pancreatic insufficiency include cystic fibrosis, Johanson-Blizzard syndrome (severe steatorrhea, aplasia of alae nasi, deafness, hypothyroidism, scalp defects), Pearson bone marrow syndrome (sideroblastic anemia, variable degree of neutropenia, thrombocytopenia), isolated pancreatic enzyme deficiency (lipase, colipase, trypsinogen, amylase, lipase-colipase), and autoimmune polyendocrinopathy-ectodermal dystrophy (APCED) (autosomal recessive disorder, chronic mucocutaneous candidiasis associated with failure of parathyroid glands, adrenal cortex, pancreatic β cells, gonads, gastric parietal cells, and thyroid gland).

Cystic fibrosis: See Section 18.13.

Bai J. Malabsorption Syndromes. Digestion 1998; 59(5): 530–46.

Cooper R, Oliver M. Pediatric function tests. In: Walker WA, Goulet O, Kleinman RE, Sherman PM, Schneider BL, Sanderson IR (eds). *Pediatric Gastrointestinal Disease.* Vol. 1. 4th edn. Hamilton, Ontario BC: Decker Inc., 2004;1816–9.

Sood MR. Disorders of malabsorption. In: Kliegman RM, Behrman RE, Jenson HB, Stanton BF (eds). *Nelson Textbook of Pediatrics.* 18th edn. Vol. 2. Philadelphia: Saunders, 2007;1587–602.

16.10 DIARRHEAL DISEASES IN CHILDREN

Diarrhea is usually defined as passage of 3 or more loose or watery stools in a 24-hour period, a loose stool being one that would take the shape of a container. However, for practical purposes, it is the recent change in consistency and character of stool and its water content rather than the number of stools that is important. Infants who are exclusively breast-fed normally pass several soft or semi-liquid stools each day; for them it is practical to define diarrhea as an increase in stool frequency or liquidity that is considered abnormal by mother.

Clinical presentation: Three clinical syndromes of diarrhea have been defined, each reflecting a different pathogenesis and requiring different approach to treatment. *Acute watery diarrhea* refers to diarrhea that begins acutely, lasts for less than 14 days, with passage of frequent loose or watery stools without visible blood. Vomiting may occur and fever may be present. Loss of large volume of water and electrolytes can result in dehydration and dyselectrolytemia. *Dysentery* is the term used for diarrhea with visible blood and mucus. Dysentery is often associated with fever and tenesmus. Common clinical features of dysentery include anorexia, rapid weight loss and complications like renal failure and encephalopathy. Persistent diarrhea, presumed to be caused by infectious agents, begins acutely but is of usually longer duration (more than 14 days). The episode may begin either as acute watery diarrhea or as dysentery. Marked weight loss is common. Diarrheal stool volume may also be great, with a risk of dehydration. *Persistent diarrhea* should not be confused with *"chronic diarrhea"*, which is recurrent or long lasting diarrhea due to non-infectious causes such as sensitivity to gluten or inherited metabolic disorder.

Risk factors and etiology: Most of the diarrheal episodes occur during the first 2 years of life (incidence is highest in 6–11 months), low socioeconomic status, in non-breast-fed infants, and in association with measles, severe malnutrition, and immunodeficiency. In developing countries, the organisms most frequently associated with acute watery diarrhea include rotavirus, enterotoxigenic *Escherichia coli* (ETEC), enteropathogenic *Escherichia coli* (EPEC), shigella and *Campylobacter jejuni*. *Vibrio cholerae* is an important organism in endemic areas and during epidemics. Non-typhoidal salmonella is a common organism in areas where commercially processed foods are widely used and in hospital outbreaks. Most of these organisms produce watery diarrhea. The main causes of acute dysentery are *Shigella, Campylobacter jejuni* and infrequently enteroinvasive *Escherichia coli* (EIEC) or *Salmonella*. Epidemics of dysentery are usually caused by *S. dysentery type 1. Entamoeba histolytica* can cause dysentery in adults but is a less common cause in young children.

Diarrhea may also be caused by a number of antibacterial agents like ampicillin, cotrimoxazole, chloramphenicol, amoxicillin, clindamycin, etc. Pseudomembranous colitis is the most severe form of antibiotic associated diarrhea (*see* Chapter 14).

Pathophysiology of infectious diarrhea: Most enteropathogens can cause diarrhea by more than one mechanism. Hence, the clinical presentation depends upon the underlying pathophysiological changes taking place in the gastrointestinal tract. Various mechanisms which have been suggested include: (i) increased secretion of fluid and electrolytes, (ii) decreased digestion and absorption of nutrients, and (iii) abnormal transit due to aberrations of intestinal motility.

i. *Increased secretion:* Increased secretion of fluid and electrolytes may occur due to the effect of enterotoxins liberated by microorganisms which mediate through cyclic AMP or cyclic GMP thereby disturbing the sodium pump and leading to (a) increased secretion from crypt cells, (b) poor absorption of water and electrolytes from the villi, and (c) increased passive flow of water and electrolytes from ECF to small bowel lumen through intercellular channels. *Secretory diarrhea* is characterized by acute watery diarrhea with profound losses of water and electrolytes due to sodium pump failure as a result of the action of identified toxins. This group is at risk for rapid development of dehydration and electrolyte imbalance. Common causes are ETEC and *V. cholerae*.

ii. *Invasion of intestinal mucosa:* Intestinal mucosal cells are actually invaded by the microorganisms (*Shigella, Salmonella, enteroinvasive Escherichia coli* (EIEC), *Campylobacter jejuni, rota virus, E. histolytica*), which set up an inflammatory reaction clinically presenting as *dysentery* with blood and mucus in the stools. This group is prone to develop other complications like intestinal perforation, toxic megacolon, rectal prolapse, convulsions, septicemia and hemolytic uremic syndrome.

iii. *Decreased digestion and absorption:* Decreased digestion and absorption of nutrients particularly carbohydrates can take place as a consequence of (a) disorganized epithelial cell renewal, i.e. villus atrophy and crypt hyperplasia with failure of normal enterocyte maturation during migration from the crypt to villus or (b) damage to absorptive surface as a result of brush border damage (*Giardia lamblia*, EPEC, *Y. enterocolitica*) and destruction leading to decreased mucosal disaccharidase activity (*Y. enterocolitica*). These cases manifest as *persistent diarrhea or osmotic diarrhea*. The clinical presentation in these cases is characterized by passing of large, frothy, explosive and acidic stools. High osmolar solutions given orally (e.g. carbonated soft drinks and ORS with high sugar content) can also result in osmotic diarrhea. Besides worsening in the hydration status of the child there is also a serious danger of developing hypernatremia in these cases.

iv. *Disordered transit:* Abnormal intestinal myoelectrical activity initiated by non-invasive organisms and their enterotoxins as well as by invasive enteropathogens can result in disordered transit not only as secondary response to disordered mucosal transport but may also occur independently as a primary pathophysiological mechanism.

Consequences of Diarrhea

Dehydration: The immediate consequence of diarrheal disease, is a frequent and a serious consequence of acute watery diarrhea including cholera, but some cases of dysentery and persistent diarrhea may also present with variable degree of dehydration. Young children are more susceptible to develop dehydration due to limited urinary concentration capacity of the kidneys, more insensible losses of water through skin and lungs owing to large surface area and rapid breathing, and their dependence on adults to replace their fluid losses. Loss of water and electrolytes in the diarrheal stool results in depletion of the extra cellular fluid volume (ECFV), electrolyte imbalance and clinical manifestation of dehydration. Even though intracellular and extracellular fluid compartments are equally depleted in diarrhea, the measurements of ECFV show mostly a depletion of this compartment. The reason is that ECFV contracts in "two directions"—out in the stools and into the cell, so that the net measured loss of volume appears to come chiefly from the ECFV. Continued ECFV contraction is at the root of all the physiological changes taking place in dehydration and reversion to normal is more readily accomplished by solutions more nearly approximating that of the extracellular fluid.

In the past, higher mortality, which was reported soon after admission, was mostly due to uncorrected volume depletion or electrolyte imbalance. These observations highlight the importance of the "first day" in the fluid therapy of severe dehydration and the need for prompt replacement of losses particularly in severe secretory diarrhea like cholera which results in rapidly progressing dehydration, metabolic acidosis and other electrolyte imbalances. The first symptom of dehydration appears after fluid loss of about 5% of body weight. When fluid loss reaches 10%, shock often sets in. and the cascade of events that follows can culminate in death unless there is immediate intervention. Without treatment, severe episodes literally bring out body fluids from the victim faster than they can be replaced. Rehydration, orally or intravenously, is the only effective therapy.

Compensatory mechanisms: Contraction of the ECFV consequent upon loss of water and electrolytes in diarrheal stools, leads to increase in renin, angiotensin, aldosterone and antidiuretic hormone (ADH), and fall of GFR. All these changes lead to compensatory retention of salt and water but proportionately more of the latter. The first palpable response to ECFV contraction is thirst and if water is administered, it will be mostly retained due to the effect of ADH. In addition, water may also be generated internally by steroids and catacholamines. Therefore, retention of water by these mechanisms results in isotonic or hypotonic dehydration. Pre-existing or uncorrected potassium deficiency can also perpetuate hypotonicity. Comparison of various intravenous regimens containing high or low sodium have shown that rational treatment should reverse all the compensatory events by restoring volume quickly, correcting acidosis and reducing potassium deficit with solutions approximating the composition of the extracellular fluid. The more hypotonic the fluid is with respect to sodium, the less well it can quickly correct the ECFV contraction.

Malnutrition: Diarrhea is a major cause of malnutrition in children, owing to low food intake during the illness (poor appetite, vomiting, oral thrush/stomatitis, diluting/withholding of food, etc.), reduced nutrient absorption in the intestines, and increased requirements as a result of infection. Prolonged and recurrent episodes of diarrhea adversely affect the nutritional status of a child and thereby significantly contribute to vicious cycle of malnutrition and infection, which may culminate in growth failure, complications associated with severe malnutrition and even death.

Case Management

Principles of standard case management: Standard case management of diarrhea includes: (i) assessment of hydration status, (ii) administration of appropriate fluids for prevention and treatment of dehydration, including continuing appropriate feeding and supplementation to provide normal nutritional requirements, (iii) treatment of associated problems like dysentery and persistent diarrhea, (iv) assessment for concurrent illnesses like pneumonia, otitis media, meningitis, etc. (v) nutritional rehabilitation, (vi) health education for prevention of diarrhea and (vii) zinc sulfate tablet for 14 days; children <6 year 10 mg and >6 year 20 mg per day.

i. *Assessment of dehydration:* Loss of water and electrolytes in the stools can produce varying degree of dehydration. Thirst and irritability are the earliest symptoms, which appear by the time an infant has already lost almost 4–5% of body weight. Extreme degree of dehydration presents with alteration in consciousness, shock, acidosis and renal failure. A number of clinical signs and symptoms can help in detecting dehydration. However, a simple assessment chart, revised in the guidelines for IMNCI, can be referred for quick assessment of dehydration (Table 16.4). According

Table 16.4: Assessment of hydration status in a patient with diarrhea			
Clinical signs			
General condition	Well alert	Restless, irritable	Lethargic, unconscious
Eyes	Normal	Sunken	Sunken
Thirst*	Drinks normally, not thirsty	Drinks eagerly, thirsty	Drinks poorly, not able to drink
Skin pinch	Goes back quickly	Goes back 'slowly'	Goes back 'very slowly'
Decide hydration status			
	The patient has NO signs of dehydration	If the patient has two or more signs, there is **some** dehydration	If the patient has two or more signs, there is **severe** dehydration
Treatment plan	Plan A	Plan B	Plan C

* In a young infant less than 2 months of age, thirst is not assessed and decision regarding 'some' or 'severe dehydration' is made if 'two' of the three signs are present.

to the assessment chart, a patient may be grouped as 'no dehydration' (when there are no signs of dehydration), 'some dehydration' (which includes signs of mild and moderate dehydration- identified by the presence of at least two of the signs in this category in the chart) and 'severe dehydration' (cases with two or more signs suggestive of severe losses of fluid and electrolytes). Depending upon the state of hydration, patients with 'no dehydration' (Plan A, Table 16.5) or 'some' dehydration (Plan B, Box 16.2) can be successfully treated with oral rehydration therapy (ORT) and the ones with 'severe dehydration' should be initially rehydrated by intravenous therapy (Plan C, Table 16.6) and supplemented by/changed over to ORT as soon as the child is able to take orally (Tables 16.7 and 16.8). ORT alone may not successful to rehydrate a child with 'some dehydration' in certain situations like high rates of purging (watery stools > 15 ml/kg/hour), persis-

tent vomiting, (4 or more episodes of vomiting / hour), inability to drink (due to severe stomatitis, fatigue, central nervous system depression induced by antiemetics or antimotility drugs) and glucose malabsorption. Such cases need to be rehydrated with intravenous therapy as per Plan C (Table 16.6).

ii. *Oral rehydration therapy:* Oral Rehydration Therapy (ORT) has radically changed the treatment of diarrheal diseases. The term ORT includes (a) ORS solution of WHO recommended composition, (b) solution made from sugar and salt (if prepared correctly), (c) food based solutions (with appropriate concentration of salt) given (d) along with continued feeding.

The use of oral rehydration salts (ORS) to treat diarrhea stems from the discovery during 1960s of the coupled active transport of glucose and sodium in the small bowel resulting in the passive absorption of water and other electrolytes even during copious diarrhea. WHO and UNICEF recommend low osmolarity ORS with a total osmolarity of 245 mOsm/L (Tables 16.7 and 16.8), replacing the earlier ORS (dextrose 111, sodium 90, potassium 20, chloride 80, citrate 10, osmolarity 311 mOsm/L) (Table 16. 9). In neonates breast feeding should always be offered. In electrolyte depletion states rice syrup formula can be given (Table 16.10).

iii. *Intravenous fluid therapy:* Ringer's lactate given rapidly as 30 mL/kg followed by 70 ml/kg for deficit therapy is considered the treatment of choice for severe dehydration (Plan C, Table 16.6). However, in order to encourage oral feeding, the child

Table 16.5: Guidelines for replacement of fluid and electrolytes in children with 'No Dehydration' (Plan A)

Age	After each loose stool, offer*:
< 6 months	Quarter glass or cup (50 ml)
7 months–2 years	Quarter to half glass or cup (50 ml–100 ml)
2–5 years	Half to one glass or cup (100–200 ml)
Older children	As much as the child can take

* Fluids which can be offered include ORS, lemon water, butter milk, rice kanji, lentil soup, light tea, etc

---

Box 16.2: Guidelines for replacement of fluid and electrolytes in children with 'Some Dehydration' (Plan B)

Objective: To treat dehydration and electrolyte imbalance, and to continue feeding.
Plan B: Rehydration with ORS under supervision in a health facility.

Correction of dehydration

- For correction of fluid and electrolyte deficit administer 50–100 ml/kg body weight (75 ml/kg) of ORS, over a period of 4 hours. If the child wants more, give more ORS. Breastfeeding should be continued.
- For infants less than 6 months who are fed on artificial milk, 100–200 ml of plain water should be given in addition to ORS.
- Older children should have free access to plain water.
- Acceptance of ORS, purge rate and vomiting should be closely monitored.
  Reassess after 4 hours
- If still dehydrated, repeat deficit therapy and also offer milk/food.
- If rehydrated, treat as 'no dehydration' with maintenance therapy with ORS as in Plan A.
- If ORT is not successful, treat as 'severe dehydration' with intravenous fluids as per Plan C.

Resume feeding as early as possible

- Resume feeding after correction of dehydration (after first 4 hours of rehydration even if the child still has signs of dehydration).
- Continue feeding while correcting the dehydration in severely malnourished children.
- Breastfeeding should always be continued.

Table 16.6: Deficit fluid therapy for 'Severe Dehydration' (Plan C)

	Infants (< 1 year)	Older child (> 1 year)
Volume of Ringer's lactate	30 ml/ kg body weight within first 1 hour followed by 70 ml/kg body weight over next 5 hours	30 ml/ kg body weight within ½ hour, followed by 70 ml/kg body weight over next 2½ hours
Monitoring	*Assess for improvement every 1–2 hours*	

Under Monitoring:

Assess for improvement every 1–2 hours
- If not improving, give IV infusion more rapidly
- Encourage oral feeding by giving ORS 5 ml/kg/hour, along with IV fluids, as soon as the child is able to drink

Reassess hydration status
- After 6 hours (infants) and 3 hours (older children) assess hydration status and choose appropriate plan for hydration (Plan A, B or C)

should be offered ORS (5 ml/kg/hour) along with intravenous infusion as soon as he/she is able to drink orally. It is imperative to closely watch the child for passage of urine after plasma expansion has been achieved by rapid intravenous therapy. If the child fails to pass urine even after 2 hours of giving Ringer's lactate, he/she should be consi-

dered to have developed acute renal failure and managed accordingly.

iv. ***Rehydration of severely malnourished children:*** Rehydration of severely malnourished children deserves special attention owing to certain pathophysiological changes in water and electrolyte balance peculiar to protein energy malnutrition (PEM). Children with severe PEM have an increase in total body water and sodium while potassium stores in the body are depleted. The renal concentrating capacity is poor and thus they cannot conserve water efficiently. Moreover, they cannot handle excessive fluid and salt load and can develop fluid retention. Hence, malnourished children are more prone to diarrheal dehydration, and if given excessive fluids run a risk of

Table 16.7: Oral rehydration salt base on WHO formula (powder 21.80 g of electoral)

Constituents	Quantity
Sodium chloride	2.6 g
Potassium chloride	1.5 g
Sodium citrate	2.9 g
Dextrose	13.5 g

Table 16.8: Oral rehydration salt based on WHO formula (21.80 g of electoral in 1 litre of water supplies electrolytes in the concentration mentioned in the table)

Electrolytes	mOsm/litre
Sodium	75
Potassium	20
Chloride	65
Citrate	10
Dextrose	75
Total osmolarity	**245**

Table 16.10: Composition of Rice syrup formula (Ricelyt)

Composition	Rice syrup formula
Sodium chloride (gram)	3.5
Trisodium citrate (gram)	2.9
Potassium chloride (gram)	1.5
Extruded rice (gram)*	50.0
Osmolality (mOsm/L)	311

*Cooked rice base.
Indication: Electrolyte depletion states. Dose: Daily dose should be equivalent to patient's fluid requirement for maintenance and replacement of losses. Formulation: Sachet: 59 g.

Table 16.9: Composition of new and old WHO–ORS formula

Composition	New WHO–ORS formula	Old WHO–ORS formula
Sodium chloride (in gram)	2.6*	3.5
Trisodium citrate "	2.9	2.9
Potassium chloride "	1.5	1.5
Glucose, anhydrous "	13.5*	20.0
Osmolality (mOsm/L)	245*	311

*Denotes the recent change in composition.

developing cardiac failure. This risk is further increased by the fact that it is often difficult to judge the extent of dehydration in these children owing to absence of subcutaneous fat. Assessment of hydration status is also difficult because a number of the signs that are normally used are unreliable. Marasmic children normally have sunken eyes, and the diminished skin turgor may be masked by edema in children with kwashiorkor. In both types of patients, irritability or apathy makes assessment of mental state difficult. Signs that remain useful for assessing hydration status in severe PEM include: eagerness to drink (signs of some dehydration) and weak or absent radial pulse (signs of severe dehydration). It is often difficult to distinguish between some and severe dehydration in severely malnourished children and it is best to assume at least some dehydration in them if they have acute watery diarrhea.

Several workers have reported a high incidence of hyponatremic dehydration with ORS containing 90 mmol/L of sodium in malnourished children but satisfactory results have been reported by others. Low osmolarity ORS is safer in these children. However, it is recommended that rehydration of severely malnourished children should be carefully monitored and preferably take place in a hospital. Rehydration with ORS solution should be preferred because IV fluids can easily cause over hydration and heart failure. Rehydration should take place slowly in children with severe malnutrition giving 70–100 ml of ORS solution per kg body weight over 8–12 hours (5 ml/ kg every 30 minutes for first 2 hours, then 5–10 ml/ kg/hour for the next 4–10 hours). The exact amount depends on how much the child wants, volume of stool loss and whether the child is vomiting. For hospitalized children with severe malnutrition rehydration solution for malnourished children (ReSoMal, Table 16.11) is a preferred dehydrating

fluid (1 litre WHO–ORS packet dissolved in 2 litres of water with addition of 50 g sucrose and 40 ml of mineral mix solution).

Feeding should begin as soon as possible and supplemental potassium should be given with food for 2 weeks. A single mega dose of vitamin A (50,000 IU in infants less than 6 months, 100,000 IU between 6 and 12 months and 200,000 IU in children > 2 years) and zinc sulfate 20 mg daily for 14 days should also been given.

v. *Nutritional rehabilitation:* Nutritional management during and after each diarrheal episode is the corner stone of standard case management of diarrhea. Each diarrheal episode has a detrimental effect on the nutritional status of a child. Therefore, food intake should never be restricted during or following diarrhea. Rather, the goal should be to maintain the intake of energy and other nutrients at as high a level as possible. When this is done, even with only 80–95% carbohydrates, 70% of fat and 75% of nitrogen being actually absorbed during acute diarrhea, sufficient nutrients can be absorbed to support continued growth and weight gain. Continued feeding also speeds the recovery of normal intestinal function, including the ability to digest and absorb various nutrients. In contrast, children whose food is restricted or diluted usually lose weight, have diarrhea of longer duration, and recover intestinal function more slowly.

During an episode of diarrhea specific recommendations for feeding are determined by the child's age and feeding pattern before the illness and the state of hydration. In children with 'no dehydration' feeding is continued while as in 'some dehydration' normal feeding is usually resumed after rehydration is completed. However, in severely malnourished children, even with dehydration, some food should be offered as soon as possible during the rehydration period. Breastfeeding should always be continued. After the rehydration phase the dietary management during an episode of diarrhea includes continuing breastfeeding, undiluted animal milk for young non-breastfed infants and energy rich mixture of soft complementary foods in addition to breast-milk or animal milk in older children (Table 16.12). In young children these foods should be particularly well cooked and soft or mashed to aid digestion. Owing to loss of appetite or vomiting, children may need considerable encouragement to eat. It is helpful to give food frequently in small amounts, i.e. 6 times per day or more.

Table 16.11: Composition of solution for severely malnourished children (ReSoMal) compared with ORS		
Component	*ReSoMal (mOsm/L)*	*WHO–ORS (mOsm/L)*
Glucose	125	75
Sodium	45	75
Potassium	40	20
Chloride	70	65
Citrate	7	10
Magnesium	3	–
Zinc	0.3	–
Copper	0.045	–
Osmolarity	**300**	**245**

After an episode of diarrhea, a child should receive more food than usual for at least two weeks after diarrhea stops. During this period, the child may consume up to 150 kcal/kg of body weight per day. A practical approach to help in nutritional rehabilitation of these children is to give the child one extra meal at least for 2 weeks after an episode of acute diarrhea and for at least one month after persistent diarrhea, stressing the need for 'catch up growth.'

vi. *Use of antimicrobial agents:* Antibiotic therapy should be reserved only for cases of dysentery and suspected cholera (Table 16.13). Every case of diarrhea needs to be carefully evaluated for the presence of blood in the stools which indicates dysentery and to identify cases of suspected cholera (high purge rate with severe dehydration in a child above 2 years in an area where cholera is known to be present). Associated non-gastrointestinal infections like pneumonia, meningitis, urinary tract infection, etc. should also be carefully looked for and appropriately treated. In severe malnutrition, the usual sign of infection such as fever is often absent, yet multiple infections are common in these children. Therefore, it is assumed that all severely malnourished children may have an underlying infection, which should be treated with broad spectrum parenteral antibiotics.

vi. *Management of persistent diarrhea:* Management of persistent diarrhea involves a broad based therapeutic approach to take care of some of the problems associated with prolonged episodes which include: (i) impaired absorption of nutrients, particularly lactose and other disaccharides, (ii) persistent gut infection, and (iii) presence of associated non-gastrointestinal infections. Broad

Table 16.12: Feeding during diarrhea

Stage of hydration	Recommended schedule of feeding
During rehydration phase	
• Breastfed infants	• Continue Breastfeeding
• Non-breastfed infants	• Should be preferable given only ORS till they are rehydrated
	• Animal milk/food should be offered, if rehydration takes longer than 4 hours
• Severely malnourished children	• Offer some food as soon as possible
After rehydration phase	
• Breastfed infants	• Breastfeed more frequently
• Nonbreastfed infants	• Offer undiluted milk as before
• Infants 6–12 months	• Give easily digestible energy rich complementary foods in addition to breast/ animal milk
	• Encourage to eat at least 3 times a day in breastfed infants and 2 times in a nonbreastfed infants
• For Older children	• Give thick preparation of staple food with extra vegetable oil or animal fats, rich in potassium (legumes, banana), carotene (dark green leafy vegetables, red palm oil, carrot, pumpkin)
	• Encourage to eat at least 6 times a day

Table 16.13: Antimicrobials used to treat specific causes of diarrhea in children

Causes	Drugs of choice	Doses
Cholera	Doxycycline OR	Single dose of 5 mg/kg (max 200 mg)
	Furazolidone OR	5–8 mg/kg/day in 4 divided doses × 3 days
	Trimethoprim (TMP)-sulfamethoxazole (SMX)	TMP 10 mg/kg and SMX 50 mg/kg in 2 divided doses × 3 days
Dysentery	Trimethoprim (TMP)-sulfamethoxazole (SMX) OR	TMP 10 mg/kg and SMX 50 mg/kg in 2 divided doses × 5 days
	Nalidixic acid	60 mg/kg/day in 4 divided doses × 5 days
Amebic dysentery	Metronidazole	30 mg/kg/day in 3 divided doses × 5–10 days
Acute giardiasis	Metronidazole OR	15 mg/kg/day in 3 divided doses × 5 days
	Tinidazole	10–15 mg /kg/day in 3 divided doses × 5 days

principles of management of persistent diarrhea include the following: Assess hydration status and manage dehydration as discussed, investigate stool (pH, reducing substances, ova or cyst, RBC), continue breastfeeding, offer low lactose diet for non breastfed babies, treat dysentery (if visible blood in stool), treat amebiasis or giardiasis (if cysts or trophozoites of these parasites are detected in the stool), and hospitalize (if age less than 6 months, dehydration , severe malnutrition, associated infections and severe lactose malabsorption).

In the hospital, management of persistent diarrhea is based on following guidelines: (i) investigate and treat for associated infections (ARI, UTI, septicemia, etc. (ii) treat persistent infection due to enteropathogens, if diagnosed, and (iii) dietary manipulations (Table 16.10): Offer low lactose diet (kheer, "dalia", "phirni", yoghurt, "khichri" with yoghurt etc.) if there is evidence of lactose malabsorption. If there is no improvement in 2–3 days change over to lactose free diet (lactose free commercial formula in artificially fed young infants less than 6 months of age and "khichri (mixture of rice and pulse)" with egg in older children). If there is no response to lactose free diet, change over to disaccharide free feeding (chicken- glucose puree). Most of the hospitalized cases respond satisfactorily to lactose reduced or lactose free dietary formulation.

Prevention of diarrhea: Diarrheal diseases can be prevented to a great extent by improving infant feeding practices and personal and domestic hygiene. Some of the interventions which are feasible and cost-effective include: (i) promotion of exclusive breastfeeding up to 6 months of age, (ii) improved complementary feeding practices, (iii) use of clean drinking water and sufficient water for personal hygiene, (iv) hand washing, (v) use of sanitary toilets, (vi) safe disposal of the stool of young children, (vii) measles and rota virus vaccination, and (viii) use zinc tablet 20 mg/day and 10 mg/day in children less than 6 yr for 14 days along with ORS.

Diarrhea Training and Training Units (DTTU) and ORT Corners

Standard case management of diarrheal diseases (SCMD) is the most effective strategy to reduce diarrhea-related mortality and its consequences such as malnutrition. Diarrhea case management is very simple and can be easily carried out at the community level by a health worker. In fact, the success of the diarrhea case management lies with the important role-played by the mothers/caretakers who can manage children with diarrhea at home. However, hospital based referral facilities are essential for the management of more severe and complicated cases.

Establishment of Diarrhea Training and Training Units (DTTUs) have been proposed as a cost-effective strategy for promotion of appropriate case management of diarrheal diseases. Setting up of these units in medical colleges and large referral hospitals help to: (i) practice and promote SCMD on routine basis, (ii) train faculty members and other health personnel, (iii) train medical students in SCMD, and (iv) encourage and educate mothers/caretakers about home management of diarrhea by providing information and demonstration.

Treatment areas for managing children with diarrhea need to be identified within the existing set up of these health facilities which can be later expanded or scaled up depending upon the availability of space, manpower and resources. These identified areas serve to shorten the waiting time of the patients, screen patients with diarrhea who need to be referred/hospitalized, provide ORS, practice SCMD on routine basis and educate mothers/caretakers about home management of diarrhea. Depending upon the patient load, available space and other facilities, this identified area may function as a full-fledged DTTU or smaller service units. In a large referral hospital where inflow of diarrhea patients is large, the unit may be assigned a permanent area in the hospital as a DTTU. In smaller referral hospitals such as a District Hospital, 'Mini DTTU' (one room multipurpose assessment and treatment area for mothers and children with diarrhea as well as other problems) and in a first level health facility like a Primary Health Centre an 'ORT Corner' (extension of outpatient department with facilities of providing ORS, rehydration under observation and educating mothers) can be set up during diarrhea season.

DTTU is a service unit which does not require sophisticated infrastructure. Nevertheless, some of the essential characteristics of DTTUs include: (i) easy access and direct inflow of patients to reduce the waiting time, (ii) health staff readily available to receive and assess the patients (reception and triage area), (iii) facilities to rehydrate children under close monitoring with ORS/IV fluids (ORT area/diarrhea ward for IV fluids) depending upon the degree of dehydration, and (iv) mothers are educated on home management of diarrhea, preparation and administration of ORS, when to return immediately to the health facility and how to prevent diarrhea, before they leave the DTTU.

Establishment of DTTUs has resulted in a significant improvement in SCMD across the world and in India these units have demonstrated significant reduction in diarrhea related case fatality rates, hospital admissions, and average expenditure on antimicrobial agents.

Guidelines for Management of Diarrhea in Children. Report of Task Force on Diarrheal Diseases, Indian Academy of Pediatrics and Govt. of India, 2000; 1–62.

Integrated Management of Neonatal and Childhood Illness. Training Module for First Level Health Providers. Govt.of India, WHO and UNICEF. New Delhi, 2002.

Jelliffe DB, Jelliffe EFP. Dietary management of Young Children with Acute Diarrhea. 2nd edn. Geneva: WHO/UNICEF, 1991.

Patwari AK, Anand VK, Aneja S, et al. Persistent Diarrhea: Management in a Diarrhea Treatment Unit. *Indian Pediatr* 1995; 32:281–8.

Patwari AK. Cost effective strategy for promotion of appropriate case management of diarrheal diseases-Establishment of DTUs. *Indian J Pediatr* 1991;58:783–7.

Patwari AK, Kumar H, Anand VK, Aneja S, Sharma D. Diarrhea training and Treatment Unit: Experience from a teaching hospital. *Indian J Pediatr* 1991;58:775–81.

Patwari AK. Experiences in Case Management of Diarrhea in Large Hospitals. JIMA 1995;93:243–4.

Patwari AK. Diarrheal Diseases in Children. In: Mathur GP, Mathur Sarla (eds). *Current Trends in Pediatrics*. Vol 1. Delhi: Academa Publishers, 2005;381–92.

World Health Organization. Integrated Management of Childhood illness. WHO/CHD/97.3.A , WHO, Geneva, 1997.

World Health Organization. Training in diarrhea. In: Division of Diarrheal and Acute Respiratory Disease Control Program- Interim Report 1994, WHO, Geneva, 1995;16–17.

World Health Organization. New Formula for Oral Dehydration Salts will save millions of lives. Press Release WHO/35, 8 May 2002.

World Health Organization. Management of the child with a serious infection or severe malnutrition. WHO/FCH/CAH/00.1, WHO, Geneva, 2000;1–146.

16.11 CLINICAL APPROACH TO A CHILD WITH INTRA-ABDOMINAL MASS

Abdominal masses in the pediatric age group include a spectrum of lesions of diverse origin and significance. They may occur at any age—from the newborn period through adolescence, and have a wide range of clinical presentations. One must first exclude some of the normal abdominal masses in children. The liver is often palpable in infants and children up to the age of 3–4 years. A constipated child may have a fecaloma presenting as a palpable mass in the iliac fossa. A full bladder may also mimic a cystic mass in the suprapubic region.

Neonatal Abdominal Masses

Neonatal abdominal masses include *hydronephrosis; multicystic dysplastic kidney; infantile polycystic kidney disease; adult polycystic kidney disease; renal vein thrombosis; neonatal adrenal hemorrhage; teratoma:* (sacrococcygeal); gastrointestinal masses (duplication, omental and mesenteric cysts, malrotation with midgut volvulus, meconium peritonitis and intestinal atresia with cystic dilatation of fluid or gas filled proximal bowel); hepatobiliary masses (choledochal cyst, hemangioendothelioma, solitary liver cysts, hepatoblastoma, hydrops of the gall bladder); genital masses: hydrometrocolpos, ovarian cysts.

Abdominal Masses in Infants and Children

Abdominal masses in infants and children include *Wilms tumor* (*see* Chapter 34); neuroblastoma (*see* Chapter 34); *rhabdomyosarcoma* (*see* Chapter 34); *Appendicular mass or appendicular abscess* (*see* Chapter 16, page 464); *hepatoblastoma* (*see* Chapter 34); *choledochal cyst* (*see* Chapter 17, page 479); Teratoma forming the most common ovarian tumor presenting in the adolescent age group (*see* Figs 16.5 to 16.7 in CD).

Caty MG, Shamberger RC. Abdominal tumors in infancy and childhood. Pediatr Clin North Am 1993; 40(6):1253–71.

Pearl RH, Irish MS, Caty MG, Glick PL The approach to common abdominal diagnosis in infants and children. Pediatr Clin North Am 1998;45(6):1287–26.

Sinha Shalini, Sarin YK. Clinical approach to a Child with Intra-abdominal Mass. In: Mathur GP, Mathur Sarla (eds). Current Trends in Pediatrics. Vol 3. Delhi: Academa Publishers, 2007;183–98.

16.12 RECURRENT ABDOMINAL PAIN IN CHILDREN

Recurrent abdominal pain (RAP) has been recognized as an important clinical condition for a long time. Despite its seemingly benign nature, this disorder has been associated with increased school absenteeism, frequent visits to doctors, family disruption and significant anxiety and depression.

Investigatory approach: It is critical to thoroughly assess the overall physical and psychological condition of the child in order to make a clinical diagnosis without losing sight of early stages of functional bowel disorders and presence/ association of psychosomatic factors.

Treatment: Treatment of RAP essentially depends upon overall assessment of the child (and the family) and identifying any underlying cause after eliciting a detailed history, conducting a thorough physical examination supported by the results of base line investigations. Depending upon the physical and psychological assessment, specific interventions are recommended on a case to case basis. Various approaches in managing children with RAP include behavioral techniques, dietary interventions, pharmacological therapy or a combination of these approaches. Fiber supplementation and restriction of lactose in the diet have been two major dietary interventions to treat RAP. Medications are used in RAP primarily to offer symptomatic relief. Medications are used in RAP primarily to offer symptomatic relief. Systematic review of treatment suggests that therapies which target specific functional GI disorders (famotidine for dyspepsia, peppermint oil for irritable bowel syndrome) have been used.

Long-term prognosis: The current practice of recognizing RAP as a 'functional' disorder, after excluding possible organic causes, is that of support and empathy for the family with reassurance that no serious disease is present and that the children are likely to outgrow it. With this approach, approximately 30–40% of children do have resolution of pain. However, the remainder continues to exhibit symptoms and go on to be adults with abdominal pain, anxiety, or other somatic disorders. Many children may continue as irritable colon and peptic ulcer/gastritis in later life.

Balani B, Patwari AK, Bajaj P et al. Recurrent abdominal pain-A Reappraisal. Indian Pediatr 2000;37:876–81.

Bansal D, Patwari AK, Malhotra VL et al. Helicobacter pylori infection in recurrent abdominal pain. Indian Pediatr 1998;35:329–35.

Dutta S, Mehta M, Verma IC. Recurrent abdominal pain in Indian children and its relation with school and family environment. Indian Pediatr 1999;36:917–20.

16.13 ACUTE ABDOMEN IN CHILDREN

The term 'Acute abdomen' is applied to any condition that gives rise to acute abdominal pain. It may be a potentially life-threatening intra-abdominal emergency, often requiring immediate surgical intervention; the pathological process usually originating in the gastrointestinal system and involves inflammation, obstruction, perforation of a viscus, hemorrhage, or vascular compromise.

Clinical evaluation of a child with acute abdomen: In evaluating a child with abdominal pain, a thorough history is required to identify the most likely cause. An initial evaluation of the history is followed by a physical examination and a reassessment of certain points of the history. Age is a critical factor in the evaluation of a child with abdominal pain as many conditions are commoner in certain age groups (Table 16.14).

Acute Appendicitis

Etiology and clinical features: Appendicitis is the most common acute surgical condition of the abdomen. Approximately 7% of the population will have appendicitis in their lifetime, with a peak incidence occurring between 10 and 30 years. Obstruction of the narrow appendiceal lumen initiates the clinical illness of acute appendicitis. This may be due to lymphoid hyperplasia (due to a viral illness including upper respiratory illness, infectious mononucleosis, and gastroenteritis), fecoliths, parasites, foreign bodies and Crohn's disease. Lymphoid hyperplasia is the most common cause of appendicitis.

Abdominal pain is the most common symptom of appendicitis. Anorexia, nausea and vomiting are symptoms that are commonly associated with acute appendicitis with the classic history of pain beginning in the periumbilical region and migrating to the right lower quadrant. Occasionally, the pain may start at the McBurney point without the earlier visceral component. In 1889, McBurney described the classic point of localized tenderness in acute appendicitis, which is the junction of the lateral and middle thirds of the line joining the right anterior–superior iliac spine and the umbilicus, but the tenderness can also to any of the aberrant locations of the appendix. When the appendix is hidden from the anterior peritoneum, the usual symptoms and signs of acute appendicitis may not be present. A retrocecal appendix in a retroperitoneal location may cause flank pain and may be suspected by stretching the psoas muscle. The psoas sign is elicited with active right thigh flexion or passive extension of the hip. In contrast, a patient with pelvic appendix may not show any abdominal signs, but a rectal examination may elicit extreme tenderness. In addition, stretching of the obturator muscle may elicit the pain in a child with pelvic appendix. The obturator sign is demonstrated by adductor pain after internal rotation of the flexed sign. Tenesmus may be present in patients with pelvic appendicitis. Localized abdominal tenderness is the single most reliable finding in the diagnosis of acute appendicitis. Rebound tenderness and referred rebound tenderness (Rovsing sign) are also consistent findings in acute appendicitis

Table 16.14: Common etiologies for acute abdomen by age groups		
Neonates	*< 2 Years*	*>2 years*
Neonatal necrotizing enterocolitis	Incarcerated hernia	Appendicitis
Hirschsprung's disease, *see* Section 8.19	Intussusception	Meckel's diverticulitis, *see* Section 16.6
Incarcerated hernia	Meckel's diverticulitis	Intestinal perforation
Malrotation/volvulus	Malrotation/volvulus	Primary peritonitis
Intestinal perforation	Liver abscess, *see* Section 17.5	

but not always present. Rebound tenderness is elicited by deep palpation of the abdomen followed by the sudden release of the examining hand.

Children with appendicitis tend to lie still in the bed and the demonstration of localized tenderness in the right iliac fossa is the cornerstone for the diagnosis of appendicitis. With progression of the disease, the signs become more generalized and may lead to peritonitis from a perforated appendix.

Laboratory and radiological evaluation: The white blood cell count is elevated greater than $10,000/mm^3$ in 80% cases of acute appendicitis. Since the WBC may be elevated in other causes of right lower quadrant pain, an elevated WBC has a low predictive value. However, serial WBC measurements over a period to 6–8 hours in suspected cases may increase the specificity as the WBC count often increases in acute appendicitis.

Recently, it has been suggested that laboratory determination of the C-reactive protein level (CRP greater than 0.8 mg/dl) is common in appendicitis. Thus, an elevated C-reactive protein level in combination with an elevated WBC count and neutrophilia are highly sensitive (up to 100%). Therefore, if all three findings are absent, the chances of appendicitis are less than 1%.

Ultrasonography is the most widely used modality for confirming the diagnosis of acute appendicitis in equivocal cases. Graded-compression sonography of the right lower quadrant using a high resolution transducer has been shown to be a useful technique for diagnosing appendicitis, with sensitivity between 80–95%. A normal appendix (6 mm or less in diameter) must be identified to rule out appendicitis. An inflamed appendix usually measures greater than 6 mm in diameter and is non-compressible and tender on focal compression. Recently, color Doppler examination of the appendix has been used to diagnose appendicitis and an attempt has been made to identify complicated appendicitis with perforation. Acute appendicitis is accompanied by inflammatory hypervascularity with increased color signals and higher diastolic Doppler shifts which is visible on Doppler sonography. Patients with acute necrotic appendicitis with perforation demonstrate no signals in the necrotic area of the tip.

Computerized tomography has been used to diagnose appendicitis. A technique of appendiceal CT is used which consists of a focused, helical appendiceal CT after gastrograffin-saline enema and can be performed and interpreted within an hour. Appendiceal CT is more accurate than ultrasonography especially due to its ability to identify a normal appendix better than ultrasonography. In cases with atypical history with equivocal physical findings, diagnostic laparoscopy serves as a diagnostic tool with a definitive therapeutic capability.

Treatment: The standard management of non-perforated appendix remains appendectomy. Non-operative management has been attempted but 40 percent of these patients eventually required appendectomy. Appendicectomy is usually performed by laparotomy through a limited right lower quadrant incision. Laparoscopic appendicectomy is now accepted as a reasonable alternative to open appendicectomy. The advantages include shortened hospital stay and a quicker return to full activity. However, the procedure requires a longer operating time and higher costs as compared to traditional appendicectomy.

Typhoid Fever and Intestinal Bleeding

The most serious complication, intestinal bleeding or perforation, occurs in about 5% of patients. Bleeding usually is noted after the second week of illness, but perforation may occur unexpectedly after the patient has started to improve, usually after the third week of illness. The child with bowel perforation presents with a history of constitutional symptoms like fever, chills, headache, sore throat, muscle pain, and weakness. The abdominal pain usually begins 2–3 weeks after the onset of symptoms. Nausea, vomiting, anorexia, diarrhea, and constipation are also associated. About half the patients demonstrate relative bradycardia. Clinical examination of the child demonstrates features of generalized peritonitis.

Laboratory and radiological investigations: Laboratory findings may demonstrate anemia and thrombocytopenia. Blood, urine, and stool cultures may demonstrate the growth of Salmonella. Widal test may be positive. Abdominal radiographs demonstrate free gas in the abdomen suggestive of perforation.

Treatment: The child with typhoid perforation requires urgent laparotomy. The patient may have single or multiple perforations, usually near the terminal ileum. The perforation may be closed primarily or the child may require resection of an involved segment with re-anastomosis of the bowel. Very sick children with delayed presentation may be better served by an ileostomy. Ceftriaxone is the drug of choice for children in the treatment of typhoid fever. Older children or patients sensitive to ceftriaxone may be administered ciprofloxacin. Chloramphenicol is generally reserved for resistant cases.

Intussusception

Etiology and clinical features: Intussusception is telescoping or invagination of one segment of bowel into another. An intussusception has an identifiable lesion that serves as a lead point, drawing the proximal bowel into the distal by peristaltic activity. The usual location is the ileocecal valve (ileocolic), but other regions of the bowel may rarely be also involved. It occurs most commonly between 3 and 12 months of age with a peak incidence at 9 months of age. The cause is usually unknown, although there is a definite relationship to adenovirus infections, summer infectious diarrhea (rotavirus, reovirus, and echovirus) and winter respiratory infection. In almost every patient at operation, there is a marked hypertrophy of the lymphoid tissue of the ileal wall. It is generally believed that viral infections (adenovirus, rotavirus, reovirus, and echovirus) lead to hypertrophy of Payer's patches, which act as lead point for intussusception. About 2–12% of cases have a definitive anatomical lead point, which includes Meckel's diverticulum, the appendix, polyps, carcinoid tumors, sub-mucosal hemorrhage, lymphoma, ectopic gastric mucosa, etc. The incidence of anatomic lead point increases in proportion to age.

Intussusception produces acute crampy abdominal pain in a previously comfortable infant. Pain is recurrent in nature, with an asymptomatic interval of 5–30 minutes. Vomiting is almost universal and usually follows the onset of pain and may contain bile. A few normal bowel movements are followed by the passage of "currant jelly" stools with bloody mucus. An early physical examination may be normal. A later examination reveals fever, tachycardia, and lethargy. A sausage shaped mass may be felt, usually in the right upper quadrant with a characteristic emptiness of the right lower quadrant (le dance's sign). In advanced cases, an abdominal examination reveals exquisite tenderness or rigidity from peritonitis. The child becomes grossly toxic with severe dehydration.

Laboratory and radiological evaluation: Laboratory examination is mainly used to confirm the metabolic and electrolyte status of the patient. Severe bleeding per rectally may lead to severe anemia and the differential leukocyte count shows moderate leucocytosis. The diagnosis of intussusception may be made on the basis of suggestive radiographic abnormalities (show a density in the area of the intussusceptions) on a plain abdominal radiograph.

Recently, however, ultrasound examination of the abdomen with hydrostatic reduction with air is being used widely both for diagnosis and treatment. Ultrasonography of the abdomen reveal the characteristic signs of intussusception namely the "target" lesion (on transverse section) and the "pseudo-kidney" sign (on longitudinal section). The virtue of sonography is that it minimizes exposure to ionizing radiation and pneumatic reduction or reduction with saline can be performed under ultrasound guidance after the diagnosis has been reached. This can be supplemented with color Doppler imaging that has sometimes proven useful in predicting gangrene of the intestinal segment and whether a non-operative reduction is likely to be successful.

Treatment: The treatment consists of either non-operative measures or operative measures for reduction of the intussusception.

1. **Non-operative measures:** a. Controlled hydrostatic reduction is done by saline or by water soluble isotonic contrast e.g. meglumine diatrizoate. b. In pneumatic reduction the maximum safe pressure is between 80 mmHg (for young infants) and 120 mmHg (for older infants and children). Successful reduction is seen in around 75–94% patients, which is higher than those achieved using hydrostatic reduction.
2. **Operative treatment:** Surgical treatment is required whenever the medical or non-operative methods fail to reduce the intussusception.

Incarcerated Inguinal Hernia

Clinical features: Incarceration is the entrapment of viscera in the hernial pouch. It is usually seen in children below 3 years. Almost one-third of incarcerations become strangulated, posing an immediate danger of vascular interruption. These children present with a firm, often tender, irreducible mass in the inguinal canal. Erythema and edema over the mass suggests strangulation. Untreated, it evolves to intestinal obstruction with pain abdomen. The pain is generally diffused and poorly localized and is associated with abdominal distension. In girls, the ovary may get incarcerated.

Laboratory investigation and radiography: Plain abdominal radiographs demonstrate air-fluid levels with distended small bowel loops with a relatively gasless rectum. Laboratory findings are unremarkable except may reflect the electrolytes imbalances and dehydration.

Treatment: Initial treatment of incarceration without strangulation, is sedation followed by wait and watch for spontaneous reduction. Reduction of incarcerated bowel is usually successful if strangulation has not occurred. If reduction is successful, a surgical repair should be done within 48 hours so as to permit edema resolution. A failed reduction necessitates an urgent surgical repair after adequate hydration.

Malrotation and Volvulus

Clinical features: Commonly, these patients have a malpositioned cecum and are also associated with band running from it and going across the second part of the duodenum. The mesentery of the midgut also has a correspondingly small base, making the bowel prone to volvulus. Up to 2/3rd of patients of malrotation, who become symptomatic; do so within the first month of life. Almost all patients present within the first year of life.

The symptoms with which patients with malrotation present generally result from either partial duodenal obstruction or midgut volvulus. Duodenal obstruction commonly occurs as a result of compression of the duodenum by Ladd's peritoneal bands and generally results in a post-ampullary obstruction and therefore, bilious vomiting is characteristic presenting feature.

Midgut volvulus occurs when the whole midgut undergoes torsion and leads to a compromise in the superior mesenteric arterial supply leading to an acute vascular insufficiency of the midgut and may rapidly lead to intestinal necrosis. These children present with bilious vomiting, abdominal distension, hypotension, acidosis, severe systemic sepsis and thrombocytopenia. A delay of a few hours may lead to massive bowel loss.

Diagnosis: A plain abdominal radiograph usually demonstrates a dilated stomach and duodenum with a paucity of gas in the distal small bowel. However, a child with midgut volvulus may have a normal plain radiograph. An upper GI contrast study is necessary for the diagnosis and shows dilated proximal duodenum with appearance of extrinsic compression. The duodenojejunal junction is usually on the right side. "Corkscrew" appearance is seen in cases of volvulus. A contrast enema was earlier used as part of the diagnostic workup of a child with malrotation, but has been proven to be less reliable and is no longer used. Ultrasonography has also been successfully used for the diagnosis of malrotation and volvulus and demonstrate "whirlpool" flow pattern in the superior mesenteric vein and by demonstrating the presence of the mesentery around the superior mesenteric artery. Computerized tomography has also been used to diagnose malrotation.

Treatment: The Ladd's procedure corrects the fundamental problems associated with malrotation with or without midgut volvulus. This procedure consists of an evisceration of the midgut with counterclockwise derotation of the midgut volvulus. The bowel viability should be assessed and the Ladd's bands are lysed and the C-loop is straightened with a widening of the mesenteric base. Appendicectomy is then performed and the cecum is placed in the left lower quadrant. Non-salvageable bowel requires resection and may require long-term parental hyperalimentation and may require subsequent bowel transplantation. Laparoscopic Ladd's procedure has also been successfully used recently.

Primary Peritonitis

Clinical features and etiology: Primary peritonitis is a term given to the condition where the infectious process of the peritoneal cavity that has no intra-abdominal source. Bacterial access to the peritoneal cavity is difficult to trace, although hematogenous, lymphatic, and ascending genitourinary route has been implicated. In girls, retrograde spread of infection by way of the fallopian tube is possible and may result in "swimming pool" peritonitis or an ascending vulvovaginitis. Primary peritonitis is also common in children with nephrotic syndrome, hepatic dysfunction, chronic renal failure or following steroid administration and the term spontaneous bacterial peritonitis (SBP) is often used in these conditions and is postulated to be due to enteric bacterial translocation in a setting of pre-existing ascites. The common offending organisms in SBP are enteric gram-negative bacteria like *E. coli*. The children with primary peritonitis present with acute abdominal pain associated with abdominal pain. It is associated with vomiting, nausea, and diarrhea. The pain is diffuse with a lack of localization.

Diagnosis: A plain radiograph may demonstrate ileus pattern or may demonstrate the presence of ascites. When free fluid is present, diagnostic paracentesis is usually helpful. In cases of primary peritonitis, there will be more than 500 leukocytes/mm^3 with predominant granulocyte count. The pH is usually less than 7.35, and the lactate levels will usually be more than 25 mg/dl. Cultures of the fluid usually demonstrate gram-positive organisms like Pneumococcus or Streptococcus. Primary pneumococcal peritonitis occurs typically in undernourished girls between 3 and 6 years, but may also occur in boys. In females, ascending genitourinary infection is the predominant cause, whereas in males, it is usually blood-borne from respiratory infections and middle ear infections. It is associated with lower abdominal pain with profuse diarrhea, which is occasionally blood stained. The peritoneal exudate is typically odorless and sticky. Primary streptococcal peritonitis is commoner and here the exudate is thin, cloudy that contains flakes of fibrin.

Treatment: These patients are usually managed conservatively with intravenous antibiotics and fluids. Exploration may be required in case the child does not improve on medical management or there is a diagnostic difficulty. Laparoscopic evaluation may also be performed in these cases.

Gastrointestinal tuberculosis: See Section 14.3.

Pelvic inflammatory disease (PID): PID is a disease of sexually active adolescent girl and is diagnosed with difficulty as many patients deny sexual activity. The usual history is that of acute abdominal pain that began shortly after the onset of her menstrual period and is associated with vaginal discharge. Severe cases may have right upper quadrant pain due to peri-hepatic inflammation (Fitz Hugh-Curtis syndrome). The patient usually has diffuse tenderness on abdominal examination. Local signs of peritoneal inflammation are less common. Pelvic examination reveals cervical discharge and adnexal tenderness. Treatment is by antibiotics and analgesics.

Ectopic pregnancy: Any post-pubertal female patient with severe acute abdominal pain should have a urine pregnancy test performed, because ectopic pregnancy may cause acute abdomen. Ectopic pregnancy is rare, occurring in less than 1% of all pregnancies. The history reveals symptoms of early pregnancy such as missed or scanty menstrual period, morning sickness, and breast tenderness. Uterine enlargement may be demonstrated. Vaginal examination may reveal adnexal masses in more than half the patients. Associated vaginal bleed suspiciously points towards the diagnosis of ectopic pregnancy. The treatment is by an urgent laparotomy and salpingectomy.

Small bowel obstructions: Infants and young children with intestinal obstruction present with pain, irritability, vomiting and abdominal distension. Small bowel obstructions progress to decreased or even no bowel movements. Intussusception, incarcerated hernia, malrotation, volvulus, and necrotizing entero-colitis can lead to acute intestinal obstruction in children. Abdominal tuberculosis, Hirschsprung's disease, abdominal masses like duplication cysts are important causes of chronic partial intestinal obstruction.

Initial treatment consists of decompression of the bowel by keeping the child nil by mouth along with intravenous fluid replacement of the third space losses and correction of shock. Antibiotics are administered against enteric gram-negative bacteria and against anaerobes. Emergent laparotomy is required after initial stabilization to prevent development of complications.

Other causes of acute abdominal pain in children include a variety of conditions such as urolithiasis, hydronephrosis, acute pyelonephritis and pyoneph-rosis. The diagnosis is usually obvious on history and confirmed on ultrasonography of the abdomen. Acute pancreatitis and pseudocyst especially following trauma are quite rare and a high index of suspicion is required.

Aiken JJ, Oldham KT. Acute appendicitis. In: Kliegman RM, Behrman RE, Jenson HB, Stanton BF (eds). *Nelson Textbook of Pediatrics.* 18th edn. Vol. 2. Philadelphia: Saunders, 2007;1628–35.

Sinha Arvind, Sarin Yogesh Kumar. Acute Abdomen in Children. In: Mathur GP, Mathur Sarla (eds). *Current Trends in Pediatrics.* Vol 2. Delhi: Academa Publishers, 2006;342–55.

16.14 ANORECTAL MALFORMATIONS

Anorectal malformations (ARMs) form a major group of the most common congenital anomalies dealt by pediatric surgeons worldwide. The worldwide incidence of the anomaly is 1 : 5000 live births. Low anomalies are more common in girls while high anomalies are more frequent in males. The exact etiology is still unknown but these malformations are thought to be the result of arrests or abnormalities in the embryological development of the anus, rectum and urogenital tract. Genetic predisposition has been seen rarely in some families. Sex linked and autosomal dominant inheritances have been suggested.

Krickenbeck classification: The standards for diagnosis-international classification (Krickenbech) are depicted in Table 16.15.

Clinical Manifestations

Local examination: The anomaly is usually characterized by the absence of anal opening at its normal site though a varied spectrum of anomalies is seen depending upon the extent of anorectal agenesis and the presence or absence of associated genitourinary fistula. The key to successful clinical diagnosis in a case of anorectal malformation is very careful examination, which may need to be repeated in babies seen only few hours after birth as it takes 12–18 hours for swallowed air to reach the terminal part of the colon.

Table 16.15: Standards for diagnosis: International classification (Krickenbech)

Major clinical groups	Rare/regional variants
Perineal (cutaneous) fistula	Pouch colon
Rectourethral fistula	Rectal atresia/stenosis
• Prostatic	Rectovaginal fistula
• Bulbar	H-fistula
Rectovesical fistula	Others
Vestibular fistula	
Cloaca	
No fistula	
Anal stenosis	

Source: Holschneider A, Hutson J, Pena A, et al. Preliminary report on the International Conference for the Development of Standards for the Treatment of Anorectal Malformations. *J Pediatr Surg* 2005;40:1521–6.

A visible abnormal anal opening: If there is a visible opening in the perineum near the normal site of anus, it has to be examined in detail carefully.

Anal stenosis: The anal opening may be small and at the normal anal site. It may be covered by a bridge of skin resembling a bucket handle. Bowel of normal caliber is generally found close to the surface, but occasionally it may be higher up with a long narrow tract when it is named anorectal stenosis.

Ectopic anus: The anal opening may be sited anteriorly. In boys, it is generally found between the normal anal site and the posterior limit of the scrotum, but may extend anteriorly on the penile shaft. Rarely the anus may be located posteriorly in the midline. It may be in the midline or slightly deviated.

Anocutaneous fistula: The anal opening may be ectopic and stenotic and a meconium filled tract may be seen in the midline behind it. The meconium may be milked out on applying pressure over the tract. On passing a bougie, it is felt almost horizontally backwards and bowel of normal caliber is usually found fairly close to the surface.

Rectoperineal fistula: The bougie in the visible opening passes more vertically upwards and bowel of normal caliber is higher up. In girls, the opening may be in the perineum, but is more commonly seen in the vestibule. The anatomy can be recognized in the same manner with the help of a bougie after identifying three separate openings in the vestibule.

Anovestibular fistula: The opening is in the vestibule and on passing a metallic bougie, it takes a posterior route towards the normal anal site and it can be felt percutaneously.

Rectovestibular fistula: The opening is in the vestibule and on passing a metallic bougie, it takes a cranial route towards the vagina and it cannot be felt percutaneously

Vulval anus: It is lined by mucosa anteriorly and by skin posteriorly. However, there are shades of gray between the classical types in both sexes. Clinically, if the baby is symptomatic with straining at stools or remains constipated, the opening is inadequate and possibly a fistula exists requiring a preliminary colostomy.

No visible anal opening: In boys, the passage of meconium through the urethra may sometimes be noted. The bowel commonly terminates in either the prostatic or the bulbar urethra, but it may terminate blindly or at the bladder base. Thus, the anomaly in males may be: ARM with rectoprostatic urethral fistula; ARM with rectobulbar urethral fistula; ARM with bladder neck fistula; ARM without fistulous connection.

In girls, meconium may be seen emerging from the orifice of the vagina or of a common urethrovaginal canal or cloaca. The level of the terminal bowel can be established by ultrasonography, invertogram, CT scan and MRI scan as described above or by a lateral vaginogram or a cloacogram if there is a large fistula. The anatomy of the pelvic organs of girls who have normal urethral and vaginal orifices is relatively easy to unravel, but if there is a common urethrovaginal canal, the anatomy can be bizarre.

If there are three openings in the vestibule, the lesion may be: (i) rectovaginal fistula; (ii) anorectal agenesis without fistula; (iii) anal agenesis without fistula.

If there is one opening in the vestibule, the lesion may be rectocloacal fistula.

Congenital pouch colon (CPC): Congenital pouch colon is a condition associated with anorectal agenesis, seen particularly in Asia. The condition is defined as an anomaly in which all or part of the colon is replaced by a pouch-like dilatation, which communicates distally with the urogenital tract via a large fistula. In this condition, a supralevator anorectal malformation (ARM) is associated with a colonic pouch of variable size (5–15 cm in diameter). The mesentery of this pouch is short and poorly developed, the wall is very thick, the taenia coli are absent or ill defined, and haustration and the appendices epiploicae are absent. The main pouch is supplied by the branches arising from the superior mesenteric artery, which form a leash of vessels around it. This condition is more common in the northern Indian population and neighboring nations like Pakistan and Nepal, although sporadic reports have also come from other parts of the world. Its management involves a diversion colostomy at birth with or without the excision of the pouch followed by a pull-through.

Rectal atresia: Rectal atresia is characterized by the presence of the proximal rectum, which ends at or above the pubococcygeal (PC) line, and a well-formed distal anus that is in its normal location and has a normal appearance, which is about 1–3 cm in depth. The two pouches may be connected to each other by a fibrous strand that may be hugged by the puborectalis sling. Unlike other ARM, the anal canal and lower rectum are well surrounded by the sphincter complexes and hence the outcome after surgery is good.

Systemic examination: Complete physical examination, including passage of a nasogastric tube to rule out an esophageal atresia should be done in all cases. The abdomen should be examined for any palpable enlargement of the kidneys or bladder, other associated congenital anomalies like major cardiac malformations, major vertebral and craniocerebral defects and Down syndrome. Associated anomalies that need to be identified before the infant is discharged include: (a) obstructive uropathies and severe vesicoureteric reflux; (b) ambiguous external genitalia and deformities of male and female genitalia; (c) other renal, limb and ocular anomalies.

Investigations: The gold standard Wangensteen and Rice invertogram whether done in the standard head down position or the prone cross table lateral position is still the most widely used investigation of choice. It is reliable only after at least 18–20 hours after birth as it takes this much time for the swallowed gas to reach the lower rectal pouch. Once filled with air or contrast, the blind rectal pouch is located in relation to the pubo-coccygeal line or the I-point of ischium. If the sacrum is poorly developed, the (P-C) line may be determined by commencing from the midpoint of the pubis anteriorly and transecting the junction of the upper and lower three quarters of ischium.

Supralevator lesions are identified when the blind rectal pouch ends above the P-C line. The bowel in intermediate lesions extends to a line drawn through the most inferior portion of the ischium (I-point), parallel to the P-C line.

A gap of 1 cm between gas shadow and skin usually represents a high anomaly. A gap < 5 mm usually represents a low lesion.

The level of the terminal bowel can be also be determined by ultrasonography. A pouch perineal distance of less than 1 cm is suggestive of a low anomaly. The relation of the terminal bowel to the sacrum, the urogenital organs and the surface can thus be visualized.

A large loop of bowel with single air fluid level occupying more than half of the total width of abdomen and displacing the small bowel to one side (usually right) is the classical picture in a case of congenital pouch colon. An early perforation in cases of high ARM is suggestive of pouch colon, especially if the baby comes from an area where CPC is commonly seen.

A lateral X-ray taken after instillation of radio-opaque dye through a catheter in the urethra will delineate the terminal bowel if there is a relatively large urethral fistula. Voiding cystogram may be obtained to demonstrate a fistula, ureteral reflux, urethral stricture or connection between the ureter and vas deferens. This is usually not done in the newborn period as the main criteria to decide at that time is whether or not a colostomy will be required.

In cases that have undergone colostomy in the newborn period, a distal cologram is performed to delineate the fistulous communication.

The newer imaging modalities, namely CT scan and MRI scan are not really essential for managing a neonate, though their information is valuable in delineating the anatomy in complicated cases or those requiring a redo surgery.

A detailed work up of the baby at the time of definitive surgery should include ultrasound of the abdomen, intravenous urogram, and voiding cystourethrography and echocardiography to evaluate for associated anomalies. Spiral computed tomography with three-dimensional reconstruction of the pelvic musculature, or magnetic resonance imaging of the pelvis are optional for studying the pelvic musculature.

Treatment

Anorectal agenesis has a varied spectrum of anomalies. Each case should be examined carefully with a wide knowledge of the anatomical variations and identification of rare anomalies so that the best possible treatment option can be adopted to achieve the optimal results. Colostomy is performed in most neonates with ARM presenting after 48 hrs or so with distension of abdomen. However, if the baby presents early without gross distension of abdomen, perforation and sepsis, the authors prefer a single stage PSARP in the newborn period without a covering colostomy. Perineal procedures can be carried out safely on all neonates with a very low lesion.

Anal stenosis: Dilatations—minimal stenosis can be cured by repeated dilatations.

Y-V plasty—a posterior V flap of sensitive perianal skin is sutured into the posterior wall of the anal canal after this is opened up.

Anal transposition: A circumferential incision is made around the opening; the bowel is separated posteriorly and laterally from the surrounding levator sling, and anteriorly from the posterior surface of the vagina until bowel of normal caliber is reached. Separation is easily achieved in the relatively low lesions but is difficult if there is a long tract adherent to the whole length of the vagina and dissection has to be continued up to the level of the peritoneal reflection.

Colostomy: It is usually performed as a first stage in a newborn with high anomaly. Colostomy should be urgently performed on the neonate who presents without a visible opening of the bowel, with low birth weight, with bilious vomiting and abdominal distension and with a life threatening associated anomaly.

Anorectal reconstruction: The treatment plan is for intermediate and high anorectal malformations advocated by the authors.

Follow-up: It is mandatory to ensure a regular follow-up so that a good quality life may be provided to the patients in terms of functional and cosmetic results.

Chatterjee SK. Anorectal Malformations—problems in the neonate. In: Gupta DK (ed). *Textbook of Neonatal Surgery.* 1st edn. New Delhi: Modern Publishers, 2000;228–32.

Gupta DK. Anorectal Malformation - A pictorial depiction. In: Gupta DK (ed). Textbook of Neonatal Surgery. 1st edn. New Delhi: Modern Publishers, 2000;233–9.

Gupta Devendra K. Anorectal malformations - Wingspread to Krickenbeck. JIAPS 2005;10:75–77.

Gupta DK, Sharma Shilpa. Recta duplication and anal duplication. In: Holschneider A, Hutson J (eds). *Anorectal Malformations in children.* 1st edn. Germany: Springer Publishers, 2006;231–8.

Gupta DK, Sharma Shilpa. Congenital Pouch Colon. In: Holschneider A, Hutson J (eds). Anorectal Malformations in children.1st edn. Germany: Springer Publishers, 2006; 211–22.

Gupta DK, Sharma Shilpa. Rectal Atresia and Rectal Ectasia. In: Holschneider A, Hutson J (eds). Anorectal Malformations in children. 1st edn. Germany: Springer Publishers, 2006; 223–30.

Gupta Devendra K, Sharma Shilpa. Current Trends in Anorectal Malformations. In: Mathur GP, Mathur Sarla (eds). Current Trends in Pediatrics. Vol 3. Delhi: Academa Publishers, 2007;161–73.

16.15 HERNIA IN CHILDREN

Hernia is classically defined as protrusion of a viscus or a part of viscus through the defect in the walls of cavity containing it. It is one of the most common indications of surgical intervention in pediatric age group. Hernia can be external or internal (Box 16.3).

Inguinal hernia: The inguinal hernia can be direct or indirect. Indirect hernias are more common on the right side because of delayed descent of the right testicle. The patient is examined in both supine and standing positions. Physical examination of a child with an inguinal hernia typically reveals a palpable smooth mass originating from the external ring lateral to the pubic tubercle. The mass may only be noticeable after coughing or performing a Valsalva maneuver and it should be reduced easily. Occasionally, the examining physician may feel the loops of intestine within the hernia sac. When the hernia sac is palpated over the cord structures, the sensation may be similar to that of rubbing two layers of silk together. This finding is known as the 'silk sign' and is highly suggestive of an inguinal hernia (incarcinated inguinal hernia, *see* Section 16.13 and Fig. 16.8 in CD).

Box 16.3 Causes of hernia

External hernia: Inguinal hernia, femoral hernia; umbilical hernia; epigastric hernia; lumbar hernia; spigelian hernia; perineal hernia, incisional hernia. *Internal hernia:* Diaphragmatic hernia; hiatal hernia; lung hernia; internal hernia

---

Direct inguinal hernia: These hernias are rare in children. Direct hernias appear as groin masses that extend toward the femoral vessels with exertion or straining. The etiology is from a muscular defect or weakness in the floor of the inguinal canal medial to the epigastric vessels. The causes of direct hernia include a prior indirect hernia repair on the side of the direct hernia, Ehlers-Danlos syndrome, Marfan syndrome, and Hunter-Hurler syndrome.

Femoral hernia: They are more common in girls than in boys, with a ratio of 2 : 1. Femoral hernia represents a protrusion through the femoral canal. Its location is below the inguinal ligament, and typically projects toward the medial aspect of the thigh.

Umbilical hernia is one of the most common conditions seen in the childhood. Umbilical hernias are more common in the low birth-weight babies. Umbilical hernias are more commonly associated with Down's syndrome, trisomy 18, trisomy 13, mucopolysaccharidosis and congenital hypothyroidism. These may also form a component of Beckwith-Wiedeman syndrome. Most umbilical hernias present shortly after birth. Most complain of swelling that increases on crying or straining. The concerned parent should be counseled that strangulation is rare and continued observation is safe. Any interventions in the form of pressure dressings or strapping are avoided.

Hernias with a diameter greater than 2.0 cm are unlikely to resolve on their own. A thicker and more rounded fascial edge is predictive of increased chances of spontaneous closure. If the hernia persists as the child approaches school age, it should be repaired. Earlier repair is advised if the symptoms of incarceration or recurrent pain are present. Most umbilical hernias do not cause any symptoms and do not require surgical repair until approximately 5 years of age.

Epigastric hernias are common in children and frequently present in infancy. Epigastric hernias occur due to defect in the decussating fibres of the linea alba. These can be multiple. The defect typically contains only the properitoneal, which protrudes through the defect.

Lumbar hernia mostly occurs in otherwise normal children but an association has been noted with lumbocostovertebral deficiency syndrome. A lumbar hernia presents as a bulge, mostly due to protruding retroperitoneal fat. Palpation usually reveals a reducible soft swelling.

Spigelian hernia develops at the intersection of the linea semilunaris, the lateral border of rectus abdominis muscle and the caudal termination of the posterior sheath of rectus muscle, the linea semicircularis. The hernia presents as a tender mass near the umbilicus.

Perineal hernia: Perineal hernia presents as a perineal, gluteal or labial mass that is reducible and demonstrates impulse on coughing. The child may present with constipation and soft tissue mass.

Incisional hernia: Hernia formation occurs at the site of a previous laparotomy. Factors associated with an increased risk of incisional hernia include increased intra-abdominal pressure, wound infection, and midline incision.

Diaphragmatic hernia: A diaphragmatic hernia is defined as communication between the abdominal and thoracic cavities with or without abdominal contents in the thorax. The etiology may be congenital or traumatic. The defect may be at the esophageal hiatus (hiatal), paraesophageal (adjacent to the hiatus), retrosternal (Morgagni) or at the posterolateral (Bochdalek) portion of the diaphragm.

Congenital Diaphragmatic Hernia (Bochdalek)

The term congenital diaphragmatic hernia (CDH) typically refers to the Bochdalek form. These lesions may cause significant respiratory distress at birth, can be associated with other congenital anomalies and mortality and morbidity. The Bochdalek hernia accounts for up to 90% of the hernias seen in the newborn period, with 85% occurring on the left side and occasionally (<5%) bilateral. The incidence of CDH is between 1/2,000 and 1/5,000 live births, with females affected twice as often as males. Pulmonary hypoplasia and malrotation of the intestine are part of the lesion, not associated anomalies. Associated anomalies have been reported in up to 30% of cases; these include central nervous system lesions, esophageal atresia, omphalocele, and cardiovascular lesions. CDH is associated with chromosomal syndromes: trisomy 21, trisomy 13, trisomy 18, Fryn, Brachmann-de Lange, Pallister-Killan, and Turner.

Clinical presentation: Respiratory distress is a cardinal sign in babies with CDH. This may occur immediately or there may be a "honeymoon" period of up to 48 hr when the baby is relatively stable. Early respiratory distress within 6 hr of life is thought to be a poor prognostic sign. The clinical signs of respiratory distress include tachypnea, grunting, use of accessory muscles, and cyanosis. Children with CDH will also have scaphoid abdomen and increased chest wall diameter. Bowel sounds may also be heard in the chest with decreased breath sounds bilaterally. The point of maximal cardiac impulse may be displaced away from the side of hernia if mediastinal shift has occurred.

Diagnosis: A chest radiograph and nasal gastric tube is all that is usually required to confirm the diagnosis.

CDH can be diagnosed on prenatal ultrasound (between 16 and 24 wk) in over 50% of cases. High-speed magnetic resonance imaging can further define the lesion. Findings on ultrasound may include polyhydramnios, chest mass, mediastinal shift, gastric bubble or a liver in the thoracic cavity, and fetal hydrops. Lung size to head size ratio (LHR) may predict the outcome.

Treatment: Aggressive respiratory support is often needed in children with CDH. The ideal time to repair the diaphragmatic defect is under debate. Most centers will wait at least 48 hr after stabilization and resolution of the pulmonary hypertension. A subcostal surgical approach is the most frequently used. Gastroesophageal reflux disease (GERD) is reported in more than 50% of children with CDH.

Foramen of Morgagni hernia: The anteromedial diaphragmatic defect through the foramen of Morgagni accounts for 2–6% of diaphragmatic hernia. Failure of sternal or crural portions of the diaphragm to meet and fuse produces this defect. These defects more commonly right sided (90%), but may be bilateral. The transverse colon, or small intestine or liver is usually contained in the hernia sac. The diagnosis is usually made on the chest X-ray when the children are evaluated for another reason. The chest X-ray shows a structure behind the heart and a lateral film localizes the mass to the retrosternal area. A chest CT will confirm the diagnosis. When symptoms occur, they can be recurrent respiratory tract infections, cough, vomiting, or reflux; incarceration may occur in rare instances. Repair is recommended for all patients.

Paraesophageal hernia is differentiated from hiatal hernia in that the gastroesophageal junction is in the normal location. The herniation of the stomach alongside or adjacent to the gastrointestinal junction is prone to incarceration with strangulation and perforation. A previous Niseen fundoplication and other diaphragmatic surgeries are risk factors. The usual diaphragmatic hernia should be repaired promptly after diagnosis.

Hiatal hernia: Herniation of the stomach through the esophageal hiatus can occur as a common sliding hernia, in which the gastroesophageal junction slides into the thorax or it can be paraesophageal, in which a portion of the stomach (usually the fundus) is insinuated next to the esophagus inside the gastroesophageal junction in the hiatus. Sliding hernias are frequently associated with gastroesophageal reflux, especially in developmentally delayed children. Gastroesophageal reflux should be treated in these children.

Internal hernia: Intestinal obstructions can be caused by defects in the mesentery ("intestinal hernias") through which loop of small bowel may pass and become trapped. Vascular engorgement of the trapped bowel results in intestinal ischemia and gangrene unless promptly relieved. Symptoms include bilious vomiting, abdominal distension and abdominal pain. Peritoneal signs suggest ischemic bowel. Plain radiographs will show signs of small bowel obstruction or free air if the bowel is perforated. Supportive management includes intravenous fluids, antibiotics and nasogastric aspiration. Prompt surgical intervention is indicated to relieve obstruction. This will prevent the development of the intestinal gangrene.

Lung hernia: A lung hernia is a protusion of the lung beyond its normal thoracic boundaries. About 20% are congenital and the other 80% cases are seen after chest trauma or thoracic surgery or in patients with pulmonary diseases such as cystic fibrosis or asthma, which cause frequent cough and generate high intrathoracic pressure. The presenting sign of a cervical hernia ("Sibson hernia") is usually a neck mass noticed while straining or coughing. Some lesions are asymptomatic and detected only when a chest film is taken for another reason. Surgical treatment for lung hernia is occasionally justified for cosmetic reasons.

Aiken JJ, Oldham KT. Inguinal hernias. In: Kliegman RM, Behrman RE, Jenson HB, Stanton BF (eds). *Nelson Textbook of Pediatrics*. 18th edn. Vol. 2. Philadelphia: Saunders, 2007; 1644–50.

·Al-Shanafey S, Giacomantonio M. Femoral hernia in children. *J Pediatr Surg* 1999;34:1104–6.

Ehrlich PF, Coran AG. Diaphragmatic hernia. In: Kliegman RM, Behrman RE, Jenson HB, Stanton BF (eds). *Nelson Textbook of Pediatrics*. 18th edn. Vol. 1. Philadelphia: Saunders, 2007;746–50.

Ehrlich PF, Coran AG. Foramen of Morgagni hernia. In: Kliegman RM, Behrman RE, Jenson HB, Stanton BF (eds). *Nelson Textbook of Pediatrics*. 18th edn. Vol. 1. Philadelphia: Saunders, 2007; 749.

Ehrlich PF, Coran AG. Paraesophageal hernia. In: Kliegman RM, Behrman RE, Jenson HB, Stanton BF (eds). *Nelson Textbook of Pediatrics*. 18th edn. Vol. 1. Philadelphia: Saunders, 2007; 749.

Finder JD, Michelson. Congenital disorders of the lung. In: Kliegman RM, Behrman RE, Jenson HB, Stanton BF (eds). *Nelson Textbook of Pediatrics*. 18th edn. Vol. 1. Philadelphia: Saunders, 2007; 1783–1787.

Mohta A, Jain N, Irniraya K P., Saluja SS, Sharma S, Gupta A: Non-ligation of hernial sac during herniotomy: A prospective study. *Pediatr Surg Int* 2003; 19: 451–452

Mohta Anup. Hernia in Children. In: Mathur GP, Mathur Sarla (eds). *Current Trends in Pediatrics*. Vol 3. Delhi: Academa Publishers, 2007; 174–182.

Mohta A, Bhargava SK. Congenital perineal hernia: a case report. *Surg Today* 2004; 34:630–631.

Orenstein S, Peters J, Khan S, Youssef N, Hussain SZ. Hiatal hernia. In: Kliegman RM, Behrman RE, Jenson HB, Stanton BF (eds). *Nelson Textbook of Pediatrics*. 18th edn. Vol. 2. Philadelphia: Saunders, 2007; 1546.

Wakhlu A, Wakhlu AK.Congenital lumbar hernia. *Pediatr Surg Int* 2000; 16:146–148.

16.16 DISORDERS OF EXOCRINE PANCREAS

Acute Pancreatitis

Acute pancreatitis is the most common pancreatic disorder in children defined by sudden onset of abdominal pain associated with rise in digestive enzymes in blood and urine.

Causes of pancreatitis: The most common causes of pancreatitis in children include trauma, drug toxicity and infections (especially mumps). The causes are enumerated in Table 16.16.

Table 16.16: Causes of pancreatitis	
Causes	*Name of diseases/drugs/toxins*
Trauma	Blunt injury, burns, child abuse, hypothermia, surgical trauma, total body cast
Drug and toxins	acetaminophen overdose, alcohol, azathioprine, erythromycin, enalapril, estrogen, sulfonamide, thiazide diuretic, tetracycline, valproate, venom, vincristine
Infections	Ascaris, mumps, rubella, *Mycoplasma pneumoniae*, coxsackie B virus, hepatitis A, B, influenza A, B, post-varicella, human immunodeficiency virus (HIV), leptospirosis, malaria
Anatomical abnormalities	Pancreas divisum, annular pancreas, choledochal cyst, choledocholithiasis
Metabolic causes	Hyperlipoproteinemia type 1, type 4, type 5, cystic fibrosis, hyperparathyroidism, refeeding
Vascular causes	Hemolytic uremic syndrome, systemic lupus erythematosus (SLE), Henoch-Schönlein purpura
Tubercular causes idiopathic	

Clinical manifestations: Patient of acute pancreatitis presents with acute excruciating epigastric pain, persistent vomiting and high-grade fever. The abdominal pain is dull and steady in the beginning which radiates to the flanks and often increases in intensity over the next 24 to 48 hours with progressively increasing vomiting. The child on examination appears anxious, restless, dehydrated and likes to sit in a knee chest position in an attempt to relieve pain. The abdomen is distended and tender to palpation with no definite guarding or rigidity. In severe cases a bluish discoloration may be seen around the umbilicus (*Cullen sign*) or in the flanks (*Grey Turner sign*).

Periostitis, nodular skin lesions, and synovial fat necrosis may develop as a result of lipases released during pancreatitis. In patients with acute pancreatitis, elevated serum lipase and amylase levels, periosteal new bone formation, and abnormal findings on bone scintigraphy (revealing fat-induced infarcts) may be found.

Diagnosis: Various biochemical parameters and radiological findings are helpful in arriving at diagnosis. Serum amylase (normal 17–115 IU/L), serum lipase (normal 13–60 IU/L) are elevated. Abdominal erect X-ray may show evidence of regional small bowel ileus most commonly in left upper quadrant (sentinel loop sign), dilation of transverse colon (colon cut off sign), absence of air in descending colon, generalized ileus, blurring of left psoas margin, pancreatic calcifications or diffuse abdominal haziness. CT Scan is useful in demonstrating an enlarged pancreas when the diagnosis of pancreatitis is uncertain. It helps in detecting pseudocysts and in differentiating pancreatitis from other possible intra abdominal catastrophes.

Differential diagnosis: Acute pancreatitis must be differentiated from an acute cholecystitis, acute intestinal obstruction and renal colic.

Treatment: The mainstay of treatment of acute pancreatitis in children include pain relief, pancreatic rest, and to manage complications. Most children do well with supportive conservative approach. Patient is kept nil orally, intravenous fluids and electrolytes infusion is started and pethidine/morphine is given as analgesic. Frequent monitoring of vital signs and clinical examination of the child are important for treatment. Non-invasive monitoring of vital parameters is of great value in assessing the child frequently. It is better to treat the child in ICU setting. Asepsis must be ensured as these patients are prone to contract nosocomial infection. Role of prophylactic antibiotics to prevent local complications may be justified. Children with uncomplicated cases do well and recover over a period of 2–5 days. Surgical therapy of acute pancreatitis is rarely required, but may include drainage of necrotic material or abscesses.

Prognosis: Children with uncomplicated acute pancreatitis recover within 4–5 days. When pancreatitis is associated with trauma or systemic disease, the prognosis is typically related to the associated medical condition.

Das S, Arora NK, Gupta DK, Gupta AK, Mathur P, Ahuja A. Pancreatic Diseases in children in a north Indian referral hospital. Indian Pediatr 2004 41:704–11.

Lerner A. Acute pancreatitis in children and adolescents. In: Lebenthal E (ed). *Textbook of Gastroenterology and Nutrition in Infancy.* 2nd edn. New York: Raven Press Ltd., 1989;897–908.

Miller ML. Miscellaneous conditions associated with arthritis. In: Kliegman RM, Behrman RE, Jenson HB, Stanton BF (eds). Nelson Textbook of Pediatrics. 18th edn. Vol. 1. Philadelphia: Saunders, 2007;1051–2.

Werlin SL. Exocrine pancreas. In: Kliegman RM, Behrman RE, Jenson HB, Stanton BF (eds). *Nelson Textbook of Pediatrics.* 18th edn. Vol. 2. Philadelphia: Saunders, 2007;1650–7.

16.17 PERITONEUM

Ascites is an accumulation of serous fluid within the peritoneal cavity. The causes of ascites have been described in Box 16.4. In children, hepatic, renal, cardiac diseases are the most common causes. The clinical feature of ascites is abdominal distension but this may also be caused by other conditions, including gaseous distension, fecal retention, tumor masses, peritoneal hemorrhage, extreme bladder distension, pregnancy, and obesity (5F, fat, fluid, flatus, fetus, fetus/tumor masses/bladder distension). Ascites is detected by the five classic physical signs: bulging flanks, flank dullness, shifting dullness, fluid wave,

---

Box 16.4: Causes of ascites

Hepatic: Cirrhosis; congenital hepatic fibrosis; portal vein obstruction; fulminant hepatic failure; Budd-Chiari syndrome; lysosomal storage disease
Gastrointestinal: Infected bowel; perforation
Renal: Nephrotic syndrome; obstructive uropathy; perforation of urinary tract; peritoneal dialysis
Pancreatic: Pancreatitis; ruptured pancreatic duct
Cardiac: Heart failure; constrictive pericarditis; inferior vena cava web
Infectious: Tuberculosis; abscess; chlamydia; schistosomiasis
Gynecologic: Ovarian tumors; ovarian torsion, rupture
Neoplastic: lymphoma; neuroblastoma
Miscellaneous: Systemic lupus erythematosus; ventriculoperitoneal shunt; eosinophilic ascites; chylous ascites; hypothyroidism

and the "puddle sign" (decreased auscultation of high-frequency vibrations in central abdomen when flicking side of abdomen with patient on hands and knees). Umbilical herniation may be associated with tense ascites. Ultrasound examination can detect small amount of ascites. For diagnostic and therapeutic purposes ascitic fluid is obtained via paracentesis.

The course, prognosis, and treatment of ascites depend entirely on the cause. Patients are at increased risk for spontaneous bacterial peritonitis.

Chylous ascites can result from an anomaly, injury or obstruction of the intra-abdominal portion of thoracic duct. The causes are congenital malformations, peritoneal bands, generalized lymphangiomatosis, chronic inflammatory processes of the bowel, tumors, enlarged lymph nodded, previous abdominal surgery and trauma. Congenital anomalies of the lymphatic system are associated with Turner, Noonan, yellow nail, and Klippel-Trénaunay-Weber syndromes. Diagnosis of chylous ascites depends on the demonstration of milky ascitic fluid obtained via paracentesis after a fat-containing feeding. Fluid analysis will reveal a high protein content, elevated triglycerides, and lymphocytosis. Treatment includes the provision of a high protein, low-fat containing diet supplemented with medium-chain triglycerides (MCT) that are absorbed directly into the portal circulation. Parenteral alimentation may be needed in case nutrition remains impaired on oral feedings and also in order to decrease lymph flow to facilitate sealing at the point of lymph leakage. Octerotide, a somatostatin analog, has been used. Paracentesis should be repeated only if abdominal distension causes respiratory distress. Laparotomy may be indicated to search for the site of the leak if a trial of dietary management has been unsuccessful.

Alami AO, Allen DB, Organ CH. Chylous ascites: A collective review. Surgery 2000;128:761–8.

Hymas JS. Ascites. In: Kliegman RM, Behrman RE, Jenson HB, Stanton BF (eds). *Nelson Textbook of Pediatrics*. 18th edn. Vol. 2. Philadelphia: Saunders, 2007;1614.

16.18 ENDOSCOPIC EXAMINATION OF GASTROINTESTINAL TRACT

Endoscopy provides direct method of inspection in a variety of primary or secondary gastrointestinal conditions. Endoscopic examination of gastrointestinal tract has both diagnostic and therapeutic uses and can be broadly divided into two groups:

1. Upper gastrointestinal endoscopy (esophagogastroduodenoscopy).
2. Lower gastrointestinal endoscopy (colonoscopy).

Upper Gastrointestinal Endoscopy

Indications for upper gastrointestinal (UGI) endoscopy: The indications can be divided into two groups: diagnostic and therapeutic.

Diagnostic: 1. Upper gastrointestinal hemorrhage (hemetemesis); 2. Portal hypertension; 3. Chronic diarrhea; 4. Recurrent abdominal pain when an organic gastrointestinal cause is suspected; 5. Failure to thrive/short stature and 6. Dysphagia/odynophagia and caustic ingestion.

Therapeutic: 1. Endoscopic variceal ligation and sclerotherapy; 2. Stricture dilatation; 3. Foreign body removal; and 4. Placement of feeding tubes (*see* Figs 16.18.1 to 16.1.8.11 in CD).

Diagnostic Indications for UGI Endoscopy

1. *Upper GI hemorrhage:* Endoscopy is undertaken to find out the cause of hemetemesis after stabilizing the patients. Nasopharynx should be carefully examined as a cause of bleeding before endoscopy is performed. Primary aim of endoscopy is to differentiate variceal and nonvariceal hemorrhages as treatment varies considerably. Variceal bleeding is often assumed in the context of a patient with portal hypertension and presence of esophageal varices on endoscopy. Other sources of hemorrhage such as gastric and duodenal varices, congestive gastropathy, or a bleeding ulcer/erosions should also be looked for. Non-variceal bleeding may be due to erosive esophagitis, gastric erosions, peptic ulcer, and vascular malformations.

2. *Suspected portal hypertension:* Upper GI endoscopy provides most reliable diagnostic modality for visualization of esophageal varices in children presenting with features suggestive of portal hypertension or cirrhosis (ascites/icterus/hepatosplenomegaly).

3. *Unexplained recurrent abdominal pain:* Endoscopy is useful in cases who present with unexplained abdominal pain or chest pain. Gastroesophageal reflux and reflux esophagitis are common causes of organic pain in abdomen in pediatric age group. Although 24 hr pH monitoring is the single best test for gastroesophageal reflux, diagnostic yield increases with endoscopy and biopsy. Endoscopy also gives opportunity to look for peptic or duodenal ulcer in children who present with recurrent pain abdomen. Nodular antritis is a typical endoscopic finding suggestive of *H. pylori* colonization, often confirmed by histological evidence.

4. *Chronic diarrhea:* Chronic diarrhea is another common problem for which endoscopy is indicated. Multiple duodenal biopsies can be easily

obtained from the duodenum during endoscopy. Histopathological examination of duodenal biopsies is useful for diagnosing conditions like celiac disease, tropical sprue and giardiasis. Endoscopic brush cytology further increases diagnostic yield for giardiasis.

5. *Dysphagia:* Dysphagia may be the clinical manifestation in the setting of esophagitis or stricture. Endoscopic evaluation includes biopsies for identification and characterization of inflammatory changes.

6. *Caustic ingestion:* UGI endoscopy can be useful for differentiating mucosal injury from extensive esophagogastric necrosis. The severities of changes correlate well with chances of subsequent stricture formation and serial endoscopic examination is useful in defining the extent of healing.

Therapeutic UGI Endoscopy

1. *Endoscopic variceal ligation and sclerotherapy:* Extrahepatic portal hypertension is the most common cause of upper GI hemorrhage in children in India. Sclerotherapy and variceal ligation are done for esophageal varices in cases with history of hematemesis.

Endoscopic sclerotherapy (EST): Sclerotherapy has been used as endoscopic therapy for managing esophageal variceal hemorrhage. Endoscopic sclerotherapy (EST) has been found successful in controlling active bleeding in over 90% of patients and it also has been found useful in reducing the frequency and severity of recurrent variceal hemorrhage (secondary prophylaxis). Esophageal EST may also be appropriate in a patient in whom acute bleeding has ceased, when no other cause for hemorrhage can be identified. Esophageal EST is not indicated in patients without a history of variceal bleeding. Gastric varices which are in continuity with esophageal varices may be treated with EST below the esophagogastric junction. Isolated gastric varices, however, tend to form an intermingling network and are therefore less amenable to EST.

Sclerotherapy may be performed by injection of the sclerosant directly into the varix (intravariceal) to produce thrombosis, or adjacent to the varix (paravariceal) to induce submucosal fibrosis and obliteration of deeper perforating vessels. In practice, a combination of both techniques may be utilized during the same session. Several sclerosants (sodium tetradecyl sulfate, ethanolamine oleate, polidocanol and ethanol) have been employed at varying concentrations and volumes.

Fever, retrosternal discomfort and dysphagia frequently occur as complication of sclerotherapy which usually resolve within 48 hours. Injection-induced bleeding, post-injection esophageal ulceration and esophageal perforation may also occur rarely. Dysphagia may occur after EST due to esophageal ulceration, or a stricture. Dysphagia related to post-sclerotherapy strictures usually improves with esophageal dilatation. Other potential complications include mediastinitis, pleural effusion, and bronchoesophageal fistula.

Endoscopic variceal ligation (EVL): Endoscopic variceal ligation, initially introduced by Steigmann in 1986, has been found superior to EST in terms of eradicating varices more rapidly with less rebleeding and with fewer complications. Recurrence of esophageal varices may occur more frequently in those treated with EVL and regular endoscopic surveillance is required. Gastric varices should not be treated with EVL alone. Other practical problems associated with the use of EVL include the difficulty of performing the procedure in the presence of active hemorrhage related to poor visibility.

Sometimes combined use—sclerotherapy for lesser grades and ligation for advanced varices may be more useful.

2. *Stricture dilatation:* Endoscopic dilatation has revolutionized the management of esophageal stricture secondary to caustic ingestion, esophagitis or sclerotherapy. Endoscopic dilatation involves serial passage of dilators through the stricture segment over a guide wire introduced through the side channel of endoscope. Availability of sialistic catheters and the angioplasty balloon catheters has made the procedure safer as compared to metallic dilators.

3. *Foreign body removal:* More than 80% of swallowed foreign bodies are likely to pass GI tract without the need for intervention. Most complications occur due to esophageal impaction. The most common site of esophageal impaction is at the thoracic inlet where about 70% of blunt foreign bodies that lodge in the esophagus do so at this location. Another 15% become lodged at the mid esophagus, in the region where the aortic arch and carina overlap the esophagus on chest radiograph. The third typical location is at the lower esophageal sphincter (LES) where remaining 15% are likely to get stuck.

Most ingested foreign bodies are best treated with flexible endoscopes. However, rigid esophagoscopy may be helpful for proximal foreign bodies impacted at the level of upper esophageal sphincter.

Once a swallowed foreign body reaches stomach of a child with a normal GI tract, it is likely to pass without any complications. However, retained foreign bodies may cause GI mucosal erosion, abrasion, local scarring, or perforation. Objects wider than 2.5 cm are less likely to pass the pylorus and so endoscopic removal is recommended. Objects that fails to pass beyond the stomach by 4 weeks should also be removed endoscopically.

Lower Gastrointestinal Endoscopy (Colonoscopy)

Colonoscopy provides opportunity of direct visual inspection of the mucosa of rectum and throughout the length of colon till ileocecal junction.

Indications for colonoscopy: Colonoscopy is performed for (i) diagnostic: 1. Rectal bleeding; 2. Occult GI hemorrhage; 3. Unexplained chronic diarrhea; 4. Inflammatory bowel disease and (ii) therapeutic: 1. Polypectomy.

1. *Rectal bleeding:* Hematochezia is the most common indication to perform colonoscopy in infants and children. A recurrent episode of minor bleeding is the most common condition where colonoscopy is helpful. If there is active bleeding it is advisable to do RBC scan (technetium-99m-labelled red blood cells scans) before colonoscopy to localize areas of bleeding. Lesions such as juvenile, adenomatous or hemartomatous polyps, vascular malformations, mucosal ulcerations may be identified by colonoscopy. If polyps are found to be the cause of bleeding, polypectomy is done in the same sitting. Prior to the development of colonoscopic polypectomy, surgical polypectomy was the only means available for the removal of polyp situated out of reach of the sigmoidoscope.

2. *Colitis:* The endoscopic appearance of the colonic mucosa in conjunction with the histological features on biopsy is a tool which aid in the diagnosis of a number of inflammatory processes of the colon. Inflammatory bowel diseases, infectious colitis, tuberculosis, pseudomembranous colitis are conditions with features of colitis where multiple endoscopic biopsies and the histological picture confirm the diagnosis.

Contraindications of colonoscopy: Suspected perforation and signs of peritonitis is an absolute contraindication of colonoscopy. Severe acute colitis and acute lower GI hemorrhage are other contraindications.

Complications: Hemorrhage and perforation are major complications which may occur due to direct manipulation of the tip of the instrument, by pneumatic pressure or by biopsy instrumentation. Fluid and electrolyte disturbance can occur due to bowel preparation.

Fox VL. Endoscopy. In: Walker WA, Durie PR, Hamilton JR, Walker-Smith JA, Watkins JB (eds). *Pediatric Gastrointestinal disease: Pathophysiology, diagnosis, management*. 2nd edn. Vol 2. St Louis, USA: Mosby, 1996;1513–33.

Kumar Praveen, Patwari AK. Endoscopic Examination of Gastrointestinal Tract. In: Mathur GP, Mathur Sarla (eds). *Current Trends in Pediatrics*. Vol 3. Delhi: Academa Publishers, 2007;79–83.

Mittal SK, Kalra KK, Aggarwal V. Diagnostic upper GI endoscopy for hemetemesis in children: Experience from a pediatric gastroenterology centre in north India. *Indian J Pediatr* 1994;61:651–4.

Patwari AK et al. Brush cytology: an adjunct to diagnostic upper GI endoscopy. *Indian J Pediatr* 2001;68:515–8.

17 Liver and Biliary System

17.1 MANIFESTATIONS OF LIVER DISEASE

Clinical Manifestation

Normal liver and hepatomegaly: Normal liver size estimations are based on age-related clinical indices, such as: the degree of extension of the liver edge below the costal margin, the span of dullness to percussion; or the length of the vertical axis of the liver, as estimated from imaging techniques. In children, the normal liver edge can be felt up to 2 cm below the right costal margin. In newborn infant, extension of liver edge >3.5 cm below the costal margin in the midclavicular line suggests hepatic enlargement. Measurement of liver span is carried out by percussing the upper margin of dullness and by palpating the lower edge in the right midclavicular line. The liver span increases linearly with body weight and age in both sexes, ranging from ~4.5 to 5.0 at 1 wk of age to ~7–8 cm in boys and ~6–6.5 cm in girls by 12 yr of age. The lower edge of the right lobe of the liver extends downward (Riedel lobe) and is palpable as a broad mass in some normal people. An enlarged left lobe of the liver is palpable in the epigastrium of some patients in cirrhosis. *Downward displacement of liver by the diaphragm (hyperinflation) or thoracic organs is not hepatomegaly.* Enlargement of the liver can be due to several mechanisms (Table 17.1).

Examination of the liver should note the consistency, contour, tenderness, or the presence of any masses, bruits, ascites or any stigmata of chronic liver disease, as well as assessment of spleen size and lymphadenopathy. Tender liver is associated with infective hepatitis, amebic hepatitis, liver abscess, congestive heart failure.

Biochemical tests commonly used to screen for or to confirm a suspicion of liver disease include measurements of:

i. Serum aminotransferase
ii. Bilirubin (total and fractionated)
iii. Alkaline phosphatase (AP)
iv. Prothrombin time (PT) or international normalized ratio (INR) and albumin level.

Ultrasonography is useful in assessment of liver size and consistency, as well as gallbladder size. Hyperechogenic parenchyma can be seen with metabolic disease (glycogen storage disease) or fatty liver (obesity, malnutrition, hyperalimentation, corticosteroids).

Gallbladder length normally varies from 1.5 to 5.5 cm (average 3.0 cm) in infants to 4–8 cm in adolescents; width ranges from 0.5 to 2.5 cm for all ages. Gallbladder distension may be seen in infants with sepsis. The gallbladder is often absent in infants with biliary atresia.

Ask the patient to breathe in deeply and palpate for the gallbladder in the normal way; at the height of inspiration the breathing stops with a gasp as the mass is felt. This represents *Murphy's sign*. The sign is not found in chronic cholecystitis or uncomplicated of gallstones.

478

Table 17.1: Mechanisms and causes of hepatomegaly

A. Increase in the number or size of the cells intrinsic to the liver

Storage	*Causes*
Fat	Malnutrition, obesity, metabolic liver disease (e.g. diseases of fatty acid oxidation and Reye syndrome-like diseases), lipid infusion (total parenteral nutrition), cystic fibrosis, diabetes mellitus, medication related, pregnancy
Specific lipid storage diseases	Gaucher, Niemann-Pick, Wolman disease
Glycogen	Glycogen storage diseases (multiple enzyme defects), total parenteral nutritionInfant of diabetic mother, Beckwith syndrome
Miscellaneous	α_1-antitrypsin deficiency, Wilson disease, hypervitaminosis A, neonatal iron storage disease

Inflammation	**Causes**
Hepatocyte enlargement (hepatitis)	Viral—acute or chronic; Bacterial—sepsis, abscess, cholangitis; Toxic—drugs
Autoimmune	chronic hepatitis, sarcoidosis, systemic lupus erythematosus, sclerosing cholangitis

B. Infiltration of cells

Primary liver tumors	**Causes**
Benign	Focal nodular hyperplasia, nodular regenerative hyperplasia, hepato-cellular adenoma, infantile hemangioendothelioma, mesenchymal hamartoma, cystic masses (choledochal cyst, hepatic cyst, hematoma, parasitic cyst, amebic abscess, pyogenic abscess)
Malignant	Hepatoblastoma, hepatiocellular carcinoma, angiosarcoma, undifferen-tiated embryonal sarcoma
Secondary or metastatic processes	Lymphoma, leukemia, histiocytosis, neuroblastoma, Wilms' tumor

C. Increased size of vascular space

Intrahepatic obstruction to hepatic vein outflow	Veno-occlusive disease, hepatic vein thrombosis (Budd-Chiari syndrome), hepatic vein web
Suprahepatic	Congestive heart failure, pericardial disease, tamponade
Constrictive pericarditis	
Hematopoietic	Sickle cell anemia, thalassemia

D. Increased size of biliary space

Congenital hepatic fibrosis	Autosomal recessive disorder characterized by diffuse and perilobular fibrosis in broad bands that contain distorted bile duct-like structures and that often compress or incorporate central or sublobular veins. Irregularly shaped islands of liver parenchyma contain normal-appearing hepatocytes. Caroli disease and choledochal cysts have been associated.
Caroli disease	Cystic dilatation of the intrahepatic bile ducts
Extrahepatic obstruction	

E. Idiopathic (? "Benign")

Courvoisier's law states that in the presence of jaundice a palpable gallbladder makes gallstone obstruction of the common bile duct an unlikely cause (because it is likely that the patient will have had gallstones for some time, and these will have rendered the wall of the gallbladder relatively fibrotic and therefore nondistensible).

Choledochal cysts are congenital dilatations of the common bile duct that can cause progressive biliary obstruction and biliary cirrhosis. Approximately 75% of cases appear during childhood.

Jaundice (icterus): Yellow discoloration of sclera, skin, and mucous membranes is assign of hyperbili-rubinemia. Clinically apparent jaundice in children and adults occurs when the serum concentration of bilirubin reaches 2–3 mg/dl (34–51 µmol/L); the neonate may not become icteric until the bilirubin is >5 mg/dl (85 µmol/L). Jaundice may be the earliest and only sign of hepatic dysfunction. Liver disease must be suspected in the infant who appears only mildly jaundiced but has dark urine or acholic (light-colored) stools. Measure the total serum bilirubin concentration.

Bilirubin occurs in plasma in four forms:

1. *Unconjugated bilirubin* tightly bound to bilirubin
2. *Free or unbound bilirubin*, the form responsible for kernicterus, because it can cross cell membranes
3. *Conjugated bilirubin* the only fraction which appears in urine; and

---

Box 17.1: Differential diagnosis of unconjugated hyperbilirubinemia

Increased production of unconjugated bilirubin from heme
  i. Hemolytic disease (hereditary or acquired):
     a. Isoimmune hemolysis (neonatal acute or delayed transfusion reaction; autoimmune)—Rh incompatibility, ABO incompatibility, other blood group incompatibilities
     b. Congenital spherocytosis; hereditary elliptocytosis
     c. Infantile piknocytosis
     d. Erythrocyte enzyme defects
     e. Hemoglobinopathy (sickle cell anemia, thalassemia, other disease); sepsis; microangiopathy [(hemolytic uremic syndrome, hemangioma, mechanical trauma (heart valve)]
  ii. Ineffective erythropoiesis
  iii. Drugs
  iv. Infection
  v. Enclosed hematoma
  vi. Polycythemia [diabetic mother, fetal transfusion (recipient), delayed cord clamping]

Decreased delivery of unconjugated bilirubin (in plasma) to hepatocyte
  i. Right-sided congestive heart failure
  ii. Portacaval shunt

Decreased bilirubin uptake across hepatocyte membrane
  i. Presumed enzyme transporter deficiency
  ii. Competitive inhibition [(breast milk jaundice, Lucey-Driscoll syndrome, drug inhibition (radiocontrast material)];
  iii. Miscellaneous (hypothyroidism, hypoxia, acidosis)

Decreased storage of unconjugated bilirubin in cytosol (decreased Y and Z proteins)
  i. Competitive inhibition
  ii. Fever

Decreased biotransformation (conjugation)
  i. Neonatal jaundice (physiologic)
  ii. Inhibition (drugs)
  iii. Hereditary [(Crigler-Najjar syndrome, Type 1 (complete enzyme deficiency), Type II (partial deficiency)]
  iv. Gilbert disease
  v. Hepatocellular dysfunction

Enterohepatic recirculation
  i. Intestinal obstruction (ileal atresia, Hirschsprung's disease, cystic fibrosis, pyloric stenosis)
  ii. Antibiotic administration

Breast milk jaundice

---

4. *Delta (δ) fraction* bilirubin covalently bound to albumin, which appears in serum when hepatic excretion of conjugated bilirubin is impaired in patients with hepatobiliary disease. The δ fraction permits conjugated bilirubin to persist in circulation and delays resolution of jaundice. The terms *direct* and *indirect* bilirubin is used equivalently with *conjugated* and *unconjugated* bilirubin are not quantitatively correct, because the direct fraction includes both conjugated bilirubin and δ bilirubin. An elevation of serum bile acids is frequently seen in the presence of any form of cholestasis.

Investigations of jaundice must include determination of the accumulation of both unconjugated and conjugated bilirubin. *Unconjugated hyperbilirubinemia* may indicate increased production, hemolysis, reduced hepatic removal or altered metabolism of bilirubin (Box 17.1). *Conjugated hyperbilirubinemia* reflects decreased excretion by damaged hepatic parenchymal cells or disease of the biliary tract, which may be due to obstruction, sepsis, toxins, inflammation, and genetic or metabolic disease (*see* Fig. 17.1 in CD).

Pruritus: Intense generalized itching, often with skin excoriation, can occur in patients with cholestasis (conjugated hyperbilirubinemia). Pruritus is unrelated to the degree of hyperbilirubinemia; deeply jaundiced patients can be asymptomatic. The cause is multifactorial including retained components of bile (the most important cause), as evidenced by the symptomatic relief of pruritus after administration of various therapeutic agents such as bile-acid binding agents (cholestyramine), choleretic agents (ursodeoxycholic acid), opiate antagonists, antihistamines, and antibiotics (rifampin)., and surgical diversion of bile (partial external biliary diversion) has provided relief for medically refractory pruritus.

Spider angiomas: Vascular spiders (telengiectasias), characterized by central pulsating arterioles from which small, wiry venules radiate, may be seen in patients with chronic liver disease; these are usually most prominent over the face and chest. They are presumably due to altered estrogen metabolism in the presence of hepatic dysfunction.

Palmar erythema: Blotchy erythema, most noticeable over the thenar and hypothenar eminences and on the tips of the fingers, is also noted in patients with chronic liver disease. This may be due to vasodilatation and increased blood flow.

Xanthomas: The marked elevations of cholesterol levels (> 500 mg/dl) associated with chronic cholestasis can cause the deposition of lipid in the dermis and subcutaneous tissue. Brown nodules may develop, 1st over the extensor surface of the extremities; rarely, xanthelasma of the eyelids develops.

Portal hypertension: Section 17.9.

Ascites: The onset of ascites in the child in chronic liver disease means that the two prerequisite conditions for ascites are present: Portal hypertension and hepatic insufficiency. Factors favoring the intra-abdominal accumulation of fluid include: Decreased plasma colloid osmotic pressure, increased capillary hydrostatic pressure, increased ascetic colloid osmotic fluid pressure, and decreased ascetic fluid hydrostatic pressure.

Visceral hemorrhage: Gastroesophageal varices are the more clinically significant portosystemic collaterals because of their propensity to rupture and cause life-threatening hemorrhage. Variceal hemorrhage results from increased pressure within the varix (an enlarged tortuous vein), which leads to changes in the diameter of the varix and increased wall tension. When the variceal wall strength is exceeded, physical rupture of the varix results and bleeding occurs.

Encephalopathy: Hepatic encephalopathy can involve any neurologic function, and it can be prominent or present in subtle forms such as deterioration of school performance, depression, or emotional outbursts. It can be recurrent and precipitated by recurrent illness, drugs, bleeding, or electrolyte and acid–base disturbances. The appearance of hepatic encephalopathy depends on the presence of portosystemic shunting, alterations in the blood–brain barrier, and the interactions of toxic metabolites with the central nervous system. Postulated causes include altered ammonia metabolism, synergistic neurotoxins, or false neurotransmitters with plasma amino acid imbalance.

Endocrine abnormalities: Endocrine abnormalities are most common in adults with hepatic disease than in children. They reflect alterations in hepatic synthetic, storage, and metabolic functions including those concerned with hormonal metabolism in the liver. Proteins that bind hormones in plasma are synthesized in the liver, and steroid hormones are conjugated in the liver and excreted in the urine; failure of such functions can have clinical consequences. Endocrine abnormalities can also result from malnutrition or specific deficiencies.

Renal dysfunction: Systemic disease or toxins can affect the liver and kidney simultaneously, or parenchymal liver disease can produce secondary impairment of renal function. Hepatorenal syndrome (HRS) is defined as functional renal failure in patients with end-stage liver disease. In this condition there is intense renal vasoconstriction (mediated by hemodynamic, humoral or neurogenic mechanisms) with coexistent systemic vasodilation. The diagnosis is supported by the findings of oliguria (<1 ml/kg/day), a characteristic pattern of urine electrolyte abnormalities (urine sodium of <10 mEq/L, fractional excretion of sodium of <1%, urine: plasma creatinine ratio <10, and normal urinary sediment), absence of hypovolemia, and exclusion of other kidney pathology. The best treatment of HRS is timely liver transplantation, as complete recovery can be expected.

Pulmonary involvement: Hepatopulmonary syndrome is characterized by the typical triad of hypoxemia, intrapulmonary vascular dilations, and liver disease. There is intrapulmonic right-to-left shunting of blood, which results in systemic desaturation. It should be suspected and investigated in the child with chronic liver disease with history of shortness of breath or exercise intolerance and clinical findings of cyanosis (particularly of the lips and fingers), digital clubbing, and oxygen saturations <96%, particularly in the upright position. Treatment is timely liver transplantation; successful pulmonary resolution follows.

Recurrent cholangitis: Ascending infection of the biliary system is often seen in pediatric cholestatic disease, due most commonly to gram-negative enteric organisms, such as *Escherichia coli*, *Klebsiella*, *Pseudomonas* and *Enterococcus*. Liver transplantation is the effective treatment in the child with chronic cholestatic liver disease, especially when medical treatment is not effective.

Miscellaneous manifestations of liver dysfunction: Nonspecific signs of acute and chronic liver disease include: anorexia, which often affects patients with anicteric hepatitis and with cirrhosis associated with chronic cholestasis: abdominal pain or distension resulting from ascites, spontaneous peritonitis, or visceromegaly; malnutrition and growth failure; and bleeding, which may be due to altered synthesis of coagulation factors (biliary obstruction with vitamin K deficiency or excessive hepatic drainage) or to portal hypertension with hypersplenism. In the presence of hypersplenism, there can be decreased synthesis of specific clotting factors, production of qualitatively abnormal proteins, or alterations in platelet number and function. Altered drug metabolism may prolong the biologic half-life of commonly administered medications.

Boamah L, Balistreri WF. Manifestations of liver disease. In: Kliegman RM, Behrman RE, Jenson HB, Stanton BF (eds). *Nelson Textbook of Pediatrics*. 18th edn. Vol. 2. Philadelphia: Saunders, 2007;1661–8.

Bezerra JA, Balistreri WF, Cholestatic syndromes of infancy and childhood. *Semin Gastrointes Dis* 2001;12:54–65.

17.2 CHOLESTASIS

Neonatal Cholestasis

Neonatal cholestasis is defined as prolonged elevation of serum levels of conjugated bilirubin beyond the first 14 days of life. Jaundice that appears after 2 wk of age, progresses after this time, or does not resolve at this time should be evaluated and a direct bilirubin should be determined. Cholestasis in a newborn may be due to infectious, genetic, metabolic, or undefined abnormalities giving rise either to mechanical obstruction of bile flow or to functional impairment of hepatic excretory function and bile secretion. Neonatal cholestasis may be divided into.

i. *Extrahepatic* (extrahepatic biliary atresia) and
ii. *Intrahepatic* [hepatocyte injury (metabolic disease, viral disease, idiopathic neonatal hepatitis); bile duct injury (intrahepatic bile duct hypoplasia or paucity)].

The two pathogenic mechanisms are virus-induced liver injury or metabolic liver disease. Metabolic liver disease caused by inborn errors of bile acid metabolism is associated with accumulation toxic primitive bile acids and failure to produce normal choleretic and trophic bile acids.

Neonatal hepatitis syndrome (intrahepatic cholestasis): There are various forms: (i) idiopathic neonatal hepatitis which can occur in either a sporadic or a familial form, and the cause is unknown, (ii) infectious hepatitis in a neonate may be due to a specific virus such as herpes simplex, enteroviruses, cytomegalovirus (CMV), or, rarely hepatitis B, (iii) congenital defects in hepatic excretory function in a neonate resulting in intrahepatic cholestasis.

Intrahepatic bile duct paucity: Some syndromes characterized morphologically by intrahepatic cholestasis may be clinically manifested either as neonatal hepatitis or as cholestasis in an older child. Certain cases are associated with bile duct "paucity", which designates an absence or marked reduction in the number of interlobular bile ducts in the portal triads, with normal-sized branches of portal vein and hepatic arteriole.

Alagille syndrome (arteriohepatic dysplasia) has unusual facial characteristics (broad forehead; deep-set, widely-spaced eyes; long, straight nose; and an under-developed mandible. Other clinical features may be present include ocular abnormalities, cardiovascular abnormalities (peripheral pulmonary stenosis, tetralogy of Fallot), vertebral arch defect, tubulointerstitial nephropathy, growth retardation and defective spermatogenesis. The prognosis for prolonged survival is good, but patients are likely to have pruritus, xanthomas with markedly elevated serum cholesterol levels and neurologic complications of vitamin E deficiency if untreated.

Byler disease, a severe form of progressive intrahepatic cholestasis (PFIC type 1), is characterized by unique structural abnormalities in the bile canalicular membrane. Affected patients present with failure to thrive, steatorrhea, pruritus, rickets, and low γ-glutamyl transpeptidase levels. Cirrhosis gradually develops. The major clinical differentiation from Alagille syndrome is the absence of bile duct paucity and extrahepatic features.

Aagenaes syndrome is a form of idiopathic familial intrahepatic cholestasis associated with lymphedema of the lower extremities. Affected patients usually present with episodic cholestasis with elevation of serum aminotransferases, alkaline phosphatase, and bile acids. Between the episodes the patients are usually asymptomatic and the biochemical indices improve. The locus for Aagenaes syndrome is mapped to a 6.6-cM interval on chromosome 15q.

Zellweger (cerebrohepatorenal) syndrome is a rare autosomal recessive genetic disorder marked by progressive degeneration of the liver and kidneys. The incidence is estimated to be 1/100,000 births. Affected infants have severe generalized hypotonia and markedly impaired neurologic function with psychomotor retardation. Patients have an abnormal head shape and unusual facies, hepatomegaly, renal cortical cysts, stippled calcifications of the patellas and greater trochanter, and ocular abnormalities. Hepatic cells on ultrastructural examination show an absence of peroxisomes. This is due to the inherited absence of peroxisomes in all tissues. The disease is usually fatal in 6–12 mo.

Table 17.2: Differential diagnosis of biliary atresia and idiopathic neonatal hepatitis

Biliary atresia	*Idiopathic neonatal hepatitis*
Unlikely to recur within the same family	Familial incidence of ~20%
A few infants with fetal onset have an increased incidence of other abnormalities, such as the polysplenia syndrome with abdominal heterotaxia, malrotation, levocardia, and intra-abdominal vascular anomalies	More common in premature or small for gestational age infants
Persistently acholic stools	Transient bile excretion in severe cases only
Consistently pigmented stools and bile-stained fluid on duodenal intubation excludes biliary atresia	
Abnormal size or consistency of liver in patients with extrahepatic biliary atresia	Abnormal size or consistency of liver is less common
USG may detect abdominal polysplenia and vascular malformations; gallbladder is either not recognized or a micro-gallbladder; triangular cord (TC) sign, which represents a cone-shaped fibrotic mass cranial to the bifurcation of the portal vein	
*Hepatic uptake of the agent is normal, but excretion into the intestine is absent	*Hepatic uptake may be impaired in neonatal hepatitis, excretion into the bowel will eventually occur
Percutaneous liver biopsy: Bile ductular proliferation, the presence of bile plugs, and portal or perilobular edema and fibrosis, with the basic hepatic lobular architecture intact	Percutaneous liver biopsy: Severe, diffuse hepatocellular disease, with distortion of lobular architecture, marked infiltration with inflammatory cells, and focal hepatocellular necrosis; the bile ductules show little alteration

Hepatobiliary scintigraphy with technetium-labeled iminodiacetic acid derivatives

Neonatal iron storage disease (NISD) (*see* Section 17.3, page 485)

Inborn errors of bile acid biosynthesis: An inborn errors of bile acid biosynthesis is a cause of acute and chronic liver disease. Early recognition allows institution of bile acid replacement, which reverses the hepatic injury.

Biliary Atresia

In biliary atresia there is progressive obliterative cholangiopathy. It is of two types:
  i. Distal segmental bile duct obliteration with patent extrahepatic ducts up to the porta hepatis, a surgically correctable lesion, but it is uncommon;
  ii. Obliteration of the entire extrahepatic biliary tree at or above the porta hepatis, accounting for ~85% of the cases, presents a much more difficult problem in surgical management.

85–90% patients with biliary atresia have a postnatal onset; embryonic fetal onset presents at birth and is associated with other congenital anomalies within the polysplenia spectrum (biliary atresia splenic malformation [SASM]). Differential diagnosis of biliary atresia and idiopathic neonatal hepatitis is mentioned in Table 17.2.

Incidence: Biliary atresia has been detected in 1/10,000–15,000, idiopathic neonatal hepatitis in 1/5,000–10,000, and intrahepatic bile duct paucity in about 1/50,000–75,000 live births.

Management of patients with suspected biliary atresia: Exploratory laparotomy and direct cholangiography should be performed in all patients suspected of having biliary atresia to determine the presence and the site of obstruction. Direct drainage can be accomplished in a few patients with a correctable lesion. For patients in whom no correctable lesion is found, the hepatoportoenterostomy (Kasai) procedure should be performed. The short-term benefit of hepatoportoenterostomy is decompression and damage sufficient to forestall the onset of cirrhosis and sustain growth until a successful liver transplantation can be done (Section 17.10).

Management of chronic cholestasis: The various forms of neonatal cholestasis, affected patients are at increased risk for chronic complications. These reflect various degrees of residual hepatic functional capacity and are due directly or indirectly to diminished bile flow. Treatment of such patients (Table 17.3) is empirical, and is guided by careful monitoring. No therapy is known to be effective in halting the progression of cholestasis or in preventing further hepatocellular damage and cirrhosis.

Prognosis: In sporadic cases with idiopathic neonatal hepatitis, 60–70% recovers with no evidence of hepatic structural or functional impairment; 5–10% has persistent fibrosis or inflammation and a smaller percentage have more severe disease, such as cirrhosis. Death of infants occurs early, owing to hemorrhage

Table 17.3: Suggested medical management of patients with persistent cholestasis

Clinical Impairment	Management
Malnutrition resulting from malabsorption of dietary long-chain triglycerides	Replace with dietary formula or supplements containing medium-chain triglycerides
Vitamin A deficiency (night blindness, thick skin)*	Replace with 10,000–15,000 IU/day as Aquasol A
Vitamin E deficiency (neuromuscular degeneration)*	Replace with 50–400 IU/day as oral α-tocopherol
Vitamin D deficiency (metabolic bone disease)*	Replace with 5,000–8,000 IU/day of D$_2$ or 3–5 µg/kg/day of 25-hydroxycholecalciferol
Vitamin K deficiency (hypoprothrombinemia)*	Replace with 2.5–5.0 mg every other day as water soluble derivative of menadione
Micronutrient deficiency	Calcium phosphate or zinc supplementation
Deficiency of water soluble vitamins	Supplement with twice the recommended daily allowance
Retention of biliary constituents such as cholesterol (itch or xanthomas)	Administer choleretic bile acids and ursodeoxycholic acid, 15–20 mg/kg/day
Progressive liver disease; portal hypertension (variceal bleeding, ascites, hypersplenism)	Interim management (control bleeding, salt restriction, spironolactone
End-stage liver disease (liver failure)	Transplantation

*Fat-soluble vitamin malabsorption.

or sepsis. In infants with idiopathic neonatal hepatitis of the familial variety only 20–30% recover; 10–15% acquires chronic liver disease with cirrhosis. Liver transplantation may be required.

Cholestasis in the Older Child

Most cases of cholestasis with onset after the neonatal period are due to acute viral hepatitis or hepatotoxic drugs. Many of the conditions causing neonatal cholestasis can also cause chronic cholestasis in older patients. Adolescents with conjugated hyperbilirubinemia should be evaluated for acute and chronic hepatitis, α$_1$-antitrypsin deficiency, Wilson disease, liver disease associated with inflammatory bowel disease, autoimmune hepatitis, syndromes of intrahepatic cholestasis, and obstruction caused by cholelithiasis, abdominal tumors, enlarged lymph nodes, or hepatic inflammation resulting from drug ingestion. Management of cholestasis in the older child is similar to that proposed for neonatal cholestasis (Table 17.3).

A-Kader HH, Balistreri WF. Cholestasis. In: Kliegman RM, Behrman RE, Jenson HB, Stanton BF (eds). *Nelson Textbook of Pediatrics*. 18th edn. Vol. 2. Philadelphia: Saunders, 2007;1668–75.

17.3 METABOLIC DISEASES OF THE LIVER

Inherited deficient conjugation of bilirubin (familial nonhemolytic unconjugated hyperbilirubinemia): Bilirubin is the metabolic end product of heme. Before excretion into bile, it is 1st glucuronidated by the enzyme bilirubin uridinediphosphoglucuronate glucuronosyltransferase (UDPGT). UDPGT activity is deficient or altered in three genetically and functionally distinct disorders (Crigler-Najjar syndromes type I and II and Gilbert syndrome), producing congenital nonobstructive, nonhemolytic, unconjugated hyperbilirubinemia.

Inherited conjugated hyperbilirubinemia: Inherited conjugated hyperbilirubinemia are autosomal recessive disorders characterized by mild jaundice. The transfer of bilirubin and other organic anions from liver to bile is defective. Chronic mild conjugated hyperbilirubinemia is usually detected during adolescence or early adulthood but can occur as early as the 2nd yr of life. The results of routine liver function tests are normal. Jaundice can be exacerbated by infection, pregnancy, oral contraceptives, alcohol consumption and surgery. There is no morbidity and the life expectancy is normal.

Dubin-Johnson syndrome: Dubin-Johnson syndrome is an autosomal recessive inherited defect in hepatocyte secretion of bilirubin glucuronide. Bile acid excretion and serum bile acid levels are normal. Total urinary coproporphyrin excretion is normal in quantity but coproporphyrin I excretion increases to ~ 80% with a concomitant decrease in coproporphyrin III excretion. Normally, coproporphyrin III is >75% of the total. Cholangiography fails to visualize the biliary tract and roentgenography of the gallbladder is also abnormal. The liver cells contain black pigment similar to melanin.

Rotor syndrome: These patients have an additional deficiency in organic anion uptake. Total urinary coproporphyrin excretion is elevated, with a relative increase in the amount of the coproporphyrin I isomer. The gallbladder is normal by roentgenography and the liver cells contain no black pigment. In both Dubin-

Johnson syndrome and Rotor syndromes, sulfo-bromphthalein excretion is also abnormal.

Wilson Disease

Wilson disease (hepatolenticular degeneration) is an autosomal recessive disorder. The incidence is 1/500,000 to 1/100,000 births. The abnormal gene for Wilson disease is localized to long arm of chromosome 13(13q14.3). The Wilson disease gene encodes a copper transporting P-type ATPase, ATP7B. ATP7B is mainly but not exclusively expressed in hepatocytes and is thought to be critical for biliary copper excretion and for incorporation into ceruloplasmin. Absence or malfunction of ATP7B results in decreased biliary copper excretion and diffuse accumulation of copper in the cytosol of hepatocytes. When liver cells are overloaded, copper is redistributed to other tissues including the brain and kidneys, to which it is toxic, primarily as a potent inhibitor of enzymatic processes. Ionic copper inhibits pyruvate oxidase in brain and ATPase in membranes leading to decreased ATP-phosphocreatine and potassium content of tissue.

Clinical manifestations: Wilson disease is characterized by degenerative changes in the brain, liver disease, and Kayser-Fleischer rings in the cornea. Forms of Wilsonian hepatic disease include asymptomatic hepatomegaly (with or without splenomegaly), subacute or chronic hepatitis, and fulminant hepatic failure. Neurological disorders can develop insidiously or precipitously, with intention tremor, dysarthria, dystonia, lack of motor coordination, deterioration in school performance, or behavioral changes. Kayser-Fleischer rings may be absent in young patients with liver disease but are always present in patients with neurologic symptoms. Coombs' negative hemolytic anemia may be an initial manifestation, possibly related to the release of large amounts of copper from damaged hepatocytes. During hemolytic episodes, urinary copper excretion and serum copper levels are markedly raised. Manifestations of renal Fanconi syndrome and progressive renal failure with alterations in tubular transport of amino acids, glucose, and uric acid may be present. Unusual manifestations include arthritis, cardiomyopathy, and endocrinopathies (hypoparathyroidism).

Diagnosis: Serum ceruloplasmin level is decreased. Serum copper level may be elevated and urinary copper excretion (usually <40 µg/day) is increased to >100 µg/day and often up to 1,000 µg or more per day. Liver biopsy for measurement of the hepatic copper content (normal <10 µg/g dry weight), which is elevated (>250 µg/g dry weight). Kayser-Fleischer rings in the cornea are demonstrated in a slit-lamp examination. Family members of patients with proven cases should be screened for determination of the serum ceruloplasmin level and urinary copper excretion to exclude Wilson disease.

Treatment: Restriction in copper intake to <1 mg/day is important in the management of Wilson disease. Foods such as liver, shellfish, nuts, and chocolate should be avoided. If the copper content of the drinking water exceeds 0.1 mg/L, it may be necessary to demineralize. Oral administration of D-penicillamine (chelation therapy) in a dose of 1 g/day in two doses before meals in adults and 20 mg/kg/day for pediatric patients, increases urinary copper excretion resulting to normal urinary copper level, marked improvement of hepatic and neurologic function and the disappearance of Kayser-Fleischer rings. Additional amount of vitamin B_6 should be added because penicillamine is an antimetabolite of vitamin B_6. For those patients who are unable to tolerate penicillamine, triethylene tetramine dihydrochloride at a dose of 0.5–2 g/day for adults and 20 mg/kg/day for children should be used.

Prognosis: Untreated patients die of hepatic, neurologic, renal or hematologic complications. Liver transplantation should be considered in patients with fulminant hepatic disease, decompensated cirrhosis, or progressive neurologic disease. In asymptomatic siblings of affected parents, early institution of chelation therapy can prevent expression of the disease.

Indian childhood cirrhosis: Indian childhood cirrhosis (ICC) occurs predominantly in rural areas in India and presents with jaundice, pruritus, lethargy, and hepatosplenomegaly. Histologically it is characterized by hepatocyte necrosis, Mallory bodies, intralobular fibrosis, and inflammation. There is an increased hepatic copper content, usually > 700 µg/g dry weight. ICC has been linked to excess dietary ingestion of copper primarily through the use of contaminated utensils used to feed babies animal milk and a genetic susceptibility to copper toxicosis. Administration of penicillamine early in the course of disease (20 mg/kg/day), increases urinary copper excretion and decreases the mortality to half.

Neonatal iron storage disease (NISD): NISD, also known as neonatal hemochromatosis, is a rare form of fulminant liver disease that presents in 1st few days of life. Clinically, NISD is a rapidly fatal, progressive illness characterized by hepatomegaly, hypoglycemia, hypoprothrombinemia, hypoalbuminemia, hyperferritinemia, and hyperbilirubinemia. The coagulopathy is refractory to therapy with vitamin K. The diagnosis can be confirmed through documentation of extrahepatic hemosiderosis (biopsy material of buccal mucosal glands is laden with iron) or MRI determination of iron storage in organs such as pancreas. Some patients with NISD can be treated with iron chelating agent (deferoxamine) combined with aggressive antioxidant therapy, if initiated very early. Liver transplantation should also be an early consideration.

α₁-antitrypsin deficiency: A small percentage of individuals homozygous for deficiency of the major serum protease inhibitor α_1-antitrypsin manifest neonatal cholestasis or later onset childhood cirrhosis. α_1-antitrypsin, a protease inhibitor synthesized by the liver, protects lung alveolar tissues from destruction by neutrophil elastase. Liver transplantation has been curative.

Ala A, Walker AP, Ashkan K, et al. Wilson's disease. *Lancet* 2007;369:397–408.

Carey RG, Balistreri WF. Metabolic diseases of the liver. In: Kliegman RM, Behrman RE, Jenson HB, Stanton BF (eds). *Nelson Textbook of Pediatrics.* 18th edn. Vol. 2. Philadelphia: Saunders, 2007;1675–80.

Grabhon E, Richter A, Burdelski M, et al. Neonatal hemochromatosis: Long term experience with favorable outcome. *Pediatrics* 2006;118:2060–5.

Tanner MS. Role of copper in Indian childhood cirrhosis. *Am J Clin Nutr* 1998;67:S1074–81.

17.4 VIRAL HEPATITIS

Viral hepatitis is a worldwide major health problem. This disorder is caused by 5 pathogenic hepatotropic viuses: hepatitis A, B, C, D, and E viruses. Many other viruses can cause hepatitis, usually as one component of a multisystem disease; these include herpes simplex virus (HSV), cytomegalovirus (CMV), Epstein-Barr virus (EBV), varicella-zoster virus, HIV, rubella, adenoviruses, enteroviruses, parvovirus B19, and arboviruses. Hepatitis G virus (GBV) and transfusion transmissible virus (TTV) often infect the liver as a co-infection with another hepatotropic virus, and may produce acute or chronic viremia but rarely produce hepatocellular injury on their own.

Hepatitis A

Hepatitis A virus (HAV) is the most prevalent of the five viruses in India and worldwide. HAV is an RNA virus, a member of the picornavirus family. This virus is also responsible for most forms of acute and benign hepatitis. The mean incubation period is 30 days. HAV is highly contagious. Transmission of HAV is by person-to-person contact. Spread is predominantly by the fecal-oral route; percutaneous or sexual transmission occurs rarely. HAV infection during pregnancy or at the time of delivery does not appear to result in increased complications of pregnancy or increased clinical disease in the newborn.

Clinical manifestations: It is characteristically an acute febrile illness with an abrupt onset of anorexia, nausea, malaise, vomiting, and jaundice (*see* Fig. 17.2 in CD). The typical duration of illness is 7–14 days. Other organ systems can be affected during acute HAV infection include regional lymph nodes and spleen may be enlarged; bone marrow may be moderately hypoplastic and aplastic anemia may occur; ulceration of the gastrointestinal tract; acute pancreatitis and myocarditis; nephritis, arthritis, vasculitis, and cryoglobulinemia can result from circulating immune complexes. Although most patients achieve full recovery; two distinct complications: (i) acute liver failure (LF) and (ii) prolonged cholestatic syndrome rarely occur.

Diagnosis: The virus is excreted in stools from 2 wk before to 1 wk after the onset of illness. Acute HAV infection is diagnosed by detecting antibodies to HAV, specifically, anti-HAV [immunoglobulin (Ig) M] by radioimmunoassay. Rises in ALT, AST, bilirubin, ALP, 5' nucleotidase, and γ-glutamyl transpeptidase (GTT) are found but do not help to differentiate the cause of hepatitis.

Treatment: There is no specific treatment for hepatitis A. Supportive treatment consists of intravenous hydration, and antipruritic agents and fat soluble vitamins for the prolonged cholestatic form of disease. Serial monitoring for signs of acute liver failure and early referral to a transplantation center can be life saving.

Prevention: Patients infected with HAV are contagious for 2 wk before about 7 days after the onset of jaundice and should be excluded from school, child care, or work during this period. Careful hand washing is necessary, particularly after changing and before preparing or serving food. In hospital settings, contact and standard precautions are recommended for 1 wk after onset of symptoms. Vaccine is administered intramuscularly in two doses schedule, with a 2nd dose given 6–12 months after the first dose in children >1 yr of age. Indications for intramuscular administration of immunoglobulin (Ig) include pre-exposure and post-exposure prophylaxis.

Prognosis: The prognosis is excellent, with no long-term sequelae. The only feared complication is ALF.

Hepatitis B

HBV has a world wide spread, with an estimated 400 million persons chronically infected. HBV is a member of the Hepadinaviridae family, which includes a hepatotropic group of DNA viruses. Four genes have been identified: S (surface), C (core), X, and P (polymer) genes. The inner portion of the virion contains hepatitis B core antigen (HBcAg), the nucleocapsid that encodes the viral DNA, and a nonstructural antigen called hepatitis Be antigen (HbeAg), a nonparticulate soluble antigen derived from HBcAg by proteolytic self-cleavage. HBeAg serves as a marker of active viral replication and usually correlates with HBV DNA levels. Replication of HBV occurs predominantly in the liver but also occurs in the lymphocytes, spleen, kidneys, and the pancreas. The incubation period ranges from 45 to 160 days, with a mean of about 120 days. HBV is present in higher concentrations in blood, serum, and serous exudates and in moderate concentrations in saliva, vaginal fluid, and semen; efficient transmission occurs through blood exposure and sexual contact. Risk factors for HBV infection in children and adolescents include intravenous acquisition by drugs or blood products, acupuncture or tattoos, sexual contact, institutional care, and intimates contact with carriers. The risk of transmission is greatest if the mother is also HBeAg positive.

HBsAg is inconsistently recovered in human milk of infected mothers. Breast-feeding of nonimmunized infants by infected mothers does not confer a greater risk of hepatitis than does formula feeding.

HBV has eight genotypes (A–H). A is pandemic, B and C are prevalent in Asia, D is seen in Southern Europe, E in Africa, F in the United States, G in the United States and France, and H in Central America.

Clinical manifestations: In many asymptomatic cases serum markers are present. The usual acute asymptomatic episode is similar to HAV and HCV infections but may be more severe and is more likely to include involvement of skin and joints and extrahepatic conditions. The risk of developing chronic HBV infection defined as being positive for HBsAg for > 6 mo, is inversely related to age of acquisition and is associated with complications. The risk of chronic infection is 90% in children < 1 yr; the risk is 30% for those 1–5 yr and 2% for adults. Immune-mediated mechanisms are also involved in the extrahepatic conditions that can be associated with HBV infections. Circulating immune complexes containing HBsAg can occur in patients who develop associated polyarteritis nodosa, membranous or membranoproliferative glomerulonephritis, poly-myalgia rheumatica, leukocytoclastic vasculitis, and Guillain-Barré syndrome. On physical examination, symptomatic infection results in icteric skin and mucous membranes. The liver is usually enlarged and tender to palpation and percussion. Splenomegaly and lymphadenopathy are common. Clinical signs of altered sensorium and hyper-reflexivity should be carefully looked for, as they mark the onset of encephalopathy and ALF.

Diagnosis: Routine screening for HBV infection requires assay of at least serologic markers (HBsAg, anti-HBc, anti-HBs). HBsAg is the 1st serologic marker of infection to appear and is found in almost all infected persons; its rise closely coincides with the onset of symptoms. The 1st biochemical evidence of HBV infection is elevation of ALT levels, which begin to rise just before development of lethargy, anorexia, and malaise, which occurs about 6–7 wk after exposure. The serologic profile of HBV infection differs depending on whether the disease is acute or chronic.

Complications: ALF occurs more frequently with HBV than with the other hepatotropic viruses. The risk of ALF is further increased when there is co-infection or super-infection with HDV. HBV infection can also result in chronic hepatitis, which can lead to cirrhosis, end-stage liver disease complications, and primary hepatocellular carcinoma. Membranous glomerulo-nephritis with deposition of complement and HBeAg in glomerular capillaries is a rare complication of HBV infection.

Treatment: The treatment of acute infection is supportive. Interferon-α-2b (IFN- α2b) and lamivudine [children and adolescents: 12 mg/kg/day PO divided q 12 hr (maximum dose: 150 mg); adults: 300 mg/day PO divided q 12 hr] are for the treatment of chronic hepatitis B in adults >18 yr of age with compensated liver disease and HBV replication. IFN-α2b has also been used in children, with long-term eradication rates similar to the 25% rate reported in adults. The goal of treatment is cessation of active replication as manifested by HBeAg seroconversion; HBsAg seroconversion occurs in a minority of untreated patients.

Prevention: Preventive measures include hepatitis B vaccine and hepatitis B immunoglobulin, and educational advice. Two recombinant DNA vaccines are available and highly immunogenic in children. The most reported side effects of vaccination are pain at the injection site and fever. Patients should be advised about the perinatal and intimate contact risk of transmission of HBV. HBV is not spread by breast-feeding, kissing, hugging, or sharing water or utensils. Children with HBV should not be excluded from school, play, child care, or work, unless they are prone to biting. Hepatitis B immunoglobulin (HBIg) is indicated only for specific postexposure circumstances and provides only temporary protection (3–6 mo).

Infants born to HBsAg-positive women should receive HIB vaccine at birth, 6 wk, and 14 wk of age (at birth, 1–2 mo, and 6 mo of age in many countries other than India). The first dose is accompanied by administration of 0.5 ml of HBIg (hepatitis B immunoglobulin) as soon after delivery as possible, because the effectiveness decreases rapidly with increased time after birth. Post-vaccination testing for HBsAg and anti-HBs should be at 9–15 months. If the result is positive for anti-HBs, the child is immune to HBV. If the result is positive for HBsAg only, the parent should be counseled and the child should be evaluated later. If the result is negative for both HBsAg and anti-HBs, a second complete hepatitis B vaccine series should be administered, followed by testing for anti-HBs to determine if subsequent doses are needed. Infants born to HBsAg-negative women should receive the vaccine at 0–2 mo, 1–4 mo, and at 6–18 mo of age. Routine postvaccination testing of immunized infants born to HBsAg-negative women or with anti-HBs is not recommended. The three-dose series can be completed even if the interval between doses is longer than recommended.

Prognosis: In general, the outcome after HBV infection is favorable, despite the risk of ALF after acute HBV infection, and the risk of developing chronic infection and liver cirrhosis and hepatocellular carcinoma. HBV infection and its complications are effectively controlled with vaccination.

Hepatitis C

HCV is the cause of most cases previously known as "transfusion-related non-A, non-B hepatitis." HCV is a single stranded RNA virus, classified as a separate genus within the Flaviviridae family, with marked genetic heterogeneity. It has six major genotypes and genotype 1b is the least responsive to the available medications. The mean incubation period is 7–9 wk. The risk factors of HCV transmission are blood transfusion, multiple sexual partners, imprisonment and occupational exposure; ~10% of new infections have no known transmission source. In children, perinatal transmission is the most prevalent mode of transmission. Vertical transmission occurs in up to 5% of infants born to viremic mothers, may increase to 20%, when there is high viremia titers (HCV RNA positive) in the mother.

Clinical manifestations: Acute HCV infection tends to be mild and insidious in onset. Acute liver failure rarely occurs. Chronic infection is common leading to chronic hepatitis. About 25% of infected patients ultimately progress to cirrhosis, liver failure, and occasionally primary hepatocellular carcinoma (HCC) within 20–30 yr of the acute infection. Chronic HCV infection can be associated with small vessel vasculitis and is a common cause of essential mixed cryoglobulinemia. Other extrahepatic manifestations predominantly seen in adults include cutaneous vasculitis, peripheral neuropathy, cerebritis, membranoproliferative glomerulonephritis and nephrotic syndrome. Antibodies to smooth muscle, antinuclear antibodies, and low thyroid levels may also be present.

Diagnosis: The diagnosis of HCV infection is made by serologic test to detect anti-HCV or by PCR to detect HCV–RNA in serum and tissue samples.

Complications: The risk of acute liver failure (ALF) due to HCV is low, but the risk of chronic hepatitis is the highest of all the hepatotropic viruses.

Treatment: IFN-α2b and ribavirin are used in children >3 yr of age with HCV hepatitis. Higher response is in children <12 yr, genotypes 2 and 3 and poor response in genotype 1b virus..

Prevention: No vaccine is available to prevent HCV. Vaccinating the affected patient against HAV and HBV will prevent superinfection with these viruses and the increased risk of developing severe liver failure.

Prognosis: Viral titers should be checked yearly to document spontaneous remission. Most patients develop chronic hepatitis.

Hepatitis D

HDV, the smallest known animal virus (36 nm diameter virus), is considered defective because it cannot produce infection without a concurrent HBV infection. Liver pathology in HDV hepatitis has no distinguishing features except that damage is usually quite severe. The mean incubation period is 2–4 mo. Transmission usually occurs by intrafamilial or intimate contact in areas of high prevalence, which are primarily developing countries. In areas of low prevalence, the percutaneous route is far more common.

Clinical manifestations: The symptoms of hepatitis D infection are similar to but usually more severe than those of the other hepatotropic viruses. In co-infection, acute hepatitis, which is much more severe than for HBV alone, is common but the risk of developing chronic hepatitis is low. In superinfection, acute illness is rare and chronic hepatitis is common. The risk of ALF is highest in superinfection. Hepatitis D should be considered in any child who experiences acute liver failure.

Diagnosis: The diagnosis is made by detecting IgM antibody to HDV; the antibodies to HDV develop ~2–4 wk after co-infection and ~10 wk after a super-infection.

Complications: HDV must be considered in all cases of ALF. Co-infection with HBV can also result in a more severe chronic disease.

Treatment: The treatment is based on supportive measures once an infection is identified. The treatment is mostly based on controlling and treating HBV infection, without which HDV can not induce hepatitis.

Prevention: There is no vaccine for hepatitis D. Because HDV replication cannot occur without hepatitis B co-infection, immunization against HBV also prevents HDV infection.

Hepatitis E

HEV has not been isolated but has been cloned using molecular techniques. Hepatitis E is the epidemic form of what was formally called non-A, non-B hepatitis. The mean incubation period is 40 days. Transmission occurs by fecal-oral route. The pathologic findings are similar to those of the other hepatitis viruses. The highest prevalence of HEV infection has been reported in the Indian subcontinent, the Middle East, Southeast Asia, and Mexico, especially in areas with poor sanitation.

Clinical manifestations: The clinical illness associated with HEV infection is similar to HAV but is more severe. Chronic illness does not occur. HEV tends to affect older patients with a peak age between 15 and 34 yr. HEV is a major pathogen in pregnant women, in whom it causes ALF with a high fatality incidence.

Complication: HEV is associated with a high risk of death in pregnant women.

Diagnosis: IgM antibody to viral antigen can be detected by recombinant DNA technology after 1 week of illness. Viral RNA can be detected in serum and stool by PCR.

Treatment and prevention: Treatment is supportive. A recombinant hepatitis E vaccine is highly effective in adults.

Aggarwal R, Ranjan P. Preventing and treating hepatitis B infection. *Br Med J* 2004;329:1080–6.

Beeching NJ. Hepatitis B infection. *Br Med J* 2004;329:1059–60.

Elisofon SA, Jonas MM. Hepatitis B and C in children: Current treatment and future strategies. *Clin Liver Dis* 2006; 10:133–48.

Flamm SL. Chronic hepatitis C virus infection. N Engl J Med 2002;347:975–82.

Kelly D, Skidmore S. Hepatitis C-Z: Recent advances. *Arch Dis Child* 2002;86:339–43.

Temte JL. Should all children be immunized against hepatitis A? *Br Med J* 2006;332:715–8.

Yang HI, Lu SN, Liaw YF, et al. Hepatitis Be antigen and the risk of hepatocellular carcinoma. *N Engl J Med* 2002;347:168–74.

Yazigi N, Balistreri WF. Viral hepatitis. In: Kliegman RM, Behrman RE, Jenson HB, Stanton BF (eds). *Nelson Textbook of Pediatrics.* 18th edn. Vol. 2. Philadelphia: Saunders, 2007;1680–90.

17.5 LIVER ABSCESS

Clinical features and etiology: Liver abscesses are usually classified as pyogenic or amoebic. Pyogenic liver abscess may occur in infancy in association with sepsis or may follow umbilical vein cannulation. Beyond infancy, pyogenic abscesses are seen in immunocompromised patients like AIDS, leukemia, and chronic granulomatous diseases. Bacteria and other organisms may enter the liver through various routes like the biliary tract, portal vein, or the hepatic artery. Pyogenic hepatic abscess may arise from the portal circulation in patients with intra-abdominal sepsis like appendicitis or may follow generalized sepsis. Cholangitis following biliary tract obstructions like choledochal cysts or choledocholithiasis may also cause liver abscesses. *Staphylococcus aureus, Escherichia coli, Salmonella* or anaerobes are the common offenders in pyogenic liver abscess.

Amoebic liver abscess is a serious complication of disseminated infection by *Entamoeba histolytica*. It is believed to be a complication of intestinal amoebiasis with the trophozoites traveling to the liver via the portal vein. Males are more commonly affected. Fever is the hallmark of liver abscess in children. It is associated with severe abdominal pain, distention and an enlarged and tender liver. These symptoms are much more common in amoebic liver abscess, whereas pyogenic liver abscess may be present in the setting of sepsis and is often missed due to low index of suspicion.

Laboratory and radiological investigations: Laboratory findings include mild leucocytosis, mild anemia with almost normal liver function tests. Radiological diagnosis is best established by using either ultrasonography or CT scan. Ultrasound demonstrates thin walled lesions that are hypoechoic and may contain air. CT scan demonstrates low-density lesions, with well-defined fluid collection and an enhancing rim with or without internal septations. The diagnosis of an amoebic liver abscess can be confirmed by appropriate serologic testing for entamoeba (indirect hemagglutination or agar-gel immunodiffusion).

Treatment: Pyogenic liver abscess are best treated with systemic antibiotics and closed continuous percutaneous drainage. Surgical drainage may be required in case of failed percutaneous drainage or a technically non-feasible percutaneous drainage. Amoebic liver abscess are usually treated with oral metronidazole. Large abscesses may require multiple needle aspirations. Surgical therapy is not required except in cases of complications like secondary infection or rupture.

Xanthakos SA, Balistreri WF. Liver abscess. In: Kliegman RM, Behrman RE, Jenson HB, Stanton BF (eds). *Nelson Textbook of Pediatrics.* 18th edn. Vol. 2. Philadelphia: Saunders, 2007; 1690–2.

17.6 AUTOIMMUNE AND CHRONIC HEPATITIS

Autoimmune hepatitis is a chronic hepatic inflammatory process manifested by elevated serum aminotransaminase concentrations and liver-associated serum autoantibodies and hypergammaglobulinemia. The inflammatory process can affect both hepatocytes and bile duct epithelium. The chronic stage is determined either by duration of liver disease (more than 3–6 months) or by evidence of either severe liver disease or physical stigmata of chronic disease (clubbing, spider telangiectasia, hepatosplenomegaly).

Chronic hepatitis can be caused by persistent viral infection (Section 17.4), drugs (Section 17.7), metabolic diseases (Section 17.3) or unknown factors. Drugs commonly used in children that can cause chronic liver injury include isoniazid, methyldopa, pemoline, nitrofurantoin, dantrolene, minocycline, pemoline, and the sulphonamides. In most cases, the cause of chronic hepatitis is unknown; in many, an autoimmune mechanism is suggested by the finding of serum antinuclear and anti-smooth muscle antibodies and by multisystem involvement (arthropathy, thyroiditis, rashes, and Coombs' positive hemolytic anemia).

Autoimmune hepatitis may be the result of an imbalance between CD4 and CD8 T-lymphocyte activity. Genetic predisposition may play an important role in the development of autoimmune hepatitis, although viral infection or drug exposure may initiate the process.

Clinical manifestations: The clinical features and course of autoimmune hepatitis are extremely variable. In 25–30% of patients, particularly in children, the illness mimics acute viral hepatitis. In most, the onset is insidious. Patients can be asymptomatic or have fatigue, malaise, behavioral changes, anorexia, and amenorrhea, sometimes for many months before jaundice or stigmata of chronic liver disease are recognized. Some patients' initial clinical features reflect cirrhosis. Extrahepatic manifestations include arthritis, vasculitis, nephritis, thyroiditis, Coombs' positive anemia, and rash. There is usually mild to moderate jaundice. Spider telangiectasias and palmar erythema may be present. The liver is often tender and slightly enlarged but may not be felt in patients with cirrhosis. The spleen is enlarged. Edema and ascites may be present in advance cases. Evidence of involvement of other organ systems may be found.

Diagnosis: Important positive features include female gender, primary elevation in transaminases and not ALP, elevated gammaglobulin levels, the presence of autoantibodies (most commonly antinuclear, smooth muscle or liver-kidney microsomes) and characteristic histologic findings. Liver biopsy in autoimmune hepatitis includes fibrous expansion of the portal tracts with moderate portal lymphocytic infiltrates rich in plasma cells and extensive interface hepatitis. Important negative features include the absence of viral markers (hepatitis B, C, D) of infection, absence of a history of drug or blood product exposure, and negligible alcohol consumption. All other conditions

Table 17.4: Drug induced liver disease	
Disease/pathologic finding	*Drug*
Centrilobular necrosis of hepatocytes	Acetaminophen, halothane
Microvesicular steatosis	Tetracycline
Macrovesicular steatosis	Ethanol
Cholestatic hepatitis	Erythromycin estolate, chlorpromazine
Cholestasis without inflammation	Estrogens, anabolic steroids
Acute hepatitis	Isoniazid
Chronic hepatitis	Methyldopa
General hypersensitivity	Sulphonamide, phenytoin
Fibrosis	Methotrexate
Veno-occlusive disease	Irradiation plus busulfan, cyclophosphamide
Portal and hepatic vein thrombosis	Estrogens, androgens
Biliary sludge	Ceftriaxone
Hepatic adenoma or hepatocellular carcinoma	Oral contraceptives, anabolic steroids

that might lead to chronic hepatitis should be excluded.

Treatment: Prednisolone with or without azathioprine or 6-mercaptopurine, improves the clinical, biochemical, and histologic features in most patients with autoimmune hepatitis and prolongs survival in most patients with severe disease. The choleretic agent ursodeoxycholic acid may be particularly useful in patients with biliary features of their disease.

Prognosis: The initial response to therapy in autoimmune hepatitis is generally prompt, with a >75% rate of remission. Transaminases and bilirubin fall to near-normal levels often in the 1st 1–3 mo. Corticosteroid therapy in fulminant autoimmune disease may be useful, although it should be administered with caution, given the predisposition of these patients to systemic bacterial and fungal infection. Orthotopic liver transplantation has been successful in patients with end-stage liver disease associated with autoimmune hepatitis.

Krawitt EL. Autoimmune hepatitis. *N Engl J Med* 2006;354: 54–66.

Shneider BL, Suchy FJ. Autoimmune and chronic hepatitis. In: Kliegman RM, Behrman RE, Jenson HB, Stanton BF (eds). *Nelson Textbook of Pediatrics.* 18th edn. Vol. 2. Philadelphia: Saunders, 2007;1698–701.

Squires RH. Autoimmune hepatitis in children. *Curr Gastroenterol Rep* 2004;6:225–30.

17.7 DRUG- AND TOXIN-INDUCED LIVER INJURY

The liver is the main site of drug metabolism and is particularly susceptible to structural and functional injury after ingestion, parenteral administration, or inhalation of chemical agents, drugs, plant derivatives (home remedies), or environmental toxins. Chemical hepatotoxicity can be predictable or idiosyncratic. Predictable hepatotoxicity implies a high incidence of hepatic injury in exposed individuals, with dose dependence. Idiosyncratic hepatotoxicity is infrequent and unpredictable but accounts for the majority of adverse reactions. The likelihood of injury is not dose dependant and may occur at any time during exposure to the agent. An idiosyncratic reaction can also be immunologically mediated as a result of prior sensitization (hypersensitivity); extrahepatic manifestations of hypersensitivity can include fever, rash, arthralgia and eosinophilia. Duration of exposure before reaction is generally 1–4 wk, with prompt recurrence of injury on re-exposure. The pathologic spectrum of drug-induced liver disease is extremely wide, is rarely specific, and can mimic other liver diseases (Table 17.4). Some herbal supplements are associated with hepatic failure, such as kava, chaparral, Ma Huang, comfrey leaves, germander extracts, valerian with skullcap, mushroom (Amantia phalloides, Galerina) and lipokinelix.

Clinical manifestations: The clinical manifestations can be mild and nonspecific, such as fever and malaise. Fever, rash, and arthralgia may be prominent in cases of hypersensitivity. In ill, hospitalized patients, the signs and symptoms of hepatic drug toxicity may be difficult to separate from the underlying illness.

Diagnosis: Hepatocyte damage can lead to elevations of serum aminotransferase activities and serum bilirubin levels and to impaired synthetic function as evidenced by decreased serum coagulation factors and albumin. Hyperammonemia can occur with liver failure or with selective inhibition of the urea cycle (sodium valproate). Toxicologic screening of blood and urine specimens can aid in the detection of drug or toxin exposure. Percutaneous liver biopsy may be necessary to distinguish drug injury from complications of an underlying disorder or from intercurrent infection. Slight elevation of aminotransferase activities may occur during therapy with drugs, particularly anticonvulsants, capable of inducing microsomal pathways for drug metabolism. Liver test abnormalities often resolve with continued drug therapy.

Treatment: The treatment of drug or toxin-related liver injury is mainly supportive. Contact with the offending agent should be avoided. Corticosteroids may have a role in immune-mediated disease. N-acetylcysteine therapy, by stimulating glutathione synthesis is effective in preventing hepatotoxicity when administered within 16 hr after an acute overdose of acetaminophen (*see* Section 36.3). Orthotopic liver transplantation may be required for treatment of drug or toxin induced hepatic failure.

Prognosis: Injury is usually completely reversible when the hepatotoxic factor is withdrawn. With continued use of certain drugs, such as methotrexate, effects of hepatotoxicity can proceed insidiously to cirrhosis. Neoplasia can follow long-term androgen therapy.

Estes JD, Stolpman D, Olyaei A, et al. High prevalence of potentially hepatotoxic herbal supplement use in patients with fulminant hepatic failure. *Arch Surg* 2003;138:852–8.

Leeder JS. Pharmacogenesis and pharmacogenomics. *Pediatr Clin North Am* 2001;48:765–81.

Navarro VJ, Senior JR. Drug related hypertoxicity. *N Engl J Med* 2006;354:731–9.

Suchy FJ. Drug- and toxin-induced liver injury. In: Kliegman RM, Behrman RE, Jenson HB, Stanton BF (eds). *Nelson Textbook of Pediatrics.* 18th edn. Vol. 2. Philadelphia: Saunders, 2007; 1701–3.

17.8 FULMINANT HEPATIC FAILURE

Fulminant hepatic failure is defined as a clinical syndrome resulting from massive necrosis of hepatocytes or from severe functional impairment of hepatocytes. Synthetic, excretory and detoxifying functions of the liver are all severely impaired. In adults, hepatic encephalopathy is an essential diagnostic feature. In infants and children, it is difficult to detect early hepatic encephalopathy, hence, the currently accepted definition in children includes:

1. Biochemical evidence of acute liver injury (usually <8 wk duration)
2. No evidence of chronic liver disease; and
3. Hepatic based encephalopathy defined as a prothrombin time (PT) >15 sec or international normalized ratio (INR) >1.5 not corrected by vitamin K in the presence of clinical hepatic encephalopathy, or a PT >20 sec or INR >2 regardless of the presence of clinical hepatic encephalopathy.

Etiology: Fulminant hepatic failure can be due to viral hepatitis and other causes listed in Table 17.5. There is high risk of fulminant hepatic failure in young people who have combined infections with hepatitis B virus (HBV) and hepatitis D virus (HDV). An idiopathic form of fulminant hepatic failure accounts for 40–50% of cases in children.

Pathology: Liver biopsy usually reveals patchy or confluent massive necrosis of hepatocytes. Multi-lobular or bridging necrosis can be associated with collapse of the reticulin framework of the liver. There may be little or no regeneration of hepatocytes. Centrilobular damage is associated with aceta-minophen hepatotoxicity or with circulatory shock. Severe hepatocyte dysfunction rather than cell necrosis may be occasionally seen in histologic finding (e.g. microvesicular fatty infiltrate of hepatocytes is observed in Reye syndrome, β-oxidation defects and tetracycline toxicity).

Pathogenesis: The mechanisms that lead to fulminant hepatic failure are poorly understood. Whatever the initial cause of hepatocyte injury, various factors may contribute to the pathogenesis of liver failure, including impaired hepatocyte regeneration, altered parenchymal perfusion, endotoxemia, and decreased hepatic reticuloendothelial function. One-third to one half of patients with HIV-induced liver failure become negative for serum hepatitis B surface antigen within a few days of presentation and often have no detectable HBV antigen or HBV DNA in serum. These findings suggest a hyperimmune response to the virus that underlines the massive liver necrosis. The pathogenesis of hepatic encephalopathy may relate to increased serum levels of ammonia, false neurotransmitters, amines, increased γ-aminobutyric acid (GABA) receptor activity, or increased circulating levels of endogenous benzodiazepines-like compounds. Decreased hepatic clearance of these substances may produce marked central nervous system dysfunction.

Clinical manifestations: Fulminant hepatic failure may complicate previously known acute liver disease or be the presenting feature of liver disease. A history of developmental delay and/or neuromuscular dysfunction may indicate an underlying mitochondrial or β-oxidation defect. Fulminant hepatic failure may occur in a previously healthy child, having no risk factors for liver disease such as hepatitis or blood product exposure. Progressive jaundice, fetor hepaticus, fever, anorexia, vomiting and abdominal pain are common; hemorrhagic diathesis and ascites may develop. A rapid decrease in liver size without clinical improvement is an ominous sign. Patients should be

Table 17.5: Causes of fulminant hepatic failure	
Viral hepatitis	*Hepatitis A, B, C, D, E viruses*
Other viruses	Epstein-Barr virus, herpes simplex virus, adenovirus; enterovirus, cytomegalovirus, parvovirus B19, and varicella-zoster
Hepatotoxic drugs and chemicals	Acetaminophen overdose; sodium valproate; halothane; carbon tetrachloride; *Amanita phalloides* mushroom
Autoimmune hepatitis	
Ischemia and hypoxia	Hepatic vascular occlusion; congestive heart failure; cyanotic congenital heart disease; circulatory shock
Metabolic disorders	Wilson disease; acute fatty liver of pregnancy; galactosemia; hereditary tyrosinemia; hereditary fructose intolerance; neonatal iron storage disease; defects in β-oxidation of fatty acids; deficiencies of mitochondrial electron transport
Idiopathic	
Herbal supplements	Kava, chaparral, Ma Huang, comfrey leaves, germander extracts, valerian with skullcap, mushroom (*Amantia phalloides*, Galerina), lipokinelix

Table 17.6: Stages of hepatic encephalopathy

Stages	Symptoms	Signs	Electroencephalogram
I	Periods of lethargy, euphoria, reversal of day-night sleeping, may be alert	Trouble drawing figures, performing mental tasks	Normal
II	Drowsiness, inappropriate behavior, agitation, wide mood swings, disorientation	Asterixis, fetus hepaticus, incontinence	Generalized slowing, q waves
III	Stupor but arousable, confused, incoherent speech	Asterixis, hyper-reflexia, extensor reflexes, rigidity	Markedly abnormal, triphasic waves
IV	Coma, IVa. Responds to noxious stimuli; IVb. No response	Areflexia, no asterixis, flaccidity	Markedly abnormal bilateral slowing, δ waves, electrocortical silence

observed for hepatic encephalopathy, which is initially associated with minor disturbances of unconsciousness or motor function. Patients may rapidly progress to deeper stages of coma in which extensor responses and decerebrate and decorticate posturing appear. Irritability, poor feeding, and a change in sleep rhythm may be the only findings in infants; asterixis may be seen in older children. Respirations are usually increased early but later respiratory failure may occur in stage IV coma (Table 17.6).

Laboratory findings: Serum direct and indirect bilirubin, serum aminotransferase (may decrease when patient deteriorates) and blood ammonia (may be normal in hepatic coma) levels are markedly elevated. Prothrombin time is prolonged, often does not improve after parenteral administration of vitamin K. Hypoglycemia, hypokalemia, hyponatremia, metabolic acidosis, or respiratory alkalosis may develop. Investigations to determine the cause of fulminant hepatic failure are shown in Box 17.2.

Anti-hepatitis B core (anti-HBc); anti-hepatitis A virus (anti-HAV); anti-hepatitis E virus (anti-HEV); anti-hepatitis C virus (anti-HCV); cytomegalovirus (CMV); Epstein-Barr virus (EBV); Anti-hepatitis B core (HBc); anti-hepatitis A (anti-HAV); antinuclear factor (ANF); anti-smooth muscle antibodies (ASMA); liver, kidney, microsomal (LKM) antibodies.

Treatment: The treatment is supportive and the patient should be treated in an intensive care unit where continuous monitoring of vital functions is possible (Box 17.3). Endotracheal intubation is required to prevent aspiration, to reduce cerebral edema by hyperventilation and to facilitate pulmonary toilet. Mechanical ventilation and supplemental oxygen are often necessary in advanced coma. Electrolyte and glucose solutions should be administered intravenously to maintain urine output, to correct or to prevent hypoglycemia (2 mL/kg of 10% dextrose), and to maintain normal serum potassium concentrations. Hyponatremia is common but is usually dilutional and is not as a result of sodium depletion. Parenteral supplementation with calcium, phosphorus, and magnesium may be required. Hypovolemia should be avoided and treated with intravenous of fluids (D5 ½ NS + 20 mEq/L KCl) and blood products. Coagulopathy should be treated with parenteral administration of vitamin K and may require fresh plasma; disseminated intravascular coagulation may also occur. Plasmapheresis may be useful in temporary correction of the bleeding diathesis without resulting fluid overload. Continuous hemofiltration is useful for the treatment of fluid overload and acute renal failure. Antacids or H2 receptor blockers (ranitidine continuous 24 hr IV infusion 2–5 mg/kg/24 hr) or both

Box 17.2: Investigations to determine the cause of fulminant hepatic failure

- Toxicology screen of blood and urine
- IgM anti-HBc
- IgM anti-HAV
- Anti-HEV, HCV, CMV, EBV, herpes simplex
- Ceruloplasmin, serum copper, urinary copper
- Autoantibodies: ANF, ASMA, LKM
- Ultrasound of liver and Doppler of hepatic veins

Box 17.3: Observations in fulminant hepatic failure

Neurological: Conscious level; Pupils—size, equality, reactivity; Fundi—papilledema; plantar response

Cardiorespiratory: Pulse; blood pressure (BP); central venous pressure; respiratory rate

Fluid balance: Input—oral, intravenous; output—hourly urine output, 24-hour sodium output, vomiting, diarrhea

Blood analysis: Arterial blood gases; peripheral blood count (including platelets); creatinine, urea; sodium, potassium, bicarbonate, calcium, magnesium; glucose (2-hourly in acute phase); prothrombin time

Infection surveillance: Cultures—blood, urine, throat, sputum, cannula sites; chest radiograph; temperature

should be considered because of the high risk of gastrointestinal bleeding. Renal dysfunction may result from dehydration, acute tubular necrosis or functional renal failure (hepatorenal syndrome). Monitor patients for evidence of infection, including sepsis, pneumonia, peritonitis and urinary tract infections. The most common pathogens are gram-positive organisms (*Staphylococcus aureus, S. epidermidis*), but infections can also occur due to gram negative bacteria and fungi (administer broad spectrum antibiotics). Cerebral edema is an extremely serious complication that responds poorly to corticosteroid administration and osmotic diuresis (mannitol used as a rapid bolus of 0.5 g/kg/dose as a 20% solution over a 15 minute period). The outcome is reported has worsened in-patients treated with corticosteroids. Immunosuppressive therapy may be effective in cases of autoimmune hepatitis. N-acetylcysteine therapy may improve outcome, particularly in-patients with fulminant liver failure due to paracetamol poisoning. The antiviral drug pleconaril is effective in the treatment of fulminant enteroviral hepatitis in the neonate. Plasmapheresis is used to assist the liver in removing neuroactive toxins to improve encephalopathy but this does not improve survival of the patient. Cultured hepatocytes or liver cell lines are now used experimentally in an effort to allow regeneration of a patient's liver or to delay until a suitable organ donor is available. *Liver transplantation* includes orthotopic liver transplantation (OLT), partial auxiliary arthotopic, heterotopic, reduced-size allografts, and living donor transplantation that is done in-patients depending upon the age and availability of the liver transplant. OLT should not be done in-patients suffering from liver failure and neuromuscular dysfunction secondary to a mitochondrial disorder.

Gastrointestinal hemorrhage, infection, constipation, sedatives, electrolyte imbalance, and hypovolemia may precipitate encephalopathy and should be identified and corrected. The gut should be purged with several enemas. Lactulose should be given every 2–4 hourly orally or by nasogastric tube in doses (10–50 ml) sufficient to cause diarrhea (acidic stool). Lactulose syrup diluted with 1–3 volumes of water may also be given as a retention enema every 6 hour. Lactulose, a nonabsorbable disaccharide is metabolized to organic acids by colonic bacteria; it probably lowers the ammonia levels by decreasing microbial ammonia production and by trapping of ammonia in acidic intestinal contents. Oral or rectal administration of a nonabsorbable antibiotic such as neomycin may reduce enteric bacteria responsible for ammonia production. Treat seizures with phenytoin

(15–18 mg/kg IV). Flumazenil, a benzodiazepine antagonist, may reverse early hepatic encephalopathy.

Complications: Complications of fulminant hepatic failure are encephalopathy, cerebral edema, infection, bleeding, respiratory failure, hypotension, hypothermia, pancreatitis, renal failure, and metabolic disturbances (hypoglycemia, hypokalemia, hypocalcemia, hypomagnesemia, acid–base disturbance).

Prognosis: The mortality is more than 70% and depends upon the cause of liver failure and stage of hepatic encephalopathy. Major complications such as sepsis, severe hemorrhage or renal failure increase the mortality. Aplastic anemia, jaundice for more than 7 days before the onset of encephalopathy, prothrombin time more than 50 seconds, serum bilirubin level more than 17.5 mg/dl (300 mmol/L), liver necrosis and multiorgan failure indicate a poor prognosis. Patients who recover from fulminant hepatic failure with only supportive care do not usually develop cirrhosis or chronic liver disease.

Dhawan A, Cheeseman P, Mieli-Vergani G. Approaches to acute liver failure in children. *Pediatr Transplant* 2004;8:584–8.

Gines P, Guevara M, Arroyo V, Rodes J. Hepatorenal syndrome. *Lancet* 2003;362:1819–26.

Keays R, Harrison PM, Wendon JA, et al. Intravenous acetylcysteine in paracetamol induced fulminant hepatic failure: a prospective controlled trial. *BMJ* 1991;303:1026–9.

Lee WM. Management of acute liver failure. *Semin Liver Dis* 1996;16:369–738.

Mathur GP, Kushwaha KP, Mathur Sarla. Fulminant hepatic failure. In: Mathur GP, Mathur Sarla (eds). *Current Trends in Pediatrics*. Vol 3. Delhi: Academa Publishers, 2007;56–63.

Shawcross D, Jalan R. Dispelling myths in the treatment of hepatic encephalopathy. *Lancet* 2005;265:431–3.

Singer AL, Olthoff KM, Kim H, et al. Role of plasmapheresis in the management of acute hepatic failure in children. *Ann Surg* 2001;234:418–24.

Squires RH, Shneider BL, Bucuvalus J, et al. Acute failure in children: the first 348 patients in the pediatric acute liver failure study group. *J Pediatr* 2006;148:652–8.

Suchy FJ. Fulminant hepatic failure. In: Kliegman RM, Behrman RE, Jenson HB, Stanton BF (eds). *Nelson Textbook of Pediatrics*. 18th edn. Vol. 2. Philadelphia: Saunders, 2007;1703–5.

Suchy FJ. Fulminant hepatic failure. . In: Kliegman RM, Stanton BF, St.Geme JW, Schor NF, Behrman RE. *Nelson Textbook of Pediatrics*. 19th edn. New Delhi: Elsevier, 2011; 1412–5.

17.9 PORTAL HYPERTENSION

Etiopathogenesis: Portal hypertension is defined as an elevation of portal pressure >10–12 mm Hg. The normal portal venous pressure is ~7 mm Hg. The portal vein drains the splanchnic area (abdominal portion of the gastrointestinal tract, pancreas, and spleen) into the hepatic sinusoids. Normal portal pressure gradient, the pressure difference between the portal vein and the systemic veins (hepatic veins or inferior vena cava), is 3–6 mm Hg. The portal hypertension exists when the pressure exceeds 10 mm Hg. Portal hypertension can result from obstruction to portal blood flow any where along the course of the portal venous system. The various disorders associated with portal hypertension are listed in Box 17.4.

Clinical manifestations: Bleeding from esophageal varices is the most common presentation. In patients with underlying hepatic disease physical examination may show jaundice and stigmata of cirrhosis (palmar erythema, vascular telangiectasias), ascites, and growth retardation. Dilated cutaneous collateral vessels carrying blood from the portal to systemic circulation may be apparent in the periumbilical region known as **caput medusae**. Ascites may be present in patients with intrahepatic causes of portal hypertension and may transiently occur with portal vein obstruction. With a liver of normal size along with absence of clinical or biochemical features of liver disease, portal hypertension is the most likely cause. Coughing during a respiratory illness can also increase intravariceal pressure; bleeding may become apparent with hematemesis or with melena. Gastrointestinal hemorrhage can also originate from portal hypertensive

---

Box 17.4: Various disorders associated with portal hypertension

1. *Extrahepatic portal hypertension*
   1. Portal vein agenesis, atresia, stenosis
   2. Portal vein thrombosis or cavernous malformation
   3. Splenic vein thrombosis
   4. Increased portal flow
   5. Arteriovenous fistula

2. *Intrahepatic portal hypertension*

2a. *Hepatocellular disease*
1. Acute and chronic viral hepatitis
2. Cirrhosis
3. Congenital hepatic fibrosis
4. Wilson disease
5. α_1-Antitrypsin deficiency
6. Glycogen storage disease type IV
7. Hepatotoxicity (methotrexate, parenteral nutrition)

2b. *Biliary tract disease*
1. Extrahepatic biliary atresia
2. Cystic fibrosis
3. Choledochal cyst
4. Sclerosing cholangitis
5. Intrahepatic bile duct paucity

2c. *Idiopathic portal hypertension*

2d. *Postsinusoidal obstruction*
1. Budd-Chiari syndrome
2. Veno-occlusive disease

---

gastropathy or from gastric, duodenal, peristomal, or rectal varices. Splenomegaly, sometimes with hypersplenism, is a common presenting feature in portal vein obstruction and may be detected 1st on routine physical examination. Children with portal hypertension, regardless of the underlying cause, may have recurrent bouts of life-threatening hemorrhage.

Another serious complication of portal hypertension is the hepatopulmonary syndrome, which develops in some patients with cirrhosis. It is defined as an arterial oxygenation defect induced by intrapulmonary microvascular dilatation, resulting from release of mediators such as nitric oxide in to the venous circulation.

Diagnosis: Ultrasonography will demonstrate the patency of portal vein. In addition, the use of Doppler flow ultrasonography can demonstrate the direction of flow with in the portal system. The pattern of flow correlates with the severity of cirrhosis and encephalopathy. Reversal of portal vein blood flow (hepatofungal flow) is more likely to be associated with variceal bleeding. Ultrasonography can also demonstrate esophageal varices and cavernous transformation of the portal vein, in which an extensive complex of small collateral vessels form in the paracholedochal and epicholedochal venous system to bypass the obstruction. Other imaging techniques such as contrast enhanced CT, and magnetic resonance angiography will contribute to portal vein anatomy and selective arteriography in precise mapping of the extrahepatic vascular anatomy, such as the celiac axis, superior mesenteric artery, and splenic vein, but are not required to establish a diagnosis.

In a patient with hypoxia (hepatopulmonary syndrome), intrapulmonary microvascular dilatation is demonstrated with contrast-enhanced echocardiography that will demonstrate delayed appearance in the left heart of microbubbles from a saline bolus injected into a peripheral vein.

Endoscopy is the most reliable method for detecting esophageal varices and for identifying the source of gastrointestinal bleeding (*see* Section 16.20). Red spots apparent over varices at the time of endoscopy are a strong predictor of imminent hemorrhage.

Treatment: The therapy of portal hypertension can be divided in to emergency treatment of potentially life-threatening hemorrhage and prophylaxis directed at prevention of initial or subsequent bleeding. Treatment of patients with variceal hemorrhage must include fluid resuscitation, initially in the form of crystalloid infusion, followed by the replacement of red blood cells. Correction of coagulopathy by administration of vitamin K or the infusion of platelets or fresh frozen plasma, or both therapies, may be required. A nasogastric tube should be placed to document the presence of blood within the stomach and to monitor for ongoing bleeding. An H_2 receptor blocker such as ranitidine should be given intravenously to reduce the risk of bleeding from gastric erosions. In most patients, particularly those with extrahepatic hypertension and with normal hepatic synthetic function, bleeding usually stops spontaneously. Fluid resuscitation should be monitored in children after bleeding to avoid producing an excessively high venous pressure and an increased risk for further bleeding.

To decrease portal pressure **vasopressin** is administered initially with a bolus of 0.33 U/kg over 20 min, followed by a continuous infusion of the same dose on an hourly basis or a continuous infusion of 0.2 U/L 73 m^2/min. The side effects of vasoconstriction, can impair cardiac function and perfusion to the heart, bowel, and kidneys, and exacerbate fluid retention. **Nitroglycerine**, usually given as a portion of a skin patch to decrease portal pressure, and when used in conjunction with vasopressin may ameliorate some of its untoward effects. **Somatostatin** analog octreotide administered by continuous intravenous infusion of 1.0–5.0 µg/kg/hr, has been used in adults, its use and efficacy in children have not been well evaluated.

Endoscopic sclerosis or elastic band ligations of esophageal varices are other options to control bleeding. Treatment with endoscopic sclerosis may be associated with further bleeding, bacteremia, esophageal ulceration, and stricture formation. Therefore, most centers do not perform endoscopic sclerotherapy of varices prophylactically but use the procedure as a bridge to the time of liver transplantation or until collateral circulation develops in extrahepatic portal vein obstruction. Endoscopic elastic band ligation of varices has been shown to be more effective and associated with fewer complications than is sclerotherapy (*see* Section 16.18).

In patients who continue to bleed despite pharmacologic and endoscopic methods to control hemorrhage, a Sengstaken-Blakemore tube can be placed to stop hemorrhage by mechanically compressing esophageal and gastric varices. The device may be the only option to control life-threatening hemorrhage but carries a risk of pulmonary aspiration, bleeding when the device is removed and tube not well tolerated in children without sedation.

Various surgical procedures have been devised to divert portal blood flow and to decrease portal pressure.

Orthotopic liver transplantation is a much better therapy for portal hypertension resulting from intrahepatic disease.

Long-term treatment with β blockers such as propranolol has been used in adults with portal hypertension. Propranolol may reduce the incidence of variceal hemorrhage and improve long term survival. There is limited published data regarding the use of this therapy in children.

Prognosis: This is a major cause of morbidity and mortality in children with liver disease. Portal hypertension secondary to intrahepatic disease has a poor prognosis. Portal hypertension is usually progressive in these patients and is often associated with deteriorating liver function. In patients, with portal vein obstruction, episodes of bleeding may become less frequent and severe with age as a collateral circulation develops. Most patients can be treated conservatively with endoscopic sclerotherapy therapy, when necessary. During adolescence some children may continue to experience significant bleeding and may eventually require a portosystemic shunting procedure.

Narayanan Menon KV, Shah V, Kamath PS. The Budd-Chiari syndrome. *N Engl J Med* 2004;350:578–84.

Orenstein S. Esophageal varices. In: Kliegman RM, Behrman RE, Jenson HB, Stanton BF (eds). *Nelson Textbook of Pediatrics.* 18th edn. Vol. 2. Philadelphia: Saunders, 2007;1552.

Ryckman FC, Alonso MH. Causes and management of portal hypertension in the pediatric population. *Clin Liver Dis* 2001;5:789–18.

Sarin SK, Agarwal SR. Extrahepatic portal vein obstruction. *Semin Liver Dis* 2002;22:43–58.

Suchy FJ. Portal hypertension and varices. In: Kliegman RM, Behrman RE, Jenson HB, Stanton BF (eds). *Nelson Textbook of Pediatrics.* 18th edn. Vol. 2. Philadelphia: Saunders, 2007; 1709–12.

17.10 LIVER TRANSPLANTATION

Liver transplantation is the standard therapy for children with end-stage liver disease. The indication for liver transplantation is extrahepatic biliary atresia after a failed portoenterostomy (Kasai) procedure, metabolic liver disease (α_1-antitrypsin deficiency, tyrosenemia, Wilson disease, urea cycle defects), acetaminophen or mushroom mediated hepatic failure, localized cancers of the liver and acute hepatic necrosis.

Early referral to a transplant center is important so that patients and their families can be evaluated and treated well in time. Medical and psychological issues are assessed to determine the appropriateness of transplant, optimal management and urgency. Age (<1 yr), growth failure (defined as height or weight 2 standard deviations below normal), hyperbilirubinemia, hypoalbuminemia, and coagulopathy (as indicated by prolonged international normalized ratio (INR) have been predictive of increased morbidity and mortality and are used to determine the urgency for liver transplantation. Other variables that also indicate the need for liver transplantation are ascites, encephalopathy, visceral bleeding, renal failure and fulminant hepatic failure (prompt referral).

The areas of major importance include nutrition, immunization and medical management. Caloric requirements may be as high as 150 kcal/kg/day. Nocturnal nasogastric tube feedings and intravenous nutrition, especially lipids, may be required because of the anorexia and malabsorption. Fat-soluble vitamins (A, D, E, K) deficiencies must be prevented by providing vitamin supplements. Immunization should be given for hepatitis A and B to avoid additional hepatic injury caused by these infections. Immunizations containing live viruses (measles-mumps-rubella, varicella) should be given on schedule because immunosuppression after transplantation may prevent administration.

Medical management should include control of variceal bleeding, ascites, encephalopathy, coagulopathy and sepsis. The success of transplantation depends on better preservation of the organ (up to 18 hr *ex vivo* with <2% primary nonfunction), surgical techniques, and advancement in immunosuppressive therapy. Steroids and either cyclosporin or tacrolimus are standard therapies to prevent rejection. Hirsutism and gingival hyperplasia are specific side-effects of cyclosporin.

Early complications in the postoperative period include fluid shifts, electrolyte imbalance, renal dysfunction, and hypertension. Primary nonfunction of graft or vascular complications, such as thrombosis of graft vessels that often results in death unless the graft is replaced within 48 hrs. Infection and organ rejection are the most frequent problems. When rejection has required high doses of cyclosporine or tacrolimus and/or continued use of steroids, azathioprine, sirolimus, or mycophenolate mofetil may control rejection and allow reduction of the doses of these more toxic drugs.

Post-transplant lymphoproliferative disease (PTLD) may occur in those children who are associated with high-dose immunosuppression and EBV infection. The morbidity and mortality has been reduced by the use of intravenous ganciclovir in the post-transplant period for high-risk patients, and lowering or discontinuing immunosuppression as soon as EBV infection is detected. Hypertension and renal failure are common long-term complications, especially in children on high doses of cyclosporine or tacrolimus.

The prognosis for 1 and 5 survival rates have improved with immunosuppressant and surgical techniques. In most children there is improvement in growth and development and the stigmata of the chronic liver disease resolve. However, close follow-up of medical and psychosocial issues is necessary.

Cherqui D, Soubrane O, Husson E, et al. Laparoscopic living donor hepatectomy for liver transplantation in children. *Lancet* 2002;359:392–6.

Hurwitz M, Cox KL. Liver transplantation. In: Kliegman RM, Behrman RE, Jenson HB, Stanton BF (eds). *Nelson Textbook of Pediatrics*. 18th edn. Vol. 2. Philadelphia: Saunders, 2007; 1712–13.

McDiarmid SV. Liver transplantation: The pediatric challenge. *Clin Liver Dis* 2000;4:879–927.

18 Respiratory System

18.1 RESPIRATORY PATHOPHYSIOLOGY AND REGULATION

In children, the age and growth-dependent changes take place in physiology and anatomy of the respiratory control mechanism, airway dynamics, and lung parenchyma. These changes have direct influence on the pathophysiologic manifestations of the diseases in children.

Lung volumes: Lung volumes are traditionally measured with a spirogram. *Tidal volume* (V_T) is the amount of air moved in and out of the lungs during each breath. At rest V_T is usually 6–7 ml/kg body weight. *Inspiratory capacity* (IC) is the amount of air inspired by maximum inspiratory effort after tidal expiration. *Expiratory reserve volume* (ERV) is the amount of air inhaled by maximum expiratory effort after tidal expiration. The volume of gas remaining in the lungs after maximum expiration is *residual volume* (RV). *Vital capacity* (VC) is defined as the amount of air moved in and out of the lungs with maximum inspiration and expiration. VC, IC, and ERV are decreased in lung pathology but are also effort dependent. Total lung capacity (TLC) is the volume of gas occupying the lungs after maximum inhalation. *Functional residual capacity* (FRC) is the amount of air left in the lungs after tidal expiration. FRC is abnormally increased in intrathoracic airway obstruction, which results in incomplete exhalation, and abnormally decreased alveolar interstitial diseases. Alveolar PO_2 (PaO_2) increases and alveolar PCO_2 $(PaCO_2)$ decreases during inspiration as fresh atmospheric gas enters the lungs. During inhalation alveolar PO_2 (PaO_2) decreases and alveolar PCO_2 $(PaCO_2)$ increases as pulmonary capillary blood continues to remove oxygen from and add carbon dioxide into the alveoli. FRC acts as a buffer minimizing the changes in PaO_2 and $PaCO_2$ during inspiration and expiration. The major pathophysiologic consequence of decreased FRC is hypoxemia.

Since most of the oxygen in the blood is combined with hemoglobin, it is the percentage of *oxyhemoglobin* (SO$_2$) that gets averaged rather than the PO$_2$. The adverse pathophysiologic consequences of decreased FRC are ameliorated by application of *positive end expiratory pressure* (PEEP) and increasing the inspiratory time during the mechanical ventilation.

Interpretation of clinical signs to localize the site of pathology: Respiratory distress can occur without respiratory disease, and severe respiratory failure can be present without significant respiratory distress. Diseases characterized by CNS excitation (encephalitis, neuroexcitatory drugs) are associated with central neurogenic hyperventilation. Similarly, diseases that produce metabolic acidosis such as diabetic keto-acidosis, salicylism, and shock, result in hyperventilation as a compensatory response.

The rate and depth of respiration and the presence of retractions, stridor, wheezing, and grunting are valuable signs in localizing the site of respiratory pathology. Rapid and shallow respirations (*tachypnea*) are characteristic of parenchymal pathology. Chest wall, intercostals, and suprasternal *retractions* are most striking during inspiration in extrathoracic airway obstruction. Expiratory *wheezing* is characteristic of intrathoracic airway obstruction, either extrapulmonary or intrapulmonary. *Grunting* is produced by expiration against a partially closed glottis and is seen in pulmonary edema, hyaline membrane disease, pneumonia, and bronchiolitis.

Gas exchange: The main function of the respiratory system is to remove carbon dioxide from and add oxygen to the systemic venous blood brought to the lung. Oxygen delivery to the tissues is a product of oxygen content and cardiac output. When hemoglobin is near 100% saturated, the blood contains = 20 ml oxygen/100 ml or 200 ml/L. In a healthy adult, the cardiac output is = 5 L/min, oxygen delivery 1,000 ml/min, and oxygen consumption 250 ml/min. Mixed venous blood returning to the heart has PO$_2$ of 40 torr and is 75% saturated with oxygen.

Pulmonary vasculature: Up to 90% of the systemic venous return is shunted away from the pulmonary arterial circulation to the systemic arterial circulation through the foramen ovale and the ductus arteriosus. After birth, with functional closure of the foramen ovale, and the ductus arteriosus, and dilatation of the pulmonary arterial circulation with consequent decrease in *pulmonary vascular resistance* (PVR), all of the right ventricular output passes through the lung. Failure of the pulmonary arterial circulation to dilate after birth results in *persistent pulmonary hypertension of the newborn* (PPHN).

Pulmonary hypertension can develop without a well defined cause (primary pulmonary hypertension) or as a consequence of an underlying disease (secondary pulmonary hypertension). Adverse effects of hypertension are related to an increased right ventricular afterload, decreased cardiac output, and heart failure characterized by increased systemic venous pressure, hepatomegaly, and edema.

Regulation of respiration: The main function of respiration is to maintain normal blood gas homeostasis to match the metabolic needs of the body with the least amount of energy expenditure. Respiratory rate and tidal volume are regulated by a complex interaction of controllers, sensors and effectors.

Carskadon MA, Dement WC. Normal human sleep: A review. In: Kryger MH, Roth T, Dement WC (eds). *Principles and Practice of Sleep Medicine.* 3rd edn. Philadelphia: WB Saunders, 2000:15–25.

Feldman JL, Mitchell GS, Nattie EE. Breathing, rhythmicity, plasticity, chemosensitivity. *Annu Rev Neurosci* 2003;26:239–66.

Gozal D. New concepts in abnormalities of respiratory control in children. *Curr Opin Pediatr* 2004;19:305–8.

Sarnaik AP, Heidemann SM. Respiratory pathophysiology and regulation. In: Kliegman RM, Behrman RE, Jenson HB, Stanton BF (eds). *Nelson Textbook of Pediatrics.* 18th edn. Vol. 2. Philadelphia: Saunders, 2007;1719–31.

18.2 DIAGNOSTIC APPROACH TO RESPIRATORY DISEASE

The appropriate diagnosis of a child presenting with respiratory signs and symptoms depend on a careful history, and physical examination and investigations wherever required.

History

The history should include questions about respiratory symptoms (dyspnea, cough, pain, wheezing, snoring, apnea, and cyanosis), chronicity, timing during day or night, and associations with activities such as exercise or food intake. Relevant questions related to cardiac, gastrointestinal, central nervous, hematologic, and immune system should also be asked. The family history should include similar symptoms or any chronic disease with respiratory system involvement in siblings and other close relatives.

Physical Examination

An examination of the respiratory system is incomplete without a simultaneous general assessment (including ear, nose, and throat examination (*see* Chapter 29). Points to be noted are physique, voice, breathlessness, clubbing, cyanosis or pallor, intercostal recession, use of accessory respiratory muscles, venous pulses, lymph nodes.

Inspection: The normal chest is bilaterally symmetrical and elliptical in shape. Note scars, lumps, lesions in the skin wall, ribs and vertebrae and chest wall abnormalities, kyphosis, scoliosis, flattening, overinflated, and barrel-shaped chest. Look at the chest movements: symmetrical, diminished on one side, intercostal recession, and rate of respiration. Respiratory rate (breaths/min) varies with the age: newborn—40–70, 0–3 mo, 35–55; 1–6 mo—30–45, 6–12 mo—25–40, 1–3 yr—20–30, 3–6 yr—20–25, 6–12 yr—14–22, and 12 yr—12–18.

Digital clubbing is a sign of chronic hypoxia, but may be due to nonpulmonary etiologies (Box 18.1). In clubbing of the fingers the tissue at the base of the nail is thickened, and the angle between the nail base and adjacent skin of the finger is obliterated. The nail itself looses its longitudinal ridges and becomes convex from above downwards as well as from side to side. In extreme cases the terminal segment of the finger is bulbous, like the end of a drumstick. The toes may also be affected and should be examined for evidence for clubbing. In hypertrophic pulmonary osteo-arthropathy, besides clubbing of fingers, there is thickening of the periosteum of the radius, ulna, tibia, and fibula. This gives rise to swelling above the wrist and ankle. For bedside clinical assessment, the Schamroth sign (Schamroths' window test) is useful. The dorsal surfaces of the terminal phalanges of similar fingers are placed together. With clubbing, the normal diamond-shaped aperture or "window" at the bases of the nail beds disappears, and a prominent distal angle forms between the ends of the nails. In normal subjects, the angle is minimal or nonexistent.

Hypertrophic osteoarthropathy: Some children with chronic disease, especially pulmonary or cardiac disease develop clubbing, which is hypervascularization and soft tissue proliferation about the terminal phalanges, especially the fingers. There may be associated arthritis of the distal interphalangeal joints, as well as tender periosteal new bone formation along tubular long bones and in bones of the hand. This complication, *hypertrophic osteoarthropathy*, is found in children with chronic pulmonary disease (cystic fibrosis), congenital heart disease, gastrointestinal diseases (malabsorption syndrome, biliary atresia, and inflammatory bowel disease), and malignancies (nasopharyngeal sarcoma, osteosarcoma, Hodgkin disease). The cause is unknown, but studies suggest that platelet precursors fail to fragment into platelets within the pulmonary vascular bed before entering the systemic circulation. These clumps are trapped in the peripheral vasculature and interact with peripheral endothelial cells, resulting in release of platelet-derived growth factor and vascular endothelial growth factor, which induces proliferation of vascular endothelial cells, smooth muscle cells, and fibroblasts. Symptoms may improve if the underlying condition can be treated successfully.

Palpation: The lymph nodes in the supraclavicular fossae, cervical and axillary regions should be palpated. Palpate the swelling and areas of pain on the chest wall. Palpate tactile vocal fremitus and exclude asymmetry of the chest wall. The position of the cardiac impulse and trachea should be determined. Displacement of cardiac impulse or trachea or of both together suggests that the position of the mediastinum has been altered by disease of the lungs or pleura. The mediastinum may be pushed away from the affected side by a pleural effusion or pneumothorax. Fibrosis or collapse of the lung will pull the mediastinum towards the affected side. Displacement of the cardiac impulse without displacement of the trachea may be due to scoliosis, to a congenital funnel depression of the sternum or to enlargement of the left ventricle.

Percussion: Points to note on percussion of the chest are dullness, resonance and pain and tenderness. Percussion is dull in pleural effusion, pneumonia, and atelactasis, and tympanic in pneumothorax, emphysema, and asthma.

Auscultation: Points to note on auscultation of the chest are vesicular breath sounds, bronchial breath

---

Box 18.1: Diseases associated with clubbing

Pulmonary: Severe chronic cyanosis; emphysema; chronic suppuration in the lungs (bronchiectasis, empyema); pulmonary tuberculosis; chronic fibrosing alveolitis; carcinoma of the bronchus

Cardiac: Cyanotic congenital heart disease; subacute bacterial endocarditis; chronic congestive heart failure

Gastrointestinal: Crohn's disease; ulcerative colitis; chronic dysentery; sprue; polyposis coli; severe gastrointestinal hemorrhage; small bowel lymphoma; liver cirrhosis (including α_1-antitrypsin deficiency)

Hematologic: Thalassemia; congenital methemoglobinemia (rare)

Other: Thyroid deficiency (thyroid acropachy); chronic pyelonephritis (rare); toxic (e.g. arsenic, mercury, beryllium); lymphomatoid granulomatosis; Fabry disease; Raynaud disease, scleroderma

Congenital (rare)

Unilateral clubbing: Vascular disorders (e.g. subclavian arterial aneurysm, brachial arteriovenous fistula); subluxation of shoulder; median nerve injury; local trauma

sounds, vocal fremitus and resonance, and abnormal or adventitious sounds. Vesicular breathing has a rustling quality, lower pitched, the inspiration is more than expiration and there is no gap between inspiration and expiration. Bronchial breathing is high pitched breath sound with a hollow or blowing quality with similar in length and intensity in inspiration and expiration and a pause between the inspiration and expiration. Bronchial breathing is heard over the trachea or larynx during tidal breathing, lung consolidation, and localized pulmonary fibrosis, at the top of a pleural fluid, collapsed lung (where the underlying major bronchus is patent and cavity in the lung. In addition, it often detects abnormal or adventitious sounds such as *stridor* (a predominant inspiratory monophasic noise); *crackles* (high pitch, interrupted sounds found during inspiration and more rarely during early expiration, which denote opening of previously closed air spaces), *fine crackles* (high pitched, low amplitude, short duration), *coarse crackles* (low pitched, high amplitude, long duration); *rhonchi* are coarse rattling sound (derives from the French word râle meaning rattle); *wheezes* (musical, continuous sounds usually caused by development of turbulent flow in narrow airways); *pleural rub*, creaking or rubbing character.

Blood Gas Analysis

An arterial blood gas analysis is the single most useful rapid test of pulmonary function. Blood gas exchange is evaluated most accurately by the direct management of arterial PO_2, PCO_2, and pH. The blood specimen is best collected anaerobically in a heparinized syringe containing only enough heparin solution to displace the air from the syringe. The syringe should be sealed, placed in ice, and carried to the laboratory for immediate analysis. The age and clinical condition of the patient need to be taken into account when interpreting blood gas tensions. The arterial PO_2 <85 mmHg is abnormal in a child (except in neonates) breathing room air at sea level. Values of arterial PCO_2 >45 mmHg usually indicate hypoventilation or a severe ventilation-perfusion mismatch, unless they reflect respiratory compensation for metabolic alkalosis.

Radiographic Techniques

Radiographic techniques include chest roentgeno-grams; upper airway film; sinus and nasal films; chest CT and MRI; fluoroscopy; barium swallow; broncho-graphy; pulmonary arteriography and aortogram; radionuclide lung scans; spiral reconstruction CT.

Investigative Procedures

Investigative procedures include pulmonary function testing; microbiology: examination of lung secretions; exercise testing; sleep studies; sweat testing.

Lung Visualization and Lung Specimen-based on Diagnostic Tests

These tests include laryngoscopy; bronchoscopy and bronchoalveolar lavage (BAL); thoracoscopy; thoracentesis; lung tap; lung biopsy.

Ansell BM. Hypertrophic osteoarthropathy in the paediatric age. *Clin Exp Rheumatol* 1992;10 (Suppl 7):15–18.

ChemickV, Boat TF. *Kendig's Disorders of the Respiratory tract in Children.* 6th edn. Philadelphia: WB Saunders, 1998; 102.

Haddad GG, Green TP. Diagnostic approach to respiratory disease. In: Kliegman RM, Behrman RE, Jenson HB, Stanton BF (eds). *Nelson Textbook of Pediatrics.* 18th edn. Vol. 2. Philadelphia: Saunders, 2007;1731–36.

Schechter MS. Snoring: Investigations guidelines. *Pediatr Pulmonol Suppl* 2004;26:172–4.

18.3 SUDDEN INFANT DEATH SYNDROME

Sudden infant death syndrome (SIDS) is the most common cause of post-neonatal infant mortality (1 mo to 1 yr of age). SIDS is defined as the sudden death of an infant that is unexpected by history and unexpected by a thorough postmortem examination, which includes a complete autopsy, investigation of the scene of death, and review of the medical history. An autopsy is essential to identify natural causes of sudden, unexpected death such as congenital anomalies or infection and to diagnose traumatic child abuse. The autopsy cannot reliably distinguish between SIDS and intentional suffocation, but the scene investigation and medical history may be of help if inconsistencies are evident.

Reducing the risk of SIDS: The components of the educational programme are as follows:

1. Full-term and premature infants should be placed for sleep in the supine position. There are no adverse health outcomes from supine sleeping. Side sleeping is not recommended.

2. Infants should not be put to sleep on waterbeds, sofas, soft mattresses or other soft surfaces.

3. Soft materials in the infant's sleep environment should be avoided, either over, under, or near the infant. These include pillows, comforters (pacifier), quilts, sheepskin, and stuffed toys. Blankets should be tucked in around the crib mattress. Sleeping clothing (such as a sleep sack) may be used in place of blankets.

4. Bed sharing or co-sleeping may be hazardous under certain conditions. Adults (other than parents) and

children or other siblings should not share a bed with an infant. The parents should not share a bed with their infant if they smoke or use substances such as drugs or alcohol that impair parental arousal.

5. Avoid overheating or over bundling. The infant should be lightly clothed for sleep and the thermostat sat at a comfortable temperature.

6. Infants should have some time in the prone position while awake and observed. Alternating the placement of the infant's head as well as his or her orientation can also minimize the risk of head flattening from supine sleeping.

7. Devices advertised to maintain sleep position or reduce the risk of rebreathing are not recommended.

Hunt CE, Hauck ER. Sudden infant death syndrome. In: Kliegman RM, Behrman RE, Jenson HB, Stanton BF (eds). *Nelson Textbook of Pediatrics*. 18th edn. Vol. 2. Philadelphia: Saunders, 2007;1736–42.

Li DK, Willinger M, Pettiti DB, et al. Use of dummy (pacifier) during sleep and risk of sudden infant death syndrome (SIDS): Population based case control study. *Br Med J* 2006;332:18–21.

18.4 ACUTE RESPIRATORY TRACT INFECTION (ARI) CONTROL PROGRAM

Acute lower respiratory tract infections (LRTIs) are a leading cause of mortality in children below 5 yr of age. The common bacteria causing LRTI in preschool children include *H. influenzae, S. pneumoniae*, staphylococci. All these are sensitive to antibacterials like cotrimoxazole. Hence, judicious use of cotrimoxazole in children with LRTI may prevent deaths due to pneumonia. The World Health Organization (WHO) has recommended certain criteria for diagnosis of pneumonia in children at primary health care level for control of LRTI deaths in countries where the infant mortality is more than 40/1000 live births. The clinical criteria for diagnosis of pneumonia include rapid respiration with or without difficulty in respiration. Rapid respiration (RR) is defined as respiratory rate of more than 60, 50, 40 per minutes in children below 2 mo of age, 2 mo to 1 yr and 1 to 5 yr of age respectively. Difficulty in respiration is defined as lower chest in drawing. The WHO recommends that in a primary care setting if a child between 2 mo to 5 yr of age presents with cough he should be examined for rapid respiration and difficulty in breathing along with presence of cyanosis or difficulty in feeding (Table 18.1). In future these drugs may be replaced with amoxicillin and penicillin.

In children below 2 mo of age, the presence of any of the following indicates severe disease: fever (38°C or more), convulsions, abnormally sleepy or difficult to wake, stridor in calm child, wheezing, not feeding, tachypnea, chest indrawing, altered sensorium, central cyanosis grunting, apneic spells or distended abdomen. Such children should be referred to the hospital for admission and treated with ampicillin and gentamicin and supportive care.

Home care advice for mother include:

1. *Increase fluids:* increase breastfeeding and offer the child extra to drink
2. *Feed the child:* feed the child during illness and increase feeding after illness
3. *Clear the nostril* if it interferes with feeding
4. *Most important:* watch for signs of pneumonia. Bring child back quickly to health worker if: breathing becomes difficult, breathing becomes fast, child is not able to drink, and child becomes more sick.

Mishra S, Kumar H, Anand VK, Patwari AL, Sharma D. ARI control programme: results in hospitalized children. *J Trop Pediatr* 1993;39(5):288–92.

Technical basis for WHO recommendations on the management of pneumonia in children at first level health facilities. WHO/ARI/91.20 Geneva: World Health Organization, 1991.

Table 18.1: Children aged 2 mo to 5 yr with cough or difficult breathing: Clinical classification to facilitate treatment decisions recommended by WHO

Signs and symptoms	Classification	Therapy	Where to treat
Cough or cold No fast breathing No chest indrawing No indicators of severe illness	No pneumonia	Home remedies	Home
RR/minute: Age	Pneumonia	Cotrimoxazole	Home
60 or more: < 2 months			
50 or more: 2–12 months			
40 or more: 12–60 months			
Chest indrawing	Severe pneumonia	IV/IM Penicillin	Hospital
Cyanosis, severe chest indrawing, inability to feed	Very severe pneumonia	IV Chloramphenicol	Hospital

18.5 WHEEZING, BRONCHIOLITIS, AND BRONCHITIS

Wheezing in Infants

Definitions: A *wheeze* is a musical and continuous sound that originates from oscillations in narrowed airways. Wheezing is mostly heard in expiration as a result of critical airway obstruction. Wheezing is *polyphonic* when there is widespread narrowing of the airways causing various pitches or levels of obstruction to airflow as seen in asthma. *Monophonic* wheezing refers to a single-pitch sound that is produced in the larger airways during expiration as in distal tracheomalacia or bronchomalacia. When obstruction occurs in the extrathoracic airways during inspiration, the noise is referred to as *stridor*.

Etiology: In infants wheezing mostly is caused by inflammation (generally bronchiolitis), but many other entities can cause wheezing. **Chronic infectious** causes of wheezing should be considered in those infants who do not have a normal clinical course. Cystic fibrosis is one such entity. **Allergy and asthma** are important causes of wheezing. Risk factors for persistent wheezing are maternal asthma, maternal smoking, persistent rhinitis (apart from upper respiratory tract infections), and eczema at <1 yr of age. **Other causes** include congenital malformations of the respiratory tract, foreign body aspiration, gastroesophageal reflux, and trauma and tumors.

Clinical manifestations: Initial **history** of a wheezing infant should include onset, duration, and other factors. *Birth history* includes weeks of gestation, neonatal intensive care unit admission, and history of intubation or oxygen requirement, maternal complications including infection, herpes simplex virus (HSV) status, HIV status, and prenatal smoke exposure. *Past medical history* includes any co-morbid conditions including syndromes or associations. *Family history* of cystic fibrosis, immunodeficiencies, asthma in a first degree relative, or any other recurrent respiratory conditions should be obtained. *Social history* should include an environmental history including any smokers at home, inside or out, day care exposure, number of siblings, occupation of inhabitants of the home, pets, tuberculosis exposure, and concerns regarding home environment (i.e. dust mites, construction dust, heating and cooling techniques, mold, and cockroaches).

On **physical examination**, evaluation of the patient's vital signs with special attention to the respiratory rate and the pulse oximetry reading for oxygen saturation is an important initial step. Patient's growth chart should be reviewed for signs of failure to thrive. Wheezing produces an expiratory whistling sound that can be polyphonic or monophonic in nature. Prolonged expiratory time may be present. Biphasic wheezing can occur if there is a central, large airway obstruction. A trial of a bronchodilator to evaluate for any change in wheezing after treatment should be carried out. Listening to breath sounds over the neck will help differentiate upper airway from lower airway sounds. The presence or absence of stridor should be noted during inspiration. Signs of respiratory distress include tachypnea, increased respiratory effort, nasal flaring, tracheal tugging, subcostal and intercostal retractions, and excess use of accessory muscles. In the upper airway, signs of atopy, including boggy turbinates and posterior oropharynx cobblestoning, can be evaluated in older infants. Note on the skin for eczema, and significant hemangiomas; midline lesions may be associated with an intrathoracic lesion. Digital clubbing should be noted.

Acute Bronchiolitis

Acute bronchiolitis is caused by viruses (respiratory syncytial virus (RSV) in >50% of the cases. Other agents include parainfluenza virus, metapneumovirus, adenovirus, influenza, rhinovirus) and mycoplasma. Bacterial infections do not cause acute bronchiolitis. Acute bronchiolitis is more common in males, in those who have not been breastfed, and in those who live in crowded conditions.

Acute bronchiolitis is characterized by bronchiolar obstruction with edema, mucus, and cellular debris. Even minor bronchiolar wall thickening significantly affects airflow because resistance is inversely proportional to the 4th power of the radius of the bronchiolar passage. Resistance in the small air passages is increased during both inspiration and exhalation, but because the radius of an airway is smaller during expiration, the resultant respiratory obstruction leads to early air trapping and overinflation. If obstruction becomes complete, there will be resorption of trapped distal air, and the child will develop atelectasis. Hypoxemia develops due to ventilation-perfusion mismatch early in the course. With severe obstructive disease and tiring of respiratory effort, hypercapnia may develop.

Acute bronchiolitis is usually preceded by exposure to an older contact with minor respiratory syndrome with in the previous week. The infant first develops a mild upper respiratory tract infection with sneezing and clear rhinorrhea. This may be accompanied by diminished appetite and fever of 38.5–39°C (101–102°F), although the temperature may range from subnormal to markedly elevated. Gradually, respiratory distress ensues, with paroxysmal wheezy cough, dyspnea, and irritability. The infant is often tachypneic, which may interfere with feeding. Diarrhea or vomiting is usually absent. Apnea may be more prominent than wheezing early in the course of the disease, particularly with very young infants (<2 mo old) or former premature infants. The *physical examination* is characterized by wheezing, rapid breathing, nasal flaring and retractions. Auscultations may reveal fine crackles or wheezes, with prolongation of expiratory phase of breathing. Hyperinflation of the lungs may permit palpation of liver and spleen.

Diagnosis: Physical findings include grunting, decreased breath sounds, prolonged inspiratory to expiratory ratio, and crackles. In acute bronchiolitis, chest radiography reveals hyperinflated lungs with patchy atelectasis, the white blood cell and differential counts are usually normal. A trial of bronchodilator may be diagnostic as well as therapeutic because these medications can reverse conditions such as bronchiolitis (occasionally) and asthma. Bronchodilators may potentially worsen a case of wheezing caused by tracheal or bronchial malacia. A sweat test to evaluate for cystic fibrosis and evaluation of base line immune status should be considered in infants with recurrent wheezing. Further evaluation such as upper gastrointestinal (GI) contrast X-rays, chest CT, bronchoscopy, infant pulmonary function testing, video swallow study, and pH probe can be considered second-tier diagnostic procedures in complicated patients.

Viral testing (usually rapid immunofluorescence, polymerase chain reaction, or viral culture) is helpful if the diagnosis is uncertain or for epidemiologic purposes. The diagnosis is clinical, particularly in a previously healthy infant presenting with a first-time wheezing episode during a community outbreak. Because concurrent bacterial infection (sepsis, pneumonia, meningitis) is highly unlikely, sepsis evaluation in a febrile infant is not required.

Treatment: Treatment of an infant with wheezing depends on the underlying etiology. It is appropriate to administer salbutamol or albuterol aerosol and observe the response. For infants < 3 yr of age continue to administer inhaled medications through a metered-dose inhaler (MDI) with mask and spacer if a therapeutic benefit is demonstrated. Therapy should be continued in all patients with asthma exacerbations from a viral illness.

The use of ipratropium bromide appears to be some what effective, but it appears to be somewhat effective as an adjunct therapy. It is also useful in infants with significant tracheal and bronchial malacia who may be made worse by β₂-agonists such as salbutamol or albuterol because of the subsequent decrease in smooth muscle tone.

A trial of inhaled steroids may be warranted in a patient who has responded to multiple courses of oral steroids, has moderate to severe wheezing or has significant history of atopy including food allergy or eczema. Inhaled steroids are also indicated in patients with known reactive airways, but are controversial when used for episodic or acute illnesses.

Oral steroids should be used in atopic wheezing infants thought to have asthma that is refractory to other medications. Their use in first-time wheezing infants or those infants that do not warrant hospitalization is controversial.

Infants with *acute bronchiolitis* who are experiencing respiratory distress should be hospitalized. The main treatment is supportive. If hypoxemic, the child should receive cool humidified oxygen. Sedatives are to be avoided because they may depress respiratory drive. Keep the infant in comfortable position; sometimes most comfortable with head and chest elevated at a 30-degree angle with neck extended. The risk of aspiration oral feedings may be high in infants with bronchiolitis, owing to tachypnea and increased work of breathing. The infant may be fed through a nasogastric tube. If there is any risk for further respiratory decompensation potentially necessitating tracheal intubation, the infant should not be fed orally but be maintained with parenteral fluids. Frequent suctioning of nasal and oral secretions will provide relief of distress or cyanosis. Oxygen is indicated in all infants with hypoxia.

A number of agents have been proposed as adjunctive therapy for bronchiolitis, such as bronchodilators, and corticosteroids. *Nebulized epinephrine may be more effective than β-agonists and should be tried and further therapy will depend on response on individual patient.* Corticosteroids (parenteral, oral, or inhaled) have been used for bronchiolitis, despite conflicting and often negative studies. Corticosteroids are not recommended in previously healthy infants with RSV. Antibiotics have no value unless there is secondary bacterial pneumonia. There is also no role for RSV immunoglobulin administration during acute episodes of RSV bronchiolitis.

Prognosis: Infants with acute bronchiolitis are at higher risk for further respiratory compromise in the first 48–72 hr after onset of cough and dyspnea; the child may be desperately ill with air hunger, apnea, and respiratory acidosis. After this critical period the symptoms persist. The median duration of symptoms in ambulatory patients is ~12 days. The case fatality rate is <1%, with death due to apnea, uncompensated respiratory acidosis, or severe dehydration. Infants with congenital heart disease, bronchopulmonary dysplasia, and immunodeficiency often have more severe disease, with higher morbidity and mortality. There is higher incidence of wheezing and asthma in atopic syndromes. It is unclear whether bronchiolitis incites an immune response that manifests as asthma later or whether infants have an inherent prediction for asthma that is merely unmasked by their episode of RSV. Approximately 60% of infants who wheeze will stop wheezing.

Bronchiolitis Obliterans

Bronchiolitis obliterans (BO) is a rare, chronic lung disease of the bronchioles and smaller airways. The BO most commonly occurs after respiratory infections (adenovirus, *Mycoplasma*, measles, legionella, influenza, pertussis), and less commonly occurs due to inflammatory diseases (juvenile rheumatoid arthritis, systemic lupus erythematosus, scleroderma, Stevens-Johnson syndrome), toxin fume inhalation (NO_2, NH_3), and after lung and bone marrow transplantation. Bronchiolitis obliterans organizing pneumonia (BOOP) is a fibrosing lung disease that includes the features of BO with extension of inflammatory process from distal alveolar ducts into alveoli and proliferation of fibroblasts.

Clinical manifestations: Cough, fever, cyanosis, dyspnea, chest pain, and respiratory distress followed by initial improvement may be the initial signs of BO. In this phase, BO is easily confused with pneumonia, bronchitis, or acute bronchiolitis. Physical examination findings are usually nonspecific and may include wheezing and crackles.

Laboratory findings: Chest radiographs may be normal or may demonstrate hyperlucency and patchy infiltration. Chest CT often shows patchy areas of hyperlucency and bronchiectasis. The diagnosis of BO or bronchiolitis obliterans organizing pneumonia (BOOP) is established by open lung biopsy or transbronchial biopsy. Pulmonary function tests typically show signs of airway obstruction.

Treatment: There is no definitive therapy for BO; corticosteroids may be beneficial. For BOOP, use of oral corticosteroids for up to 1 yr has been advocated as first-line therapy for symptomatic and progressive disease.

Prognosis: Some patients with BO experience rapid deterioration in their condition and die within week of initial symptoms; most nontransplant patients survive with chronic disability. In patients with BOOP total recovery is reported in 60–80% of patients.

Bronchitis

Bronchitis refers to nonspecific bronchial inflammation. *Acute bronchitis* is a syndrome, usually viral in origin, with cough as a prominent feature. *Acute tracheobronchitis* is a term used when the trachea is prominently involved. It is associated with nasopharyngitis, and a variety of viral and bacterial agents, such as those causing influenza, pertussis, and diphtheria, may be responsible. These infectious agents lead to activation of inflammatory cells and release to cytokines. The tracheobronchial epithelium may become significantly damaged or hypersensitized, leading to a protracted cough lasting 1–3 wk.

Acute Bronchitis

Acute bronchitis is commonly preceded by a viral upper respiratory tract infection. It is more common in the winter when respiratory viral syndromes predominate. The child first has rhinitis. Three to four days later, a frequent dry, hacking cough develops which may or may not be productive. After several days the sputum may become purulent, indicating leukocyte migration but not necessarily bacterial infection. Many children may swallow their sputum and this may produce emesis. Chest pain may be a prominent complaint in older children, exacerbated by coughing. The mucus gradually thins, usually within 5–10 days, and then the cough gradually abates. The entire episode usually lasts about 2 wk and seldom longer than 3 wk.

The findings on physical examination vary with age of the patient and stage of the disease. In the early stage of the disease there is low grade fever and upper respiratory signs such as nasopharyngitis, conjunctivitis, and rhinitis. As the disease progresses and cough worsens, the breath sounds become coarse, with coarse and fine crackles and scattered high-pitched wheezing. Chest radiographs are normal or may have increased bronchial markings. The principle objective is to exclude pneumonia, which is more likely caused by bacterial agents, requiring antibiotic therapy. In adults, the chances of pneumonia are less likely in the absence of abnormality of vital signs (tachycardia, tachypnea, fever) and a normal physical examination of the chest.

Differential diagnosis: If the symptoms persist or there is recurrence of symptoms other causes of cough as a prominent symptom should be considered (Table 18.2).

Treatment: There is no specific therapy and the disease is self-limited. Frequent shifts in position may facilitate pulmonary drainage in infants. Older children are sometimes more comfortable with humidity. Antibiotics though frequently prescribed, do not hasten

Table 18.2: Disorders with cough as a prominent finding	
Category	*Diagnoses*
Chronic pulmonary disorders	Asthma, bronchopulmonary dysplasia, postinfectious bronchiectasis, cystic fibrosis, tracheo or bronchomalacia, ciliary abnormalities
Other chronic diseases/congenital disorders	Swallowing disorders, gastroesophageal reflux, air-way compression (such as a vascular ring or hemangioma), laryngeal cleft, congenital heart disease
Infectious/immune disorders	Tuberculosis, sinusitis, tonsillitis or adenoids, pertussis, *Mycoplasma pneumoniae*, immunodeficiency, allergy, chlamydia/ureaplasma infection (infants)
Acquired	Foreign body aspiration

improvement. Cough suppressants may produce symptomatic relief, but there is also increased risk of suppuration and inspissated secretions, and should not be prescribed. Antihistamines dry secretions and are not helpful. Expectorants are also not indicated.

Chronic Bronchitis

Chronic bronchitis disease may develop insidiously, with episodes of acute obstruction alternating with quiescent periods. A number of predisposing factors can lead to progression of airflow obstruction or chronic obstructive pulmonary disease (COPD), such as smoking (approximately 80% of patients have a smoking history), air pollution, occupational exposures, and repeated infections. In cases of children, cystic fibrosis, bronchopulmonary dysplasia, and bronchiectasis must be ruled out. The existence of chronic bronchitis as a distinct entity is controversial. Thus, children with chronic or recurring cough should be reviewed and investigated for underlying pulmonary or systemic disorders.

Cigarette Smoking and Air Pollution

Exposure to environmental irritants, such as tobacco smoke and air pollution, can incite or aggravate cough. There is a well established association between tobacco exposure and pulmonary disease, including bronchitis and wheezing. This can occur through cigarette smoking or by exposure to passive smoke. Marijuana smoke is another irritant. A number of pollutants compromise lung development and likely precipitate lung disease including particulate matter, ozone, acid vapor, and nitrogen dioxide.

Boas S. Other distal airway diseases. In: Kliegman RM, Behrman RE, Jenson HB, Stanton BF (eds). *Nelson Textbook of Pediatrics.* 18th edn. Vol. 2. Philadelphia: Saunders, 2007;1781–83.

Goodman DM. Bronchitis. In: Kliegman RM, Behrman RE, Jenson HB, Stanton BF (eds). *Nelson Textbook of Pediatrics.* 18th edn. Vol. 2. Philadelphia: Saunders, 2007;1777–8.

Kurland G, Michelson P. Bronchiolitis obliterans in children. *Pediatr Pulmonol* 2005;39:193–208.

Morton RL, Sheikh S, Corbett ML, Eid NS. Evaluation of the wheezy infant. *Ann Allergy Asthma Immunol* 2002;86:251–6.

Smyth RL, Openshaw PJM. Bronchiolitis. *Lancet* 2006;368:312–22.

Subcommittee on Diagnosis and Management of Bronchitis: Diagnosis and management of bronchitis. *Pediatrics* 2006;118:1774–93.

Watts KD, Goodman DM. Wheezing in infants: Bronchiolitis. In: Kliegman RM, Behrman RE, Jenson HB, Stanton BF (eds). *Nelson Textbook of Pediatrics.* 18th edn. Vol. 2. Philadelphia: Saunders, 2007;1773–7.

18.6 EMPHYSEMA AND OVERINFLATION

Pulmonary emphysema is distension of air spaces with irreversible disruption of the alveolar septa. It can be generalized or localized, involving part or all of a lung.

Overinflation is distension with or without alveolar rupture and is often reversible. It is obstructive or compensatory. *Obstructive overinflation* results from partial obstruction of a bronchus or bronchiole, when it becomes more difficult for air to leave the alveoli than to enter. This results in a gradual accumulation of air distal to the obstruction, which is so-called bypass, ball valve or check valve type of obstruction. *Compensatory overinflation* can be acute or chronic and occurs in normally functioning pulmonary tissue when, for any reason a sizable portion of the lung is removed or becomes partially or completely airless, which can occur with pneumonia, atelectasis, empyema, and pneumothorax.

LOCALIZED OBSTRUCTIVE OVERINFLATION

When a ball-valve type of obstruction partially occludes the main stem bronchus, the entire lung becomes overinflated. Individual lobes are affected when the obstruction is in lobar bronchi and segments and subsegments are affected when their individual bronchi are blocked. Localized obstruction results from foreign bodies, endobronchial tuberculosis or tuberculosis of the tracheobronchial lymph nodes, abnormally thick mucus in cases of cystic fibrosis, and endobronchial or mediastinal tumors. The distended lung may extend across the mediastinum into the opposite hemithorax.

Unilateral hyperlucent lung can be associated with cardiac and pulmonary diseases or without demonstrable underlying active disease; commonest is pneumonia, and rarely Swyer-James or Macleod syndrome (hyper-resonance lung and a small lung shifted toward the more abnormal lung).

Congenital lobar emphysema (CLE) can result in severe respiratory distress in early infancy and can be caused by obstruction. In 50% cases, a cause of CLE is identified including congenital deficiency of the bronchial cartilage, external compression by aberrant vessels, bronchial stenosis, redundant mucosal flaps, and kinking of the bronchus caused by herniation in the mediastinum. Familial occurrence has been reported.

Overinflation of all three lobes of the right lung has been produced by anomalous location of the left pulmonary artery, which impinges on the right main stem bronchus. Hyperinflation also occurs in patients with the absent pulmonary valve type of tetralogy of Fallot and secondary aneurismal dilatation of the pulmonary artery, which partially compresses the main stem bronchi. A number of newborn infants have lobar overinflation while being treated for hyaline membrane disease with assisted ventilation, suggesting an acquired cause.

Clinical manifestations: The clinical manifestations usually become apparent in the neonatal period but are delayed for as long as 5–6 mo in a few patients. Signs vary from mild tachypnea and wheeze to severe dyspnea with cyanosis. CLE affects the upper and middle lobes; with the left upper lobe is the most common site. The affected lobe is essentially nonfunctional because of the overdistension, and atelectasis of the ipsilateral lung may ensue. With further distension, the mediastinum is shifted to the contralateral side with impaired function seen as well.

Diagnosis: Radiographic examination will often reveal a radiolucent lobe and a mediastinal shift. A CT scan may demonstrate the aberrant anatomy of the lesion, and MRI/MRA will demonstrate any vascular lesions, which might be causing extraluminal compression. Nuclear imaging studies are useful to demonstrate perfusion defects in the affected lobe. The differential diagnosis includes pneumonia with or without an effusion and cystic adenomastoid malformation.

Treatment: Immediate surgery and excision of the lobe may be life-saving when cyanosis and severe respiratory distress are present, but some patients respond to medical treatment. Medical management with selective intubation of the unaffected bronchus or high frequency ventilation has occasionally been successful and lobectomy avoided. Some children with apparent CLE have reversible overinflation, without the classic alveolar septal rupture.

Generailzed Obstructive Overinflation

Acute generalized overinflation of the lung results from widespread involvement of the bronchioles and is usually reversible. It occurs more commonly in infants than in children and may be secondary to asthma, cystic fibrosis, acute bronchiolitis, interstitial pneumonitis, atypical forms of acute laryngotracheo-bronchitis, aspiration of zinc stearate powder, chronic passive congestion secondary to a congenital cardiac lesion, and miliary tuberculosis. In *chronic overinflation*, many of the alveoli are ruptured and communicate with one another, producing distended saccules. Air may also enter the interstitial tissue (i.e. interstitial emphysema), resulting in pneumomediastinum and pneumothorax.

Clinical manifestations: Generalized obstructive overinfation is characterized by dyspnea, with difficulty on exhaling. Cyanosis is more common in the severe cases. The lungs become increasingly overdistended, and the chest remains expanded during exhalation. An increased respiratory rate and decreased respiratory excursion result from the overdistension of the alveoli and their inability to be emptied normally through the narrowed bronchioles. Air hunger is responsible for forced respiratory movements. Overaction of the accessory muscles of respiration results in retraction at the suprasternal notch, the supraclavicular spaces, the lower margin of the thorax, and the intercostals spaces. Unlike the flattened chest during inspiration and exhalation in cases of laryngeal obstruction, minimal reduction in the size of the overdistended chest during exhalation is observed. The percussion note is hyperresonant. On auscultation, the inspiratory phase is usually less prominent than the expiratory phase, which is prolonged and roughened. Fine or medium crackles may be heard. Cyanosis is present in severe cases.

Diagnosis: Radiographic and fluoroscopic examinations of chest will show that both leaves of the diaphragm are low and flattened, the ribs are farther apart than usual, and the lung fields are less dense. The movement of the diaphragm during exhalation is decreased, and the excursion of the low, flattened diaphragm in severe cases is barely discernible. The anteroposterior diameter of the chest is increased, and the sternum may be bowed outward.

Bullous emphysema: Bullous emphysematous blebs or cysts (pneumatocele) result from overdistension and rupture of alveoli during birth or shortly thereafter, or they may be sequelae of pneumonia and other infections including tuberculous lesions during antituberculous therapy. The emphysematous areas rupture forming a single or multiloculated cavity. The cysts may become large and may contain some fluid; an air-fluid level may be demonstrated on the radiograph. The cysts should be differentiated from pulmonary abscesses. In most cases cysts disappear spontaneously within a few months but may persist for a year or more in some cases. Aspiration or surgery is indicted in cases of severe respiratory and cardiac compromise.

Subcutaneous emphysema: Subcutaneous emphysema results from any process that allows free air to enter into the subcutaneous tissue. The causes include pneumomediastinum, pneumothorax, complication of fracture of the orbit which permits free air to escape from the nasal sinuses, tracheostomy, deep ulceration in the pharyngeal region, esophageal wounds or any perforating lesion of the larynx and trachea, a complication of thoracocentesis, asthma, or abdominal surgery, and gas producing bacteria.

Tenderness over the site of emphysema and a "crepitant" quality on palpation of the skin are the classic signs. Subcutaneous emphysema is usually a self-limited process and requires no specific treatment. Resolution occurs by resorption of subcutaneous air after elimination of its sources. The activities that may increase airway pressure such as cough, performance of high-pressure pulmonary function testing maneuvers should be minimized. Rarely, surgical intervention is required when dangerous compression of the trachea by air in the surrounding soft tissue occurs.

Boas S, Winnie GB. Emphysema and overinflation. In: Kliegman RM, Behrman RE, Jenson HB, Stanton BF (eds). *Nelson Textbook of Pediatrics.* 18th edn. Vol. 2. Philadelphia: Saunders, 2007;1778–80.

ChaoMC, Karamzadeh AM, Ahuja G. Congenital lobar emphysema: An otolaryngologic perspective. *Int J Pediatr Otorhinolaryngol* 2005;69:549–54.

Cumming GR, Macpherson RI, Chernick V. Unilateral hyperlucent lung syndrome in children. *J Pediatr* 1971;78:250–60.

Horak E, Bodner J, Gassner I, et al. Congenital lobar emphysema: Diagnostic and therapeutic considerations. *J Pediatr Surg* 1994;34:1347–51.

Mura M, Zompatori M, Mussoni A, et al. Bullous emphysema versus diffuse emphysema: A functional and radiologic consideration. *Respir Med* 2005;99:171–8.

18.7 PULMONARY EDEMA

Pulmonary edema is an excessive accumulation of fluid in the interstitium and air spaces of the lung, resulting in oxygen desaturation and respiratory distress. Pulmonary edema is separated into two categories according to cause i) *cardiogenic* such as left ventricular failure and ii) *noncardiogenic* as in pulmonary veno-occlusive disease, pulmonary venous fibrosis, mediastinal tumors.

Clinical manifestations: The earliest clinical signs include increased work of breathing in the form of tachypnea and dyspnea. With the accumulation of fluid in the alveolar space, auscultation reveals crackles and wheezing, especially in dependent lung fields. In cardiogenic pulmonary edema, a gallop may be present as well as peripheral edema and distended jugular veins.

Laboratory findings: Early radiographic signs including peribronchial and perivascular cuffing, indicate accumulation of interstitial edema. Diffuse streakiness reflects interlobular edema and distended pulmonary lymphatics. Diffuse patchy densities (due to alveolar filling) and the "butterfly" appearance are late signs. Cardiomegaly and increased pulmonary vascular markings are seen with causes involving left ventricular dysfunction. Pleural effusion, peribronchial cuffing and septal lines may be present in cardiogenic edema. In noncardiogenic pulmonary edema, heart size is usually normal and air bronchogram may be present. Brain natriuretic peptide (BNP) level >500 pg/ml suggests heart disease; <100 pg/ml suggests lung disease.

Treatment: The treatment of a patient with noncardiogenic pulmonary edema is supportive (adequate ventilation and oxygenation) and therapy of the underlying cause. Patients should receive supplemental oxygen in order to increase alveolar oxygen tension and decrease pulmonary vasoconstriction. Patients with cardiogenic causes should be managed with inotropic agents and systemic vasodilators to produce afterload reduction. Judicious use of diuretics is valuable in the treatment of pulmonary edema associated with total body fluid overload (sepsis, renal insufficiency). Morphine is often useful as a vasodilator and a mild sedative.

High altitude pulmonary edema (HAPE) (*see* Section 7.12).

Bahk T, Mazor R, Green TP. Pulmonary edema. In: Kliegman RM, Behrman RE, Jenson HB, Stanton BF (eds). *Nelson Textbook of Pediatrics.* 18th edn. Vol. 2. Philadelphia: Saunders, 2007;1787–9.

Perina DG. Noncardiogenic pulmonary edema. *Emerg Med Clin North Am* 2003;21:385–93.

Ware LB, Matthay MA. Acute pulmonary edema. *N Engl J Med* 2005;353:2788–96.

18.8 ASPIRATION SYNDROMES

Aspiration syndromes can be arbitrarily divided into two types:
1. Acute aspiration syndrome, and
2. Chronic recurrent aspiration.

1. Acute Aspiration Syndrome

Acute aspiration syndrome may result from aspiration of large volumes of gastric contents or from toxic aspiration.

1a. *Gastric Contents*

Aspiration of large volumes of gastric contents most commonly occurs after vomiting. It is an infrequent complication of general anesthesia, gastroenteritis, and an altered level of consciousness. Increased clinical severity is noted with volumes greater than approximately 0.8 ml/kg and/or pH < 2.5. Hypoxemia, hemorrhagic pneumonitis, atelactasis, intravascular fluid shifts, and pulmonary edema all occur rapidly with massive aspiration. Most clinical changes are present within minutes to 1–2 hr after aspiration. Over the next 24–48 hr there is a marked increase in lung parenchymal neutrophil infiltration, mucosal sloughing and alveolar consolidation that often correlates with increasing infiltrates on chest roentgenograms. Infection usually does not have a role in initial lung injury after aspiration of gastric contents but such aspiration may impair pulmonary defenses, predisposing the patient to secondary bacterial pneumonia. In the patient who has shown clinical improvement but then develops clinical worsening, especially with fever and leukocytosis, secondary bacterial pneumonia should be suspected.

Treatment: If a patient has had large volume or highly toxic substance aspiration, and already has an artificial airway in place, it is important to perform immediate suctioning of the airway. Patient's oxygenation should be measured by oximetry or blood-gas analysis, and chest radiograph taken, even if asymptomatic. If the chest radiograph and oxygen saturation are normal, and the patient remain asymptomatic, home observation, after a period of observation in the hospital is adequate. No treatment is indicated, but the caregivers are instructed to bring the child back in for medical attention should respiratory symptoms or fever develops.

For those patients who present with or develop abnormal findings during observation, oxygen therapy is given to correct hypoxemia. Endotracheal intubation and mechanical ventilation are often necessary for more severe cases. Bronchodilators may be tried but are usually of limited benefit. Cortico-steroids do not appear to have any benefit; their use may increase the risk of secondary infection. Prophylactic antibiotics are not indicated except in serious cases for early antibiotic coverage. If used, antibiotics should be used that cover for anaerobic microbes. If the aspiration event occurs in hospitalized patients or chronically ill patient, coverage of *Pseudomonas* and enteric gram-negative organisms should be considered. Mortality is high if three or few lobes are involved. Most patients, in whom complications such as infection or barotraumas do not develop, recover in 2–3 wk, although prolonged damage may persist, with scarring and bronchiolitis obliterans.

Prevention: Prevention of aspiration should be the aim when airway manipulation is necessary for intubation or other invasive procedures. Feeding with enteral tubes passed beyond the pylorus and elevating the head of the bed in mechanically ventilated patients have been shown to reduce the incidence of aspiration complications in the intensive care unit.

1b. *Hydrocarbon Aspiration*

The most dangerous consequence of acute hydro-carbon ingestion is usually aspiration and resulting pneumonitis. Hydrocarbons with lower surface tensions (kerosene oil, petrol, turpentine, naphthalene) have more potential for aspiration toxicity than heavier mineral or fuel oils. Ingestion of >30 ml (approximate volume of adult swallow) of hydrocarbon is associated with an increased risk of severe pneumonitis. Clinical findings of chest retractions, grunting, cough, and fever may occur as soon as 30 min after aspiration, or may be delayed for several hours. Lung radiograph changes usually occur within 2–8 hr, peaking in 48–72 hr. Pneumatoceles and pleural effusions may occur. Patients presenting with cough, shortness of breath, or hypoxemia are at high risk of pneumonitis. Persistent pulmonary function abnormalities can be present many years after hydrocarbon aspiration. Other organ systems also may suffer serious injury, especially the liver, central nervous system, and heart. Cardiac dysrhythmias may occur and be exacerbated by hypoxia and acid–base or electrolyte disturbances.

Treatment: Gastric emptying is always contraindicated because the risk of aspiration is greater than any systemic toxicity. Treatment is generally supportive with oxygen, fluids, and ventilatory support as necessary.
1. The child who has no symptoms and a normal chest radiograph should be observed for 6–8 hr to ensure safe discharge.
2. Certain hydrocarbons have more inherent systemic toxicity. The pneumonic CHAMP refers collectively

to these: camphor, halogenated carbons, aromatic hydrocarbons, and those associated with metals and pesticides. Patients who ingest these compounds in volumes >30 ml, such as might occur with intentional overdose, may benefit from gastric emptying. This is a dangerous procedure that can result in further aspiration. If a cuffed endotracheal tube can be placed without inducing vomiting, this should be considered, especially in the presence of altered mental status.

3. Other substances that are particularly toxic and occasionally aspirated, causing significant lung injury, when aspirated or inhaled include baby powder, chlorine, shellac, beryllium, and mercury vapors. Repeated exposures to lower concentrations of these agents may lead to chronic lung disease, such as interstitial pneumonitis and granuloma formation. Corticosteroids may help reduce fibrosis development and improve pulmonary function.

2. Chronic Recurrent Aspiration

The recurrent aspiration of gastric, nasal, or oral contents can lead to several clinical presentations, including recurrent bronchitis or bronchiolitis, recurrent pneumonia, atelectasis, wheezing, cough, apnea or laryngospasm. Pathologic outcomes include granulomatous inflammation, interstitial inflammation, fibrosis, lipoid pneumonia, and bronchiolitis obliterans. The disorders that are frequently associated with recurrent aspiration are listed in Box 18.2. The most common underlying problem include oropharyngeal incoordination and gastroesophageal reflux (GER).

Box 18.2: Conditions frequently associated with recurrent aspiration

Anatomical and mechanical: Gastroesophageal reflux disease (GERD); cleft palate; tracheoesophageal fistula; laryngeal cleft; vascular ring; micrognathia; macroglossia; achalasia; esophageal foreign body; tracheostomy; endotracheal tube; nasoenteric tube; collagen vascular disease (scleroderma, dermatomyositis); obesity

Neuromuscular: Altered consciousness; immaturity of swallowing/prematurity; cerebral palsy; dysautonomia; increased intracranial pressure; hydrocephalus; vocal cord paralysis; muscular dystrophy; myasthenia gravis; Guillain-Barré syndrome; Werdnig-Hoffmann disease; ataxia-telangiectasia; cerebral vascular accident

Miscellaneous: Poor feeding techniques (bottle propping, overfeeding, inappropriate foods for toddlers); poor oral hygiene; gingivitis; prolonged hospitalization; gastric outlet or intestinal obstruction; bronchopulmonary dysplasia; viral infection

---

Clinical manifestations: The timing of symptoms in relation to feedings, positional changes, spitting, vomiting, arching or gastric discomfort in an older child and nocturnal symptoms with coughing or wheezing are characteristic clinical manifestations. Coughing or gagging may be minimal or absent in a child with a depressed cough or gag reflex. Observation of a feeding is essential when considering a diagnosis of recurrent aspiration and particular attention should be given to nasopharyngeal reflux, difficulty with sucking or swallowing and associated coughing and choking. Oral cavity should be examined for gross abnormalities and stimulated to assess the gag reflex. Drooling or excessive accumulation of secretions in the mouth suggests dysphagia. Transient wheezes or crackles after feeding are heard on auscultation, particularly in the dependent lung segments.

Over 50% of children with chronic asthma and/or recurrent pneumonia also have excessive gastroesophageal reflux (GER). In addition to these disorders, GER has been associated with apnea (both central and obstructive), stridor, and recurrent cough. It is also associated with bronchopulmonary dysplasia and cystic fibrosis.

Laboratory findings: A plain chest radiograph may reveal segmental or lobar infiltrates, diffuse infiltrates, bronchial wall thickening, hyperinflation or normal findings. CT scan may show infiltrates with decreased attenuation suggestive of lipoid pneumonia. A modified barium swallow with videofluoroscopy is done to evaluate the swallowing mechanism as it occasionally detects aspiration in patients without abnormal respiratory findings. The child should be seated in a normal eating position and consistencies of barium or barium impregnated foods are offered.

Treatment: If chronic aspiration is associated with another underlying medical condition, treatment should be directed toward that problem. Mild dysphagia can be treated with alteration of feeding position or giving thicker foods. Nasogastric tube feedings can be temporarily utilized during periods of transient vocal cord dysfunction or other dysphagia. Postpyloric feedings may also be helpful, especially when GER is the cause. Medical treatment with anticholinergics such as glycopyrrolate or scopolamine, or botulism toxin may significantly reduce salivation and morbidity from salivary aspiration but often has side effects. Surgical procedures may be considered for the most severe cases, such as tracheostomy, fundoplication with gastrostomy or jejunostomy feeding tube, salivary gland excision, ductal ligation, laryngotracheal separation, esophagogastric disconnection.

Bynum L, Pierce A. Pulmonary aspiration of gastric contents. *Am Rev Respir Dis* 1976;114:1129–36.

Celedon JC. Litonuja L, Ryan L, et al. Bottle feeding on the bed or crib before sleep time and wheezing in early childhood. *Pediatrics* 2002;110: e77.

Colombo JL. Aspiration syndromes. In: Kliegman RM, Behrman RE, Jenson HB, Stanton BF (eds). *Nelson Textbook of Pediatrics.* 18th edn. Vol. 2. Philadelphia: Saunders, 2007;1789–90.

Colombo JL. Chronic recurrent aspiration. In: Kliegman RM, Behrman RE, Jenson HB, Stanton BF (eds). *Nelson Textbook of Pediatrics.* 18th edn. Vol. 2. Philadelphia: Saunders, 2007; 1790–2.

Marik PE, Aspiration pneumonitis and aspiration pneumonia. *N Engl J Med* 2001;144:665–71.

Mickiewicz M, Gomez HF. Hydrocarbon toxicity: General review and management guidelines. *Air Med J* 2001;20:8–11.

18.9 EOSINOPHILIC LUNG DISEASE (FORMERLY LÖFFLER SYNDROME)

Eosinophilic lung diseases are heterogeneous disorders linked by the common findings of pulmonary infiltrates and circulating or tissue eosinophilia. Now *pulmonary infiltrates with eosinophilia* (PIE) is considered more accurate label for these disorders. PIE syndromes can be divided into simple pulmonary eosinophilia (Löffler syndrome), prolonged pulmonary eosinophilia, tropical pulmonary eosinophilia, pulmonary eosinophilia with asthma, polyarteritis nodosa, chronic eosinophilic pneumonia, acute eosinophilic pneumonia, Churg-Strauss syndrome, allergic bronchopulmonary aspergillosis (ABPA), and idiopathic hypereosinophilia syndrome.

Löffler syndrome, the most common PIE syndrome in children, is characterized by migrating pulmonary infiltrates accompanied by peripheral blood eosinophilia but minimal respiratory symptoms. This term is rarely used now, because it is most likely that most patients with this diagnosis have allergic bronchopulmonary helminthiasis (parasitic), medication reactions, or ABPA. Age at presentation ranges from infancy to adolescence. Other PIE syndromes are much less common.

Etiology: In the pediatric age group, the most common etiology of PIE syndromes includes parasite infection and drug reactions. The most common parasites causing PIE syndromes are *Ascaris lumbricoides*, *Ancylostoma* species, the filarial worms (*Wuchereria bancrofti*, and *Brugia malayi*), *Strongyloides* species, *Toxocara canis* (dog round worm, and visceral larva migrans).

Drugs reported to cause PIE syndromes include sulfasalazine, penicillin, ampicillin, ibuprofen, and cromolyn. These drugs cause intense pulmonary inflammatory reactions by immunologic mechanisms.

Clinical manifestations: Patients with PIE syndromes caused by parasites or drugs present with malaise, chronic cough, intermittent fevers, dyspnea, wheezing, and occasionally abdominal pain, rash, and weight loss. In acute eosinophilic pneumonia, symptoms are usually present for less than a month and do not recur once treated. In chronic eosinophilic pneumonia, symptoms are present for more than 6 months and often recur despite successful treatment. The physical findings include tachypnea, crackles and wheezing.

Diagnosis: The diagnosis of PIE syndrome is made by clinical manifestations with associated blood eosinophila and chest radiologic findings. Radiologic findings include nonspecific interstitial, alveolar, or mixed infiltrates; the infiltrates tend to be bilateral and diffuse. Patients with chronic eosinophilic pneumonia demonstrate peripheral infiltrates with central sparing. In addition, eosinophilic lung diseases can be diagnosed by the presence of pulmonary infiltrates and eosinophilia on brochoalveolar lavage or the presence of parasitic larvae in bronchoscopic or gastric lavage. Lung biopsy can be used to make the diagnosis.

Treatment: Parasitic and drug-induced PIE syndromes have a good prognosis and resolve spontaneously with supportive care and removal of exposure. Medications to eradicate the parasites may be warranted. Patients with other forms of eosinophilic lung diseases including acute eosinophilic pneumonia and chronic eosinophilic pneumonia may require a course of corticosteroids. Prognosis for patients with most forms of eosinophilic lung disease is good except acute eosinophilic pneumonia patients.

Allen JN, Margo CM, King MA. The eosinophilic pneumonias. *Semin Respir Crit Care Med* 2002;23:127–43.

Ceviz N, Kaynar H, Olgun H, et al. Pigeon breeder's lung in childhood: is family screening necessary? *Pediatr Pulmonol* 2006;41:279–82.

Knutsen AP, Sotelo-Avila C, Albers GM. Hypersensitivity pneumonitis in children. *Pediatr Asthma Allergy Immunol* 2003; 16:247–64.

Lasker A. Parenchymal disease with prominent hypersensitivity, eosinophilic infiltration, or toxin mediated injury. In: Kliegman RM, Behrman RE, Jenson HB, Stanton BF (eds). *Nelson Textbook of Pediatrics.* 18th edn. Vol. 2. Philadelphia: Saunders, 2007;1792–5.

18.10 PNEUMONIA

Pneumonia is an inflammation of the parenchyma of lungs. It is an important cause of morbidity and mortality in childhood (particularly among children <5 yr of age) throughout the world.

Etiology: Pneumonia is caused by infectious and noninfectious causes. The causes of infectious

---

Box 18.3: Causes of infectious pneumonia

Bacterial (common): Streptococcus pneumoniae, Haemophilus influenzae type b, Group B streptococci; Group A streptococci, *Staphylococcus aureus, Mycoplasma pneumoniae*, *Chlamydia pneumoniae*, *Chlamydia trachomatis,* Mixed anaerobes, gram-negative enteric

Bacterial (uncommon): Moraxella catarrhalis, Neisseria meningitidis, Francisella tularensis, Nocardia species, *Chlamydophila psittaci*, Yersinia pestis, Legionella* species*

Mycobacterial: Mycobacterium tuberculosis, Atypical mycobacterium

Viral (common): Respiratory syncytial virus (RSV), parainfluenza types 1-3, influenza A, B, adenovirus, metapneumovirus

Viral (uncommon): Rhinovirus, enterovirus, herpes simplex, cytomegalovirus, measles, varicella, hantavirus, SARS agent

Fungal: Histoplasma capsulatum, Cryptococcus neoformans, aspergillus species, Mucormycosis, *Coccidioides immitis, Blastomyces dermatitidis*

Rickettsial: Coxiella burnetti, Rickettsia rickettsiiae*

Parasitic: Pneumocystis carinii, Ascaris, *Strongyloides* species, filarial worms

*Atypical pneumonia syndrome: Atypical in terms of extrapulmonary manifestations; low grade fever; patchy diffuse infiltrates; poor response to penicillin type of antibiotic and negative sputum Gram stain.
SARS : Severe acute respiratory syndrome

Table 18.3: Etiologic agents grouped by age of the patient	
Age group	Pathogens
Neonates (< 1 mo)	Group B Streptococcus, *Escherichia coli,* other gram-negative bacilli, *Streptococcus pneumoniae, Haemophilus influenzae (type b* nontypable)
1–3 mo	*Febrile pneumonia:* RSV, other respiratory viruses (parainfluenza viruses, influenza viruses, adenoviruses), *S. pneumoniae, H. influenzae (type b* nontypable)*
	Afebrile pneumonia: Chlamydia trachomatis, Mycoplasma hominis, Ureaplasma urealyticum, cytomegalovirus
3–12 mo	RSV, other respiratory viruses (parainfluenza viruses, influenza viruses, adenoviruses), *S. pneumoniae, H. influenzae (type b* nontypable), Chlamydia trachomatis, Mycoplasma pneumoniae,* group A Streptococcus
2–5 yr	Respiratory viruses (parainfluenza viruses, influenza viruses, adenoviruses), *S. pneumoniae, H. influenzae (type b* nontypable), Mycoplasma pneumoniae, Chlamydophila pneumonia, S. aureus,* Group A Streptococcus
5–18 yr	*M. pneumoniae, S. pneumoniae, C. pneumoniae, H. influenzae (type b* nontypable),* influenza viruses, adenoviruses, other respiratory viruses
≥18 yr	*M. pneumoniae, S. pneumoniae, C. pneumoniae, H. influenzae (type b* nontypable),* influenza viruses, adenoviruses, *Legionella pneumophila*

H. influenzae type b is uncommon with universal *H. influenzae* type b immunization; RSV: Respiratory syncytial virus

---

pneumonia are listed in Box 18.3 and Table 18.3. The noninfectious causes include aspiration of food or gastric acid, foreign bodies, hydrocarbons, and lipoid substances, hypersensitivity reactions, and drugs or radiation-induced pneumonitis. The causes of lung infection in neonates (*see* Section 8.18) are distinct from those affecting otherwise normal infants and children.

Pathogenesis: The lower respiratory tract is normally sterile. Viral pneumonia is accompanied by direct injury of the respiratory epithelium, resulting in airway obstruction from swelling, abnormal secretions, and cellular debris. The small caliber of airways in young infants makes them particularly susceptible to severe infection. The pathologic process varies according to invading bacterial infection. In case of *M. pneumoniae* the infection spread along the bronchial tree. *S. pneumoniae* produces local edema and characteristic focal lobar involvement. Group A Streptococcus infection of the lower respiratory tract results in more diffuse infection with interstitial pneumonia. *S. aureus* pneumonia manifests in confluent bronchopneumonia, which is often unilateral and associated with pneumatoceles, empyema, or at times, bronchopulmonary fistulas.

Recurrent pneumonia is defined as 2 or more episodes in a single year or 3 or more episodes ever, with

Box 18.4: Differential diagnosis of recurrent pneumonia

Hereditary disorders: Cystic fibrosis; sickle cell disease

Disorders of immunity: AIDS; Bruton agammaglobulinemia; selective IgG subclass deficiencies; common variable immunodeficiency syndrome; severe combined immunodeficiency syndrome

Disorders of leukocytes: Chronic granulomatous disease; hyperimmunologic E syndrome; leukocyte adhesion defect

Disorders of cilia: Immobile cilia syndrome; Kartagener syndrome

Anatomic disorders: Sequestration; lobar emphysema; esophageal reflux; foreign body
Tracheoesophageal fistula (H type); gastroesophageal reflux; bronchiectasis
Aspiration (oropharyngeal incoordination)

radiographic clearing between occurrences. An underlying disorder should be considered if a child experiences recurrent bacterial pneumonia (Box 18.4). Additional factors that promote pulmonary infection include trauma, anesthesia, and aspiration.

Slowly revolving pneumonia refers to the persistence of symptoms, and radiographic abnormalities beyond the expected time course. The time course varies, depending on the organism involved, the extent of disease, and the presence of associated complicating conditions.

Clinical manifestations: Viral and bacterial pneumonias are often preceded by several days of symptoms of an upper respiratory tract infection, usually rhinitis and cough. In viral pneumonia, fever is usually present; but temperatures are usually lower than in bacterial pneumonia. Tachypnea is the most consistent clinical finding of pneumonia. Increased work of breathing accompanied by intercostal, subcostal, and suprasternal retractions, nasal flaring and use of accessory muscles is common. Severe infection may be accompanied by cyanosis. Auscultation of the chest may reveal crackles and wheezing. It is often not possible to distinguish viral pneumonia clinically from diseases caused by *Mycoplasma* and other bacterial pathogens.

In older children and adolescents, a brief upper respiratory tract illness is followed by the abrupt onset of shaking chills and high fever accompanied by drowsiness with intermittent periods of restlessness, rapid respirations, a dry, hacking unproductive cough, anxiety and occasionally delirium. Circumoral cyanosis may be seen. Many children may lie on the affected side with their knees drawn up to their chest to minimize pleuritic pain.

Physical findings depend on the stage of pneumonia. Early in the course of illness, diminished breath sounds, scattered crackles are commonly heard over the affected lung field. Dullness on percussion and diminished breath sounds is noted over consolidation, effusion, or empyema. Abdominal distension may be prominent because of gastric dilation from swallowed air or ileus. Abdominal pain is common in lower lobe pneumonia. Nuchal rigidity, in the absence of meningitis, may also be prominent, especially with involvement of the right upper lobe.

Diagnosis: The chest radiograph confirms the diagnosis of pneumonia and may indicate a complication such as pleural effusion or empyema. Viral pneumonia is usually characterized by hyperinflation with bilateral interstitial infiltrates and peribronchial cuffing. Lobar consolidation is typically seen with pneumococcal pneumonia (*see* Fig. 18.1 in CD).

The peripheral white blood cell (WBC) can differentiate viral from bacterial pneumonia. In viral pneumonia, the WBC count can be normal or elevated but is usually not higher than 20,000/mm^3, with a lymphocyte predominance. Bacterial pneumonia (occasionally, adenovirus pneumonia) is often associated with an elevated WBC count in the range of 15,000–40,000/mm^3 and a predominance of granulocytes.

A large pleural effusion, lobar consolidation, and a high fever at the onset of the illness are also suggestive of a bacterial etiology. Atypical pneumonia due to *C. pneumonia* or *M. pneumonia* is difficult to distinguish from pneumococcal pneumonia by X-ray and other laboratory investigations, although pneumococcal pneumonia is associated with a higher WBC count, erythrocyte sedimentation rate (ESR), and C-reactive protein (CRP), there is considerable overlap.

Rapid detection of RSV, parainfluenza, influenza, and adenoviruses is done by DNA or RNA tests. Serologic testing is valuable as an epidemiologic tool to define the incidence and prevalence of the various respiratory viral pathogens.

The definitive diagnosis of a bacterial infection requires isolation of an organism from the blood, pleural fluid, or lung. Culture of sputum is of little value in the diagnosis of pneumonia in young children. Blood cultures are positive in only 10% of children with pneumococcal pneumonia. *M. pneumonia* can be diagnosed on the basis of a positive PCR test or seroconversion in an IgG assay; cold agglutinins at titers of >1 : 64 found in the blood in ~50% of patients are nonspecific, because other pathogens such as influenza virus may also increase cold agglutinins. Anti-streptolysin O (ASO) titer may be useful in the diagnosis of group A streptococcal pneumonia.

Treatment: The treatment of suspected bacterial pneumonia is based on the presumptive cause and the clinical appearance of the child. For mildly ill children who do not require hospitalization, amoxicillin (80–90 mg/kg/24 hr) should be prescribed. Therapeutic alternatives include cefuroxime axetil or amoxicillin/clavulanate. For school aged children and in those in whom infection with *M. pneumonia* or *C. pneumonia* (atypical pneumonia) is suggested, a macrolide antibiotic such as azithromycin is an important choice to be considered. In adolescents, a respiratory fluoroquinolone (levofloxacin, gatifloxacin, moxifloxacin, gemifloxacin) may be considered for atypical pneumonia.

The empirical treatment of suspected bacterial pneumonia in a hospitalized child depends on the clinical manifestations at the time of presentation. Parenteral cefuroxime (150 mg/kg/24 hr), cefotaxime, or ceftriaxone is the main therapy when bacterial pneumonia is suggested. If clinical features suggests staphylococcal pneumonia (pneumatoceles, empyema), initial antimicrobial therapy should also include vancomycin or clindamycin. If viral pneumonia is suspected in patients who are mildly ill with no respiratory distress, it is reasonable to withhold antibiotics. Up to 30% of patients with known viral infection may have coexisting bacterial pathogens, deterioration in clinical status indicates the possibility of superimposed bacterial infection and antibiotic therapy should be initiated. Oral zinc (20 mg/day) helps accelerate recovery from pneumonia. The factors suggesting need for hospitalization of children include age <6 mo, toxic appearance, severe respiratory distress, vomiting, dehydration, multiple lobe involvement, immunocompromised state, sickle cell anemia with acute chest syndrome, no response to appropriate oral antibiotic therapy, and noncompliant parents.

Response to treatment: Typically patients with uncomplicated community-acquired bacterial pneumonia respond to therapy with improvement in clinical symptoms (fever, cough, tachypnea, chest pain) within 48–96 hr of initiation of antibiotics. Radiographic evidence of improvement substantially lags behind clinical improvement. When the patient does not improve on appropriate antibiotic therapy **(slowly resolving pneumonia)** the following factors should be considered:

1. Complications, such as empyema
2. Bacterial resistance
3. Nonbacterial etiologies such as viruses, and aspiration of foreign bodies or food

4. Bronchial obstruction from endobronchial lesions, foreign body or mucus plug
5. Pre-existing diseases such as immunodeficiencies, ciliary dyskinesia, cystic fibrosis, pulmonary sequestration, or cystic adenomatoid malformation; and
6. Other noninfectious causes (including bronchiolitis obliterans, hypersensitivity pneumonitis, eosinophilic pneumonia, aspiration, and Wegener granulomatosis). A repeat chest X-ray should be done in determining the reason for delay in response to treatment before further investigating the patient.

Complications: Complications of pneumonia are usually the result of direct spread of bacterial infection within the thoracic cavity (pleural effusion, empyema, pericarditis) or bacteremia and hematologic spread of pneumococcal or *H influenzae* type b infection (rarely cause meningitis, suppurative arthritis and osteomyelitis). *S. aureus*, *S. pneumonia*, and *S. pyogenes* are the most common causes of parapneumonic effusions and of empyema. The main treatment of empyema is antibiotic therapy and drainage with tube thoracostomy. Additional approaches include the use of fibrinolytic therapy (urokinase, streptokinase) and selected video-assisted thoracoscopy (VATS) to debride, lyse adhesions, and drain loculated areas of pus.

Bhutta ZA. Childhood pneumonia in developing countries. *BMJ* 2006;333:612–3.

Duke T. Neonatal pneumonia in developing countries. *Arch Dis Child Fetal Neonatal Ed* 2005;90:F211–9.

Panitch HB. Evaluation of recurrent pneumonia. *Pediatr Infect Dis J* 2005;24:265–6.

Sectish TC, Prober CG. Pneumonia. In: Kliegman RM, Behrman RE, Jenson HB, Stanton BF (eds). *Nelson Textbook of Pediatrics.* 18th edn. Vol. 2. Philadelphia: Saunders, 2007; 1795–1800.

18.11 BRONCHIECTASIS

Bronchiectasis is a disease characterized by irreversible abnormal dilatation of the bronchial tree. In the developing countries infection and in the developed countries cystic fibrosis is the most important cause.

Etiology: The causes of bronchiectasis include: infections especially pertussis, measles, rubella, respiratory syncytial virus and tuberculosis; cystic fibrosis; ciliary dyskinesia; immune deficiency syndromes; right middle lobe syndrome (chronic extrinsic compression of right middle lobe bronchus by hilar lymph nodes); yellow nail syndrome (pleural effusion, lymphedema, discolored nails); Williams-Campbell syndrome (there is absence of annular bronchial cartilage); Marnier-Kuhn syndrome (congenital tracheobronchomegaly).

Pathogenesis and pathology: Three basic mechanisms are involved in the pathogenesis of bronchiectasis include obstruction, chronic inflammation, and infections. The common problem in the bronchiectasis is difficulty in clearing secretions and recurrent infections with a "vicious cycle" of infection and inflammation resulting in airway injury and remodeling. Bronchiectasis can present in any combination of three pathologic forms, cylindrical, varicose, and saccular (cystic) bronchiectasis. Saccular (cystic) is the most severe form of bronchiectasis.

Clinical manifestations: Cough and copious purulent sputum production are the most common complaints. Younger children may swallow the sputum. Hemoptysis, fever, anorexia and poor weight gain is also observed. Physical examination typically reveals crackles localized to the affected area, but wheezing and digital clubbing may also occur.

Diagnosis: Chest radiographs tend to be nonspecific; typical findings can include increase in size and loss of bonchovascular markings, crowding of bronchi, and loss of lung volume. CT provides information on disease location, presence of mediastinal lesions, and the extent of segmental involvement. The CT findings in patients with bronchiectasis typically include cylindrical ("tram lines," "signet ring appearance"), varicose (bronchi with "beaded contour"), cystic (cysts in "strings and clusters"), or mixed forms. The lower lobes are most commonly affected. Pulmonary function studies may demonstrate an obstructive, restrictive, or mixed pattern; impaired diffusion capacity is a late finding.

Treatment: The initial treatment is medical and aims at decreasing airway obstruction and controlling infection. Chest physiotherapy (postural drainage), antibiotics and bronchodilators are essential. Two to four weeks antibiotics are often necessary to manage acute exacerbations adequately. The choice of antibiotics depends on the identification and sensitivity of organisms found on deep throat, sputum (induced or spontaneous), or bronchoalveolar lavage fluid cultures. Chronic prophylactic oral (macrolide antibiotics include erythromycin, clarithromycin and azithromycin) or nebulized antibiotics may be beneficial. Any underlying disorder (immunodeficiency or aspiration) that may be contributing must be treated. When localized bronchiectasis becomes more severe or resistant to medical management, segmental or lobar resection may be performed. Lung transplantation can also be performed in patients with bronchiectasis.

Prognosis: Earlier recognition or prevention of predisposing conditions, more powerful and wide-spectrum antibiotics, and improved surgical outcomes are likely reasons for improved prognosis.

Barker AF. Bronchiectasis. *N Engl J Med* 2002;346:1383–93.

Lakser O. Bronchiectasis. In: Kliegman RM, Behrman RE, Jenson HB, Stanton BF (eds). *Nelson Textbook of Pediatrics.* 18th edn. Vol. 2. Philadelphia: Saunders, 2007; 1800–1.

Morrissey BM, Evans SJ. Severe bronchiectasis. *Clin Rev Allergy Immunol* 2003;25:233–48.

18.12 PULMONARY ABSCESS

Pulmonary abscesses are localized areas composed of thick-walled purulent material formed as a result of lung infection that lead to destruction of lung parenchyma, cavitation, and central necrosis. A *primary lung abscess* occurs in a previously healthy patient with no underlying disorders. A *secondary lung abscess* occurs in a patient with underlying or predisposing conditions. The conditions that predispose children to the development of pulmonary abscesses, including aspiration, pneumonia, cystic fibrosis, gastroesophageal reflux, tracheoesophageal fistula, immunodeficiencies, postoperative complications of tonsillectomy and adenoidectomy, seizures and a variety of neurological diseases. In children, aspirations of infected materials or a foreign body is the predominant source of the organisms causing abscesses.

Both anaerobic and aerobic organisms cause lung abscesses. Fungi can also cause lung abscesses, particularly in immunocompromised patients. Common anaerobic bacteria are *Bacteroides* spp., *Fusobacterium* spp., and *Peptostreptococcus* spp., and aerobic bacteria are *Streptococcus* spp., *Staphylococcus aureus, Escherichia coli, Klebsiella pneumoniae,* and *Pseudomonas aeruginosa.* In all patients with a lung abscess aerobic and anaerobic cultures should be performed.

Clinical manifestations: The most common symptoms include cough, fever, tachypnea, dyspnea, chest pain, vomiting, sputum production, weight loss, and hemoptysis. Physical examination reveals tachypnea, dyspnea, and retractions with accessory muscle use, decreased breath sounds, and dullness to percussion in the affected area. Crackles and, occasionally, a prolonged expiratory phase may be heard on auscultation.

Diagnosis: Chest radiograph shows a parenchymal inflammation with a cavity containing an air-fluid level. Pneumatoceles, with thin and smooth walled localized air collections with or without an air-fluid level should be distinguished from an abscess (a thick-walled lesion and an air-fluid level). Pneumatoceles, often resolve spontaneously with the specific treatment of pneumonia.

The etiologic bacteria (helpful in guiding the antibiotic choice) can be determined by methods, such as Gram stain of sputum (sputum cultures typically yield mixed bacteria and are unreliable), or from direct lung puncture and percutaneous (aided by CT guidance), bronchoscopic, and transtracheal aspiration. In previously normal hosts, empiric therapy can be initiated in the absence of cultural material.

Treatment: In uncomplicated cases, 2–3 wk course of parenteral antibiotics, followed by a course of oral antibiotics to complete a total of 4–6 wk. Antibiotic choice should be guided by gram stain and culture but initially should include aerobic and anaerobic coverage typically with clindamycin or amoxicillin/clavulinic acid. If gram-negative bacteria are suspected or isolated, an aminolycoside should be added. For severely ill patients or those who fail to improve after 7–10 days of appropriate antimicrobial therapy, surgical intervention should be considered.

Prognosis: Most children become asymptomatic within 7–10 days, although the fever can persist for as long as 3 wk. Radiologic abnormalities usually resolve in 1–3 mo but can persist for years.

Brook I. Anaerobic pulmonary infections in children. *Pediatr Emerg Care* 2004;20:636–40.

De A, Varaiya A, Mathur M. Anaerobes in pleuropulmonary infections. *Indian J Med Microbiol* 2002;20:150–2.

Lakser O. Pulmonary abscess. In: Kliegman RM, Behrman RE, Jenson HB, Stanton BF (eds), *Nelson Textbook of Pediatrics,* 18th edn. Vol. 2. Philadelphia: Saunders, 2007;1801–03.

18.13 CYSTIC FIBROSIS

Cystic fibrosis (CF) is an inherited multisystem disorder of children and adults, characterized chiefly by obstruction and infection of airways and maldigestion and its consequences. CF is inherited as an autosomal recessive trait. The CF gene codes for a protein of 1,480 amino acids called *CF transmembrane regulator (CFTR).* CF occurs most frequently in white populations of Northern Europe, North America, and Australia/New Zealand.

Clinical Manifestations

Respiratory tract: Cough may be dry and hacking, but eventually it becomes loose and productive. Expectorated mucous is usually purulent. Viral infections occur frequently. Acute sinusitis is infrequent, although the paranasal sinuses are virtually always opacified radiographically. Nasal obstruction and rhinorrhea are common, caused by inflamed, swollen mucus membranes or in some cases polyposis. Nasal polyps are most commonly occurring between 5 and 20 yr of age.

Intestinal tract: In newborn infants with CF meconium ileus and meconium peritonitis may occur. Abdominal distension, emesis, and failure to pass meconium appear in the 1st 24–48 hr of life. More than 85% of affected children show evidence of maldigestion from exocrine pancreatic insufficiency. Symptoms include frequent, bulky, greasy stools (and stool contains droplets of fat) and failure to gain weight even when food intake appears to be large. Less common gastrointestinal manifestations include epigastric pain owing to duodenal inflammation, acid or bile reflux with esophagitis symptoms, intussusception, fecal impaction of the cecum with an asymptomatic right lower quadrant mass, subacute appendicitis and periappendiceal abscess, and rectal prolapse. Occasionally, hypoproteinemia with anasarca appears in malnourished infants, especially if children are fed soy-based preparations.

Neurologic dysfunction (dementia, peripheral neuropathy) and hemolytic anemia may occur because of vitamin E deficiency. Hypoprothrombinemia owing to vitamin K deficiency may result in a bleeding diathesis. Clinical manifestations of other fat-soluble vitamin deficiencies, such as decreased bone densities and night blindness, have been noted. Rickets is rare.

Biliary tract: Evidence of liver dysfunction is most often detected in the 1st 15 yr of life. Biliary cirrhosis is observed in 2–3% of patients and the clinical findings include icterus, ascites, hematemesis from esophageal varices and evidence of hypersplenism. Biliary colic secondary to cholelithiasis may occur in 2nd decade or later.

Pancreas: In addition to exocrine pancreatic insufficiency, evidence for hyperglycemia and glycosuria including polyuria and weight loss may appear especially in the 2nd decade of life. Ketoacidosis usually does not occur, but eye, kidney, and other vascular complications have been noted in patients living ≥ 10 yr after the onset of hyperglycemia. Recurrent, acute pancreatitis occurs occasionally in individuals who have residual exocrine pancreatic function and may be the sole manifestation of two CFTR mutations.

Genitourinary tract: Sexual development is often delayed but only by an average of 2 yr. More than 95% of males are azoospermic because of failure of development of Wolffian duct structures, but sexual function is generally unimpaired. The incidence of inguinal hernia, hydrocele and undescended testis is higher than expected. Adolescent females may experience secondary amenorrhea, especially with exacerbations of pulmonary disease. Cervicitis and accumulation of tenacious mucus in the cervical canal have been noted. The female fertility rate is diminished.

Sweat glands: Excessive loss of salt in the sweat predisposes young children to salt depletion episodes, especially during episodes of gastroenteritis and during warm weather. These children present with *hypochloremic alkalosis*. Frequently, parents notice salt "frosting" of the skin or a salty taste when they kiss the child. A few genotypes (3849 + 10 kb C>T) are associated with normal sweat chloride values.

Diagnosis: The diagnosis of CF has been based on a positive quantitative sweat test ($Cl^- \geq 60$ mEq/L) in conjunction with 1 or more of the following: typical obstructive pulmonary disease, documented exocrine pancreatic insufficiency, or a positive family history. Diagnostic criteria have been recommended to include additional testing procedures (Box 18.5).

Sweat testing: The sweat test, using pilocarpine iontophoresis to collect sweat and chemical analysis of its chloride content is the standard approach to diagnosis. A 3 mA electric current is used to carry pilocarpine into the skin of the forearm and locally stimulate the sweat glands. After washing the arm with distilled water, sweat is collected on filter paper or gauze (or in capillary tube) that has been placed on the stimulated skin and covered to prevent evaporation. After 30 min, the filter paper is removed, weighed, and eluted in distilled water. Analysis of chloride in these samples is done by chloridometer. For reliable results, at least 75 mg and preferably 100 mg of sweat should be collected. Testing may be difficult in the 1st 2 wk of life because of low sweat rates but is recommended any time after 1st 48 hr of life. More than 60 mEq/L of chloride in sweat is diagnostic of CF if 1 or more other criteria are present. False-negative test results may be encountered in children with hypoproteinemic edema; false-positive results can occur when testing is performed on skin affected by eczema or contaminated with skin creams or lotions.

Non-CF conditions associated with elevated concentrations of sweat electrolytes include untreated adrenal insufficiency, ectodermal dysplasia, hereditary nephrogenic diabetes insipidus, glucose-6-phosphate deficiency, hypothyroidism, hypoparathyroidism, familial cholestasis, pancreatitis, mucopolysaccharidoses, fucosidosis, and malnutrition. Most of these conditions can be distinguished from CF by clinical criteria.

Box 18.5: Diagnostic criteria for cystic fibrosis (CF)

Presence of typical clinical features (respiratory, gastrointestinal, or genitourinary) or a history of CF in a sibling or a positive newborn screening test plus laboratory evidence of CFTR dysfunction: two elevated sweat chloride concentrations obtained on separate days or identification of two CF mutations or an abnormal nasal potential difference measurement CFTR, CF transmembrane regulator

---

DNA testing: DNA testing identifies $\geq 90\%$ individuals who carry 2 CF mutations. Some children with typical CF manifestations have 1 or no detectable mutations by this methodology. Some laboratories perform comprehensive mutation analysis, screening for all the >1,500 identified mutations.

Newborn screening: Most newborns with CF can be identified by determination of immunoreactive trypsinogen and limited DNA testing on blood spots, coupled with confirmatory sweat analysis. This screening test is ~95% sensitive.

Treatment

1. *General approach to care:* Initial efforts after the diagnosis should be intensive and include baseline assessment, initiation of treatment, clearing of pulmonary involvement, education of patient and parents and 2–3 monthly follow-up. Immunoprophylaxis especially against measles, pertussis and influenza is essential. For children, who have episodic acute or low grade chronic lung infection ≥ 2 wk of intensive inhalation and physical therapy and intravenous antibiotics are indicated. Intravenous antibiotics may be required infrequently or as often as every 2–3 mo. Because therapy is medication-intensive, monitoring of iatrogenic problems is also an important part of management

2. *Nutritional therapy:* Up to 90% of patients have loss of exocrine pancreatic function and inadequate digestion and absorption of fats and proteins. They require dietary adjustments, pancreatic enzyme replacement, and supplementary vitamins. Children with CF need to exceed the required caloric intake to grow (130 kcal/kg), along with daily supplement of the fat-soluble vitamins (A, D, E, and K) and minerals especially zinc and iron. Now a days normal fat, high protein and high-caloric diet is recommended. With the advent of improved pancreatic enzyme products, normal to increased amount of fat is well tolerated. With advance lung disease, weight stabilization or gain sometimes requires nocturnal feeding via nasogastric tube or percutaneous enterostomy or by short-term intravenous hyperalimentation. Three times a week

human recombinant growth hormone therapy has improved nutritional outcomes, including positive effects on nitrogen balance and improved height and weight velocities.

Pancreatic enzyme replacement should not exceed 2,500 lipase units/kg/meal in most circumstances. One to 3 capsules/meal is sufficient for most patients; infants need 2,000–4,000 lipase units per feeding.

3. *Pulmonary therapy:* The object is to clear secretions and to control infection.

Inhalation therapy: Aerosol therapy is used to deliver medications and hydrate the lower respiratory tract. The basic aerosol solution is 0.9% saline. In patients with reactive airways, salbutamol or other β-agonists are added. Human recombinant DNase (2.5 mg), given as a single daily aerosol dose, improves pulmonary function, decreases numbers of pulmonary exacerbations, and promotes a sense of well-being in patients who have moderate disease and purulent secretions.

Airway clearance therapy: This treatment usually consists of chest percussion combined with postural drainage, because the cough clears mucous from large airways, but chest vibrations are required to move secretions from small airways where expiratory flow rates are low. Chest physical therapy (PT) is recommended 1–4 times a day, depending on the severity of lung dysfunction. Cough, huffing, or forced expirations are encouraged after each lung segment is "drained."

Antibiotic therapy: Wherever possible the choice of antibiotic should be guided by in vitro sensitivity. Tetracycline should be avoided in children <9 yr of age. Although many patients improve within 7 days, it is usually advisable to extend the period of treatment to at least 14 days.

Nasal polyps: Nasal polyps are most prevalent in the 2nd decade of life. Local corticosteroids and nasal decongestants occasionally provide some relief. When the polyps completely obstruct the nasal airway, rhinorrhea becomes constant, or widening of the nasal bridge is noticed, surgical removal is indicated. Polyps after surgical removal may recur promptly or after a symptom-free interval of months to year or inexplicably stop developing in many adults.

Rhinosinusitis: Acute or chronic sinus-related symptoms are treated initially with antibiotics, with or without maxillary sinus aspiration for cultures. Functional endoscopic sinus surgery has provided benefit.

4. *Intestinal complications:* A number of intestinal complications including meconium ileus, distal intestinal obstruction syndrome (DIOS, meconium ileus equivalent), gastroesophageal reflux, rectal prolapse, hepatobiliary disease require extra attention or special measures.

5. *Pancreatitis:* Pancreatitis can be precipitated by fatty meals, alcohol ingestion, or tetracycline therapy. Serum amylase and lipase levels may remain elevated for long periods. Treatment is discussed in Chapter 16.

6. *Hyperglycemia:* Onset of hyperglycemia occurs most frequently after the 1st decade. Prevalence is greater in females and in "F508 homozygotes. With persistent glycosuria and symptoms, insulin treatment should be instituted. Oral hypoglycemic agents may also be effective. Exocrine pancreatic insufficiency and malabsorption make strict dietary control of hyperglycemia difficult. Corticosteroid therapy should be avoided. The development of significant hyperglycemia favors acquisition of *P. aeruginosa* and *B. cepacia* in the airways and may adversely affect pulmonary function. Long-term vascular complications of diabetes occur, hence a good control of blood sugar levels are essential.

7. *Salt depletion:* Sweat salt losses can be high, especially in warm arid climates. Children should have free access to salt, and precautions against over-dressing infants should be observed. Hyperchloremic alkalosis should be suspected in any infant who has symptoms of gastroenteritis, and prompt fluid and electrolyte therapy should be instituted as needed.

Prognosis: CF remains a life-limiting disorder, although survival has improved. Children with CF usually have good school attendance records and should not be restricted in their activities. With appropriate medical and psychosocial support, children and adolescents with CF generally cope well in life.

Boat TF, Acton JD. Cystic fibrosis. In: Kliegman RM, Behrman RE, Jenson HB, Stanton BF (eds). *Nelson Textbook of Pediatrics.* 18th edn. Vol. 2. Philadelphia: Saunders, 2007; 1803–17.

Kabra SK, Kabra M, Lodha R, et al. Cystic fibrosis in India. Pediatric Pulmonology 2007;42:1087–94.

18.14 PULMONARY EMBOLISM, INFARCTION, AND HEMORRHAGE

Pulmonary Embolus and Infarction

Embolic disease occurs in children and adolescents, although the risk of development of venous thromboembolic disease (VTE) is less in children than adults. Embolic disease has variable etiologies in children. An embolus can contain thrombus, air, amniotic fluid, septic material, or metastatic neoplastic tissue; however, thromboemboli are most commonly encountered. Children with deep venous thrombosis (DVT) and pulmonary embolism (PE) are much more likely to have 1 or more identifiable conditions or circumstances placing them at risk. A commonly encountered risk factor for DVT and PE in the pediatric population is the presence of a central venous catheter. The presence of a catheter in a vessel lumen as well as instilled medications can induce endothelial damage and favor thrombus formation. Thrombotic disease can also present in older infants and children. Disease can be congenital or acquired; DVT/PE may be the initial presentation. Septic emboli are rare in children but may be caused by osteomyelitis, cellulitis, urinary tract infection, jugular vein or umbilical thrombophlebitis, and right-sided endocarditis.

In the neonatal period thromboembolic disease and PE are often related to indwelling catheters used for parenteral nutrition and medication delivery. Emboli in this age group may occasionally reflect maternal risk factors, such as diabetes or toxemia of pregnancy. Infants with congenitally acquired homozygous deficiencies of antithrombin, protein C, and protein S are also likely to present in the neonatal period.

Clinical manifestations: Presentation is variable and many pulmonary emboli are silent. Common symptoms and signs of PE include hypoxia (cyanosis), tachypnea, dyspnea, cough, diaphoresis, and chest pain. Localized crackles may occasionally be appreciated on examination.

Laboratory findings and diagnosis: Patients with septic emboli may have multiple areas of modularity and cavitation, which are typically located peripherally in both lung fields. A review of complete blood count (CBC), urinalysis, and coagulation profile is warranted.

Electrocardiographs may reveal ST segment changes or evidence of pulmonary hypertension with right ventricular failure (cor pulmonale), but these changes are nonspecific and nondiagnostic. Echocardiograms may be warranted to assess ventricular size and function. A transthoracic echocardiogram is required if there is any suspicion of intracardiac thrombi or endocarditis. Noninvasive venous ultrasound with Doppler flow can be used to confirm DVT in the lower extremities. In patients with significant venous thrombosis, D-dimers are usually elevated. When a high level of suspicion exists, confirmatory testing with venography should be pursued. Helical or spiral CT with intravenous contrast is valuable and the diagnostic test of choice to detect a PE. CT studies detect emboli in lobar and segmental vessels.

Treatment: Initial treatment should be directed toward stabilization of the patient, which includes ventilation, fluid resuscitation, and inotropic support. After the patient with a PE has been stabilized, the next therapeutic approach is anticoagulation. Treatment is generally initiated with heparin. Anticoagulation is usually achieved when the activated partial thromboplastin time (PTT) is 1.5–2 times the control. Long-term therapy with heparin should be avoided whenever possible. Thrombolytic agents (urokinase, streptokinase, and recombinant tissue plasminogen activator) can be combined with anticoagulants in early stages of treatment. Combined therapy may reduce the incidences of progressive thromboembolism, pulmonary embolus, and postphlebitic syndrome. The use of thrombolytic agents in patients with active bleeding, recent cerebrovascular accidents, or trauma is contraindicated. Surgical embolectomy should be considered in patients who are refractory to standard therapy. Mortality in pediatric patients with PE is likely to be attributable to an underlying disease process rather than to the embolus itself.

Pulmonary Hemorrhage and Hemoptysis

Conditions that can present with pulmonary hemorrhage or hemoptysis in children are listed in Box 18.6. Hemoptysis must always be separated from episodes of hemetemesis or epistaxis, as all can present similarly in the young patient.

Clinical manifestations: Older children and young adults with a focal hemorrhage may complain of warmth or a 'bubbling" sensation in the chest wall; this may aid the clinician in locating the area. Rapid and large volume of blood loss presents with symptoms of cyanosis, respiratory distress, and shock. Chronic, subclinical blood loss may present with anemia, fatigue, dyspnea, or altered activity tolerance. Less commonly, patients present with persistent infiltrates on chest radiograph or symptoms of chronic illness such as failure to thrive.

Laboratory findings and diagnosis: Every patient with suspected hemorrhage should have a laboratory evaluation with CBC and coagulation studies. The CBC finding may demonstrate a microcytic, hypochromic anemia. The classic finding, which defines pulmonary hemorrhage, is that of hemosiderin-laden macrophages in pulmonary secretions. These can be obtained by sputum analysis with Prussian blue staining. Chest X-rays may demonstrate fluffy bilateral densities. Alveolar infiltrates on chest radiograph, often symmetric and diffuse may be seen with recent bleeding. CT may be indicated to assess for underlying disease processes. Flexible bronchoscopy with

Box 18.6: Etiology of pulmonary hemorrhage (hemoptysis)

Focal hemorrhage

1. Bronchitis and bronchiectasis (especially cystic fibrosis related)
2. Infection (acute or chronic)
3. Tuberculosis
4. Trauma
5. Pulmonary arteriovenous malformation
6. Foreign body (chronic)
7. Neoplasm including hemangioma
8. Pulmonary embolus with or without infarction

Diffuse hemorrhage

1. Idiopathic of infancy
2. Congenital heart disease (including pulmonary hypertension, veno-occlusive disease)
3. Prematurity
4. Cow's milk hyperactivity (Heiner syndrome)
5. Goodpasture syndrome
6. Collagen vascular diseases (SLE rheumatoid arthritis)
7. Henoch-Schönlein purpura and vasculitic disorder
8. Granulomatous disease (Wegener)
9. Celiac disease
10. Coagulopathy (congenital or acquired)
11. Malignancy
12. Immunodeficiency
13. Exogenous toxins
14. Idiopathic pulmonary hemosiderosis
15. Tuberous sclerosis
16. Lymphangiomyomatosis or lymphangioleiomyomatosis
17. Physical injury or abuse

bronchoalveolar lavage is frequently utilized to obtain pulmonary secretions in a child or young adult who is not able to expectorate secretions. Lung biopsy is indicated if the bleeding is chronic or an etiology is unavailable by other methods.

Treatment: In patients with massive blood loss, volume resuscitation and transfusion of blood products are necessary. Maintenance of adequate ventilation and circulatory function are necessary. Rigid bronchoscopy is used for removal of debris or the application of topical vasoconstrictive agents. In patients with diffuse hemorrhage, corticosteroids and other immunosuppressive agents have been shown to be of benefit. Prognosis depends largely on the underling disease process.

Godfrey S. Pulmonary hemorrhage/ hemoptysis in children. *Pediatr Pulmonol* 2004;17:476–84.

Goldhaber SZ. Pulmonary embolism. *Lancet* 2004;363:1295–305.

Johnson AS, Bolte RG. Pulmonary embolism in pediatric patient. *Pediatr Emerg Care* 2004;20:555–60.

Nevin MA. Pulmonary Embolism, Infarction, and Hemorrhage. In: Kliegman RM, Behrman RE, Jenson HB, Stanton BF (eds). *Nelson Textbook of Pediatrics.* 18th edn. Vol. 2. Philadelphia: Saunders, 2007;1826–30.

Robinson GV. Pulmonary embolism in hospital practice. *Br Med J* 2006;332:156–60.

18.15 ATELECTASIS

Atelectasis, the incomplete expansion or complete collapse of air bearing tissue results from obstruction of air intake into the alveolar sacs. Segmental, lobar, or whole lung collapse is associated with the absorption of air contained in the alveoli, which are no longer ventilated.

Pathophysiology: The causes of atelectasis can be divided into five groups (Table 18.4). Viral infections in young children, specifically respiratory syncytial virus can cause multiple areas of atelectasis.

Clinical manifestations: A small area is likely to be asymptomatic. When a large area of normal lung becomes atelectatic, especially if it occurs suddenly, dyspnea accompanied by rapid shallow respirations, tachycardia, cough, and often cyanosis occurs. If the obstruction is removed, the symptoms disappear rapidly. Massive atelectasis usually presents with

Table 18.4: Anatomic causes of atelectasis	
Cause	*Clinical examples*
External compression on the pulmonary parenchyma	Pleural effusion, pneumothorax, intrathoracic tumors, diaphragmatic hernia
Endobronchial obstruction completely obstructing air entry	Enlarged lymph node, tumor, cardiac enlargement, foreign body, mucoid plug, broncholithiasis
Intraluminal obstruction of a bronchus	Foreign body, granulomatous tissue, tumor, secretions, including mucus plugs, bronchiectasis, pulmonary abscess, asthma, chronic bronchitis, acute laryngotracheobronchitis
Intrabronchiolar obstruction	Bronchiolitis, interstitial pneumonitis, asthma
Respiratory compromise or paralysis	Neuromuscular abnormalities, osseous deformities, overly restrictive casts and surgical dressings, defective movement of the diaphragm or restriction of respiratory effort

dyspnea, cyanosis, and tachycardia. An affected child is extremely anxious and, if old enough, complains of chest pain.

Physical findings include limitation of chest movement, decreased breath sound intensity, and coarse crackles. Breath sounds are decreased or absent over extensive atelectatic areas. When massive atelectasis occurs the chest appears flat on the affected side, where decreased respiratory movement, dullness on percussion, and feeble or absent breath sounds are also noted. Postoperatively, atelectasis usually presents within 24 hr after operation but may not occur for several days.

In contrast to adult patients in whom the lower lobes and, in particular, the left lower lobe are most often involved, upper lobes, especially the right upper lobe are involved in children. There is also a high incidence of upper lobe atelectasis and especially right upper lobe collapse in neonatal intensive care units. This may be due to the endotracheal tube moving into the right main stem bronchus and obstructing or causing inflammation of the bronchus to the right upper lobe.

Diagnosis: The typical findings on chest radiograph include volume loss and displacement of fissures. Atypical presentations include atelectasis presenting as a mass-like opacity and atelectasis in an unusual location. Lobar atelectasis may be associated with pneumothorax. The typical findings of massive collapse on chest X-ray include elevation of diaphragm, narrowing of the intercostals spaces, and displacement of mediastinal structures and heart toward the affected side (*see* Fig. 18.2 in CD). In foreign body aspiration, the site of atelectasis usually indicates the site of foreign body in the chest X-ray. Atelectasis is more common when patients have a delay in diagnosis of > 2 wk duration. Bronchoscopic examination reveals a collapsed main bronchus when the obstruction is at the tracheobronchial junction and may also disclose the nature of obstruction.

Treatment: Treatment depends on the cause of the collapse. If effusion or pneumothorax is responsible, the external pressure must be removed. Bronchoscopic examination is immediately indicated if atelectasis is the result of a foreign body or any other bronchial obstruction. For bilateral atelectasis, bronchoscopic aspiration should also be performed immediately. If no anatomic basis for atelectasis is found and no material can be obtained by suctioning, the introduction of a small amount of saline followed by suctioning brings out bronchial secretions for culture and, possibly, for cytologic examination.

Frequent changes in the child's position, deep breathing, and chest physiotherapy may be beneficial. Oxygen therapy is indicated when there is dyspnea or desaturation. In some conditions, such as asthma, bronchodilator and corticosteroid treatment may accelerate atelectasis clearance.

Atelectasis can occur in patients with neuromuscular diseases. These patients tend to have ineffective cough and difficulty expelling respiratory tract secretions, which leads to pneumonia and atelectasis. There are devices to assist patients with neuromuscular diseases, including intermittent pressure breathing.

Birnkrant DJ. The assessment and management of the respiratory complications of pediatric neuromuscular diseases. *Clin Pediatr* 2002;41:301–8.

Rozenfeld RA. Atelectasis. In: Kliegman RM, Behrman RE, Jenson HB, Stanton BF (eds). *Nelson Textbook of Pediatrics.* 18th edn. Vol. 2. Philadelphia: Saunders, 2007;1830–2.

Tokar B, Ozkan R, Ilhan H. Tracheobronchial foreign bodies in children: Importance of accurate history and plain chest radiography in delayed presentation. *Clin Radiol* 2004;59:609–15.

18.16 PLEURISY, PLEURAL EFFUSIONS AND EMPYEMA

Dry or Plastic Pleurisy

Etiology: Plastic pleurisy may be associated with acute bacterial or viral pulmonary infections or may develop during the course of an acute upper respiratory tract illness. The condition is also associated with tuberculosis and connective tissue diseases such as rheumatic fever.

Pathogenesis: Visceral pleura are primarily involved, with small amounts of yellow serous fluid and adhesions between the visceral and parietal pleural surfaces. In tuberculosis, the adhesions develop rapidly, and pleura are often thickened. Occasionally, fibrin deposition and adhesions are severe enough that markedly inhibits the movement of the lung.

Clinical manifestations: Pain is the principal symptom, and is exaggerated by deep breathing, coughing, and straining. The pain is often localized over the chest wall, or is referred to the shoulder or the back. The child often lies on the affected side in an attempt to decrease respiratory movements. A leathery, rough, inspiratory and expiratory friction rub may be audible, early in illness, but this usually disappears rapidly. Increased dullness on percussion and decreased breath sounds are heard if the layer of exudates is thick. Chronic pleurisy is occasionally encountered with conditions such as atelectasis, pulmonary abscess, connective tissue diseases, and tuberculosis.

Laboratory findings: Chest radiograph will demonstrate a diffuse haziness at the pleural surface or a dense, sharply demarcated shadow, which may be indistinguishable from small amounts of pleural exudates. Chest radiographs may be normal, but ultrasonography or CT will be positive (*see* Fig. 18.3 in CD).

Differential diagnosis: Plastic pleurisy must be distinguished from other diseases such as epidemic pleurodynia, trauma to the rib cage (rib fracture), lesions of the dorsal root ganglia, tumors of the spinal cord, herpes zoster, gallbladder disease, and the trichinosis. Patients with pleurisy and pneumonia should always be screened for tuberculosis.

Treatment: When pneumonia is present immobilization of chest wall with adhesive plaster and cough suppressant medications are not indicated. If pneumonia is not present or is under good therapeutic control, strapping of the chest wall to restrict expansion may afford relief of pain. Nonsteroidal anti-inflammatory agents should be prescribed for relief of pain.

Serofibrinous or Serosanguineous Pleurisy

Etiology: Serofibrinous pleurisy is defined by fibrinous exudates on the pleural surface and an exudative effusion of serous fluid into the pleural cavity. It is most commonly associated with infections of the lung (including tuberculosis) or with inflammatory conditions of the abdomen or mediastinum, and less commonly with connective tissue diseases (lupus erythematosus, rheumatoid arthritis, or periarteritis), and with primary or metastatic neoplasms (commonly associated with a hemorrhagic pleurisy)

Pathogenesis: In health, pleural fluid originates from the capillaries of the parietal pleura and is absorbed from the pleural space via pleural stromas and the lymphatics of the parietal pleura. Normally, only 4–12 ml of fluid is present in the pleural space, but if formation exceeds clearance, fluid accumulates. Pleural inflammation increases the permeability of the pleural surface, with increased proteinaceous fluid formation; there may also be some obstruction to lymphatic absorption.

Clinical manifestations: Serofibrinous pleurisy is often preceded by the plastic type, early signs and symptoms may be those of plastic pleurisy. As fluid accumulates, pleuritic pain may disappear and the patient may become asymptomatic if the effusion remains small, or there may be only signs and symptoms of the underlying disease. Large fluid collections may produce cough, dyspnea, retractions, tachypnea, orthopnea, or cyanosis.

Dullness to flatness may be found on percussion. There are decreased or absent breath sounds, a diminution in tactile fremitus, a shift of the mediastinum away from the affected side, and occasionally fullness of the intercostal spaces. If the fluid is not loculated, these signs may shift with changes in position. The process is usually unilateral. In infants, physical signs are less definite. If extensive pneumonia is present, crackles and rhonchi may also be audible. Friction rubs are usually detected only during the early or late plastic stage.

Laboratory findings: Radiographic examination shows a more or less homogeneous density obliterating the normal markings of the underlying lung. Small effusions may cause obliteration of only the costophrenic or cardiophrenic angles or a widening of the interlobar septa. Radiologically, with the patient in the supine and upright positions will demonstrate a shift of the effusion with a change in position: the decubitus position may be helpful. Ultrasonographic examinations are useful, and may guide thoracentesis if the effusion is loculated. Thoracentesis should be performed when pleural fluid is present, unless the effusion is small and the patient has a classic lobar pneumococcal pneumonia. Examination of fluid is essential to differentiate exudates from transudates, and to determine the type of exudates (Table 18.5). Depending on the clinical findings, pleural fluid is sent for cultures; antigen testing; Gram stain; Ziehl-Neelsen stain; and chemistries including protein, lactic dehydrogenase and glucose, amylase, specific gravity, total cell count and differential, cytologic examination, and pH. The fluid of serofibrinous pleurisy is clear or slightly cloudy and contains relatively few leukocytes and, occasionally, some erythrocytes.

Treatment: Therapy should treat the underlying disease, although with draining the large effusions to make the patient more comfortable. When a diagnostic thoracentesis is performed, as much fluid as possible should be removed for therapeutic purposes. Rapid removal of ≥ 1 L pleural fluid should not be done because it may be associated with the development of re-expansion pulmonary edema. If the underlying disease is adequately treated further drainage is usually not needed, but if sufficient fluid reaccumulates to cause respiratory embarrassment, chest tube drainage should be performed. In older children with parapneumonic effusion, tube thoracostomy is considered necessary if pleural fluid pH is < 7.20 or the pleural fluid glucose level is < 50 mg/dl. If the fluid is clearly purulent, tube drainage is indicated. Patients with pleural effusions may need analgesia, particularly after thoracentesis or insertion of a chest tube. Those with acute pneumonia often need supplemental oxygen in addition to specific antibiotic treatment.

Table 18.5: Differentiation of pleural fluid

	Serofibrinous	Exudate#	Empyema#&
Appearance	Clear	Cloudy	Purulent
Cell count	Normal	Increased	> 100,000/µl
Cell type*	Few leukocytes and occasionally erythrocytes	Many small lymphocytes	Neutrophils
LDH	<200 IU/l	> 200 IU/l	> 200 IU/l
Pleural fluid/serum LDH ratio	<0.6	> 0.6	> 0.6
Protein	<3 g/dl	> 3 g/dl	> 3 g/dl
Pleural fluid/serum protein ratio	<0.5	> 0.5	> 0.5
Glucose*	Normal	< 60 mg/dl	< 60 mg/dl
pH*	Normal	< 7.20	< 7.20
Gram stain	-	Occasionally show bacteria	Bacteria are present
Acid-fast stain	-	Rarely demonstrates tubercle bacilli	-

*Glucose is usually < 60 mg/dl in malignancy, rheumatoid disease (e.g. systemic lupus erythematosus), and tuberculosis; many small lymphocytes and pH < 7.20 suggest tuberculosis; LDH: Lactate dehydrogenase.
#Blood cultures have a high yield than that of pleural fluid
&leukocytosis and an elevated sedimentation rate

Pleural thickening may develop and is occasionally mistaken for small quantities of fluid or for persistent infiltrates. Pleural thickening may persist for months, but usually disappears completely.

Purulent Pleurisy or Empyema

Etiology: Empyema is the accumulation of pus in the pleural space. Empyema is produced by bacterial infection (*Staphylococcus aureus, Streptococcus pneumonia, Haemophilus influenzae*, Group A *Streptococcus*, gram-negative organisms), tuberculosis, fungi, malignancy, rupture of a lung abscess, contamination introduced from trauma or thoracic surgery, mediastinitis, or by the extension of intra-abdominal abscesses.

Pathology: Empyema has 3 stages: exudative, fibrinopurulent, and organizational. During the *exudative stage*, fibrinous exudates form on the pleural surface. In the *fibrinopurulent stage*, fibrinous septae form, causing loculation of the fluid with thickening of the parietal pleura. In case the pus is not drained, it may dissect through the pleura into lung parenchyma, producing bronchopleural fistulas and pyopneumothorax, or into the abdominal cavity. The pus may dissect through the chest wall known as empyema necessitatis. During the *organizational stage*, fibroblast proliferation occurs and pockets of loculated pus may eventually develop into thick-walled abscess cavities or the lung may collapse and become surrounded by a thick, inelastic envelope (peel).

Clinical manifestations: The initial signs and symptoms are primarily those of bacterial pneumonia. Children treated inadequately or with inappropriate antibiotic agents may have an interval of few days between the clinical pneumonia phase and the evidence of empyema. Patients are febrile, appear ill and have respiratory distress. Physical findings are similar to those described for serofibrinous pleurisy. The two conditions are differentiated only by thoracentesis. Thoracentesis must be performed when empyema is suspected.

Laboratory findings: Radiologically, all pleural effusions appear similar, but no shift of fluid with a change of position indicates a loculated empyema; this may be confirmed by ultrasonography or CT scan. The maximal amount of fluid obtainable should be withdrawn by thoracentesis. The effusion is empyema if bacteria are present on Gram stain, the pH is <7.20, and there are >100,000 neutrophils/µl. Pus cultures should be obtained to find out bacteria. Blood cultures should be done, because of higher yield of bacteria than from pleural fluid. In patients with negative culture for pneumococcus, the pneumococcal PCR is most helpful in making the diagnosis. Leukocytosis and an elevated sedimentation rate may be found.

Complications: With staphylococcal infections, bronchopleural fistulas and pyopneumothorax commonly develop. Other local complications include purulent pericarditis, pulmonary abscesses, peritonitis secondary to rupture through the diaphragm, and osteomyelitis of the ribs. Septic complications such as meningitis, arthritis, and osteomyelitis may also occur. Septicemia is often encountered in *H. influenzae* and *S. pneumoniae*.

Treatment: Various treatment options include antibiotics, thoracentesis, chest tube drainage with or without a fibrinolytic agent, video-assisted thoracoscopic surgery (VATS), or open decortication. When pus is obtained by thoracentesis, closed chest tube drainage should be instituted immediately and controlled by an under water seal or continuous suction (*see* Fig. 18.4 in CD). The maximal amount of pus obtainable should be withdrawn by thoracentesis. Closed drainage is usually continued for about 1 wk, even though small amounts of material continue to drain after this time, probably in response of the tube in the pleural cavity. Chest tubes that are no longer draining should be removed. Controlling empyema by multiple aspirations of the pleural cavity should not be attempted. If the condition is diagnosed early, thoracentesis and antibiotic therapy alone can bring about complete cure. The selection of the antibiotic should be based on the in-vitro sensitivities of the responsible microorganism. With staphylococcal infections, resolution of the process is very slow, and systemic antibiotic therapy is required for 3–4 wk. Clinical response in non-staphylococcal empyema is also slow, little improvement may occur for as long as 2 wk. In patients with inadequately treated empyema, extensive fibrinous changes may take place over the surface of the collapsed lungs, but surgical decortication procedures are rarely indicated. In the child who remains febrile and dyspneic longer than 72 hr after initiation of therapy with intravenous antibiotics and thoracostomy tube drainage, surgical decortication via video-assisted thoracoscopic surgery or open thoracostomy may be needed for speedy recovery. Pneumatoceles usually resolve spontaneously in time. No attempt should be made to treat them surgically or by aspiration, unless they reach sufficient size and causing respiratory embarrassment or become secondarily infected.

Instillation of fibrinolytic agents into the pleural cavity may promote drainage, decrease fever, lessen need for surgical intervention, and shorten hospitalization, but there is risk of hemorrhage and other complications. Streptokinase 15,000 U/kg in 50 ml of 0.9% saline daily for 3–5 days, and urokinase 40,000 U in 40 ml saline every 12 hr for 6 doses are used in children. Antibiotics should not be instilled in to the pleural cavity because they do not improve results and are associated with local reactions.

Prognosis: The long-term clinical prognosis for adequately treated empyema is excellent, and follow-up pulmonary function studies suggest that residual restrictive disease is uncommon with or without surgical intervention.

Jaffe A, Cohen G. Thoracic empyema: A role of primary video assisted thoracoscopic surgery? *Arch Dis Child* 2003; 88: 839–41.

McColley SA. Pleurisy, Pleural Effusions and Empyema. In: Kliegman RM, Behrman RE, Jenson HB, Stanton BF (eds).

Nelson Textbook of Pediatrics. 18th edn. Vol. 2. Philadelphia: Saunders, 2007;1832–5.

Singh M, Mathew JL, Chandra S, et al. Randomized controlled trial of intrapleural streptokinase in empyema thoracis in children. *Acta Paediatr* 2004;93:1443–5.

Thompson AH, Hull J, Kumar MR, et al. Randomized trial of intrapleural urokinase in the treatment of childhood empyema. *Thorax* 2002;57:556–71.

18.17 HYDROTHORAX, HEMOTHORAX, AND CHYLOTHORAX

Hydrothorax

Hydrothorax is a transudative pleural effusion usually caused by abnormal pressure gradients in the lung. Hydrothorax is associated with cardiac, renal or hepatic disease, severe nutritional edema, ventriculo-peritoneal shunt and venous obstruction. Venous obstruction is caused by neoplasms, enlarged lymph nodes, or adhesions.

Clinical manifestations: Hydrothorax is usually bilateral, but in cardiac disease, it can be limited to the right side, or greater on the right than on the left side. The physical signs are the same as those described for serofibrinous pleurisy, but in hydrothorax, there is more rapid shifting of the level of dullness with changes in position. It is usually associated with an accumulation of fluid in other parts of the body. A pleural fluid associated with a pneumothorax is called *hydropneumothorax.*

Laboratory findings: The fluid has few cells and has a lower specific gravity (<1.015) than that of a serofibrinous exudate. The ratio of the pleural fluid to serum total protein is <0.5, the ratio of pleural fluid to serum lactic dehydrogenase is <0.6 and the pleural fluid lactic dehydrogenase is less than T, the upper limit of the normal serum lactic dehydrogenase.

Treatment: Therapy is for the underlying disorder; aspiration may be necessary when pressure symptoms are notable.

Hemothorax

Hemothorax is an accumulation of blood in the pleural cavity. Bleeding into the pleural cavity (hemothorax) may occur in inflammatory processes such as tuberculosis and empyema causing erosion of a blood vessel; congenital anomalies such as sequestration, patent ductus arteriosus, and pulmonary arterio-venous malformation; intrathoracic neoplasms, blood dyscrasias; bleeding diatheses; thrombolytic therapy; thoracic trauma, including surgical procedures or venous line insertion; rupture of an aneurism; blunt chest trauma; and spontaneously in neonates and older children. A pleural hemorrhage associated with a pneumothorax is called *hemopneumothorax*.

Clinical manifestations: In addition to the symptoms and signs of pleural effusion, hemothorax is associated hemodynamic compromise related to the amount and rapidity of bleeding.

Diagnosis: The diagnosis of a hemothorax can be made only by thoracentesis. In every case, determine the cause.

Treatment: Initial therapy is tube thoracostomy. Surgical intervention may be required to control active bleeding, and transfusion is necessary if blood loss is excessive. Inadequate removal of blood in extensive hemothorax may lead to substantial restrictive disease secondary to organization of fibrin. In such cases fibrinolytic therapy or a decortication procedure may then be necessary.

Chylothorax

Chylothorax results from the escape of chyle from the thoracic duct or lymphatics into the thoracic cavity. The causes of chylothorax include operative complication resulting from rupture of the thoracic duct (about 50% cases), chest injury, primary or metastatic intrathoracic malignancy, particularly lymphoma as a result of pressure of enlarged lymph nodes or tumor, lymphangiomatosis, restrictive pulmonary diseases, thrombosis of the duct, superior venacava or the subclavian vein, congenital anomalies of the duct system, child abuse and idiopathic (no specific cause in some patients, especially newborns).

Clinical manifestations: Chylothorax usually occurs on the right side and is rarely bilateral. The signs and symptoms are the same as due to pleural effusion of similar size. Chyle is not irritating, so pleuritic pain is uncommon. Onset is often gradual; after trauma to the thoracic duct, chyle may accumulate in the posterior mediastinum for days and then rupture into the pleural space with sudden onset of dyspnea, hypotension, and hypoxemia. Newborns with chylothorax may present with respiratory distress in the first day of life. The loss of T lymphocytes is associated with increased risk of infection in neonates; otherwise clinical problems of infection are uncommon.

Laboratory findings: The diagnosis is established when thoracentesis demonstrates a chylous effusion, a milky fluid containing fat, protein, lymphocytes, and other constituents of chyle; fluid may be yellow or bloody. In newborn infants who have not yet been fed, the fluid may be clear. In chylothorax, the fluid triglyceride is >110 mg/dL, pleural fluid to serum triglyceride ratio is >1.0, and pleural fluid to serum

cholesterol ratio is <1.0; lipoprotein analysis reveals chylomicrons. The cells are primarily T lymphocytes.

Chest radiograph shows an effusion; CT scan shows normal pleural thickness and may reveal a lymphoma as the etiology of the chylothorax. A lymphangiogram may localize the site of the leak in refractory cases when surgical ligation is contemplated.

Treatment: Spontaneous recovery occurs in >50% in infants younger than 1 yr of age. Therapy include diet containing low fat (or medium-chain triglycerides), high protein diet along with various vitamins especially the fat soluble vitamins, low salt and greater total calories than the average requirements, and diuretic. Repeated thoracentesis is done as needed to relieve presser symptoms; tube thoracostomy is often performed. If fluid continues to reaccumulate over 1–2 wk, total parenteral nutrition should be instituted, and if unsuccessful, locate and ligate the thoracic duct. Lack of resolution of chylothorax can lead to inanition, infection and death.

Ambrogi MC, Lucchi M, Dini P, et al. Videothorascopy for evaluation and treatment of hemothorax. *J Cardiovasc Surg* 2002; 43:109–12.

Beghetti M, La Scala G, Belli D, et al. Etiology and management of pediatric chylothorax. *J Pediatr* 2000;136:653–58.

Platis IE, Nwogu CE. Chylothorax. *Thoracic Surg Clin* 2006; 16(3):209–14.

Winnie GB. Hydrothorax. In: Kliegman RM, Behrman RE, Jenson HB, Stanton BF (eds). *Nelson Textbook of Pediatrics.* 18th edn. Vol. 2. Philadelphia: Saunders, 2007;1839.

Winnie GB. Hemothorax. In: Kliegman RM, Behrman RE, Jenson HB, Stanton BF (eds). *Nelson Textbook of Pediatrics.* 18th edn. Vol. 2. Philadelphia: Saunders, 2007; 1839.

Winnie GB. Chylothorax. In: Kliegman RM, Behrman RE, Jenson HB, Stanton BF (eds). *Nelson Textbook of Pediatrics.* 18th edn. Vol. 2. Philadelphia: Saunders, 2007;1839–40.

18.18 PNEUMOTHORAX

Pneumothorax is the accumulation of extrapulmonary air within the chest. Pneumothorax most commonly results from leakage of air from within the lung. Air leaks can be primary or secondary and can be spontaneous, traumatic, iatrogenic or catamenial (Box 18.7). Pneumothorax may be associated with a serous effusion (hydropneumothorax) or a purulent effusion (pyoneumothorax). Bilateral pneumothorax is rare beyond the neonatal period but has been reported after lung transplantation, and with *Mycoplasma pneumoniae* infection.

Iatrogenic: Thoractomy; Thoracoscopy thoracentesis; Tracheostomy; tube or needle puncture; mechanical ventilation.

Pathophysiology: When air enters the pleural space, the lung collapses. Hypoxemia occurs due to alveolar hypoventilation, ventilation-perfusion mismatch, and intrapulmonary shunt. In simple pnemothorax, intrapleural pressure is atmospheric, and the lung collapses up to 30%. In complicated or tension pneumothorax, continuing leak causes increasing positive pressure in the pleural space, with further compression of lung, shift of the mediastinal structures toward the contralateral side, decreased venous return, and decreased cardiac output.

Clinical manifestations: The onset is usually abrupt and the severity of symptoms depends on the extent of the lung collapse and on the amount of pre-existing lung disease. Pneumothorax may cause pain, dyspnea, and cyanosis. Moderate pneumothorax may cause little displacement of the intrathoracic organs and few or no symptoms. In tension pneumothorax there is respiratory distress, retractions, and markedly decreased breath sounds over the involved lung. The percussion note over the involved area is tympanitic. The larynx, trachea and heart may be shifted toward the unaffected side. When fluid is present there is usually a sharply limited area of tympany above a level of flatness to percussion. The presence of amphoric (resembling the sound made by blowing across the neck of a bottle) breathing or, when fluid is present in the pleural cavity, of gurgling sounds synchronous with respirations suggests an open fistula connecting with air-containing tissues.

It is important to determine whether the pneumothorax is under tension (tension pneumothorax) because this condition limits expansion of the contralateral lung and may compromise venous return. In tension pneumothorax there is shift of mediastinal structures away from the side of air leak. A shift may be absent in the case of bilateral pneumothorax.

Diagnosis: The diagnosis can be established by radiographic examination (*see* Fig. 18.5 in CD). On expiratory film, the pnemothorax becomes obvious as the lung has deflated and become more opaque. Ultrasound can also be used to establish the diagnosis. Evidence of tension pneumothorax includes shift of mediastinal structures away from the side of air leak.

Differential diagnosis: Pneumothorax must be differentiated from localized or generalized emphysema, an extensive emphysematous bleb, large pulmonary cavities, or other cystic formations, diaphragmatic hernia, compensatory overexpansion with contralateral atelectasis, and gaseous distension of the stomach. A chest radiograph or CT will differentiate among these conditions.

Treatment: A small or even moderate-sized pneumothorax in an otherwise normal child may resolve without specific treatment, usually within about 1 week. A small (<5%) pneumothorax complicating asthma may also resolve spontaneously. Administration of 100% oxygen may hasten resolution. Pleural pain can be controlled with nonsteroidal anti-inflammatory agents, if not then codeine, morphine or meperidine will be needed. If there is more than 5% collapse or if the pneumothorax is recurrent or under tension definitive treatment is necessary.

Closed thoracotomy (simple insertion of a chest tube) and drainage of the trapped air through a catheter, the external opening of which is kept in a dependent position under water, is adequate to re-expand the lung in most patients. When there have been previous pneumothoraces, it may be indicated to induce the formation of strong adhesions between the lung and the chest wall by a sclerosing procedure to prevent recurrence. This can be carried out by the introduction of doxycycline or talc into the pleural space (chemical pleurodesis).

Kuhn JP, Slovis TL, Haller JD. Caffey's Pediatric Diagnostic Imaging. Vol 1. 10th edn. Philadelphia: Mosby, 2004; 885.

Liu CM, Hang LW. Chen WK, et al. Pigtail tube drainage in the treatment of spontaneous pneumothorax. *Am J Emerg Med* 2003;21:241–4.

O'Connor AR, Morgan WE. Radiological review of pneumothorax. *Br Med J* 2005;330:1493–7.

Ruddy RM. Trauma and the paediatric lung. *Paediatr Resp Rev* 2005;6:61–67.

Whitle GB. Pneumothorax. In: Klegman RM, Behrman RE, Jenson HB, Stanton BF (eds). *Nelson Textbook of Pediatrics.* 18th edn. Vol. 2. Philadelphia. Saunders, 2007,1835–7.

18.19 PNEUMOMEDIASTINUM

Etiology: Pneumomediastinum is the presence of air or gas in the mediastinum and results from respiratory (usually results from alveolar rupture during acute or chronic pulmonary disease), non-respiratory entities or may occur in an apparently normal child (no underlying cause). Acute asthma is the most common cause of pneumomediastinum in older children and teenagers. Pneumomediastinum has been reported after dental extractions, normal menses, obstetric delivery, diabetes mellitus with ketoacidosis, acupuncture, acute gastroenteritis, esophageal perforation, and penetrating chest trauma.

Pathogenesis: After intrapulmonary alveolar rupture, air can dissect through the perivascular sheaths and other soft tissue planes toward the hilum and enter the mediastinum. In older children the mediastinum can be depressurized by escape of air into the neck or abdomen, but in newborn, the rate at which air can leave the mediastinum is limited. Pneumomediastinum can lead to dangerous cardiovascular compromise or pneumothorax.

Clinical manifestations: There is transient stabbing pain in the chest that may radiate to the neck. Isolated abdominal pain and sore throat also occur. The patient may have dyspnea and cough. Subcutaneous emphysema, if present is diagnostic. Cardiac dullness on percussion may be decreased and a mediastinal "crunch" (Hamman sign) on auscultation (confused with a friction rub) may be present. In older children, pneumomediastinum is rarely a major problem, because the mediastinum can be depressurized by escape of air into the neck or abdomen. In the case of newborn, the rate at which air can leave the mediastinum is limited, and pneumomediastinum can lead to cardiovascular compromise or pneumothorax.

Laboratory findings: Chest radiography reveals mediastinal air with a more distinct cardiac border than normal. On the lateral projection, the posterior mediastinal structures are clearly defined, there may be a lucent ring around the right pulmonary artery, and a retrosternal air can usually be seen. Subcutaneous air, seen radiographically, confirms the pneumomediastinum.

Treatment: This is directed primarily at the underlying obstructive pulmonary disease or other precipitating condition. For the relief of chest pain analgesics are needed occasionally. Rarely, subcutaneous emphysema can cause sufficient tracheal compression to justify

---

Box 18.7: Causes of pneumothorax in children

A. *Spontaneous*
A1. *Primary idiopathic:* Usually resulting from ruptured subpleural
A2. Secondary blebs
Congenital lung disease: Congenital cystic adenomastoid malformation; bronchogenic cysts; pulmonary hypoplasia
Conditions associated with increased intrathoracic pressure: Asthma; bronchiolitis; air block syndrome in neonates; cystic fibrosis; airway foreign body
Infection: Pneumatocele; lung abscess; bronchopleural fistula
Diffuse lung disease: Langerhans' cell histiocytosis; tuberous sclerosis; Marfan syndrome; Ehlers-Danlos syndrome
Metastatic neoplasm: Osteosarcoma

B. *Traumatic*
Noniatrogenic: Penetrating trauma; blunt trauma; loud music (air pressure)
Iatrogenic: Thoractomy; thoracoscopy thoracentesis; tracheostomy; tube or needle puncture; mechanical ventilation

---

tracheotomy; the tracheotomy also decompresses the mediastinum. Collar mediastinotomy and percutaneous drainage catheter placement are other treatment modalities.

Chalumeau M, Le Clainche L, Sayeg N, et al. Spontaneous pneumomediastinum in children. *Pediatr Pulmonol* 2001; 31: 67–75.

Chapdelaine J, Beaunoyer M, Daigneault P, et al. Spontaneous pneumomediastinum: Are we overinvestgating? *J Pediatr Surg* 2004;39:681–4.

Winnie GB. Pneumomediastinum. In: Kliegman RM, Behrman RE, Jenson HB, Stanton BF (eds). *Nelson Textbook of Pediatrics.* 18th edn. Vol. 2. Philadelphia: Saunders, 2007; 1837–39.

18.20 SKELETAL DISEASES INFLUENCING PULMONARY FUNCTION

Chest wall abnormalities can lead to restrictive or obstructive pulmonary disease, impaired respiratory muscle strength, and decreased ventilatory performance in response to physical stress. The congenital chest wall deformities include pectus excavatum, pectus carinatum and sternal cleft, asphyxiating thoracic dystrophy, achondroplasia, kyphoscoliosis, and congenital rib anomalies.

Pectus Excavatum (Funnel Chest)

Pectus excavatum (funnel chest) is the commonest cause and accounts for >90% of congenital chest wall anomalies. The incidence is ≈1/300 births with a 9 : 1 male preponderance. The cause is unknown or may be associated with a connective tissue disorder (i.e. Marfan syndrome, Ehlers-Danlos syndrome), or rickets, or may be acquired secondarily to chronic lung disease, neuromuscular disease or trauma.

Clinical manifestations: The deformity is present at or shortly after birth but is usually not associated with any symptoms at that time. Over time, decreased exercise tolerance, chest pain, palpitations, recurrent respiratory infections, wheezing, stridor, and cough may be present. Many children experience significant psychological stress because of the cosmetic nature of this deformity. Physical examination may reveal sternal depression (a narrowed anteroposterior diameter), protracted shoulders, kyphoscoliosis, inferior rib flares, rib cage rigidity, forward head tilt, scapular winging, and loss of vertebral contours, left shift of the cardiac impulse, and an innocent systolic murmur.

Laboratory findings: Lateral chest radiograms demonstrate the depression. Use of the Haller index on chest CT (maximal internal transverse diameter of the chest divided by the minimal anteroposterior diameter at the same level) compared to age and gender-appropriate normative values for determining the extent of depression of the chest wall anomaly has become useful in determining the extent of the anatomic abnormality. An electrocardiogram may show a right-axis deviation or Wolff-Parkinson-White syndrome. An echocardiogram may demonstrate a mitral valve prolapse and ventricular compression. Results of the pulmonary function tests may be normal but commonly show an obstructive defect in the lower airways and, less commonly, a restrictive defect, if the pectus deformity is severe.

Treatment: Therapeutic options include physical therapy to address musculoskeletal compromise, and corrective surgery. Corrective surgery is beneficial for individuals with restrictive lung disease. Surgery is often performed for psychological or cosmetic reasons.

Pectus Carinatum

Pectus carinatum (pigeon breast) is an uncommon sternal deformity accounting for 5–15% of congenital chest wall anomalies. Males are affected more often than females. A high familial occurrence, mild to moderate scoliosis and mitral valve disease and coarctation of the aorta, is observed with this anomaly.

On physical examination, a marked increase in the anteroposterior chest diameter is seen, with resultant reduction in chest movement and expansion. Chest radiographs show an increased anteroposterior diameter of the chest wall, emphysematous-appearing lungs, and a narrow cardiac shadow. Surgical correction in symptomatic patient results in improvement of the clinical symptoms. Surgery is often performed for cosmetic and psychological reasons.

Sternal Clefts

Sternal clefts are either partial (more common) or complete sternal clefts with complete failure of sternal fusion (rare). This disorder may occur in isolation or may be associated with other congenital anomalies. Surgery is required early in life before fixation and immobility take place.

Asphyxiating Thoracic Dystrophy

Physical examination reveals a narrowed thorax that at birth is much smaller than the head circumference. The ribs are horizontal and these children have short extremities. Chest radiographs demonstrate a bell-shaped chest cage with short horizontal and flaring ribs and high clavicles. No specific treatment exists. Children younger than 1 yr often succumb to respiratory infection and failure.

Achondroplasia (*see* Section 31.11)

Scoliosis (*see* Section 31.8)

Congenital Rib Anomalies

Isolated defects of the highest and lowest ribs have minimal pulmonary symptoms, Missing mid-thoracic ribs are associated with the absence of the pectoralis muscle, and lung function can become compromised. Kyphoscoliosis and hemivertebrae may accompany this defect. When 2nd to 5th ribs are absent anteriorly, lung herniation and significant abnormal respiration ensue. Complicating sequelae include severe lung restriction (secondary to scoliosis), cor pulmonale, and congestive heart failure.

Chest radiographs demonstrate the deformed and absent ribs with secondary scoliosis.

If symptoms are severe or significant lung herniation, then homologous rib grafting can be performed. Rib-expanding procedures are also of great value. Adolescent girls may require cosmetic breast surgery.

Boas SR. Skeletal diseases influencing pulmonary function. In: Kliegman RM, Behrman RE, Jenson HB, Stanton BF (eds). *Nelson Textbook of Pediatrics*. 18th edn. Vol. 2. Philadelphia: Saunders, 2007; 1841–4.

Goretsky MJ, Kelly RE, Croitoru D, Nuss D. Chest wall anomalies: Pectus excavatum and pectus carinatum *Adolesc Med Clin* 2004;15:455–71.

Mehta MH, Patel RV, Mehta LV, et al. Congenital absence of ribs. *Indian Pediatr* 1992;29:1149–52.

18.21 CHRONIC SEVERE RESPIRATORY INSUFFICIENCY

Infants, children and adolescents with chronic severe respiratory insufficiency disorders may develop hypercarbic and/or hypoxemic chronic respiratory failure. Various causes are:

1. Obstructive sleep apnea (OSA) (*see* Section 27.5)
2. Children with myelomeningocele, hydrocephalus, and Arnold-Chiari malformation, and survivors of brainstem tumors.
3. Lung diseases including bronchopulmonary dysplasia (BPD) and children recuperating from adult respiratory distress syndrome (ARDS).
4. Conditions associated with airway malacia include tracheoesophageal fistula, innominate artery compression, or pulmonary artery sling after surgical repair.
5. Neuromuscular weakness include spinal muscular atrophy, neurodegenerative diseases, myasthenia gravis, spinal cord injuries, post-infectious neurologic diseases (such as poliomyelitis and Guillain-Barré syndrome), children recuperating

from severe illness, and children with neuro-muscular diseases.

Evaluation: The evaluation should include a complete physical examination, radiologic studies, pulmonary tests, nutritional evaluation, developmental assessment, and analysis of family dynamics. Many children with severe chronic respiratory insufficiency have combination of factors contributing their overall clinical status.

Long-term mechanical ventilation: Some children with chronic severe pulmonary insufficiency benefit from chronic ventilatory support. The goal of such support is to maintain normal oxygenation and ventilation and minimize work of breathing. Long-term ventilation in the home is an expensive process for the family and for society. The prognosis of the disease is a critical factor in deciding whether long-term ventilation should be initiated. The discharge process on ventilator support should start as soon as the child is medically stable on equipment that can be maintained in the home.

Corrado A, Gorini M. Long term negative pressure ventilation. *Respir Care Clin N Am* 2002;8:545–7.

Noah Z, Budek C. Chronic severe respiratory insufficiency. In: Kliegman RM, Behrman RE, Jenson HB, Stanton BF (eds). *Nelson Textbook of Pediatrics.* 18th edn. Vol. 2. Philadelphia: Saunders, 2007;1847–9.

19 Cardiovascular System

19.1 FETAL-TO-NEONATAL CIRCULATORY TRANSITION

Fetal circulation: In the fetal circulation, the right and left ventricles exist in a parallel circuit, as opposed to the series circuit of a newborn or adult. In the fetus, the placenta provides for gas and metabolite exchange.

The lungs do not provide gas exchange, and the vessels in the pulmonary circulation are vasoconstricted. Three cardiovascular structures in the fetus are important for maintaining this parallel circulation: *ductus venosus, foramen ovale*, and *ductus arteriosus*. Oxygenated blood returning from the placenta flows to the fetus through the umbilical vein with a PO_2 of about 30–35 mm Hg. Approximately 50% of the umbilical venous blood enters the hepatic circulation, whereas the rest bypasses the liver and joins the inferior vena cava via *ductus venosus*, where it partially mixes with poorly oxygenated inferior vena cava blood derived from the lower part of the fetal body. This combined lower body plus umbilical venous blood flow (PO_2 of about 26–28 mm Hg) enters the right atrium and is preferentially directed across the *foramen ovale* to the left atrium. The blood then flows into the left ventricle and is ejected into the ascending aorta. Fetal superior vena cava blood, which is less oxygenated (PO_2 of 12–14 mm Hg), enters the right atrium and preferentially traverses the tricuspid valve, rather than the foramen ovale, and flows primarily to right ventricle.

From the right ventricle, only about 10% of the blood is ejected into the pulmonary artery (because of vasoconstriction) and enters the lungs. The major portion (about 90%) of the right ventricular blood, which has a PO_2 of about 18–22 mm Hg bypasses the lungs and flows through the *ductus arteriosus* into the descending aorta to perfuse the lower part of the fetal body, after which it returns to the placenta via the two umbilical arteries. Thus, the upper part of the fetal body (including coronary and cerebral arteries and those to the upper extremities) is perfused exclusively from the left ventricle with blood that has a slightly higher PO_2 than the blood perfusing the lower part of the fetal body which is derived mostly from the right ventricle. Only a small volume of blood from the ascending aorta (10% of fetal cardiac output) flows across the aortic isthmus to the descending aorta. The total fetal cardiac output (output of both the right and left ventricles) amounts to about 450 ml/kg/min. Approximately 65% of descending aortic blood flow returns to the placenta; the remaining 35% perfuses the fetal organs and tissues. During fetal life the right ventricle is not only pumping against systemic blood pressure but is also performing a greater volume of work than the left ventricle.

Transitional circulation: At birth, mechanical expansion of the lungs and an increase in arterial PO_2 result in a rapid decrease in pulmonary vascular resistance. The output from the right ventricle now flows entirely into the pulmonary circulation, and because pulmonary vascular resistance becomes lower than systemic vascular resistance, the shunt through the ductus arteriosus reverses and becomes left to right. The high arterial PO_2 constricts the ductus arteriosus and it closes, eventually becoming the ligamentum arteriosum. The increased volume of pulmonary blood flow returning to the left atrium increases left atrial volume and pressure sufficiently to close the foramen ovale functionally, although the foramen may remain probe patent. Removal of the placenta from the circulation also results in closure of the *ductus venosus* eventually becoming the ligamentum venosum. The left ventricle is now getting adjusted to high-resistance systemic circulation, and its wall thickness and mass begin to increase. In contrast, the right ventricle is now getting adjusted to the low-resistance pulmonary circulation, and its wall thickness and mass decrease slightly. The left ventricle, which in the fetus pumped blood only to the upper part of the body and brain, now will deliver the entire systemic cardiac output (approximately 350 ml/kg/min), an almost 200% increase in output. This marked increase in left ventricular performance is achieved through a combination of hormonal and metabolic signals, including an increase in the level of circulating catecholamines and the myocardial receptors (β-adrenergic) through which catecholamines have their effect.

Neonatal circulation: At birth, the fetal circulation must immediately adapt to extrauterine life as gas exchange is transferred from placenta to the lung. Significant differences between the neonatal circulation and that of older infants includes: (i) right-to-left or left-to-right shunting may persist across the patent foramen ovale; (ii) in the presence of cardiopulmonary disease, continued patency of ductus arteriosus may allow left-to-right, right-to-left, or bidirectional shunting; (iii) the neonatal pulmonary vasculature constricts more vigorously in response to hypoxemia, hypercapnia and acidosis; (iv) the wall thickness and muscle mass of the neonatal left and right ventricles are almost equal; and (v) newborn infants at rest have relatively high oxygen consumption, which is associated with relatively high cardiac output. The newborn cardiac output (about 350 ml/kg/min) falls over the 1st two months of life to about 150 ml/kg/min and then more gradually to the normal adult cardiac output of about 75 ml/kg/min. The presence of high percentage of fetal hemoglobin in the newborn may actually interfere with the delivery of oxygen to tissues in the neonate, so increased cardiac output is needed for delivery of oxygen.

The foramen ovale is functionally closed by the third month of life, although it is possible to pass a probe through the overlapping flaps in a large percentage of children and 15–20% of adults. Functional closure of the ductus arteriosus is usually complete by 10–15 hr in a normal neonate, although the ductus may remain patent much longer in the presence of congenital heart disease, especially when associated with cyanosis. During fetal life, patency of the ductus arteriosus appears to be maintained by the effects of low oxygen tension and the endogenously produced prostaglandins, specifically prostaglandin E_2. In a full-term neonate when the PO_2 of the blood passing through the ductus reaches about 50 mm Hg, the ductal wall constricts. The ductus of a premature infant is less responsive to oxygen.

Persistent pulmonary hypertension of the newborn (persistent fetal circulation): PPHN occurs in term and post-term babies. Persistence of the fetal circulatory pattern of right to left shunting through the PDA and foramen ovale after birth is due to excessively high pulmonary vascular resistance (PVR). Infants with PPHN become ill in the delivery room or within the 1st 24 hr of life. PPHN is related to polycythemia, idiopathic causes, hypoglycemia, or asphyxia may result in severe cyanosis with tachypnea, although initial signs of respiratory distress may be minimal. Infants who have PPHN associated with meconium aspirtin, group B streptococcal pneumonia, diaphragmatic hernia, or pulmonary hypoplasia usually exhibit cyanosis, grunting, flaring, retractions, tachycardia, and shock. Multiple organ involvement may be present.

PPHN should be suspected in all term infants who have cyanosis with or without a history of fetal distress, intrauterine growth restriction, meconium-stained amniotic fluid, hypoglycemia, polycythemia, diaphragmatic hernia, pleural effusions, and birth asphyxia. Hypoxia is universal and is unresponsive to 100% oxygen given by oxygen hood, but it may respond transiently to hypoxic hyperventilation administered after endotracheal intubation or to the application of a bag and mask.

Therapy is directed toward correcting any predisposing condition (hypoglycemia, polycythemia) and improving poor tissue oxygenation. The response to therapy is usually unpredictable, and complicated by the adverse effects of drugs or mechanical ventilation. Initial management includes oxygen administration and correction of acidosis, hypotension, and hypercapnia. Persistent hypoxemia should be managed with intubation and mechanical ventilation.

Ambalavanan N, Carlo WA. Persistent pulmonary hypertension of the newborn (Persistent fetal circulation). In: Kliegman RM, Stanton BF, St.Geme JW, Schor NF, Behrman RE. Nelson Textbook of Pediatrics. 19th edn. New Delhi: Elsevier, 2011;592–4.

Bernstein Daniel. The fetal to neonatal circulatory transition. In: Kliegman RM, Behrman RE, Jenson HB, Stanton BF (eds). Nelson Textbook of Pediatrics. 18th edn. Vol. 2. Philadelphia: Saunders, 2007;1855–7.

Konduri GG. New approaches for persistent pulmonary hypertension of newborn. Clin Perinatol 2004;31:591–611.

19.2 EVALUATION OF THE CARDIOVASCULAR SYSTEM

History and Physical Examination

History: The cardiac history starts with details of the perinatal period, including the presence of cyanosis, respiratory distress, or prematurity. Maternal history regarding gestational diabetes, medications, systemic lupus erythematosus, or substance abuse should be noted. Many of the symptoms of congestive heart failure in infants and children are age specific. In infants *feeding difficulties* such as often takes less volume per feeding and become dyspneic or diaphoretic while sucking and *respiratory distress* (rapid breathing, nasal flaring, cyanosis, and chest retractions) are common symptoms and signs. In older children, heart failure may be manifested as *exercise intolerance*, difficulty keeping up with peers during sports, getting fatigue in age-specific activities such as stair climbing, walking, bicycling riding, *growth failure*, and *orthopnea* and *nocturnal dyspnea*. Presence of *swelling* (edema) over the body is an indication of cardiac failure. Cyanosis at rest or during crying or exercise is noted and should be differentiated from breath-holding spells (blue around the lips) and acrocyanosis (cyanotic extremities) from congenital cyanotic heart disease. *Chest pain* is an unusual manifestation of cardiac disease in pediatric patients. A careful history, physical examination, and laboratory or imaging tests will assist in identifying the cause of chest pain. Musculoskeletal, pulmonary, anxiety, hyperventilation and panic disorder are common causes and cardiac is less common cause of pain. A careful *family history* may also reveal early coronary artery disease, stroke, generalized muscle disease (muscular dystrophy, dermatomyositis, familial or metabolic cardiomyopathy), or relatives with congenital heart disease.

Physical examination: Examine first extra-cardiac findings: weight, height/length, head circumference, vital signs (pulse, blood pressure, respiratory rate, and temperature), cyanosis, clubbing (fingers and toes), cardiac failure (edema, neck veins, tender hepatic enlargement), infective endocarditis and extra-cardiac malformations (which may be noted in about 20–45% of infants and children with congenital heart disease; approximately 5 to 10% of patients have a known chromosomal abnormality).

Growth failure is usually manifested by poor weight gain; both cardiac failure and chronic cyanosis result in failure to thrive. If length or head circumference is also affected, additional congenital malformations or metabolic disorders may be present. Cyanosis is best observed over the nail beds, lips, tongue, and mucus membranes. *Differential cyanosis*, manifested as blue lower extremities and pink upper extremities (usually the right arm), is seen with right-to-left shunting across a ductus arteriosus in the presence of coarctation, or an interrupted aortic arch. Circumoral cyanosis or blueness around the forehead may be the result of prominent venous plexuses in these areas rather than decreased arterial oxygen saturation. Cyanosis should be differentiated from breath-holding spells (blue around the lips) and acrocyanosis (cyanotic extremities) of infants often turn blue, when the infant is unwrapped and cold from congenital cyanotic heart disease, in which cyanosis is present in the lips, tongue and mucous membranes.

The *heart rate* of newborn is rapid and wide fluctuations are seen. The average rate ranges from 120 to 140 beats/min and may increase to 170 + beats/min during crying and activity or drop to 70–90 beats/min during sleep. As the child grows older, the average pulse rate decreases and may be as low as 40 beats/min in athletic adolescents. Persistent tachycardia (> 200 beats/min in neonates, 150 beats/min in infants, or 120 beats/min in older children), bradycardia, or an irregular heartbeat other than sins arrhythmia requires investigation to exclude pathologic arrhythmias.

The *arterial pulses* should be palpated for evaluation of rate, rhythm, character and symmetry. Rate and rhythm by convention, both are assessed by palpation of the right radial pulse (*see* Fig. 19.1 in CD). Rate is expressed in beats per minute. Normal sinus rhythm is regular, but in children may show phasic variation in rate during respiration (sinus arrhythmia). An irregular rhythm indicates atrial fibrillation, frequent ectopic beats, or paroxysmal arrhythmias. "Pulse deficit" is noted in atrial fibrillation because beats that follow very short diastolic intervals do not generate sufficient pressure to be palpable at the radial artery, but heard on auscultation, leading to heart rate more than pulse rate. Character should be evaluated at the right carotid artery (the pulse closest to the heart). The character of the pulse such as wide pulse pressure with bounding pulses may suggest an aortic runoff lesion (patent ductus arteriosus, aortic insufficiency, an arterial-venous communication or increased cardiac output secondary to anemia, anxiety, or conditions associated with increased catecholamine or thyroid hormone secretion. The presence of diminished pulses in all extremities is associated with pericardial tamponade, left ventricular outflow obstruction, or cardiomyopathy. In coarctation of the aorta the femoral pulses are also diminished. Paradoxical pulse-an inspiratory decline in systolic pressure greater than 10 mm Hg- occurs in cardiac tamponade, and less frequently in constrictive pericarditis and obstructive

pulmonary disease. Symmetry of the radial, brachial, carotid, femoral, popliteal, and dorsalis pedis should be confirmed. The radial and femoral pulses should be palpated simultaneously. Normally, the femoral pulses should be appreciated immediately before the radial pulse. In coarctation of the aorta blood flow to the descending aorta may channel through collateral vessels and result in the femoral pulse being delayed until after the radial pulse (radial-femoral delay).

Blood pressure can be measured with the patient either seated or supine; infants may be held in the lap of the parent. Cuff size is necessary to avoid over diagnosis. The cuff should completely encircle the upper part of the arm to ensure uniform compression; the inflatable bladder should cover at least two thirds of the upper arm length and three quarters of the circumference. A cuff that is too short or narrow artificially increases blood pressure readings, where there is a cough that is too large records slightly decreased pressure. The different sizes of cough including 3, 5, 7, 12, and 18 cm cuffs can accommodate large number of pediatric patient sizes. Blood pressure should be obtained in all the four extremities to detect coarctation of the aorta; in the legs on at least one occasion to exclude coarctation of the aorta, because palpation of the femoral or dorsalis pedis pulse or both is not reliable alone to exclude coarctation of aorta.

Systolic pressure is indicated by appearance of the 1st Korotkoff sound. True diastolic pressure probably lies between the muffling and the disappearance of Korotkoff sounds; muffling may be difficult to appreciate in small children. Palpation is useful for rapid assessment of systolic blood pressure, although the palpated pressure is generally about 10 mm Hg less than that obtained via auscultation. For lower extremity blood pressure determination, the stethoscope is placed over the popliteal artery. The blood pressure recorded in the legs with the cuff technique is about 10 mm Hg higher than that in the arms. In infants, blood pressure can be determined by auscultation, palpation, or an oscillometric (Dinamap) device.

Blood pressure gradually increases with age and is closely related to height and weight. The blood pressure in the arms is about 65/45 in the newborn, 75/50 at 1 yr, 45/60 at 4 yr, 95/65 at 8 yr and 100/70 at 10 yr of age. Significant increases occur during adolescence, and temporary variations take place before the more stable levels of adult life is attained. Exercise, excitement, coughing, crying, and struggling may raise the systolic blood pressure of infants and children as much as 40–50 mm Hg greater than usual levels. Serial measurements should always be obtained when evaluating a patient with hypertension. Quick formula for determining expected blood pressure (BP) is as follows:

- *Systolic BP:* 1–7 yr (age in yr + 90)
- *Systolic BP:* 8–18 yr (2 × age in yr + 83)
- *Diastolic BP:* 1–5 yr: 56
- *Diastolic BP:* 6–18 yr: Age in yr + 52

Inspection of jugular *venous pulse* wave provides information about central venous and right atrial pressure. The neck veins should be inspected with the patient sitting at a 90-degree angle. The external jugular vein should not be visible above the clavicles unless central venous pressure is elevated. Increased venous pressure transmitted to the internal jugular vein may appear as venous pulsations without visible distension; such pulsation is not seen in normal children reclining at an angle of 45 degrees. Because great veins are in direct contact of right atrium, changes in the pressure and the volume of this chamber are also transmitted to the veins, except in superior vena cava obstruction, in which venous pulsations are absent.

Heart failure in infants and children results in some degree of hepatomegaly (usually tender) and occasionally splenomegaly and edema. The sites of peripheral edema are age dependent. In infants the edema, is usually seen around the eyes and over the flanks, especially after first waking in the morning. Older children and teenagers manifest both periorbital edema and pedal edema.

Cardiac examination: The heart should be examined after completing the extracardiac examination, starting with inspection and palpation. *Precordium* is the chest wall area covering the heart. A *precordial bulge* to the left of the sternum with precordial activity suggests cardiac enlargement; it is best appreciated in the child lying supine and the examiner is looking up from the child's feet. A *substernal thrust* indicates the presence of right ventricular enlargement; where as *apical heave* is due to left ventricular hypertrophy. A *hyperdynamic precordium* suggests a volume overload that is with left-to-right shunt although it may be normal in a thin patient. A *silent precordium* with a barely detectable apical impulse suggests pericardial effusion or severe cardiomyopathy; it may be normal in obese patient. The apical impulse lies in the left fourth or fifth intercostal space internal to midclavicular line. A relationship of the apical impulse to the midclavicular line is helpful in the estimation of cardiac size and shifting of cardiac impulses. The apical impulse moves laterally and inferiorly with enlargement of left ventricle. Left-sided shift of the apical impulses occur in right-sided tension pnemothorax, or right-sided

massive pleural effusion, right-sided apical impulses signify dextrocardia, left- sided tension pnemothorax, massive pleural effusion, and thoracic space occupying lesions (e.g. diaphragmatic hernia), or right lung collapse. Shifting of the trachea on the same side along with moving of the cardiac impulses also may be palpated.

Thrills are the palpable equivalent of murmurs and correlate with the area of maximal auscultatory intensity of murmur. It is important to palpate the suprasternal notch and the neck for aortic bruits which may indicate the presence of aortic stenosis, or when faint, pulmonary stenosis. Apical systolic thrills are present in mitral insufficiency, whereas systolic thrills at the right lower sternal border indicates ventricular septal defect. Diastolic thrills are occasionally palpable in the presence of atrioventricular valve stenosis.

For *auscultation*, the diaphragm of the stethoscope is placed firmly on the chest for high-pitched sounds and the bell is lightly placed for low-pitched sounds. Initially concentrate on the characteristics of the individual heart sounds and their variation with respirations and later concentrate on murmurs. The patient should be supine, lying quietly, and breathing normally. There are four heart sounds (S1, S2, S3, S4). The first heart sound (S1) is best heard at the apex, whereas the second heart sound at the upper left and right sternal borders. The 1st heart sound (S1) 'lub' is caused by closure of atrioventricular valves (mitral and tricuspid); the 2nd heart sound (S2) 'dup' is caused by closure of the semilunar valves at the onset of ventricular systole (pulmonary and aortic). During inspiration, the decrease in intrathoracic pressure results in increased filling of the right side of the heart, which leads to an increased right ventricular ejection time and thus delayed closure of the pulmonary valve; consequently, splitting of the second heart sound increases during inspiration and decreases during expiration. Often, the second heart sound appears to be single during expiration. The presence of a normally split 2nd sound is against the diagnosis of atrial septal defect, defects associated with pulmonary arterial hypertension, severe pulmonary valve stenosis, aortic and pulmonary atresia, and truncus arteriosus. Wide splitting is noted in atrial septal defect, pulmonary stenosis, Ebstein anomaly, total anomalous pulmonary venous return, and right bundle branch block. An accentuated pulmonary component of the 2nd sound with narrow splitting is a sign of pulmonary hypertension. A single second sound occurs in pulmonary or aortic atresia or severe stenosis, truncus arteriosus and transposition of great arteries.

A 3rd heart sound (S3) is best heard with the bell at the apex in mid-diastole. A 4th heart sound (S4) occurring in conjunction with atrial contraction may be heard just before the 1st heart sound in late diastole.

The 3rd sound may be normal in an adolescent with a relatively slow heart rate, but in a patient with clinical signs of heart failure and tachycardia, it may be heard as a gallop rhythm and may merge with a 4th heart sound, this is known as summation gallop. A gallop rhythm is due to poor compliance of the ventricle and exaggeration of the normal 3rd sound is associated with ventricular filling.

Ejection clicks, which are heard in early systole, may be related to dilatation of the aorta or pulmonary artery or to a mildly to moderately stenotic semilunar valve. They are heard so close to the 1st heart sound that they may be mistaken for a split 1st sound. The *split 1st heart sounds* are usually heard best at the lower left sternal border. *Aortic ejection* clicks are best heard at the left middle to right upper sternal border and are constant in intensity; they occur in aortic stenosis and in dilated aorta (tetralogy of Fallot, truncus arteriosus). *Pulmonary ejection* clicks are best heard at the left middle to upper sternal border, vary with respirations, often disappearing with inspiration are associated mild to moderate pulmonary stenosis. A midsystolic click heard at the apex, often preceding a late systolic murmur, suggests mitral valve prolapse.

Murmurs should be described according to their intensity, pitch, timing (systolic or diastolic), variation in intensity, time to peak intensity, area of maximal intensity, and radiation to other areas. Auscultation for murmurs should be carried out across the upper precordium, down to the left or right sternal border, and out to the apex and left axilla. Auscultation should also be performed in the right axilla and over the back. *Systolic murmurs* are classified as ejection, pansystolic or late systolic according to the timing of the murmur in relation to the 1st and 2nd heart sounds. The intensity of systolic murmurs is graded from I to VI; I, barely audible; II, medium intensity; III, loud but not thrill; IV, loud with a thrill; V, very loud but still requiring positioning of stethoscope at least partly on the chest; and VI, so loud that the murmur can be heard with the stethoscope off the chest.

Systolic ejection murmurs start a short time after 1st heart sound, increase in intensity, peak, and then decrease in intensity; they usually end before the 2nd sound. However, in patients with severe aortic or pulmonary stenosis, the murmur may extend beyond the 1 st component of the 2nd sound, thus obscuring it. *Systolic ejection murmurs* indicate increased flow or stenosis across one of the ventricular outflow tracts (aortic or pulmonary). Systolic ejection murmurs indicate increased flow or stenosis across one of the ventricular outflow tracts (aortic or pulmonary). *Pansystolic or holosystolic murmurs* begin almost simultaneously with the 1st heart sound and continue throughout systole. Pansystolic murmurs are related to blood exiting the contracting ventricle via either an abnormal opening (ventricular septal defect) or atrioventricular (mitral or tricuspid) valve insufficiency. A *continuous murmur* is a systolic murmur that continues or "spill" into diastole and indicates continuous flow and is associated with patent ductus arteriosus or other aortopulmonary communication. This murmur should be differentiated from a to and fro murmur, which indicates that the systolic component of the murmur ends at or before the 2nd sound and the diastolic murmur begins after semilunar valve closure (e.g. aortic or pulmonary stenosis combined with insufficiency). A late systolic murmur begins well beyond the 1st heart sound and continues until the end of systole; such murmurs may be heard after a midsystolic click in patients with mitral valve prolapse and insufficiency.

Diastolic murmurs can also be graded from I–IV. A *decrescendo diastolic murmur* is a blowing murmur along the left sternal border that begins with 2nd heart sound and diminishes toward mid-diastole. When high-pitched, this murmur is associated with aortic valve insufficiency or pulmonary insufficiency related to pulmonary hypertension. A low pitched decrescendo diastolic murmur is typically noted after surgical repair of the pulmonary outflow tract in defects such as tetralogy of Fallot or in patients with absent pulmonary valves. A *rumbling mid-diastolic murmur* at the left middle and lower sternal border may be due to increased blood flow across the tricuspid valve, such as occurs with an atrial septal defect or stenosis of valve. When the murmur is heard at thc apex, it is caused by increased flow across the mitral valve, such as occurs with large left-to-right shunts at the ventricular level (ventricular septal defects), at the great vessel level (patent ductus arteriosus, aortopulmonary shunts), or with increased flow because of mitral insufficiency. When an apical diastolic rumbling murmur is longer and is accentuated at the end of diastole (presystolic), it usually indicates mitral valve stenosis.

Friction rub occurs in pericarditis. It is a high-pitched scratching noise audible during any part of the cardiac cycle and over any part of the left precordium.

The absence of a precordial murmur does not rule out congenital or acquired heart disease. A murmur is not heard in congenital pulmonary or tricuspid valve atresia and transposition of the great vessels until the ductus arteriosus closes. Murmur may seem insignificant in making the diagnosis of severe aortic stenosis, atrial septal defects, anomalous pulmonary venous return, atrioventricular septal defects, coarctation of the aorta, or anomalous insertion of a coronary artery. In these cases other physical findings such as growth failure, cyanosis, clubbing, peripheral pulses, heart sounds, and extracardiac congenital malformations increases the index of suspicion of congenital heart defects in these cases. In contrast, loud murmurs may be present in the absence of structural heart disease in patients with a large noncardiac arteriovenous malformation, myocarditis or severe anemia.

Innocent murmurs: Many murmurs are not associated hemodynamic abnormalities. These murmurs are referred to as functional or innocent (preferred name) murmur. During routine random auscultation more than 30% of children may have an innocent murmur at one time in their lives; this percentage increases when auscultation is carried out under nonbasal circumstances (high cardiac output because of fever, infection, anxiety). (i) *Medium-pitched*, vibratory or musical short systolic ejection murmur is the most common innocent murmur, which is heard best along the left lower and midsternal border and has no significant radiation to the apex, base or back. The intensity of the murmur often changes with respiration and position and may be attenuated in the sitting or prone position. It is most frequently heard in children between 3 and 7 yr of age. (ii) *Innocent pulmonic* murmurs originate from normal turbulence during ejection into the pulmonary artery, are common in children and adolescents. They are higher pitched, blowing, brief early systolic murmurs of grade I–II in intensity and are best detected in the 2nd left parasternal space with patient in supine position. (iii) *Venous hums* are produced by turbulence of blood in the jugular venous system, may be heard in the neck or anterior portion of the upper part of the chest during childhood. A venous hum consists of a soft humming sound heard in both systole and diastole; it can be exaggerated or made to disappear by varying the position of the head, or it can be decreased by lightly compressing the jugular venous system in the neck. These maneuvers differentiate a venous hum from the murmurs from a patent ductus arteriosus. Features suggestive of heart disease include murmurs that are pansystolic, grade III or higher, harsh, located at the left upper sternal border, and associated with an early or midsystolic click or an abnormal 2nd heart sound.

The physician should explain to the child's parents and older children and adolescents that an innocent murmur is simply a "noise" and does not indicate the presence of a significant cardiac defect. Therefore, it does not matter whether it "goes away" or "not". However, with growth, innocent murmurs are less well heard and often disappear completely.

Nada's criteria: The assessment of a child for the presence or absence of heart disease can be done with the help of "Nada's criteria", guidelines suggested by The criteria are divided into major and minor criteria. Presence of one major and two minor are essential for indicating the presence of heart disease (Table 19.1).

Bernstein Daniel. Evaluation of cardiovascular system. In: Kliegman RM, Behrman RE, Jenson HB, Stanton BF (eds). *Nelson Textbook of Pediatrics*. 18th edn. Vol. 2. Philadelphia: Saunders, 2007;1857–64.

Biancaniello T. Innocent murmurs. *Circulation* 2005;111:e20–22.

Steinberger J, Moller JH, Berry JM, et al. Echocardiographic diagnosis of heart disease in apparently healthy adolescents. *Pediatrics* 2000;105:815–8.

Laboratory Evaluation

Radiologic assessment: The chest roentgenogram may provide information about cardiac size and shape, pulmonary blood flow (vascularity), pulmonary edema, and associated lung and thoracic anomalies that may be associated with congenital syndromes (skeletal dysplasias, extra or deficient number of ribs, abnormal vertebrae, previous cardiac surgery). Cardiac size is the maximal width of the cardiac shadow in a posteroanterior (PA) chest film taken during midinspiration with the patient in an upright position. A vertical line is drawn down the middle of the sternal shadow, and perpendicular lines are drawn from the sternal line to the extreme right and left borders of the heart; the sum of the length of these lines is the *maximal cardiac width. The maximal chest width* is obtained by drawing a horizontal line between the right and left inner borders of the rib cage at the level of the top of the right diaphragm. When the maximal cardiac width is more than half the maximal chest width (*cardiothoracic ratio >50%*), the heart is

Table 19.1: Nada's criteria	
Major	*Minor*
i. Systolic murmur Grade 3 or more	i. Systolic murmur less than Grade 3 in ntensity
ii. Diastolic murmur	ii. Abnormal second heart sound (S2)
iii. Cyanosis	iii. Abnormal blood pressure (BP)
iv. Congestive cardiac failure	iv. Abnormal electrocardiogram (ECG)
	v. Abnormal X-ray chest

usually enlarged. The diagnosis of cardiac enlargement on expiratory or prone films is not correct and should never be made. The cardiothoracic ratio is a less useful index of cardiac enlargement in infants than older children because the horizontal position of the heart may increase the ratio to more than 50% in the absence of true enlargement and the thymus may overlap not only the base of the heart but the entire mediastinum obscuring the true cardiac silhouette.

A lateral chest roentgenogram may be helpful in infants and children with pectus excavatum or other conditions that result in a narrow anteroposterior chest dimension; the heart may appear small and suggest that the apparent enlargement in the posteroanterior projection was either due to thymic image (anterior mediastinum only) or flattening of the cardiac chambers as a result of a structural chest abnormality.

In the posteroanterior view (*see* Fig. 19.2 in CD), the left border of the cardiac shadow consists of three convex shadows produced from above downward, by the aortic knob, the main and left pulmonary arteries, and the left ventricle. In cases of moderate to marked left atrial enlargement, the atrium may project between the pulmonary artery and the left ventricle. The side of the aortic arch (right or left) can often be inferred as being opposite the side of the midline from which the air filled trachea is visualized. Right-sided aortic arch is often present in cyanotic congenital heart disease, particularly the tetralogy of Fallot. Three structures contribute to the right border of the cardiac silhouette; from above downward these are the superior vena cava, the ascending aorta, and the right atrium. Enlargement of cardiac chambers or major arteries and veins are prominent in the areas in which these structures are normally outlined on the chest roentgenogram. However, the electrocardiogram (ECG) is a more sensitive and accurate index of ventricular hypertrophy. Pulmonary vascularity should also be evaluated; hilar shadows are mainly vascular. *Pulmonary overcirculation* (pulmonary plethora) is usually associated with left-to-right shunt lesions, whereas *pulmonary undercirculation* is associated with obstruction of the outflow tract of the right ventricle. The esophagus is closely related to the great vessels, and a barium esophagogram can help delineate these structures in the initial evaluation of the suspected vascular rings. However, echocardiographic examination best defines the morphologic features of intracardiac chambers, and CT and MRI best define extracardiac vascular morphology.

Electrocardiography: The electrocardiogram (ECG) records the electrical activity of the heart at the skin surface. A 12-lead ECG (3 limb leads—L1, L2, L3 and 9 chest leads—aVR, aVL, aVF, V1–V6) is essential for the evaluation of cardiac patients, but in pediatric patients ECG is performed with 13 leads. Lead I–III are the standard bipolar leads, which each measure the potential difference between two limbs: Lead I: left arm to right arm, lead II: left leg to right arm, lead III: left leg to left arm. The remaining leads are unipolar connected to the limb (aVR, aVL, aVF) or to the chest wall (V1–V6). An electrocardiogram (ECG) consists of P, QRS, T waves and P-R and Q-T intervals. In some patients a small U wave can be seen following the T wave. Its orientation (positive or negative) is the same as the T wave but its cause is unknown. The ECG deflection produced by the depolarization of the atria (P wave) is smaller than that produced by the depolarization of the more muscular ventricles (QRS complex). Ventricular repolarization produces the T wave. Any positive deflection after the Q wave is termed an R wave and a negative deflection before the R wave is termed a Q wave (this must be the first deflection of the complex), while a negative deflection after the R wave is termed an S wave. *The electrical axis* shows a wide range of normality in QRS pattern (from −30° to 90°). The QRS pattern is abnormal in 90° and +120°. Thus, correct interpretation of the ECG must take account of the electrical axis. The mean frontal plane QRS axis is determined by identifying the limb lead in which the net QRS deflection (positive and negative) is least pronounced (in leads 1 to aVF) (*see* Fig. 19.9 in CD).

Reasons for using electrocardiogram in pediatrics: The most common reasons for obtaining ECGs in children are chest pain, suspected dysrhythmias, seizures, syncope, drug exposure, electrical burns, electrolyte abnormalities, and abnormal physical examination findings. Of all of these, the most life-threatening findings are those caused by electrolyte disturbances, drug exposure and burns. For a complete ECG interpretation, it is advisable to use a systematic approach, with special attention to rate, rhythm, axis, ventricular and atrial hypertrophy, and the presence of any ischemia or repolarization abnormalities. More specifically, it is essential to interpret pediatric ECG's based on age-specific rates and intervals. The ECG can be evaluated further for rhythm, chamber size, and T-wave morphology.

Hematologic data: In acyanotic patients with large left-to-right shunts, the onset of heart failure often coincides with the nadir of the normal physiologic anemia. In cyanotic patients polycythemia is frequently noted in cyanotic patients with right to left shunts. Patients with severe polycythemia are in a delicate balance between the risks of intravascular thrombosis and a bleeding diathesis. Because of the high viscosity of polycythemic blood (hematocrit

> 60%), patients with cyanotic congenital heart disease are at risk for the development of vascular thrombosis, especially of cerebral veins. Dehydration increases the risk of thrombosis. The most frequent abnormalities include accelerated fibrinolysis, thrombocytopenia, abnormal clot retraction, hypofibrinogenemia, prolonged prothrombin time, and prolonged partial thromboplastin time. Severely cyanotic patients should have periodic determination of hemoglobin and hematocrit. In cyanotic patients with inoperable conditions, phlebotomy may be required to treat individuals whose hematocrit has risen to the 65–70% level, usually when the polycythemia is associated with symptoms such as headache.

Echocardiography: Echocardiography reduces the requirement for invasive studies such as cardiac catheterization in certain common congenital anomalies. The echocardiographic examination can be used to evaluate cardiac structure in congenital heart lesions, estimate intracardiac pressures and gradients across stenotic valves and vessels, quantitative cardiac contractile function (both systolic and diastolic), determine the direction of flow across a defect, examine the integrity of the coronary arteries, and detect the presence of vegetations from endocarditis and presence of pericardial fluid, cardiac tumors and chamber thrombi. Echocardiography may also be used to assist pericardiocentesis, balloon atrial septostomy, and endocardial biopsy and in the placement of flow-directed pulmonary artery (Swan-Ganz) monitoring catheters. A complete echocardiographic examination usually entails a combination of M mode, two dimensional and three-dimensional imaging, as well as pulsed, continuous, and color Doppler flow studies. Trasesophageal echocardiography is used to confirm the presence of sinus venosus ASD (which is often not definitely possible with the trans thoracic echo study), to assess the size of secundum atrial septal defect (for suitability for a 'device closure'), to assess the suitability of the mitral valve for 'balloon mitral valvotomy' in severe mitral stenosis and to monitor ventricular function in patients during difficult surgical procedures and can provide an immediate assessment of the results of surgical repair of congenital heart lesions. Fetal echocardiography can detect the presence of many congenital heart lesions, often as early as 17–19 wk of gestation, and is especially valuable in evaluating fetal cardiac arrhythmias (*see* Figs 19.4 to 19.7 in CD).

Ventricular function: M-mode and two-dimensional echocardiographic methods of assessing left ventricular systolic and diastolic function (e.g. end-systolic wall stress and dobutamine stress echocardiography) are useful in serial assessment of patients at risk (patients on anthracycline drugs for cancer chemotherapy, patients for iron overload and patients being monitored for rejection or coronary artery disease after heart transplantation) for the development of ventricular dysfunction.

Exercise testing: Exercise testing plays an important role in evaluating symptoms, quantitating the severity of cardiac abnormalities, and assisting in the management of these patients, including prescribing physical activity schedule. In older children, exercise studies are generally performed on a graded treadmill apparatus with timed intervals of increasing grade and speed. In younger children, exercise studies are performed on a bicycle ergometer. Dynamic exercise testing defines not only endurance and exercise capacity but also the effect of such exercise on myocardial blood flow and cardiac rhythm. Significant ST segment depression reflects abnormalities in myocardial perfusion, for example, the subendocardial ischemia that commonly occurs during exercise in children with hypertrophied left ventricles. The exercise ECG is considered abnormal if the ST segment depression is greater than 2 mm and extends for at least 0.06 sec after J point (onset of the ST segment) in conjunction with a horizontal-, upward-, or downward-sloping ST segment. Provocation of rhythm disturbances during an exercise study is an important method of evaluating selected patients with known or suspected rhythm disturbances. The effect of pharmacologic management can also be tested in this manner.

MRI, electron beam CT, and radionuclide studies. MRI is helpful in the diagnosis and management of patients with congenital heart disease. MRI is particularly useful in evaluating areas that are less well visualized by echocardiography. Computer processing of MRA images allow the noninvasive visualization of the cardiovascular system from inside of the heart or vessel, *e* technique known as fly through imaging. Electron beam CT (EBCT) scanning images is especially useful in evaluating branch pulmonary arteries, anomalies in systemic and pulmonary venous return, and great vessel anomalies such as coarctation of aorta. Radionuclide angiography may be used to detect and quantify shunts and to analyze the distribution of blood flow to each lung, and is particularly useful in evaluating patients after a shunt operation (Blalock-Taussig or Glenn), balloon angioplasty and intravascular stenting operations.

Cardiac catheterization is an important tool in the diagnosis of congenital heart disease. During catheterization, blood samples are obtained for measuring oxygen saturation and calculating shunt volumes, pressures are measured for calculating gradients and valve areas, and contrast is injected to delineate structures. The major indications for cardiac catheterization include: (i) presurgical evaluation of cardiac anatomy or shunt size, or both, in children with congenital lesions when echocardiographic evaluation is incomplete; (ii) evaluation of the pulmonary vascular resistance and its response to vasodilators or oxygen; (iii) follow-up after surgical repair or palliation of complex congenital heart lesions; (iv) myocardial biopsy for the diagnosis of cardiomyopathy or screening for cardiac rejection after transplantation; (v) interventional cardiac catheterization; and (vi) electrocardiographic study or transcathetor ablation, or both.

Thermodilution measurement of cardiac output is performed with a flow-directed, thermistor-tipped, pulmonary artery (Swan-Ganz) catheter. Monitoring cardiac output by thermodilution method is useful in managing critically ill infants and children in an intensive care setting after cardiac surgery or in the presence of shock.

Angiocardiography: The major blood vessels and individual cardiac chambers may be visualized by selective angiocardiography, or the injection of contrast material into specific chambers or great vessels. This method allows identification of structural abnormalities with out interference from the superimposed shadows of normal chambers. Rapid injection of contrast medium under pressure into the circulation is not without risk. Contrast agents consist of hypertonic solutions, with some containing organic iodides, which can cause complications, including nausea, a generalized burning sensation, central nervous symptoms, and allergic reactions. Hypertonicity of contrast medium can transiently increase the symptoms of heart failure in critically ill patients.

Interventional catheterization: Nonsurgical treatment of certain cardiac defects is performed with interventional cardiac catheterization. Interventional techniques include balloon dilatation of stenotic valves and arteries, embolization of abnormal vascular connections, and catheter closures of both intracardiac and extracardiac defects. *Balloon valvuloplasty* is performed in valvular pulmonary stenosis and aortic stenosis. A special catheter with a sausage-shaped balloon at the distal end is passed through an obstructed valve. Rapid filling of the balloon with a mixture of contrast material and saline solution results in tearing of the stenotic valve tissue, usually at the site of inappropriately fused raphe. One complication of both valvuloplasty and surgery is the creation of valvular insufficiency. *Balloon angioplasty* is the

procedure of choice for patients with re-stenosis of coarctation of the aorta after earlier surgery. Other applications of balloon angioplasty technique include amelioration of mitral stenosis, dilatation of surgical conduits (Mustard), relief of branch pulmonary artery narrowing, dilatations of venous obstructions, and the long used balloon atrial septostomy (Rashkind procedure) for transportation of the great arteries.

Interventional cardiac catheterization techniques using metal coils have been developed for obliteration of arteriovenous shunts and pulmonary collateral vessels. Coils have been used to close small and medium-sized PDAs. Patients with branch pulmonary artery stenosis are treated with both balloon angioplasty and intravascular stents.

Catheter introduced devices (clamshell, Helex, button) are used for closure of small to moderate-sized ASDs. Umbrella or bag devices may also be introduced to close a large PDA not amenable to coil closure.

Andrews RE, Tulloh RMR. Interventional cardiac catheterization in congenital heart disease. *Arch Dis Child* 2004;89: 1168–73.

Bernstein Daniel. Laboratory Evaluation. In: Kliegman RM, Behrman RE, Jenson HB, Stanton BF (eds). *Nelson Textbook of Pediatrics*. 18th edn. Vol. 2. Philadelphia: Saunders, 2007;1864–78.

Frommelt MA, Frommelt PC. Advances in Echocardiographic diagnostic modalities for the pediatrician. *Pediatr Clin North Am* 1999;46:427–39.

Nienaber CA, Rehders TC, Frarz S. Detection and assessment of congenital heart disease with magnetic resonance techniques. *J Cardiovasc Magn Reson* 1999;1:169–84.

Nixon PA, Joswiak ML, Fricker FJ. A six-minute walk test for assessing exercise tolerance in severely ill children. *J Pediatr* 1996;129:362–6.

Stevenson JG. Role of intraoperative transesophageal echocardiography during repair of congenital cardiac defects. *Acta Paediatr Suppl* 1995;410:23–33.

Strife JL, Sze RW. Radiologic evaluation of the neonate with congenital heart disease. *Radiol Clin North Am* 1999;37:1093–107.

Todros T. Prenatal diagnosis and management of fetal cardiovascular malformations. *Curr Opin Obstet Gynecol* 2000; 12:105–9.

Walsh KP. Interventional paediatric cardiology. *Br Med J* 2003;327:385–8.

Van Der Velde ME, Perry SB. Transesophageal echocardiography during interventional catheterization in congenital heart disease. *Echocardiography* 1977;14:513–28.

19.3 EVALUATION OF THE INFANT OR CHILD WITH CONGENITAL HEART DISEASE

The evaluation of suspected infant or child with congenital heart disease involves a systemic approach: (i) presence or absence of cyanosis, which can be determined by physical examination aided by pulse oximetry; the character of the heart sounds and the presence and character of any murmurs helps in the differential diagnosis; (ii) the two groups (cyanotic and acyanotic) can be further subdivided according to whether the chest radiograph shows evidence of increased, normal, or decreased pulmonary vascular markings; and (iii) Electrocardiogram will determine whether right, left, or biventricular hypertrophy exists. The final diagnosis is then confirmed by echocardiography, CT or MRI, or cardiac catheterization.

Acyanotic congenital heart lesions: Acyanotic congenital heart lesions can be classified according to the predominant physiologic load that they place on the heart: increased volume load or increased pressure load. The lesions resulting in increased volume load are those that cause left-to-right shunting (atrial septal defect, ventricular septal defect, AV septal defects and patent ductus arteriosus), regurgitant lesions (pulmonary valvular insufficiency and congenital absence of the pulmonary valve, congenital mitral insufficiency, mitral valve prolapsed, tricuspid regurgitation) and cardiomyopathies. In contrast to left-to-right shunts, in which intrinsic cardiac muscle function is generally either normal or increased, heart muscle function is decreased in the cardiomyopathies. In lesions resulting in *increased pressure* load there is an obstruction in normal blood flow; most frequent are obstructions to ventricular outflow: valvular pulmonic stenosis, valvular aortic stenosis, and coarctation of the aorta. Less common are obstruction to ventricular inflow: tricuspid or mitral stenosis and cor triatriatum.

Cyanotic congenital heart lesions: Cyanotic congenital heart lesions can also be further divided according to pathophysiology: whether *pulmonary blood flow is decreased* (tetralogy of Fallot, pulmonary atresia with an intact septum, tricuspid atresia, total anomalous pulmonary venous return with obstruction without obstruction) or increased (transposition of the great vessels, single ventricle, truncus arteriosus, total anomalous pulmonary venous return without obstruction).

Bernstein Daniel. Evaluation of the child with congenital heart disease. In: Kliegman RM, Behrman RE, Jenson HB, Stanton BF (eds). Nelson Textbook of Pediatrics. 18th edn. Vol. 2. Philadelphia: Saunders, 2007;1881–3.

19.4 ACYANOTIC CONGENITAL HEART DISEASE: THE LEFT-TO-RIGHT SHUNT LESIONS

Atrial Septal Defect

Atrial septal defects (ASD) can occur in any portion of the atrial septum (secundum, primum, or sinus venosus), depending on which embryonic septal structure has failed to develop normally. Isolated secundum ASDs account for 7% of congenital heart defects. The majority of cases are sporadic; autosomal dominant inheritance is reported in the cases of Holt-Oram syndrome (hypoplastic or absent radii, 1st-degree heart block, ASD) or in families with secundum ASD and heart block. An isolated valve-incompetent patent foramen ovale (PFO) is a common echocardiographic finding during infancy. It is usually of no hemodynamic significance and is not considered ASD; a PFO may play an important role if other structural heart defects are present.

Ostium Secundum Defect

An ostium secundum defect in the region of the fossa ovalis is the most common form of ASD and is associated with structurally normal atrioventricular (AV) valves. Secundum ASDs may be single or multiple (fenestrated atrial septum), and openings ≥ 2 cm in diameter are common in symptomatic older children. Larger defects may extend inferiorly towards the inferior vena cava and ostium of the coronary sinus, superiorly toward the superior vena cava, or posteriorly. In larger defects, a considerable shunt of oxygenated blood flows from the left to the right atrium, and the ratio of pulmonary to systemic blood flow (Qp : Qs) is usually between 2 : 1 and 4 : 1. Secundum atrial septal defect occurs more commonly in females than males, with a female to male ratio of 3 : 1.

Clinical manifestations: Patients are acyanotic and may have a slender build. An isolated secundum atrial septal defect very seldom causes significant symptoms in pediatric patients, regardless of defect size. Physical findings: mild left precordial bulge; right ventricular systolic lift palpable at the left sternal border; a loud 1st heart sound and sometimes a pulmonic ejection click; the 2nd heart sound is widely split and fixed in splitting in all phases of respiration; systolic ejection murmur, medium pitched, seldom accompanied by thrill, best heard at the left middle and upper sternal border; a short, rumbling mid-diastolic murmur produced by the increased volume of blood flow tricuspid valve is often audible at the lower left sternal border.

Diagnosis: Chest roentgenogram: enlargement of right ventricle and atrium of varying degree depending on the size of the shunt; large pulmonary artery and increased pulmonary vascularity. *Electrocardiogram:* shows volume overload of the right ventricle; QRS axis normal or exhibit right axis deviation, and a minor right ventricular conduction delay (rsR pattern in the right precordial leads). *Echocardiogram:* characteristic findings of right ventricular volume overload, including an increased right ventricular end-diastolic dimension and flattening and abnormal motion of the ventricular septum. A normal ventricular septum moves posteriorly during systole and anteriorly during diastole. With right ventricular overload and normal pulmonary vascular resistance, septal motion is reversed—that is anterior movement in systole, or the motion may be intermediate so that the septum remains straight. The location and size of the atrial defect are appreciated by two-dimensional scanning, with a characteristic brightening of the echo image seen at the edge of the defect (T-artifact). The shunt is confirmed by pulsed and color flow Doppler. Cardiac catheterization: not done before surgical closure, except in the older patient in whom pulmonary vascular resistance is suspected. At catheterization, the oxygen content of blood from the atrium will be much higher than that from the superior vena cava (*see* Figs 19.8 to 19.11 in CD).

Complications: Secundum ASD is usually isolated, rarely associated with partial anomalous pulmonary venous return, pulmonary valvular stenosis, VSD, pulmonary artery branch stenosis, persistent left superior vena cava, mitral valve prolapse and insufficiency and autosomal dominant Holt-Oram syndrome.

Treatment: Surgical or transcatheter device closure is advised for all symptomatic patients and also for asymptomatic patients with a Qp : Qs ratio of at least 2 : 1. The timing for elective closure is usually after the 1st year and before entry into school. Mortality is < 1% if closure is carried out at open heart surgery.

Prognosis: ASDs detected in term infants may close spontaneously. Secundum ASDs are well tolerated during childhood. Pulmonary hypertension, atrial dysrhythmias, tricuspid or mitral insufficiency, and heart failure are late manifestations; these symptoms may initially appear during the increased volume of pregnancy. Infective endocarditis is not a risk with this lesion and the antibiotic prophylaxis is not recommended.

Atrioventricular Septal Defects (Ostium Primum and Atrioventricular Canal or Endocardial Cushion Defects)

An ostium primum defect is situated in the lower portion of the atrial septum and overlies the mitral and tricuspid valves. An AV septal defect, also known as an AV canal defect or an endocardial cushion defect, consists of contiguous atrial and ventricular septal defects with markedly abnormal AV valves. The basic abnormality in patients with ostium primum defects is the combination of a left-to-right shunt across the atrial defect and mitral (or occasionally tricuspid) insufficiency.

Clinical manifestations: Many children with ostium primum defects are asymptomatic, and the anomaly is discovered during a general physical examination. In patients with moderate shunts and mild mitral insufficiency, the physical signs are similar to those of the secundum ASD, and with an additional apical murmur caused by mitral insufficiency.

A history of exercise intolerance, easy fatigability, and recurrent pneumonia may be obtained, especially in infants with larger left-to-right shunts and severe mitral insufficiency. With complete AV septal defects, heart failure and intercurrent pulmonary infection usually appear in infancy. During these episodes, minimal cyanosis may be evident. Cardiac enlargement is moderate to marked, and a systolic thrill is frequently palpable at the lower left sternal border. A precordial bulge and lift may be present. The 1st heart sound is normal or accentuated. The 2nd heart sound is widely split if the pulmonary flow is massive. A low-pitched, mid-diastolic rumbling murmur is audible at the lower left sternal border, and a pulmonary systolic ejection murmur is produced by the large pulmonary flow. A harsh apical holosystolic murmur of mitral insufficiency may also be present.

Diagnosis: Chest roentgenogram: moderate to severe cardiac enlargement, large pulmonary artery and increased pulmonary vascularity. *Electrocardiogram:* biventricular hypertrophy or isolated right ventricular hypertrophy; right ventricular delay (RSR pattern in V3R and V1); normal or tall P waves; occasional prolongation of P-R interval. Echocardiogram: signs of right ventricular enlargement with encroachment of the mitral valve echo on the left ventricular outflow tract; the abnormally low position of the AV valves results in a "gooseneck" deformity of the left ventricular outflow tract on both echocardiography and angiography. *Doppler echocardiography will demonstrate left-to-right shunting at the atrial, ventricular, or ventricular to atrial levels. Cardiac catheterization and angiocardiography:* catheterization demonstrates the magnitude of the left-to-right shunt, the degree of elevation of pulmonary vascular resistance, and the severity of insufficiency of the common AV valve.

Treatment: Surgical intervention must be performed during infancy because of the risk of pulmonary vascular disease developing as early as 6–12 mo of age. The atrial and ventricular defects are patched and the AV valves reconstructed. Complications include surgically induced heart block requiring placement of a permanent pacemaker, excessive narrowing of the left ventricular outflow tract requiring surgical revision, and eventual worsening of mitral regurgitation requiring replacement with a prosthetic valve.

Prognosis: Most patients with ostium primum defects and minimal AV valve involvement are asymptomatic or have only minor, nonprogressive symptoms until they reach the 3rd–4th decade of life, similar to the course of patients with secundum ASD. Death occurs during infancy from heart failure and patients who survive without surgery, pulmonary vascular disease or more rarely pulmonary stenosis usually develops.

Ventricular Septal Defect

Ventricular septal defect (VSD) is the most common cardiac defect and accounts for 25% of congenital heart disease. The ventricular septum consists of an inferior muscular and superior membranous portion. Defects may occur in any portion of the ventricular septum, but most are of the membranous type. VSDs between the crista supraventricularis and the papillary muscle of the conus may be associated with pulmonary stenosis and other malformations of the tetralogy of Fallot. VSDs superior to the crista supraventricularis (supracrystal) are found just beneath the pulmonary valve and may impinge on an aortic sinus and cause aortic insufficiency. VSDs in the midportion or apical region of the ventricular septum are muscular in type and may be single or multiple (Swiss cheese septum). Congenital VSDs are frequently associated with other congenital conditions such as Down syndrome.

Clinical manifestations: Small VSDs with trivial left-to-right shunts and normal pulmonary arterial pressure are the most common. These patients are asymptomatic, and the cardiac lesion is usually found during routine physical examination. A loud harsh or blowing holosystolic murmur is present and herd best over the lower left sternal border and is frequently accompanied by a thrill. A short, harsh systolic murmur localizes to the apex in a neonate is a sign of a tiny muscular VSD. In the immediate neonatal period, the systolic murmur may not be audible during the first few days, as the left-to-right shunt is minimal because of higher right sided pressure. In premature infants, the murmur may be heard early because pulmonary vascular resistance decreases more rapidly. Large VSDs with increased pulmonary blood flow and pulmonary hypertension are associated with dyspnea, feeding difficulties, poor growth, profuse perspiration, recurrent pulmonary infections, and cardiac failure in infancy. Prominence of the left precordium, palpable parasternal lift, a laterally displaced apical impulse and apical thrust, and a systolic thrill is present along with the holosystolic murmur and increased pulmonic component of the 2nd heart sound. The presence of a mid-diastolic, low-pitched rumble at the apex is caused by increased blood flow across the mitral valve and indicates a Qp:Qs ratio of $\geq 2 : 1$. When the ratio

of pulmonary to systemic resistance approaches 1 : 1, the shunt becomes bidirectional, the signs of heart failure abate, and the patient becomes cyanotic (Eisenmenger syndrome).

Diagnosis: In patients with small VSDs, the chest roentgenogram is usually normal, although minimal cardiomegaly and a borderline increase in pulmonary vasculature may be observed. The ECG is generally normal but may suggest left ventricular hypertrophy with small VSD. The presence of right ventricular hypertrophy suggests that the defect is not small and that the patient has pulmonary hypertension or an associated lesion such as pulmonic stenosis. In large VSDs, the chest roentgenogram shows gross cardiomegaly with prominence of both ventricles, the left atrium, and the pulmonary artery; pulmonary vascular markings are increased, and frank pulmonary edema, including pleural effusions may be present. The ECG in large VSD shows biventricular hypertrophy; P waves may be notched or peaked. The two-dimensional echocardiogram shows the position and size of the VSD. Small defects, especially those of the muscular septum are visualized only by color Doppler examination. The echocardiogram can also be useful to determine the presence of aortic valve insufficiency or leaflet prolapse in the case of supracristal VSDs. Cardiac catheterization is performed only when the size of the shunt is uncertain or when pulmonary vascular disease is suspected. Oximetry demonstrates increased oxygen content in the right ventricle (*see* Figs 19.12 to 19.16 in CD).

Treatment: Treatment is either conservative or surgical. A significant number (30–50%) of small defects close spontaneously, most frequently during the 1st 2 yr of life (vast majority before the age of 4 yr). Small muscular VSDs are more likely to close (up to 80%) than membranous VSDs are (up to 35%). In patients with small VSDs, parents should be reassured of the relatively benign nature of the lesion, and the child should be encouraged to live a normal life with no restrictions on physical activity. Antibiotic prophylaxis is indicated as there is risk of infective endocarditis.

In infants with a large VSD, medical management includes, to control heart failure and prevent the development of pulmonary vascular disease. Severe pulmonary vascular disease is a contradiction to closure of a VSD.

Indications for surgical closure of a VSD include patients at any age with large defects in whom clinical symptoms and failure to thrive cannot be controlled medically; infants between 6 and 12 mo of age with large defects associated with pulmonary hypertension, even if the symptoms are controlled by medication; patients older than 24 mo with a Qp : Qs ratio greater than 2 : 1; and patients with supracristal VSD of any size because of the high risk for aortic valve regurgitation.

Prognosis: The results of primary surgical repair are excellent, and complications leading to long-term problems (residual ventricular shunts requiring reoperation or heart block requiring a pacemaker) are rare. After surgical obliteration of the left-to-right shunt, the hyperdynamic heart becomes quiet, cardiac size decreases towards normal, thrills and murmurs are abolished, and pulmonary artery hypertension regresses. Catch-up growth occurs in most patients within the next 1–2 yr.

Patent Ductus Arteriosus

Patent ductus arteriosus (PDA) is the persistence of a normal fetal structure between the left pulmonary artery and the descending aorta. Persistence of this fetal structure beyond 10 days of life is considered abnormal. The aortic end of the ductus is just distal to the origin of the left subclavian artery, and the ductus enters the pulmonary artery at its bifurcation. PDA is more in females than males in the ratio of 2 : 1. As a result of the higher aortic pressure, the blood shunts left-to-right through the ductus, from the aorta to pulmonary artery.

Clinical manifestations: A small patent ductus does not usually have any symptoms associated with it. A large PDA will result in important physical signs attributable to the wide pulse pressure, most prominently, bounding peripheral arterial pulses. The heart is normal in size when the ductus is small, but moderately or grossly enlarged in cases with a large communication. The apical impulse is prominent and is heaving with cardiac enlargement. A thrill, maximal in the 2nd left intercostal space is often present and may radiate towards the left clavicle, down the left sternal border, or toward the apex. The thrill is usually systolic but may also be palpated throughout the cardiac cycle. The classic continuous murmur is described as being like machinery murmur or rolling thunder in quality. It begins soon after onset of the 1st sound, reaches maximal intensity at the end of systole, and wanes in late diastole. It may be localized to the 2nd left intercostal space or radiate towards the left clavicle, or radiate down the left sternal border. The diastolic component of the murmur is less prominent or absent, when pulmonary vascular resistance is increased. In patients with a large left-to-right shunt, a low-pitched mitral mid-diastolic murmur may be audible at the apex as a result of the increased volume of blood flow across the mitral valve.

Diagnosis: Chest roentgenogram: a large PDA will show a prominent pulmonary artery with increased intrapulmonary vascular markings, and cardiomegaly. *Electrocardiogram:* normal if the left-to-right is small; if the ductus is large left ventricular or biventricular hypertrophy is present. *Echocardiogram: cardiac* chambers are normal if the ductus is small; with large shunts, the left atrial and left ventricular dimensions are increased; size of the left atrium is usually quantitated by comparison to the size of the aortic root, known as the LA : Ao ratio; scanning from the suprasternal notch allows direct visualization of the ductus. Color and pulsed Doppler examinations demonstrate systolic or diastolic (or both) retrograde turbulent flow in the pulmonary artery and aortic retrograde flow in diastole (*see* Figs 19.17 and 19.18 in CD).

Treatment: Irrespective of age, patients with PDA require surgical or catheter closure, because it will prevent bacterial endarteritis and other late complications such as heart failure, pulmonary hypertension (*Eisenmenger syndrome*). In infants with low birth weight (weighing <1500 g), oral ibuprofen (10 mg/kg initially followed an interval of 24 hr by two doses of 5 mg/kg) is as effective as intravenous indomethacin (0.2 mg/kg initially followed by two doses at 24 hr intervals) for closing symptomatic PDA.

19.5 ACYANOTIC CONGENITAL HEART DISEASE: OBSTRUCTIVE LESIONS

Pulmonary Valve Stenosis with Intact Ventricular Septum

Pulmonary valve stenosis is the most common isolated obstructive lesion, which accounts for 7–10% of all congenital heart defects. The valve cusps (may be bicuspid or tricuspid) are deformed to various degrees and, as a result the valve opens incompletely during systole. Pulmonary stenosis is an associated finding in Noonan syndrome and in Alagille syndrome (patients with arteriohepatic dysplasia). In severe pulmonic stenosis, mild to moderate cyanosis may be noted in patients with an interatrial communication (atrial septal defect or patent foramen ovale); hepatic enlargement and peripheral edema indicate right ventricular failure; jugular venous pressure is elevated and is caused by a large presystolic jugular a wave. Heart is moderately or greatly enlarged, and a conspicuous parasternal right ventricular lift is present and frequently extends to the left midclavicular line. The pulmonary component of the 2nd sound is usually inaudible. A loud, long, and harsh systolic ejection murmur, usually accompanied by a thrill, is maximally audible in the pulmonic area and may radiate over the entire precordium, to both lung fields, into the neck, and to the back. Chest roentgenogram confirms cardiac enlargement with prominence of the right ventricle and right atrium and pulmonary artery segment; intrapulmonary vascularity is decreased. Electrocardiogram shows gross right ventricular hypertrophy, frequently accompanied by a tall, spiked P wave. Two-dimensional echocardiogram shows severe deformity of the pulmonary valve and right ventricular hypertrophy, systolic dysfunction of the right ventricle and tricuspid regurgitation. Doppler studies demonstrate a large gradient (> 60 mmHg) across the pulmonary valve. Cardiac catheterization: is undertaken as part of a balloon valvuloplasty.

Treatment: Patients with moderate or severe isolated pulmonary stenosis require relief of the obstruction. Balloon valvuloplasty is the initial treatment of choice for the majority of patients. Patients with severely thickened pulmonic valves, especially common in those with Noonan syndrome, may require surgical intervention. Children with mild stenosis can lead a normal life, but their progress should be evaluated at regular intervals.

Aortic Stenosis

Congenital aortic stenosis occurs in approximately 5% of cardiac malformations. Aortic stenosis is more frequent in males (3 : 1). It is of three types: *(i) valvular aortic stenosis* (most common type), *(ii) subvalvular (subaortic) stenosis*, and *(iii) supravalvular aortic stenosis*.

Symptoms in patients with aortic stenosis depend on the severity of the obstruction. Severe aortic stenosis that occurs in early infancy is termed *critical aortic stenosis*, and is associated with left ventricular failure and signs of low cardiac output. In *mild stenosis*, the pulses, the heart size, and apical impulses are all normal. *Mild to moderate* valvular aortic stenosis is usually associated with an early systolic ejection click, best heard at the apex and left sternal edge. If the stenosis is *severe*, the first heart sound may be diminished because of decreased compliance of the thickened left ventricle. Normal splitting of the 2nd heart sound is present in mild to moderate obstruction; and in patients with severe obstruction, the 2nd sound may be split paradoxically (becoming wider in expiration), and 4th heart sound may be audible. Systolic ejection murmur is audible maximally at the right upper sternal border and radiates to the neck and the left sternal border and is usually accompanied by a thrill in the suprasternal notch. In patients with subvalvular aortic stenosis, the murmur may be maximal along the left sternal border or even at the apex. The other murmurs that are heard include a soft decrescendo diastolic murmur indicative of aortic

insufficiency when the obstruction is subvalvular, or in patients with a bicuspid aortic valve; and an apical short mid-diastolic rumbling murmur, even in the presence of normal mitral valve. Graded exercise testing is useful in evaluating the severity of the left ventricular outflow tract obstruction in older children. *Chest roentgenogram* shows a prominent ascending aorta with normal aortic notch, normal heart size and valvular calcification. *Electrocardiogram* is normal even with more severe obstruction, but evidence of left ventricular hypertrophy and strain (inverted T waves in the left precordial leads) in severe stenosis of long standing. *Echocardiogram* identifies both the site and the severity of the obstruction; shows left ventricular hypertrophy and the thickened and domed aortic valve, the number of valve leaflets and their morphology and a subaortic membrane or supravalvular stenosis, if present. Left heart catheterization demonstrates the magnitude of the pressure gradient from the left ventricle to aorta.

Treatment: Balloon valvuloplasty is indicated for children with moderate to severe valvular aortic stenosis. For more rapidly progressive subaortic obstructive lesions surgery is indicated. Regardless of whether surgical or catheter treatment has been carried out, aortic insufficiency or calcification with re-stenosis is likely to occur later and eventually require reoperation and often aortic valve replacement.

Coarctation of the Aorta

Constrictions of the aorta of varying degrees may occur at any point from the transverse arch to the iliac bifurcation, but 98% occur just below the origin of the ductus arteriosus (juxtaductal coarctation). The coarctation of the aorta is more frequent in males (2 : 1).

Coarctation of the aorta may be a feature of Turner syndrome. Mitral valve abnormalities (a supravalvular mitral ring or parachute mitral valve) and subaortic stenosis are associated lesions in patients with coarctation of the aorta.

Clinical manifestations: Coarctation of the aorta recognized after infancy is not usually associated with significant symptoms. Some children or adolescents complain about weakness or pain (or both) in the legs after exercise or have hypertension detected on routine physical examination. The classic sign of coarctation of the aorta is a disparity in pulsation and blood pressure in the arms and legs. The femoral, popliteal, posterior tibial, and dorsalis pedis pulses are weak (or absent in up to 40% of patients), in contrast to the bounding pulses of the arm and carotid vessels. The radial and femoral pulses should always be palpated simultaneously for the presence of a radial-femoral delay. Normally, the femoral pulse occurs slightly before the radial pulse. In normal persons (except neonates), systolic blood pressure in the legs obtained by the cuff method is 10–20 mm Hg higher than that in the arms. In coarctation of the aorta, blood pressure in the legs is lower than that in the arms. Occasionally, the right subclavian artery may arise anomalously from below the area of coarctation and results in a left arm pressure that is higher than the right, therefore it is important to determine the blood pressure in each arm. With exercise, a more prominent rise in systemic blood pressure occurs, and the upper-to-lower extremity pressure gradient will increase.

The precordial impulse and heart sounds are usually normal. The presence of a systolic ejection click or thrill in the suprasternal notch suggests a bicuspid aortic valve (present in 70% of cases). A short systolic is often heard along the left sternal border at the 3rd and 4th intercostals spaces, transmitted to the left infrascapular area and occasionally to the neck. Other murmurs heard including systolic ejection murmur of aortic stenosis, low pitched mid-diastolic murmur at the apex of the mitral valve stenosis, and systolic or continuous murmurs over the left and right sides of the chest laterally and posteriorly in patients with well developed collateral blood flow.

Diagnosis: Chest roentgenogram shows cardiac enlargement and pulmonary congestion are noted in infants with severe coarctation; during childhood the findings include mildly or moderately enlarged heart, enlarged left subclavian artery, notching of the inferior border of the ribs from pressure erosion by enlarged collateral vessels, and an area of poststenotic dilatation of the descending aorta. *Electrocardiogram* is usually normal in young children, but reveals evidence of left ventricular hypertrophy in older patients. *Echocardiogram* shows segment of coarctation and associated anomalies of the mitral and aortic valve and hypopulsatile descending aorta. *Color Doppler demonstrates* the specific site of obstruction. Pulsed and continuous wave Doppler studies determine the pressure gradient directly at the area of coarctation. *Cardiac catheterization* with selective left ventriculography and aortography is useful in detecting additional anomalies and visualizing collateral blood flow. CT and MRI are valuable tools for evaluation of coarctation when the echocardiogram is equivocal.

Treatment: In neonates with severe coarctation of the aorta an infusion of prostaglandin E_1 should be given to reopen the ductus and re-establish adequate lower extremity blood flow. Once a diagnosis has been confirmed and the patient stabilized surgical repair should be performed. In the immediate postoperative course, "rebound" hypertension is common and requires medical management. Postcoarctectomy syndrome characterized by postoperative mesenteric arteritis associated with acute hypertension and abdominal pain occurs in the immediate postoperative period. Relief is usually obtained with antihypertensive drugs (nitroprusside, esmolol, captopril) and intestinal decompression; surgical exploration is rarely required for bowel obstruction or infarction.

19.6 CYANOTIC CONGENITAL HEART DISEASE: LESIONS ASSOCIATED WITH DECREASED PULMONARY BLOOD FLOW

Tetralogy of Fallot

Tetralogy of Fallot (TOF) consists of (i) pulmonary stenosis, (ii) VSD, (iii) right ventricular hypertrophy, and (iv) dextroposition of the aorta with override of the ventricular septum. Complete obstruction of the right ventricular outflow (pulmonary atresia with VSD) is classified as an extreme form of tetralogy of Fallot. The degree of right ventricular outflow obstruction determines the timing of the onset of symptoms, the severity of cyanosis and the degree of right ventricular hypertrophy. When the obstruction to the right ventricular outflow is mild to moderate and a balanced shunt is present across the VSD, the patient may not be visibly cyanotic (acyanotic or "pink" tetralogy of Fallot). When obstruction is severe, cyanosis will be present from birth and worsen when the ductus begins to close.

Clinical manifestations: Cyanosis is often not present at birth, but with increasing hypertrophy of the right ventricular infundibulum, and patient growth, the cyanosis occurs later in the 1st year of life. Cyanosis is the most prominent in the mucus membranes of the lips and mouth and in the fingernails and toenails. In infants with severe degrees of right ventricular outflow obstruction, neonatal cyanosis is noted immediately. Older children with long-standing cyanosis who have not undergone surgery may have dusky blue skin, grey sclerae with engorged blood vessels, and marked clubbing of the fingers and toes. Dyspnea occurs on exertion. Infants and toddlers play actively for a shot time and then sit or lie down. The older children may be able to walk before stopping to rest. Characteristically, children assume a squatting position for the relief of dyspnea caused by physical effort; the child is usually able to resume physical activity within a few minutes. These findings occur in patients with significant cyanosis at rest (*see* Figs 19.19 and 19.20 in CD).

Paroxysmal hypercyanotic attacks (hypoxic, "blue" or "tet" spells) occur during the 1st 2 yr of life. The infant becomes hyperpneic and restless, cyanosis increases, gasping respirations ensue, and syncope may follow. The spells occur most frequently in the morning on initially awakening or after episodes of vigorous crying. The spells last from a few minutes to a few hours but are rarely fatal. Spells are associated with reduction of an already compromised pulmonary blood flow, which when prolonged, results in severe systemic hypoxia and metabolic acidosis. Infants who are mildly cyanotic at rest are often more to the development of hypoxic spells because they have not acquired the homeostatic mechanisms to tolerate rapid lowering of the arterial oxygen saturation such as polycythemia.

Growth and development may be delayed in patients with severe untreated tetralogy of Fallot, particularly when oxygen saturation is chronically <70%. Puberty may also be delayed in patients who do not undergo surgery. The pulse is normal. The left anterior hemithorax may bulge anteriorly because of right ventricular hypertrophy. Systolic thrill may be felt along the left sternal border in the 3rd and 4th parasternal spaces. The 2nd heart sound is either single or the pulmonic component is soft. The systolic murmur is usually loud and harsh, may be preceded by a click, transmitted widely, especially to the lungs, but is most intense at the left sternal border. The murmur is ejection in quality at the upper sternal border but it may sound more holosystolic toward the lower sternal border. The murmur is caused by turbulence through the right ventricular outflow tract. The murmur tends to become louder, longer, and harsher as the severity of pulmonary stenosis increases from mild to moderate, but becomes less prominent with severe obstruction, especially during a hyper-cyanotic spell. Infrequently, a continuous murmur may be audible, especially if prominent collaterals are present.

Diagnosis: Chest roentgenogram: the anteroposterior view consists of a narrow base, concavity of the left heart border in the area usually occupied by the pulmonary artery, and normal heart size. The hypertrophied right ventricle caused the rounded apical shadow to be uplifted so that it is situated higher above the diaphragm than normal. The cardiac silhouette looks like that of a boot or wooden shoe ("Coeur en sabot") (Fig. 19.1). The hilar areas and lung fields are relatively clear because of diminished pulmonary blood flow or the small size of the pulmonary arteries, or both. The aorta is usually large and in 20% of patients it arches to the right. *Electrocardiogram* demonstrates right axis deviation and evidence of right ventricular hypertrophy (Fig. 19.2). A dominant R wave appears in the right

precordial chest leads (Rs, R, qR, qRS) or an RSR′ pattern. In some cases the only sign of right ventricular hypertrophy may be a positive T wave in leads V3R and V1. The P wave is tall and peaked or sometimes bifid. *Two-dimensional echocardiography* establish the diagnosis and provides information about the extent of aortic override of the septum, the location and degree of the right ventricular outflow tract obstruction, the size of the proximal branch pulmonary arteries, and the site of the aortic arch and also in determining whether a PDA is supplying a portion of the pulmonary blood. In a patient without pulmonary atresia catheterization before surgical repair is not required. *Cardiac catheterization* demonstrates a systolic pressure in the right ventricle equal to systemic pressure; *selective right ventriculography* demonstrates the anatomy of the tetralogy of Fallot and *left ventriculography* the size of the left ventricle, position of the VSD, overriding of aorta and mitral-aortic continuity, thereby ruling out a double-outlet right

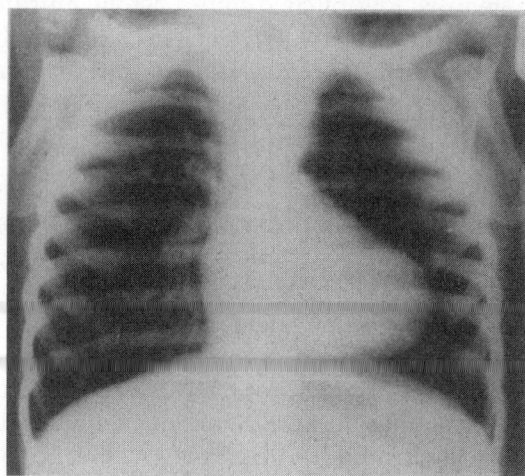

Fig. 19.1: Uplifted apex and absence of pulmonary artery segment typifies the "Coeur en sabot" (i.e. boot-shaped heart) of tetralogy of Fallot (*see* Fig. 19.21 in CD)

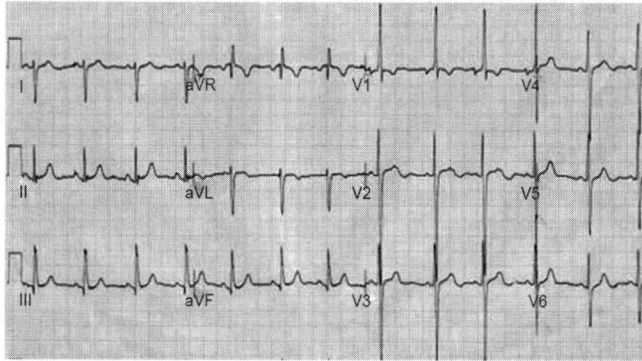

Fig. 19.2: ECG in tetralogy of Fallot (TOF) showing right ventricular hypertrophy (*Courtesy:* Dr Vivek Kumar) (*see* Fig. 19.22 in CD)

ventricle; *aortography or coronary angiography* outlines the course of the coronary arteries (*see* Fig. 19.23 in CD).

Complications: Before correction, patients with the tetralogy of Fallot are susceptible to serious complications such as cerebral thromboses, brain abscess, polycythemia, bacterial endocarditis, and heart failure.

Associated anomalies include PDA, multiple VSDs, congenital absence of the pulmonary valve, absence of a branch pulmonary artery most often the left, and CATCH 22 (cardiac defects, abnormal facies, thymic hypoplasia, cleft palate, and hypocalcemia).

Treatment: Depending on the frequency and severity of hypercyanotic attacks, one or more of the following procedures should be instituted in sequence: (i) placement of the infant on the abdomen in the knee-chest position, (ii) administration of oxygen, and (iii) injection of morphine subcutaneously in a dose not in excess of 0.2 mg/kg. Because metabolic acidosis develops when arterial PO_2 is < 40 mmHg, rapid correction (within several minutes) with intravenous administration of soda bicarbonate is necessary if the spell is unusually severe and the child shows a lack of response to the foregoing therapy. Recovery from the spell is rapid once a pH has returned to normal. β-Adrenergic blockade by the administration of propranolol (0.1 mg/kg given slowly to a maximum of 0.2 mg/kg) is also useful.

Neonates with marked right ventricular outflow tract obstruction may deteriorate rapidly because, as the ductus arteriosus begins to close, pulmonary blood flow is further compromised. Prostaglandin E_1 (0.01–0.20 μg/kg/min), a potent and specific relaxant of ductal smooth muscle, should be administered intravenously until a surgical procedure is performed. Infants with less severe right ventricular outflow tract obstruction who are stable and awaiting surgical intervention require prevention or prompt treatment of dehydration to avoid hemoconcentration and thrombotic episodes, iron therapy to decrease paroxysmal dyspneic attacks, and oral propranolol (0.5–1 mg/kg every 6 hr) to decrease the frequency and severity of hypercyanotic spells.

Infants with symptoms and severe cyanosis in the 1st month of life have marked obstruction of the right ventricular outflow tract or pulmonary atresia require either a palliative systemic-to-pulmonary artery shunt to augment pulmonary artery blood flow or corrective heart surgery (electively performed at between 4 and 6 mo of age). The modified Blalock-Taussig shunt is the aortopulmonary shunt procedure. After a successful shunt procedure, cyanosis diminishes. The development of a continuous murmur over the lung fields after the operation indicates a functioning anasto-

mosis. Postoperative complications after the Blalock-Taussig shunt include chylothorax, diaphragmatic paralysis, and Horner syndrome.

Corrective surgical therapy consists of relief of the right ventricular outflow tract obstruction and by patch closure of the VSD. The surgical risk of total correction is <5%. Increased bleeding in the immediate postoperative period may be a complicating factor in extremely polycythemic patients.

Prognosis: After a successful total correction, patients are generally asymptomatic and are able to lead unrestricted lives. Follow-up of patients 5–20 yr after surgery indicates that the marked improvement in symptoms is generally maintained. Uncommon immediate postoperative problems include right ventricular failure, transient heart block, residual VSD with let-to-right shunting, and myocardial infarction from interruption of an aberrant coronary artery. Postoperative heart failure may require diuretics and a positive inotropic agent such as digoxin. A number of children have premature ventricular beats after repair of tetralogy of Fallot and some also suffer from complex ventricular arrhythmias and may require antiarrhythmic therapy.

Pulmonary Atresia with Ventricular Septal Defect

Tetralogy of Fallot with pulmonary atresia is the most extreme form of the tetralogy of Fallot. The pulmonary valve is atretic, rudimentary, or absent, and the pulmonary trunk is atretic or hypoplastic. The entire right ventricular output is ejected into the aorta. Pulmonary blood flow is then dependent on a PDA or on collateral vessels. Patients have findings similar to those in patients with severe tetralogy of Fallot.

Tricuspid Atresia

In tricuspid atresia, no outlet from the right atrium to the right ventricle is present; the entire systemic venous return enters the left side of the heart by means of a foramen ovale or an associated ASD. Left ventricular blood usually flows into the right ventricle via a VSD. Pulmonary blood flow depends on the size of the VSD and the presence and severity of pulmonary stenosis. Cyanosis is usually evident at birth. The diagnosis is made on the findings of chest roentgenogram, electrocardiogram, echocardiogram and cardiac catheterization. Management of patients with tricuspid atresia depends on the adequacy of pulmonary blood flow. Severely cyanotic neonates should be maintained on an intravenous infusion of prostaglandin E_1 until a surgical aortopulmonary shunt procedure can be performed to increase pulmonary blood flow. Various aortopulmonary shunt procedures include Blalock-Taussig procedure, Rashkind balloon atrial septostomy, bidirectional Glenn shunt, and modified Fontan operation. Heart transplantation is a treatment option for pediatric patients with "failed" Fontan circuits.

Ebstein Anomaly of the Tricuspid Valve

Ebstein anomaly consists of downward displacement of an abnormal tricuspid valve into the ventricle. The severity of symptoms and the degree of cyanosis are highly variable and depend on the extent of displacement of the tricuspid valve and the severity of right ventricular outflow tract obstruction. *Chest roentgenogram:* heart size varies from the normal to massive, box shaped cardiomegaly caused by enlargement of the right atrium and ventricle. The pulmonary vasculature can be normal or decreased. *Electrocardiogram* usually shows a right bundle branch block, normal or tall and broad P waves and a normal or prolonged PR interval. Wolff-Parkinson-White syndrome may be present. Echocardiogram shows the degree of displacement of the tricuspid valve leaflets, a dilated right atrium and any right ventricular outflow tract obstruction. *Pulsed* and *color Doppler examination* demonstrates the degree of tricuspid regurgitation. *Cardiac catheterization* confirms the presence of a large right atrium, an abnormal tricuspid valve, and any right-to-left shunt at the atrial level (*see* Fig. 19.24 in CD).

Treatment: Neonates with severe cyanosis should be maintained on an intravenous infusion of prostaglandin E_1 until a surgical aortopulmonary shunt procedure can be performed to increase pulmonary blood flow. In older children with mild or moderate disease, control of supraventricular dysrhythmias is done; surgical treatment may not be necessary until adolescence or young adulthood. In patients with severe tricuspid regurgitation, repair or replacement of the abnormal tricuspid valve along with closure of the ASD is then carried out.

19.7 CYANOTIC CONGENITAL HEART DISEASE: LESIONS ASSOCIATED WITH INCREASED PULMONARY BLOOD FLOW

D-Transposition of the Great Arteries

Transposition of great vessels, a common congenital anomaly accounts for 5% of all congenital heart disease. In the anomaly, the systemic veins return normally to the right atrium and the pulmonary veins return to the left atrium. The connections between the atria and ventricles are also normal (atrioventricular concordance). The aorta arises from the right ventricle and the pulmonary artery from the left ventricle. In normally related great vessels, the aorta is posterior and to the right of the pulmonary artery, whereas in

d-transposition of the great arteries (*d*-TGA), the aorta is anterior and to the right of the pulmonary artery (the d-indicates a dextroposition of aorta). Desaturated blood returning from the body to the right side of the heart goes to the aorta and back to the body again, whereas the oxygenated pulmonary venous blood returning to the left side of the heart is returned directly to the lungs. Survival in these newborns is provided by the foramen ovale and the ductus arteriosus, which permit some mixture of oxygenated and deoxygenated blood. TGA is more common in males (3 : 1) and infants born from diabetic mothers. Other factors associated with this disease include rubella or other viral illness in the mother during pregnancy, poor nutrition in the mother during pregnancy (prenatal nutrition), alcoholism, mother's age over 40, and deletion of chromosome 22q11 (CATCH 22 [cardiac defects, abnormal facies, thymic aplasia, cleft palate, hypoplasia], DiGeorge syndrome). Mortality is >90% in the 1st yr of life without corrective or palliative surgery (*see* Fig. 19.25 in CD).

D-Transposition of the Great Arteries with Intact Ventricular Septum

Cyanosis and tachypnea are most often recognized within the 1st hr of life. Untreated, the vast majority of these infants would not survive the neonatal period. The precordial may be normal, or a parasternal heave may be present. The second heart sound is usually single and loud, although occasionally it may be split. Murmurs may be absent, or a soft systolic ejection murmur may be noted at the midleft sterna border. The ECG shows the normal neonatal right-sided dominant pattern. Roentgenograms of the chest may show mild cardiomegaly, a narrow mediastinum (an egg-shaped heart), and normal to increased pulmonary blood flow. Echocardiography confirms the transposed ventricular-arterial connections. When transposition is suspected, an infusion of prostaglandin E_1 (dosage, 0.01–0.20 μg/kg/min) should be initiated immediately to maintain patency of the ductus arteriosus and improve oxygenation. Infants who remain severely hypoxic or acidotic despite prostaglandin infusion should undergo *Rashkind balloon arterial septostomy.*

Transposition of the Great Arteries with Ventricular Septal Defect

The clinical manifestations, laboratory findings, and treatment are similar to those described previously for transposition with an intact ventricular septum, if the VSD associated with TGA is small. When the VSD is large the clinical manifestations of cardiac failure are seen. The onset of cyanosis may be subtle and frequently delayed and can be generally recognized within the 1st month of life. The murmur is holocystic and generally indistinguishable from that produced by a large VSD with normally related great arteries. The heart is usually significantly enlarged. Chest roentgenogram demonstrates cardiomegaly, a narrow mediastinal waist and increased pulmonary vascularity. ECG shows prominent *P waves* and isolated right ventricular hypertrophy or biventricular hypertrophy. The diagnosis can be confirmed by echocardiography. Surgical treatment is advised soon after diagnosis, usually within the first months of life.

L-Transposition of the Great Arteries (Corrected Transposition)

In L-transposition, the atrioventricular relationships are discordant with the right atrium connected to the left ventricle and the left atrium to the right ventricle (ventricular inversion). The great arteries are also transposed, with the aorta arising from the right ventricle and the pulmonary artery from the left. The aorta arises to the left of the pulmonary artery (hence the designation L for levotransposition). The aorta may be anterior to the pulmonary artery; usually, they are nearly side by side. Symptoms and signs are widely variable and are determined by the associated lesions. The clinical signs are similar to those of an isolated VSD, if pulmonary outflow is unobstructed, whereas if the TGA is associated with pulmonary stenosis and a VSD, the clinical signs are similar to those of tetralogy of Fallot. Chest roentgenogram: may suggest the abnormal position of the great arteries; the ascending aorta occupies the upper left border of the cardiac silhouette and has a straight profile. *Electrocardiogram:* shows atrioventricular conduction disturbances, abnormal P waves, absent Q waves in V6, abnormally present Q waves in leads III, aVR, aVF, V1, and upright T waves across the precordium. *Echocardiogram* is diagnostic. Arterial switch operation (double switch operation) is the treatment of choice.

Double-Outlet Right Ventricle with Transposition of the Great Arteries (Taussig-Bing Anomaly)

In double-outlet right ventricle with TGA, the VSD is located above the crista supraventricularis (subarterial VSD) and is either directly subpulmonary or related to both the pulmonary and aortic valves (doubly committed VSD). Clinical manifestations include cyanosis, cardiac failure in early infancy, cardiomegaly, and a parasternal systolic ejection murmur and loud closure of the pulmonary valve. Chest roentgenogram demonstrates cardiomegaly, a large left atrium, and prominence of the pulmonary artery and pulmonary vasculature. Electrocardiogram shows right axis deviation, and right, left, or biventricular hypertrophy. The anatomic features of the anomaly and associated abnormalities are demonstrated by a combination of echocardiography and selective right and left ventriculography. In infancy pulmonary artery banding and surgical correction at a later stage by a Rastelli procedure or by an arterial switch procedure.

Total Anomalous Pulmonary Venous Return

Total anomalous pulmonary venous return (TAPVR) allows total mixing of systemic venous and pulmonary venous blood flow within the heart and thus produces cyanosis.

Chest roentgenogram demonstrates a large supracardiac shadow which together with the normal cardiac shadow forms a *"snowman"* appearance (or *figure 8 configuration*) in older children, but this shadow in early infancy is not helpful in diagnosis because of the presence of thymus. ECG shows right ventricular hypertrophy (usually a qR pattern in V3R and V1 and the P waves are frequently tall and spiked). Echocardiogram demonstrates a large right ventricle and identifies the pattern of abnormal pulmonary venous connections. The demonstration of a vessel in the abdomen with Doppler venous flow away from the heart is pathognomonic of TAPVR below the diaphragm. Cardiac catheterization shows that the oxygen saturation of blood in both atria, both ventricles, and the aorta is more or less similar, indicative of total mixing lesion. An increase in systemic venous saturation occurs at the site of entry of the abnormal pulmonary venous channel. Selective pulmonary arteriography shows the anatomy of the pulmonary veins and their point of entry into the systemic venous circulation. MRI and CT may be used for confirming the diagnosis (*see* Fig. 19.26 in CD).

Treatment: Obstructed TAPVR is a pediatric cardiac emergency because prostaglandin therapy is usually not effective. Surgical correction of TAPVR is indicated during infancy. If surgery cannot be performed urgently, extracorporeal membrane oxygenation (ECMO) may be required to maintain oxygenation. Long-term prognosis in these patients is poor and heart-lung transplantation may be the only option.

Truncus Arteriosus

In truncus arteriosus, a single arterial trunk (truncus arteriosus) arises from the heart and supplies the systemic, pulmonary, and coronary circulation. A VSD is always present, with the truncus overriding the defect and receiving blood from both the right and left ventricles. In the newborn period, signs of heart failure are absent. A murmur and minimal cyanosis are the initial signs. In most older infants the clinical picture is dominated by heart failure. Cyanosis is minimal. Runoff blood from the truncus to the pulmonary circulation may result in a wide pulse pressure and bounding pulses. The heart is usually enlarged, and the precordium is hyperdynamic. The 2nd heart sound is loud and single. A systolic ejection murmur, sometimes accompanied by a thrill is generally audible along the left sternal border. In older children with restricted pulmonary blood flow secondary to pulmonary vascular obstruction disease, progressive cyanosis, polycythemia, and clubbing develops.

Diagnosis: Chest roentgenogram shows cardiac enlargement, prominent truncus that follows the normal course of the ascending aorta and aortic knob, aortic arch to the right in 50% of patients, and increased pulmonary vascularity after the 1st few weeks of life. ECG shows right, left or combined ventricular hypertrophy. Echocardiogram demonstrates the large truncal artery overriding the VSD and the pattern of origin of the branch pulmonary arteries. Pulse and Doppler studies are used to evaluate truncal valve regurgitation. Cardiac catheterization shows a left-to-right shunt at the ventricular level, with right-to-left shunting into the truncus. Systolic pressure in both ventricles and the truncus is similar. Angiography reveals the large truncus arteriosus and more precisely defines the origin of pulmonary arteries.

Treatment: In the 1st few weeks of life, many of these infants can be managed with anticongestive medications. But as the pulmonary vascular resistance falls heart failure symptoms worsens and surgery is indicated usually in the next few weeks. Delay of surgery much beyond 4–8 wk may increase the likelihood of pulmonary vascular disease. Without surgery, many of these patients succumb during infancy or by the 1st or 2nd yr of life.

Abnormal Positions of the Heart and the Heterotaxy Syndromes (Asplenia, Polysplenia)

The classification and diagnosis of abnormal positions of the heart is based first on the position of the viscera and atria and then the ventricles followed by the great vessels. The atrial situs is related to the situs of the viscera and lungs. In *situs solitus*, the viscera are in their normal positions (stomach and spleen on the left and liver in the right), the three lobed right lung is on the right, and the two lobed left lung on the left; the right atrium is on the right, and the left atrium is on the left. When the abdominal organs and lung lobulation are reversed, the left atrium is on the right and the right atrium on the left, it is known as situs

inversus. If the visceroatrial situs cannot be determined, a condition known as *situs indeterminus* or *heterotaxia exists*. The heterotaxia syndromes are usually associated with severe congenital heart lesions: The two major variations are: (i) *asplenia syndrome*, which is associated with a centrally located liver, absent spleen and two morphologic right lungs; and (ii) *polysplenia syndrome*, which is associated with multiple small spleens, absence of the intrahepatic portion of the inferior vena cava, and bilateral left lung morphology (in both lungs).

Dextrocardia occurs when the heart is in the right side of the chest; levocardia (the normal situation) is present when the heart is in the left side of the chest. Dextrocardia without associated situs inversus and levocardia in the presence of situs inversus are often complicated by severe cardiac malformations. Dextrocardia with situs inversus and normally related great arteries ("mirror image" dextrocardia) is often associated with a functionally normal heart, although congenital heart disease of a less severe nature is common (*see* Figs 19.27 and 19.28 in CD).

Anatomic or functional abnormalities of lungs, diaphragm and thoracic cage may result in displacement of the heart to the right (dextroposition), but in this case the cardiac apex is pointed normally to the left.

The treatment and prognosis of patients with one of the positional anomalies are determined by the underlying defects. There is increased risk of serious infections such as bacterial sepsis in patients with asplenia and therefore, such patients require daily antibiotic prophylaxis.

19.8 OTHER CONGENITAL HEART AND VASCULAR MALFORMATIONS

Anomalies of the Aortic Arch

Two types of anomalies of the aortic arch are right aortic arch and *vascular rings*. In the right aortic arch abnormality, the aorta curves to the right and if it descends on the right side of the vertebral column, is usually associated with other cardiac malformations. It is found in cases of tetralogy of Fallot (in 20% cases) and truncus arteriosus. A right aortic arch without other cardiac anomalies is not associated with symptoms. The trachea is deviated to the left of the midline rather to the right, as in the presence of a normal left arch. Chest roentgenogram shows the anomalies of the aortic arch. Barium esophagogram shows the esophagus indented on its right border at the level of the aortic arch.

Congenital abnormalities of the aortic arch and its major branches result in the formation of *vascular rings* around the trachea and esophagus with varying degrees of compression. Associated congenital heart disease may be present in 5–50% of patients. Clinical manifestations of compression of the vascular ring appear during infancy include vomiting, brassy cough and pneumonia, and chronic wheezing exacerbated by crying, feeding, and flexion of the neck; extension of the neck tends to relieve the noisy respiration, Sudden death occurs from aspiration. Chest roentgenograhic examination of the barium-filled esophagus and aortography identify the anomaly. The diagnosis is confirmed by two-dimensional echocardiography, MRI, or CT. Cardiac catheterization is performed in patients with associated cardiac anomalies and bronchoscopy is done to determine the extent of airway narrowing. Surgery is advised for symptomatic patients.

Anomalous Origin of the Coronary Arteries

1. In anomalous origin of the left coronary artery from the pulmonary artery (ALCAPA), the blood supply to the left ventricular myocardium is severely compromised. Heart failure becomes apparent with in the first few months of life and is often precipitated by respiratory infection. A gallop rhythm is common. Murmurs may be of the nonspecific, ejection type or may be holosystolic due to mitral insufficiency. Untreated, death often occurs from heart failure within the 1st 6 mo. Surgical treatment consists of detaching the anomalous coronary artery from the pulmonary artery and anastomosing it to the aorta to establish normal myocardial perfusion.
2. Anomalous origin of the right coronary artery is from the pulmonary artery: The left coronary artery is enlarged, whereas the right is thin walled and mildly enlarged. In early infancy, perfusion of the right coronary artery is from the pulmonary artery, and later perfusion is from collaterals of the left coronary vessels. Angina and sudden death can occur in adolescence or adulthood. When recognized, the anomaly should be repaired by re-anastomosis of the right coronary artery to the aorta.
3. Ectopic origin of the coronary artery is from the aorta with aberrant proximal course: The aberrant artery may be a left, right, or major branch coronary artery. Patients with this rare abnormality are often initially seen with severe myocardial infarction, ventricular arrhythmias, angina pectoris or syncope; sudden death may occur especially in young athletes. The diagnosis of anomalous origin of the coronary arteries should include an electrocardiogram, stress testing, two-dimensional echocardiography, CT or MRI, and cardiac catheterization with selective coronary angiography.

Treatment is indicated for obstructed vessels and consists of aortoplasty with re-anastomosis of the aberrant vessel or occasionally, coronary artery bypass grafting.

19.9 EISENMENGER SYNDROME

The term Eisenmenger syndrome refers to patients with a VSD in which blood is shunted partially or totally from right to left as a result of the development of pulmonary vascular disease. This physiologic abnormality can also occur with ASD, atrioventricular septal defect, PDA, or any other communication between the aorta and pulmonary artery. The pathologic changes of Eisenmenger syndrome occur in the small pulmonary arterioles (<300 mm).

Clinical manifestations: Symptoms do not usually develop until the 2nd or 3rd decade of life, although a more fulminant course may occur. Cyanosis and dyspnea, fatigue and dysrhythmias occur. In the late stages heart failure, chest pain, headaches, syncope, and hemoptysis are noted. Physical examination reveals a right ventricular heave, palpable pulmonary artery pulsation at the left upper sternal border, a narrowly split 2nd heart sound with a loud pulmonary component, and a holosystolic murmur of tricuspid regurgitation and an early decrescendo diastolic murmur of pulmonary insufficiency audible along the left sternal border.

Diagnosis: Cyanotic patients have various degrees of polycythemia. Chest roentgenogram shows from normal to greatly enlarged heart size, prominent main pulmonary artery and pulmonary vessels enlarged in the hilar areas and taper rapidly in caliber in the peripheral branches. ECG shows marked right ventricular hypertrophy with tall and spiked P waves. Echocardiogram shows a thick walled right ventricle and demonstrates the underlying congenital heart disease; pulmonary valve shows a characteristic early midsystolic closure, the "W sign." Cardiac catheterization: usually shows a bidirectional shunt at the site of the defect.

Treatment: Medical treatment is primarily symptomatic. Benefits from calcium channel blocker such as nifedipine or intravenous prostacyclin therapy has been reported. Symptomatic polycythemia in older children and adolescents may be improved by repeated phlebotomies with volume replacement. Patients who are at risk for the development of late pulmonary vascular disease, prevention is the best management by early surgical elimination of large intracardiac or great vessels communications during infancy. Infants with trisomy 21 have a propensity for earlier development of pulmonary vascular disease. Combined heart-lung or bilateral lung transplantation is the only surgical option for many of these patients of Eisenmenger syndrome.

19.10 GENERAL PRINCIPLES OF TREATMENT OF CONGENITAL HEART DISEASE

Most patients who have *mild congenital heart disease* require no treatment. The parents and child should made aware that a normal life is expected and that no restriction of the child's activities. General health maintenance, including the well balanced diet, aerobic exercise, and avoidance of smoking, should be encouraged. Even *patients with moderate to severe heart disease* need not be markedly restricted in physical activity.

1. *Physical education* should be modified appropriately to the child's capacity to participate. Competitive sports for most of these patients should be discouraged.
2. *Routine immunizations* should be given, with the inclusion of influenza vaccine. Patients who might be considered candidates for heart or heart-lung transplantation should not receive live-virus vaccinations just before transplantation.
3. *Bacteria infections* should be treated vigorously.
4. *Prophylaxis against infective endocarditis* should be carried out during dental procedures, during instrumentation of the urinary tract, and before gastrointestinal tract manipulation.
5. *Cyanotic patients* need to be monitored for noncardiac manifestations of oxygen deficiency such as iron deficiency anemia, polycythemia (hematocrit >65%).

Postoperative care: Immediate postoperative care should be provided in an intensive care unit. Preparation for postoperative monitoring begins in the operative room, where anesthesiologist or surgeon places an arterial catheter to allow direct arterial pressure measurements and arterial sampling for blood gas determination. A central venous catheter is also placed for measuring central venous pressure and for infusions of cardioactive medications. In more complex cases, left atrial, or pulmonary artery catheters and used for pressure monitoring purposes. Flow-directed thermodilution monitoring (Swan-Ganz) catheters are sometimes used for monitoring pulmonary wedge pressure and the cardiac index. Temporary pacing wires are placed on the atrium or ventricle, or both, in case temporary heart block occurs. Transcutaneous oximetry provides for continuous monitoring of arterial oxygen saturation.

Serious postoperative complication encountered after open heart surgery include respiratory failure, cardiac rhythm disorders, heart failure, acidosis secondary to low cardiac output, renal failure or hypovolemia, neurological abnormalities especially in the neonatal period (seizures, thromboembolism and stroke), postcardiotomy syndrome, hemolysis of mechanical origin seen after repair of certain cardiac defects (such as atrioventricular septal defects, or after the insertion of a mechanical prosthetic valve) and infection. It is important that these complications are identified and treated.

The Adult with Congenital Heart Disease

All individuals born with congenital heart defects require both primary medical care and routine cardiac follow-up. The coordination of care between primary and specialty providers is particularly important during adolescence, because of new medical and social issues that arise and affect medical care. Physical fitness and exercise are generally recommended for all patients. Restrictions may be placed on certain patients with respect to competitive athletics and high-intensity aerobic activities. Competitive athletic participation should not be approved without recommendations from the cardiologist.

Issues of contraception and pregnancy should be discussed with all adolescent patients at the appropriate age and in the proper setting. Intrauterine devices should be avoided due to increased risk of infective endocarditis. Successful pregnancy is possible for most young women with congenital heart disease. However, there are conditions in which the risks of pregnancy are significantly increased, such as persistent cyanotic heart disease or pulmonary hypertension. Anticipatory counseling and education are key aspects to care of the adolescent with regard to contraception and pregnancy. There is also a tendency for young adults to avoid medical care and cardiac follow-up due to lack of education, denial, or difficulty with access to the medical care system.

American Academy of Pediatrics: A consensus statement of health care transitions for young adults with special health care needs. *Pediatrics* 2002;110:1304–6.

Bernstein D. Congenital heart disease. In: Kliegman RM, Behrman RE, Jenson HB, Stanton BF (eds). *Nelson Textbook of Pediatrics*. 18th edn. Vol. 2. Philadelphia: Saunders, 2007; 1878–940.

Consensus on timing of intervention of common congenital heart diseases. Working group on management of congenital heart diseases in India. *Indian Pediatr* 2008;45:117–26.

Lee CH, Chen HN, Tsao LY, Hsiao CC, Lee ML. Oral ibuprofen versus intravenous indomethacin for closure of patent ductus arteriosus in very low birth weight infants. *Pediatrics and Neonatology* 2012;53:346–53.

Murphy D. The adult with congenital heart disease. In: Kliegman RM, Behrman RE, Jenson HB, Stanton BF (eds). *Nelson Textbook of Pediatrics*. 18th edn. Vol. 2. Philadelphia: Saunders, 2007;1940–2.

19.11 CARDIAC ARRHYTHMIAS (DISTURBANCES OF THE RATE AND RHYTHM OF THE HEART)

Despite the infrequency and vague presenting symptoms, it is critical to identify and appropriately manage these disorders. When left unrecognized and untreated, dysrhythmias can lead to cardiopulmonary compromise and arrest. The overall incidence of arrhythmias is 13.9 per 100,000 and 55.1 per 100,000 pediatric ED visits (children under 18 yr of age). Among children with arrhythmias, the most common dysrhythmias are sinus tachycardia (50%), supraventricular tachycardia (13%), bradycardia (6%), and atrial fibrillation (4.6%).

Sinus Arrhythmias

Sinus arrhythmia represents a normal physiologic variation in impulse discharges from the sinus node related to respirations. The heart rate slows during expiration and accelerates during inspiration. Occasionally, if the sinus rate becomes slow enough, an escape beat arises from the atrioventricular (AV) junction region. Irregularities in sinus rhythm, especially bradycardia associated with periodic apnea, are commonly seen in premature infants. Sinus arrhythmia is exaggerated during febrile illness and by drugs that increase vagal tone such as digitalis; it is usually abolished by exercise.

Extrasystoles

Extrasystoles are produced by the discharge of an ectopic focus that may be situated anywhere in atrial, junctional, or ventricular tissue. Usually, isolated extrasystoles are of no clinical or prognostic significance. Under certain circumstances, however, premature beats may be due to organic heart disease (inflammation, ischemia, fibrosis) or to drug toxicity, especially from digitalis.

Tachydysrhythmias

Tachycardia is defined as a heart rate beyond the upper limit of normal for the patient's age. In adults, the heart rate is greater than 100 beats per minute (BPM). Tachycardias can be classified broadly into those that originate form loci above the atrioventricular (AV) node (i.e. supraventricular), from the AV node (AV node reentrant tachycardias), and from the ventricle. The majority of tachycardians are supraventricular (SVT) in origin. Those that are ventricular in origin are associated typically with hemodynamic compromise. When tachycardia is recognized, stepwise questioning can help evaluate the ECG tracing. Is it regular or irregular? Is the QRS complex narrow or wide? Does every P wave results in a single QRS complex? Once these have been established, the treatment options are considered according to whether the patient has a pulse and the presenting rhythm on ECG.

Sinus tachycardia can be differentiated from other tachycardians by a narrow QRS axis and a P wave that precedes every QRS complex. The rate is usually greater than 140 beat per minute (BPM) in children and greater than 160 BPM in infants. Sinus tachycardia is typically benign. The pulse rate has been shown to increase linearly with temperature in children older than 2 months of age. For every 1°C (1.8°F) increase in body temperature, the pulse rate increase by an average of 9.6 BPM. Sinus tachycardia can also be associated with such underlying conditions as hypoxia, anemia, hypovolemia, shock, myocardial ischemia, pulmonary edema, hyperthyroidism, medications (catecholamine), hypocalcemia, and illicit drug use. Most commonly, it is the result of dehydration and hypovolemia. Treatment aimed at correcting the heart rate alone may be harmful to the patient because the tachycardia is a compensatory response to sustain adequate cardiac output. For this reason, the treatment of sinus tachycardia is largely targeted at treating the underlying disorder, rather than treating the tachycardia itself.

Ventricular tachycardia is an important rhythm to recognize and treat promptly. Nonperfusing ventricular rhythms are seen in up to 19% of pediatric cardiac arrests, when sudden infant death syndrome (SIDS) cases are excluded. Furthermore, ventricular tachycardia can decompensate into ventricular fibrillation, which is a nonperfusing, terminal arrhythmia. Ventricular tachycardia may result from electrolyte disturbances (hyperkalemia, hypokalemia, and hypocalcemia), metabolic abnormalities, congenital heart disorders, myocarditis, or drug toxicity. Other causes include cardiomyopathies, cardiac tumors, acquired heart disease, prolonged QT syndrome, and idiopathic causes.

On electrocardiogram the QRS complex has a wide configuration. The QRS duration is prolonged, ranging from 0.06 to 0.14 seconds. Complexes may appear monomorphic with a uniform contour and absent or retrograde P waves. Alternatively, the QRS complexes may appear polymorphic or vary randomly as is seen in torsades de pointes. EKG findings that further support the presence of ventricular tachycardia include the presence of AV dissociation with the ventricular rate exceeding the atrial rate (*see* Fig. 19.29 in CD).

In a patient who has ventricular tachycardia, the urgency of treatment depends on the patient's clinical status. Initially, the airway, breathing and circulation (ABCs) must be maintained, and it must be determined whether the patient has a pulse and is hemodynamically stable.

Ventricular tachycardia with a pulse in an unstable patient warrants immediate synchronized cardioversion at 0.5 to 1 J/kg. It is important to pretreat conscious patients with light sedation (e.g. midazolam, 0.1 mg/kg). Pharmacologic interventions include amiodarone (5 mg/kg intravenously over 20–60 min; maximum single dose, 150 mg; maximum daily dose, 15 mg/kg/d), procainamide (15 mg IV over 30–60 min), or lidocaine (1 mg kg IV bolus, repeat every 5–10 min, with max total dose of 3 mg/kg).

After cardioversion, the return to normal sinus rhythm is usually transient. The medication used to achieve sinus rhythm must be given as a continuous infusion using lidocaine (20–50 g/kg/min), amiodarone (7–15 mg/kg/day), or procainamide (20–80 g/kg/min [maximum dose of 2 g/24 h]). In polymorphic ventricular tachycardia, temporary atrial or ventricular pacing may be required. Overall, the treatment goal is to keep the heart rate at less than 150 BPM in infants and less than 130 BPM in older children.

If pulseless ventricular tachycardia is refractory to defibrillation, antiarrhythmic drugs are indicated, such as amiodarone (5 mg/kg, IV bolus) or lidocaine (1 mg/kg, IV bolus, and repeated to a maximum of 3 mg/kg). Although the pediatric dosing of amiodarone has not been clearly establishing, the recommended loading dose of 5 mg/Kg IV may be given over 20–60 minutes. If rate control is not achieved, the dose may be repeated in increments of 5 mg/kg IV, to a maximum of 15 mg/kg/d IV. For polymorphic ventricular tachycardia (*torsades de pointes)* the mainstay of treatment is magnesium (20–50 mg/kg, IV).

Premature ventricular contractions: A premature ventricular contraction (PVC) is a premature, wide QRS complex that has a distinct configuration and is not preceded by a P wave. They may appear in a pattern of two consecutive PVCs (couplet), alternating PVC with a normal QRS complex (bigeminy) or in which every third beat is PVC (trigeminy). The occurrence of three or more consecutive is considered ventricular tachycardia. Although most children who have PVCs are otherwise healthy, PVCs can also be associated with congenital heart disease, mitral valve prolapse, prolonged QT syndrome, and cardiomyopathies (dilated and hypertrophic) (*see* Fig. 19.30 in CD).

For the most part, patients who have PVCs are asymptomatic. However, when they are unrecognized and untreated, there is a risk of developing ventricular tachycardia in patients who have a serious underlying cause. When they are examined, 50 to 75% of otherwise normal children may have PVCs seen on Holter monitoring.

Supraventricular tachycardia: SVT is the most common symptomatic dysrhythmias in infants and children. In newborns and infants who have SVT, the heart rate is greater than 220 BPM. In older children, it is defined as having a heart rate of more than 180 BPM. The ECG shows a narrow complex tachycardia, either without discernible P waves or with retrograde P waves with an abnormal axis. The QRS duration is normal but is occasionally increased with aberrancy. It is further characterized by little or no variation in the heart rate. AV re-entrant tachycardia uses a bypass tract that may either be able to conduct antegrade (Wolff-Parkinson-White [WPW] syndrome) or remain concealed (*see* Fig. 19.31 in CD).

In newborns and infants, most patients do not have an underlying cause to account for the tachycardia, such as fever, dehydration, fluid or blood loss, anxiety, or pain. Infants often present with nonspecific complaints such as "fussiness," lethargy, poor feeding, pallor, sweating with feeds, or simply "not acting right". If congestive heart failure (CHF) develops there may be pallor, cough, and respiratory distress. Although many infants can tolerate SVT well for 24 hr, within 48 hr, 90% of them will develop heart failure and may deteriorate rapidly. In contrast, CHF rarely occurs in older children, who are usually able to describe palpitations, chest pain, dizziness, or shortness of breath. Important historical factor include a relationship to exercise, meals stress, color changes, neurologic changes or syncope. A medical history significant for cardiac problems, current medications, allergies, or a family history of sudden death or cardiac disease should be investigated.

The management of SVT always begins with ensuring that the patient maintaining, airway, breathing and cardiovascular status. It is important to promptly administer oxygen and to obtain a 12-lead ECG with a rhythm strip. It is of utmost importance to expeditiously differentiate between patients who are stable and those who are unstable. In a child presenting with unstable SVT with severe heart failure and poor perfusion synchronized cardioversion is initiated at 0.5 J/kg and can be increased up to 1 J/kg. Adenosine may be given before cardioversion if intravenous access has already been established. In unstable patients, cardioversion should not be delayed for attempts at IV access or sedation.

In children who present with asymptomatic SVT or with mild heart failure, vagal stimulation maneuvers such as placing ice bag over the face on an infant and child or blowing through a straw to abort the attack; the other vagotonic maneuvers include Valsalva maneuver, straining, breath holding, and drinking ice water. If that is unsuccessful, adenosine is administered through an IV that is preferable close to the heart. Because of its extremely short half-life adenosine must be pushed and flushed (with 5 ml normal saline) quickly, to be effective. The initial dose of adenosine is 0.1 mg/kg (up to 6 mg) and can be increased to 0.2 mg/kg/dose (up to 12 mg), if the first dose is ineffective. An effective response is a brief period of asystole on ECG, with the return of normal sinus rhythm. Failure to terminate the dysrhythmia after the second dose of adenosine in a stable patient should prompt consultation with a pediatric cardiologist. Adenosine can be therapeutic as well as diagnostic; however, it is not effective with no reciprocating atrial tachycardia, atrial flutter, atrial fibrillation, or ventricular tachycardia. There are minimal hemodynamic consequences associated with adenosine administration. Contraindications include a deinnervated heart (e.g. transplant) and second- or third-degree heart block. Additional, adenosine can worsen bronchospasm in asthmatics and an increase heart block or precipitate ventricular arrhythmias in those taking carbamazepine, verapamil, or digoxin (alterative medication include procainamide).

The evaluation of SVT includes attempts at elucidating the cause of SVT to prevent future episodes. Laboratory studies may include electrolytes (especially potassium, calcium, magnesium, and glucose), complete blood count, toxicology screen, and blood gas and thyroid function tests.

Once stabilized, the majority of patients who present with SVTs will need to be admitted to a hospital, to investigate the underlying cause of SVT and the potential for long-term medical management or radiofrequency ablation.

Atrial flutter is an uncommon rhythm presenting in the pediatric population. Atrial rates may present in the range of 240 to 450 BPM, with the ventricular response depending on the A V nodal conduction. The pacemaker lies in an ectopic focus. Causes of atrial flutter in children are attributed largely to structural heart disease, including a dilated atria, myocarditis, or acute infection. It is associated most notably with postoperative complications of congenital heart disease repairs, such as atrial septal detect (ASD) repairs, the Mustard procedure for D-transposition of the great arteries, or the Fontan procedure for single ventricle.

These procedures cause atrial futter through disruption in the conduction system as happens when there is suturing through the atrial septum.

On an electrocardiogram, the hallmark pattern is "saw-toothed" flutter waves, which is best, viewed in leads II, III, and VI. The atrial rate is, on average, approximately 300 atrial BPM. Because the AV node cannot respond this quickly, there is an AV node which can resent as a 2 : 1, 3 : 1, or 4 : 1 block. The QRS complex is generally normal in configuration. The clinician must recognize whether the patient is hemodynamically stable. An unstable patient may warrant electrical cardioversion with the consideration of adding heparin to prevent embolization. In patients who are receiving digoxin, it is advisable to avoid electrical cardioversion, unless the condition is life-threatening because the combination is associated with malignant ventricular arrhythmias. For patients who are thermodynamically stable, digoxin is administered to increase AV blockade, thereby slowing the ventricular rate. Propranolol 1.0 to 4.0 mg/kg/day, orally divided three to four times daily, may also be added. Recurrences are then prevented by administering quinidine (*see* Fig. 19.32 in CD).

Atrial fibrillation is defined as disorganized rapid atrial activity with atrail rates ranging from 350 to 600 BPM. The ventricular rate is variable and depends on a varying AV block. The rhythm of atrial fibrillation is described as being "irregularly irregular" alternating between fast and slow rates. On electrocardiography, the hallmark features are irregular atrail waves, with beat to beat variability of the atrial size and shape. This is best recognized in lead VI. The QRS complexes appear normal. Children at an increased risk of developing atrial fibrillation include those who have an underlying structural heart defect (such as congenital mitral valve disease and hyperthyroidism) and those who have undergone intra-atrail operative procedures. Atrial fibrillation is also associated with decreased cardiac output and in patients with WPW syndrome (*see* Fig. 19.33 in CD).

When the child presents to the emergency department, the clinician must promptly recognize whether he or she is hemodynamically stable or has cardiac compromise. Hemodynamically unstable patients warrant immediate cardioversion. However, in patients who are hemodynamically stable, digoxin can be administered for ventricular rate control allowing for a 24 hour time period to ineffective; a second medication may be added such as propranolol, and procainamide. Digoxin is not given when WPW syndrome is present. During admission, cardioverted patients are often started on an agent to keep them in normal-sinus rhythm (e.g. amiodarone, procainamide).

Ventricular fibrillation is an uncommon rhythm in the pediatric population but is certainly life threatening. The hallmark is chaotic, irregular ventricular contractions without circulation to the body. On the electrocardiogram, the rhythm is one of bizarre QRS complexes with varying sizes and configurations and a rapid, irregular rate. Cause of ventricular fibrillation includes postoperative complication from congenital heart disease repair, severe hypoxemia, hyperkalemia, medications (digitalis, quinidine, catecholamines, and anesthesia), myocarditis, and myocardial infarction.

Because ventricular fibrillation is a nonperfusing rhythm, CPR must be initiated immediately. Ventricular fibrillation is treated the same way as ventricular tachycardia without a pulse. Defibrillation is initiated at 2 J/kg, increased from 2 to 4 J/kg, and then followed by a third shock at 4 J/kg. If defibrillation is unsuccessful, epinephrine (0.01 mg/kg, 1:10,000 solution) should be given and repeated every 3 to 5 minutes as necessary.

Bradydysrhythmias

Bradycardia is defined as a heart rate slower than the lower limit of normal for the patient's age. Mechanisms of bradycardia include depression of the pacemaker in the sinus and conduction system blocks. Complete heart block is a common cause of significant bradycardia in pediatric patients and may be acquired or congenial.

Bradycardia in children may be attributable to vagal stimulation, hypoxemia, acidosis, or an acute elevation of intracranial pressure. The most common cause of bradycardia in the pediatric population is hypoxemia. It is important to correct hypoxemia before increasing the heart rate in children.

Sinus bradycardia includes a heart rate less than the lower limit of normal for the patient's age, with P waves preceding each QRS complex on an ECG. Usually, the heart rate is less than 80 BPM in infant and less than 60 BPM in older children. Sinus bradycardia is a predominantly benign entity, seen most often in athletes and during sleep.

Sinus bradycardia can also be associated with underlying causes. One such ominous cause is an acute one of increased intracranial pressure as part of Cushing's triad of bradycardia, hypertension, and irregular respirations. An important cause of bradycardia is respiratory compromise. Therefore, the adequacy of the patient's oxygenation and ventilation should be assessed rapidly. Bradycardia can also be associated with hyperkalemia, hypercalcemia, hypoxia, hypothermia, hypothyroidism, and medications (e.g. digitalis and β-blockers). As with sinus tachycardia, the treatment of sinus bradycardia is targeted at the treatment of the underlying cause.

An important distinction must be made between sinus bradycardia and junctional (nodal) bradycardia. On electrocardiography, junctional bradycardia has either no P waves or inverted P waves after QRS complexes. QRS complexes have a normal configuration and generally have rates between 40 and 60 BPM.

Junctional bradycardia may occur in an otherwise nom1al heart or postoperatively, in cases of digitalis toxicity, or with increased vagal tone. If the patient is asymptomatic no treatment is indicated. However, if the patient has signs of decreased cardiac output, atropine or pacing may be indicated.

Atrioventricular Block (AV Block)

First-degree atrioventricular (AV) block is an abnormal delay in conduction through the AV node. In this type there is a disturbance in the conduction between the normal sinus impulse and its eventual ventricular response. This manifests as a prolonged PR interval on electrocardiography. Meanwhile, the heart is maintained in sinus rhythm with a normal QRS configuration. There are no dropped beats.

First-degree heart block can be an incidental finding on an otherwise normal ECG reading. Common causes include otherwise healthy children with an infectons disease. It may further be associated with myocarditis (e.g. rheumatic fever and lyme disease), cardiomyopathies, and congenital heart disease. (Atrial septal detect and Ebstein anomaly) (*see* Fig. 19.34 in CD).

Second-degree atrioventricular block: Mobitz type I (Wenckebach type) and Mobitz type II. In the Mobitz type I heart block also known as the Wenckebach phenomena, the PR interval lengthens progressively until a QRS complex is dropped. This usually occurs over three to six cardiac cycles, followed by a long diastolic pause and then the cycle resumes. There are occasional and frequent P waves that conduct refractory period at the level of the AV node.

The Mobitz type II second-degree heart block is known as the all-or-none phenomena. There is either AV conduction with a normal PR interval or a completely blocked conduction. The failure of conduction is at the level of the bundle of His, with a prolongation of the refractory period in the Pukinje system, because some of the atrial impulses are not conducted (*see* Figs 19.35 and 19.36 in CD).

Third-degree heart block: The third degree heart block is also known as complete heart block, occurs when none of the atrial impulses is conducted to the ventricles. There is a complete loss of rhythm conduction from a working atrial pacemaker, thereby allowing the ventricular pacemaker to take over. On electrocardiograph, the dissociated, both the atrial and ventricular rhythms are regular, maintaining regular PP and RR intervals, respectively (*see* Fig. 19.37 in CD).

Children presenting with first-degree heart block are largely asymptomatic but have the potential to progress to further heart block, including second- and third degree heart blocks. Those presenting with second-degree type I (Wenckebach type), rarely progress to complete heart block, whereas second-degree, type II block frequently progresses to complete heart block. Those children who present with complete heart block, most notably in infancy may present with signs of congestive heart failure. Older children may present with syncopal attacks, otherwise own as Stokes-Adams attacks with heart rates less than 40 to 45 BPM or even sudden death.

Patients who have complete heart block may present with symptoms related to hypoperfusion, including fatigue, dizziness, impaired exercise tolerance syncope, confusion and even sudden death. No treatment is indicated for a first-degree heart block. However, if suspicious features are present patients may require evaluation for treatment that is directed at the underlying cause. In patients who have Mobitz type II second-degree heart block pacemaker may be warranted because there is a risk of progressing to complete heart block. For those who present with a complete heart block, the mainstay of therapy is a pacemaker. While awaiting pacemaker insertion, it may be necessary to administer atropine or isoproterenol, which temporarily increases the heart rate.

Long QT syndrome: (LQTS) is a disorder of delayed ventricular depolarization characterized by prolongation of the QT interval, as seen on electrocardiography. Prolongation of the QT interval may be either hereditary or acquired. Jervell-Lange-Nielsen syndrome is an autosomal recessive from of prolonged QT syndrome associated with congenital deafness, whereas Romano-Ward syndrome (RWS) is an autosomal dominant form that is not associated with deafness.

Drugs may prolong the QT interval directly (terfenadine, astemizole) or more often when drugs such as erythromycin or ketoconazole inhibit their metabolism.

Patients with LQTS commonly present between the ages of 9 and 15 yr of age. In children with LQTS there is most often a syncopal episode often brought on by exercise, fright, or a sudden startle; some events occur during sleep. Patients can initially be seen with seizures, presyncope and palpitations and about 10% are initially in cardiac arrest. The diagnosis is based on electrocardiographic and clinical criteria. A heart rate-corrected QT interval of greater than 0.47 sec is highly indicative, whereas a QT interval greater than 0.44 sec is suggestive. Other features include notched T waves, T wave alternans, a low heart rate for age, a history of syncope (especially with stress), and a familial history of either LQTS or unexplained sudden death. Twenty-four-hour Holter monitoring and exercise testing are adjuncts to the diagnosis.

Treatment of LQTS includes the use of propranolol (β-blocker) at doses (1–4 mg/kg/24 hr q 6 h, increase to 16 mg/kg/24 hr) that blunt the heart rate response to exercise. Some patients may require pacemaker because of drug-induced profound bradycardia.

Once a patient is diagnosed with LQTS, an EKG should be performed on all other family members. All affected individuals regardless of age should be restricted from competitive sports but not necessarily recreational spots. Patients should be educated to avoid triggering factors such as certain medications, loud noise, emotionally stressful situation, and dehydration. Because of the high risk of unexpected cardiac events, family members and close friends should be instructed in CPR.

Sinus Node Dysfunction

Sinus arrest and sinoatrial block may cause a sudden pause in the heartbeat. The sinus arrest is caused by failure of impulse formation within the sinus node and sinoatrial block is caused by a block between the sinus impulse and the surrounding atrium. These arrhythmias are manifested in digitalis toxicity or in patients who have had extensive atrial surgery.

Sick sinus syndrome is the result of abnormalities in the sinus node or atrial conduction pathways or both. Most commonly seen after surgical correction of congenital heart defects, especially the atrial switch (Mustard or Senning) operation for the transposition of great arteries. Pacemaker therapy is indicated in patients who experience symptoms such as dizziness and syncope.

Patients with sinus node dysfunction may also have episodes of bradycardia–tachycardia syndrome with symptoms of palpitation, exercise intolerance, or dizziness. For symptomatic patients a pacemaker in conjunction of drug therapy (propranolol, quinidine, procainamide) is usually necessary.

Dubin A. Cardiac arrhythmias. In: Kliegman RM, Behrman RE, Jenson HB, Stanton BF (eds). Nelson Textbook of Pediatrics. 18th edn. Vol. 2. Philadelphia: Saunders, 2007;1942–50.

Gera Rani, Arora A. Pediatric Arrhythmias In: Mathur GP, Mathur Sarla (eds). Current Trends in Pediatrics. Vol 3. Delhi: Academa Publishers, 2007;249–55.

Goldberger Z, Lampert R. Implantable cardioverter-defibrillators. JAMA 2006;295:809–18.

Goodacre S, MacleodK. Paediatric electrocardiography. Br Med J 2002;324:1382–5.

Kaultman H, Shah M. Evaluation of the child with an arrhythmia. Pediatr Clin North Am 2004;51:1537–51.

19.12 RHEUMATIC FEVER

Etiology: There is considerable evidence to support the link between Group A Streptococcus (GAS) upper respiratory tract infections and acute rheumatic fever and rheumatic heart disease. About 2/3 of the patients with an acute episode of rheumatic fever have a history of upper respiratory tract infection several weeks before, and the peak age and seasonal incidence of acute rheumatic fever closely parallel those of GAS infections. Not all but certain serotypes of GAS (M types 1, 3, 5, 6, 18, 24) are more frequently isolated from patients with acute rheumatic fever than are other serotypes.

Epidemiology: Worldwide, rheumatic heart disease remains the most common form of acquired heart disease in all age groups, accounting for as much as 50% of all cardiovascular disease and as much as 50% of all cardiac admissions in many developing countries. A number of studies have suggested that poverty and crowding contributes to the spread of GAS infections and is most closely associated with the incidence of acute rheumatic fever. The decline in incidence of acute rheumatic fever in industrialized countries over the past four decades has also been attributable to the greater availability of medical care and to the wide spread use of antibiotics. Antibiotic therapy of GAS pharyngitis has been important in preventing initial attacks, and, particularly recurrences of the disease. The incidence of both initial attacks and recurrences of rheumatic fever peaks in the children 5–15 yr of age, the age of greatest risk of pharyngitis. In addition, there is genetic predisposition to acute rheumatic fever. Studies in twins have shown a higher concordance rate of acute rheumatic fever in monozygotic than in dizygotic twin pairs.

Pathogenesis: Two theories of the pathogenesis of acute rheumatic fever and rheumatic heart disease have been proposed: the cytotoxic theory and the immunologic theory. The cytotoxic theory suggests that a GAS toxin may be involved in the pathogenesis of acute rheumatic fever and rheumatic heart disease. GAS produces several enzymes that are cytotoxic for mammalian cardiac cells, such as streptolysin O, which has a cytotoxic effect on mammalian cells in tissue culture. However, one of the major problems with the cytotoxic hypothesis is its inability to explain the latent period between GAS pharyngitis and the onset of acute rheumatic fever.

An *immune-mediated pathogenesis* for acute rheumatic fever and rheumatic heart disease has been suggested by the clinical similarity of acute rheumatic fever to other illnesses produced by immunopathogenic processes and by the latent period between the GAS infection and the acute rheumatic fever (*immunologic theory*). Common antigenic determinants are shared between certain components of GAS (M protein, protoplast membrane, cell membrane, cell wall Group A carbohydrate, capsular hyaluronate) and specific mammalian tissues (e.g. heart, brain, joint). For example, certain M proteins (M1, M5, M6, and M19) share epitopes with human tropomyosin and myosin. The involvement of GAS superantigens such as pyrogenic exotoxins in the pathogenesis of acute rheumatic fever has been also proposed.

Clinical manifestations and diagnosis: There is no clinical or laboratory finding that is pathognomic for acute rheumatic fever. T. Duckett Jones in 1944 proposed guidelines to aid in diagnosis and to limit over diagnosis. The Jones criteria, as revised in 1992 by the American Heart Association are intended only for the diagnosis of the initial attack of acute rheumatic fever and not for recurrences. There are 5 *major* and 4 *minor* criteria and an absolute requirement for *evidence (microbiologic or serologic) of recent GAS infection.* The diagnosis of acute rheumatic fever can be established by the Jones criteria when a patient fulfills 2 major criteria or 1 major and 2 minor criteria and meets the absolute requirement. There are 3 circumstances in which the diagnosis of acute rheumatic fever can be made without strict adherence to the Jones criteria: (i) chorea may occur as the only manifestation of acute rheumatic fever; (ii) indolent carditis may be the only manifestation in patients who 1st come to medical attention after the onset of acute rheumatic fever; and (iii) although most patients with recurrences of acute rheumatic fever fulfill the Jones criteria, some may not.

A. *Major manifestations:* There are 5 major criteria. The presence of 2 major criteria with evidence (microbiologic or serologic) of recent Group A Streptococcus (GAS) infection fulfils the Jones criteria.

   1. *Migratory polyarthritis:* Arthritis occurs in about 75% of patients with acute rheumatic fever and typically involves large joints, particularly the knees, ankles, wrists, and elbows. Involvement of the spine, small joints of the hands and feet, or hips is uncommon.

Rheumatic joints are generally hot, red, swollen and exquisitely tender; even the friction of bedclothes is uncomfortable. The pain can precede and can appear to be disproportionate to the other findings. The joint involvement is characteristically migratory in nature; a severely inflamed joint can become normal within 1–3 days without treatment, as one or more other large joints become involved. Severe arthritis can persist several weeks in untreated patients. Monoarticular arthritis is unusual unless anti-inflammatory therapy is instituted prematurely, aborting the progression of the migratory polyarthritis. If a child with fever and arthritis is suspected having acute rheumatic fever, salicylates should be withheld and observe for migratory progression. A dramatic response to even small doses of salicylates is another characteristic feature of the arthritis, and the absence of such a response should suggest an alternative diagnosis. There is no deformity in the joint. Synovial fluid in acute rheumatic fever usually contains 10,000 to 100,000 white blood cells/mm^3 with a preponderance of neutrophils, about 4 g/dl protein, normal glucose level, and forms a good mucus clot. Frequently, arthritis is the earliest manifestation of acute rheumatic fever and may correlate with peak antistreptococcal antibody titers temporarily. There is an apparent inverse relationship between the severity of arthritis and the severity of cardiac involvement.

2. Carditis occurs in about 50–60% of all cases of acute rheumatic fever. Rheumatic carditis is characterized by pancarditis, with severe inflammation of myocardium, pericardium, and endocardium. Cardiac involvement during acute rheumatic fever varies in severity from fulminant, potentially fatal exudative pericarditis to mild, transient cardiac involvement. Endocarditis (valvulitis), which manifests by one or more cardiac murmurs, is the constant finding in rheumatic carditis, whereas the presence of pericarditis or myocarditis is variable. Myocarditis and/or pericarditis without evidence of endocarditis are rare due to rheumatic heart disease. Most cases have either isolated mitral valvular disease or combined aortic and mitral valvular disease. Isolated aortic or right-sided valvular involvement is uncommon. Serious and long-term illness is entirely related to valvular heart disease as a consequence of a single attack or recurrent attacks of acute rheumatic fever.

Valvular insufficiency is characteristic of both acute and convalescent stages of acute rheumatic fever, whereas valvular stenosis usually appears several years or even decades after the acute illness. In developing countries rheumatic fever often occurs at a younger age and mitral stenosis and aortic stenosis may develop sooner after acute rheumatic fever than in developed countries and can occur in young children.

Acute rheumatic carditis usually presents as tachycardia and cardiac murmurs, with or without evidence of myocardial or pericardial involvement. Moderate to severe carditis can result in cardiomegaly and congestive heart failure with hepatomegaly and peripheral and pulmonary edema. Echocardiographic findings include pericardial effusion, decreased ventricular contractibility, and aortic and/or mitral regurgitation. Mitral regurgitation is characterized by a high-pitched apical holosystolic murmur radiating to the axilla. In patients with significant mitral regurgitation, this may be associated with an apical mid-diastolic murmur of relative mitral stenosis. Aortic insufficiency is characterized by high-pitched decrescendo diastolic murmur at the upper left sternal border. The major consequence of acute rheumatic carditis is chronic progressive valvular disease particularly valvular stenosis, which can require valve replacement and predispose to infective endocarditis.

3. Chorea (rheumatic chorea, St. Vitus' Dance, Sydenham chorea): It has been recognized for three centuries (Thomas Sydenham 1684). Sydenham chorea occurs in about 10–15% of patients with acute rheumatic fever and usually presents as an isolated, frequently subtle neurologic behavior disorder. The three major features of Sydenham's chorea include chorea, hypotonia and emotional lability. Emotional lability, incoordination, poor school performance, uncontrollable movements, and facial grimacing, exacerbated by stress and disappearing with sleep are characteristic features in children with Sydenham chorea. Chorea rarely, if ever, leads to permanent neurologic sequelae, although the acute illness is distressing. Chorea occasionally is unilateral. The latent period from acute GAS infection to chorea is usually longer than for arthritis or carditis and can be months. In patients who have history of rheumatic fever, the chorea tends to develop between 1 and 6 months later. Clinical maneuvers to elicit features of chorea

include: 1. *Milkmaid's grip*—relaxing and tightening handshake; 2. *Choreic hand*—spooning of the extended hand by flexion at the wrist and extension of the fingers; 3. *Darting tongue*—tongue cannot be protruded for longer than a few seconds; 4. *Pronator sign*—arms and palms turn outward when held above the head; and 5. *Handwriting*—examination of handwriting to evaluate fine motor movements. Diagnosis is based on clinical findings with supportive evidence of GAS antibodies. However, in patients with a long latent period from the inciting streptococcal infection, antibody levels may have declined to normal. Sydenham's chorea may persist for several months and as long as 1–2 yr. About 20% of children suffer from a recurrence of chorea within 2 yr of the initial episode.

4. *Erythema marginatum* is a characteristic rash, which occurs in <3% of patients with acute rheumatic fever. It consists of erythematous, serpiginous, macular lesions with pale centers that are not pruritic. It occurs primarily on the trunk and extremities, but not on the face and it can be accentuated by warming the skin.

5. *Subcutaneous nodules* are rare (≤1%) in patients with acute rheumatic fever. Subcutaneous nodules are firm nodules approximately 1 cm in diameter, which are present along the extensor surfaces of tendons near bony prominences. There is a correlation between the presence of these nodules and significant rheumatic heart disease.

B. *Minor manifestations:* There are 2 clinical and 2 laboratory minor manifestations. The 2 clinical minor manifestations are arthralgia (in the absence of polyarthritis as a minor criterion) and fever (typically temperature ≥102°F and occurring early in the course of illness). The 2 laboratory minor manifestations are elevated acute phase reactants (e.g. C-reactive protein, erythrocyte sedimentation rate) and prolonged PR interval on electrocardiogram (1st degree heart block). However, a prolonged PR interval alone does not constitute evidence of carditis or predict long term cardiac sequelae.

C. *Recent Group A streptococcal infections:* An absolute requirement for the diagnosis of acute rheumatic fever is supporting evidence of a recent Group A streptococcus (GAS) infection. Acute rheumatic fever typically develops 2–4 wk after an acute episode of GAS pharyngitis at a time when clinical findings of pharyngitis are not present and only 10–20% of the throat culture or rapid streptococcal antigen test results are positive. One third of patients have no history of an antecedent pharyngitis. Therefore, evidence of an antecedent GAS infection is usually based on elevated or increasing serum antistreptococcal antibody titers. If only a single antibody is measured (antistreptolysin O), only 80–85% of patients with acute rheumatic fever have an elevated titer; however, 95–100% have an elevation if 3 different antibodies (antistreptolysin O, anti-DNase B, antihyaluronidase) are measured. Therefore, when acute rheumatic fever is suspected clinically, multiple antibody tests are performed. Except for patients with chorea, clinical findings of acute rheumatic fever generally coincide with peak antistreptococcal antibody responses. Most patients with chorea have elevation of antibodies to 1 or more GAS antigens although these antibodies may be waning. The diagnosis of acute rheumatic fever should not be made in patients with elevated or increasing streptococcal antibody titers who do not fulfill the Jones criteria because such titer changes may be coincidental.

Differential diagnosis: The differential diagnoses of rheumatic fever include many infectious and noninfectious illnesses (Table 19.2).

Treatment

Bed rest: All patients with acute rheumatic fever should be placed on bed rest and monitored closely

Table 19.2: Differential diagnosis of rheumatic fever		
Arthritis	*Carditis*	*Chorea*
Rheumatoid arthritis	Viral myocarditis	Huntington's chorea
Reactive arthritis (e.g. *Shigella, Salmonella, Yersinia*)	Viral pericarditis	Wilson disease
Serum sickness	Infective endocarditis	Systemic lupus erythematosus
Sickle cell anemia	Kawasaki disease	Cerebral palsy
Malignancies	Congenital heart disease	Tics
Systemic lupus erythematosus	Mitral valve prolapse	Hyperactivity
Lyme disease	Innocent murmurs	
Gonococcal infection		

for evidence of carditis. They can be allowed to ambulate as soon as the signs of acute inflammation have subsided; patients with carditis require longer periods of bed rest.

Antibiotic therapy: Patient should receive 10 days of orally administered penicillin or erythromycin, or a single intramuscular injection of benzathine penicillin to eradicate GAS from the upper respiratory tract. After this initial course of antibiotic therapy, the patient should be started on long-term antibiotic prophylaxis.

Anti-inflammatory therapy: Antiinflammatory agents (e.g. salicylates, corticosteroids) should be withheld if arthralgia or atypical arthritis is the only clinical manifestation of presumed acute rheumatic fever. Premature treatment with one of these agents may interfere with the development of the characteristic migratory polyarthritis and thus obscure the diagnosis of acute rheumatic fever. Agents such as acetaminophen can be used to control pain and fever while the patient is being observed for more definite signs of acute rheumatic fever or for evidence of another disease.

Patients with typical migratory polyarthritis and those with carditis without cardiomegaly or congestive heart failure should be treated with oral salicylates. The usual dose of aspirin is 100 mg/kg/day in 4 divided doses PO for 3–5 days, followed by 75 mg/kg/day in 4 divided doses PO for 4 wk. Determination of salicylate level is indicated when the arthritis does not respond or signs of salicylate toxicity (tinnitus, hyperventilation) develop. Patients with carditis or cardiomegaly or congestive heart failure should receive corticosteroids. The usual dose of prednisolone is 2 mg/kg/day in 4 divided doses for 2–3 wk followed by a tapering of the dose that reduces the dose by 5 mg/24 hr every 2–3 days. At the beginning of the tapering of the prednisolone dose, aspirin should be started at 75 mg/kg/day in 4 divided doses for 6 wk. Supportive therapies for patients with moderate to severe carditis include digoxin, fluid and salt restriction, diuretics and oxygen. The cardiac toxicity of digoxin is enhanced with myocarditis. Termination of the anti-inflammatory therapy may be followed by the reappearance of clinical manifestations or of laboratory abnormalities. These "rebounds" are best left untreated unless the clinical manifestations are severe; salicylates or steroids should be reinstated in such cases.

Sydenham chorea: Chorea often occurs as an isolated manifestation after resolution of acute phase of the disease; therefore, anti-inflammatory agents are usually not indicated. Sedatives may be helpful early in the course of disease; phenobarbital (16–32 mg every 6–8 hr PO) is the drug of choice. If phenobarbital is ineffective, then haloperidol (0.01–0.03 mg/kg/24 hr divided bid PO) or chlorpromazine (0.5 mg/kg every 4–6 hr PO) should be started. Approximately 20% of patients who present with "pure" chorea who are not given secondary prophylaxis develop rheumatic heart disease within 20 yr. Therefore, patients with chorea, even in the absence of other manifestations of rheumatic fever, require long-term antibiotic prophylaxis.

Complications: The arthritis and chorea of acute rheumatic fever resolve completely without sequelae. Therefore, the long-term sequelae of rheumatic fever are usually due to heart. Patients with cardiac valvular disease secondary to acute rheumatic fever are at increased risk for developing infective endocarditis during episodes of transient bacteremia. Patients require short-term antibiotic prophylaxis before surgical or dental procedures that are associated with transient bacteremia. The importance of good dental hygiene in the prevention of infective endocarditis should also be stressed. Patients who have had rheumatic fever but have no evidence of residual valvular disease do not require endocarditis prophylaxis.

Prognosis: The prognosis for patients with acute rheumatic fever depends on the clinical manifestations present at the time of the initial episode, the severity of the initial episode, and the presence of recurrences. Approximately 70% of the patients with carditis during the initial episode of rheumatic fever recover with no residual heart disease. However, the more severe the initial cardiac involvement, the greater is the risk for residual heart disease. Patients without carditis during the initial episode are unlikely to have carditis with recurrences. In contrast, patients with carditis during the initial episode are likely to have carditis with recurrences, and the risk for permanent heart damage increases with each recurrence. Patients who have had acute rheumatic fever are susceptible to recurrent attacks following reinfection of the upper respiratory tract with GAS. Therefore, these patients require long-term continuous chemoprophylaxis. Patients with chorea, even in the absence of other manifestations of rheumatic fever, require long-term antibiotic prophylaxis because of the development of rheumatic heart disease.

Prevention

Prevention of both initial and recurrent episodes of acute rheumatic fever depends on controlling GAS infections of the upper respiratory tract.

Primary prevention: Appropriate antibiotic therapy instituted before the 9th day of symptoms of acute GAS pharyngitis is highly effective in preventing 1st attacks of acute rheumatic fever from that episode.

Secondary prevention: Secondary prevention is directed at preventing GAS pharyngitis in patients who are at substantial risk for recurrent acute rheumatic fever. Secondary prevention requires continuous antibiotic prophylaxis, which should begin as soon as the diagnosis of acute rheumatic fever has been made and immediately after a full course of antibiotic therapy has been completed. Because patients who have had carditis with their initial episode of acute rheumatic fever are at a relatively higher risk for having carditis with recurrences and for sustaining additional cardiac damage, they should receive antibiotic prophylaxis into adulthood and perhaps for life. Patients who did not have carditis with their initial episode of acute rheumatic fever have a relatively low risk for carditis with recurrences. The duration of prophylaxis is noted in Table 19.3.

The regimen of choice for secondary prevention is a single intramuscular injection of benzathine penicillin G (1.2 million IU) every 4 wk (Table 19.4). In certain high risk patients and in certain areas of the world where the incidence of rheumatic fever is particularly high, use of benzathine penicillin every 3 wk may be necessary because levels of penicillin may decrease to marginally effective amounts after 3 wk. In compliant patients, continuous oral antimicrobial

prophylaxis can be used. Penicillin V given twice daily and sulfadiazine given once daily are equally effective when used in such patients. For the exceptional patient who is allergic to both penicillin and sulfonamides, erythromycin given twice daily may be used.

Dajani A, Taubert K, Ferrieri P, et al. Guidelines for the diagnosis of rheumatic fever: Jones criteria, 1992 update. *JAMA* 1992;268:2069–73.

Gerber MA. Group A *Streptococcus*. In: Kliegman RM, Behrman RE, Jenson HB, Stanton BF (eds). *Nelson Textbook of Pediatrics*. 18th edn. Vol. 1. Philadelphia: Saunders, 2007;1135–45.

Grover A, Vijayvergia R, Thingam ST. Burden of rheumatic and congenital heart disease in India: Lowest estimate based on the 2001 census. *Indian Heart J* 2002;54:104–7.

Padmawati S. Present status of rheumatic fever and rheumatic heart disease in India. *Indian Heart J* 1995;47:395–8.

Saxena Anita. Rheumatic fever and rheumatic heart disease-current status. In: Mathur GP, Mathur Sarla (eds). *Current Trends in Pediatrics*. Vol 3. Delhi: Academa Publishers, 2007; 238–48.

Rheumatic Heart Disease

Rheumatic involvement of the valves and endocardium is the most important manifestation of rheumatic fever. The valvular lesions begin as small verrucae composed of fibrin and blood cells along the borders of one or more of the heart valves. As the inflammation subsides, the verrucae tend to disappear and leave scar tissue. With repeated attacks of rheumatic fever, new

Table 19.3: Duration of prophylaxis

Category	Duration
Rheumatic fever without carditis	5 yr or until 21 yr of age, whichever is longer
Rheumatic fever with carditis but without residual heart disease (no valvular disease*)	10 yr or well into adulthood, whichever is longer
Rheumatic fever with carditis and residual heart disease (persistent valvular disease*)	At least 10 yr since last episode and at least until 40 yr of age, sometimes lifelong prophylaxis

*Clinical or echocardiographic evidence

Source: American Academy of Pediatrics. *Red Book 2006 Report of the Committee on Infectious Diseases*, 27th edn. Elk Grove Village, IL: American Academy of Pediatrics, 2006;619.

Table 19.4: Chemoprophylaxis for recurrences of acute rheumatic fever

Drug	Dose	Route
Penicillin G benzathine, or	1.2 million U every 4 wk*	Intramuscular
Penicillin V, or	250 mg twice a day	Oral
Sulfadiazine or Sulfsoxazole	0.5 g once a day for patients ≤27 kg (≤60 lb)	Oral
	1 g once a day for patients >27 kg (>60 lb)	
For people who are allergic to penicillin and sulfonamide		
Erythromycin	250 mg twice a day	Oral

*In high risk situations, administration every 3 wk is recommended

Source: American Academy of Pediatrics. *Red Book 2006 Report of the Committee on Infectious Diseases*, 27th edn. Elk Grove Village, IL: American Academy of Pediatrics, 2006;619.

verrucae form near the previous ones, and the mural endocardium and chordae tendineae get involved. The mitral valve is affected most often, followed in frequency by the aortic valve. The right sided heart manifestations are rare.

Mitral Insufficiency

Mitral insufficiency is the result of structural changes that usually include some loss of valvular substance and shortening and thickening of the chordae tendineae. The resultant chronic lesion is mild, moderate or severe in severity. In patients with severe chronic mitral insufficiency, pulmonary arterial pressure becomes elevated, the right ventricle and atrium becomes enlarged, and the right sides heart failure subsequently develops.

Clinical manifestations: The physical signs of mitral insufficiency depend on its severity. In mild disease, high-pitched holosystolic murmur (pansystolic murmur) at the apex, radiating to the axilla is present, but the signs of heart failure are absent. In severe *mitral insufficiency* there is enlarged heart, heaving apical left ventricular impulse, apical systolic thrill, accentuated 2nd heart sound, prominent 3rd heart sound, holosystolic murmur (pansystolic murmur) at the apex radiating to the axilla, and short mid-diastolic rumbling murmur.

Laboratory findings: The electrocardiogram (ECG) and roentgenograms are normal in *mild lesions*. With severe *mitral insufficiency* the ECG shows bifid P wave, signs of left ventricular hypertrophy, and associated right ventricular hypertrophy, in the presence of pulmonary hypertension. X-ray chest in severe insufficiency shows prominent left atrium and left ventricle, congestion of perihilar vessels (a sign of pulmonary venous hypertension), and rarely calcification of the mitral valve. Echocardiography shows enlargement of the left atrium and left ventricle, and Doppler studies demonstrate the severity of the mitral regurgitation. Invasive studies such as heart catheterization and left ventriculography are considered only if diagnostic questions are not totally resolved by noninvasive assessment.

Complications: Severe mitral insufficiency may result in cardiac failure, atrial fibrillation, other atrial and ventricular arrhythmias and infective endocarditis.

Treatment: Prophylaxis against recurrences of rheumatic fever (Benzathine penicillin G 1,200,000 units every 3 wk) is the only treatment that is required in mild cases. Severe cases may need treatment for heart failure, arrhythmias, infective endocarditis, and afterload reducing agents (captopril, hydralazine) to reduce the regurgitant volume and to preserve left

ventricular function. Surgical treatment (annuloplasty or valve replacement) is indicated for patients who despite adequate medical therapy have recurrent episodes of heart failure, dyspnea with moderate activity, and progressive cardiomegaly, often with pulmonary hypertension. In these cases prophylaxis against infective endocarditis should be done for dental or other surgical procedures, because the routine antibiotics taken by theses patients for rheumatic fever prophylaxis are insufficient to prevent endocarditis.

Mitral Stenosis

Mitral stenosis of rheumatic origin results from fibrosis of the mitral ring, commissural adhesions, and contracture of valve leaflets, chordae, and papillary muscles. It takes 10 yr or more for the lesions to become fully established, although the process may occasionally be accelerated. In significant mitral stenosis there is increased pressure and enlargement and hypertrophy of the left atrium, pulmonary venous hypertension, increased pulmonary vascular resistance, and pulmonary hypertension. Right ventricular and atrial dilatation and hypertrophy ensue and are followed by right-sided heart failure.

Clinical manifestations: Patients with mild mitral stenosis are asymptomatic. Patients with severe mitral stenosis are associated with exercise intolerance and dyspnea, loud 1st heart sound, opening snap, long, low pitched, rumbling, mitral diastolic murmur with presystolic accentuation at the apex, functional tricuspid insufficiency (pansystolic murmur), heart failure, hepatomegaly, ascitis, edema, atrial fibrillation, and hemoptysis. An elevated left atrial pressure causes forceful opening of the thickened valve leaflets; this generates a snap (opening snap) early in the diastole which precedes the mid-diastolic murmur. Hemoptysis is caused by rupture of bronchial or pleurohilar veins and occasionally by pulmonary infarction.

Laboratory findings: The electrocardiogram (ECG) and roentgenograms are normal in mild lesions. In severe insufficiency ECG shows notched P wave, right ventricular hypertrophy. X-ray chest in severe insufficiency shows left atrial enlargement and prominence of the pulmonary artery and right-sided heart chambers; calcification of mitral valve may be present. Echocardiography shows distinct narrowing of the mitral orifice during diastole and left atrial enlargement and Doppler can estimate the transmitral pressure gradient. Cardiac catheterization quantitates the diastolic gradient across the mitral valve and the degree of elevation of pulmonary arterial pressure.

Treatment: Prophylaxis against recurrence of rheumatic fever (benzathine penicillin G 1,200,000 units every 3 wk), and no other treatment is required in mild cases. In severe disease surgical valvotomy or balloon catheter mitral valvuloplasty is usually performed and valve replacement is only done when it is absolutely necessary.

Aortic Insufficiency

Combined mitral and aortic insufficiency is more common than aortic involvement alone. Patients with combined lesions during the episode of acute rheumatic fever may have only aortic involvement 1–2 yr later. Mild and moderate lesions are well tolerated and many individuals with severe regurgitation are symptoms free and tolerate advanced lesions upto 30–40 yr of age. In chronic aortic rheumatic insufficiency, sclerosis of the aortic valve results in distortion and retraction of the cusps.

Clinical manifestations: Dyspnea on exertion can progress to orthopnea. The large stroke volume and forceful left ventricular contractions may result in palpitations. Excessive sweating and heat intolerance are due to vasodilation. The physical signs are as follows: 1. Increased stroke volume and pulse pressure (systolic blood pressure is elevated and the diastolic pressure is low) in chronic aortic insufficiency lead to many physical signs. These signs may be absent in acute aortic insufficiency because compensatory increases in end-diastolic volume and stroke volume have not yet occurred. (a) Corrigan's pulse: The carotid pulse has a rapid rise and full upstroke with a rapid fall in diastole. (b) Hill's sign refers to a disproportionate (i.e. 20 mm Hg) increase of systolic blood pressure taken in the leg as compared to systolic blood pressure measured in the arm. Its presence suggests severe aortic insufficiency. (c) Pistal-shot femoral pulses. Auscultation over the femoral arteries reveals a pistal-shot pulse. (d) Duroziez's sign: A stethoscope is placed over the femoral artery with enough pressure to produce a systolic bruit. The concomitant occurrence of diastolic bruit constitutes Duroziez's sign. (e) de Musset's sign refers to a bobbing movement of the head caused by the increased stroke volume and pulse pressure. (f) Quincke's pulse is systolic blushing and diastolic blanching of the nail bed when gentle upward traction is placed on the nail. 2. The heart is enlarged with a left ventricular apical heave, which is displaced downward and to the left and diastolic thrill may be palpable. 3. The typical diastolic murmur has a high-pitched blowing quality, easily audible in full expiration with the diaphragm of the stethoscope placed firmly on the chest and the patient leaning forward, begins immediately with the 2nd heart sound and continues until late in diastole. The murmur is heard over the upper and mid-left sternal border with radiation to the apex and the aortic area. 4. A systolic ejection murmur because of the increased stroke volume and an apical presystolic murmur (Austin Flint murmur) as a result of the large regurgitant aortic flow in diastole that prevents the mitral valve from opening fully can also be heard.

Laboratory findings: ECG may be normal, but in advanced cases it shows left ventricular hypertrophy and strain with prominent P waves. X-Ray chest shows enlargement of the left ventricle and aorta. The echocardiogram shows a large left ventricle and diastolic mitral valve flutter or oscillation caused by regurgitant flow hitting the valve leaflets. Doppler studies demonstrate the degree of aortic runoff into the left ventricle. Cardiac catheterization is indicated only when the echocardiographic data are equivocal.

Treatment: The treatment consists of afterload reducers (e.g. captopril, hydralazine) and prophylaxis against recurrence of acute rheumatic fever and the development of infective endocarditis. Surgery (valve replacement) is considered when early symptoms are present, ST-T wave changes are seen on the ECG, or evidence of decreasing left ventricular fraction is noted and should be carried out before the onset of heart failure, pulmonary edema, or angina, and increasing left ventricular distension on the echocardiogram.

Tricuspid Valve Disease

Primary tricuspid valve disease is rare after rheumatic fever. *Tricuspid insufficiency* is more common secondary to right ventricular dilatation resulting from unrepaired left-sided lesions. The signs produced by tricuspid insufficiency include prominent pulsations in the jugular veins, systolic pulsations of the liver and blowing holosystolic murmur (pansystolic murmur) at the lower left sternal border that increases in intensity during inspiration; concomitant signs of mitral or aortic valve disease with or without atrial fibrillation are frequently seen. Signs of tricuspid insufficiency decrease or disappear when heart failure produced by left-sided lesions is treated. Tricuspid valvuloplasty may be required in rare cases.

Pulmonary Valve Disease

Pulmonary insufficiency usually occurs on a functional basis secondary to pulmonary hypertension and is a late finding with severe mitral stenosis. The diastolic murmur (Graham Steell murmur) is similar to that of aortic insufficiency, but peripheral arterial signs (bounding pulses) are absent. The diagnosis is confirmed by two-dimensional echocardiography and Doppler studies.

Bernstein Daniel. Rheumatic heart disease. In: Kliegman RM, Behrman RE, Jenson HB, Stanton BF (eds). *Nelson Textbook of Pediatrics*. 18th edn. Vol. 2. Philadelphia: Saunders, 2007; 1961–3.

Cilliers A.Treating acute rheumatic failure.*Br Med J* 2003; 127:631–2.

Holmes DR, Nishimura RA, Reeder GS. Aortic and mitral balloon valvuloplasty: Emergence of a new percutaneous technique. *Int J Cardiol* 1987;16:227–33.

Narula J, Chandrasekhar Y, Rahimtoola S. Diagnosis of active rheumatic carditis. *Circulation* 1999;100:1576–81.

Stollerman GH. Rheumatic fever in the 21st century. *Clin Infect Dis* 2001;33:806–14.

19.13 DISEASES OF THE MYOCARDIUM

Cardiomyopathies

Cardiomyopathies are divided on the basis of etiology into primary or idiopathic (those with unknown cause) and secondary (those are due to infections, endocrine disorders, metabolic and nutritional diseases, neuromuscular diseases, blood diseases, and tumors. Cardiomyopathies can be classified on the basis of predominant structural and functional abnormalities: dilated cardiomyopathy, hypertrophic cardiomyopathy, and restrictive cardiomyopathy. For making the diagnosis ECG, chest roentgenogram, echocardiogram and Doppler studies are performed. The prognosis of cardiomyopathies is generally poor; clinical deterioration can be rapid.

Dilated Cardiomyopathy

Dilated cardiomyopathy is characterized by cardiomegaly secondary to extensive dilatation of the ventricles most prominently the left. Varying degrees of ventricular hypertrophy is also present. The cause in majority cases is unknown (idiopathic dilated cardiomegaly), but may have a genetic basis; a remote history of viral illness. All age groups are affected. Usually the onset is insidious, but sometimes the symptoms of heart failure occur suddenly.

Neuromuscular diseases: Heart disease is common in patients with Friedreich ataxia, Duchenne muscular dystrophy, and Becker dystrophy.

Kawasaki disease: The arteries associated with Kawasaki disease initially involve small arterioles, but in the second or third week of illness, medium sized arteries become inflamed and aneurysmal dilatation of the coronary arteries. During the healing phase, areas of both coronary dilatation and stenosis may result and can lead to myocardial infarction and death.

Autoimmune diseases: Rheumatic carditis and cardiovascular involvement occur in cases of juvenile rheumatoid arthritis, systemic lupus erythematosus, periarteritis nodosa, dermatomyositis, and scleroderma.

Endocrine disorders: Hyper and hypothyroidism produces cardiac enlargement. Diabetic cardiomyopathy is rare in children; however, infants of diabetic mothers can have cardiac hypertrophy and dilatation. Cardiomyopathy may be caused by chronic exposure to elevated catecholamines in patients with pheochromocytoma.

Metabolic and nutritional diseases: Cardiomyopathy may develop in children suffering from beriberi, kwashiorkor, selenium, and taurine and carnitine deficiency and those suffering from malabsorption.

Hematologic diseases: In infants and children, severe anemia may be associated with cardiac involvement. Although cardiac output increases when the hemoglobin content is less than about 7 g/dl, significant cardiac enlargement occurs with an extreme reduction in hemoglobin (3–4 g or less).

Disorders of the coronary arteries: Anomalous origin of the left coronary artery from the pulmonary artery, and one of the coronary arteries from the aorta ("suicide coronary"), coronary calcinosis and coronary artery malformations such as coronary ostial stenosis and coronary artery stenosis in the setting of supravalvular aortic stenosis. Patients with homozygous familial hypercholesterolemia may have a propensity for coronary atherosclerosis at an early age. Patients who have undergone heart transplantation are at risk for the development of graft coronary artery disease.

Doxorubicin (Adriamycin) cardiotoxicity: This chemotherapeutic agent can cause acute myocarditis but more often results in chronic dilated cardiomyopathy. Cardiomyopathy may become manifested months or even years after doxorubicin treatment. Cardiomegaly is principally due to left ventricular and left atrial enlargement.

Ipecac cardiac toxicity: Cardiac toxicity can occur with chronic intentional ipecac abuse secondary to anorexia nervosa or bulimia.

Hypertrophic Cardiomyopathy

Hypertrophic cardiomyopathies in children may be secondary to obstructive congenital heart disease (aortic stenosis, coarctation of aorta) or to an inborn error of metabolism or it may be idiopathic. Massive ventricular hypertrophy with principal involvement of the ventricular septum characterizes the disease, but all portions of the left ventricle and sometimes the right ventricle can be affected; varying degrees of myocardial fibrosis is also present.

Hypertrophic cardiomyopathy in infants of diabetic mothers: In infants of diabetic mothers, a transient form of hypertrophic cardiomyopathy may be encountered with or without left ventricular outflow tract obstruction. The increased left ventricular mass usually regress within several months (*see* Chapter 8).

Corticosteroids in premature infants: Premature infants who are receiving corticosteroids for chronic lung disease may also suffer from transient hypertrophic cardiomyopathy, which usually resolves rapidly with cessation of steroid therapy.

Glycogen storage disease: Cardiac as well as skeletal muscles are involved in the generalized form of glycogen storage disease known as type II or Pompe disease (*see* Section 26.4).

Restrictive Cardiomyopathy

Restrictive cardiomyopathy is associated with poor ventricular compliance and inadequate filling of the ventricular cavities during diastole and results in clinical manifestations that closely simulate those of constrictive pericarditis. In its full blown form, restrictive cardiomyopathy results in dyspnea, edema, ascites, hepatomegaly, increased venous pressure, and pulmonary congestion.

Löffler hypereosinophilic syndrome: This disorder produces severe multisystem dysfunction (skin, liver, lungs, nervous system), and the predominant cause of death in restrictive cardiomyopathy with endocardial fibrosis of the mitral and tricuspid valves and the right and left ventricles.

Mucopolysaccharidosis: In this disorder, most commonly Hurler syndrome, mucopolysaccharides accumulate in many organs, including the heart and great vessels (*see* Section 26.5). The most pronounced lesions are found in the valves and coronary arteries. The heart may be moderately enlarged, with electrocardiographic signs of left ventricular hypertrophy.

Isolated noncompaction of the left ventricle: This cardiomyopathy of unknown cause results in both left ventricular restriction and dilatation. The condition may be diagnosed at any age, from infancy to young adulthood, and the severity of congestive heart failure varies. The electrocardiogram is diagnostic and shows left ventricular hypertrophy. Patients may be at risk for ventricular arrhythmias and sudden death, as well as mural thromboses and stroke.

Myocarditis

Myocarditis refers to inflammation, necrosis, or myocytolysis and is caused by many infectious (viral or nonviral agents), connective tissue (including rheumatic myocarditis), granulomatous, toxic, or idiopathic processes affecting the myocardium with or without associated systemic manifestations of the disease process or involvement of the endocardium or pericardium. Coronary pathology is uniformly absent. The most common manifestation is heart failure, although arrhythmias and sudden death may be the first detectable signs. Viral infections are the most common cause.

Viral Myocarditis

This is the commonest type of myocarditis. Viral myocarditis is typically a sporadic, but occasionally an epidemic illness. The most common causative agents are coxsackie virus B and adenovirus, although many other known viral agents are implicated. In early infancy, viral myocarditis often occurs as an acute fulminant illness; a neonate may initially have fever, heart failure, arrhythmias, respiratory distress, and cyanosis and may have evidence of viral hepatitis, aseptic meningitis, and an associated rash. In toddlers and young children an acute but less fulminant myopericarditis occur. Whereas, in older children and adolescents, viral myocarditis is asymptomatic, may be seen with gradual onset of congestive heart failure (rarely with acute congestive heart failure) or a sudden onset of ventricular arrhythmias or manifested as a precursor to idiopathic dilated cardiomyopathy.

Diagnosis: The sedimentation rate and heart enzymes (creatine phosphokinase, lactic dehydrogenase) may be elevated in acute or chronic myocarditis. Serum viral titers are positive, but negative titers do not eliminate the diagnosis. *Echocardiography* demonstrates poor ventricular function and often a pericardial effusion, mitral valve regurgitation, and the absence of coronary artery or other congenital heart lesions. Myocarditis can be confirmed by endomyocardial biopsy, which is performed during cardiac catheterization and can also be used to detect other causes of cardiomyopathy (storage disease, mitochondrial defects). PCR can identify specific viral RNA or DNA.

The *differential diagnosis* of myocarditis include idiopathic dilated cardiomyopathy, pericarditis, fibroelastosis of the endocardium, anomalous origin of the left coronary artery disease, carnitine deficiency, and hereditary mitochondrial defects.

Treatment: The role of corticosteroids is controversial. Treatment with prednisolone (2 mg/kg daily, tapered to 0.3 mg/kg daily over a period of 3 months) is effective in reducing myocardial inflammation and improving cardiac function. Relapse has been reported when immunosuppression is discontinued. The role of specific treatments of viral myocarditis is controversial. Intravenous immunoglobulin (IVIG) has been used at 2 g/kg. Trials with antiviral therapy for enterovirus (pleconaril) or Epstein-Barr virus (acyclovir) may be effective. Supportive measures for the treatment of congestive heart failure include dopamine or epinephrine which may be helpful in those with poor cardiac output and systemic hypotension. Digoxin should be used with caution, is often started half the normal dose, because of the arrhythmogenic properties. Arrhythmias should be treated aggressively and may require intravenous amiodarone to achieve adequate control. Extracorporeal membrane oxygenation (ECMO) may be indicated for infants and children with cardiogenic shock. In larger children and adolescents with refractory heart failure implantation of a left ventricular assist device (LVAD) has been performed, usually as a bridge to heart transplantation, which is the treatment of choice.

Prognosis: The outcome of symptomatic neonates with acute viral myocarditis has been poor. Patients with lesser symptoms have a better prognosis. Spontaneous resolution has been reported.

Nonviral Causes of Myocarditis

Nonviral myocarditis occurs due to bacterial, fungal and parasitic infections and rickettsial diseases.

Bacterial infections: In *diphtheria* the toxin of the *Corynebacterium diphtheriae* may produce peripheral circulatory failure or toxic myocarditis which is characterized by atrioventricular block, bundle branch block or extrasystoles within first 2 wk of disease. Heart failure occurs later with cardiac enlargement. Treatment includes bed rest (until all signs of myocarditis have disappeared), therapy for diphtheria, as well as management of cardiogenic shock, and arrhythmias including cardiac pacing. Digitalis is reserved with frank congestive heart failure and is used with care, because of the possibility of increased myocardial sensitivity.

In many systemic bacterial infections, cardiovascular involvement is manifested as peripheral circulatory collapse or toxic myocarditis. A myocardial depressant factor may produce an acute toxic cardiomyopathy. The treatment includes control of primary infection and cardiovascular problems. The prognosis depends on the effective control of infection and cardiovascular abnormalities.

Fungal infections: Lesions in the myocardium have been described in association with *histoplasmosis, coccidioidomycosis, toxoplasmosis, and trichinosis,* but clinical signs of myocarditis are rarely seen. *Actinomycosis* may involve the pericardium and myocardium by direct contiguity to a pulmonary abscess.

Parasitic infections: Hydatid cysts present in the pericardium, usually produce symptoms only when they rupture, and are detected on routine roentgenograms of the chest. *Schistosomiasis* may result in pulmonary hypertension and cor pulmonale. Chagas' disease, caused by *Trypanosoma cruzi* may produce either acute or subacute myocarditis and can lead to sudden death.

Rickettsial diseases: Rocky Mountain spotted fever may be complicated by hypotension and peripheral vascular collapse has been attributed to the general vasculitis but acute myocarditis may be a contributing factor.

Endocardial Fibroelastosis

Endocardial Fibroelastosis (EFE) also called fetal endocardiosis, is either primary EFE or secondary EFE. In primary endocardial fibroelstosis (EFE), no apparent predisposing valvular lesion or other congenital hear abnormality can be found. In secondary EFE, severe congenital heart disease of the left sided obstructive type (aortic stenosis or atresia, forms of hypoplastic left heart syndrome, or severe coarctation of the aorta) is present. Pathologically, a white, opaque fibroelastic thickening of the endocardium is present, usually in the left ventricle, and it frequently obscures the trabeculation of the inner surface of the cardiac chamber. The lesion may spread to involve the valves.

Infants, usually those younger than 6 mo, experience severe congestive heart failure, often precipitated by a respiratory infection. Chronic heart failure can be controlled for some time by digitalis and diuretics, however, most patients eventually succumb. Infants in whom valvular lesions or associated congenital cardiovascular defects are predominant usually expire in the first month of life. Chest X-ray shows enlargement of the heart, without a distinctive contour and clear lung fields. ECG is indicative of left atrial and left ventricular hypertrophy with strain. The echocardiogram shows a bright-appearing endocardial surface and a dilated, poorly functioning left ventricle. MRI may also delineate the fibrotic endomyocardial surface. Treatment consists of management of congestive heart failure and prevention of intercurrent infections. Children with signs of heart failure despite maximal medical treatment are indication for heart transplantation.

Batra AS, Lewis AB. Acute myocarditis. Curr Opin Pediatr 2001;13:234–9.

Bernstein Daniel. Diseases of the myocardium. In: Kliegman RM, Behrman RE, Jenson HB, Stanton BF (eds). *Nelson Textbook of Pediatrics.* 18th edn. Vol. 2. Philadelphia: Saunders, 2007; 1963–72.

Elliott P, Mckenna WJ. Hypertrophic cardiomyopathy. Lancet 2004;363:1881–91.

Kushwaha SS, Fallon JT, Fuster V. Restrictive cardiomyopathy. N Engl J Med 1997;336:267.

Levi D, Alejos J. Diagnosis and treatment of pediatric viral myocarditis. Curr Opin Cardiol 2001;16:77–83.

19.14 PERICARDITIS, CARDIAC TAMPONADE AND CONSTRICTIVE PERICARDITIS

The pericardium (pericardial complex) consists of an outer fibrous layer and an inner serous layer. The fibrous pericardium is a flask-shaped, tough outer sac with attachments to the diaphragm, sternum, and costal cartilage. The serous layer is thin and is adjacent to the surface of the heart. The potential space produced by these layers contains 10–15 ml fluid in a healthy child (approximately 20 cc of fluid in an adult) with electrolyte and protein profiles similar to plasma. Approximately 120 cc of additional fluid can accumulate in the pericardium without an increase in pressure. Further fluid accumulation can result in marked increases in pericardial pressure, eliciting decreased cardiac output and hypotension (cardiac tamponade). The rapidity of fluid accumulation influences the hemodynamic effect. The pericardium disease includes pericarditis, cardiac tamponade and constrictive pericarditis.

Pericarditis is broadly divided clinically in to 3 types. 1. *Acute pericarditis (<6 wk):* Fibrinous; effusive (serous or sanguineous); 2. *Subacute pericarditis (6 wk to 6 months):* Effusive-constrictive; constrictive; 3. *Chronic pericarditis (<6 months):* Constrictive; effusive; adhesive (nonconstrictive). Acute pericarditis is the most common pathologic process involving the pericardium. Pericardial effusions can be serous, serosanguineous, hemorrhagic, chylous or purulent. The etiologic classification is mentioned in Box 19.1.

Acute Pericarditis

During less than 6 wk the inflammation of pericardium is known as acute pericarditis. It may be fibrinous or effusive (serous or sanguineous). The first symptom of pericardial disease is often precordial pain. There is a sharp *stabbing* sensation over the precordium and often the left shoulder and back; the pain may be exaggerated by lying supine and relieved by sitting, especially leaning forward. As there is no sensory innervation of the pericardium, the pain is probably referred from diaphragmatic and pleural irritation. Cough, dyspnea, abdominal pain, vomiting, and fever may also occur. Patients can present with acute abdominal pain. Cardiac arrhythmias including premature atrial and ventricular contractions occasionally are present. Tachypnea and dyspnea is a frequent complaint and it may be severe with myocarditis, pericarditis, and tamponade. Fevers usually are low grade, but they occasionally reach 104°F. The presence of symptoms or signs associated with other organs depends on the cause of pericarditis. Many of the findings on physical examination are related to the degree of fluid accumulation in the pericardial sac.

Pericardial friction rub, the most important physical sign of acute pericarditis, may have up to three components per cardiac cycle and is high pitched, scratching, and grating. It can sometimes be elicited only when firm pressure with the diaphragm of the stethoscope is applied to the chest wall at the left lower sternal border. It is heard most frequently during expiration with the patient in the sitting position. Pleural rub is often inconstant, and the loud to and fro leathery sound may disappear within a few hours, then may reappear again the following day. The electrocardiogram (ECG) in acute pericarditis with out massive effusion is secondary to acute subepicardial inflammation. There is wide spread elevation of the ST segments, often with upward concavity, involving two or three standard limb leads and V_2–V_6, with reciprocal depressions only in aVR and sometimes V_1. Generalized T wave inversion occurs as a consequence of associated myocardial inflammation. The ST segment and T waves changes are more generalized than those seen with myocardial infarction, and ST segment elevations tend to precede the T wave changes. Usually there are no significant changes in QRS complexes. In pericarditis, the pericardium may have a normal appearance, without evidence of fluid accumulation in echocardiography.

Treatment: Treat the underlying cause (see differential diagnosis).

Box 19.1: Etiologic classification of pericardial disease

1. *Infectious.* 1a. Viral: Coxsackievirus B, Epstein-Barr virus, influenza, adenovirus, HIV infection; 1b. Bacterial: Streptococcus, Pneumococcus, Staphylococcus, Meningococcus, *H. influenzae*, Mycoplasma, *Mycobacterim tuberculosis*; 1c. Fungal: Histoplasmosis, Actinomycosis; 1d. Parasitic: Toxoplasmosis, Echinococcus

2. *Connective tissue diseases:* Rheumatic fever; rheumatoid arthritis; systemic lupus erythematosus (SLE); systemic sclerosis; sarcoidosis

3. *Metabolic–Endocrine:* Hypothyroidism; uremia; chylopericardium

4. *Hematology–Oncology:* Bleeding and coagulation disorders; malignancy (primary, metastatic); radiotherapy-induced

5. *Traumatic:* Penetrating or blunt injury

6. *Drugs:* Hydralazine, procainamide, isoniazid, minoxidil

7. *Others:* Iatrogenic (catheter-related); postpericardiotomy (cardiac surgery); aortic dissection; familial Mediterranean fever; idiopathic pericarditis

8. *Congenital anomalies:* Absence (partial, complete); cysts; congenital pericardial thickening and constriction

Percardial Effusion

When pericardial effusion is larger muffled heart sounds may be the only auscultatory finding, narrow pulses, tachycardia, neck vein distension and increased pulsus paradoxus suggest significant fluid accumulation. Cardiac tamponade, which occurs when the amount of pericardial fluid reaches a level that, compromises cardiac function. In an adolescent with pericarditis an excess of 1,000 ml of fluid may accumulate (pericardial fluid in healthy child: 10–15 ml).

Investigations: Pericardial fluid examination is done to find out the cause of effusion. X-ray chest will show enlarged cardiac shadow "water bottle-shaped". *ECG* will show low voltage of the QRS complexes which results from a damping effect of the pericardial fluid. *Echocardiogram* is used in evaluating the size and progression of pericardial effusions. A posterior effusion is recorded behind the left ventricular epicardium and ends at the junction of the left ventricle and left atrium. An anterior effusion will be recorded between the chest wall and the anterior right ventricular wall. The presence of both an anterior and posterior effusion generally indicates a larger collection of fluid. Flattening of septal motion and collapse of the right ventricular outflow during diastole are signs of pericardial tamponade (*see* Figs 19.38 to 19.40 in CD).

Treatment: Treat the underlying cause (*see* differential diagnosis).

Postpericardiotomy syndrome: Pericardial effusions may be seen 1–2 wk or longer after open heart surgery. The syndrome is a nonspecific hypersensitivity reaction to trauma to the pericardium and the epicardial surface of the heart. High titers of antiheart antibodies have been reported. Patients may have low-grade fever, lethargy, loss of appetite, or abdominal, precordial or pleural chest pain. Tamponade can occur if not treated. In most children, the syndrome responds to aspirin or other non-steroidal anti-inflammatory agents. Corticosteroids may be required for more severe cases. Treatment is continued for 1–3 months, but recurrences may be seen as long as one year postoperatively and require reinstitution of therapy.

Cardiac Tamponade

Cardiac tamponade is a clinical syndrome caused by the accumulation of fluid in the pericardial space, resulting in reduced ventricular filling and subsequent hemodynamic compromise. Cardiac tamponade is a medical emergency. In children, cardiac tamponade is more common in boys than in girls, with a male to female ratio of 7 : 3. Approximately 2% of penetrating injuries are reported to result in cardiac tamponade.

Pathophysiology: The underlying pathophysiologic process for the development of tamponade is markedly diminished diastolic filling because transmural distending pressures are insufficient to overcome the increased intrapericardial pressures.

Systemic venous return is also altered during tamponade. Because the heart is compressed throughout the cardiac cycle due to the increased intrapericardial pressure, systemic venous return is impaired and right atrial collapse occurs. During inspiration, intrapericardial and right atrial pressures decrease because of negative intrathoracic pressure. This results in augmented systemic venous return to right-sided chambers and a marked increase in the right ventricular volume. Because the pulmonary vascular bed is a vast and compliant circuit, blood preferentially accumulates in the venous circulation, at the expense of left ventricular (LV) filling. This results in a reduced cardiac output.

The amount of pericardial fluid needed to impair the diastolic filling of the heart depends on the rate of fluid accumulation and the compliance of the pericardium. Rapid accumulation of as little as 150 ml of fluid can result in a marked increase in pericardial pressure and can severely impede cardiac output, whereas 1000 ml of fluid may accumulate over a longer period without any significant effect on diastolic filling of the heart. This is due to adaptive stretching of the pericardium over time. A more compliant pericardium can allow considerable fluid accumulation over a longer period without hemodynamic insult.

Clinical manifestations: Symptoms vary with the underlying cause and the acuteness of the tamponade. Patients with acute tamponade may present with dyspnea, tachycardia, and tachypnea. Cold and clammy extremities from hypoperfusion are also observed in some patients. A comprehensive review of the patient's history usually helps identify the probable etiology of a pericardial effusion, which may result in cardiac tamponade. Patients with systemic or malignant disease present with weight loss, fatigue, or anorexia. Symptoms of night sweats, fever, and weight loss, may be indicative of tuberculosis. Inquire about chest wall radiation (i.e. for lung, mediastinal, or esophageal cancer). Chest pain may be the presenting symptom in patients with pericarditis or myocardial infarction. Musculoskeletal pain or fever may be present in patients with an underlying connective tissue disorder. A history of renal failure can lead to a consideration of uremia as a cause of pericardial effusion. Careful review of a patient's medications may indicate drug-related lupus leading to a pericardial effusion. Recent cardiovascular surgery, coronary intervention, or trauma can lead to the rapid accumulation of pericardial fluid and tamponade. Recent pacemaker lead implantation or central venous catheter insertion can lead to the rapid accumulation of pericardial fluid and tamponade. Consider HIV-related pericardial effusion and tamponade if the patient has a history of intravenous drug abuse or opportunistic infections.

Physical examination: Distended neck veins are a common feature in patients with tamponade. Evidence of chest wall injury may be present in trauma patients. Tachycardia, tachypnea, and hepatomegaly are observed in more than 50% of patients with cardiac tamponade, and diminished heart sounds and a pericardial friction rub are present in approximately one-third of patients.

The Beck triad or acute compression triad was described in 1935, this complex of physical findings refers to increased jugular venous pressure, hypotension, and diminished heart sounds, is usually observed in patients with acute cardiac tamponade.

Pulsus paradoxus or paradoxical pulse: Patient is asked to breathe normally while the mercury manometer is allowed to fall slowly, the first Korotkoff sound will initially be heard intermittently (varying with respirations). This first point is noted, and the manometer is then further allowed to fall until the first Korotkoff sound is heard continuously. The difference between the two systolic pressures is the pulsus paradoxus. (Pulsus paradoxus: >20 mm Hg indicates cardiac tamponade; 10–20 mmHg equivocal).

An increased pulsus paradoxus may also be observed in patients with severe dyspnea of any cause, with pulmonary disease (emphysema or asthma), in obese individuals or in patients being ventilated with a positive-pressure respirator. In these patients, the paradoxical pulse is due to a marked increase in intrathoracic pressure. The cause of a paradoxical pulse in a child on a ventilator after heart surgery may therefore be difficult to assess.

A pulsus paradoxus may be absent in patients with markedly elevated LV diastolic pressures, atrial septal defect, pulmonary hypertension, and aortic regurgitation.

Kussmaul sign: This was described by Adolph Kussmaul as a paradoxical increase in venous distension and pressure during inspiration. This sign is usually observed in patients with constrictive pericarditis but occasionally is observed in patients with effusive-constrictive pericarditis and cardiac tamponade.

Ewart sign: It is also known as the Pins sign; this is observed in patients with large pericardial effusions.

It is described as an area of dullness, with bronchial breath sounds and bronchophony below the angle of the left scapula.

The y descent: The y descent is abolished in the jugular venous or right atrial waveform. This is due to an increase in intrapericardial pressure, preventing diastolic filling of the ventricles.

Investigations: X-ray chest in cardiac tamponade (or large effusions), may demonstrate an enlarged cardiac silhouette after 200–250 ml of fluid accumulation. This occurs in patients with slow fluid accumulation, compared to a normal cardiac silhouette seen in patients with rapid accumulation and tamponade. Thus, the chronicity of the effusion may be suggested by the presence of a huge cardiac silhouette.

Electrical alternans is pathognomonic of cardiac tamponade and is characterized by alternating levels of ECG voltage of the P wave, QRS complex, and T waves in electrocardiography. This is a result of the heart swinging in a large effusion.

A swinging heart may be present in *echocardiography*. This is characterized as counterclockwise rotational movement, which occurs in addition to the triangular movement of the heart, producing a dance like motion. A dilated inferior vena cava (IVC) without inspiratory collapse (plethora) is highly suggestive of tamponade. Transthoracic echocardiography is the initial test of choice for detecting pericardial effusions and diagnosing tamponade.

Differential diagnosis: The differential diagnosis includes: cardiogenic shock, pericarditis, constrictive pericarditis, constrictive effusive, pulmonary embolism, and tension pneumothorax.

Management: The management will include pericardiocentesis, treatment of the underlying cause and further outpatient care. Thoracotomy and pericardiotomy may be required in the emergency department if the patient has rapid deterioration or cardiac arrest. After pericardiocentesis, leave the intrapericardial catheter in place after securing it to the skin using sterile procedure and attaching it to a closed drainage system via a 3-way stopcock. Periodically check for reaccumulation of fluid, and drain as needed. The catheter can be left in place for 1–2 days and can be used for pericardiodesis. Serial fluid cell counts can be useful for helping discover an impending bacterial catheter infection, which could be catastrophic. If the white blood cell (WBC) count rises significantly, the pericardial catheter must be removed immediately.

Pericardiocentesis: (a) The traditional approach is the subxiphoid technique. This technique avoids injury to the coronary arteries. The chest is prepared with betadine and a 16- to 18-gauge catheter is introduced between the xiphoid and the left subcostal margin. The catheter is directed toward the inferior tip of the left scapula with slow advancement and with negative pressure. If fluid is found, the catheter is advanced and the needle is withdrawn. Fluid is removed via the catheter. The catheter may be sutured in place for subsequent use. Alternatively, a 16- to 18-gauge spinal needle may be employed for onetime drainage.

(b) Echocardiographically guided pericardiocentesis now is considered the procedure of choice for removal of pericardial fluid. The technique for echocardiographically guided pericardiocentesis differs from traditional blind pericardiocentesis primarily in the site of needle entry.

Further outpatient care: A follow-up echocardiogram and chest radiograph should be performed at a monthly follow-up examination to check for recurrent fluid accumulation.

Prognosis: Prognosis depends on prompt recognition and management of the condition and the underlying cause of the tamponade. For penetrating injuries, the prognosis depends heavily upon the rapid identification of tamponade.

Constrictive Pericarditis

It commonly occurs months or years after the initial pericarditis, but occasionally during acute phase.

Clinical manifestations: The clinical findings occur as a result of impairment of diastolic ventricular filling, compromise of myocardial contractility, and resultant depression of cardiac function. Hepatomegaly, ascites, neck vein distension, narrow pulses, quiet precordium, distant heart sounds, pericardial friction rub, and increased pulsus paradoxus are observed. Congestive hepatomegaly is more pronounced and may impair hepatic function. Ascites is usually more prominent than dependent edema. In about half of patients the heart is normal in size. The apical pulse is reduced and retracts in systole. The heart sounds may be distant; an early third heart sound, i.e. a pericardial knock, occurring 0.09 to 0.12 seconds after aortic valve closure often conspicuous. Protein-loosing enteropathy with hypoproteinemia and lymphopenia may be present.

Diagnosis: Constrictive pericarditis may be difficult to distinguish from chronic restrictive cardiomyopathy. Impaired myocardial function occurs with both conditions. The myocardial disease of constrictive pericarditis is usually reversible with pericardiectomy. Presence of calcification of pericardium in the chest roentgenograms is diagnostic.

Treatment: In addition to treatment the underlying cause, radical pericardiectomy with decortication of the pericardium over a wide area of the heart, including the systemic and pulmonary veins is the effective treatment for constrictive pericarditis. In most patients, surgical intervention elicits a rapid response characterized by increased cardiac output and prompt diuresis. The long-term prognosis is usually good.

Bernstein Daniel. Diseases of pericardium. In: Kliegman RM, Behrman RE, Jenson HB, Stanton BF (eds). *Nelson Textbook of Pediatrics*. 18th edn. Vol. 2. Philadelphia: Saunders, 2007; 1972–76.

Braunwald E. Pericardial disease. In: Kasper DL, Braunwald E, Fauci AS, Hauser SL, Longo DL, Jameson JL (eds). Harrison's Principles of Internal Medicine. 16th edn. Vol I and Vol II. Newyork: McGraw-Hill, 2005;1414–20.

Goldstein JA. Cardiac tamponade, constrictive pericarditis, and restrictive cardiomyopathy. *Curr Probl Cardiol* 2004;29: 503–67.

Mathur Sarla, Singhal PK, Mathur GP, Sharma Anya. Pericarditis and Cardiac Tamponade. In: Mathur GP, Mathur Sarla (eds). *Current Trends in Pediatrics*. Vol 2. Delhi: Academa Publishers, 2006;186–94.

Salem K, Mulji A, Lonn E. Echocardiographically guided pericardiocentesis—the gold standard for the management of pericardial effusion and cardiac tamponade. *Can J Cardiol* 1999; 15(11):1251–5.

19.15 SYSTEMIC HYPERTENSION

Blood pressure is the product of cardiac output and peripheral vascular resistance. An increase in either cardiac output or peripheral resistance results in an increase in blood pressure; if one of these factors increases while the other decreases, blood pressure may not increase. When hypertension is the result of another disease process, it is referred to as *secondary hypertension*. When no identifiable cause can be found, it is referred to as *primary or essential hypertension*. In infants and younger children systemic hypertension is uncommon, but if present it is usually indicative of an underlying disease process (secondary hypertension). Adolescents may have primary (essential) or secondary hypertension.

For early detection of hypertension, accurate blood pressure measurements should be part of the routine physical examination of all children 3 yr or older. A complete family history of hypertension should be elicited.

Etiology and pathophysiology: Many factors, including heredity, diet, stress, and obesity may play a role in the development of essential hypertension. Many childhood diseases may be responsible for both acute and chronic elevation of blood pressure. Consider first the most likely causes of hypertension that varies with age, before considering other conditions: (a) newborn: umbilical artery catheteri-

> **Box 19.2:** Conditions associated with transient or intermittent and chronic hypertension in children

Renal causes

Transient or intermittent: Acute postinfectious glomerulonephritis; anaphylactoid (Henoch-Schönlein) purpura with nephritis; hemolytic-uremic syndrome; acute tubular necrosis; after renal transplantation (immediately and during episodes of rejection); after blood transfusion in patients with azotemia; hypervolemia; after surgical procedures on the genitourinary tract; pyelonephritis; renal trauma; leukemic infiltration of the kidney; obstructive uropathy associated with Crohn's disease

Chronic: Chronic pyelonephritis; chronic glomerulonephritis; hydronephrosis; congenital dysplastic; kidney; multicystic kidney; solitary renal cyst; vesicoureteral reflux nephropathy; segmental hypoplasia (Ask-Upmark kidney); ureteral obstruction; renal tumors; renal trauma; rejection damage following transplantation; postirradiation damage; systemic lupus erythematosus (other connective tissue diseases)

Vascular causes

Chronic: Coarctation of thoracic or abdominal aorta; Renal artery lesions (stenosis, fibromuscular dysplasia, thrombosis, aneurism); umbilical artery catheterization with thrombus formation; Neurofibromatosis (intrinsic or extrinsic narrowing of the vascular lumen); renal vein thrombosis; vasculitis; arteriovenous shunt; Williams-Beuren syndrome; Moyamoya disease

Endocrine causes

Chronic: Hyperthyroidism; hyperparathyroidism; congenital adrenal hyperplasia (11β-hydroxylase and 17-hydroxylase defect); Cushing syndrome; Primary aldosteronism; Dexamethasone-suppressible hyperaldosteronism; pheochromocytoma; other neural crest tumors (neuroblastoma, ganglioneuroblastoma, ganglioneuroma); diabetic nephropathy; Liddle syndrome

Central and autonomic nervous system causes

Transient or intermittent: Increased intracranial pressure; encephalitis; poliomyelitis; posterior fossa lesions; Guillain-Barré syndrome; familial dysautonomia; burns; Stevens-Johnson syndrome; porphyria

Chronic: Intracranial mass; hemorrhage; residual following brain injury; quadriplegia

Drugs and poisons causes

Transient or intermittent: Corticosteroids and adrenocorticotropic hormone; oral contraceptives; sympathomimetic agents; amphetamine; phencyclidine; cyclosporine or sirolimus treatment post-transplantation; licorice (glycyrrhizic acid); antihypertensive withdrawal (clonidine, methyldopa, propranolol); vitamin D intoxication; cocaine; lead, mercury, cadmium, thallium

Miscellaneous causes

Transient or intermittent: Pre-eclampsia; fractures of long bones; hypercalcemia; after coarctation repair; white cell transfusion; extracorporeal membrane oxygenation; chronic upper airway obstruction

Essential hypertension causes

Chronic: Low rennin; normal rennin; high rennin

zation and renal artery stenosis; (b) early childhood: renal disease, coarctation of the aorta, endocrine disorders, or medications; (c) adolescents: essential hypertension. Conditions associated with transient or intermittent and chronic hypertension in children are listed in Box 19.2. Regardless of the cause, end-organ (cardiac and renal) dysfunction occurs in the face of marked hypertension.

Clinical manifestations: Children and adolescents with essential hypertension are usually asymptomatic; there is mild elevation of blood pressure, which is detected during a routine examination or evaluation before athletic participation. These children may have mild to moderate obesity. The growth failure in children with chronic renal disease is the most frequent reasons for detecting the hypertension. With substantial hypertension, headache, dizziness, epistaxis, anorexia, visual changes and seizures may occur. Hypertensive encephalopathy is suggested by the presence of vomiting, temperature elevation, ataxia, stupor and seizures.

Diagnosis: The diagnosis of essential hypertension is suggested by the patient's age (usually adolescent; uncommon in children less than 10 yr), level of blood pressure elevation (usually mild), weight (mild to moderate obesity), positive family history, and the paucity of signs and symptoms of underlying disease. If blood pressure continues to rise over several weeks or months of observation, additional diagnostic studies to exclude secondary hypertension are indicated. The diagnosis of secondary hypertension is suggested by the patient's age (younger), level of blood pressure elevation (varying from mild to severe), and presence of symptoms and signs of underlying conditions associated with hypertension.

Screening tests should include a complete blood count, urinalysis, and determination of serum electrolyte, blood urea nitrogen, serum ceatinine, calcium, and uric acid levels. Urine culture should be performed. A lipid panel is indicated if the family history is suggestive or if primary hypertension is suspected. Echocardiography is helpful in assessing the chronicity of the hypertension, which if long-standing, should lead to left ventricular hypertrophy. Renal ultrasonography provides a comparison of kidney size and a view of the anatomy of the collecting system. Renal Doppler ultrasonography and angiography can demonstrate lesions in the main arteries or in the segmental branches; if angiography is performed, venous blood samples should be collected from both renal veins and the inferior vena cava for assay of plasma renal activity. Doppler ultrasonography may demonstrate abnormal arterial and venous blood flow. A radionuclide scan is helpful in distinguishing variation in perfusion or scarring of the two kidneys.

Peripheral plasma renal activity is useful screening test for both renovascular and renal parenchymal disease. Normal values gradually decrease with age. A suppressed value suggests excess mineralocorticoid effect, and an elevated value is associated with renal or renovascular involvement. Urinary catecholamines and plasma and urinary steroids should also be measured. A pregnancy test is useful in a sexually active female who is noted to be hypertensive (pre-eclampsia).

Treatment: The goal of treatment for hypertension should be to reduce blood pressure below the 95th percentile for age. Both *nonpharmacologic and pharmacologic approaches* should be used. *Nonpharmacologic approaches* should focus on the risk factors, include: (i) weight reduction in obese patients may result in a 5–10 mm Hg reduction in systolic pressure; (ii) reduction in salt intake often lowers pressure by a similar amount; (iii) aerobic exercises to reduce blood pressure in patients in mild essential hypertension and; (iv) counseling for not to use tobacco and alcohol, because of their adverse effects on blood pressure. In view of benefits and the undesirable effects of many hypertensive drugs, nonpharmacologic therapy should be prescribed for most young patients with essential hypertension. When the patient is unable to cooperate with the nonpharmacologic approach or the reduction in blood pressure is insufficient antihypertensive agents should be prescribed. However,

adolescents who are poorly compliant with changes in lifestyle are also unlikely to be complaint with a long-term drug regimen.

Pharmacologic therapy is required for many children with secondary hypertension and for selected patients with essential hypertension (Box 19.3). In most hypertensive emergencies the drug of choice are intravenous labetalol or nitroprusside or sublingual nifedipine. In general, the pressure should be reduced by about one-third of the total planned reduction during the first 6 hr and the remaining amount over the following 48–72 hr, in cases of hypertensive emergencies, because too rapid a reduction in blood pressure may interfere with adequate organ perfusion. Most children with hypertensive crisis have chronic or acute renal disease; in these patients in addition to the management of blood pressure, fluid balance and diuresis should be reviewed. Intravenous fursemide is usually effective, even though glomerular filtration is impaired.

In selecting a drug regimen for long-term use, therapy can be tailored to the specific pathologic condition, as the drugs with different sites and mechanisms of action are available. For example, excessive activity of the rennin-angiotensin-aldosterone system may be treated effectively with a β-blocking drug (e.g. propranolol) for suppression of rennin secretion, an ACE inhibitor (e.g. captopril) or rarely, an aldosterone antagonist (e.g. spironolactone). Excess angiotensin production is the probable cause of most hypertension in neonates after partial occlusion of a renal vessel by thrombus; captopril is an effective agent in most patients. α-adrenergic blocking agents (phentolamine, phenoxybenzamine) are beneficial in patients in neural crest tumors who have high circulating levels of catecholamines; labetalol may also be used. Labetalol is also effective in patients who experience marked stimulation of cardiovascular system from high doses of cocaine.

ACE inhibitors and calcium channel blockers may be considered for initial therapy in an adolescent patient with essential hypertension, who requires drug therapy. Enalapril instead captopril is now commonly used, which has a longer duration of action, and requires less frequent administration.

Patients with long-standing or poorly controlled hypertension, frequently require trials of combinations of antihypertensive drugs with different sites and mechanism of action, to gain control of markedly elevated or labile pressure. The drug regimen should be as simple as possible and should take advantage of longer acting agents that can be administered once or twice daily when available. Compliance is a problem; therefore, drug calendars, parental supervision, and

---

Box 19.3: Antihypertensive drugs

Arterial vasodilators

Hydralazine (relax arteriolar smooth muscle): 0.1–0.4 mg/kg/dose; IV; 2–4 hr; 0.25–1 mg/kg/dose and increase to max of 200 mg/24 hr; PO; 6–8 hr. Adverse events: Tachycardia, nausea; drug induced lupus.

Diazoxide (relax smooth muscle): 1–3 mg/kg/dose and max of 150 mg/24 hr; IV; 6–24 hr. Adverse events: Tachycardia, hypotension, hyperglycemia.

Nitroprusside (dilatation of arterioles and venules): 0.5–8.0 µg/kg/min; IV with infusion. Adverse events: Thiocyanate production, rarely hypothyroidism.

Minoxidil (dilatation of arterioles): 0.1–0.2 mg/kg/dose, max of 50 mg/24 hr; PO; 12–24 hr. Adverse events: Hypertrichosis, fluid retention.

Adrenergic blockers

Phentolamine (α-receptor blockade): 0.05–0.1 mg/kg/dose, max of 5 mg ; IV; 1–2 hr. Adverse events: Reflex tachycardia

Phenoxybenzamine (α-receptor blockade): 0.2–1.2 mg/kg/24 hr, max single dose of 10 mg; PO; 6–12 hr. Adverse events: Tachycardia may progress to arrhythmia.

Prazosin (α-receptor blockade): 0.005–0.1 mg/kg/dose; PO; 6–12 hr. Adverse events: First dose, orthostatic hypotension.

Propranolol (β-receptor blockade): 0.01–0.1 mg/kg/dose; IV slow push; 6–8 hr; (reduces rennin release). 0.5–0.6 mg/kg/24 hr, max of 16 mg/kg/24 hr or 60 mg/24 hr; PO. Adverse events: Bronchospasm, bradycardia, vivid dreams.

Labetalol (α and β-receptors blockade): 0.2–1.0 mg/kg/dose, max of 20 mg dose; IV bolus; with infusion 0.25–2.0 mg/kg/hr; IV continuous; 6–12 hr 1–3 mg/kg/24 hr; PO. Adverse events: Orthostasis, dizziness, bronchospasm.

Clonidine (CNS α$_2$-agonist): 0.005–0.025 mg/kg/24 hr initially, max of 9 mg/24 hr; PO; 6–12 hr. Adverse events: Sedation, constipation, rebound withdrawal, hypertension.

Renin-angiotensin inhibitors

Captopril (ACE inhibition): Neonates <2 mo: 0.05–0.1 mg/kg/dose up to 0.5 mg/kg/dose ; PO; 6–24 hr. Infants and children: 0.15–0.5 mg/kg/dose up to 6 mg/kg/24 hr; PO; 8–12 hr. Older children and adolescents: 6.25–12.5 mg/kg up to 450 mg/24 hr; PO; 8–12 hr. Adverse events: Proteinuria, neutropenia, rash, dysuria, chronic cough.

Enalaprilat (ACE inhibition): Children: 0.005–0.010 mg/kg/dose; IV; 8–24 hr; adults: 0.625–1.25mg/dose; IV; over 5 min. Adverse events: Transient hypotension.

Enalapril (ACE inhibition): Children: 0.2–1 mg/kg/24 hr; PO; 12–24 hr; adolescents: 2.5–5 mg/24 hr up to 40 mg/24 hr; PO; 24 hr. Adverse events: Hypotension.

Calcium channel blockers

Nifedipine (calcium channel blocker): Infants and children: Hypertensive emergency PO/sublingual 0.25–0.5 mg/kg/dose 4–6 hr (max 10 mg); hypertrophic cardiomyopathy: PO: 0.2–0.3 mg/kg q 8 hr. Adverse events: Facial flushing, tachycardia.

Diuretic agents

Hydrochlorothiazide (diuresis): 1–2 mg/kg/dose, max of 100 mg/24 hr; PO; 12–24 hr. Adverse events: Hypokalemia, hyeruricemia, hypercalcemia.

Frusemide (furosemide) (diuresis): 1 mg/kg/dose; IV; 4–6 hr; 1–2 mg/kg/dose, up to 6 mg/24 hr; PO; 6–12 hr. Adverse events: Hypokalemia, alkalosis.

Bumetanide (diuresis): 0.015–0.1 mg/kg/dose, max 10 mg/24 hr; PO; 6–24 hr. Adverse events: Hypokalemia, hyperglycemia, hyeruricemia.

ACE : angiotensin converting enzyme; SL : sublingual.

---

close patient–physician communication help ensure compliance.

In patients with renal artery stenosis secondary to fibromuscular dysplasia, percutaneous balloon angioplasty may cure some patients. Angioplasty is not successful for renal artery stenosis because of atherosclerotic plaques. If angioplasty is unsuccessful, placement of an intravascular stent or surgery may be indicated.

Prevention: Prevention of hypertension may be viewed as part of cardiovascular disease and stroke. Risk factors for cardiovascular disease include hypertension, obesity, elevated serum cholesterol levels, high dietary sodium intake, a sedentary life style, and alcohol and tobacco use. Smoking should be discouraged because of the pulmonary and cardiovascular consequences and increase in arterial wall rigidity and blood viscosity. Reduction in sodium intake and increase in physical activity are other preventive measures that should be implemented through school based programs.

Course and prognosis: In children and adolescents with essential hypertension drug therapy has been shown to be beneficial in reducing the incidence of congestive heart failure, renal failure and stroke. The prognosis of a child with secondary hypertension is primarily determined by the nature of the underlying disease and its responsiveness to specific therapy.

Bartosh SM, Aronson AJ. Childhood hypertension. An update on etiology, diagnosis, and treatment. *Pediatr Clin North Am* 1999;46:235–52.

Bernstein Daniel. Systemic hypertension. In: Kliegman RM, Behrman RE, Jenson HB, Stanton BF (eds). *Nelson Textbook of Pediatrics.* 18th edn. Vol. 2. Philadelphia: Saunders, 2007; 1988–95.

Sinaico AR. Hypertension in children. *N Engl J Med* 1996: 335:1968–73.

Tyagi S, Kaul UA, Satsangi UK, et al. Percutaneous trans-luminal angioplasty for renovascular hypertension in children: Initial and long-term results. *Pediatrics* 1997;99:44–49.

19.16 INFECTIVE ENDOCARDITIS

Infective endocarditis includes acute and subacute bacterial endocarditis and nonbacterial endocarditis caused by bacterial, viral, and mycotic infectious agents. Infective endocarditis is often a complication of congenital or acquired heart disease but can also occur in children without any abnormal valves or cardiac malformations. Endocarditis is rare in infancy; in this age group it usually follows open heart surgery or is associated with a central venous line. Patients with congenital heart lesions in which blood is ejected at a high velocity through a hole or stenotic orifice are most susceptible to endocarditis. Vegetations usually form at the site of the endocardial or intimal erosion that result from the turbulent flow. Children with ventricular

septal defect (VSD), left-sided valvular disease, systemic-pulmonary arterial communications (including palliative shunts), tetralogy of Fallot, aortic stenosis, patent ductus arteriosus, transposition of great arteries, congenital bicuspid aortic valves, mitral valve prolapse, Blalock-Taussig shunts, and valve replacement or valve conduit repair are most frequently associated with endocarditis. Surgical correction of congenital heart disease may reduce but does not eliminate the risk of endocarditis with the exception of simple atrial septal defect (ASD) or patent ductus arteriosus. *Predisposing factors* include a surgical or dental procedure, poor dental hygiene with congenital cyanotic heart disease are of a greater risk for endocarditis. The occurrence of endocarditis directly after heart surgery is low.

Etiology: The commonest micro-organisms responsible for endocarditis in children are: Viridans-type streptococci (α-hemolytic streptococci) and *Staphylococcus aureus.* Other organisms cause endocarditis less frequently, and in approximately 6% of cases, blood cultures are negative for any organisms (Box 19.4).

Clinical manifestations: Early manifestations are usually mild, especially when infecting organisms are viridans group streptococci. Many of the classic findings develop late in the course of disease; they are seldom seen in appropriately treated patients. Such manifestations include *Osler nodes* (tender pea-sized intradermal nodules in the pads of the fingers and toes), *Janeway lesions* (painless small erythematous or hemorrhagic lesions on the palms and soles), *splinter hemorrhages* (linear lesions beneath the nails), and *Roth spots* (hemorrhages with white centers). These lesions may represent vasculitis produced by circulating antigen-antibody complexes (Table 19.5).

Diagnosis: The index of suspicion should be high when evaluating infection in a child with an underlying contributing factor. The information for

---

Box 19.4: Microbiological agents in pediatric infective endocarditis

Common: Native valve or other cardiac lesions: *Viridans-type streptococci (S. mutans, S. sanguis, S. mitis); Staphylococcus aureus;* Group D *Streptococcus* (enterococcus) *(S. bovis, S. faecalis).*

Uncommon: Native valve or other cardiac lesions: *Streptococcus pneumoniae; Haemophilus influenzae; Staphylococcus epidermidis; Coxiella burnetti* (Q fever*); *Neisseria gonorrhoeae; Brucella*; Chlamydia psittaci*; Chlamydia trachomatis*; Chlamydia pneumoniae*;* Legionella*; Bartonella*; HACEK group; *Streptobacillus moniliformis*; Pasteurella multocida*; Campylobacter fetus;* Culture negative (6% of cases).

Prosthetic valve: *Staphylococcus epidermidis; Staphylococcus aureus;* Viridans group *Streptococcus; Pseudomonas aeruginosa; Serratia marcescens;* Diphtheroids; *Legionella* species*; HACEK group; Fungi#

*These fastidious bacteria plus some fungi may produce culture-negative endocarditis. Detection may require special media, incubation for more than 7 days, or serologic tests.
HACEK group includes: *Haemophilus* species (*H. paraphrophilus, H. parainfluenzae, H. aphrophilus*), *Actinobacillus actinomycetem-comitans, Cardiobacterium hominis, Eikenella corrodens,* and *Kingella* species.
#Fungi includes: *Candida* species, *Aspergillus* species, *Pseudallescheria boydii, Histoplasma capsulatum.*

Table 19.5: Manifestations of infective endocarditis

History: Prior congenital or rheumatic heart disease; Preceding dental, urinary tract or intestinal procedure; Intravenous drug use; central venous catheter; prosthetic heart valve

Symptoms: Fever; chills; chest and abdominal pain; arthralgia; myalgia; dyspnea; malaise; night sweats; weight loss; CNS manifestations (stroke, seizures, headache)

Signs: Elevated temperature; tachycardia; embolic phenomena (Roth spots, petechiae, splinter nail bed hemorrhages, Osler nodes, CNS or ocular lesions); Janeway lesions; new or changing murmur; splenomegaly; arthritis; heart failure; arrhythmias; metastatic infection (arthritis, meningitis, mycotic arterial aneurism, pericarditis, abscesses, septic pulmonary emboli); clubbing

Laboratory investigations: Positive blood culture; elevated ESR (may be low with heart or renal failure); elevated C-reactive protein; anemia; leukocytosis; immune complexes; hypergammaglobulinemia; hypocomplementemia; cryoglobulinemia; rheumatoid factor; hematuria; renal failure: azotemia, high creatinine (glomerulonephritis); chest radiograph: bilateral infiltrates, nodules, pleural effusions; echocardiographic evidence of valve vegetations, prosthetic valves dysfunction or leak, myocardial abscess, new-onset valve insufficiency

appropriate treatment of infective endocarditis is obtained from blood cultures. Blood specimens for culture should be obtained as promptly as possible, even if the child feels well and has no other physical findings. Three to five separate blood collections should be obtained after careful preparation of the phlebotomy site. Contamination should be avoided because bacteria found on the skin may themselves cause infective endocarditis. The laboratory should be notified that endocarditis is suspected so that if necessary, the blood can be cultured on enriched media for longer than usual (>7 days) to detect nutritionally deficient and fastidious bacteria and fungi. Antibiotic pretreatment of the patient reduces the yield of blood cultures to 50–60 %. Echocardiography helps in the diagnosis of endocarditis and cardiac lesions. The absence of vegetations does not exclude endocarditis, and vegetations are often not visualized in the early phases of the disease or in patients with complex congenital heart lesions.

Duke criteria help the diagnosis of endocarditis (Box 19.5). Two major criteria, one major and three minor, or five minor criteria suggest definite endocarditis.

Complications: Heart failure is caused by vegetations (most common cause) involving the aortic or mitral valve, myocardial abscesses and toxic myocarditis. Systemic emboli, often involve central nervous system. Pulmonary emboli occur in children with VSD or tetralogy of Fallot. Other complications include heart block as a result of involvement (abscess) of the conduction system, mycotic aneurysm, rupture of a sinus of Valsalva, obstruction of a valve secondary to large vegetations, and acquired VSD. Additional complications include: meningitis, osteomyelitis, arthritis, renal abscess, and immune complex-mediated glomerulonephritis.

Treatment: Antibiotics should be instituted immediately. A total of 4–6 wk treatment is recommended, in some cases more prolonged treatment is required (Table 19.6).

Resolution in staphylococcal disease takes longer. Digitalis, salt restriction and diuretic therapy should be used for the treatment of heart failure. Surgical intervention for infective endocarditis is indicated for severe aortic or mitral valve involvement with intractable heart failure. Fungal endocarditis is difficult to manage and has a poor prognosis. The drugs of choice are amphotericin B and 5-fluorocytosine.

Box 19.5: Duke criteria for the clinical diagnosis of infective endocarditis

Major criteria: 1. Positive blood cultures: Two separate cultures for a usual pathogen, two or more for less typical pathogens; 2. Evidence of endocarditis on echocardiography: Intracardiac mass on a valve or other site, regurgitant flow near a prosthesis, abscess, partial dehiscence of prosthetic valves, or new valve regurgitant flow

Minor criteria: 1. Predisposition: Predisposing heart condition or injection drug use 2. Fever ≥ 38.0°C (≥ 100.4°F); 3. Embolic-vascular signs: Major arterial emboli, septic pulmonary infarcts, mycotic aneurysm, intracranial hemorrhage, conjunctival hemorrhages, Janeway lesions; 4. Immune complex phenomena: Glomerulonephritis, rheumatoid factor, Osler nodes, Roth spots; 5. Micobiologic evidence: A single positive blood culture or serologic evidence of infection; 6. Echocardiographic signs not meeting the major criteria.

Table 19.6: Treatment of infective endocarditis				
Etiologic agent	*Drug*	*Dose*	*Route*	*Duration of therapy (wk)*
Streptococcus viridans, *S. bovis* (MIC ≤ 0.1 µg/ml)	(1) Penicillin G Or	200,000–300,000 U/kg/24 hr q 4 h, not to exceed 20 million U/24 hr	IV	4–6
	(2) Penicillin G plus gentamicin	As above no1 plus 3–7.5 mg/ kg/24 hr q 8 h not to exceed 240 mg/24 hr	IV IV	2–4 2
S. viridans, S. bovis (MIC ≥ 0.1 µg/ml)	(3) Penicillin G plus gentamicin	As above no. 2 As above no. 2	IV IV	4–6 2
S. viridans, or enterococci (*S. bovis* or *Streptococcus faecalis* (MIC ≥ 0.5 µg/ml)	(4) Penicillin G Or Ampicillin plus gentamicin	As above no. 2 300 mg/kg/24 hr q 4–6 h, not to exceed 12 g/24 hr As above no. 2	IV IV	4–6 4–6
S. viridans, S. bovis* (penicillin allergy†)	(5) Vancomycin Plus (6) Gentamicin if resistant*	40–60 mg/kg/24 hr q 8–12h, not to exceed 12 g/24 hr As above no. 2	IV IV	4–6 4–6
Staphylococcus aureus	(7) Nafcillin Or Oxacillin plus optional gentamicin	200 mg/kg/24 hr q 4–6 h, not to exceed 12 g/24 hr As above no 2	IV IV	6–8 1–2
S. aureus (methicillin resistant) (penicillin allergy)	(8) Vancomycin plus optional trimethoprim sulfamethoxazole	As above no. 5 12 mg/kg/24 hr trimethoprim q 8 h not to exceed 1 g/24 hr	IV IV, PO	6–8 4–8
S. aureus (with prosthetic device, methicillin sensitive ‡)	(9) Nafcillin plus gentami- cin plus optional rifampin	As above no. 7 As above no. 2 10–20 mg/kg/24 hr q 12 h not to exceed 600 mg/24 hr	IV IV PO	6–8 2 ≥6
S. aureus (with prosthetic device, methicillin resistant)	(10) Vancomycin plus gentamicin plus optional rifampin	As above no. 5 As above no. 9 As above no. 9	IV IV PO	6–8 2 ≥6
S. epidermidis	(11) Vancomycin plus optional rifampin	As above no. 5 As above no. 9	PO IV	6–8 6–8
Haemophilus species	(12) Ampicillin plus optional gentamicin	As above no. 4 As above no. 2	IV IV	4–6 2–4
Unknown Postoperative	(13) Vancomycin plus gentamicin	As above no. 5 As above no. 2	IV IV	6–8 2–4
Nonoperative	(14) Nafcillin Or Vancomycin plus gentamicin plus optional ampicillin	As above no. 7 As above no. 5 As above no. 2 As above no. 4	IV IV IV IV	6–8 6–8 2–4 6–8

*Add gentamicin for relatively resistant organisms. Monitor vancomycin peaks 1 hr after infusion (30–45 µg/ml). Adjust the dose according to vancomycin.

†Consider desensitization for patients allergic to penicillin. Cephalosporins are not recommended.

‡May require valve replacement.

IV: intravenous; PO: oral.

Prevention: Proper general dental care and oral hygiene are most important in decreasing the risk of infective endocarditis in susceptible individuals. Continuing education regarding prophylaxis is important, especially in teenagers and young adults, who often have poor knowledge of their own congenital lesion. Antimicrobial prophylaxis prior to various procedures, including dental and oral procedures, surgery and instrumentation in respiratory tract, gastrointestinal tract and genitourinary tract, reduces the incidence of infective endocarditis in susceptible patients (Tables 19.7 and 19.8). Vigorous treatment of sepsis and local infections and asepsis during heart surgery and catheterization reduce the incidence of infective endocarditis.

Prognosis: The mortality remains high, approximately 20–25%, despite the use of antibiotic agents. Serious morbidity has been reported in 50–60% of children with documented infective endocarditis; the most common is heart failure caused by vegetations involving the aortic or mitral valve.

Bernstein Daniel. Infective Endocarditis. In: Kliegman RM, Behrman RE, Jenson HB, Stanton BF (eds). *Nelson Textbook of Pediatrics.* 18th edn. Vol. 2. Philadelphia: Saunders, 2007; 1953–61.

Dajani AS, Taubert KA, Wilson W, et al. Prevention of bacterial endocarditis. Recommendations by the American Heart Association. *JAMA* 1997; 277:1794–801.

Houpikian P, Raoult D. Blood culture-negative endocarditis in a reference centre: Etiologic diagnosis of 348 cases. *Medicine (Baltimore)* 2005;84:162–73.

Table 19.7: Recommendations of the American Heart Association for prophylaxis against bacterial endocarditis

Dental and oral procedures and surgery of the upper respiratory tract or esophagus		*Gastrointestinal and genitourinary tract surgery and instrumentation*	
For most patients	Oral amoxicillin Children 50 mg/kg; adults 2.0 g, 1 hr before procedure	**High-risk patients**	IM or IV ampicillin Children 50 mg/kg; adults 2.0 g, plus
For patients unable to take oral medicine	IM or IV ampicillin Children 50 mg/kg; Adults 2.0 g, given within 30 min before procedure		IM or IV gentamicin 1.5 mg/kg (maximal dose, 120 mg) given within 30 min before procedure plus 6 hr later
Ampicillin and amoxicillin allergic patients	Oral clindamycin Children 20 mg/kg; adults 600 mg, 1 hr before procedure, or		IM or IV ampicillin or oral amoxicillin Children 25 mg/kg; Adults 1.0 g
	Oral cephalexin* or cefadroxil* Children 50 mg/kg; adults, 2.0 g, 1 hr before procedure or	**High-risk patients allergic to ampicillin and amoxicillin**	IV vancomycin Children 20 mg/kg; adults 1.0 g, given over 1–2 hr plus
	Oral azithromycin or clarithromycin Children 15 mg/kg; adults 500 mg, 1 hr before procedure given within 30 min before		IM or IV gentamicin 1.5 mg/kg (maximal dose, 120 mg) complete injection/infusion starting procedure
Ampicillin and amoxicillin allergic patients unable to take oral medications	IV clindamycin Children 20 mg/kg; adults 600 mg, given within 30 min before procedure or IV cefazolin Children 25 mg/kg; adults 1.0 g, given within 30 min before procedure	**Moderate risk patients**	Oral amoxicillin Children 50 mg/kg; Adults, 2.0 g, 1 hr before procedure
		Moderate risk patients who are allergic to ampicillin and amoxicillin	IM or IV ampicillin Children 50 mg/kg; adults 2.0 g, given within 30 min before procedure IV vancomycin Children 20 mg/kg; adults 1.0 g, given over 1–2 hr, complete infusion within 30 min of starting procedure

Table 19.8: Procedures and endocarditis prophylaxis

*Endocarditis prophylaxis recommended**	*Endocarditis prophylaxis not recommended*
Dental	**Dental**
Tooth extractions	Restorative dentistry‡ (operative and prosthodontic) with or without retraction cord§
Periodontal procedures including surgery, scaling and root planning, probing, and recall maintenance	Local anesthesia injections (non-intraligamentary)
Dental implant placement and re-implantation of avulsed teeth	Intracanal endodontic treatment, after placement and buildup
Endodontic (root canal) instrumentation or surgery only beyond the apex	Placement of rubber dams
Subgingival placement of antibiotic fibers or strips	Postoperative suture removal
Initial placement of orthodontic bands but not brackets	Placement of removable prosthodontic or orthodontic appliances
Intraligamentary local anesthesia injections	Taking of oral impressions
Prophylactic cleaning of teeth or implants when bleeding is anticipated	Fluoride treatments
	Taking of oral radiographs
Respiratory tract	Orthodontic appliance adjustment
Tonsillectomy or adenoidectomy or both	Shedding of primary teeth
Surgical operations that involve respiratory mucosa	
Bronchoscopy with a rigid bronchoscope	**Respiratory tract**
	Endotracheal intubation
Gastrointestinal tract†	Bronchoscopy with a flexible bronchoscope, with or without biopsy§
Sclerotherapy for esophageal varices	Tympanostomy tube insertion
Esophageal stricture dilatation	
Endoscopy retrograde cholangiography with biliary obstruction	**Gastrointestinal tract**
Biliary tract surgery	Transesophageal echocardiography§
Surgical operations that involve intestinal mucosa.	Endoscopy with or without gastrointestinal biopsy§
	Genitourinary tract
Genitourinary tract	Vaginal delivery§
Cystoscopy	Cesarean section
	In uninfected tissue:
	Urethral catheterization
	Uterine dilatation and curettage
	Therapeutic abortion
	Sterilization procedures
	Insertion or removal of intrauterine devices
	Other
	Cardiac catheterization, including balloon angioplasty
	Implanted cardiac pacemakers, implanted defibrillators, and coronary stents
	Incision or biopsy of surgically scrubbed skin
	Circumcision

*Prophylaxis is recommended for patients with high or moderate-risk heart conditions.
†Prophylaxis is recommended for high-risk; optional for medium-risk patients.
‡Includes restoration of decayed teeth (filling cavities) and replacement of missing teeth.
§Prophylaxis is optional for high-risk patients.

Karcher AW. Infective endocarditis. In: KasperDL, Braunwald E, Fauci AS, Hauser SL, Longo DL, Jameson JL (eds). *Harrison's Principles of Internal Medicine*. 16th edn. Vol I. New York: McGraw-Hill, 2005; 731–740.

19.17. HEART FAILURE

Heart failure is a term used to describe the state that develops when the heart cannot maintain an adequate cardiac output or can do so only at the expense of an elevated filling pressure. In the mildest forms of heart failure, cardiac output is adequate at rest and becomes inadequate only when the metabolic demand increases only during exercise or some other form of stress.

Pathophysiology: The cardiac output is a function of the preload (the volume and pressure of blood in the ventricle at the end of diastole), the afterload (the arterial resistance) and myocardial contractility. In patients without valvular disease the primary abnormality in heart failure is impairment of ventricular function resulting in a fall of cardiac output. This activates counter-regulatory neurohormonal mechanisms, which in normal physiological would support cardiac function, but in the setting of impaired ventricular function can lead to a deleterious increase in both afterload and preload. A vicious circle is thus established because any additional fall in cardiac output will cause further neurohormonal activation and increasing peripheral vascular resistance.

Stimulation of the renin-angiotensin-aldosterone system leads to vasoconstriction, salt and water retention and sympathetic activation mediated by angiotensin II, which is a potent vasoconstrictor of efferent arterioles of both in the kidney and systemic circulation. Activation of sympathetic system may initially maintain cardiac output through an increase in myocardial contractility, heart rate, and peripheral vasoconstriction. But prolonged sympathetic stimulation leads to cardiac myocyte apoptosis (cell death), hypertrophy, and focal myocardial necrosis. Salt and water retention is promoted by the release of aldosterone and in severe heart failure, antidiuretic hormone (ADH). Natriuretic peptides are released from the atria, in response to atrial stretch, and act as physiological antagonists to the fluid conserving effect of aldosterone; however, they have a short life in circulation. The onset of pulmonary and/or peripheral edema is due to high atrial pressures compounded by salt and water retention caused by impaired renal perfusion and secondary aldosteronism.

Types of Heart Failure

Heart failure is described or classified as follows: Acute and chronic heart failure, left, right and biventricular heart failure, forward and backward heart failure, diastolic and systolic dysfunction, and high-output failure.

Acute and chronic heart failure: Heart failure may develop suddenly, as in myocardial infarction, or gradually, as in progressive valvular heart disease. When there is gradual impairment of cardiac function, a variety of compensated changes may take place. A patient with impaired cardiac function in whom adaptive changes have prevented the development of overt heart failure is said to be suffering from 'compensated heart failure'. In such patients factors that may precipitate overt or acute heart failure are listed in Box 19.6. Patients with chronic heart failure commonly experience a relapsing or remitting course.

Left heart failure: The left heart comprises left atrium, left ventricle, mitral and aortic valves. In this condition there is a reduction in the left ventricular output and/or an increase in the left atrial or pulmonary venous pressure. An acute increase in left atrial pressure may cause pulmonary congestion or pulmonary edema; a more gradual increase in left atrial pressure instead may cause reflex pulmonary vasoconstriction and increasing pulmonary hypertension without producing pulmonary edema.

Right heart failure: The right heart comprises right atrium, right ventricle, tricuspid and pulmonary valves. In this condition there is a reduction in right ventricular output for any given right atrial pressure. Causes of isolated heart failure include chronic lung disease (cor pulmonale), multiple pulmonary emboli, and pulmonary valvular stenosis.

Biventricular heart failure: Failure of the left and right heart failure my develop in diseases which affect both ventricles (e.g. dilated cardiomyopathy or ischemic heart disease), or when disease of the left heart leads to chronic elevation of the left atrial pressure, pulmonary hypertension, and subsequent heart failure.

Forward and backward heart failure: In some patients with heart failure the predominant problem is an inadequate cardiac output (forward failure), whereas other patients may have a normal or near-normal

---

Box 19.6: Factors that may precipitate or aggravate heart failure in patients with pre-existing heart disease

1. Intercurrent illness (e.g. infection)
2. Arrhythmia (e.g. atrial fibrillation)
3. Conditions associated with increased metabolic demand (e.g. anemia, pregnancy, thyrotoxicosis)
4. Intravenous fluid overload (e.g. during treatment of a case with diarrhea with dehydration, postoperative IV infusion)
5. Pulmonary embolism
6. Inappropriate reduction of therapy
7. Administration of a drug with negative inotropic properties (e.g. non-steroidal anti-inflammatory drugs (NSAID), corticosteroids)
8. Myocardial ischemia or infarction (e.g. Kawasaki disease)

cardiac output with marked salt and water retention causing pulmonary and systemic venous congestion (backward failure).

Diastolic and systolic dysfunction: Heart failure may develop as a result of impaired myocardial contraction (systolic dysfunction) but can also result from poor ventricular filling and high filling pressures caused by abnormal ventricular relaxation (diastolic dysfunction). The latter is commonly found in patients with left ventricular hypertrophy and occurs in cases of hypertension and ischemic heart disease. Systolic and diastolic dysfunction often coexist, particularly in patients with coronary artery disease.

High-output failure: Conditions that are associated with a very high cardiac output (e.g. severe anemia, thyrotoxicosis, large AV shunt, beriberi) can occasionally cause heart failure. In such cases additional causes of heart failure are often present.

Clinical manifestations: The clinical findings will depend on the nature of the underlying heart disease, the type of heart failure that it has evoked and the neural and endocrine that has developed (Box 19.7, Table 19.9).

A low cardiac output causes fatigue, listlessness and poor effort intolerance; the peripheries are cold and the blood pressure is low. Poor renal perfusion may lead to oliguria and uremia.

Left heart failure due pulmonary edema may present with breathlessness, orthopnea, paroxysmal nocturnal dyspnea, and inspiratory crepitations over the lung bases. In contrast, right heart failure produces a high jugular venous pressure, hepatic congestion (enlarged and tender liver) and dependent peripheral edema. In ambulant patients the edema affects the ankles, whereas in bed-bound patients it collects around the sacrum and thighs. Massive accumulation of fluid may cause ascites or pleural effusion.

Chronic heart failure is sometimes is associated with marked weight loss (cardiac cachexia) caused by a combination of anorexia and impaired absorption due to gastrointestinal congestion; poor tissue perfusion due to a low cardiac output; and skeletal muscle atrophy due to immobility. An increased level of cytokine tumor necrosis factor is also found.

Box 19.7: Etiology of heart failure

Fetal: Severe anemia (hemolysis-Rh incompatibility, fetal-maternal transfusion, parvovirus B19-induced anemia, hypoplastic anemia); supraventricular tachycardia; ventricular tachycardia; complete heart block.

Neonate: Asphyxial cardiomyopathy; arteriovenous malformation (vein of Galen, hepatic); left-sided-obstructive lesions (coarctation of aorta, hypoplastic left side of the heart); large mixing cardiac defects (single ventricle, truncus arteriosus); viral myocarditis; fluid overload; patent ductus arteriosus; ventricular septal defect; cor pulmonale (bronchopulmonary dysplasia); hypertension.

Infant-Toddler: Left-to-right cardiac shunts (ventricular septal defect); hemangioma (arteriovenous malformation); anomalous left coronary artery; metabolic cardiomyopathy; acute hypertension (hemolytic-uremic syndrome); Supraventricular tachycardia; Kawasaki disease.

Child-adolescent: Rheumatic fever; acute hypertension (glomerulonephritis); viral myocarditis; thyrotoxicosis; hemochromatosis-hemosiderosis; cancer therapy (radiation, doxorubicin); sickle cell anemia; endocarditis; cor pulmonale (cystic fibrosis); cardiomyopathy (hypertrophic, dilated)

Table 19.9: Symptoms and signs in heart failure

Symptoms	Signs
Dyspnea	Cachexia and muscle wasting
Orthopnea	Tachycardia
Paroxysmal nocturnal dyspnea	Pulsus alternans
Reduced exercise tolerance, lethargy, fatigue	Elevated jugular venous pressure
Nocturnal cough	Displaced apex beat
Wheeze	Right ventricular heave
Ankle swelling	Crepitations or wheeze
Anorexia	Third heart sound
	Edema
	Hepatomegaly (tender)
	Ascites

In Children

Symptoms: Fatigue, effort intolerance, anorexia, abdominal pain, cough, and dyspnea (due to pulmonary congestion).

Signs: Orthopnea, elevation of jugular venous pressure, liver enlargement, basal rales, edema over the dependent portions of the body, or anasarca, cardiomegaly, auscultatory findings include gallop rhythm, and findings specific to the basic cardiac lesion.

In Infant

Symptoms: Tachypnea, feeding difficulties, poor weight gain, excessive perspiration, irritability, weak cry, and noisy, labored respirations with intercostal and subcostal retractions as well as flaring of alae nasi. Signs: wheezing, pneumonitis (with or without atelectasis, especially the right middle and lower lobes, due to bronchial compression by the enlarged heart), hepatomegaly, tachycardia, gallop rhythm, auscultatory signs produced by the underlying cardiac lesion; edema is generalized, usually involving the eyelids, as well as the scrotum, and less often the legs and feet. Differential diagnosis: The differential of peripheral edema is listed in Box 19.8.

Complications of heart failure: The complications of heart failure are listed in Table 19.10.

Laboratory findings: The chest radiological findings of heart failure will show enlarged cardiac silhouette, enlarged hilar vessels, ground glass appearance of alveolar edema, prominence of upper lobe blood vessels, and septal or 'Kerley B' lines, as horizontal lines in the costophrenic angles (interstitial edema causes thickened interlobular septa and dilated lymphatics, which are evident as horizontal lines in the costophrenic angles).

The ECG is the best tool for evaluating cardiac arrhythmias as a potential cause of heart failure. Chamber hypertrophy, cardiomyopathies, left or right ventricular ischemic changes noted by ECG may be helpful in assessing the cause of heart failure, but does not establish the diagnosis. Low-voltage QRS findings along with ST-T wave abnormalities are seen in myocardial inflammatory disease and in pericarditis.

Echocardiographic techniques are useful in assessing ventricular function such as fractional shortening (normal between 28 and 40%; normal ejection fraction (which measures volume 55–65%) as measured by angiography; pre-ejection: ejection period ratio as measured by M-mode echocardiography (less than 40%). A long pre-ejection time with a short ejection time usually denotes myocardial failure. Doppler studies can be used to calculate cardiac output.

Arterial oxygen levels may be decreased when ventilation-perfusion inequalities occur secondary to pulmonary edema. When heart failure is severe, respiratory or metabolic acidosis, or both, may be

---

Box 19.8: Differential diagnosis of peripheral edema

- Cardiac failure (right or combined left and right heart failure, pericardial constriction, cardiomyopathy)
- Hypoalbuminemia (nephrotic syndrome, liver disease (cirrhosis of liver), protein loosing enteropathy, Kwashiorkor, marasmus with edema)
- Beriberi
- Chronic venous insufficiency (varicose veins)
- Chronic lymphatic obstruction
- Drugs—sodium retention (corticosteroids, non-steroidal anti-inflammatory drugs); increasing capillary permeability (nifedipine, amlodipine)
- Idiopathic

Table 19.10: Complications and clinical manifestations of heart failure

Complications	Clinical manifestations
Cardiovascular	Arrhythmias (atrial fibrillation; ventricular arrhythmias [ventricular tachycardia, ventricular fibrillation]; bradyarrhythmias); acute myocardial infarction; cardiogenic shock
Thromboembolism	Stroke; peripheral embolism; deep venous thrombosis; pulmonary embolism
Gastrointestinal	Hepatic congestion and hepatic dysfunction; malabsorption, mesenteric insufficiency
Musculoskeletal	Muscle wasting
Respiratory	Pulmonary congestion; respiratory muscle weakness; pulmonary hypertension (rare)
Electrolyte disturbances	
Digitalis intoxication	Hypokalemia is common in patients receiving frusemide

present. In infants with heart failure hyponatremia occur as a result of renal water retention.

B-type natriuretic peptide (BNP) is elevated in adult patients in cases of dyspnea due to congestive failure but normal in other causes of dyspnea.

Treatment

The underlying cause of cardiac failure must be removed or alleviated if possible (congenital heart disease; cardiomyopathy, myocarditis).

A. *General measures:* 1. Education to parents about the nature of disease and treatment plan. 2. Vaccination: Influenza and pneumococcal vaccination should be considered. 3. Rest: Child should rest often and rest adequately. Strict bed rest in extreme cases. Most patients feel better sleeping in a semi-upright position. Restrictions on activities can be modified after the child responds to treatment. Competitive and strenuous sports are usually contraindicated. 4. Patients admitted in an intensive care unit (ICU) may require positive pressure ventilation (in patients with severe pulmonary edema), β-adrenergic agonists (dopamine, dobutamine, epinephrine), phospho-diesterase inhibitors, and afterload reducing agents (e.g. nitroprusside, captopril, enalapril).

B. *Diet:* Good general nutrition and avoidance of high salt foods and "no added salt", especially for patients with severe congestive heart failure.

C. *Drug therapy:* Cardiac function can be improved by increasing contractility, optimizing preload or decreasing afterload. Drugs that reduce preload are most appropriate in patients with high end-diastolic filling pressures and evidence of pulmonary or systemic venous congestion (backward failure); drugs that reduce afterload or increase myocardial contractility are particularly valuable in patients with signs and symptoms of a low cardiac output (forward failure) (Box 19.9).

Digoxin: This should be used as the first line of treatment in patients with heart failure and atrial fibrillation, when it will usually provide adequate control of the ventricular rate together with a small positive inotropic effect. The role of digoxin in the treatment of patients with heart failure and sinus rhythm is less certain. Digoxin is used most often in pediatric patients. Hypokalemia is common in patients receiving frusemide.

Diuretics: These agents interfere with reabsorption of water and sodium by kidneys, which results in a reduction in circulating blood volume and thereby reduce pulmonary fluid overload and ventricular filling pressure. Diuretics are most often used in conjunction with digitalis. Frusemide is the most commonly used diuretic (PO, IV: 1–2 mg/kg). Potassium chloride supplementation is usually required unless the potassium-sparing diuretic spironolactone is given concomitantly. When frusemide is administered every other day, dietary potassium supplementation may be adequate to maintain normal serum potassium levels. Chronic administration of frusemide causes fluid loss without bicarbonate, thus the total body bicarbonate is contained in a smaller total body fluid compartment and result in "contraction alkalosis." Which produces metabolic alkalosis.

Spironolactone is an inhibitor of aldosterone and enhances potassium retention. Combinations of spironolactone and chlorothiazide are commonly used. Chlorothiazide is used occasionally for diuresis in children with less severe chronic heart failure.

Afterload-reducing agents and angiotensin-converting enzyme (ACE) inhibitors: ACE inhibitors are especially useful in children with heart failure caused by cardiomyopathy, severe mitral or aortic insufficiency and left to right shunts. They are not generally used in the presence of stenotic lesions of the left ventricular outflow tract. They are used in conjunction with other anticongestive drugs such as digoxin and diuretics. Enalapril, an ACE inhibitor is the drug of choice because of its longer action. Captopril (ACE inhibitor) is associated with adverse reactions such as neutropenia, renal toxicity and chronic cough in addition to hypotension, and maculopapular pruritic rash.

Nitroprusside is administered intravenously is critically ill patients in an intensive care unit for shorter period; contraindicated in patients with pre-existing hypotension. When high doses of nitroprusside are administered for several days, blood thiocyanate levels should be monitored; values greater than 10 g/dl are consistent clinical symptoms of toxicity (fatigue, nausea, disorientation, acidosis, and muscular spasm).

Angiotensin II receptor antagonists have been used in adults with heart failure. Intravenous nesiritide is a recombinant human brain (B-type) natriuretic peptide that has venous, arterial and coronary vasodilatory effects. Nesiritide infusion in adults with decompensated heart failure improves hemodynamic function and clinical manifestations of heart failure.

Chronic treatment with β-blockers: β-blockers (metoprolol) are used for the chronic treatment of patients with heart failure and should not be administered when patients are still in the acute stage of heart failure (i.e. in the intensive care unit and receiving intravenous adrenergic agonists infusions).

α and β-adrenergic agonists: Dopamine, dobutamie and isoproterenol are useful drugs in treating low cardiac output. Dopamine has fewer chronotropic and arrhythmogenic effects than has isoproterenol. In addition, it results in selective renal vasodilatation, which is particularly useful in patients with the compromised kidney function that is often associated with low cardiac output. At a dose of 2–10 µg/kg/min, dopamine results in increased contractility with little peripheral vasoconstrictive effects, but if the dose is increased beyond 15 µg/kg/min, its peripheral α-adrenergic effects may result in vasoconstriction. At high doses, dopamine may potentially cause an increase in pulmonary vascular resistance.

Dobutamine, a derivative of dopamine can be used as an adjunct to dopamine therapy in order to avoid the vasoconstrictive effects of high-dose dopamine. Dobutamine is also less likely to cause cardiac rhythm disturbances.

Isoproterenol has both central and peripheral β-adrenergic effects and therefore enhances myocardial contractility and also reduces cardiac afterload. Because isoproterenol has a marked chronotropic effect, it should not be used in patients who already have significant tachycardia.

Epinephrine, a mixed α- and β-adrenergic receptor agonist is usually used for patients with cardiogenic shock and low arterial blood pressure. Because epinephrine raises blood pressure as well as increases systemic vascular resistance, and therefore, increases the afterload against which the heart has to work.

Phosphodiesterase inhibitors: They are useful in treating patients with low cardiac output who are refractory to standard therapy, and work by inhibition of phosphodiesterase, preventing the degradation of intracellular cyclic adenosine monophosphate. *Milrinone* has both positive inotropic effects on the heart and significant peripheral vasodilatory effects

---

Box 19.9: Dosage of drugs for the treatment of congestive heart failure

Digoxin: *Digitalization:* PO (1/2 initially, followed by ¼ every 8–12 hr × 2): Full term neonate (up to 1 mo): 20–30 µg/kg; infant or child: 25–40 µg/kg; adolescent or adult: 0.5–1 mg in divided doses IV dose is 75% of PO dose.
Maintenance: 5–10 µg/kg/24 hr, divided q 12 hr; trough serum level: 1.5–3 ng/ml, < 6 mo old; 1–2 ng/ml > 6 mo old; IV dose is 75% of PO dose

Diuretics
Frusemide: IV 1–2 mg/dose, prn; PO 1–4 mg/kg/24 hr, divided qd–qid
Bumetanide: IV 0.01–0.1 mg/kg/dose; PO 0.05–0.1 mg/kg/24 hr, divided q 6–8 hr
Chlorothiazide: PO 20–50 mg/kg/24 hr, divided bid or tid
Spironolactone: PO 1–3 mg/kg/24 hr, divided bid or tid

β-adrenergic agonists IV
Dobutamine 2–20 µg/kg/min, dopamine 2–50 µg/kg/min, isoproterenol 0.01–0.5 µg/kg/min; epinephrine 0.05–0.1 µg/kg/min; norepinephrine 0.1–2.0 µg/kg/min

Phosphodiesterase inhibitors IV
Amrinone 3–10 µg/kg/min; milrinone 0.25–1 µg/kg/min

Aafterload-reducing agents
Captopril: PO infants: 0.1–0.5 mg/kg/dose, q 8–12 hr (max: 4 mg/kg/24 hr); prematures: Start at 0.01 mg/kg/dose; Children: 0.1–2 mg/kg/24 hr, q 8–12 hr (Adult dose: 6.25–25 mg/dose}
Enalapril: PO: 0.08–0.5 mg/kg/dose q 12–24 hr (max: 1 mg/kg/24 hr)
Hydralazine: IV or IM : 0.1–0.5 mg/kg/dose (max: 20 mg); PO: 0.25–1.0 mg/kg/dose, q 6–8 hr (max: 200 mg/24 hr)
Nitroglycerin: 0.25–5 µg/kg/min
Nitroprusside: IV: 0.5–8 µg/kg/min
Prazosin: 0.005–0.05 mg/kg/dose q 6–8 hr (max: 0.1 mg/kg/dose)

β-Adrenergic blockers
Carvedilol: PO: Initial dose 0.1 mg/kg/day (0.5 mg/kg) divided bid increase gradually (usually 2 wk intervals) to maximum of 0.5–1 mg/kg/day over 8–12 wk is tolerated; adult maximal dose is 50–100 mg/day
Metoprolol: PO: Non-extended release form: 0.2 mg/kg/day divided bid, increase gradually (usually 2 wk intervals) to maximum dose 1–2 mg/kg/day PO: Extended release form: Given once daily; adult dose 25 mg/day, maximum dose is 200 mg/day

Note: Pediatric doses based on weight should not exceed adult doses. As recommendations may change, these doses should always be double checked. Doses may also need to be modified in any patient with renal or hepatic dysfunction.
PO : by mouth; IV : intravenously; prn : as necessary; qd : everyday; bid : twice daily; tid : three times per day; qid : four times per day.

and is generally used as an adjunct to dopamine or dobutamine therapy. A major side effect is hypotension secondary to peripheral vasodilatation. The hypotension can usually be managed by the administration of intravenous fluids to restore adequate intravascular volume. Amrinone can cause thrombocytopenia; the severity appears to be related to both the rate of infusion and the duration of therapy. It is reversible when the drug is discontinued.

D. *Surgical procedures:* If the cause is amenable to surgical procedures such as (i) heart valve repair or replacement; (ii) pacemaker insertion; (iii) correction of congenital heart defects; (iv) coronary artery bypass surgery; (v) mechanical assistance devices; (vi) heart transplantation, medical treatment is indicated to prepare the patient for surgery.

Prognosis: Results of initial treatment are usually good, regardless of cause. Long-term prognosis is variable. Mortality rates range from 10% in patients with mild symptoms to 50% with advanced, progressive symptoms. Sudden death may be related to ventricular arrhythmias, although asystole is a common terminal event in severe heart failure.

Patient education: 1. Provide instructions to patients discharged home to return to the ED for recurrence or changes in severity of symptoms. 2. Provide specific instructions to patients discharged regarding dietary restrictions and compliance with medical therapy. 3. Require patients to promptly follow-up with their primary care physician or cardiologist.

Bernstein Daniel. Heart Failure. In: Kliegman RM, Behrman RE, Jenson HB, Stanton BF (eds). *Nelson Textbook of Pediatrics.* 18th edn. Vol. 2. Philadelphia: Saunders, 2007;1976–81.

Boon N A, Fox KAA, Bloomfield P, et al. Cardiovascular disease. In: Haslett C, Chilvers ER, Boon NA, Colledge NR, Hunter JAA (eds). *Davidson's Principles and Practice of Medicine.* 19th edn. Edinburgh: Churchill Livingstone, 2002; 357–481.

McMurphy JJV. Heart failure. *Lancet* 2005;365:1877–89.

20 Blood Disorders

20.1 ANEMIAS

Anemia is defined as a reduction of the red blood cell (RBC) volume or hemoglobin concentration below the range of values occurring in healthy persons (Tables 20.1 and 20.2). Anemia is not a specific entity but results from many underlying pathologic processes. The clinical disturbance such as pallor becomes evident in the skin and mucous membranes when the hemoglobin level falls below 7–8 g/dl. A number of physiologic adjustments to anemia include increased cardiac output, increased oxygen extraction (increased arteriovenous oxygen difference), and a shunting of blood flow toward vital organs and tissues.

Anemia is not a specific entity but, rather the result of many underlying pathologic processes. RBC size

Table 20.1: Hematological values during infancy and childhood

Age	Hemoglobin (g/dl) Mean	Range	Hematocrit (%) Mean	Range	Reticulocytes (%) Mean	MCV(fl) Lowest
Cord blood	16.8	13.7–20.1	55	45–65	5.0	110
2 wk	16.5	13.0–20.0	50	42–66	1.0	–
3 mo	12.0	9.5–14.5	36	31–41	1.0	–
6 mo–1 yr	12.0	10.5–14.0	37	33–42	1.0	70–74
7–12 yr	13.0	11.0–16.0	38	34–40	1.0	76–80
Adult						
Female	14	12.0–16.0	42	37–47	1.6	80
Male	16	14.0–18.0	47	42–52		80

fl : femtoliters; MCV : mean corpuscular volume

Table 20.2: Hematological values (leukocytes) during infancy and childhood

Age	Leukocytes (WBC/mm³) Mean	Range	Neutrophils (%) Mean	Range	Lymphocytes (%) Mean	Eosinophils (%) Mean	Monocytes (%) Mean
Cord blood	18,000	(9,000–30,000)	61	(40–80)	31	2	6
2 wk	12,000	(5,000–21,000)				63	39
3 mo	12,000	(6,000–18,000)				48	25
6 mo–1 yr	10,000	(6,000–15,000)				48	25
7–12 yr	8,000	(4,5000–13,500)				38	25
Adult Female and Male	7,500	(5,000–10,000)	55	(35–70)	35	3	7

WBC : white blood cells

changes with age; and before an anemia can be specifically characterized with respect to RBC size, normal developmental changes in the mean corpuscular volume (MCV) must be understood (see Table 20.1). It is essential to review the appearance of RBC on a peripheral blood smear. Specific morphologic features may point to the underlying diagnosis. The presence of *polychromatophilia*, which generally correlates with the degree of reticulocytosis, indicates that the marrow is able to respond to RBC loss or destruction. Use of the complete blood count, reticulocyte count, and blood smear is used in the diagnosis of anemia. Normal ranges for differential counts on aspirate bone marrow is documented in Table 20.3 (*see* Figs 20.1 to 20.24 in CD).

Anemias can be arbitrarily divided into four groups:
1. Anemias of inadequate production
2. Hemolytic anemias
3. Pancytopenia
4. Hemorrhagic and thrombotic diseases

An approach to assess the common causes of anemia in children is discussed.

Is anemia associated with other hematologic abnormalities? The presence of thrombocytopenia, abnormalities in white blood cell (WBC) numbers, or the presence of abnormal leukocytes often indicates

Table 20.3: Normal ranges for differential counts on aspirate bone marrow

Myeloblasts 0–3%, promyelocytes 3–12%, myelocytes (neutrophil) 2–13%

Metamyelocytes 2–6%, neutrophils 22–46%, myelocytes (eosinophil) 0–3%

Eosinophils 0.3–4%, basophils 0–0.5%, lymphocytes 5–20%, monocytes 0–3%

Plasma cells 0–3.5%, erythroblasts 5–35%, megakaryocytes 0–2%, macrophages 0–2%

From Kliegman RM, Marcdante Kj, Jenson HJ, et al. Nelson Essentials of Pediatrics. 5th edn. Philadelphia: Elsevier/Saunders, 2006;694.

bone marrow failure caused by aplastic anemia, leukemia, or other malignant marrow disease.

Is anemia associated with reticulocytosis? In anemic children with an appropriate reticulocyte response, the anemia usually is a consequence of bleeding or ongoing hemolysis. The most characteristic feature of hemolytic anemia is reticulocytosis with indirect hyperbilirubinemia and often, increased serum lactate dehydrogenase as indicators of accelerated erythrocyte destruction. The peripheral blood smear will show abnormal RBC morphology (e.g. spherocytes, sickle forms, microangiopathy) and is often helpful in ascertaining the cause of hemolysis.

Is anemia associated with reticulocytopenia? If yes anemia in children with a less than appropriate reticulocyte response reflects an impairment of normal erythropoiesis; in this group the analysis of MCV is particularly helpful.

Are red blood cells microcytic? Almost all children with anemia and reticulocytopenia have defects in hemoglobin synthesis from iron deficiency, thalassemia trait, hemoglobin E disorders or hemoglobin C. A distinguishing feature of thalassemia trait conditions and hemoglobin E is that the RBC count is higher than normal despite the presence of mild anemia and microcytosis, in contrast to iron deficiency anemia in which the RBC count usually decreases along with the reduced hemoglobin and MCV.

Are red blood cells macrocytic? The anemia sometimes is megaloblastic as a result of impaired DNA synthesis and nuclear development and the formation of other blood cells also is affected. The peripheral blood smear in megaloblastic anemias contains large macrovalocytes and nuclear hypersegmentation of the neutrophils. The causes of megaloblastic anemia include folate deficiency, vitamin B_{12} deficiency and inborn errors of metabolism. In cases of Diamond-Blackfan anemia, congenital dyserythropoietic anemia and Pearson syndrome macrocytic anemia is not megaloblastic.

Are red blood cells normocytic? Normocytic anemia, low reticulocyte count, and normal bilirubin levels is associated with anemia of chronic disease, renal failure, hypothyroidism and acquired pure red cell aplasia.

Glader B. The anemias. In: Kliegman RM, Behrman RE, Jenson HB, Stanton BF (eds). *Nelson Textbook of Pediatrics.* 18th edn. Vol. 2. Philadelphia: Saunders, 2007;2003–6.

Greer JP, Foerster J, Lukens J, et al. *Wintrobe's Clinical Hematology.* 11th edn. Baltimore: Williams & Wilkins, 2004.

Nathan DG, Orkin SH, Ginsburg O, Look AT. *Nathan and Oski's Hematology of Infancy and Childhood.* 6th edn. Philadelphia: WB Saunders, 2003.

20.2 PHYSIOLOGIC ANEMIA OF INFANCY

Normal full-term newborn infants have higher hemoglobin and hematocrit levels with larger red blood cells (RBCs) than older children and adults. Within the first week of life, a progressive decline in hemoglobin level begins and persists for 6–8 wk. The result of this decline is referred to as *physiologic anemia of infancy.* Several factors are involved. With the onset of respiration at birth, considerably more oxygen is available for binding to hemoglobin, and the hemoglobin oxygen saturation increases from 50 to 95% or more. The normal developmental switch from fetal to adult hemoglobin synthesis actively replaces high-oxygen-affinity fetal hemoglobin with lower-oxygen-affinity adult hemoglobin, which can deliver a greater fraction of hemoglobin-bound oxygen to tissues. Immediately after birth the increase in blood oxygen content and tissue oxygen delivery down-regulates erythropoietin (EPO) production, and as a consequence, erythropoiesis is suppressed. In the absence of erythropoiesis, hemoglobin levels decrease, because the aged RBCs are not replaced as they are normally removed from the circulation. Iron from degraded RBCs is stored for future hemoglobin synthesis. The hemoglobin concentration continues to decrease until tissue oxygen needs are greater than oxygen delivery. Normally, this point is reached between 8–12 wk of age, when the hemoglobin concentration is 9–11 g/dl. Hypoxia is detected by renal or hepatic oxygen sensors, EPO production increases and erythropoiesis resumes. The iron previously stored in reticuloendothelial tissues can then be used for hemoglobin synthesis. The supply of stored iron is sufficient for hemoglobin synthesis, even in the absence of dietary iron intake, until approximately 20 wk of age. This 'anemia' should be viewed as a physiologic adaptation to extrauterine life, reflecting the excess capability for oxygen delivery relative to tissue oxygen requirements. There is no hematologic problem, and no therapy is required.

Premature infants also develop a physiologic anemia but the decline in hemoglobin is both more extreme and more rapid. Minimal hemoglobin levels of 7–9 g/dl commonly reached by 3–6 wk of age, and levels may be even lower in very small premature infants. The cause of this anemia is multifaceted. The same factors are operative as in term infants, but they are exaggerated. An important component in the first few weeks of life is blood loss as a result of sampling for the many laboratory tests necessary to stabilize the clinical status of these infants, particularly those with cardiorespiratory problems. The erythropoietic response to anemia is also suboptimal, due to inadequate synthesis of EPO in response to hypoxia and there is shorter survival of RBCs of premature infants (40–60 days instead of the 120 days in adults) and the rapid expansion of RBC mass that accompanies growth. The spontaneous resolution of the anemia that occurs by approximately 40 wk gestational age is in keeping with a developmental switch from the relatively insensitive hepatic oxygen sensor to the renal oxygen sensor, which is sensitive to hypoxia, because by this time the predominant site of EPO synthesis is shifted to the kidneys.

Treatment: Physiologic anemia requires no therapy beyond ensuring that the diet of the infant contains essential nutrients for normal hematopoiesis, especially folic acid and iron. Premature infants who are feeding well and growing normally rarely need transfusion unless iatrogenic blood loss has been significant. In otherwise healthy premature infants, hemoglobin levels as low as 6.5 g/dl usually are well tolerated. When transfusions are necessary, an RBC volume of 10–15 ml/kg is recommended. The number of donors for an infant should be minimized. In early premature infants (<1,250 g), the half life of of transfused RBCs is about 30 days.

Anemia in very low birthweight preterm infants may be related to a relative deficiency of EPO, and clinical trials indicate that premature infants who do not have severe illnesses and are treated with recombinant human EPO (rHuEPO) and iron (oral iron 4–6 mg/kg/day) during the first 6 wk of life require few transfusions.

Glader B. Anemias of inadequate production. In: Kliegman RM, Behrman RE, Jenson HB, Stanton BF (eds). *Nelson Textbook of Pediatrics*. 18th edn. Vol. 2. Philadelphia: Saunders, 2007; 2006–18.

Ohis RK. The use of erythropoietin in neonates. *Clin Perinatol* 2000;27:681–96.

20.3 IRON DEFICIENCY ANEMIA

Anemia resulting from lack of sufficient iron for synthesis of hemoglobin is the most common cause of anemia in infancy and childhood. It is estimated that 30% of the global population suffers from iron deficiency anemia; most of those affected live in developing countries. It is important to note that to maintain positive iron balance in childhood, about 1 mg of iron must be absorbed everyday. The body of a newborn infant contains about 0.5 g of iron, whereas the adult content is estimated to be 5 g. Absorption of dietary iron is assumed to be about 10%, a diet containing 8–10 mg of iron daily is necessary for optimal nutrition. Iron is absorbed in the proximal small intestine, mediated in part by a variety of duodenal proteins. Formulas with 7–12 mg/liter of iron for full term infants and formulas with 15 mg/liter for premature infants less than 1800 g at birth are effective. Exclusively breastfed infants should receive iron supplementation from 4 months of age. As the high hemoglobin concentration of newborn infant falls during the first 2–3 mo of life, considerable iron is reclaimed and stored. These reclaimed iron stores usually are sufficient for blood formation in the first 6–9 mo of life in term infants.

Adolescents also are susceptible to iron deficiency because of high requirements due to growth spurt, dietary deficiencies, and menstrual blood loss.

Etiology: In term infants, anemia caused solely by inadequate dietary iron is unusual before 6 mo and usually occurs at 9–24 mo of age because reclaimed iron stores usually are sufficient for blood formation in the first 6–9 mo of life. Therefore, it is relatively uncommon. Low birth weight and unusual perinatal hemorrhage are associated with decreases in neonatal hemoglobin mass and stores of iron. Stored iron may be depleted earlier, and dietary sources become of paramount importance. Delayed clamping of the umbilical cord (~2 min) may reduce the incidence of iron deficiency. The usual *dietary pattern* observed in infants with iron-deficiency anemia is prolonged consumption of large amounts of cow's milk (>24 oz/day) and of foods not supplemented with iron.

Blood loss must be considered as a possible cause in every case of iron-deficiency anemia, particularly in older children. Chronic iron-deficiency anemia from occult bleeding may be caused by a lesion of the gastrointestinal tract, such as milk protein-induced inflammatory colitis, peptic ulcer, Meckel diverticulum, polyp, or hemangioma, or by inflammatory bowel disease. Other causes are hookworm infestation, *Helicobacter pylori* infection, pulmonary hemosiderosis, chronic diarrhea.

Intense exercise conditioning, as occurs in competitive athletics in school may result in iron depletion in girls; this occurs less commonly in boys.

Clinical manifestations: Pallor is the most important sign of iron deficiency. World Health Organization recommends use of palmar pallor as a screening measure for anemia. There are, however, high rates of false-positive and false-negative results from palmar, nailbed and conjunctival pallor, which vary according to the degree of anemia. In mild to moderate iron deficiency (i.e., hemoglobin levels of 6–10 g/dl), compensatory mechanisms, including levels of 2,3-diphosphoglycerate (2,3-DPG) and a shift of the oxygen dissociation curve may be so effective that few symptoms of anemia are noted, although affected children may be irritable. *Pagophagia*, the desire to ingest unusual substances such as ice or dirt, may be present. In some children, ingestion of lead-containing substances may lead to concomitant plumbism. When the hemoglobin level falls to <5 g/dl, irritability and anorexia are prominent. Tachycardia and cardiac dilation occur, and systolic murmurs are often present.

Children with iron-deficiency anemia may be obese or may be underweight, with other findings of poor nutrition. The irritability and anorexia characteristics of advanced cases is due to deficiency in tissue iron. Iron therapy often produces improvement in behavior before significant hematologic improvement is noted.

Iron deficiency may have effects on neurologic and intellectual function. Iron-deficiency affects attention span, alertness, and learning in both infants and adolescents. Adolescent girls with serum ferritin levels of ≥ 12 ng/L but without anemia have demonstrated improved verbal learning and memory after taking iron for 8 wk.

Laboratory findings: In progressive iron deficiency, a sequence of biochemical and hematologic events occur. First, the tissue iron stores represented by bone marrow hemosiderin disappear. The level of serum ferritin is decreased (normal: μg/L or ng/ml newborn: 25–200; 1 mo: 200–600; 2–5 mo: 50–200; 6 mo: 15 yr: 7–140). Next, serum iron level (normal: 22–184 μg/dl or 4–33 μmol/L) decreases, serum transferring increases, transferring saturation falls below normal and free erythrocyte protoporphyrin (FEP) accumulate. As the deficiency progresses, the red blood cells (RBCs) become smaller than normal and their hemoglobin content decreases. The morphologic characteristics of RBCs are best quantified by the determination of mean corpuscular hemoglobin (MCH), mean corpuscular volume (MCV) (Table 20.1). With increasing deficiency, the RBCs become deformed and misshapen and present characteristic microcytosis, poikilocytosis, and elevated RBC distribution width (RDW). Nucleated RBCs occasionally seen in the peripheral blood if the anemia is severe. White blood cell counts are normal. Sometimes there is thrombocytosis, which is believed to be caused by increased erythropoietin. Very severe iron deficiency anemia occasionally may be associated with thrombocytopenia.

Differential diagnosis: Iron deficiency anemia must be differentiated from other hypochromic microcytic anemias. The most important is to differentiate iron deficiency anemia from α- and β-thalassemia trait and Hb E syndromes. In latter conditions, the RBC often is elevated above normal despite the presence of a mild anemia and microcytosis; in iron deficiency anemia, RBC count is decreased along with reduced hemoglobin and MCV. Another difference between α- and β-thalassemia trait and iron deficiency anemia is that the RDW is elevated in iron deficiency.

The anemia of chronic disorders (ACD) and infection is usually normocytic, although occasionally it may be slightly microcytic. Serum iron level and iron-binding capacity, total iron-binding capacity (TIBC, normal: infant 100–400 μg/dl and thereafter 250–400 μg/dl) are reduced, and serum ferritin levels are normal or elevated. The serum transferring receptor (TfR) level is useful in the distinction between iron-deficiency anemia and anemia of chronic disease because it is not affected by inflammation. The concentration of TfR is elevated in iron deficiency and is within the normal range in anemia of chronic disease.

Lead poisoning and iron deficiency anemia both are associated with elevated FEP though it is more marked in lead intoxication. Coarse basophilic stippling of the RBCs is frequently predominant in lead intoxication. Elevated blood lead, FEP, and urinary coproporphyrin levels are seen (*see* Section 35.3).

Sideroblastic anemias result from acquired (idiopathic or secondary to drugs, alcohol, or myelodysplastic disorders) and hereditary disorders of heme synthesis. The anemias are characterized by hypochromic microcytic red blood cells (RBCs) mixed with normal RBCs and marrow nucleated RBCs with iron granules that have a perinuclear distribution (ringed sidero-blasts). The serum iron concentration usually elevated and total iron-binding capacity (TIBC) is increased. *Congenital sideroblastic anemia* has an X-linked pattern of inheritance, usually occurs in males, although rarely affected in females. Clinical findings include pallor, icterus, and moderate splenomegaly and/or hepatomegaly.

Treatment: Oral administration of ferrous salts (sulphate, fumarate, gluconate) in 4–6 mg/kg of elemental iron in three divided doses is quite effective. Within 72–96 hr after administration of iron to an anemic child, peripheral reticulocytosis is noted (Table 20.4). Reticlocytosis is followed by a rise in the hemoglobin level, which may increase as much as 0.5 g/24 hr. Iron medication should be continued for 8 wk after blood values are normal. The response to iron therapy in iron deficiency anemia is presented in Table 20.4. Intolerance to oral iron is not frequent in small children, although older children and adolescents sometimes have gastrointestinal complaints. Common side effect of oral iron is constipation. A parenteral iron preparation (iron dextran) can be used when the patient is refractory to oral iron. However, there is

Table 20.4: Response to iron therapy in iron deficiency anemia	
Time after iron administration	*Response*
12–24 hr	Replacement of intracellular iron enzymes; subjective improvement; decreased irritability; increased appetite
36–48 hr	Initial bone marrow response; erythroid hyperplasia
48–72 hr	Reticulocytosis, peaking on 5–7 days
4–30 days	Increase in hemoglobin level
1–3 mo	Repletion of stores

increased risk of anaphylaxis. The risk of anaphylaxis is much less with ferric gluconate given IV. Milk consumption should be limited to a reasonable quantity, preferably 500 mL (1 pint)/24 hr or less during iron therapy. This reduction of milk has a dual effect: The iron rich food is increased, and blood loss from intolerance to cow's milk proteins are reduced. Iron deficiency in adolescent females secondary to abnormal uterine bleeding is treated with iron and hormone therapy. Blood transfusion is indicated in severe anemia or when superimposed infection interferes with the response. Packed or sedimented RBCs should be transfused slowly. When hemoglobin level is less than 4 g/dl, only 2–3 ml/kg of packed cells are given at one time along with diuretics. If congestive cardiac failure is present, a modified exchange transfusion using fresh-packed RBCs may be considered, although diuretics followed by slow infusion of packed RBCs usually suffice.

Alcindor T, Bridges KR. Sideroblastic anemias. *Br J Hematol* 2002;116:733–43.

Dallman PR, Slimes MA, Stekel A. Iron deficiency anemia in infancy and childhood. *Am J Clin Nutr* 1980;33:86–118.

Dallman PR, Yip R, Oski FA. Iron deficiency and related nutritional anemias. In: Nathan DG, Oski FA (eds). *Hematology of infancy and childhood.* 4th edn. Philadelphia: WB Saunders Co., 1993:428.

Das BK, Shrestha Pramod. Microcytic Anemia. In: Mathur GP, Mathur Sarla (eds). *Current Trends in Pediatrics.* Vol 3. Delhi: Academa Publishers, 2007;219–27.

Fomon SJ, Ziegler EE, Nelson SE, Edwards BB. Cow's milk feeding in infancy, gastrointestinal blood loss and iron nutritional status. *J Pediatr* 1981;98:540–5.

Glader B. Anemias of inadequate production. In: Kliegman RM, Behrman RE, Jenson HB, Stanton BF (eds). *Nelson Textbook of Pediatrics.* 18th edn. Vol. 2. Philadelphia: Saunders, 2007; 2006–18.

Nathan WG, Orkin SH. *Nathan and Oski's Hematology of Infancy and Childhood.* 5th edn. Philadelphia: WB Saunders, 2002.

20.4 MEGALOBLASTIC ANEMIAS

The RBCs in megaloblastic anemias are large (increased mean corpuscular volume (MCV) and often oval. Neutrophils are hypersegmented with many neutrophils having > 5 lobes. Almost all cases of childhood megaloblastic anemia result from a deficiency of folic acid or vitamin B_{12}; rarely may be caused by inborn errors of metabolism. Both vitamin B_{12} and folate are required in the synthesis of nucleoproteins; deficiencies result in defective synthesis of DNA and to lesser extent, RNA and protein.

Folic Acid Deficiency

Folates are abundant in many foods, including green vegetables, fruits and animal organs (e.g., liver, kidney). Human breast milk, pasteurized cow's milk, and infant formulas provide adequate amounts of folic acid. Goat's milk is deficient, so folic acid supplementation must be given when it is the child's main food. Folates are heat labile and water soluble, and consequently boiling or heating folate sources leads to decreased amount of vitamin. Megaloblastic anemia occurs after 2–3 mo on a folate free diet.

Etiology: Folic acid deficiency can occur as a consequence of inadequate folate intake, decreased folate absorption, or acquired and congenital disorders of folate metabolism.

Inadequate folate intake: Folate requirements increased markedly during pregnancy, in part to meet fetal needs, growth in infancy and in chronic hemolysis. The normal daily infant's requirement is 25–35 µg/day. Folate supplementation of at least 400 µg/day is recommended from the start of pregnancy to prevent neural tube defects and to meet growth needs of the developing fetus.

Decreased folate absorption: Malabsorption due to chronic diarrheal states or diffuse inflammatory disease can lead to folate deficiency. Certain anti-convulsant drugs (e.g., phenytoin, primidone, phenobarbital) can impair absorption of folic acid.

Congenital abnormalities in folate metabolism: Congenital dihydrofolate reductase deficiency and methylene tetrahydrofolate reductase deficiency is rarely reported.

Drug-induced abnormalities in folate metabolism: A number of drugs have anti-folic acid activity such as methotrexate, pyrimethamine, and trimethoprim.

Clinical manifestations: Mild megaloblastic anemia has been reported in very low birth weight infants. Megaloblastic anemia due to folate deficiency has its peak incidence at 4–7 mo of age, somewhat earlier than iron deficiency anemia, although both conditions may be present concomitantly in infants with poor nutrition. Affected infants with folic acid deficiency have in addition to clinical features of anemia are irritable, have inadequate weight gain and chronic diarrhea. Hemorrhages from thrombocytopenia occur in advanced cases. Folic acid deficiency may be associated with Kwashiorkor, marasmus, or sprue.

Laboratory findings: The anemia is macrocytic (mean corpuscular volume >100 fl). Large, abnormal neutrophilic forms (giant metamyelocytes) with cytoplasmic vacuolation are also seen (Table 20.3).

Treatment: In established cases of folate deficiency, folic acid may be administered orally or parenterally at 0.5–1 mg/day. In doubtful cases, smaller doses of folate (0.1 mg/day) may be used for 1 wk as a diagnostic test, because hematologic response can be expected within 72 hr. Doses of folate > 0.1 mg can correct the anemia of vitamin B_{12} deficiency but may aggravate any associated neurologic abnormalities. Folic acid therapy (0.5–1.0 mg/day) should be continued for 3–4 wk until a definite hematologic response has occurred. Maintenance therapy with a multivitamin (containing 0.2 mg of folate) is adequate. Transfusions are indicated only when the anemia is severe or the child is very ill.

Vitamin B_{12} (Cobalamin) Deficiency

Vitamin B_{12} is derived from cobalamin in food mainly (mainly animal sources) secondary to the production by microorganisms. Humans cannot synthesize vitamin B_{12}. The cobalamins are released by the acidity of the stomach and combine there with R proteins and intrinsic factor (IF); traverses the duodenum, where pancreatic proteases break down the R proteins; and are absorbed in the distal ileum via specific receptors for IF-cobalamin. In the plasma, cobalamin binds to a transport protein transcobalamin II (TC-II), which carries the vitamin B_{12} to the liver, bone marrow, and other tissue storage sites. Plasma also contains two other vitamin B_{12}-binding proteins, transcobalamin I and III (TC-I and TC-III). In contrast to folate stores, older children and adults have sufficient vitamin B_{12} stores to last 3–5 yr. In infants born to mothers with low vitamin B_{12} stores, clinical signs of cobalamin deficiency can become apparent in the first 6–18 mo of life.

Etiology: Vitamin B_{12} deficiency may result from inadequate dietary intake of vitamin, lack of IF-secretion by the stomach, impaired intestinal absorption of IF-cobalamin, or absence of vitamin B_{12} transport protein.

Inadequate vitamin B_{12} intake: It may occur in strict vegetarians or vegans, in which case no animal products are consumed. Vitamin B_{12} deficiency may be seen in cases of Kwashiorkor or infantile marasmus. In children, megaloblastic anemia from inadequate of vitamin B_{12} occurs in breastfed infants whose mothers are vegans or themselves have pernicious anemia.

Lack of intrinsic factor: Congenital pernicious anemia is a rare autosomal recessive disorder due to an inability to secrete gastric intrinsic factor (IF) or secretion of functionally abnormal IF. It differs from the typical disease of adults in that the stomach secretes acid normally and is histologically normal. There are no antibodies to parietal cells and no associated endocrine disorders. The symptoms of juvenile pernicious anemia become prominent at around 1 yr of age. The tongue is smooth, red and painful. Neurological manifestations include ataxia, parasthesias, hyporeflexias, Babinski responses, and clonus. Juvenile pernicious anemia is another rare disorder occurring in older children. It is an immunologic disorder akin to that of adult-type pernicious anemia.

Impaired vitamin B_{12} absorption: It occurs in patients with inflammatory disorders such as regional enteritis or neonatal necrotizing enterocolitis, surgically removed terminal ileum (if there is evidence that vitamin B_{12} is not absorbed), overgrowth of intestinal bacteria within diverticula or duplication of small intestine (vitamin B_{12} deficiency by consumption of or competition for the vitamin or by splitting of its complex with IF), and infestation of fish tapeworm *Diphyllobothrium latum* in the upper small intestine. In these cases serum vitamin B_{12} level is low, the gastric juice contains intrinsic factor, and the abnormal Schilling test result is not corrected by addition of exogenous IF. Megaloblastic anemia due to vitamin B_{12} deficiency has been reported as a result of defects of the receptor for IF-B_{12} in the intestinal ileum, in some instances associated with proteinuria (Imerslund-Grasbeck syndrome, an autosomal recessive disorder with involvement of chromosome 10p12.1).

Absence of vitamin B_{12} transport protein: Transcobalamin II (TC-II) deficiency is a rare cause of megaloblastic anemia due to decreased utilization of cobalamin. Serum vitamin B_{12} levels are normal because the storage forms of cobalamin TC-I and TC-III are not affected. This disorder usually manifests in the first weeks of life with failure to thrive, diarrhea, vomiting, glossitis, neurologic abnormalities, and megaloblastic anemia. The diagnosis is made by specific tests for TC-II. The serum vitamin B_{12} levels must be kept high to utilize cobalamin. Larger parenteral doses of vitamin B_{12} are given twice a week for life.

Clinical manifestations: Children with cobalamin deficiency often presents with weakness, fatigue, failure to thrive, irritability, pallor, glossitis, vomiting, diarrhea, icterus, and neurologic symptoms (paresthesias, sensory deficits, hypotonia, seizures, developmental delay, developmental regression, and neuropsychiatric changes). Neurologic problems from vitamin B_{12} deficiency can occur in the absence of any hematologic abnormalities.

Laboratory findings: The hematologic manifestations of folate and cobalamin deficiency are identical. The anemia resulting from cobalamin deficiency is macrocytic, with prominent macro-ovalocystosis of the RBCs (Table 20.5).

Table 20.5: Laboratory findings of folate and cobalamin deficiency

Laboratory findings	Folate deficiency	Cobalamin deficiency
Red blood cells (RBCs)	Macrocytic, macro-ovalocystosis	Macrocytic, macro-ovalocystosis
Neutrophils	Large, some with hypersegmented nuclei	Large, some with hypersegmented nuclei
Neutropenia	Present	Present
Thrombocytopenia	Present	Present
Serum folic acid level (normal 5–20 ng/ml); RBC folate level (normal 150–600 ng/ml of packed cells)	Low (<3 ng/ml) RBC folate level	Normal or elevated
Seum iron level	Normal or elevated	Normal or elevated
Serum vitamin B_{12} level	Normal or elevated	Low
LDH	Markedly elevated	Markedly elevated
Seum bilirubin	Normal	Moderately elevated (2–3 mg/dl)
Methylmalonic acid in urine (normal 0–3.5 mg/24 hr)	Normal	Elevated (reliable and sensitive index)

Diagnosis: The specific cause of vitamin B_{12} deficiency often is apparent from the clinical history. Administration of a minidose (physiologic requirement for vitamin B_{12} is 1–5 µg/day) may be used as a therapeutic test when the diagnosis of vitamin B_{12} deficiency is in doubt. If there is no obvious cause for serum vitamin B_{12} deficiency, absorption of vitamin B_{12} can be assessed by the Schilling test. When a normal person ingests a small amount of vitamin B_{12} into which cobalt 57 has been incorporated, the radioactive vitamin combines with the IF in stomach secretions and passes to the terminal ileum, where absorption occurs. Because the absorbed vitamin is bound to TC-II and incorporated into tissues, little or none normally is excreted in the urine. If a large dose (1 mg) of nonradioactive vitamin B_{12} is injected parenterally after 2 hr (flushing dose), 10–30% of the previously absorbed radioactive vitamin appears in the urine in 24 hr. Children with pernicious anemia usually excrete ≤ 2% under these conditions. IF is given with a second dose of radioactive vitamin B_{12} to confirm its malabsorption. When vitamin B_{12} malabsorption results from absence of ileal receptor sites or other intestinal causes, no improvement in absorption occurs with IF. The Schilling test results remain abnormal in the patients with pernicious anemia, even when therapy has completely reversed the hematologic and neurologic manifestations of the disease.

Treatment: After parenteral administration of 1 mg of vitamin B_{12} prompt hematologic response occurs, usually with reticulocytosis in 2–4 days, unless there is concurrent inflammatory disease. Hematologic responses have been observed with small doses. In cases of neurologic involvement, 1 mg should be injected intramuscularly daily for at least 2 wk.

Maintenance therapy (1 mg monthly intramuscular injection) is necessary throughout life. Oral therapy is not advisable, owing to uncertainty of absorption.

Glader B. Anemia of inadequate production. In: Kliegman RM, Behrman RE, Jenson HB, Stanton BF (eds). *Nelson Textbook of Pediatrics.* 18th edn. Vol. 2. Philadelphia: Saunders, 2007; 2006–2018.

Rasmussen SA, Fernhoff PM, Scanlon KS. Vitamin B_{12} deficiency in children and adolescents. *J Pediatr* 2001;138:10–17.

Rosenblatt DS, Whitehead VM. Cobalamin and folate deficiency: Acquired and hereditary disorders in children. *Semin Hematol* 1999;36:19–34.

20.5 HEMOLYTIC ANEMIAS

Definition and Classification of Hemolytic Anemias

Hemolysis is defined as the premature destruction of red blood cells (RBCs). Normal RBC survival time is 110–120 days (half-life, 55–60 days), and approximately 0.85% of the most senescent RBCs are removed and replaced each day. Anemia results when the rate of destruction exceeds the capacity of the marrow to produce RBCs. During hemolysis, RBC survival is shortened, the RBCs count falls, erythropoietin is increased, and the stimulation of marrow activity results in heightened RBCs production. This results in increased percentage of reticulocytes in the blood. Thus, *hemolysis should be suspected as a cause of anemia if elevated reticulocyte count is present.* The reticulocyte count may also be elevated as a response to acute blood loss or for a short period after replacement therapy for iron, vitamin B_{12}, or folate deficiency.

Hemolytic anemias may be classified as either (i) *cellular,* resulting from intrinsic abnormalities of the membrane, enzymes, or hemoglobin, or (ii) *extracellular*, resulting from antibodies, mechanical factors, or plasma factors. Most cellular defects are inherited (paroxysmal nocturnal hemoglobinuria is acquired), and most extracellular defects are acquired (abetalipoproteinemia with acanthocytosis is inherited).

Hereditary Spherocytosis

Hereditary spherocytosis is a common cause of hemolysis and hemolytic anemia. It is the most common inherited abnormality of the red blood cell (RBC) membrane. Hereditary spherocytosis usually is transmitted as an autosomal dominant, less frequently, as an autosomal recessive disorder.

Clinical manifestations: Hereditary spherocytosis may be a cause of hemolytic disease in the newborn and may present as anemia and hyperbilirubinemia sufficiently severe to require phototherapy or exchange transfusions. The severity of symptoms in infants and children is variable. Some children remain asymptomatic into adulthood, but others may have severe anemia, with pallor, jaundice, fatigue, and exercise intolerance. Severe cases may be marked by expansion of diploe of the skull and the medullary region of other bones. After infancy, the spleen is usually enlarged, and pigmentary (bilirubin) gallstones may form as early as age 4–5 yr. Because of the high RBC turnover and heightened erythroid marrow activity, children with hereditary spherocytosis are susceptible to aplastic crisis, primarily as a result of parvovirus B19 infection, and to hypoplastic crisis associated with various other infections. The erythroid marrow failure may result rapidly in profound anemia (hematocrit <10%), high output heart failure, hypoxia, cardiovascular collapse, and death. White blood cell and platelet counts may also fall.

Laboratory findings: The laboratory findings include evidence of hemolysis [reticlocytosis (reticulocyte count 6–20%, mean approximately 10%) and indirect hyperbilirubinemia], 6–10 g/dl hemoglobin levels, normal mean corpuscular volume (MCV), increased (36–38 g/dl RBC) mean corpuscular hemoglobin concentration (MCHC), and presence of polychromatophilic reticulocytes and spherocytes. The spherocytes are smaller in diameter and hyperchromic on the blood film as a result of the high hemoglobin concentration. The central pallor is less conspicuous, than the normal cells. The presence of spherocytes in the blood can be confirmed with an osmotic fragility test; exposure to hypotonic saline causes the RBCs to swell, and the spherocytes lyse more readily than biconcave cells in hypotonic solutions. Erythroid hyperplasia is evident in the marrow aspirate or biopsy. Marrow expansion may be evident on routine radiologic studies. Gallstones are seen on ultrasonography.

The diagnosis of hereditary spherocytosis usually is established clinically from the blood film, which shows many spherocytes and reticulocytes, from the family history, and from splenomegaly.

Treatment: Splenectomy markedly improves RBC life span and cures the anemia. For patients whose hemoglobin values exceed 10 g/dl and reticulocyte count <10%, folic acid 1 mg daily should be administered to prevent deficiency and the resultant decrease in erythropoiesis and splenectomy is not recommended. Splenectomy is recommended for patients with more severe anemia and reticulocytosis or those with hypoplastic or aplastic crisis, poor growth, or cardiomegaly, after age 5–6 yr to avoid the heightened risk of postsplenectomy sepsis in younger children. Laparoscopic splenectomy decreases the length of hospital stay and has replaced open splenectomy for many patients. Vaccines (conjugated and/or capsular) for encapsulated organisms such as pneumococcus, meningococcus, and *Haemophilus influenzae* type b, should be administered before splenectomy, and prophylactic oral penicillin V (age <5 yr, 125 mg twice daily; age 5 yr through adulthood, 250 mg twice daily) administered thereafter. Postsplenectomy thrombocytosis is commonly observed, but no treatment is required as it usually resolves spontaneously. Partial splenectomy also may be useful in children younger than 5 yr.

Segel GB. Definitions and classification of hemolytic anemias. In: Kliegman RM, Behrman RE, Jenson HB, Stanton BF (eds). *Nelson Textbook of Pediatrics.* 18th edn. Vol. 2. Philadelphia: Saunders, 2007; 2018–20.

Segel GB. Hereditary spherocytosis. In: Kliegman RM, Behrman RE, Jenson HB, Stanton BF (eds). *Nelson Textbook of Pediatrics.* 18th edn. Vol. 2. Philadelphia: Saunders, 2007; 2020–3.

Sickle Cell Disease

Hemoglobin S (HbS) is the result of a single base pair change, thymine for adenine, at the 6th codon of the β-globin gene. This change encodes valine instead of glutamine in the 6th position in the β-globin molecule. *Sickle cell anemia*, homozygous HbS, occurs when both β-globin genes have the sickle cell mutation. *Sickle cell disease* refers not only to individuals with sickle cell anemia, but also to compound heterozygotes where one β-globin gene mutation includes the sickle cell mutation and the 2nd β-globin includes a gene mutation in the β-globin gene other than the sickle cell mutation such as mutations associated with Hb C, Hb β-thalassemia, HbD, and HbO Arab. In sickle cell anemia, HbS is commonly as high as 90% of the total hemoglobin. In sickle cell disease, HbS is > 50% of all hemoglobin.

Sickle Cell Anemia (Homozygous Hemoglobin S) or S β-Thalassemia

Clinical manifestations and treatment: Infants with sickle cell anemia have *abnormal immune function.* As early as 6 months of age, some children, and by 5 yr of age, most children have functional asplenia. Children with sickle cell anemia also have deficient levels of serum opsonins against pneumococci. Regardless of age, all patients with sickle cell anemia are at increased risk for infection and death as a result of bacterial infection, particularly with encapsulated organisms, such as *Streptococcus pneumoniae* and *Haemophilus influenzae* type b. Children with sickle cell anemia should receive prophylactic oral penicillin at least until 5 yr of age (125 mg twice daily up to age 3 yr, then 250 mg twice daily). No established guidelines exist for penicillin prophylaxis beyond 5 yr of age. Some clinicians continue penicillin prophylaxis, whereas others recommend discontinuation. Penicillin prophylaxis should be considered for children beyond 5 yr of age, when there is previous diagnosis of pnemococcal infection due to the increased risk of recurrent infection. To children allergic to penicillin, erythromycin ethyl succinate 10 mg/kg twice daily should be prescribed. In addition to penicillin prophylaxis, routine childhood immunizations and annual administration of influenza vaccine are recommended.

Human parvovirus B19 infection in patients with sickle cell anemia limits the production of reticulocytes. Any child with reticulocytopenia should be considered as having parvovirus B 19 until proven otherwise. Acute infection with parvovirus B 19 is usually associated with red cell aplasia (aplastic episode), fever, and pain in addition to splenic sequestration, acute chest syndrome (ACS), glomerulonephritis, and stroke. Treatment requires packed red cell transfusion for hemodynamic instability.

The *management of fever* in a child with sickle cell anemia requires prompt medical evaluation and administration of antibiotics because of high risk of bacterial infection and high mortality rate when infected. A paraneural long-acting 3rd generation cephalosporin antibiotic should be given before a positive blood culture report is available. If *Salmonella* or *Staphylococcus* bacteremia occurs, osteomyelitis with a bone scan or an MRI should also be considered.

Dactylitis, often referred to as *hand–foot syndrome,* is frequently the first manifestation of pain in children with sickle cell anemia, occurring in 50% of children by 2 yr of age. Dactylitis often presents with symmetric swelling of the hands and/or feet. Unilateral dactylitis can be confused with osteomyelitis and requires careful evaluation, because the former requires palliation with pain medication (paracetamol with codeine), whereas osteomyelitis requires at least a 4–6 wk course of IV antibiotics.

Acute *splenic sequestration* is a life-threatening complication, occurring primarily in infants, and may occur as early as 5 wk of age. The etiology of splenic sequestration episodes is unknown. There is engorgement of spleen with a subsequent increase in spleen size, evidence of hypovolemia, and decline in hemoglobin of at least 2.0 g/dl from baseline, reticulocytosis and a decrease in platelet count. These events can be accompanied by upper respiratory tract bacterial or viral infections. Treatment consists of administration of isotonic fluid or blood transfusions to maintain hemodynamic stability. Repeated episodes of splenic sequestration are common, usually occurring 6 mo of the previous event. Prophylactic splenectomy performed after the acute episode has resolved is the only strategy for prevention of future life-threatening episodes.

The pain from *vaso-occclusive episode* is characterized as unremitting discomfort that may occur in any part of the body, but most often occurs in the chest, abdomen, or extremities. These painful episodes are often abrupt and can disrupt daily life activities. The pathogenesis of pain is disruption of blood flow in the microvsculature by sickle cells, resulting in tissue ischemia. The precipitating cases of painful episodes can include physical stress, infection, dehydration, hypoxia, local or systemic acidosis, exposure to cold, and swimming in nonheated water for prolonged period. The treatment of painful episodes requires education of both the parents and the patient regarding the symptoms and management strategy. The therapies of pain generally include the use of acetaminophen or a nonsteroidal agent early in the course of pain, followed by acetaminophen with codeine and short or long acting oral opioids, or hospitalization with IV administration of morphine or morphine derivatives. Hydroxyurea, a myelo-suppressive agent is given 15–20 mg/kg daily, with an increase in dose every 8 wk of 2.5–5.0 mg/kg, if no toxicities occur, up to a maximum dose of 35 mg/kg. Hydroxyurea raises the level of HbF and the hemoglobin level and usually decreases the rate of painful episodes by 50%.

Priapism, a common problem in sickle cell anemia is an involuntary penile erection lasting longer than 30 min. Priapism occurs in 2 patterns, *stuttering* and *refractory. Stuttering priapism* is defined as self-limiting intermittent bouts of priapism with several episodes over a defined period. *Refractory priapism* is defined as prolonged priapism beyond several hours. For treatment of priapism, supportive therapy such as a sitz bath or pain medication, is commonly used. If the priapism lasts longer than 4 hr, then aspiration of blood from the corpora cavernosa, followed by irrigation with dilute epinephrine, is effective in producing immediate and sustained detumescence.

Neurologic complications include strokes, headaches, seizures, cerebral venous thrombosis and reversible posterior leukoencephalopathy syndrome (RPLS). CT to exclude cerebral hemorrhage should be done as soon as possible; if available MRI of the brain with diffusion-weighed imaging should be done to distinguish between ischemic infarcts and RPLS. *Treatment* of stroke includes oxygen administration to maintain oxygen saturation at >96% and simple blood transfusion therapy as quickly and safely as possible with a goal of transfusion with in 1 hr of presentation, with a goal of increasing the hemoglobin to a maximum of 11.0 g/dl.

Lung disease in children with sickle cell anemia is the 2nd most common reason for admission to the hospital and a common cause of death. *Acute chest syndrome* (ACS) consists of a new radiodensity on chest radiograph, fever, respiratory distress, and pain that often occurs in the chest, but may include only the back and/or the abdomen. Even when no respiratory symptoms are present, all patients with fever should receive a chest radiograph to identify ACS. Radiographs may show single lobe involvement, most often the left lower lobe, and when multiple lobes are involved, usually both lower lobes are affected. Pleural effusions, either unilateral or bilateral, may not be present initially (or may be minimal in size), but may progress rapidly. A wide range of therapeutic strategies have been used because of clinical overlap between ACS and common pulmonary complications, such as bronchiolitis, asthma (which is also common in children with sickle cell anemia), and pneumonia. The most common illness preceding ACS is a painful episode requiring opioids, and infection is believed to be the most common identifiable cause. *Treatment* of the ACS includes oxygen administration and simple or exchange blood transfusion therapy. Oxygen should be administered when the oxygen saturation is <90%. Blood transfusion is given, when at least one of the following clinical features is present: decreasing oxygen saturation; increasing work of breathing; rapid change in respiratory effort, with or without a worsening chest radiograph; or a history of severe ACS requiring admission to the intensive care unit. As a result of clinical overlap between pneumonia and ACS, all episodes should be treated promptly with antimicrobial therapy that includes at least a macrolide and a 3rd-generation cephalosporin to treat the most common pathogens associated with ACS (*S. pneumoniae*, *Mycoplasma pneumoniae*, *Chlamydia pneumoniae*). A previous diagnosis of asthma should prompt treatment with steroids and bronchodilators, even when the patient does not have evidence of wheezing.

Pulmonary hypertension, associated with sickle cell anemia, and other chronic hemolytic anemias (thalassemia, hereditary spherocytosis, paroxysmal nocturnal hemoglobinuria), is a major risk factor for death in adults. The natural history of pulmonary hypertension in children with sickle cell anemia is unknown; therefore, the optimal diagnostic and therapeutic strategy for pulmonary hypertension has not been identified.

Renal disease in patients with sickle cell anemia is a major comorbid condition that can lead to premature death. The clinical manifestations of renal disease include hematuria, proteinuria, renal insufficiency, concentrating defects, and hypertension. Angiotensin-converting enzyme (ACE) inhibitors are useful in the management of patients with proteinuria. Suspicion of *renal medullary carcinoma* should be kept in mind.

The other complications include *sickle cell retinopathy*, *delayed onset of puberty*, *avascular necrosis of the femoral head* and *humerus*, and *leg ulcers*.

As with any child with a chronic illness, good health maintenance must include psychologic and social assessment. Children with sickle cell anemia are at great risk for academic failure.

Surgical preparation for children with sickle cell anemia requires management of ACS and pain, blood transfusion before surgery to raise the hemoglobin level preoperatively to 10.0 g/dl is desirable.

Laboratory findings: Sickle cell disease should be suspected in all patients who have the clinical manifestations of sickle cell disease. A complete blood cell count usually reveals an increased reticulocyte count (5–15%), upper limit of normal or greater leukocyte count (12,000–20,000/mm^3), normal mean corpuscular volume (MCV) (unless a thalassemic hemoglobin is present), mild to moderate anemia (5–9 g/dl), normal to increased platelet count, and a normal differential (or predominance of neutrophils), if severe anemia is present, nucleated red cells can be found. A diagnosis of sickle disease can be suspected by examination of the blood smear for target cells, poikilocytes, polychromasia, sickle red cells, nucleated RBCs, and Howell-Jolly bodies and confirmed by hemoglobin electrophoresis or high pressure liquid chromatography (HPLC). Bone marrow is markedly hyperplastic with ertythroid predominance. Radiologic studies may reveal characteristic bony findings of sickle cell disease in the vertebral bodies, mild expansion of marrow cavities, osteoporosis and possibly sclerosis of the long bones and femoral heads. Renal concentrating capacity is usually decreased.

Diagnosis: Sickle test is simple and detects both sickle cell traits and patients with sickle cell anemia. Red cells containing HbS take on a sickle shape, when mixed with a freshly prepared solution of the reducing agent, sodium metabisulphite. Sickle cell disease is diagnosed at birth through newborn screening program. These programs use hemoglobin electrophoresis or HPLC to define abnormal hemoglobins. Confirmatory studies for HbS or variants are performed after birth. Prenatal diagnosis is also possible for parents who both have sickle cell trait.

Differential diagnosis: The various clinical manifestations of sickle cell disease, including limb pain, heart murmurs, hepatosplenomegaly, and anemia may suggest a number of other diagnoses, including rheumatic fever or rheumatoid arthritis, osteomyelitis, and leukemia.

Prevention: All children who have sickle cell disease should be immunized with the conjugate pneumococcal vaccine and all other routine vaccines of childhood. All children should receive penicillin prophylaxis. Because of the thrombotic nature of the sickle hemoglobins and the high red cell turnover, folate supplementation is recommended as well. Treatment in sickle cell disease is directed toward the prevention of complications and optimization of health and healthy coping strategies.

Sickle Cell Trait

The prevalence of sickle cell trait varies throughout the world. The amount of HbS in individuals with sickle cell trait is <50%; life span of people with sickle cell trait is normal and serious complications are very rare. Hemoglobin analysis is diagnostic, revealing a predominance of HbA_2 typically >50%. Complications of sickle cell trait include sudden death during rigorous exercise, splenic infarct at high altitude, hematuria, hyposthenuria, and bacteriuria, susceptibility to eye injury with formation of a hyphema, and renal medullary carcinoma. Children with sickle cell trait should not have any restriction on activities.

Adhikari RC. Sickle Cell Anemia. In: Mathur GP, Mathur Sarla (eds). *Current Trends in Pediatrics.* Vol 1. Delhi: Academa Publishers, 2005;279–83.

Claster S, Vichinsky FP. Managing sickle cell disease. *BMJ* 2003;327:1151–5.

DeBaun MR, Vichinsky. Hemoglobinopathies. In: Kliegman RM, Behrman RE, Jenson HB, Stanton BF (eds). *Nelson Textbook of Pediatrics.* 18th edn. Vol. 2. Philadelphia: Saunders, 2007; 2025–38.

Lehmann H, Cutbush M. Sickle cell trait in Southern India. *BMJ* 1952;1:404–05.

Mandot S, Khurana VL, Sonesh JK. Sickle cell anemia in Garasia tribals of Rajasthan. *Indian Pediatr* 2009; 46: 239–240.

Shukla RM, Solanki BR. Sickle cell trait in Central India. *Lancet* 1985;1:297–8.

Stuart MJ, Nagel RL. Sickle cell disease. *Lancet* 2004;364:343–60.

Thalassemia Syndromes

Thalassemia refers to genetic disorders in globin chain production. In individuals with β-thalassemia, there is either a complete absence of β-globin production (β-thalassemia major) or a partial reduction in β-globin production (β-thalassemia minor). In α-thalassemia, there is an absence of or partial reduction in α-globin production.

Epidemiology: There are more than 200 mutations for β-thalassemia. About 20 common alleles constitute 80% of the known thalassemia worldwide. 3% of the world's population carries genes for β-thalassemia, and in Southeast Asia 5–10% of the population carries genes for α-thalassemia. In India the carrier frequency of β-thalassemia varies from 1 to 17% (mean 3.3%) in different ethnic groups. Overall, three crore population is carrier of this gene in India and approximately 7600 children with transfusion dependent β-thalassemia are born in India every year (Kabra, 2005).

Pathophysiology: Two related features contribute to the sequelae of β-thalassemia: inadequate β-globin gene production leading to decreased levels of normal hemoglobin (HbA) and unbalanced α- and β-globin gene production. In the bone marrow, thalassemia mutations disrupt the maturation of erythrocytes, resulting in ineffective erythropoiesis; the marrow is hyperactive, but there are relatively few reticulocytes and severe anemia exists. In β-thalassemia, there is an excess of α-globin chains relative to β- and γ-globin chains, and α-globin tetramers (α_4) are formed. These inclusions interact with the red cell membrane and shorten red cell survival, leading to anemia and increased erythroid production. The γ-globin chains are produced in increased amounts leading to an elevated HbF ($\alpha_2\gamma_2$). The δ-globin chains are also produced in increased amounts, leading to an elevated HbA_2 ($\alpha_2\delta_2$) in β-thalassemia.

In α-thalassemia there are relatively fewer α-globin chains and an excess of β- and γ-globin chains. These excess chains form Bart's hemoglobin (γ_4) in fetal life and HbH (β_4) after birth. These abnormal tetramers are not lethal but lead to extravascular hemolysis. Prenatally, a fetus with α-thalassemia can become symptomatic because HbF requires sufficient of α-globin gene production, whereas postnatally infants with β-thalassemia becomes symptomatic because HbA requires sufficient production of β-globin genes.

Homozygous β-thalassemia (Thalassemia Major, Cooley Anemia)

Clinical manifestations: Children with β-thalassemia, if not treated usually become symptomatic as a result of progressive hemolytic anemia, with marked weakness and cardiac decompensation during the second 6 months of life. The classic presentation of children with severe disease includes thalassemic facies (maxilla hyperplasia, flat nasal bridge, frontal bossing), pathologic bone fractures, marked hepatosplenomegaly, and cachexia. The spleen can become so enlarged that it causes mechanical discomfort and secondary hyperslenism. The features of ineffective erythropoiesis include expanded medullary spaces (with massive expansion of the marrow of the face and skull producing the characteristic thalassemic facies), extramedullary hematopoiesis, and higher caloric need. Pallor, hemosiderosis and jaundice may combine to produce a greenish brown complexion (*see* Figs 20.25 and 20.26 in CD). As a result of the anemia there is also an increase in iron absorption from the gastrointestinal tract, with toxicity leading to further complications.

Many of these features become less severe and less infrequent with blood transfusion. But excessive iron stores associated with transfusional iron overload is a real problem. Many of the complications of thalassemia seen in developed countries are as a result of increased iron deposition. Most of these complications can be avoided by the consistent use of an iron chelator. But chelation therapy also has associated complications, such as hearing loss, peripheral neuropathy, and poor growth. Endocrine and cardiac problems are often associated with excessive iron stores who are chronically transfused. Endocrine dysfunction may include hypothyroidism, hypoparathyroidism, gonadal failure and diabetes mellitus. Congestive heart failure and cardiac arrhythmias are potentially lethal complications of excessive iron stores.

Laboratory findings: The infant is born only with HbF or, in some cases, HbF and HbE (heterozygosity for β-thalassemia). There is severe anemia, reticulocytopenia, numerous nucleated erythrocytes, and microcytosis with almost no normal-appearing erythrocytes on the peripheral smear. The hemoglobin level falls progressively to <5 g/dl unless transfusions are given. The reticulocyte count is commonly <8%, which is inappropriately low when compared to the degree of anemia due to ineffective erythropoiesis. The unconjugated serum bilirubin level is usually elevated. Even if the child does not receive transfusions, eventually there is iron accumulation with elevated serum ferritin level and saturation of transferrin. Bone marrow hyperplasia can be seen on radiographs. X-ray skull lateral view can show "hair-on-end appearance" in a child with thalassemia (Fig. 20.27 in CD).

Treatment: Before initiating chronic transfusions, the diagnosis of β-thalassemia major should be confirmed and parents counseled concerning this lifelong therapy. Before beginning transfusion therapy, a red cell phenotype is obtained; blood products that are leukoreduced and phenotypically matched for the Rh and Kell antigens are required for transfusion. If a bone marrow transplant is a possibility, the blood for transfusion should be negative for cytomegalovirus and irradiated. A transfusion program generally requires monthly transfusions, with the pretransfusion hemoglobin level >9.5 and <10.5 g/dl. In patients with cardiac disease, higher pretransfusion hemoglobin levels may be beneficial. Transfusion therapy promotes general health and well-being and avoids the consequences of ineffective erythropoiesis. Where blood centres have donor programs, pairing donors and recipients, decreases the exposure to multiple red cell antigens.

Excessive iron stores from transfusion cause many of the complications of β-thalassemia major. Accurate assessment of excessive iron stores is essential to optimal therapy. The serum ferritin level is useful in assessing iron balance trends but does not accurately predict quantitative iron stores. Undertreatment or overtreatment of presumed excessive iron stores can occur in managing a patient based on serum ferritin level alone. Measurement of the iron level by liver biopsy is the standard method for accurately determining the iron stores. A specialized MRI software is now used to estimate iron stores in the liver in patients with β-thalassemia major.

Transfusional hemosiderosis can be prevented by the use of deferoxamine (Desferal 500 mg vial). Deferoxamine chelates iron and some other divalent cations allowing their excretion in the urine and the stool. Deferoxamine infusion of 15 mg/kg/hr (max 6 g/24 hr) is given subcutaneously (SC) over 10–12 hr, 5–6 days a week.

The side effects include ototoxicity with high frequency hearing loss, retinal changes, and bone dysplasia with truncal shortening. High dose, short-term infusions increase toxicity with little efficacy. Plasma non-transferrin bound iron (NTBI) is most likely responsible for serious iron injury. When deferoxamine is infusing, it binds NTBI. When deferoxamine is stopped, there are rebound increases in NTBI levels and risk for injury. In patients with excessive iron stores in the heart resulting in symptomatic congestive heart failure, 24-hr deferoxamine has been shown to reverse cardiomyopathy.

Hematopoietic stem cell transfusion has cured patients who have β-thalassemia major. Most success has been in children younger than 15 yr of age without excessive iron stores and hepatomegaly who undergo sibling HLA-matched allogeneic transplantation. All children who have an HLA-matched sibling should be offered the option of bone marrow transplantation.

Other β-Thalassemia Syndromes

The β-thalassemia syndromes are broken into six groups: β-thalassemia, δβ-thalassemias, γ-thalassemias, δ-thalassemias, εγδβ-thalassemias and the HPFH syndrome. Most of these thalassemias are rare. The β-thalassemias can also be classified clinically as thalassemia trait and as minima, minor, intermedia, and major, reflecting the degree of anemia. The genetic classification does not necessarily define the phenotype. The degree of anemia does not always predict the genetic classification.

Thalassemia intermedia can be any combination of β-thalassemia mutations (b°/b⁺, b°/b$_{variant}$, E/b°) resulting in a phenotype of microcytic anemia with hemoglobin of about 7 g/dl. They will certainly develop a degree of medullary hyperplasia, nutritional hemosiderosis perhaps requiring chelation, splenomegaly, and other complications of β-thalassemia associated with excessive iron stores. Extramedullary hematopoiesis can occur in the vertebral canal, which will lead to the compression of spinal cord and causing neurologic symptoms; this is a medical emergency requiring immediate local radiation therapy to stop erythropoiesis. Transfusion alleviates the thalassemic manifestations. The decision to transfuse must be balanced against the future need for chelation therapy. Splenectomy may be indicated for patients with thalassemia intermedia who have a falling steady-state hemoglobin and for transfused patients with rising transfusion requirements. All patients should be fully immunized against encapsulated bacteria before splenectomy and subsequently should be on long-term penicillin prophylaxis. They need appropriate instructions if fever develops.

Thalassemia minima and minor are usually heterozygotes (b°/b, b⁺/b⁺), having a phenotype more severe than trait but not as severe as intermedia. These children should be investigated for their genotype and monitored for iron accumulation. Often patients require transfusions in adolescence or adulthood; some may be candidates for chemotherapy such as hydroxyurea.

Thalassemia trait is often misdiagnosed as iron deficiency in children because the two produce similar hematologic abnormalities on CBC, and iron deficiency is more prevalent. A short course of iron and re-evaluation is required to identify children who will need further evaluation. Children with β-thalassemia trait have on hemoglobin analysis an elevated HbF and elevated HbA$_2$.

α-thalassemia

Infants are identified in the newborn period by the increased production of Bart's hemoglobin (γ₄) during fetal life and its presence at birth. The α-thalassemia occur most commonly in Southeast Asia. Deletion mutations are common in α-thalassemia. There are four α-globin genes and four deletional α-thalassemia phenotypes.

Children with deletion of 2α-globin genes result in **α-thalassemia trait**. α-thalassemia trait children manifest as microcytic anemia (both low MCV and MCH) that can be mistaken for iron-deficiency anemia. The simplest way to distinguish between iron deficiency and α-thalassemia trait is with a good dietary history. Children with iron-deficiency anemia often have a diet low in iron. Alternatively, a brief course of iron supplementation, along with monitoring of the red blood cell parameters, may make the diagnosis of iron deficiency, or α-globin gene deletion analysis may be necessary.

The deletion of three α-globin genes leads to the diagnosis of **HbH disease**. During the neonatal period the disease can be diagnosed when excess in ξ-tetramers are present and Hb Bart's is commonly >25%. Later in childhood, there is an excess in β-globin chain tetramers that results in HbH. A definitive diagnosis of HbH disease requires DNA analysis with supportive evidence. Patients with HbH disease have a marked microcytosis, anemia, mild splenomegaly, and occasionally, sclera icterus or cholelithiasis. In these cases transfusion is not commonly used for therapy because the range of hemoglobin is 7–11 g/dl, with MCV 51–73 fl.

The deletion of all four α-globin genes causes profound anemia during fetal life, resulting hydrops fetalis; the ξ-globin gene must be present for fetal survival. There are no normal hemoglobins present at birth (primarily Hb Bart's, with Hb Gower 1, Gower 2, and Portland). If the fetus survives, immediate exchange transfusion is indicated. These infants with α-thalassemia major are transfusion dependent, and hematopoietic stem cell transplant is the only cure.

The presence of a nondeletional α-globin mutation with α₂-gene deletion results in a more severe anemia, increased hepatomegaly, increased jaundice, and a much more severe clinical course than HbH disease. HbH constant spring is the most common form.

Treatment of the α-thalassemia deletion syndromes consists of folate supplementation, possible splenectomy (with the attendant risks). Intermittent transfusion during severe anemia for non-deletional HbH diseases, and chronic transfusion therapy or bone marrow transplant for survivors of hydrops fetalis is required. These children should not be exposed to oxidative medications.

Agarwal MB. Hydroxyurea therapy in management of severe thalassemia—A dream or reality? *Proceedings of 4th National Thalassemia Conference* 2003 (May 17th–18th);32–36.

Chandra J. Adult thalassemics: Problems and solutions. *Proceedings of "Symposium on thalassemia"*. 2005 (May 8th); 31–38.

Chandra Jagdish. Diagnosis and Management of Thalassemia. In: Mathur GP, Mathur Sarla (eds). *Current Trends in Pediatrics*. Vol 2. Delhi: Academa Publishers, 2006;240–252.

Choudhry VP, Kotwal J, Saxena R. Thalassemia screening & control programme. *Pediatrics Today* 1998;1:283–9.

Choudhry VP. Current management of thalassemia. *Proceedings of symposium on thalassemia.* New Delhi. 2003 (May 8th);39–47.

DeBaun MR, Feri-Jones M, Vichinsky E.Thalassemia syndromes. In: Kliegman RM, Stanton BF, St.Geme JW, Schor NF, Behrman RE. *Nelson Textbook of Pediatrics.* 19th edn. New Delhi: Elsevier, 2011;1674–77.

Guidelines for the clinical management of thalassemia. *Publication of Thalassemia International Federation.* April 2000.

Kabra M. Prevention and control of thalassemia. *Proceedings of "Symposium on Thalassemia",* 2005 (May 8th); 53–59.

Kumar R. Iron chelation. Proceedings of "Symposium on thalassemia" 2005 (May 8th);6–17.

Pyruvate Kinase (PK) Deficiency

Congenital hemolytic anemia occurs in persons homozygous for an autosomal recessive gene that causes either a marked reduction in RBC PK or production of an abnormal enzyme with decreased activity. There are 2 mammalian PK genes, but only the PKLR gene is expressed in red cells. The human PKLR gene is located on chromosome 1q21.

Clinical manifestations: The clinical manifestations vary from severe neonatal hemolytic anemia to mild, well compensated hemolysis first noted in adulthood. Severe jaundice and anemia may occur in the neonatal period; kernicterus has been reported. The hemolysis in older children and adults varies in severity, with hemoglobin values ranging from 8 to 12 g/dl associated with some pallor, jaundice, and splenomegaly.

Laboratory findings: Polychromatophilia and mild macrocytosis reflect the elevated reticulocyte count. Spherocytes are uncommon, but a few spiculated *pyknocytes* are found. Non-incubated osmotic fragility

is normal. Diagnosis is based on a demonstration of a marked reduction of RBC PK activity or an increase in the Michaelis-Menten dissociation constant (K_m) for its substrate, phosphoenolpyruvate. Other RBC activity is normal or elevated, reflecting the reticulocytosis. No abnormalities of hemoglobin are noted. The white cells have normal PK activity and must be rigorously excluded from the hemolysate used to measure PK activity. Heterozygous carriers usually have moderately reduced levels of PK activity.

Treatment: Exchange transfusions may be indicated for hyperbilirubinemia in newborns. Transfusions of packed RBCs are necessary for severe anemia or for aplastic crisis. If the anemia is persistently severe or if frequent transfusions are required, splenectomy should be performed after 5–6 yr of age. Death resulting from overwhelming pneumococcal sepsis has followed splenectomy; thus, immunization with vaccines for encapsulated organisms should be given before splenectomy, and prophylactic penicillin should be administered after splenectomy.

Glucose-6-Phosphate Dehydrogenase (G6PD) and Related Deficiencies

Glucose-6-phosphate dehydrogenase (G6PD) deficiency is the most important disease of the hexose monophosphate pathway and is responsible for 2 clinical syndromes, episodic hemolytic anemia, and spontaneous chronic nonspherocytic hemolytic anemia. This X-linked enzyme deficiency affects more than 200 million people worldwide.

1. *Episodic or Induced Hemolytic Anemia*

Etiology: G6PD catalyzes the conversion of glucose 6-phosphate to 6-phosphogluconic acid to produce nicotinamide-adenine dinucleotide phosphate (NADPH) and maintain glutathione in the reduced state. Synthesis of RBC G6PD is determined by a gene on the X chromosome. Diseases involving this enzyme therefore occur more frequently in males than in females. Episodic hemolytic anemia is induced by infections, certain drugs (aspirin, sulfonamides, and antimalarials such as primaquine), or rarely fava beans (Box 20.1).

Clinical manifestations: Symptoms develop 24–48 hr after a patient has ingested a substance that has oxidant properties (Box 20.1). In some patients, ingestion of fava beans, a Mediterranean dietary staple, may also produce an acute, severe hemolytic syndrome called *favism.* In severe cases, hemoglobinuria and jaundice result, and the hemoglobin concentration may fall precipitously and may be life-threatening. When a pregnant woman ingests oxidant drugs, they may be

Adapted from Asselin BL, Segel GB. In: Rakel R (ed). *Conn's Current Therapy.* Philadelphia: WB Saunders, 1994; 341.

transmitted to her G6PD-deficient fetus, and hemolytic anemia and jaundice may be apparent at birth.

Diagnosis can be suspected when G6PD activity is within the low-normal range in the presence of a high reticulocyte count. G6PD variants also can be detected by electrophoretic analysis.

Prevention and treatment: If possible, males belonging to ethnic groups with a significant incidence of G6PD deficiency (e.g. Greeks, Southern Italians, Sephardic Jews, Filipinos, Southern Chinese, Americans of African descent, and Thais) should be tested for the defect before known oxidant drugs are given. When hemolysis has occurred, supportive therapy may require blood transfusions, although recovery is the rule when the oxidant agent is discontinued.

2. Chronic Nonspherocytic Hemolytic Anemia

Chronic nonspherocytic hemolytic anemia has been associated with profound deficiency of G6PD caused by enzyme variants, particularly those defective in quantity, activity or stability. The gene defects leading to chronic hemolysis are located primarily on the region of the NADP binding site near the carboxyl terminus of the protein. Mild, chronic nonspherocytic anemia has been reported in association with decreased RBC GSH resulting from γ-glutamylcysteine or glutathione synthetase deficiencies. Deficiency of 6-posphogluconate dehydrogenase (6PDG) has been associated primarily with drug induced hemolysis, and hemolysis with hyperbilirubinemia has been related to a deficiency of glutathione peroxidase in newborn infants.

Hemolytic Anemias Resulting from Extracellular Factors

Autoimmune hemolytic anemias: Hemolytic anemias as a result of extracellular factors may occur due to premature destruction of red blood cells (RBCs). In this group of diseases there is a positive direct antiglobulin (Coombs') test, which detects a coating of immunoglobulin or components of complement on the RBC surface. The most important immune hemolytic disorder is hemolytic disease of the newborn (erythroblastosis fetalis), caused by transplacental transfer of maternal antibody active against the RBCs of the fetus, that is isoimmune hemolytic anemia. Various other immune hemolytic anemias are autoimmune (Box 20.2) and may be *idiopathic* or related to various *infections:* Epstein-Barr virus, HIV, cytomegalovirus, and mycoplasma; *immunologic diseases:* SLE, rheumatoid arthritis; *immunodeficiency diseases:* agammaglobulinemia, autoimmune lymphoproliferative disorder, dysagammaglobulinemia; *neoplasms:* lymphoma, leukemia, and Hodgkin disease; or *drugs:* methyldopa, L-dopa. *Other drugs:* penicillins, cephalosporins cause immune hemolysis that is not "autoimmune." The antibodies are "drug dependent" and usually have no "specificity" for RBC membrane antigens.

Autoimmune hemolytic anemias associated with "warm" antibodies: In the autoimmune hemolytic anemias, abnormal antibodies are directed against RBCs, but the pathogenic mechanisms are uncertain. In most instances of warm antibody hemolysis, no underlying cause can be found (Box 20.2).

Clinical manifestations: Autoimmune hemolytic anemias present in either acute or chronic form. An acute transient type lasting 3–6 mo and occurring predominantly in children ages 2–12 yr in approximately in 70–80% patients. It is frequently preceded by an infection, usually respiratory. Onset may be acute with prostration, pallor, jaundice, pyrexia, and hemoglobinuria. The spleen is usually enlarged and is the primary site of destruction of immunoglobulin G (IgG)-coated RBCs. Underlying systemic disorder is unusual. They respond to glucocorticoid therapy, a low mortality rate and full recovery occur. The other is the prolonged and chronic form, which is more frequent in infants and in children older than 12 yr. Hemolysis may continue for many months or years. Abnormalities involving other blood elements are common, and the response to glucocorticoids is variable and inconsistent. The mortality rate is approximately 10%, and death is often attributable to an underlying systemic disease.

Laboratory findings: In many cases, anemia is profound, with hemoglobin levels < 6g/dl, spherocytosis, polychromatophilia, nucleated RBCs, and > 50% of the circulating RBCs may be reticulocytes, and nucleated RBCs are usually present. Leukocytosis is common. Platelet count is usually normal, but concomitant immune thrombocytopenic purpura sometimes occurs (*Evans syndrome*). Direct antiglobulin test is strongly positive (direct Coombs' test) and free antibody can sometimes be demonstrated in the serum (indirect Coombs test) at 35–40°C ("warm" antibodies) and most often belongs to the Ig G class.

Treatment: Transfusions usually are only of transient benefit, but may be required initially because of the severity of anemia until the effect of other treatment is observed. Patients with mild disease and compensated hemolysis may not require any treatment. If the hemolysis is severe and results in significant anemia or symptoms, treatment with glucocorticoids is initiated. Glucocorticoids decrease the rate of hemolysis by blocking macrophage function by downregulating Fcγ receptor expression, decreasing the production of the autoantibody and perhaps by enhancing the elution of antibody from the RBCs. Prednisolone is administered at a dose of 2 mg/kg/24 hr. In some patients with severe hemolysis, doses of prednisolone of up to 6 mg/kg/24 hr may be required to reduce the rate of hemolysis. Treatment should be continued until the rate of hemolysis decreases, and then the dose is gradually is reduced. If relapse occurs, resumption of the full dosage may be necessary. The disease tends to remit spontaneously within a few wk or mo. The Coombs' test result may remain positive, even after hemolysis has subsided. IV immunoglobulin, rituximab, a monoclonal antibody that targets B lymphocytes and plasmapheresis has been used in refractory cases. Splenectomy may be beneficial, but is complicated by a heightened risk of infection with encapsulated organisms particularly in patients younger than 2 yr. Prophylaxis is indicated with appropriate vaccines (pneumococcal, meningococcal, and *Haemophilus influenzae* type b) before splenectomy and with oral penicillin after splenectomy.

Course and prognosis: Acute idiopathic autoimmune hemolytic disease in childhood varies in severity, but is self limited and the prognosis is good. Patients with chronic hemolysis are often associated with underlying disease such as SLE, lymphoma or leukemia. Mortality in chronic cases depends on the primary disorder.

Autoimmune hemolytic anemias associated with "cold" antibodies: Cold agglutinin disease is less common in children than in adults, and it more frequently results in an acute, self limited episode of hemolysis. "Cold" antibodies are RBC antibodies that are more active at low temperatures and agglutinate RBCs at temperatures <37°C. They are primary of IgM class and require complement for activity. The range of temperature associated with RBC agglutination is called *thermal amplitude*. Higher thermal amplitude results in hemolysis with less severe exposure to a cold

environment. High antibody titers are associated with high thermal amplitude.

Cold antibodies may occur in primary or idiopathic cold agglutinin disease, secondary to infections such as those from *Mycoplasma pneumoniae* and Epstein-Barr virus, or secondary to lymphoproliferative disorders (Box 20.2). Glucocorticoids are much less effective in cold agglutinin disease than in disease with warm antibodies. Patients should avoid exposure to cold and should be treated for underlying disease. Treatment for patients with severe hemolytic disease includes immunosuppression, plasmapheresis and rituximab. Splenectomy is not useful in cold agglutinin disease.

Paroxysmal cold hemoglobinuria: This form of hemolytic anemia is mediated by the Donath-Landsteiner hemolysin, which is an IgG cold-reactive autoantibody with anti-P specificity. This antibody fixes large amounts of complement in the cold and the RBCs lyse as the temperature is increased. Most reported cases are self-limited and usually are associated with nonspecific viral infections (Box 20.2). This disorder may account for 30% of immune hemolytic episodes among children. Treatment includes transfusion for severe anemia and avoidance of cold ambient temperatures.

Box 20.2: Diseases characterized by immune mediated red blood cell destruction

Autoimmune hemolytic anemia due to warm reactive antibodies
Primary (idiopathic)
Secondary
   Lymphoproliferative disorders
   Connective tissue disorders [especially systemic lupus erythematosus (SLE)]
   Nonlymphoid neoplasms (e.g. ovarian tumors)
   Chronic inflammatory diseases (e.g. ulcerative colitis)
Autoimmune hemolytic anemia due to cold reactive antibodies (cryopathic hemolytic syndromes)
Primary (idiopathic) cold agglutinin disease
Secondary cold agglutinin disease
   Lymphoproliferative disorders
   Infectious (*Mycoplasma pneumoniae*, Epstein-Barr virus)
Paroxysmal cold hemoglobinuria
   Primary (idiopathic)
   Congenital or tertiary syphilis
   Viral syndromes (most common)
Drug induced hemolytic anemia
   Hapten/drug absorption (e.g. penicillin)
   Tertiary (immune) complex (e.g. quinine or quinidine)
   True autoantibody induction (e.g. methyldopa)

Modified from Packman CH. Autoimmune hemolytic anemias. In: Rakel R (Ed). Conn's Current Therapy. Philadelphia: WB Saunders, 1995; 306.

Hemolytic Anemias Secondary to other Extracellular Factors

Fragmentation hemolysis: Red blood cell (RBC) destruction may occur in hemolytic anemias because of mechanical injury as the cells traverse a damaged vascular bed. Damage may be microvascular during intravascular coagulation, hemolytic–uremic syndrome or thrombotic thrombocytopenic purpura. Large vessels may be involved in Kasabach-Merritt syndrome (giant hemangioma and thrombocytopenia) or when a replacement heart valve is poorly epithelialized. The blood film shows many "spherocytes," or fragmented cells, polychromatophilia, reflecting the reticulocytosis. Secondary iron deficiency may complicate the intravascular hemolysis because of urinary hemoglobin and hemosiderin iron loss. Treatment should be directed toward the underlying condition, and the prognosis depends on the effectiveness of treatment. Temporary improvement is observed from transfusion, because the transfused cells are destroyed as quickly as those produced by the patient.

Thermal injury: Excessive burns may directly damage the RBCs and cause hemolysis that result in the formation of spherocytes. Blood loss and marrow suppression are responsible for anemia and require blood transfusion. Erythropoietin (EPO) is used in cases of diminished RBC production.

Renal disease: The anemia of uremia is multifactorial in origin and may be due to decreased EPO production, marrow suppression by toxic metabolites, and shortened RBC lifespan owing to retention of metabolites and organic acidemia. The use of EPO in chronic renal disease has markedly decreased the need for blood transfusion.

Liver disease: A change in the ratio of cholesterol to phospholipids in the plasma may result in changes in the composition of the RBC membrane and shortening of the RBC lifespan. Some patients with liver disease have many target RBCs, whereas others have a preponderance of spiculated cells on the blood film.

Toxins and venoms: Hemolytic anemia has been observed due to bacterial sepsis due to *Haemophilus influenzae*, staphylococci, streptococci and clostridial infections, and spherocytes may be complicated by accompanying hemolysis. Spherocytic hemolysis also may occur after bites by various snakes, including cobras, vipers, and rattle snakes, which have phospholipases in their venom. Large number of bites by insects, such as bees, wasps, and yellow jackets also may cause spherocytic hemolysis by a similar mechanism.

Wilson disease: An acute and self-limited episode of hemolytic anemia may precede by years the onset of hepatic or neurologic symptoms in Wilson disease. This results from the toxic effect of free copper on the RBC membrane. The blood film often shows large numbers of spherocytes, and the Coombs' test result is negative.

Beutler E. Glucose-6-phosphate dehydrogenase (G6PD) deficiency. *N Engl J Med* 1994;331:169–71.

Segel GB. Enzymatic defects. In: Kliegman RM, Behrman RE, Jenson HB, Stanton BF (eds). *Nelson Textbook of Pediatrics.* 18th edn. Vol. 2. Philadelphia: Saunders, 2007;2038–42.

Segel GB. Hemolytic anemias resulting from extracellular factors. In: Kliegman RM, Behrman RE, Jenson HB, Stanton BF (eds). *Nelson Textbook of Pediatrics.* 18th edn. Vol. 2. Philadelphia: Saunders, 2007;2042–44.

Segel GB. Hemolytic anemias secondary to other extracellular factors. In: Kliegman RM, Behrman RE, Jenson HB, Stanton BF (eds). *Nelson Textbook of Pediatrics.* 18th edn. Vol. 2. Philadelphia: Saunders, 2007;2044–45.

20.6 POLYCYTHEMIA (ERYTHROCYTOSIS)

When the red blood cell (RBC) count, hemoglobin level, and total RBC volume all exceed the upper limits of normal, it is known as polycythemia. In postpubertal individuals an RBC mass > 25% above the mean normal value (based on body surface area) or hematocrit > 60 (in males) or > 56 (in females) indicates absolute erythrocytosis. A decrease in plasma volume such as occurs in acute dehydration and burns, may result in high hemoglobin value. These situations are more accurately designated as hemoconcentration, because the RBC mass is not increased and normalization of the plasma volume restores hemoglobin to normal levels.

Primary Polycythemia (Polycythemia Rubra Vera)

Polycythemia vera, a panmyeloproliferative disorder has been reported in only a few children. Serum erythropoietin levels are normal or low. Diagnostic criteria are listed in Box 20.3.

Clinical manifestations: Patients with polycythemia vera usually have hepatosplenomegaly. Erythrocytosis may cause hypertension, headache, shortness of breath, or neurologic symptoms. Granulocytosis may cause diarrhea or pruritus from histamine release. Thrombocytosis (with or without platelet dysfunction) may cause thrombosis or hemorrhage.

Treatment: Phlebotomy is the initial treatment of choice. Iron supplementation, to prevent viscosity problems from microcytosis and aspirin (antiplatelet agent) to reduce the risk of thrombosis and abnormal bleeding is given. If this is unsuccessful antiproliferative treatments (hydroxyurea, interferon-α) may be

Box 20.3: Diagnosis of polycythemia vera

Major criteria

1. Increased red blood cell mass > 25% above the mean normal value;
2. Arterial oxygen saturation of ε 92*;
3. Palpable splenomegaly

Minor criteria

1. Platelet count of > 400 × 10^9/L
2. Leukocytosis of >12 × 10^9/L
3. Increased leukocyte alkaline phosphatase
4. Increased vitamin B$_{12}$ (> 900 pg/ml) or unbound B$_{12}$ binding capacity (> 2,200 pg/ml)

Diagnosis: All 3 major criteria or; 1, 2, major and 2 minor criteria

*Absent causes of secondary polycythemia

helpful. Discontinuation of the use of alkylating agents and radioactive phosphorus has diminished the risk of transformation of the disease into myelofibrosis or acute leukemia. Prolonged survival is now possible.

Secondary Polycythemia

Secondary polycythemia is diagnosed when true polycythemia is caused by other physiologic process (Box 20.4). Polycythemia may be present in any clinical situation associated with chronic arterial oxygen desaturation. Cardiovascular defects involving right-to-left shunts and pulmonary diseases interfering with proper oxygenation are the most common causes of hypoxic polycythemia. Clinical findings usually include cyanosis, hyperemia of the sclerae and mucous membranes and clubbing of the fingers. Living at high

Box 20.4: Differential diagnosis of polycythemia

1. *Polycythemia rubra vera*
2. *Secondary:*
   2a. *Familial*
   2b. *Hemoglobinopathy:* High oxygen affinity variants, methemoglobin reductase deficiency, chronic carbon monoxide exposure
   2c. *Hormonal:* Adrenal disease (virilizing hyperplasia, Cushing syndrome); anabolic steroid therapy; malignant tumors (adrenal, cerebellar, hepatic, other); renal disease (cysts, hydronephrosis)
   2d. *Hypoxia:* Altitude, cardiac disease, lung disease; central hypoventilation
   2e. *Metabolic:* 2,3-Diphosphoglycerate deficiency
   2f. *Neonatal:* Normal intrauterine environment; twin-twin or maternal-fetal hemorrhage; infants of diabetic mothers; intrauterine growth retardation; trisomy 13, 18, or 21; adrenal hyperplasia; thyrotoxicosis
3. *Spurious (plasma volume decrease)*

altitudes also causes hypoxic polycythemia; the hemoglobin level increases approximately 4% for each rise of 1,000 M in altitude. Partial obstruction of a renal artery rarely results in polycythemia. Congenital methemoglobinemia may cause cyanosis and polycythemia. Cyanosis may occur in the presence of as little as 1.5 g/dl of methemoglobin, but is uncommon in other hemoglobin variants unless hyperviscosity results in localized hypoxemia. Polycythemia has been associated with benign and malignant tumors that secrete erythropoietin, and exogenous or endogenous anabolic steroids.

Treatment: For mild disease observation is sufficient. As the hematocrit rises to >65%, clinical manifestations of hyperviscosity, such as headache and hypertension may require phlebotomy. Periodic assessment of iron status, with treatment of iron deficiency should be performed.

Burns K, Camitta BM. Polycythemia (Erythrocytosis). In: Kliegman RM, Behrman RE, Jenson HB, Stanton BF (eds). *Nelson Textbook of Pediatrics.* 18th edn. Vol. 2. Philadelphia: Saunders, 2007;2045–7.

Cario H. Childhood polycythemias/erythrocytosis: Classification, diagnosis, clinical presentation and treatment. *Ann Hematol* 2005;84:137–45. Epub 2004 Dec 15.

Pappas A, Delancy-Black V. Differential diagnosis and management of polycythemia. *Pediatr Clin North Am* 2004;51: 1063–86.

Spivak JL. Polycythemia vera: Myths, mechanisms, and management. *Blood* 2002;100:4272–90.

20.7 PANCYTOPENIAS

Pancytopenia is a loss of all marrow elements. Pancytopenia can result from a failure of production of hematopoietic progenitors, their destruction, or replacement of the bone marrow by tumor or fibrosis. Pancytopenias are broadly classified in to constitutional and acquired pancytopenias. The clinical consequences include anemia, neutropenia, and thrombocytopenia, and depending on the degree and duration of their impairment, can lead to serious illness and death.

Constitutional Pancytopenias

Constitutional pancytopenia arises as a consequence of an inherited genetic defect affecting hematopoietic progenitors. Common disorders include Fanconi (aplastic) anemia, dyskeratosis congenital, Shwachman-Diamond syndrome, and amegakaryocytic thrombocytopenia.

Clinical manifestations: Various physical abnormalities accompany most of the congenital pancytopenias, including hand/arm, particularly Fanconi anemia and dyskeratosis congenita. Fanconi anemia have hyperpigmentation and café au lait spots, skeletal abnormalities (especially absent or hypoplastic thumb), short stature, and a wide array of integumentary and organ abnormalities. Dyskeratosis congenita is also very commonly associated with hyperpigmentation, nail dystrophy of the hands and feet, leukoplakia, and a number of ocular abnormalities, including epiphora, blepharitis, and cataracts.

Laboratory findings: Depending on the specific disorder, thrombocytopenia, leukopenia, lymphopenia, or anemia generally precedes the onset of pancytopenia. The age at onset of hematologic abnormalities ranges from infancy to adolescence. Additional laboratory examination should include skeletal radiographs and examination of genitourinary tract, eyes, gastrointestinal tract, heart, teeth, and gonads.

Diagnosis: The presence of characteristic skeletal and cutaneous abnormalities coupled with short stature should suggest the diagnosis of congenital pancytopenia even in the absence of hematologic problems. When a child presents with evidence of bone marrow failure, a genetic or familial defect should always be considered and evaluated by cytogenetic examination, including chromosomal breakage studies.

Complications: The major complications include the consequences of bone marrow failure, increased risk for leukemia and other cancers and organ complications that are specific to the primary defect (e.g. liver problems in Fanconi syndrome, malabsorption in Shwachman-Diamond syndrome). Infection and bleeding can lead to life-threatening complications.

Treatment: The traditional backbone of therapy for patients with congenital anemias has been steroids and androgens (especially oxymethalone or nandrolone) alone or in combination. Although 50–75% of patients show some evidence of improvement with androgens, relapse is common and complications (especially hepatic tumors or obstructive liver disease) occur. Improvements in RBCs generally precede those in white blood cells, and it may take months to achieve the maximum benefit. However, these therapies prolong life by approximately 2 yr, and hence, can only be considered palliative. The only "curative" therapy is bone marrow transplantation (BMT).

Prognosis: When marrow failure develops, the prognosis is guarded, although bone marrow transplantation and hematopoietic growth factor offer some hope.

Genetic counseling: Once an index case is identified genetic counseling is important and must be oriented to the patterns of inheritance and the prospect for prenatal diagnosis.

Acquired Pancytopenias

Acquired pancytopenia is usually characterized by anemia, leucopenia, and thrombocytopenia. Etiology of acquired aplastic anemia is listed in Box 20.5. A specific cause cannot be identified in most cases of acquired marrow failure in childhood, and these cases are termed "idiopathic". Patients with evidence of bone marrow failure should also be evaluated for paroxysmal nocturnal hemoglobinuria (PNH) and collagen vascular diseases. PNH is an acquired disorder of hematopoiesis characterized by a defect in proteins of the cell membrane that renders the red blood cells (RBCs) and other cells susceptible to damage by normal plasma complement protein. The hallmark of aplastic anemia is peripheral pancytopenia coupled with hypoplastic or aplastic bone marrow. The severity of the clinical course is related to the degree of myelosuppression. Severe aplastic anemia is defined as a condition in which two or more cell components have become seriously compromised (i.e., an absolute neutrophil count $<500/mm^3$, a platelet count $<20,000/mm^3$, a reticulocyte count $<1\%$ after correction for the hematocrit) in a patient whose bone marrow biopsy material is moderately or severely hypocellular.

Clinical manifestations, differential diagnosis and laboratory findings: The pancytopenia results in increased risks of fatigue, cardiac failure, infection, and bleeding. Other treatable disorders such as cancer, collagen vascular disorders, PNH, or infections that may respond to specific therapies (e.g. intravenous immune globulin for parvovirus) should be considered in differential diagnosis. Examination of the peripheral blood smear for RBC, leukocyte, and platelet morphology is important. A reticulocyte count should be performed to assess erythropoietic activity. In children, the possibility of congenital pancytopenia must always be considered and chromosomal breakage analysis should be performed to evaluate for Fanconi anemia. The presence of fetal hemoglobin suggests a congenital pancytopenia. Bone marrow examination should be done to evaluate for morphology, cellularity, and cytogenetics.

Complications: The major complications of severe pancytopenia are bleeding from prolonged thrombocytopenia or to infection (bacterial and fungal) secondary to protracted neutropenia.

Treatment: The treatment includes supportive care coupled with an attempt to treat the underlying marrow failure. For patients with a human leukocyte antigen (HLA)-identical sibling marrow donor, allogeneic bone marrow transplantation offers a 90% chance of long-term survival. The problem of graft failure has diminished with the incorporation of antithymocyte globulin (ATG) and cyclophosphamide into the transplant conditioning regimen. For those without a sibling donor the therapy is immuno-suppression with ATG and cyclosporine combined with a hematopoietic colony-stimulating factor (e.g. granulocyte-stimulating factor, granulocyte-macrophage colony-stimulating factor). Response to this combination therapy is in the range of 60–80%, but a few responders will relapse.

Prognosis: In untreated severe pancytopenia cases, the mortality rate is about 50% within 6 months of diagnosis with infection and hemorrhage in majority of cases. The majority of children respond to allogeneic marrow transplantation or immunosuppression, but those who fail to respond, prognosis remains poor.

Pancytopenia caused by marrow replacement: Processes that either infiltrate or replace the bone marrow can present as acquired pancytopenia. This can occur either before or during malignancy (classically, neuroblastoma or leukemia) or as a consequence of myelofibrosis, myelodysplasia, or osteoporosis. Morphologic examination of the peripheral blood and the bone marrow as well as marrow cytogenetic studies are important in making the diagnoses of leukemia, myelofibrosis, and myelodysplasia.

Myelodysplasia (MDS) in children is very rare but the clinical course is more aggressive than the same category of MDS in adults. About 50% children with MDS had clonal abnormalities involving chromosome 7 (usually monsomy 7). The transition time from pediatric MDS to leukemia is short at 14 to 26 months, so aggressive treatment such as bone marrow transplantation (BMT) must be considered shortly after

diagnosis. With conventional chemotherapy there is a 20–25% long-term survival, but with allogeneic BMT the survival increases to about 50%. But in MDS/acute myelocytic leukemia in children with Down syndrome, because this disease in this specific population is very responsive to conventional chemotherapy with long-term survival rates of greater than 80%.

Ades L, Mary JY, Robin M, et al. Long-term outcome after bone marrow transplantation for severe aplastic anemia. *Blood* 2004;103:2490–7.

Broddsky RA, Jones RJ. Aplastic anemia. *Lancet* 2005;365:1647–6.

Damodar Sharat. Pediatric Aplastic Anemia—Bone Marrow Transplantation. In: Mathur GP, Mathur Sarla (eds). Current Trends in Pediatrics. Vol 3. Delhi: Academa Publishers, 2007;28–38.

Freedman MH. The constitutional pancytopenias. In: Kliegman RM, Behrman RE, Jenson HB, Stanton BF (eds). *Nelson Textbook of Pediatrics.* 18th edn. Vol. 2. Philadelphia: Saunders, 2007;2047–53.

Hord JD. The acquired pancytopenias. In: Kliegman RM, Behrman RE, Jenson HB, Stanton BF (eds). *Nelson Textbook of Pediatrics.* 18th edn. Vol. 2. Philadelphia: Saunders, 2007;2053–55.

20.8 HEMOSTASIS

Hemostasis is the dynamic process that clots blood in areas of blood vessel injury, yet simultaneously limits the clot size only to the areas of injury. Over time, the clot is lysed by the fibrinolytic system, and normal blood flow is restored. The main components of the hemostatic process are the *vessel wall, the platelet, coagulation proteins, anticoagulant proteins, and fibrinolytic system.* Most components of hemostasis are multifunctional; fibrinogen serves as the ligand between platelets during platelet aggregation and also serves as the substrate for thrombin that forms the fibrin clot. Platelets provide the reaction surface on which clotting reactions occur, from the plug at the site of vessel injury, and contract to constrict and limit clot size. The intact vascular endothelium is the primary barrier against hemorrhage. The endothelial cells that line the vessel wall normally inhibit coagulation and provide a smooth surface that permits rapid blood flow.

Process of hemostasis: After vascular injury, vasoconstriction occurs and flowing blood comes in contact with the subendothelial matrix. In flowing blood, when exposed to subendothelial matrix proteins, von Willebrand factor (vWF) changes conformation and provides the glue to which the platelet vWF receptor binds. After adhesion, platelets are activated and release storage granules containing

---

Box 20.5: Etiology of acquired aplastic anemia

Radiation

Drugs and chemicals: Predictable (chemotherapy, benzene); idiosyncratic (chloramphenicol, antiepileptics, gold)

Viruses: Cytomegalovirus; Epstein-Barr; hepatitis B; hepatitis C; human immunodeficiency (HIV)

Immune diseases: Eosinophilic fascitis; hypoimmuno-globulinemia; thymoma

Pregnancy

Paroxysmal nocturnal hemoglobinuria (PNH)

Marrow replacement: Leukemia; myelodysplasia; myelo-fibrosis

adenosine diphosphate (ADP), thromboxane A$_2$, and other stored proteins. These trigger the aggregation and recruitment of other platelets to form the platelet plug. Aggregation involves the interaction of specific receptors on the platelet surface with plasma hemostatic proteins, primarily fibrinogen.

Just as exposed subendothelial matrix proteins bind vWF, tissue factor, another subendothelial matrix protein is also exposed, binds to factor VII, and activates the clotting cascade. Virtually all procoagulant proteins are balanced by an anticoagulant protein that regulates or inhibits procoagulation function. There are four clinically important, naturally occurring anticoagulants that regulate the extension of the clotting process. These include antithrombin III (AT-III), protein C, protein S, and tissue factor pathway inhibitor (TFPI).

Once a stable fibrin-platelet plug is formed, the fibrinolytic system limits its extension and also lyses the clot (fibrinolysis) to re-establish vascular integrity. Plasmin, generated from plasminogen by either urokinase-like or tissue-type plasminogen activator, degrades the fibrin clot. In the process of dissolving the fibrin clot, fibrin degradation products are produced. The fibrinolytic pathway is regulated by plasminogen activator inhibitors and α$_2$-antiplasmin. Finally, the flow of blood in and around the clot is crucial as flowing blood returns to the liver, where activated clotting factor complexes are removed and new pro- and anticoagulant proteins are synthesized to main homeostasis of the hemostatic system. The coagulation factors and their disorders are mentioned in Table 20.6.

Developmental hemostasis: The normal newborn infant has a reduced level of most procoagulants and anticoagulants (Table 20.6). In general, there is a more marked abnormality in the preterm infant. During, gestation, there is progressive maturation and increase of the clotting factors synthesized by the liver. The extremely premature infant will have prolonged PT and PTT as well as marked reduction in anticoagulant proteins (protein C, protein S, and AT-III).Levels of fibrinogen, factor V and VIII, vWF, and platelets are near normal throughout the later stages of gestation. Because protein C and protein S are physiologically reduced, the normal factors V and VIII are not balanced with their regulatory proteins. In contrast, the physiologic deficiency of vitamin- K dependent procoagulant proteins (factors II, VII, IX, and X) is partially balanced by the physiologic reduction of AT-III. The net effect is that newborns (especially premature infants) are at increased risk for complications of bleeding, clotting or both.

Pathology: Congenital deficiency of an individual precoagulant protein leads to a bleeding disorder, whereas deficiency of an anticoagulant (clotting factor inhibitor) predisposes the patient to excessive thrombosis. In acquired hemostatic disorders, there are frequently multiple problems with homeostasis that perturb and dysregulate hemostasis. A primary illness (sepsis) and its secondary effects (shock and acidosis) activate coagulation and fibrinolysis and impair the host's ability to restore normal hemostatic function. When sepsis triggers disseminated intravascular coagulation, procoagulant clotting factors and anticoagulant proteins are consumed, leaving the hemostatic system unbalanced and prone to bleeding or clotting.

Clinical evaluation: The clinical **history** provides the most useful information. For a hemorrhagic condition, the history should determine the site or sites of bleeding, the severity and duration of hemorrhage, bleeding occurs spontaneous or after trauma, bruising occurs spontaneously, lumps and bruises for trauma and the age at onset. If the child or an adolescent has

Clotting factor	Synonym	Disorder
I	Fibrinogen	Congenital deficiency (afibrinogenemia) and dysfunction (dysfibrinogenemia)
II	Prothrombin	Congenital deficiency or dysfunction
V	Labile factor or proaccelerin	Congenital deficiency (parahemophilia)
VII	Stable factor or proconvertin	Congenital deficiency
VIII	Antihemophilic factor (AHF)	Congenital deficiency—hemophilia A
IX	Christmas factor	Congenital deficiency—hemophila B
X	Stuart-Prower factor	Congenital deficiency
XI	Plasma thromboplastin antecedent	Congenital deficiency—hemophilia C
XII	Hageman factor	Congenital deficiency—not associated with clinical symptoms
XIII	Fibrin stabilizing factor	Congenital deficiency

Table 20.6: Blood coagulation factors and disorders

Adapted: Scot JP, Montgomery RR. Hemorrhagic and thrombotic diseases. In: Behrman RE, Kliegman RM, Jenson HB (eds). *Nelson Textbook of Pediatrics.* 18th edn. Vol. 2. Philadelphia: Saunders, 2008;2060–6.

had surgery affecting the mucosal surfaces such as a tonsillectomy or major dental extractions, the absence of bleeding usually rules out a hereditary bleeding disorder. Delayed or slow healing of superficial injuries may suggest a hereditary bleeding disorder. In postpubertal females menstrual disorder is abnormal (menorrhagia) in von Willebrand disease (vWD).

The **physical examination** should focus on whether bleeding symptoms are primarily associated with the mucous membranes or skin (mucocutaneous bleeding) or the muscles and joints (deep bleeding). The examination should determine the presence of petechiae, ecchymoses, hematomas, hemarthroses, or mucous membrane bleeding. Patients with vWD or platelet function defects usually have mucocutaneous bleeding, which may include epistaxis, menorrhagia, petechiae, ecchymoses, occasional hematomas, and less commonly hematuria and gastrointestinal bleeding. Patients with hemophilia (factor VIII or factor IX deficiency) have symptoms of deep bleeding into muscles and joints with more extensive ecchymoses and hematoma formation. Individuals with Ehlers-Danlos syndrome are associated with easy bruising.

Patients undergoing evaluation for thrombotic disorders should be asked about swollen, warm, tender extremities or internal organs (venous thrombosis), unexplained dyspnea or persistent "pneumonia," especially in the absence of fever (pulmonary emboli), and varicosities and post-phlebitic changes. Arterial thrombi usually cause an acute impairment of organ function, such as stroke, myocardial infarction, or a painful, white, cold extremity.

Laboratory tests: Patients who have a positive bleeding history or who are actively hemorrhaging should have a platelet count, prothrombin time (PT), partial thromboplastin time (PTT). If the results are normal, a thrombin time to evaluate fibrinogen function and vWF testing should be considered. In individuals with abnormal screening test results, further specific factor should be undertaken.

Chalmers EA. Neonatal coagulation problems. *Arch Dis Child Fetal Neonatal Ed* 2004;89:F475–8.

Esmon CT. Blood coagulation. In: Nathan DG, Orkin SH, Ginsburg D, et al (eds). *Hematology of Infancy and Childhood.* 6th edn. Philadelphia: WB Saunders, 2003;1475–96.

Scot JP, Montgomery RR.Hemorrhagic and thrombotic diseases. In: Kliegman RM, Behrman RE, Jenson HB, Stanton BF (eds). *Nelson Textbook of Pediatrics.* 18th edn. Vol. 2. Philadelphia: Saunders, 2007;2060–66.

HEREDITARY CLOTTING FACTOR DEFICIENCIES (BLEEDING DISORDERS)

Factor VIII or Factor IX Deficiency (Hemophilia A or B)

Deficiencies of factors VIII and IX are the most common severe inherited bleeding disorders. Hemophilia occurs in approximately 1:5,000 males, with 85% having factor VIII deficiency and 10–15% having factor IX deficiency. The severity of hemophilia is classified on the basis of the patient's baseline level of factor VIII or factor IX because factor levels usually correlate with the severity of bleeding symptoms. By definition, 1 international unit (IU) of each factor is defined as that amount in 1 ml of normal plasma referenced against a standard established by the World Health Organization (WHO); thus, 100 ml of normal plasma has 100 IU/dl (100% activity) of each factor (severe hemophilia).

Genetics: The genes for factors VIII and IX are carried near the terminus of the long arm of the X chromosome and are therefore X-linked traits. The majority of patients have a reduction in the amount of clotting factor protein: 5–10% of those with hemophilia A and 40–50% of those with hemophilia B make a dysfunctional protein. Mildly affected patients have normal or near normal levels of factor VIII, because in the newborn factor VIII levels may be artificially elevated due to acute phase response elicited by the birth process. Patients with severe hemophilia will not have detectable levels. In contrast, factor IX levels are physiologically low in the newborn. If severe hemophilia is present in the family, an undetectable level of factor IX is diagnostic of severe hemophilia B.

Through lyonization of the factor X chromosome, some female carriers of hemophilia A or B have sufficient reduction of factor VIII or factor IX to produce mild bleeding disorders. Levels of these factors should be determined in all known carriers to assess the need for treatment in the event of surgery or clinical bleeding. Because factor VIII is carried in the plasma by von Willebrand factor, the ratio of factor VIII to von Willebrand factor is sometimes used to diagnose carriers of hemophilia (*see* von Willebrand disease).

Pathophysiology: After injury, the initial hemostatic event is formation of the platelet plug, together with the generation of the fibrin clot that prevents further hemorrhage. In hemophilia A or B, clot formation is delayed and is not robust. Inadequate thrombin generation leads to failure to form a tightly cross-linked fibrin clot to support the platelet plug. Patients with hemophilia slowly form a soft, friable clot. When untreated bleeding occurs in a closed space such as a joint, cessation of bleeding may be the result of tamponade. With open wounds, in which tamponade cannot occur, profuse bleeding may result in significant blood loss. The clot that is formed may be friable, and rebleeding occurs during the physiologic lysis of clots or with minimal new trauma.

Classification: In males 85% have factor VIII deficiency and 10–15% have factor IX deficiency. The severity of hemophilia is classified on the basis of patient's baseline level of factor VIII or factor IX. By definition 1 international unit (IU) of each factor is defined as that amount in 1 ml of normal plasma referred against a standard established by the World Health Organization (WHO); thus, 100 ml of normal plasma has 100 IU/dl (100% activity) of each factor. **Severe hemophilia** is characterized by having <1% activity of the specific clotting factor and bleeding is often spontaneous. Patients with **moderate hemophilia** have levels of 1–5% and require mild trauma to induce bleeding. Individuals with **mild hemophilia** have levels of >5% may go many years before the condition is diagnosed and bleeding occurs after significant trauma. The hemostatic level for factor VIII is >30–40%, and for actor IX, it is >25–30%. The lower limit of levels for factors VIII and IX in normal individuals is approximately 50%.

Clinical manifestations: Bleeding symptoms may be present from birth or may occur in the fetus because factor VIII and factor IX do not cross placenta. Only about 2% of neonates with hemophilia may sustain intracranial hemorrhages and 30% of male infants with hemophilia bleed with circumcision. Obvious symptoms of easy bruising, minor traumatic lacerations of the mouth (a torn frenulum), intramuscular hematomas, and hemarthroses begin when the child "begins to cruise". Even in patients with severe hemophilia, only 90% have evidence of increased bleeding by 1 yr of age. Although bleeding may occur in any area of the body, the important finding of hemophilia is hemarthrosis. Bleeding in to the joints may be induced by minor trauma; many hemarthroses are spontaneous. The earliest joint hemorrhages appear most commonly in the ankle; hemorrhages of the knees and elbows are also common in the older child and adolescent. Patients complain of a warm, tingling sensation in the joint as the first sign of an early joint hemorrhage. After repeated bleeding episodes into the same joint, patients with severe hemophilia may develop a *target* joint. Recurrent bleeding may become spontaneous because of pathologic changes in the joint that had repeated bleeding episodes.

Although most muscular hemorrhages are clinically evident owing to localized pain or swelling, a vague area of referred pain in the groin is complained by the patient in the case of bleeding into the *iliopsoas muscle*. The diagnosis is made clinically by the inability to extend the hip, but must be confirmed with ultrasonography or CT scan. Life-threatening bleeding in the patient with hemophilia is caused by bleeding into vital structures (central nervous system, upper airway) or by exsanguination (external, gastrointestinal, or iliopsoas hemorrhage).

Patients with mild hemophilia who have factor VIII or factor IX levels of > 5 IU/dl usually do not have spontaneous hemorrhages. These individuals may experience prolonged bleeding after dental work, surgery or injuries from moderate trauma.

Laboratory findings and diagnosis: The laboratory screening test that is affected by a reduced level of factor VIII or factor IX is PTT. In severe hemophilia, PTT is usually 2–3 times more than normal. Results of the other screening tests of the hemostatic mechanism (platelet count, bleeding time, prothrombin time, and thrombin time) are normal. Unless the patient has an inhibitor of factor VIII or IX, the mixing of normal plasma with patient plasma results in correction of PTT. The specific assay for factors VIII or IX will confirm the diagnosis of hemophilia. If correction does not occur on mixing, an inhibitor may be present. In 25–35% of patients with hemophilia who receive infusions of factor VIII or factor IX, a factor-specific antibody may develop. These antibodies are directed against the active clotting site and are termed *inhibitors*.

Differential diagnosis: In young infants with severe bleeding manifestations, the differential diagnosis includes severe thrombocytopenia; severe platelet function disorders, such as Bernard-Soulier syndrome and Glanzmann thrombasthenia; type 3 (severe) von Willebrand disease; and vitamin K deficiency. Hemostatic screening tests differentiates these entities from hemophilia.

Treatment: Treatment should be started early (Table 20.7). When mild to moderate bleeding occurs, levels of factor VIII or factor IX must be raised to hemostatic levels in the 35–50% range. For life-threatening or major hemorrhages, the dose should aim to achieve levels of 100% activity. Calculation of the dose of recombinant factor VIII (FVIII) or recombinant factor IX (FIX) is as follows:

Dose of FVIII (IU) = % desired (rise in FVIII) × body weight (kg) × 0.5
Dose of FIX (IU) = % desired (rise in plasma FIX) × body weight (kg) × 1.4

Table 20.7: Treatment of hemophilia

Type of hemorrhage	Hemophilia A	Hemophilia B
Hemarthrosis*	40 IU/kg factor VIII concentrate on\ day 1; then 20 IU/kg on days 2, 3, 5 until joint function is normal or back to baseline. Consider additional treatment every other day for 7–10 days. Consider prophylaxis	60–80 IU/kg factor IX concentrate on day 1; then 40 IU/kg on days 2, 4. Consider additional treatment every other day for 7–10 days. Consider prophylaxis
Muscle or significant sub-cutaneous hematoma	20 IU/kg factor VIII concentrate; may need every other day treatment until resolved	40 IU/kg factor IX concentrate; may need treatment every 2–3 days until resolved
Mouth, deciduous tooth or tooth extraction	20 IU/kg factor VIII concentrate; anti-fibrinolytic therapy; remove loose deciduous tooth	40 IU/kg factor IX concentrate; antifibrino-lytic therapy; remove loose deciduous tooth
Epistaxis	Apply pressure for 15–20 min, pack with petrolatum gauze, give anti-fibrinolytic therapy; 20 IU/kg factor VIII concentrate if this treatment fails	Apply pressure for 15–20 min, pack with petrolatum gauze, give antifibrinolytic therapy; 30 IU/kg factor IX concentrate if this treatment fails
Major injury, life-threatening hemorrhage	50–75 IU/kg factor VIII concentrate, then initiate continuous infusion of 2–4 IU/kg/hr to maintain factor VIII >100 IU/dl for 24 hr, then give 2–3 IU/kg/hr continuously for 5–7 days to maintain the level at >50 IU/dl and an additional 5–7 days at a level of >30 IU/dl	120 IU/kg factor IX concentrate, then 50–60 IU/kg every 12–24 hr to maintain factor IX at > 40 IU/dL for 5–7 days and then >30 IU/dl for 7 days
Iliopsoas hemorrhage	50 IU/kg factor VIII concentrate, then 25 IU/kg every 12 hr until-asymptomatic, then 20 IU/kg every other day for a total of 10–14 days	120 IU/kg factor IX concentrate; then 50–60 IU/kg every 12–24 hr to maintain factor IX at >40 IU/dl until asymptomatic, then 40–50 IU/kg every other day for a total of 10–14 days
Hematuria	Bed rest; 11/2 × maintenance fluids; if not controlled in 1–2 days, 20 IU/kg factor VIII concentrate; if not controlled, give prednisolone (unless HIV infected)	Bed rest; 11/2 × maintenance fluids; if not controlled in 1–2 days, 40 IU/kg factor IX concentrate; if not controlled, give prednisolone (unless HIV infected)
Prophylaxis	20–40 IU/kg factorVIII concentrate every other day to achieve a trough level of ≥ 1%	30–50 IU/kg factor IX concentrate every 2–3 days to achieve a trough level of ≥ 1%

*For hip hemarthrosis, orthopedic evaluation for possible aspiration is advisable to prevent avascular necrosis of the femoral head.

For factor VIII, the correction factor is based on the volume of distribution of factor VIII. For factor IX, the correction factor is based on the volume of distribution and the observed rise in plasma level after infusion of recombinant factor IX. The treatment of some common types of hemorrhage in a patient with hemophilia is mentioned in Table 20.8. A concentrated intranasal form of desmopressin acetate (D-void; Stimate) can also be used to treat with mild hemophilia A (dose: 150 μg (1 puff) for children weighing <50 kg and 300 μg (2 puffs) for young adults weighing >50 kg). Desmopressin is not effective in factor IX-deficient hemophilia.

Prophylaxis: Many patients are now given lifelong prophylaxis to prevent spontaneous joint bleeding. Usually such programs are initiated with the first joint hemorrhage. Young children often require the insertion of a central catheter to ensure venous access. Treatment is usually provided every 2–3 days to maintain a measurable plasma level of clotting factor (1–2%) when assayed just before the next infusion (trough level). If moderate arthropathy develops, prevention of future bleeding will require higher plasma levels of clotting factors. In the older child who is not given primary prophylaxis, secondary prophylaxis is frequently initiated if a target joint develops.

Supportive care: Parents are advised that their child should avoid trauma. Toddlers are active, are curious about everything, and injure themselves. Effective measures include anticipatory guidance, including the use of car seats, seatbelts, and bike helmets, and importance of avoiding high-risk behaviors. Older boys should be counseled to avoid violent contact sports. Early psychosocial intervention helps the family to achieve a balance between overprotection and permissiveness. Patients with hemophilia should avoid aspirin and other nonsteroidal anti-inflammatory drugs that affect platelet function. The child with a bleeding disorder should receive the appropriate vaccinations against hepatitis B, even though recombinant products may avoid exposure to transfusion-transmitted diseases. Patients exposed to plasma derived products should be screened periodically for hepatitis B and C, HIV, and abnormalities in liver function.

Chronic complications: Long-term complications of hemophilia A and B include chronic arthropathy, the development of an inhibitor of either factor VIII or factor IX, and the risk of transfusion-transmitted infectious diseases such as hepatitis B and C and HIV.

Comprehensive care: Patients with hemophilia are best treated through comprehensive hemophilia care centres. Such centres provide patient care and family education as well as the prevention and/or treatment of the complications of hemophilia, including chronic joint disease and inhibitor development as well as infection such as hepatitis C and HIV.

Factor XI Deficiency (Hemophilia C)

Factor XI deficiency is an autosomal deficiency associated with mild to moderate bleeding symptoms. It is frequently encountered in Ashkenazi Jews, but is reported in many other ethnic groups. In Israel, 1–3/1,000 are homozygous for this deficiency.

The deficiency of factor XI can be confirmed by specific factor XI assays. The bleeding associated with factor XI deficiency is not correlated with the amount of factor XI. At the time of major surgery replacement therapy should be given preoperatively. The physician must use fresh frozen plasma (FFP). Bleeding during minor surgery can be controlled with local pressure; patients undergoing dental extractions can be monitored closely and treated only if hemorrhage occurs. Plasma infusions of 1 IU/kg usually increase the plasma concentration by 2%. Thus, infusion of plasma at 10–15 ml/kg will result in a plasma level of 20–30%, a level usually sufficient to control moderate hemorrhage. Frequent infusions of plasma would be necessary to achieve higher levels of factor XI. Because the half-life of factor XI is usually ≥ 48 hr, maintaining adequate levels of factor XI usually is not difficult.

Chronic joint bleeding is rarely a problem. For most patients factor XI deficiency is a concern only at the time of major surgery unless there is a second underlying hemostatic defect (e.g. von Willebrand disease).

Deficiencies of the contact factors (nonbleeding disorders): Deficiency of the "contact factors" (factor XII, prekallikrein, and high molecular weight kininogen) causes prolonged PTT, but no bleeding symptoms. In this condition PTT is extremely prolonged, but there is no evidence of clinical bleeding. These individuals do not need treatment, even for major surgery.

Factor VII deficiency: Factor VII deficiency is a rare bleeding disorder that is usually detected in the homozygous state. Individuals with this deficiency may have spontaneous intracranial hemorrhage and frequent mucocutaneous bleeding. Such patients have markedly prolonged PT but normal PTT. Factor VII assays show a marked reduction of factor VII. Because the plasma-half life of factor VII is 2–4 hr, therapy with FFP is difficult and is often complicated by fluid overload.

Factor X deficiency is a rare autosomal disorder that results in mucocutaneous and post-traumatic bleeding. Factor X deficiency is the result of either a quantitative deficiency or a dysfunctional molecule. Both PT and PTT are prolonged in factor X deficiency. These patients can be treated by using either FFP or prothrombin complex concentrate. The half-life of factor X is approximately 30 hr, and its volume of distribution is similar to that of factor IX. Thus, 1 IU/kg will increase the plasma level of factor X by 1%. In the case of patients associated with systemic amyloidosis transfusion therapy often is not successful because of the rapid clearance of factor X.

Prothrombin (Factor II) deficiency is caused either by a markedly reduced prothrombin level (hypoprothrombinemia) or by functionally abnormal prothrombin (dysprothrombinemia). Factor II or prothrombin, assays show a markedly reduced prothrombin level. In homozygous patients PT and PTT is prolonged. Patients are treated with either prothrombin complex concentrates or FFP. In prothrombin deficiency FFP is useful, because the half life of prothrombin is 3.5 days. Administration of 1 IU/kg of prothrombin will increase the plasma activity by 1%.

Factor V deficiency is an autosomal recessive mild or moderate bleeding disorder that has also been termed *parahemophilia*. Hemarthrosis occur rarely; mucocutaneous bleeding and hematomas are the most common symptoms. Severe menorrhagia is a frequent symptom in women. Specific assays for factor V show a reduction in factor V levels. PT and PTT are prolonged. Patients are treated with FFP that contains factor V. Factor V is lost rapidly from stored FFP. Patients with severe factor V deficiency are treated with infusions of FFP at 10 mL/kg every 12 hr.

Combined deficiency of factors V and VIII occurs secondary to the absence of an intracellular transport protein, FRGIC-53, that is responsible for transporting factors V and VIII from the endoplasmic reticulum to the Golgi compartments. ERGIC-53 is encoded on chromosome 18. The deficiencies of factors V and VIII is not related to defective genes for this protein, but is secondary to a deficiency of a transport protein.

Fibrinogen deficiency (Factor I): Congenital afibrogenemia is a rare autosomal recessive disorder in which there is an absence of fibrinogen. Affected patients may present in the neonatal period with gastrointestinal hemorrhage or hematomas after vaginal delivery. These patients do not bleed as frequently as patients with hemophilia, and they rarely have hemarthroses. In addition to marked prolongation of PT and PTT, thrombin time is prolonged. In the absence of consumptive coagulopathy, an unmeasurable fibrinogen level is diagnostic. In addition to the quantitative deficiency of fibrinogen, a number of dysfunctional fibrinogens have been reported (dysfibrinogenemia). Treatment with either FFP or cryoprecipitate is effective, because the plasma half-life of fibrinogen is 2–4 days. The hemostatic level of fibrinogen is > 60 mg/dl. Each bag of cryoprecipitate contains 100–150 mg of fibrinogen.

Factor XIII deficiency (fibrin stabilizing factor or transglutaminase deficiency): Factor XIII is responsible for the cross-linking of fibrin to stabilize the fibrin clot; the symptoms of delayed hemorrhage are secondary to instability of the clot. Patients have mild bruising, delayed separation of the umbilical stump beyond 4 wk, poor wound healing, and recurrent spontaneous abortions in women. Results of the usual screening tests for hemostasis are normal. The normal clot remains insoluble in the presence of 5 M urea, whereas in a patient with XIII deficiency, the clot dissolves. Because the plasma half-life of factor XIII is 5–7 days and the hemostatic level is 2–3% activity, infusion with either FFP or cryoprecipitate will correct the deficiency in these patients. Plasma contains 1 IU/dl, and the cryoprecipitate contains 75 IU/bag. In patients with sufficient bleeding symptoms, prophylaxis can be achieved with infusion of cryoprecipitate every 3–4 wk.

Antiplasmin or plasminogen activator inhibitor deficiency: Deficiency of either antiplasmin or plasminogen activator inhibitor, which are antifibrinolytic proteins, results in increased plasmin generation and premature lysis of fibrin clots. Patients have mucocutaneous bleeding, but rarely have joint hemorrhages. Usual hemostatic tests are normal. Specific assays for α_2-antiplasmin and plasminogen activator inhibitor are available. Patients are treated with FFP.

Bollton-Maggs PH, Stobart K, Smyth RL. Evidence-based treatment of haemophilia. *Haemophilia* 2004;10 (Suppl 4):20–24.

Manco-Jhnson M. Hemophilia management: Optimizing treatment based on patient needs. *Curr Opin Pediatr* 2005;17: 3–6.

Montgomery RR, Gill JC, Scott JP. Hemophilia and von Willebrand disease. In: Nathan DG, Orkin SH, Ginsburg D, et al (eds). *Hematology of Infancy and Childhood.* 6th edn. Philadelphia: WB Saunders, 2003;1547–76.

Scot JP, Montgomery RR. Hemorrhagic and thrombotic diseases. In: Kliegman RM, Behrman RE, Jenson HB, Stanton BF (eds). *Nelson Textbook of Pediatrics.* 18th edn. Vol. 2. Philadelphia: Saunders, 2007;2060–6.

von Willebrand Disease

von Willebrand disease (vWD) is the most common hereditary bleeding disorder and is present in 1–2% of the general population. vWD is inherited autosomally. Chromosome 12 contains the gene for vWF. vWD is classified on the basis of whether the protein is quantitatively reduced, but not absent (type I); qualitatively abnormal (type II); or absent (type III). Mutations in different loci that code for different functional domains of the von Willebrand factor (vWF) protein cause the different variants of vWD.

Pathophysiology: A large multimeric glycoprotein that is synthesized in megakaryocytes and endothelial cells, vWF is stored in platelet α-granules and endothelial cell Weibel-Palade bodies. The highest molecular weight multimers of vWF are responsible for the normal interaction of vWF with the subendothelial matrix and platelets. During normal hemostasis, vWF adheres to the subendothelial matrix after vascular damage. When vWF binds to the subendothelial matrix, the conformation of vWF is changed so that it causes platelets to adhere to vWF through their glycoprotein IB (GPIb) receptor. These platelets are then activated, causing the recruitment of additional platelets and exposing phosphatidylserine, which is an important regulatory step for factors V- and VIII-dependent steps in the clotting cascade. vWF also serves as the carrier protein for plasma factor VIII. A severe deficiency of vWF causes a secondary deficiency in factor VIII, even though the gene for factor VIII is normal. This is the cause of autosomal deficiency of factor VIII, now known to be a molecular abnormality of vWF and known as *type 2N vWD*.

Clinical manifestations: Patients with vWD usually have symptoms of mucocutaneous hemorrhage, including excessive bruising, epistaxis, menorrhagia, and postoperative hemorrhage, particularly after mucosal surgery, such as tonsillectomy or wisdom tooth extraction. Because vWF is an acute-phase protein, stress will increase its level. Thus, patients may not bleed with procedures that incur major stress, such as appendicectomy and childbirth, but may bleed excessively at the time of cosmetic or mucosal surgery. Bruising symptoms may diminish during pregnancy because vWF levels may double or triple during pregnancy.

Laboratory findings: Patients with vWD have a long bleeding time and a long partial thromboplastin time, these findings are usually normal in patients with type 1 vWD. If the history is suggestive of a mucocutaneous bleeding disorder, vWD testing should be undertaken, including a quantitative assay for vWF antigen, testing for vWF activity (ristocetin cofactor activity), testing for plasma factor VIII activity, determination of vWF structure (vWF multimers), and a platelet count. Though the platelet count is usually normal in most patients, those with type 2B disease or platelet-type disease (pseudo-vWD) may have life long thrombocytopenia. Because factor VIII is carried in the plasma by von Willebrand factor, the ratio of factor VIII to von Willebrand factor is sometimes used to diagnose carriers of hemophilia.

Treatment: The treatment of vWD is directed toward increasing the plasma level of vWF and factor VIII. Because the gene for factor VIII is normal in patients with vWD, elevating the plasma concentration of vWF permits normal recovery and survival of endogenously produced factor VIII. Desmopressin acetate (DDAVP, Stimate) is effective in type 1 and in some patients of type 2 vWD variants. Both vWF and factor VIII are required for normal hemostasis. If only vWF is replaced, endogenous correction of factor VIII level takes 12–24 hr. Dental extractions and sometimes nosebleeds can be managed with both DDAVP and an antifibrinolytic agent such as ε-aminocaproic acid (Amicar).

Gill JC. Diagnosis and treatment of von Willebrand disease. *Hematol Oncol Clin North Am* 2004;18:1277–99.

Mannucci PM. Treatment of von Willebrand disease. *N Engl J Med* 2004;351:683–94.

Montgomery RR, Gill JC, Scott JP. Hemophilia and von Willebrand Disease. In: Nathan DG, Orkin SH, Ginsburg D, et al (eds). *Hematology of Infancy and Childhood.* 6th edn. Philadelphia: WB Saunders, 2003;1547–76.

Scot JP, Montgomery RR.Hemorrhagic and thrombotic diseases. In: Kliegman RM, Behrman RE, Jenson HB, Stanton BF (eds). *Nelson Textbook of Pediatrics.* 18th edn. Vol. 2. Philadelphia: Saunders, 2007;2060–6.

Hereditary Predisposition to Thrombosis

Thromboses in children are frequently associated with a hereditary or acquired prothrombotic state. The sick newborn infant is particularly at risk because interventions to provide support often include placement of large indwelling catheters into major veins or arteries. Homozygous deficiency of protein C presents with purpura fulminants in the first few hr of life. After the neonatal period, if a thrombus is identified in the young child, particularly when the family history is abnormal, a thrombotic evaluation should be initiated. In children and teenagers, thromboses are often triggered by major medical or surgical problems. Children have an increased frequency of venous thrombosis. Young women are at increased risk for venous thrombosis during pregnancy or while receiving oral contraceptive agents. There is also increased risk of recurrent abortions.

Etiology: A hereditary predisposition to thrombosis can be caused by deficiencies of the regulatory proteins, protein C, protein S, antithrombin III, and plasminogen; synthesis of procoagulant protein; prothrombin mutation (G20210A); elevated levels of a toxic organic acid, homocystinemia. In young adults with thrombosis, factor V Leiden (hereditary mutation of factor V) and prothrombin mutation (G20210A) are the most common abnormalities. Heterozygous deficiency of anticoagulant proteins, protein C, protein S, or antithrombin III, induces a tendency toward venous thromboembolic disease at an early age.

Laboratory findings: There are no screening tests for a hereditary predisposition to thrombosis; thus, specific testing is required for protein C, protein S, antithrombin III, factor V Leiden, and prothrombin 20210. Molecular testing for the factor V Leiden and the prothrombin mutation (G20210A) genes is more sensitive and specific than clotting-based tests.

Treatment: Amelioration of symptoms of plasma fulminans usually requires (providing protein C) 10–15 ml/kg of fresh frozen plasma (FFP) every 8–12 hr. A recombinant activated protein C concentrate (drotrecogin-α) has been approved for adult sepsis but not for treating hereditary deficiency. When the infant is beyond the neonatal period, high-dose warfarin (to achieve an International Normalized Ratio of 3–5) may prevent most of the thrombotic problems, but acute intermittent thromboses require additional FFP or protein concentrate. Patients who sustain a thrombosis associated with a hereditary predisposition of clotting should be treated with anticoagulants. Individuals with homocystinuria should receive anticoagulation in addition to management of their primary disease.

Esmon CT. Blood coagulation. In: Nathan DG, Orkin SH, Ginsburg D, et al (eds). *Hematology of Infancy and Childhood.* 6th edn. Philadelphia: WB Saunders, 2003;1475–96.

Heller C, Nowak-Gottel U. Maternal thrombophilia and neonatal thrombosis. *Best Pract Res Clin Haematol* 2003;16:333–45.

Hoppe C, Matsunaga A. Pediatric thrombosis. *Pediatr Clin North Am* 2002;49:1257–83.

Monagle P, Andrew M. Acquired disorders of hemostasis. In: Nathan DG, Orkin SH, Ginsburg D, et al (eds). *Hematology of Infancy and Childhood.* 6th edn. Philadelphia: WB Saunders, 2003;1631–68.

Scot JP, Montgomery RR. Hemorrhagic and thrombotic diseases. In: Kliegman RM, Behrman RE, Jenson HB, Stanton BF (eds). *Nelson Textbook of Pediatrics.* 18th edn. Vol. 2. Philadelphia: Saunders, 2007;2060–6.

Acquired Thrombotic Disorders

Acquired thrombotic and embolic events are uncommon in otherwise healthy children, thromboembolism is a common complication in sick newborns and in with specific diseases. Occlusion of a blood vessel with a platelet plug or fibrin clot may occur in vessels of any size.

Etiology: Occlusion of arterial or venous vessels of diverse caliber may occur to vessel injury and mechanics that lead to thrombosis.

A. *Vessel injury*

1. Systemic disorders associated with occlusion such as systemic lupus erythematosus and Kawasaki disease; metabolic defects such as homocystinuria; and hemoglobinopathies such as sickle cell anemia and polycythemia.

2. Activation of clotting as a complication disseminated intravascular coagulation can cause microvascular and macrovascular thrombosis.

3. Medical interventions can cause a predisposition to thrombosis such as when sick newborns having indwelling catheters placed in major vessels or when children with acute lymphoblastic leukemia receive the chemotherapeutic agent L-asparaginase, which depletes anticoagulant proteins.

B. *Mechanisms that lead to thrombosis*

1. Abnormal platelet adheseveness-aggregation
2. An activated coagulation mechanism
3. A defective or deficient coagulation system
4. A dysfunctional fibrinolytic mechanism; and
5. Reduced blood flow.

Arterial thrombosis appears to depend on vascular injury and platelet activation under high flow (high shear), whereas venous thrombosis generally occurs in low-flow (low shear) conditions associated with activation of the coagulation mechanism or with an impaired inhibitor-fibrinolytic system.

Clinical manifestations: Arterial thrombosis usually present with organ dysfunction due to ischemia (cold, pulseless extremity). Such findings can be triggered by thrombi formed at the site of vascular damage or caused by emboli. Venous events usually present as a warm, swollen, or distended tender organ or extremity. A deep venous thrombosis (DVT) may be asymptomatic, and present only after the development of pulmonary emboli. In general, vascular occlusion events in children have an acute or sudden onset.

Diagnosis: The diagnosis of thrombosis is made by Doppler ultrasonography or magnetic resonance angiography. In special cases (upper extremity thrombosis), radiocontrast angiography may be necessary. Routine coagulation screening studies are rarely helpful in diagnosing a thromboembolic event.

Treatment

Venous thrombosis and thrombophlebitis: Superficial thrombophlebitis is treated with anti-inflammatory drugs (nonsteroidal anti-inflammatory agents), heat compresses, rest, and elevation of the affected part. Patients with DVT (deep vein thrombosis) or thrombophlebitis are treated with anticoagulation and rarely with thrombolytic agents. Heparin [low molecular weight (LMW)] should be used in a full dose (1.0–1.5 mg/kg q 12 hr SC) for 3–5 days with warfarin added for an additional 6 months in patients with proximal (above the knee) venous thrombosis. The use of thrombolytic therapy should probably be limited to life- or limb-threatening situations. The treatment of patients with calf vein thrombosis is short-term anticoagulation, which may hasten recovery and prevent progression.

Pulmonary embolism: The patient with acute pulmonary embolism can be treated with heparin or, less often, with thrombolytic drugs. Most patients should receive heparin and later warfarin. Thrombolytic therapy should be reserved for life-threatening pulmonary emboli, because thrombolytic therapy in adults produces more rapid clinical improvement than heparin therapy, but overall survival and long-term pulmonary function abnormalities appear to be the same in both treatment groups. Embolectomy is used rarely when there is a large embolism and no benefit is derived from thrombolytic or anticoagulant therapy.

Arterial thrombosis: Fibrinolytic therapy with recombinant tissue-type plasminogen activator, followed by heparin anticoagulation is the treatment of acute arterial thrombosis of recent onset. Rarely, surgical removal of the clot is performed if lytic therapy is unsuccessful or if the thrombosis affects a major organ or limb. Thrombolytic therapy should not be used if there has been recent surgery or central nervous system thrombosis or hemorrhage.

Stroke: Ischemic stroke commonly presents with hemiparesis, loss of consciousness, or seizures. Arterial occlusion in the brain may occur as a component of a systemic disorder (sickle cell disease) or after embolization either from a damaged vessel (carotid aneurysm after trauma) or from venous thrombi that enter the arterial circulation via a patent foramen ovale. Often stroke are idiopathic. Venous thrombosis of the cerebral vessels (sinovenous thrombosis) occurs with cyanotic heart disease, inflammatory or infectious lesions of the brain or surrounding tissues, hyperviscosity states, or congenital thrombophilia. Antiplatelet therapy with aspirin is safe. Heparin therapy may improve the outcome of stroke in adults, although the risk of hemorrhagic infarction may be increased. Sinovenous thrombosis in the absence of hemorrhage is usually treated with heparin. The presence of a hemorrhagic infarct is a contraindication to anticoagulant therapy. Thrombolytic therapy, if used in nonhemorrhagic strokes, should only be instituted in patients within 3 hr of the onset of symptoms.

Anticoagulant and Thrombolytic Therapy

The commonly used anticoagulant agents are unfrationated (standard) heparin, low molecular weight heparin, warfarin, and thrombolytic therapy.

Unfractionated (standard) heparin enhances the rate by which antithrombin III neutralizes the activity of several clotting proteins, especially factor Xa and thrombin. Anticoagulation with heparin is contraindicated in the following circumstances: A recent central nervous system hemorrhage; bleeding from inaccessible sites; malignant hypertension; bacterial endocarditis; recent surgery of the eye, brain, or the spinal cord; current administration of regional or lumbar block anesthesia; and a pre-existing coagulation defect or bleeding abnormality (a relative contraindication).

Low molecular weight (LMW) *heparin* is an effective, convenient alternative to standard heparin therapy. Adult patients receiving LMW heparin rarely need to have their heparin levels monitored, but in pediatric patients, there is more diversity of response. A specific assay should be used to monitor LMW heparin. Once a therapeutic range is achieved, monitoring is required only infrequently. When LMW heparin is used for prophylaxis against thrombosis, the dose is 0.5 mg/kg q 12 hr subcutaneously, with the goal of achieving a level of 0.3 unit/ml 4 hr after injection.

Warfarin an oral anticoagulant drug, probably acts by competitively inhibiting vitamin K metabolism. After the administration of warfarin, levels of factors II (3.5 days), VII (2–4 hr), IX, and X (30 hr) decreases gradually, according to each factor's plasma half life. Because factor VII has the shortest half-life, its level is first to decrease, followed by factors IX and X, and finally factor II. It generally takes 4–5 days to reduce the levels of all 4 coagulation factors consistent with effective coagulation. Prothrombin time (PT) is the clotting test used to assess warfarin anticoagulation. The most serious side effect of warfarin is hemorrhage. Warfarin-induced bleeding is treated by discontinuation of the drug and oral administration of vitamin K. Vitamin K is given equal to the amount of the daily warfarin dose. Vitamin K can be administered orally, subcutaneously, or IV (not IM), but the parenteral forms have much longer half-life and may overshoot the correction. Correction of the coagulopathy begins within 6–8 hr and should be complete in 24–48 hr. If a patient has a significant or life-threatening hemorrhage, fresh frozen plasma (15 ml/kg) should be given when vitamin K is administered.

The addition or removal of certain drugs in the patient's therapeutic regimen can have significant effects on oral anticoagulation. The effects of warfarin can be enhanced by the administration of antibiotics, salicylates, anabolic steroids, chloral hydrate, laxatives, allopurinol, vitamin E, and methylphenidate hydrochloride; its effects can be diminished by barbiturates, vitamin K, oral contraceptives, phenytoin, and other agents.

Contraindications to warfarin (coumarin anticoagulant), is the same as those for hepatic therapy. The oral anticoagulants are teratogenic, cross the placenta, and should not be given during pregnancy, particularly during the first trimester. Although breastmilk contains warfarin, the quantity is insignificant and the drug can be used to treat the lactating mother without a significant effect on the infant.

Thrombolytic agents such as recombinant tissue-type plasminogen activator (rTPA), activate plasminogen to lyse blood clots by enzymatic digestion; rTPA is most often used in pediatrics for *thrombolytic therapy.* For the therapy to be effective, the patient should have a relatively fresh clot (< 3–5 days old), the clot must be accessible to the lytic agent, and there must be an adequate amount of plasminogen. Once plasmin has been formed, it lyses fibrin. Relatively more fibrin-specific than the older thrombolytic agents (urokinase and streptokinase), rTPA activates plasminogen within or on a fibrin clot. rTPA rarely produces a systemic hyperfibrinolytic state. The initial dose of rTPA is 0.1 mg/kg/hr. It may be useful to monitor for a therapeutic effect by looking for an increase in the concentration of D-dimers or fibrin degradation products. Higher doses or more prolonged courses of thrombolytic therapy are likely to be associated with an increased risk of bleeding complications. Low doses of rTPA have been efficacious in restoring patency in occluded vascular access catheters.

Prevention: Children with known prothrombotic conditions who are going to be immobilized for a protracted time probably should receive prophylactic treatment with enoxaparin 0.5 mg/kg q 12 hr while immobile. Use of such therapy is controversial for children who are immobilized for a prolonged period due to a severe medical illness, especially if it is associated with inflammation or trauma.

Nowak-Gottl U, Straeter R, Sebire G, et al. Antithrombotic drug treatment of pediatric patients with ischemic stroke. *Paediatr Drugs* 2003;5:167–75.

Sutor AH, Chan AK, Massicotte P. Low molecular weight heparin in pediatric patients. *Semin Thromb Hemost* 2004;30 (Suppl 1):31–39.

Scot JP, Montgomery RR.Hemorrhagic and thrombotic diseases. In: Kliegman RM, Behrman RE, Jenson HB, Stanton BF (eds). *Nelson Textbook of Pediatrics.* 18th edn. Vol. 2. Philadelphia: Saunders, 2007;2060–66.

Postneonatal Vitamin K Deficiency

The causes of vitamin K deficiency occurring after the neonatal period are as follows: (i) "late" hemorrhagic disease in breastfed children; (ii) secondary to a lack of oral intake of vitamin K, alterations in the gut flora due to the long-term use of broad spectrum antibiotics, or malabsorption of vitamin K; (iii) intestinal malabsorption of fats may accompany cystic fibrosis or biliary atresia and result in a deficiency of fat-soluble dietary vitamin, with reduced synthesis of vitamin K-dependent clotting factors (factors II, VII, IX, and X, and protein C and protein S); and (iv) patients with advanced cirrhosis, synthesis of many of the clotting factors may reduced because of hepatocellular damage.

Prophylactic administration of water-soluble vitamin K orally is indicated (not in patients with advanced cirrhosis) in the dosage of 2–3 mg/24 hr for children and 5–10 mg/24 hr in adolescents and adults. In patients with advanced cirrhosis, vitamin K may be ineffective.

Monagle P, Andrew M. Acquired disorders of hemostasis. In: Nathan DG, Orkin SH, Ginsburg D, et al (eds). *Hematology of Infancy and Childhood.* 6th edn. Philadelphia: WB Saunders, 2003;1631–68.

Disseminated Intravascular Coagulation

Consumption coagulopathy refers to a heterogeneous group of conditions including disseminated intra-vascular coagulation (DIC), that result in consumption of clotting factors, platelets, and anticoagulant proteins. Consequences of this process include wide spread intravascular deposition of fibrin, leading to tissue ischemia and necrosis, a generalized hemorrhagic state, and hemolytic anemia.

Etiopathogenesis: Conditions associated with DIC include septic shock (especially meningococcemia), incompatible blood transfusion, rickettsial infection, snake bite, purpura fulminans, giant hemangioma, and malignancy, especially acute promyelocytic leukemia. Any life-threatening pathologic process associated with hypoxia, acidosis, tissue necrosis, shock, and/or endothelial damage may trigger DIC.

The initiating event is usually excessive activation of clotting that consumes both the physiologic anticoagulants (protein C, protein S, and antithrombin III) and procoagulants, resulting in a deficiency of factor V, factor VIII, prothrombin, fibrinogen, and platelets. Commonly, the clinical result of this sequence of events is hemorrhage. In addition, because the fibrinolytic mechanism is activated, fibrinogen degradation products (FDPs, D-dimers) appear in the blood. Anemia caused by hemolysis may develop rapidly owing to microangiopathic hemolytic anemia. The hemostatic dysregulation may also result in thromboses in the skin, kidneys, and other organs.

Clinical manifestations: Usually, DIC accompanies a severe systemic disease process associated with bleeding and anemia. Bleeding frequently first occurs from the sites of venipuncture or surgical incision. The skin may show petechiae and ecchymoses. Tissue necrosis may involve many organs and can be seen as infarction of large areas of skin, subcutaneous tissue, or kidneys.

Laboratory findings: Prothrombin, partial thrombo-plastin, and thrombin times are prolonged. Platelet counts may be markedly decreased. The blood smear may contain fragmented, burr-, and helmet-shaped red blood cells (schistocytes). The D-dimer is formed by fibrinolysis of a cross-linked fibrin clot. The D-dimer is sensitive and more specific for activation of coagulation and fibrinolysis.

Treatment: The management is directed to treat the trigger that caused DIC, and to restore normal homeostasis by correcting the shock, acidosis, and hypoxia that usually complicate DIC. If the underlying problem can be controlled, bleeding quickly ceases, and there is improvement of the abnormal laboratory findings. Blood components are used for replacement therapy in patients with hemorrhage. This may consist of platelet infusions (for thrombocytopenia), cryoprecipitate (for hypofibrinogenemia), and/or fresh frozen plasma (for replacement of other coagulation factors and natural inhibitors). Patients who have vascular thrombosis in association with DIC should be treated as outlined (*see* Acquired thrombotic disorders).

The *prognosis* of patients with DIC is primarily dependent on the outcome of the treatment of the primary diseases and prevention of end-organ damage.

Franchini M, Manzato F. Update on the treatment of disseminated intravascular coagulation. *Hematology* 2004; 9: 81–85.

Liebman HA, Weitz IC. Disseminated intravascular coagulation. In: Hoffman R, Benz EJ, Shattil SJ, et al (eds). *Hematology: Basic Principles and Practice.* 4th edn. Philadelphia: Elsevier Churchill Livingstone, 2005;2169–82.

Monagle P, Andrew M. Acquired disorders of hemostasis. In: Nathan DG, Orkin SH, Ginsburg D, et al (eds). *Hematology of Infancy and Childhood.* 6th edn. Philadelphia: WB Saunders, 2003;1631–68.

Scot JP, Montgomery RR. Hemorrhagic and thrombotic diseases. In: Kliegman RM, Behrman RE, Jenson HB, Stanton BF (eds). *Nelson Textbook of Pediatrics.* 18th edn. Vol. 2. Philadelphia: Saunders, 2007;2060–6.

Platelet and Blood Vessel Disorders

Idiopathic Thrombocytopenic Purpura

The most common cause of acute onset of thrombocytopenia in an otherwise well child is (autoimmune) idiopathic thrombocytopenic pupura (ITP). There is a recent history of viral illness. Most common infectious viruses described in association with ITP include Epstein-Barr virus and HIV. Epstein-Barr virus-related ITP is usually of short duration and follows the course of infectious mononucleosis. HIV-associated ITP is usually chronic. 1–4 wk after exposure to a viral infection, an autoantibody directed against the platelet develops. After binding of the antibody to the platelet surface, circulating antibody-coated platelets are recognized by the Fc receptor on the splenic macrophages, ingested, and destroyed.

Clinical manifestations: The classic presentation of ITP is that of a previously healthy 1–4 yr old child who has sudden onset of generalized petechiae and purpura. Often there is bleeding from the gums and mucous membrane, particularly with profound thrombocytopenia (platelet $< 10 \times 10^9/L$). There is a history of a preceding viral infection 1–4 wk before

the onset of thrombocytopenia. An easy classification system is proposed from the UK to characterize the severity of bleeding in ITP on the basis of symptoms and signs but not platelet count:
1. No symptoms
2. Mild symptoms: Bruising and petechiae, occasional minor epistaxis, very little interference with daily living
3. Moderate: More severe skin and mucosal lesions, more troublesome epistaxis and menorrhagia
4. Severe: Bleeding episodes-menorrhagia, epistaxis, malena-requiring transfusion or hospitalization, symptoms interfering seriously with the quality of life

In 70–80% of children who present with acute ITP, spontaneous resolution occurs within 6 months. Less than 1% of patients have intracranial hemorrhage. Approximately 20% of children who present with acute ITP go on to have chronic ITP.

Laboratory findings and differential diagnosis: Severe thrombocytopenia (platelet count $< 20 \times 10^9/L$) is common and platelet size is normal or increased, reflective of increased platelet turnover. In acute ITP, the hemoglobin value, white blood cell (WBC) count, the differential count should be normal. Hemoglobin may be decreased if there have been profuse nosebleeds or menorrhagia. Indications for bone marrow aspiration include an abnormal WBC count or differential or unexplained anemia as well as findings suggestive of bone marrow disease on history and physical examination.

In adolescents with new onset ITP, an antinuclear antibody test should be done to evaluate SLE. HIV studies should be done in at-risk populations, especially sexual active teens. A Coombs' test should be done if there is unexplained anemia to rule out Evans syndrome (autohemolytic–hemolytic anemia and thrombocytopenia).

Treatment: Platelet transfusion is usually contra-indicated unless life-threatening is present. Initial approaches to the management of ITP include the following:
1. *No therapy* other than education and counseling of the family and patient for patients with minimal, mild, and moderate symptoms.
2. *Intravenous immunoglobulin (IVIG):* IVIG at a dose of 0.8–1.0 g/kg/day for 1–2 days induces a rapid rise in platelet count (usually $> 20 \times 10^9/L$) in 95% patients within 48 hr. After infusion, there is high frequency of headaches and vomiting, suggestive of IVIG-induced aseptic meningitis.
3. *Intravenous anti-D therapy:* For Rh positive patients, IV anti-D at a dose of 50–75 µg/kg causes a rise in

platelet count to > 20 × 10⁹/L in 80–90% of patients within 48–72 hr. IV anti-D induces mild hemolytic anemia in Rh positive individuals. RBC-antibody complexes bind to macrophage Fc receptors and interfere with platelet destruction, thereby causing a rise in platelet count. IV anti-D is ineffective in Rh negative patients.

4. *Corticosteroid therapy:* Prednisolone in the dose 1–4 mg/kg/24 hr induces a more rapid rise in platelet count than in untreated patients with ITP. Corticosteroid therapy is usually continued for 2–3 wk or until a rise in platelet count to > 20 × 10⁹/L has been achieved, with a rapid taper to avoid the long term side effects of corticosteroid therapy, especially growth failure, diabetes mellitus, and osteoporosis.

Each of these medications may be used to treat exacerbations of ITP, which commonly occur several wk after an initial course of therapy. In the case of intracranial hemorrhage, multiple modalities should be used, including platelet transfusion, IVIG, high dose corticosteroids, and prompt surgical consultation, with plans for emergency splenectomy.

Splenectomy should be reserved in older child (≥ 4yr) with severe ITP that has lasted > 1 yr (chronic ITP) and whose symptoms are not controlled with therapy. Splenectomy must also be considered when life-threatening hemorrhage (intracranial hemorrhage) complicates acute ITP, if the platelet count cannot be corrected rapidly with transfusion of platelets and administration of IVIG and corticosteroids. Splenectomy is associated with a lifelong risk of overwhelming postsplenectomy infection caused by encapsulated organisms.

Chronic idiopathic thrombocytopenic purpura: Approximately 20% of patients who present with acute ITP have persistent thrombocytopenia for > 6 mo and are said to have chronic ITP. The causes of chronic ITP includes SLE, HIV, and nonimmune causes of chronic thrombocytopenia such as type 2B and platelet-type von Willebrand disease, X-linked thrombocytopenia, autoimmune lymphoproliferative syndrome, common variable immunodeficiency syndrome, autosomal macrothrombocytopenia, and WAS (also X-linked). *Therapy* should be aimed at controlling symptoms and preventing serious bleeding. Splenectomy should be considered in children with chronic ITP. Before splenectomy, the child should receive pneumococcal and meningococcal vaccines, and after splenectomy, the child should receive penicillin prophylaxis for a number of years. Whether penicillin prophylaxis should be lifelong is controversial.

Drug-induced thrombocytopenia: A number of drugs are associated with immune thrombocytopenia as the result of either an immune process or megakaryocyte injury. Some common drugs that cause thrombocytopenia include valproic acid, phenytoin, sulphonamides, and trimethoprim-sulfamethoxazole.

Nonimmune platelet destruction: The syndromes of DIC, HUS, and thrombotic thrombocytopenic purpura (TTP) share the hemolytic picture of a thrombotic microangiopathy in which there is RBC destruction and consumptive thrombocytopenia caused by platelet and fibrin deposition in the microvasculature. The microangiopathic hemolytic anemia is characterized by the presence of RBC fragments, including helmet cells, schistocytes, spherocytes, and burr cells.

Hemolytic–uremic syndrome (HUS): HUS, an acute disease of infancy and early childhood, usually follows an episode of acute gastroenteritis, often triggered by *Escherichia coli* 0157:H7. Shortly thereafter, signs and symptoms of hemolytic anemia, thrombocytopenia, and acute renal failure ensue. Sometimes neurologic symptoms are associated with these findings. The hemolytic anemia is characterized by morphologically abnormal RBCs, with the presence of helmet cells, spherocytes, schistocytes, burr cells, and other distorted forms. Thrombocytopenia despite normal numbers of megakaryocytes in the marrow indicates excessive platelet destruction. Urine examination shows protein, RBCs and casts. Anuria and severe azotemia indicate grave renal damage (*see* Chapter 21, Nephrology).

Treatment of most cases of HUS includes careful fluid management and prompt appropriate dialysis. Plasmapheresis is usually reserved for patients with HUS associated with major neurologic complications.

Thrombotic thrombocytopenic purpura (TTP): TTP is a rare pentad of fever, microangiopathic hemolytic anemia, thrombocytopenia, abnormal renal function and central nervous changes that is clinically similar to HUS, although TTP usually presents in adults and occasionally in adolescents. The treatment of TTP is plasmapheresis (plasma exchange). Corticosteroids and splenectomy are reserved for refractory cases.

Kasabach-Merritt syndrome: The association of a giant hemangioma with localized intravascular coagulation causing thrombocytopenia and hypofibrinogenemia is called Kasabach-Merritt syndrome. In most patients, the site of hemangioma is obvious but retroperitoneal and intra-abdominal hemangiomas may require body imaging for detection. The peripheral blood smear shows microangiopathic changes. Treatment includes surgical excision of hemangioma (if possible), laser photocoagulation, high-dose corticosteroid, local radiation therapy, and antiangiogenic agents such as interferon α_2. Treatment of the associated coagulopathy may benefit from a trial of antifibrinolytic therapy with ε-aminocaproic acid.

Sequestration: Thrombocytopenia develops in individuals with massive splenomegaly because the spleen acts as a sponge for platelets and sequesters large numbers. Most such patients also have mild leukopenia and anemia. In such patients, the splenomegaly should be investigated to find out the cause and treated on the basis of the underlying disease process.

Congenital Thrombocytopenic Syndromes

Congenital amegakaryocytic thrombocytopenia is caused by a rare defect in hematopoiesis that usually manifests within the first few days to wk of life, when the child presents with petechiae and purpura caused by profound thrombocytopenia. Bone marrow transplantation is curative.

Thrombocytopenia-absent radius **(TAR)** *syndrome* consists of thrombocytopenia (absence or hypoplasia of megakaryocytes) that presents in early infancy with bilateral radial anomalies of variable severity, ranging from mild changes to marked limb shortening. The thrombocytopenia of TAR syndrome frequently remits over the first few yr of life.

Wiskott-Aldrich syndrome **(WAS)** is characterized by thrombocytopenia, with tiny platelets, eczema, and recurrent infection due to immune deficiency. WAS is inherited as an X-linked disorder. Splenectomy often corrects the thrombocytopenia, suggesting that the platelets formed in WAS have accelerated destruction. After splenectomy, these patients are at increased risk for overwhelming infection and require lifelong antibiotic prophylaxis against encapsulated organisms. Approximately 5% of patients develop lymphoreticular malignancies. Bone marrow transplantation cures WAS.

Neonatal thrombocytopenia: Neonatal thrombocytopenia occurs: (i) in various fetal and neonatal infections (congenital viral infections, especially rubella and cytomegalovirus; protozoal infection such as toxoplasmosis; syphilis; and bacterial infection, especially those caused by gram-negative bacilli); (ii) in antibody mediated thrombocytopenia [neonatal alloimmune thrombocytopenic purpura (NATP); and children born to mothers with ITP (maternal ITP)]; and in two syndromes of congenital failure of platelet production (amegakaryocytic thrombocytopenia; and TAR syndrome). There may be spontaneous bleeding. The *treatment* includes prenatal administration of corticosteroids to the mother and administration of

IVIG and sometimes corticosteroids to the infant after delivery. Thrombocytopenia in an infant, due to NATP or maternal ITP usually resolves within 2–4 mo after delivery.

Acquired disorders of platelet function: Systemic illnesses associated with platelet dysfunction include liver disease, kidney disease (uremia), and disorders that trigger increased amount of fibrin degradation products. These disorders frequently cause prolonged bleeding time and are often associated with other abnormalities of the coagulation mechanism. The management is directed to treat the primary illness. If treatment of the primary process is not feasible, infusions of desmopressin or transfusions of platelets and/or cryoprecipitate have been helpful in improving hemostasis and correcting bleeding time. Many drugs alter platelet function. Acetylsalicylic acid (aspirin) commonly used in adults alters platelet function. Aspirin irreversibly acetylates the enzyme cyclooxygenase, which is critical in the formation of thromboxane A_2. Other commonly used drugs that affect platelet function include other nonsteroidal antiinflammatory drugs, valproic acid, and high-dose penicillin. When a patient is being evaluated for possible platelet dysfunction it is important to exclude the presence of other exogenous agents and if possible, stop all medications for 2 wk.

Congenital Abnormalities of Platelet Function

Severe platelet function defects usually present with petechiae and purpura shortly after birth, especially after vaginal delivery. Defects in the platelet GPIb complex (the vWF receptor) or the GPIIb-IIIa complex (the fibrinogen receptor) cause severe congenital platelet dysfunction.

Bernard-Soulier syndrome inherited as an autosomal recessive disorder is caused by absence or severe deficiency of the vWF receptor (GPIb complex) on the platelet membrane. This syndrome is characterized by thrombocytopenia, with giant platelets and markedly prolonged bleeding time.

Glanzmann thrombasthenia an autosomal recessive disorder is characterized by normal platelet count, platelets with normal size and morphology and prolonged bleeding time. The disorder is caused by deficiency of platelet fibrinogen receptor GPIIb-IIIa, an integrin complex on the platelet surface that undergoes conformational changes when platelets are activated. Fibrinogen binds to this complex when the platelet is activated and causes platelets to aggregate. Aggregation studies show abnormal or absent aggregation with all agonists used except ristocetin.

Other hereditary disorders of platelet function: Abnormalities in the pathways of platelet activation and release of granular contents cause a heterogeneous group of platelet function defects that are usually manifested as increased bruising, epistaxis, and/or menorrhagia. Bleeding time is variable and closure time as measured by the PFA-100 is frequently, but not always prolonged. Platelet aggregation studies show deficient aggregation with 1 or 2 agonists and/or abnormal release of granular contents.

Treatment of platelet function defects: In all but severe platelet function defects desmopressin 0.3 µg/kg IV may be used for mild to moderate bleeding disorders. In addition to its effect on stimulating levels of vWD and factor VIII, desmopressin corrects bleeding time and provides normal hemostasis in many individuals with mild to moderate platelet function defects. For individuals with Bernard-Soulier syndrome and Glanzmann thrombasthenia, platelet transfusions of 1 U/5–10 kg corrects the defect in hemostasis and may be lifesaving.

Disorders of the Blood Vessels

Henoch- Schönlein purpura (HSP) is characterized by the sudden development of a purpuric rash, arthritis, abdominal pain, and renal involvement. The characteristic rash consisting of petechiae and often palpable purpura, usually involves the lower extremities and buttocks (*see* Section 12.12). Results of coagulation studies and platelet count are normal. The pathologic studies in the skin, intestines, and synovium are leukocytoclastic angitis, inflammatory damage to the endothelium of the capillary and postcapillary venules mediated by WBCs and macrophages. The trigger for HSP is unknown. In the kidney, the lesion is focal glomerulonephritis with deposition of immunoglobulin A.

Ehlers-Danlos syndrome is a common disorder of collagen structure that causes easy bruising and poor wound healing. The characteristic physical findings include soft, velvety skin that is hyperelastic; lax joints that are easily subluxed; and unusual scarring. Results of coagulation screening studies are usually normal, although bleeding time may be mildly increased. Results of platelet aggregation studies are either normal or mildly abnormal.

Acquired disorders such as scurvy, chronic corticosteroid therapy, and severe malnutrition are associated with "weakening" of the collagen matrix that supports the blood vessels. Therefore, these factors are associated with easy bruising, and particularly in the case of scurvy, bleeding gums and loosening of the teeth. Petechiae and purpura may be seen in vasculitis syndrome such as SLE on the skin.

Blanchette V. Childhood chronic immune thrombocytopenic purpura (ITP). *Blood Rev* 2002;16:23–26.

Kokame K, Miyata T. Genetic defects leading to hereditary thrombotic thrombocytopenic purpura. *Semin Hematol* 2004; 41:34–40.

Ramasamy I. Inherited bleeding disorders: Disorders of platelet adhesion and aggregation. *Crit Rev Oncol Hematol* 2004; 49: 1–35.

Roberts I, Murray NA. Neonatal thrombocytopenia: Causes and management. *Arch Dis Child Fetal Neonatal Ed* 2003;88: F359–64.

Scot JP, Montgomery RR. Hemorrhagic and thrombotic diseases. In: Kliegman RM, Behrman RE, Jenson HB, Stanton BF (eds). *Nelson Textbook of Pediatrics.* 18th edn. Vol. 2. Philadelphia: Saunders, 2007;2060–6.

20.9 BLOOD TRANSFUSION

Blood transfusions often are needed for trauma victims due to accidents and burns, heart surgery, organ transplants, intensive care of premature neonates, and patients receiving treatment for leukemia, cancer or other diseases such as sickle cell disease and thalassemia.

Typically, each donated unit of blood, referred to as whole blood is separated into multiple components such as red blood cells, plasma, platelets, and cryoprecipitated AHF (antihemophilic factor).

Patients scheduled for surgery may be eligible to donate blood for themselves, a process known as **autologous** blood donation. In the weeks before non-emergency surgery, an autologous donor may be able to donate blood that will be stored until the surgical procedure.

In an emergency, any individual can receive type O red blood cells, and type AB individuals can receive red blood cells of any ABO blood group type. Therefore, people with type O blood group are known as "universal donors," and those with type AB blood group are known as "universal recipients." In addition, AB plasma donors can donate to all blood types.

Although donated blood is free but there are significant costs associated with collecting, testing, preparing components, labeling, storing and transporting blood as well as recruiting and educating donors and quality assurance. As a result, processing fees are charged to recover costs. Processing fees for individual blood components vary considerably.

1. Whole Blood and Whole Blood Components

Description: Whole blood contains the red blood cells and plasma components of donor blood. Most of the platelets and/or white blood cells may have been

Box 20.6: Guidelines for pediatric RBC transfusions

Children and adolescents
Acute loss > 25% circulating blood volume (i.e., > 17 ml/kg body weight)
Hemoglobin < 8.0 g/dl* in perioperative period
Hemoglobin < 13.0 g/dl and severe cardiopulmonary disease
Hemoglobin < 8.0 g/dl and symptomatic chronic anemia
Hemoglobin < 8.0 g/dl and marrow failure

Infants within first 4 months of life
Hemoglobin < 13.0 g/dl and severe pulmonary disease
Hemoglobin < 10.0 g/dl and moderate pulmonary disease
Hemoglobin < 13.0 g/dl and severe cardiac disease
Hemoglobin < 10.0 g/dl and major surgery
Hemoglobin < 8.0 g/dl and symptomatic anemia

*Hematocrit estimated by Hb g/dl × 3.

removed during processing; those remaining in stored blood are usually nonviable after a few days.

Actions: Whole blood provides oxygen to tissues through RBCs. It is also a blood volume expander and source of proteins and certain coagulation factors.

Indications: Whole blood is indicated only for those patients who have a symptomatic deficit of oxygen carrying capacity combined with hypovolemia of sufficient degree to be associated with shock. If only the former is present, the component of choice is RBCs. Whole blood, less than 7 days old may be used for exchange transfusion. Whole blood cannot be considered a source of viable platelets or white cells or of therapeutic levels of labile coagulation factors V and VIII.

Contraindications: Do not use whole blood or other RBC components if anemia can be treated with specific medications such as iron, vitamin B_{12}, recombinant erythropoietin or folic acid, and if the clinical condition of the patient permits sufficient time for these agents to promote erythropoiesis. Do not use whole blood when blood volume can be safely and adequately replaced with other volume expanders such as 0.9% sodium chloride, lactated Ringer's; albumin; or plasma protein fraction. Do not use whole blood to correct coagulation deficiencies when they can be treated better by appropriate components and derivatives.

Side effects and hazards: See Box 20.10.

Dosage and administration: The usual dose of whole blood is 10–15 ml/kg, but transfusion volumes vary greatly depending on clinical circumstances (e.g. continued vs arrested bleeding, hemolysis, etc) (Box 20.6).

Exchange blood transfusion: Blood for exchange transfusion should be as fresh as possible. Heparin or adenosine-citrate-phosphate-dextrose may be used as an anticoagulant. If the blood is obtained before delivery, it should be taken from a type O, Rh negative donor with a low titer of anti-A and anti-B and should be compatible with the mother's serum by indirect Coombs' test. After delivery, blood should be obtained from an Rh negative donor whose cells are compatible with both the infant's and the mother's serum; when possible, type O donor cells are usually used, but cells of the infant's ABO blood type may be used when the mother has the same type. A complete cross-match, including indirect Coombs' test should be performed before the second and subsequent transfusions.

Using strict aseptic technique, the umbilical vein is cannulated with a polyvinyl catheter to distance no greater than 7 cm in a full-term infant. Alternatively, the exchange may be performed through placement of peripheral arterial and venous lines. Exchange should be carried out over a 45-to 60-minute period, alternating aspirations of 20 ml of infant blood and infusions of 20 ml of donor blood. Smaller aliquots (5–10 ml) may be indicated for sick and preterm infants. The goal should be an isovolumetric exchange of approximately two blood volumes of the infant (2X 85 ml/kg).

2. Red Blood Cell Components
2a. Red Blood Cells

Description: Red blood cells are prepared by centrifugal or gravitational separation of the red cells from the plasma. The usual 300 cc unit has a hematocrit of 0.65–0.80 (65–80%).

Actions: This component increases the oxygen-carrying capacity of the blood by increasing the circulation red blood cell mass. If the patient is not bleeding, 1 unit of packed red blood cells should increase the patient's hemoglobin (Hg) 1 g/dl and increase the hematocrit (Hct) by 3%.

Indications: Red blood cells are the component of choice for virtually all patients with a symptomatic deficit of oxygen-carrying capacity. This component may be used for exchange transfusion and to help restore blood volume following significant hemorrhage. Hypovolemia without significant red cell mass deficit is best managed with other volume expanders. When used for exchange transfusions, red blood cells should be less than 7 days old.

Contraindications: Do not use red blood cells when anemia can be corrected with specific medications.

Side effects and hazards: See Box 20.10.

Dosage and administration: The dosage and administrations of red blood cells are similar to those for whole blood. Because of the minimal amounts of plasma and ABO alloantibodies, red blood cells can be used when compatible but not ABO identical. Immediately before infusion, 60–100 cc of 0.9% sodium chloride may be added to the unit of red blood cells. When diluted in this manner, the flow rate is approximately the same as for whole blood.

2b. Red Blood Cells, Leukocytes Removed (Washed RBCs)

Description: Red blood cells (or whole blood) may be modified by centrifugation, filtration, addition of sedimenting agents or a combination of these procedures to remove the leukocytes.

Action: The febrile condition results from a reaction to antigens on the WBC. The cytomegalovirus (CMV) is usually found in white cells. Leukocyte poor red cells are considered as CMV negative. Neonates should be given only CMV negative cells.

Indications: Washed RBCs may be desirable to reduce the risk of non-hemolytic, febrile transfusion reactions and are indicated for patients who have had febrile reactions following transfusions. Caution should be noted that all the filtration procedures still leave some leukocytes, they cannot be totally removed. Usually 70–80% are removed but some filters currently available can achieve significantly higher levels of leukocyte removal. When leukocytes are removed from the red blood cells by using a sedimenting agent, the laboratory will indicate which agent was used. This is because small amounts of the agent will remain in the red blood cell component and allergic reactions are possible. However, the known side effects of these agents are minor.

Dosage and administration: The dosage, administration, and hazards of this component is similar to those indicated for red blood cells.

3. Plasma Components

3a. Plasma and Liquid Plasma

Description: Plasma and liquid plasma consist of the anticoagulated clear portion of blood that is separated by centrifugation or sedimentation no later than 5 days after the expiry date of the whole blood. Plasma is stored frozen, while liquid plasma is refrigerated. These components generally contain between 180–300 cc of anticoagulated plasma, with the volume indicated on the label. Plasma can be prepared from whole blood.

Actions: Plasma and liquid plasma contain plasma proteins, including nonlabile clotting factors such as fibrinogen and factor IX.

Indications: This component may be indicated for the treatment of clotting factor deficiencies when no concentrates are otherwise available. Plasma may also be indicated when clotting factor concentrates are available, e.g. to keep the number of donor exposures to a minimum in a patient with a mild factor IX deficiency.

Contraindications: Do not use plasma and liquid plasma for the replacement of labile coagulation factors such as factors V and VIII. Do not use these components when blood volume can be safely and adequately replaced with other volume expanders such as 0.9% sodium chloride, lactated Ringer's, albumin, and plasma protein fraction.

Side effects and hazards: See Box 20.10.

Dosage and administration: Compatibility tests before transfusion is not necessary. Plasma should be ABO compatible with the recipient's red cells; Rh typing is not necessary. The volume transfused depends on the clinical situations and the patient's size, and may be guided by serial laboratory assays of coagulation function.

3b. Fresh Frozen Plasma

Description: Fresh frozen plasma (FFP) is separated and frozen within 8 hrs after collection of whole blood. A bag of FFP contains about 200 units of factor VIII plus the other labile plasma coagulation factor, factor V.

Action: In short, FFP contains water, electrolytes, proteins (principally albumin), globulin, and coagulation factors.

Indications: The use of FFP is limited. Widely used for temporary volume replacement in patients depleted of whole blood or colloids. Also in those who need replacement of labile plasma coagulation factors with simultaneous blood volume expansion. FFP is also indicated for patients with thrombotic thrombocytopenic purpura.

Contraindications: Do not use FFP when a coagulation problem can be corrected more effectively with other therapies such as vitamin K, cryoprecipitated antihemolytic factor, or antihemophilic factor VIII concentrates. Do not use FFP when blood volume can be safely replaced with other volume expanders like 0.9% sodium chloride, lactated Ringer's, albumin, and plasma protein fraction.

Side effects and hazards: See Box 20.10.

Dosage and administration: FFP should be used as soon as possible but no more than 24 hr after thawing (stored at 1–6°C). FFP may not be refrozen. For thawed blood components, it is important to communicate with the blood bank since there is a long time needed for preparation and a short shelf-life (Box 20.7).

4. Platelet Components

4a. Platelets, Pooled

Description: To obtain platelets (PLTs), whole blood is collected from donors, the plasma is separated from whole blood through the process of centrifugation, then the platelets are separated from the plasma through slow centrifugation. The plasma is not completely separated, therefore the collection of platelets is suspended in plasma. There may also be lymphocytes and red blood cells (which gives it a pink to salmon color) in the plasma suspension, depending on centrifugation speed. A unit of platelets contains no less than 5.5×10^{10} platelets in 40–70 ml of plasma if stored in 20–24°C or 20–30 ml if plasma is stored at 1–6°C. The volume should be indicated in the label. The label will also indicate the number of bags of platelets in the pool. The expiratory date is determined by the temperature in which it is stored and the type of container it is stored in.

Actions: Platelets (thrombocytes) are required for hemostasis. They take their action by occluding breaks in blood vessels to stop bleeding (coagulation). Platelet transfusion is used for treatment of severe decrease in platelet (PLT) production or abnormally functioning platelets that cannot prevent the escape of blood. Clotting factors V and VIII are bound to platelets. Variable amounts of these factors are contained in a unit of platelets.

Indications: Thrombocytopenic bleeding (bleeding due to low amounts of platelets because of abnormal production) or bleeding related to abnormal functions of platelets are the indications for infusions. Platelet infusion can be given as a prophylactic for low platelet counts resulting from 10×10^9/L (10,000–20,000/(L). In postoperative bleeding, a count of less than 50×10^9/L (50,000/(L) cancer or chemotherapy or postoperative bleeding. A low platelet count is considered less than is considered low.

Contraindications: Do not give platelets to patients with bleeding that is not associated with low count or abnormal platelet function. Do not use in patients with idiopathic thrombocytopenic purpura (ITP), in which there is endogenous platelet destruction, and drug-induced thrombocytopenia. For these patients, platelets are transfused only if they have a life-threatening bleeding.

Side effects and hazards: *See* Box 20.10.

Dosage/administration: It is not necessary to test compatibility. The plasma of the donor and red blood cells of the recipient should be ABO compatible. The number of bags administered is individualized by each patient's situation. The adult dose is usually 6 to 8 bags if the platelet count is lower than 20×10^9/L (20,000/L). Since platelets have only a lifespan of 3–4 days, it may be necessary to repeat this dose in 1–3 days (Box 20.8). An alternative way of calculating dosage is to infuse one unit of plasma per 10 kg of patient's weight. One bag of platelets should raise the platelet count to $5–12 \times 10^9$/L (5,000–12,000/L) in a 70 kg adult. It should raise the platelet count to 20×10^9 (20,000/L) in an 18 kg child. Transfusion time should not be more than 4 hr and transfusion can proceed as fast as patient can tolerate. Concentration of platelets may be done right before infusion and should be administered one by one using special administration sets. Flush the container and filter per hospital protocol or manufacturer's recommendations. The container filter may be flushed with 0.9% sodium chloride. Monitor for refractory reactions. A count of less than 2.5×10^9/L/M^2 (2500/(L/M^2) may mean that there is refractory reaction from unmatched donors. This can be done by platelet count in 1 to 2 hr after infusion.

Nursing implications: Watch patient for side effects. As ordered by physician, premedicate with antihistaminics and antipyretics if the patient has a history of transfusion reaction. Avoid administering platelets if the patient has fever because the platelets will be rapidly destroyed. Follow the manufacturer's instructions or hospital protocol for administration.

4b. Platelet Apheresis

Description: It is the same process as used to obtain pooled platelets except that the platelets are obtained from one donor and once the platelets are separated the remainder of plasma is transfused back to the donor. This concentration should have a content of at least 3×10^{11} platelets and the plasma volume is between 200 and 500 ml. This comes in a large plastic pack or in two connected packs; this increases the life of the platelet by providing a greater surface area for gas exchange. Anticoagulant solutions presently being used for preservation are ACD-A, ACD-B, and CPD and 2–3% sodium citrate. The label indicates the type, volume, and sedimentation agent (usually HES) contained in the bag.

Action: The action of these platelets is the same as pooled platelets.

Indications: This is used more on patients who has had refractory reaction to platelets from unmatched donors. In this case, a patient who is HLA-matched with a donor will receive these platelets since they are compatible.

Contraindications: These are the same as for pooled platelets.

Side effects and hazards: See Box 20.10.

Dosage and administration: This is similar to pooled platelets, except that only one bag is used. The volume of platelets in the plasma can be requested from the faculty collecting the platelet concentration or the manufacturer if not indicated on the label. When measured 10 minutes to an hour after infusion, the platelet count should be at least $30–60 \times 10^9$/L (30,000–60,000/(L) for a 70 kg adult. Compatibility testing must be done before transfusion if there appears to be a large amount of RBCs (giving it a red color) in the plasma.

Nursing implications: These are the same as mentioned for pooled platelets.

5. Autologous Blood Transfusion

Rationale for autologous blood transfusions: It is based on three assumptions:

1. RBC transfusions are needed (in some cases) during and after surgery
2. Autologous blood is safer than allogeneic blood, and
3. That it is possible for some patients to donate blood.

Methods of autologous transfusion

 i. Preoperative blood donation
 ii. Acute normovolaemic haemodilution
iii. Intraoperative blood salvage
iv. Postoperative blood salvage

i. Preoperative blood donation—prerequisites
- Realistic chance (> 50%) that blood transfusion will be needed
- Realistic chance that at least 2 units of blood will be required
- More than 4 units will not be required
- Adequate time to collect the units required
- Patient fit to donate

Preoperative blood donation
- Planning, co-ordination and consent
- Fitness to donate
- Allow 3 to 7 days between collections
- A minimum of 3 days between last collection and surgery
- Iron supplements—before, during and after
- Blood grouping serology and infectious disease screening
- Labeling and storage
- Cross-match before issue
- Release for general issue?

ii. Acute normovolaemic haemodilution
Consider
- Surgical blood loss is expected to be more than 20% of blood volume or 1 L
- Hemoglobin is greater than 10 g/dl
- No significant heart disease

Advantages
- Red cell loss reduced
- Improved tissue oxygenation due to reduced viscosity
- No testing needed
- Risk of incompatible transfusion due to clerical errors reduced
- Risk of bacterial contamination reduced
- Time and money saved

Efficiency increases with
- Higher preoperative hematocrit
- Greater surgical blood loss
- Lower post-ANH hematocrit

iii. Intraoperative blood salvage
Requirements
- No malignant cells
- No bacteria
- No other contaminants (e.g. amniotic fluid)
- Cardiac, orthopedic or abdominal surgery

Techniques
- Direct transfusion after anticoagulation and filtration (e.g. Solcotrans)
- Transfusion after anticoagulation, filtration and washing (e.g. Hemonetics Cell-Saver)

Problems
- Transfusion of activated complement components and coagulation factors and hemolysed blood—

avoid high aspiration pressure and surface suctioning
* Air embolism

iv. Postoperative blood salvage
* From drainage tubes after cardiac and orthopedic surgery
* Defibrinogenated blood—does not require anticoagulation before transfusion.

Problems include: Hemolysed RBCs—renal failure; dilutional coagulopathy; RBC volume of the collected fluid is low—doubtful clinical benefit; cardiac enzymes may confuse picture after cardiac surgery.

Autologous Transfusions—Advantages and Disadvantages

* Prevents transfusion transmitted infections BUT does not prevent bacterial contamination of the unit
* Prevents RBC allo-immunization BUT does not eliminate ABO incompatibility due to administrative errors
* Supplements the blood supply BUT costs more
* Provides compatible blood for patients with allo-antibodies BUT results in the wastage of unused units
* Prevents some adverse transfusion reactions BUT causes peri-operative anaemia and the likelihood of transfusion
* Cost effectiveness of autologous transfusions will depend on the current perceived risks associated with autologous/allogeneic transfusions
* Other applications of autologous donations:
  i. Frozen RBCs—for patients with rare blood groups or those with allo-antibodies to high incidence antigens
  ii. Plasma
  iii. Cryoprecipitate; and
  iv. Hematopoietic stem cell
* Alternatives to transfusion including methods to improve O_2 supply relative to demand, crystalloids and colloids, colony stimulating factors (e.g. erythropoietin, G-CSF, etc.), stroma-free hemoglobin, and perfluorocarbons.

ABO Compatibility

Cryoprecipitate: No ABO or Rh typing needed. All can be pooled together.

Granulocyte: Because RBC contamination is often significant, the red donor cells should be ABO compatible with the recipients plasma. Please notice that the recipient/donor match is different between blood cells and plasma. This is really important. They are functionally the opposite (Box 20.9).

Table 20.8: Donor's blood cells should be ABO compatible	
Recipient	*Donor*
O	O
A	A, O
B	B, O
AB	AB, O, A, B

Blood cells: Donor's blood cells should be ABO compatible with the recipient's plasma (antibody) (Table 20.8).

If possible only give Rh negative to Rh negative. Never give Rh positive to a Rh negative young woman. For babies (up to 3 months) the donor's blood cells should be ABO compatible with the baby's mother's plasma because the baby has not produced her own antibodies yet. They still have the mother's antibodies. *For a baby and for emergency transfusions give O negative.

Fresh frozen plasma: The donor's plasma should be ABO compatible with the recipient's red cells (Table 20.9).

Specimens for crossmatching: For patients who have been, within the previous 3 months, pregnant or received transfusions, the sample used for compatibility testing should be no more than 2 days old. For all others, the sample must be no more than 7 days old. In a hospital setting this should not be a problem but in a rural clinic, it could present some difficulty if transportation of the sample to a blood typing center is deficient. Additionally, the sample should be whole blood and without hemolysis.

Prior to transfusion: Two qualified persons must check the component unit. One person reading the patient's arm band (and nothing else). The other person reading the invoice of the blood product. They must check the Medical ID Number, the name and the correct product.

Box 20.9: Guidelines for pediatric granulocyte transfusions

Children and adolescents
Neutrophils $<0.5 \times 10^9/L$ and bacterial infection unresponsive to appropriate antimicrobial therapy
Qualitative neutrophil defect and infection (bacterial or fungal) unresponsive to appropriate antimicrobial therapy

Infants within first 4 months of life
Neutrophils $<3.0 \times 10^9/L$ (1st wk of life) or $<1.0 \times 10^9/L$ (thereafter) and fulminant bacterial infection

---

*Usually there is no need to worry about Rh type unless the patient is a known anti-D, then give Rh negative to Rh negative.

Table 20.9: Donor's plasma should be ABO compatible

Recipient	Donor
O	O, AB, A, B
A	A, AB
B	B, AB
AB	AB

Always Transfuse Only One Patient at A Time

It is too easy to get two patients mixed up on a busy day. It could cost them their life. If there is any doubt whatsoever, get someone else to help or call the lab to verify.

Always give blood products one unit at a time unless in the emergency room where several units could be infused at once for severe volume depletion or profuse bleeding. Sign for only one unit at a time from the blood bank section of the laboratory if in a hospital setting. It sometimes takes several hours to infuse one unit. It only takes 10–20 minutes for bacteria to begin forming inside a bag sitting at room temperature. Nurses cannot store an extra unit in their medication refrigerator. Do not even think about this! It is not of the correct temperature or humidity. When one unit is completed or nearly completed then retrieve the next unit for multiple unit transfusions.

Nursing care should include careful monitoring of cardiac and pulmonary function along with amount of fluid intake and output in addition to complications (hazards) of blood transfusion (Box 20.10).

Blood Transfusion Guidelines for International Travelers

There is growing public awareness of the AIDS epidemic, and a concern about acquiring the AIDS virus through blood transfusions. Blood transfusion is not free of risk, even in the best of conditions. Therefore, blood should be transfused only when absolutely indicated. When urgent resuscitation is necessary, the use of plasma expanders rather than blood should always be considered. When blood transfusion cannot be avoided, the attending physician should make every effort to ensure that the blood has been screened for transmissible diseases, including HIV.

Points to be Remembered

1. We must promote the reasonable use of blood products (right indications, right dose, right time)
2. All transfusions, whether autologous or allogeneic pose hazards, but autologous transfusions may be a safer option in some situations
3. Follow blood transfusion guidelines for international travelers

Box 20.10: Hazards of blood transfusions

Immunological: Hemolytic transfusion reaction; febrile non-hemolytic transfusion reaction; hypersensitivity reactions esp. in IgA deficient patients; transfusion associated acute lung injury; transfusion associated graft-versus-host disease; allo-immunization to HLA antigens; post-transfusion purpura; refractoriness to platelet transfusions; immunomodulation

Nonimmunolgical: (i) Transfusion transmitted infections: Hepatitis B; hepatitis C; other hepatitis viruses; HIV I and II; HTLV I and II; cytomegalovirus; malaria; filariasis; leptospirosis; syphilis. (ii) other problems: Volume overload; iron overload; air embolism

4. If it is suspected that a transfusion reaction is occurring, the nurse should stop the transfusion and notify the doctor immediately. The following steps are taken so that a diagnosis may be made regarding the type and severity of the reaction:
5. The transfusion set is disconnected, but the IV line is kept open with a saline solution in case intravenous medication should be needed rapidly.
6. The blood component container and tubing are saved, not discarded. They should be sent to the blood bank for repeat typing and culture.
7. The patient's blood is drawn for plasma hemoglobin, culture, and retyping.
8. A urine sample is collected as soon as possible and sent to the laboratory for a hemoglobin determination. Subsequent voiding of urine should be observed.
9. The blood bank is notified that a suspected transfusion reaction has occurred.

Anderson KC, Ness PM (eds). Scientific Basis of Transfusion Medicine, Implications for Clinical Practice. Philadelphia: Saunders, 1999.

Dodd RY. The risk of transfusion-transmitted infection. New Engl J Med 1992;327:419–20.

Dzieczkowski JS, Anderson KC. Transfusion Biology and Therapy. In: Braunwald E, Fauci AS, Kasper DL, Hauser SL, Longo DL, Jameson JL (eds). *Harrison's Principles of Internal Medicine.* 15th edn. New York: McGraw-Hill, 2001;733–9.

Khare Vandana. Blood Transfusion. In: Mathur GP, Mathur Sarla (eds). *Current Trends in Pediatrics.* Vol 1. Delhi: Academa Publishers, 2005;332–44.

Saran RK, Makroo RN (eds). In: *Transfusion Medicine Technical Manual.* Sponsored by world Health Organization. Directorate General of Health services. New Delhi: ANB Communications Private Limited, 1991;1–295.

Smeltzer SC, Bare BG. Assessment and management of patients with hematologic disorders. In: Brunner and Suddarth (eds). *Textbook of Medical-Surgical Nursing.* 7th edn. Philadelphia: Lippincott, 1992;813–6.

Strauss RG. Blood component transfusions. In: Kliegman RM, Behrman RE, Jenson HB, Stanton BF (eds). *Nelson Textbook of Pediatrics.* 18th edn. Vol. 2. Philadelphia: Saunders, 2007;2055–60.

20.10 SPLEEN

The spleen performs reservoir, filtering, and immunologic functions. The spleen receives 5–6% of the cardiac output, but normally contains only 25 ml of blood. It can retain much more blood when it enlarges. Hematopoiesis is a major splenic function at 3–6 mo of fetal life, but then it disappears. Splenic hematopoiesis can be resumed in patients with severe hemolytic anemia or myelofibrosis. The spleen is the primary site for destruction of old RBCs; this function is assumed by other reticuloendothelial cells after splenectomy. Immunoglobulins are produced in the spleen. Nonimmune or hyposplenic individuals are at increased risk for sepsis caused by pneumococci and other encapsulated bacteria. The spleen can also use phagocytosis to trap and destroy intracellular parasites. The spleen may be an important site of antibody production in immune thrombocytopenic purpura.

Splenomegaly: A soft, thin spleen may be palpable in 15% of neonates, 10% of normal children, and 5% of adolescents. The spleen is increased 2–3 times from its normal size before it is palpable. Superficial abdominal venous distension may be present when splenomegaly is due to portal hypertension.

Common causes of splenomegaly (typhoid fever, malaria, kala-azar, military tuberculosis, infectious mononucleosis, congestive heart failure, cirrhosis or hepatic fibrosis, hepatic portal or splenic vein obstruction, hemolytic anemia, thalassemia, osteopetrosis, myelofibrosis, rheumatoid arthritis, SLE, leukemia, lymphoma) should be kept in mind before considering other causes such as storage diseases (Gaucher disease, Niemann-Pick disease, infantile GH1 gangliosidosis, Hurler, Hunter-type, galactosemia, fructose intolerance).

Hypersplenism: Increased splenic function (sequestration or destruction of circulating cells) results in peripheral blood cytopenia, increased bone marrow activity, and splenomegaly. It is usually secondary to another disease and may be cured by treating the underlying condition or, if absolutely necessary splenectomy should be performed.

Congestive splenomegaly (Banti syndrome): Splenomegaly may result from obstruction in the hepatic, portal, or splenic veins. Congenital abnormalities of the portal (absent or hypoplastic) or splenic veins may cause vascular obstruction. Wilson disease, galactosemia, biliary atresia, and α-antitrypsin deficiency may result in hepatic inflammation, fibrosis, and vascular obstruction. Septic omphalitis or thrombophlebitis may be spontaneous or may occur as a result of umbilical venous catheterization in neonates and may also result in secondary obliteration of these vessels. Splenic venous flow may be obstructed by masses of sickled erythrocytes. When the spleen is the site of vascular obstruction, splenectomy cures hypersplenism. If the obstruction is in the hepatic or portal system, portocaval shunting may be more helpful in these cases, because both portal hypertension and thrombocytopenia contribute to variceal bleeding.

Hyposplenism: Splenic hypofunction is characterized by RBC inclusions in peripheral blood smears, "pits" on interference microscopy, and poor uptake of technetium on spleen scan. Patients with functional hyposplenism or asplenia are at increased risk for sepsis from encapsulated bacteria. Congenital absence of spleen is associated with complex cyanotic heart defects, dextrocardia, bilateral trilobed lungs, and heterotopic abdominal organs (Ivemark syndrome). Splenic function is usually normal in children with congenital polysplenia. Functional hyposplenism may occur in normal neonates, especially premature infants, and in children with sickle cell hemoglobinopathies, malaria, after irradiation to the left upper quadrant, severe hemolytic anemia, metabolic storage disease, vasculitis, nephritis, inflammatory bowel disease, celiac disease, Pearson syndrome, Fanconi anemia and graft-vs-host disease.

Splenic trauma: Injuries to the spleen may occur with abdominal trauma. Small splenic capsular tears may cause abdominal or referral left shoulder pain as a result of peritoneal irritation by blood. Larger tears result in more severe blood loss, with similar pain and signs of hypovolemia. Enlarged spleen, especially due to infectious mononucleosis is more likely to rupture with minor trauma. CT scan with IV contrast is used to assess for splenic trauma. Treatment of a small capsular injury should include observation for vital signs, abdominal findings, and serial hemoglobin determinations and prompt surgical intervention should a patient's condition deteriorate. RBC transfusion requirements should be minimal (< 25 ml/kg/48 hr). These patients are usually hospitalized for 10–14 days and have their activities restricted for months. Laparatomy, with or without splenectomy, is indicated for more marked abdominal bleeding, in patients who have clinical instability, or deterioration, or when other organ damage is suspected. When feasible, partial splenectomy and splenic repair should be substituted for total splenectomy.

Splenectomy: The indications for splenectomy include traumatic splenic rupture, anatomic defects, severe hemolytic anemia, immune cytopenia, metabolic storage disease and secondary hypersplenism.

Splenectomy should be performed where medical therapy is (or has been) ineffective. The major long-term risk of splenectomy is sudden overwhelming bacterial infection (sepsis or meningitis), which is especially high in children less than 5 yr of age at the time of surgery. Encapsulated bacteria such as *Streptococcus pneumoniae*, (> 60% of cases), *Haemophilus influenzae*, and *Neisseria meningitidis* account for 80% of postsplenectomy sepsis. Pneumococcal, meningococcal, and *H. influenzae* vaccines given before splenectomy may reduce postsplenectomy sepsis. The efficacy of unconjugated vaccine is lower in children younger than 2 yr of age and in immunosuppressed patients. Febrile splenectomized patients should be treated promptly with an antibiotic. Cefotaxime (50 mg/kg q 8 hr) or vancomycin (10 mg/kg q 6 hr) to cover penicillin-resistant pneumococci is recommended, until specific antibiotic susceptibility is known. Splenectomized patients are also at increased risk for contracting protozoal infections such as malaria.

In patients with traumatic injury, splenic repair or partial splenectomy should be considered to preserve splenic function. Partial splenectomy or partial splenic embolization may be sufficient to ameliorate some forms of hemolytic anemia. Up to 50% of children whose spleen is removed because of trauma have spontaneous splenosis; surgical splenosis (distributing small pieces of spleen throughout the abdomen) may decrease the risk of sepsis in patients whose splenectomy is necessitated by trauma. But the splenic tissue that grows has inadequate function.

Prophylaxis with oral penicillin V (125 mg twice daily in children younger than 5 yr; 250 mg twice daily for children 5 yr or older) should be given for at least 2 yr after splenectomy (to at least 6 yr of age). Prophylaxis may be continued into adulthood for higher risk patients. Other postoperative measures include patient and family education, use of a medical information bracelet, prompt evaluation, and treatment of fevers.

Camitta BM. The spleen. In: Kliegman RM, Behrman RE, Jenson HB, Stanton BF (eds). *Nelson Textbook of Pediatrics*. 18th edn. Vol. 2. Philadelphia: Saunders, 2007;2089–92.

Castagnola E, Fioredda F. prevention of life-threatening infections due to encapsulated bacteria in children with hyposplenia or asplenia: A brief review of current recommendations for practical purposes. Eur J Haemotol 2003;71:319–26.

Subhasis RC, Rajiv C, Kumar SA, et al. Surgical treatment of massive splenomegaly and severe hypersplenism secondary to extrahepatic portal venous obstruction in children. Surg Today 2007;37:19–23.

Upadhyaya P. Conservative treatment of splenic trauma: History and current trends. Pediatr Surg Int 2003;19:617–27.

20.11 LYMPHATIC SYSTEM

The lymphatic system includes circulating lymphocytes, lymphatic vessels, lymph nodes, spleen, tonsils, adenoids, Peyer patches, and thymus. Lymph, an ultrafiltrate of blood is collected by lymphatic capillaries that are present in all organs except brain and the heart. During their course, the lymphatic vessels carry lymph to the lymph nodes. In the nodes, lymph is filtered through sinuses, where particulate matter and infectious organisms are phagocytosed, processed, and presented as antigens to surrounding lymphocytes. These actions stimulate antibody production, T cell responses, and cytokine secretion. The composition of lymph can vary with the site of lymph drainage. Lymph is usually clear, but drained from the intestinal tract may be milky (chylous) because of the presence of fats. The protein content is intermediate between that of exudates and that of transudate. The protein level may be increased with inflammation and in lymph drained from the liver or intestines. Lymph contains variable numbers of lymphocytes.

Abnormalities of the Lymphatic Vessels

Abnormalities of the lymph vessels include lymphangiectasia, lymphangiomas and cystic hygromas and lymphatic dysplasia includes lymphedema, chylous ascites, chylothorax, and lymphangiomas of the bone, lung, or other sites. Abnormalities of the lymph vessels may be congenital or acquired. Signs and symptoms may result from increased lymphatic tissue mass or from leakage of lymph. Lymphangiectasia is dilation of lymphatics, involves, the lung lymphatics (pulmonary lymphangiectasia) causes respiratory distress and the intestinal lymphatics causes hypoproteinemia and lymphocytopenia secondary to loss of lymph into the intestines. Lymphangiomas and cystic hygromas are lymphatic malformations or a mass of dilated lymphatics. Some of these lesions also have a hemangiomatous component. Lymphatic dysplasia includes lymphedema, chylous ascites, chylothorax, and lymphangiomas of the bone, lung, or other sites (*see* Fig. 20.28 in CD).

Lymphadenopathy

Most lymph nodes are not usually palpable in the newborn. With antigenic exposure, lymphoid tissue increases in volume so that the cervical, axillary, and inguinal nodes are often palpable in childhood. They are not considered enlarged until their diameter exceeds 1 cm for cervical and axillary nodes and 1.5 cm for inguinal nodes. Other lymph nodes usually not palpable are visualized with radiographs. Lymph node enlargement is caused by proliferation of normal lymphoid elements or by infiltration with malignant or phagocytic cells. In most patients, a careful history and complete physical examination suggest the proper diagnosis. Acutely infected nodes are usually tender there may also be erythema and warmth of the overlying skin. Fluctuance suggests abscess formation. Tuberculosis nodes may be matted. In cases of chronic lymphnoditis many of the above signs are absent. Tumor-bearing lymph nodes are usually firm and nontender, and may be matted or fixed to the skin or underlying structures. Generalized adenopathy (enlargement of > 2 noncontiguous node regions) is caused by systemic disease and is often accompanied by abnormal physical findings in other systems (Box 20.11). In contrast, regional adenopathy is most frequently the result of infection in the involved node and/or its drainage area (Box 20.12).

Treatment: Evaluation and treatment of lymphadenopathy is guided by the probable etiologic factor, as determined by the history and physical examination. The sizes of involved nodes should be documented before treatment. Failure to decrease in size within 10–14 days also suggests the need for further evaluation. This may include a complete blood count with differential; tuberculosis, Epstein-Barr virus, cytomegalovirus, Toxoplasma, and cat scratch disease titers; antistreptolysin O or anti-DNase serologic tests; tuberculin test; and chest radiograph. Biopsy should

---

Box 20.11: Causes of systemic generalized lymphadenopathy

Infants: Common causes: Syphilis; toxoplasmosis; CMV; HIV. Rare causes: Congenital tuberculosis; congenital leukemia; reticuloendotheliosis; lymphoproliferative disease; Chagas' disease (congenital); histiocytic disorders; metabolic storage disease

Children and adolescents: Common causes: Viral infections: EBV, CMV, HIV; tuberculosis; syphilis; toxoplasmosis. Rare causes: Serum sickness; SLE, RA; leukemia/lymphoma/Hodgkin disease; lymphoproliferative disease; histoplasmosis; sarcoidosis; fungal infection; plague; drug reaction

EBV: Ebstein-Barr virus; CMV: cytomegalovirus; HIV: human immunodeficiency virus; SLE: systemic lupus erythematosus; JRA: juvenile rheumatoid arthritis

Adapted with some modification from Kliegman RM, Greenbaum LA, Lye PS. Practical Strategies in Pediatric Diagnosis and Therapy. 2nd edn. Philadelphia: Elsevier, 2004; 864.

Box 20.12: Sites for local lymphadenopathy and associated diseases

Cervical: Oropharyngeal infection; scalp infection; mycobacterial lymphnoditis (tuberculosis and nontubercular mycobacteria); viral infection (EBV, CMV, HHV-6); cat-scratch disease; toxoplasmosis; Kawasaki disease; thyroid disease; Kikuchi disease; situs histiocytosis; autoimmune lymphoproliferative disease
Anterior auricular: Conjunctivitis; other eye infection; oculoglandular infections; facial cellulitis
Posterior auricular: Otitis media; viral infection (especially rubella, parvoinfection)
Submaxillary: Tuberculosis; Hodgkin and non-Hodgkin lymphoma; histoplasmosis
Supraclavicular: Infection or malignancy in the mediastinum (right); tuberculosis; metastatic malignancy from the abdomen (left); lymphoma
Epitrochlear: Hand and arm infection; lymphoma; sarcoid; syphilis
Inguinal: Urinary tract infection; venereal disease (especially syphilis, lymphogranuloma venereum); other perineal infection; infections of the leg, groin; plague
Popliteal: Knee joint, skin of the lateral lower leg and foot
Hilar (not palpable, found on chest radiograph or CT): Tuberculosis; histoplasmosis; blastomycosis; coccidioidomycosis; leukemia/lymphoma; Hodgkin disease; metastatic malignancy; sarcoidosis; Castleman disease
Axillary: Arm or chest wall infection; cat-scratch disease; malignancy of chest wall; leukemia/lymphoma; brucellosis
Abdominal (lymphadenopathy-unilateral or bilateral): Mesenteric adenitis (measles, tuberculosis, yersinia, Group A streptococci); malignancies

EBV: Ebstein-Barr virus; CMV: cytomegalovirus; HHV-6: human herpes virus-6; CT: computed tomography
Adapted with some modification from Kliegman RM, Greenbaum LA, Lye PS. Practical Strategies in Pediatric Diagnosis and Therapy. 2nd edn. Philadelphia: Elsevier, 2004; 863.

---

be considered if there is persistent or unexplained fever, weight loss, night sweats, hard nodes, or fixation of the nodes to surrounding tissues.

Camitta BM. The lymphatic system. In: Kliegman RM, Behrman RE, Jenson HB, Stanton BF (eds). *Nelson Textbook of Pediatrics.* 18th edn. Vol. 2. Philadelphia: Saunders, 2007; 2092–5.

Dispenzieri A, Gertz MA. Treatment of Castleman's disease. Curr Treat Options Oncol 2005;6:255–66.

Nield LS, Kamar D. Lymphadenopathy in children: When and how to evaluate. Clin Pediatr 2004;43:25–33.

Twist CJ, Link MP. Assessment of lymphadenopathy in children. Pediatr Clin North Am 2002;49:1009–25.

21 Nephrology

21.1 ANATOMY OF GLOMERULUS AND GLOMERULAR FILTRATION

Anatomy of Glomerulus

The kidneys lie in the retroperitoneal space slightly above the level of umbilicus. The range in length and weight respectively, from approximately 6 cm and 24 g in a full term newborn to 12 cm or more and 150 g in an adult. The kidney has an outer layer, the cortex, that contains glomeruli, proximal and distal convoluted tubules, and collecting ducts and an inner layer the medulla, that contains the straight portions the tubules, the loops of Henle, the vasa recta, and the terminal collecting ducts.

The blood supply of each kidney usually consists of a main renal artery that arises from the aorta; multiple renal arteries may occur. The main renal artery divides into segmental branches within the medulla and these into interlobar arteries that pass through the medulla to the junction of the cortex and medulla. At this point, the interlobar arteries branch to form the arcuate arteries, which run parallel to the surface of the kidney. Interlobular arteries originate from the arcuate arteries and give rise to the afferent arterioles of the glomeruli. Specialized muscle cells in the wall of the afferent arteriole and the macula densa within the distal tubule next to the glomerulus form the juxtaglomerular apparatus that controls the secretion of renin. The afferent arteriole divides into the glomerular capillary network, which then merges into the efferent arteriole. The efferent arterioles of glomeruli next to the medulla (juxtamedullary glomeruli) are larger than those in the outer cortex and provide the blood supply (vasa recta) to the tubules and medulla.

Each kidney contains approximately one million nephrons (glomeruli and associated tubules). In humans, formation of nephrons is complete at birth, but functional maturation with tubular growth and elongation continues during the first decade of life.

630

New nephrons cannot be formed after birth; therefore, progressive loss of nephrons may lead to renal insufficiency.

The glomerular network of specialized capillaries serves as the filtering mechanism of the kidney. The glomerular capillaries are lined by endothelial cells and have very thin cytoplasm that contains many holes (fenestrations). The glomerular basement membrane (GBM) forms a continuous layer between the endothelial and mesangial cells on one side and the epithelial cells on the other. The membrane has three layers: (i) a central electron-dense lamina densa; (ii) the lamina rara interna, which lies between the lamina densa and the endothelial cells; and (iii) the lamina rara externa, which lies between the lamina densa and epithelial cells. The visceral epithelial cells cover the capillary and project cytoplasmic "foot processes," which attach to the lamina rara externa. Between the foot processes are spaces or filtration slits. The mesangium (mesangial cells and matrix) lies between the glomerular capillaries on the endothelial cell side of the GBM and forms the medial part of the capillary wall. The mesangium may serve as a supporting structure for the glomerular capillaries and probably has a role in the regulation of glomerular blood flow and filtration and in the removal of macromolecules (such as immune complexes) from the glomerulus, either through intracellular phagocytosis or by transport through intercellulular channels to the juxtaglomerular region. Bowman's capsule, which surrounds the glomerulus, is composed of (i) a basement membrane, which is continuous with the basement membranes of the glomerular capillaries and the proximal tubules, and (ii) the parietal epithelial cells, which are continuous with the visceral epithelial cells.

Glomerular Filtration

As the blood passes through the glomerular capillaries, the plasma is filtered through the glomerular capillary walls. The ultrafiltrate, which is cell free, contains all the substances in the plasma (electrolytes, glucose, phosphate, urea, creatinine, peptides, low molecular weight proteins) except proteins (such as albumin and globulins) having a molecular weight of ≥ 68 kd. The filtrate is collected in Bowman's space and enters the tubules, where its composition is modified by solute and fluid secretion and absorption in accordance with rightly regulated tubular homeostatic mechanisms until it leaves the kidney as urine. Glomerular filtration begins around the 9th wk of fetal life, but it is the placenta that serves as the major fetal excretory organ. After birth, the glomerular filtration rate (GFR) increases until growth ceases toward the end of the second decade of life. The GFR is standardized to the surface area (1.73 m^2) of a 70 kg adult for comparing the GFR of a child. The GFR may be estimated by measurement of the serum creatinine level. Nowadays GFR is estimated by the clearance of endogenous creatinine because the inulin technique is cumbersome. The changes in renal function should be monitored by serum creatinine concentration when the serum creatinine level exceeds 2.0 mg/dL (180 μmol/L).

Davis ID, Avner ED. Glomerular disease. In: Kliegman RM, Behrman RE, Jenson HB, Stanton BF (eds). *Nelson Textbook of Pediatrics*. 18th edn. Vol. 2. Philadelphia: Saunders, 2007; 2163–2167.

Fogo A. Renal pathology. In: Avner ED, Harmon WE, Niaudet P (eds). *Pediatric Nephrology*, 5th edn. Baltimore: Lippincott Williams and Wilkins, 2004; 475–500.

Stevens LA, Corsh J, Greene T, Levey AS. Assessing kidney function- measured and estimated glomerular filtrate rate. *N Engl J Med* 2006; 354: 2473–2483.

21.2 CONDITIONS PARTICULARLY ASSOCIATED WITH HEMATURIA

Clinical Evaluation of the Child with Hematuria

Normal children may excrete 500,000 RBCs per 12hr.; this increases with fever and/or exercise. Microscopic analysis of 10–15 mL of freshly centrifuged urine is essential in confirming the diagnosis of hematuria. Evaluation of the child with hematuria begins with a detailed history, physical examination, and urinalysis. Red urine without RBCs is seen in a number of conditions listed in Box 21.1. Causes of hematuria in children are described in Box 21.2.

IgA Nephropathy (Berger Nephropathy)

IgA is the most common chronic glomerular disease worldwide. IgA nephropathy is an immune complex disease that appears to be caused by abnormalities in the IgA immune system. The linkage of IgA nephropathy is 6q22–23.

Pathology: Focal and segmental mesangial proliferation and increased mesangial matrix are seen in the glomerulus.

Box 21.1: Causes of red urine without RBCs

Heme-positive: Hemoglobin; Myoglobin
Heme-negative: (i) Drugs: Chloroquine; Deferoxamine; Ibuprofen; Iron sorbitol; Metronidazole; Nitrofurantoin; Phenazopyridine (pyridium); Phenolphthalein; Phenothiazines; Rifampin; Salicylates; Sulphasalazine. **(ii) Dyes (vegetables/fruits):** beets, black berries, food coloring. **(iii) Metabolites:** Homogentisic acid; Melanin; Methemoglobin; Porphyrin; Tyrosinosis; Urates.

Box 21.2: Causes of hematuria in children

Glomerular hematuria
Isolated renal disease: *IgA nephropathy; *Alport syndrome; *Thin glomerular basement membrane nephropathy; *Postinfectious glomerulonephritis; *Membranous nephropathy; *Membranoproliferative GN; *Focal segmental glomerulonephritis; Anti-glomerular basement membrane disease.
Multisystem diseases: *Systemic lupus erythematosus nephritis; *Henoch-Schönlein purpura nephritis; Wegener granulomatosis; Polyarteritis nodosa; Goodpasture syndrome; Hemolytic-uremic syndrome; Sickle cell glomerulopathy; HIV nephropathy.
Extraglomerular hematuria
Upper urinary tract: *Tubulointerstitial:* *Pyelonephritis, Interstitial nephritis, Acute tubular necrosis, Papillary necrosis, Nephrocalcinosis; *Vascular:* Arterial/venous thrombosis, Malformations (aneurysms, hemangiomas), Nutcracker syndrome; *Cystalluria:* Calcium, Oxalate, Uric acid ; *Hemoglobinopathy:* Sickle cell trait/disease, SC Hemoglobin; *Anatomic abnormalities:* Hydronephrosis, Cystic kidney disease, Polycystic disease, Multicystic dysplasia; *Tumor:* Wilms, rhabdomyosarcoma, angiomyolipoma; *Trauma*
Lower urinary tract: Inflammation (infectious and noninfectious): Cystitis, Urethritis; *Urolithiasis; *Trauma; *Coagulopathy; Heavy exercise; Munchausen/Munchausen by proxy syndrome.*

GN = glomerulonephritis; *Common causes of gross hematuria

Clinical manifestations: More often seen in males than in females. A majority of children present with gross hematuria, whereas microscopic hematuria and/or proteinuria is a more common presentation. Other types of presentation include acute nephritic syndrome, nephrotic syndrome or a combined nephritic-nephrotic syndrome. Mild to moderate hypertension is most often seen in patients with nephritic or nephrotic syndrome.

Laboratory diagnosis: Normal serum levels of C3 in IgA nephropathy help to distinguish this disorder from poststreptococcal glomerulonephritis. Serum IgA levels have no diagnostic value, because they are elevated in only 15% of patients.

Treatment: The treatment includes proper blood pressure control, use of fish oil (contains omega-3, decreases the rate of renal progression), and immunosuppressive therapy with alternate-day corticosteroids or more intensive multidrug regimens may be beneficial in some patients. Angiotensin-converting enzyme inhibitors and angiotensin II receptor antagonists are effective in reducing proteinuria and retarding the rate of renal progression when used as single agents or in combination. Tonsillectomy may reduce the frequency of gross hematuria and the rate of renal disease progression.

Prognosis: IgA nephropathy does not lead to significant kidney damage in most children; progressive disease develops in 20–30% of children in 15–20 yr after disease onset.

Alport Syndrome (AS)

AS is a hereditary nephritis disease. Approximately 85% of patients have X-linked disease and the rest are autosomal recessive (10%) and autosomal dominant (5%) form.

Pathology: Kidney biopsy specimens during the 1st decade of life may show a few changes, latter, the glomeruli may develop mesangial proliferation and capillary wall thickening, leading to progressive glomerular sclerosis, and tubular atrophy, interstitial inflammation and fibrosis and foam cells.

Clinical manifestations: AS children have asymptomatic microscopic hematuria, which may be intermittent in girls and younger boys, or single or recurrent episodes of gross hematuria commonly occurring 1–2 days after an upper respiratory infection. Proteinuria is frequently seen in males but may be absent, mild, or intermittent in females. Progressive proteinuria, often exceeding 1 g/24 hr is common in 2nd decade of life and can be severe enough to cause nephrotic syndrome. In addition to renal manifestations, extrarenal manifestations include hearing defects, ocular abnormalities, leiomyomatosis of the esophagus, tracheobronchial tree, and female genitals and platelet abnormalities.

Diagnosis: A family history, a screening urinalysis of first-degree relatives, an audiogram, and an ophthalmologic examination are helpful in the diagnosis of AS. The presence of anterior lenticonus (extrusion of the central portion of the lens into the anterior chamber) is pathognomic. Prenatal diagnosis is available for families with X-linked AS individuals, who carry an identified mutation.

Treatment: No specific therapy is available to treat AS, although some studies suggest that cyclosporine and angiotensin-converting enzyme inhibitors may slow the rate of renal progression.

Prognosis: The risk of progressive renal dysfunction leading to renal end disease (ESRD) is highest among hemizygotes and autosomal recessive homozygotes.

Risk factors for progression are gross hematuria during childhood, nephrotic syndrome, and prominent GBM thickening.

Acute Poststreptococcal Glomerulonephritis

Etiology: Acute poststreptococcal glomerulonephritis follows infection of the throat or skin by certain "nephritogenic" strains of group A β-hemolytic streptococci. Poststreptococcal glomerulonephritis commonly follows streptococcal pharyngitis during cold weather months with serotype 12, and streptococcal skin infections or pyoderma, during warm weather months with serotype 49.

Pathology: The kidneys appear symmetrically enlarged. All glomeruli appear enlarged and relatively bloodless and show diffuse mesangial cell proliferation with an increase in mesangial matrix. Polymorphonuclear leukocytes are common in glomeruli during the early disease and crescents and interstitial inflammation may be seen in severe cases. Immunofluorescence microscopy reveals lumpy-bumpy deposits of immunoglobulin and complement on the glomerular basement membrane (GBM) and in the mesangium. On electron microscopy, electron-dense deposits, or "humps," are observed on the epithelial side of the GBM.

Pathogenesis: The morphologic studies and a depression in the serum complement (C3) level strongly suggest that poststreptococcal glomerulonephritis is mediated by immune complexes, but the precise mechanisms by which nephritogenic streptococci induce complex formation remain to be determined.

Clinical manifestations: Poststreptococcal glomerulonephritis is most common in children aged 5–12 yr and uncommon before the age of 3 yr. Acute poststreptococcal glomerulonephritis is characterized by the sudden onset of gross hematuria, edema, hypertension, and renal insufficiency. This is a classic example of acute nephritic syndrome. Acute nephritic syndrome develops 1–2 wk after an antecedent streptococcal pharyngitis or 3–6 wk after a streptococcal pyoderma. Patients may develop encephalopathy and/or heart failure owing to hypertension or hypervolemia. Encephalopathy may also result from the direct toxic effects of streptococcal bacteria on the central nervous system. Edema results from salt and water retention. The acute phase generally resolves within 6–8 wk, although urinary protein excretion and hypertension usually normalize by 4–6 wk after onset, persistent microscopic hematuria may persist for 1–2 yr after the initial presentation.

Diagnosis: Urine examination demonstrates red blood cells, (frequently RBC casts), proteinuria, and polymorphonuclear leukocytes. The serum C3 is usually reduced in the acute phase and returns to normal 6–8 wk after onset. A mild normochromic anemia may be present from hemodilution and mild hemolysis. Confirmation of the diagnosis requires evidence of invasive streptococcal infection such as a positive throat culture report (may simply represent the carrier state), and a rising antibody titer to streptococcal antigen(s) confirms a recent streptococcal infection. The antisteptolysin O (ASO) titer is commonly elevated after a pharyngeal infection but rarely increases after streptococcal skin infections; for streptococcal skin infection the best single test is antideoxyribonuclease (DNase) B level. The streptozyme test is a diagnostic test that detects antibodies to streptolysin O, DNase B, hyaluronidase, streptokinase and nicotinamide-adenine dinucleotidase using a slide agglutination test. The clinical diagnosis of poststreptococcal glomerulonephritis is quite likely in a child presenting with acute nephritic syndrome, evidence of recent streptococcal infection, and a low C3 level. Renal biopsy should be considered only in the presence of acute renal failure, nephrotic syndrome, absence of evidence of streptococcal infection, or normal complement level and when hematuria and proteinuria, diminished renal function, and/or a low C3 level persist more than 2 month after onset.

Differential diagnosis: The differential diagnosis of poststreptococcal glomerulonephritis includes many causes listed in Box 21.2. Acute glomerulonephritis may occur due to coagulase-positive and coagulase-negative staphylococci, *Streptococcus pneumoniae*, gram-negative bacteria, bacterial endocarditis, fungal, rickettsial, and viral disease, particularly influenza.

Complications: Acute complications of this disease result from hypertension and acute renal dysfunction. Other potential complications include heart failure, hyperkalemia, hyperphosphatemia, hypocalcemia, acidosis, seizures, and uremia.

Prevention: Early systemic antibiotic therapy for streptococcal sore throat and skin infections does not eliminate the risk of glomerulonephritis. Family members of patients with acute glomerulonephritis should be cultured for group A β-hemolytic streptococci and treated if culture is positive.

Treatment: The patient should be managed for the acute effects of renal insufficiency and hypertension. Sodium restriction, diuresis with frusemide, and calcium channel antagonists, vasodilators, or angiotensin converting enzyme (ACE) inhibitors are used to treat hypertension. A ten-day course of systemic antibiotic therapy with penicillin is recommended to limit the spread of the nephritogenic organisms, but antibiotic therapy does not affect the natural history of glomerulonephritis.

Prognosis: In more than 95% of children with acute poststreptococcal glomerulonephritis there is complete recovery. Recurrences are extremely rare. Mortality in the acute phase can be avoided by appropriate management of acute renal failure, cardiac failure, and hypertension. Infrequently acute phase may be severe and lead to glomerular hyalinization and chronic kidney disease.

Other Chronic Infections

Glomerulonephritis has been recognized during the course of various chronic infections, including bacterial endocarditis caused by viridans streptococcus and other organisms, ventrioatrial shunts for hydrocephalus infected with *Staphylococcus epidermidis*, syphilis, hepatitis B virus, hepatitis C virus, candidiasis, and parasitic infections including malaria, schistosomiasis, leishmaniasis, filariasis, hydatid disease, trypanosomiasis, and toxoplasmosis. In each condition, the infective organism has low virulence and the host is chronically infected with foreign antigen. In the presence of high levels of circulating antigen, the host's antibody response leads to formation of immune complexes that deposit into kidneys and initiate glomerular inflammation.

The histologic findings may resemble poststreptococcal, membranous or membranoproliferative glomerulonephritis. The clinical manifestations are generally those of an acute nephritic or nephrotic syndrome. The complement C3 level is frequently depressed. Eradication of the infection before severe glomerular injury occurs usually results in resolution of the glomerulonephritis. Progression to end-stage renal failure is uncommon.

Membranous Glomerulopathy (Glomerulonephritis)

Membranous glomerulopathy typically presents as an isolated renal disease, but it may be associated with systemic illnesses, including autoimmune diseases such as SLE or chronic immune thrombocytopenic purpura, sarcoidosis, neuroblastoma, gonadoblastoma, gold or penicillamine therapy, syphilis, hepatitis B and C virus infections.

Pathology: The glomeruli show diffuse thickening of the glomerular basement membrane (GBM), without significant proliferative changes. Morphologic studies suggest that membranous glomerulopathy is an immune complex-mediated disease.

Clinical manifestations: Membranous nephropathy is most common in the 2nd decade of life. The disease usually presents as nephrotic syndrome and accounts for 2–6% of childhood nephrotic syndrome cases. Most patients have microscopic hematuria and occasionally demonstrate gross hematuria. Approximately 20% patients present with hypertension. C3 levels are normal except in cases of SLE, in which levels may be depressed.

Diagnosis: The diagnosis of membranous nephropathy is confirmed only by kidney biopsy. The indications for biopsy include the presentation of nephrotic syndrome in a child, usually older than 10 yr, or the presence of unexplained hematuria and proteinuria.

Treatment: The nephrotic syndrome is controlled with salt restriction and diuretic agents. Proteinuria may be decreased by ACE inhibitors or angiotensin II receptor antagonists (alone or in combination), immunosuppressive therapy with prednisolone in conjunction with chlorambucil or cyclophosphamide may be beneficial in adults in slowing the rate of progressive renal disease, particularly in patients, with severe or prolonged proteinuria, renal insufficiency or hypertension, but there is no controlled data on the use of these agents in children. Rituximab has been effective therapy in a small number of adult patients.

Prognosis: Children presenting with asymptomatic low-grade proteinuria may achieve a spontaneous remission. 20% of children progress to chronic renal disease, whereas 40% continue with active disease Identification of the secondary causes of membranous glomerulopathy is important because treatment of these diseases may lead to resolution of the glomerular lesions. Patients with membranous glomerulopathy are at an increased risk of renal vein thrombosis.

Membranoproliferative (Mesangiocapillary) Glomerulonephritis

Clinical manifestations: Membranoproliferative glomerulonephritis (MPGN) is the most common cause of chronic glomerulonephritis in older children and young adults.

Majority of patients present with nephrotic syndrome, others present with an acute nephritic syndrome characterized by gross hematuria or asymptomatic microscopic hematuria and proteinuria. Renal function may be normal or decreased. Hypertension is common. The serum C3 complement level may be decreased.

Diagnosis and differential diagnosis: The diagnosis MPGN is made by renal biopsy. The indications for biopsy include nephrotic syndrome in a child, usually older than 10 yr, with significant proteinuria, microscopic hematuria, and hypocomplementemia lasting longer than 8 wk in a child with acute nephritis. Both MPGN and poststreptococcal glomerulonephritis may be associated with gross hematuria, hypertension, low C3 levels, and elevated antistreptococcal antibody titers. Patients with poststreptococcal glomerulonephritis improve within 2 months of onset, whereas clinical manifestations persist in patients with MPGN.

Treatment: No definitive therapy exists, although stabilization of the clinical course has been reported in patients receiving 3–7 yr of alternate-day prednisolone therapy.

Prognosis: Although some patients recover completely, approximately 50% of patients with MPGN progress to end-stage renal disease 10 yr after their initial presentation.

Glomerulonephritis Associated with Systemic Lupus Erythematosus

Kidney disease, one of the most common features of systemic lupus erythematosus (SLE) in childhood, may occasionally be the only manifestation. The World Health Organization (WHO) has classified lupus nephritis into 5 classes: class I—no histologic abnormalities; class II—mesangial lupus nephritis, mild (class II A) or moderate mesangial hypercellularity and increased matrix (class II B); class III—focal segmental lupus glomerulonephritis; class IV—diffuse proliferative lupus nephritis; and class V—membranous lupus nephritis. Transformation of the histologic lesion from one class to another is common.

Clinical manifestations: The majority of children with SLE are adolescent females. Clinical evidence of renal disease occurs in 30–70% of children. The clinical findings having the mild forms (all class II, some class III) of lupus nephritis include hematuria, proteinuria of < 1g/24 hr, and normal renal function. Some patients with class III and all patients with class IV nephritis have hematuria and proteinuria, reduced renal function, nephritic syndrome or acute renal failure. Patients with class V nephritis commonly present with nephrotic syndrome.

Diagnosis: The diagnosis of SLE is suggested by the detection of circulating antinuclear antibodies. In most patients with active disease, C3 and C4 levels are depressed. Renal biopsy should be performed in all cases and the results are used to guide the selection of immunosuppressive therapies.

Treatment: Therapy is initiated in all patients with prednisolone at a dose of 1–2 mg/kg/day divided into 2 or 3 doses followed by slow steroid taper over 4–6 months beginning 4–6 wk after achieving a serologic remission, defined as normalization of anti-DNA, C3, and C4 levels. For patients with WHO classes III and IV, 6 consecutive monthly intravenous infusions of cyclophosphamide at a dose of 500–1,000 mg/m^2 followed by dosing every 3 mo for 18 mo appears to reduce the risk of progressive renal dysfunction. With WHO class I and II lupus nephritis azathioprine at a single daily dose of 1.5–2 mg/kg may be used as a steroid-sparing agent. Rituximab, a chimeric monoclonal antibody and mycophenolate mofetil have been used with beneficial effect in some cases.

Prognosis: Aggressive immunosuppressive therapy improves the prognosis of SLE in childhood. Patients with WHO class IV lupus nephritis exhibit the highest risk for progression to end-stage renal disease.

Henoch-Schönlein Purpura Nephritis

Henoch-Schönlein purpura (HSP) nephritis (anaphylactoid purpura) is small vessel vasculitis characterized by a purpuric rash, arthritis, abdominal pain, and glomerulonephritis (*see* Section 12.12). HSP nephritis and IgA nephropathy demonstrate identical renal pathologic findings, but systemic findings are only seen in HSP nephritis. The symptoms and signs of HSP nephritis typically appear 1–3 wk after an upper respiratory tract infection. Renal manifestations of HSP nephritis occur up to 12 wk after the initial presentation of HSP. Patients may present with microscopic hematuria, hematuria, hematuria and proteinuria, acute nephritic syndrome, nephrotic syndrome, and acute renal insufficiency are less common. The prognosis in HSP nephritis is generally favorable.

Rapidly Progressive (Crescentic) Glomerulonephritis

The clinical course of several forms of glomerulonephritis (GN) is rapidly progressive whose common abnormality is the histopathologic finding of crescents in the majority of the glomeruli. Crescents may be found in several well-defined types of GN including(1) the immune complex-mediated forms of GN: poststreptococcal GN, lupus nephritis, membranoproliferative GN, and Henoch-Schönlein purpura/IgA nephritis; (2) anti-glomerular basement membrane-mediated GN such as Goodpasture disease; and (3) antineutrophil cytoplasmic antibody (ANCA)-mediated GN; microscopic polyarteritis nodosa and Wegener granulomatosis. Most patients develop acute renal failure associated with acute nephritic and/or nephrotic syndrome. Progression to end-stage renal failure usually occurs within weeks to months after onset. The diagnosis is confirmed by kidney biopsy.

Goodpasture Disease

Goodpasture disease is characterized by pulmonary hemorrhage and glomerulonephritis associated with antibodies. Patients usually present with hemoptysis associated with pulmonary hemorrhage. Renal manifestations include acute nephritic syndrome with hematuria, proteinuria, and hypertension. Progressive renal dysfunction occurs within days to weeks. The serum complement C3 level is normal.

The diagnosis is suggested by kidney biopsy. The changes on light microscopy resemble those of rapidly progressive glomerulonephritis. Patients who survive pulmonary hemorrhage commonly progress to end-stage renal failure. Rates of survival and recovery of renal function have improved with pulse methyl prednisolone, oral cyclophosphamide, and plasma-pheresis therapy.

Hemolytic–Uremic Syndrome

Etiology: Acute enteritis with diarrhea caused by Shiga-like toxin-producing *Escherichia coli* 0157 : H7 precedes 80% or more of hemolytic–uremic syndrome (HUS) cases in developed countries. The organism produces a Shiga-like verotoxin that is absorbed from the intestines and initiates endothelial cell injury. HUS is also associated with Shigella and less commonly with other bacterial (*Salmonella, Compylobacter, Streptococcus pneumoniae, Bartonella*) and viral (coxsackievirus, echovirus, influenza, varicella, HIV, Epstein-Barr) infections. HUS may also develop with the use of oral contraceptives, mitomycin, cyclosporine.

Pathology: Initial glomerular changes include thickening of the capillary walls, narrowing of the capillary lumens, and widening of the mesangium. These changes take place as a result of subendothelial and mesangial deposition of a granular, amorphous material of unknown origin. Fibrin thrombi can be found in glomerular capillaries and arterioles and may lead to cortical necrosis. Severely involved glomeruli progress to partial or total sclerosis.

Clinical manifestations: It is characterized by the triad of microangiopathic hemolytic anemia, thrombocy-topenia, and uremia. HUS is most common in children younger than 4 yr of age. The onset is usually preceded by a gastroenteritis characterized by fever, vomiting, abdominal pain, and diarrhea that is initially watery but then becomes bloody. Less commonly, patients may present after an upper respiratory tract infection. Sudden onset of pallor, irritability, weakness, lethargy, and oliguria usually occurs 5–10 days after the initial gastrointestinal or respiratory illness. Physical examination may reveal dehydration, edema, petec-hiae, hepatosplenomegaly, and marked irritability.

Diagnosis and differential diagnosis: The diagnosis is supported by the findings of a microangiopathic hemolytic anemia, thrombocytopenia, and acute renal failure. The hemoglobin value varies from 5–9 g/dl; blood peripheral smear reveals helmet cells, burr cells, and fragmented RBCs; reticulocytes moderately elevated, and the Coombs' test result is negative; leukocytosis; and thrmbocytopenia (20,000–100,000/mm³). Urinalysis consists of microscopic hematuria and proteinuria. Renal manifestations vary from mild renal insufficiency to acute oliguria or anuric renal failure requiring dialysis. HUS should always be considered in the child with a sudden onset of acute renal failure. Other causes of acute renal failure should be excluded.

Complications: Complications include anemia, acidosis, hyperkalemia, fluid overload, heart failure, hypertension, and uremia. Extrarenal complications of CNS, GIT, heart, and skeletal muscles may be life threatening.

Treatment: The treatment includes administration of fluid and electrolytes, control of hypertension, nutrition, and early institution of dialysis. Antibiotics should be avoided in patients with acute enteritis secondary to *E. coli* 0157:H7 as they may increase of developing HUS. Peritoneal dialysis controls fluid and electrolyte abnormalities, maintains a normal intravascular volume and provides opportunity for aggressive nutritional support and may contribute to the dissolution of vascular thrombi by removing fibrinolysis inhibitors.

Prognosis: With aggressive management of acute renal failure more than 90% of patients survive the acute phase of HUS with a diarrheal prodrome.

Upper Urinary Tract Causes of Hematuria

The upper urinary tract causes of hematuria include interstitial nephritis, toxic nephropathy, cortical necrosis, pyelonephritis, nephrocalcinosis, vascular abnormalities, renal vein thrombosis, idiopathic hypercalciuria, sickle cell nephropathy, coagulopathies and thrombocytopenia, congenital renal anomalies, autosomal recessive polycystic kidney disease, autosomal dominant polycystic kidney disease, trauma, and renal tumors.

Vascular abnormalities such as hemangiomas, angiomyomas, and arteriovenous malformations of the kidney and lower urinary tract are rare causes of hematuria. The diagnosis is confirmed by Doppler ultrasonography, CT, or magnetic resonance angio-graphy.

Renal vein thrombosis (RVT) occurs in two distinct clinical situations. In newborns and infants, RVT is commonly associated with asphyxia, dehydration, shock, sepsis, congenital hypercoagulable states, and infants born to mothers with diabetes mellitus. In older children, RVT is seen in patients with nephrotic syndrome, cyanotic heart disease, inherited hypercoagulable states, and following exposure to angiographic contrast agents. The typical *clinical manifestations* of RVT are the sudden onset of gross hematuria and unilateral or bilateral flank masses. Patients may also present with microscopic hematuria, flank pain, hypertension, or oliguria. RVT is usually unilateral; bilateral RVT results in acute renal failure. The *diagnosis* is suggested by the development of hematuria and flank masses in a patient with predisposing clinical factors. Patients may also have a microangiopathic hemolytic anemia and thrombocytopenia. Ultrasonography shows marked enlargement, whereas radionuclide studies reveal a little or no renal function in the affected kidney (s). Doppler flow studies of the inferior vena cava and renal vein confirm the diagnosis. The *differential diagnosis* of RVT includes other causes of hematuria that are associated with microangiopathic hemolytic anemia or renal enlargement, such as hemolytic-uremic syndrome, hydronephrosis, polycystic kidney disease, Wilms' tumor, abscess, or hematoma. The primary *treatment* of RVT consists of supportive care including correction of fluid and electrolyte imbalance and treatment of renal insufficiency. Treatment with streptokinase, urokinase, or recombinant tissue plasminogen activator is common but remains controversial. Patients with thrombosis of the inferior vena cava may require surgical thrombectomy. Nephrectomy is indicated in those children with severe hypertension, who are refractory to antihypertensive medications.

Idiopathic hypercalciuria is an autosomal dominant disorder may present as recurrent gross hematuria, persistent microscopic hematuria, dysuria, or abdominal pain in the absence of stone formation. The causes of hypercalciuria include hypercalcemia (caused by hyperparathyroidism, vitamin D intoxication, immobilization, and sarcoidosis), Cushing syndrome, corticosteroid therapy, tubular dysfunction secondary to Fanconi syndrome (Wilson disease, oculocerebrorenal syndrome), Williams syndrome, distal tubular renal acidosis, Bartter syndrome, and Dent disease (an X-linked form of nephrolithiasis associated with hypophosphatemic rickets). Hypercalciuria is diagnosed by a 24-hr urinary calcium excretion exceeding 4 mg/kg. A screening test may be performed on a random urine specimen by measuring the calcium and creatinine concentration. A spot urine calcium to creatinine ratio (mg/mg) exceeding 0.2 suggests hypercalciuria, although

normal ratios may be as high as 0.8 in infants younger than 7 mo of age. In patients with persistent gross hematuria or dysuria, *treatment* is initiated with hydrochlorothiazide at a dose of 1–2 mg/kg/24 hr as a single morning dose. The dose is titrated upward until the 24-hr urinary calcium excretion is < 4 mg/kg and the clinical manifestations resolve. After 1 yr of treatment hydrochlorothiazide is usually discontinued but may be resumed if gross hematuria, nephrolithiasis, or dysuria recurs. During hydrochlorothiazide therapy, the serum potassium level should be monitored periodically to avoid hypokalemia. Potassium citrate at a dose of 1 mEq/kg/24 hr may also be given, particularly in patients with low urinary citrate excertion and symptomatic dysuria. Dietary calcium restriction is not recommended (except in children with massive calcium intake by dietary history) because of the obligate requirement for growth and lack of evidence demonstrating a relationship between decreased calcium intake and decreased urinary calcium levels. If untreated, hypercalciuria leads to nephrolithiasis in approximately 15% cases.

Sickle cell nephropathy: Gross or microscopic hematuria may be seen in children with sickle cell disease or sickle trait. Signs and symptoms resolve spontaneously in majority of cases. The hematuria presumably results from microthrombosis secondary to sickling in the relatively hypoxic, acidic, hypertonic renal medulla where vascular stasis is present. ACE inhibitors, such as enalapril, are often used to reduce in urine protein excretion in patients who are excreting daily more than 500 mg protein. Sickle cell nephropathy may eventually lead to hypertension and renal insufficiency that may progress to end-stage renal disease.

Coagulopathies and thrombocytopenia: Gross or microscopic hematuria may be associated with inherited or acquired disorders of coagulation (hemophilia, disseminated intravascular coagulation, thrombocytopenia). In these cases hematuria develops after other manifestations of the disease.

Congenital renal anomalies: Gross or microscopic hematuria may be associated with many types of different malformations of the urinary tract (see Chapter 22).

Autosomal recessive polycystic kidney disease: Autosomal recessive polycystic kidney disease (ARPKD) is also known as infantile polycystic disease is an autosomal recessive disorder. Both kidneys are markedly enlarged and grossly show innumerable cysts throughout the cortex and medulla. The child presents with bilateral flank masses during the neonatal period or early infancy with pulmonary hypoplasia, oligohydramnios, and hypertension and the absence of renal cysts by sonography of the parents. Markedly enlarged and uniformly hyperechogenic kidneys with poor corticomedullary distinction are seen on ultrasonography. ARPKD presents beyond with renal insufficiency, hypertension, or hepatomegally related to hepatic fibrosis. The treatment of ARPKD is supportive. Ventilatory support is often necessary in the neonatal period along with treatment of hypertension, fluid and electrolyte abnormalities, and clinical manifestations of renal insufficiency. Neonatal respiratory support and renal replacement therapies have improved survival of children. Morbidity and mortality in the older child are related to complications from chronic renal failure and liver disease.

Autosomal dominant polycystic kidney disease: Autosomal dominant polycystic kidney disease (ADPKD) is the most common hereditary human kidney disease, occurring with an incidence of 1:500 to 1,000. The kidneys are enlarged and show cortical and medullary cysts originating from all regions of the nephron. Although symptomatic ADPKD commonly presents in the 4th or 5th decade of life, symptoms including gross or microscopic hematuria, bilateral flank pain, abdominal masses, hypertension, and urinary tract infection may be seen in children and neonates. Renal ultrasonography usually demonstrates multiple bilateral macrocytes, although unilateral disease may be seen in the early phase of disease. ADPKD is a systemic disorder affecting many organ systems. Cysts may be present within the liver, pancreas, spleen and ovaries. Intracranial aneurysms, mitral valve prolapse, hernias and intestinal diverticula may also occur in these children. Treatment of ADPKD is primarily supportive and the control of blood pressure is most important because the rate of disease progression correlates with the presence of hypertension. ACE inhibitors and/or angiotensin II receptor antagonists are agents of choice. Neonatal ADPKD may be lethal, but long term patient and renal survival is possible for children surviving the neonatal period. The presentation of ADPKD in older children has a favorable prognosis.

Trauma: Infants and children are more susceptible to renal injury following blunt or penetrating injury to the back or abdomen due to the decreased muscle mass protecting the kidney. Gross or microscopic hematuria, flank pain, and abdominal rigidity may occur along with associated injuries. Urethral trauma is suspected when gross blood appears at the external urethral meatus, which may result from crush injury, frequently associated with a fractured pelvis or from direct injury.

Lower Urinary Tract Causes of Hematuria

The lower urinary tract causes of hematuria include infectious causes of cystitis and urethritis, hemorrhagic cystitis, heavy exercise, and Munchausen/Munchausen-by-proxy syndrome.

Infectious causes of cystitis and urethritis: Gross or microscopic hematuria may be associated with bacterial, mycobactrial, or viral infections of the bladder. Urethritis may be present as gross or microscopic hematuria, associated with urgency and pyuria. Urine cultures occasionally reveal bacteria. The disorder frequently resolves spontaneously. In children older than 8 yr of age, a 10-day course of doxycycline is the treatment of choice, in conjunction with a urinary analgesic such as phenazopyridine for relief of pain. Cystoscopy may be required to determine the nature of any underlying abnormality such as ulceration or inflammation, in children in whom conservative management fails, hemorrhagic cystitis is defined as acute or chronic bleeding of the bladder. Hemorrhagic cystitis may occur in response to chemical toxins (cyclophosphamide, penicillin, busulfan, thiotepa, dyes, and insecticides), viruses (adenovirus types 11 and 21, polyoma BK virus (BKV), influenza A), radiation, and amyloidosis. Hydration and the use of MESNA disulfide (350 mg/m^2 every 6 hr), which inactivates cyclophosphamide metabolites, helps to protect the bladder from the chemical irritation related to the use of IV cyclophosphamide. Administration of oral cyclophosphamide in the morning followed by oral aggressive hydration throughout the remainder of the day is very effective in reducing the risk of hemorrhagic cystitis. Bladder irrigation with saline, alum, silver nitrate, or aminocaproic acid may be needed in more severe cases. Gross hematuria associated with viral hemorrhagic cystitis usually resolves in 1 wk.

Heavy exercise: Gross or microscopic hematuria may follow vigorous exercise. Exercise hematuria is rare in females. The color of urine may vary from red to black. Blood clots may be present in the urine. Urine culture and other laboratory investigations are normal. The condition is benign and resolve within 48 hr after cessation of exercise.

Bergstein J, Leiser J, Andreoli S. The clinical significance of asymptomatic, gross, and microscopic hematuria in children. *Arch Pediatr Adolesc Med* 2005; 159: 353–355.

Davis ID, Avner ED. Conditions particularly associated with hematuria. In: Kliegman RM, Behrman RE, Jenson HB, Stanton BF (eds). *Nelson Textbook of Pediatrics.* 18th edn. Vol. 2. Philadelphia: Saunders, 2007; 2168–2188.

Meyers KE. Evaluation of hematuria in children. *Urol Clin North Am* 2004; 3: 559–573.

Shin JI, Park JM, Lee SM, et al. Factors affecting spontaneous resolution of hematuria in childhood nutcracker syndrome. *Pediatr Nephrol* 2005; 20: 609–613.

Walters S, Levine M. Infectious diseases and the kidney. In: Barratt TM, Avner ED, Harmon WE (eds). *Pediatric Nephrology*. 4th edn. Baltimore: Lippincott Williams and Wilkins, 1999; 1079–1102.

21.3 CONDITIONS PARTICULARLY ASSOCIATED WITH PROTEINURIA

Transient Proteinuria

The upper limit of normal protein excretion in healthy children is 150 mg/24 hr. A normal protein excretion is defined as ≤ 4 mg/m^2/hr; abnormal is defined as 4–40 mg/m^2/hr; and nephrotic range is defined as > 40 mg/m^2/hr. Of the 10% of children found to have proteinuria by a single dipstick measurement, only 1% had persistent proteinuria when measured on 4 separate occasions. This phenomenon is known as transient proteinuria. The causes are fever (temperature >38.3°C (101°F), exercise, dehydration, cold exposure, congestive heart failure, seizures, stress. The proteinuria does not exceed 2+ on the dipstick. The mechanism of transient proteinuria is unknown. No evaluation or treatment is needed for children with this benign condition.

Orthostatic (Postural) Proteinuria

Orthostatic proteinuria is the most common cause of persistent proteinuria in school-aged children and adolescents, occurring in up to 60% of children with persistent proteinuria. Children with this condition are usually asymptomatic and the condition is discovered on routine urinalysis. Individuals with orthostatic proteinuria excrete normal or minimally increased amounts of protein in the supine position, whereas in the upright position, urinary excretion of protein is increased up to 10-fold, up to 1,000 mg/24 hr (1g/24 hr). Hematuria, hypertension, hypoalbuminemia, edema, and renal dysfunction are absent.

The cause of orthostatic proteinuria is unknown, although altered renal hemodynamics and partial vein obstruction in the upright position are possible causes. Long-term follow-up of children with orthostatic proteinuria is prudent to monitor for evidence of renal disease, including hematuria, hypertension, edema, diminished renal function, or proteinuria exceeding 1,000 mg/24 hr.

Fixed Proteinuria

Individuals found to have significant proteinuria on a first morning urine sample on 3 consecutive days (> 1+ on dipstick, or protein/creatinine ratio > 0.2) have fixed proteinuria. Fixed proteinuria indicates renal disease and may be caused by glomerular or tubular disorders (Box 21.3).

Box 21.3: Causes of proteinuria

1. *Transient proteinuria:*
2. *Orthostatic (postural) proteinuria*
3. *Glomerular diseases characterized by isolated proteinuria:* Focal segmental glomerulosclerosis; Mesangial proliferative glomerulonephritis; Membranous nephropathy; Membranoproliferative glomerulonephritis; Amyloidosis; Diabetic nephropathy; Sickle cell nephropathy
4. *Glomerular diseases with proteinuria as a feature:* Acute postinfectious glomerulonephritis; IgA nephropathy; Henoch-Schönlein purpura (HSP) nephritis; Lupus nephritis; Alport syndrome
5. *Tubular diseases:* Cystinosis; Wilson disease; Lowe syndrome; Galactosemia; Tubulointerstitial nephritis; Heavy metal poisoning; Acute tubular necrosis; Renal dysplasia; Polycystic kidney disease; Reflux nephropathy

---

Nephrotic Syndrome

The nephrotic syndrome is characterized by heavy proteinuria (> 3.5 g/24 hr in adults or 40 mg/m^2/24 hr in children), hypoalbuminemia, edema, and hyperlipidemia. The incidence is 2–3/100,000 children per year; and the majority of the affected children will have steroid sensitive minimal change disease.

Etiology: Most children (90%) with nephrotic syndrome have idiopathic nephrotic syndrome. Causes of idiopathic nephrotic syndrome include minimal change disease (85%), mesangial proliferation (5%), and focal segmental glomerulosclerosis (10%). The remaining 10% of children with nephrotic syndrome have secondary nephrotic syndrome related to systemic or glomerular diseases such as membranous nephropathy or membranoproliferative glomerulonephritis.

Pathophysiology: The underlying abnormality in nephrotic syndrome is an increase in permeability of the glomerular capillary wall, which leads to massive proteinuria and hypoalbuminemia. The cause of the increased permeability is not well understood. In minimal change disease, it is possible that T-cell dysfunction leads to alteration of cytokines, which causes a loss of negatively charged glycoproteins within the glomerular capillary wall. In focal segmental glomerulosclerosis, a plasma factor, perhaps produced by lymphocytes, may be responsible for the increase in capillary wall permeability. Alternately, mutations in podocyte proteins (podocin, α-actinin 4) are associated with focal segmental glomerulo-sclerosis. Steroid-resistant nephrotic syndrome is associated with mutations in *NPHS2* (podocin) and *WT1* genes.

The mechanism of edema formation in nephrotic syndrome is incompletely understood. It seems likely that, in most instances, massive urinary protein loss leads to hypoalbuminemia, which may cause a decrease in the plasma oncotic pressure and transu-dation of fluid from the intravascular compartment to the interstitial space. The reduction in intravascular volume decreases renal perfusion, activating the renin-angiotensin-aldosterone system, which stimulates tubular reabsorption of sodium. The reduced intravascular volume also stimulates the release of antidiuretic hormone, which enhances the reabsorp-tion of water in the collecting duct. However, this theory does not apply to all patients with nephrotic syndrome because some patients actually have increased intravascular volume with diminished plasma levels of renin and aldosterone. Therefore, other factors, such as a primary renal avidity for sodium and water, may be involved in the formation of edema in some patients with nephrotic syndrome.

In the nephrotic state, serum lipid levels (cholesterol, triglycerides) are elevated for two reasons: (1) hypoalbuminemia stimulates generalized hepatic protein synthesis, including synthesis of lipoproteins; and (2) lipid catabolism is diminished, as a result of reduced plasma levels of lipoprotein lipase, related to increased urinary losses of this enzyme.

Idiopathic Nephrotic Syndrome

Approximately 90% of children with nephrotic syndrome have idiopathic nephrotic syndrome. Idiopathic nephrotic syndrome includes 3 histologic types: minimal change disease, mesangial prolifera-tion, and focal glomerulosclerosis. These 3 disorders may represent 3 separate diseases with a similar presentation.

Pathology: In *minimal change nephrotic syndrome* (MCNS) (85% of total cases), the glomeuli appear normal or show a minimal increase in mesangial cells and matrix on light microscopy. Findings on immunofluorescence microscopy are typically negative and electron microscopy reveals effacement of the epithelial cell foot processes. More than 95% of children with minimal change disease respond to corticosteroid therapy.

The histologic findings of *mesangial proliferation* (5% of total cases) consists of a diffuse increase in mesangial cells and matrix on light microscopy; trace to 1+ mesangial IgM and/or IgA staining on immunofluo-rescence microscopy; increased numbers of mesangial cells and matrix as well as effacement of the epithelial cell foot processes. Approximately 50% of patients with histologic lesion respond to corticosteroid therapy.

In *focal segmental glomerulosclerosis (FSGS)* (10% of total cases) glomeruli show mesangial proliferation and segmental scarring on light microscopy; immunofluorescence microscopy shows IgM and C3 staining in the areas of segmental sclerosis; electron microscopy shows segmental scarring of the glomeruli tuft with obliteration of the glomerular capillary lumen. A similar lesion may be seen with HIV infection, vesicoureteral reflux, and intravenous heroin abuse. Only 20% of patients with FSGS respond to corticosteroid therapy. The disease is frequently progressive, ultimately involving all glomeruli and leads to end-stage renal disease in most patients.

Clinical manifestations: The idiopathic nephrotic syndrome commonly occurs in males than in females (2:1) and between the ages of 2 and 6 yr. It has been reported as early as 6 mo and throughout adulthood. MCNS is present in 85–90% of patients < 6 yr. FSGS develops in older children. 20–30% of adolescents have MCNS. The initial episode and subsequent relapses may follow minor infections and, occasionally, reactions to insect bites, bee stings, or poison ivy. Children with nephrotic syndrome initially present with mild edema, which is initially noted around the eyes and in lower extremities. With times, the edema becomes generalized, with the development of ascites, pleural effusions, and genital edema. Anorexia, irritability, abdominal pain and diarrhea are common. A diagnosis other than MCNS should be considered in the presence of age < 1yr, a family history, extrarenal findings (arthritis, rash, anemia), hypertension or pulmonary edema, acute or chronic renal insufficiency, and hematuria (*see* Figs 21.1 and 21.2 in CD).

Diagnosis: The urinalysis reveals 3+ or 4+ proteinuria; microscopic hematuria may be present in 20% of children. Spot urine protein/creatinine ratio exceeds 2.0 and urinary protein excretion exceeds 3.5 g/24 hr in adults and 40 mg/m²/24 hr in children. The serum creatinine level is usually normal, but it may be increased because of decreased renal perfusion resulting from contraction of the intravascular volume. The serum albumin level is generally < 2.5 g/dl and the serum cholesterol and triglyceride levels are elevated. C3 and C4 levels are normal. Renal biopsy is not required for diagnosis in most children.

Differential diagnosis: The differential diagnosis of the child with marked edema includes congestive heart failure, hepatic failure, protein loosing enteropathy, acute or chronic glomerulonephritis, and protein malnutrition.

Treatment: Children having first episode of nephrotic syndrome and mild to moderate edema should have reduced intake of salt (low sodium diet) and may be normalized when the child enters remission. Diuretic use should be reserved for patients with severe symptoms and must be closely monitored because of the possibility of increasing the risk of thromboembolic complications.

Children with severe symptomatic edema, including large pleural effusions, ascites, or severe genital edema should be hospitalized. In addition to salt restriction, fluid restriction may be necessary if the child is hyponatremic. A swollen scrotum may be elevated with pillows to enhance the removal of fluid by gravity. Diuresis may be augmented by administration of chlorothiazide (10 mg/kg/dose IV every 12 hr) or metolazone (0.1 mg/kg/dose PO bid) followed by frusemide 30 min later (1–2 mg/kg/dose IV q12 hr).

IV administration of 25% human albumin (0.5 g/kg/dose q6–12 hr administered over 1–2 hr) followed by frusemide (1–2 mg/kg/dose IV) is often necessary when fluid restriction and parenteral diuretics are not effective. During this therapy a close monitoring of volume status, serum electrolyte balance, and renal function is required. Symptomatic volume overload, with hypertension and heart failure, is a potential complication of parenteral albumin therapy, particularly in rapid infusions.

Children with onset of nephrotic syndrome between 1 and 4 yr of age are likely to have steroid responsive MCNS and steroid therapy may be initiated without renal biopsy. Children with features that make MCNS less likely (hematuria, hypertension, renal insufficiency, hypocomplementemia, age < 1yr or > 8yr) should be considered for renal biopsy before treatment.

In children with presumed MCNS, prednisolone should be administered (after confirming a negative PPD test) at a dose of 60 mg/m^2/day (maximum daily dose). 80 mg divided into 2–3 doses for at least 4 consecutive weeks. However, an initial 6 wk course of daily steroid treatment may lead to a lower relapse rate, although the frequency of steroid-induced side effects is higher. Eighty to 90% of children will respond to steroid therapy (urine trace or negative for protein for three consecutive days), by 2 wk. The vast majority of children who will respond to prednisolone therapy will do so within the first 4 wk of treatment.

After the initial 6-wk course, the prednisolone dose should be tapered to 40 mg/m^2/day given every other day as a single morning dose. The alternate-day dose is then slowly tapered and discontinued over the next 2–3 mo. Children who continue to have proteinuria (2+ or greater) after 8 wk of steroid therapy are considered *steroid resistant* and a diagnostic renal biopsy should be performed.

Many children with nephrotic syndrome will experience one *relapse* (3–4+ proteinuria plus edema). The relapse rate in children treated with longer initial steroid courses may be as low as 30–40%. Relapse should be treated with daily divided-dose prednisolone at the doses noted earlier (initial doses) until the child enters remission (urine trace or negative for proteins for 3 consecutive days). The prednisolone dose is then changed to alternate day dosing and tapered over 1–2 mo.

A number of patients will relapse while on alternate-day steroid therapy or within 28 days of stopping prednisolone therapy. Such patients are termed *steroid dependent*. Patients who respond well to prednisolone therapy, but relapse ≥ 4 times in a 12 mo period are termed *frequent relapsers*. Children who fail to respond to prednisolone therapy within 8 wk are termed *steroid resistant*. Steroid resistant nephrotic syndrome is usually FSGS (80%), MCNS (20%), and rarely mesangial proliferative.

Steroid dependent patients, frequent relapsers, and steroid-resistant patients may be candidate for alternative agents, particularly if the child suffers severe corticosteroid toxicity (cushingoid appearance, hypertension, cataracts, and/or growth failure). *Cyclophosphamide* prolongs the duration of remission and reduces the number on relapses in children with *frequently relapsing and steroid-dependent* nephrotic syndrome. The potential side effects of the drug (neutropenia, disseminated varicella, hemorrhagic cystitis, alopecia, sterility, increased risk of future malignancy) should be reviewed with the family before initiating therapy. The dose of cyclophosphamide is 2–3 mg/kg/24 hr given as a single dose, for a total duration of 8–12 wk. Alternate prednisolone therapy is often continued during the course of cyclophosphamide administration. During cyclophosphamide therapy, the white blood cell count must be monitored weekly and the drug should be withheld if the count falls below 5,000/mm^3.

An additional option for the child with complicated nephrotic syndrome is *high-dose pulse methylprednisolone*. Methylprednisolone is usually given as a 30-mg/kg bolus (maximum 1,000 mg), with the first six doses given every other day, followed by a tapering regimen for periods up to 18 mo. Cyclophosphamide may be added to this regimen in selected patients.

Cyclosporine (3–6 mg/kg/24 hr divided q 12 hr) or *tacrolimus* (0.15 mg/kg/24 hr divided q 12 hr) are also effective in maintaining prolonged remission in children with nephrotic syndrome and are useful as steroid-sparing agents. Children must be monitored for side effects, including hypertension, nephrotoxicity, hirsutism, and gingival hyperplasia.

Mycophenolate may maintain remission in children with steroid-dependent or frequently relapsing nephrotic syndrome. Most children who respond to cyclosporine, tacrolimus, or mycophenolate therapy tend to relapse when the medication is discontinued. ACE inhibitors and angiotensin II blockers may be helpful as adjunct therapy to reduce proteinuria in steroid-resistant patients.

Complications: Infection is the major complication of nephrotic syndrome. Children in relapse have increased susceptibility to bacterial infections because of urinary losses of immunoglobulins and properdin factor B, defective cell mediated immunity, immunosuppressive therapy, malnutrition, and edema/ascites acting as a potential "culture medium". Spontaneous bacterial peritonitis, sepsis, pneumonia, cellulites, urinary tract infection are frequent types of infection that occur in children with nephrotic syndrome. The common bacteria responsible for infection are *Streptococcus pneumoniae*, and gram negative bacteria such as *Escherichia coli*. The role of prophylactic antibiotic therapy during nephrotic syndrome relapse is controversial.

All nonimmunized children with nephrotic syndrome should receive pnemococcal vaccine, varicella vaccine (nonimmunized children in relapse within 72 hr of exposure with varicella should receive varicella-zoster immunoglobulin) and influenza vaccine (on a yearly basis).

Children with nephrotic syndrome are also at an increased risk of thromboembolic events with an incidence of 2–5%. Both arterial and venous thromboses may be seen, including renal vein thrombosis, pulmonary embolus, sagittal sinus thrombosis, and thrombosis of indwelling arterial and venous catheters. The risk of thrombosis is related to increased prothrombotic factors (fibrinogen, thrombocytosis, hemoconcentration, relative immobilization) and decreased fibrinolytic factors (urinary losses of antithrombin III, proteins C and S). Prophylactic anticoagulation is not recommended unless they have had a previous thromboembolic event. Overaggressive diuresis should be avoided and use of indwelling catheters should be limited because these factors may increase the likelihood of clotting complications.

Hyperlipidemia, particularly in complicated patients with nephrotic syndrome, may be a risk factor for a CVS disease, and myocardial infarction. 3-hydroxy-3-methylglutaryl coenzyme A (HMG-CoA)

reductase-inhibiting drugs may be considered to treat the hyperlipidemia seen in nephrotic syndrome.

Prognosis: The majority of children with steroid-responsive nephrotic syndrome have repeated relapses, which generally decrease in frequency as the child grows older. Those children who respond steroid rapidly and those who have on relapses during the first 6 mo after diagnosis are likely to follow an infrequently relapsing course. The family should be informed that the child with steroid-responsive nephrotic syndrome is unlikely to develop chronic kidney disease, that the disease is generally not hereditary and that the child (in the absence of prolonged cyclophosphamide therapy) will remain fertile.

Children with steroid resistant nephrotic syndrome, most often caused by FSGS, generally have a much poorer prognosis. These children develop progressive renal insufficiency, ultimately leading to end-stage renal disease requiring dialysis or renal transplantation. Recurrent nephrotic syndrome develops in 30–50% of transplant recipients with FSGS. Plasmapheresis, high dose cyclosporine or tacrolimus, and ACE inhibitors may reduce proteinuria in these cases.

Secondary Nephrotic Syndrome

Nephrotic syndrome also occurs as a secondary feature of many glomerular diseases, such as membranous nephropathy, membranoproliferative glomeruonephritis, postinfectious glomerulonephritis, lupus nephritis and Henoch-Schönlein purpura nephritis. Secondary nephrotic syndrome should be suspected in patients with age > 8 yr, hypertension, hematuria, renal dysfunction, extrarenal symptomatology (rash, arthralgia, fever) or depressed serum complement levels. The causes of secondary nephrotic syndrome are listed in Box 21.4.

Box 21.4: Causes of secondary nephrotic syndrome

1. *Infectious:* Malaria; Schistosomiasis; Leprosy; Filaria; Hepatitis B virus; Hepatitis C virus; HIV
2. **Drugs and Chemicals**
   2.1 *Membranous glomerulopathy:* Penicillamine; Captopril; Gold; Nonsteroidal anti-inflammatory drugs; Mercury compounds
   2.2 *Minimal change nephritic syndrome (MCNS):* Probenecid; Ethosuximide; Methimazole; Lithium
   2.3 *Proliferative Glomeruonephritis:* Procainamide; Chlorpopamide; Phenytoin; Trimethdione; Paramethadione
3. **Malignancy** (particularly in adult population)
   3.1 *Membranous glomerulopathy:* Carcinoma lung; Carcinoma gastrointestinal tract
   3.2 *Minimal change nephritic syndrome (MCNS):* Lymphomas particularly Hodgkin lymphoma

Congenital Nephrotic Syndrome

Infants who develop nephrotic syndrome within the first 3 mo of life are considered to have congenital nephrotic syndrome. The most common cause of this syndrome is Finnish-type congenital nephrotic syndrome, an autosomal recessive disorder seen commonly in population of Scandinavian descent (1:8,000 incidence). Other causes of congenital nephrotic syndrome include congenital infections such as syphilis, toxoplasmosis, rubella, cytomegalovirus, HIV, hepatitis B, and diffuse mesangial sclerosis.

Bagga A, Srivastava RN. Nephrotic syndrome. In: Srivastava RN, Bagga A (eds). *Pediatric Nephrology* 4th edn. New Delhi: Jaypee, 2005; 114–136.

Pais P, Avner ED. Nephrotic syndrome. In: Kliegman RM, Stanton BF, St.Geme JW, Schor NF, Behrman RE. *Nelson Textbook of Pediatrics.* 19th edn. New Delhi: Elsevier, 2011; 1801–1804.

Pais P, Avner ED. Idiopathic nephrotic syndrome. In: Kliegman RM, Stanton BF, St.Geme JW, Schor NF, Behrman RE. *Nelson Textbook of Pediatrics.* 19th edn. New Delhi: Elsevier, 2011; 1804–1806.

Pais P, Avner ED. Secondary nephrotic syndrome. In: Kliegman RM, Stanton BF, St.Geme JW, Schor NF, Behrman RE. *Nelson Textbook of Pediatrics.* 19th edn. New Delhi: Elsevier, 2011; 1806.

Pais P, Avner ED. Congenital nephrotic syndrome. In: Kliegman RM, Stanton BF, St.Geme JW, Schor NF, Behrman RE. *Nelson Textbook of Pediatrics.* 19th edn. New Delhi: Elsevier, 2011; 1807.

Vogt BA, Avner ED. Conditions particularly associated with proteinuria. In: Kliegman RM, Behrman RE, Jenson HB, Stanton BF (eds). *Nelson Textbook of Pediatrics.* 18th edn. Vol. 2. Philadelphia: Saunders, 2007; 2188–2195.

21.4 TUBULAR DISORDERS

Renal Tubular Acidosis

Renal tubular acidosis (RTA) is characterized by a normal anion gap metabolic acidosis resulting from either impaired bicarbonate reabsorption or impaired urinary acid (hydrogen ion) excretion. Both inherited and acquired primary and secondary forms exist. There are three main forms of RTA: proximal (type II) RTA, distal (type I) RTA, and hyperkalemic (type IV) RTA. Mixed lesions (those with elements of type I and II) in patients with inherited carbonic anhydrase deficiency, are designated as type III RTA.

Proximal (Type II) Renal Tubular Acidosis

Proximal RTA results from impaired proximal tubule bicarbonate reabsorption. The causes of proximal RTA and Fanconi syndrome are listed in Box 21.5.

Clinical manifestations of proximal RTA and Fanconi syndrome: There is growth failure in the first year of life.

Box 21.5: Causes of proximal RTA and Fanconi syndrome

Isolated: Sporadic; Hereditary
Fanconi syndrome: *Primary:* Sporadic, Hereditary, Cystinosis, Lowe syndrome, Galactosemia; Tyrosinemia; Fructosemia, Fanconi-Bickel syndrome, Wilson disease, Mitochondrial diseases, Dent disease (X-linked nephrolithiasis)
Secondary: Heavy metals, Outdated tetracycline, Gentamicin, Ifosfamide, Cyclosporine/tacrolimus

Additional symptoms include polyuria, dehydration, anorexia, vomiting, constipation, and hypotonia. Patients with primary Fanconi syndrome will have in addition secondary to phosphaturia (phosphate wasting) such as rickets. Those with systemic diseases will present with additional signs and symptoms specific to their underlying disease. A non-anion gap metabolic acidosis will be present.

Laboratory investigations: Urinalysis in patients with isolated proximal RTA is normal except that urine pH is acidic (pH <5.5). Urinary findings in patients with Fanconi syndrome demonstrate varying degrees of proteinuria, glycosuria, phosphaturia, aminoaciduria, uricosuria, and elevated urinary sodium or potassium. Depending on the nature of the underlying disorder, laboratory evidence of chronic renal insufficiency, including elevated serum creatinine, may be present.

Treatment: The treatment includes correcting the metabolic abnormalities associated with Fanconi syndrome or chronic renal failure. In addition, oral cysteamine therapy, which binds to cystine and coverts it to cysteine. This facilitates lysosomal transport and decreases tissue cystine. For ocular tissues, an additional therapy cysteamine eye drops are required, because oral cysteamine does not achieve adequate levels in ocular tissues. Early initiation of the drug may prevent or delay deterioration of renal function. Patient with growth failure who does not respond may benefit with growth hormone. Depending on the nature of the underlying disorder, treatment should be administered.

Lowe syndrome (*Oculocerebrorenal syndrome of Lowe*) is a rare X-linked recessive disorder characterized by congenital cataracts, mental retardation, and Fanconi syndrome. Patients with Lowe syndrome present in infancy with cataracts, progressive growth failure, hypotonia, and Fanconi syndrome. There is no specific therapy for the renal disease or neurologic deficits. Cataract removal is done to improve vision.

Distal (Type I) Renal Tubular Acidosis

Distal RTA occurs as the result of impaired distal urinary acidification (hydrogen ion secretion). Primary and secondary causes of distal RTA are listed in Box 21.6. Because of impaired hydrogen ion excretion the urine pH cannot be reduced below 5.5, despite the presence of severe metabolic acidosis. Loss of sodium bicarbonate results in hyperchloremia and hypokalemia. Hypercalciuria is usually present and may lead to nephrocalcinosis or nephrolithiasis. Chronic metabolic acidosis also impairs urinary citrate excretion. Hypocitraturia further increases the risk of calcium deposition in the tubules. Bone disease is common, resulting from mobilization of organic components from bone.

Clinical manifestations: Patients with distal RTA share common features with those of proximal RTA, including non-anion gap metabolic acidosis and growth failure. The distinguishing features of distal RTA include nephrocalcinosis and hypercalciuria.

Hyperkalemic (Type IV) Renal Tubular Acidosis

Type IV RTA occurs as a result of impaired aldosterone production (hypoaldosteronism) or impaired renal responsiveness to aldosterone (pseudohypoaldosteronism). The causes of hyperkalemic (type IV) RTA is listed in Box 21.7.

Clinical manifestations: Patients with type IV RTA may present with growth failure (in the first few years of life), polyuria and dehydration (from salt wasting).

Rarely, patients (especially those with pseudohypoaldosteronism) will present with life threatening hyperkalemia. Patients with obstructive uropathies may present acutely with signs and symptoms of pyelonephritis, such as fever, vomiting, and fowl-smelling urine.

Laboratory investigations: Laboratory tests reveal a hyperkalemic non-anion gap metabolic acidosis. Urine may be alkaline or acidic. Elevated urine sodium levels with inappropriately low urine potassium levels reflect the absence of aldosterone effect.

Diagnostic approach to RTA: The first step in the evaluation of patient with suspected RTA is to confirm the presence of a normal anion gap metabolic acidosis, identify electrolyte abnormalities, assess renal function, and rule out other causes of bicarbonate loss such as diarrhea. Other investigations depend on the type of RTA.

Treatment of RTA: The main treatment of all forms of RTA is bicarbonate replacement. Patients with proximal RTA often require large quantities of bicarbonate, up to 20 mEq/kg/24 hr in the form of sodium bicarbonate or sodium citrate solution. The base requirement for distal RTAs is generally in the range of 2–4 mEq/kg/24 hr, although patient requirements may vary. Patients with Fanconi syndrome usually require phosphate supplementation. Patients with distal RTA should be monitored for the development of hypercalciuria (recurrent episodes of gross hematuria), nephrocalcinosis, or nephrolithiasis may require thiazide diuretics to decrease urine calcium excretion. Patients with type IV RTA may require chronic treatment for hyperkalemia with sodium–potassium exchange resin (Kayexalate).

Prognosis of RTA: Prognosis is dependent to a large part on the nature of underlying disease. Patients with treated isolated proximal or distal RTA will generally show improvement in growth, provided serum bicarbonate levels can be maintained in the normal range. Patients with systemic illness and Fanconi syndrome may have ongoing morbidity with growth failure, rickets, and signs and symptoms related to their underlying cause.

Rickets Associated with Renal Tubular Acidosis

Rickets may be present in primary RTA, particularly in type II (proximal) RTA. Hypophosphatemia and phosphaturia are common in these syndromes, which are also characterized by hyperchloremic metabolic acidosis, various degrees bicarbonaturia, and frequently, hypercalciuria and hyperkaluria. Bone demineralization without overt rickets usually is

---

Box 21.6: Causes of distal (type I) RTA

Primary: Sporadic; Hereditary.
Secondary: *Interstitial nephritis:* Obstructive uropathy, Vesicoureteral reflux, Pyelonephritis, Transplant rejection, Sickle cell nephropathy, Ehlers-Danlos syndrome, Lupus nephritis, Nephrocalcinosis, Medullary sponge disease, Hepatic cirrhosis.
Toxins/Medications: Amphotericin B, Lithium, Toluene, Cisplatin.

Box 21.7: Causes of hyperkalemic (type IV) renal tubular acidosis

Primary: Sporadic; Hereditary.
Secondary: Hypoaldosteronism, Addison disease, Congenital adrenal hyperplasia, Prolonged heparinization, Pseudohypoaldosteronism (type I or II), Obstructive Uropathy, Pyelonephritis, Interstitial nephritis, Diabetes mellitus, Sickle cell nephropathy, Trimethoprim/sulfamethoxazole, Angiotensin-converting enzyme inhibitors, Cyclosporine.

detected in type I (distal) RTA. This metabolic bone disease may be characterized by bone pain, growth retardation, osteopenia, and occasionally pathological fractures.

Administration of sufficient bicarbonate to reverse acidosis stops bone dissolution and the hypercalciuria that is common in distal RTA. Proximal RTA is treated with both bicarbonate and oral phosphate supplements to heal rickets. Vitamin D is indicated to offset the secondary hyperparathyroidism that complicates oral phosphate therapy. Following treatment, growth in patients with type II (proximal) RTA is greater than in patients with primary Fanconi syndrome.

Chesney RW. Rickets associated with renal tubular acidosis. In: Kliegman RM, Behrman RE, Jenson HB, Stanton BF (eds). *Nelson Textbook of Pediatrics*. 18th edn. Vol. 2. Philadelphia: Saunders, 2007; 2200.

Dell KM, Avner ED. Renal tubular acidosis. In: Kliegman RM, Behrman RE, Jenson HB, Stanton BF (eds). *Nelson Textbook of Pediatrics*. 18th edn. Vol. 2. Philadelphia: Saunders, 2007; 2197–2200.

Gahl WA. Early oral cysteamine therapy for nephrogenic cystinosis. *Eur J Pediatr* 2003; 162 (suppl 1): S38–S41.

Wuhl E, Haffner D, Offner, et al. Long-term treatment with growth hormone in short children with nephrogenic cystinosis. *J Pediatr* 2001; 138: 880–887.

Bartter/Gitelman Syndromes

Bartter syndrome: Bartter syndrome is a rare form of hypokalemic metabolic alkalosis with hypercalciuria, with an autosomal recessive pattern of inheritance. There are two distinct clinical subtypes: *antenatal Bartter syndrome* (also called hyperprostaglandin E syndrome), severe phenotype, typically presents in infancy and *classic Bartter syndrome*, milder phenotype, presents in childhood.

A history of polyhydramnios may be elicited. Dysmorphic features, including triangular facies, protruding ears, large eyes with strabismus, and drooping mouth may be present. Consanguinity suggests the presence of an autosomal recessive disorder. Older children may have a history of recurrent episodes of dehydration, failure to thrive and the classic biochemical abnormalities of hypokalemic metabolic alkalosis. Urinary calcium, potassium, and sodium levels are elevated. Serum renin, aldosterone, and prostaglandin E levels are often markedly elevated, particularly in the antenatal form. Blood pressure is usually normal, although patients with the antenatal form may have severe salt wasting, resulting in dehydration and hypotension. Renal function is typically normal. Nephrocalcinosis, resulting from hypercalciuria, may be seen on ultrasound examination.

Treatment of Bartter syndrome includes preventing dehydration, maintaining nutritional status, and correcting hypokalemia. Potassium supplementation, often at very high doses, is required. Infants and young children may require sodium supplementation as well. Indomethacin, a prostaglandin inhibitor may be effective.

The long term prognosis is generally good if proper attention is paid in maintaining electrolyte balance, volume status, and growth. However, in a small minority of patients, chronic hypokalemia, nephrocalcinosis, and indomethacin therapy can lead to chronic interstitial nephritis, and chronic renal failure.

Gitelman syndrome: Gitelman syndrome (often called a Bartter syndrome variant) is a rare autosomal recessive disorder present at a later age than those with Bartter syndrome. Patients often have a history of recurrent muscle cramps and spasms, presumably caused by low serum magnesium levels. They do not have a history of recurrent episodes of dehydration. Biochemical abnormalities include hypokalemia, metabolic alkalosis, and hypomagnesemia. The urinary calcium level is usually very low (in contrast to the elevated urinary calcium level often seen in Bartter syndrome), and the urinary magnesium level is elevated. Renin and aldosterone levels are usually normal, and prostaglandin E secretion is not elevated. Growth failure is less prominent in Gitelman syndrome than in Bartter syndrome.

The diagnosis of Gitelman syndrome is suggested in an adolescent or adult presenting with hypokalemia, metabolic alkalosis, hypomagnesemia, and hypocalciuria.

Treatment is directed at correcting hypokalemia and hypomagnesemia with supplemental potassium and magnesium.

Other inherited tubular transport abnormalities

Cystinuria is an autosomal recessive disorder and is characterized by recurrent stone formation.
X-linked nephrolithiasis (Dent disease) is a disease characterized by recurrent stone formation and progresses to Fanconi syndrome, and is seen exclusively in males.

Dell KM, Avner ED. Bartter/Gitelman syndromes and other inherited tubular transport abnormalities. In: Kliegman RM, Behrman RE, Jenson HB, Stanton BF (eds). *Nelson Textbook of Pediatrics*. 18th edn. Vol. 2. Philadelphia: Saunders, 2007; 2201–2202.

21.5 RENAL FAILURE

Acute Renal Failure

Acute renal failure (ARF) is a clinical syndrome in which a sudden deterioration in renal function results in the inability of the kidneys to maintain fluid and electrolyte homeostasis.

Pathogenesis: ARF has been conventionally classified into 3 categories: prerenal, intrinsic renal and postrenal (Box 21.8).

Prerenal ARF is characterized by diminished effective circulating arterial volume which leads to inadequate renal perfusion and a decreased glomerular filtration rate (GFR). If the underlying cause of the renal hypoperfusion is reversed promptly, renal function returns to normal. If hypoperfusion is sustained, intrinsic renal parenchymal damage may develop.

Intrinsic renal ARF is characterized by renal parenchymal damage, including sustained hypoperfusion/ischemia.

Extrinsic is characterized by obstruction of the urinary tract. Relief of the obstruction usually results in recovery of renal function except in patients with associated renal dysplasia or prolonged urinary tract obstruction.

Clinical manifestations and diagnosis: A history is helpful in defining the cause of ARF, such as (1) an infant with a history of diarrhea and vomiting most likely has prenatal ARF caused by volume depletion; (2) a child with a recent pharyngitis presents with priorbital edema, hypertension and gross hematuria most likely has intrinsic ARF related to postinfectious glomerulonephritis; (3) a critically ill child with

hypotension and exposure to nephrotoxic drugs most likely has acute tubular necrosis (ATN); or (4) a neonate with a history of hydronephrosis on prenatal ultrasound and a palpable bladder and prostate most likely has congenital urinary tract obstruction, probably related to posterior urethral valves.

Laboratory findings: The presence of hematuria, proteinuria, and red blood cell or granular urinary casts suggests intrinsic ARF, in particular glomerular disease. The presence of white blood cells, and white blood cell casts with low grade hematuria and proteinuria suggests tubulointerstitial disease. Urinary eosinophils may be present in children with drug-induced tubulointerstitial nephritis. Urinary indices useful in differentiating prerenal ARF from intrinsic ARF is described in Table 21.1. Renal biopsy may ultimately be required to determine the precise cause of ARF in patients who do not have clearly defined prerenal or postrenal ARF.

Chest radiography may reveal cardiomegaly and pulmonary congestion (fluid overload). Renal ultrasonography may reveal hydronephrosis and/or hydroureter, which are suggestive of urinary tract obstruction.

Treatment

Medical treatment: In a newborn with urinary tract obstruction with suspected posterior urethral valves, a bladder catheter should be placed immediately for adequate drainage. The placement of a bladder catheter may also be considered in nonambulatory older children and adolescents to accurately monitor urine output during ARF.

If there is no evidence of volume overload or cardiac failure, intravascular volume should be expanded by intravenous administration of isotonic saline, 20 ml/kg over 30 min. Severe hypovolemia may require additional fluid boluses. In the absence of blood loss or hypoproteinemia, colloid containing solutions are not required for volume expansion. After volume resuscitation, hypovolemic patients generally void within 2 hr; failure to do so indicates the presence of

---

Box 21.8: Common causes of acute renal failure

Prerenal: Dehydration, hemorrhage, sepsis, hypoalbuminemia, cardiac failure.

Intrinsic renal: Glomerulonephritis (postinfectious, poststreptococcal, lupus erythematosus, Henoch-Schönlein purpura, membroproliferative, anti-glomerular basement membrane), hemolytic uremic syndrome (HUS), acute tubular necrosis, renal cortical necrosis, renal vein thrombosis, rhabdomyolysis, acute interstitial nephritis, tumor infiltration, tumor lysis syndrome.

Postrenal: Posterior urethral valves, ureteropelvic junction obstruction, ureterovesical junction obstruction, ureterocele, tumor, urolithiasis, hemorrhagic cystitis, neurogenic bladder.

Table 21.1: Laboratory indices for prenatal vs intrinsic acute renal failure		
Laboratory indices	*Prerenal*	*Intrinsic renal*
Specific gravity	> 1020	< 1010
Urine osmolality (mOsm/kg)	> 500	< 350
Urine sodium (mEq/L)	< 20	> 40
FENa (%)	< 1(< 2.5% in neonates)	> 2 (> 10% in neonates)
Blood urea nitrogen/creatinine	> 20	< 20

FENa: fractional excretion of sodium; PCr: plasma creatinine; PNa: plasma sodium; UCr: urea creatinine; UNa: urea sodium

$$FENa\ (\%) = \frac{UNa \times PCr}{PNa \times UCr} \times 100$$

intrinsic or postrenal ARF. Determination of central venous pressure may be helpful if adequacy of blood volume is in question.

Diuretic therapy should be considered only after the adequacy of the circulating blood volume has been established. Mannitol (0.5g/kg) and frusemide (2–4 mg/kg) may be administered as a single IV dose. Bumetanide (0.1 mg/kg) may be given as an alternative to frusemide. If urine output is not improved, then a continuous diuretic infusion may be considered. To increase renal cortical blood flow, many clinicians administer dopamine (2–3 μg/kg/min) in combination with diuretic therapy, although no controlled data supports this practice. There is a little evidence that diuretics or dopamine can prevent ARF or hasten recovery. Mannitol may be effective in pigment (myoglobin, hemoglobin)-induced renal failure.

If there is no response to diuretic therapy, diuretics should be discontinued and fluids should be restricted. Patients with a relatively normal intravascular volume should initially be limited to 400 mL/m^2/24 hr (insensible losses) plus an amount of fluid equal to the urine output for that day. Extrarenal (blood, gastrointestinal) fluid losses should be replaced, milliliter for milliliter, with appropriate fluids. Markedly hypervolemic patients may require further fluid restriction, omitting the replacement of insensible fluid losses, urine output, and extrarenal losses to diminish the expanded intravascular volume. Fluid intake, stool and urine output, body weight, and serum chemistries should be monitored on a daily basis.

In ARF rapid development of *hyperkalemia* (serum potassium level > 6 mEq/L) occurs; the earliest electrocardiographic change seen is the appearance of peaked T waves and this may be followed by widening of the QRS intervals, ST segment depression, ventricular arrhythmias, and cardiac arrest. Procedures to deplete body potassium stores should be initiated when the serum potassium value rises above 6.0 mEq/L. Exogenous sources of potassium (dietary, intravenous fluids, total parenteral nutrition) should be eliminated. Sodium polystyrene sulfonate resin (Kayexalate), 1 g/kg should be given orally or by retention enema. Resin therapy may be repeated every 2 hr, the frequency being limited primarily by the risk of sodium overload. This resin exchanges sodium for potassium and a single dose of 1 g/kg can lower the serum potassium level by about 1 mEq/L.

If the serum potassium is still elevated (> 7 mEq/L), especially if accompanied by electrocardiographic changes, in addition to Kayexalate, the following agents should be administered: calcium gluconate (10% solution, 1 ml/kg IV, over 3–5 min), sodium bicarbonate (1–2 mEq/kg IV, over 1–10 min), and regular insulin (0.1 U/kg with glucose 50% solution, 1 ml/kg, IV over 1 hr). Calcium gluconate counteracts the potassium-induced increase in myocardial irritability, but does not lower the serum potassium. Sodium bicarbonate and insulin and glucose lower the serum potassium level by shifting potassium from the extracellular to the intracellular compartment. Because the duration of action of these emergency measures is just a few hours, persistent hyperkalemia should be managed by dialysis. In adults a β-adrenergic agonist administration has been reported to lower the serum potassium level as an emergency measure, but there are no controlled data in pediatric patients.

Mild *metabolic acidosis* is common in ARF because of retention of hydrogen ions, phosphate, and sulfate, but it rarely requires treatment. If acidosis is severe (arterial pH < 7.15; serum bicarbonate < 8 mEq/L) or contributes to hyperkalemia, treatment is required. The acidosis should be corrected partially by intravenous route, generally giving enough bicarbonate to raise the arterial pH to 7.20 (which approximates a serum bicarbonate level of 12 mEq/L). The remainder of the correction may be accomplished by oral administration of sodium bicarbonate after normalization of the serum calcium and phosphorus levels. Correction of metabolic acidosis with intravenous bicarbonate may precipitate tetany in patients with renal failure as rapid correction or acidosis reduces the ionized calcium concentration.

Hypocalcemia is primarily treated by lowering the serum phosphorus level. Calcium should not be given intravenously, except in cases of tetany, to avoid deposition of calcium salts into tissues. Patients should take a low phosphorus diet and phosphate binders such as calcium carbonate or calcium acetate orally.

Hyponatremia is most commonly a dilutional disturbance that must be corrected by fluid restriction rather than sodium chloride administration. Hypertonic (3%) saline should only be administered in patients with symptomatic hyponatremia (seizures, lethargy) or with the serum sodium level < 120 mEq/L. Acute correction of the serum sodium to 125 mEq/L (mmol/L) should be accomplished using the following formula:

mEq/L NaCl required = 0.6 × weight (kg) × [125 – serum sodium (mEq/L)].

ARF patients are predisposed to *gastrointestinal bleeding* because of uremic dysfunction, increased stress, and heparin exposure if on hemodialysis or continuous renal replacement therapy. Oral or intravenous H$_2$ blockers such as ranitidine should be administered to prevent this complication.

Hypertension may result from hyperreninemia associated with primary disease process and/or expansion of the extracellular fluid volume and is most common in ARF patients with acute glomerulonephritis or HUS. Salt and water restriction and diuretics should be used along with antihypertensive therapy. Nifedipine (0.025–0.5 mg/kg PO, maximum dose 10 mg q 2–6 hr) may be administered for relatively rapid reduction of blood pressure. Longer acting antihypertensive agents such as calcium channel blockers (amlodipine, 0.1–0.6 mg/kg/24 hr qd or divided bid) or β-blockers (propranolol, 0.5–8 mg/kg/24 hr divided bid or tid; labetalol, 4–40 mg/kg/24 hr divided bid or tid) may be helpful in maintaining control of blood pressure. Patients with severe symptomatic hypertension (hypertensive emergency) should be treated with continuous infusions of sodium nitroprusside (0.5–10 µg/kg/min), labetalol (0.25–3.0 mg/kg/hr), or esmolol (150–300 µg/kg/min) and converted to intermittently dosed antihypertensives when more stable.

Neurologic symptoms may include headache, seizures, lethargy and confusion. Potential etiologic factors responsible for neurologic symptoms include hyponatremia, hypocalcemia, hypertension, cerebral hemorrhage, cerebral vasculitis, and the uremic state. Diazepam should be used to control seizures and therapy should be directed toward the precipitating cause.

Anemia of ARF is generally mild (hemoglobin 9–11 g/dl) and primarily results from volume expansion. Children with HUS, SLE, active, or prolonged ARF may require transfusion of packed red blood cells if their hemoglobin falls below 7 g/dl. Slow (4–6 hr) transfusion with packed red blood cells (10 ml/kg) diminishes the risk of hypervolemia. The use of fresh, washed red blood cells minimizes the risk of hyperkalemia. In the presence of hypervolemia or hyperkalemia, blood transfusions are most safely administered during dialysis/ultrafiltration.

Nutrition: In most cases, sodium, potassium, and phosphorus should be restricted. Protein should be restricted moderately while maximizing caloric intake to minimize the accumulation of nitrogenous wastes. In critically ill patients, parenteral hyperalimentation with essential amino acids should be considered.

Dialysis: (*See* Section 21.5 on Dialysis in children).

Prognosis: The mortality rate in children depends entirely on the nature of the underlying cause rather than on the renal failure itself; low mortality rate (< 1%) in renal limited condition such as postinfectious glomerulonephritis and a very high mortality rate (> 90%) in ARF related to multiorgan failure.

Chronic Kidney Disease

Chronic Kidney Disease (CKD) is defined as either renal injury (proteinuria) and/or a glomerular filtration rate < 60 ml/min/1.73 m^2 for > 3 months. The standardized terminology to describe the stages of chronic kidney disease is shown in Table 21.2.

Etiology: In children CKD may be the result of congenital, acquired, inherited, or metabolic renal disease. The underlying cause correlates closely with the age of the patient at the time when the CKD is first detected. CKD in children younger than 5 yr is most commonly the result of congenital abnormalities, whereas in children after 5 yr of age acquired diseases. The causes of CKD are listed in Box 21.9.

Clinical manifestations: The clinical presentation of CKD is quite varied and dependent on the underlying renal disease. Children and adolescents with chronic glomerulonephritis (membranoproliferative glomerulonephritis) may present with edema, hypertension, hematuria, and proteinuria. Infants and children with congenital disorders such as renal dysplasia and obstructive uropathy may present in neonatal period with failure to thrive, polyuria, dehydration, urinary tract infection, or overt renal insufficiency. Many infants with congenital kidney disease are identified with prenatal ultrasonography, allowing early diagnostic and therapeutic intervention.

Table 21.2: Standardized terminology for stages of chronic kidney disease

Stage	Description	GFR (ml/min/1.73 m^2)
Stage 1	Kidney damage with normal or increased GFR	> 90
Stage 2	Mild decrease in glomerular filtration rate (GFR)	60–89
Stage 3	Moderate decrease in GFR	30–59
Stage 4	Severe decrease in GFR	5–29
Stage 5	Kidney failure	< 15 or on dialysis

Box 21.9: Causes of chronic kidney disease (CKD) in relation to age of the patient

Children younger than 5 yr: renal hyperplasia, renal dysplasia, obstructive uropathy, congenital nephrotic syndrome, Prune belly syndrome, renal cortical necrosis, focal segmental glomerulonephritis, polycystic kidney disease, renal vein thrombosis, hemolytic uremic syndrome.

Children older than 5 yr: various forms of glomerulonephritis including lupus nephritis, inherited disorders (familial juvenile nephronophthisis, Alport syndrome, polycystic kidney disease), metabolic disorders (cystinosis, hyperoxaluria).

The physical examination with CKD may reveal pallor and a shallow appearance. Patients with long standing untreated CKD may have short stature and the bony abnormalities of renal osteodystrophy. Children with CKD due to chronic glomerulonephritis (or children with advanced renal failure from any cause) may have edema, hypertension, and other signs of extracellular fluid volume overload.

Laboratory findings: Laboratory findings reveal elevations in blood urea nitrogen and serum creatinine and may also show hyperkalemia, hypocalcemia, hyperphosphatemia, hypoalbuminemia and an elevation in cholesterol, triglyceride and uric acid levels. In children with CKD caused by glomerulonephritis, the urinalysis shows hematuria and proteinuria and in cases of renal dysplasia low specific gravity and minimal abnormalities. The degree of renal dysfunction may be determined by applying the following formula, which provides an estimation of the patient's GFR:

$$GFR \ (mL/min/1.73 \ m^2)$$
$$= \frac{k \times height \ (cm)}{Serum \ creatinine \ (mg/dL)}$$

(where k is 0.33 for low birth weight infants younger than 1 yr, 0.45 for term AGA infants younger than 1 yr, 0.55 for children and adolescent females, and 0.70 for adolescent males).

Treatment: The management of CKD requires close monitoring of a patient's clinical laboratory status including serum electrolytes, blood urea nitrogen, creatinine, calcium, phosphorus, albumin, alkaline phosphatase, and hemoglobin levels. Periodic measurement of parathyroid hormone (PTH) levels and roentgenographic studies of bone may be helpful in early diagnosis of renal osteodystrophy. Echocardiography should be performed periodically to identify left ventricular hypertrophy and cardiac dysfunction. The aim of treatment of CKD is (1) replacing absent/diminished renal functions and (2) slowing the progression of renal dysfunction.

Fluid and electrolyte management: Most children with CKD maintain their normal sodium and water balance with an appropriate diet. Children with high blood pressure, edema or heart failure may require sodium restriction and diuretic therapy. Hyperkalemia may develop in patients with moderate renal insufficiency, who have excessive dietary potassium intake, severe acidosis, or hyporeninemic hypoaldosteronism (related to the destruction of the renin-secreting juxtaglomerular apparatus). Hyperkalemia may be treated by restriction of dietary potassium intake, administration of oral alkalizing agents, and/or treatment with sodium polystyrene sulfonate (Kayexalate).

Acidosis: Metabolic acidosis develops in almost all children with CKD as a result of decreased acid excretion by the failing kidneys. Either sodium citrate (1 mEq/ml) or sodium bicarbonate tablets (650 mg equals 8 mEq of base) may be used to maintain the serum bicarbonate level >22 mEq/L.

Nutrition: Patients with CKD usually require progressive restriction of various dietary components as their renal functions deteriorates, such as dietary phosphorus, potassium and sodium. In infants with CKD, formulas containing a reduced amount of phosphate are commonly used. Protein intake should be 2.5 g/kg/24 hr and should consist of proteins of high biologic value that are metabolized primarily to usable amino acids rather than to nitrogenous waste. The proteins of high biologic value are those of eggs and milk, followed by meat, fish, and fowl. The optimal caloric intake in patients with CKD is unknown. If oral caloric intake remains inadequate and/or weight gain, and growth velocity suboptimal, enteral tube-feedings should be considered. Children with CKD may become deficient in water soluble vitamins either because of inadequate dietary intake or dialysis losses, which should be continuously supplied. Zinc and iron supplements should be added only if deficiencies are confirmed.

Growth: Children with CKD have growth hormone (GH) resistance with elevated GH levels and decreased insulin-like-growth factor I levels and major abnormalities of insulin-like growth factor-binding proteins. Children with CKD who remain less than –2 SD for height despite optimal medical support (adequate caloric intake and effective treatment of renal osteodystrophy, anemia, and metabolic acidosis) may benefit from treatment with pharmacologic doses of recombinant human GH (rHuGH).

Renal osteodystrophy: The skeletal pathologic finding in this condition is osteitis fibrosa cystica. The clinical manifestations of renal osteodystrophy include muscle weakness, bone pain, and fractures with minor trauma. In growing children, rachitic changes, varus and valgus deformities of the long bones, and slipped capital femoral epiphyses may be seen. Laboratories studies may demonstrate a decreased serum calcium level, increased serum phosphorus level, increased alkaline phosphatase, and a normal PTH level. Radiographs of the hands, wrists, and knees show subperiosteal resorption of bone with widening of the metaphyses.

Children and adolescents should follow a low phosphorus diet, and infants should be provided low phosphorus formula. Because it is impossible to fully restrict phosphorus intake, phosphate binders are used to enhance fecal phosphate excretion. Calcium carbonate and calcium acetate have been the most commonly used phosphate binders, newer, non-calcium based binders such as sevelamer (Renagel) are increasing in use, particularly in patients prone to hypercalcemia.

Vitamin D therapy is indicated in patients with (1) 25-hydroxy-vitamin D levels below the established goal range or (2) PTH levels above the established goal range for CKD stage. Patients with low 25-hydroxy-vitamin D levels should be treated with ergocalciferol. Patients with a normal25-hydroxy-vitamin D level but elevated PTH level should be treated with 0.01–0.05 μg/kg/24 hr of calcitriol (0. 25 μg capsules or 1 μg/ ml suspension). Phosphate binders and vitamin D should be adjusted to maintain the PTH level within the designated goal range and serum calcium and phosphorus levels within the normal range for age. It is better to maintain the calcium/phosphorus product $(Ca \times PO_4)$ at < 55 to minimize the possibility of tissue deposition of calcium phosphorus salts.

Adynamic bone disease: Children have osteomalacia associated with oversuppression of PTH, perhaps related to the widespread use of calcium-containing phosphate binders and vitamin D analogues.

Anemia: Anemia is primarily the result of inadequate erythropoietin production by the failing kidneys and usually becomes manifest in patients with stages 3–4 CKD. Other contributory factors include iron deficiency, folic acid or B_{12} deficiency, and decreased erythrocyte survival. Recombinant human erythropoietin (rHuEPO) therapy has decreased the need for transfusion. Erythropoietin is usually initiated when the patient's hemoglobin concentration falls below 10 g/dL, at a dose of 50–150 mg/kg/dose subcutaneously 1–3 times weekly, and the dose is adjusted to maintain the hemoglobin concentration between 12 and 13 g/dL. All patients receiving rHuEPO therapy should be provided with either oral or intravenous iron supplementation. Patients who appear to be resistant to rHuEPO should be evaluated for iron deficiency, occult blood loss, chronic infection/inflammatory state, vitamin B_{12} or folate deficiency, and bone marrow fibrosis related to secondary hyperparathyroidism. An alternative option is darbopoietin alfa (Aranesp), a longer acting agent administered at a dose of 0.45 μg/kg/wk; may be given once weekly to once monthly.

Hypertension: Hypertensive children with suspected volume overload should follow a salt restricted diet (2–3 g/24 hr) and should receive thiazide diuretics (hydrochlorothiazide 2 mg/kg/24 hr divided bid) if having mild renal dysfunction (CKD stages 1–3), and frusemide (1–2 mg/kg/dose bid or tid) if GFR falls into stage 4 CKD. ACE inhibitors (enalapril or lisinopril) and angiotensin II blockers (losartan) are the antihypertensive medications of choice in children with proteinuria, because of their potential ability to slow the progression to ESRD. Calcium channel blockers (amlodipine), β blockers (propranolol, arenolol), and centrally acting agents (clonidine) may be useful as adjunctive agents in children whose blood pressure cannot be controlled using dietary sodium restriction, diuretics, and ACE inhibitors.

Immunizations: Children with CKD should receive all the standard immunizations according to the schedule used for healthy children and a yearly influenza vaccine. Live vaccines should not be administered in children with CKD related to glomerulonephritis during immunosuppressive therapy. It is important, to administer live virus vaccines [MMR (measles, mumps, rubella), varicella] before renal transplantation because these vaccines are not advised for use in immunosuppressed patients. Children with CKD may respond suboptimally to immunizations.

Adjustment in drug dose: Drugs that are excreted by kidneys, their dosing may need to be adjusted to maximize effectiveness and minimize the risk of toxicity. The dose adjustment includes lengthening the interval between doses, decreasing the absolute dose, or both.

Progression of disease: There are no definitive treatments to improve renal functions in children or adults with CKD, but slowing the rate of progression of renal dysfunction is possible. (1) Optimal control of hypertension (maintaining blood pressure at lower than the 75th percentile and if possible even lower). (2) Serum phosphorus should be maintained within the normal range for age and the calcium-phosphorus product < 55 to minimize renal calcium-phosphorus deposition. (3) Prompt treatment of infectious complications and dehydration to minimize additional loss of renal parenchyma. (4) Correction of anemia with erythropoietin or darbopoietin alfa therapy. (5) Control of hyperlipidemia, avoidance of cigarette smoking, prevention of obesity, and minimum use of nonsteroidal anti-inflammatory medicine. (6) Dietary protein restriction is generally not suggested for children because of the concern of adverse effects on growth and development.

End-Stage Renal Disease

End-stage renal disease (ESRD) represents the state in which the renal dysfunction of the patient has progressed to the point at which homeostasis and survival can no longer be sustained with native kidney function and maximal medical management. At this point renal replacement therapy (dialysis or renal transplantation) becomes necessary.

Chan JCM, William DM, Roth KS. Kidney failure in infants and children. *Pediatr Rev* 2002; 23: 47–59.

Phadke K, Vasudevan A, IyengarA. Pediatric Renal Transplantation. In: Mathur GP, Mathur Sarla (eds). *Current Trends in Pediatrics.* Vol 3. Delhi: Academa Publishers. 2007; 39–55.

Urizar RE. Renal transplantation. In: Kliegman RM, Behrman RE, Jenson HB, Stanton BF (eds). *Nelson Textbook of Pediatrics.* 18th edn. Vol. 2. Philadelphia: Saunders, 2007; 2214–2219.

Vogt BA, Avner ED. Renal failure. In: Kliegman RM, Behrman RE, Jenson HB, Stanton BF (eds). *Nelson Textbook of Pediatrics.* 18th edn. Vol. 2. Philadelphia: Saunders, 2007; 2206–2214.

Dialysis in Children

A wide variety of dialysis modalities are available for management of patients with acute renal failure (ARF) and end stage renal disease (ESRD). The recent development of continuous therapies, including hemofiltration and related techniques, has facilitated the provision of dialysis to more complicated and unstable patients than in the past. Such therapies are finding increasing use in the treatment of children with renal failure all across the world.

Indications of dialysis: **(a) Acute renal failure (ARF):** The indications for initiating dialysis in ARF include uremic pericarditis or encephalopathy, fluid overload associated with congestive heart failure or hypertension, uncontrolled hyperkalemia, metabolic acidosis, and hyperphosphatemia.

(b) End-stage renal disease (ESRD): Although no predetermined threshold level of serum creatinine or blood urea nitrogen has been established above which dialysis should be started, regular dialysis is usually considered when the creatinine clearance has decreased below 10 ml/min/1.73 m^2. Children with advanced renal disease may present with nonspecific symptoms such as decreased appetite, nausea and vomiting, easy fatigability, reduced exercise tolerance, and poor school performance, which may prompt dialysis initiation. Young children with poor growth may also be considered for dialysis. In addition, regular dialysis should be considered when nutritional requirements cannot be maintained because of severe fluid limitations.

Principle of various dialysis modalities: Dialysis procedures remove nitrogenous end-products of catabolism and begin the correction of the salt, water, and acid-base derangements associated with renal failure. Dialysis is an imperfect treatment for the myriad abnormalities that occur in renal failure, as it does not correct the endocrine functions of the kidney. All forms of readily available dialysis depend on diffusion of small molecules across a semipermeable membrane; extracorporeal with a synthetic cellulose membrane in hemodialysis and intracorporeal with a biologic membrane in peritoneal dialysis. Dialysis works on the principles of the diffusion and osmosis of solutes and fluid across a semipermeable membrane. Blood flows by one side of a semipermeable membrane, and dialysis fluid flows by the opposite side. Smaller solutes and fluid pass through the membrane. The concentrations of undesired solutes (for example, potassium, calcium, and urea) are high in the blood, but low or absent in the dialysis solution and constant replacement of the dialysate ensures that the concentration of undesired solutes is kept low on this side of the membrane. The dialysis solution has levels of minerals like potassium and calcium that are similar to their natural concentration in healthy blood. For bicarbonate, dialysis solution level is set at a slightly higher level than in normal blood, to encourage diffusion of bicarbonate into the blood, to neutralize the metabolic acidosis that is often present in these patients (Table 21.3).

Peritoneal Dialysis

Acute peritoneal dialysis (PD): Acute PD has been the renal replacement therapy of choice for decades in ARF because of its simplicity and safety and the relative ease with which the procedure can be performed in very small patients. The technique has no serious hemodynamic consequences and no vascular access is needed (which is often the limiting factor in the dialysis of small children and infants). However, the acute PD catheter needs careful attention, because catheter-related infections continue to be the most common complication of acute PD in children and infants and the most frequent cause of catheter removal. Traditionally, the catheters that have most commonly been used for acute PD in infants and children are the non-cuffed, rigid acute catheter and the surgically placed cuffed silicone Tenckhoff catheters. Once inserted, a stiff catheter can be used safely for a maximum of 72 hours beyond which there is an increasing risk of peritonitis. Thus when one anticipates that the patient will need PD for more than one week, a permanent catheter or a single-cuff Tenckhoff soft catheter should be inserted. Easy and safe bedside placement of a single-cuff soft Tenckhoff peritoneal catheter may lead to favorable outcomes of PD treatment in children and infants with ARF.

Table 21.3: Constituents of dialysis solutions used in PD and HD

Constituent	Peritoneal dialysis	Hemodialysis
pH	5.8	
Dextrose (g/dl)	1.7	0.1
Sodium (mEq/L)	130	135–140
Potassium (mEq/L)	0	0–3
Chloride (mEq/L)	100	108
Acetate/lactate (mEq/L)	35	35–40
Magnesium (mEq/L)	1.5	0.5–1.5
Calcium (mEq/L)	3.0	2.5–3.2
Osmolality (mOsm/kg)	355	

Note: Icodextrin, amino acid and neutral PD fluids also used in ESRD

Acute PD prescription: After insertion of an acute or (preferably) chronic peritoneal catheter, the dialysis prescription must be individualized to the patient's clinical situation. The infusion volume, commonly 0.5 L – 2 L, must be adjusted to the size of the patient's peritoneal cavity and to the severity of the uremic syndrome. In children, a fluid volume of 20 – 50 mL/kg is typical starting volume. The exchange time (combined time for inflow, dwell, and drain) most commonly used is 1 hour (inflow 10 minutes, dwell 30 minutes, outflow 20 minutes). Usually 2 L hourly exchanges of a solution with 1.5% glucose usually give an ultrafiltration rate of 50–150 ml/hr, which equals 1200–3600 ml/24 hr; higher glucose concentrations (2.5–4.25%) can result in the removal of larger volumes of fluid (200 – 400 ml/hr). Furthermore, by reducing the dwell time (the time from the end of inflow to the beginning of outflow) to 15 minutes from 30 minutes, the dialysate flow rate can be increased to about 4 L/hr and thus achieve more efficient dialysis that might be used for short periods in hypercatabolic and hyperkalemic patients. The length of the session depends on the dose of acute PD that must be delivered. A patient with ARF requires continuous removal of fluids and solutes, especially when oliguric, hypercatabolic, and in need of ongoing nutritional and therapeutic support. In such a case, PD sessions regularly last from 24 hours to 72 hours with hourly 2 L exchanges, but the PD dose would be considered efficient if it can meet the daily protein and energy requirements of the patient and maintain stable, near-normal fluid and electrolyte homeostasis.

Chronic peritoneal dialysis (PD): The three types of chronic peritoneal dialysis differ mainly in the schedule of exchanges. In *continuous ambulatory peritoneal dialysis* (CAPD), the patient empties a fresh bag of dialysis solution into the abdomen. After 4 to 6 hours of dwell time (during the day), the patient returns the solution containing wastes to the bag. The patient then repeats the cycle with a fresh bag of solution. CAPD does not require a machine; the process uses gravity to fill and empty the abdomen. A typical prescription for CAPD requires three or four exchanges during the day and one long (usually 8 to 10 hours) overnight exchange as the patient sleeps. For added clearance, a mini-cycler machine can be used to exchange the dialysis solution once or several times overnight as the patient sleeps.

Continuous cycler-assisted peritoneal dialysis (CCPD) uses a machine to fill and empty the abdomen three to five times during the night while the child sleeps. In the morning, the CCPD patient performs one exchange with a dwell time that lasts the entire day. Sometimes one additional exchange is done in the mid-afternoon to increase the amount of waste removed and to prevent excessive absorption of fluid.

Nocturnal intermittent peritoneal dialysis (NIPD) is like CCPD, only the number of overnight exchanges is greater (six or more), and the patient does not perform an exchange during the day. Peritoneal dialysis is associated with complications; that may occur as a result of catheter placement or the procedure per se. The advantages and disadvantages and complications of peritoneal are listed in Tables 21.4 and 21.5 respectively.

Hemodialysis

Achieving venous access in infants and young children is a challenging task even for pediatricians. In hemodialysis (HD), a patient's blood is pumped into a dialyzer containing two fluid compartments configured as bundles of hollow fiber capillary tubes. Blood is pumped along one side of a semipermeable membrane while the dialysate is pumped along the other side, in a separate compartment, in the opposite direction. Concentration gradients of solute between blood and dialysate lead to desired changes in the patient's serum solutes, such as a reduction in urea nitrogen and creatinine; an increase in HCO_3; and equilibration of Na, Cl, K, and Mg. The dialyzed blood is then returned to the patient. The dialysate compartment is under negative pressure relative to the blood compartment to prevent filtration of dialysate into the bloodstream and to remove the excess fluid from the patient. There are three methods of accessing the bloodstream: 1. Arteriovenous fistula (AVF), 2. Arteriovenous graft (AVG), 3. Temporary venous dialysis catheter.

Hemodialysis in children is performed under carefully controlled circumstances, with close and frequent monitoring of vital signs, blood pressure, physical examination, and assessment of body weight before, during (if available, within bed scales) and after treatments. The extracorporeal blood volume can often be maintained at < 8 – 10% of the intravascular volume. Blood flow rates generated by the dialysis peristaltic pump usually range from 3 to 5 ml/kg body weight/minute, often starting at the lower blood flow rate and slowly increasing the rate during the procedure. Heparinization is provided during the HD procedure, typically with a pre-dialysis infusion of 10 – 20 U/kg/dose with bedside monitoring of the activated clotting time (ACT). The decision on the amount of ultrafiltration (fluid volume to be removed from the patient during the dialysis process) depends on the extent of the pre-dialysis volume status (including the presence of edema), blood pressure, and the weight gain noted between dialysis procedures. The advantages and disadvantages and complications of hemodialysis are shown in Tables 21.4 and 21.5 respectively.

Continuous Renal Replacement Therapy (CRRT)

Continuous renal replacement therapies (CRRT) are dialysis treatments that are provided as a continuous 24 hour per day therapy. The major difference between intermittent and continuous therapies is the speed at which water and wastes are removed. Intermittent hemodialysis removes large amounts of water and wastes in a short period of time (usually over 2–4 hours), whereas continuous renal replacement therapies remove water and wastes at a slow and steady rate. While intermittent dialysis allows chronic renal failure patients to limit the amount of time that they are connected to a machine, the rapid removal of water and wastes during intermittent treatments may be poorly tolerated by hemodynamically unstable patients.

Originally it was proposed as a simple method of filtration powered by arteriovenous circuits and known as CAVH (continuous arteriovenous hemofiltration). Now several technical modifications has been developed to enhance the efficiency of the treatment. These include the addition of a diffusive component to solute removal, known as CAVHD (continuous arteriovenous hemodialysis), and the development of specialized machines for providing continuous pumped filtration allowing for a new set of extremely efficient techniques that do not require arterial access and that are no longer dependent on the variability of the patient's changing blood pressure e.g. CVVH (continuous venovenous hemo-filtration), CVVHD (continuous venovenous hemodialysis), and CVVHDF (continuous venovenous hemo-diafiltration).

Table 21.4: Advantages and disadvantages of peritoneal dialysis as compared to hemodialysis	
Advantages	*Disadvantages*
1. Widely available and easy to perform	1. PD catheters cannot be inserted in patients with multiple intra-abdominal adhesions
2. Low risk of disequilibrium syndrome	2. Provides relatively small quantity of dialysis in catabolic patients with ARF
3. Minimal cardiovascular stress due to gradual fluid removal	3. Cannot correct severe hyperkalemia rapidly peritonitis
4. Safe in patients with poor cardiac function	
5. No vascular access, anticoagulation needed	

Table 21.5: Complications of peritoneal dialysis and hemodialysis	
Peritoneal dialysis	*Hemodialysis*
Visceral perforations of bowel, bladder or aorta	Hemorrhage
Pain on inflow of dialysis solution	Dialysis disequilibrium
Bloody dialysate	Catheter related infections
Dialysate leakage	Back, chest pain, leg cramps
Catheter malfunction	Fever, chills (infected catheter related bacteremia)
Peritonitis	Headache, light-headness, nausea, vomiting
Surgical wound infection	Hypotension
Ultra-filtration failure	

The continuous renal replacement therapy has several potential advantages over intermittent dialytic techniques (Table 21.6). The most obvious is that the treatment is continuous, allowing for a constant readjustment of fluid and electrolyte therapy and the administration of large amounts of parenteral nutrition without the risk of interdialytic volume overload. Second among the advantages at least for the hemofiltration-based treatments (CAVH, CVVH) is its convective mode of solute transport, known to increase middle molecule clearance when compared with diffusion-based dialytic techniques. When compared with peritoneal dialysis, CRRT is not contraindicated in patients with prior abdominal surgery and offers iso-volumetric fluid removal without the risk of peritonitis. The major drawbacks are the need for continuous anticoagulation and that the patient must remain bedridden during the treatment.

Choice of modality of treatment: From a clinical standpoint, the two most-important factors that influence choice of a dialysis modality are the indication for dialysis and the overall clinical status of the patient. Table 21.7 shows the various dialysis modalities and their specific indications. Both hemodialysis (HD) and peritoneal dialysis (PD) are effective in the management of ARF. The choice of procedure depends on (i) the age and size of the patient, (ii) cardiovascular status, (iii) the availability of vascular access, or integrity of peritoneal membrane and abdominal cavity, and (iv) the expertise available. Most children with ARF who require dialyses are treated with PD. PD is easier to perform and does not require much equipment. Moreover, the gradual rates of fluid removal and correction of metabolic derangements provided by PD is often an advantage in critically sick children or small infants. PD is also the most effective treatment for severe hyperphosphatemia. Children with cardiovascular compromise also tolerate this procedure better than HD. The wide range of acute PD catheters available and their ease of insertion make PD technically feasible even in the smallest infant. Hemodialysis should be considered (1) if rapid removal of toxins is desired, (2) if the size of the patient makes hemodialysis less technically cumbersome and hemodynamically well tolerated, or (3) if impediments to efficient peritoneal dialysis are present (e.g. ileus, adhesions). Furthermore, if vascular access and usage of anticoagulation are not impediments, a slow, continuous hemodialytic process (continuous renal replacement treatment) may be applied specially in hemodynamically unstable patients in an intensive care unit.

Alarabi AA, Petersson T, Danielson BG, Wikstrom B. Continuous peritoneal dialysis in children with acute renal failure. *Adv Perit Dial* 1994; 10:289–293.

Table 21.6: Advantages and disadvantages of continuous renal replacement therapy

Advantages of using CRRT	*Disadvantages of using CRRT*
1. Suitable for use in hemodynamically unstable patients.	1. Extremely costly.
2. Precise volume control, which is immediately adaptable to changing circumstances.	2. Anticoagulation—to prevent extracorporeal circuit from clotting.
3. Very effective control of uremia, hypophosphatemia and hyperkalemia.	3. Complications of line insertion and sepsis.
4. Available 24 hours a day with minimal training.	4. Risk of line disconnection.
5. May have an effect as an adjuvant therapy in sepsis.	5. Hypothermia.
6. Probable advantage in terms of renal recovery.	6. Severe depletion of electrolytes—particularly potassium and phosphate.

Table 21.7: Selection of dialysis modality in ARF

Indication of dialysis	*Dialysis Modality* *Hemodynamically stable*	*Hemodynamically unstable*
Fluid overload	Intermittent hemodialysis (IHD) with isolated ultrafiltration	Continuous venovenous hemofiltration (CVVH) or Peritoneal dialysis (PD)
Uremia	IHD or PD	CVVH or PD
Hyperkalemia	IHD	IHD
Metabolic acidosis	IHD or CVVH or PD	CVVH or PD
Hyperphosphatemia	CVVH	CVVH

Flynn JT. Causes, management approaches, and outcome of acute renal failure in children. *Curr Opin Pediatr* 1998; 10: 184–189.

Flynn JT. Choice of dialysis modality for management of pediatric acute renal failure. Pediatr Nephrol 2002; 17: 61–69.

Harvey EA. Peritoneal access in children. *Perit Dial Int* 2001; 21(Suppl 3):S218–22.

Kuizon BD, Salusky IB. End stage renal disease. In: Rudolph AM (Ed). *Rudolph's Pediatrics*. New York: McGraw-Hill;, 2003; 1345–1346.

Latta K, Krull F, Wilken M, Burdelski P, Rodeck B, Offiner G. Continuous arteriovenous hemofiltration in critically ill children. *Pediatr Nephrol* 1994; 8: 334–337.

Mendoza SA, Griswold WR, Peterson BM, et al. Acute peritoneal dialysis in critically ill infants and children. *Dial Transplant* 1993; 22:129–132.

Passadakis PS, Oreopoulos DG. Peritoneal Dialysis in Patients with Acute Renal Failure. *Advances in Peritoneal Dialysis* 2007; 23:7–16.

22 Urologic Disorders

22.1 URINARY TRACT INFECTIONS

Urinary tract infections (UTIs) occur in 3–5% of girls and 1% of boys. The prevalence of UTIs varies with age. During the first year of life, the male : female ratio is 2.8–5.4:1. Beyond 1–2 yr, there is a female preponderance with a male : female ratio 1:10.

Etiology: UTIs is mainly caused by colonic bacteria. In females 75–90% of all infections are caused by *Escherichia coli*, followed by *Klebsiella* spp. and *Proteus* spp. In males older than 1 yr of age, *Proteus, E. coli* and gram-positive organisms are responsible for UTIs. *Staphylococcus saprophyticus* and *Enterococcus* are pathogens in both sexes. Viral infections, particularly adenovirus, also may occur, especially as a cause of cystitis.

Clinical manifestations: The three basic forms of UTI are pyelonephritis, cystitis, and asymptomatic bacteriuria. *Pyelonephritis* is characterized by any or all of the following: abdominal or flank pain, fever, malaise, nausea, vomiting, and occasionally diarrhea. Newborns may show nonspecific symptoms such as poor feeding, irritability, and weight loss. Involvement of the renal parenchyma is termed acute pyelonephritis, whereas if there is no parenchymal involvement, the condition may be termed pyelitis. Acute pyelonephritis may result in renal injury, termed *pyelonephritic scarring*. *Acute lobar nephronia (acute lobar nephritis)* is a localized renal bacterial infection involving >1 lobe that represents either a complication of pyelonephritis or an early stage in the development of *renal abscess* (usually caused by *S. aureus*). *Perinephric abscesses* may

be secondary to contiguous infection in the perirenal area (e.g. vertebral osteomyelitis, psoas abscess) or pyelonephritis that dissects to the renal capsule.

Cystitis indicates that there is bladder involvement; symptoms include dysuria, urgency, frequency, suprapubic pain, incontinence, and malodorous urine. Fever is absent in cystitis and does not result in renal injury.

Asymptomatic bacteriuria refers to a condition that results in a positive urine culture without any manifestations of infection. It is most common in girls. The incidence is 1–2% in preschool and school girls and 0.03% in boys. The condition is benign and does not cause renal injury, except in pregnant woman, in whom asymptomatic bacteriuria, if left untreated, can result in a symptomatic UTI.

Pathogenesis and pathology: All UTIs, virtually are ascending infections. The bacteria arise from the fecal flora, colonize the perineum, and enter the bladder via the urethra. In uncircumcised boys, the bacterial pathogens arise from the flora beneath the prepuce. In some cases, the bacteria causing cystitis ascend to the kidney to cause pyelonephritis. Rarely renal infection may occur by hematogenous spread, as in endocarditis or in some neonates. Host risk factors for UTI are listed in Box 22.1.

Box 22.1: Risk factors for urinary tract infection

Female gender; Uncircumcised male; Vesicoureteral reflux; toilet Training; Voiding dysfunction; Obstructive uropathy; Urethral instrumentation; Wiping from back to front in females; Tight clothing (underwear); Pinworm infestation; Constipation; Bubble bath; Bacteria with P fimbriae; Anatomic abnormality (labial adhesion); Neuropathic bladder; Sexual activity; Pregnancy.

Diagnosis: A UTI may be suspected based on symptoms or findings on urinalysis or both. A urine culture is necessary for confirmation and appropriate therapy. The correct diagnosis of UTI depends on having the proper sample of urine. In *toilet-trained children*, a midstream urine sample is usually satisfactory. If the culture shows >100,000 colonies of a single pathogens, or if there are 10,000 colonies and the child is symptomatic, the child is considered to have a UTI. In uncircumcised males, the prepuce must be retracted; if the prepuce is not retractable, this method of urine collection is unreliable. In *infants*, the application of an adhesive, sealed, sterile collection bag after disinfection of the skin of the genitals can be useful, particularly if the culture is negative. A positive culture may reflect a contaminant, particularly in girls and uncircumcised boys. In such cases, if the culture is positive, the patient is symptomatic, and there is a single organism cultured with a colony count greater than 100,000, there is a presumed UTI. If any of these criteria are not met, confirmation of infection with a catheterized sample is recommended. Proper skin preparation and good catheterization technique are important in obtaining the specimen. Use of a No. 5 French polyethylene feeding tube in infants or a No. 8 French tube with proper lubrication in older children minimizes the chance of urethral trauma and contamination. Only a few milliliters need to be aspirated with a syringe to obtain the urine sample. Catheterization shortly after spontaneous voiding produces a measure of the residual urine in the bladder. Prompt plating of the urine culture is important, because if the urine sits in room temperature for more than 60 minutes, overgrowth of a minor contaminant may suggest a UTI, when the urine may not, in fact, be infected. Refrigeration is a reliable method of storing the urine until it can be cultured.

A urinalysis should be obtained from the same specimen that was cultured. Pyuria (leukocytes in the urine) suggests infection, but infection can occur in the absence of pyuria. Nitrites and leukocyte esterase usually are positive in infected urine. Microscopic hematuria is common in cystitis. White blood cell casts in the urinary segment suggest renal involvement. If the child is symptomatic, a UTI is possible even if the urinalysis result is negative.

Imaging studies: In children with a UTI imaging studies are needed to identify anatomic abnormalities that predispose the infection. In children with clinical pyelonephritis (febrile UTI), a renal sonogram should be obtained to rule out hydronephrosis and structural urinary abnormalities; sonography also may suggest acute pyelonephritis by demonstrating an enlarged kidney. Voiding cystourethrogram (VCUG) is recommended in a febrile UTI in girls who have had 2 or 3 UTIs in a period of 6 months, and for boys with more than one UTI. When the diagnosis of acute pyelonephritis is uncertain, renal scanning with technetium-labeled DMSA or glucoheptonate is useful. The presence of photopenia supports the diagnosis of pyelonephritis and also it is possible to differentiate between the acute and chronic process. A DMSA scan is the most sensitive and accurate method for demonstrating scarring in the presence of vesico-ureteral reflux. CT scanning also has been used to evaluate the upper urinary tract, because it is effective in demonstrating renal scarring (*see* Fig. 22.1 in CD).

Treatment: Acute cystitis should be treated to prevent possible progression to pyelonephritis. If the treatment is initiated before the results of a culture and sensitivities are available, a 3 to 5-day course of therapy with trimethoprim-sulfamethoxazole against *E. coli* or nitrofurantoin (5–7 mg/kg/24 hr in 3 or 4 divided doses) against *Klebsiella*—*Enterobacter* organisms or amoxicillin (50 mg/kg/24 hr) is effective.

In acute febrile infection suggestive of pyelonephritis, a 10 to 14 day course of broad-spectrum antibiotics should be used. Children, who are dehydrated, or vomiting, or unable to drink fluids, are 1 month of age, or in whom urosepsis is a possibility should be admitted in the hospital for intravenous rehydration and intravenous antibiotic therapy. Parenteral treatment with ceftriaxone (50–75 mg/kg/24 hr, not to exceed 2 g), or ampicillin (100 mg/kg/24 hr) with an aminoglycoside such as gentamicin (3–5 mg/kg/24 hr in 1 to 3 divided doses) is preferable. The potential ototoxicity and nephrotoxicity of aminoglycosides should be considered and serum creatinine and trough gentamicin must be obtained before starting the treatment. Treatment with aminoglycosides is particularly effective against *Pseudomonas* spp., and alkalization of urine with sodium bicarbonate increases their effectiveness in the urinary tract. The other options for treatment of UTI include: oral 3rd generation cephalosporins such as cefixime effective in gram-negative organisms other than *Pseudomonas;* intramuscular injection of a loading dose of ceftriaxone followed by oral therapy with a 3rd generation cephalosporin; oral fluoroquinolone ciprofloxacin effective against resistant *Pseudomonas*, in patients older than 17 yr (used occasionally for short course therapy in children). The safety and efficacy of fluoroquinolone in children is under study because of potential cartilage damage that has been seen in research in immature animals, thus its clinical use should be restricted. Nitrofurantoin should not be used routinely in children with a febrile UTI because it does not achieve significant renal tissue levels. A urine culture 1 wk after termination of treatment of a UTI ensures that the urine is sterile.

Children with a renal or perirenal abscess or with infection in obstructed urinary tracts often require surgical or percutaneous drainage in addition to antibiotic therapy and other supportive measures.

In a child with UTIs, predisposing factors should be identified such as voiding dysfunction, neurogenic bladder, urinary tract stasis and obstruction, reflux, and calculi may require long-term prophylaxis. Voiding dysfunction in school-aged girls or voiding infrequently and severe constipation in children may require for treatment and counseling of parents and patients in controlling recurrences. Prophylaxis against reinfection, using trimethoprim-sulfamethoxazole, trimethoprim, or nitrofurantoin at ½ of the normal therapeutic dose once a day, often is effective. Prophylaxis with amoxicillin or cephalexin also may be effective, but the risk of breakthrough UTI may be higher because resistance may be induced. The main consequences of chronic renal damage caused by pyelonephritis are arterial hypertension and renal insufficiency.

Craig JC, Hodson EM. Treatment of acute pyelonephritis in children. *BMJ* 2004; 328: 179–180.

Elder JS. Urinary Tract Infections. In: Kliegman RM, Behrman RE, Jenson HB, Stanton BF (eds). *Nelson Textbook of Pediatrics*. 18th edn. Vol. 2. Philadelphia: Saunders, 2007; 2223–2228.

Modgil G, Baverstock A. Should bubble baths be avoided in children with urinary tract infections? *Arch Dis Child* 2006; 91: 863–865.

Shah G, Upadhyay J. Controversies in the diagnosis and management of urinary tract infections in children. *Paediatr Drugs* 2005; 7: 339–346.

Singh-Grewal D, Macdessi J, Craig J. Circumcision for the prevention of urinary tract infection in boys: A systematic review of randomized trials and observational studies. *Arch Dis Child* 2005; 90: 853–858.

22.2 OBSTRUCTION OF THE URINARY TRACT

Ureteropelvic junction obstruction (UPJ): UPJ obstruction is usually caused by intrinsic stenosis and rarely by an accessory artery to the lower pole of the kidney (extrinsic obstruction). The male : female ratio is 2 : 1. The diagnosis is usually established by ultrasonography (*see* Figs 22.2 and 22.3 in CD).

Midureteral obstruction: The causes include congenital ureteral stenosis or a ureteral valve in the midureter, retrocaval ureter (right ureter travels posterior to inferior vena cava, causing extrinsic compression and obstruction), retroperitoneal tumors, fibrosis caused by surgical procedures, inflammatory processes (granulomatous diseases), and radiation therapy. Congenital ureteral stenosis or a ureteral valve in the midureter is corrected by excision of the strictured segment and re-anastomosis of the normal upper and lower segments. Surgical treatment of retrocaval ureter consists of transaction of the upper ureter, moving it anterior to the vena cava, and reanastomosing the upper and lower segments. Repair is necessary only when obstruction is present.

Ectopic ureters: A ureter that drains outside the bladder is referred to as an ectopic ureter. This anomaly is three times more common in girls than in boys and is usually detected prenatally. The ectopic ureter usually drains the upper pole of a duplex collecting system (two ureters). In girls, these ureters enter the- urethra at the bladder neck, urethrovaginal septum, vagina, cervix, uterus, Gartner duct, or a urethral diverticulum. Evaluation includes a renal sonogram, VCUG, and renal scan, which demonstrates whether the affected segment has significant function. If there is satisfactory function, ureteral reimplantation into the bladder or ureterenterostomy (anastomosing the ectopic upper pole ureter into the normally inserting lower pole ureter) is indicated. If function is poor, partial or total nephrectomy is indicated.

Prune-belly syndrome: Prune-belly syndrome, also called triad syndrome or Eagle-Barrett syndrome, is characterized by deficient abdominal muscles, undescended testes, and urinary tract abnormalities, probably results from severe urethral obstruction in fetal life. It occurs in approximately in 1 in 40,000 births, 95% individuals are male. Oligohydramnios and pulmonary hypoplasia are common complications in the perinatal period. When no obstruction is present, prevention of urinary tract infection, with antibiotic prophylaxis should be done. When obstruction of the ureters or urethra is demonstrated, temporary drainage procedures, such as vesicostomy may help to preserve renal function until the child is old enough for surgery.

Bladder neck obstruction: Bladder neck obstruction usually is secondary to ectopic ureterocele, bladder calculi or a tumor of the prostate (rhabdomyosarcoma). The clinical manifestations include difficulty voiding, urinary retention, urinary tract infection, and bladder distension with overflow incontinence.

Posterior urethral valves: Affect one in 8,000 boys. The prostatic urethra dilates and the bladde muscle undergoes hypertrophy. The diagnosis is established with a VCUG or by perineal ultrasonography.

Urethral atresia: Urethral atresia is the most severe form of obstructive uropathy in boys. Some boys with prune-belly syndrome also have urethral atresia.

Urethral construction is difficult and most patients are managed with continent urinary diversion.

Urethral strictures: Urethral strictures in males usually results from urethral trauma, either iatrogenic (catheterization, septic procedures, previous urethral reconstruction) or accidental (straddle injuries, pelvic fractures). The obstruction most commonly causes symptoms of bladder instability, hematuria, or dysuria and decrease in force of the urinary stream is seldom noticed by the child or parents because these lesions develop gradually. Catheterization of the bladder usually is impossible. The diagnosis is made by a voiding film obtained during intravenous urography or retrograde urethrography, or by ultrasonography and endoscopy is confirmatory. Endoscopic treatment of short strictures by direct vision urethrotomy is often successful, but longer strictures surrounded by periurethral fibrosis often require urethroplasty.

Elder JS. Obstruction of the urinary tract. In: Kliegman RM, Behrman RE, Jenson HB, Stanton BF (eds). *Nelson Textbook of Pediatrics*. 18th edn. Vol. 2. Philadelphia: Saunders, 2007; 2234–2243.

Fefer S, Ellsworth P. Prenatal hydronephrosis. *Pediatr Clin North Am* 2006; 53: 429–447.

Sty JR, Pan CG. Genitourinary imaging techniques. *Pediatr Clin North Am* 2006; 53: 339–361.

22.3 ANOMALIES OF THE BLADDER

Bladder exstrophy: Exstrophy of the urinary bladder occurs about once in every 15,000–40,000 births. The male: female ratio is 2:1. The severity ranges from simple epispadias to complete exstrophy of the cloaca involving exposure of the entire hindgut and the bladder. The umbilicus is displaced downward, the pubic rami are widely separated in the midline, and the rectus muscles are separated. In *males*, there is complete epispadias with dorsal chordee, and the overall penile length is approximately half of unaffected boys. The scrotum typically is separated slightly from the penis and undescended testes and inguinal hernias are common. In *females*, there are two halves of the clitoris and wide separation of the labia. The anus is displaced anteriorly in both sexes, and there may be rectal prolapse. The genital deformities can produce sexual disabilities in both sexes particularly in males. The wide separation of the pubic rami causes broad based gait, but no significant disability. In classic bladder exstrophy, the upper urinary tracts are usually normal (*see* Figs 22.4 and 22.5 in CD).

Management of the bladder exstrophy should start at birth. The bladder should be covered with plastic wrap to keep the bladder mucosa moist. The infant should be transferred promptly to a centre equipped for the treatment of such anomalies. Prompt closure of the exstrophic bladder is the preferred treatment. Total reconstruction includes closure of the bladder, closure of the abdominal wall, and in boys, correction of epispadias. The final stage of reconstruction involves creation of a sphincter muscle for bladder control and correction of the vesicoureteral reflux. At this point the child is 3–6 yr old, the bladder capacity should be at least 80–90 mL, and the child must have gained rectal control. Fertility has been low, possibly because of iatrogenic injury to the secondary sexual organs.

Urachal anomalies: Urachal abnormalities are more common in males than in females. 1. A *patent urachus* can occur as an isolated anomaly or may be associated with prune-belly syndrome or posterior urethral valves. In this condition there is continuous urinary drainage from the umbilicus. The tract should be excised. 2. *Urachal cyst*, which can become infected; the clinical findings include suprapubic pain, fever, irritative voiding symptoms and an infraumbilical mass, which may be erythematous. Diagnosis is made by ultrasonography or CT. Treatment is intravenous antibiotic, drainage and excision. 3. *Urachal diverticulum*, which is a diverticulum of the bladder dome, and external urachal sinus, which is a blind external sinus that opens at the umbilicus. These lesions should be excised.

Elder JS. Anomalies of the bladder. In: Kliegman RM, Behrman RE, Jenson HB, Stanton BF (eds). *Nelson Textbook of Pediatrics*. 18th edn. Vol. 2. Philadelphia: Saunders, 2007; 2243–2246.

Mitchell ME. Bladder exstrophy repair: Complete primary repair of exstrophy. *Urology* 2005; 65: 5–8.

22.4 NEUROPATHIC BLADDER

Neuropathic bladder dysfunction is usually congenital (neural tube defects or other spinal anomalies), acquired diseases and traumatic lesions of the spinal cord are less common. Central nervous tumors, sacrococcygeal teratoma, and spinal abnormalities associated with imperforate anus also can result in abnormal innervation of the bladder or sphincter or both. Patients with neuropathic bladder are associated with various problems such as renal damage, urinary incontinence, and latex allergy.

Neural tube defects: *See* Section 24.2.

Occult spinal dysraphism: Occult spinal dysraphism is seen in 1/4,000 patients that includes lipomeningocele, intradural lipoma, diastematomyelia, tight filum terminale, dermoid cyst sinus, aberrant nerve roots, anterior sacral meningocele, and cauda equina tumor. More than 90% of patients have a cutaneous abnormality overlying the lower spine, including a small dimple, tuft of hair, dermal vascular malformation, or a subcutaneous lipoma. Management of the urinary tract is similar to that described earlier for neural tube defects.

Sacral agenesis: Sacral agenesis is defined as the absence of part or all of two or more lower vertebral bodies. Palpation of the coccygeal area detects the absent vertebrae. These children have a flattened buttock and a low, short gluteal cleft, and some have high arched feet. This condition is more common in the offspring of women with diabetes. Most children need clean intermittent catheterization and pharmacotherapy to stay dry.

Imperforate anus: Children with a high imperforate anus may have a neuropathic bladder, often because of sacral agenesis.

Cerebral palsy: Children with cerebral palsy have reasonable bladder control, but they achieve continence at a later age than unaffected children.

Elder JS. Neuropathic bladder. In: Kliegman RM, Behrman RE, Jenson HB, Stanton BF (eds). *Nelson Textbook of Pediatrics.* 18th edn. Vol. 2. Philadelphia: Saunders, 2007; 2246–2249.

Elder JS. Latex allergy: Time for a change. *J Urol* 2006; 175: 1193–1104.

Joseph DB. Bladder rehabilitation in children with spina bifida: State of art. *J Urol* 2005; 173: 1850–1851.

Kaufman BA. Neural tube defects. *Pediatr Clin North Am* 2004; 51: 389–419.

Thomas J, Elder JS. Neuropathic bladder in children. *AUA Update Series* 2007.

22.5 VOIDING DYSFUNCTION

Normal voiding and toilet training: The fetus voids by reflex contraction in concert with simultaneous contraction of the bladder and relaxation of sphincter. The infant has coordinated voiding as often as 15–20 times per day. Over time the bladder capacity increases. In children up to the age of 14 yr, the mean bladder capacity in ounces is equal to the age (in years) plus 2. At 2–4 yr, the child is developmentally ready to begin toilet training. Girls acquire bladder control before boys, and bowel control is achieved before urinary control. By 5 yr of age, 90–95% of children are nearly completely continent during the day and 80–85% are continent at night.

Nocturnal enuresis: See Section 5. 12.

Diurnal incontinence: Daytime incontinence is common in children who do not have neurologic abnormalities. At 5 yr 92% and at 12 yr 99% are dry during the day. The most common cause of daytime incontinence is a pediatric unstable bladder. The history should be obtained regarding the frequency of voiding, nocturnal enuresis, UTIs, reflux, neurologic disorders, bowel habits (constipation, encopresis or both), and sexual abuse in girls. Physical examination should identify signs of organic causes of incontinence such as short stature, hypertension, enlarged kidneys or bladder or both, constipation, labial adhesion, ureteral ectopy, back or sacral anomalies and neurologic abnormalities. A urinalysis or culture or both should be performed to exclude infection. A renal ultrasonogram with or without a voiding cystourethrogram is indicated in children who have significant physical findings, a family history of urinary tract anomalies, UTIs, or those who do not respond to therapy appropriately.

Pediatric unstable (overactive) bladder: A pediatric unstable bladder is smaller than normal and exhibits strong uninhibited contractions. These children typically exhibit urinary infrequency, urgency and urge incontinence and constipation. Often girls will squat down on their foot to try to prevent incontinence ("Vincent curtsy"). In females a history of urinary tract infection is common. In girls, voiding cystourethrography (VCUG) often shows a dilated urethra and narrowed bladder neck with bladder wall hypertrophy.

Initial therapy is timed voiding every 1.5–2 hr and anticholinergic therapy with oxybutynin chloride, hyoscyamine or tolterodine. Constipation and UTI must be treated. In addition to chemotherapy biofeedback, in which children are taught pelvic floor exercises, because there is evidence that such exercises may reduce or eliminate unstable bladder contractions.

Non-neurogenic neurogenic bladder (Hinman syndrome): Hinman syndrome (also called detrusor-sphincter dyssynergia) is a more serious but less common disorder, in which there is failure of the external sphincter to relax during voiding in children without neurologic abnormalities. The pathogenesis of this syndrome is thought to involve learning abnormal voiding habits during toilet training; the syndrome is rarely seen in infants. In severe cases hydronephrosis, renal insufficiency, and even end-stage renal disease may occur. The treatment includes anticholinergic and alpha blocker therapy, timed voiding, treatment of constipation and UTI, behavioral modification and biofeedback in older children.

Infrequent voiding: Infrequent voiding is a common disorder of micturition, usually associated with UTIs. The disorder is behavioral. Affected children, usually girls, void only twice a day rather than normal four to seven times. With bladder over distension and prolonged retention of urine, growth of bacteria can lead to recurrent UTIs. Some of these children are constipated;

others have episodes of incontinence due to overflow or urgency. The treatment of children with UTIs is antibacterial prophylaxis, and encouragement of frequent voiding and complete emptying of the bladder by double voiding until a normal pattern is re-established.

Vaginal voiding: In girls with vaginal voiding, incontinence typically occurs after urination after the girl stands up. Usually the volume is 5–10 ml. The most common cause is labial adhesion, which is treated by topical application of estrogen cream to the adhesion or lysis. Some girls, usually overweight, experience vaginal voiding because they do not separate their legs widely during urination, while other girls do not pull their underwear down to their ankles when they urinate. Such girls are advised to separate the legs as widely as possible during urination; the most effective way to do this is to have child sit backward on the toilet seat during micturition.

Voiding disorders without incontinence: Some children have the abrupt onset of severe urinary infrequency, voiding as often as every 10–15 min during the day without dysuria, UTI, daytime incontinence, or nocturia. The most common age for these symptoms to occur is 4–6 yr, after the child is toilet-trained and is more common in boys. This condition is termed the *daytime frequency syndrome of childhood or pollakiuria*. The condition is functional; no anatomic problem is detected. The condition is self-limited, and the symptoms generally resolve within 2–3 months.

Elder JS. Voiding Dysfunction. In: Kliegman RM, Behrman RE, Jenson HB, Stanton BF (eds). *Nelson Textbook of Pediatrics.* 18th edn. Vol. 2. Philadelphia: Saunders, 2007; 2249–2253.

Feldman AS, Bauer SB. Diagnosis and management of dysfunctional voiding. *Curr Opin Pediatr* 2006; 18: 139–147.

Robson WL, Leung AK, Van Howe R. Primary and secondary nocturnal enuresis: Similarities in presentation. *Pediatrics* 2005; 115: 956–959.

Yagci F, Kibar Y, Akay O, et al. The effect of biofeedback treatment on voiding and urodynamic parameters in children with voiding dysfunction. *J Urol* 2005; 174: 1994–1997.

22.6 ANOMALIES OF THE PENIS AND URETHRA

Hypospadias: The term hypospadias refers a urethral opening that is on the ventral surface of the penile shaft, a condition affects 1 in 250 male newborns. Hypospadias is classified according to the position of the urethral meatus after taking into account the presence of chordae. The deformity is described as glandular (on the glans-penis), coronal, subcoronal, midpenile, penoscrotal, scrotal, or perineal. Approximately 60% of cases are distal, 25% subcoronal or midpenile, and 15% are proximal. Circumcision should

be avoided, because the foreskin is often used in the repair of hypospadias. The ideal age for repair in a healthy infant is 6–12 months. With the exception of proximal hypospadias, usually all cases are repaired in a single operation (*see* Fig. 22.6 in CD).

Phimosis: Phimosis refers to the inability to retract the prepuce. At birth, phimosis is physiologic. Over time, the adhesions between the prepuce and glans lyse and the distal phimotic ring loosens. In 90% of uncircumcised males the prepuce becomes retractable by the age of 3 yr. Accumulation of the epithelial debris under the infant prepuce is physiologic and is not an indication for circumcision. In older boys, phimosis may be physiologic or pathologic from inflammation and scarring at the tip of the foreskin or may occur after circumcision. Boys with a large hydrocele or hernia are at particular risk for secondary phimosis. In boys with persistent physiologic or pathologic phimosis, application of the corticosteroid cream to the foreskin three times daily for one month will loosen the phimotic ring in two-thirds of the cases. If there is ballooning of the foreskin during voiding or phimosis beyond 10 yr of age and topical steroid therapy is ineffective, circumcision is recommended.

Paraphimosis occurs when the foreskin is retracted past the coronal sulcus and the prepuce cannot be pulled back over the glans. Painful venous stasis in the retracted foreskin results, with edema leading to severe pain and inability to reduce the foreskin (pull it back over the glans). Treatment includes lubricating the foreskin and glans and then simultaneously compressing the glans and placing distal traction on the foreskin to try to push the phimotic ring past the coronal sulcus. In rare cases, emergency circumcision under general anesthesia is necessary.

Circumcision: In India and many countries, circumcision usually is performed for cultural reasons. The reasons given in support of circumcision include reducing the risk of UTI and sexually transmitted infections and prevention of penile cancer, phimosis, HIV infection and balanitis. When performing a neonatal circumcision, local analgesia, such as a dorsal nerve block or application of lidocaine cream is recommended. Many recommend circumcision in infants who are predisposed to UTI, such as those with congenital hydronephrosis and vesicoureteral reflux.

Complications after neonatal circumcision include bleeding, wound infection, meatal stenosis, secondary phimosis, removal of insufficient skin and dense penile adhesions. Potentially serious complications include sepsis, amputation of the distal part of the glans, removal of an excessive amount of foreskin, and urethrocutaneous fistula. Circumcision should not be performed in neonates with hypospadias, chordee without hypospadias or a dorsal hood deformity (relative contraindication) or in those with a small penis.

Micropenis: Micropenis is defined as a normally formed penis that is at least 2.5 standard below the mean in size. Typically, the ratio of the length of the penile shaft to its circumference is normal. The pertinent measurement is the stretched penile length, which is measured by stretching the penis and measuring the distance from the penile base under the pubic symphysis to the tip of the glans. The mean length of the term newborn penis is 3.5 ± 0.7 cm and the diameter is 1.1 ± 0.2 cm. The diagnosis of micropenis is made if the stretched length is less than 1.9 cm. Micropenis results from a hormonal abnormality that occurs after 14 wk of gestation. Common causes include hypogonadotropic hypogonadism, hypergonadotropic hypogonadism (primary testicular failure), and idiopathic micropenis. Neonatal hypoglycemia occurs if there is deficiency of growth hormone. The most common cause of micropenis is failure of the hypothalamus to produce an adequate amount of gonadotropin-releasing hormone, as occurs in Kallmann syndrome, Prader-Willi syndrome and Lawrence-Moon-Biedl syndrome. Primary testicular failure may result from gonadal dysgenesis or rudimentary testes syndrome and also occurs in Robinow syndrome (characterized by hypoplastic genitalia, shortening of the forearms, frontal bossing, hypertelorism, wide palpebral fissures, short broad nose, long philtrum, small chin, brachydactyly, and a normal karyotype). Evaluation of a child with micropenis includes a karyotype, assessment of the anterior pituitary and testicular function, and MRI to determine the anatomic integrity of the hypothalamus, anterior pituitary gland and the midline structure of the brain. Some men with micropenis, but not all have satisfactory sexual function, and the use of androgen therapy is controversial to stimulate penile growth.

American Academy of Pediatrics, Task Force on Circumcision: Circumcision policy statement. *Pediatrics* 1999; 103: 686–693.

Elder JS. Anomalies of the penis and urethra. In: Kliegman RM, Behrman RE, Jenson HB, Stanton BF (eds). *Nelson Textbook of Pediatrics*. 18th edn. Vol. 2. Philadelphia: Saunders, 2007; 2253–2260.

Lee PA, Hook CP. Outcome studies among men with micropenis. *J Pediatr Endocrinol Metab* 2004; 17: 1043–1053.

22.7 DISORDERS AND ANOMALIES OF THE SCROTAL CONTENTS

Scrotal swelling: Scrotal swelling may be acute or chronic, and painful or painless. Abrupt onset of painful scrotal swelling is due to conditions such as testicular torsion and incarcerated inguinal hernia require emergency surgical management. Painful scrotal masses include testicular torsion, torsion of appendix testis, epididymitis, trauma (ruptured testis, hematocele); inguinal hernia (incarcerated); mumps orchitis. Painless scrotal masses include hydrocele, inguinal hernia, varicocele, spermatocele, testicular tumor, Henoch-Schönlein purpura, idiopathic scrotal edema. *Differential diagnosis* of scrotal masses include hydrocele, inguinal hernia (reducible), inguinal hernia (incarcerated), testicular torsion, scrotal hematoma; testicular tumor, meconium peritonitis, and epididymitis.

Cryptorchidism

Undescended testis (UDT), also known as cryptorchidism, is defined as a condition in which testis cannot be made to reach the bottom of the scrotum. The testis may be arrested at any level along the path of descent of testis from the retroperitoneal to the scrotum. Cryptorchidism is the most common genital anomaly identified at birth (approximately 4.5%) in boys. 30% premature male infants and 3.4% in term infants have undescended testes, because testicular descent occurs late in gestation. The majority of undescended testes descend spontaneously during the first three months of life and by 6 months the incidence decreases to 0.8%. If the testis has not descended by 4 months, it will remain undescended. Prevalence of cryptorchidism in prepubertal boys is reportedly 1.7 to 4%. True undescended testis is more common on the right side and is unilateral in 2/3rd cases. Cryptorchidism is bilateral in 10% cases.

Clinical manifestations: Location of the undescended testes has been found to be abdominal (10%); inguinal (68%); prescrotal (24%) and ectopic (11.5%). A more useful classification is whether testes are palpable upon physical examination. If palpable, testes may be undescended, ectopic, or retractile. A testis may be impalpable because of obesity, intra-abdominal location, ectopic site or an absent testis (vanishing testis syndrome). Best way to evaluate the impalpable testis is physical examination in a calm child. Once located, the size and consistency of testis should be noted.

Unilateral or bilateral undescended testis associated with hypospadias should alert the clinician about the possibility of intersex disorder and further investigations should be carried out at the earliest for confirming or excluding the diagnosis. Undescended testes can be classified as: (1) spontaneously descending testis—a testis that was not present in the scrotum at birth but has descended with time without any hormonal or surgical manipulation; (2) truly undescended testis—a testis that is arrested along the path of migration from the retroperitoneum to the scrotum; (3) retractile testis—retractile testis is (i) normal in shape and size;(ii) can be brought down to the base of scrotum; (iii) stays in the scrotum for some time after the pull is released and (iv) the scrotum is normally developed; (4) ectopic testis—a testis that has emerged from the external inguinal ring but fails to reach the scrotum is labeled as ectopic testis and can be found in perineum, femoral area or contralateral scrotum. (5) ascended testis—ascended testis, also known as acquired undescended testis, is one that has been documented to be present in the scrotum once, has attained a higher position at a subsequent examination and cannot be brought down into the scrotum. An ascended testis can be either primary (without antecedent inguinal surgery) or secondary (ascent of testis after inguinal cord manipulation for hernia or hydrocele repair); and (6) gliding testis—an inguinal testis that can moved down to the upper scrotum under tension and retracts to the original position once the pull is released.

Ectopic and undescended testes have been considered to be variants of same congenital anomaly and this spectrum of abnormal testicular position with associated pathological conditions and complications are referred to as 'undescended testis sequence.'

The consequences of cryptorchidism include infertility, malignancy, associated hernia, torsion of the cryptorchid testis, and psychological effects of an empty scrotum.

Treatment: Optimal goals of treatment of undescended testis include improve fertility, decrease potential for malignancy, repair of associated hernia, decrease incidence of spontaneous torsion, and minimize psychological trauma of empty scrotum. The congenital undescended testis should be treated surgically no later than 9–15 mo; at 6 mo is the appropriate time, because spontaneous descent of testis do not occur after 4 mo of age. *Laparoscopic management* is superior to open technique regarding morbidity, complication rate and length of stay. *Hormonal treatment* is used infrequently. Examination for neoplasia at the time of primary orchiopexy is recommended for intra-abdominal testis, abnormal external genitalia or known abnormal karyotype. Placement of *testicular prosthesis* may be considered in

a case of congenital anorchia or removal of testis for normal psychological development of the boy. This is better done at puberty. The child should be evaluated at regular intervals for testis location, size, and viability. When the child reaches puberty, the physician should readdress the potential issues of fertility and testicular cancer and give instructions concerning the boy's monthly testicular self-examination.

Testicular (spermatic cord) torsion: Testicular torsion is the most common cause of testicular pain in boys 12 yr and older and is uncommon in boys younger than 10 yr. It is caused by inadequate fixation of the testis within the scrotum, resulting from a redundant tunica vaginalis, allowing excessive mobility of the testis. The abnormal attachment is termed a *bell clapper deformity* and often is bilateral. Shortly after erosion occurs, venous congestion begins; subsequently, arterial flow is interrupted. The testis survival depends on the duration and severity of torsion; within 4–6 hr of absent blood flow to the testis, irreversible loss of spermatogenesis may occur.

Testicular torsion produces acute pain and swelling of the scrotum. On examination, the scrotum is swollen and the testis is tender and often difficult to examine. The cremasteric reflex usually is absent. The condition can be differentiated from an incarcerated hernia because swelling in the inguinal area often is absent.

Testicular torsion requires prompt treatment, which includes prompt surgical exploration and detorsion. If the pain has lasted less than 4–6 hr, manual detorsion should be attempted. In 2/3rd of cases the torsed testis rotates inward, so detorsion should be attempted in the opposite direction (e.g. the left testis is rotated clockwise). Successful manual detorsion results in the relief of pain. If the testis is explored within 6 hr of torsion, as many as 90% of the gonads will survive. Survival decreases rapidly with a delay of more than 6 hr. If the degree of torsion is 360 degree or less, the testis may have sufficient arterial flow to allow the gonad to survive, even after 24–48 hr. The testis then fixed in the scrotum with unabsorbable sutures, termed *scrotal orchiopaxy* to prevent torsion in the future. The contralateral testis also should be fixed to the scrotum because the anatomical condition is often bilateral. If the testis appears nonviable, orchidectomy is performed.

When torsion occurs in utero, the baby is usually born with a large, firm, nontender testis. Usually the ipsilateral hemiscrotum is ecchymotic. It is recommended to explore to establish the diagnosis, remove the necrotic testis, and anchor the contralateral testis.

Epididymitis: Acute inflammation of the epididymis is an ascending retrograde infection from the urethra, through the vas into the epididymis. There is acute scrotal pain, erythema, and swelling. If it occurs before puberty, a congenital abnormality of the wolffian duct, such as an ectopic ureter entering the vas should be suspected. The common causative organism is *Escherechia coli*, others are gonococcus and chlamydia. Other etiologies include Henoch-Schönlein purpura, familial Mediterranean fever, enterovirus, and adenoviruses. Treatment consists of bed rest and antibiotics. If there is difficulty in distinguishing from torsion, surgical exploration is required in children.

Varicocele: A varicocele is a congenital condition in which there is abnormal dilation of the pampiniform venous plexus in the scrotum as a result of valvular incompetence of the spermatic vein. A varicocele is found in 5–15% of adolescent boys, and rarely diagnosed in boys below 10 yr old, because the varicocele becomes distended only after the increased blood flow associated with puberty occurs. Varicocele predominantly occurs on the left side, bilateral in 10% cases and rarely on the right side. A varicocele in a boy < 10 yr or on the right side may be indicative of an abdominal or retroperitoneal mass, an abdominal sonogram or CT scan should be performed in such cases.

A varicocele is a painless paratesticular mass (occasionally patients complain of dull ache in the affected testis), often described as a "bag of worms." Usually the varicocele is not apparent when the patient is supine, because it is decompressed; in contrast the varicocele becomes prominent when the patient is standing and enlarges with Valsalva maneuver. Varicocele is graded from 1 to 3: **grade 1** is palpable only with Valsalva; **grade 2** is palpable without Valsalva but is not visible on inspection; and **grade 3** varicocele is visible with inspection. Boys with a grade 3 varicocele are at greatest risk for testicular growth arrest. If the affected left testis is significantly is smaller than the right testis, spermatogenesis probably has been adversely affected.

Varicocelectomy (surgical treatment of varicoceles) in children and adolescents is indicated in boys with a significant disparity in testicular size or pain in the affected testis, or if the contralateral testis is diseased or absent, or grade 3 varicocele, even without a disparity in testicular size. Laparoscopic repair is becoming more popular.

Spermatocele: A spermatocele is a cystic lesion containing sperm that is attached to the upper pole of the sexually mature testis. Spermatoceles usually are painless swelling. Enlargement of the spermatocele or pain is an indication for removal.

Hydrocele: A hydrocele is an accumulation of fluid in the tunica vaginalis. 1–2% of male neonates have a hydrocele. In most cases the hydrocele is noncommunicating (the processus vaginalis was obliterated during development). In such cases, the hydrocele fluid disappears by 1 yr of age. If there is a persistently patent processus (communicating), the hydrocele persists and becomes progressively larger during the day and is small in the morning. The long-term risk of a communicating hydrocele is the development of an inguinal hernia. In some older boys, a non-communicating hydrocele may result from an inflammatory condition within the scrotum such as testicular torsion, torsion of the appendix testis, epididymitis or testicular tumor. Some older boys and male adolescents develop hydrocele acutely after an episode of scrotal trauma or epididymo-orchitis, whereas others develop more insidiously. On examination, hydroceles are smooth and nontender. Transillumination of the scrotum confirms the fluid-filled nature of the mass. Palpate the testis, as some young men develop a hydrocele in association with a testis tumor. If compression of the fluid-filled mass completely reduces the hydrocele, an inguinal hernia/hydrocele is the likely diagnosis.

Most congenital hydroceles resolve by 1 yr of age following reabsorption of the hydrocele fluid. Hydroceles persisting beyond 12–18 months usually communicating and should be repaired. If the hydrocele is large and tense early surgical correction should be considered, because it is difficult to verify that the child does not have a hernia, and large hydroceles rarely develop spontaneously.

Inguinal hernia: Inguinal hernia is discussed in Section 16.15.

Bica DTG, Hadziselimovic F. Buserlin treatment of cryptorchidism: A randomized double blind placebo controlled study. *J Urol* 1992; 148: 617–621.

Elder JS. Urinary Tract Infections. In: Kliegman RM, Behrman RE, Jenson HB, Stanton BF (eds). *Nelson Textbook of Pediatrics.* 18th edn. Vol. 2. Philadelphia: Saunders, 2007; 2260–2261.

Elder JS. Anomalies of the penis and urethra. In: Kliegman RM, Behrman RE, Jenson HB, Stanton BF (eds). *Nelson Textbook of Pediatrics.* 18th edn. Vol. 2. Philadelphia: Saunders, 2007; 2260–2265.

Mohta A. Cryptorchidism. In: Mathur GP, Mathur Sarla (eds). *Current Trends in Pediatrics.* Vol 2. Delhi: Academa Publishers, 2006; 356–364.

22.8 TRAUMA TO THE GENITOURINARY TRACT

Trauma to the genitourinary tract in children usually results from blunt trauma during falls, athletic activities, or motor vehicle accidents. In more than half of cases there also are major injuries to the brain, spinal cord, skeleton, lungs, or abdominal organs. Children are at greater risk of blunt renal injury than are adults, because they have less body fat and because the kidneys are not located directly behind the ribs. Children with a pre-existing renal anomaly also are at increased risk for renal injury. Blunt abdominal or flank trauma often causes a renal injury. Straddle injuries usually are associated with trauma to the bulbous urethra.

Clinical manifestations: Symptoms and signs of urinary tract injury include gross or microscopic hematuria, bleeding from the urethral meatus, abdominal or flank pain, a flank mass, fractured lower ribs or lumbar transverse processes, a perineal or scrotal trauma.

Diagnosis: Evaluation of the patient begins after an adequate airway has been established and the patient is hemodynamically stable. Renal imaging is indicated in patients with significant abdominal injury, gross hematuria or > 50 red blood cells per high-power field, or suspicion of renal injury. Minor renal injuries are more common.

Treatment: Minor renal injuries such as contusions are managed by bed rest and monitoring of vital signs until abdominal or flank discomfort and gross hematuria has resolved. Children with a major renal injury usually are admitted to an intensive care unit for continuous monitoring of vital signs and urine output. Intravenous antibiotics are also administered. These injuries also are managed nonoperatively, because Gerota's fascia often causes tamponade of bleeding from the kidney, and dramatic healing of the injured parenchyma can occur even with significant urinary extravasation. The kidney can be salvaged by emergency renal revascularization only if the kidney is explored within 2–3 hr of injury. All penetrating injuries of the kidneys should be explored. In addition to loss of renal function, the main long term complication of renal injury is renin-mediated hypertension. Children who sustain renal injuries must have periodic measurement of blood pressure. Ureteral, bladder, and urethral injuries should be identified and treated. Penile and testicular injuries are relatively uncommon in children. Ultrasonography demonstrates rupture of the tunica albuginea, which is the capsule of the testis, and surrounding hemorrhage. Prompt surgical treatment of the testicular injuries increases the salvage rate. Zipper injury, which can affect either to scrotum or foreskin, is an uncommon injury. This problem generally occurs in boys who do not wear underwear. The zipper can be cut with either bone or metal cutters.

Buckley JC, McAninch JW, The diagnosis, and outcome of pediatric renal injuries. *Urol Clin North Am* 2006; 33: 33–40.

Elder JS. Anomalies of the penis and urethra. In: Kliegman RM, Behrman RE, Jenson HB, Stanton BF (eds). *Nelson Textbook of Pediatrics*. 18th edn. Vol. 2. Philadelphia: Saunders, 2007; 2265–2267.

Murum D, Levitt CJ, Frazier LD, et al. Genital injuries. *J Pediatr Adolesc Gynecol* 2003; 16: 149–155.

22.9 URINARY LITHIASIS

Stones in children occur in the entire urinary tract including calyces, renal pelvis, ureter (upper, middle and lower), vesico-ureteric junction, bladder and urethra. Renal stones as per the stone characteristics are broadly classified into: (i) Primary stones—appear in apparently healthy urinary tract and without any pre-existing urinary tract infection. The stones formed are composed of calcium, oxalate, uric acid, cystine and xanthine; and (ii) Secondary stones—appear as a result of infection and inflammation and are triple phosphate or mixed calculi. The approximate frequency of renal stone types in the pediatric age group is calcium with phosphate or oxalate (57%), struvite (24%), uric acid (8%), cystine (6%), endemic (2%), mixed (2%), and other (1%). It must be differentiated from nephrocalcinosis in which there is deposition of calcium salts in the renal parenchyma (*see* Figs 22.7 to 22.10 in CD).

Etiology and risk factors: Renal stone disease is multifactorial in origin. Diet and environmental factors play a major role in formation of renal stones. These include low urine volumes, high ambient temperatures, low fluid intake, dietary pattern (high protein, sodium, and calcium intake), high sodium, calcium, oxalate, and urate excretion and low citrate excretion.

1. Several **congenital renal system** morpho-anatomic factors also play a role in stone formation, secondary to factors which cause stasis of urine, e.g. obstruction at pelvi-ureteric junction or uretero-vesical junction, megaureter, calyceal diverticula, renal duplication, horseshoe kidney, megacalycosis, ureterocele, neurogenic bladder, exstrophy bladder, and vesical diverticula. Pelvi-ureteral junction abnormalities are found to be the most common cause of stone formation.

2. **Metabolic risk factors** include hypocitraturia, hypercalciuria, hyperoxaluria, hyperuricosuria and xanthinuria. The incidence of metabolic factors causing stones ranges from 30 to 50% in various studies and are a leading etiologic factor of calculus formation.

3. **Drugs** such as ceftriaxone, diuretics (fursemide, triamterene), steroids, chemotherapeutic agents, protease inhibitors (indinavir for HIV infection)

have all been implicated in the formation of renal stones.

4. **Urinary tract infections** most often *Proteus* spp., and occasionally *Klebsiella* spp., *Escherichia coli*, *Pseudomonas* spp. *result* in urinary alkalization and excessive production of ammonia, which can lead to the precipitation of magnesium ammonium phosphate (**struvite**) and calcium phosphate. In the kidney, the calculi often have a staghorn configuration, filling the calyces. The calculi cause obstruction, perpetuating infection, and causing gradual renal damage.

5. **Medical conditions** like malabsorption syndromes, hyperparathyroidism, prolonged immobilization, etc. could also be a cause of renal stones.

6. A **low urine volume** is a crucial determinant of risk of urinary stones. The risk of calcium stone formation is substantially increased with urine output of less than 15 ml/kg/day in children. A supersaturated urine is associated with low urine volumes and thus is a major predisposing factor for stone formation.

7. **Nephrocalcinosis** refers to calcium deposition within the renal tissue. Often nephrocalcinosis is associated with urolithiasis. The most common causes are frusemide, (administered to premature neonates), distal RTA, hyperparathyroidism, medullary sponge kidney, hypophosphatemic rickets, sarcoidosis, cortical necrosis, hyperoxaluria, prolonged immobilization, Cushing syndrome, hyperuricosuria, and renal candidiasis.

Clinical manifestations: The symptoms and signs of renal stones are related to the size of the stone, the location either in the pelvis or the calyces, presence or absence of outflow obstruction and infection. In children less than five years old, the most common mode of presentation is irritability, vomiting, diarrhea, and other non-specific symptoms. The classical flank pain of renal colic is usually not present. Older children present with flank or abdominal pain as a typical renal colic or as a dull-aching abdominal pain, nausea, vomiting, and dysuria, with or without hematuria. In the presence of urinary tract infection, fever with chills would be associated. Tenderness at the renal angle may be present on physical examination and rarely with obstruction at pelvi-ureteral junction; a palpable kidney may be found.

Investigations: The child suspected to have renal stone has to be investigated for: (a) Confirmation of the presence, location of stone and effects of stone; (b) the etiologic factor of the renal stone; and (c) the possibilities of recurrence.

Confirmation of the stone can be done on a plain X-ray, ultrasonography, intravenous pyelography, computed tomography (CT) and magnetic resonance imaging (MRI). A non-enhanced CT-scan provides a very high stone pick-up rate, especially the ureteral stones, due to the higher attenuation of the stones as compared to the surrounding tissues regardless of the stone chemical composition.

Laboratory evaluation is mandatory for children with renal stone disease for appropriate therapy and prevention of recurrence. A 24-hour urine sample is studied for stone-risk profile and detection of metabolic abnormalities. Urinary volume, pH, calcium, sodium, protein, phosphorus, magnesium, citrate, oxalate, uric acid, creatinine and cystine including a saturation study of the salts in urine have to be estimated. Chemical analysis for stone composition is important to diagnose the type and etiology of the stone and to decide the future dietary and medical therapy.

In view of a high incidence of recurrence of renal stones in children as high as 40%, the evaluation of genetic/hereditary factors (cystinuria, primary hyperoxaluria, familial hyperuricosuria) and the presence of syndromes (renal tubular syndromes, Lesch-Nyhan syndrome) causing stones need to be evaluated.

Management of renal stones: The most important factor in long term management and prevention of recurrence is adequate fluid intake and dietary recommendations. The various factors which need to be considered before outlining the treatment for a particular patient include: 1. Stone factors—site (pelvic or calyceal), size, number, composition; 2. Renal anatomic factors—presence of obstruction, calyceal configuration, anatomical renal abnormalities; and 3. Patient characteristics—body habitus, associated infection, coagulation defects, renal function, associated co-morbidity. Various treatment options are available.

Treatment Options

1. *Spontaneous passage of stone with or without hydrotherapy:* In children a high percentage (about 50%) of renal stones pass spontaneously, the chances of spontaneous passage are inversely proportional to the size of the stone. More than 5 mm. stone rarely passes down the ureter in a child. Spontaneous passage of the stone can be assisted by hydrotherapy either through the oral or through intravenous route. Hydrotherapy must be instituted only when there is no obstructive uropathy or uncontrolled pain and vomiting, i.e. when the stone is not impacted.

Other conservative measures necessary for overall management and prevention of recurrence of stones are: adequate fluid intake, low salt and animal protein diet, various dietary modifications as per the type of stone.

Alpha-adrenergic blockers (tamsulosin, terazosin, and doxazosin) and calcium channel blocking agents with or without steroids have been shown to facilitate stone passage by decreasing ureteral pressure below the stone in adults and also in children with ureteral calculi, but their safety and efficacy in children have not been demonstrated.

2. *Chemolysis:* Several oral medications to dissolve the stone or reduce the size are available, so that there is spontaneous passage of the stone. Urinary alkalinization by potassium citrate or sodium bicarbonate and allopurinol in patients with hyperuricemia acts as chemolytic agents in uric acid stones.

3. *Extra-corporeal shock wave lithotripsy (ESWL):* ESWL is a non-invasive procedure in which an externally applied, focused, high-intensity acoustic pulse is used to break the stone into particles which can pass down the ureter with minimal collateral damage. Success rates of treatment with ESWL are acceptable, though not the best as chances of residual and recurrent stones are higher. Short hospital stay, least morbidity, rapid recovery and high safety profile has made ESWL the preferred first line of treatment for children with stones, especially renal stones. Usually, stones 1–2 cm. can be treated by ESWL. The success rate with monotherapy is about 50–90%, the complication rates being 5–20%.

4. *Percutaneous nephrolithotomy (PCNL):* PCNL is a minimally invasive procedure wherein a nephroscope is passed through the kidney into the pelvis and the stone is either extracted or broken up with an ultrasonic probe, electrohydraulic probe or a holmium laser lithotripter. This technique is good for larger stones more than 1cm; the success rates of this technique are approximately 95–98%. Hence, it is considered to be a superior technique of managing renal stones, though the complication rates are between 5–7%; hypothermia and blood loss being the main concerns especially in small children.

5. *Open pyelolithotomy:* The rates of residual stones and thereby recurrence is very minimal with this technique. In children with large staghorn calculi, it is still preferable to remove the stone by open technique to minimize the complications of treatment.

6. *Laparoscopic and robotic/robot assisted laparoscopic nephrolithotomy:* The role of laparoscopy with or without robotic surgery in the management of renal stones is still evolving and has their own limitations.

Recurrence: Residual particulate matter or small stones are a nidus for stone recurrence and must be avoided at all costs. The fragments which are small and thought of as clinically insignificant have been shown to form clinically significant stones in about 50% of patients. Residual stone should be treated by conservative as well as by other noninvasive and minimally invasive techniques. ESWL has been found to be an effective treatment modality for residual renal stone after any form of primary treatment.

The incidence of stone recurrence is high in children due to the pre-existing metabolic abnormalities. To prevent recurrence, an identification of the etiologic and risk factors for stone development must be studied and corrected. The most common risk factors are high levels of minerals such as calcium, oxalate, uric acid in the serum, urine or both, low urine output due to inadequate fluid intake or due to obstructive uropathy, urinary tract infections, low levels of citrate in the urine which is necessary to prevent stone formation and an abnormal urine pH.

Potassium citrate or potassium citrate and magnesium citrate oral solution reduces the chances of recurrence by approximately 85%.

Apart from metabolic abnormalities, the children with infective calculi should have prophylactic antibiotics to prevent urinary tract infection and thus reformation of stones. Evaluation and management of the cause of infection should be instituted. Those with idiopathic renal stones also need to be closely followed. Those children with a family history of urinary stones should be followed and evaluated regularly for recurrence.

Ureteral Stones

The ureteral stones are secondary to renal calculi which have dislodged from the renal pelvis. Ureteral stones can be in the proximal, mid, or distal ureter, the most common site being the distal ureter. Ureteric calculi are almost always symptomatic and present as ureteric colic. Spontaneous passage of ureteral stones occurs, but is dependant on the size of the stone. Most of the treatment modalities remain the same as in renal stones. *Ureteroscopy (US)* for extraction of renal stones is another technique of stone removal endoscopically. The results of treatment of urinary calculi with ESWL is 75.4%, endourologic procedures 93.3%, and 100% with open surgery (Muslumanoglu and coworkers, 2006).

Bladder Stones

The common factors identified were low socio-economic status, diet low in proteins, consisting mainly of vegetables and starches. The most common cause of stones in the bladder is idiopathic, also known as endemic stones. These stones are more common in boys less than 11 years mostly belonging to low socio-economic groups. These are formed primarily in the bladder due to a nidus and once treated do not generally recur.

Currently, the treatment options for removal of bladder stone in children are open cystolithotomy, transurethral lithotripsy and percutaneous cystolithotripsy. Small bladder stones may pass spontaneously or following hydrotherapy. Sometimes while passing through the urethra, the stone could get obstructed in the urethra causing retention of urine and would require emergency treatment. The stone could either be pushed back into the bladder and child catheterized or stone extracted via a cystoscope from the urethra (*see* Fig. 22.11 in CD).

Prevention: Prevention of stone formation by proper diet, adequate fluid intake is the most important step in reducing the morbidity and mortality of the affected children. A thorough metabolic evaluation and further management of the abnormality is essential for stone free long-term outcome.

Elder JS. Urinary lithiasis. In: Kliegman RM, Behrman RE, Jenson HB, Stanton BF (eds). *Nelson Textbook of Pediatrics*. 18th edn. Vol. 2. Philadelphia: Saunders, 2007; 2207–2271.

Gupta NP, Kesarwani P. Current approaches in the medical management of urolithiasis: A review article. *Indian J Urol* 2002; 19. 20–28.

Khanna PC, Karnik ND, Jankharia BG, Merchant SA, Joshi AR, Kukreja KU. Magnetic resonance urography (MRU) versus intravenous urography (IVU) in obstructive uropathy: a prospective study of 30 cases. *J Assoc Physicians India* 2005; 53:527–534.

Muslumanoglu A, Tefekli A, Altunrende F, Karadag M, Baykal M, Akcay M. Efficacy of extracorporeal shock wave lithotripsy for ureteric stones in children. *Int Urol Nephro* 2006; 38: 225–229.

Shokeir AA, Sheir KZ, El-Nahas AR, El-Assmy AM, Eassa W, El-Kappany HA. Treatment of Renal Stones in Children: A Comparison between Percutaneous Nephrolithotomy and Shock Wave Lithotripsy. *J Urol* 2006:176: 706–710.

22.10 VESICOURETERAL REFLUX

Vesicoureteric reflux (VUR) is defined as retrograde flow of urine from the bladder to the upper urinary tracts. VUR is usually asymptomatic but when complicated by urinary tract infection (UTI) in childhood. VUR is an important cause of symptomatic ill health, which, if undiagnosed and untreated can result in failure to thrive. In the longer term, renal scarring (reflux nephropathy) poses threats of late morbidity which includes hypertension, complications of pregnancy, renal impairment and end-stage renal failure.

Grading of reflux: In 1981, the International Reflux Study Committee proposed a system of five grades of reflux that remains in current use today (Table 22.1).

Presentation of VUR

Symptomatic: Symptomatic UTI remains by far the commonest form of clinical presentation. Pain is not generally regarded as a symptom of primary VUR. However, loin pain is a well recognized feature of pyelonephritis and the occurrence of pain may also signal the presence of secondary pelviureteric junction obstruction. VUR occasionally comes to light for the first time in individuals presenting with renal insufficiency and/or hypertension who have a little, if any, history of urinary infection.

Asymptomatic: Antenatally detected fetal hydronephrosis especially when it is bilateral warrants a postnatal work up, which includes VCUG. Variable hydronephrosis during one examination or between examinations should always raise the suspicion of reflux and prompt postnatal evaluation. Primary VUR (usually of moderate to high grade) accounts for 15–20% of clinically significant prenatally detected uropathies. Asymptomatic VUR also comes to light during the course of sibling screening.

Diagnosis and Evaluation of Vesicoureteral Reflux

Confirmation of urinary tract infection: Reflux nephropathy results because of a combined effect of UTI and reflux. Hence confirmation plus documentation of true UTI is paramount in the appropriate management of a patient with reflux.

Grade	Description
I	Into a non-dilated ureter
II	Into the pelvis and calyces without dilatation
III	Mild to moderate dilatation of the ureter, renal pelvis, and calyces with minimal blunting of the fornices
IV	Moderate ureteral tortuosity and dilatation of the pelvis and calyces
V	Gross dilatation of the ureter, pelvis, and calyces; loss of papillary impressions; and ureteral tortuosity

Table 22.1: International Reflux Study Committee classification

Renal sonography: Ultrasonography is the imaging modality of choice to monitor renal status over time.

Renal scintigraphy: 99mTc-labeled dimercapto-succinic acid (DMSA) is the most sensitive modality for visualizing scarring and quantifying differential renal function (*see* Fig. 22.12 in CD).

Voiding cystourethrography (VCUG): Although invasive, the conventional radiological contrast study remains the gold standard investigation for the diagnosis and evaluation of VUR. It permits accurate grading of the severity of VUR, which is important when assessing prognosis and planning treatment.

Management

The essential tenants of reflux management are: (i) Spontaneous resolution of reflux is very common; (ii) High-grade reflux is less likely to resolve spontaneously; (iii) Sterile reflux is benign; (iv) Extended use of prophylactic antibiotics is benign; and (v) The success rate with surgical correction is very high. A guideline of the Indian Society of Pediatric Nephrology (ISPN) for management of VUR is described in Table 22.2.

Conservative or 'medical' management: The conventional approach to medical management comprises:

- **Continuous antibiotic prophylaxis:** typically, trimethoprim 1–2 mg/kg/day, usually as a single night-time dose. The prophylactic dose is typically one-third to one-fourth the therapeutic dose used to treat conventional cystitis.

- **Urine surveillance:** The availability of reagent strips which test for nitrites and leucocytes make it much easier for parents or physicians to make a provisional diagnosis. Nevertheless, wherever possible, a freshly collected midstream urine specimen should be examined by microscopy and culture.

- **Treatment of any underlying bladder dysfunction:** A regular voiding regimen, including double voiding where there is evidence of significant postvoid residual on bladder ultrasound. Anticholinergics, e.g. oxybutynin, should be considered if there are symptoms suggesting detrusor instability.

- **Treatment of constipation:** Similar to other forms of habitual constipation.

- **Commitment:** Parental commitment is vital to ensure compliance with the medical regimen. Older children must be motivated to modify their voiding habits to correct voiding dysfunction. Effective arrangements are needed to ensure that urine samples are collected and examined promptly to facilitate diagnosis and treatment of breakthrough infections. If this commitment is lacking, surgical intervention may be preferable.

Surgical intervention: Indications for surgery are relative rather than absolute (Table 22.2). Parents are increasingly supporting early endoscopic treatment for low to moderate grade VUR as an alternative to long-term continuous antibiotic prophylaxis. It is recommended that patients should initially receive antibiotic prophylaxis while awaiting spontaneous resolution of VUR. A close follow up is required for occurrence of breakthrough UTI. Repeat imaging is required after 18–36 months in patients with grade III–V VUR. Multiple surgical techniques have been described to effectively correct VUR include open surgical procedure, endoscopic, laparoscopic, and robotic surgery.

Baker R, Maxted W, Maylath J, Shuman I: Relation of age, sex, and infection to reflux: Data indicating high spontaneous cure rate in pediatric patients. *J Urol* 1966; 95:27.

Duckett JW, Bellinger MF: A plea for standardized grading of vesicoureteral reflux. *Eur Urol* 1982; 8:74–77.

Kaefer M, Curran M, Treves ST, et al: Sibling vesicoureteral reflux in multiple gestation births. *Pediatrics* 2000; 105:800–804.

Indian Society of Pediatric Nephrology, Vijayakumar M, Kanitkar M, Nammalwar BR, Bagga A. Revised statement on management of urinary tract infections. *Indian Pediatr* 2011; 48:709–17.

Ransley PG, Risdon RA: The pathogenesis of reflux nephropathy. *Contrib Nephrol* 1979; 16:90–97.

22.11 GENITOURINARY TUMORS IN CHILDREN

The tumors of the kidney, ureter, bladder, urethra, ovaries and testis and paratesticular region are included here. The common tumors in the genitourinary tract of children include Wilms' tumor (WT), rhabdomyosarcoma (RMS), testicular tumors and ovarian tumors (*see* Figs 22.13 to 22.15 in CD).

Tumors of the female genital tract: The most common malignant tumor of the genital tract of the female is RMS. The various sites of RMS are vulva, vagina, cervix and uterus. The most common primary tumor

Table 22.2: Guidelines of the Indian Society of Pediatric Nephrology (ISPN) for management of VUR-2011	
VUR Grade	*Management*
Grades I and II	Antibiotic prophylaxis until 1 yr old. Restart antibiotic prophylaxis if breakthrough febrile UTI.
Grades III to V	Antibiotic prophylaxis up to 5 yr of age. Consider surgery if breakthrough febrile TI. Beyond 5 yr: Prophylaxis continued if there is bowel bladder dysfunction.

of the vagina is the RMS. Vaginal RMS presents as usually a polypoidal mass protruding out of the vagina with muco-sanguinous discharge. Frank bleeding may also occur. Uterine/cervix RMS present as pelvic mass with or without vaginal discharge. Vulvar RMS present as a palpable mass involving the labia and is commonly mistaken as Bartholin's gland infections.

The treatment options for the RMS of the female genital tract remain the same, except that the histologic subtype of RMS differs, thus offering a better long-term prognosis in spite of incomplete resection. Botryoid RMS is the most commonly seen in the female genital tract and is usually completely resectable. The other common subtype of RMS of female genital tract is the embryonal RMS. As compared to the bladder and prostate RMS, the tumors of the female genital tract seem to have a better prognosis in spite of incomplete resection.

Paratesticular rhabdomyosarcoma: Paratesticular RMS account for 4% of the entire RMSs and is the commonest paratesticular tumor seen in the prepubertal boys. The paratesticular region consists of spermatic cord, epididymis, vestigial remnants, and tunica vaginalis. 40% of paratesticular RMS occur in spermatic cord. Like all testicular tumors, the paratesticular RMS also presents as a painless scrotal mass. The mass in the early stages can be felt separate from the testis, but in the advanced stages invades the testis and the surrounding structures, including the scrotal skin which is when the inguinal lymph nodes become enlarged. The paratesticular RMS metastasizes to the para-aortic and paracaval lymph nodes. The diagnosis can be achieved by an ultrasound of the scrotum, and/or CT-Scan/MRI and FNAC of the mass. Multimodality treatment with radical orchiectomy via inguinal approach, retroperitoneal lymph node dissection, and aggressive adjuvant chemotherapy is required as all RMS are rapidly progressing. Postoperative radiotherapy is necessary for positive retroperitoneal lymph nodes. Paratesticular RMS has a better prognosis as compared to the RMS at other genitourinary sites; the long term survival to be more than 90% (*see* Figs 22.16 to 22.18 in CD).

Testicular tumors: 1–2% of all pediatric solid tumors are testicular tumors. The peak age incidence occurs at 2–3 years of age. The major factor increasing the risk of testicular malignancy in children is cryptorchidism. The 2 main groups of testicular tumors are: Germ cell tumors (endodermal sinus tumor, followed by testicular teratomas) and non-germ cell tumors, which could be benign or malignant. About 75% of testicular tumors are malignant (*see* Fig. 22.19 in CD).

Ovarian tumors: Mature teratomas are the most common germ cell tumors of ovary and they are benign. The most common neoplasms are germ cell tumors, followed by epithelial tumors, stromal tumors, and then miscellaneous tumors such as Burkitt's lymphoma (*see* Fig. 22.20 in CD).

Agarwal PK, Palmer JS. Testicular and paratesticular neoplasms in prepubertal males. *J Urol* 2006; 176:875–881.

Bhatnagar S. Management of Wilms' tumor: NWTS vs SIOP. *J Indian Assoc Pediatr Surg* 2009;14:6–14.

Broecker B. Non-Wilms' renal tumors in children. *Urol Clin North Am* 2000;27:463–69.

Kaefer M, Rink RC. Genitourinary rhabdomyosarcoma treatment options. *Urol Clin North Am* 2000;27:471–87.

23 Endocrinology

23.1 DISORDERS OF THE HYPOTHALAMUS AND PITUITARY

The pituitary gland is composed of an anterior (adenohypophysis) and a posterior (neurohypophysis) lobe. The anterior lobe constitutes about 80% of the gland. The posterior lobe of the pituitary is part of a functional unit, the neurohypophysis that consists of the neurons of the supraoptic and paraventricular nuclei of the hypothalamus; neuronal axons, which form the pituitary stalk; and neuronal terminals in the median eminence or in the posterior lobe. Arginine vasopressin (AVP; Antidiuretic hormone [ADH]) and oxytocin are the two hormones produced by the neurosecretion in the hypothalamic nuclei and released from the posterior pituitary.

Hormones of the Hypothalamus and Pituitary

The pituitary gland is the major regulator of an elaborate hormonal system. The pituitary gland receives signals from the hypothalamus and responds by sending pituitary hormones to target glands. The target glands produce hormones that provide negative feedback at the level of hypothalamus and pituitary. This feedback mechanism enables the pituitary to regulate the amount of hormone released into the bloodstream by the target glands.

Hormones Produced by Anterior Pituitary Cell Types

Five anterior pituitary cell types (somatotropes, lactotropes, thyrotropes, corticotropes, gonadotropes) in the anterior pituitary produce six peptide hormones (growth hormone, prolactin, thyroid stimulating hormone, adrenocorticotropic hormone, luteinizing, and follicle-stimulating hormone).

Growth hormone: Human GH is a 191-amino acid single-chain polypeptide that is synthesized, stored, and secreted by *somatotropes* in the pituitary. GH is secreted in a pulsatile fashion under the regulation of hypothalamic hormones. The alternating secretion of growth hormone-releasing hormone (GHRH), which stimulates GH release, and somatostatin, which inhibits GH release, accounts for the rhythmic secretion of GH. Peaks of GH occur when peaks of GHRH coincide with troughs of somatostatin. Ghrelin, a peptide produced in the arcuate nucleus of the hypothalamus and is much greater quantities by the stomach, also stimulates GH secretion. Sleep, exercise, physical stress, trauma, acute illness, puberty, fasting, and hypoglycemia stimulate the release of GH, whereas hyperglycemia, hyperthyroidism, and glucocorticoids inhibit GH release.

The biologic effects of GH include increases in linear growth, bone thickness, soft tissue growth, protein synthesis, fatty acid release from adipose tissue, insulin resistance, and blood glucose levels.

Prolactin: PRL is a 199-amino acid peptide made in pituitary lactotropes. Prolactin (PRL) is consistently secreted unless it is actively inhibited by dopamine, which is produced by neurons in the hypothalamus. Disruption of the hypothalamus or pituitary stalk can result in elevated PRL levels. Dopamine antagonists, primary hypothyroidism, administration of thyrotropin releasing hormone (TRH), physiologic stress (shock), and pituitary tumors result in increased serum levels of PRL. Dopamine agonists and processes causing destruction of the pituitary cause reduced levels of PRL.

The primary physiologic role of PRL is the initiation and maintenance of lactation. PRL prepares the breasts for lactation and stimulates milk production postpartum. During pregnancy, PRL stimulates the development of the milk secretary apparatus, but lactation does not occur because of the high levels of estrogen and progesterone. After delivery, the estrogen and progesterone levels drop and physiologic stimuli such as suckling and nipple stimulation signal PRL release and initiate lactation.

Thyroid-stimulating hormone: TSH is stored in secretory granules and released into circulation primarily in response to thyrotropin-releasing hormone (TRH), which is produced by the hypothalamus. TRH is released from the hypothalamus into the hypothalamic-pituitary portal system, ultimately stimulating TSH release from pituitary thyrotropes. TSH stimulates release of thyroxine (T_4) and tri-iodothyronine (T_3) from the thyroid gland through the formation of cyclic adenosine monophosphate (CAMP) and the G-protein second messenger system. In addition to the negative feedback inhibition by T_3, the release of TRH and TSH are also inhibited by dopamine, somatostatin, and glucocorticoids. Deficiency of TSH results in inactivity and atrophy of the thyroid gland, whereas excess TSH results in hypertrophy and hyperplasia of thyroid gland.

Adrenocorticotropic hormone: Secretion of ACTH is regulated by corticotropin-releasing hormone (CRH), a 41-amino-acid peptide found predominantly in the median eminence but also in other areas in and outside the brain. ACTH is secreted in a diurnal pattern. It acts on the adrenal cortex to stimulate corisol synthesis and secretion. ACTH and cortisol levels are highest in the morning at the time of waking, and low in the late afternoon and evening and reach their nadir 1–2 hr after the beginning of sleep. ACTH also is the principal pigmentary hormone in humans. CRH and ACTH function through the formation of cyclic adenosine monophosphate (CAMP) and the G-protein second messenger system. Although CRH is the primary regulator of ACTH secretion, other hormones have a role. Arginine vasopressin (AVP), oxytocin, angiotensin II, and cholecystokinin stimulate release of CRH and ACTH, whereas atrial natriuretic peptide (ANP) and opioids inhibit release of CRH and ACTH. Cortisol inhibits CRH and ACTH. Physiologic conditions such as stress, fasting, hypoglycemia also stimulate release of CRH and ACTH.

Luteinizing hormone and follicle-stimulating hormone: Gonadotropic hormones include 2 glyco-proteins: LH and FSH. Receptors for FSH on the ovarian granulose cells and on testicular Sertoli cells mediate FSH stimulation of follicular development in the ovary and of gametogenesis in the testis. On binding to specific receptors on ovarian theca cells and testicular Leydig cells, LH promotes luteinization of the ovary and Leydig cell function of the testis.

Luteinizing hormone-releasing hormone, a decapeptide, has been isolated, synthesized, and used therapeutically. Because it leads to release of LH and FSH from the same gonadotropic cells, it appears that there is only one gonadotropin-releasing hormone.

Secretion of LH is inhibited by androgens and estrogens, and secretion of FSH is suppressed by gonadal production of inhibin, a 31-kd glycoprotein produced by the Sertoli cells. Inhibin consists of α- and β- subunits joined by disulfide bonds. The β-β dimer (activin) also occurs; its biologic effect is to stimulate FSH secretion. In addition to its endocrine effect, activin has paracrine effects in the testis. It facilitates LH-induced testosterone production, indicating a direct effect of Sertoli cells on Leydig cells.

Hormones Produced by Posterior Pituitary Cell Types

Antidiuretic hormone: ADH regulates water conservation at the level of the kidney by increasing the permeability of the renal collecting duct to water. ADH stimulates translocation of water channels through its interaction with vasopressin 2 (V2) receptors in the collecting duct, which act through G-proteins to increase adenylyl cyclase activity and increase permeability to water. V2 receptors also mediate the von Willebrand factor and tissue plasminogen activator. At higher concentrations, ADH activates V1 receptors in smooth muscle cells and hepatocytes and exerts pressure and glycogenolytic effects through mobilization of intracellular calcium stores. Separate V3 receptors mediate stimulation of ACTH secretion.

ADH and its accompanying protein, neurophysis II, are encoded by the same gene. A preprohormone is cleaved and the two are transported to neurosecretory vesicles in the posterior pituitary. The two are released in equimolar amounts.

ADH has a short half-life and responds quickly to changes in hydration. The stimuli for its release are increased plasma osmolality, perceived by osmoreceptor in the hypothalamus, and decreased blood volume, perceived by baroreceptors in the carotid sinus of the aortic arch.

Oxytocin: Oxytocin stimulates uterine contractions at the time of labor and delivery in response to distension of the reproductive tract, and it stimulates smooth muscle contraction in the breast during suckling, which results in milk let-down.

Hypopituitarism

Hypopituitarism denotes underproduction of growth hormone (GH) alone or in combination with deficiencies of other pituitary hormones. The incidence of hypopituitarism is between 1 in 4,000 and 1 in 10,000 live births.

Clinical Manifestations

Congenital hypopituitarism: The child with hypopituitarism is usually of normal size and weight at birth. Delayed closure of the epiphyses permits growth beyond the normal age when growth should be complete. Infants with congenital defects of the pituitary or hypothalamus usually present with neonatal emergencies such as apnea, cyanosis, or severe hypoglycemia with or without seizures. Deficiency of GH may be accompanied by hypoadrenalism and hypothyroidism. Prolonged neonatal jaundice is common.

The head of the toddler is round, and the face is short and broad. The frontal bone is prominent, and the bridge of the nose is depressed and saddle-shaped. The nose is small and the nasolabial folds are well developed. The eyes are somewhat bulging. The mandible and chin are underdeveloped, and the teeth, which erupt late, are frequently crowded. The neck is short, and the larynx is small. The voice is high-pitched and remains high after puberty. The extremities are well proportioned, with small hands and feet. Weight for height is usually normal, but an excess of body fat and a deficiency of muscle mass contributes to a pudgy (short and stout) appearance. The genitals are usually small for age, and sexual maturation may be delayed or absent. Microphallus in boys may be present. Facial, axillary, and pubic hair is usually deficient, and the scalp hair is fine. Mainly the length is affected, giving toddlers a pudgy appearance. Intelligence is usually normal. Symptomatic hypoglycemia, usually after fasting, occurs in 10–15% of children with panhypopituitarism.

Acquired hypopituitarism: The child initially is normal, but growth slows. When complete or almost complete destruction of the pituitary gland occurs, signs of pituitary insufficiency are present. Atrophy of the adrenal cortex, thyroid and gonads results in loss of weight, asthenia, sensitivity to cold, dullness, laziness, and absence of sweating. Sexual maturation fails to take place, or regress if already present. There may be atrophy of the gonads and genital tract with amenorrhea, and loss of pubic and axillary hair. There is a tendency to hypoglycemia. Diabetes insipidus may be present early.

If the lesion is an expanding tumor, symptoms such as headache, vomiting, visual disturbances, pathologic sleep patterns, decreased school performance, seizures, polyuria, and growth failure may occur. Slowing of growth may antedate neurologic signs and symptoms, especially with craniopharyngiomas. In children with craniopharyngiomas, visual field defects, optic atrophy, papilledema, and cranial nerve palsy are common.

Laboratory findings: The diagnosis of GH deficiency is suspected in children with moderate to severe postnatal growth failure. Criteria for growth failure include height below the 1% for age and sex or height more than 2 SD below sex-adjusted mid-parent height. Acquired GH deficiency can occur at any age, when it is of acute onset, height may be within the normal range.

The definitive diagnosis of GH deficiency requires demonstration of absent or low levels of GH. In addition to establishing the diagnosis of GH deficiency, it is necessary to examine other pituitary functions. Levels of TSH, thyroxine (T_4), ACTH, cortisol, gonadotropins, and gonadal steroids may provide evidence of other pituitary hormonal deficiencies. The defect can be localized to the hypothalamus if there is a normal response to the administration of hypothalamic-releasing hormones for TSH, ACTH or gonadotropins.

Radiologic findings: Computed tomography (CT) and magnetic resonance imaging (MRI) are now used and not X-ray films of the skull. CT is appropriate for recognizing suprasellar calcification associated with craniopharyngiomas and bony erosions accompanying histiocytosis. MRI provides a much more detailed view of hypothalamic and pituitary anatomy. Craniopharyngiomas are common and pituitary adenomas are rare in children with hypopituitarism.

Differential Diagnosis

There are many causes of growth disorders. Systemic conditions such as inflammatory bowel disease, celiac disease, occult renal disease, and anemia must be considered. Patients with systemic conditions often have greater loss of weight than length.

Constitutional growth delay: Constitutional growth delay is a common variant of normal growth. Length and weight measurements of affected children are normal at birth, and growth is normal for the first 4–12 mo of life. Height is sustained at a lower percentile during childhood. The pubertal growth spurt is delayed, so their growth rates continue to decline after their classmates have begun to accelerate. There are often other family members (frequently one or both parents) with histories of short stature in childhood, delayed puberty, and eventual normal stature. Insulin-like growth factor-I (IGF-I) levels tend to be low for chronological age but within the normal range for bone age. Growth hormone responses to provocative testing tend to be lower than in children with a more typical timing of puberty. The prognosis of normal adult height in these children is guarded. Boys with more than 2 yr of pubertal delay may benefit from a short course of testosterone therapy to hasten puberty after 14 yr of age. The cause of this variant of normal growth is thought to be persistence of the relatively hypogonadotropic state of childhood.

Primary hypothyroidism: Primary hypothyroidism is more common than GH deficiency. Low total or free T_4 and elevated TSH levels establish the diagnosis. Pituitary hyperplasia recedes during treatment with thyroid hormone. Because thyroid hormone is a necessary prerequisite for normal GH synthesis, it must always be assessed before GH evaluation.

Psychosocial dwarfism: Emotional deprivation is an important cause of retardation of growth and mimics hypopituitarism. The condition is known as psychosocial dwarfism. Puberty may be normal or even premature in its appearance. Appropriate history and careful observations reveal disturbed mother-child or family relations and provide clues to the diagnosis. Emotionally deprived children frequently have perverted or voracious appetites, enuresis, encopresis, insomnia, crying spasms, and sudden tantrums. Children tend to show catch-up growth when placed in a less stress environment.

Treatment: In children with classic GH deficiency, treatment should be started as soon as possible to narrow the gap in height between patients and their classmates during childhood and to have the greatest effect on mature height. The recommended dose of hGH is 0.18–0.3 mg/kg/wk during childhood. Higher doses have been used during puberty. Recombinant GH is administered subcutaneously in 6 or 7 divided doses. Maximal response in GH occurs in the 1st year of treatment; growth velocity in the 1st yr is above the 95th percentile. With each successive year of treatment, the growth rate tends to decrease. If the growth rate drops below the 25th percentile, compliance should be evaluated before the dose is increased. Criteria for stopping treatment include a decision by the patient that he or she is tall enough, a growth rate less than 1 inch/yr and a bone age >14 yr in girls and >16 yr in boys. During treatment with GH, some patients develop either primary or secondary hypothyroidism. There is also a risk of developing adrenal insufficiency; if unrecognized, this can be fatal. Periodic evaluation of thyroid and adrenal function is indicated for all patients treated with GH.

GH is also used for treatment of children with growth failure as a result of Turner syndrome, end-stage renal failure before kidney transplantation, Prader-Willi syndrome, intrauterine growth restriction (IUGR), and idiopathic short stature.

In children with multiple pituitary hormone deficiency (MPHD), replacement should also include other hormonal deficiencies. For infants with microphallus, one or two 3-month courses of monthly intramuscular injections of 25 mg of testosterone cypionate or testosterone enanthate may bring the penis to normal size without an inordinate effect on the osseous maturation.

Side effects reported in patients treated with GH include pseudotumor cerebri, slipped capital femoral epiphysis, gynecomastia, and worsening of scoliosis. Treatment does not increase the risk of type 1 diabetes, but it may increase the risk of type 2 diabetes.

Amar AP, Weiss MH. Pituitary anatomy and physiology. *Neurosurg Clin North Am* 2003; 14 (1): 11–23.

Badaru A, Wilson DM. Alternatives to growth hormone stimulation testing in children. *Trends Endocrinol Metab* 2004; 15 (6): 252–258.

Dattani MT, Preece M. Growth hormone deficiency and related disorders: Insights into causation, diagnosis, and treatment. *Lancet* 2004; 363: 1977–1986.

Parks JS, Felner E I. Disorders of the hypothalamus and pituitary. In: Kliegman RM, Behrman RE, Jenson HB, Stanton BF (eds). *Nelson Textbook of Pediatrics*. 18th edn. Vol 2. Philadelphia: Saunders, 2007; 2291–2293.

Parks JS, Felner E I. Hypopituitarism. In: Kliegman RM, Behrman RE, Jenson HB, Stanton BF (eds). *Nelson Textbook of Pediatrics*. 18th edn. Vol 2. Philadelphia: Saunders, 2007; 2293–2299.

Diabetes Insipidus

Diabetes insipidus (DI) presents clinically with polyuria and polydipsia and may result from either vasopressin deficiency (central DI) or vasopressin insensitivity at the level of the kidney (nephrogenic DI). Both central DI and nephrogenic DI can arise from inherited defects of congenital or neonatal onset or can be secondary to a variety of causes.

Approach to the patient with polyuria, polydipsia, and hypernatremia: Patients with suspected diabetes insipidus (DI) should have a careful history taken, which should include the child's daily fluid intake and output, voiding pattern, nocturia, and primary and secondary enuresis. Infants may present with irritability, failure to thrive, and intermittent fever. A detailed physical examination should be done to establish the hydration status, visual and central nervous dysfunction, and other pituitary hormone deficiencies.

Central diabetes insipidus: Central diabetes insipidus (central DI) can result from multiple etiologies. (i) In approximately 10% of children with central DI, the etiology is idiopathic. Other pituitary hormone deficiencies may be present. (ii) Autosomal dominant central DI usually presents within the first 5 yr of life and results from mutations in the vasopressin gene. *Wolfarian syndrome,* which includes DI, diabetes mellitus, optic atrophy, and deafness, also results from vasopressin deficiency. Congenital brain abnormalities such as *septo-optic dysplasia* with agenesis of corpus callosum, the *Kabuki syndrome,* holoprosencephaly, and posterior pituitary hypoplasia with absent stalk may be associated with central DI, and defects in thirst perception. Empty sella syndrome, possibly due to unrecognized infarction can be associated with DI in children. (iii) Trauma (to the base of the brain) and neurosurgical intervention (in the region of hypothalamus and pituitary) are common causes of central DI. The *triphasic response* following surgery refers to an initial phase of transient DI, lasting 12–48 hr, followed by a 2nd phase of syndrome of inappropriate antidiuretic hormone secretion, lasting up to 10 days, which may be followed by permanent DI (results if more than 90% of the neurons have been destroyed). (vi) Tumors that causes central DI are germinomas, pineolomas, craniopharyngiomas, and optic gliomas. Hematologic malignancies, as with acute myelocytic leukemia can cause DI via infiltration of the pituitary stalk and sella. Langerhans cell histiocytosis and lymphocytic hypophysitis are common types of infiltrative disorders causing central DI. (v) Infections involving the base of the brain, including meningitis (meningococcal, tubercular, cryptococcal, listerial, and toxoplasmal), congenital cytomegalovirus infection, and nonspecific inflammatory diseases of the brain may give rise to central DI that is often transient. (vi) Drugs associated with the inhibition of vasopressin release includes ethanol, phenytoin, opiate antagonists, halothane, and α-adrenergic agents.

Nephrogenic diabetes insipidus: Nephrogenic diabetes insipidus (NDI) can result from genetic or acquired conditions. Genetic (X-linked, autosomal recessive, autosomal dominant) causes are less common but more serious than acquired forms of NDI. Acquired NDI can result from hypercalcemia, hypokalemia; drugs; kidney disease.

Treatment of central diabetes insipidus: Neonates and young infants should be treated with *fluid therapy,* given their requirement for large volumes ($3L/m^2/24$ hr) of nutritive fluids. The use of vasopressin analogs in patients with obligate high fluid intake is contraindicated because of the risk of life-threatening hyponatremia.

Older children are best treated by the long-acting *vasopressin analog* dDAVP (desmopressin), available in an intranasal preparation (onset 5–10 min) and as tablets (onset 15–30 min). The intranasal preparation of dDAVP ($10\,\mu g/0.1$ ml) can be administered by rhinal tube (allowing dose titration) or by nasal spray. The appropriate dose is determined empirically based on the desired length of antidiuresis. The nasal spray delivers ($10\,\mu g/0.1$ ml) per spray is used in the treatment of primary enuresis in older children, but it is a temporary measure and should be used with caution. Oral doses of 25–$300\,\mu g$ every 8–12 hr of dDAVP tablets is safe and effective in children.

Central DI of acute onset following neurosurgery is managed with continuous administration of synthetic *aqueous vasopressin* (pitressin). Total fluid intake must be limited to $1\,L/m^2/24$ hr during antidiuresis. Vasopressin is administered intravenously 1.5 mU/kg/hr, which results in a blood vasopressin concentration of approximately 10 pg/ml. Post-neurosurgical patients treated with vasopressin infusion should be switched from intravenous to oral fluids as soon as possible to allow thirst sensation, if intact, to help regulate osmolality.

Treatment of nephrogenic diabetes insipidus: The treatment of acquired NDI mainly is on elimination of the underlying disorder, such as offending drugs, hypercalcemia, hypokalemia and ureteral obstruction. The main treatment of congenital NDI is to ensure the intake of adequate calories for growth and to avoid severe dehydration. Despite early therapy, growth failure and mental retardation are common. The use of thiazide diuretics for the treatment of NDI is intended to decrease the overall urine output. Indomethacin and amiloride may be used in combination with thiazide to further reduce polyuria. High-dose dDAVP therapy, in combination with indomethacin may be useful in patients with genetic defects in the V2 receptor associated with a reduced binding affinity for vasopressin.

Other Abnormalities of Arginine Vasopressin Metabolism and Action

Hyponatremia (serum sodium<130 mEq/L) in children is usually associated with severe systemic disorders and is most often due to: (1) Intravascular volume depletion, (2) excessive salt loss, or (3) hyponatremic fluid overload, especially in infants.

First of all is to determine the volume status in a patient with hyponatremia. A careful history, physical examination, including changes in weight, and vital signs helps in determining whether the patient is hypovolemic or hypervolemic. Laboratory data such as serum electrolytes, blood urea nitrogen, creatinine, uric acid, urine sodium, specific gravity and osmolality will support the diagnosis (Table 23.1).

Causes of Hyponatremia

Syndrome of inappropriate antidiuretic hormone secretion: SIADH is characterized by hyponatremia, an inappropriately concentrated urine (>100 mOsm/kg), normal or slightly elevated plasma volume, normal-to-high urine sodium and low serum uric acid. SIADH is uncommon in children, with most cases resulting from excessive administration of vasopressin in the treatment of central diabetes insipidus. It can also occur with encephalitis, pneumonia, tuberculous meningitis, brain tumors, head trauma, AIDS and psychiatric disease and in the postictal period after generalized seizures, and after prolonged nausea. SIADH is the cause of the hyponatremic second phase of the triphasic response seen after hypothalamic-pituitary surgery.

Cerebral salt wasting: Cerebral salt wasting appears to be the result of hypersecretion of atrial natriuretic peptide and is seen primarily with central nervous system disorders including brain tumors, head trauma,

hydrocephalus, neurosurgery, cerebral vascular accidents, and brain death. Hyponatremia is accompanied by elevated urinary sodium excretion (often > 150 mEq/L), excessive urine output, hypovolemia, normal or high uric acid, suppressed vasopressin, and elevated atrial natriuretic peptide concentrations (> 20 pmol/L). Thus, it is distinguished from SIADH, in which normal or decreased urine output, euvolemia, low uric acid, modestly elevated urine sodium concentration, and an elevated vasopressin level occur.

Treatment of Hyponatremia

Patients with hyponatremia due to primary salt loss require supplementation with sodium chloride and fluids. Initially, intravenous replacement of urine volume with fluid containing sodium chloride, 150–450 mEq/L depending on the degree of salt loss, may be necessary; oral supplementation is required subsequently (note the difference in the treatment of SIADH).

Treatment of SIADH: In the treatment of SIADH, water restriction without sodium supplementation is the mainstay. Oral fluid intake is limited to 1,000 ml/m^2/24 hr to avoid hyponatremia. In young children this degree of fluid restriction may not provide adequate calories for growth. In this situation, the creation of nephrogenic diabetes insipidus using demeclocycline therapy may be indicated to allow sufficient fluid intake for normal growth. Conivaptan, a V2-receptor antagonist, decreases permeability of the collecting duct to water producing an aquaresis. It has been effective in the treatment of SIADH in adults.

Breault DT, Majzoub JA. Diabetes insipidus. In: Kliegman RM, Behrman RE, Jenson HB, Stanton BF (eds). *Nelson Textbook of Pediatrics.* 18th edn. Vol 2. Philadelphia: Saunders, 2007; 2299–2301.

Breault DT, Majzoub JA. Other abnormalities of arginine vasopressin metabolism and action. In: Kliegman RM, Behrman RE, Jenson HB, Stanton BF (eds). *Nelson Textbook of Pediatrics.* 18th edn. Vol 2. Philadelphia: Saunders, 2007; 2301–2303.

Knoers N, Monnems LH. Nephrogenic diabetes insipidus: Clinical symptoms, pathogenesis, genetics and treatment. *Pediatr Nephrol* 1992; 6: 476–482.

Muglia LJ, Majzoub JA. Disorders of the posterior pituitary. In: Sperling MA (Ed). *Pediatric Endocrinology.* 2nd edn. Philadelphia: WB Saunders, 2002.

Table 23.1: Clinical parameters to distinguish between SIADH, cerebral salt wasting, and central diabetes insipidus			
Clinical parameter	*SIADH*	*Cerebral salt wasting*	*Central DI*
Serum sodium	Low	Low	High
Urine output	Normal or low	High	High
Urine sodium	High	Very high	Low
Intravascular volume status	Normal or high	Low	Low
Serum uric acid	Low	Normal or high	High
Vasopressin level	High	Low	Low

Hyperpituitarism

Primary hypersecretion of pituitary hormones are rarely seen in children and if occurs it is due to a pituitary adenoma. Secondary hyperpituitarism occurs due to target hormone deficiencies resulting in decreased hormonal feedback, such as in hypogonadism, hypoadrenalism, or hypothyroidism. The most commonly seen adenoma during childhood is prolactinoma, followed by corticotropinoma, and then somatotropinoma, which secrete prolactin, corticotropin, and growth hormone, respectively.

Prolactinoma: Prolactin-secreting pituitary adenomas are the most common tumors of the pituitary in adolescents. The most common presenting manifestations are headache, amenorrhea, and galactorrhea. Girls are affected two times more than boys. Most patients have undergone normal puberty before becoming symptomatic. Prolactin levels may be moderately (40–50 ng/ml) or markedly (10,000–15,000 ng/ml) elevated. Most prolactinomas in children are large (macroadenomas), cause the sella to enlarge, and in some cases produce visual field defects. Approximately 1/3rd of patients with macroadenomas develop hypopituitarism, particularly GH deficiency. Treatment of prolactinoma for most children is surgical resection by transfrontal or transsphenoidal approach. Medical treatment of prolactinoma is by bromocriptine or long-acting cabergoline; about 80% of adult patients respond with shrinkage of the tumor and marked decreases in serum prolactin levels.

Corticotropinoma: Corticotropinomas are the most common adenomas seen prepubertally although they occur at all ages. Adenomas causing Cushing's disease, refers specifically to an ACTH-producing pituitary adenoma that stimulates excess cortisol secretion. Adenomas causing Cushing's disease are significantly smaller than all other types of adenomas at the time of presentation. The indicator of excess glucocorticoid secretion in children is growth failure, which generally precedes other manifestations. Patients develop weight gain that tends to be centripetal rather than generalized. Pubertal arrest, fatigue, and depression are other clinical features.

Growth hormone oversecretion: In young persons with open epiphyses, overproduction of growth hormone (GH) results in gigantism, whereas in persons with closed epiphyses in acromegaly. Gigantism features consist of longitudinal growth acceleration secondary to GH excess and coarse facial features, and enlarging hands and feet. In young children rapid growth of head may precede linear growth. Some patients have behavioral and visual problems. Giants have rarely been reported to grow to a height of over 8 ft.

Acromegalic features consist chiefly of enlargement of the distal parts of the body, but manifestations of abnormal growth involve all portions. The circumference of the skull increases, the nose becomes broad, and the tongue is often enlarged, with coarse facial features. The mandible grows excessively, and the teeth become separated. Visual field defects and neurologic abnormalities are common; signs of intracranial pressure appear later. The fingers and toes grow chiefly in thickness. There may be dorsal kyphosis. Fatigue and lassitude are early symptoms. Approximately 20% patients with gigantism are those with McCune-Albright syndrome (MAS), commonly consisting of a triad of precocious puberty, café-au-lait spots, and fibrous dysplasia.

Diagnosis: Failure to suppress serum GH levels to less than 5 mg/dl after a 1.75 g/kg oral glucose challenge (maximum 75 g) is diagnostic of GH excess. This test measures the ability of insulin-like growth factor (IGF-1) to suppress GH secretion because the glucose load results in insulin secretion, leading to suppression of insulin-like growth factor binding protein (IGFBP-1), which results in an acute increase in free IGF-1 levels. The increased free IGF-1 suppresses GH secretion within 30–90 min. This test can be abnormal in diabetic patients. A single measurement of GH is inadequate because GH is secreted in a pulsatile manner. If laboratory findings suggest GH excess, the presence of a pituitary adenoma should be confirmed by MRI.

Treatment: Transsphenoidal surgery is the treatment of choice for well-circumscribed adenomas and may be curative. At times a transcranial approach may be necessary. The primary goal of treatment is to normalize GH levels. GH levels (< 1 ng/ml within 2 hr after a glucose load) and serum IGF-1 levels (age adjusted normal range) are the best tests to define a biochemical cure. If GH secretion is not normalized by surgery, the options include pituitary irradiation and medical therapy. Hypopituitarism is a predictable outcome, occurring in 40–50% of patients 10 yr after irradiation. The medical treatment is effective with long-acting somatostatin analogs, dopamine agonists and novel GH antagonists.

Clemmons DR. Role of insulin-like growth factor-I in diagnosis and management of acromegaly. *Endocr Pract* 2004; 10: 362–371.

Cohen P, Shim M. Hyperpituitarism, tall stature, and overgrowth syndromes. In: Kliegman RM, Behrman RE, Jenson HB, Stanton BF (eds). *Nelson Textbook of Pediatrics*. 18th edn. Vol 2. Philadelphia: Saunders, 2007; 2303–2307.

Daughaday WH. Pituitary gigantism. *Endocrinol Metab Clin North Am* 1992; 21: 633–647.

Feenata J, de Herder WW, Van der Beld AW, et al. combined therapy with somatostatin analogues and weekly pegvisomant in active acromegaly. *Lancet* 2005; 365: 1644–1646.

Kane LA, Leinung MC, Scheithaver BW, et al. Pituitary adenomas in childhood and adolescence. *J Clin Endocrinol Metab* 1994; 79: 1135–1140.

Tall Stature

Tall stature and excessive overgrowth syndromes represent physical development in excess of 2 standard deviations (SD) above the mean for the person's age and gender. The causes of tall stature are shown in Table 23.2. Assessment of the child or adolescent with tall stature requires repeated height measurements. The combination of careful history-taking and physical examination will exclude the need for laboratory investigations in most cases. Procedures needed for the clinical assessment of child are given in Table 23.3.

If the physical examination is completely normal and the child comes from a tall family, investigations are usually not indicated. Regular height measurements will be sufficient. In presence of any abnormal history or physical examination indicates some investigations, as shown in Table 23.4.

Constitutional tall stature: This is the most common cause of excessive height. Height of these individuals has been above ninety-fifth percentile since early childhood, and their height velocity is within normal limits. Physical examination is normal but bone age is moderately advanced .One or both parents are usually tall. Puberty will be early in this entity, so that the final height will not be out of normal range, although height during childhood was greater than normal. Diagnosis can be made from history including family history, physical examination and bone age, and growth record.

Table 23.2: Causes of tall stature

1. **Variations of normal**
   - 1a. Constitution
   - 1b. Exogenous obesity
2. **Tall stature of endocrine origin**
   - 2a. GH secreting pituitary tumor
   - 2b. Hyperthyroidism
   - 2c. Precocious puberty
3. **Syndromes associated with tall stature**
   - 3a. Chromosomal defects: Klinefelter syndrome (XXY), XXXY, XYY syndromes
   - 3b. Marfan's syndrome
   - 3c. MEN 2B
   - 3d. ACTH/cortisol deficiency/resistance
   - 3e. Homocystinuria
   - 3f. Sotos syndrome (cerebral gigantism)
   - 3g. Overgrowth in the fetus: Maternal diabetes mellitus, Weaver syndrome, Marshall-Smith syndrome, Beckwith-Wiedemann syndrome, Other IGF-II excess syndrome

Table 23.3: Clinical assessment of tall stature

Height, weight, height velocity, heights of parents, siblings and final height prediction
Birth weight, length, head circumference
History of previous growth, past medical history
History s/o mental retardation
History s/o systemic illness
Dysmorphology assessment
Systematic examination
Tanner staging

Table 23.4: Investigations

Chromosome karyotype
Thyroxine (T$_4$), thyroid stimulation hormone (TSH)
Insulin-like growth factor-1 (IGF-I)
Bone age X-rays
Further investigations will be dictated by the results of baseline tests, including amino acid screen (homocystinuria)

Exogenous obesity is a common condition in adolescence and may be associated with rapid linear growth and early maturation; adult height is typically normal.

GH-secreting pituitary tumor: A GH-secreting tumor causes tall stature and gigantism. Suppression of GH secretion may require treatment consist of pituitary surgery; radiotherapy and medical therapy (somatostatin analogs, dopamine agonists or GH-receptor antagonist) (*see* Section 23.1 on Hyperpituitarism).

Hyperthyroidism in adolescents is associated with rapid growth but normal adult height. It is almost always caused by Graves' disease and is much more common in females.

Precocious puberty (*see* Section 23.2).

Klinefelter syndrome (*see* Chapter 9).

XXY syndrome is associated with tall stature and behavioral and mental problems.

Marfan syndrome (*see* Section 31.11).

Multiple endocrine neoplasia, Type IIB: MEN 2B is characterized by multiple neuromas, tall stature, with arachnodactyly and a Marfan-like appearance. Total thyroidectomy is indicated for all children.

ACTH/cortisol deficiency/resistance: Patients mainly have hypoglycemia, seizures, and increased pigmentation during the 1st decade of life. The disorder affects both sexes equally and is inherited in an autosomal recessive manner.

ACTH resistance occurs in association with achalasia of the gastric cardia and alacrima (triple A or Allgrove syndrome). These patients often have a progressive neuropathic disorder that includes autonomic dysfunction, mental retardation, deafness, and motor neuropathy. This syndrome is inherited in an autosomal recessive fashion, and the AAAS gene has been mapped in chromosome 12q13 (*see* Section 23.5).

Homocystinuria (*see* Section 26.2)

Sotos syndrome (Cerebral gigantism): Rapid growth is common during the first five years of life. Thereafter, growth continues to parallel the 97th percentile or above. Head circumference has been documented well above the 98th percentile. The presence of a high arched palate (roof of the mouth is narrow and arched upward), poor suck, and low muscle tone often produces feeding problems. Jaundice occurs frequently. Craniofacial abnormality and advanced bone age is common. The hands and feet may be large in comparison with the rest of the body. Hypotonia, developmental delay, behavioral problem, enlarged ventricles of brain can be present.

Maternal diabetes constitutes the most common cause of infants who are large for gestational age (LGA). The birth of an excessively large infant should lead to evaluation for maternal (or gestational) diabetes.

Overgrowth syndromes: A group of disorders associated with excessive growth and growth of specific organs has been described and is collectively referred to as overgrowth syndromes. These disorders appear to be caused by excess availability of insulin-like growth factor-II (IGF-II) encoded by the gene. The best described of these syndromes is the *Beckwith-Wiedemann syndrome* (BWS). Increased birth weight and lengths are present and growth velocity and bone age is advanced during first 4–6 years of life. Macroglossia, hemihypertrophy, ear-signs, earlobe creases, hypoglycaemia, omphalocoele, malignancies (e.g. Wilms' tumor and adrenocortical carcinoma) and learning difficulties are some of the features of this syndrome. Mutations in GPC3, a glypican gene (which codes for an IGF-II neutralizing membrane receptor), cause the related *Simpson-Golabi-Behmel* overgrowth syndrome.

Treatment of familial (constitutional) tall stature: Reassurance of the family and the patients is the key to the management of familial (constitutional) tall stature. The use of the bone age to predict adult height may provide some comfort. Occasionally, the degree of anxiety surrounding advanced growth, usually in girls, is so great that treatment is indicated to try to slow down growth and therefore, reduce final height. Two forms of therapy are currently used: sex-steroid therapy and somatostatin analog therapy.

Sex-steroid therapy: In girls, ethinylestradiol 0.15–0.5 mg/day orally until cessation of growth occurs. If necessary, a progestational agent can be added after 1 yr of unopposed estrogen. Short-term side effects of estrogen treatment for tall stature include menstrual irregularities, weight gain, nausea, limb pain, galactorrhea, benign breast disease, cholelithiasis, hypertension, and thrombosis. Reduced fertility later in life may be a potential long-term complication. If used relatively early, reduced final height is up to 7 cm. In boys, testosterone enanthate is used at the dose of 250–1000 mg IM every 2 wk for 6 months cause a similar reduction. The optimal dose of sex steroids is not known. For late maturing individuals, it is advisable to initially prescribe a reduced dose with subsequent gradual increments.

An early age of onset of treatment (bone age 10 years in girls, 12.5 years in boys) is associated with the best results. In an extensive inquiry, 10 years after final height, no significant adverse affects were identified.

In conclusion, it is recommended first to refer constitutionally tall children in the late prepubertal period (8–10 yr) to secure proper pretreatment evaluation of growth and bone maturation. Second, is to restrict treatment to excessive tallness or a very outspoken professional desire where height forms a clear limitation (e.g. pilot, ballet dancer). Third, treatment should be initiated at an early 'bone age, psychosocial constraints permitting'. Treatment should not start before an age corresponding to the 10th percentile of the first stage of pubertal development. Moreover, although retrospective studies have not provided hard evidence of testicular damage, it should be realized that in boys' androgen treatment might interfere with pubertal testicular development. Finally, treatment should be continued until complete closure of the epiphyses has been established radiologically.

Somatostatin analog therapy: The somatostatin analogs are highly effective in the treatment of patients with GH excess.

Some facts: 1. As tall stature is better tolerated by society, there seems to be less indication for therapy. 2. Rare conditions, such as GH secreting pituitary tumors, are very infrequently seen in pediatric practice. These patients must be managed jointly with an adult endocrine unit.

Potential pitfalls: 1. Failure to consider the diagnosis of or examine the patient carefully enough for dysmorphic features suggestive of Marfan's syndrome. This diagnosis may have serious consequences as these patients need lifelong cardiovascular surveillance. 2. Failure to appreciate that tall statue and delayed puberty are an unusual combination. An important differential diagnosis is Klinefelter syndrome, which should be considered.

Specialist centre consultation will be required in certain situations: 1. Dysmorphic syndromes associated with tall stature; 2. Tall stature associated with excess GH secretion; 3. Difficult cases of tall stature associated with hyperthyroidism or precocious puberty; 4. GH receptor antagonist treatment is likely to become established as the treatment of choice for constitutional tall stature.

Cohen P, Shim M. Hyperpituitarism, tall stature, and overgrowth syndromes. In: Kliegman RM, Behrman RE, Jenson HB, Stanton BF (eds). *Nelson Textbook of Pediatrics*. 18th edn. Vol 2. Philadelphia: Saunders, 2007;2303–07.

Lamberts SWJ. Somatostatin analogs: Their role in the treatment of growth hormone hypersecretion and excessive body growth. *Growth Regulators* 1991;1:3–10.

Lee JM, Howell JD. Tall girls: The social shaping of a medical therapy. *Arch Pediatr Adolesc Med* 2006;160:1035–9.

Opitz JM, Weaver DW, Reynolds JF. The syndromes of Sotos and Weaver: reports and review. *Am J Med Genet* 1998;79:294–304.

Sotos JF. Overgrowth genetic syndromes and other disorders associated with overgrowth. *Clin Pediatr* 1997; 36: 157–170.

Tanner JM, Whitehouse RH. Longitudinal standards for height, weight-height, height velocity and stages of puberty. *Arch Dis Childhood* 1976; 51: 170–179.

Short Stature

The child is considered to be short stature, if the length or height of the child is >3 standard deviation (SD) below the mean for age. The recumbent length or height of 95 percent of normal children lies between the 5th and 95th percentiles. Short statue is usually normal. Adult height is influenced by polygenic inheritance and has a normal distribution. Any significant illness in childhood will have an impact on the rate of growth.

Etiology: Short stature can be due to variety of causes (Box 23.1). Amongst the pathological causes, undernutrition and systemic illness are the common etiological factors followed by growth hormone deficiency and hypothyroidism.

Box 23.1: Causes of short stature

1. **Familial**
2. **Constitutional delay**
3. **Systemic disorders**
   Endocrine. Primary hypothyroidism (cretin), hypopituitarism; congenital adrenal hyperplasia; Cushing syndrome, pseudohypoparathyroidism.
   Chronic infections: tuberculosis; malaria; leishmaniasis; syphilis; HIV.
   Alimentary: Malabsorption including gluten enteropathy, Crohn's disease, cystic fibrosis
   Liver-biliary disease
   Cardiorespiratory: Congenital heart disease; asthma; suppurative lung disease.
   Renal: renal failure
   Hematological: Anemia
   Locomotor (skeletal abnormality): Primary chondrodystrophy (metaphyseal dysplasia) .
   With short limbs: Achondroplasia; deformities due to rickets and osteogenesis imperfect; dystrophic dysplasia; disorders involving cartilage matrix protein; cartilage hair hypoplasia (CHH).
   With short trunk: Mucopolysaccharidoses; severe scoliosis; Pott disease; hemivertebra.
4. **Genetic and chromosomal disorders:** Turner syndrome; Down syndrome.
5. **Nutritional:** Intrauterine growth restriction; marasmus; Kwashiorkor; vitamin D deficiency rickets.
6. **Psychosocial:** Failure to thrive.

Assessment of a child with short stature: A clinical examination of child will provide useful information in making the clinical diagnosis.

1. *Accurate height measurement:* For children below 2 years, supine length should be measured using an infantometer. For older children, height should be measured with a stadiometer.

2. *Assessment of body proportion:* Children may be proportionate and disproportionate types. Disproportionate children are those who have short limbs or trunk. The proportionality is assessed by upper segment (US) and lower segment (LG) ratio and comparison of arm span with height. Normally US: LS ratio is 1.7 at birth, 1.3 at 3 years, 1.1 by 6 years, 1 by 10 years and 0.9 in adults. Increase in US: LS ratio is seen in rickets, achondroplasia, and untreated congenital hypothyroidism. Decrease in US: LS ratio is seen in spondyloepiphyseal dysplasia and vertebral anomalies. Arm span is shorter than length by 2.5 cm at birth, equals height at 11 years and thereafter greater than height.

3. *Assessment of height velocity:* Height velocity is the rate of increase in height over a period of time expressed as cm/year. It varies with the age of the child. If height velocity is low, the child is more likely to be suffering from a pathological cause of short stature.

4. *Comparison with population norms:* The height should be plotted on appropriate growth charts and expressed in percentiles.

5. *Comparison with child's own genetic potential:* Parent's height significantly affects the child's height. Mid parental height (MPH) gives an approximate estimate of the child's genetically determined potential. This value is then plotted on the growth chart at 18–20 years (adult equivalent) of age. This gives an estimate of the target height for the child and the percentile that he/she is likely to follow.

MPH for boys

$$= \frac{\text{Mother's height (cm)} + \text{Father's height (cm)}}{2} + 6.5$$

MPH for girls

$$= \frac{\text{Mother's height (cm)} + \text{Father's height (cm)}}{2} - 6.5$$

6. *Sexual maturity rating (SMR):* SMR stage should be assessed in older children. Height spurt is seen in early puberty in girls and mid puberty in boys. Precocious puberty can lead to early height spurt followed by premature epiphyseal fusion and ultimate short stature. On the other hand, delayed puberty can also be present with short stature in adolescents as the height spurt is also delayed. This is common in children with constitutional delay in growth.

Diagnosis: Diagnosis is based on a detailed clinical history, examination and laboratory evaluation (Box 23.2).

Investigations: The investigative workup will be based on the history and clinical examination (Box 23.3).

Bone age: Assessment of bone age should be done in all children with short stature. Bone age is studied from radiograph of hand and wrist. The appearance of various epiphyseal centres and fusion of epiphyses with metaphyses tells about the skeletal maturity of the child. Bone age also gives an idea as to what proportion of the adult height has been achieved by the child and what is the remaining potential left for gaining in height.

Bone age is delayed compared to chronological age in almost all causes of short stature. A few exceptions to this are familial short stature, in which bone age equals chronological age and precocious puberty, in which bone age exceeds chronological age. In case of constitutional delay, undernutrition and systemic illness, bone age is less than chronological age and equals height age. In cases of growth hormone deficiency and hypothyroidism, bone age may be even less than height age if the endocrine condition is diagnosed late.

Box 23.2: Clinical assessment of short stature

Height, weight, height velocity, heights of parents, siblings and final height prediction
Birth weight, length, head circumference
History of previous growth, past medical history
History s/o mental retardation
History s/o systemic illness
Dysmorphology assessment
Systematic examination
Tanner staging

Box 23.3: Investigations

Essential investigations
Complete hemogram with ESR
Urine examination
Stool examination for parasites, steatorrhea and occult blood
Blood-urea, creatinine, calcium, phosphate, alkaline phosphatase, fasting glucose, albumin and transaminases
Bone age X-rays
Other investigations based on clinical and results of baseline tests
Chromosome karyotype
Thyroxine (T$_4$), thyroid stimulation hormone (TSH)
Insulin-like growth factor-1 (IGF-I)

Differential Diagnosis

Familial-genetic short stature: Since familial and genetic influences strongly determine how a child grows, most children with short parents will have short children. This is termed familial short stature. While children with familial short stature may be at or near or just below the 3rd or 5th percentile on their growth chart for their height, their growth curve or channel will run parallel to the normal growth curves and they have a normal rate of growth. They also have a bone age that is close to their chronological age. Although growing normally, children with familial short stature will usually be short as adults, with a similar height to their parents. Familial-genetic short stature is usually found in other family members. The level of skeletal maturation is consistent with chronologic age in genetic short stature but not in constitutional growth delay. Hormones related to growth are normal.

Constitutional growth delay: Constitutional growth delay is one of the variants of normal growth. Length and weight measurements of affected children are normal at birth and growth is normal for the first 4–12 months of life. Growth then decelerates to near or below the 5th percentile for height and weight. By 2–3 years of age growth resumes at a normal rate of 5 cm/yr or more. Growth hormone secretion is normal. Bone age is closure to height age than to chronological age. There is often other family members (frequently one or both parents) have histories of short stature in childhood, delayed puberty, and eventual normal stature. Boys with unusual degrees of delayed puberty may benefit from a short course of testosterone therapy to hasten puberty after 14 years of age. The cause of this variant of normal growth is perhaps due to the persistence of the relatively hypogonadotropic state of childhood. The prognosis of these children to achieve normal adult height is good.

Systemic conditions: Patients with systemic conditions often have greater loss of weight than length. A few otherwise normal children are short (i.e. > 3 SD below the mean for age) and grow 5 cm per year or less but have normal levels of GH in response to provocative tests and normal spontaneous episodic secretion. Systemic conditions such as inflammatory bowel disease, celiac disease, occult renal disease, and anemia must be considered. Treat the underlying cause.

Primary hypothyroidism: Primary hypothyroidism is more common than GH deficiency. Low total or free T_4 and elevated TSH levels establish the diagnosis (*see* Section 23.3).

Hypopituitarism: The child with hypopituitarism is usually of normal size and weight at birth. Prolonged neonatal jaundice is common. The head of the toddler is round, and the face is short and broad. The frontal bone is prominent, and the bridge of the nose is depressed and saddle-shaped. The nose is small and the nasolabial folds are well developed. The eyes are somewhat bulging. The mandible and chin are underdeveloped, and the teeth, which erupt late, are frequently crowded. The neck is short, and the larynx is small. The voice is high-pitched and remains high after puberty. The extremities are well proportioned, with small hands and feet. Weight for height is usually normal, but an excess of body fat and a deficiency of muscle mass contributes to a pudgy (short and stout) appearance. The genitals are usually small for age, and sexual maturation may be delayed or absent. Microphallus in boys may be present. Facial, axillary, and pubic hair is usually deficient, and the scalp hair is fine. Mainly the length is affected, giving toddlers a pudgy appearance. Intelligence is usually normal (*see* Section 23.1).

Cushing syndrome: It is frequently suspected in children with obesity, particularly when striae and hypertension is present. Purplish striae on the hips, abdomen, and thighs are common.

Pseudohypoparathyroidism: Affected children have a short, stocky build and a round face. Brachydactyly with dimpling of the dorsum of the hand is usually present. The second metacarpal and second metatarsal are least affected. As a result, index finger and second toe may occasionally be longer than the middle finger and third toe respectively (short metacarpals, especially the fourth and fifth are found). There may be short and wide phalanges, bowing, exostosis, and thickening of the calvaria. Tetany is often the presenting sign. These patients frequently have calcium deposits and metaplastic bone formation subcutaneously. Moderate degree of mental retardation, calcification of basal ganglia, and lenticular cataracts are common in patients who are diagnosed late (*see* Section 23.4).

Intrauterine growth restriction (IUGR): IUGR is often classified as reduced growth that is symmetric (head circumference, length and weight equally affected) or asymmetric (with relative sparing of head growth).

Primary chondrodystrophy (metaphyseal dysplasia): In this autosomal dominant condition, bowing of the legs, short stature, and a waddling gait appear in the absence of abnormalities of serum levels of calcium and phosphate, alkaline phosphatase activity, or vitamin D metabolites.

Silver-Russell syndrome is characterized by short stature, frontal bossing, small triangular facies, sparse subcutaneous tissue, shortened and incurred 5th fingers and in many cases hemihypertrophy. Affected children have low birth weight for gestational age.

Pott disease: The classic manifestation of tuberculous spondylitis is progression to Pott disease, in which destruction of vertebral bodies leads to gibbus deformity and kyphosis.

Seckel syndrome: Seckel syndrome, sometimes called "bird-headed dwarfism," is an autosomal recessive developmental disorder characterized by marked growth failure and mental deficiency, microcephaly, a hypoplastic face, with a prominent nose, and low-set and/or malformed ears. Approximately 25% of patients have aplastic anemia or malignancies.

Mauriac syndrome: One of the complications in type 1 diabetic children is dwarfism associated with a glycogen-laden enlarged liver (Mauriac syndrome). Clinical features of Mauriac syndrome include moon face, protuberant abdomen, proximal muscle wasting, and enlarged liver due to fat and glycogen infiltration. The Mauriac syndrome is related to under-insulinization.

Cartilage hair hypoplasia (CHH) occurs predominantly among the Pennsylvania Amish, but non-Amish patients have been described. Clinical features include short, pudgy hands; redundant skin; hyperextensible joints of hands and feet but an inability to extend the elbows completely; and fine, sparse, light hair and eyebrows. The bones radiographically show sclerotic or cystic changes in the metaphyses and flaring of the costochondral junctions of the ribs.

Y-linked inheritance: These demonstrate only male-male transmission, and only males are affected and are associated with infertility.

Psychosocial dwarfism: Appropriate history and careful observations reveal disturbed mother-child or family relations and provide clues to diagnosis. Emotionally deprived children frequently have perverted or voracious appetites, enuresis, encopresis, insomnia, crying spasms, and sudden tantrums (*see* Section 6.7).

Treatment: Providing emotional support is an important part of treatment. Children may be teased by classmates and friends. Parents should be counseled to highlight the positive aspects of the child's other skills and strengths and not give undue emphasis on stature. Intake of a balanced diet containing recommended amount of macro- and micronutrients should be based on three—3 meals, 3 breakfasts, and 3 varieties. The specific management depends on the underlying cause. For familial and constitutional growth delay reassurance, annual monitoring of height and weight is sufficient. Dietary rehabilitation for undernutrition and treatment of underlying condition such as celiac disease or renal tubular acidosis are generally associated with good catch up growth. For hypothyroidism, the treatment is levothyroxine given orally. Children of short stature who are found to have a lack of growth hormone in their body will usually be treated with growth hormone injections.

Chesney RW. Metabolic bone diseases. In: Kliegman RM, Behrman RE, Jenson HB, Stanton BF (eds). *Nelson Textbook of Pediatrics*. 18th edn. Vol 2. Philadelphia: Saunders, 2007; 2893–2898.

Greenbaum LA. Rickets and hypervitaminosis D. In: Kliegman RM, Behrman RE, Jenson HB, Stanton BF (eds). *Nelson Textbook of Pediatrics*. 18th edn. Vol 1. Philadelphia: Saunders, 2007; 253–263.

Ghai OP, Jain V, Sankhyan N, Agarwal R. Normal growth and its disorders. In: Ghai OP, Paul VK, Bagga A (eds). *Ghai Essential Pediatrics*. 7th edn. New Delhi: CBS Publishers & Distributors Pvt Ltd, 2009; 1–21.

Horton WA, Hecht JT. The skeletal dysplasia: General considerations. In: Kliegman RM, Behrman RE, Jenson HB, Stanton BF (eds). *Nelson Textbook of Pediatrics*. 18th edn. Vol 2. Philadelphia: Saunders, 2007; 2869–2873.

Horton WA, Hecht JT. Disorders involving cartilage matrix proteins. In: Kliegman RM, Behrman RE, Jenson HB, Stanton BF (eds). *Nelson Textbook of Pediatrics*. 18th edn. Vol 2. Philadelphia: Saunders, 2007; 2873–2877.

LaFranchi S. Disorders of thyroid gland. In: Kliegman RM, Behrman RE, Jenson HB, Stanton BF (eds). *Nelson Textbook of Pediatrics*. 18th edn. Vol 2. Philadelphia: Saunders, 2007; 2316–2340.

Marini JC. Osteogenesis imperfect. In: Kliegman RM, Behrman RE, Jenson HB, Stanton BF (eds). *Nelson Textbook of Pediatrics*. 18th edn. Vol 2. Philadelphia: Saunders, 2007; 2887–2890.

Parks JS, Felner EI. Hypopituitarism. In: Kliegman RM, Behrman RE, Jenson HB, Stanton BF (eds). *Nelson Textbook of Pediatrics*. 18th edn. Vol 2. Philadelphia: Saunders, 2007; 2293–2299.

23.2 PUBERTY AND DISORDERS OF PUBERTY

Puberty

Puberty is a biological process in the continuum of life which is characterized by the appearance of secondary sex characteristics and the achievement of reproductive capacity. Puberty is a gradual process culminating in ovulatory menstrual cycling in the female and fully mature spermatogenesis in the male. The reawakening of gonadal function at puberty is known as gonadarche, and the increased adrenal androgen secretion of puberty is known as adrenarche, and development of pubic hair is pubarche. These processes are temporally related in the average child, i.e. adrenarche, pubarche and gonadarche occurs. The pubertal development involves a cascade of hypothalamic-pituitary-gonadal axis activation. Hypothalamic-pituitary gonadotropin-gonadal control via feedback mechanisms is acquired in fetal life; hypothalamic gonadotropin releasing hormone (GnRH) and pituitary luteinizing hormone (LH) and follicle stimulating hormone (FSH) are present in the early fetus.

Age of onset of puberty: The age of onset and tempo of puberty varies considerably. The normal age at onset of puberty is 9 to 14 years in boys and 8 to 13 years in girls and this has not changed appreciably in the last several decades. The average age at onset of puberty in boys is 10.5 years and completes in 2 to 4.5 years with a mean of 3.5 years. The average age of onset of puberty in girls is 10 years and is complete in 1.5 to 6 years with a mean of 4.2 years. The secular trends occurring over the last century towards earlier puberty is continuing but at a much reduced rate.

In girls accelerated growth rate is the usual first evidence of puberty, but thelarche is usually the first evidence to be noted. The mean age of breast development (Tanner stage 2) among girls, not considering race, is between 9.5 and 10 years of age with 5% girls having breast development by their eighth birthday with full maturity at 14 years. The interval between pubertal onset and menarche is variable; the average interval is 2 years. Ovulation may occur before menarche or later. There is considerable variation in the tempo of puberty, with earlier onset, the tempo is slower.

In males, increased testicular size, i.e. testicular volume of more than 4 ml or the long axis dimension of 2.5 cm or more is the earliest physical evidence of onset of puberty. In the average boy without regard to race, testicular growth begins before his twelfth birthday and may be present as young as 9.5 years of age. Pubic hair is the most frequently noted change of puberty, although testicular growth precedes this. It proceeds with genital growth and maturity and pubic hair growth and progression to male pattern of hair distribution. Among boys accelerated growth occurs during mid puberty, rather than at pubertal onset, as among girls. Peak growth velocity is usually at 14 years of age, during Tanner stage 3 and 4. Onset of spermarche is also a mid pubertal event, usually during Tanner stage 3, occurring at age 13.5 to 14 years. Other mid pubertal events include voice deepening, acne, and axillary hair growth, facial hair growth begins approx 3 years after the onset of pubic hair growth. There is progressive increase in total body bone mineral content and lean body mass.

Sexual maturity rating: The physical changes of puberty are widely known as Sex Maturity Rating (SMR) (*see* Chapter 2).

Disorders of Puberty

Disorders of puberty include precocious puberty, incomplete (partial) precocious puberty, medicational precocity and delayed puberty.

Precocious Puberty

Precocious puberty is defined as early onset of physical findings of puberty followed by progression and the demonstration of pubertal physiology or abnormal sex steroid stimulation at an age younger than the age range for pubertal onset. When a girl has signs of puberty before 7 years or 6 years in Afro-Americans, and boys develop secondary sexual characteristics before 9 years, the condition is sexual precocity. Central precocious puberty (CPP) or true or gonadotropin-releasing dependent (GnRH-dependent) occurs from early onset of pubertal hypothalamic-pituitary-gonadal activity. Incomplete precocious puberty or pseudo precocious or peripheral (PPP) or gonadotropin independent (GnRH-independent) is due to autonomous secretion of sex steroids in boys or girls. The source of sex steroid is exogenous or endogenous, gonadal or extragonadal. Patients of both the categories will have rapid growth and skeletal maturation; investigations are warranted to discern the cause. The tall child seen on presentation will later cease to grow because of premature epiphyseal fusion and finally becomes a short child.

Central precocious puberty: Majority of girls present with central precocious puberty with an underlying CNS lesion seen only in 5% of girls. It is less common among males who are more likely to have a demonstrable CNS lesion, in 20%.

Constitutional precocious puberty: Some children will normally begin puberty somewhat before the lower age limits of normal pubertal development without evidence of any organic lesion. The sequence and progression is the same as in normal puberty. A family history is likely to be present. Early onset of puberty must be considered a disorder until proven otherwise.

Idiopathic precocious puberty: These patients have all the findings of normal puberty at an earlier age. The progress may be normal and continuous or slow and waxing and waning. Girls are brought more often for evaluation than boys. Boys have a symmetrical and progressive testicular enlargement.

Central nervous system disorders: In all cases of CPP, a CNS tumor must be considered as an etiology. Hamartomas of tuber cinereum are composed of ectopic hypothalamic tissue and usually contain GnRH in the neurons. They function as supplemental hypothalamus that operates outside of the normal inhibitory effects of the CNS on GnRH secretion. They are tumor masses and because of their sensitive location not amenable to surgical removal. CNS tumors include astrocytomas, ependymomas, and gliomas. There are CNS lesions causing increased intracranial pressure including inflammatory granulomas, suprasellar cysts, hydrocephalus or head trauma.

Peripheral precocious puberty: In girls incomplete isosexual precocious puberty may develop because of ovarian or adrenal secretion or ingestion of estrogen, estrogen secreting tumors like granular cell tumors (the most common) gonadoblastomas, lipoid tumors and ovarian carcinomas. Serum gonadotropins are suppressed and serum estradiol concentrations are elevated. Ovarian follicular cysts can secrete enough estrogen to cause breast development and when the cyst resolves withdrawal bleeding can occur. Cysts are small and limited, but may secrete high concentrations of estrogen or may be recurrent. Surgical intervention is rarely indicated. Peripheral precocious puberty is more common among boys and can develop by autonomous secretion of sex steroids by gonadal or adrenal tumors. In adrenal source of androgens, testis may be small such as in congenital virilizing adrenal hyperplasia or androgen secreting tumors. In human chorionic gonadotropin secreting tumors and LH receptor activating mutation or in Leydig cell tumors, testis are enlarged.

McCune-Albright syndrome: McCune-Albright syndrome, involves several endocrinopathies, including peripheral precocious puberty, which occurs more frequently in females than males. Originally it is described as triad of hyperpigmented skin macules (Café au lait spots), fibrous dysplasia and precocious puberty. This syndrome may manifest with precocious puberty, hyperthyroidism, hyperadrenocorticism, pituitary gigantism and hypophosphatemia along with increase in sex steroids without gonadotropin stimulation. There is no ideal therapy, medroxy progesterone, aromatase inhibitors and antiestrogens have been used with equivocal results. If secondary CPP occurs GnRH becomes a therapeutic option. The treatment of choice is surgery.

Primary hypothyroidism: Very rarely, prepubertal children with primary hypothyroidism develop pubertal changes as a consequence of an overlap phenomenon of trophic hormones—FSH due to excess TSH. There is breast development in females and bilateral testicular enlargement among males. Thyroid replacement therapy is followed by regression of the changes of puberty.

Evaluation: The history relates to progress of pubertal growth, ages of parental puberty, exposure to androgens, symptoms related to elevated intracranial pressure, neurological, ophthalmological presentations, hypothyroidism, and skin lesions. Clinical examination includes anthropometric measurements, with data plotted on growth charts, pubertal staging, skin lesions, thyroid, neurological and fundus examination. In girls look for features of estrogenization and in boys do careful examination of testis. Radiograph of hand wrist for estimation of skeletal maturity. Normal estimation of LH and FSH either basal or after stimulation with GnRH, estradiol and testosterone levels.

In case of suspected CNS lesions MRI or CT and pelvic ultrasound or abdominal CT for adrenal or gonadal tumors should be done.

Treatment of precocious puberty: In a child with precocious puberty the accelerated growth rate and skeletal maturation, will result in diminished growth potential and final adult height, sexual and reproductive characteristics advance, and the child is capable of sexual function and is at risk of sexual abuse or other age inappropriate sexual behavior. Therefore, therapy is considered to alter or reclaim growth and skeletal maturity as well as to prevent or help psychosocial and psychological issues.

Gonadotropin releasing hormone analogue (GnRH-As) are extremely potent and suppress gonadotropin secretion, sex steroid secretion decreases, rate of bone age advancement and rate of rapid growth decreases and the height prognosis of treated patients improves. On discontinuation, there is increase in gonadotropin secretion to pubertal values and the patterns of normal puberty follows.

In peripheral precocious puberty (PPP) the aim is to diminish the synthesis or metabolic effects of the sex steroid. Aromatase inhibitors, testolactone may be effective in suppressing estrogens. Medroxyprogesterone acetate has been used in McCune Albright syndrome with variable success and also in familial gonadotropin independent Leydig cell and germ cell maturation. Ovarian cysts usually regress spontaneously requiring watchful follow up.

Psychological support and counseling are helpful to both the child and parents.

Incomplete (Partial) Precocious Development

They include premature thelarche, i.e. isolated early breast development or premature adrenarche, i.e. mild androgen effect leading to sexual hair growth.

Premature thelarche: It is a benign condition of unilateral or bilateral breast development, usually seen before 3 to 4 years. There are no other signs of estrogen effect and no linear growth. Serum estradiol values and LH are pre-pubertal, FSH may be slightly higher when compared with normal age matched children. Ovarian follicular cysts may be present which regress spontaneously. The condition requires reassurance but continued follow-up and observation at 3 to 6 months interval is necessary.

Bilateral breast hypertrophy may occur in a newborn as a result of elevated circulating maternal endogenous steroid hormone in late gestation (*see* Fig. 23.1 in CD). It may be associated with discharge from the nipples known as 'which's milk.' Repeated manipulation of the breast can exacerbate the condition. On occasion the hypertrophy is associated with mastitis caused by staphylococcal infection, antibiotics should be administered.

Premature adrenarche: It is a benign, self-limited appearance of small amount of pubic hair or axillary hair usually occurring after 6 years. There is slight increase in adrenal androgens DHEA and its sulfate. The rest of the pubertal development occurs at a normal age. There may be slight increase in growth rate or advancement of bone age. Late onset congenital adrenal hyperplasia may have an initial appearance like this. Thus, clinical follow-up is mandatory.

Premature menarche: This is a rare entity and is a diagnosis of exclusion. In girls with isolated vaginal bleeding in the absence of other secondary sexual characteristics, more common causes such as vulvovaginitis, a foreign body, or sexual abuse, and uncommon causes such as urethral prolapse and sarcoma botryoides must be excluded. The majority of girls with idiopathic premature menarche have only 1–3 episodes of bleeding; puberty occurs at the usual time, and menstrual cycles are normal. Plasma levels of gonadotropins are normal, but estradiol levels may be elevated, probably owing to episodic ovarian estrogen secretion. Occasionally patients may have ovarian follicular cysts on ultrasound.

Medicational Precocity

Precocious pseudopuberty has occurred in both boys and girls from the accidental ingestion of estrogens (including contraceptive pills) and from the administration of anabolic steroids. Estrogens in cosmetics, hair creams, and breast augmentation creams have caused breast development in girls and gynecomastia in boys; estrogens are readily absorbed from the skin. Exogenous estrogens may produce an intense, dark brown color in the areola of the breasts that is not usually seen in endogenous types of precocity. The precocious changes disappear after cessation of exposure to the hormones. The use of testosterone gels or creams, which are applied to the skin for treatment of male hypogonadism, has resulted in virilization of children and women following skin contact.

Delayed Puberty

Delayed puberty is defined as the onset of puberty after the age of 13 years in girls and 14 years in boys. Most of these young adolescents have simple, constitutional delay of puberty (CDP). Pathologic causes of delayed puberty are less frequent. However, in some situations, further investigations are warranted.

Constitutional delay of puberty: Patients who are healthy but have a slower rate of development than average are said to have constitutional delay. They are shorter for their age matched peers throughout childhood and their height is appropriate for bone age. The skeletal age is delayed, body habitus is thin, mental development is appropriate for age. There often is a family history of delay. Both adrenarche and gonadarche are delayed. After elimination of any neurological or chronic illness, one can consider the diagnosis.

Hypogonadotropic hypogonadism: Abnormalities of the hypothalamus or pituitary gland leading to lack of gonadotropins results in lack of onset of pubertal development. In gonadotropin deficiency the patient will have normal height, may be with eunuchoid proportions (i.e. US: LS ratio is below 0.9) and if associated with the GH deficiency the patient's growth rate is also decreased during childhood.

Isolated gonadotropin deficiency: Patients with isolated gonadotropin deficiency are of normal height, till adolescence, when they neither go into puberty nor have pubertal height spurt; however, they may continue to grow and have normal adult height with eunuchoid proportions. They may have midline defects. They may present with non-initiation or progress of puberty or failure to reach maturity or later as infertility. They may present as abnormalities in GnRH function like Kallmann syndrome, associated with anosmia/hyposmia or as receptor defects or mutations of FSH, LH or adrenal hypoplasia gene defects.

Central nervous system tumors: CNS tumors or cysts in the region of hypothalamus or pituitary can present with delayed puberty. These may be associated with other signs of pan hypopituitarism or hypothalamic dysfunction or visual defects. Craniopharyngiomas is one of the common varieties and there may be others like germinomas, astrocytomas, gliomas, etc. Inflammatory granulomas, histiocytosis, trauma, surgery, cranial irradiation and hydrocephalus may cause hypothalamic pituitary deficiency.

Idiopathic hypopituitarism can present with GH deficiency, microphallus, and cryptorchidism.

Systemic diseases: Pubertal delay is typically seen in a wide range of systemic diseases like malnutrition, malabsorption, chronic renal failure, hematological disorders like thalassemia and eating disorders.

Hypergonadotropic hypogonadism: Primary gonadal failure resulting from a range of chromosomal and syndromic causes, disorders of steroid and androgen synthesis or any insult to gonads can result in impaired pubertal development. Boys will present with lack of virilization and girls will present with lack of feminization and amenorrhea. Serum gonadotropins are elevated because of lack of feedback inhibition from the gonads.

Turner syndrome (TS) is the most common form of primary gonadal failure in females and Klinefelter (KS) and its variants in males. Noonan Syndrome is a dominantly inherited condition with some features similar to Turner's and some different from Turner (normal karyotype) triangular shaped face, pectus excavatum, right-sided heart disease, mental retardation, affected boys may have undescended testes.

Mixed gonadal dysgenesis results from 46XY/45X mosaicism and usually presents with ambiguous genitalia at birth or as pubertal failure later. The streak gonads should be removed.

Assessment and investigation of delayed puberty: Children who present with delayed puberty require a thorough assessment and physical examination to exclude many physical and functional causes of delayed puberty. Height and puberty ratings should be recorded. Testicular volumes can be measured with an orchidometer. A hand radiograph to assess skeletal age to determine the delay is required. The pelvic ultrasonography is done to assess the internal gonads. Baseline blood counts, blood chemistry, celiac screen, thyroid functions, and a karyotype are required for evaluation. Basal gonadotropins are raised in most children with gonadal failure, but normal or low levels do not reliably differentiate constitutional delay in puberty from hypogonadotropic hypogonadism (HH). GnRH stimulation tests or hCG stimulation might support the diagnosis of HH if the response is poor. Imaging of the brain, hypothalamus and pituitary can help with CNS defects.

Treatment of pubertal delay and pubertal failure: Children with pubertal delay who are worried about their development can be treated with low doses of sex steroids for a short period of time, with the aim of inducing sexual development, and stimulating activation of the child's own HPG axis so that puberty continues once the administration is stopped and the further progress pubertal development is then monitored. Counseling with psychological support is required. Continuation of sex steroids treatment may be needed when endogenous puberty is not established or in cases of permanent gonadotropin insufficiency or gonadal failure.

Garibaldi L. Physiology of puberty. In: Kliegman RM, Behrman RE, Jenson HB, Stanton BF (eds). *Nelson Textbook of Pediatrics*. 18th edn. Vol 2. Philadelphia: Saunders, 2007; 2308.

Garibaldi L. Disorders of pubertal development. In: Kliegman RM, Behrman RE, Jenson HB, Stanton BF (eds). *Nelson Textbook of Pediatrics*. 18th edn. Vol 2. Philadelphia: Saunders, 2007; 2309–2316.

Prescovitz OH, Eugster EA. *Pediatric Endocrinology*. Philadelphia: Lippincott, Williams and Wilkins, 2004; 316–348.

Sanfilippo TS. Breast disorders. In: Behrman RE, Kliegman RM, Jenson HB (eds). *Nelson Textbook of Pediatrics*. 17th edn. Philadelphia: Saunders, 2004; 1833–1835.

Styne DM. *Pediatric Endocrinology*. Philadelphia: Lippincott, Williams and Wilkins, 2004; 159–195.

Yadav Sangeeta. Puberty and Disorders of Pubertal Development. In: Mathur GP, Mathur Sarla (eds). *Current Trends in Pediatrics*. Vol 2. Delhi: Academa Publishers, 2006; 404–410.

23.3 THYROID DISORDERS

Thyroid physiology: The thyroid is regulated by thyroid-stimulating hormone (TSH), a glycoprotein produced and secreted by the anterior pituitary. The main function of thyroid gland is to synthesize T_4 and T_3. The physiologic role of iodine is in the synthesis of these hormones. The recommended dietary allowance of iodine is 30 µg/kg/24 hr for infants, 90–120 µg/kg/24 hr for children, and 150 µg/kg/24 hr for adolescents and adults. Thyroid tissue has avidity for iodine and is able to trap, transport, and concentrate it in the follicular lumen for synthesis of thyroid hormone. Before trapped iodide can react with tyrosine, it must be oxidized; this reaction is catalyzed by *thyroidal peroxidase*. The thyroid cells also elaborate a specific thyroprotein, a globulin with approximately 120 tyrosine units, *thyroglobulin*. Iodination of tyrosine forms monoiodotyrosine and diiodotyrosine; 2 molecules of diiodotyrosine then couple to form 1 molecule of T_4 or 1 molecule of diiodotyrosine and 1 of monoiodotyrosine to form T_3. Once formed, hormones are stored as thyroglobulin in the lumen of the follicle (colloid) until ready to be delivered to the body cells. T_4 and T_3 are liberated from thyroglobulin by activation of proteases and peptidases.

The thyroid hormones are transported in plasma bound to *thyroxine-binding globulin* (TBG), a glycoprotein synthesized in the liver. Thyroid hormones increase oxygen consumption, stimulate protein synthesis, influence growth and differentiation, and affect carbohydrate, lipid, and vitamin metabolism.

Hypothyroidism

Hypothyroidism results from deficient production of thyroid hormone or a defect in thyroid hormonal receptor activity. The disorder may be manifested from birth or acquired. When symptoms appear after a period of apparently normal thyroid function, the disorder may be truly "acquired" or may only appear due to a variety of congenital defects in which the manifestation of the deficiency is delayed. The term cretinism often used synonymously with congenital hypothyroidism and endemic iodine deficiency should be avoided (*see* Fig. 23.2 in CD).

Congenital Hypothyroidism

Most cases of congenital hypothyroidism result from thyroid dysgenesis and are not hereditary (Table 23.5). The prevalence of congenital hypothyroidism based on nationwide programs for neonatal screening is 1/4,000 infants worldwide. Girls are affected two times more than boys.

Clinical manifestations: Most infants with congenital hypothyroidism are asymptomatic at birth, even if there is complete agenesis of the thyroid gland. This situation is due to the transplacental passage of moderate amounts of maternal T_4 which provides fetal levels that are approximately 33% of normal at birth. Low serum levels of T_4 and elevated levels of TSH make it possible to screen and detect hypothyroid neonates.

Congenital hypothyroidism is twice as common in girls as in boys. Before neonatal screening programs, congenital hypothyroidism was rarely recognized in the newborn because the signs and symptoms are usually not significantly developed. Symptoms appear gradually, the clinical diagnosis is often delayed. Birth weight and length are normal. Head size may be slightly increased because of myxedema of the brain. Prolongation of physiological jaundice, caused by delayed maturation of glucuronide conjugation, may be the earliest sign. Feeding difficulties, choking spells during nursing, respiratory difficulties are present during the 1st mo of life. Characteristically the infant cry little, sleep much, have poor appetites, sluggish, and constipated (considered a goody-goody child). Abdomen is large and an umbilical hernia is usually present. The temperature is subnormal; temperature often less than 35°C (95°F). Skin of extremities may be cold and mottled. Edema of genitals and extremities may be present. The pulse is slow, and heart murmurs, cardiomegaly, and asymptomatic pericardial effusion are common. Macrocytic anemia is often present and is refractory to treatment with hematinics. Approximately 10% of infants with congenital hypothyroidism have associated congenital anomalies, including cardiac anomalies (most common), and anomalies of the nervous system and eye.

When there is only partial deficiency of thyroid hormone, the symptoms may be milder and the onset

---

Table 23.5: Etiologic classification of congenital hypothyroidism
Central (Hypopituitary) Hypothyroidism
PIT-1 mutations: Deficiency of thyrotropin (TSH), growth hormone, and prolactin
PROP-1 mutations: Deficiency of thyrotropin (TSH), growth hormone, prolactin, LH, FSH, ±ACTH
Thyrotropin releasing hormone (TRH) deficiency: Isolated; multiple hypothalamic deficiencies (e.g. septo-optic dysplasia)
TRH unresponsiveness: Mutations in TRH receptor
TSH deficiency: Mutations in β-chain
Multiple pituitary deficiencies: Craniopharyngioma
TSH unresponsiveness: G-α mutations (type IA pseudohypoparathyroidism); mutation of TSH receptor
Primary Hypothyroidism
Defect of fetal thyroid development: Aplasia, hypoplasia, ectopia (dysgenesis)
Defect in thyroid hormone synthesis (e.g. goitrous hypothyroidism): Iodide transport defect; thyroid peroxidase defect; thyroid oxidase mutations, homozygotic-permanent, homozygotic transient; thyroglobulin synthesis defect; deiodination defect
Defect in thyroid hormone transport: Thyroid oxidase mutations; homozygotic-permanent; homozygotic transient, deiodination defect
Defect in thyroid hormone transport
Iodine deficiency (endemic goiter): Neurologic type; myxedematous type
Maternal antibodies: Thyrotropin receptor-blocking antibody (TRBAb, also termed thyrotropin binding inhibitor immunoglobulin)
Maternal medications: Radioiodine; iodides; propylthiouracil; methimazole; amiodarone

ACTH, adrenocorticotropic hormone; FSH, follicle-stimulating hormone; LH, luteinizing hormone.

is delayed. Although breast milk contains significant amounts of thyroid hormones, particularly T_3, it is inadequate to protect the breast-fed infants with congenital hypothyroidism and it has no effect on neonatal thyroid screening tests.

If congenital hypothyroidism goes undetected and untreated, retardation of physical and mental development becomes greater during the following months, and by 3–6 months of age the clinical picture is fully developed. The child's growth will be stunted. Extremities are short and hands are broad and fingers short. Head size is normal or increased; the anterior and posterior fontanels are open widely (only in 3% of normal newborn infants posterior fontanel is larger than 0.5 cm). The eyes appear far apart and the bridge of the broad nose depressed. The palpebral fissures are narrow and the eyelids are swollen. The mouth is kept open and the thick, broad tongue protrudes. Dentition will be delayed. The scalp is thickened and hair is coarse, brittle and scanty. The hairline reaches far down on the forehead, which usually appears wrinkled, especially when the infant cries. The neck is short and thick and there may be deposits of fat above the clavicles and between the neck and shoulders. The skin is dry and scaly, and there is a little perspiration. The skin shows generalized pallor with a sallow complexion. Carotenemia may cause a yellow discoloration of the skin, but the scleras remain white. Myxedema is manifested, particularly in the skin of the eyelids, the back of the hands, and the external genitals.

Development is usually retarded. Hypothyroid infants appear lethargic and are late in learning to sit and stand. The voice is hoarse, and they do not learn to talk. The degree of physical and mental retardation increases with age. Sexual maturation may be delayed or may not take place at all.

The muscles are usually hypotonic. But in rare instances generalized muscular pseudohypertrophy occurs (*Kocher-Debré-Sémélaigne syndrome*), the pathogenesis of which is unknown. Affected older children may have an athletic appearance because of pseudohypertrophy, particularly in the calf muscles. Boys are more to development of the syndrome, observed in siblings born to a consanguineous mating. Affected patients have hypothyroidism of longer duration and severity.

Laboratory findings: Neonatal screening test to measure T_4 (low) and THS (elevated) is used for the diagnosis of congenital hypothyroidism and primary hypothyroidism. X-ray of the knee joint shows absence of distal femoral epiphysis (normally present at birth). In undetected and untreated patients, the discrepancy between chronological age and osseous development increases. The epiphyses often have multiple foci of ossification (epiphyseal dysgenesis); deformity ("beaking") of the 12th thoracic or 1st or 2nd lumbar vertebra is common. Roentgenograms of the skull show large fontanels, wide sutures, and intersutural (wormian) bones. The sella turcica is often enlarged and round and erosion and thinning is seen in rare instances. Delays in formation and eruption of teeth may occur. Cardiac enlargement or pericardial effusion may be present.

Scintigraphy can help to pinpoint the underlying cause in infants with congenital hypothyroidism, but the treatment should not be unduly delayed for this study. ^{123}I sodium iodide is superior to ^{99m}Tc-sodium pertechnetate for this purpose. Ultrasonography of the thyroid gland is useful, but may miss some ectopic glands shown by scintigraphy. Serum levels of thyroglobulin are low with agenesis and elevated with ectopic glands and goiter. Demonstration of ectopic thyroid tissue is diagnostic of thyroid dysgenesis and establishes the need for life-long treatment with T_4. Failure to demonstrate any thyroid tissue suggests thyroid aplasia, but this also occurs in neonates with TRBAb and in infants with the iodide-trapping defect. A normally situated thyroid gland with a normal or avid uptake of radionuclide indicates a defect in thyroid hormone biosynthesis. Patients with goitrous hypothyroidism can now be evaluated by genetic studies looking for defects in the steps along the thyroxine biosynthetic pathway.

The electrocardiogram may show low-voltage P and T waves with diminished amplitude of QRS complexes and suggest poor left ventricular function and pericardial effusion. The electroencephalogram frequently shows low voltage. In children older than 2 yr of age, the serum cholesterol level is usually elevated.

Treatment: Levothyroxine [sodium-L-thyroxine (100 µg) tablet] given orally is the treatment of choice, because 80% of circulating T_3 is formed by monodeiodination of T_4, serum levels of T_4 and T_3 in treated infants return to normal. This also happens in the brain, where 80% of required T_3 is produced locally from T_4. In neonates, the recommended initial starting dose is 10–15 µg/kg (37.5 to 50 µg/24 hr). Newborns with more severe hypothyroidism, as judged by a serum $T_4 < 3$ µg/dl, should be started at the higher end of the dosage range. Thyroxin tablets should not be mixed with soy protein formulas or iron, because these can bind T_4 and inhibit its absorption. Levels of T_4 or free T_4 and TSH should be monitored at recommended intervals (approximately monthly in the Ist 6 mo of life, and then every 2–3 mo between 6 mo and 2 yr) and maintained in the normal range for age. Children with hypothyroidism require about 4 µg/kg/24 hr, and adults require only 2 µg/kg/24 hr.

To rule out the possibility of transient hypothyroidism confirmation of the diagnosis may be required for some infants, but not in infants with proven thyroid ectopia or in those who manifest elevated levels of TSH after 6–12 mo of therapy because of poor compliance or an inadequate dose of T$_4$. Discontinuation of therapy at about 3 yr of age for 3–4 wk results in marked increase of TSH levels in children with permanent hypothyroidism.

Over treatment may risk craniosynostosis and temperamental problems. An older child (8–13 yr) with acquired hypothyroidism occasionally may experience pseudotumor cerebri within the first 4 mo of treatment. In older children, after catch-up growth is complete, the growth rate provides a good index of the adequacy of therapy.

Prognosis: Early diagnosis and adequate treatment from the first weeks of life result in normal linear growth and intelligence comparable with that of unaffected siblings. Severely affected infants as judged by the lowest T$_4$ levels and retarded skeletal maturation, have reduced (5–10 points) IQs and other neuropsychological sequelae, such as incoordination, hypotonia or hypertonia, short attention span, and speech problems. Brain damage occurs when there is inadequate treatment and poor compliance in the first 2–3 yr of life. When onset of hypothyroidism occurs after 2 yr of age, the outlook for normal development is much better.

Acquired Hypothyroidism

Epidemiology: Acquired hypothyroidism occurs in approximately 0.3% (1/333) of school-aged children. 6% of children aged 12–19 yr have evidence of autoimmune thyroid disease, which occurs with a 2:1 female to male preponderance.

Etiology: Acquired hypothyroidism is most commonly a result of chronic lymphocytic thyroiditis (Table 23.6). Autoimmune thyroid disease may be part of polyglandular syndromes; children with Down, Turner, and Klinefilter syndromes and celiac disease

or diabetes are at higher risk for associated autoimmune thyroid disease (*see* Section 23.3 on Lymphocytic Thyroiditis). Additional autoimmune diseases with an increased risk of hypothyroidism include Sjögren syndrome, multiple sclerosis, pernicious anemia, Addison disease, and ovarian failure.

Clinical manifestations: Deceleration of growth is usually the first clinical manifestation. Goiter, which may be a presenting, typically is non-tender and firm, with a rubbery consistency and a pebbly surface. Myxedematous changes of the skin, constipation, cold intolerance, decreased energy, and an increased need for sleep develop insidiously. School work and grades usually do not suffer. Osseous maturation is delayed, which is an indication of the duration of the hypothyroidism. Adolescents have delayed puberty, whereas younger children may present with galactorrhea or pseudoprecocious puberty. Additional features include ataxia, muscle weakness or cramps, menstrual disturbances, bradycardia, weight gain, and abnormal laboratory studies (hyponatremia, macrocytic anemia, hypercholesterolemia, elevated CPK, hyperprolactenemia).

Complications seen in severe hypothyroidism include heart failure, ventilatory failure, hyponatremia, ileus, medication sensitivity, hypothermia and lack of febrile response to sepsis, delirium, dementia, seizures, stupor and coma, adrenal insufficiency, and coagulopathy.

Diagnostic studies and treatment is the same as described for congenital hypothyroidism. Measurement of antithyroglobulin and antiperoxidase antibodies may pinpoint autoimmune thyroiditis as the cause. In case of goiter resulting from autoimmune disease ultrasound examination shows diffuse enlargement with scattered hypoechogenecity. During the 1st yr of treatment, deterioration of school work, poor sleeping habits, restlessness, short attention span, and behavioral problems may ensue, but these are transient. These may be partially ameliorated by starting at sub-replacement T$_4$ doses and advancing slowly.

Table 23.6: Etiologic classification of acquired hypothyroidism
Autoimmune (acquired hypothyroidism): Hashimoto thyroiditis; polyglandular autoimmune syndrome, type I and II
Iatrogenic: Drugs (propylthiouracil; methimazole; iodides; lithium; amiodarone); Irradiation of the area of thyroid; Radioiodine; Thyroidectomy
Systemic disease: Cystinosis; Langerhans' cell histiocytosis; histiocytic infiltration of thyroid
Hemangiomas (large) of the liver (type 3 iodothyronine deiodinase activity)
Resistance to thyroid hormone (only occasional clinical manifestations of hypothyroidism)

Lymphocytic Thyroiditis

Lymphocytic thyroiditis (Hashimoto thyroiditis, autoimmune thyroiditis) is the commonest cause of thyroid disease in children and adolescents. The typical organ-specific autoimmune disease is characterized histologically by lymphocytic infiltration of the thyroid.

Clinical manifestations: Lymphocytic thyroiditis is 2–4 times more frequent in girls than in boys. The disorder is more common after 6 yr, the peak incidence during adolescence, but may occur during the first 3 yr of life. The most common clinical manifestations are goiter and growth retardation. The thyroid is diffusely enlarged, firm, and non-tender; the gland is lobular and may seem to be nodular in 30% of patients. Most of the affected children are clinically euthyroid and asymptomatic; some may have symptoms of pressure in the neck. Some children have clinical signs of hypothyroidism, but others who appear clinically euthyroid have laboratory evidence of hypothyroidism. A few children have manifestations suggestive of hyperthyroidism, such as nervousness, irritability, increased sweating, and hyperactivity, but laboratory findings are not necessarily suggestive of hyperthyroidism. Occasionally the disorder may coexist with Graves' disease. Ophthalmopathy may occur in the absence of Graves' disease. The clinical course is variable. The goiter may become smaller or may disappear spontaneously, or it may persist unchanged for years while the patient remains euthyroid. Thyroiditis is the cause of most cases of nongoitrous (atrophic) hypothyroidism Autoimmune thyroiditis is associated with hypoparathyroidism, Addison disease, Turner syndrome and Klinefelter syndrome.

Laboratory findings: Thyroid function tests are often normal, although thyroid stimulating hormone (TSH) may be slightly or moderately elevated in some individuals, (normal T_4 or free T_4, elevated TSH) termed subclinical hypothyroidism. When both tests (antibodies to TPO and thyroglobulin) are used, approximately 95% of patients with thyroid autoimmunity are detected. Thyroid scans and ultrasonography usually are not needed. Thyroid scans in 50% of children reveal irregular and patchy distribution of the radioisotope and in about 60% or more, the administration of perchlorate results in a greater than 10% discharge of iodide from the thyroid gland. Thyroid ultrasonography shows scattered hypoechogenicity in most patients. The definitive diagnosis can be established by biopsy of thyroid, but is rarely indicated.

Antithyroid antibodies may also be found in almost 1/2 of siblings of affected patients and also in some mothers of children with Down syndrome or Turner syndrome without demonstrable thyroid disease. They are also found in 20% of children with diabetes mellitus and in 23% of children with the congenital rubella syndrome.

Treatment: If there is evidence of hypothyroidism treat with sodium-L-thyroxine (50–150 µg daily). The goiter usually shows some decrease in size but may persist for years. Because the disease may be self-limited in some patients, the need for continued therapy requires periodic re-evaluation. Children with subclinical hypothyroidism (normal T_4 or free T_4, elevated TSH) should be treated until growth and puberty are complete and then reevaluate their thyroid function. Prominent nodules that persist despite suppressive therapy should be examined histologically, since thyroid lymphoma or carcinoma has occurred in patients with lymphocytic thyroiditis.

Goiter

A goiter is an enlargement of the thyroid gland. Persons with enlarged thyroids may have normal function of the gland (euthyroidism), thyroid deficiency (hypothyroidism), or overproduction of the hormones (hyperthyroidism). Goiter may be congenital or acquired, endemic, or sporadic. The goiter may result from: 1. Increased pituitary secretion of thyroid-stimulating hormone (TSH) in response to decreased circulating levels of thyroid hormones; 2. Infiltrative processes that may be inflammatory or neoplastic; and 3. Thyrotropin receptor-stimulating antibodies (TRSAbs) in patients with Graves' disease and thyrotoxicosis. Estimation of thyroid size by palpatory method, described by WHO is mentioned in Box 23.4.

1. **Congenital goiter:** Congenital goiter is usually sporadic and may result from a variety of causes as follows: 1. Fetal thyroxine (T_4) synthetic defect; 2. Administration of antithyroid drugs or iodides during pregnancy for the treatment of thyrotoxicosis; 3. Iodides for the treatment of asthma; 4.

Box 23.4: Estimation of thyroid size by palpation

Stage 0 No goiter.
Stage 1 A Goiter detectable only by palpation and not visible even when the neck is fully extended.
Stage 1 B Goiter palpable but visible only when the neck is fully extended (this stage also includes nodular glands even if not goitrous).
Stage 2 Goiter visible when the neck is in normal position; palpation not needed for diagnosis.
Stage 3 Very large goiters, which can be recognized at a considerable distance.

Administration amiodarone containing 37% iodine content; 5. Iodine deficiency; 6. Propylthiouracil drug therapy to the pregnant woman with Graves disease; 7. Teratoma within or in the vicinity of the thyroid, when the goiter is lobulated, asymmetric, firm or large. *Goiter is almost always present in the congenitally hyperthyroid infant.* Enlargement of the thyroid at birth may cause respiratory distress that interferes with nursing and may cause death.

2. **Endemic goiter and cretinism:** See Section 37.5.
3. **Acquired goiter:** Lymphocytic thyroiditis is the most common cause. Other causes include excess iodide ingestion and certain drugs, including amiodarone and lithium. Patients are usually euthyroid but may be hypothyroid.

Toxic goiter (Hyperthyroidism)

4. **Intratracheal goiter:** Goitrous enlargement of scotopic thyroid located within the trachea causes obstruction. If obstructive symptoms are mild, treatment with sodium L-thyroxine usually causes the goiter to decrease in size. When symptoms are severe, surgical removal of the endotracheal goiter is indicated.

Hyperthyroidism

Hyperthyroidism results from excessive secretion of thyroid hormone. The causes of hyperthyroidism include Graves' disease (an autoimmune disorder), McCune-Albright syndrome, toxic uninodular goiter (Plummer disease), hyperfunctioning thyroid carcinoma, thyrotoxicosis factitia, subacute thyroiditis, and acute suppurative thyroiditis. Suppression of plasma TSH indicates that the hyperthyroidism is not pituitary in origin. Hyperthyroidism due to excess thyrotropin secretion is rare and, in most cases, is caused by pituitary resistance to thyroid hormone. In infants born to mothers with Graves' disease, hyperthyroidism is almost always a transitory phenomenon; classic Graves' disease during the neonatal period is rare. The symptoms and signs of hyperthyroidism are listed in Table 23.7.

Graves' Disease

Graves' disease (an autoimmune disorder) occurs in approximately 0.02% of children. It has a peak incidence in the 11–15 yr old and 5:1 is female to male ratio. Symptoms develop gradually; the usual interval between onset and diagnosis is 6–12 months and may be longer in prepubertal children compared with adolescents. The earliest signs in children may be emotional disturbances accompanied by motor hyperactivity. On physical examination, signs of hyperthyroidism include diffused goiter, exophthalmos, tremor, hyperreflexia, and tachycardia (*see* Fig. 23.3 in CD). As there

is no standardization of goiter size in children, it has to be estimated by palpation (*see* Table 23.4 for estimation of thyroid size by palpation). The major symptoms and signs have been enumerated in Table 23.7.

Thyroid "crisis" or "storm" is a form of hyperthyroidism manifested by an acute onset, hyperthermia, severe tachycardia, heart failure and restlessness. There may be rapid progression to delirium, coma, and death. Precipitating events include trauma, parturition, infection or surgery. "Apathetic" or "masked," is another variety of hyperthyroidism which is characterized by extreme restlessness, apathy, and cachexia. A combination of both forms may also occur. These symptom complexes are rare in children.

Laboratory findings: Serum levels of thyroxine (T_4), triiodothyronine (T_3), free T_4 and free T_3 are elevated. In some patients T_3 may be elevated more than those of T_4. Levels of thyroid stimulating hormone (TSH) are less than the normal levels. Antithyroid antibodies, including thyroid peroxidase antibodies, are often present. The presence of thyrotropin receptor-stimulating antibody (TRSAb) establishes the cause as Graves' disease and its disappearance predicts remission of the disease. A radio-isotope uptake scan of the thyroid gland will show diffusely increased uptake in Graves' disease but decreased uptake in Hashimoto disease. Scan helps to detect multinodular goiter and toxic adenoma. Ultrasound scanning is useful to determine the size of the goiter, and the echogenicity of the thyroid tissue may suggest either Graves' or Hashimoto disease. Ultrasonography can also be used to investigate a nodule or nodular goiter and is useful in conditions like McCune-Albright syndrome. Very young children or those congenitally affected with Graves' disease often have advanced skeletal maturation and craniostenosis. Bone density may be reduced at diagnosis but returns to normal with treatment. Fine needle aspiration (FNA) of thyroid cytology is particularly useful whenever there is multinodularity and possibility of thyroid neoplasia.

Differential diagnosis: Once hyperthyroidism is suspected, elevated levels of thyroxine (T_4), triiodothyronine (T_3), free T_4 and free T_3 in association with suppressed levels of TSH are usually diagnostic. The presence of TRSAb establishes the cause as Graves' disease. If a thyroid nodule is palpable, or if T_3 is preferentially elevated, a functional thyroid nodule must be considered. Radionuclide study is diagnostic, with uptake in the nodule and absent uptake in the rest of the gland ("hot nodule"). If precocious puberty, polyostotic fibrous dysplasia, or café au lait pigmentation is present, the autonomous thyroid

Table 23.7: Major symptoms and signs of hyperthyroidism, Graves' disease and conditions associated with Graves' disease

Manifestations of hyperthyroidism

Symptoms
Hyperactivity, irritability, altered mood, insomnia, anxiety
Heat intolerance, increased sweating
Palpitations
Fatigue, weakness
Dyspnea
Weight loss with increased appetite (weight gain in 10% of patients)
Pruritus
Increased stool frequency
Thirst and polyuria
Oligomenorrhea or amenorrhea, loss of libido

Signs
Sinus tachycardia, supraventricular tachycardia, atrial fibrillation (rare in children)
Fine tremor, hyperkinesis, hyperreflexia
Warm, moist skin
Palmar erythema, onycholysis
Hair loss
Osteoporosis
Hypercalcemia
Muscle weakness and wasting
High-output heart failure
Chorea
Periodic (hypokalemic) paralysis
Psychosis (rare)

Manifestations of Graves' disease
Diffuse goiter
Ophthalmopathy: Feeling of grittiness and discomfort in the eye; retrobulbar pressure and pain; eyelid lag and retraction; periorbital edema, chemosis, scleral injection; exophthalmos (proptosis); extraocular muscle dysfunction; exposure keratitis; optic neuropathy
Localized dermopathy
Lymphoid hyperplasia
Thyroid acropachy

Conditions associated with Graves' disease
Type 1 diabetes mellitus; Addison disease; vitiligo; pernicious anemia; alopecia areata; myasthenia gravis; celiac disease

Adapted from Weetman AP. Graves' disease. *N Engl J Med* 2000; 343: 1236–1248.

disorder of McCune-Albright syndrome is likely. When hyperthyroxinemia is caused by exogenous thyroid hormone, levels of free T_4 and TSH are the same as those seen in Graves' disease, but the level of thyroglobulin is very low, whereas in patients with Graves' disease, it is elevated.

Treatment: The initial recommended treatment is medical therapy using antithyroid drugs rather than radioiodine or subtotal thyroidectomy.

Drug therapy: There are three antithyroid drugs: propylthiouracil, methimazole, carbimazole. Propylthiouracil (PTU) and methimazole are in widest use, carbimazole is commonly used in India. Carbimazole acts largely by getting converted to methimazole in the body. These drugs inhibit incorporation of trapped inorganic iodide into organic compounds, and they may also suppress TRSAb levels by directly affecting intrathyroidal autoimmunity. Methimazole is at least 10 times more potent than PTU on a weight basis and has a longer serum half-life (6–8 hr vs 0.5 hr); PTU is administered 3 times daily, but methimazole can be given once daily. PTU is protein-bound and has a lesser ability to cross the placenta and to pass into breast-milk; theoretically, PTU is the preferred drug during pregnancy and for nursing mothers. PTU, more than methimazole inhibits extrathyroidal conversion of T_4 to T_3; this may be advantageous in the treatment of neonatal thyrotoxicosis.

Adverse reactions occur with these drugs; minor adverse effects in approximately 10–20% while more severe side effects occur in 2–5% of children. Reactions are unpredictable and can occur after therapy of any duration. These reactions are reported to be fewer in patents treated with methimazole. Transient granulocytopenia ($< 2,000/mm^3$) is common, asymptomatic and it usually is not a reason to discontinue treatment. Transient urticarial rashes are common, and can be managed by a short period of therapy, restarting with the alternate antithyroid drug. The most severe reactions are hypersensitive and include agranulocytosis (0.1–0.5%), hepatitis (0.2–1%), hepatic failure, a lupus-like polyarthritis-like syndrome, glomerulonephritis, and an ANCA antibodies to nuclear cytoplasmic antigens-positive vasculitis involving the skin and other organs.

The initial dose of propylthiouracil (PTU) is 5–10 mg/kg/24 hr PO, given three times a day, and that of methimazole (5 mg tablet) 0.25 –1.0 mg/kg/24 hr PO given once or twice daily (preferred). Smaller initial doses should be used in early childhood. Rising serum levels of TSH to greater than normal indicates overtreatment and leads to increased size of the goiter. Clinical response becomes apparent in 3–6 wk, and adequate control is evident in 3–4 mo. The dose is decreased to the minimal level required to maintain a euthyroid state. The duration of therapy is for 5 yr or longer, because there appears to be a remission rate of about 25% every 2 yr. If a relapse occurs, it usually appears within 3 mo and almost always within 6 mo after therapy has been discontinued. Therapy may be resumed in case of relapse.

Propranolol, a β-adrenergic blocking agent (0.5–2.0 mg/kg/24 hr PO, given three times a day) is a useful supplement in the management of severely toxic patients.

Ophthalmopathy remits gradually and usually independently of the hyperthyroidism. Severe ophthalmopathy may require treatment with high-dose prednisolone, orbital radiotherapy (of questionable value), or orbital decompression surgery. Cigarette smoking is a risk factor of thyroid eye disease and should be avoided or discontinued to avoid progression of eye involvement.

Surgery is indicated when adequate cooperation for medical management is not possible, when adequate trial of medical treatment has failed to provide permanent remission, or when severe side effects preclude further use of antithyroid drugs.

Radioiodine is an effective, relatively safe first or alternative therapy for Graves' disease in children over 10 yr of age. Pretreatment with antithyroid drugs is unnecessary; if the patient is taking these drugs, they should be stopped a week before radioiodine administration. A dose of radioiodine of 300 µCi/g of thyroid tissue, or a total dose of approximately of 15 mCi, will achieve the goal. Essentially all patients treated with this dose will become hypothyroid; the time course to hypothyroidism averages 11 wk, with a range of 9 wk to 28 wk. because the full effects of treatment may take 1–6 mo, adjunctive therapy with propranolol and lower doses of antithyroid drugs are recommended.

Congenital Hyperthyroidism

Neonatal Graves' disease is caused by transplacental passage of TRSAb, but the clinical onset, severity, and course may be modified by the concurrent presence of TRBAb and by the transplacental passage of antithyroid drugs taken by the mother. The mothers of these infants have active Graves' disease, Graves' disease in remission, or rarely hypothyroidism and a history of lymphocytic thyroiditis. Neonatal hyperthyroidism occurs in only about 2% of infants to mothers with a history Graves' disease. Prenatal diagnosis can be made regarding the occurrence of an affected infant if there is presence of very high levels of TRSAb in the mothers and fetal tachycardia and goiter.

Clinical manifestations: Neonatal hyperthyroidism affects boys as often as girls. The disorder usually remits spontaneously within 6–12 wk but may persist longer, depending on the levels of TRSAb. Many of the infants are premature and appear to have intrauterine growth restriction. Most have goiters. The infant is extremely restless, irritable, and hyperactive, and appears anxious and unusually alert. Microcephaly and ventricular enlargement may be present. The eyes are opened widely and appear exophthalmic. There may be extreme tachycardia and tachypnea, and the temperature is elevated. In severely affected infants there is progression of symptoms: weight loss despite vigorous appetite, hepatosplenomegaly increases, jaundice appears, and cardiac decompensation and hypertension. Advanced bone age, frontal bossing with triangular facies and cranial synostosis are common, especially in infants with persistent clinical manifestations of hyperthyroidism. The serum level of T_4 is markedly elevated, and TSH is suppressed.

Treatment of the neonate consists of oral administration of propranolol (1–2 mg/kg/24 hr orally in 3 divided doses) and PTU (5–10 mg/kg/24 hr orally given 8 hourly) or methimazole (0.25–1.0 mg/kg/24 hr orally given every 12 hr); Lugol solution (1 drop every 8 hr) may be added. When propranolol is used during pregnancy to treat thyrotoxicosis, it crosses the placenta and may cause respiratory depression in the newborn infant. If the thyrotoxic state is severe, parenteral fluid therapy and corticosteroids may be indicated. If heart failure occurs, digitalization is indicated. After a euthyroid state is reached, only antithyroid drug treatment is necessary. The dose should be gradually tapered to keep the infant euthyroid. Most cases remit by 3–4 mo of age. Occasionally, neonatal hyperthyroidism does not remit but persists into childhood. Hyperthyroidism recurs when antithyroid drugs are discontinued. Therefore, these children must be treated with radioiodine or surgery.

Prognosis: Advanced bone age, microcephaly and mental retardation occur when treatment is delayed. Intellectual development is normal in most treated infants with neonatal Graves' disease. Some may show injury from in utero hyperthyroidism, requiring lifelong thyroid hormone treatment.

Ahluwalia A I. Thyrotoxicosis in Children and Adolescents. In: Mathur GP, Mathur Sarla (eds). *Current Trends in Pediatrics.* Vol 2. Delhi: Academa Publishers, 2006; 253–259.

Brix TH, Kyvik KO, Christensen K, et al. Evidence for a major role of heredity in Graves' disease: a population-based study of two Danish twin cohorts. *J Clin Endocrinol Metab* 2001; 86:930–934. Cavalieri RD. Iodine metabolism and thyroid physiology: current concepts [Review]. *Thyroid* 1997; 7: 177–181.

Cavalieri RD. Iodine metabolism and thyroid physiology: current concepts [Review]. *Thyroid* 1997; 7: 177–181.

Desai MP, Karandikar S. Autoimmune thyroid disease in childhood: a study of children and their families. *Indian Pediatr* 1999; 36(7):659–668.

De Vijlder JJ. Primary congenital hypothyroidism: defects in iodine pathways. *Eur J Endocrinol* 2003; 149: 247–256.

Eugster EA, LeMay D, Xerin JM, et al. Definitive diagnosis in children with congenital hypothyroidism. *J Pediatr* 2004; 144:643–647.

Jaruratanasirikul S, Leethanaporn K, Khuntigij P, et al. The clinical course of Hashimoto's thyroiditis in children and adolescents: 6 years longitudinal follow-up. *J Pediatr Endocrinal Metab* 2001; 14: 177–184.

LaFranchi S. Disorders of thyroid gland. In: Kliegman RM, Behrman RE, Jenson HB, Stanton BF (eds). *Nelson Textbook of Pediatrics.* 18th edn. Vol 2. Philadelphia: Saunders, 2007; 2316–2340.

Lavard L, Ranlov R, Perrild H, et al. Incidence of juvenile thyrotoxicosis in Denmark, 1982–1988, A nationwide study. *Eur J Endocrinol* 1994; 130:565–568.

Madison LD, LaFranchi S. Screening for congenital hypothyroidism: current controversies. *Curr Opin Endocrinol Metabol* 2005; 12: 32.

Marwaha RK, Sen S, Tandon H, et al. Familial aggregation of autoimmune thyroiditis in the first-degree relatives of patients with juvenile autoimmune thyroid disease. *Thyroid* 2003; 13: 297–300.

Menon PS, Singh GR. Hyperthyroidism in children: an Indian experience. *J Pediatr Endocrinol Metab* 1996;9(4):441–446.

Roberts CG, Landenson PW. Hypothyroidism. *Lancet* 2004; 363: 793–803.

Rovet J. Congenital hypothyroidism. Treatment and outcome. *Curr Opin Endocrinol Diabetes* 2005; 12: 42.

Teng W, Shan Z, Teng X, et al. Effect of iodine intake in thyroid diseases in China. *N Engl J Med* 2006; 354:2783–2792.

Tietgens ST, Leinung MC. Thyroid storm. *Med Clin North Am* 1995; 79:169–185.

Tripathi KD. Essentials of Medical Pharmacology. 6 th edn. New Delhi: Jaypee Brothers Medical Publishers (P) Ltd, 2008; 1–940.

Vade A, Gottschalk ME, Yetter EM, et al. Sonographic measurements of the neonatal thyroid gland. *J Ultrasound Med* 1997; 16: 395–399.

Vicens-Calver E, Potau N, Carreras E, et al. Diagnosis and treatment in utero of goiter with hypothyroidism caused by iodine overload. *J Pediatr* 1998; 133: 147–148.

WHO, UNICEF, and ICCIDD. Assessment of the iodine deficiency disorders and monitoring their elimination. Geneva, WHO publ.WHO/NHD/01.1, 2001; 1–107.

23.4 PARATHYROID DISORDERS

Parathyroid hormone (PTH) and vitamin D are the principal regulators of calcium homeostasis. Calcitonin (CT) and PTH-related peptide (PTHrP) are important primarily in the fetus.

Hypoparathyroidism

Hypocalcemia is common between 12 and 72 hr of life, especially in premature infants, in infants with asphyxia, and in infants of diabetic mothers (early neonatal hypocalcemia). After the 2nd to 3rd day and during the 1st wk of life, the type of feeding also is a determinant of the level of serum calcium (late neonatal hypocalcemia). It is possible that the functional immaturity is a manifestation of a delay in development of the enzymes that convert glandular PTH to secreted PTH; other mechanisms are possible.

The etiologic classification of hypocalcemia include parathyroid deficiency (hypoparathyroidism); pseudoparahypothyroidism; mitochondrial DNA mutations (Kearns-Sayre syndrome, Pearson marrow pancreas syndrome, mutation of long-chain 3-hydroxyacylcoenzyme a dehydrogenase); magnesium deficiency (renal magnesium loss, magnesium malabsorption, aminoglycoside therapy); exogenous inorganic phosphate excess (laxatives, soft drinks with phosphoric acid); and vitamin D deficiency [nutritional, vitamin D deficiency [rickets], mutation of 1α-(OH)ase (P450)].

Parathyroid deficiency occurs due to (i) aplasia or hypoplasia of the parathyroid glands; (ii) surgical hypoparathyroidism: removal or damage of the parathyroid glands; (iii) X-linked excessive hypoparathyroidism; (iv) autosomal dominant hypoparathyroidism; (v) autosomal recessive hypoparathyroidism with dysmorphic features include microcephaly, deepset eyes, beaked nose, micrognathia, and large floppy ears; (vi) HDR syndrome (hypoparathyroidism, sensorineural deafness, and renal anomaly); (vii) suppression of neonatal PTH secretion due to maternal hyperparathyroidism; (viii) hypoparathyroidism associated with mitochondrial disorders in Kearns-Sayre syndrome and in mitochondrial trifunctional protein; (ix) deposition of iron pigment in thalassemia or of copper in Wilson disease in the parathyroid glands; (x) autoimmune hypoparathyroidism (parathyroid antibodies and by its frequent association with Addison disease and chronic mucocutaneous candidiasis); (xi) idiopathic hypoparathyroidism.

Clinical manifestations: Mild deficiency may be revealed only by appropriate laboratory studies. Muscular pain and cramps are early manifestations; they progress to numbness, stiffness, and tingling of the hands and feet. There may be only a positive Chvostek or Trousseau sign or laryngeal or carpopedal spasms. Convulsions with or without loss of consciousness may occur at intervals of days, weeks, or months. These episodes may begin with abdominal pain, followed by tonic rigidity, retraction of the head, and cyanosis.

In patients with long-standing hypocalcemia (i) teeth erupt late and irregularly with irregular enamel formation and the teeth may be unusually soft; (ii) skin may be dry and scaly, and the nails of the fingers and toes may have horizontal lines; (iii) mucocutaneous candidiasis, candidal infection most often involves the nails, the oral mucosa, the angles of the mouth, and less often the skin; (iv) cataracts in patients with long standing untreated disease; (v) permanent physical and mental deterioration occur if initiation of treatment is long delayed.

Laboratory findings: The serum calcium level is low (5–7 mg/dL), and the phosphorus level is elevated (7–12 mg/dL). Blood levels of ionized calcium (usually approximately 45% of the total) more nearly reflect physiologic adequacy but also are low. The serum level of alkaline phosphatase is normal or low, and the level of $1,25[OH]_2D_3$ is usually low. The level of serum magnesium is normal but should always be checked in hypocalcemic patients. Levels of PTH are low when measured by immunometric assay. Radiographs of the bones occasionally reveal an increased density limited to the metaphyses, suggestive of heavy metal poisoning. Radiographs or CT scan of the skull may reveal calcifications in the basal ganglia. There is a prolongation of the QT interval on the electrocardiogram, which disappears when the hypocalcemia is corrected. The electroencephalogram usually reveals widespread slow activity; the tracing returns to normal after serum calcium concentration has been within the normal range for a few weeks, unless irreversible brain

damage has occurred or unless the parathyroid insufficiency is associated with epilepsy. When hypoparathyroidism occurs concurrently with Addison disease, the serum level of calcium may be normal, but hypocalcemia appears after effective treatment of adrenal insufficiency.

Differential diagnosis: Hypocalcemic tetany has to be differentiated from seizures. Magnesium deficiency must be considered in patients with unexplained hypocalcemia. Hypomagnesemia impairs release of PTH and induces resistance to the effects of the hormone. Concentration of serum magnesium less than 1.5 mg/dL (1.2 mEq/L) is usually abnormal. Hypomagnesemia occurs in malabsorption syndromes such as Crohn disease and cystic fibrosis, autoimmune polyglandular disease type I and hypoparathyroidism and therapy with aminoglycosides, which causes hypomagnesemia by increasing urinary losses.

Treatment: Emergency treatment of neonatal tetany consists of intravenous injections of 5–10 ml of a 10% solution of calcium gluconate at a rate of 0.5–1 ml/minute while the heart rate is monitored. Additionally 1,25-dihydroxycholecalciferol (calcitriol) should be given in 2 equal divided doses. The initial dose is 0.25 µg/24 hr; the maintenance dosage ranges from 0.01 to 0.10 µg/24 hr to a maximum of 1–2 µg/24 hr. An adequate intake of calcium should be ensured. Supplemental calcium can be given in the form of calcium gluconate or calcium glubionate to provide 800 mg of elemental calcium daily, which may be rarely required. Foods with high phosphorus content such as milk, eggs, and cheese should be reduced in the diet.

Pseudohypoparathyroidism (Albright Hereditary Osteodystrophy)

In pseudohypoparathyroidism (PHP) the parathyroid glands are normal or hyperplastic and they can synthesize and secrete parathyroid hormone (PTH). Serum levels of immunoreactive PTH are elevated even when the patient is hypocalcemic and may be elevated when the patient is normocalcemic. Neither endogenous nor administered PTH raises the serum levels of calcium or lowers the levels of phosphorus.

Tetany is often the presenting sign. Affected children have a short stocky build and a round face. Brachydactyly with dimpling of the dorsum of the hand is usually present. The 2nd metacarpal is involved least often. As a result the index finger may occasionally longer than the middle finger. Likewise, the 2nd metatarsal is only rarely affected. There may be other skeletal abnormalities such as short and wide phalanges, bowing, exostoses, and thickening of the calvaria. These patients frequently have calcium deposits and metaplastic bone formation subcutaneously. Moderate degrees of mental retardation, calcification of the basal ganglia, and lenticular cataracts are common in patients who are diagnosed late.

Serum calcium level is low and serum phosphorus and alkaline phosphatase are elevated. Clinical diagnosis can be confirmed by demonstration of a markedly attenuated response in urinary phosphate and cyclic AMP after intravenous infusion of the synthetic 1–34 fragment of human PTH (teriparatide acetate). Definitive diagnosis is established by demonstration of the mutated G-protein.

Hyperparathyroidism

Excessive production of parathyroid hormone (PTH) may result from a primary defect of the parathyroid glands such as an adenoma or hyperplasia (primary hyperparathyroidism). More often, the increased production of PTH is compensatory, usually aimed at correcting the hypocalcemic states, such as vitamin D-deficient rickets and the malabsorption syndromes, pseudohypoparathyroidism, and in advanced stages of renal failure, including after renal transplantation (secondary hyperparathyroidism). The etiologic classification of hypercalcemia include parathyroid hormone (PTH) excess; vitamin D excess [iatrogenic, ectopic production (sarcoidosis, tuberculosis, granulomatous lesions, subcutaneous fat necrosis)]; unknown cause [Williams syndrome (7q11.23 deletion)]; and other causes [hypophosphatasea (mutation of tissue-nonspecific alkaline phosphatase gene), prolonged immobilization, thyrotoxicosis, hypervitaminosis, leukemia, acquired hypocalciuric hypercalcemia autoantibodies to calcium-sensing receptor].

Childhood hyperparathyroidism is rare. Onset during childhood is usually the result of a single benign adenoma. It usually becomes manifested after 10 yr of age. There have been a number of kind reds in which multiple members have hyperparathyroidism transmitted in an autosomal dominant fashion. Most of the family members are adults, but children have been involved in approximately in 1/3 of the pedigrees. Some of the affected patients in these families are asymptomatic, while in other kindreds hyperparathyroidism occurs as part of the constellation known as the multiple endocrine neoplasia (MEN) syndromes or of the hyperparathyroidism/jaw tumor syndrome.

Neonatal severe hyperparathyroidism is a rare disorder. Symptoms develop shortly after birth and consist of anorexia, irritability, lethargy, constipation, and failure to thrive. Radiographs reveal subperiosteal bone resorption, osteoporosis, and pathologic fractures. Symptoms may be mild, resolving without treatment, or may have a rapidly fatal course if diagnosis and treatment are delayed.

Transient neonatal hyperparathyroidism has occurred in a few infants born to mothers with hyperparathyroidism (idiopathic or surgical) or with pseudohypoparathyroidism. The maternal disorder had been undiagnosed or inadequately treated during pregnancy. The cause of the condition is chronic intrauterine exposure to hypocalcemia with resultant hyperplasia of the fetal parathyroid glands. in the newborn, bones are primarily involved and healing occurs between 4 and 7 mo of age.

Clinical manifestations: The clinical manifestations of hypercalcemia of any cause include muscular weakness, fatigue, headache, anorexia, abdominal pain, nausea, vomiting, constipation, polydipsia, polyuria, loss of weight, and fever. When hypercalcemia is of long duration, calcium may be deposited in the renal parenchyma (nephrocalcinosis) with progressively diminished renal function. Renal calculi may occur and may produce renal colic and hematuria. Osseous changes may produce pain in the back or extremities, disturbances of gait, genu valgum, fractures, and tumors. Height may be decreased from compression of vertebrae; the patient may become bedridden. Abdominal pain is occasionally severe and may be associated with acute pancreatitis. Parathyroid crisis may occur, when serum calcium level is greater than 15 mg/dL, and is manifested by progressive oliguria, azotemia, stupor, and coma. In infants, failure to thrive, poor feeding and hypotonia are common. Mental retardation, convulsions, and blindness may occur as sequelae of long-standing hypercalcemia.

Laboratory findings: Serum calcium level is elevated; when the total serum calcium level is borderline or only slightly elevated, and ionized calcium levels are often increased. The serum phosphorus level is reduced to about 3 mg/dl or less, and serum magnesium level is low. Serum phosphatase levels are elevated in patients with adenoma who have skeletal involvement, but in infants with hyperplasia the levels of alkaline phosphatase may be normal even when there is extensive involvement of bone. Serum levels of PTH measured by carboxyterminal antisera are elevated, especially in relation to the level of calcium. Calcitonin levels are normal. Acute hypercalcemia can stimulate calcitonin release; but with prolonged hypercalcemia, hypercalcitoninemia does not occur. The urine may have a low and fixed specific gravity, and serum levels of non-protein nitrogen and uric acid may be elevated.

The most consistent and characteristic radiographic finding is resorption of subperiosteal bone, best seen along the margins of the phalanges of the hands. In the skull there may be gross trabeculation or granular appearance resulting from focal rarefaction; the lamina dura may be absent. In more advanced disease, there may be generalized rarefaction, cysts, tumors, fractures, and deformities. About 10% patients have radiographic signs of rickets. Radiographs of the abdomen may reveal renal calculi or nephrocalcinosis.

Differential diagnosis: Other causes of hypercalcemia may result in a similar clinical pattern and must be differentiated from hyperparathyroidism. A low serum phosphorus level with hypercalcemia is characteristic of primary hyperparathyroidism; elevated levels of PTH are also diagnostic. With hypercalcemia of any cause except hyperparathyroidism and familial hypocalciuric hypercalcemia, PTH levels are suppressed. Pharmacologic doses of corticosteroids lower the serum calcium level to normal in patients with hypercalcemia from other causes but generally do not affect the calcium level in patients with hyperparathyroidism.

Treatment: Surgical exploration is indicated in all patients of hyperparathyroidism. If an adenoma is discovered, it should be removed; very few instances of carcinoma are reported in children. Most neonates with severe hypercalcemia require total parathyroidectomy; less severe hypercalcemia may remit spontaneously in others. A portion of a parathyroid gland may be autografted into the forearm. The patient should be carefully observed postoperatively for the development of hypocalcemia and tetany; intravenous administration of calcium gluconate may be required for a few days. The serum calcium level then gradually returns to normal, and under ordinary circumstances, a diet high in calcium and phosphorus must be maintained for only several months after operation.

Prognosis: The prognosis is good if the disease is recognized early and there is appropriate surgical treatment. When extensive osseous lesions are present, deformities may be present. Nephrocalcinosis may develop if hypercalcemia persists.

Other Causes of Hypercalcemia

Familial hypocalciuric hypercalcemia; Hypophosphatasia; Idiopathic hypercalcemia of infancy; Hypervitaminosis D resulting in hypercalcemia from drinking milk that has been incorrectly fortified with vitamin D; Prolonged immobilization; Granulomatous diseases (tuberculosis, sarcoidosis); Hypercalcemia of malignancy (malignant rhabdoid tumors of kidney, neuroblastoma, medulloblastoma, leukemia, Burkitt

lymphoma, dysgerminoma and rhabdomyosarcoma). Patients with Williams syndrome (in 10% cases), also inconsistently exhibit associated infantile hypercalcemia and is characterized by feeding difficulties, slow growth, elfin facies (small mandible, prominent maxilla, upturned nose), renovascular disorders, and a gregarious "cocktail party" personality. Cardiac lesions include supravalvular aortic stenosis, peripheral pulmonary stenosis, aortic hypoplasia, coronary artery stenosis, and atrial or ventricular septal defects.

Cook JS, Stone MS, Hansen JR. Hypercalcemia in association with subcutaneous fat necrosis of the newborn: Studies of calcium-regulating hormones. *Pediatrics* 1992; 90: 93–96.

Doyle DA, DiGeorge AM. Disorders of the parathyroid. In: Kliegman RM, Behrman RE, Jenson HB, Stanton BF (eds). *Nelson Textbook of Pediatrics*. 18th edn. Vol 2. Philadelphia: Saunders, 2007; 2340–2348.

Irvin GL, Carneiro DM. Management changes in primary hyperparathyroidism. *JAMA* 2000; 284: 934–936.

McKay C, Furman WL. Hypercalcemia complicating childhood malignancies. *Cancer* 1993; 72: 256–260.

Toft AD. Surgery for primary hyperparathyroidism–sooner rather than later *Lancet* 2000; 355: 1478–1479.

23.5 DISORDERS OF THE ADRENAL GLAND

Physiology of the Adrenal Gland

The adrenal gland consists of 2 endocrine tissues: The cortex and the medulla. The adrenal cortex consists of 3 zones: zona glomerulosa, the outermost zone located immediately beneath the capsule, zona fasciculata, the middle zone; and zona reticularis, the innermost zone, lying next to the adrenal medulla. Zona glomerulosa synthesizes aldosterone, zona fasciculata produces cortisol, and both zona fasciculata and zona reticularis synthesize adrenal androgens. The *adrenal medulla* consists mainly of neuroendocrine (chromaffin) cells and glial (sustentacular) cells with some connective tissue and vascular cells. The principal hormones of the adrenal medulla are the physiologically active catecholamines: dopamine, norepinephrine and epinephrine.

Cushing Syndrome

Cushing syndrome is the result of abnormally high blood levels of cortisol or other glucocorticoids. This can be iatrogenic or the result of endogenous cortisol secretion, due either to an adrenal tumor or to hypersecretion of corticotropin (adrenocorticotropic hormone [ACTH]) by the pituitary (Cushing disease) or by a tumor (Table 23.8). The most common cause of Cushing syndrome is prolonged *exogenous administration of glucocorticoid hormones*, especially at the high doses used to treat lymphoproliferative

Table 23.8: Etiologic classification of adrenocortical hyperfunction

Excess Cortisol (Cushing syndrome)	• Bilateral adrenal hyperplasia
	  Hypersecretion of corticotrophin (Cushing disease)
	  Ectopic secretion of corticotropin
	  Exogenous corticotropin
	• Adrenocortical nodular dysplasia
	• Potential nodular adrenocortical disease (Carney complex)
	• Tumor

Excess Androgens	• Congenital adrenal hyperplasia
	  21-Hydroxylase deficiency
	  11β-Hydroxylase deficiency
	  3β-Hydroxysteroid dehydrogenase defect (deficiency or dysregulation)
	• Tumor

Excess Mineralocorticoid	• Primary hyperaldosteronism
	  Aldosterone-secreting adenoma
	  Bilateral micronodular adrenocortical hyperplasia
	  Glucocorticoid-suppressible aldosteronism
	  Tumor
	• Deoxycorticosterone excess
	  Congenital adrenal hyperplasia
	    11β-Hydroxylase
	    17α-Hydroxylase
	Tumor
	• Apparent mineralocorticoid excess (deficiency of 3β-hydroxysteroid dehydrogenase type 2)

Excess Estrogen	• Tumor

disorders. *Endogenous Cushing syndrome* is most often caused in infants by a functioning adrenocortical tumor (benign adenoma or malignant carcinoma).

Clinical manifestations: The disorder is more severe and very obvious in infants than older children. The face is rounded, with prominent cheeks and a flushed appearance (moon facies). Generalized obesity is common in younger children. Signs of abnormal masculization occur frequently in children with adrenal tumors; there may be hirsutism on the face and trunk, pubic hair, acne, deepening of the voice, and enlargement of clitoris in girls. Growth is impaired with length falling below 3rd percentile; however, significant virilization produces normal or even accelerated growth. Hypertension is a common finding and may occasionally lead to heart failure. There is increased susceptibility of infection, which may also lead to sepsis.

In older children, in addition to obesity, short stature is a characteristic feature. The more severe obesity is present on the face and trunk compared with the extremities. Purplish striae on the hips, abdomen, and thighs are common. Pubertal development may be delayed, or amenorrhea may occur in girls past menarche. Weakness, headache, and emotional lability may be seen. Hypertension and hyperglycemia usually occur. Hyperglycemia may progress to frank diabetes mellitus. Osteoporosis is common and may cause pathologic fractures.

Differential diagnosis: Cushing syndrome is frequently suspected in children with obesity, particularly when striae and hypertension are present. Children with simple obesity are usually tall, whereas those with Cushing syndrome are short or have a decelerating growth rate. Although urinary excretion of cortisol is often elevated in simple obesity, salivary night-time levels of cortisol are normal and cortisol secretion is suppressed by oral administration of low doses of dexamethasone.

Elevated levels of cortisol and ACTH without clinical evidence of Cushing syndrome occur in patients with generalized glucocorticoid resistance. Affected patients may be asymptomatic or there is hypertension, hyperkalemia, and precocious pseudopuberty; these manifestations are caused by increased mineralocorticoid and adrenal androgen secretion in response to elevated ACTH levels.

Laboratory findings: Cortisol levels in blood are usually elevated at 8 am and decrease to less than 50% by midnight except in infants and young children in whom the diurnal rhythm is not always established. In patients with Cushing syndrome this circadian rhythm is lost; midnight cortisol levels > 4.4 µg/dl strongly suggest the diagnosis. Elevated night-time salivary cortisol levels raise suspicion for Cushing syndrome. Urinary excretion of free cortisol is increased. This is best obtained in a 24 hr urine sample and is expressed as a ratio of micrograms of cortisol excreted per gram of creatinine.

A single-dose dexamethasone suppression test is often helpful; a dose of 25–30 µg/kg (maximum of 2 mg) given at 11 pm results in a plasma cortisol level of less than 5 µg/dl at 8 am the next morning in normal individuals but not in patients with Cushing syndrome.

A glucose tolerance test is often abnormal. Levels of serum electrolytes are usually normal but potassium may be decreased, especially in patients with tumors that excrete ACTH ectopically.

After the diagnosis of Cushing syndrome has been established, then it is necessary to determine whether it is caused by a pituitary adenoma, an ectopic ACTH-secreting tumor, or a cortisol-secreting adrenal tumor. ACTH concentrations are usually suppressed in patients with cortisol-secreting tumors, are very high in patients with ectopic ACTH-secreting pituitary adenomas. After an intravenous bolus of corticotrophin-releasing hormone (CRH), patients with ACTH-dependent Cushing syndrome have an exaggerated ACTH and cortisol response, whereas those with adrenal tumors show no response in ACTH and cotisol. 2-step dexamethasone suppression test consists of administration of dexamethasone 30 and 120 µg/kg/24 hr in 4 divided doses on consecutive days. In children with pituitary Cushing syndrome, the larger dose, but not smaller dose, suppresses serum levels of cortisol. Patients with ACTH-independent Cushing syndrome do not show suppressed cortisol levels with dexamethasone.

CT detects all adrenal tumors larger than 1.5 cm in diameter. MRI may detect ACTH-secreting pituitary adenomas, but many are too small to be seen; the addition of gadolinium contrast increases the sensitivity of detection. Bilateral inferior petrosal blood sampling to measure concentration of ACTH before and after CRH administration may be required to localize the tumor, when a pituitary adenoma is visualized.

Treatment: Transsphenoidal pituitary microsurgery is the treatment of choice in pituitary Cushing disease in children. Relapses are treated with re-operation or pituitary irradiation.

Inhibitors of adrenal steroidogenesis (metyrapone, ketoconazole, aminoglutethimide, etomidate) have been used preoperatively to normalize circulating cortisol levels and reduce perioperative morbidity and mortality.

If a pituitary adenoma does not respond to treatment or if ACTH is secreted by an ectopic metastatic tumor, the adrenal glands may need to be removed. Adrenalectomy may lead to increased ACTH secretion by an unresected pituitary adenoma, evidenced mainly by marked hyperpigmentation. This condition is termed Nelson syndrome. Patients undergoing adrenalectomy requires adequate preoperative and postoperative replacement therapy with a corticosteroid.

Adrenal Insufficiency

In primary adrenal insufficiency, congenital or acquired lesions of the adrenal cortex prevent production of cortisol and often aldosterone. Acquired primary adrenal insufficiency is termed Addison disease. Dysfunction of the hypothalamus or anterior pituitary gland can cause a deficiency of corticotropin (ACTH) and lead to hypofunction of the adrenal cortex; this is termed secondary adrenal insufficiency. The causes of adrenal insufficiency are listed in Table 23.9.

Primary Adrenal Insufficiency

Clinical manifestations: Primary adrenal deficiency leads to cortisol and often aldosterone deficiency. Hyperglycemia is a prominent feature of adrenal insufficiency. It is often accompanied by ketosis as the body uses fatty acids as an alternative energy source. Ketosis is aggravated by anorexia, nausea, and vomiting. Orthostatic hypotension is present in children and can progress to shock. Hypovolemia, hyponatremia and hyperkalemia are other important findings. Pigmentation may be more prominent in skin creases, mucosa, and scars. In patients with a fair skin complexion, the skin has a bronze cast. In dark-skinned patients, it may be appreciated in the gingival and buccal mucosa.

Laboratory findings: Hypoglycemia, ketosis, hyponatremia, and hyperkalemia are present. An ECG is useful in quickly detecting hyperkalemia in a critically ill child. Acidosis, elevated blood urea nitrogen occurs in a dehydrated child. Cortisol levels are low. ACTH levels are high in primary adrenal insufficiency. The most definitive test for adrenal insufficiency is measurement of serum levels of cortisol before and after administration of ACTH; resting levels are low and do not increase normally after administration of ACTH. Traditionally this test has been performed by measuring cortisol levels before and 30 or 60 min after giving 0.25 mg of cosyntropin (ACTH 1–24) by rapid intravenous infusion. Aldosterone will transiently increase in response to this dose of ACTH and may also be measured.

Differential diagnosis: Addison disease needs to be distinguished from more acute illnesses such as gastroenteritis with dehydration or sepsis, congenital adrenal hyperplasia, autoimmune Addison disease. Additional testing is directed at identifying the specific

Table 23.9: Causes of adrenal insufficiency

A. Primary adrenal insufficiency

1. *Autoimmune adrenalitis:* Isolated autoimmune adrenalitis; Autoimmune adrenalitis as part of APS (APS type 1, APS type 2, APS type 4)
2. *Infections adrenalitis:* Tuberculous adenitis; AIDS; Fungal adenitis
3. *Genetic disorders leading to adrenal insufficiency:* Adrenoleukodystrophy; Adrenomyeloneuropathy; Congenital lipoid adrenal hypoplasia; CYP oxireductase deficiency; Smith-Lemli-Opitz syndrome; Pallister-Hall syndrome; IMAGe syndrome; Kearns-Sayre syndrome; ACTH insensitivity syndrome (familial glucocorticoid deficiency [Type 1, Type 2; Triple A syndrome (Allgrove's syndrome)]
4. *Congenital adrenal hypoplasia:* 21-hydoxylase deficiency; 11 β-hydroxylase deficiency; 3 β-hydroxysteroid dehydrodenase deficiency; 17 α- hydroxylase deficiency
5. *Adrenal hypoplasia congenital:* X-linked; Xp21 contiguous gene syndrome; SF-1 linked
6. *Other causes:* Bilateral adrenal hemorrhage; Adrenal infiltration; Bilateral adrenalectomy; Drug-induced adrenal insufficiency (treatment with ketokenazole, suramin, mitotane, aminoglutethimide, mifepristone, etomidate)

B. Secondary adrenal insufficiency

1. *Pituitary tumors*
2. *Other tumors of the hypothalamic-pituitary region:* Craniopharyngioma; Meningioma; Ependymoma; Germinoma; Intrasellar or surasellar metastases
3. *Pituitary irradiation*
4. *Lymphocytic hypophisitis: Isolated; As part of APS*
5. *Isolated congenital ACTH deficiency*
6. *Pro-opiomelanocortin deficiency syndrome*
7. *Combined pituitary hormone deficiency*
8. *Pituitary apoplexy (Sheehan's syndrome)*
9. *Pituitary infiltration or granuloma*
10. *Head trauma*
11. *Previous chronic glucocorticoid excess*

ACTH, adrenocorticotropin hormone; APS, autoimmune polyendocrinopathy; CVP, cytochrome P-450; FSH, follicle stimulating hormone; GH, growth hormone; LH, luteinizing hormone; P-450 scc, cytochrome P-450 side chain cleavage enzyme; PRL, prolactin; TSH, thyrotropin.
Source: Arit W, Allolio B. Adrenal insufficiency. *Lancet* 2003; 361: 1881–1892.

cause for adrenal insufficiency. Ultrasonography, CT, or MRI can help define the size of adrenal gland.

Treatment: The treatment of acute adrenal insufficiency must be immediate and vigorous. If the diagnosis of adrenal insufficiency has not been established, a blood sample should be obtained before therapy to determine electrolytes, glucose, ACTH, cortisol, aldosterone, and plasma renin activity. If the patient's condition permits, an ACTH stimulation test can be performed while initial fluid resuscitation is underway. An intravenous solution of 5% glucose in 0.9% saline should be administered to correct hypoglycemia, hypovolemia, and hyponatremia. Avoid giving hypotonic fluids. If hyperkalemia is severe, it can require treatment with intravenous calcium and/or bicarbonate, intrarectal potassium-binding resin (Kayexalate) or intravenous infusion of glucose and insulin. A water soluble hydrocortisone, such as hydrocortisone sodium succinate should be given intravenously (10 mg for infants; 25 mg for toddlers; 50 mg for older children; 100 mg for adolescents). Administer first as a bolus and a similar total amount given in divided doses at 6 hr intervals for the first 24 hr. These doses may be reduced during the next 24 hr if progress is satisfactory.

In a rare patient with concomitant adrenal insufficiency and hypothyroidism, adrenal crisis may be precipitated if hypothyroidism is treated without first ensuring adequate glucocorticoid replacement, because thyroxine can increase cortisol clearance.

After the acute manifestations are under control, most patients require chronic replacement therapy for their cortisol and aldosterone deficiencies. Hydrocortisone (cortisol) may be given orally in daily doses of 10 mg/m^2/24 hr in 3 divided doses; some patients require 15 mg/m^2/24 hr to minimize fatigue, especially in the morning. Equivalent doses (20–25% of the hydrocortisone dose) of prednisolone or prednisone may be used and divided and given twice daily. ACTH levels may be used to monitor adequacy of glucocorticoid replacement in primary adrenal insufficiency; in congenital adrenal hyperplasia, levels of precursor hormones are used instead of ACTH. Blood samples for monitoring should be obtained at a consistent time of day and in a consistent relation to (i.e. before or after) the hydrocortisone dose. Normalizing ACTH levels is not needed. Generally morning ACTH levels high in the normal range to 2–3 times normal are satisfactory.

During situations of stress, such as periods of infection or minor operative procedures, the dose of hydrocortisone should be increased 2- to 3-fold. Major surgery under general anesthesia requires high intravenous doses of hydrocortisone similar to those used for acute adrenal deficiency.

If aldosterone deficiency is present, fludrocortisones (Florinef), a synthetic mineralocorticoid, is given orally in doses of 0.05–0.2 mg daily. Measurements of plasma renin activity are useful in monitoring the adequacy of mineralocorticoid replacement.

Chronic overdosage with glucocorticoids leads to obesity, short stature, and osteoporosis, whereas overdosages with fludrocortisones results in tachycardia, hypertension, and occasionally hypokalemia.

Additional therapy might be needed for the underlying cause of the adrenal insufficiency in regard to infections and certain metabolic defects.

Secondary Adrenal Insufficiency

Clinical manifestations: Secondary adrenal insufficiency most commonly occurs when the hypothalamic-pituitary-adrenal axis is suppressed by prolonged administration of high doses of a potent glucocorticoid and that agent is suddenly withdrawn or the dose is tapered too quickly. Aldosterone secretion is unaffected in secondary adrenal insufficiency, because the adrenal gland is intact and the renin-angiotensin system is not involved. Thus, signs and symptoms are those of cortisol deficiency. Newborns often have hypoglycemia. Older children can have orthostatic hypotension or weakness; hyponatremia may be present.

When secondary adrenal insufficiency is due to an inborn or acquired anatomic defect involving the pituitary, there may be signs of associated deficiencies or other pituitary hormones. The penis may be small in male infants if gonadotropins are also deficient. Infants with secondary hypothyroidism are often jaundiced. Children with associated growth hormone deficiency grow poorly after the 1st yr of life.

Some children with pituitary abnormalities have hypoplasia of the midface. Children with optic nerve hypoplasia have visual impairment and characteristic wandering nystagmus.

Laboratory findings: The most commonly used test to diagnose secondary adrenal insufficiency is low-dose ACTH stimulation testing (1 µg/1.73 m^2 of cosyntropin given intravenously), the rationale being that there will be some degree of atrophy of the adrenal cortex if normal physiologic ACTH stimulation is lacking. Thus, this test may be falsely negative in cases of acute compromise of the pituitary (e.g. injury or surgery). Such circumstances rarely pose a diagnostic problem; in general, this test provides excellent sensitivity and specificity. A cortisol level of 18–20 µg/dl 30 minutes after cosyntropin administration may be used to dichotomize normal and abnormal responses.

Treatment: Iatrogenic secondary insufficiency (caused by chronic glucocorticoid administration) is best avoided by use of the smallest effective doses of systemic glucocorticoids for the shortest possible time. When a patient is thought to be at risk, taper the dose rapidly to a level equivalent to or slightly less than physiologic replacement (~10mg/m^2/24 hr of hydrocortisone) and further tapering over several wk can allow the adrenal cortex to recover without development of signs of adrenal insufficiency. Patients with anatomic lesions of the pituitary should be treated with glucocorticoids indefinitely; mineralocorticoid replacement is not required. In patients with panhypopituitarism, treating cortisol deficiency can increase free water excretion, unmasking central diabetes insipidus. Electrolytes must be monitored when initiating cortisol therapy in patients with panhypopituitarism.

Primary Aldosteronism

Primary aldosteronism includes disorders caused by excessive aldosterone secretion independent of the renin-angiotensin system. These disorders are characterized by hypertension, hypokalemia, and suppression of the renin-angiotensin system. These conditions are thought to be rare in childhood, but they may account for 5–10% cases of hypertension in adults. Chronic hypokalemia if present may lead to polyuria, nocturia, enuresis, polydipsia, and muscle weakness, tetany and growth failure. Primary aldosteronism should be distinguished from glucocorticoid suppressible hyperaldosteronism. Plasma levels of aldosterone may be normal or elevated. Aldosterone concentrations in 24-hr urine collections are always increased. Plasma levels of renin are persistently low. The ratio of plasma aldosterone concentration to renin activity is always high.

Treatment of an aldosterone-producing adenoma is surgical removal. Hyperaldosteronism due to bilateral adrenal hyperplasia is treated with the mineralo-corticoid antagonists, spironolactone, often normalizing blood pressure and serum potassium levels. In patients who do not improve with drugs, unilateral adrenalectomy may be considered.

Congenital Adrenal Hyperplasia and Related Disorders

Congenital adrenal hyperplasia (CAH) is a family of autosomal recessive disorders of cortisol biosynthesis. In this condition cortisol deficiency increases secretion of corticotropin (ACTH), this in turn leads to adrenal hyperplasia and overproduction of intermediate metabolites. Depending on the enzymatic step that is deficient, there may be signs, symptoms, and laboratory findings of mineralocorticoid deficiency or excess; incomplete virilization or premature puberty in affected males; and virilization or sexual infantilism in affected females. More than 90% of CAH cases are caused by 21-hydroxylase deficiency. Other disorders include 11-hydroxylase deficiency (5–8% cases); 3β-Hydroxysteroid dehydrogenase deficiency (<2% cases); 17α-hydroxylase deficiency (<1% cases); Lipoid congenital adrenal hyperplasia (rare disorder); Aldosterone synthase deficiency (rare disorder); Glucocorticoid-suppressible hyperaldosteronism (Autosomal dominant mode of inheritance) (rare disorder); P450 Oxidoreductase deficiency (Antley-Bixler syndrome) (rare disorder).

21-Hydroxylase Deficiency

Affected gene is CYP21; and chromosome 6p21.3.
Signs and symptoms: Salt-wasting crisis; Female pseudohermaphroditism; Postnatal virilization in males and females; Precocious pubarche; Disordered puberty; Menstrual irregularity, Hirsutism; Acne; Infertility. *Laboratory findings:* Markedly raised baseline and ACTH-stimulated 17-OH progesterone and pregnanetriol; markedly elevated serum androgens, urinary metabolites, ACTH. Suppression of elevated adrenal steroids after glucocorticoid administration. *Prenatal diagnosis: Prenatal diagnosis* of 21-hydroxylase deficiency is possible late in the first trimester by analysis of DNA obtained by chorionic villus sampling or during the second trimester by amniocentesis. This is usually done because parents already have an affected child. Most often, the *CYP21* gene is analyzed. *Newborn screening:* Analysis of 17-hydroxyprogesterone levels in dried blood obtained by heel-stick and absorbed on filter paper cards. The same cards are screened in parallel for other congenital conditions such as hypothyroidism and phenylketonuria. Potentially affected infants are quickly recalled for additional testing. *Prenatal treatment* of affected females is done by administration of dexamethasone, in an amount of 20 g/kg prepregnancy maternal weight daily in two or three divided doses. This suppresses secretion of steroids by the fetal adrenal, including secretion of adrenal androgens. If started by 6 wk of gestation, it ameliorates virilization of the external genitals in affected females. Chorionic villus biopsy is then performed to determine the sex and genotype of the fetus; therapy is continued only if the fetus is an affected female. DNA analysis of fetal cells isolated from maternal plasma for sex determination and CYP21 gene analysis will provide earlier identification of the affected female fetus. No specific deleterious effects have been observed in children exposed to this therapy. Maternal side effects of prenatal treatment have included edema, excessive weight gain, hypertension, glucose intolerance, cushingoid facial features, and severe striae.

Treatment

Glucocorticoid replacement: This often requires larger glucocorticoid doses than are needed in other forms of adrenal insufficiency. Hydrocortisone 15–20 mg/m^2/24 hr daily administered orally in three divided doses. Double or triple doses are indicated during periods of stress, such as infection or surgery. Treatment must be continued indefinitely in all patients with classic 21-hydroxylase deficiency, but may not be required in nonclassic disease in all cases.

Mineralocorticoid replacement: Patients with salt-wasting disease (i.e. aldosterone deficiency) require mineralocorticoid replacement with fludrocortisone. Infants may have very high mineralocorticoid requirements in the first few months of life, usually 0.1–0.3 mg daily in two divided doses but occasionally up to 0.4 mg daily, and often require sodium supplementation (sodium chloride, 1–3 g) in addition to the mineralocorticoid. Older infants and children are usually maintained with 0.05–0.1 mg daily of fludrocortisone. Therapy is evaluated by monitoring of vital signs: tachycardia and hypertension are signs of overtreatment with mineralocorticoids. Serum electrolytes should be measured frequently in early infancy as therapy is adjusted. Plasma renin activity is a useful way to determine adequacy of therapy and should be maintained in or near the normal range but not suppressed.

Antihypertensive therapy: Nifedipine (calcium channel blocker) is the drug of choice.

Children: 0.25–0.5 mg/kg/dose maximum of 10 mg/dose and 1–2 mg/kg/24 hr PO, Sublingual (SL); repeat q4–6 hr. Adolescents: 10–30 mg (capsules) PO 6–8 hr or 30–120 mg qd (sustained release) PO 24 hr.

Surgical management of ambiguous genitalia: Surgery is done between 2 and 6 months of age in significantly virilized females. The clitoris in cases of marked clitoromegaly is reduced in size, with partial excision of the corporal bodies and preservation of the neurovascular bundle. Vaginoplasty and correction of the urogenital sinus usually are performed at the same time of clitoral surgery; revision in adolescence is often required.

Adrenal Tumors and Adrenal Masses

Adrenal Tumors

Adrenocortical tumors are rare in childhood; most commonly occur in children younger than 10 yr of age. Symptoms of endocrine hyperfunction are present in more than 90% of children with adrenal tumors. Tumors may be associated with hemihypertrophy, Beckwith-Wiedemann syndrome and other congenital defects, particularly genitourinary tract and central nervous system abnormalities and hamartomatous defects. Adrenal tumors are of two types: virilizing adrenocortical tumors and feminizing adrenal tumors.

Adrenal Masses

Adrenal incidentaloma: The unexpected recovery of adrenal masses in patients undergoing abdominal imaging for reasons unrelated to the adrenal gland is described as adrenal incidentoloma. The differential diagnosis of adrenal incidentoloma includes benign lesions such as cysts, hemorrhagic cysts, hemartomas, and myelolipomas. These lesions can usually be identified on CT or MRI. Functional tumors require removal.

Adrenal calcifications are often detected as incidental findings in radiographic studies of the abdomen in infants and children. There may be history of anoxia or trauma at birth. Hemorrhage into the adrenal gland at or immediately after birth is probably the most common factor that leads to subsequent calcification.

Neuroblastomas, ganglioneuroma, cortical carcinomas, pheochromocytomas, and cysts of the adrenal gland may be responsible for calcifications, particularly if hemorrhage has occurred within the tumor. Calcification in such lesions is almost always unilateral. Tuberculosis is also a cause both of calcification within the adrenals and of Addison disease. Calcifications may also develop in adrenal glands of children who recover from Waterhouse-Friderichsen syndrome. Infants with Wolman disease, a rare lipid disorder due to deficiency of lysosomal acid lipase, have extensive bilateral calcifications of the adrenal glands.

Pheochromocytoma

Pheochromocytomas, catecholamine-secreting tumors, arise from chromaffin cells of the adrenal medulla in approximately 90% of cases. Other sites include abdominal sympathetic chain and are likely to be located near the aorta at the level of the mesenteric artery or its bifurcation, periadrenal area, urinary bladder or ureteral walls, thoracic cavity, and cervical region. Ten percent occur in children, most frequently between 6 and 14 yr of age. Tumors vary from 1 to 10 cm in diameter and found more often in affected children on right than on the left, bilateral in more than 20%, and in 30–40% both the adrenals and extra-adrenal area or only in an extra-adrenal area. Pheochromocytomas may be inherited as an autosomal dominant trait. Pheochromocytomas may also be associated with other syndromes such as neurofibromatosis, von Hippel-Lindau disease, tuberous sclerosis, Sturge-Weber syndrome, ataxia-telangiectasia, and as a component of multiple endocrine neoplasia (MEN) syndromes MEN-2A and MEN-2B.

Clinical manifestations: The clinical features of pheochromocytomas result from excessive secretion of epinephrine and nonepinephrine. Paroxysmal hypertension is suggestive of pheochromocytoma as a diagnostic possibility. The hypertension in children is more often sustained rather than paroxysmal in contrast to adults. Between attacks of hypertension, the patient may be free of symptoms. During attacks, the patient complains of headache, palpitations, abdominal pain, and dizziness; pallor, vomiting, and sweating also occur. In severe cases, precordial pains radiate into the arms; pulmonary edema and cardiac and hepatic enlargement may develop. Convulsions and other manifestations of hypertensive encephalopathy may occur. Symptoms may be exaggerated by exercise. The child has a good appetite but because of hypermetabolism does not gain weight, and severe cachexia may develop. The blood pressure may range from 180 to 260 mm Hg systolic and from 120 to 210 mm Hg diastolic and the heart may be enlarged. Ophthalmoscopic examination may reveal papilledema, hemorrhages, exudates, and arterial constriction.

Laboratory findings: There is elevated blood or urinary levels of catecholamines and their metabolites; total urinary catecholamine excretion usually exceeds 300 μg/24 hr; increased urinary excretion of vanillylmandelic acid (VMA).

Major tumors in the area of the adrenal gland are readily localized by ultrasonography or by CT or MRI. ^{131}I-metaiodobenzylguanidine (MIBG) is taken up by chromaffin tissue anywhere in the body and is useful for localizing small tumors.

Differential diagnosis: Various causes of hypertension in children include renal or renovascular disease; coarctation of the aorta; hyperthyroidism; Cushing syndrome; deficiencies of 11β-hydroxylase, 17α-hydroxylase, or 11β-hydroxysteroid dehydrogenase; primary aldosteronism; aderocortical tumors; and essential hypertension.

Neuroblastoma, ganglioneuroblastoma, and ganglioneuroma frequently produce catecholamines. Secreting neurogenic tumors commonly produce hypertension, excessive sweating, flushing, pallor, rash, polyuria, and polydipsia. Chronic diarrhea may be associated with these tumors, particularly with ganglioneuroma.

Treatment: Removal of these tumors results in cure, but the operation is high-risk. Preoperative α- and β-adrenergic blockade and fluid loading are required.

Barzon L, Boscaro M. Diagnosis and management of adrenal incidentaloma. *J Urol* 2000; 163: 398–407.

Brunt LM, Moley JF. Adrenal incidentaloma. *World J Surg* 2001; 25: 905–913.

Grim CE. Evolution of diagnostic criteria for primary aldosteronism: Why is it more common in "drug resistant" hypertension today? *Curr Hypertens Rep* 2004; 6: 485–492.

John M, Shah NS. Approach to a child with adrenal dysfunction. In: Mathur GP, Mathur Sarla (eds). *Current Trends in Pediatrics*. Vol 3. Delhi: Academa Publishers, 2007; 264–274.

Merke DP, Bornstein SR. Congenital adrenal hyperplasia. *Lancet* 2005; 365: 2125–2136.

Miller WL. The adrenal cortex and its disorders In: Brook CGD, Hindmarsh PC (eds). *Clinical Pediatric Endocrinology*. 4th edn. London: Blackwell Science Ltd, 2001; 321–376.

Prys-Roberts C. Pheochromocytoma-recent progress in the management. *Br J Anaesth* 2000; 85: 44–57.

Ribeiro RC, Figueiredo B. Childhood adrenocortical tumors. *Eur J Cancer* 2004; 40: 1117–1126.

Ross JH. Pheochromocytoma: Special considerations in children. *Urol Clin North Am* 2000; 27: 393–402.

Schnitzer JJ, Donahoe PK. Surgical treatment of congenital adrenal hyperplasia. *Endocrinol Metab Clin North Am* 2001; 30: 137–154.

Stewart PM. The adrenal cortex. In: Larsen, Kronenberg, Melmed, Polonsky (eds). *Williams Textbook of Endocrinology*. 10th edn. Philadelphia: Saunders, 2003; 491–551.

Therrell BL. Newborn screening for congenital adrenal hyperplasia. *Endocrinol Metab Clin North Am* 2001; 30: 15–30.

White PC. Disorders of the adrenal glands. In: Kliegman RM, Behrman RE, Jenson HB, Stanton BF (eds). *Nelson Textbook of Pediatrics*. 18th edn. Vol 2. Philadelphia: Saunders, 2007; 2349–2374.

23.6 DISORDERS OF THE GONADS

Hypofunction of the Testes

Testicular hypofunction may be primary in the testis (primary hypogonadism) or secondary to deficiency of pituitary gonadotropic hormones (secondary hypogonadism). Patients with primary hypogonadism have elevated levels of gonadotropin (hypergonadotropic); those with secondary hypogonadism have low or absent levels (hypogonadotropic).

Noonan Syndrome

Etiology: The disorder is autosomal dominant; sporadic and autosomal recessive occurrence has been reported. Noonan syndrome occurs in 1: 1000–2000 live births.

Clinical manifestations: The most common abnormalities are short stature, webbing of the neck, pectus carinatum or pectus excavatum, cubitus valgus, right sided congenital heart disease (pulmonary valvular stenosis, hypertrophic cardiomyopathy, or atrial septal defect), and characteristic facies. Hypertelorism, epicanthus, downward slanted palpebral fissures, ptosis, micrognathia, and ear abnormalities. Other abnormalities such as clinodactyly, hernias, and vertebral anomalies occur less frequently. The mean IQ of school-aged children is 86, with a range of 53 to 127. High-frequency hearing loss is common. Hepatosplenomegaly and several hematologic diseases are noted. Males frequently have cryptorchidism and small testes; they may be hypogonadal or normal. Puberty is delayed 2 yr; adult height is achieved by the end of the 2nd decade and usually reaches the lowest limit of the normal population. Prenatal diagnosis should be suspected in fetuses with normal karyotype, edema, or hydrops and short femur length.

Treatment: Human growth hormone treatment has resulted in improvement in growth velocity without adverse effects on cardiac ventricular wall thickness.

Klinefelter Syndrome (*see* Chapter 9)

Hypogonadotropic Hypogonadism in the Male (Secondary Hypogonadism)

In hypogonadotropic hypogonadism, there is deficiency of FSH or LH or both. The primary defect may lie in the anterior pituitary or in the hypothalamus as a deficiency of GnRH. The testes are normal but remain in the prepubertal state because stimulation by gonadotropins is lacking. The disorder may be recognized in infancy, around the time of puberty, or rarely in adulthood.

Etiology: The causes of hypogonadotropic hypogonadism (HHG) include hypopituitarism, isolated deficiency of gonadotropin, Kallmann syndrome (X-linked disorder [KAL1] associated with anosmia or hyposmia), X-linked congenital adrenal hypoplasia, genetic defects involving the hypothalamic-pituitary-gonadal-axis, and polyglandular autoimmune syndrome.

Diagnosis: Levels of gonadotropins and gonadal steroids remain in the prepubertal range, and nocturnal pulsatile secretion of LH does not occur. The gonadotropin response to stimulation with GnRH or a more potent analog of GnRH is markedly blunted. These findings are also observed in normal adolescents with the variant known as constitutional delayed puberty; it is difficult to distinguish between the two conditions. Gonadotropin deficiency is likely if the patient has evidence of another pituitary deficiency, such as a deficiency of growth hormone, particularly if it is associated with corticotropin (adrenocortico-tropic hormone [ACTH]) deficiency. The presence of *anosmia* usually indicates permanent gonadotropin deficiency. *Prolactinomas* are recognized as a cause of delayed puberty and should be excluded by determination of serum levels of prolactin. Probes are available to establish the diagnosis in heterozygotes and newborn infants with the X-linked form of Kallmann syndrome.

Treatment: Constitutional delayed puberty should be ruled out before a diagnosis of isolated deficiency of GnRH is established and treatment is indicated. If by 15 yr of age no clinical evidence of puberty is beginning and the testosterone level is less than 50 ng/dl, testosterone enanthate, 100 mg intramuscularly once monthly for 4–6 mo, usually results in an increase in the signs of secondary sexual characteristics and an increase in growth velocity; it may initiate puberty and may differentiate constitutional delay in puberty from isolated gonadotropin deficiency.

Patients with established deficiency of gonadotropins should be treated in the same way as that used for those with primary testicular deficiency. With this therapy, the testes will remain small. Treatment with hCG, given subcutaneously or intramuscularly in doses of 500–1,000 IU, three times weekly, stimulates growth of the testes and spermatogenesis.

Gynecomastia

Gynecomastia, the occurrence of mammary tissue in the male, is a common condition. True gynecomastia (the presence of granular breast tissue) should be differentiated from pseudogynecomastia (consisting of only adipose tissue) seen in overweight boys. Gynecomastia is usually a sign of estrogen-androgen imbalance; its cause is obscure.

Gynecomastia occurs in many newborn males as a result of a normal stimulation by maternal hormones; the effect disappears in a few weeks. During early to midpuberty, approximately two-thirds of boys develop various degrees of subareolar hyperplasia of the breasts. *Physiologic pubertal gynecomastia* may involve only one breast, but occasionally both breasts are enlarged at disproportionate rates or at different times. Tenderness of the breast is common but transitory. Spontaneous regression may occur within

a few months; it may rarely persist longer than 2 yr. When levels are correlated with stage of puberty, a decreased ratio of testosterone to estradiol is found in boys with gynecomastia. Treatment usually consists of reassuring the boy and his family of the physiologic and transient nature of the phenomenon. When the enlargement is striking and persistent and serious emotional disturbances occur, treatment may be justified. The medical treatment is aimed at decreasing the estrogen/androgen ratio. Danazol or anastrozole may be used. Occasionally, breast development may mimic female breast development (to Tanner stages 3–5) and fail to regress. In such cases, surgical removal of the enlarged breast tissue may be indicated.

Benign, self-limited and usually transient gyneco-mastia has been reported in prepubertal children during the initiation of therapy with human growth hormone.

Familial gynecomastia has occurred in several kindreds as an X-linked or autosomal dominant sex-limited trait. Increased peripheral conversion of C–19 steroids to estrogens (increased aromatization) has been found in familial and sporadic cases of gynecomastia and may explain some instances of this condition.

In prepubertal children with gynecomastia, an exogenous source of estrogens must be sought. Accidental or therapeutic exposure to small amounts of exogenous estrogens by inhalation, percutaneous absorption, or ingestion may cause gynecomastia. Several other pathologic conditions may cause gynecomastia such as 11β-hydroxylase deficiency, Leydig cell tumors of the testis, feminizing tumors of the adrenal gland, Klinefelter syndrome, Reifenstein syndrome, prolactinoma, fibrolamellar carcinoma of the liver, and hyperthyroidism.

Hypofunction of the Ovaries

Hypofunction of the ovaries may be caused by conge-nital failure of development, postnatal destruction (primary or hypergonadotropic hypogonadism), or lack of stimulation by the pituitary and or hypo-thalamus (secondary or tertiary hypogonadotropic hypogonadism).

Hypergonadotropic Hypogonadism in the Female (Primary Hypogonadism)
Turner Syndrome (*see* Chapter 9)
Noonan syndrome

Girls with Noonan syndrome show certain anomalies that also occur in girls with 45, XO Turner syndrome, but they have normal 46, XX chromosomes. The most common abnormalities are the same as those described for males with Noonan syndrome. The phenotype differs from Turner syndrome in several aspects. Mental retardation is often present, the cardiac defect is most often pulmonary valvular stenosis or an atrial septal defect rather than an aortic defect, normal sexual maturation usually occurs but is delayed by 2 yr on average, and premature ovarian failure has been reported.

Hypogonadotropic Hypogonadism in the Female (Secondary Hypogonadism)

Hypofunction of the ovaries can result from failure to secrete normal levels of gonadotropins. The defect may lie in the anterior pituitary or, more commonly, in the hypothalamus.

Etiology: Hypopituitarism: Congenital or acquired lesions in or near the pituitary almost always result in impaired secretion of gonadotropins and other pituitary hormones. Isolated deficiency of gonadotropins: In most children the pituitary is normal, with the defect residing in the hypothalamus, GnRH test is helpful in distinguishing the two conditions. Gonadotropin hormone deficiency is reported in Kallmann syndrome (in anosmic hypogonadal females), Laurence-Moon-Biedl, multiple lentigines, Carpenter syndrome, Prader-Willi syndrome, severe thalassemia, and anorexia nervosa.

Diagnosis: The diagnosis may be apparent in patients with other deficiencies of pituitary tropic hormones, but it is difficult to differentiate isolated hypogonadotropic hypogonadism from physiologic delay of puberty. Repeated measurements of FSH and LH, particularly during sleep, may reveal the rising levels that herald the onset of puberty. Stimulation testing with GnRH or one of its analogs may help establish the diagnosis.

Polycystic Ovary Syndrome (Stein-Leventhal Syndrome): See Section 33.6

Bondy CA. Care of girls and women with Turner syndrome: A guideline of Turner syndrome study group. *J Clin Endo Metab* 2007; 92:10–25.

Braunstein GD. Gynecomastia. *N Engl J Med* 1993; 328: 490–495.

Hardelin J. Kallmann syndrome: Towards molecular pathogenesis. *Mol Cell Endocrinol* 2001; 179: 75–81.

Noonan JA. Noonan syndrome revisited. *J Pediatr* 1999; 135: 667–668.

Rapaport R. Disorders of the gonads. In: Kliegman RM, Behrman RE, Jenson HB, Stanton BF (eds). *Nelson Textbook of Pediatrics.* 18th edn. Vol 2. Philadelphia: Saunders, 2007; 2374–2403.

Ross JL, Roeltgen D, Feuillan, et al. Use of estrogen in young girls with Turner syndrome. *Neurology* 2000; 54:164–170.

Intersex

An intersexual or intersex person is one who is born with genitalia and/or secondary sex characteristics determined as neither exclusively male nor female, or in whom there are combine features of the male and female sexes. There is a move to drop the term "intersex" in medical usage, replacing it with "Disorders of Sex Development" (DSD) in order to avoid conflicting anatomy with identity. However, this has been met with criticism from some activists who consider **intersex to be a third gender**. The phrase "ambiguous genitalia" refers specifically to external genital appearance, but not all intersex conditions result in atypical external genital appearance. In cases in whom genitalia are unambiguous at birth, it may be years before the presence of an intersex disorder is recognized. Patients presenting with intersex disorders can be classified into two types: A. Neonatal infant presenting with ambiguous genitalia. B. Other children/adolescents presenting with virilization, premature pubarche/ thelarche, primary amenorrhoea or absence of secondary sexual characteristics.

Intersex occurs when the appearance of the internal or external genitalia is at variance with normal development for either sex. In the neonatal period, the first question asked by, and of new parents in relation to their offspring is often "Is it a boy or a girl"? A rational approach, based on knowledge of normal prenatal sexual development, and based on a careful physical examination to guide further investigation, is required to reach a diagnosis. In 46, XX individuals, the commonest cause of genital ambiguity is congenital adrenal hyperplasia due to 21-hydroxylase deficiency; however, in 46, XY individuals the differential diagnosis is wide, and may remain unexplained, even after extensive investigation. In childhood or adolescence, the presenting symptoms may include virilization of a female, or absence of secondary sexual characteristics in a male or female.

Incidence: According to the highest estimates perhaps 1 percent of live births exhibit some degree of sexual ambiguity and that between 0.1% and 0.2% of live births are ambiguous enough to become the subject of specialist medical attention, including surgery to disguise their sexual ambiguity. Other sources create a narrower definition of "true intersexual conditions" and estimate the incidence as far lower, at approximately 0.018%.

Sexual differentiation: Before about 6 weeks' gestation, male and female embryos develop undifferentiated gonadal tissue and have primordial structures with the potential to produce either male or female genitalia. The genital appearance of the newborn is largely determined by the presence or absence of genetic and hormonal influences responsible for the active process of male differentiation. The fetus tends to develop as a female in the absence of these male influences. Intersex conditions arise because of an abnormality along the male pathway that interferes with complete masculinization or, in the case of a genetic female, some virilizing influence that acts on the developing embryo.

Male sexual differentiation is initiated by the SRY gene on the short arm of the Y chromosome. Under the influence of SRY, the undifferentiated gonad forms a testis, which produces the hormonal milieu that results in male sexual differentiation: testosterone stimulates the Wolffian structures (epididymis, vas deferens, and seminal vesicles), and anti-Mullerian hormone suppresses the development of the Mullerian structures (fallopian tubes, uterus, and upper vagina). The conversion of testosterone to dihydrotestosterone occurs in the skin of the external genitalia and masculinizes the external genital structures. Most of this male differentiation takes place by about 12 weeks, after which the penis grows and the testes descend into the scrotum. In the absence of SRY, female sexual differentiation occurs. An error in genital morphogenesis may occur at any step in this developmental pathway.

A. The Neonatal Infant with Ambiguous Genitalia

It is important that a definitive diagnosis be determined in the newborn with abnormal genital development as quickly as possible so that an appropriate treatment plan can be established to minimize medical, psychological, and social complications. Principal causes of ambiguous genitalia according to gonadal histology include: **Ovary:** Congenital Adrenal Hyperplasia(CAH); Placental aromatase deficiency; Maternal source of virilization; **Testis:** Leydig cell hypoplasia; Testosterone biosynthesis defect; 5-α-reductase deficiency; Androgen insensitivity; **Ovary and Testis:** True hermaphroditism; **Dysgenetic gonads:** Gonadal dysgenesis; Denys-Drash and Frasier syndromes; Smith-Lemli-Opitz syndrome; Camptomelic dwarfism.

The two most likely causes of ambiguous genitalia are CAH (21-hydroxylase deficiency) and mixed gonadal dysgenesis. Partial androgen insensitivity syndrome and 17 β-hydroxysteroid dehydrogenase deficiency (a defect in testosterone biosynthesis) are next in order of prevalence.

These guidelines for investigation permit most newborns with an underlying intersex condition to be recognized promptly after birth. Other children with intersex disorders, however, may not be diagnosed until childhood or adolescence when virilization, premature pubarche or thelarche, or primary amenorrhea is investigated.

History and examination in a case of ambiguous genitalia: Evaluation begins with an obstetric history to include any evidence of endocrine disturbance during pregnancy. A family history should be sought of unexplained neonatal deaths or genital anomalies, abnormal pubertal development, or infertility in close relatives. The clinical findings in a newborn infant that raise the possibility of intersexuality are shown in Table 23.10. The physical examination begins with a search for any features suggestive of a malformation syndrome. The external genitalia are then inspected to determine the degree of masculinization. The size of the phallus is assessed by rolling the corporeal bodies between the fingers to appreciate their true length and girth, as both ventral curvature (chordee), which is almost always present, and an abundance of prepubic fat often mask the true size of the penis. In full-term newborns the stretched penile length should measure at least 2 cm. The extent to which the urogenital sinus has closed is then determined by identifying the position of the urethral meatus, which sometimes requires waiting until the baby voids. The fullness, symmetry, and rugosity of the labioscrotal folds are then noted. When these folds are asymmetrical, a gonad is frequently palpable on the more virilized side and is often associated with an inguinal hernia. An attempt should be made to palpate the

---

Table 23.10: Clinical findings in a newborn infant that raise the possibility of intersexuality

Apparent male
1. Bilateral nonpalpable testes in a full-term infant
2. Hypospadias associated with separation of the scrotal sacs
3. Undescended testis with hypospadias

Indeterminate
1. Ambiguous genitalia

Apparent female
1. Clitoral hypertrophy of any degree
2. Foreshortened vulva with single opening
3. Inguinal hernia containing a gonad

gonads on each side by sweeping the examining fingers down along the line of the inguinal canal toward the labium or scrotum while the other hand grasps any possible gonad. This maneuver requires warm hands.

It is generally unwise at this stage to make a definitive diagnosis based on the physical findings alone, as the appearance of the external genitalia can vary widely, even among patients with the same underlying condition. There is only one deduction that can confidently be made, namely, that if a gonad is palpable the diagnosis is not a female infant with CAH in which the gonads are normal ovaries situated in the abdominal cavity. Some clues to help establish a diagnosis, however, may be found. For example, a well-developed phallus indicates that significant levels of circulating testosterone were present in utero, whereas asymmetry of the scrotum suggests the secretion of testosterone by the gonad on the better developed side. Other findings include dark skin pigmentation associated with high circulating levels of adrenocorticotropic hormone, suggesting CAH, or a virilized appearance of the mother resulting from placental aromatase deficiency or a maternal endocrine tumor.

Biochemical tests and imaging: Ambiguous genitalia in the newborn need immediate and rational management. This complex situation requires a strategy of clinical, hormonal, genetic, molecular, and radiographic investigation to determine the etiology of the intersex state and orient the therapeutic approach. Physical examination is the key to diagnosis. Careful palpation to locate gonads at the genital folds or in the inguinal region provides the first element for diagnostic orientation. If gonads are absent, a diagnosis of female pseudohermaphroditism seems advisable; if gonads are palpated, a diagnosis of male pseudohermaphroditism is more appropriate. Karyotyping reports are available after a few days, while polymerase chain reaction (PCR) analysis of the SRY gene provides information about the presence of a Y chromosome within one day. Hormonal investigation should be based on clinical and genetic orientation. Substantially elevated plasma 17-OH progesterone will confirm the diagnosis of congenital adrenal hyperplasia due to deficiency in 21-hydroxylase. Testicular stimulation with human chorionic gonadotropin (hCG) will determine the functional value of testicular tissue. Other tests, such as ACTH stimulation test, testosterone trial test or serum 11- deoxy-cortisol may be required in individual cases. Exploration of the genitourinary axis is principally carried out by ultrasound and genitography.

By the end of these investigations, the medical team should be able to give a precise diagnosis.

- Female pseudohermaphroditism may be due to excess fetal androgens (congenital adrenal hyperplasia), increased androgen production of maternal origin, or placental androgen excess.
- In male pseudohermaphroditism, if testosterone rises normally after hCG stimulation, androgen resistance is indicated. If it does not rise after this test, either testicular dysgenesis or disturbance in testosterone biosynthesis may be responsible.
- The assignment of sex for rearing must be guided by the etiology of the genital malformation, the anatomic condition, and family considerations.
- In cases of female pseudohermaphroditism, the newborn should always be declared to be of female sex at birth.
- In cases of male pseudohermaphroditism, great care should be taken in the declaration of male sex: the potential for reconstructive surgery and the pubertal "programmed" response of the external genitalia to endogenous and exogenous testosterone are determinant.
- Management of ambiguous genitalia in the newborn requires an entire multidisciplinary team in every step of the diagnostic procedure, the choice of sex assignment, and the treatment strategy.

Etiological diagnosis of a newborn with intersex disorder: An approach to the etiological diagnosis of a newborn with intersex disorder is presented in Table 23.11.

Common Conditions Presenting as Ambiguous Genitalia

1. *Congenital adrenal hyperplasia (CAH) (21-hydroxylase deficiency):* If a patient has XX karyotype and ambiguous genitalia, then the most likely diagnosis is 21-hydroxylase deficiency. In the classic salt-losing form (accounting for 75% of cases of 21 hydroxylase deficiency), the activity of the enzyme is reduced to practically zero, as a result of which mineralocorticoid activity is interrupted. Signs of hyponatremic dehydration and hyperkalemia occur requiring prompt management with intravenous rehydration, replacement of electrolytes, hydrocortisone and mineralocorticoid. Synthesis of adrenal androgens is increased, leading to virilization and ambiguous genitalia in the female. The development of ovaries and Muellerian structures is unaffected. Hyperpigmented (due to increased ACTH) male-appearing external genitalia, nonpalpable gonads, clitoromegaly, common urogenital sinus and hypospadias are some of the prominent features. In severe cases, complete fusion of the labia

Table 23.11: Differential diagnosis on the basis of gonad(s) palpable or not palpable

Features identified	Differential diagnosis
No gonads palpable, uterus present, hyperpigmentation present	Congenital adrenal hyperplasia (CAH) (a) 21 hydroxylase deficiency (hyponatremia and hyperkalemia with raised 17 OHP levels) (b) 11β-hydroxylase deficiency (hypertension with hypokalemia with raised 11 DOC levels)
Gonad(s) palpable, no uterus	(a) Partial androgen insensitivity syndrome (b) Defect in testosterone biosynthesis (17β-hydroxy steroid dehydrogenase deficiency, 5α-reductase deficiency)
Gonads palpable, uterus present, asymmetrical labioscrotal folds	(a) Mixed gonadal dysgenesis (b) True hermaphroditism

DOC: 11-deoxycorticosterone; 17-OHP: 17-hydroxyprogestirone.

may occur. In male newborns, the condition may go unrecognized. Non-classic and simple virilizing varieties of the disorder may present later in childhood with precocious puberty. Raised serum levels of 17-hydroxyprogesterone are diagnostic of 21-hydroxylase deficiency.

Ambiguous genitalia with hyperpigmented skin may also be seen in rare conditions like 11β-hydroxylase deficiency (associated with hypertension and hypokalemia), 3α-hydroxysteroid dehydrogenase deficiency and lipoid adrenal hyperplasia. Features of various forms of congenital adrenal hyperplasia (CAH) are mentioned in Section 23.5 on congenital adrenal hyperplasia and related disorders.

2. *Mixed gonadal dysgenesis (45,X/46,XY karyotype):* This is the second most common cause of ambiguous genitalia. It results from incomplete differentiation of the bipotential gonad into either ovary or testes. The clinical clue is presence of at least one palpable gonad with asymmetric labioscrotal folds. 33% of these neonates have Turner phenotype. At puberty, testes secrete androgen causing virilization, but testes lack germinal elements, therefore, they become infertile men. The risk of malignancy (gonadoblastoma) is high.

3. *True hermaphroditism:* In this rare condition, when the gonads in one individual are composed of both ovarian and testicular elements, it is called true hermaphroditism. The gonad found is ovotestes. 80% are XX, 10% are mosaic and 10% are XY. Any testicular tissue is dysgenetic. The ovarian tissue is normal. So if raised as females, these neonates may be fertile, but if raised as male they are never fertile. External genitalia exhibit all gradation from male to female spectrum.

4. *Partial androgen insensitivity syndrome (PAIS):* In this condition, there is a fault at the androgen receptor level. HCG stimulated ratio of androstenedione to testosterone is normal. At least one gonad is palpable. There is no uterus. The testes enlarge at puberty and patient undergoes considerable virilization and inevitably experiences gynecomastia. 17β-hydroxysteroid dehydrogenase (17β-HSD) deficiency resembles PAIS in phenotype, but HCG test reveals abnormally high ratio of androstenedione to testosterone in the serum.

5. *5α-Reductase deficiency:* In this autosomal recessive condition testosterone is not able to convert to the more potent dihydrotestosterone (DHT). Affected XY subjects are born with ambiguous genitalia, at least one palpable testis and may have severe perineoscrotal hypospadias. There is no uterus or fallopian tube. Wolffian structures are present. Breast development is absent though female habitus and pubarche are present. They are usually identified as female in childhood but undergo striking virilization at puberty but the stretched penile length is less than 6 cm.

B. Intersex Conditions Presenting in Adolescence/Childhood

Four different phenotypes are described: XY female, XX male, 46 XY male with persistent Muellerian structures and 46XX female with Mullerian agenesis.

1. XY Female: (a) Complete 46, XY gonadal dysgenesis (Swyer syndrome). Complete 46XY gonadal dysgenesis is diagnosed when a healthy girl of normal stature presents with delayed puberty. FSH and LH levels in the serum are raised, whereas plasma estradiol levels are low, indicating primary gonadal failure. XY karyotype is diagnostic. Bone age is delayed and eunuchoid skeletal proportions may be found. Pelvic ultrasound shows small uterus; ovaries may not be visualized. In 10–15% cases, this condition is caused by a mutation in the SRY gene or by a Yp deletion. In the remaining 85–90% of XY females, the cause of gonadal dysgenesis remains unknown. Mutations in genes including WT-1 (Wilms' tumor suppressor gene) and SOX-9 have been described, but they are unlikely to explain more than a small proportion of cases. Two syndromes have been associated with WT-1 gene mutation: Denys-Drash Syndrome and Frasier syndrome. Wilms' tumor is described in the former, but the latter is not associated with increased risk of Wilms' tumor.

(b) Complete androgen insensitivity syndrome (CAIS). These XY females present with female external genitalia, short blind ending vagina and no uterus. In infancy or childhood, these girls may present with bilateral inguinal hernias containing testes. Pubic hair is completely absent or very sparse. Vagina is about 2/3 of normal length. In adult patients, serum testosterone levels are in male range or higher; LH is normal or elevated. Serum estradiol levels are between normal male and female ranges.

(c) Defects in steroid hormone biosynthesis. 17α-hydroxylase deficiency and lipoid adrenal hyperplasia are rare causes which may present as XY female phenotype in adolescence.

2. XX Males: In this rare condition, the phenotype resembles Klinefelter syndrome. (47XXY). In this the testes are small (pea-like) and dysgenetic and infertility is inevitable. Patients can be normal males or somewhat eunuchoid with gynecomastia. Mullerian structures are absent.

3. 46,XY Male with Persistent Mullerian Structures: Patients with this syndrome have normal male genitalia and the testes are usually undescended. The presence of uterus and fallopian tubes is often discovered by the surgeon at operation. The testes secrete normal amounts of testosterone and therefore should never be removed.

4. 46 XX Female with Mullerian Agenesis: This condition presents with primary amenorrhoea. In some cases the entire Müllerian tract is absent, whereas in others there is partial agenesis. The alternative name, Meyer-Rokitansky-Kuster-Hauser syndrome, is widely used.

Deciding the Sex of Rearing

The decision as to the appropriate sex of rearing of a baby born with ambiguous genitalia is based on a number of considerations that have an impact on the infant's future.

Fertility potential: All female infants virilized because of CAH or maternal androgens are potentially fertile and should therefore be raised as girls. In most other intersex conditions the potential for fertility is either reduced or absent.

Capacity for normal sexual function: The size of the phallus and its potential to develop at puberty into a sexually functional penis are of paramount importance when one is considering male sex of rearing. In infants with partial androgen insensitivity, a trial of testosterone injections should be given in equivocal cases and the infant is raised as a boy only when there is a very good response. The severity of the hypospadias should not be a deciding factor in the sex of rearing. The presence of a capacious, low-lying vagina, is advantageous if assignment as a female is being considered.

Endocrine function: Among the intersex disorders the ovaries of virilized genetic females can be assumed to be normal. Ovaries of true hermaphrodites may also produce adequate levels of estrogen. However, the testes of true hermaphrodites and those of infants with mixed gonadal dysgenesis may initially show good function that declines during childhood, so that testosterone supplements may be necessary for the establishment of puberty or in adult life.

Malignant change: The potential for malignant degeneration in a retained gonad with a Y chromosome-bearing cell line must be considered. Such changes are common in streak gonads in patients with a 46, XY cell line; streak gonads, therefore, should be removed at the time of diagnosis. Similarly, testes that show dysgenetic features on biopsy also need to be excised. The incidence of tumors is increased in histologically normal undescended testes, particularly those residing in the abdomen. However, a case can be made for retaining such a testis in patients with mild androgen insensitivity, true hermaphroditism, or mixed gonadal dysgenesis provided biopsy results show normal testicular tissue, the testis can easily be brought down into the scrotum, and the patient can be kept under long-term observation.

Testosterone imprinting: Testosterone imprinting of the fetal brain may play a role in determining male sexual orientation. Until further data become available, caution should be exercised when a recommendation is made that the sex of rearing should differ from the chromosomal sex. Such cases warrant careful individual consideration. Psychological counseling of affected individuals and their parents may be beneficial.

Timing of surgery: Infants raised as girls will usually require clitoral reduction which, with current techniques, will result not only in a normal-looking vulva but preservation of a functional clitoris. In girls with CAH, surgery can usually be performed once hormone replacement therapy is begun. A low-lying vagina can be exteriorized at the initial surgery, but in other cases this is best deferred until 1 year of age and often later. Additional surgery is often necessary. The testes should be removed soon after birth in infants with partial androgen insensitivity or testicular dysgenesis in whom a very small phallus mandates a female sex of rearing. In boys, an undescended testis that is to be retained is best brought down into the scrotum at the time of initial gonadal biopsy. Correction of chordee and urethroplasty in boys with hypospadias is usually performed between 6 and 18 months of age, usually in one stage as an outpatient procedure.

Gender Assignment and Family Centered Management Recommendations

1. Genetic females recognized in the neonatal period should be raised as females. No change in sex assignment should be made after two years of age.
2. It is easy to convert an intersex child to female rather than to male. This is because the female genotype with intersexuality may be fertile but a male genotype with intersexuality has low fertility.
3. All dysgenetic testes must be removed latest by 12 years of age.
4. Neonates with overtly ambiguous genitalia should have sex assignment deferred.
5. Parental notification should be made in careful terms. Suggested language may include the following: the genitalia are unfinished in their development and we will need a few days to perform some studies to determine which sex your baby was intended to be.
6. Recognize that the birth of a neonate with ambiguous genitalia is a major traumatic event for the family.
7. The delivery room is not an appropriate location for an in-depth discussion. Meet with parents together if possible and re-examine the neonates' genitalia in the presence of the parents. Show them the abnormalities in a calm and professional manner. Assure the family that when data from tests are available, the correct sex will be known and discussed with them.
8. Discourage the use of intersex names.
9. Do not complete the birth certificate or make any reference to gender in the mother and/or newborn's permanent medical record.
10. All female pseudohermaphrodites should be raised as females. On the other hand, in the case of male pseudohermaphrodites, gender assignment policy varies. Severe androgen resistant cases should be raised as females. If there is hypospadias

only, raise as a male. In cases of 5α-reductase deficiency, raise as a male with nandrolene supplementation. True hermaphrodites should be raised as females if phallus length is less than 2 cm with no response to testosterone.

Brown J, Warne G. Practical management of the intersex infant. *J Pediatr Endocrinol Metab* 2005; 18:3–23.

Diamond M, Sigmundson HK. Management of intersexuality: Guidelines for dealing with persons with ambiguous genitalia. *Arch Pediatr Adolesc Med* 1997; 151: 1046–1050

Donahoe PK, Schnitzer JJ. Evaluation of the infant who has ambiguous genitalia, and principles of operative management. *Semin Pediatr Surg* 1996; 5: 30–40.

Evaluation of the newborn with developmental anomalies of the external genitalia. American Academy of Pediatrics. Committee on Genetics. *Pediatrics* 2000; 106: 138–142.

Lee PA, Mazur T, Danish R. Micropenis: Criteria, etiologies and classification. *Johns Hopkins Med J* 1980; 146: 156–163.

Sax L. How common is intersex? A response to Anne Fausto-Sterling. *J Sex Res* 2002; 39(3):174–178.

Yadav S, Krishnamurthy S. Intersex. In: Mathur GP, Mathur Sarla (eds). *Current Trends in Pediatrics*. Vol 3. Delhi: Academa Publishers, 2007; 275–284.

Zdravkovic D, Milenkovic T, Sedlecki K, Guc-Scekic M, Rajic V. Causes of ambiguous external genitalia in neonates. *Srp Arh Celok Lek* 2001; 129: 57–60.

23.7 DIABETES MELLITUS IN CHILDREN

Diabetes mellitus (DM) is a common, chronic metabolic syndrome, characterized by hyperglycemia. The major forms of diabetes are classified according to those caused by deficiency of insulin secretion due to pancreatic β-cell damage (type 1DM or T1DM) and those that are as a result of insulin resistance occurring at the level of skeletal muscle, liver, and adipose tissue with various degrees of β-cell impairment (type 2 DM, or T2DM).

Type 1 Diabetes Mellitus (Immune Mediated)

Epidemiology: T1DM accounts for about 10% of all diabetes affecting over 1.5 million in the world. While it accounts for most cases of diabetes in childhood, it is not limited to this age group; cases continue to occur in adult life and approximately 50% of individuals with T1DM present in adults. India is home to 50.8 million people with diabetes, the highest in the world, followed by China with 43.2 million. India and China are ahead because of their huge population. Girls and boys are almost equally affected. There is no correlation with socioeconomic status. The onset occurs predominantly in childhood, with median age of 7 to 15 yr, but it may present at any age. Peaks of presentation occur in 2 age groups: at 5–7 yr of age and at the time of puberty. The 1st peak may correspond to the time of increased exposure to infections coincident with the beginning of school; the 2nd peak may correspond to the pubertal growth spurt induced by gonadal steroids and the increased pubertal growth hormone secretion, which antagonizes insulin.

Genetics: Genes for T1DM may provide susceptibility to, or protection from the disease. The most important genes are located within the MHC HLA class II region on chromosome 6p21, formerly termed (IDDM1), accounting for about 60% genetic susceptibility for the disease. T1DM represents a heterogeneous and polygenic disorder. About 20 non-HLA loci contributing to disease susceptibility have been identified. There is a clear familial clustering of T1DM, with prevalence in siblings approaching 6% while the prevalence in the general population in the USA is only 0.4%. Risk of diabetes is also increased when a parent has diabetes and this risk differs between the two parents; the risk is 2% if the mother has diabetes, but 7% when the father has diabetes. In monozygotic twins, the concordance rate ranges from 30–65%, whereas dizygotic twins have a concordance rate of 6–10%.

Environmental Factors

Virus infections and vaccinations: Role of viral infections in human T1DM is controversial; Coxsackie B3, Coxsackie B4, cytomegalovirus, rubella, and mumps can infect human? cells. Only congenital rubella infection is associated with diabetes in later life. It is estimated that 10–12% of patients infected with congenital rubella develop T1DM and up to 40% develop impaired glucose tolerance. There has been no convincing correlation between childhood vaccination and risk of T1DM.

Seasonal associations: Seasonal and long-term cyclic variations occur in the incidence of IDDM. Seasonal variations are most apparent in the adolescent years.

 Puberty: The pubertal peak in onset of type 1 DM occurs earlier in girls than in boys. The sex difference might be due to impart, by estrogen or by genes regulated by estrogen, such as the interleukin-6 (IL6) gene and suggests that pubertal changes may contribute to accelerated onset of type 1DM in genetically susceptible females.

Early infant diet: There appears to be a strong relationship between cow's milk consumption and national incidence of diabetes in children, the role of cow's milk in human T1DM is controversial. Delaying introduction of cereals, and increasing the duration of breastfeeding are all potentially beneficial.

Body mass index: There may be greater risk of T1DM among individuals who were heavier as young children.

Chemicals: Drugs such as alloxan, streptozotocin (STZ), pentamidine, and Vector are directly cytotoxic to β cells and cause diabetes in experimental animals and humans.

Pathogenesis

Autoimmune injury: T1DM is a chronic, T cell-mediated autoimmune disease that results in the destruction of the pancreatic islets. Genetic predisposition and environmental factors lead to initiation of an autoimmune process against the pancreatic islets. The autoimmune attack on the pancreatic islets leads to a gradual and progressive destruction of β cells, with loss of insulin secretion. It is estimated that, at the onset of clinical diabetes, 80–90% of the pancreatic islets are destroyed. Regeneration of new islets has been detected at onset of T1DM and it is thought to be responsible for the honeymoon phase (a transient decrease in insulin requirement associated with improved β-cell function). In young diabetic children, especially those of DR3/DR4 haplotypes, the destruction of β-cells is almost complete during the 1st 3 yr after the onset of hyperglycemia, whereas in older patients complete β-cell destruction may take up to 10 yr.

Psychosocial stress stemming from serious life events may also constitute a trigger mechanism for T1DM or the autoimmune process behind the disease.

Pathophysiology: Insulin performs a critical role in the storage and retrieval of cellular fuel. Its secretion in response to feeding is modulated by the interplay of neural, hormonal, and substrate-related mechanisms to permit controlled disposition of ingested foodstuffs as energy for immediate or future use. Insulin levels must be lowered in order to mobilize stored energy during the fasted state. Thus, in normal metabolism, there are regular swings between the postprandial, high-insulin metabolic state and the fasted, low insulin catabolic state that affect liver, muscle, and adipose tissue. T1DM is a progressive low-insulin catabolic state in which feeding does not reverse but rather exaggerates these catabolic processes. With moderate insulinopenia, glucose utilization by muscle and fat decreases and post-prandial hyperglycemia appears. At even lower insulin levels, the liver produces excessive glucose via glycogenolysis and gluconeogenesis, and fasting hyperglycemia begins. Hyperglycemia produces an osmotic dieresis (glycosuria) when the renal threshold is exceeded (180 mg/dl; 10 mmol/L). The resulting loss of calories and electrolytes, as well as the persistent dehydration, produce a physiologic stress with hypersecretion of stress hormones (epinephrine, cortisol, growth hormone, and glucagon). The hormonal interplay of insulin deficiency and glucagon excess shunts the free fatty acids into ketone body formation; the rate of formation of these ketone bodies, principally β-hydroxybutyrate and acetoacetone, exceeds the capacity for peripheral utilization and renal excretion. Accumulation of these ketoacids results in metabolic acidosis (diabetic ketoacidosis, DKA) and complementary rapid deep breathing on an attempt to excrete excess CO_2 (Kussmaul respiration). Acetone, formed by nonenzymatic conversion of acetoacetone, is responsible for the characteristic fruity odor of the breath. Ketones are excreted in the urine in association with cations and thus further increase losses of water and electrolyte. With progressive dehydration, acidosis, hyperosmolality, and diminished cerebral oxygen utilization, consciousness becomes impaired, and the patient ultimately becomes comatose.

Clinical manifestations: As diabetes develops, symptoms increase steadily, reflecting the decreasing of β-cell mass, worsening insulopenia, progressive hyperglycemia and eventual ketoacidosis. The clinical features include polyuria (often with nocturnal enuresis), polydipsia, hyperglycemia, glycosuria, hyperphagia, and weight loss (including loss of body fat). Female patients may develop monilial vaginitis due to chronic glycosuria. When extremely low insulin levels are reached, ketoacids accumulate and the child quickly deteriorates. Ketoacids produce abdominal discomfort, nausea, and emesis, and dehydration. Kussmaul respirations (deep, heavy, rapid breathing), fruity breath odor (acetone), prolonged corrected Q-T interval (QTc), diminished neurocognitive function, and coma. About 20–40% of children, with new-onset diabetes progress to diabetic ketoacidosis (DKA) before diagnosis. The entire progression happens much more quickly (over a few weeks) in younger children, owing to more aggressive autoimmune destruction of β-cells.

Diagnosis: The most important clue for the diagnosis of T1DM is an inappropriate polyuria in a child with dehydration, poor weight gain, or respiratory illness. In such children hyperglycemia, glycosuria, and ketonuria can be determined quickly. Nonfasting blood glucose greater than 200 mg/dl (11.1 mmol/L) with typical symptoms is diagnostic with or without ketonuria. In the obese child, T2DM must be considered. Once hyperglycemia is confirmed it is prudent to determine whether DKA is present (especially if ketonuria is found) and to evaluate electrolyte abnormalities-even if signs of dehydration are minimal. A baseline hemoglobin A1C (HbA1C) allows an estimate of the duration of hyperglycemia and provides an initial value by which to compare the effectiveness of subsequent therapy.

Diabetic ketoacidosis: DKA is the end result of the metabolic abnormalities resulting from a severe deficiency of insulin or insulin effectiveness. DKA occurs in 20–40% of children with new onset diabetes and in children with known diabetes who omit insulin doses or who do not successfully manage an intercurrent illness. DKA may be arbitrarily classified as mild, moderate or severe (Table 23.12).

Treatment: Therapy depends on to the degree of insulinopenia at presentation—without ketoacidosis or with ketoacidosis.

A. New-onset diabetes without ketoacidosis

Insulin therapy: Children with long-standing diabetes and no insulin reserve require about 0.7 U/kg/day if prepubertal, 1.0 U/kg/day at midpuberty, and 1.2 U/kg/day by the end of puberty. In a newly diagnosed child the dose is about 60–70% of the full replacement dose based on pubertal status (Tables 23.13 and 23.14). The optimal dose can only be determined empirically, with frequent self-monitored blood glucose levels and insulin adjustment by the diabetes team. The initial insulin schedule should be directed toward the optimal degree of glucose control. Frequent blood glucose monitoring and insulin adjustment are necessary in the 1st week as the child returns to routine activities and adapts a new nutritional schedule, and as the total daily insulin requirements are determined. The major physiologic limit to tight control is hypoglycemia. Intensive control no doubt reduces the risk of long-term vascular complications; it is associated with a 3-fold increase in severe hypogly-

	Normal	Mild	Moderate	Severe
CO_2 (mEq/L), Venous	20–28	16–20	10–15	< 10
pH Venous	7.35–7.45	7.25–7.35	7.15–7.25	< 7.15
Clinical	No change	Oriented, alert but fatigued	Kussmaul respirations, oriented but sleepy, arousable	Kussmaul or depressed respirations; sleepy to depressed sensorium to coma

Table 23.12: Classification of diabetic ketoacidosis

cemia. Use of insulin analogs moderates but does not eliminate this problem.

Some families may be unable to administer 4 daily injections with insulin syringe. In these cases, a compromise may be needed. A 3-injection regimen combining NPH with a rapid analog bolus at breakfast, a rapid-acting analog bolus at supper (evening meal), and NPH at bedtime may provide fair glucose control. Further compromise to a 2-injection regimen (NPH and rapid analog at breakfast and supper) may occasionally be needed. However, such a schedule would provide poor coverage for lunch and early morning, and would increase the risk of hypoglycemia at midmorning and early night.

Other Methods of Administration of Insulin Therapy

Insulin pump therapy: Continuous subcutaneous insulin infusion (CSII) via battery-powered pumps provides a closer approximation of normal plasma insulin profiles and increased flexibility regarding timing of meals and snacks compared with conventional insulin injection regimens. One benefit of pump therapy may be reduction in severe hypoglycemia and associated seizures.

Inhaled and oral insulin therapies: Preprandial inhaled insulin is being evaluated in adults with T1DM and T2DM. The preliminary metabolic data are promising. Patients taking pre-meal inhaled insulin in combination with once daily bedtime long-acting insulin (Ultralente) injection achieved similar metabolic control compared with patients taking 2–3 daily injections of insulin.

Amylin-based adjunct therapy: Pramlintide acetate, a synthetic analog of amylin, may be of therapeutic value combined with insulin therapy. In adolescents it has been shown to decrease postprandial hyperglycemia, insulin dosage, gastric emptying, and HbA1c levels. It is given as a subcutaneous dose before meals.

Table 23.13: Insulins				
Type	*Onset (hr)*	*Peak (hr)*	*Duration (hr)*	*Can be mixed with*
Short Acting/Rapid Acting				
Regular (soluble) insulin	0.5–1	2–4	6–8	All preparations
Prompt insulin zinc suspension (amorphous) or semilente	1	3–6	12–16	Regular, Lente preparations
Intermediate Acting				
Insulin zinc suspension or Lente (Ultra: Semi: 7:3)	1–2	8–10	20–24	Regular, Semilente
Neutral protamine hagedom (NPH) or isophane insulin	1–2	8–10	20–24	Regular
Long Acting				
Extended insulin zinc suspension (Crystalline) or (Ultralente)	4–6	14–18	24–36	Regular, Semilente
Protamine zinc insulin (PZI)	4–6	14–20	24–36	Regular

Appearance: is clear of regular (soluble) insulin and cloudy of other insulins.

Table 23.14: Subcutaneous insulin dosing					
Age (Yr)	*Target Glucose (mg/dl)*	*Total daily insulin in (U/kg/day*)*	*Basal insulin in % of total Daily dose*	*Bolus^ insulin Units added Per 100 mg/dL above target*	*Bolus^ insulin units added per 15 g at meal*
0–5	100–200	0.6–0.7	25–30	0.50	0.50
5–12	80–150	0.7–1.0	40–60	0.75	0.75
12–18	80–130	1.0–1.2	40–50	1.0–2.0#	1.0–2.0

*Newly diagnosed children in the "honeymoon" may only need 60–70% of a full replacement dose. Total daily dose per kg increases with puberty.

^Newly diagnosed children who do not use carbohydrate dosing should divide the nonbasal portion of the daily insulin dose into equal doses for each meal. A dosing scale is then added for each dose. For example, a 6 yr old child who weighs 20 kg needs about (0.7U/kg/24 hr × 20 kg) = 14 U/24 hr with 7U (50%) as basal and 7 U as total daily bolus. Give basal as glargine at bedtime. Give 2 U lispro or aspart before each meal if the blood glucose is within target; substract 1 U if below target; add 0.75 U for each 100 mg/L above target (round the dose to the nearest 0.5 U).

#For finer control, extra insulin may be added in 50 mg/L increments.

Basic and advanced diabetes education: Treatment consists not only of initiation and adjustment of insulin dose but also of education of the patient and family. In the acute phase, the family must learn the "basics" which includes monitoring the child's blood glucose and urine ketones, preparing and injecting the correct insulin dose subcutaneously at the proper time, recognizing and treating low blood glucose reactions, and having a basic meal plan. Written materials covering these basic topics help the family during the 1st few days. Children and their families are also required to complete advanced self-management classes in order to facilitate implementation of flexible insulin management. These educational classes will help patients and their families acquire skills for managing diabetics during athletic activities and sick days.

B. Ketoacidosis

Severe insulinopenia (or lack of effective insulin action) results in 3 general pathways: (i) Excessive glucose production coupled with reduced glucose utilization raises serum glucose, which produces an osmotic diuresis with loss of fluid and electrolytes, dehydration, and potassium loss. Excessive potassium loss is due to activation of the renin-angiotensin aldosterone axis. If glucose elevation and dehydration are severe and persist for several hours, the risk of cerebral edema increases. (ii) Increased catabolic processes result in cellular losses of sodium, potassium, and phosphate. (iii) Increase release of free fatty acids from peripheral fat stores supplies substrate for hepatic keto acid production. When keto acids accumulate, buffer systems are depleted and metabolic acidosis results. Therapy must address both the initiating event (insulinopenia) and the subsequent physiologic disruptions. Reversal of DKA is associated with inherent risks that include hypoglycemia, hypokalemia, and cerebral edema. Any protocol for treatment of DKA must be used with caution (Table 23.15) and close monitoring of the patient.

Hyperglycemia and dehydration: Insulin must be given at the beginning of therapy to accelerate movement of glucose into cells, to control hepatic glucose production, and to stop the movement of fatty acids from the periphery to the liver. An initial insulin bolus does not speed recovery and may increase the risk of hypokalemia and hypoglycemia. Therefore, *insulin infusion is begun without a bolus at a rate of 0.1U/kg/hr.* Rehydration also lowers glucose levels by improving renal perfusion and enhancing renal excretion. The combination of these therapies usually causes a rapid initial decline in serum glucose levels. Once glucose level goes below 180 mg/dl (10 mmol/l), the osmotic diuresis stops and rehydration accelerates without further increase in the infusion rate.

Table 23.15: Diabetic ketoacidosis (DKA) treatment protocol

Time	Therapy	Comments
1st hr	10–20 mL/kg IV bolus 0.9 NaCl or LR insulin drip at 0.05 to 0.10 µ/kg/hr	Quick volume expansion; may be repeated NPO. Monitor I/O, neurologic status. Use flow sheet: Have mannitol at bedside: IV push for cerebral edema.
2nd hr until DKA	0.45% of NaCl plus continue insulin drip	$\text{IV rate} = \dfrac{85\,\text{mL/kg} + \text{maintenance} - \text{bolus}}{23\,\text{hr}}$
resolution	20 mEq/L KPhos and 20 mEq/L KAc 5% glucose if blood sugar >250 mg/dL (14 mmol/L)	If K < 3 mEq/L, give 0.5 to 1.0 mEq/kg as oral K solution OR increase IV K to 80 mEq/L
Variable	Oral intake with subcutaneous insulin	No emesis: $CO_2 \geq 16$ mEq/L; normal electrolytes

Note that the initial IV bolus is considered part of the total fluid allowed in the 1st 24 hr and is substracted before calculating the IV rate.

Maintenance (24 hr) = 100 ml/kg (for the 1st 10 kg) + 50 ml/kg (for the 2nd 10 kg) + 25 ml/kg (for all remaining kg)

Sample calculation of a 30 kg child:

1st hr + 300 ml IV bolus 0.9% NaCl or LR

(85 ml × 30) + 1750 ml–300 ml 175 ml

$$\text{2nd and subsequent hours} = \frac{(85\,\text{ml} \times 30) + 1750\,\text{ml} - 300\,\text{ml}}{23\,\text{hr}} = \frac{175\,\text{ml}}{\text{hr}}$$

(0.45% NaCl with 20 mEq/L Kphos and 20 mEq/L KAC)

I/O: input and output (urine, emesis); KAc: potassium acetate; KPhos: potassium phosphate; LR: Lactated Ringer solution; NaCl: Sodium chloride.

Insulin infusion must continue without causing hypoglycemia for correction of acidosis; glucose as a 5% solution should be added when the serum glucose has decreased to about 250 mg/dl (14 mmol/L) so that there is sufficient time to adjust the infusion before the serum glucose falls further. The insulin infusion can also be lowered from the initial maximal rate once hyperglycemia has resolved. There is potential risk of cerebral edema with the correction of fluid deficit. It is prudent to approach any child in any hyperosmotic state with cautious rehydration.

DKA treatment protocol: Even though DKA can be of variable severity, a common approach to all cases simplifies the therapeutic regimen, and can be used in most children (Table 23.18). Fluids should be calculated on weight. The Milwaukee protocol is designed to restore most electrolyte deficits, to reverse the acidosis and to rehydrate the moderately ill child in about 24 hr. A standard water deficit (85 ml/kg) is assumed. This amount when added to maintenance yields about 4 L/m^2 for children of all sizes. Children with milder DKA recover in 10–20 hr (and need less total IV fluid before switching to oral intake), whereas those with more severe DKA require 30–36 hr with this protocol. Any child can be easily transitioned to oral intake and subcutaneous insulin when DKA has essentially resolved (total CO$_2$>15 mEq/L; pH >7.30; sodium stable between 135 and 145 mEq/L; no emesis). The IV is capped, and the 1st dose of subcutaneous insulin is given with a meal. Children with mild DKA can be discharged after a few hours of therapy in the emergency department, if adequate follow-up can be provided.

A flow sheet is mandatory for accurate monitoring of changes in acidosis, electrolytes, fluid balance, and clinical status, especially if the patient is transferred to the inpatient. Blood testing should occur every 1–2 hr for children with severe DKA and every 3–4 hr for those with mild to moderate DKA.

Cerebral edema: Cerebral edema complicating DKA remains the major cause of morbidity and mortality in children and adolescents with T1DM. The etiology is unknown. The risk factors include acidosis, abnormalities of sodium, potassium, BUN, early administration of insulin and high volumes of fluid. Children with moderate to severe DKA have a higher overall risk and should be treated in an intensive care environment. Mannitol must be used at the earliest sign of cerebral edema (such as change of consciousness, depressed respiration, worsening headache, bradycardia, apnea, pupillary changes, papilledema, posturing, and seizures).

Nonketotic hyperosmolar coma: The syndrome is characterized by severe hyperglycemia (blood glucose > 800 mg/dl), absence of or only slight ketosis, nonketotic acidosis, severe dehydration, depressed sensorium, or frank coma, and various neurologic signs that may include grand mal seizures, hyperthermia, hemiparesis, and positive Babinski signs. Respirations are usually shallow, but coexistent metabolic acidosis is manifested by Kussmaul breathing. Serum osmolality is commonly 350 mOsm/kg or greater. This condition is uncommon in children; among adults, mortality rates have been high. The low production of ketones is attributed mainly to the hyperosmolality.

The goals of treatment of nonketotonic hyperosmolar coma are rapid repletion of the vascular volume deficit and very slow correction of the hyperosmolar state. One-half isotonic saline (0.45% NaCl) is administered at a rate estimated to replace 50% of the volume deficit in the first 12 hr; and the remainder is administered during the ensuing 24 hr. When the blood glucose concentration approaches: 300 mg/dL, the hydrating fluid should be changed to 5% dextrose in 0.2 normal saline. Approximately 20 mEq/L of potassium chloride should be added to prevent hypokalemia. Serum potassium and plasma glucose composition should be monitored at 2 hr intervals for 1st 12 hr and at 4 hr intervals for the next 24 hr to permit appropriate adjustments of administered potassium and insulin.

Insulin can be given by continuous IV infusion beginning with the 2nd hr of fluid therapy. Blood glucose may decrease with fluid therapy alone. The IV insulin dosage should be 0.05 U/kg/hr of regular rather than 0.1 U/kg/hr as advocated for patients with DKA.

Nutritional management: In outlining nutritional requirements for the child on the basis of age, sex, weight and activity, food preferences, including cultural and ethnic ones, must be considered. The caloric mixture should comprise approximately 55% carbohydrate, 30% fat, and 15% protein. Approximately 70% of the carbohydrate content should be derived from complex carbohydrates such as starch; intake of sucrose and highly refined sugars should be limited. Glucose from refined sugars, including carbonated beverages is rapidly absorbed and may cause wide swings in the metabolic pattern; carbonated beverages should be sugar free. Each carbohydrate exchange unit is 15 g. Diets with high fiber content are useful in improving control of blood sugar. The total daily caloric intake is divided to provide 20% at breakfast, 20% at lunch, and 30% at dinner, leaving 10% for each of the midmorning, midafternoon, and evening snacks, if they are desired. In older children, the midmorning snack may be omitted and its caloric equivalent added to lunch. The caloric needs (Kcal required/kg) for children include 120: 0–12 mo; 100–75: 1–10 yr; 35: 11–15 yr (female); 30: ≥ 16 yr (female); 80–55 (average 65): 11–20 yr (male).

Monitoring: Self-monitoring of blood glucose (SMBG) is essential component of managing diabetes. Parents and patients should be taught to use glucose measuring instrument (strips impregnated with glucose oxidase that permit blood glucose measurement from a drop of blood) and measure blood glucose at least 4 times daily—before breakfast, lunch, and supper, and at bedtime. A reliable index of long-term glycemic control is provided by measurement of glycosylated hemoglobin (HbA1c). The formation HbA1c is a slow reaction that is dependent on the prevailing concentration of blood glucose; it continues irreversibility throughout the red blood cell's life span approximately 120 days. Therefore, HbA1c should be performed 3–4 times per year to obtain a profile of long-term glycemic control.

Exercise: No form of exercise, including competitive sports, should be forbidden to the diabetic child. A major complication of exercise in diabetic patients is the presence of a hypoglycemic reaction during or within hours after exercise. Therefore, each patient, guided by the physician, should develop an appropriate regimen for regularly planned exercise.

Somogyi phenomenon, Dawn phenomenon, and Brittle diabetes: There are several reasons that blood glucose levels increase in the early morning hours before breakfast. The dawn phenomenon is thought to be due mainly to overnight growth hormone secretion and increased insulin clearance. It is normal physiologic process seen in most nondiabetic adolescents, who compensate with more insulin output. A child with T1DM cannot compensate and may actually have declining insulin levels if using NPH or Lente. The *dawn phenomenon* is usually recurrent and modestly elevates most morning glucose levels.

Rarely, high morning glucose is due to the Somogyi phenomenon, a theoretical rebound from late night or early morning hypoglycemia, thought to be due to an exaggerated counter-regulatory response. It is unlikely to be a common cause, in that most children remain hypoglycemic (do not rebound) once night-time glucose levels decline. Continuous glucose monitoring system will help clarify the cause of elevated morning glucose levels.

The term brittle diabetes has been used to describe the child, usually an adolescent female, with unexplained wide fluctuations in blood glucose, often with recurrent DKA, who is taking large doses of insulin. An inherent physiologic abnormality is rarely present; rather psychosocial or psychiatric problems, including eating disorders, and disturbed family are usually present. Hospitalization is usually needed, where the patient will show normal insulin responsiveness in changed environment.

Nonadherence: Nonadherence to instructions regarding nutritional and insulin therapy and in noncompliance with self monitoring is usually seen where there is family conflict, denial, and feeling of anxiety. Many of these problems can be averted through continued emphatic counseling.

Sick-day management: Infections can often disrupt glucose control and may precipitate DKA. In addition, the diabetic child is at increased risk of dehydration if hyperglycemia causes an osmotic dieresis or if ketosis causes emesis. If anorexia occurs, lack of caloric intake increases the risk of hypoglycemia. There is no need to admit the child each time the child gets unwell. Parents should be educated in sick day management. Insulin should not be stopped even when the child is not eating much.

Blood glucose and urine for ketones should be checked 4 hrly at home by parents. When blood glucose is more than 250 mg/dl, an extra dose of short acting insulin should be given. If the regular meals are not consumed, then semisolids or liquids are given. If blood glucose is less than 100 mg/dl sweet liquids can be given but insulin should not be stopped.

Child may need hospitalization if after doing all the above any of the following appears: vomiting; oliguria; ketones rising in the urine; child becomes drowsy or breathless.

Management during surgery: Surgery can disrupt glucose control in the same way as can intercurrent infections. Stress hormones associated with the underlying condition as well as with surgery itself decrease insulin sensitivity. This increase glucose levels exacerbates fluid losses, and may initiate DKA. On the other hand, caloric intake is usually restricted, which decreases glucose levels. The net effect is as difficult to predict as during an infection. Monitoring and frequent insulin adjustments are required to maintain euglycemia and avoid ketosis. Maintaining glucose control and avoiding DKA are best accomplished with IV-insulin and fluids (Table 23.16). IV insulin is continued after surgery as the child begins to take oral fluids; the IV fluids can be steadily decreased as oral intake increases. When full oral intake is achieved, the IV may be capped and subcutaneous insulin begun. When surgery is elective, it is best performed early in the day, allowing the patient maximal recovery time to restart oral intake and subcutaneous insulin therapy.

Long-term complications: The increasing prolonged survival of the diabetic child is associated with an increasing prevalence of complications. Complications of DM can be divided into 3 major categories: (1) microvascular complications, specifically, retinopathy and nephropathy; (2) macrovascular complications, particularly accelerated coronary artery disease, cerebrovascular disease, and peripheral vascular disease; and (3) neuropathies, both peripheral and autonomic. In addition, cataracts may occur more frequently. Therefore, children with type 1DM should be screened as stated in Table 23.17.

Prevention: Delaying the introduction of cow's milk protein, delaying introduction of cereals, and increasing the duration of breastfeeding are all potentially beneficial.

Prognosis: T1DM is a serious, chronic disease. The average life span of individuals with diabetes is about 10 yr shorter than that of nondiabetic population. Although diabetic children eventually attain a height within the normal adult range, puberty may be delayed, and the final height may be less than the genetic potential.

Pancreas and islet transplantation and regeneration: In an attempt to cure T1DM, transplantation of a segment of the pancreas or of isolated islets has been performed. But transplantation of pancreas is not recommended in children and islets of Langerhans for transplantation is considered now. Regeneration of islets is an approach that could cure T1DM.

Type 2 Diabetes Mellitus (T2DM)

T2DM, formerly known as non-insulin dependent diabetes or adult-onset diabetes, is a heterogeneous disorder, characterized by peripheral insulin resistance and failure of β-cell to keep up with increasing insulin demand. These patients have relative rather than absolute insulin deficiency. T2DM is considered a polygenic disease aggravated by environmental factors, such as low physical activity and excessive caloric intake. Most patients are obese though the disease can occasionally be seen in normal weight individuals. Asians in particular appear at risk for T2DM at lower degrees of total adiposity. The epidemic of T2DM in children and adolescents parallel the emergence of the obesity epidemic. Although obesity itself is associated with insulin resistance, diabetes does not develop until there is some degree of failure of insulin secretion. Insulin secretion in response to glucose or other stimuli is always lower in persons with T2DM than in control subjects matched for age, sex, weight, and equivalent glucose concentration.

Table 23.16: Guidelines for intravenous insulin coverage during surgery

Blood glucose level (mg/dL)	Insulin infusion (units/kg/hr)	Blood glucose monitoring
<120	00	1 hr
121–200	0.03	2 hr
200–300	0.06	2 hr
300–400	0.08	1 hr*
400	0.10	1 hr*

An infusion of 5% glucose and 0.45% saline solution with 20 mEq/L of potassium acetate is given as 1.5 times maintenance rate.
*Check urine ketones.

Table 23.17: Screening guidelines

	When to commence screening	Frequency
Retinopathy	After 5 yr duration in prepubertal children, after 2 yr in pubertal children	1–2 yearly
Nephropathy	After 5 yr duration in prepubertal children, after 2 yr in pubertal children	Annually
Neuropathy	Unclear	Unclear
Macrovascular disease	After age 2 yr	Every 5 yr
Thyroid disease	At diagnosis	Every 2–3 yr
Celiac disease	At diagnosis	Every 2–3 yr

Source: Modified from Glastras SJ, MohsinF, Donaghue KC. Complications of diabetes mellitus in childhood. *Pediatr Clin North Am* 2005; 52:1735–1753.

Genetics: T2DM has a strong genetic component; concordance rates among identical twins are virtually 100% for type 2 and only 30–50% for type 1DM. The genetic basis for type 2DM is complex and incompletely defined; no single defect predominates as does the HLA association with T1DM. Acanthosis nigrans may be a marker for insulin resistance, hyperinsulinemia, and eventually type 2DM. Hirsutism, associated with the polycystic ovary syndrome, premature adrenarche, or mild mutations in steroidogenic enzymes, is frequently associated with insulin resistance in children and adolescents and may be a forerunner of the future development of type 2 DM.

Environmental and lifestyle-related risk factors: Obesity is the most important lifestyle factor associated with development of diabetes associated with the intake of high-energy foods, physical inactivity, and TV viewing.

Clinical features: T2DM children are highest in the 15–19 yr of age group while cases may be seen as young as 6 yr of age. Family history of T2DM is present in practically all cases. Typically these patients are obese and present with mild symptoms of polyuria and polydipsia, or are asymptomatic and detected on screening tests. Presentation with diabetic ketoacidosis occurs in up to 10% of cases. Physical examination frequently reveals the presence of acanthocytosis nigricans, most commonly on the neck and in other flexural areas. Other findings may include striae and an increased waist-hip ratio. Laboratory testing reveals elevated HbA1c levels and HbA1c values are higher at diagnosis among minority youth. Hyperlipidemia characterized by elevated triglycerides and low density lipoprotein (LDL) cholesterol levels are commonly seen in patients with T2DM at diagnosis. Since hyperglycemia develops slowly and patients may be asymptomatic for months or years after they develop T2DM, screening for T2DM is recommended in high-risk children (Table 23.18).

Treatment: Type 2 diabetes is a progressive syndrome that gradually leads to complete insulin deficiency during the patient's life. A systemic approach for treatment of T2DM should be implemented, including adding insulin when hypoglycemic oral agent failure occurs. Lifestyle modification (diet and exercise) is an essential part of the treatment regimen and consultation with a dietitian is usually necessary. Most physicians recommend a low-calorie, low-fat diet and 30–60 minutes of physical activity at least 5 times per week. Screen time should be limited to 1–2 hr per day. When lifestyle interventions fail to normalize blood glucose, oral hypoglycemic agents are introduced for management of persistent hyperglycemia. Patients who present with DKA or with markedly elevated HbA1c (> 9.0%) will require treatment with insulin using protocols similar to those used for treating T1DM. Once blood glucose levels are under control most cases can be managed with oral hypoglycemic agents and lifestyle changes, but some patients will continue to require insulin therapy.

The most commonly used oral hypoglycemic agent is *metformin*. Renal function must be assessed before starting metformin as impaired renal function has been associated with potentially fatal lactic acidosis in adults. Significant hepatic dysfunction is also a contraindication, though mild elevations in liver enzymes may not be an absolute contraindication. The usual starting dose is 500 mg bid and this may be increased to a maximum dose of 2,500 mg per day. Abdominal symptoms are common early in the course of treatment, but in most cases will resolve with time.

Complications: 92% of the patients with T2DM have 2 or more elements of the metabolic syndrome

Table 23.18: Testing for type 2 diabetes in children
Criteria*
• Overweight (BMI > 85th percentile for age and sex, weight for height > 85th percentile or weight > 120% of ideal for height)
Plus
Any 2 of the following factors:
• Family history of T2DM in 1st or 2nd degree relative
• Race/ethnicity
Signs of insulin resistance or conditions associated with insulin resistance (acanthosis nigrans, hypertension, dyslipidemia, polycystic ovary syndrome)
Age of initiation: Age at 10 yr or at onset of puberty if puberty occurs at a younger age
Frequency: Every 2 yr
Test: Fasting plasma glucose

*Clinical judgement should be used to test for diabetes who do not meet these criteria in high-risk patients.
Source: American Diabetes Association: Type 2 diabetes in children and adolescents. *Diabetes Care* 2000; 23: 386.

(hypertension, hypertriglyceridemia, decreased HDL, increased waist circumference), including 70% with hypertension. In addition, the incidence of micro-albuminuria and diabetic nephropathy appears to be higher in T2DM than it is in T1DM. Complications associated with all forms of diabetes and recommendations for screening are noted in Table 23.17 while Table 23.19 shows lists of additional conditions particularly associated with T2DM.

Prevention: There are difficulties in achieving good glucose control and preventing diabetes complications that is particularly true for T2DM, which is clearly linked to modifiable risk factors (obesity, a sedentary lifestyle). However, lifestyle intervention or drug intervention in adult individuals with impaired glucose tolerance (IGT) prevented or delayed the onset of T2DM. Lifestyle intervention reduced diabetes incidence by 58%; metformin reduced the incidence by 31% compared with placebo. Life-style interventions have similar beneficial effects in obese adolescents with IGT.

Impaired Glucose Tolerance

The term impaired glucose tolerance (IGT) is suggested as a replacement for terms such as asymptomatic diabetes, chemical diabetes, subclinical diabetes, borderline diabetes, and latent diabetes in order to avoid the stigma associated with the term diabetes mellitus. Such diagnostic labels may influence the choice of vocation, eligibility for health or life insurance, and self image. Although IGT refers to a metabolic stage that is intermediate between normal glucose homeostasis and diabetes, but only a few children with IGT go on to acquire diabetes; estimates range from zero to 10%. There is disagreement about whether the degree of glucose intolerance is useful as a prognostic index of the likelihood of progression, the insulin response during glucose tolerance testing is severely impaired. Islet cell or insulin autoantibodies as well as the HLA-DR3 or -DR4 haplotype are commonly found in those who go on to develop clinical diabetes. Now most obese children with IGT, insulin responses during oral glucose tolerance test are higher than the mean for age-adjusted but not weight-adjusted control objects; these individuals have some resistance to the effects of insulin rather than a total inability to secrete it. In healthy nondiabetic children, the glucose response during an oral glucose tolerans test is similar at all ages. But plasma insulin responses during the test increase progressively within the age span of about 3–15 yr and are significantly higher during puberty. Therefore interpretation of these responses requires comparison with age- and puberty-adjusted responses.

The performance of the glucose tolerance test should be standardized according to currently accepted criteria. These include at least 3 days of a well-balanced diet containing approximately 50% of calories from carbohydrates, fasting from midnight until the time of the test in the morning, and a dose of glucose for the test of 1.75 g/kg but not more than 75 g plasma samples are obtained before ingestion of the glucose and at 1, 2, and 3 hr thereafter. The arbitrarily designated response to the test that identifies IGT is a fasting plasma glucose value of less than 125 mg/dl and a value of 2 hr of more than 140 mg/dl but less than 200 mg/dl (Table 23.20). A fasting glucose concentration of 99 mg/dl (5.5 mmol/L) is the upper limit of "normal". In the absence of pregnancy, IGT is not a clinical entity but rather a risk factor for future diabetes and cardiovascular disease. This may be observed as an intermediate stage in any of the diseases (T1DM, T2DM, other specific types of secondary diabetes, insulin resistance syndrome). IGT is often associated with the insulin resistance syndrome (also known as syndrome X or the metabolic syndrome), which consists of insulin resistance, compensatory hyperinsulinemia to maintain glucose homeostasis, obesity (especially abdominal, or visceral obesity), dyslipidemia of the high-triglyceride or low- or high-density lipoprotein type, or both, and hypertension.

Table 23.19: Monitoring for complications and co-morbidities	
Condition	Screening test
Hypertension	Blood pressure
Fatty liver	AST, ALT, possibly ultrasound
Polycystic ovary syndrome	Menstrual history, assessment for androgen excess with free/total testosterone, DHEA
Microalbuminuria	Urine albumin concentration and albumin/creatinine ratio
Dyslipidemia*	Fasting lipid profile (Total, LDL, HDL, cholesterol, triglycerides)
Sleep apnea	Sleep study to assess overnight oxygen saturation

*Obtain at diagnosis and every 2 yr.
Source: Hironaka K, PihokerC: Type 2 diabetes in youth. *Curr Probl Pediatr Adolesc Health Care* 2004; 34: 249–280.

Table 23.20: Diagnostic criteria for impaired glucose tolerance and diabetes mellitus

Impaired glucose tolerance test (IGT)	Diabetes mellitus (DM)
Fasting glucose 110–125 mg/dl (6.1–7.0 mmol/L) 2hr plasma glucose during the OGTT < 200 mg/dl (11.1 mmol/L) but ≤ 140 mg/dl	Symptoms* of DM plus random plasma glucose ≥ 200 mg/dl (11.1 mmol/L) or Fasting plasma glucose ≥ 126 mg/dl (7.0 mmol/L) or 2–hr plasma glucose during the OGTT ≥ 200 mg/dl

*Symptoms include polyuria, polydipsia, and unexplained weight loss with glycosuria and ketonuria; OGTT, oral glucose tolerance test.

From Report of the Expert Committee on the diagnosis and classification of diabetes mellitus care 1999; 201 (Suppl 1): S5.

Diabetic Cheiroarthropathy

Diabetic cheiroarthropathy, or arthropathy of the joints of the hands and fingers, is a complication of juvenile-onset diabetes mellitus. The soft tissues of the hands and fingers undergo progressive thickening and tightening, leading to contractures of the small joints in the hand, but without fingertip tapering and loss of digital pulp characteristic of sclerodactyly in scleroderma.

Diabetes Mellitus of the Newborn

Transient: Neonatal diabetes is rare, with an estimated incidence of 1 per 100,000 newborns. Onset of classic autoimmune TNDM before the age of 6 mo is most unusual.

The syndrome of transient DM in the newborn has its onset in the 1st wk of life and persists several weeks to months before spontaneous resolution. Median duration is 12 wk. It occurs most often in infants who are small for gestational age and is characterized by hyperglycemia and glycosuria, resulting in severe dehydration, and at times metabolic acidosis, but with only minimal or no ketonemia or ketonuria. *Abnormalities of chromosome 6q24 are common* in transient neonatal DM (TNDM). This syndrome of TNDM should be distinguished from the severe hyperglycemia that may occur in hypertonic dehydration; that usually occurs in infants beyond the neonatal period and responds promptly to rehydration with minimal or no requirement for insulin.

Administration of insulin is mandatory during the active phase. One to 2 U/kg/24 hr of an intermediate-acting insulin in 2 divided doses usually results in dramatic improvement and accelerated growth and gain in weight. Insulin dose should be gradually reduced as soon as recurrent hypoglycemia becomes manifested or after 2 mo of age. Genetic testing is now available for 6q24 abnormalities.

Permanent: DM in the newborn period may be permanent if associated with the rare syndrome of pancreatic agenesis. Majority of these infants were small at birth. Almost one half had permanent diabetes, one third had transient diabetes, and about one fourth had transient diabetes that recurred when they were 7–20 yr old.

Alemzadeh R, Ali O. Introduction and classification: Diabetes Mellitus. In: Kliegman RM, Stanton BF, St.Geme JW, NF Schor NF, Behrman RE. *Nelson Textbook of Pediatrics*. 19th edn. New Delhi: Elsevier, 2011; 1968.

Amiel SA, Alberti KGMM. Inhaled insulin. *Br Med J* 2004; 228. 1215–1216.

Deneman D. Type 1 diabetes. Lancet 2006; 367: 847– 858.

Dhabadgaon P, Bhatia E, Bhatia V, Colman P. Islet-cell antibodies in malnutrition related diabetes from North India. *Diabetes Res Clin Prac* 1996; 34:73–78.

Litton J, Rice A, Friedman N, et al. Insulin pump therapy in toddlers and preschool children with type 1 diabetes mellitus. *J Pediatr* 2002; 141: 490–495.

Report of the Expert Committee on the Diagnosis and Classification of Diabetes Mellitus. American Diabetic Association: Clinical practice recommendation. *Diabetes Care* 2000; 23 (Suppl): S4–S19.

The diabetes control and complications trial research group. The effect of intensive treatment of diabetes on the development and progression of long-term complications in insulin dependent diabetes mellitus. *N Engl J Med* 1993; 329: 977–986.

24.1 NEUROLOGICAL EVALUATION

The central nervous system (CNS) should be examined by means of a through history, physical examination, and ancillary studies to determine the location (and causes) of abnormal function. The most important component of a neurologic history is a child's *developmental assessment* (*see* Chapter 2). A loss of skills (regression) over time strongly suggests an underlying degenerative disease of the CNS (*see* Section 24.11). Table 24.1 provides some guidelines regarding the upper range of normal skills that are usually recalled by the parents and that, if not present, should alert the physician.

Age (mo)	Gross motor	Fine motor	Social skills	Language
3	Supports weight on forearms	Opens hands spontaneously	Smiles	Coos, Laughs
6	Sits momentarily	Transfers objects	Shows likes and dislikes	Babbles
9	Pulls to stand	Pincer grasp	Plays pat-a-cake, peek-a-boo	Imitates sounds
12	Walks with one hand held	Releases an object on command	Comes when called	1–2 meaningful words
18	Walks upstairs with assistance	Feeds from a spoon	Mimics actions of others	At least 6 words
24	Runs	Builds a tower of 6 blocks	Plays with others	2–3 word sentences

Table 24.1: Guidelines regarding the upper range of normal skills

Neurological Examination

Neurologic examination of a child begins at the outset of the interview. *Observe* during interaction with parents, while playing, or during the time when little attention is directed to the child as it can provide useful information. The child has characteristic facies, an unusual posture, or an abnormality of motor function manifested by a gait disturbance or hemiparesis. Also observe the child's *behavior* during the interview. A normally inquisitive child or toddler may play independently but soon wishes to become involved with interview process. A child with an attention disorder may display inappropriate behaviors in the examination room, whereas a neurologically abnormal child may appear lethargic or disinterested or may show complete lack of awareness of the environment. The interaction between the parent and child should also be noted.

The examination should be conducted in a setting where a child is comfortable. Children may be most comfortable on a parent's lap or interacting on the floor of the examination room. Cooperation is essential for a comprehensive neurologic examination. First find out whether the child is right or left handed. *Handedness* is usually established by the 3rd year. Also note the particular *odors/smells* noted by the parents or the examiner, as they point to certain metabolic disorders (the "musty" smell of phenylketonuria or the "sweety feet" smell of isovaleric academia). If a hearing assessment is considered necessary, it should be performed first before other examination.

Examination of the head: Correct measurement of the head circumference is important. An infant has two fontanels at birth: a diamond shaped open anterior fontanel that is situated at the midline at the junction of the coronal and the sagittal sutures and a posterior fontanel placed between the intersection of the occipital and parietal bones that may be closed at birth or, at the most, admit the tip of a finger. The posterior fontanel is usually closed and no palpable after the first 6 to 8 weeks of life; its persistence suggests underlying hydrocephalus or the possibility of congenital hypothyroidism. The anterior fontanel varies greatly in size but the usual normal measurement is 20 ± 10 mm. The fontanel is normally slightly depressed and pulsatile and is best evaluated when an infant is held upright and is asleep or feeding. The average time of closure is 18 months, but the fontanel may normally close as early as 9–12 months. A bulging fontanel indicates increased intracranial pressure, but vigorous crying can cause a protuberant fontanel in a normal infant. Large anterior fontanel is associated with hydrocephalus and prematurity. A very small or absent anterior fontanel at birth may indicate premature fusion of the sutures or microcephaly. Auscultation of the skull is an important adjunct to a neurologic examination. Cranial bruits are most prominent over the anterior fontanel, temporal region, or the orbits and are best heard through the diaphragm of the stethoscope. Bruits may be discovered in normal children younger than 4 yr, febrile illness, severe anemia, arteriovenous malformations of the middle cerebral artery or vein of Galen, and murmurs arising from the heart or great vessels.

Cranial nerves: There are 12 cranial nerves: Olfactory (1); Optic (2); Oculomotor (3); Trochlear (4); Trigeminal Nerve (5); Abducens (6); Facial Nerve (7); Auditory Nerve (8); Glossopharyngeal Nerve (9); Vagus Nerve (10); Accessory Nerve (11); Hypoglossal Nerve (12). The 3rd to 12th cranial nerves arise from the brainstem and innervate facial, cranial and cervical tissues. The 1st and 2nd cranial nerves actually consist of central nervous tissue rather than peripheral nerves. All the 12 cranial nerves may be involved in disease processes in their intracranial and extracranial courses, and at their sites of origin within the brain and brainstem. The cranial nerves are examined in numerical order, except III, IV, and VI because of their similar function (*see* Fig. 24.1 in CD).

Motor examination: The motor examination includes testing of strength (power), muscle bulk, tone, posture, locomotion and motility, superficial and deep tendon reflexes, and the presence of primitive reflexes, when applicable (*see* Figs 24.2 and 24.3 in CD).

Sensory examination: Apart from the special senses of vision, hearing, taste and smell, there are six main sensory modalities that can be tested at the bedside: pain, temperature, tactile sensibility (this includes light touch and pressure, and tactile localization and discrimination), vibration, position sense (the appreciation of passive movement), stereognosis (recognition of the size, shape, weight and form of objects).

Gait: During the neurological examination observe the gait. The *spastic gait* is characterized by stiffness and by stepping like a tin soldier. Spastic children may walk on tip toes because of tightness or contractures of the Achilles tendons. *Hemiparesis* is associated with a decreased arm swing on the affected side and a lateral circular motion of the leg (*circumduction gait*). Extrapyramidal movements, such as dystonia or chorea, may become apparent while the child is walking or running. *Cerebellar ataxia* produces a broad-based unsteady gait and if, severe, the child requires support to prevent falling. Heel-to-toe or tandem walking is performed poorly in parents with abnormalities of the cerebellum. A *waddling gait* results from weakness of the proximal hip-girdle (e.g. Duchene and Becker muscular dystrophies). Affected children often develop a compensatory lordosis and have difficulty in climbing stairs. Weakness or hypotonia of the lower extremities may result in genu recurvatum and flat feet, which causes a clumsy-*tentative gait*. Scoliosis may cause an abnormal gait and can result from disorders of muscle and spinal cord.

Cerebellar lesions: The clinical signs of cerebellar lesions are cerebellar ataxia, intention tremor, and involvement of limbs, trunk and external ocular movements (nystagmus), past-pointing, rebound, impaired ability to generate alternating rhythmic movements (dysdiadochokinesia).

Child with Paralysis

1. **Hemiplegia** is paralysis of the arm, leg, and trunk on the same side of the body. Hemiplegia is more severe than hemiparesis, wherein one half of the body has less marked weakness. Hemiplegia and Hemiparesis may be congenital, or they might be acquired conditions resulting from an illness, an injury, or a stroke. Common causes by etiology: (i) *Vascular:* cerebral hemorrhage, stroke (*see* Section 24.6); (ii) *Infective:* encephalitis, meningitis, brain abscess; (iii) *Neoplastic:* glioma-meningioma; (iv) *Demyelination:* disseminated sclerosis, lesions to the internal capsule; (v) *Traumatic:* cerebral lacerations,

subdural hematoma rare cause of hemiplegia is due to local anaesthetic injections given intra-arterially rapidly, instead of given in a nerve branch; (vi) *Congenital:* cerebral palsy; (vii) *Disseminated:* multiple sclerosis; (viii) Psychological: parasomnia (nocturnal hemiplegia).

2. **Paraplegia** is an impairment in motor or sensory function of the lower extremities. It is usually caused by spinal cord injury or a congenital condition such as spina bifida that affects the neural elements of the spinal canal. The area of the spinal canal that is affected in paraplegia is either the thoracic, lumbar, or sacral regions. If all four limbs are affected by paralysis, quadriplegia is the proper terminology. If only one limb is affected, the correct term is monoplegia. *Spastic paraplegia* is a form of paraplegia defined by spasticity of the affected muscles, rather than flaccid paralysis.

3. **Flaccid paralysis** is a clinical manifestation characterized weakness or paralysis and reduced muscle tone. Flaccid paralysis can be associated with a lower motor neuron lesion. This is in contrast to an upper motor neuron lesion, which often presents with spastic paralysis, although early on this may present with flaccid paralysis. This abnormal condition may be caused by disease or by trauma affecting the nerves associated with the involved muscles. For example, if the somatic nerves to a skeletal muscle are severed, then the muscle will exhibit flaccid paralysis. When muscles enter this state, they become limp and cannot contract. This condition can become fatal if it affects the respiratory muscles, posing the threat of suffocation. The term acute flaccid paralysis (AFP) is often used to describe a sudden onset, as might be found with polio. AFP is the most common sign of acute polio, and used for surveillance during polio outbreaks. Causes of flaccid paralysis include poliomyelitis, enteroviruses, echoviruses, and adenoviruses, transverse myelitis, Guillain-Barré syndrome, traumatic neuritis, Reye's syndrome, botulism, curare, and venomous snakes (kraits, mambas, and cobras).

Specific Diagnostic Procedures
Lumbar Puncture and Cerebrospinal Fluid Examination

Examination of cerebrospinal fluid (CSF) is essential in confirming the diagnosis of meningitis, encephalitis, subarachnoid hemorrhage, pseudotumor cerebri, demyelinating, degenerative, and collagen vascular diseases and the presence of tumor cells within the subarachnoid space.

Preparation of the patient: The skin is thoroughly prepared with a cleansing agent and the patient is placed in the lateral recumbent position. An assistant has a vital role in positioning, restraining, and comforting the patient. The physician should wear mask, gloves and gown. The patient should be draped. The neck and legs of the patient are flexed by an assistant to enlarge the intervertebral spaces. The ideal interspace for lumbar puncture (LP) is L3–L4 or L4–L5, which is determined by drawing an imaginary horizontal line from one superior iliac spine of the ileum to the other. The skin and underlying tissue are anesthetized with a local anesthetic. A 22-gauge, 1–2 inches, sharp, beveled spinal needle with a properly fitting stylet is introduced into the midsagittal plane, directed slightly in the cephalic direction. The stylet is removed frequently as the needle is slowly advanced to determine whether CSF is present. A pop (short, sharp, explosive sound) is felt as the needle penetrates the dura and enters the subarachnoid space. A manometer and a three-way stopcock may be attached to obtain an opening pressure. The opening pressure in the recumbent and relaxed position averages 100 mm of fluid; the range in the flexed lateral decubitus position is 60–180 mm of fluid. The pressure is recorded with a child positioned comfortably with the head and legs extended. The pressure is elevated in a crying, uncooperative and struggling patient. Sick neonates should be placed in the upright position for a spinal tap, because decreased ventilation and perfusion abnormalities leading to respiratory arrest are more common in the recumbent position in this age group.

Contraindications for performing an LP are listed in the Box 24.1. Transtentorial herniation or herniation of the cerebellar tonsils may develop after the procedure, therefore, the eyes should be examined for the presence of pailledema, and obtaining a head CT are mandatory before proceeding with an LP.

Cerebrospinal fluid examination: Normal CSF is the color of water (Table 24.2). Normal CSF does not contain RBCs. The presence of RBCs indicates a

Table 24.2: Normal CSF findings

Pressure	60–180 mm of fluid (average 100 mm of fluid) in the recumbent and relaxed position
Color	Color of water
Cells	Up to 5/mm^3 WBCs (normal newborn may have as many as 15/mm^3).
Protein	10–40 mg/dl in a child and in a neonate as high as 120 mg/dl
Glucose	About 60% of the blood glucose

traumatic tap or a subarachnoid hemorrhage. CSF containing blood should be centrifuged immediately. The supernatant of a bloody tap is clear, but it is xanthochromic in the presence of a subarachnoid hemorrhage.

Subdural Tap

Subdural tap is performed to establish the diagnosis of a subdural effusion or hematoma. A blunt, short-beveled 20-gauge needle and stylet are used for the procedure. The subdural space is approached at the lateral border of the anterior fontanel or along the upper margin of the coronal suture at least 2–3 cm from the midline to prevent injury to the underlying sagittal sinus. After adequate cleansing and preparation of the skull, including shaving of the hair from the operative site, the patient is placed in the supine position and is firmly held by an attendant. After a local anesthetic, the needle and stylet are slowly advanced through the skin and underlying tissue with a z-like movement until the dura is entered with a sudden popping sensation. Now prevent advancement of the needle into the cerebral cortex, which in infant is ≈ 1.5 cm from the skin surface. A hemostat attached ≈ 5–7 mm from the beveled end of the needle should provide adequate safeguard. The subdural fluid, which may squirt out under pressure, is collected and sent for protein analysis, cell count and culture. The color of the fluid may be xanthochromic, bright red or oily brown (depending on the age of the subdural collections). Bilateral subdural taps may be indicated, because subdural collections are bilateral in most cases. The amount of fluid removed with each tap should be limited to a total of 15–20 ml from each side in order to prevent rebleeding from a sudden shift of the intracranial contents. At the termination of the procedure, a sterile dressing is applied. The child is placed in a sitting position that tends to prevent leakage of fluid from the puncture site.

Ventricular Tap

A ventricular tap is used for the removal of CSF in the management of life-threatening increased intracranial pressure (ICP) associated with hydrocephalus, when

Box 24.1: Contraindications for performing lumbar puncture

1. Elevated intracranial pressure (ICP) owing to a suspected mass lesion of the brain or spinal cord
2. Symptoms and signs of pending cerebral herniation in a child with probable meningitis
3. Critical illness
4. Skin infection at the site of the LP
5. Thrombocytopenia (platelet count < 20 × 10^9/L)

the conservative methods have failed. For an infant, the procedure is similar to a subdural tap. A 20-gauge ventricular needle with a stylet is placed in the lateral border of the anterior fontanel and is directed toward the inner canthus of the ipsilateral eye. The needle is advanced slowly and, the stylet is removed frequently to determine the presence of CSF. The ventricle is usually encountered about 4 cm from the skin surface.

Neurologic Procedures

Skull roentgenogram may demonstrate fractures, intracranial calcification, craniosynostosis, congenital anomalies, or bony defects and evidence of increased ICP. Acute increased ICP is characterized by separation of the sutures, whereas erosion of the posterior clinoid processes, enlargement of the sella turcica, and an increase in convolutional markings indicate long-standing intracranial hypertension.

Computed tomography (CT) scanning is a noninvasive and rapid procedure. Sedation is usually required for infants and young children because a lack of head movement is essential during the study. Phenobarbitone, 4 mg/kg intramuscularly 10 min before the CT scan, with a supplementary dose of 2 mg/kg intramuscularly 1–1½ hr later if necessary, is usually effective. Chloral hydrate, 50–75 mg/kg orally 45 min before the procedure, is an alternative method of sedation. CT scan is useful in demonstrating congenital malformations of brain, including hydrocephalus and porencephalic cysts, subdural collections, cerebral atrophy, intracranial calcification, intracerebral hematoma, brain tumors and areas of cerebral edema, infarction, and demyelination.

Magnetic resonance imaging (MRI) is a noninvasive procedure and is especially well suited for the study of neoplasms, cerebral edema, acute stroke (diffusion-weighted MRI, demyelination, degenerative diseases, and congenital anomalies, particularly of the posterior fossa and spinal cord. MRI can detect small plaques in patients with multiple sclerosis and areas of local gliosis in children with uncontrolled seizures. MRI is routinely used in the evaluation of children who are potential candidates for epilepsy surgery. Intracerebral calcifications are not detected by MRI. The contrast agent, gadolinium-DTPA, is useful during MRI, especially to highlight lesions associated with a disrupted blood–brain barrier. *MR angiography* **(MRA)** and *venography* **(MRV)** provide detailed images of major intracranial vasculature structures and assist in the diagnosis of diseases such as stroke, vascular malformations, and cerebral vascular thrombosis. *Functional* **MRI (fMRI)** is a noninvasive technique for detecting and mapping with high resolution the hemodynamic changes produced by localized brain activity during specific cognitive and/or, sensory-motor functions. It is useful for presurgical localization of critical brain functions.

Single-photon emission computed tomography **(SPECT)**, using 99mTc hexamethyl propylenamine oxime (Tc99m-HMPAO), is to study regional cerebral flow. SPECT is particularly useful in investigating cerebral vascular disease in children (systemic lupus erythematosus), herpes encephalitis and for localization of focal epileptiform discharges and recurrent brain tumors. *Cerebral angiography* is reserved for the study of vascular disorders. The procedure requires a general anesthetic in most children. MRA may reduce the need for contrast invasive angiography. *Cranial ultrasonography* is performed for the detection of periventricular leukomalacia, intracranial hemorrhage, hydrocephalus, and intracranial tumors in infants with a patent fontanel. The procedure is used intraoperatively in older children for placing shunts, locating small tumors, and directing needle biopsies. *Myelography* was used in the past for demonstrating congenital anomalies, tumors and vascular malformations of the spinal cord are not used now. MRI is superior in most cases to contrast myelography and is not associated with arachnoiditis, which occasionally complicates injection of contrast material into the subarachnoid space.

Electroencephalography

An electroencephalogram (EEG) provides a continuous recording of electrical activity between reference electrodes placed on the scalp. Electrical activity most likely originates from postsynaptic potentials in the dendrites of cortical neurons; not all potentials are recorded because there is a buffering effect of the scalp, muscles, bone, vessels, and subarachnoid fluid. The EEG waves are classified according to their frequency as delta (1–3/sec), theta (4–7/sec), alpha (8–12/sec), and beta (13–20/sec). These EEG waves are altered by many factors, including age, state of alertness, eye closure, drugs, and disease states. High-voltage slow and sharp waves (K complexes) and sleep spindles (regular 12–14/sec waves) confined to the central regions occurs during sleep in a normal EEG. Abnormalities of waveform include spikes and slow waves. Spikes are paroxysmal, sharp, and of high voltage followed by a slow wave. Spikes and slow waves are associated with epilepsy, but some normal patients may have this EEG finding. Focal spikes are often associated with irritative lesions, including cysts, slow-growing tumors, and glial scar tissue. Epileptiform activity may be enhanced by activation procedures, including hyperventilation, photic stimulation, and sleep deprivation. Slow waves may be focal, in which case, a circumscribed lesion such as a hematoma, tumor, infarction, or a localized infectious process may be considered; whereas generalized slow waves suggest a metabolic, inflammatory, or more widespread process.

EEG/polygraphic/video monitoring demonstrates precise characterization of seizure types, which helps to undertake specific medical or surgical management.

EEG/polygraphic/video monitoring provides more accurate differentiation of epileptic seizures from paroxysmal events that mimic epilepsy (including pseudoseizures), and efficacy of various therapeutic regimens. EEG/polygraphic/video monitoring also simultaneously records physiologic and EEG changes, which is particularly useful in neonates in whom the characterization of seizures is difficult.

Magnetic source imaging **(MSI)** is an advanced neurophysiologic technique that is particularly useful for the investigations of patients who may be for epilepsy surgery.

Evoked Potentials

An evoked potential is an electrical response that follows stimulation of the CNS by a specific stimulus of the visual, auditory or sensory system. Stimulation of the visual system by a flash or patterned stimulus, such as a black-and-white checkerboard produces *visual-evoked potentials* **(VEPs)**, which are recorded over the occiput and averaged in a computer. **Brainstem auditory-evoked potentials (BAEPs)** may be used for objective measurement of hearing acuity, particularly in a neonate or uncooperative child when routine hearing assessment techniques have failed. *Somatosensory evoked potentials* **(SSEPs)** are obtained by stimulating a peripheral nerve (peroneal, median) and by recording the electrical response over the cervical region and contralateral parietal somatosensory cortex.

Gilman S. Imaging the brain. *N Engl J Med* 1998; 338: 812–820

Haslam RHA. Neurologic evaluation. In: Kliegman RM, Behrman RE, Jenson HB, Stanton BF (eds). *Nelson Textbook of Pediatrics*. 18th edn. Vol. 2. Philadelphia: Saunders, 2007; 2433–2443.

McAuley J, Swash M. Nervous system. In: Swash M, Glynn M (eds). *Hutchison's Clinical Methods*. 22nd edn. Edinburgh: Saunders, 2007; 178–247.

Rennie JM. Assessment of the neonatal nervous system. In: Rennie JM (Ed). *Roberton's Textbook of Neonatology*. 4th edn. London: Elsevier Churchill Livingstone, 2005; 1093–1105.

Taylor MJ. Evoked potentials in paediatrics. In: Halliday AM (Ed). *Evoked potentials in Clinical Testing*. 2nd edn. Edinburgh: Churchill Livingstone, 1993; 489.

24.2 CONGENITAL ANOMALIES OF THE CENTRAL NERVOUS SYSTEM

Neural tube defects (dysraphism): Neural tube defects (NTDs) account for most congenital anomalies of the central nervous system (CNS) and result from failure of the neural tube to close spontaneously between the 3rd and 4th wk of in utero development. The precise cause of neural tube defects remains unknown; evidence suggests that many factors, including hyperthermia, drugs, malnutrition, chemicals, maternal obesity or diabetes and genetic determinants (mutations in folate-responsive or folate-dependent pathways) may adversely affect normal development of the CNS from the time of conception. In some cases, an abnormal maternal nutritional state or exposure to radiation before conception may increase the likelihood of a CNS congenital malformation. Failure of closure of the neural tube allows excretion of fetal substances (α-fetoprotein [AFP], acetylcholinesterase) into the amniotic fluid, serving as biochemical markers for a neural tube defect. Prenatal screening of maternal serum for AFP in the 16th–18th wk of gestation is used for identifying pregnancies at risk for fetuses with neural tube defects in utero. The major neural tube defects include spina bifida occulta, meningocele, myelomeningocele, encephalocele, anencephaly, dermal sinus, tethered cord, syringomyelia, diastematomyelia, and lipoma involving the conus medullaris and/or filum terminale.

Spina bifida occulta: This anomaly consists of a midline defect of the vertebral bodies without protrusion of the spinal cord or meninges. Most individuals are asymptomatic (no neurologic signs) but in some cases, patches of hair, a lipoma, discoloration of skin, or a dermal sinus in the midline of the lower back suggests a more significant malformation of the spinal cord. Dermoid sinuses occur in the midline at the site of where meningoceles or encephaloceles may occur: the lumbosacral region or occiput. Recurrent meningitis of occult origin should prompt clinical examination for a small sinus tract in the posterior midline region, including the back of the head. A roentgenogram of the spine in spina bifida occulta shows a defect in closure of the posterior vertebral arches and laminae, typically involving L5 and S1; there is no abnormality of the meninges, spinal cord or nerve roots. Spina bifida occulta is occasionally associated with syringomyelia, diastematomyelia, and a tethered cord. These abnormalities are identified with MRI.

Meningocele: A meningocele is formed when the meninges herniated through a defect in the posterior vertebral arches. The spinal cord is usually normal and assumes a normal position in the spinal canal, although there may be tethering, syringomyelia, or diastematomyelia. A fluctuant midline mass that may transilluminate occurs along the vertebral column, usually in the lower back. Surgery may be delayed if meningoceles are well covered with skin, with normal neurologic findings. Before surgical correction of the defect, the patient must be thoroughly examined with the use of plain roentgenograms, ultrasonography, and MRI to determine the extent of neural tissue involvement, if any or associated anomalies and CT scan of the head because of the association with hydrocephalus. Urologic evaluation, usually including cystometrogrm (CMG), will identify those children with neurogenic bladder who are at risk for renal deterioration. Patients with leaking CSF or a thin skin covering should be treated immediately surgically in order to prevent meningitis.

An *anterior meningocele* projects into the pelvis through a defect in the sacrum. Symptoms of constipation and bladder dysfunction develop due to the increasing size of the lesion. Female patients may have associated anomalies of the genital tract, including a rectovaginal fistula and vaginal septa. Plain roentgenograms demonstrate a defect in the sacrum; and the CT scanning or MRI outlines the extent of the meningocele.

Myelomeningocele

Myelomeningocele represents the most severe form of dysraphism involving the vertebral column and occurs with an incidence of $\approx 1/4,000$ live birth. Maternal periconceptional use of folic acid supplementation reduces the incidence of NTDs in pregnancies at risk by at least 50%. To be effective, folic acid supplementation should be initiated before conception and continued until at least 12th wk of gestation when neurulation is complete. The utero diagnosis can be made by maternal serum α-fetoprotein screening and by fetal ultrasonography.

Clinical manifestations: This condition produces dysfunction of many organs and structures, including the peripheral nervous system, CNS, skeleton, skin, and gastrointestinal and genitourinary tracts. A myelomeningocele may be located anywhere along the neuraxis, but the lumbosacral region accounts for at least 75% of the cases. The extent and degree of the neurologic deficit depends on the location of the myelomeningocele and the associated lesions. A lesion in the low sacral region causes bowel and bladder incontinence associated with anesthesia in the perineal area but with no impairment of motor function. Newborns with a defect in the midlumbar region have a sac-like cystic structure covered by a thin layer of partially epithelialized tissue. Remnants of neural tissue are visible beneath the membrane, which may occasionally rupture and leak CSF. The infant, on examination, shows flaccid paralysis of the lower extremities, and absent touch and pain sensation and deep tendon reflexes. There is a high incidence of lower extremity deformities (clubfeet, subluxation of deformities). Constant urinary dribbling and a relaxed anal sphincter may be evident. In some children there is a high-pressure bladder and sphincter dyssynergy. Thus, a myelomeningocele in the midlumbar region tends to produce lower motor neuron signs due to abnormalities and disruption of the conus medullaris. Infants with myelomeningocele typically have an increasing neurologic deficit as the myelomeningocele extends higher into the thoracic region. Patients with a myelomeningocele in the upper thoracic or cervical region usually have a very minimal neurologic deficit and in most cases, do not have hydrocephalus (*see* Fig. 24.4 in CD).

Hydrocephalus in association with a type II Chiari defect develops in at least of 80% of patients with myelomeningocele. Generally, lower the deformity in the neuraxis (sacrum), the less likely the risk of the development of hydrocephalus. About 15% of infants with hydrocephalus and Chiari II malformation develop symptoms of hindbrain dysfunction, including difficulty feeding, choking, stridor, apnea, vocal cord paralysis, pooling of secretions, and spasticity of the upper extremities, which if untreated, can lead to death. This *Chiari crisis* is due to downward herniation of the medulla and cerebellar tonsils through the foramen magnum.

Treatment: Management and supervision of a child and family with a myelomeningocele require a multidisciplinary team approach, including surgeons, physicians, and therapists, with one individual (often a pediatrician) acting as the advocate and coordinator of the treatment program. Surgery is often done within a day or so of birth, but can be delayed for several days except when there is a CSF leak. Regular catheterization of a neurogenic bladder is taught to parents and ultimately the patient. Incontinence of fecal matter is common. Many children can be bowel-trained with a regimen of timed enemas or suppositories that allows evacuation at a predetermined time once or twice a day.

Functional ambulation may be possible, depending on the level of the lesion and on intact function of iliopsoas muscles. Almost every child with a sacral or lumbosacral lesion obtains functional ambulation. A utero-surgical closure of a spinal lesion has been possible. The mortality rate is ≈ 10–15% in a child who is born with myelomeningocele and who is treated aggressively. Most deaths occur before 4 yr of age.

Prevention: The US public health service has recommended that all women of childbearing age and who are capable of becoming pregnant take 0.4 mg of folic acid daily. If a pregnancy is planned in high-risk women (previously affected child), supplementation should be started with 4 mg of folic acid daily, beginning 1 month before the time of the planned conception. Certain drugs, including drugs that antagonize folic acid such as trimethoprim and anticonvulsants (carbamazepine, phenytoin, phenobarbitone, and primidone) increase the risk of myelomeningocele. Valproic acid causes NTDs in ≈1–2% of pregnancies, if the drug is administered during pregnancy. Some epilepsy clinicians recommend folic acid supplements to all female patients of child bearing potential who are taking anticonvulsant medications.

Encephalocele: Two major forms of dysraphism affect the skull, resulting in protrusion of tissue through a bony midline defect, called *cranium bifidum*. 1. A *cranial meningocele* consists of a CSF-filled meningeal sac only. 2. A *cranial encephalocele* contains the sac plus cerebral cortex, cerebellum, or portions of the brainstem (*see* Fig. 24.5 in CD). The cranial defects occur most commonly in the occipital region at or below the inion, but frontal or nasofrontal encephaloceles are more common in certain parts of the world. The etiology is presumed to be similar to that for encephalocele and myelomeningocele (*see* Fig. 24.6 in CD).

Anencephaly: An anencephalic infant presents a distinctive appearance with a large defect of the calvarium, meninges, and scalp associated with the primitive brain, which results from failure of closure of the rostral neuropore, the opening of the neural tube. The cerebral hemispheres and cerebellum are usually absent, and only a residue of the brainstem can be identified. The pituitary gland is hypoplastic. Additional anomalies include folding of the ears, cleft palate, and congenital heart defect in 10–20% of cases. Affected infants are stillborn or die shortly after birth. The incidence of anencephaly approximates 1/1,000 live births, the greatest frequency is in Ireland, Wales, and Northern China. The recurrence risk is ≈ 4% and increases to 10% if a couple has had two previously affected pregnancies. Approximately 50% of cases of anencephaly have associated polyhydroamnios. Successive pregnancies should be monitored, including amniocentesis, determination of AFP levels, and ultrasound examination between the 14th and 16th wk of gestation.

Fernandes ET, Reinberg Y, Vernier R, et al. Neurogenic bladder dysfunction in children: Review of pathophysiology and current management. *J Pediatr* 1994; 124:1–7.

Guggisberg D, Hadj-Rabia S, Vinay C, et al. Skin markers of occult spinal dysraphism in children. *Arch Dermatol* 2004; 140: 1109–1115.

Ickowicz V, Ewin D, Maugay-Laudom B, et al. Meckel-Gruber syndrome, sonography and pathology. *Ultrasound Obstat Gynecol* 2006. 27:296–300.

Kinsman SL, Johnston MV. Congenital anomalies of the central nervous system. In: Kliegman RM, Behrman RE, Jenson HB, Stanton BF (eds). *Nelson Textbook of Pediatrics*. 18th edn. Vol. 2. Philadelphia: Saunders, 2007; 2443–2448.

Mitchell IE, Adzick NS, Melchionne J, et al. Spina bifida. *Lancet* 2004; 364: 1885–1895.

Microcephaly

Microcephaly is defined as a head circumference that measures more than three standard deviations below the mean for age and sex. Microcephaly may be subdivided into two main subgroups: Primary (genetic) microcephaly and secondary (nongenetic) microcephaly. *Primary microcephaly* is either autosomal recessive (typical appearance with slanted forehead, prominent nose and ears, severely mentally retarded and seizures) or dominant (nondistinctive facies, up-slanting palpebral fissures, mild forehead slanting and prominent ears, normal linear growth, seizures can be readily controlled and mild or borderline mental) or is present in various syndromes (Down syndrome [trisomy 21], Edward syndrome [trisomy 18], Cri-du-chat (5p-), Cornelia de Lange, Smith-Lemli-Opitz).

Secondary microcephaly results from a large number of noxious agents (radiation, congenital infections [cytomegalovirus, rubella, toxoplasmosis], fetal alcohol, fetal hydantoin, meningitis and encephalitis, malnutrition, metabolic [maternal diabetes mellitus and maternal hyperphenylalaninemia] hyperthermia, hypoxic-ischemic encephalopathy) that may affect a fetus in utero or an infant during periods of rapid brain growth, particularly the 1st 2 yr of life.

Clinical manifestations: A family history should be taken regarding additional cases of microcephaly, or disorders affecting the nervous system. It is important to measure a patient's head circumference at birth. A very small head circumference implies a process that began early in embryonic or fetal development. If an insult to the brain occurs later in life, particularly beyond the age of 2 yr, severe microcephaly is less likely to occur. Serial head circumference measurements are more meaningful than a single determination, particularly when the abnormality is minimal. The head circumference of each parent and sibling should also be recorded.

Diagnosis: If the cause of the microcephaly is unknown, the mother's serum phenylalanine level should be determined. High phenylalanine serum levels in an asymptomatic mother can produce marked brain damage to her infant. A karyotype is obtained if a chromosomal syndrome is suspected or if the child has abnormal facies, short stature, and additional congenital anomalies. MRI is useful in identifying structural abnormalities of the brain. CT scanning is performed to detect intracerebral calcification. Additional studies include a fasting plasma and urine aminoacid analysis; serum ammonia determination; toxoplasma, rubella, cytomegalovirus, and herpes simplex (TORCH) titers as well as HIV testing of the mother and child; a urine sample for the culture of cytomegalovirus.

Treatment: After establishing the cause of microcephaly, the physician must provide accurate and supportive genetic and family counseling. The physician must assist with placement in an appropriate program that will provide for maximum development of the child, because many children with microcephaly are also mentally retarded.

Barkovich AJ, Kuzniecky RI, Jackson MD, et al. Classification system for malformations of cortical development. *Neurology*. 2001; 57: 2168–2178.

Barr M, Cohen MM. Holoprosencephaly survival and performance. *Am J Med Genet* 1999; 89: 116–120.

Clark GD. The classification of cortical dysplasias through molecular genetics. *Brain Dev* 2004; 26: 351–362.

Kinsman SL, Johnston MV. Congenital anomalies of the central nervous system. In: Kliegman RM, Behrman RE, Jenson HB, Stanton BF (eds). *Nelson Textbook of Pediatrics*. 18th edn. Vol. 2. Philadelphia: Saunders, 2007; 2443–2448.

Hydrocephalus

Hydrocephalus is a condition in which excess cerebrospinal fluid (CSF) builds up in the brain causing abnormal enlargement of the ventricles in the brain. It results from impaired circulation and absorption of CSF or, in rare circumstances from increased production of CSF by a choroid plexus papilloma. Excess CSF in the ventricles can put too much pressure on the brain, potentially damaging the brain. Hydrocephalus can develop at birth (congenital hydrocephalus) or can develop later (acquired hydrocephalus).

Etiology: (i) Obstructive or noncommunicating hydrocephalus develops because of an abnormality of the aqueduct or a lesion in the 4th ventricle. Aqueductal stenosis results from an abnormally narrow aqueduct of Sylvius that is often associated with branching or forking. (ii) Nonobstructive or communicating hydrocephalus most commonly follows a subarachnoid hemorrhage, which is usually a result of intraventricular hemorrhage in a premature infant.

Clinical manifestations: In an infant, an accelerated rate of enlargement of the head is the most prominent sign; the anterior fontanel is wide open and bulging, and the scalp veins are dilated. The forehead is broad, and the eyes might deviate downward because of impingement of the dilated suprapineal recess on the tectum, producing the setting-sun eye sign (*see* Fig. 24.7 in CD). Long-tract signs such as brisk tendon reflexes, spasticity, clonus (particularly in the lower extremities), and Babinski sign are common owing to stretching and disruption of the corticospinal fibers originating from the leg region of the motor cortex. *In an older child,* the cranial sutures are partially closed so that the signs of hydrocephalus may be subtler. Irritability, lethargy, poor appetite, and vomiting are common to both age groups. Headache is a prominent symptom in older patients. A gradual change in personality and deterioration in academic performance suggest a slowly progressive form of hydrocephalus. Serial measurements of the head circumference often indicate an increased velocity of growth. Percussion of the skull might produce a cracked pot sound or Macewen sign, indicating separation of the sutures. A foreshortened occiput suggests Chiari malformation, and a prominent occiput suggests the Dandy-Walker malformation. Papilledema, abducens nerve palsies, and pyramidal tract signs, most evident in lower extremities, are seen in many cases. Chiari malformation consists of two major subgroups. Type I typically produces symptoms during adolescence or adult life and is usually not associated with hydrocephalus. Type II *Chiari malformation* is characterized by progressive hydrocephalus with a myelomeningocele. The *Dandy-Walker malformation* consists of a cystic expansion of the 4th ventricle in the posterior fossa and midline cerebellar hypoplasia, which results from a developmental failure of the roof of the 4th ventricle during embryogenesis. Approximately 90% of patients have hydrocephalus, and associated anomalies, including agenesis of the posterior cerebellar vermis and corpus callosum. Infants present with a rapid increase in head size and a prominent occiput.

Diagnosis and differential diagnosis: Examination should include skull and spine. The occipitofrontal head circumference is recorded and compared with previous measurements. The size and configuration of the anterior fontanel are noted and the back is inspected for abnormal midline skin lesions, including tufts of hair, lipoma, or angioma that might suggest spinal dysraphism. A cranial bruit is audible in cases of Galen arteriovenous malformation. Transillumination of the skull is positive with massive dilatation of the ventricular system or in the Dandy-Walker syndrome. Eye examination is mandatory because the finding of chorioretinitis suggests an intrauterine infection, such as toxoplasmosis, as a cause of the hydrocephalus. Papilledema is present in older children, but is rarely present in infants because the cranial sutures separate as a result of the increased pressure. Plain skull films show separation of the sutures, erosion of the posterior clinoids in an older child, and an increase in convolutional markings (beaten silver appearance) with long-standing increased ICP. The CT scan and/or MRI along with ultrasonography in an infant are the most important studies to identify the specific cause and severity of hydrocephalus. The head might appear enlarged and can be confused with hydrocephalus secondary to a thickened cranium resulting from chronic anemia, rickets, osteogenesis imperfect, and epiphyseal dysplasia. Chronic subdural collections can produce parietal bone prominence. Various metabolic and degenerative disorders of the CNS produce megencephaly. Sotos syndrome (cerebral gigantism) is the most common megalencephalic syndrome. Hydranencephaly may be confused with hydrocephalus. The cerebral hemispheres are absent or represented by membranous sacs with remnants of frontal, temporal, or occipital cortex dispersed over the membrane. The midbrain and brainstem are relatively intact. MRI can demonstrate the defect.

Treatment: Therapy for hydrocephalus depends on the cause. Medical management including the use of acetazolamide and furosemide (fursemide) can provide temporary relief by reducing the rate of CSF production. Most cases of hydrocephalus require extracranial shunts, particularly a ventriculoperitoneal shunt. The major complications of shunting are occlusion (headache, emesis, mental status changes and papilledema) and bacterial infection (fever, headache, meningism) usually due to *Staphylococcus epidermidis*. Endoscopic third ventriculostomy (ETV) is an alternative procedure to shunt for some individuals with hydrocephalus. In this procedure, a hole is made in the bottom of the third ventricle. This lets CSF flow toward the base of the brain, where normal absorption occurs.

Prognosis: Treatment for hydrocephalus can be lifesaving and life sustaining. Lifelong follow-up examinations are needed to evaluate changes in developmental, intellectual, neurological and physical impairments and to maintain proper functioning of a shunt system.

Bindal AK, Storrs BB, McLone DG. Management of the Dandy-Walker syndrome. *Pediatr Neurosurg* 1990;16:163–9.

Cutler RWP, Page, L, Galicich J. Formation and absorption of cerebrospinal fluid in man. *Brain* 1968;91:707–20.

Desai Somesh, Purohit AK. Pediatric Hydrocephalus. In: Mathur GP, Mathur Sarla (eds). *Current Trends in Pediatrics*. Vol 2. Delhi: Academa Publishers, 2006;333–41.

Kinsman SL, Johnston MV. Congenital anomalies of the central nervous system. In: Kliegman RM, Behrman RE, Jenson HB, Stanton BF (eds). *Nelson Textbook of Pediatrics*. 18th edn. Vol. 2. Philadelphia: Saunders, 2007;2443–8.

Kinsman SL, Johnston MV. Hydrocephalus. In: Kliegman RM, Stanton BF, St.Geme JW, Schor NF, Behrman RE. *Nelson Textbook of Pediatrics*. 19th edn. New Delhi: Elsevier, 2011;2008–2011.

Craniosynostosis

Craniosynostosis is defined as premature closure of the cranial sutures and is classified as primary and secondary. **Primary craniosynostosis** is the closure of one or more sutures due to abnormalities of skull development, whereas **secondary craniosynostosis** results from failure of brain growth and expansion. The incidence of primary craniosynostosis is approximately 1/2,000 births. The cause of craniosynostosis is unknown, but the prevailing hypothesis suggests that abnormal development of the base of the skull creates exaggerated forces on the duramater that act to disrupt normal suture development.

Clinical manifestations: Most cases of craniosynostosis are evident at birth and are characterized by a skull deformity that is a direct result of premature suture fusion. Palpation of the suture reveals a prominent bony ridge, and fusion of the suture may be confirmed by plain roentgenograms or bone scan in ambiguous cases.

A. PREMATURE FUSION OF SUTURES

Scaphocephaly, the most common form of craniosynostosis is due to premature closure of the sagittal suture. Scaphocephaly is characterized by a long and narrow skull, prominent occiput, broad forehead and a small or absent anterior fontanel. The condition is sporadic, more common in males, and often causes difficulties during labor because of cephalopelvic disproportion. Scaphocephaly does not cause increased ICP or hydrocephalus and neurologic examination is normal.

Frontal plagiocephaly is the next most common form of craniosynostosis and is the result of premature fusion of a coronal and sphenofrontal suture. It is characterized by unilateral flattening of the forehead, elevation of the ipsilateral orbit and eyebrow, and a prominent ear on the corresponding side. The condition is more common in females.

Occipital plagiocephaly is most often a result of positioning in infancy and is more common in an immobile or handicapped child, but fusion or sclerosis of the lambdoid suture can cause unilateral occipital flattening and bulging of the ipsilateral frontal bone.

Trigonocephaly is a rare form of craniosynostosis due to premature fusion of the metopic suture. These children have a keel shaped forehead and hypotelorism and are at risk for associated developmental abnormalities of the forebrain.

Turricephaly is characterized by a cone-shaped head due to premature fusion of the coronal and often sphenofrontal and frontoethmoidal sutures.

Kleeblattschädel deformity resembles a cloverleaf. Affected children have very prominent temporal bones, and the remaining of the cranium is constricted. Hydrocephalus is a common complication.

B. GENETIC DISORDERS

Crouzon syndrome is characterized by premature craniosynostosis and is inherited as an autosomal dominant trait. Brachycephaly head due to bilateral closure of the coronal sutures, underdeveloped orbits, prominent ocular proptosis, hypoplasia of the maxilla and orbital hypertelorism are typical features.

Apert syndrome is usually a sporadic condition, although autosomal dominant inheritance may occur. It is associated with premature fusion of multiple sutures, including the coronal, sagittal, squamosal, and lambdoid sutures. The facies tend to be asymmetric and the eyes are proptotic. Syndactyly of the 2nd, 3rd, and 4th fingers, which may be joined to the thumb and the 5th finger. Similar abnormalities often occur in the feet. All patients have progressive calcification and fusion of the bones of the hands, feet, and cervical spine.

Carpenter syndrome is inherited as an autosomal recessive condition and the many fusions of the sutures tend to produce the Kleeblattschädel skull deformity. Soft tissue syndactyly of the hands and feet is always present, and mental retardation is common. Additional but less common abnormalities include congenital heart disease, corneal opacities, coax valga, and genu valgum.

Chotzen syndrome is characterized by asymmetric craniosynostosis and plagiocephaly. It is associated with facial asymmetry, ptosis of the eyelids, shortened fingers, and soft tissue syndactyly of the 2nd and 3rd fingers. The condition is the most prevalent of the genetic syndromes and is inherited as an autosomal dominant trait.

Pfeiffer syndrome is most often associated with turricephaly. The eyes are prominent and widely spaced, and the thumbs and great toes are short and broad. Partial soft tissue syndactyly may be present. Most cases are usually sporadic, although autosomal dominant inheritance may occur.

Treatment: Premature fusion of one suture rarely causes a neurologic deficit. In this situation, the sole indication for surgery is to enhance the child's cosmetic appearance, and the prognosis depends on the suture involved and on the degree of disfigurement. Surgical intervention cosmetically improves the outlook of the patient suffering from frontal plagiocephaly. Neurologic complications, including hydrocephalus and increased ICP, are more likely to occur when two or more sutures are prematurely fused, in which case operative intervention is essential. Craniectomy is mandatory for management of increased ICP. A multidisciplinary craniofacial team is essential for the long term follow up of affected children. Craniosynostosis may be surgically corrected with good outcomes and relatively low morbidity and mortality especially for nonsyndromic infants.

Kinsman SL, Johnston MV. Congenital anomalies of the central nervous system. In: Kliegman RM, Behrman RE, Jenson HB, Stanton BF (eds). *Nelson Textbook of Pediatrics.* 18th edn. Vol. 2. Philadelphia: Saunders, 2007; 2443–2448.

Losse JE, Mason AC. Deformational plagiocephaly: Diagnosis, prevention and treatment. *Clin Plast Surg* 005; 32: 52–64.

Ridgway ER, Weiner HL. Skull deformities. *Pediatr Clin North Am* 2004; 51: 359–387.

24.3 HEADACHES

Headache is a common problem in children. A headache may occasionally indicate a severe underlying disorder (brain tumor), and thus careful evaluation of children with recurrent, severe, progressive, or unconventional headaches is mandatory. Most toddlers cannot communicate the characteristics of headache; rather they become irritable and cranky, vomit, prefer a darkened room because of photophobia, or repeatedly rub their eyes and head. Children cannot describe the headache correctly and its associated symptoms. The most important causes of headache in children include migraine, psychogenic factors or stress, and increased intracranial pressure (ICP). Refractive errors, strabismus, sinusitis, and malocclusion of the teeth are much less common causes of significant headaches in children. Headaches are often an associated manifestation of common head and neck infections in children.

1. **Migraine:** Migraine is the most important and frequent type of headache. **Cortical spreading depression (CSD)**, a phenomenon thought to be responsible for the aura of migraine, is associated with elevation of CNS hydrogen and potassium ions, with the release of glutamate and nitrous oxide. Migraine may occur without an aura or with an aura. **Hemiplegic migraine** is considered a migraine aura and is characterized by the onset of

unilateral sensory or motor signs during an episode of migraine. In **basilar type migraine** the brainstem signs predominate because of vasoconstriction of the basilar and posterior cerebral arteries. The major symptoms include vertigo, tinnitus, diplopia, blurred vision, scotoma, ataxia, and an occipital headache. **Childhood periodic syndromes that are common precursors of migraine** include cyclic vomiting, abdominal migraine, and benign paroxysmal vertigo. **Abdominal migraine** is a recurrent disorder characterized by mid-abdominal pain with pain free periods between each attack.

Treatment: Most migraine headaches are not severe and are readily managed by conservative measures without requiring medical treatment. Migraine may be prevented or ameliorated by avoiding certain initiating stimuli, such as stress, fatigue, and anxiety. An affected child may be under undue stress because of difficulties at home or school, particularly when unrealistic pressures or demands are placed on the patient. Certain foods are implicated as a cause of migraine, particularly nuts, chocolate, cola drinks, citrous fruits, fried foods, cheese, yogurt, hot dogs, spicy meats and processed meats, kippers, and Chinese food (monosodium glutamate).

Management of an acute attack of migraine should include the use of analgesics and antiemetics. Most headaches can be treated by acetaminophen (15 mg/kg) or ibuprofen (7.5–10 mg/kg), particularly if the headaches are mild, infrequent, and of short duration. An antiemetic such as dimenhydrinate by rectal suppository, 5 mg/kg/24 hr in four divided doses is the treatment of choice when vomiting is the major problem. Parenteral metoclopramide is very effective as an antiemetic agent. Children may develop severe intractable migraine attacks or status migrainous (persistent headache lasting longer than 3 days) that are unresponsive to conventional drug regimens, intravenous prochlorperazine 0.15 mg/kg (max 10 mg) is highly effective in aborting intractable migraine in children who have not responded to acute management of the headache.

The decision to use continuous daily medication (prophylactic therapy) is based on the severity and frequency of the headaches and on the impact of the migraine on the child's daily activities, including school attendance and performance as well as participation in recreation. Propranolol, a β blocker is used as a prophylactic medication in the dose of 10–20 mg tid (beginning with 10 mg/24 hr and gradually increasing the drug to the maximum dose or until the desired therapeutic effect is achieved)

in children 7–8 yr or older. Additional drugs that are useful for the prophylaxis of pediatric migraine include sodium valproate, topiramate, gabapentin, cyproheptadine, and amitriptyline. Cyclic vomiting is treated with injected antiemetics, such as ondansetron and fluid replacement if the vomiting is excessive.

Behavior management is an effective method for the treatment of migraine in some children and adolescents. Biofeedback and self-hypnosis is used. Biofeedback can be mastered by most children older than 8 yr.

2. **Organic headaches:** An organic headache may be the earliest symptom of increased intracranial pressure (ICP). The onset is insidious, increased by any activity that elevates the ICP. Early morning vomiting is present. Headache may be diffuse and generalized but is more prominent over the frontal and occipital region. Physical examination may show CNS involvement. Papilledema may be present on fundoscopic examination. EEG may be abnormal. Neuroradiologic findings present depending on the underlying cause. The management of organic headaches depends on the cause.

3. **Tension or stress headaches:** Tension or stress headaches are common in pediatric age group, particularly after the onset of puberty. Infrequently appear in the morning hours, but most apparent during the school day, coinciding with a test or similarly anxiety provoking circumstances. Headache is present in the frontal region, may localize over the vertex or the occipital area. It is hurting or aching in character, but rarely perceived as throbbing. Not associated with nausea and vomiting. CNS examination, fundus examination, neuroradiologic procedures and EEG are normal. Family history of headache is absent. Headache is to be differentiated from migraine. The diagnosis of tension headache is made by exclusion. Daily ingestion of cola or coffee may produce headaches. Gradual withdrawal eliminates the caffeine-induced chronic headaches. **Treatment** of tension headaches begins with reassurance and an explanation about how stress may cause an headache. Anxiety and stress may unconsciously produce constant isometric contraction of temporalis, masseter, or trapezius muscles, which leads to the characteristic dull, aching headache. Steps should be taken to remove obvious anxiety-provoking situations. Acetaminophen and other mild analgesics are required to treat a tension headache. Sedatives and antidepressants are rarely necessary. Biofeedback and self-hypnosis exercises are

effective in the treatment of some patients with tension headaches.

Fuller G, Kaye C. Headaches. *BMJ* 2007; 334: 254–256.
Haslam RHA. Headaches. In: Kliegman RM, Behrman RE, Jenson HB, Stanton BF (eds). *Nelson Textbook of Pediatrics.* 18th edn. Vol. 2. Philadelphia: Saunders, 2007; 2479–2483.
Silberstein SD. Migraine. *Lancet* 2004; 363: 381–391.

24.4 CENTRAL NERVOUS SYSTEM INFECTIONS

Infection of the central nervous system (CNS) is the most common cause of fever associated with signs and symptoms of CNS disease in children. Viral infections of CNS are much more common than bacterial infections. Fungal, parasitic, rickettsial, and *Mycoplasma* spp. infections are less common. ***Common symptoms*** include headache, nausea, vomiting, anorexia, restlessness, altered state of unconsciousness, and irritability. ***Common signs*** of CNS infection, in addition to fever include photophobia, neck pain and rigidity, obtundation, stupor, coma, seizures, and focal neurologic deficits. Infection of the CNS may be diffuse or focal. Meningitis and encephalitis are examples of diffuse infection. Brain abscess is the example of a focal infection of CNS. The diagnosis of diffuse CNS infections depends on examination of cerebrospinal fluid (CSF) obtained by lumbar puncture (LP). Table 24.3 provides expected CSF abnormalities with various CNS disorders.

Table 24.3: Cerebrospinal fluid findings in cases of meningitis

Condition	Pressure (mm of H₂O)	Leukocytes (mm³)	Protein (mg/dl)	Glucose (mg/dl)	Comments
Acute bacterial meningitis	Usually elevated (100–300)	100–10,000 or more, usually 300–2,000, PMNs predominate	Usually 100–500	Decreased usually < 40 (or serum < 50% serum glucose)	Organisms usually seen on Gram stain and recovered by culture
Partially treated bacterial meningitis	Normal or elevated	5–10,000; PMNs usual but mononuclear cells may predominate if treated for extended period of time	Usually 100–500	Normal or decreased	Organisms may be seen on Gram stain. CSF may become sterile after pretreatment. Antigen may be detected by agglutination test
Viral meningitis or meningoencephalitis	Normal or slightly elevated (80–150)	Rarely>1,000 cells	Usually 50–200	Generally normal,; may be decreased to <40 in some viral diseases, particularly mumps (15–20% of cases)	HSV and enteroviruses may be detected by PCR of CSF
Tuberculous meningitis	Usually elevated	10–500, PMNs early, but lymphocytes predominate through most of the course	100–3,000, may be higher in the presence of block	<50 in most cases	*M.tuberculosis* may be detected by PCR of CSF
Fungal meningitis	Usually elevated	5–500; PMNs early but mononuclear cells predominate	25–500	<50; decreases with time if not treated	Budding yeast may be seen
Syphilis (acute) and leptospirosis	Usually elevated	50–500; lymphocytes predominate	50–200	Usually normal	Positive CSF serology; dark field examination may be positive for spirochetes
Amebic meningo-encephalitis	Elevated	1,000–10,000 or more; PMNs predominate	50–500	Normal or slightly decreased	Mobile amebae may be seen by hanging-drop examination of CSF at room temperature

PMN: polymorphonuclear neutrophils; CSF: cerebrospinal fluid; EEG: electroencephalogram; HSV: herpes simplex virus; PCR: polymerase chain reaction.

Acute Bacterial Meningitis beyond the Neonatal Period

The most important cause of bacterial meningitis in **children 2 mo to 12 yr of age** is *Neisseria meningitidis, Streptococcus pneumoniae,* and *Haemophilus influenzae* type b. Those with certain underlying immunologic (HIV infection, IgG subclass deficiency) or anatomic (splenic dysfunction, cochlear defects or implants) disorders also may be at increased risk of infection caused by these bacteria. The causes of bacterial meningitis in the *neonatal period* (0–28 days) include groups streptococci (enterococcus), gram-negative enteric bacilli (*E. coli, Klebsiella*), and *Listeria monocytogenes.*

Epidemiology: A major risk factor for meningitis is the lack of immunity to specific pathogens associated with young age. Congenital or acquired CSF leak across a mucocutaneous barrier, such as cranial or midline facial defects are associated with an increased risk of pneumococcal meningitis. Defects of the complement system (C5–C8) and defects of the properdin system have been associated with a significant risk of meningococcal disease. Splenic dysfunction (sickle cell anemia) or asplenia (due to trauma or congenital defect) is associated with an increased risk of pneumococcal, *H. influenzae* type b, and rarely meningococcal sepsis and meningitis. T-lymphocyte defects (congenital or acquired by chemotherapy, AIDS, or malignancy) are associated with increased risk of *L. monocytogenes* infections of the CNS.

Pathogenesis and pathology: Bacterial meningitis most commonly results from hematogenous dissemination of microorganisms from a distant site of infection; bacteremia usually precedes meningitis or occurs concomitantly. Bacterial colonization of the nasopharynx with a potentially pathogenic microorganism is the usual source of the bacteremia. Prior or concurrent viral upper respiratory tract infection may enhance the pathogenicity of bacteria producing meningitis.

The meningeal purulent exudates of varying thickness may be distributed around the cerebral veins, venous sinuses, and convexity of the brain and the cerebellum and in the sulci, sylvian fissures, basal cisterns and spinal cord. Inflammation of spinal nerves and roots produces meningeal signs, and inflammation of the cranial nerves produces cranial neuropathies of optic, oculomotor, facial and auditory nerves. Increased ICP also produces oculomotor nerve palsy due to the presence of temporal lobe compression of the nerve during tentorial herniation. Abducens nerve palsy may be a nonlocalizing sign of elevated ICP. The syndrome of inappropriate antidiuretic hormone secretion (SIADH) may produce excessive water retention and potentially increase the risk of elevated ICP.

Clinical manifestations: The onset of acute meningitis has two predominant patterns. (i) More often, meningitis is preceded by several days of fever accompanied by upper respiratory tract or gastrointestinal symptoms, followed by nonspecific signs of CNS infection such as increasing lethargy and irritability. (ii) Less common presentation is sudden onset with rapidly progressive manifestations of shock, purpura, disseminated intravascular coagulation (DIC), and reduced levels of consciousness, often resulting in progression to coma or death within 24 hr.

Nonspecific findings include fever, anorexia, and poor feeding, headache, symptoms of respiratory tract infection, myalgias, arthralgias, tachycardia, hypotension, and various cutaneous signs, such as petechiae, purpura, or an erythematous macular rash. *Meningeal irritation* is manifested as nuchal rigidity, back pain, Kernig sign and Brudzinski sign. *Increased ICP* is suggested by headache, emesis, bulging fontanel or diastasis (widening) of the sutures, oculomotor (anisocoria, ptosis) or abducens nerve paralysis, hypertension with bradycardia, apnea or hyperventilation, decorticate or decerebrate posturing, stupor, coma, or signs of herniation. *Papilledema* is uncommon in uncomplicated meningitis and should suggest a more chronic process, such as the presence of an intracranial abscess, subdural empyema, or occlusion of a dural venous sinus. *Cranial neuropathies* of the optic, oculomotor, abducens, facial, and auditory nerves may also be due to focal inflammation. Seizures (focal or generalized) due to cerebritis, infarction or electrolyte disturbances may occur in meningitis and if persist after 4th day of illness and those that are difficult to treat may be associated with a poor prognosis. Alterations of mental status are common among patients with meningitis and may be due to elevated ICP, cerebritis, or hypotension; manifestations include irritability, lethargy, stupor, obtundation, and coma. Comatose patients have a poor prognosis. Additional manifestations of meningitis include photophobia and tache cérébrale, which is elicited by stroking the skin with a blunt object and observing a raised red streak within 30–60 sec.

Diagnosis: The diagnosis of acute pyogenic meningitis is confirmed by analysis of the CSF (*see* Table 24.3). Blood cultures should be performed in all patients with suspected meningitis. Blood cultures reveal bacteria responsible for meningitis in up to 80–90% cases. CSF obtained from children with bacterial meningitis, after the initiation of antibiotics, may be negative on Gram stain and culture. Pleocytosis with a predominance of neutrophils, elevated protein level, and a reduced concentration of CSF glucose usually persists for several days after the administration of appropriate intravenous antibiotics. Therefore, despite negative cultures, the presumptive diagnosis of bacterial meningitis can be made. In case of traumatic LP, it is prudent to rely on the bacteriologic results rather than attempt to interpret the CSF leukocytes and protein level.

Determining the specific cause of CNS infection is facilitated by careful examination of the CSF with specific stains (Ziehl Neelsen stain for mycobacteria, Gomori methenamine silver stain for fungi), cytology, antigen detection (Cryptococcus), serology (syphilis, Westnile virus, arboviruses, herpes simplex), viral culture (enteroviruses) and polymerase chain reaction (herpes simplex, enterovirus, and others). Other diagnostic tests include blood cultures, CT or MRI of the brain, serologic tests, and rarely brain biopsy.

Acute viral meningoencephalitis is the most likely infection to be confused with bacterial meningitis. Although classic CSF profiles associated with bacterial versus viral infection tend to be distinct.

Treatment: The treatment of patients presumed to be suffering from bacterial meningitis depends on the nature of the initial manifestations of illness. 1. A child with rapidly progressing disease of less than 24 hr duration, in the absence of increased ICP, should receive antibiotics as soon as possible after an LP is performed. 2. If there are signs of increased ICP or focal neurologic findings, antibiotics should be given without performing an LP and before obtaining a CT scan. Increased ICP should be treated simultaneously. Immediate treatment of associated multiple organ system failure, shock, acute respiratory distress syndrome is also indicated. If no signs of increased ICP are evident, an LP should be performed.

Initial antibiotic therapy: The initial (empirical) choice of therapy for meningitis in *immunocompetent infants and children* is primarily influenced by the antibiotic susceptibilities. Due to resistance of *S. pneumoniae* to b-lactam drugs, vancomycin (60 mg/kg/24 hr, given every 6 hr) is recommended as part of initial empirical therapy. Because of the efficacy of 3rd-generation cephalosporins in the therapy of meningitis caused by sensitive *Streptococcus pneumoniae, Neisseria meningitidis,* and *Haemophilus influenzae* type b, cefotaxime (200 mg/kg/24 hr, given every 6 hr) or ceftriaxone (100 mg/kg/24 hr administered once per day or 50 mg/kg/dose, given every 12 hr) should also be used in empirical therapy. If *L. monocytogenes*

infection is suspected ampicillin (200 mg/kg/24 hr, given every 6 hr) also should be given, because cephalosporins are inactive against *L. monocytogenes.* Intravenous trimethoprim-sulfamethoxazole is an alternative treatment for *L. monocytogenes.*

If the patient is immunocompromised and gram-negative bacterial meningitis is suspected, initial therapy might include ceftazidime and an aminoglycoside.

Duration of antibiotic therapy: (i) Therapy for uncomplicated penicillin-sensitive *S. pneumoniae* meningitis should be completed in 10 to 14 days with a 3rd-generation cephalosporin or intravenous penicillin (400,000 U/kg/24 hr, given every 4–6 hr). If the isolate is resistant to penicillin and the 3rd-generation cephalosporin, therapy should be completed with vancomycin. (ii) Intravenous penicillin (400,000 U/kg/ 24 hr) for 5–7 days is the treatment of choice for uncomplicated *N. meningitidis meninigitis.* (iii) Uncomplicated *H. influenzae* type b meningitis should be treated for $\approx$ 7–10 days. (iv) Patients who receive intravenous or oral antibiotics before LP and who do not have an identifiable pathogen but do have evidence of an acute bacterial infection on the basis of their CSF profile should continue to receive therapy with ceftriaxone or cefotaxime for 7–10 days. If focal signs are present or the child does not respond to treatment, a parameningeal focus may be present and a CT or MRI scan should be performed. The CSF should be sterile within 24–48 hr after initiation of appropriate antibiotic therapy.

Most isolates of *E. coli* are sensitive to cefotaxime or ceftriaxone, and most isolates of *P. aeruginosa* are sensitive to ceftazidime. Gram-negative bacillary meningitis should be treated for 3 wk or for at least 2 wk after CSF sterilization, which may occur after 2–10 days of treatment.

Side effects of antibiotic therapy of meningitis include phlebitis, drug fever, rash, emesis, oral candidiasis, and diarrhea. Ceftriaxone may cause reversible gall bladder pseudolithiasis, detectable by abdominal ultrasonography. This is usually asymptomatic but may be associated with emesis and upper right quadrant pain.

Corticosteroids: Children older than 6 wk with acute bacterial meningitis caused by *H. influenzae* type b, receiving corticosteroid (intravenous dexamethasone, 0.15 mg/kg/dose given every 6 hr for 2 days) in the treatment have a shorter duration of fever, lower CSF protein and lactate levels, and a reduction in sensorineural hearing loss. Benefit, if any, of corticosteroids in the treatment of meningitis caused by other bacteria are inconclusive. Corticosteroids appear to have maximum benefit if given 1–2 hr before antibiotics are initiated. They also may be effective if given concurrently with or soon after the 1st dose of antibiotics. *Complications* of corticosteroids include gastrointestinal bleeding, hypertension, hyperglycemia, leukocytosis, and rebound fever after the last dose.

Supportive care: Repeated medical and neurologic assessments of patients with bacterial meningitis are essential to identify early signs of cardiovascular, CNS, and metabolic complications. Temperature, pulse rate, blood pressure, and respiratory rate (TPBPR) should be monitored frequently. Neurologic assessment, including pupillary reflexes, level of consciousness, motor strength, cranial nerve involvement and seizures should be made frequently in the 1st 72 hr when the risk of neurologic complications is greatest. Important laboratory studies include an assessment of blood urea nitrogen, serum sodium, chloride, potassium, and bicarbonate levels; urine output and specific gravity; complete blood and platelet counts, and, in the presence of petechiae, purpura, or abnormal bleeding, coagulation function tests (fibrinogen, prothrombin, and partial thromboplastin times).

Initially the patient is not given anything orally. If the patient is judged to be normovolemic, with normal blood pressure, intravenous fluid administration should be restricted to one half to two thirds of maintenance, or 800–1,000 ml/m²/24 hr, until it can be established that increased ICP or SIADH is not present. Fluid administration may be returned to normal (1,500–1,700 ml/m²/24 hr), when serum sodium levels are normal. Shock (systemic hypotension) must be treated aggressively to prevent brain and other organ dysfunction (renal tubular necrosis, acute respiratory syndrome). Patients with septic shock may require fluid restriction and therapy with vasoactive agents such as dopamine and epinephrine. Patients with shock, a markedly elevated ICP, coma, and refractory seizures require intensive monitoring with central arterial and venous access and frequent vital signs should be admitted in a pediatric intensive care unit.

Signs of increased ICP should be treated emergently with endotracheal intubation and hyperventilation (to maintain the pCO₂ at ≈ 25 mm Hg), intravenous furosemide (Lasix, 1 mg/kg) and mannitol (0.5–1.0 mg/kg) to reduce ICP. Furosemide reduces brain swelling by venodilation and diuresis without increasing intracranial blood volume, whereas mannitol produces an osmolar gradient between the brain and plasma, thus shifting fluid from the CNS to plasma, with subsequent excretion during an osmotic diuresis. For seizures diazepam (0.1–0.2 mg/kg/dose) or lorazepam (0.05–0.10 mg/kg/dose) should be given.

Serum glucose, calcium, and sodium levels should be monitored. After immediate management of seizures, patients should receive phenytoin (15–20 mg/kg loading dose, 5 mg/kg/24 hr maintenance) to reduce the likelihood of recurrence. Phenytoin is preferred to phenobarbitone because it produces less CNS depression and permits assessment of a patient's level of consciousness. Serum phenytoin levels should be monitored to maintain them in the therapeutic range (10–20 µg/ml).

Complications: During the treatment *acute CNS complications* can include seizures, increased ICP, cranial nerve palsies, stroke, cerebral or cerebellar herniation, and thrombosis of the dural venous sinuses. *Subdural effusions* are especially common in infants. SIADH occurs in some patients resulting in hyponatremia and reduced serum osmolality; this may exacerbate cerebral edema or result in hyponatremic seizures. *Prolonged fever* (>10 days) is usually due to intercurrent viral infection, nosocomial or secondary bacterial infection, thrombophlebitis, or drug reaction. Secondary fever refers to the recrudescence of elevated temperature after an afebrile illness. *Blood disorders* (thrombocytosis, eosinophilia, anemia and DIC) may also occur.

Prognosis: Appropriate antibiotic therapy and supportive care have reduced the mortality. The prognosis is poorest among infants younger than 6 months. The most common neurologic sequelae include hearing loss (sensorineural hearing loss), mental retardation, recurrent seizures, and delay in acquisition of language, visual impairment, and behavioral problems.

Prevention: Vaccination and antibiotic prophylaxis of susceptible at-risk contacts can reduce the likelihood of bacterial meningitis.

Neisseria meningitidis: Close contacts of patients regardless of age or immunization status should be treated with rifampin 10 mg/kg/dose every 12 hr (maximum dose of 600 mg) for 2 days as soon as possible after identification of a case of suspected meningococcal meningitis or sepsis.

A quadrivalent (A,C,Y,W-135), conjugated vaccine (MCV-4) is recommended to 11–12 yr old adolescents, high risk children older than 2 yr, high risk patients (include those with anatomic or functional asplenia or deficiencies of terminal complement protein), and college freshmen (new students). The vaccine also may be used as an adjunct with chemoprophylaxis for exposed contacts and during epidemics of meningococcal disease.

Haemophilus influenzae type b: Rifampin prophylaxis should be given to all household contacts, if any close family member younger than 48 months has not been fully immunized or if an immunocompromised person, of any age, resides in the household. A household contact is one who lives in the residence of the index case or who has spent a minimum of 4 hr with the index case for at least 5 of the 7 days preceding the patient's hospitalization. Family members should receive rifampin prophylaxis immediately after the diagnosis is suspected in the index case because >50% of secondary family cases occur in the 1st wk after the index case has been hospitalized. The dose of rifampin is 20 mg/kg/24 hr (maximum dose of 600 mg) given once on each day for 4 days. Rifampin color's the urine and perspiration red-orange, stains contact lenses, and reduces the serum concentrations of some drugs, including the oral contraceptives. Rifampin is contraindicated in pregnancy. All children should be immunized with *H. influenzae* type b conjugate vaccine beginning at 2 mo of age.

Streptococcus pneumoniae: Routine administration of heptavalent conjugate vaccine against *S. pneumoniae* is recommended for children younger than 2 yr of age. The initial dose is given at ≈2 mo of age. Children who are at high risk of invasive pneumococcal infections, including those with functional or anatomic asplenia and those with underlying immunodeficiency (such as infection with HIV, primary immunodeficiency, and those receiving immunosuppressive therapy) should also receive the vaccine.

Viral Meningoencephalitis

Viral meningoencephalitis is an acute inflammatory process involving the meninges and, to a variable degree, brain tissue. These infections are caused by enteroviruses, arboviruses, Japanese encephalitis virus [JEV], West Nile virus [WNV], herpesviruses herpes simple virus (HSV) Type 1, 2, varicella-zoster virus (VZV), cytomegalovirus (CMV), Epstein-Barr virus (EBV), Human herpesvirus 6 (HHV-6), mumps, respiratory viruses (adenovirus, influenza virus, parainfluenza virus), rubeola, rubella, or rabies. It may follow live virus vaccinations against polio, measles, mumps, or rubella. The spread of enteroviruses infection occurs directly from person to person, with usual incubation period of 4–6 days. Viruses other than enteroviruses causing aseptic meningitis will depend on season, climatic conditions, animal exposures, and factors related to the specific antigen.

Pathogenesis and pathology: Neurologic damage is caused by direct invasion and destruction of neural tissues by actively multiplying viruses or by a host reaction to viral antigens. Characteristic changes occur in the brain tissue include meningeal congestion and mononuclear infiltration, perivascular cuffs of lymphocytes and plasma cells, some perivascular tissue necrosis with myelin breakdown, and neuronal disruption in various stages, including, ultimately neurophagia and endothelial proliferation or necrosis. Demyelination with preservation of neurons and their axons are considered predominantly "postinfectious" or "allergic" encephalitis. The cerebral cortex, especially the temporal lobe is often severely affected by herpes simplex virus (HSV). Arboviruses tend to affect the entire brain. Rabies has a predilection for the basal structures. Variable degree of involvement occurs in the spinal cord, nerve roots, and peripheral nerves.

Clinical manifestations: The onset of illness is generally acute, although the CNS signs and symptoms are often preceded by a nonspecific febrile illness of a few days duration. Some children may be initially mildly affected, but soon lapse into coma and die suddenly. The presenting manifestations in older children are headache and hyperesthesia, and in infants, irritability and lethargy. Headache is most often frontal or generalized; some complains of retrobulbar pain. Fever, nausea, and vomiting, photophobia, and pain in the neck, back, and legs are common. As body temperature increases, there may be mental dullness, progressing to stupor in combination with bizarre movements and convulsions. Focal neurologic signs may be stationary, progressive, or fluctuating. Nonpolioenteroviruses and West Nile virus may cause anterior horn cell injury and a flaccid paralysis. Loss of bowel and bladder control may occur. Examination often reveals nuchal rigidity without significant localizing neurologic findings, at least at the onset. The complications of CNS viral infection include Guillain-Barré syndrome, transverse myelitis, hemiplegia, and cerebellar ataxia.

Exanthems often precede or accompany the CNS signs, especially with echoviruses, Coxsackie viruses, Varicella zoster virus (VZV), measles, rubella, and occasionally West Nile virus.

Diagnosis: The diagnosis is usually made on the basis of nonspecific prodromal clinical presentation followed by progressive CNS symptoms, supported by examination of the CSF (*see* Table 24.3). The CSF should be cultured for viruses, bacteria, fungi and mycobacteria; in some instances, special examinations for protozoa, mycoplasma and other pathogens. A serum specimen should be obtained early in the course of illness and, if viral cultures are not diagnostic, again 2–3 wk later for serologic studies. The EEG typically shows diffuse-slow wave activity, usually without focal changes. Neuroimaging studies (CT or MRI) may show swelling of the brain parenchyma. Focal seizures or focal findings on EEG, CT, or MRI, especially involving the temporal lobes, suggest HSV encephalitis.

Differential diagnosis: Children with bacterial meningitis, paramaningeal bacterial infections (brain abscess or subdural or epidural empyema) and infections caused by *M. tuberculosis*, *T. pallidum* (syphilis), *B. burgdorferi* (Lyme disease), and *Bartonella henselae*, the bacillus associated with cat scratch disease should be differentiated from viral meningoencephalitis. Analysis of CSF and appropriate serologic tests are necessary to differentiate these various pathogens.

Treatment: Acyclovir is used for the treatment of HSV encephalitis. For the treatment of viral meningo-encephalitis the treatment is supportive. Headache and hyperesthesia are treated with rest, nonaspirin containing analgesics, and a reduction in room light, noise, and visitors. Paracetamol is recommended for fever. Intravenous fluids will be needed when there is poor oral intake. It is important to anticipate and be prepared to manage convulsions, cerebral edema, inadequate respiratory exchange, disturbed fluid and electrolyte balance, aspiration and asphyxia, and cardiac and respiratory arrest of central origin. All fluids, electrolytes, and medications are initially given parenterally. In prolonged states of coma parenteral alimentation is indicated. SIADH is common in acute CNS disorders and monitoring of serum sodium concentrations is required for early detection. Normal blood levels of glucose, magnesium, and calcium must be maintained to minimize the likelihood of convulsions. If cerebral edema or seizures become evident, vigorous treatment should be instituted.

Prognosis: Patients after recovery should be rehabilitated. The prognosis is poor if the clinical illness is severe with potential deficits being intellectual, motor, psychiatric, epileptic, visual, or auditory in nature.

Prevention: Vaccination against polio, measles, mumps, rubella, and varicella can eliminate CNS complications from these diseases. The frequency of rabies encephalitis is reduced because of domestic animal vaccination. Mosquito bites through the application of DEET-containing insect repellents on exposed skin and wearing long-sleeved shirts, long pants, and socks when outdoors, especially at dawn and dusk, can reduce the risk of arboviral infection.

Chotmongkol V, Sawanyawisuth K, Thavornpitak Y. Corticosteroids treatment of eosinophilic meningitis. *Clin Infect Dis* 2000; 31: 660–662.

Prober CG. Central nervous system infections. In: Kliegman RM, Behrman RE, Jenson HB, Stanton BF (eds). *Nelson Textbook of Pediatrics*. 18th edn. Vol. 2. Philadelphia: Saunders, 2007; 2512–2524.

Rorabaugh ML, Berlin LE, Heldrich F, et al. Aseptic meningitis in infants younger than 2 years of age: acute illness and neurologic complications. *Pediatrics* 1993; 92: 206–211.

Swartz MN. Bacterial meningitis- a view of the past 90 years. *N Engl J Med* 2004; 351:1826–1828.

24.5 BRAIN ABSCESS

Brain abscesses can occur in children of any age but are most commonly seen in children between 4 and 8 yr and in neonates. The causes of brain abscess include embolization due to congenital heart disease with right to left shunts (especially in tetralogy of Fallot), meningitis, chronic otitis media and mastoiditis, sinusitis, soft tissue infection of the face or scalp, orbital cellulitis, dental infections, penetrating head injuries, immunodeficiency states, and infection of the ventriculoperitoneal shunts.

Etiology: The bacteria responsible for producing abscesses include streptococci (*S. milleri*, *S. pyogenes* group A or B, *S. pneumoniae*, *S. fecalis*), anaerobic organisms (gram-positive cocci, *Bacteroides* spp., *Fusobacterium* spp., *Prevotella* spp., *Actinomyces* spp.), and gram-negative aerobic bacilli (*Haemophilus aphrophilus*, *H. parainfluenzae*. *H. influenzae*, *Enterobacter*, *E. coli*, *Proteus* spp.). *Citrobacter* is most common in neonates. Fungal abscesses (*Aspergillus*, *Candida*) are more common in immunosuppressed patients.

Pathology: Cerebral abscesses are evenly distributed between the two hemispheres, and ≈ 80% of cases is divided equally between the frontal, parietal, and temporal lobes. Most brain abscesses are single.

Clinical manifestations: In early stages of cerebritis and abscess formation, nonspecific symptoms including low-grade fever, headache, and lethargy are present. Generally with these symptoms an oral antibiotic is prescribed with resultant transient relief. As the inflammatory process proceeds, vomiting, severe headache, seizures, papilledema, focal neurologic signs (hemiparesis) and coma may develop. A cerebellar abscess is characterized by nystagmus, ipsilateral ataxia and dysmetria, vomiting, and headache. If the abscess ruptures into the ventricular cavity, overwhelming shock and death usually ensue.

Diagnosis: CT with contrast and MRI are the diagnostic tests for demonstrating cerebritis and abscess formation. The CT finding of cerebritis is a parenchymal low-density lesion and an abscess cavity shows a ring-enhancing lesion by contrast CT. MRI T2 weighted images indicate increased signal intensity in cerebritis. MRI also demonstrates an abscess capsule with gadolinium administration. The peripheral white blood cell count can be normal or elevated and the blood culture is positive in ≈ 10% of cases. Examination of CSF shows white blood cells and protein either minimally elevated or normal, and the glucose level may be low. CSF cultures are rarely positive. Aspiration of the abscess is much more likely to establish the bacteriologic diagnosis. The EEG shows corresponding focal slowing. The radionuclide brain scan indicates an area of enhancement due to disruption of the blood–brain barrier in > 80% cases.

Treatment: The initial management of a brain abscess includes prompt diagnosis and institution of an antibiotic regimen. When the cause is unknown, the combination of vancomycin, a 3rd-generation cephalosporin, and metronidazole is commonly used. The same regimen is initiated when otitis media, sinusitis or mastoiditis is the likely cause. If there is a history of penetrating head injury, head trauma, or neurosurgery vancomycin plus a 3rd-generation cephalosporin is appropriate. When cyanotic congenital heart disease is the predisposing factor ampicillin-sulbactum alone or a 3rd-generation cephalosporin plus metronidazole may be used. Abscesses secondary to an infected ventriculoperitoneal shunt may be initially treated with vancomycin and ceftazidime. A brain abscess can be treated with antibiotics without surgery if the abscess is < 2 cm in diameter, short duration illness (< 2 wk), no signs of increased intracranial pressure and the child is neurologically intact. If the decision is made to treat with antibiotic alone, the child should have weekly neuroimaging studies to ensure that the abscess is decreasing in size. An encapsulated abscess, particularly if the lesion is causing a mass effect or increased intracranial pressure, should be treated with a combination of antibiotics and aspiration. Surgery is indicated when the abscess is >2.5 cm in diameter, presence of gas in the abscess, lesion multiloculated and located in the posterior fossa, or a fungus is identified. Associated infectious processes, such as mastoiditis, sinusitis, or a periorbital abscess may require surgical drainage. The duration of antibiotic therapy depends on the organism and response to treatment, but is usually 4–6 wk.

Prognosis: The mortality rate associated has decreased significantly with the use of CT or MRI and due to prompt antibiotic and surgical treatment. Long-term sequelae include hemiparesis, seizures, hydrocephalus, cranial nerve abnormalities, and behavior and learning problems.

Brook I. Aerobic and anaerobic bacteriology of intracranial abscesses. *Pediatr Neurol* 1992; 8: 210–214.

Goodkin HP, Harper MB, Pomeroy SL. Intracranial abscess in children: historical trends in Children's Hospital Boston. *Pediatrics* 2004; 113: 1765–1770.

Haslam RHA. Brain abscess. In: Kliegman RM, Behrman RE, Jenson HB, Stanton BF (eds). *Nelson Textbook of Pediatrics.* 18th edn. Vol. 2. Philadelphia: Saunders, 2007; 2524–2525.

24.6 CEREBRAL STROKE IN CHILDHOOD

Hemiplegia secondary to vascular disorders occurs in different types of strokes such as arterial thrombosis/embolism, venous thrombosis, and intracranial hemorrhage.

1. **Arterial thrombosis/embolism** may involve major cerebral arteries (internal carotid or anterior, middle and posterior cerebral artery occlusion) or smaller cerebral arteries.

   Thrombosis of the internal carotid artery may result from acute angulation of the artery (roller coaster, barbershop, beauty parlor, child abuse) or blunt trauma to the posterior pharynx caused by a fall on a pencil on the child's mouth. The injury produces a scar in the intima of the vessel wall, which may lead to formation of a dissecting aneurism. Cerebral symptoms result from shedding of emboli from the thrombus. The symptoms may be delayed for up to 24 hr after the accident, but progressive flaccid hemiplegia, lethargy, and aphasia occurs if the dominant hemisphere is involved. Focal motor seizures are a common complication. Dissection of vessels in the vertebral basilar circulation can lead to acute signs of brainstem dysfunction.

   Other causes of hemiplegia are retropharyngeal abscess, embolization of cerebral vessels (arrhythmias, myxoma, paradoxical emboli through a patent foramen ovale, bacterial endocarditis, air emboli and fat emboli), cyanotic congenital heart disease, occlusive vascular disorders (basal arterial occlusion with telangiectasia or moyamoya), sickle cell disease, coagulation disorders, occlusion of small arteries, and transient cerebral arteriopathy.

2. **Venous thrombosis.** The symptoms and signs of venous sinus thrombosis may evolve over days and in neonates are characterized by diffuse neurologic signs and seizures, whereas focal neurologic signs are more prominent in children. Dilated scalp veins, a bulging anterior fontanel, and symptoms and signs of increased intracranial pressure may be present. The causes of venous sinus thrombosis are septic and aseptic.

   Septic causes of venous sinus thrombosis include encephalitis and bacterial meningitis (including tuberculous meningitis). Aseptic causes include severe dehydration, hypercoagulopathy, cyanotic congenital heart disease, iron-deficiency anemia, and leukemic infiltrates of cerebral veins, *prothrombotic disorders* and vascular *malformations* associated with impaired venous (such as Sturge-Weber syndrome).

3. **Intracranial hemorrhage** may occur in the subarachnoid space or the bleeding may be primarily

located in the parenchyma of the brain. Subarachnoid bleeding is characterized by severe headache, nuchal rigidity and progressive loss of consciousness. The intracerebral bleeding is characterized by focal neurologic signs and seizures. The causes are *arteriovenous malformations* (including arteriovenous malformation of the vein of Galen) and *cerebral aneurysms* (located at the carotid bifurcation or on the anterior and posterior cerebral arteries rather than the circle of Willis).

Differential diagnosis of stroke like events include alternating hemiplegia of childhood (occasionally associated with migraine), metabolic diseases (mitochondrial encephalomyelopathy (MELAS), ornithine transcarbamylase deficiency, pyruvate dehydrogenase deficiency and homocystinuria), Todd paralysis, cerebral tumor, encephalitis (particularly herpes), focal postviral encephalitis, and status epilepticus.

Diagnosis: A thorough history and physical examination, searching for an underlying disease process; evidence of trauma; an infectious, metabolic, or hematologic disorder; neurocutaneous syndrome; increased intracranial pressure, or hydrocephalus will help in arriving the diagnosis. Febrile children should have a septic screen including CRP, blood and urine cultures and if necessary, and if the patient's general condition permits, CSF examination should be done. Renal function tests and electrolytes give a clue to the degree of hydration and the presence of SIADH which will be useful in determining fluid therapy. Chest X-ray and ESR can give a clue to malignancies and tuberculosis. An EEG may be helpful in localizing the disease process. A CT scan can detect recent bleeding or a large area of infarction, but diffusion weighted MRI, perfusion MRI imaging and MRA and MRV are superior for early detection of cerebral ischemia and assessment of cerebral vessels. A four-vessel cerebral angiogram may be indicated in which MRI studies cannot detect vasculitis or sites of intracranial hemorrhage. Electrocardiography and echocardiography may be help to exclude intrinsic cardiac diseases or an arrhythmia as a cause of the stroke. Test for finding out metabolic disorders should include lactate, pyruvate and ammonia levels, and screening for homocystinuria.

Treatment of strokes: Treatment of childhood stroke includes management of acute emergencies, treatment of the underlying disorder (including early referral to a neurosurgical unit) and rehabilitation of function.

Emergency room management: Airway stabilisation is vital in deteriorating patients with raised intracranial pressure. Emergent measures including the usage of ventilation, osmotherapy and diuretics have to be used to decrease the intracranial tension. Supportive care also includes blood pressure and fluid management, maintenance of normoglycemia, and control of fever and seizures.

Treatment of the underlying disorder: Low molecular weight heparin is sometimes used to treat venous thrombosis. The contraindications for the use of an antithrombotic agent include significant intracerebral hemorrhage and hypertension. Regular blood transfusion therapy may prevent stroke in children with sickle cell disease. Consideration should be given for vitamin B_6 therapy for children with homocystinuria. Antibiotics should be started if meningitis, sepsis or infective endocarditis is suspected.

Rehabilitation: General nursing care in the acute stages includes monitoring and controlling temperature, fluid balance and nutrition. Rehabilitation including physiotherapy, occupational therapy, speech therapy and vocational training should be instituted in all cases as soon as possible.

Prognosis: 50–70% of cases of stroke in a child have some form of residual impairment.

deVeber G. Cerebrovascular disease in Children. In: Swaiman KF, Ashwal S (eds). *Pediatric Neurology: Principles and Practice.* 3rd edn. Louis, Missouri: Mosby, 1999:1099–124.

Johnston MV, Comi A. Acute stroke syndromes. In: Kliegman RM, Behrman RE, Jenson HB, Stanton BF (eds). *Nelson Textbook of Pediatrics.* 18th edn. Vol. 2. Philadelphia: Saunders, 2007;2508–12.

Kirkham FJ. Stroke in Childhood. *Arch Dis Child* 1999;81:85–89.

Nagaraja D, Verma A, Taly AB, Kumar MV, Jayakumar PN. Cerebrovascular disease in children. *Acta Neurologica Scandinavia* 1994;90:251–5.

Narayanan Manjith. Childhood Cerebral stroke. In: Mathur GP, Mathur Sarla (eds). Current Trends in Pediatrics. Vol 1. Delhi: *Academa Publishers,* 2005;432–41.

24.7 NEUROCUTANEOUS SYNDROMES

The neurocutaneous syndromes are characterized by abnormalities of both the integument and central nervous system (CNS). Most disorders are familial and believed to arise from a defect in differentiation of the primitive ectoderm. Disorders classified as neurocutaneous syndromes include 1. Neurofibromatosis, 2. Tuberous sclerosis, 3. Sturge-Weber Syndrome, 4. von Hippel-Lindau disease, 5. Linear nevus syndrome, 6. PHACE Syndrome, 7. Ataxia telangiectasia, 8. Hypomelanosis of Ito, 9. Incontinentia pigmenti.

1. **Neurofibromatosis** (NF), von Recklinghausen disease is an autosomal dominant disorder. There are two distinct forms of NF (NF-1 and NF-2). NF-1 is the most prevalent type, with an incidence of

1/4,000. The NF-1 gene is located on chromosome 17q11.2. NF-1 is diagnosed when any two of the following seven signs are present: (1) Six or more café au lait macules over 5 mm in greatest diameter in prepubertal individuals and 15 mm in greatest diameter in postpubertal individuals. (2) Axillary or inguinal freckling consisting of multiple hyperpigmented areas 2–3 mm in diameter. (3) Two or more iris Lisch nodules. (4) Two or more neurofibromas or one plexiform neurofibroma. (5) A distinctive osseous lesion such as sphenoid dysplasia (which may cause pulsating exophthalmos) or cortical thinning of long bones with or without pseudoarthrosis. (6). Optic gliomas. (7) A first-degree relative with NF-1 whose diagnosis was based on the aforementioned criteria. Children with NF-1 are susceptible to neurologic complications, psychologic disturbances, hypertension, neurofibrosarcoma, or malignant schwannoma, pheochromosarcoma, rhabdomyosarcoma, leukemia, Wilms' tumor and CNS tumors (optic gliomas, meningiomas of the brain, and spinal cord, neurofibromas, astrocytomas, and neurilemmomas).

NF-2 accounts for 10% of all cases of NF. The gene for NF-2 is located near the center of the long arm of chromosome 22q1.11. NF-2 may be diagnosed when one of the following two features is present: (1) Bilateral eighth nerve masses consistent with acoustic neuromas. (2) A parent, sibling, or child with NF-2 and either unilateral eighth nerve masses or any two of the following: neurofibroma, meningioma, glioma, schwannoma, or juvenile posterior subcapsular lenticular opacities.

2. **Tuberous sclerosis (TS)** is inherited as an autosomal dominant trait. *Skin lesions* include hypomelanotic macules (likened to an ash leaf on the trunk and extremities); a shagreen patch (consists of a roughened, raised lesion with an orange-peel consistency located primarily in the lumbosacral region); subungual or periungual fibromas (of the finger and toes during adolescence). *Retinal lesions* (mulberry tumors that arise from the nerve head or round, flat gray lesions in the region of the disc and hamatoma or depigmented areas). *Brain lesions* are cortical tuber located in the convolutions of the cerebral hemispheres, subependymal region, and region of the foramen of Monro (may cause obstruction of CSF flow and hydrocephalus).

3. **Sturge-Weber syndrome** consists of a facial nevus (port-wine stain), seizures, hemiparesis, strokelike episodes, intracranial calcifications, and in many cases mental retardation. The skull radiograph shows intracranial calcification in the occipito-parietal region in most patients, characteristically assumes a serpentine or railroad-track appearance.

4. **von Hippel-Lindau disease:** The neurologic features of the condition include cerebellar hemangioblastomas and retinal angiomata. The CT scan and MRI show a cystic cerebellar lesion with a vascular mural nodule.

5. **Linear nevus syndrome** is characterized by a facial nevus and neurodevelopmental abnormalities. The nevus is located on the forehead and nose and tends to be midline in its distribution. More than half of the patients have a seizure disorder and are mentally retarded.

6. **PHACE syndrome** consists of posterior fossa malformations, hemangiomas, arterial anomalies, coarctation of aorta and other cardiac defects, and eye abnormalities. The facial hemangioma is typically ipsilateral to the aortic arch. There is a female predominance. Airway hemangiomas may produce obstruction.

7. **Ataxia-telangiectasia** (Louis-Bar syndrome) is transmitted as an autosomal recessive trait. The characteristic telangiectasias develop at about 3 yr of age, 1st on the bulbar conjunctivae, and later on the nasal bridge, malar areas, external ears, hard palate, upper anterior chest, and antecubital and popliteal fossae. Additional cutaneous stigmata include café au lait spots, premature graying of the hair. Progressive cerebellar ataxia, neurologic deterioration, sinopulmonary infections (from bacteria and respiratory viruses), and malignancies (lymphoreticular type, adenocarcinomas) also occur. Unaffected relatives have an increased incidence of malignancy.

8. **Hypomelanosis of Ito** affects children of both sexes and is frequently associated with defects in various organ systems. *Skin lesions* are generally present at birth but may be acquired in the 1st 2 yr of life, and are of bizarre, patterned, hypopigmented macules arranged over the body surface in sharply demarcated whorls, streaks, and patches. The palms, soles, and mucous membranes are spared.

Other defects include central nervous system abnormalities (mental retardation, seizures, microcephaly, and muscular hypotonia), musculoskeletal system (scoliosis and thoracic and limb deformities), ophthalmologic defects (strabismus, nystagmus), and cardiac defects.

9. **Incontinentia pigmenti** (Bloch-Sulzberger disease) is a rare, heritable, multisystem ectodermal disorder with dermatologic, dental, and ocular abnormalities.

Haslam RHA. Neurocutaneous syndromes. In: Kliegman RM, Behrman RE, Jenson HB, Stanton BF (eds). *Nelson Textbook of Pediatrics*. 18th edn. Vol. 2. Philadelphia: Saunders, 2007; 2483–2488.

Morelli JG. Vascular disorders. In: Kliegman RM, Behrman RE, Jenson HB, Stanton BF (eds). *Nelson Textbook of Pediatrics*. 18th edn. Vol. 2. Philadelphia: Saunders, 2007; 2667–2674.

Morelli JG. Hyperpigmented lesions. In: Kliegman RM, Behrman RE, Jenson HB, Stanton BF (eds). *Nelson Textbook of Pediatrics*. 18th edn. Vol. 2. Philadelphia: Saunders, 2007; 2679–2682.

Morelli JG. Hypopigmented lesions. In: Kliegman RM, Behrman RE, Jenson HB, Stanton BF (eds). *Nelson Textbook of Pediatrics*. 18th edn. Vol. 2. Philadelphia: Saunders, 2007; 2682–2685.

24.8 SEIZURES IN CHILDHOOD

A seizure or convulsion is a paroxysmal, time-limited change in motor activity and or/behavior that results from abnormal electrical activity in the brain. Seizures are common in the pediatric age group and occur in ≈10% of children. Most seizures in children are provoked by somatic disorders originating outside the brain, such as high fever, infection, syncope, head trauma, hypoxia, toxins, or cardiac arrhythmias. Less than one third of seizures in children are caused by epilepsy. *Epilepsy* is a condition in which seizures are triggered recurrently from within the brain. Epilepsy is considered to be present when two or more unprovoked seizures occur at an interval greater than 24 hr apart. The cumulative lifetime incidence of epilepsy is 3%; more than half cases begin in childhood. The annual prevalence of epilepsy is 0.5–0.8% because many children outgrow epilepsy. The prognosis of children with epilepsy is generally good, but 10–20% cases have persistent seizures refractory to drugs.

Phases (parts) of seizure: The seizure has 3 phases. But all cases do not have 3 phases of seizure. The period during which the seizure actually occurs is defined as the ictus or ictal period. The aura is the earliest portion of a seizure recognized and the only part remembered by the patient; it may act as a "warning". The time immediately following a seizure is referred to as the postictal, period; the interval between seizures is the interictal period. Automatisms develop after loss of consciousness and may persist in to the post-ictal phase.

Evaluation of the First Seizure

Initial evaluation of an infant or child during or shortly after a suspected seizure should include an assessment of the adequacy of airway, breathing, and circulation, as well as measurement of temperature, blood pressure and glucose concentration. The first step in an evaluation is to determine whether the seizure has a focal onset or generalized. *Focal seizures* may be characterized by motor or sensory symptoms and include forceful turning of the head and eyes on one side, unilateral clonic movements beginning in the face or extremities or a sensory disturbance such as paresthesias or pain localized to a specific area. Focal seizures in an adolescent or adult usually indicate a localized lesion, but in children may be nondiagnostic. Motor seizures may be focal or generalized tonic-clonic, clonic, myoclonic, or atonic. *Tonic seizures* are characterized by increased tone or rigidity. *Atonic seizures* are characterized by flaccidity or lack of movement during a convulsion. *Clonic seizures* consist of rhythmic muscle contraction or relaxation. *Myoclonus* is characterized by shock-like contraction of a muscle. The duration of the seizure and state of consciousness should be documented.

Unprovoked Seizures

First unprovoked seizure: Although the occurrence of a seizure in a child without a provocative stimulus such as high fever is often considered beginning of a chronic disorder or epilepsy, only less than half of the children develop a 2nd seizure without a provocative stimulus.

Recurrent seizures: Two unprovoked seizures >24 hr apart suggest the presence of an epileptic disorder within the brain that will lead to future recurrences. It is therefore, important to perform a careful evaluation to look for the cause of seizures, need for treatment with antiepileptic drugs and response of treatment and remission of seizures in the future.

Mechanisms of Seizures

Although the precise mechanisms of seizures are unknown, several physiologic factors are responsible for the development of a seizure. To initiate a seizure, there must be a group of neurons that are capable of generating a significant burst discharge and impairment of the γ-aminobutyric acid (GABA)-ergic inhibitory system. Seizure discharge transmission ultimately depends on excitatory glutamatergic synapses. Excitatory amino acid neurotransmitters (glutamate, aspartate) may have a role in producing neuronal excitation by acting on specific cell receptors. Seizures may arise from areas of neuronal death, and these regions of the brain may promote development of novel hyperexcitable synapses that can cause seizures. Lesions in the temporal lobe (including slow-growing gliomas, hamartomas, gliosis, hippocampal sclerosis, and arteriovenous malformations) cause seizures, and when the abnormal tissue is removed surgically, the seizures are likely to cease. Two hypotheses have been suggested to explain the origin of seizures after brain injury. One suggests that inhibitory neurons are selectively damaged and remaining principal excitatory neurons become hyperexcitable. The other hypothesis suggests that aberrant excitatory circuits are formed as part of reorganization after injury.

Certain seizures are age specific (infantile spasms), because the underdeveloped brain is more susceptible to specific seizures indicating that the immature brain is more excitable than the mature brain, reflecting the greater influence of excitatory glutamate-containing circuits. The actions of GABA, the major inhibitory neurotransmitter, are often paradoxically excitatory in the immature brain.

Genetic factors account for at least 20% of all cases of epilepsy, such as benign neonatal convulsions (20q and 8q), juvenile myoclonic epilepsy (6p), and progressive myoclonic epilepsy (21q22.3).

Classification of Seizures

It is important to classify the seizure in order to understand its etiology, selecting the appropriate therapy, and providing prognosis (Box 24.2). The seizure activity is broadly divided into two types—partial (focal) and generalized. Some seizure types of neonates (neonatal seizures) and infants (infantile spasms) are classified as unclassified seizures.

Epilepsy in children has also been classified by syndrome, using the age of onset of seizures, cognitive development, seizure type and the EEG findings including the background rhythm (Box 24.3).

Parents and patient education: Cooperation and understanding among the parents, physician, teacher, and the child enhance the outlook of patients with epilepsy. The person with epilepsy must keep the Epilepsy Identity Card. It will be easy for the people to provide appropriate help during an attack of seizure. It will also be easier for the physician to provide treatment without wasting time in investigating the case.

Epilepsy Identity Card (*see* Fig. 24.8 in CD)

Name   Age   Sex   Blood group   Photo

Drug taking for epilepsy:

Type of seizure:

Dates of occurrence of seizure:

School address and class:

Home address and telephone/mobile:

Office address and telephone/mobile:

Child under the treatment of the doctor Address, Telephone/mobile:

First aid measures:

Box 24.2: International classification of seizures

Partial seizures
Simple partial (consciousness retained) [SPS]
   Motor
   Sensory
   Autonomic
   Psychic
Complex partial (consciousness impaired) [CPS]
   Simple partial, followed by impaired consciousness
   Consciousness impaired at onset
Partial seizures with secondary generalization
Generalized seizures
Absences
   Typical
   Atypical
Generalized tonic-clonic
Tonic
Clonic
Myoclonic
Atonic
Infantile spasms
Unclassified seizures

Box 24.3: Classification of epilepsy by syndromes

1. Benign myoclonic epilepsy of infancy
2. Benign partial epilepsy with centrotemporal spikes (BPEC)
3. Febrile convulsions
4. Infantile spasms (West syndrome)
5. Rasmussen encephalitis
6. Landau-Kleffner syndrome (LKS)
7. Lennox-Gastaut syndrome (LGS)
8. Juvenile myoclonic epilepsy (Jauz syndrome)
9. Progressive myoclonic epilepsy (Lafora disease)

Allen CMC, Lueck CJ: Seizures. In: Haslett C, Chilvers ER, Hunter JAA, Boon NA (eds). *Davidson's Principles and Practice of Medicine.* 18th edn. Edinburgh: Churchill Livingstone, 1999; 940–949.

Guerrini R. Epilepsy in children. *Lancet* 2006; 367: 499–524.

Johnston MV. Seizures in Childhood. In: Kliegman RM, Behrman RE, Jenson HB, Stanton BF (eds). *Nelson Textbook of Pediatrics.* 18th edn. Vol. 2. Philadelphia: Saunders, 2007; 2457–2475.

Lowenstein DH: Seizures and Epilepsy. In: Braunwald E, Fauci AS, Kasper DL, Hauser SL, Longo DL, Jameson JL (eds). *Harrison's Principles of Internal Medicine.* 15th edn. New York: McGraw-Hill, 2001; 2354–2369.

Mathur GP, Mathur Sarla. Seizures and epilepsy. In: Mathur GP, Mathur Sarla (eds). *Seizures in Children and Adolescents.* Delhi: Academa Publishers, 2005; 1–12.

Pohlmann-Eden B, Beghi E, Camfield C, Camfield P. The first seizure and its management in adults and children. *BMJ* 2006; 332: 339–342.

Puri V. EEG in clinical practice. In: Talukdar B (Ed). *Essentials of Pediatric Neurology.* New Delhi: New Age International (P) Limited, 1997; 31–44.

Partial Seizures

Partial seizures account for a larger proportion of seizures seen in children (up to 40%). Partial seizures (synonymous with focal) are those in which the seizure activity is restricted to discrete areas of the cerebral cortex. Partial seizures are often associated with structural abnormalities of the brain. Partial seizures may or may not be associated with aura. Partial seizures are classified into three subgroups. 1. If the consciousness is fully preserved during the seizure, the seizure is termed simple partial seizure (SPS). 2. If consciousness is impaired, the seizure is termed complex partial seizure (CPS). 3. Seizures that begin as partial seizures and then spread diffusely throughout the cortex are known as partial seizures with secondary generalization. The causes of partial seizures are listed in Table 24.4.

1. **Simple partial seizures (SPS):** The consciousness is preserved in simple partial seizures (SPS). Aura may or may not be present. Automatisms are absent. SPS may present as motor, sensory (somatosensory or special sensory) autonomic or psychic forms. The average seizure persists for 10–20 seconds. No postictal phenomenon follows the event. The presence of an aura always indicates a focal onset of seizure.

   Motor: Motor activity is the most common symptom of SPS. Epileptic activity arising in the precentral gyrus causes partial motor seizures affecting the contralateral face, neck, arm, trunk and leg. The movements are asynchronous clonic or tonic movements. Some attacks begin in one part (e.g. mouth, thumb, great toe) and spread gradually (Jacksonian seizures). Seizures consisting of head twisting and conjugate eye movements are particularly common in SPS due to a frontal epileptic focus involving the frontal eye field. This type of attack often becomes generalized to a tonic-

clonic seizure. SPS may be confused with tics. Tics primarily involve the face and shoulders (shoulder shrugging, eye blinking, and facial grimacing). Tic can be briefly suppressed but partial seizures cannot be controlled. EEG is normal in cases of tics and abnormal in cases with seizure disorder.

Sensory: Seizures arising in the precentral gyrus cause tingling or electric sensations in the contralateral face and limbs. A spreading pattern like a Jacksonian seizure may occur.

Psychic: Seizures, which cause alterations of mood, memory and perception usually, arise from the medial temporal lobe. This is a common form of seizure, causing both partial and secondary generalized seizures.

Autonomic: There will be flushing, sweating and piloerections.

Visual: Occipital epileptic foci cause simple visual hallucination such as ball of light or patterns of color. Formed visual hallucinations of face or scenes arise more anteriorly in the temporal lobes.

Other types of partial seizures: These include those that change in equilibrium (sensations of falling or vertigo). Simple partial seizures arising from the temporal or frontal cortex may also cause alterations in hearing, olfaction or higher cortical function (psychic symptoms).

2. **Complex partial seizures (CPS):** CPS may present in two ways. CPS may begin with a simple partial seizure (SPS) with or without an aura (i) followed by impaired consciousness or (ii) the onset of the CPS may coincide with an altered state of consciousness. The seizures frequently begin with an aura (i.e. simple partial seizure) that is stereotypic for the patient. An aura consisting of vague, unpleasant feelings, epigastric discomfort, or fear is present in approximately one third of children with SPS and CPS. The presence of an aura always

Table 24.4: Causes of partial seizures

Idiopathic

- Benign partial epilepsy with centrotemporal spikes (BPEC)

Focal structural lesions

- Genetic: Tuberous sclerosis, neurofibromatosis, von Hippel-Lindau syndrome
- Infantile hemiplegia
- Dysembryonic: cortical dysgenesis, Sturge-Weber syndrome
- Mesial temporal sclerosis (associated with febrile convulsions)
- Cerebrovascular disease: intracerebral hemorrhage, cerebral embolus, arteriovenous malformation
- Tumors
- Trauma (including neurosurgery)
- Infection: cerebral abscess (pyogenic), treated cases of tuberculous meningitis (TBM), toxoplasmosis, cysticercosis, subdural empyema, encephalitis, HIV
- Inflammatory disease: Sarcoidosis, vasculitis

indicates a focal onset of seizure. The postictal phase *after a complex partial seizure* is highly variable in length and consists of partial impairment of consciousness during which the patient may react to environmental stimuli. The reactions to external stimuli are often inappropriate and may include violent behavior if the patient is directed to do something he does not wish to do.

Automatisms are a common feature of CPS in infants and children, occurring in approximately 50–75% of cases; the older the child, the greater is the frequency of automatisms. Automatisms develop after the loss of consciousness and may persist into the postictal phase, but the child does not recall them. The automatic behavior observed in infants is characterized by alimentary automatisms, including lip smacking, chewing, swallowing, and excessive salivation. These movements can represent normal infant behavior and are difficult to distinguish from the automatisms of CPS. Prolonged and repetitive alimentary automatisms associated with a blank stare or with a lack of responsiveness almost always indicate CPS in an infant. Automatic behavior in older children consists of semipurposeful, incoordinated, and unplanned gestural automatisms, including picking and pulling at clothing or the bed sheets, rubbing or caressing objects, and walking or running in a nondirective, repetitive, and often fearful fashion.

3. *Partial seizures with secondary generalization:* Partial seizures can spread to involve both cerebral hemispheres and produce a generalized seizure, usually of the tonic-clonic variety. Secondary generalization is observed frequently following simple partial seizures, especially those with a focus in the frontal lobe, but may also be associated with partial seizures occurring elsewhere in the brain.

Conditions Associated with Partial Seizures

1. **Single small enhancing CT lesions (SSECTL) in epilepsy:** Neurocysticercosis is one of the important causes of epilepsy. The SSECTL are either inflammatory (cysticercosis, focal encephalitis, microabscesses, sarcoidosis, focal inflammation) or vascular. The treatment depends on the underlying cause.

2. **Gelastic seizure (Ictal laughter):** It is a rare symptom often associated with hypothalamic hamartoma. Seizures usually begin in infancy and childhood and later may be accompanied by cognitive decline. Brief, repetitive, stereotypical episodes of laughter are the first most common manifestation of the epileptic syndrome in patients with hypothalamic hamartomas. Gamma knife can be a safe and efficacious method for treating epilepsy related to hypothalamic hamartomas.

3. **Epilepsy in neurofibromatosis:** Neurofibromatosis 1 is the most common neurocutaneous disease and the neurologic manifestations are mainly represented by tumors such as optic gliomas, focal areas of high T2-weighted signal known as unidentified bright objects, and mental retardation or learning disabilities and epilepsy.

4. **Benign partial epilepsy with centrotemporal spikes (BPEC):** This is an idiopathic age-specific epileptic syndrome with a benign course. It is a common type of partial epilepsy in childhood seen in the ages of 2 and 14 with a peak age of onset of 9–10 years. The children are normal with normal past history and neurologic examination. There is often a positive family history of epilepsy. The seizures are usually partial and motor signs and somatosensory symptoms are often confined to the face. Oropharyngeal symptoms include tonic contractions and paresthesias of the tongue, unilateral numbness of the cheek (particularly along the gum), guttural noises, dysphagia, and excessive salivation. Unilateral tonic-clonic contractures of the lower face, and clonic movements or paresthesias of the ipsilateral extremities are frequently associated with oropharyngeal symptoms. Consciousness may be intact or impaired, and the partial seizure may proceed to secondary generalization. BPEC occurs during sleep in 75% of patients, whereas CPS tends to be observed during waking hours. The EEG pattern of BPEC is characterized by a repetitive spike focus localized in the centrotemporal or rolandic area with normal background activity. The clinical features (including BPEC occurring during sleep), EEG findings (rolandic foci), and absence of a neuropathologic lesion are characteristic and readily separate BPEC from CPS. Anticonvulsants are given in those cases that have frequent seizures. Carbamzepine is the preferred drug, which is continued for at least 2 years or until 14–16 years of age, when spontaneous remission of BPEC usually occurs. BPEC has an excellent prognosis.

5. **Rasmussen encephalitis:** This subacute inflammatory encephalitis is one cause of *epilepsia partialis continua*. A nonspecific febrile illness may have preceeded the onset of focal seizures, which may be frequent or continuous. The onset is usually before the age of 10 years. Sequelae include hemiplegia, hemianopia, and aphasia. As the seizures are refractory to conventional antiepileptic drug therapies surgery should be considered in patients of Rasmussen syndrome. The EEG reveals diffuse paroxysmal activity with a slow

background. The disease is progressive and potentially lethal but more often becomes self-limited with significant neurologic deficits. The disease may be due to autoantibodies that bind to and stimulate the glutamate receptors. Cytomegalovirus has been recognized in several surgical specimens of patients with Rasmussen encephalitis.

Investigations: The routine investigations including blood counts, Mantoux test, chest X-ray, computed tomography (CT scan) and electroencephalography (EEG) should be advised in all cases. Cerebrospinal fluid (CSF) examination is done in cases of inflammatory granuloma in whom clear distinction cannot be made out between tuberculosis and neurocysticercosis using radiological criteria (lesion more than 20 mm and irregular outline), enzyme linked immunosorbent assay in CSF for neurocysticercosis and evidence of tuberculosis elsewhere in the body. Negative tests do not exclude diagnosis of neurocysticercosis since ELISA is negative in inactive cases of neurocysticercosis. Magnetic resonance imaging (MRI) offers better resolution to detect the scolex. Positron Emission Tomography (PET) is helpful in precise localization of epileptic.

Treatment

Medical therapy: Patients should be treated with first line of antiepileptic drug, i.e. carbamazepine, phenytoin or valproic acid (*see* Table 24.6). A second drug is substituted if the highest dose of the first drug failed to achieve seizure control. Antituberculosis therapy is given to patients with tuberculosis. Children with seizures, with no hydrocephalus and with only calcified, inactive lesions on CT do not require therapy other than antiepileptic drugs. In these patients niclosamide (1 g per oral for children 4.98 kg–15.4 kg; 1.5 g per oral for children 15.9 kg or greater) is given if they are having adult worms. The parasite is expelled on the day of the administration. Active parenchymal lesions should be treated with one of the two-anticysticercal drugs (albendazole or praziquantel), which is associated with fewer residual seizures on long-term follow-up. Albendazole (15 mg/kg/24 hr divided in two doses for 28 days; maximum 400 mg/dose) is given with a fatty meal to improve absorption and praziquantal (50 mg/kg/24 hr divided in three doses for 15 days). Albendazole is the preferred drug. A worsening of symptoms can follow the use of either drug due to increased inflammation as a result of host response to dying parasite, which can be ameliorated, by the use of corticosteroid therapy. Corticosteroids (prednisolone 2 mg/kg/24 hr) are given for 2–3 days before and during drug therapy. In addition,

decongestive therapy is given to patients with granuloma showing mass effect or midline shift.

Epilepsy surgery: Seizures caused by a structural CNS lesion such as a brain tumor, vascular malformation, or brain abscess may not recur after appropriate treatment of the underlying lesion.

Vagus nerve stimulation (VNS): Vagus nerve stimulation (VNS) therapy for patients with medically refractory epilepsy, who are not candidates for resective brain surgery.

Prevention: All family members of index cases of cysticercosis, as well persons handling their food should be examined for disease or evidence of adult worms and treated. Hand washing and avoidance of fresh fruits and vegetables in areas endemic for Taenia solium (pork tapeworm) help prevent ingestion of eggs. All pork food items should be cooked thoroughly. All children and adults in close contact of a case of tubercular granuloma having infectious pulmonary tuberculosis should be tuberculin skin tested and examined to exclude tuberculosis.

Prognosis: Overall, generalized seizures are more easily controlled than partial seizures. The presence of a structural lesion makes complete control of the epilepsy less likely and the prognosis is generally worse compared to patients with idiopathic epilepsy. Children with best prognosis following AED withdrawal are those with BREC. CPS is more likely to recur. Epilepsy surgery and VNS should be considered in those patients who do not respond to long term treatment.

Aggarwal A, Aneja S, Taluja V, Kumar R, Bhardwaj K. Etiology of partial epilepsy. *Indian Pediatr* 1998; 35: 49–52.

Allen CMC, Lueck CJ. Seizures. In: Haslett C, Chilvers ER, Hunter JAA, Boon NA (eds). *Davidson's Principles and Practice of Medicine.* 18th edn. Edinburgh: Churchill Livingstone, 1999; 940–949.

Cascino GD, Andermann F, Berokvic SF, et al. Gelastic seizure and hypothalamic hamartomas: Evaluation of patients undergoing chronic intracranial EEG monitoring and outcome of surgical treatment. *Neurology* 1993; 43:747–750.

Chopra JS Sawhney IMS, Suresh N, Prabhakar S, Dhand UK, Suri S. Vanishing CT lesions in epilepsy. *J Neurol Sci* 1992; 107: 40–49.

Mathur GP, Singhal PK, Mathur Sarla. Partial seizures. In: Mathur GP, Mathur Sarla (eds). *Seizures in Children and Adolescents.* Delhi: Academa Publishers, 2005; 30–45.

Johnston MV. Seizures in Childhood. In: Kliegman RM, Behrman RE, Jenson HB, Stanton BF (eds). *Nelson Textbook of Pediatrics.* 18th edn. Vol. 2. Philadelphia: Saunders, 2007; 2457–2475.

Parkinson GM. High incidence of language disorder in children with focal epilepsies. *Dev Med Child Neurol* 2002; 44 (8): 533–537.

Generalized Seizures

Generalized seizures arise from both cerebral hemispheres simultaneously. But the existence of a focal region of abnormal activity that initiates the seizure prior to rapid secondary generalization (partial seizures with secondary generalization) cannot be entirely ruled out. For this reason, generalized seizures may be practically defined as bilateral clinical and electrographic events without any detectable focal onset.

Classification: Generalized seizures are classified as primary and secondary types. Various distinctive features distinguish primary generalized seizures into seven subgroups (Box 24.4).

Box 24.4: Classification of generalized seizures

A. Primary generalized seizures: 1. Absence (typical, atypical); 2. Tonic-clonic (grandmal); 3. Atonic; 4. Myoclonic; 5. Infantile spasms; 6. Landau-Kleffner syndrome (LKS)
B. Secondary generalized seizures: Partial seizures with secondary generalization

---

Pathogenesis: In primary generalized seizures, the abnormal activity is seen to begin synchronously throughout the cortex without an initial partial onset. It probably originates in the central diencephalic mechanisms controlling cortical activation. If the partial seizure activity spread into the diencephalon and then throughout the remainder of the cortex, it leads to secondary generalized seizure. If the abnormal electrical activity fails to affect muscle tone it will result in more restricted clinical manifestation. In this case there is an 'absence', in which consciousness is lost but the patient remains standing or sitting in an attack.

1. **Absence seizures (Petit mal)** are characterized by sudden, brief lapses of consciousness without loss of postural control. This seizure type is seen in approximately 15 to 20 percent of children with epilepsy. Absence seizures almost always begin in childhood (uncommon before age 5 years) or early adolescence, are more prevalent in girls; they are never associated with aura; the seizure typically lasts for only seconds (rarely persists longer than 30 seconds), consciousness returns, as suddenly as it was lost and they are not associated with a postictal state. These features tend to differentiate absence seizures from complex seizures. Automatic behavior frequently accompanies simple absence seizures. Hyperventilation for 3–4 minutes routinely produces an absence seizure. The seizures can occur hundreds of times per day, but the child may be unaware of or unable to convey their existence. In this situation the patient is constantly struggling to piece together experiences that have been interrupted by the seizures. Since the clinical signs of the seizures are subtle, the first clue to absence epilepsy is often unexplained "day dreaming" and a decline in school performance recognized by a teacher.

In the *typical absence seizures* there is a generalized, symmetric, 3 Hz spike-and-wave discharge that begins and ends suddenly on a normal EEG background. Periods of spike-and-wave discharges lasting more than a few seconds usually correlate with the clinical signs, but the EEG often shows many more periods of abnormal cortical activity than were suspected clinically. Hyperventilation tends to provoke these electrographic discharges and even the seizures themselves and is routinely used when recording the EEG. Typical absence seizures are not associated with other neurologic problems and respond well to treatment with specific anticonvulsants. Approximately 60 to 70 percent of such patients will have a spontaneous remission during adolescence. In the *atypical (complex) absence seizures* the lapse of consciousness is usually of longer duration and less abrupt in onset and cessation. The seizure is accompanied by more obvious motor signs consisting of myoclonic movements of the face, fingers or extremities and on occasion, loss of body tone, and may include focal or lateralizing features. Atypical absence seizures are usually associated with diffuse or multifocal structural abnormalities of the brain and may accompany other signs of neurologic dysfunction such as mental retardation. The EEG shows a generalized, slow-spike-and wave pattern with a frequency of 2.5 per second. The seizures are less responsive to anticonvulsants compared to typical absence seizures.

2. **Generalized tonic-clonic seizures (Grand mal)** seizures are extremely common and may follow a partial seizure with a focal onset (second generalization) or occurs de novo. The primarily generalized tonic-clonic seizures may be associated with an aura, suggesting a focal origin of the epileptiform discharge. The presence of an aura indicates its site of origin which may indicate the area of pathology. The initial phase is the tonic phase. Patients suddenly lose consciousness and in some cases emit a shrill, piercing cry. Their eyes roll back, their entire body musculature undergoes tonic contractions, and they rapidly become cyanotic in association with apnea. The clonic phase of the seizure is

heralded by rhythmic clonic contractions alternating with relaxation of all muscle groups. The clonic phase slows toward the end of the seizure, which usually persists for a few minutes, and patients often sigh as the seizure comes to an abrupt stop.

Tonic contraction of the muscles accounts for a number of the classic features of the event. Tonic contraction of the muscles of expiration and the larynx at the onset will produce a loud moan or emit a shrill, piercing cry. Respirations are impaired, secretions pool in the oropharynx, and the patient becomes cyanotic. Contractions of the jaw muscles may cause biting of the tongue [A severely bitten, bleeding tongue after an attack of loss of unconsciousness is pathognomic of a generalized seizure]. During the seizure, patients may bite their tongue but rarely vomit. A marked enhancement of sympathetic tone leads to increases in heart rate, blood pressure, and papillary size. The tonic phase of the seizure lasts for 10 to 20 seconds and then typically evolves into the clonic phase which usually lasts no more than one minute.

Tight clothing and jewelry around the neck should be loosened. The patient should be placed on one side and the neck and jaw should be gently hyperextended to enhance breathing. The mouth should not be opened forcibly by an object or by a finger because the patient's teeth may be dislodged, and aspirated or significant injury to the oropharyngeal cavity may result.

The postictal phase is characterized by unresponsiveness, muscular flaccidity, and excessive salivation that can cause stridorous breathing and partially airway obstruction. Loss of sphincter control (bladder or bowel incontinence) particularly, the bladder is common. Postictally, patients initially are semicomatose and typically remain in a deep sleep from 30 minutes to 2 hours. Patients may demonstrate truncal ataxia, hyperactive deep tendon reflexes, clonus, and a Babinski reflex if examined during the seizure or immediately postictally. The postictal phase is often associated with vomiting and an intense bifrontal headache. When the cause of generalized seizure cannot be ascertained it is termed idiopathic. Many factors are known to precipitate generalized tonic-clonic seizures in children, including low grade fever associated with infections, excessive fatigue or emotional stress, various drugs (including psychotropic medications, theophylline, and methylphenidate) and particularly if the seizures are poorly controlled by anticonvulsant drugs. There are many variants of the generalized tonic-

clonic seizure including pure tonic and pure clonic seizures. Brief tonic seizures lasting only a few seconds are usually associated with known epileptic syndromes having mixed seizure phenotypes, such as the Lennox-Gastaut syndrome.

The EEG during the tonic phase of the seizure shows a progressive increase in generalized low-voltage fast activity, followed by generalized high-amplitude, polyspike discharges. In the clonic phase, the high-amplitude activity is typically interrupted by slow waves to create a spike-and-wave pattern. The postictal EEG shows diffuse slowing that gradually recovers as the patient awakens. The routine investigations including blood counts, Mantoux test, chest X-ray, computed tomography (CT scan) and electroencephalography (EEG) should be advised in all cases. Magnetic resonance imaging (MRI) offers better resolution to detect the lesion than does CT.

Patients should be treated with first line of antiepileptic drug, i.e. carbamazepine, phenytoin, ethosuximide or valproic acid. A second drug is substituted if the highest dose of the first drug failed to achieve seizure control. Treat also the underlying cause in cases of symptomatic epilepsy. Overall, generalized seizures are more easily controlled than partial seizures. The complete control of the epilepsy is possible and the prognosis is generally good in patients with idiopathic epilepsy. In cases of symptomatic epilepsy also treat the underlying cause. Sometimes specific trigger factors are responsible for initiating seizures.

3. **Atonic seizures** are characterized by sudden loss of postural muscle tone lasting 1 to 2 seconds. Consciousness is briefly impaired, but there is usually no postictal confusion. Atonic seizures are usually seen in association with known epileptic syndromes. The EEG shows brief, generalized spike and wave discharges followed immediately by diffuse slow waves that correlate with the loss of muscle tone.

4. **Myoclonic seizures** are repetitive seizures consisting of brief, often symmetric muscular contractions with loss of body tone and falling or slumping forward, which tends to cause injuries of the face and the mouth. Myoclonus is one of the manifestations in the seizure disorders (partial seizures, neonatal seizures, and complex [atypical] absence seizures). Five distinct subgroups of myoclonic epilepsies have been identified.

   i. *Benign myoclonus of infancy:* Benign myoclonus begins during infancy and consists of clusters of myoclonic movements confined to the neck, trunk and extremities. EEG is normal in patients with benign myoclonus. The prognosis is good, with normal development and the cessation of myoclonus by 2 years of age. Such children do not require treatment with oral steroids or intramuscular ACTH or anticonvulsants.

ii. *Typical myoclonic epilepsy of early childhood:* Children are near normal prior to the onset of myoclonic seizures. The mean age of onset is ≈ 2 yr, but the range varies from 6 months to four years. There is a positive family history of epilepsy, in at least one-third of children. The frequency of myoclonic seizures varies, they may occur several times daily or children may be seizure free for weeks. A few patients have febrile convulsions or generalized tonic-clonic afebrile seizures that precede the onset of myoclonic epilepsy. The EEG shows fast spike wave complexes of ≥ 2.5 Hz and a normal background rhythm in most cases. Mental retardation develops in a few cases, but learning and language problems and emotional and behavioral disorders occur in a significant number of cases. The long-term outcome is relatively favorable and more than 50% cases are seizures free several years later.

iii. *Complex myoclonic epilepsies:* The focal or generalized tonic clonic seizures beginning during infancy antedate the onset of myoclonic epilepsy. Usually there is a history of hypoxic ischemic encephalopathy in the perinatal period. The children are usually microcephalic with generalized upper motor neuron and extra-pyramidal signs. Approximately one-third of the children are mentally retarded. Family history of epilepsy is absent. Patients with complex myoclonic epilepsy routinely have interictal slow spike waves in EEG. Some children display a combination of frequent myoclonic and tonic seizures along with slow spike waves in the EEG, the seizure disorder is classified as the **Lennox-Gastaut syndrome.** Cases of complex myoclonic epilepsies are refractory to anticonvulsant; the seizures are persistent. The mental retardation and behavioral problems are present in approximately 75% of all patients.

iv. *Juvenile myoclonic epilepsy (Janz Syndrome):* Juvenile myoclonic epilepsy (JME) is a generalized seizure disorder of unknown cause that appears in early adolescence and is usually characterized by bilateral myoclonic jerks that may be single or repetitive. The myoclonic seizures are most frequent in the morning after awakening and can be provoked by sleep deprivation, fatigue, or alcohol, is characteristic

at onset. Myoclonic movements on awakening may be a prominent manifestation, which make hair combing and tooth brushing difficult. As the myoclonus tends to abate later in the morning, most patients do not seek medical advice at this stage. A few years later, early morning generalized tonic-clonic seizures develop in association with myoclonus. Consciousness is preserved unless the myoclonus is especially severe. Generalized tonic-clonic (GTC) seizures occur in >90% and 30% have absence seizures. The GTC seizures are often preceded by a series of myoclonic jerks. There is often a family history of epilepsy, and genetic linkage studies suggest a polygenic cause. There is existence of JME locus on chromosome 6p21 (designated EJM1). This expresses the phenotype of classic JME. A separate susceptibility locus for JME maps to chromosome 15q14. Childhood absence epilepsy (CAE) that evolves to JME has a locus on chromosome 1p. JME has an overall prevalence of 5–10%. Individuals present JME between the ages of 8 and 26 years, but in more than >75%, initial manifestations occur between ages 12 and 18 years.

The EEG shows a generalized 4 to 6-Hz irregular spike-and-wave pattern, which is enhanced by photic stimulation. Rarely, structural brain lesions may be found, but these do not appear to influence the therapeutic response or prognosis in JME. Magnetic resonance imaging (MRI) shows an increase in cortical gray matter (especially mesial frontal lobes) in 40% patients of JME. The neurologic examination is normal. The majority of the cases responds to valproate, which is required life long as there is relapse on AED withdrawal.

v. *Progressive myoclonic epilepsies:* Progressive myoclonic epilepsies are a group of familial neurogenerative disorders characterized by myoclonus with epileptic seizures and progressive neurologic decline. These conditions include Lafora disease, myoclonic epilepsy with ragged-red fibers (MERRF), sialidosis type I, ceroid lipofuscinosis, juvenile neuropathic Gaucher disease, and juvenile neuroaxonal dystrophy. Ramsay Hunt syndrome has myoclonic epilepsy in addition to manifestations of Friedreich ataxia.

Lafora disease is an autosomal recessive disorder usually begins when the patients are between 10 and 18 years. Initially there are generalized tonic-clonic seizures, but ultimately myoclonic seizures appear which persist with progression of the disease. Mental deterioration becomes evident within one year of the onset of seizures. The myoclonic jerks are difficult to control, but a combination of valproic acid and clonazepam is effective in controlling generalized seizures.

Myoclonic epilepsy with ragged-red fibers (MERRF): Mitochondrial encephalomyelitis. Management is mainly supportive and includes prevention and treatment of catabolic stresses like infections, fever, starvation and excessive physical exertion, which may exacerbate the condition. Drugs compromising mitochondrial function (phenytoin, phenobarbital, chloramphenicol) should be avoided. Seizures should be controlled and adequate caloric intake ensured. Drug treatment includes vitamins C, E, B1 and B2. Steroids may help by increasing muscle strength.

Sialidosis is inherited as an autosomal recessive trait. Two types are found. Sialidosis type I, the cherry red spot-myoclonus syndrome, usually presents during the second decade of life, when a patient complains of visual deterioration. The myoclonus is triggered by voluntary movement, touch and sound and is not controlled with anticonvulsants. Generalized convulsions responsive to antiepileptic drugs have been reported in most patients. Sialidosis type II patients in addition to cherry red spots, have coarse facial features, corneal clouding (rarely), and dysostosis multiplex, producing anterior beaking of the lumbar vertebrae. Examination of lymphocytes shows vacuoles in the cytoplasm; biopsy of the liver demonstrates cytoplasmic vacuoles in kupffer cells; and membrane bound-vacuoles are found in Schwann cell cytoplasm, all attesting to the multiorgan nature of sialidosis type II. Patients with sialidosis have been reported to live beyond the 5th decade.

Neuronal ceroid lipofuscinoses are the most common neurodegenerative diseases in children. Three distinct disorders (infantile begins towards the end of the first year of life with myoclonic seizures, intellectual deterioration, blindness and cerebellar ataxia; late infantile begins between 2 and 4 years of age in a previously normal child with myoclonic seizures; Juvenile type (Spielmeyer-Vogt) is associated with progressive visual loss and intellectual impairment beginning between 5 and 10 years of age. These are inherited as autosomal recessive traits. The characteristic feature is the storage of an autofluoroescent substance within neurons and other tissues.

5. *Infantile spasms* are characterized by brief symmetrical contractions of the neck, trunk, and extremities and usually begin between the ages of 4 and 8 months. There are three main types of infantile spasms: flexor, extensor, and mixed flexor-extensor. Mixed forms of spasms are the most common types followed by flexor spasms while extensor spasms are the least common. The most common form of infantile spasm consists of flexion of the trunk, extension of the arms, and drawing up the legs ("salaam" posture). Clusters or volleys of seizures may persist for minutes, with brief intervals between each spasm. A cry may precede or follow an infantile spasm, which may be confused with colic. The spasms have a tendency to develop while patients are drowsy or immediately on awakening. Patients with infantile spasms are classified into two groups: symptomatic (80–90%) and cryptogenic (10–20%). The infantile spasms in the symptomatic group are directly related to prenatal, perinatal and postnatal factors. Prenatal and perinatal factors include hypoxic-ischemic encephalopathy with periventricular leukomalacia, congenital infections, inborn errors of metabolism, neurocutaneous syndromes such as tuberous sclerosis, cytoarchitectural abnormalities including lissencephaly and schizoencephaly and prematurity. Postnatal conditions include CNS infections, hypoxic-ischemic encephalopathy, and head trauma (especially subdural hematoma and intraventricular hemorrhage). In B_6 dependent cases the red blood cells are microcytic and hypochromic. B_6 dependent convulsions presumably occur as a result of errors in enzyme structure or function. The patient responds to very large amounts of pyridoxine. Implication of corticotropin-releasing hormone (CRH) is the most accepted hypothesis.

In EEG the most characteristic pattern is hypsarrhythmia, which consists of a chaotic pattern of high voltage, bilaterally asynchronous, slow-wave activity or a modified hypsarrhythmia pattern. CT scan may demonstrate focal lesions, including cerebrovascular lesions and rarely, brain tumors in addition to more diffuse congenital malformation. Diffuse cerebral atrophy is a common finding. MRI may demonstrate focal or diffuse abnormalities including neuronal migration defects. PET scan can detect cortical disturbances even when MRI and CT are normal. During investigation of infantile spasms, if no definite cerebral structural abnormalities are visualized, a full metabolic work-up is indicated.

Treatment: Identify the underlying etiology-symptomatic or cryptogenic. Initial treatment is with specific therapy-pyridoxine, ACTH/prednisolone/prednisone, vigabatrin. In case standard treatment fails, consider for surgical intervention. In case the patient is not a fit candidate for surgical intervention or if surgery fails consider the following options: valproic acid, lamotrigine, felbamate, topiramate, zonisamide, nitrazepam, clonazepam, ketogenic diet, and vagus nerve stimulation. Infants with cryptogenic infantile spasms have a good prognosis, but in the symptomatic cases the prognosis is poor and has an 80–90% risk of mental retardation.

6. *Landau-Kleffner Syndrome (LKS)* is characterized by loss of language skills in a previously normal child with seizure disorder. Age of onset is 5 ½ year. More common is in boys. Etiology is unknown. LKS is often confused with autism, because both candidates are associated with a loss of language function. Language regression may be sudden or the speech loss is protracted. The *aphasia* may be primarily receptive or regressive, and auditory agnosia may be so severe that the child is oblivious to everyday sound. Hearing is normal, but behavioral problems, including irritability and poor attention span are particularly common. The seizures are of several types, including focal or generalized tonic-clonic, atypical absence, partial complex, and, occasionally myoclonic. EEG shows high-amplitude spike and wave discharges predominate and tend to be bitemporal but can be multifocal or generalized. CT/MRI is normal. PET shows unilateral or bilateral hypometabolism or hypermetabolism. Valproic acid alone or in combination with clobazam is used to control seizures. If seizure and aphasia persists prednisolone (2 mg/kg/24 hours for 1 month, 1 mg/kg/24 hours for additional month and 0.5 mg/kg/24 hours for up to 6–12 months) should be given. Methylphenidate should be considered for patients with severe hyperactivity and inattention. Subpial transaction is the operative procedure, if medical treatment fails. Other measures include speech therapy and maintain for several years. Treatment is to continue for several years, as improvement in language function occurs over a prolonged period. Onset of LKS at an early age (less than 2 years) is associated with poor prognosis. The outcome is unpredictable. Some children experience a recurrence of aphasia and seizures after apparent recovery.

Acharya JN, Satish Chandra P, Shankar SK. Familial progressive myoclonus epilepsy: Clinical and electrophysiologic observations. *Epilepsia* 1995;36:429–34.

Gupte S, Mathur GP, Mathur Sarla. Landu-Kleffner syndrome. In: Mathur GP, Mathur Sarla (eds). *Seizures in Children and Adolescents.* Delhi: Academa Publishers, 2005;77–81.

Gupte S, Mathur GP, Mathur Sarla. Infantile spasms. In: Mathur GP, Mathur Sarla (eds). *Seizures in Children and Adolescents.* Delhi: Academa Publishers, 2005;82–92.

Ito M, Seki T, Takuma Y. Current therapy for West syndrome in Japan. *J Child Neurol* 2000;15:524–8.

Janz D. Juvenile myoclonic epilepsy. *Cleve Clin J Med* 1989; 56 (suppl): 23–33.

Kamala Vaidya, GP Mathur, Sarla Mathur. Generalized seizures. In: Mathur GP, Mathur Sarla (eds). *Seizures in Children and Adolescents.* Delhi: Academa Publishers, 2005;46–52.

Lowenstein DH: Seizures and Epilepsy. In: Braunwald E, Fauci AS, Kasper DL, Hauser SL, Longo DL, Jameson JL (eds). *Harrison's Principles of Internal Medicine.* 15th edn. New York: McGraw-Hill, 2001;2354–69.

Mathur GP, Mathur Sarla. Myoclonic epilepsy. In: Mathur GP, Mathur Sarla (eds). *Seizures in Children and Adolescents.* Delhi: Academa Publishers, 2005;57–65.

Mathur GP, Mathur S. Myoclonus. In: Mathur GP, Mathur S (eds). *Movement disorders in children and adolescents.* 1st edn. New Delhi: Jaypee Brothers Medical Publishers (P) Ltd., 2003; 48–61.

Rantala H, Putkonen T. Occurrence, outcome and prognostic factors of infantile spasms and Lennox-Gastaut syndrome. *Epilepsia* 1999;40:286–9.

Rao GP, Murthy JMK. Absence seizures. In: Mathur GP, Mathur Sarla (eds). *Seizures in Children and Adolescents.* Delhi: Academa Publishers, 2005;53–56.

So NK. Atonic phenomena and partial seizures: a reappraisal. *Adv Neurol* 1995;67:29–39.

Stodieck SRG, Thompson PD. Myoclonus. In: Brandt T, Caplan LR, Dichgans J, Diener HC, Kennard C (eds). *Neurological Disorders: Course and Treatment.* San Diego: Academic Press, 1996;843–52.

Shields WD. West's Syndrome. *J Child Neurol* 2002; 17: S76–S79.

West WJ. On a peculiar form of infantile convulsions. Lancet 1841;1:724.

Investigation of a case with Seizures

Investigations may be needed to arrive at a correct diagnosis of epilepsy before starting the treatment in addition to taking history and physical examination. Investigations are required to find out the underlying cause of seizure and type of seizure.

1. Is it epilepsy or not?
2. Type of seizure present.
3. Diagnosis of the underlying cause of seizure.
4. Laboratory tests to detect toxic effects of antiepileptic drugs.

The patient with seizures may be brought to you:

A. When a patient presents shortly after a seizure, one should look for vital signs, respiratory and cardiovascular support, and treatment of seizures if they resume along with investigations. Life threatening conditions such as CNS infection, metabolic derangement or drug toxicity must be recognized and managed appropriately.

B. When the patient is not acutely ill, history of earlier seizures present or is the patient's first seizure investigations should be directed (a) to establish whether the reported episode was a seizure rather than another paroxysmal event, (b) to determine the cause of the seizure by identifying risk factors and precipitating events, and (c) to decide whether anticonvulsant therapy is required in addition to treatment for any underlying illness.

C. When the patient is brought to you with prior seizures or a known history of epilepsy the investigations are directed towards (a) identification of the underlying cause and precipitating factors, and (b) determination of the adequacy of the patient's current therapy.

The investigations, which may be undertaken in a patient with suspected epilepsy, are shown in Box 24.5. Demonstration of paroxysmal discharges on the EEG during a clinical seizure is diagnostic of epilepsy, but seizures rarely occur in the EEG laboratory.

Electroencephalogram (EEG) assists in establishing the diagnosis: The EEG is the most useful investigation in a patient who has a possible seizure disorder. All patients who have a possible seizure disorder should be evaluated with an EEG as soon as possible. The EEG may help to establish the diagnosis of epilepsy, classify the seizure type, and provide evidence for the existence of a particular epilepsy syndrome (Box 24.6).

Determination of the adequacy of the patient's current therapy: Laboratory monitoring should be done during antiepileptic drug therapy, which should include detection of abnormal values (Box 24.7) and serum therapeutic levels of antiepileptic drugs (Table 24.5). Routine serum monitoring of anticonvulsant levels is not recommended, but there are some important indications when anticonvulsant drug monitoring should be done (Box 24.8).

Table 24.5: Serum Therapeutic levels of common antiepileptic drugs

Name of the drug	Therapeutic serum level (g/ml)
Carbamazepine	8–12
Clonazepam	> 0.013
Ethosuximide	40–100
Paraldehyde	10–40
Phenobarbital	15–40
Phenytoin	10–20
Primidone	5–12
Valproic acid	50–100

Box 24.5: List of investigations which may be undertaken in a patient with suspected seizure

- Blood for complete blood count (CBC), liver function studies, electrolytes, glucose, calcium, magnesium
- Serum prolactin
- Blood levels of anticonvulsants
- Serology for tuberculosis, cysticercosis, HIV
- Blood and urine for metabolic studies and toxicology
- CSF examination
- Mantoux (Mx) test
- EEG, EEG/polygraphic/video monitoring
- Neuroradiologic procedures (Box 24.6): X-ray skull, Cranial ultrasonography, CT scan, MRI, PET, SPECT, Cerebral angiography and X-ray chest (in suspected cases of tuberculosis)
- Determination of the adequacy of the patient's current therapy

Box 24.6: Indications for brain imaging in seizures

- MRI is indicated in a first seizure in all adolescents
- Seizures with local features clinically
- EEG shows a focal seizure source
- Difficult to control seizures
- Condition of the patient deteriorates

Box 24.7: Abnormal values during anticonvulsant therapy

- Hepatic enzymes more than 2.5 times than normal values
- Leukocytes less than 3,000/mm³
- Neutrophils less than 1500/mm³
- Platelets less than 100,000/mm³

If symptoms of complication appear perform clinical and laboratory evaluation

Source: So LE. Update on Epilepsy. MCNA 1993; 77(1): 203–213.

Box 24.8: Indications for anticonvulsant drug monitoring

1. At the onset of anticonvulsant therapy to confirm that the drug level is within the therapeutic range
2. For noncompliance patients and their families
3. During accelerated growth spurts
4. For patients who are on polytherapy, because of drug interactions
5. At the time of status epilepticus
6. For difficult to control seizures or seizures that have changed in type
7. For symptoms and signs of drug toxicity
8. For patients with hepatic or renal disease
9. For children with cognitive or physical disabilities, in whom toxicity may be difficult to evaluate

Lowenstein DH. Seizures and Epilepsy. In: Braunwald E, Fauci AS, Kasper DL, Hauser SL, Longo DL, Jameson JL (eds). *Harrison's Principles of Internal Medicine.* 15th edn. New York: McGraw-Hill, 2001; 2354–2369.

Mathur Sarla, Vandana Khare, Mathur GP. Investigations of a patient with seizures. In: Mathur GP, Mathur Sarla (eds). *Seizures in Children and Adolescents.* Delhi: Academa Publishers, 2005; 203–210.

Mathur GP, Mathur Sarla. Pitfalls in the diagnosis of seizures. In: Mathur GP, Mathur Sarla (eds). *Seizures in Children and Adolescents.* Delhi: Academa Publishers, 2005; 211–217.

Mishra V, Gahlaut DS, Kumar S, Mathur GP, Agnihotri SS, Gupta V. Value of serum prolactin in differentiating epilepsy from pseudoseizure. *JAPI* 1990; 38 (11): 846–847.

Treatment of Seizures

The treatment of a patient with seizure disorder includes treatment of the underlying conditions that cause or contribute to the seizures, avoidance of precipitating factors and suppression of recurrent seizures with antiepileptic drugs or surgery and addressing a variety of psychological and social issues. The aim is to protect patient from having seizures without interfering with normal cognitive function and without producing harmful side effects.

Treatment plans must be individualized. The first step in the management of epilepsy is to ensure that the patient has a seizure disorder and not a condition that mimics epilepsy. In a previously healthy child with the first afebrile convulsion and negative family history, normal physical examination and EEG in a cooperative family, antiepileptic should be withheld. Approximately 70% of these children will not experience another convulsion. A recurrent seizure particularly if it occurs in close proximity to the first seizure is an indication to start an anticonvulsant.

Treatment of underlying condition: This is an important step. If the sole cause of a seizure is a metabolic disturbance such as an abnormality of serum electrolytes or glucose, then treatment includes reversing the metabolic problem and preventing its recurrence rather treating with anticonvulsant. If the cause of seizure is a medication (e.g. theophylline) or illicit drug use (e.g. cocaine), then appropriate therapy is avoidance of the drug and antiepileptic is not needed unless subsequent seizures occur. In case the seizures are due to a structural CNS lesion such as a brain tumor, vascular malformation or brain abscess, these (seizures) will not recur after appropriate treatment of the underlying lesion. However, despite removal of the structural lesion, there is a risk that the seizure focus will remain in the surrounding tissue or develop de novo as a result of gliosis and other processes induced by surgery, radiation or other therapies.

Avoidance of precipitating factors: Precipitating (trigger) factors can be identified (Box 24.9), which should be avoided while treating the patient. These factors appear to lower their seizure threshold.

Box 24.9: Precipitating (trigger) factors for seizures

1. Sleep deprivation
2. Alcohol (particularly withdrawal)
3. Drugs—withdrawal of antiepileptic drugs, sedative drugs and recreational drug abuse
4. Physical and mental exhaustion
5. Inter-current infections and metabolic disturbances
6. Sex hormones, menstruation and pregnancy
7. Reflex epilepsy—flickering lights, including TV and computer screens, uncommonly loud noises, music, reading, hot baths

Restrictions: Patients should not be allowed to work or recreation above ground level, with dangerous machinery or near open fires or water until good control of seizures has been established. Patients should take only a shallow bath and that too when some relative is in the house, and should not lock the bathroom door. Cycling should be discouraged until at least the patient is free from seizures for six months. Recreations requiring prolonged proximity to water (e.g. swimming, fishing or boating) should always be in the company of someone who is aware of the chance of a seizure occurring. Any activity where loss of awareness might be very dangerous (e.g. mountaineering) should be discouraged.

Antiepileptic drug therapy is the mainstay of treatment for most patients with seizures. The antiepileptic drugs (AEDs) are required for acute management of tonic-clonic seizures or of status epilepticus, and for chronic management of cases suffering from seizures. The aim is to protect patient from having seizures without interfering with normal cognitive function and without producing harmful side effects.

Initiation of therapy: Drug treatment should be considered after more than one seizure has occurred. Treatment should only be started after convincing the patient and his family that seizure control is worthwhile. The aim is to use only one drug with the lowest possible side effects for the control of seizures. The drug is increased slowly until seizure control is accomplished or until undesirable side effects develop or blood levels touches the upper limit of the recommended therapeutic range. The steady static blood levels are reached slowly owing to the long serum half-life of most anticonvulsants. The patient's serum AED level should be monitored during this stage and the dose should be altered accordingly. A minimum of 2 seizure-free years is an adequate and safe period of treatment for a patient with no risk factors. Of patients whose epilepsy is controllable, only a single drug is necessary in 80% cases. The combination of more than two drugs is seldom necessary.

Risk of seizure recurrence: The risk of seizure recurrence in a patient with apparently unprovoked or idiopathic seizures is uncertain. Generally accepted risk factors associated with recurrent seizures are given in Box 24.10. Most patients with one or more of these risk factors should be treated.

Selection of antiepileptic drugs: Older medicines such as phenytoin, valproic acid, carbamazepine, and ethosuximide are generally used as first-line therapy for most seizure disorders, since they are effective and significantly less expensive than newer drugs (Table 24.6). The use of newer drugs such as gabapentin and lamotrigene is predominantly as add-on or alternative therapy. In addition to efficacy, other factors to be considered while selecting for an initial medication consists of the relative convenience of dosing schedule (e.g. once daily versus three or four times daily) and potential side effects. Seizure type is also an important element in designing the treatment plan.

Box 24.10: Risk factors for recurrence after withdrawal of AED

- Age greater than 12 years at onset
- Neurologic dysfunction (motor handicap or mental retardation)
- Seizures presenting as status epilepticus
- Postictal Todd's paralysis
- A very strong family history of seizures
- History of prior neonatal seizures
- Numerous seizures
- An abnormal EEG

Withdrawal of anticonvulsant therapy: Clinical studies suggest that the patients with the following profile have the greatest chance of remaining seizure-free after drug withdrawal: (i) complete medical control of seizures for 1 to 5 years; (ii) single seizure type, either partial or generalized; (iii) normal neurologic examination, including intelligence; and (iv) a normal EEG. The appropriate seizure-free interval is unknown and varies from different forms of epilepsy. If a patient meets all of the above criteria he should be motivated after 2 years to discontinue antiepileptic therapy after discussing with him the potential risks and benefits. It is preferable to reduce the drug gradually in about 3 months period. Most recurrences occur in the first 3 months after discontinuing therapy. Typical absence seizures carry the best prognosis for successful drug withdrawal, whereas juvenile myoclonic epilepsy has marked liability to recur after AED withdrawal. Seizures, which begin in adult life, particularly those with partial features, are also likely to recur, especially if there is an identified structural lesion. The overall recurrence rate of seizures is approximately 40%.

Treatment of recurrence after withdrawal of AED: If after discontinuation of AED therapy, the first relapse characterized by frequent attacks (similar in type to the previous seizures) occurs in a 24 hours period along with persistent EEG abnormality, AED should be started. Approximately more than 80% children become seizure free with AED therapy. The risk of second relapse is seen in patients who have an underlying pathology, seizure period is less than 4 years before discontinuation and multiple AEDs used and in patients in whom findings of the first relapse (occurs in a 24 hours period) persisted.

Table 24.6: Guidelines for the choice of antiepileptic drugs (AEDs)		
Seizure type	*First line AED*	*Alternatives*
Focal onset (Partial)	Carbamazepine	Lamotrigene; Gabapentin;
Simple partial	Phenytoin	Phenobarbital; Primidone
Complex partial	Valproic acid	Topiramate; Clobazam
Secondary generalized		Vigabatrin
tonic-clonic seizures		
Generalized tonic-clonic	Valproic acid	Phenobarbital; Primidone;
	Carbamazepine	Lamotrigene; Topiramate
	Phenytoin	Gabapentin
Absence	Ethosuximide	Acetazolamide; Clonazepam; Phenobarbital;
	Valproic acid	Lamotrigine
Myoclonic	Valproic acid	Clonazepam; Acetazolamide; Phenobarbital
Atonic	Valproic acid	Clonazepam
Infantile spasms	Prednisolone or ACTH	Valproic acid

Note: Preferably use one drug, or no more than two drugs, should be used at one time.

Follow-up visits: During the phase of initiating treatment the patient should be advised to visit two or three times so that dose adjustments and baseline investigations could be properly carried out. In a well-controlled patient, a three-six monthly follow-up is generally sufficient. During every follow-up visit note the following points and advise accordingly as follows: seizure frequency, dosage, formulation and trade name of AED being used, compliance, and side effects-of AED is being used.

Ketogenic diet: The ketogenic diet is an effective and safe medical treatment for refractory childhood epilepsy, but it must be judiciously applied and carefully monitored. The use of *valproic acid* is contraindicated in association with the ketogenic diet, because the risk of hepatotoxicity is enhanced. The patient should be admitted in the hospital for baseline studies and for observation for four to ten days, until it is clear that the diet is well tolerated. The baseline studies include physical and neurologic examinations, seizure frequency (obtained by calendars of the month), and EEG, CT/MRI and blood and urine studies. A number of blood studies, including fasting blood sugar, BUN, serum electrolytes, pH, calcium, phosphate, serum cholesterol and fatty acids, serum aminoacids, lactate, pyruvate and carnitine, serum proteins and liver function tests should be done. Blood anticonvulsant level should also be determined in patients who were receiving these drugs. The patients are than started on a classical ketogenic diet (fat: protein and carbohydrate ratio = 4:1) allowing 0.8–1.2 g of protein per kg of body weight. Parents should be encouraged to follow the diet for at least six weeks for optimal tolerance and seizure control. Patients should be discharged on the diet, as well as on their previous dosage of anticonvulsant medication and vitamin and calcium supplements. They should be seen as outpatients at four-week intervals as long as they remain on the diet. Repeat blood studies and EEG recording should be obtained during follow-up visits. No cases of possible long-term complications (more than two years of treatment) have been reported. Some children older than 2–3 years will not tolerate this fatty, unpalatable diet.

Surgery for epilepsy: Surgery should be considered for children with intractable seizures unresponsive to anticonvulsants. Certain children, particularly those with focal seizures, are also candidates for surgery.

Vagus Nerve Stimulation (VNS): A third modality in the form of a physiological therapy is vagus nerve stimulation (VNS) for patients with medically refractory epilepsy, who are not candidates for resective brain surgery. In this procedure a bipolar electrode is placed on the midcervical portion of the left vagus nerve. The electrode is connected to a small, subcutaneous generator located in the infraclavicular region, and the generator is programmed to deliver intermittent electrical pulses to the vagus nerve. The mechanism of action is unknown, although experimental studies have shown that stimulation of vagal nuclei leads to widespread activation of cortical and subcortical pathways and an associated increased seizure threshold. Adverse effects of the surgery are rare. The stimulation induced side effects, including transient hoarseness, cough, and dyspnea are usually mild and well tolerated by the patients.

Counseling: Most parents are initially frightened by the diagnosis of epilepsy. They need support and accurate information. Parents particularly like to know: (a) any restriction to be placed on the child or not, (b) whether the teacher should be informed, and (c) the genetic implications, including the risks for future children. Parents should be encouraged to treat their child as normally as possible. For most children with epilepsy, restriction of physical activity is unnecessary except that they must be attended by a responsible adult while bathing and swimming. Children can have cognitive and behavioral problems that may be due to epilepsy itself or because of AEDs. Cooperation and understanding among the parents, physician, teacher, and child is extremely important in the management of patients with epilepsy.

Prognosis: Overall, generalized seizures are more easily controlled than partial seizures. The presence of a structural lesion makes complete control of the epilepsy less likely and the prognosis is generally worse compared to patients with idiopathic epilepsy. Children with best prognosis following AED withdrawal are those with BPEC and those with idiopathic generalized seizures. CPS and juvenile myoclonic are more likely to recur. In a patient with complete seizure control for a minimum of 2 years and low risk factors, the chance of recurrence is approximately 20–25%, particularly during the first 6 months after the discontinuance of AED. Nearly half of the children with epilepsy have schooling difficulties and children with idiopathic generalized epilepsy have significantly lowered 10 scores than those of controls. The overall prognosis for the epilepsy is given in Box 24.11.

Box 24.11: Epilepsy outcome after 20 years

- 50% seizure free, without drugs, for the last 5 years
- 20% seizure free, for the last 5 years but continue to take medications
- 30% seizures continue in spite of antiepileptic therapy

Antiepileptic Drugs

A large number of antiepileptic drugs are available in the market. Older medicines such as phenobarbitone, phenytoin, valproic acid, carbamazepine, and ethosuximide are generally used as first-line therapy for most seizure disorders. The newer drugs are predominantly used as add-on or alternative therapy.

1. **Acetazolamide:** Indications are as an adjunctive therapy in catamenial epilepsy and in refractory seizures; Other uses: Glaucoma. Children and Adults: 8–30 mg/kg/hr PO in 1–4 divided doses (max: 1 g/24 hr); Dosing interval is 1–4 times a day. *Side effects:* Metabolic acidosis, hypochloremia, hypokalemia, renal calculi.

2. **Carbamazepine: Indications:** Generalized tonic-clonic and partial seizures. Other uses: Trigeminal neuralgia, glossopharyngeal neuralgia, idiopathic torsion dystonia (ITD), torticollis, postural and intention tremors; indicated in cases of manic-depressive psychosis as a prophylactic drug. Children: < 6 yr: Initial dose 5 mg/kg/24 hr in 2–4 divided doses; may increase q5–7days by 5 mg/kg based on effect or toxicity serum concentration. 6 –12 yr: Begin 10 mg/kg/24 hr in 2–4 divided doses; increase by 100 mg or 5 mg/kg/24 hr at weekly intervals until the therapeutic levels are achieved (usual dose: 800–1200 mg/24 hr). Therapeutic range: 8–12 g/ml. *Side effects:* Ataxia, aplastic anemia, leukopenia, hepatotoxicity, idiosyncratic rashes and thrombocytopenia.

3. **Clonazepam:** Half life: 18–150 hr. Indications: Lennox-Gastaut syndrome, myoclonic, akinetic, and absence seizures; Other uses: Myoclonus, startle syndromes, Gilles de la Tourette syndrome, idiopathic torsion dystonia (ITD), torticollis, tremor (essential, orthostatic). Children: 0.01–0.3 mg/kg/24 hr in 2–3 divided doses, then increase by 0.5 mg/24 hr q3–5days to response (max:0.3 mg/kg/24 hr). Side effects: Agitation, ataxia, behavioral abnormalities, idiosyncratic blood dyscrasias.

4. **Corticotropin, Adrenocorticotropic hormone (ACTH):** Indication: Infantile spasms.

    Other uses: Opsoclonus myoclonus, adrenal deficiency states. Dosage: ACTH, 20 units IM daily for 2 weeks, and if no response occurs the dose is increased to 30 and then 40 units IM daily for, an additional 4 weeks. Unless seizure control is complete the ACTH is replaced with oral prednisolone (prednisone) 2 mg/kg/24 hr for 2 weeks. If the seizures persist, prednisolone (prednisone) is given for an additional 4 weeks. *Side effects:* Transient brain shrinkage observed by

CT scanning, hyperglycemia, hypertension, electrolyte abnormalities, gastrointestinal disturbances, infection.

5. **Diazepam:** Half life: 30 hr. Indications: Status epilepticus (Used IV for initial management of status epilepticus), febrile seizures. Other uses: Anxiety disorders, acute alcohol withdrawal, muscle spasm, dystonia musculorum deformans, and tetanus. Children: Intravenous: 0.1–0.3/kg at a rate no longer than 2 mg/minute intravenously for a maximum of three doses; Rectal- 0.3–0.5 mg/kg is to be diluted in 3 mL with 0.9% sodium chloride and the amount is placed into the rectum by a syringe and a flexible tube; Oral: In cases of febrile seizures give at the onset of febrile illness 0.3 mg/kg 8 hourly (1 mg/kg/24 hr), then continue for the duration of illness (usually 2–3 days). = Caution: Inject IV slowly and do not mix or dilute with other solutions. *Side effects:* CNS disturbances including impaired alertness, ataxia.

6. **Ethosuximide:** Half life: 60 hr. Indication: Typical absence epilepsy. Children: begin 20 mg/kg/24 hr, increase to a maximum 40 mg/kg/24 hr or 1.5 g/24 hr, which is less, twice daily. Therapeutic range: 40–100 g/ml. *Side effects:* Ataxia, lethargic, headache.

7. **Fosphenytoin:** Indication: Treatment of acute seizures (status epilepticus). Children and Adults: Loading dose is 15–20 mg/kg phenytoin dosing equivalents (maximum rate: 150 mg/min). Each 1.5 mg fosphenytoin = 1 mg of phenytoin dosing equivalent. Therapeutic range: 30–40 g/ml. *Side effects:* Same as phenytoin.

8. **Gabapentin:** Half-life- 5–7 hours. Indications: Used as an add-on drug for patients with refractory complex partial and secondarily generalized tonic-clonic seizures; may be used as alternative therapy in focal-onset. Children 2–12 yr: 15–35 mg/kg/24 hr in 3 divided doses (max: 50 mg/kg/24 hr). Children >12 years and Adults: Start 300 mg daily, then daily increase by 300 mg to 900–3600 mg/day in 3 divided doses. *Side effects:* Somnolence, ataxia, headache, tremor, weight gain.

9. **Lamotrigine:** Half life: 22–37 hr. Indications: Used as an add-on drug for the management of complex partial and generalized tonic-clonic seizures. Lamotrigine is effective as monotherapy for some children with the focal onset, tonic-clonic, atypical absence, myoclonic, Lennox-Gastaut syndrome. Children 2–12 yr: 0.6 mg/kg/24 hr in 1–2 doses for 2 wk, then 1.2 mg/kg/24 hr in 2 doses for 2 wk, then 5–15 mg/kg/24 hr in 2 doses per response (max: 400 mg/24 hr). *If patient is on*

valproate: 0.15 mg/kg/24 hr in 1–2 doses for 2 wk, then 0.3 mg/kg/24 hr in 2 doses for 2 wk, then 1–5 mg/kg/24 hr in 2 doses (max: 200 mg/24 hr). Therapeutic range: 1–4 mg/L or 3.9–15.6 mol/L. *Side effects:* Headache, blurred vision, diplopia, sedation, and ataxia, gastrointestinal irritation (nausea, vomiting), idiosyncratic rashes and blood dyscrasias.

10. **Lorazepam: Indications:** Treatment for anxiety, sedation, and seizures (used IV for initial management of status epilepticus); adjunct to antiemetic therapy. Status epilepticus: Neonates: IV: 0.05–0.2 mg/kg/dose over 2–5 minutes, may repeat in 10 to 15 minutes. Infants and Children: IV: Begin 0.1 mg/kg load over 2–5 minutes, may give additional 0.05 mg/kg bolus in 10–15 minutes (administered slowly). Adolescents: IV: 0.07 mg/kg/dose over 2–5 minutes, may repeat in 10–15 minutes. *Side effects:* Myoclonus reported in neonates, tachycardia, paradoxical excitement, blurred vision.

11. **Midazolam:** Indications: Sedation, anticonvulsant. Neonates: IV: Continuous infusion 0.15–0.5 µg/kg/min for sedation; IV: bolus 0.05–0.15 mg/kg q2–4 hr. Infants and Children: Status epilepticus: IV load 0.15 mg/kg followed by continuous infusion 1 g/kg/min. Sedation: IV: 0.05–2 mg/kg load, then either same dose q1–2hr or continuous infusion 1–2 µg/kg/min. Intranasal: 2.5 mg (0.5 mL) in each nostril (total 5 mg) using 5 mg/mL injection. >12 yr: 0.5 mg q3–4 min to effect. Constant intravenous infusion of midazolam (0.20 mg/kg bolus, 1–5 g/kg/min infusion) has been effective in managing seizures during status epilepticus unresponsive to other anticonvulsant. *Side effects:* Myoclonus and prolonged movement disorders, withdrawal reactions may occur if abrupt discontinuation, sedation, amnesia, nasal burning, apnea, respiratory depression.

12. **Nitrazepam:** Half-life: 18–57 hours. Indications: Absence, myoclonic, infantile spasms, generalized status epilepticus. Children: Begin 0.2 mg/kg/24 hr, increase gradually to 1 mg/kg/24 hr 3 times/day. *Side effects:* Drowsiness, agitation, ataxia, behavioral abnormalities, depression, hallucinations, anorexia, excessive salivation.

13. **Oxcarbazepine:** Half-life: 10–17 hours (For active metabolite). Indication: Used in seizure disorders (except absent seizure). Children 3–17 yr: Start 8–10 mg/kg/24 hr divided bid, increase over 2 wk to 30–45 mg/kg/24 hr divided bid per response (max: 600 mg/24 hr). Children < 3 yr: Not recommended. Therapeutic range: 6–12 g/ml. *Side effects:* Ataxia, headache, aplastic anemia, leucopenia, skin rash, hyponatremia.

14. **Paraldehyde:** Indication: Used as an adjunct treatment for refractory status epilepticus, alcohol withdrawal. Children: 0.15 ml/kg/dose per oral (PO), per rectal (PR). May repeat once in 4–6 hr. Adult: 5–10 ml/per dose. Caution: Use glass syringe/tubing as drug reacts plastic. Mix rectal solution 2:1 in oil (e.g. olive oil). Therapeutic range: 10–40 g/ml. Caution: May give IM but inject remote from nerves owing to risk of damage. Use glass syringe/tubing because drug reacts with plastic. Rectal route is preferred to IM route. Mix rectal solution 2:1 oil (e.g. olive oil). *Side effects:* Sedation, gastric irritation, thrombophlebitis, smells and tastes unpleasant.

15. **Phenobarbital/Phenobarbitone:** Half-life: 48–150 hr (90 hr in adults). Indications: Generalized tonic-clonic, partial, status epilepticus. Other uses: Trigeminal neuralgia, essential tremor. Status epilepticus: Neonates: IV: 20–30 mg/kg. Children and adults: IV dose 15–20 mg/kg. Maintenance dose: Neonates: 3–4 mg/kg/24 hr PO, IV, q12–24hr. Children: 5–6 mg/kg/24 hr PO, IV, q12–24 hr. Therapeutic range: 15–40 g/ml; coma (acute) >60 g/ml. *Side effects:* Hyperactivity, irritability, short attention span, temper tantrums, altered sleep pattern, drowsiness, hangover, , idiopathic reactions (e.g. paradoxical excitement and confusion as well as hypersensitivity reactions).

16. **Phenytoin:** Half-life: 48–150 hr (90 hr in adults). Indications: All forms of epilepsy (primary and secondary generalized tonic-clonic seizures, partial seizures, status epilepticus, seizures following head injury or neurosurgery). Other uses: Trigeminal neuralgia, migraine, cardiac arrhythmias, asterixis. Status epilepticus: Loading dose Neonates: 15–20 mg/kg IV; do not exceed 0.5 mg/kg/min. Children and Adults: 15–18 mg/kg IV; do not exceed 1–3 mg/kg/min. Maintenance dose: Neonates: 5 mg/kg/24 hr PO, IV q12–24 hr. Children: 0.5–6 yr: 8–10 mg/kg/24 hr PO, IV q12–24 hr. 7–9 yr: 6–8 mg/kg/24 hr PO, IV q12–24 hr. 10–16 yr: 6–7 mg/kg/24 hr PO, IV q12–24 hr. Therapeutic range: 8–20 g/ml (if necessary measure free drug concentration: therapeutic 1–2 g/ml. *Side effects:* Ataxia, incoordination, confusion, gingival hypertrophy, hirsutism, facial coarsening, blood dyscrasias, lymphadenopathy, osteomalacia, skin rash appears, idiosyncratic (rashes, Stevens-Johnson syndrome, blood dyscrasias, hepatitis, thrombophlebitis, drug-induced lupus).

17. **Prednisolone/Prednisone:** Indication: Infantile spasms. Dose: Prednisolone (prednisone) in the

doses of 2 mg/kg/ 24 hr has equal efficacy as noted in ACTH (corticotropin 5–160 units/kg/ 24 hr as IM gel) for the treatment of crypytogenic and symptomatic infantile seizures, and in approximately 70% of patients complete control is expected. *Side effects:* Hyperglycemia, hypertension, electrolyte abnormalities, gastrointestinal disturbances, infection.

18. **Primidone:** Half-life: 10–21 hours. Indications: Generalized tonic-clonic, partial. Other uses: Essential tremors, myoclonus. Neonates: 12–20 mg/kg/24 hr PO, q8–12 hr. Children 8 years: 10–25 mg/kg/24 hr PO, q8–12 hr. Children > 8 years and adults: 125–1500 mg/24 hr, PO q8–12 hr (usual max: 2 g/24 hr). Therapeutic range: 5–12 g/ml. *Side effects:* Hyperactivity, irritability, short attention span, temper tantrums, ataxia.

19. **Propofol:** Indication: Status epilepticus unresponsive to other anticonvulsant. Sedation: Children: Constant IV infusion of propofol (1.5–3 mg/kg/ dose intravenous over 1–2 minute, 2–10 mg/kg/ hr infusion). Continuous sedation (mechanical ventilation): Children: 5.5 mg/kg for 30 min; increase to 6 mg/kg for 30 min; increase to 8 mg/ kg for 1 hr; increase to 10 mg/kg for 1 hr; increase to final infusion rate of 12.5 mg/kg/hr. *Side effects:* Hyperlipidemia, systemic acidosis, "Propofol syndrome" (lactic acidosis and systemic collapse with sustained use of propofol).

20. **Thiopental/Thiopentone:** Indication: Status epilepticus. Neonates: 2–3 mg/ kg IV, repeat doses 1 mg/kg as needed. Infants and Children: 2–3 mg/ kg IV, repeat if needed. Therapeutic range: 30–100 g/ml (for barbiturate coma). *Side effects:* Somnolence, respiratory depression, hypotension, myocardial depression, bronchospasm.

21. **Tiagabine:** Half life: 7–9 hr. Indications: Focal-onset, tonic-clonic, Lennox-Gastaut syndrome, add-on drug in complex partial seizures. Infants and Children: 1.5 mg/kg/24 hr in 2–4 divided doses. Adolescents: Start at 4 mg once daily, increase by 4–8 mg q wk until response, (max: 56 mg/day). *Side effects:* Poor attention span, tremor, psychosis.

22. **Topiramate:** Half-life: 21 hours. Indications: Used as adjunctive therapy for poorly controlled seizures, refractory complex partial seizures with or without secondary generalization. Children 2–16 yr: Start 1–3 mg/kg/24 hr PO q12 hr for 1 wk; titrate dose increases every 1–2 wk by 1–3 mg/ kg/24 hr bid; typical dose 5–10 mg/kg/24 hr divided q12hr. Reduce dose by 50% if CrCl <60 ml/min. *Side effects:* Sedation, renal stones.

23. **Valproic acid/ Sodium valproate/ Valproate:** Half-life: 6–16 hr. Indications: Many seizure types (including generalized tonic-clonic, absence, atypical absence, myoclonic, partial, akinetic). Other uses: Myoclonus, rheumatic chorea. Neonates: Refractory seizures: load 20 mg/kg orally, then 10 mg /kg/dose q12hr. Children and adults: Begin 10–15 mg/kg/24 hr in 2–3 doses; then increase weekly by 5–10 mg/kg/24 hr to effect, may need up to 100 mg/kg/24 hr in 3–4 divided doses, especially if used with concurrent enzyme inducers (e.g. phenytoin, carbamazepine). Therapeutic range: 50–100 g/ml (toxic > 150 g/ mL). *Side effects:* Tremor, alopecia, weight gain.

24. **Vigabatrin:** Half-life: 5–8 hr. Indications: Infantile spasms, particularly in children with tuberous sclerosis, as adjunctive therapy for poorly controlled seizures. Children: begin 30 mg /kg/ 24 hr, maintenance dose 30–100 mg/kg/24 hr., once daily or twice daily. Side effects: Hyperactivity, agitation, excitement, somnolence, weight gain.

25. **Zonisamide:** Half-life: 50–68 hours. Indication: Focal-onset. Children: Start with 2–4 mg/kg/ 24 hr, then increase by 2–5 mg/kg/ 24 hr, 4–20 mg/ kg/ 24 hr., once daily. *Side effects:* Metabolic acidosis, nephrolithiasis, hyperammonemia.

Prednisolone /Prednisone therapy: Prednisone therapy is a safe and effective adjunctive treatment for patients suffering from intractable generalized epilepsy who have failed conventional antiepileptic therapy. Prednisolone/ Prednisone in the dosage of 1 mg/kg/ day for 12 weeks (6 weeks daily and 6 weeks alternate days), in addition to their regular antiepileptic medications and followed for a period of 1–5 years in patients of absent epilepsy, severe myoclonic epilepsy, childhood myoclonic epilepsy, West's syndrome and Lennox Gastaut syndrome (LGS), 46% became seizure free, 40% significant decrease in seizure frequency, and 19% has no change in seizure frequency. The best results are reported in the absence group and in the Lennox Gastaut syndrome. Side effects are uncommon and include weight gain and aggression.

Polytherapy: Newly diagnosed epileptic patients require monotherapy. About 60–70% of patients may achieve an adequate seizure control with a single antiepileptic drug. However, this therapeutic approach may not be sufficient for the one-third of epileptic patients and the polytherapy must be initiated. The drug combination providing the supra-additive effect seems to be of clinical significance. Synergistic interactions have been shown for the combinations of valproate-phenytoin/ethosuximide, topiramate-carbamazepine/Phenobarbital and felbamate—all major conventional antiepileptics.

Overtreatment: Overtreatment is defined here as an unnecessary and excessive drug load in the management of epilepsy leading to a suboptimal risk-to-benefit balance. Although not well recognized, overtreatment may contribute to the long-term risks of AED treatment in patients with epileptic seizures.

Mortality: Epilepsy is not usually considered to be a fatal condition, and in children with secondary epilepsy, mortality is the result of common complications related to the underlying disorders. Epilepsy patients receiving medications such as phenytoin or phenobarbital have been noted to have an exceedingly low incidence of myocardial infarction, but children treated with carbamazepine have shown alteration in their serum lipid profile that could predispose them to atherosclerosis.

Aneja S. Combination drug therapy. In: Mathur GP, Mathur Sarla (eds). *Seizures in Children and Adolescents.* Delhi: Academa Publishers, 2005; 275–278.

Kushwha KP, Mathur GP, Mathur Sarla. Ketogenic diet. In: Mathur GP, Mathur Sarla (eds). *Seizures in Children and Adolescents.* Delhi: Academa Publishers, 2005; 296–302.

Mathur GP, Mathur Sarla. Treatment of epilepsy. In: Mathur GP, Mathur Sarla (eds). *Seizures in Children and Adolescents.* Delhi: Academa Publishers, 2005; 249–274.

Mathur GP, Mathur Sarla, Mathur GP, Tripathi VN. Tapering of antiepileptic drugs. In: Mathur GP, Mathur Sarla (eds). *Seizures in Children and Adolescents.* Delhi: Academa Publishers, 2005; 279–280.

Newman MJ, Dixon R, Toyonaga B. OC 144–093, a novel P glycoprotein (Pgp) inhibitor for the enhancement of antiepileptic therapy In: Bock G, Goode J (eds). *Mechanisms of drug resistance in epilepsy:* Lessons from oncology. Novartis Foundation Symposium 243. England: John Wiley & sons, Ltd., 2002; 213–230.

Purohit AK, Singh AK. Epilepsy Surgery. In: Mathur GP, Mathur Sarla (eds). *Seizures in Children and Adolescents.* Delhi: Academa Publishers, 2005; 303–307.

Schmidt D. Strategies to prevent overtreatment with antiepileptic drugs in patients with epilepsy. *Epilepsy Res* 2002; 52: 61–69.

Sinclair DB. Prednisone therapy in Pediatric Epilepsy. *Pediatr Neurol* 2003; 28: 194–98.

Febrile Seizures

Febrile convulsions are the most common seizures in children. A febrile seizure (FS) may be a manifestation of a serious underlying acute infectious disease such as sepsis or bacterial meningitis. Febrile seizures are age dependent, may have a family history and are either typical (simple) or atypical (complex) types. Febrile seizures are rare before 9 months and after 5 yr of age. The peak age of onset is ≈ 14–18 mo of age and the incidence approaches 3–4% of young children.

There is also a genetic predisposition; the gene is located to chromosomes 19p and 8q13–21. An autosomal dominant inheritance pattern is demonstrated in some families. Generalized epilepsy with febrile seizures+ (GEFS+) is an autosomal dominant disorder.

Clinical manifestations: A child with febrile seizure should be examined along with detailed history of seizure. By the time the child is brought to a hospital, the seizure is no longer present in most cases. The physicians' most important responsibility is to determine the cause of fever, family history of seizure and to rule out meningitis and abnormal neurological findings. Viral infections of the upper respiratory tract, roseola infantum, acute otitis media, pneumonia, and urinary tract infections are the most common causes of febrile seizures. Seizures may occur after immunization, in response to temperature elevation within 48 hours after DPT and 7–10 days after measles immunization

Febrile seizures are classified into two types: typical or simple febrile seizures and atypical or complex febrile seizures. The classification is helpful for determining the risk of recurrence and epilepsy. (1) **Simple febrile seizure** is usually associated with a core temperature that increases rapidly to ≥ 39°C. The seizures are typically generalized, tonic and clonic of a few seconds and rarely up to 15 minutes duration, followed by a brief postictal periods of drowsiness with no postictal neurological abnormalities and occurs only once in 24 hr. (2) **Atypical or complex febrile seizures** are associated with a seizure persisting for >15 minutes, repeated convulsions for several hours or days, focal seizures, and postictal neurological abnormalities including Todd paresis. Convulsive status epilepticus (one seizure lasting 30 min or multiple seizures during 30 min without regaining consciousness) is often due to central nervous system infection (viral or bacterial meningitis).

Approximately 30–50% children have *recurrent seizures* with later episodes of fever and a small number of cases have numerous recurrent febrile seizures. Factors associated with increased recurrence risk include age <12 mo, lower temperature before seizure onset, a positive family history of febrile seizures and complex features. Febrile seizures are not associated with later reduction in intellectual performance. Most children with febrile seizures have only a slightly greater risk of later epilepsy than the general population. The risk factors for development of epilepsy as a complication of febrile seizures include the presence of complex features during the seizure or postictal period, a positive family history of epilepsy, an initial febrile seizure before 12 months of age, prolonged or atypical febrile seizure, delayed developmental milestones, and abnormal neurological findings. The risk of epilepsy is much higher than in the general population in children with one or more complex febrile seizures especially if the seizures are focal in children with an underlying neurologic disorder. The incidence of epilepsy is > 9% when risk factors are present, compared with an incidence of 1% in children who have febrile convulsions and no risk factors. The type of epilepsy that develops is variable. Different types of seizures (generalized tonic-clonic, absence, complex partial) may occur in those children who develop epilepsy after previous febrile seizures. Febrile seizures can also be the initial manifestation of specific epilepsy syndromes, such as severe myoclonic epilepsy of infancy. In rare cases multiple febrile recurrences are followed by severe myoclonic epilepsy.

Investigations: Serum electrolytes, blood glucose, calcium, magnesium and blood counts are not routinely needed. Each child should be examined and investigated for the cause of associated fever and to rule out meningitis and encephalitis. If any doubt exists about the possibility of meningitis, a lumber puncture (LP) with examination of cerebrospinal fluid (CSF) is indicated. A LP is not indicated as a routine procedure in typical febrile seizures. Risk factors for meningitis in patients presenting with fever and seizures are: (i) abnormal neurological examination, especially meningeal signs; (ii) focal seizure, suspicious physical findings (rash or petechiae, cyanosis, hypotension, grunt, etc.), (iii) a physician has seen within 48 hours of fever; (iv) ongoing seizure activity at the time of arrival in the hospital. These risk factors considered together are very helpful in identifying children with meningitis. The American Academy of Pediatrics (1996) recommends LP in-patients under 12 months of age because meningeal signs may be minimal or absent in this age group. LP is to be considered in-patients 12 to 18 months of age as symptoms and signs may be subtle. LP is also to be considered in children with febrile seizures who have received antibiotics because symptoms and signs of meningitis may also be marked. The CSF may be normal in early meningitis and therefore does not rule out meningitis.

An EEG is not a guide to treatment or the prognosis and as such it is not helpful in children with first or recurrent febrile seizures. An EEG is not indicated after a simple febrile seizure. An EEG is indicated for atypical febrile seizures or for a child at risk for developing epilepsy. As the detection of epileptic discharges in EEG is unusual within the first postictal

week, it should preferably be done after a week. Neuroimaging (CT or MRI) of head is not indicated in a child with simple febrile seizure, but may be considered with atypical features, including focal neurologic signs or pre-existing neurologic deficits.

Treatment: Treatment of a normal child who has simple febrile seizures includes finding out the cause of fever, measures to control the fever including antipyretics, and reassurance of parents. Short-term anticonvulsant prophylaxis is not indicated. Prolonged anticonvulsant prophylaxis for preventing recurrent febrile seizures is controversial and is not recommended. Oral diazepam is recommended as it is an effective and safe method of reducing the risk of recurrence of febrile seizures. At the onset of each febrile illness, diazepam 0.3 mg/kg 8 hourly (1 mg/kg/24 hours) should be administered orally for the duration of illness (usually 2–3 days). For selected patients with recurrent complex febrile seizures diazepam is prescribed in the form of a gel that can be given rectally at the time of a seizure in a dose of approximately 0.5 mg/kg for children aged 2–5 yr or 0.3–0.5 mg/kg of diazepam is diluted in 3 ml with 0.9% sodium chloride and the amount is placed into the rectum by a syringe and a flexible tube. This will usually terminate the seizure and prevent recurrence over 12 hr. The side effects are usually minor and the symptoms such as lethargy, irritability and ataxia, can be reduced by adjusting the dose. Antiepileptic drugs such as phenytoin and carbamazepine have no effect on febrile seizures. Phenobarbital has been ineffective in preventing recurrent febrile seizures and may decrease cognitive function. Sodium valproate is effective in the treatment of febrile seizures, but the potential risks of the drug do not justify its use.

Paracetamol (acetaminophen) 10–15 mg/kg every 4 hourly is recommended and is not associated with many adverse effects. However, its massive overdose may produce hepatic failure. Ibuprofen 5–10 mg/kg every 6–8 hourly may cause dyspepsia, gastrointestinal bleeding, reduced renal blood flow and rarely aseptic meningitis, hepatic toxicity, or aplastic anemia.

Tepid sponge bathing in warm water is another recommended method of reducing high body temperature.

Antibiotic therapy should be administered in cases of infection (including meningitis) until a bacterial cause is excluded.

Hospitalization: Children with the slightest suspicion of meningitis, those with a first febrile seizure, and if any of the following situation is present: (i) age less than 18 months, (ii) CNS disorders such as cerebral palsy, mental retardation, (iii) lethargy beyond postictal state, (iv) unstable clinical status, (v) uncertain home situation, and (vi) unclear follow-up should be hospitalized.

Counseling and parent education: Counseling and education should be the sole treatment for the majority of children with febrile seizures. Parents should be counseled properly with emphasis that: (i) febrile seizures are benign in nature ; (ii) febrile seizures do not lead to neurological problems or developmental delay ; (iii) they should consult the doctor if the seizure lasts for more than 15 minutes or if the postical drowsiness persists for more than 30 minutes; (iv) give tepid sponge bathing with warm water for reducing high body temperature; and (v) keep two drugs handy-paracetamol and diazepam, a dose of each drug (as per dose of the drugs mentioned in the earlier prescription) is to be given to an established case of febrile seizures at the onset of each febrile illness in order to avoid seizure and to consult the doctor for future line of action.

Prognosis: Even though a vast majority of children can lead a perfectly healthy life after an attack of febrile seizures, there can be no doubt that the liability to febrile convulsions does place the child at risk of recurrence and epilepsy. The incidence of epilepsy is approximately 9% when several risk factors are present compared with an incidence of 1% in children who have febrile convulsion and no risk factors. Simple febrile seizures are benign in nature that does not have any long-term neurological sequalae. Simple febrile seizures require neither long-term daily phenobarbital nor intermittent diazepam therapy. A rational goal of therapy would be to prevent very prolonged febrile seizures.

American Academy of Pediatrics. Provisional Committee on Quality Improvement, Sub-committee on Febrile Seizures. *Pediatrics* 1996; 97: 769–775.

Freeman JM, Vining EPG, Pillas DJ. *Seizures and Epilepsy in Childhood: A Guide for parents.* 1st edn. Baltimore: The John Hopkins University, Press, 1990; 36–55.

Mathur GP, Mathur Sarla. Febrile seizures. In: Mathur GP, Mathur Sarla (eds). *Seizures in Children and Adolescents.* Delhi: Academa Publishers, 2005; 111–117.

Singhi PD, Srinivas M. Febrile Seizures. *Indian Pediatr* 2001; 38: 733–740.

Verity CM, Greenwood R, Golding J. Long term intellectual and behavioral outcomes of children with febrile convulsions. *N Engl J Med* 1998; 338: 1723–1725.

Neonatal Seizures

Neonatal seizures are a common neurological symptom. The incidence of clinical seizures varies from 0.2–1% in term babies to 20% in preterm babies. Neonatal seizures are classified on clinical manifestations and on EEG findings.

I. *Clinical Manifestations and Classification of Seizures*

(i) *Subtle seizures* constitute 50% of seizures in both term and preterm newborn infants. Subtle seizures consist of chewing motions, excessive salivation, and alterations in the respiratory rate including apnea, blinking, nystagmus, bicycling or pedaling movements, and changes in color. They most often occur in infants who manifest the other seizure types. (ii) *Focal seizures* consist of rhythmic twitching of muscle groups, particularly the extremities and face. These seizures are not associated with loss of consciousness. These seizures are often associated with localized structural lesions, infections and subarachnoid hemorrhage. The EEG is most often unifocally abnormal. (iii) *Multifocal clonic seizures* are characterized by clonic seizures affecting multiple muscle groups. The EEG is most often multifocally abnormal. (iv) *Tonic seizures* are characterized by rigid posturing of extremities and trunk and are sometimes associated with fixed deviation of the eyes. This condition is more often associated with diffuse central nervous system disease or intraventricular hemorrhage. The EEG is multifocally abnormal, has either a burst-suppression pattern, or has extremely attenuated amplitude. (v) *Myoclonic seizures* are brief focal or generalized jerks of the extremities or body that tend to involve distal muscle groups and are associated with diffuse CNS pathology. The EEG shows a burst-suppression pattern or focal sharp transient waves.

II. *EEG Classification of Neonatal Seizures*

a. Clinical seizure with a consistent EEG event includes focal clonic, focal tonic, and some myoclonic seizures. These seizures are, clearly epileptic and are likely to respond to an anticonvulsant.

b. Clinical seizures with inconsistent EEG event is observed with all generalized tonic seizures and subtle seizures and with some myoclonic seizures. These infants tend to be neurologically depressed or comatose as a result of hypoxic-ischemic encephalopathy. Seizures in this category are likely to be of nonepileptic origin and may not require or respond to antiepileptics.

c. Electrical seizures with absent clinical seizures: In this category two types of seizure activity are seen. Electrical seizures associated with a markedly abnormal background EEG may develop in comatose infants who are not on anticonvulsants. In-patients with focal tonic or clonic seizures after the introduction of an anticonvulsant, electrical seizures may persist without clinical signs.

Etiology: The causes of neonatal seizures include: 1. Hypoxic-ischemic encephalopathy (HIE); 2. Intracranial hemorrhage and CNS trauma; 3. Metabolic disorders (hypoglycemia, hypocalcemia, hypomagnesemia, hyponatremia, hypernatremia, pyridoxine dependency, inborn errors of metabolism); 4. Infections-bacterial meningitis including brain abscess, syphilis, toxoplasmosis, viral infections (cytomegalovirus, coxsackievirus, echovirus, rubella, herpesvirus, HIV); 5. Developmental problems—cerebral dysgenesis and malformations including those associated with chromosomal disorders, neurocutaneous syndromes; 6. Kernicterus; 7. Drug-associated seizures- narcotic and sedative withdrawals and unintentional administration of local anesthetic; 8. Polycythemia/hyperviscosity; 9. Focal infarcts from arterial or venous occlusion; 10. Hypertensive encephalopathy; 11. Unknown causes involved in 3 to 25% of cases; 12. Epileptic syndromes [early (neonatal) myoclonic encephalopathy (EME), early infantile epileptic encephalopathy with S-B EEG pattern, glucose transporter type 1 syndrome, neonatal myoclonus without EEG epileptiform activity, pyridoxine-dependent seizures, fifth-day fits, and genetic neonatal epilepsy syndromes].

Diagnosis: A detailed history of perinatal and neonatal events, along with a family history, seizure type and a clinical examination including neurologic examination and funduscopy will often aid in reaching an etiological diagnosis. An abnormal odor may offer an invaluable aid to the diagnosis (*see* Table 24.1).

Investigations: For initial studies blood should be obtained for determinations of glucose, calcium, magnesium, phosphorus, electrolytes, and blood urea nitrogen (BUN). If hypoglycemia is a possibility, a serum Dextrostix testing is indicated so that treatment can be initiated immediately.

Cerebrospinal fluid examination: Every neonate with seizure should have cerebrospinal fluid examination to exclude bacterial meningitis or aseptic encephalitis unless the cause is clearly related to a metabolic disorder such as hypoglycemia or hypocalcemia secondary to feeding of high concentrations of phosphate.

Electroencephalogram (EEG): EEG is used in making diagnosis and for the management of seizures. However, treatment should not be delayed till an EEG is done. Synchronised Video-EEG monitoring is used to provide basis for reinterpretation of various abnormal clinical signs. It also helps to establish an epileptic etiology in cases with abnormal clinical activity and quantitates electrical seizures following therapy.

Brain imaging techniques: Ultrasonography, CT and MRI help in diagnosing cerebral malformations, intraventricular hemorrhage, hydrocephalus and cerebral infarction. Positron emission tomography (PET) helps in detection of more specific metabolic disturbances.

Differential diagnosis: Neonatal seizures need to be distinguished from tetanus neonatorum, apnea, tetany, and jitteriness and clonus (associated with hypocalcemia, neonatal encephalopathy, and drug withdrawal).

Management: The treatment of neonatal seizures is an emergency. Recurrent or continuous seizures may lead to brain injury. The underlying disease should be treated.

Intravenous therapy: An intravenous line must be established (through an umbilical vein if necessary). The aim is to optimize ventilation, cardiac output, blood pressure, serum electrolytes, and pH. Take first blood for relevant laboratory investigations.

Lumbar puncture is to be done where necessary based on clinical findings and condition of the patient. In the presence of septicemia and meningitis, appropriate parenteral antibiotics are administered along with supportive therapy.

Consider the management when blood and CSF studies are available.

Glucose: Immediate therapy consists of an IV bolus of 200 mg/kg glucose (2 ml/kg 10% dextrose) over one minute (10% D/W= 10 gm/100 ml; 1 gm/10 ml; 200 mg/2 ml). Follow this by an infusion of glucose at a rate of. 8 mg of glucose /kg per minute (10% D/W at a rate of 110 ml/kg per day or 4.6 ml/kg/ hour gives 8 mg/kg per minute of glucose) Give this rate of 8 mg/kg per minute of glucose, and then taper off the rate of infusion as per laboratory reports of blood glucose levels. Recheck glucose level after 20 to 30 minutes and hourly until stable, to determine if additional therapy is needed. If hypoglycemia is the diagnosis (blood sugar less than 30 mg/dl in term and less than 20 mg/dl in preterms in first 48 hours of life, and less than 40 mg/dl thereafter), dextrose infusion must be than maintained at the rate of 6–8 mg/kg/ min. Most hypoglycemia will resolve in 2 to 3 days. If the glucose levels remain low, treatment with glucagon or hydrocortisone should be considered even if signs are not present. Excessive glucose however, promotes the accumulation of cerebral lactic acid, which may be damaging the brain. Thus, the serum glucose level should be maintained within physiologic levels (70 to 120 mg/dl).

Calcium: Failure of response to glucose or a normal blood sugar level (obtained by dextrostix), should suggest the possibility of hypocalcemia (serum calcium less than 7 mg/dl). If hypocalcemia is the cause of the seizure, calcium gluconate 10%, 2 ml/kg (18 mg of elemental calcium per kilogram) mixed with an equal volume of distilled water, is given intravenously over 3 minutes (at a rate not exceeding 1 mL/min). The patient's condition is checked during the administration with careful observation of the pulse or ECG rhythm using an electrocardiogram (ECG) or cardiac monitor.

Magnesium: Hypomagnesemia (serum levels less than 2 mg/dl) is treated with magnesium sulfate 50% (0.2 ml/kg IM). Half of all hypocalcemic infants also have hypomagnesemia. Associated hypomagnesemia may be responsible for poor or non- response to IV calcium.

Pyridoxine: Pyridoxine dependency/deficiency may be a cause of recurrent seizures. The diagnosis is one of exclusion of other known causes and is treated by administering 50 mg IV and observing for response, preferably under EEG monitoring for reversal of EEG changes. Seizures will cease within minutes if pyridoxine dependency or deficiency is the cause of seizures. In cases of pyridoxine dependency a dose of 10 to 100 mg by mouth daily of pyridoxine therapy is needed life long. A dose of 5 mg by mouth daily is required in pyridoxine deficiency, as the EEG does not normalize immediately when seizures cease during pyridoxine infusion. Rarely, pyridoxine therapy has been associated with hypotonia and apnea. Pyridoxine in high doses (300 mg/kg/day) has been used with some success in infants with refractory infantile spasms (*see* Section 26.2).

Anticonvulsant: If hypoglycemia or metabolic problems are not the evident cause of seizures, anticonvulsant medications should be administered.

1. *Phenobarbital:* a. If convulsions still remain uncontrolled (ongoing seizures) phenobarbital 15 to 20 mg/kg is given intravenously over several minutes for seizures. If the seizures continue after 60 minutes, a second dose of phenobarbital (10 mg/kg) may be given, usually concomitantly with loading dosages of phenytoin. But in refractory status epilepticus, one may elect to use very-high-dose phenobarbital. This can be administered in 10 mg/kg boluses every 30 minutes (usually totaling less than 60 mg/kg) until seizures cease. If the infant has intermittent seizures, without true status epilepticus, and has phenobarbital levels of 30 to 45 g/ml, then phenytoin may be administered. Cumulative loading doses of phenobarbital greater than 20 mg/kg require careful monitoring of blood pressure and respiratory status for the possible development of hypotension and more rarely,

apnea. b. Interictal: If an infant has had a seizure but is not currently having seizures, the intravenous administration of 15 to 20 mg/kg of phenobarbital will lead to therapeutic plasma levels. c. Maintenance doses range from 3.5 to 4.5 mg/kg per day of phenobarbital, given as a single dose or divided in two doses given every 12 hours intravenously or by mouth. d. Therapeutic plasma levels range from 15 to 45 g/ml, measured at least 1 hour after an intravenous dose or 2 to 4 hours after an oral dose. The goal is to maintain the lowest therapeutic level that controls seizures; this level is usually in the range of 15 to 30 g/ml. Phenobarbital can cause sedation and hypotonia in neonates, and it may increase theophylline requirement in premature infants with apnea.

2. *Phenytoin:* 15 to 25 mg/kg is given intravenously administered in normal saline at a rate not greater than 1 mg/kg per minute. Phenytoin is generally given if there has been no response to phenobarbital or if there is a critical need to monitor the level of consciousness. A maintenance dose of 4 to 8 mg/kg per day, divided into two or three doses, can be given intravenously. The therapeutic plasma level is 10 to 20 g/ml, taken at least 1 hour after IV administration. Phenytoin is poorly absorbed from the gastrointestinal tract and/or the half-life is very short when administered during the newborn period. If phenobarbitone twice given is not effective, then phenytoin loading dose 10 mg/kg is given slowly IV. It may be repeated once after ½ an hour. Monitor with ECG for heart block and ventricular fibrillations.

3. *Diazepam* is used only when immediate cessation of seizures is required (i.e. when seizures interfere with vital functions). a. If diazepam is required, it should be administered after dilution of 0.2 ml (1 mg) of diazepam with 0.8 ml of normal saline; b The initial dose should be 0.1 to 0.3 mg/kg given slowly, IV, (directly into the vein not the tubing) until the seizure stops; c. Diazepam acts synergistically with phenobarbital to increase the risk of provoking respiratory arrest. Appropriate facilities for circulatory and ventilatory support should be available; d. Diazepam contains sodium benzoate, which may interfere with the binding of bilirubin to albumin.

4. *Lorazepam* is an effective anticonvulsant and its anticonvulsant effect lasts longer than that of diazepam. The dose is 0.05 mg/kg per dose IV over 2 to 5 minutes. The dose may be repeated. The complications generally are the same as those of diazepam. On occasion, lorazepam has been associated with the triggering of myoclonic jerks and repetitive clonic activity.

Adequacy of therapy: The adequacy of therapy may be difficult to judge. Electrical seizures may be seen despite the absence of clinical seizures. The attempt should be to stop all clinical evidence of seizures, including blood pressure and heart rate changes in infants who are paralyzed. Phenobarbital is to be used to attain levels of 40 g/mL if necessary. Other drugs are used as indicated if clinical seizures continue. Do not attempt to stop all electrical epileptiform activity because of the side effects of doses required to do this.

Duration of therapy: If a baby has had a single seizure, the anticonvulsant is withdrawn before discharge. If a baby has required two anticonvulsants for control of seizures, phenobarbitone is continued and the other anticonvulsants withdrawn. Babies who have had multiple convulsions require to be maintained on phenobarbitone after discharge. At three months of age the baby is reassessed. A neurological examination and an EEG are done. If normal, phenobarbitone is omitted; if not, the drug is continued for one year when the child is reassessed. If possible, all medications except maintenance phenobarbital at 3.5 to 5 mg/kg per day should be discontinued before the infant is discharged.

Prognosis: Prognosis is better if seizures subside within 24 hours and if the neurological examination is normal. In the case of hypoglycemic infants of a diabetic mother or hypocalcemia associated with excessive phosphate feedings, the prognosis is excellent. On the other hand, children with intractable seizures due to severe hypoxic-ischemic encephalopathy or a cytoarchitectural abnormality of the brain have poor prognosis, usually do not respond to anticonvulsants and are susceptible to status epilepticus and early death. Normal EEG is the most useful prognostic indicator. Term infants with a normal interictal EEG have an 86% probability of normal development.

duPlessis AJ. Neonatal seizures. In: Cloherty JP, Stark AR (eds). *Manual of Neonatal Care*. 4th edn. Philadelphia: Lippincott-Raven, 1998; 483–498.

Johnston MV. Seizures in Childhood. In: Kliegman RM, Behrman RE, Jenson HB, Stanton BF (eds). *Nelson Textbook of Pediatrics*. 18th edn. Vol. 2. Philadelphia: Saunders, 2007; 2457–2475.

Mathur Sarla, GP Mathur GP, Singhal PK. Neonatal Seizures. In: Mathur GP, Mathur Sarla (eds). *Seizures in Children and Adolescents*. Delhi: Academa Publishers, 2005; 46–52.

Rezvani I. An approach to inborn errors of metabolism. In: Kliegman RM, Behrman RE, Jenson HB, Stanton BF (eds). *Nelson Textbook of Pediatrics*. 18th edn. Vol. 1. Philadelphia: Saunders, 2007; 527–528.

Singh M. Neonatal Seizures. In: Singh M (Ed). *Care of the newborn*. 5th edn. New Delhi: Sagar Printers and Publishers, 1999; 340–344.

Tharp BR. Neonatal seizures and syndromes. *Epilepsia* 2002; 43 (suppl 3): 2–10.

Reflex Epilepsy

The precipitation of seizures by specific external stimuli has been called 'reflex epilepsy'. A variety of sensory stimuli are recognized as causing reflex epilepsy. It is rarely encountered in children. The onset is usually between 6–15 years. There is a 3 : 2 female preponderance and greatest expression in adolescence. Reflex epilepsy in children unlike other types of epilepsy carries a good prognosis. Various reflex epilepsies include 1. Photosensitive epilepsy; 2. Reading epilepsy; 3. Startle epilepsy (Startle-induced seizures); 4. Auditory epilepsy (epilepsy evoked by sound); 5. Epilepsy evoked by an act of will or of the mind (psychogenic epilepsy); 6. Self-induced seizures; 7. Seizures induced by movements and other actions; 8. Reflex seizures involving stimulation of the gastrointestinal tract; 9. Reflex seizures induced by eating (Eating epilepsy); 10. Tactile epilepsy; 11. Hot water epilepsy; 12. Tooth brushing-induced seizures; 13. Tooth-loosing dream and the epileptic state; 14. Reflex seizures induced by defecation; 15. Somatosensory evoked epilepsy; 16. Rub epilepsy; 17. Benign early infantile reflex absence seizures; 18. Reflex seizures and nonketotic hyperglycemia.

Duncan JS, Shorvon SD, Fish DR. Reflex epilepsy. In: Duncan JS, Shorvon SD, Fish DR (eds). *Clinical Epilepsy*. Edinburgh: Churchill Livingstone, 1995; 66–69.

Mani KS, Gopalakrishnan PN, Vyas JN, Pillai MS. Hot water Epilepsy—A peculiar type of reflex epilepsy. A preliminary report. *Neurology India* 1968; 16:107–110.

Mathur GP, Mathur Sarla. Reflex epilepsy. In: Mathur GP, Mathur Sarla (eds). *Seizures in Children and Adolescents*. Delhi: Academa Publishers, 2005; R66–76.

Salas-Puig J, Mateos V, Amorin M, Calleja S, Jimenez L. Reflex epilepsies. *Rev Neurol* 2000; 30: 285–289.

Satishchandra P. Sivaramakrishna A. Klaperumal VG. Schoenberg BS. Hot Water Epilepsy. A variant of reflex epilepsy in Southern India. *Epilepsia* 1988; 29:52–56.

Status Epilepticus

Status epilepticus (SE) is defined as a continuous convulsion lasting longer than 20–30 minutes or the occurrence of serial convulsions between which there is no return of consciousness. Status epilepticus may be classified as *generalized* (tonic-clinic, absence) or *partial* (simple, complex or with secondary generalization). Generalized tonic-clonic seizures are commonly associated with status epilepticus.

Etiology: There are three major subtypes of status epilepticus: (1) prolonged febrile seizures, (2) idiopathic status epilepticus, and (3) symptomatic status epilepticus. The causes are listed in Table 24.7.

Pathophysiology: The relationship between the neurologic outcome and the duration of status

Table 24.7: Etiology of status epilepticus

1. Prolonged febrile seizures	Particularly in children less than 3 years of age
2. Idiopathic status epilepticus (No CNS lesion)	1. Sudden withdrawal of anticonvulsants (especially benzodiazepines and barbiturates); 2. Anticonvulsants given on an irregular basis to children suffering from epilepsy; 3. Noncompliance regarding taking anticonvulsants; 4. Sleep deprivation; 5. Intercurrent infection; 6. Status epilepticus may be the initial presentation of epilepsy.
3. Symptomatic status epilepticus (CNS lesion or metabolic abnormality)	1. Severe hypoxic-ischemic encephalopathy in the newborn; 2. Encephalitis; 3. Meningitis; 4. Drug intoxication; 5. Lead intoxication; 6. Extreme hyperpyrexia; 7. Brian tumors (particularly in frontal lobe); 8. Congenital malformation of brain (e.g. lissencephaly (or schizencephaly); 9. Inborn error of metabolism; 10. Electrolyte abnormalities; 11. Hypocalcemia; 12. Hypoglycemia

epilepticus is unknown in children and adults, as the findings are based on the studies conducted in animals. These studies have lead to the concept of a critical period during status epilepticus when irreversible neuronal changes may develop. This transitional period varies between 20 and 60 minutes in animals during constant seizure activity. In children, as the precise transitional period in humans is unknown, the convulsions should be controlled expeditiously. The most vulnerable areas of the brain include the hippocampus, amygdala, cerebellum, middle cortical area, and thalamus. Characteristic acute pathologic changes consist of venous congestion, small petechial hemorrhages, and edema. Prolonged generalized seizures activity may lead to dysfunction of the autonomic nervous system with hypotension and shock as well as to lactic acidosis, myoglobinuria, and acute tubular necrosis.

Treatment: The first priority in the treatment is the maintenance of vital functions by establishment of an airway and adequate ventilation. The oral airway is secured and inspected for patency. The pulse, temperature, respirations, and blood pressure are recorded. Excessive oral secretions are removed through suction, and a properly fitting mask attached to oxygen is applied. If patients do not respond to oxygen by mask or are difficult to ventilate by an Ambu bag, they require intubation and assisted ventilation. A nasogastric tube is placed in position and an IV cannula is immediately inserted. If hypoglycemia is confirmed by Dextrostix, a rapid infusion of 5 ml/kg of 10% dextrose is provided. Blood is obtained for a CBC and for determination of electrolytes (including calcium, phosphorus, and magnesium), glucose, creatinine, lactate, and anticonvulsant levels, if indicated. Blood and urine

may be obtained for metabolic studies and toxicology, because some drugs potentiate or precipitate status epilepticus (amphetamine, cocaine, phenothiazines, theophylline in toxic levels, tricyclic antidepressants). Arterial blood gases should be determined, and oxygen saturation (SaO_2) should be monitored with an oximeter. Examination of the CSF is imperative if meningitis or encephalitis is considered, unless there is a contraindication to the procedure. In this case, appropriate antibiotics should be administered, followed by imaging studies, before a lumbar puncture is attempted. If the seizures are refractory to the anticonvulsants or if the patient is paralyzed and is on respirator, continuous EEG monitoring is important to assess the frequency of seizure discharges, their location, and the response to anticonvulsant therapy.

A physical and neurologic examination should be carried out concurrently to assess the following: evidence of trauma; papilledema, a bulging anterior fontanel, or lateralizing neurologic signs suggesting increased intracranial pressure (ICP); manifestations of sepsis or meningitis; retinal hemorrhages that may indicate a subdural hematoma; Kussmaul breathing and dehydration suggestive of metabolic acidosis or irregular respirations due to brainstem dysfunction; evidence of failure to thrive, a peculiar body odor, or abnormal hair pigmentation that suggests an inborn error of metabolism; and constriction or dilatation of pupils suggesting a toxin or drugs as the cause of the status epilepticus. A detailed examination should be undertaken once the seizures are under control. Further investigations of the patient including neuroradiologic studies depends on the physical and neurologic findings and the seizure type and frequency.

If hypoglycemia is a possible or likely cause of seizure, a rapid infusion of glucose solution (2 ml/kg of 25% dextrose in sterile water) followed by 10 percent dextrose solution should be given. Metabolic acidosis is corrected with bicarbonate infusion (7.5% solution—2–3 ml/kg).

Drugs should always be delivered by intravenous (IV) route in the management of status epilepticus as the intramuscular (IM) route is unreliable because some drugs are bounded by muscle (Boxes 24.12 and 24.13; Table 24.8). Rectal diazepam- Diazepam diluted in 3 ml 0.9% normal saline is placed into the rectum by a syringe and a flexible tube at a dose of 0.3–0.5 mg/kg. Rectal lorazepam: The effective dose of rectal lorazepam is 0.05–0.1 mg/kg. Therapeutic serum levels occur within 5–10 min. Sublingual lorazepam: It may be used to treat children with serial seizures that tend to develop into status epilepticus while the children are at home. The dose of sublingual lorazepam is 0.05–0.1 mg/kg.

The use of anticonvulsant therapy after status epilepticus depends on the underlying condition. A long-term antiepileptic should not be maintained in children with a progressive neurologic disorder or with a history of recurrent seizures before the onset of status epilepticus. An anticonvulsant treatment is not necessary after an initial attack of idiopathic status epilepticus, particularly when a prolonged febrile seizure was the cause. Anticonvulsant therapy is maintained arbitrarily for 3 months in this case and is discontinued if the child remains asymptomatic.

Prognosis: Prognosis depends on the time allowed to elapse between the onset status epilepticus and initiation of effective treatment. Patients with status

---

Box 24.12: Immediate care of seizures

Aid (by relatives and witnesses)
- Move person away from danger (fire, water, machinery, furniture)
- After convulsions cease, turn into 'recovery' position (semiprone)
- Ensure airway is clear
- **Do Not** insert anything in mouth (tongue-biting occurs at seizure onset and cannot be prevented by observers)
- If convulsions continue for more than 5 minutes or recur without person regaining consciousness, summon urgent medical attention
- Person may be drowsy and confused for some 30–60 minutes and should not be left alone until fully recovered

Immediate Medical Care
- Ensure airway is clear
- Give oxygen to offset cerebral hypoxia
- Give intravenous anticonvulsant (e.g. diazepam 0.3 mg/kg in a child or 10 mg in an adult) ONLY
- If convulsions are continuous or repeated (if so, manage, as for status epilepticus)
- Take blood for anticonvulsant levels (if known epileptic)

---

epilepticus lasting < 1 hr had a lower mortality as compared with seizure duration 1 hr. The mortality rate is comparatively more in patients with partial status epilepticus than patients with generalized status epilepticus. Continuous status epilepticus has a higher mortality and morbidity rate than intermittent status epilepticus. Status epilepticus is a rare cause of mortality per se. Factors responsible for mortality in status epilepticus are listed in Box 24.14.

Box 24.13: Management of Generalized Status Epilepticus

- Immediate care
- Secure I.V. access
- Draw blood for glucose and electrolytes and save for future analysis (drug etc.).
- Give lorazepam 0.1 mg/kg IV at 2mg/minute (Additional emergency drug therapy may not be required if seizures stop and the cause of status epilepticus is rapidly corrected)_____Seizures are continuing
- Transfer to intensive care area, monitoring neurological condition, blood pressure, respiration and blood gases
- Give phenytoin (20 mg/kg IV at 50 mg/min) or fosphenytoin (20 mg/kg PE IV at 50 mg/min)_____Seizures are continuing
- Give an additional dose of phenytoin after 20 minutes(2– 10 mg/kg IV at 50 mg/min) or fosphenytoin (5–10 mg/kg PE IV)_____Seizures are continuing
- Give phenobarbital after 30 minutes (20 mg/kg IV at 50–75 mg/minute)_____Seizures are continuing
- Give additional dose of phenobarbital after 30 minutes (5–10 mg/kg IV)_____Seizures are continuing
- Constant IV infusion after 60 minutes (or patient has extreme hyperthermia) of either midazolam (0.2 mg/kg bolus, 1–5 g/kg/min infusion) or propofol (1–2 mg/kg, 2–10 mg/kg/hr infusion) has been effective in managing seizures during status epilepticus unresponsive to other anticonvulsants
- Investigate the cause

Approximate time interval—In minutes from the first dose of lorazepam
PE: Phenytoin equivalent

Table 24.8: Anticonvulsants used in status epilepticus by intravenous (IV) route

	Diazepam	*Lorazepam*	*Phenobarbital*	*Phenytoin**
Drug for IV use	10 mg/2 ml	2 mg/ml	200 mg/ml	50 mg/ml
Route	IV	IV	IV	IV
Loading dose Child	0.3 mg/kg	0.1 mg/kg	20 mg/kg (maximum 40 mg/kg)	20 mg/kg
Adult	10–20 mg (maximum 3mg/kg/ 24 hr)	0.1 mg/kg	20 mg/kg (maximum 1–2 g)	20 mg/kg
Rate				
Child	2 mg/min		50–75 mg/min	1–3 mg/kg/min
Adult	0.5 ml (2.5 mg)/30 seconds, repeated if required after 30–60 minutes			50 mg/min
Onset of effect	2 minutes	15 minutes		
Peak effect	Unknown		30 min	15–30 min
Therapeutic serum level			15–40 g/ml	10–20 g/ml
Half life (t 1/2)	30 hr	20 hr	100 hr	6–24 hr (at higher doses- up to 60 hr)
Side effects	Respiratory depression Hypotension	Respiratory depression Hypotension	Respiratory depression	Arrhythmia and bradycardia Hypotension

*Phenytoin forms a precipitate in glucose solutions and is rendered ineffective.

Box 24.14: Factors responsible for mortality in status epilepticus

- Patients with coexistent neurologic compromise—due to respiratory tract infection and aspiration
- Death resulting from injury—due to drowning
- Hyperthermia

Source: Breningstall GN. Mortality in Pediatric Epilepsy. Pediatr Neurol 2001; 25: 9–16.

Johnston MV. Seizures in Childhood. In: Kliegman RM, Behrman RE, Jenson HB, Stanton BF (eds). *Nelson Textbook of Pediatrics*. 18th edn. Vol. 2. Philadelphia: Saunders, 2007; 2457–2475.

Mathur GP, Mathur Sarla, Piyush Prasad.Nonconvulsive status epilepticus. In: Mathur GP, Mathur Sarla (eds). Seizures in Children and Adolescents. Delhi: *Academa Publishers*, 2005; 130–137.

O'Brien TJ, Cascino GD, So EL, Hanna DR. Incidence and clinical consequence of the purple glove syndrome in patients receiving intravenous phenytoin. *Neurology* 1998; 51: 1034–1039.

Prasad R, Mathur GP, Mathur Sarla. Status epilepticus. In: Mathur GP, Mathur Sarla (eds). *Seizures in Children and Adolescents*. Delhi: Academa Publishers, 2005; 118–129.

Intractable Epilepsy

Intractable epilepsy (refractory epilepsy; refractory seizures; seizures difficult to control) generally implies seizure recurrence despite adequate trial with appropriate antiepileptic drugs for an adequate length of time. Epilepsy is resistant to drug treatment in about one-third of cases. The proportion of cases resistant to drug treatment varies with the specific cause or syndrome diagnosis. A higher proportion of subjects with epilepsy due to hippocampal sclerosis (HS), malformations of cortical development (MCD) and dysembryoplastic neuroepithelial tumors (DNTs) are likely to have refractory epilepsy.

Management: Treatment options for these patients include continued polytherapy with or without novel antiepileptic drugs, epilepsy surgery, or vagus nerve stimulation. Five different strategies should be considered in the management of intractable cases of epilepsy.

1. Normal dose monotherapy—use of a single drug in pharmacologically accepted doses.
2. High dose monotherapy—use of carbamazepine in doses more than 30 mg/kg/day or valproic acid more than 60 mg/kg/day.

3. Normal dose polytherapy—where multiple drugs are used, the doses being within accepted range.
4. High dose polytherapy—where multiple drugs are used of which at least one is in high doses as given above.
5. Change of drug—change of a single drug to another single drug at therapeutic doses.

Newer antiepileptic drugs as the first line drugs are currently undesirable. The more widely used agents among them include vigabatrin, lamotrigine, gabapentin, topiramate, tiagabine, felbamate and oxcarbazepine (*see* antiepileptic drugs in Section 24.8).

Allen CMC, Lueck CJ. Epilepsy. In: Haslett C, Chilvers ER, Hunter JAA, Boon NA (eds). *Davidson's Principles and Practice of Medicine.* 18th edn. Edinburgh: Churchill Livingstone, 1999; 942–8.

Chawla S, Aneja S, Kashyap R, Mallika V. Etiology and clinical predictors of intractable epilepsy. *Pediatr Neurol* 2002; 27:186–91.

Mathur GP, Mathur Sarla. Intractable epilepsy. In: Mathur GP, Mathur Sarla (eds). *Seizures in Children and Adolescents.* Delhi: Academa Publishers, 2005;192–202.

Sinclair DB. Prednisone therapy in Pediatric Epilepsy. *Pediatr Neurol* 2003; 28:194–8.

Conditions that Mimic Seizures

Several conditions have features similar to the features of epilepsy such as altered levels of consciousness, tonic or clonic movements, or cyanosis. It is useful to consider the differential diagnosis of seizures based on age of the patient in clinical practice, as age is one of the most important factors determining the likely cause of seizures or epilepsy (Box 24.15).

Johnston MV. Conditions that mimic seizures. In: Kliegman RM, Behrman RE, Jenson HB, Stanton BF (eds). *Nelson Textbook of Pediatrics.* 18th edn. Vol. 2. Philadelphia: Saunders, 2007; 2476–2478.

Kumar Sudhir. Psychogenic non-epileptic seizures. In: Mathur GP, Mathur Sarla (eds). *Current Trends in Pediatrics.* Vol 2. Delhi: Academa Publishers, 2006; 160–164.

Mathur GP, Mathur Sarla. Pitfalls in the diagnosis of seizures. In: Mathur GP, Mathur Sarla (eds). *Seizures in Children and Adolescents.* Delhi: Academa Publishers, 2005; 211–217.

Mishra V, Gahlaut DS, Kumar S, Mathur GP, Agnihotri SS, Gupta V. Value of serum prolactin in differentiating epilepsy from pseudoseizure. *JAPI* 1990; 38 (11); 846–847.

24.9 MOVEMENT DISORDERS

Disorders of movement have been ascribed to abnormalities of the central nervous system and of basal ganglia and connecting structures in particular. A genetic basis for many of these disorders has been recognized.

1. *Asterixis* is irregular abrupt brief loss of posture, especially evident in the outstretched hands or tongue. Asterixis occurs in hepatic encephalopathy in cases of fulminant hepatic failure, uremia, and respiratory failure and with anticonvulsants, hypnotic drugs and radiographic contrast agents.
2. *Ataxia* is the inability to make smooth, accurate, and coordinated movements, usually due to a disorder of the cerebellum and/or sensory pathway in the posterior columns of the spinal cord. Ataxia of gait consists of irregularities in the rate, length, and consistency of walking movements, with veering to one side or the other.
3. *Athetosis:* The usual site of lesion is putamen. Athetosis refers to a peculiar writhing, irregular movement with increased tone in distal extremities. Athetotic movements are slower than those associated with chorea. When it is impossible to distinguish between athetosis and chorea, the movements are termed choreoathetosis.
4. *Ballismus* is uncommon in children, and some clinicians consider the violent, irregular flinging movements of the arms and legs as a severe form of chorea. Thus hemiballismus may be a severe form of hemichorea in-patients with Sydenham's chorea or following encephalitis or closed head injury. Vascular events (stroke) involving the contralateral subthalamic nucleus may result hemiballismus in children.
5. *Chorea:* Choreiform movements are rapid, random jerks affecting axial structures, such as the tongue, head and trunk, in addition to arms and legs. The movements often appear less obvious during voluntary movement, and are increased by agitation or nervousness. The site of lesion is caudate nucleus (*see* Figs 24.9 to 24.12 in CD).
6. *Cramp (spasm):* The spasm of part or whole of a muscle, especially of calf muscles is seen in normal

---

Box 24.15: Differential diagnosis of seizures in different age groups

Neonatal period: Jitteriness and clonus; Apnea (nonconvulsive); Benign Neonatal Sleep Myoclonus (BNSM).

Infancy and preschool period: Breath holding spells; Benign paroxysmal vertigo; Benign myoclonus of infancy; Benign paroxysmal torticollis of infancy; Infantile colic; Self-stimulation behavior or masturbation; Gastroesophageal reflux.

School going children and adolescents: Night terrors; Syncope; Paroxysmal kinesigenic choreoathetosis; Migraine; Narcolepsy and Cataplexy; Tic; Pseudoseizures.

people. It is a frequent feature in chronic or progressive neurogenic muscle weakness and in metabolic disorders e.g. hyponatremia (as in diarrhea, heat stroke) and hypomagnesemia. It is due to hyperconcentration of muscle fibers. The spasm is relieved by passive stretch of the affected muscle.

7. *Dyskinesia:* The word dyskinesia is particularly used to describe phenothiazine-induced involuntary movements, which predominantly affect the pharyngeal and facial perioral musculature and levodopa induced axial torsional movements.

8. *Dystonia* is characterized by sustained concentration of opposing agonist and antagonist muscles of limb and axial musculature. Major causes of dystonia include perinatal asphyxia, kernicterus, generalized primary dystonia, drugs, Wilson disease, Hallervorden-Spatz disease, and numerous other genetic mutations. Dystonia is considered a disorder of basal ganglia. The dystonia gene is at chromosome 7q34.

9. *Myoclonus* is clinically characterized as a brief, involuntary contraction of a muscle or group of muscles producing regular, often irregular, movements at a joint (such as fingers and toes, wrists, elbows, hips) and orofacial musculature.

10. *Myokymia* is a persistent twitchy and other rhythmical movement usually affecting the periorbital muscles. It may occur as a benign phenomenon in fatigued or anxious children. It is sometimes due to lesions in the facial nerve or its nucleus or a generalized disorder.

11. *Nystagmus* is characterized by an involuntary, rhythmic repetitive to and fro movements of the eyes.

12. *Opsoclonus* consists of spontaneous, nonrhythmic, multidirectional, chaotic movements of eyes. It may be a first sign of neuroblastoma. Opsoclonus is commonly associated with encephalitis.

13. *Parkinsonism* (Parkinson syndromes) is characterized clinically by bradykinesia, tremor, rigidity and abnormal postures.

14. *Tetany:* In a case of tetany the fingers and thumbs are held stiffy adducted and the hand is partially flexed at the metacarpophalangeal joints, the toes may be similarly affected (carpopedal spasm). Elicit Trousseau's sign and Chvostek's sign.

15. *Tic* is defined as sudden, rapid, recurrent, nonrhythmic, stereotypic, motor movement or vocalization. Tics are of two types: simple and complex tics. Simple tics involve one muscle group, while complex tics involve stretching of parts of the body with paroxysm of movement such as jumping up in air. Simple vocal tics may be little meaningless noises while complex vocal tics involve explosive utterances. Simple tics last for a few milliseconds while complex tics may last for a second or more. *Tourette's disorder* will have both types of tics, motor as well as vocal. This condition also causes marked distress or significant impairment in social, occupational or important areas of functioning. Tourette's syndrome starts in early childhood with various types of tics. Simple vocal tics will give way to echolalia (involuntary repetition of the phrases of others), coprolalia (involuntary and inappropriate swearing or obscene speech) and patilalia (repetition of one's own words). They may also have echokinesis (imitation of movement of others) copropraxia (obscene motor tics), and obsessive behavior, i.e. touching genital either their own or other's.

16. *Torticollis* is a form of dystonia. Spasmodic torticollis consists of a jerky or maintained rotational and abducted posture of the neck. It is usually self modified, partially by certain postural adjustments.

17. *Tremor:* Tremor is a rhythmical involuntary oscillatory movement of a body part (small-amplitude tremors may be detectable only by sensitive recording devices).

18. *Infantile tremor syndrome* is characterized by acute or gradual onset with mental and psychomotor changes, pigmentary disturbances of hair and skin, pallor and tremors. Etiologic possibilities are malnutrition, vitamin B_{12} deficiency and viral infections.

Mathur GP, Mathur Sarla (eds). Movement Disorders in Children and Adolescents. 1st edn. New Delhi: Jaypee Brothers Medical Publishers (P) Ltd, 2003; 1–224.

Weiner WJ, Lang AE. Movement Disorders: A comprehensive survey. Mount Kisco, NY: Futura, 1989. (Lang AE. Movement Disorder Symptomatology) In: Bardley WG, Daroff RB, Fenichel GM, Marsden CD (eds). *Neurology in Clinical Practice—Principles of diagnosis and management.* 2nd edn. 1996; 1733–1772.

24.10 ENCEPHALOPATHIES

Cerebral Palsy

Cerebral Palsy (CP) is a diagnostic term used to describe a group of motor syndromes resulting from disorders of early brain development. CP is caused by a broad group of developmental, genetic, metabolic, ischemic, infections, and other acquired etiologies (Table 24.9). CP has been considered a *static encephalopathy*, but this term is not entirely accurate because neurologic features of CP cases often change or progress over time. It is the most common form of chronic motor disability that begins in childhood with a prevalence of 2/1,000. CP is also associated with a spectrum of developmental disabilities, including mental retardation, epilepsy, and visual, hearing, speech, cognitive and behavioral abnormalities. Many children and adults achieve higher educational and vocational levels.

Clinical manifestations: CP is divided into four major motor syndromes that differ according to the pattern of neurologic involvement, neuropathology and etiology (Table 24.9).

1. **Spastic hemiplegia.** Infants with spastic hemiplegia have decreased spontaneous movements on the affected side and show hand preference at a very early age. The arm is involved more than the leg; growth arrest, particularly in the hand and thumb nail, especially if the contralateral parietal lobe is abnormal, because extremity growth is influenced by this area of the brain. The difficulty in hand manipulation is obvious by 1 yr of age. Walking is usually delayed until 18–24 months, and a circumductive gait is apparent. Spasticity is apparent in the affected extremities, particularly the ankle, causing an equinovarus deformity of the foot. The affected child often walks on tiptoe because of the increased tone, and the affected upper extremity assumes a dystonic posture when the child runs. Ankle clonus, Babinski sign, increased deep tendon reflexes and weakness of the hand and the foot dorsiflexors are present on physical examination. About one-third patients have seizure disorder that usually in the first year or 2; 25% have mental retardation. A CT scan or MRI study may show an atrophic cerebral hemisphere with a dilated lateral ventricle contralateral to the side of the affected extremities.

2. **Spastic diplegia.** There is bilateral spasticity of legs, which is greater than in the arms. The first indication of spastic diplegia is often noted when the affected infant begins to crawl. The child uses the arms in a normal reciprocal fashion but tends to drag the legs behind more as a rudder (commando crawl) rather than using the normal four-limb crawling movement. If the spasticity is severe, application of a diaper is difficult, because of the excessive adduction of the hips. If there is paraspinal muscle involvement, the child may be unable to sit. Examination of the child reveals spasticity in the legs with exaggerated deep tendon reflexes, ankle clonus and a bilateral Babinski sign. When the child is suspended by the axillae, a scissoring posture of the lower extremities is maintained. Walking is significantly delayed, the feet are held in a position of equinovarus, and the child walks on tiptoe. Severe spastic diplegia is characterized by disuse atrophy and impaired growth of the lower extremities and by disproportionate growth with normal development of the upper torso. Intellectual development is normal. Seizures are rare. The most common neuropathologic finding is periventricular leukomalacia, particularly in the area where fibers innervating the legs course through the internal capsule. MRI is done to evaluate the severity of white matter injury and for excluding other brain lesions (*see* Fig. 24.13 in CD).

3. **Spastic quadriplegia** is the most severe form of CP because of marked motor impairment of all extremities and the high association with mental retardation (MR) and seizures. Swallowing difficulties are common owing to supranuclear bulbar palsies often leading to aspiration pneumonia. The most common lesions seen on pathologic examination or on MRI scanning are severe PVL and multicystic cortical encephalomalacia. Neurologic examination reveals increased tone and spasticity in all the four limbs, decreased spontaneous movements, brisk reflexes and plantar extensor responses. Flexion contractures of the knees and elbows are often present by late childhood. Associated developmental disabilities, including speech and visual abnormalities are common. Children with spastic quadriplegia often have athetosis and may be classified as having mixed CP.

Table 24.9: Classification of cerebral palsy		
Motor syndrome	*Neuropathology*	*Major causes*
1. **Spastic hemiplegia**	Stroke: In utero or neonatal	Thrombophilic disorders; Infection; Genetic/developmental; Periventricular hemorrhage, infarction
2. **Spastic diplegia**	Periventricula leukomalacia [PVL]	Prematurity; Ischemia; Infection; Endocrine/Metabolic (e.g. thyroid)
3. **Spastic quadriplegia**	PVL; Multicystic encephalomalacia malformations	Ischemia; Infection; Endocrine/metabolic genetic/developmental
4. **Extrapyramidal: (athetoid, dyskinetic)**	Pathology: putamen, globus pallidus, thalamus, basal ganglia	Asphyxia; Kernicterus; Mitochondrial genetic/metabolic

4. **Athetoid CP,** also called **choreoathetoid** or **extrapyramidal** CP, is less common than spastic cerebral palsy. Affected infants are hypotonic with poor head control and marked head lag and develop increased variable tone with rigidity and dystonia over several years. There is difficulty in feeding. Tongue thrust and drooling of saliva may be prominent. Athetoid movements appear at approximately 1 yr of age. Generally upper motor neuron signs are not present, seizures are uncommon and intellect is preserved in many patients. Speech is affected because the oropharyngeal muscles are involved. Speech may be absent or sentences are slurred. Extrapyramidal CP secondary to acute intrapartum near-total asphyxia is associated with bilaterally symmetric lesions in the posterior putamen and ventrolateral thalamus. These lesions appear to be the correlate of the neuropathologic lesion called status marmoratus in the basal ganglia. MRI scan shows lesions in the globus pallidus bilaterally when extrapyramidal CP is caused by kernicterus.

Diagnosis: A thorough history and physical examination should include a progressive disorder of the CNS, including degenerative diseases, metabolic disorders, spinal cord tumor or muscular dystrophy. The possibility of anomalies at the base of the skull or other disorders affecting the cervical spinal cord should be considered in patients with a little involvement of the arms or cranial nerves. An MRI scan of the brain is indicated to determine the location and extent of structural lesions or associated congenital malformations; an MRI scan of the spinal cord is indicated if there is any possibility of spinal cord pathology. Additional studies may include EEG to evaluate seizures and tests of hearing and visual function. Genetic evaluation should be considered in patients with congenital malformations (chromosomes) or evidence of metabolic disorders. A multidisciplinary approach is most helpful in the assessment and treatment of CP children.

Treatment: There is no "cure" for CP. But a lot can be done to help people with CP to make them self-reliant. Early detection of CP cases is vital. It can often reduce developmental handicaps to a minimum. It leads to early treatment and better adjustment in life. A team consisting of physicians of various specialties, occupational and physical therapists, speech pathologists, social workers, educators and developmental psychologists will be required to manage cases of CP. Strabismus, nystagmus, and optic atrophy is common in children with CP; an ophthalmologist should be included in the initial assessment.

Parents are told: (i) Handling of daily activities such as, feeding, toileting, carrying, dressing, bathing, and playing. (ii) Exercises to prevent the development of contractures especially a tight Achilles tendon. Parents (both mother and father of the child) must strive hard to become personal physiotherapists of the child, which should be supervised by the professional physiotherapist from time to time.

Surgical interventions include operative procedure for spasticity and athetosis, orthopedic operative procedures, and surgery in GERD cases (usually fundoplication). Role of drugs is limited. Drugs used to treat spasticity include benzodiazepines, baclofen, dantrolene sodium, botulinum toxin. Patients with rigidity, dystonia and spastic quadriparesis sometimes respond to carbamazepine, trihexyphenidyl, and levodopa. Antiepileptic drugs, such as carbamazepine, phenobarbital, phenytoin, valproic acid or ethosuximide may be given singly or in combination to prevent seizures. Botulinum toxin injected into specific muscle groups for the management of spasticity shows a very positive response in many patients. Botulinum toxin injected into salivary glands may also help reduce the severity of drooling in patients with CP who has been traditionally treated with anticholinergic agents.

Parental counseling: Parental involvement right from the beginning is important in implementing the program. First of all the condition of the child should be explained to parents in a simple and honest way, with emphasis on the positive aspects of the child. Explain the need for long term treatment and instill positive attitudes and help to remove the feeling of guilt. Questions regarding the probable outcome in future are frequently raised by the parents. As the cause of the disability is clearly an accidental one in most of the cases, it will be easy to reassure them. Parents should be encouraged to send the child to special schools for children with CP for training and rehabilitation. Children with mild CP can be sent to normal school.

Outcome: Majority of the patients with CP lives to adulthood. Life expectancy of severely affected individuals is significantly less than that of the general population. Prognosis is worst with spastic quadriplegia. Prognosis is also modified by the presence of associated defects, socioeconomic status of the family and availability of rehabilitative services.

Reye Syndrome

Reye syndrome: RS is primarily a children's disease, although it can occur at any age.
Reye syndrome is a potentially fatal disease that causes numerous detrimental effects to many organs, especially the brain and liver, as well as causing

hypoglycemia. The disease causes fatty liver with minimal inflammation and severe encephalopathy (with swelling of the brain). The liver may become slightly enlarged and firm, and there is a change in the appearance of the kidneys. Jaundice is not usually present.

Etiology: The exact cause is unknown, and while it has been associated with aspirin consumption by children with viral illness; it also occurs in the absence of aspirin use. RS is a two-phase illness because it generally occurs in conjunction with a previous viral infection, such as the flu or chickenpox. The disorder commonly occurs during recovery from a viral infection, although it can also develop 3 to 5 days after the onset of the viral illness. Acquired abnormalities of mitochondrial function can be caused by several drugs and toxins, including valproic acid, cyanide, amiodarone, chloramphenicol, iron, actinomycin A, and the enteric toxin of Bacillus cereus.

Clinical manifestations: Reye syndrome progresses through five stages as mentioned in Table 24.10. Other symptoms that can occur with this disorder include double vision, hearing loss, muscle function loss or paralysis of the arms or legs, speech difficulties, weakness in the arms or legs, decerebrate posture.

Differential diagnosis: Causes for similar symptoms include various inborn metabolic disorders, viral encephalitis, drug overdose or poisoning, head trauma, hepatic failure due to other causes, meningitis, renal failure.

Investigations and diagnosis: The tests may be used to diagnose Reye syndrome includes blood chemistry tests, head CT or head MRI scan, liver function tests, serum ammonia test, spinal tap, liver biopsy. There is elevated SGOT, SGPT, and ammonia. Patients remain anicteric and serum bilirubin levels are normal. Liver biopsies show microvesicular steatosis without evidence of liver inflammation or necrosis.

Treatment: There is no cure for RS. Successful management, which depends on early diagnosis, is primarily aimed at protecting the brain against irreversible damage by reducing brain swelling, reversing the metabolic injury, preventing complications in the lungs, and anticipating cardiac arrest. During management of the child monitor the pressure in the brain, blood gases, and blood acid-base balance (pH). Treatment may include breathing support (a breathing machine may be needed during a deep coma), fluids by IV to provide electrolytes and glucose, and steroids to reduce swelling in the brain. Some evidence suggests that treatment in the end stages of RS with hypertonic IV glucose solutions may prevent progression of the syndrome.

Prevention: Never give a child aspirin unless told to do so by your doctor. When a child must take aspirin, take care to reduce the child's risk of catching a viral illness such as the flu and chickenpox. Avoid aspirin for several weeks after the child has received a varicella (chickenpox) vaccine.

Prognosis: Some people recover completely, while others may sustain varying degrees of brain damage. The complications include coma, permanent brain damage, and seizures. When RS is diagnosed and treated in its early stages, chances of recovery are excellent.

Johnston MV. Encephalopathies. In: Kliegman RM, Behrman RE, Jenson HB, Stanton BF (eds). *Nelson Textbook of Pediatrics*. 18th edn. Vol. 2. Philadelphia: Saunders, 2007; 2494–2499.

Johnston MV, Ingrid Tein. Mitochondrial Encephalopathies. In: Kliegman RM, Behrman RE, Jenson HB, Stanton BF (eds). *Nelson Textbook of Pediatrics*. 18th edn. Vol. 2. Philadelphia: Saunders, 2007; 2496–2499.

Little WJ. On the influence of abnormal parturition, difficult labor, premature birth and asphyxia neonatorum on the mental and physical condition of the child, especially in relation to deformities. Tr Obst Soc London 1861; 3: 293–302.

Table 24.10: Reye syndrome progresses through five stages	
Stages	*Clinical features*
Stage I	Persistent, heavy vomiting that is not relieved by eating; generalized lethargy; general mental symptoms, e.g. confusion; nightmares
Stage II	Stupor caused by minor brain inflammation; hyperventilation; fatty liver (found by biopsy); hyperactive reflexes
Stage III	Continuation of stages I and II symptoms; possible coma; possible cerebral edema; parely, respiratory arrest
Stage IV	Deepening coma; large pupils with minimal response to light; minimal but still present hepatic dysfunction
Stage V	Very rapid onset following stage IV; deep coma; seizures; multiple organ failure; flaccidity; extremely high blood ammonia (above 300 mg/dl of blood); death

24.11 APPROACH TO NEURODEGENERATIVE DISEASES IN CHILDHOOD

Neurodegenerative diseases or degenerative brain diseases (DBD) are disorders in which there is progressive deterioration with loss of abilities (intellectual, motor, sensory abilities) after a period of normal development. There may be involvement of other systems in addition to the central nervous system. There may be a delay in attainment of developmental milestones and the disease can manifest at any age. Most DBD's are inherited disorders, majority being autosomal recessive. These are gray and white matter diseases, but the distinction becomes obscure in late stages.

Gray Matter Diseases

Gaucher's disease (*see* Chapter 26); Niemann-Pick disease (*see* Chapter 26);

Tay-Sachs disease (TSD) (*see* Chapter 26); Sandhoff's disease (*see* Chapter 26);

GM1 gangliosidosis (*see* Chapter 26); Sialidosis and Galactosialidosis (*see* Chapter 26); Zellweger syndrome (*see* Chapter 26); Neonatal adrenoleukodystrophy and infantile refsum disease (*see* Chapter 26); Neuronal ceroid lipofuscinoses (NCL; *see* Chapter 24).

White Matter Degenerative Brain Diseases

Metachromatic Leukodystrophy (MLD) (*see* Chapter 26); X-linked adrenoleukodystrophy (*see* Chapter 26); Krabbe's disease (*see* Chapter 26).

Sjögren-Larsson syndrome: It includes a clinical triad of congenital ichthyosis, mental retardation, spastic diplegia or tetraplegia. There is deficient activity of fatty aldehyde dehydrogenase. The onset is usually before 1 year of age. Fundus examination reveals glistening dots in the fovea. MRI demonstrates periventricular white matter involvement with sparing of subcortical U fibers. Prenatal diagnosis can be performed by enzymatic detection of FALDH (Fatty aldehyde dehydrogenase) activity in 19 weeks gestation fetal skin biopsies and amniocentesis.

Pelizaeus-Merzbacher disease (PMD): It is an X-linked hypomyelinating leukoencephalopathy caused by deficiency of proteolipid protein (PLP). It has a broad clinical continuum ranging from connatal PMD, classic PMD, complicated SPG (spastic paraplegia) -2 to Pure SPG-2. Connatal PMD presents shortly after birth. They have severe hypotonia, extrapyramidal signs, stridor and feeding difficulties. Death occurs within a few months to years. Classic type begins in first months of infancy with abnormal eye movement rapid, irregular, small or large amplitude oscillations either vertical or horizontal. There is slow develop-

ment of spasticity, ataxia and involuntary movements. Later-optic atrophy and seizures are observed. Mental abilities usually much better preserved. X-linked form of spastic paraplegia occurs either as a pure form, consisting of a slowly progressive paraplegia involving only lower limbs. It may be complicated SPG-2 which has spastic paraplegia with other features of PMD like nystagmus, dysarthria and ataxia (*see* Fig. 24.18 in CD).

Alexander's disease: It is classified into 3 forms-infantile, juvenile and adult. All 3 forms have mutations in GFAP. *Infantile form is the* most common form with onset at birth or during first 2 years of life. Salient clinical features include megalencephaly, psychomotor retardation, often seizures and progressive downhill course. Sometimes features of raised ICT (intracranial tension), or hydrocephalus are seen. Juvenile form has onset from 4 yr to mid teen. Often there is no megalencephaly but bulbar and pseudobulbar signs of swallowing and/or speech difficulty are observed. Other features include spasticity and ataxia, kyphoscoliosis and slow decline in mental function. *Adult-onset form* has variable clinical features. It can resemble multiple sclerosis. The clinical features predominantly include ataxia, tetraparesis, palatal myoclonus and other brainstem signs.

Canavan's disease (*see* Section 26.2).

Freeman JM, Mc Khann GM. Degenerative disease of central nervous system. *Adv Pediatr* 1969; 16: 121 – 175.

Kabra M. Prenatal diagnosis. *Indian J. of Pediatr* 2003; 70: 81–86.

Schapira AHV. Mitochondrial disease. *Lancet* 2006; 368: 70–82.

Krivit W, Aubourg P, Shapiro E, Peters C. Bone marrow transplantation for globoid cell leukodystrophy, adrenoleuko-dystrophy, metachromatic leukodystrophy and Hurler syndrome. *Curr Opin Hematol* 1999; 6(6): 377–382.

Pastores GM, Kolodny EH. Lysosomal storage diseases In: Swaiman KF, Ashwal S, Ferriero DM (eds). *Pediatric Neurology-Principles and practice.* Vol I, 4th edn, Philadelphia: Mosby Elsevier, 2006; 659–714.

Rocco MD, Biancheri R, Rossi A, et al, Genetic disorders affecting white matter in the pediatric age. *Am J Med Genetics* 2004; 129B: 85–93.

24.12 BRAIN TUMORS IN CHILDHOOD

Primary CNS tumors are the second most frequent malignancy in childhood and adolescence. The etiology of pediatric brain tumors is not well defined. Familial and hereditary syndromes and cranial exposure to ionizing radiation are associated with a higher incidence of brain tumors. The incidence of CNS tumors is higher in infants and young children ≤ 7yr of age compared with older children and adolescents.

Clinical manifestations: Infants with open cranial sutures may present with signs of increased intracranial pressure (vomiting, lethargy and irritability), as well as the later finding of macrocephaly. The classic triad of headache, nausea, and vomiting and papilledema is associated with midline or infratentorial tumors. Disorders of equilibrium, gait, and coordination occur with infratentorial tumors. Blurred vision, diplopia, and nystagmus are also associated with infratentorial tumors. The signs and symptoms of meningeal metastatic disease from brain tumors or leukemia are similar to those of infratentorial tumors. Torticollis may be due to cerebellar tonsil herniation. Tumors of the brainstem region may be associated with gaze palsy, multiple cranial nerve palsies, and upper motor neurone deficits (e.g. hemiparesis, hyperreflexia, clonus).

Supratentorial tumors are more commonly associated with focal disorders such as motor weakness, sensory changes, speech disorders, seizures, and reflex abnormalities. Infants with supratentoreal tumors may present with hand preference. Optic pathway tumors manifest as visual disturbances such as decreased visual activity, Marcus Gunn pupil (afferent papillary defect), nystagmus, and/or visual field defects. Suprasellar region tumors and third ventricular region tumors may manifest initially as neuroendocrine deficits (diabetes insipidus, galactorrhea, precocious puberty, delayed puberty, and hypothyroidism). The diencephalic syndrome is manifested as failure to thrive, emaciation, increased appetite, and euphoric affect, and occurs in infants and young children with tumors in these regions. Parinaud syndrome is seen with pineal region tumors manifests by paresis of upward gaze, pupillary dilation reactive to accommodation but not to light, nystagmus to convergence or retraction, and eyelid retraction. Spinal cord tumors and spinal cord dissemination of brain tumors may manifest as long nerve tract motor and/or sensory deficits, bowel and bladder deficits, and back or radicular pain.

Diagnosis: Suspected brain tumor patient should be treated as an emergency case. The initial evaluation should include a history, physical (including ophthalmic) examination, and neurologic assessment with nuroimaging. For primary brain tumors, MRI is the neuroimaging standard investigation. Patients with tumors of the midline and pituitary/suprasellar/optic chiasmal region should be evaluated for neuroendocrine dysfunction. Both serum and CSF measurements of β-human chorionic gonadotropin and α-fetoprotein are helpful in the diagnosis of germ cell tumors. In tumors with a propensity for spreading to the meninges, such as medulloblastoma/PNET, ependymoma, and germ cell tumors, lumbar puncture with cytologic analysis of CSF is indicated.

Specific Tumors

1. **Astrocytomas** are a heterogeneous group of CNS tumors **(low-grade astrocytomas, malignant astrocytomas, oligodendrogliomas),** which occur throughout the CNS and account for approximately 40% of cases.

2. **Ependymal tumors** are the most common of these neoplasms accounting for 10% of childhood tumors. Approximately 70% occur in the posterior fossa. The mean age of patient is 6 yr.

3. **Choroid plexus tumors** account for 2–4% of childhood CNS tumors. They are the most common CNS tumor in children <1 yr of age.

4. **Embryonal tumors** or primitive neuroectodermal tumors (PNETs) are the most common group of malignant CNS tumors of childhood, accounting for 20–25% of pediatric CNS tumors..
   a. **Medulloblastoma,** which accounts for 90% of embryonal tumors, is a cerebellar tumor occurring predominantly in males at a median age of 5–7 yr.
   b. **Supratentorial primitive neuroectodermal tumors (SPNETs)** account for 2–3% of childhood tumors, primarily in children within a first decade of life. These tumors are similar histologically to medulloblastoma. SPNETs have had poorer outcomes than those with medulloblastoma after combined-modality therapy. Children with SPNETs are considered among the high-risk group and receive dose-intense chemotherapy with craniospinal radiotherapy.
   c. **Atypical teratoid/rhabdoid tumor** is a very aggressive embryonal malignancy that occurs predominantly in children <5 yr of age and can occur at any location in the neuraxis.

5. **Pineal parenchymal tumors** are the most common malignancies after germ cell tumors that occur in the pineal region.

6. **Craniopharyngioma** (WHO grade I) is a common tumor of childhood, accounting for 7–10% of all childhood tumors. The adamantinomatous variant of craniopharyngioma predominates in childhood. Children with craniopharyngioma often present with endocrinologic abnormalities such as growth failure and delayed sexual maturation and visual changes such as decrease acuity or visual field deficits. These tumors are often quite large and heterogenous, both solid and cystic components, and occur within the

suprasellar region. MRI demonstrates the solid tumor with cystic structures containing fluid of intermediate density. CT may show calcifications associated with the solid and cystic wall components. Surgery is the primary treatment modality, with gross total resection curative in small lesions. There is no role for chemotherapy. Controversy exists regarding the relative roles of surgery and radiation therapy in large, complex tumors. Significant morbidity (panhypopituitarism, growth failure, visual loss) is associated with these tumors and their therapy, owing to anatomic location.

7. **Meningeal tumors** arise from the arachnoid layer of the meninges and usually are very slow-growing.
8. **Germ cell tumors** of the CNS are a heterogeneous group of tumors, which arise predominantly in midline structures of the pineal and suprasellar regions. They account for 1–2% of pediatric brain tumors.
9. **Tumors of the brainstem** are a heterogeneous group of tumors that account for 10–15% of childhood primary CNS tumors. Patients with these tumors may present with motor weakness, cranial nerve deficits, cerebellar deficits, and/or signs of increased ICP.
10. **Metastatic tumors.** Metastatic spread of other childhood malignancies to the brain also occurs. Acute lymphoblastic leukemia and non-Hodgkin lymphoma can spread to the leptomeninges, causing symptoms of communicating hydrocephalus. Chloromas, which are collections of myeloid leukemic cells, can occur throughout the neuraxis. Rarely, brain parenchymal metastases occur from lymphoma, neuroblastoma, rhabdomyosarcoma, Ewing sarcoma, osteosarcoma, and clear cell sarcoma of the kidney. Treatment is based on the specific histologic diagnosis and may incorporate radiation therapy, intrathecal administration of chemotherapy, and/or systemic administration of chemotherapy.

Complications and Long-term Management

Data from the National Cancer Institute Surveillance, Epidemiology and End Results (SEER) Program indicate that >70% of patients with childhood brain tumors will be long-term survivors. At least 50% of these survivors will experience chronic problems as a direct result of their tumors and treatment. These problems include chronic neurologic deficits such as focal motor and sensory abnormalities, seizure disorders, neurocognitive deficits (e.g. hypothyroidism, growth failure, delay or absence of puberty). These patients are also at a significant risk for secondary malignancies. Supportive multidisciplinary interventions for children with brain tumors both during and after therapy may improve their ultimate outcome. Physical therapy, seizure and endocrine management with timely growth hormone and thyroid replacement therapy, educational and vocational programs may enhance the quality of life in children with brain tumor.

Epstein FJ, Farmer JP. Brain-stem glioma growth patterns. *J Neurosurg* 1993; 78: 408–412.

Garg Ajay, Suri Ashish, Gulati Sheffali. CNS Tumors. In: Mathur GP, Mathur Sarla (eds). *Current Trends in Pediatrics.* Vol 2. Delhi: Academa Publishers, 2006; 382–403.

Kuttesch JF Jr, Ater JL.Brain tumors in childhood. In: Kliegman RM, Behrman RE, Jenson HB, Stanton BF (eds). *Nelson Textbook of Pediatrics.* 18th edn. Vol. 2. Philadelphia: Saunders, 2007; 2128–2137.

Kuttesch JF Jr, Rush SZ, Ater JL. Brain tumors in childhood. In: Kliegman RM, Stanton BF, St.Geme JW, Schor NF, Behrman RE. *Nelson Textbook of Pediatrics.* 19th edn. New Delhi: Elsevier, 2011; 11746–1753.

24.13 PSEUDOTUMOR CEREBRI

Pseudotumor cerebri is a clinical syndrome, characterized by increased intracranial pressure (ICP) (> 200 mmH$_2$O in infants and 250 mmH$_2$O in children), normal CSF cell count and protein content and normal ventricular size, anatomy, and position documented by MRI, and that mimics brain tumors. The causes are (a) **Idiopathic:** intracranial hypertension; (b) **Secondary causes include:** 1.*Metabolic causes:* Galactosemia, hypoparathyroidism, pseudohypoparathyroidism, hypophosphatasia, prolonged corticosteroid therapy, too rapid corticosteroid withdrawal, growth hormone treatment, refeeding of a significantly malnourished child, hypervitaminosis A, vitamin A deficiency, Addison disease, obesity, menarche, oral contraceptives, pregnancy; 2. *Infections:* Roseola infantum, Sinusitis, Chronic otitis media and Mastoiditis, Guillain-Barré syndrome; 3. *Drugs:* Nalidixic acid, doxycycline, minocycline, tetracycline, nitrofurantoin; 4. *Acne therapy:* Isotretinoin especially when combined with tetracycline; 5. *Hematologic disorders:* Polycythemia, hemolytic anemia, Iron-deficiency anemia, Wiskott-Aldrich syndrome; 6. *Obstruction of intracranial drainage by venous thrombosis:* Lateral sinus thrombosis, Posterior sagittal sinus thrombosis; 7. *Head injury;* 8. *Obstruction of the superior vena cava.*

Clinical manifestations: The most frequent symptom is headache, although vomiting; transient visual disturbances and diplopia (secondary to paralysis of the abducens nerve) are also common complaints. Examination of infant reveals a bulging fontanel and a "cracked pot sound" or Macewen sign (percussion of the skull produces a resonant sound) due to separation of the cranial sutures. Papilledema is found on ophthalmoscopy.

Treatment: First find out the underlying cause. The obese patient should be treated with a weight loss regimen, and if a drug is thought to be responsible, it should be discontinued. The initial lumbar tap that follows a CT or MRI scan is diagnostic and may be therapeutic. The spinal needle produces a small rent in the dura that allows CSF to escape the subarachnoid space, thus reducing the intracranial pressure (ICP). Several lumbar taps may be required for removal of sufficient CSF to reduce pressure by 50%, occasionally lead to resolution of process. Acetazolamide, 10–30 mg/kg/24 hr, and corticosteroids have been effective in some patients. Anticoagulation is required to treat sinus thrombosis. Rarely, a lumboperitoneal shunt or subtemporal decompression is necessary to prevent optic nerve atrophy and optic nerve sheath fenestration to prevent further visual loss.

Digre KB. Not so benign intracranial hypertension. *Br Med J* 2003; 326: 613–614.

Haslam RHA. Pseudotumor cerebri. In: Kliegman RM, Behrman RE, Jenson HB, Stanton BF (eds). *Nelson Textbook of Pediatrics.* 18th edn. Vol. 2. Philadelphia: Saunders, 2007; 2525–2526.

24.14 SPINAL CORD DISORDERS

Cutaneous markers of occult spinal dysraphism: Occult spinal dysraphism (OSD) refers to congenital abnormalities that result from incomplete fusion of the soft tissue, bone or neural components of the spine that occur during primary and secondary neurulation. The skin lesions include lipomas, dermal sinuses, tails, patches of hair, deviation of the gluteal fold, hemangiomas, and port-wine stains. Every child with a midline lumbosacral birth-mark should have a complete neurologic examination. Mongolian spots and simple dimples within the gluteal folds are not associated with OSD. Two or more midline skin lesions are associated with the greatest incidence of OSD. MRI of the spine should be done.

Tethered cord: A tethered cord results when a thickened ropelike filum terminale persists and anchors the conus at or below the L2 level. Midline skin lesion such as a lipoma, tuft of hair, a caudal appendage, dermal sinus, a portwine stain or hyperpigmentation of the skin are found in ≈ 70% of cases. Infants may have asymmetric growth in a foot or leg associated with talipes cavus deformities and muscle wasting due to prolonged denervation. Surgical transection of the thickened filum terminale

will halt the progression of neurologic signs and prevents the development of dysfunction in asymptomatic patients.

Diastematomyelia: Diastematomyelia is division of the spinal cord into two halves by projection of a fibrocartilaginous or bony septum originating from the posterior vertebral body and extending posteriorly. The defect involves the lumber vertebrae (L1–L3) in ≈50% of cases. Patients may remain asymptomatic, but mostly patients have unilateral foot abnormalities, including talipes equinovarus, claw toes, atrophy of the gastrocnemius, and loss of pain and temperature sensation in a preschool child. A midline abnormality of the skin in the lumbosacral region provides a clue to the possibility of underlying abnormality. Excision of the bony spur or septum and lysis of the adjacent adhesions is the treatment of symptomatic patients.

Syringomyelia: Syringomyelia is a cystic cavity within the spinal cord that may communicate with the cerebrospinal fluid (CSF) pathways or remain localized and noncommunicating. Syrinobulbia exists when the cystic cavity extends into the medulla. Interruption of the anterior white commissure at the level of the cervical cord disrupts the lateral spinothalamic tracts, causing an asymmetric loss of pain and temperature sensation in the upper extremities, with preservation of light touch (dissociation of sensation). Progressive enlargement of the cavity impinges on the anterior horn cells and corticospinal tracts, resulting in muscle wasting of the hands, absent deep tendon reflexes in the upper extremities and upper motor neuron signs in the lower extremities. Scoliosis may be the initial manifestation of syringomyelia. Trophic ulcers associated with vasomotor disturbances of the hands and arms indicate the loss of appreciation of pain. T1 weighed MRI scan of the upper spinal cord shows the cystic cavity within the spinal cord. Treatment is surgical and depends on the site and cause of the syringo-myelia. Asymptomatic patients should be followed conservatively.

Spinal cord tumors: In children, spinal cod tumors account for ≈20% of neuraxial tumors and are classified according to anatomical position into intramedullary or extramedullary tumors. Intramedullary tumors include astrocytoma, ganglioglioma and ependymoma. Extramedullary intradural tumors tend to be benign include neurofibroma, ganglioneuroma, and meningioma. Extramedullary extradural tumours are metastatic lesions, particularly neuroblastoma, sarcoma, and lymphoma. Most children with spinal cord tumors present with a combination of gait disturbance, scoliosis, and back pain depending on tumor location. Tumors in the cervical cord produce lower motor neuron signs in the upper extremities and upper motor neuron signs in the legs. Denervation of the intercostal muscles decreases chest wall movement and also a weak cough. Extramedullary extradural tumors tend to cause an acute block of the CSF pathology and present with a flaccid paralysis, urinary retention, and a patulous anus. Some extramedullary tumors produce the *Brown-Séquard syndrome*, which consists of ipsilateral weakness, spasticity, and ataxia, with contralateral loss of pain and temperature sensation. Many tumors can be totally and safely surgically resected. Adjuvant therapy with radiation and/or chemotherapy depends primarily on the tumor type.

Spinal cord trauma: The degree of injury to the spinal cord is variable and includes concussion, contusion, laceration, and transection. The common causes of spinal cord injury in the child younger than 10 yr include birth injury, physical abuse, automobile and diving injuries, violence (gun-shot wounds, stabbing), falls from playground equipment. In older children most common injuries include automobile and sports related injuries. Approximately 20% of spinal cord injuries in children occur in the absence of a radiologic abnormality. SCIWORA (spinal cord injury without radiographic appearance) is most commonly found in children and may be associated with a severe injury to the cord.

Clinical manifestations: A patient with *severe cord injury* presents with *spinal shock*, consisting of flaccidity, areflexia, loss of sensation and often bradycardia and hypotension. Spinal shock may persist for up to 4 wk and results from dysfunction of synaptic activity in the pathways caudal to the injury. Ultimately, reflex flexor movements develop, followed by extensor reflex activity associated with hyperactive deep tendon reflexes, spasticity, and an automatic bladder. The *mildest injury*, which follows a concussion of the spinal cord, is transient quadriparesis evident for seconds or minutes with complete recovery in 24 hr. A *transverse injury in the high cervical cord level* (C1–C2) causes respiratory arrest and death in the absence of ventilatory support. Fracture dislocations at the C5–C6 level resulting in spinal cord injuries with flaccid quadriparesis, loss of sphincter function, and a sensory level corresponding to the upper sternum. *Fractures or dislocation in the lower thoracic* (T12–L1) region may produce the *conus medullary syndrome*, which includes a loss of urinary and rectal sphincter control, flaccid weakness, and sensory disturbances of the legs. A central cord lesion may result from contusion and hemorrhage and typically involves the

upper extremities to a greater degree than the legs. There are lower motor neuron signs in the upper extremities and upper motor neuron signs in the legs, bladder dysfunction, and loss of sensation caudal to the lesion. There may be considerable recovery, particularly in the lower extremities.

Spinal cord injuries should be *treated* by stabilization and complete immobilization of the spine at the accident site using a correctly fitting cervical collar or blocks and tape. The patient must be transported on a board designed for children so that the neck is not placed in flexed position. An adequate airway should be maintained, respiratory support provided, and shock should be treated with appropriate volume expanders and vasopressor agents if needed. A high-dose steroid should be administered for 24 hr if initiated within 3 hr of the injury and continuation of steroid therapy for 48 hr if started 3–8 hr after the spine injury. The initial dose of intravenous methylprednisolone (30 mg/kg bolus) should be started immediately even before transport, followed by 5.4 mg/kg/hr. After transport, lateral and anteroposterior roentgenograms of the spine should be obtained. CT and MRI are used if the diagnosis is uncertain. After appropriate imaging studies, surgical treatment is directed to stabilization of the vertebrae to prevent additional injury to the cord and decompression of the spinal cord if compromised by a fracture or hemorrhage. Fracture dislocations are treated with traction, immobilization, and, if the injury is unstable, vertebral fusion. Additional therapeutic measures include management of bladder and gastrointestinal disturbances, nutritional and skin care, and a multidisciplinary program. *Prevention* of spinal cord injury by the use of contemporary playground equipment, age appropriate seatbelts, and the implementation of strictly enforced age-related rules in contact sports such as hockey (body checking) and football are the most important aspect of management of spinal cord trauma.

Transverse myelitis: Transverse myelitis is characterized by abrupt onset of progressive weakness and sensory disturbances in the lower extremities. Low back or abdominal pain and paraesthesias of the legs are the symptoms present in the early stages. Leg muscles are weak and flaccid, and a sensory level is present, usually in the midthoracic region. Pain, temperature, and light touch sensation are affected, but joint position and vibration sense may be preserved. Sphincter disturbances are common, in which case catheterization of the bladder is necessary. Fever and nuchal rigidity are present early in most cases. The neurologic deficit evolves for 2–3 days, and flaccidity gradually changing to spasticity and upper motor neuron signs develops in the lower extremities. A history of a preceding viral infection (Epstein-Barr, herpes, influenza, rubella, mumps, and varicella) accompanied by fever and malaise is documented in most cases. Additional infectious agents include *Mycoplasma pneumonia* and *Borrelia burgdorferi* (Lyme disease) have been implicated. Pathologic examination of the spinal cord shows marked softening and perivascular cuffing by lymphocytes, supporting an immunologic basis for the disorder. Examination of the CSF shows moderate lymphocytic pleocytosis and a normal or slightly elevated protein level. MRI abnormalities of transverse myelitis include T2 hyperintense and T1-iso-or mildly hypointense fusiform swelling extending over at least 3–4 vertebral levels, usually located in the thoracolumbar region.

Differential diagnosis includes meningitis, Guillain-Barré syndrome, poliomyelitis, neuromyelitis optica (Devic disease), spinal cord neoplasm, epidural abscess, demyelinating disorders and a vascular malformation. *Treatment:* Spontaneous recovery occurs over a period of weeks or months and is complete in ≈40–50% of cases. High-dose methyl-prednisolone therapy early in the course is effective in shortening the duration of the disease and in improving the outcome. Residual deficits include bowel and bladder dysfunction and weakness of lower extremities.

Arteriovenous malformation: Arteriovenous malformation of the spinal cord consists of a collection of tortuous dilated veins that are usually located on the dorsal aspect of the thoracic cord. The malformation may cause neurologic symptoms by its mass effect on the cord or by the "steal" phenomenon, by which blood is shunted through the abnormal veins, bypassing the spinal cord, which produces transient and, in some cases, progressive loss of neurologic function. Patients occasionally present with acute paraparesis and a sensory deficit due to a subarachnoid bleed from the malformation. Gradual onset of gait abnormalities, low back pain and bladder and bowel dysfunction are noted. The deep tendon reflexes are absent or reduced in the lower extremities, and the Babinski reflex is present. A midline cutaneous angioma overlies the arteriovenous malformation, and a spinal bruit may occasionally be auscultated. The malformation is removed by surgical excision with the use of an operating microscope or is obliterated by embolization.

Haslam RHA. Spinal cord disorders. In: Kliegman RM, Behrman RE, Jenson HB, Stanton BF (eds). *Nelson Textbook of Pediatrics*. 18th edn. Vol. 2. Philadelphia: Saunders, 2007; 2526–2530.

Jallo GI, Freed D, Epstein F. Intramedullary spinal cord tumors in children. *Childs Nerv Syst* 2003; 19: 641–649.

McDonald JW, Sadowsky C. Spinal-cord injury. *Lancet* 2002; 359: 417–425.

25 Neuromuscular Disorders

25.1 APPROACH TO A FLOPPY CHILD

The floppy child is an infant with generalized hypotonia-poor muscle tone affecting the limbs and trunk with or without the involvement of facial musculature. The condition is identified by the infant's inability to maintain normal posture and lack of movements.

One may come across the syndrome of floppy child in the premature newborn, in the full term neonate, or in an older infant. Muscle tone develops in an orderly sequence through gestation and continues to change after birth. Hypotonia is frequently found in infants, and pathological degrees must be differentiated from normal variations. A variety of pathological conditions can influence muscle tone, and hypotonia can be an early and valuable clue to recognizing neuromuscular, CNS, metabolic, and other disease states in this age group. The neurological examination aids in localizing the site of the lesion to the central (upper motor neuron) or peripheral motor unit (LMN). The various etiologies of floppy child can be grouped under the headings of central hypotonia, peripheral hypotonia, and combined central and peripheral hypotonia (Table 25.1).

Approach to Diagnosis

Important aspects of history: The importance of a detailed pedigree, including parental age, consanguinity, a family history of neuromuscular disease and the identification of other affected siblings cannot be overemphasized. It is important to elicit a history of prenatal risk factors like drug or teratogen exposure. History of reduced fetal movements, presence of polyhydramnios, abnormal presentation and shortened umbilical cord indicate poor fetal movement and hypotonia. Details of perinatal history, including birth trauma, birth anoxia, delivery complications, and low APGAR scores findings (esp. lower scores for tone, reflexes and respiratory effort). Time of onset of hypotonia is important. Infants requiring ventilator assistance soon after birth to maintain respiration suggest significant muscle weakness. In a majority, hypotonia is often noticed at or soon after birth. CNS involvement is suggested by impairment in the level of consciousness, seizures, apneas, abnormal posturing, and abnormalities of brain stem reflexes, in addition to hypotonia. History should include abnormalities of ocular movements, repeated respiratory infections and feeding difficulties, which help in differential diagnosis. The presence of congenital malformations in other organ systems, deformations, and craniofacial dysmorphism can help in establishing a syndromic diagnosis.

Assessment of tone in an infant: Resting tone is that which is present with the subject in an awake, alert state, and is assessed by inspection. In a premature infant, tone depends on the gestational age, with increased gestational age associated with increased flexor tone. Flexion of the lower extremities develops at 30–32 wk, elbow flexion at 34–36 wk, and shoulder elevation at 37–38 wk. A normal term newborn is seen to have flexion at the hips, knees and elbows, with the hips partially internally rotated to lift knees off the

781

Table 25.1: Pattern of weakness and hypotonia and anatomical localization

Pattern of weakness and hypotonia	Anatomical localization
Central hypotonia, (may have with regional hypertonia)	Central nervous system
Axial hypotonia more prominent	
Hyperactive reflexes	
Generalized weakness	Motor neuron
Often spares the diaphragm, facial muscles, pelvis and sphincters	
Distal muscle groups involved	Nerve
Weakness with wasting	
Hypoactive/absent reflexes	
Bulbar, oculomotor muscles more involved	Neuromuscular junction
Weakness is prominent	Muscle
Proximal musculature more involved	
Hypoactive reflexes	
Joint contractures	

ground. Most hypotonic infants demonstrate a characteristic posture of full abduction and external rotation of the legs as well as a flaccid extension of the arms.

Static or passive is induced by passive movement in an otherwise cooperative, nonresistant individual, a requirement difficult to meet in an infant. Instead one can see the postural tone, which involves resistance to gravity for maintenance of stable posture. It is tested in infants by maneuvers like applying traction to the arms to pull to a sitting position from a supine position, or by axillary support in vertical suspension. A traction response is present in preterm infants of more than 33 wk of gestation, and exhibited as considerable head lag, head is consistently lifted. At term, there is only minimal head lag, one can feel the child pulling back against traction, and there is flexion at the elbows, knees and ankles. Once in the sitting position, the head may continue to lag or be momentarily kept erect before it falls forward. Floppiness is indicated in term neonates and infants by the presence of more than minimal head lag and the failure to counter traction by flexion of the limbs.

In vertical suspension, one lifts the child straight up with both hands in the child's axillae without holding the chest wall. A normal term newborn or an infant will have shoulder fixation strong enough to suspend the child vertically, and the head is held erect in the midline, with the legs flexed at the hips, knees and ankles. With hypotonia, the child needs to be grasped around the trunk to prevent falling, or the shoulders elevate excessively with internal rotation of the arms. Any sustained adduction or extension of the legs is suggestive of regional hypertonia, and therefore, a CNS disorder.

In horizontal suspension the child is suspended in the prone position. A normal newborn can inter-mittently keep his head erect and back straight, with flexion at the elbows, hips, knees and ankles; an older infant can sustain this posture. A hypotonic infant drapes over the examiner's hands, with the head and limbs hanging limply.

Assessment of muscle power: Assessment of muscle power is relevant in the setting of a floppy infant because normal muscle power in the setting of a diminished tone implies involvement of the CNS. Weakness in infants and children is best assessed in relation to developmentally appropriate skills and behaviors because maximal strength in isolated muscles may be difficult to elicit and grade according to the traditional five point measures used in older children and adults. For example, head and trunk power can be assessed by the upright head stability, traction response, independent sitting with or without hand propping, and ability to reach overhead without lateral propping and tilting head back. Proximal arm strength can be assessed by height of reach with arm outstretched at elbow, ability to take arms overhead, combat crawling, and wheelbarrow walk. Distal arm strength is reflected in the ability to grasp and elevate defined objects of various sizes and weights. Proximal leg strength is shown by the movement of legs against gravity in the supine position, kneeling, quadruple stance, crawling, Gower's maneuver, stance, gait, Trendelenburg's waddle, etc. Leg motion against gravity and a steppage gait with slapping feet are the things to look for when assessing distal leg weakness.

Assessment of muscle bulk: Severe loss of muscle bulk follows denervation and is most extreme in spinal muscular atrophy. Atrophy is also seen in some congenital myopathies. The decreases in muscle bulk seen in malnutrition are associated with generalized emaciation and with normal muscle power. Bulk may be better assessed by palpation than by inspection, due to masking effect of subcutaneous fat.

Range of movements: Infants and children with hypotonia have the appearance of joint laxity and increased range of movements; and may be misdiagnosed as connective tissue disorders like Ehler Danlos syndrome. However, the latter group of disorders is characterized by normal strength and tone in presence of pathological joint laxity.

Joint range may conversely be restricted in a floppy baby by muscle fibrosis, ligamentous restrictions, or by fibrosis of joint capsule. When acquired prenatally it is termed arthrogryposis, and that which develops later is called a contracture. Other in non-neurological causes, arthrogryposis may occur with motor unit disorders like spinal muscular atrophy, inherited myasthenic syndromes, neonatal myasthenia gravis, and fiber type disproportion myopathies. It may rarely be seen with CNS disorders like cerebral malformations and with spina bifida. Acquired contractures can be the result of either peripheral or central hypotonia, and therefore have limited utility in aiding differential diagnosis.

Muscle fatigue: Progressive conduction failure of the neuromuscular junction (NMJ) manifests as abnormal diminution of power in a muscle under continuous load. Appreciation that the weakness has a fatigable component is made difficult by the fact that infants do not exercise to the point of physical exhaustion, except possibly when crying vigorously. NMJ fatigue is only appreciated in those with difficulty in sucking, or possibly swallowing; the infant who appears hungry and alert and has normal sucking swallowing coordination, but only sucks briefly, may have NMJ fatigue. Other suggestive features include ptosis, restricted extraocular movements, and bulbar and facial weakness. Diseases of the NMJ are not common in children.

Reflexes: Keep the head in the midline when eliciting reflexes in younger infants, so as to avoid the asymmetric effects of the tonic neck reflex. Normal or exaggerated reflexes in the setting of hypotonia or weakness imply localization to the CNS. Diseases of the anterior motor horn cells or of the muscles decrease the reflexes commensurate with the loss of power, whereas those of the neuromuscular junction usually spare the tendon reflexes. On the other hand, demyelinating neuropathies usually diminish reflexes out of proportion to clinical weakness.

In newborns and young infants, the presence of a normal Moro's reflex indicates the intactness of the motor unit, while its absence suggests severe central or motor unit dysfunction. The tonic neck reflex in these children should be unsustained, variable and nonobligatory. An asymmetric tonic neck reflex suggests injury to the contralateral hemisphere; a persistent or obligatory response present bilaterally suggests bihemispheric injury.

Sensory examination: The relevance of sensory system examination in a floppy infant is in the detection of peripheral polyneuropathies and spinal injuries, wherein sensory and motor fibers are equally affected. However, it is difficult to carry out in younger children.

Assessment of the mother: In some disorders of the floppy infant, significant information can be discerned from a careful review of the mother. Maternal percussion myotonia or the inability to relax a tightly clenched fist may suggest that the infant has congenital myotonic dystrophy, while the presence in the mother of bulbar weakness, ptosis, or diplopia with sustained upgaze or early arm ptosis with sustained forward arm abduction may suggest unappreciated maternal myasthenia, with passive transfer of maternal antibodies being responsible for the neonate's floppiness. The age of first walking of both parents is often clearly remembered by the newborn's grandparents, and may provide a clue to early dominantly inherited weakness. These may include disorders like dominantly inherited congenital myopathies like central core disease of muscle fiber type disproportion syndromes, and dominantly inherited congenital myasthenia syndromes.

Relevant general and systemic examination: In utero immobility is associated with features, which include, in addition to arthrogryposis, a narrow high arched palate, mandibular underdevelopment, a short umbilical cord, and dislocated or easily dislocatable hips. Chest X-ray may reveal a thinning of ribs associated with demineralization of bones. The facies may be typically "myopathic" with a paucity of facial expression. An inverted V shaped upper lip is classically described with congenital myotonic dystrophy, while ptosis and external ophthalmoplegia suggest myasthenic syndromes. Storage disorders like Pompe's disease are associated with macroglossia and visceromegaly. The presence of fasciculations, seen best in the tongue, suggests anterior horn cell involvement as seen with spinal muscular atrophy. Ocular examination may reveal the presence of cataract or of pigmentary retinopathy, both of which are clues to peroxisomal disorders. Congenital glycosylation errors are associated with findings like lipodystrophy and inverted nipples.

Laboratory Diagnosis

Neuroimaging studies: Several abnormalities of the CNS can cause hypotonia in an infant, and these are best picked up on an MRI of the brain. These include neuronal migration defects like lissencephaly, laminin deficiency in congenital muscular dystrophy (manifests itself as altered signal characteristics of the white matter), mitochondrial cytopathies (basal ganglia abnormalities), and Joubert's syndrome and pontocerebellar hypoplasia (cerebellar abnormalities).

Karyotyping and FISH: Aneuploidies like Down's syndrome, and chromosomal duplications can be picked up on the standard karyotype analysis. The detection of microdeletions like in Prader Willi syndrome involves the use of fluorescent *in situ* hybridization (FISH) probes or more sophisticated gadgetry from the molecular armamentarium.

Electrophysiological studies: Nerve conduction studies and electromyogram (EMG) are very useful in delineating the true site of a lower motor neuron etiology. The value of the study relates directly to the skill of the person performing the procedure. In most cases of motor unit involvement, EMG is able to discern myopathic from neuropathic etiology; it is especially accurate in spinal muscular atrophy. Presence of low amplitude combined muscle axonal potentials (CMAP), and small polyphasic muscle action potentials that are rapidly recruited, favor a myopathic disorder. The duration, amplitude and configuration of the motor unit potential differentiate between a myopathy and a neuropathy. Nerve conduction study findings that suggest a neuropathy include a slow nerve conduction velocity (NCV) and presence of conduction block.

Defective neuromuscular transmission, as seen with the congenital myasthenic syndromes, is suggested on EMG by the presence of a decremental response at 2–3 Hz stimulation of more than one muscle. On the other hand, low CMAP amplitude that exhibits a 25–50% increment post-tetany is suggestive of botulism.

Muscle biopsy: Muscle biopsy must be considered in the diagnosis of congenital myopathies and dystrophies. Muscles free of myotendinous insertions, such as the deltoid, biceps, triceps, and rectus femoris are best suited for the purpose as these have equal fiber type representation. The chosen muscle should be mild to moderately weak, and not recently needled by EMG. Histochemical evaluation of quickly frozen muscle tissue is essential to the diagnosis. Immunohistochemistry employing antibodies directed against muscle proteins are especially helpful in the diagnosis of congenital muscular dystrophies and myopathies.

Nerve biopsy: Biopsy of the sural nerve is indicated in the setting of an unexplained neuropathy, and, with newer techniques of visualizing small myelinated and unmyelinated axons, in neurodegenerative disorders as well. Nerve biopsy can reveal features of primary demyelination or axonal degeneration, abnormal inflammation, or specific features within the myelin or axon, each of which may have a specific importance.

Biochemical tests: Only some muscle disorders are associated with an elevated creatine phosphokinase; these include congenital muscular dystrophy and some myopathies. The value of biochemical tests is in cases with multisystem abnormalities or clinical features suggestive of an inborn error of metabolism. Evaluation for a neurometabolic disorder would have to include: blood and CSF ammonia and lactate (in urea cycle defects, fatty acid oxidation defects, organic acidemias), urine and serum aminoacidogram (in aminoacidopathies), assays for very long chain fatty acids (VLCFA, elevated in peroxisomal disorders), tandem mass spectroscopy (in fatty acid oxidation defects, organic acidemias), transferrin (low in glycosylation disorders), and 7-dehydrocholesterol (elevated in Smith Lemli Opitz syndrome).

Individual Entities

Encephalopathies and structural CNS malformations: Usually present in the neonatal period with hypotonia associated with seizures, altered sensorium, or craniofacial dysmorphism(holoprosencephaly, agenesis of the corpus callosum). Diagnosis is often confirmed with a neuroimaging study. The hypotonia may improve or evolve into hypertonia during further follow-up.

Chromosomal disorders: This group includes, for example, Down syndrome (trisomy 21), trisomy 13, and trisomy 18 and Prader-Willi syndrome (deletion 15q11–13). Diagnosis is suggested by the presence of distinctive associated malformations (*see* Chapter 9).

Spinal muscular atrophy (SMA): Infantile spinal muscular atrophy type I (Werdnig Hoffman disease) is characterized by diffuse hypotonia and weakness, more in the legs than arms, present at birth or detected soon afterwards, associated with an alert face, poverty of spontaneous movements, normal sphincter tone, tongue fasciculations, and absent tendon reflexes. Paradoxical respiration is present, with a strong diaphragm but weak chest and abdominal musculature; this along with the involvement of bulbar muscles accounts for the respiratory distress, pneumonias, and respiratory failure. EMG shows spontaneous fibrillation potentials typical of denervation pattern, while the biopsy exhibits grouped neurogenic atrophy along with hypertrophic type I fibres suggesting reinnervation. DNA diagnosis is now available.

Hereditary motor-sensory neuropathies: Section 25.5.

Disorders of neuromuscular transmission: These are characterized by weakness of bulbar, facial, and oculomotor muscles, alone or in combination with limb weakness. Abnormal fatigue often limits the duration of sucking, followed by hungry irritability and weak attachment to the nipple. Congenital myasthenic syndromes include congenital myasthenia with episodic apnea, with a mutation in the choline acetyl transferase gene; slow channel and fast channel syndrome, with mutations affecting the AchR subunits; and endplate cholinesterase deficiency (see Section 25.2).

Congenital muscular dystrophy (CMD): Section 25.2.

Myopathies: Infants present with floppiness, hyporeflexia, and often with open bite, high arched palate and micrognathia. The diagnosis rests on muscle histology. Based on etiology, these have been variously classified; one such system groups them as: (1) Congenital myopathies due to developmental arrest: myotubular myopathy, congenital fiber type disproportion. (2) Congenital myopathies due to persistent organellar regression: focal loss of cross striation, myopathy with lysis of myofibrils, nemaline body myopathy, zebra body myopathy, spheroid body myopathy, myopathy with tubular aggregates, satellite cell myopathy. (3) Congenital myopathies due to metabolic errors: mitochondrial myopathy, mitochondria-lipid-glycogen disease. (4) Congenital myopathies due to the lack of the trophic influence of innervation: central core disease, multicore, minicore disease.

Aneja S, Sinha Aditi. The Floppy Child. In: Mathur GP, Mathur Sarla (eds). *Current Trends in Pediatrics*. Vol 2. Delhi: Academa Publishers, 2006; 178–185.

Bodensteiner J. Congenital myopathies. *Neurol Clin* 1988 Aug; 6(3): 499–518.

Crawford TJ. The floppy infant. In: Bradley WG et al (eds). *Neurology in clinical practice*. 3rd edn. Oxford: Butterworth-Heinemann, 2000.

Jaradeh SS, Ho H. Muscle, nerve and skin biopsy. *Neurol Clin* 2004; 22:539–561.

Johnston HM. The floppy weak infant revisited. *Brain Dev* 2003 (Apr); 25(3): 155–158.

Korenyi-Both A, Korenyi-Both I. Congenital myopathies with "diagnostic" pathological features. *J Med* 1987; 18(2): 93–107.

Prasad AN, Prasad C. The floppy infant: contribution of genetic and metabolic disorders. *Brain Dev* 2003 Oct; 25(7): 457–476.

Sarnat HB. Neuromuscular disorders. In: Kliegman RM, Behrman RE, Jenson HB, Stanton BF (eds). *Nelson Textbook of Pediatrics*. 18th edn. Vol. 2. Philadelphia: Saunders, 2007; 2531–2567.

25.2 MUSCULAR DYSTROPHIES

Muscular dystrophies are distinguished from all other neuromuscular diseases by four criteria (i) it is a primary myopathy, (ii) it has a genetic basis, (iii) the course is progressive, (iv) and degeneration and death of muscle fibers occur at some stage in the disease. The term dystrophy means abnormal growth, derived from the Greek *trophe*, meaning "nourishment". Six muscular dystrophies affect children and adolescents.

1. Duchenne and Becker Muscular Dystrophies

Duchenne muscular dystrophy **(DMD)** is the commonest form of muscular dystrophy, inherited as an X-linked recessive trait; the abnormal gene is at the Xp21 locus. Its characteristic clinical features are progressive weakness, intellectual impairment, hypertrophy of the calves, and proliferation of connective tissue in muscle. The incidence is 3:3, 600 live-born infant boys. *Becker muscular dystrophy* (BMD) is a similar disease as DMD, with a genetic defect at the same locus, but it clinically follows a milder and more protracted course.

Clinical manifestations: Infant boys are only rarely symptomatic at birth or in early infancy, although some are mildly hypotonic. The first sign noted in infancy is the poor head control. Walking is often accomplished at the normal age of about 12 mo, but hip girdle weakness be seen as early as in the 2nd year. Toddlers might assume a lordotic posture when standing to compensate for gluteal weakness. The disease has an onset between 3 and 5 or 6 yr (*see* Fig. 25.1 in CD). Weakness typically begins in the lower limbs affecting the pelvic girdle muscles and manifests with repeated falls, difficulty in climbing upstairs, and squatting. Patients experience a lot of difficulty in getting up from squatting position and stand up with the aid of hands pushing on knees, referred to as 'Gowers sign' (*see* Fig. 25.2 in CD). An early Gowers sign is often evident by age 3 yr and is fully expressed by age 5 or 6 yr. A Trendelenburg gait or waddling gait (hip waddle) appear at this time. The patient remains ambulatory varies greatly. Some patients are confined to a wheelchair by 7 yr of age. Most patients continue to walk with increasing difficulty until age 10 yr without orthopedic intervention, whereas with orthotic bracing, physiotherapy, and sometimes minor surgery (Achilles tendon lengthening) most are able to walk until age 12 yr.

The weakness continues in the 2nd decade. The function of distal muscles is usually relatively well preserved, allowing the child to continue to use eating utensils, a pencil and a computer keyboard. Respiratory muscles are weak and ineffective cough, frequent pulmonary infections, and decreasing respiratory reserve. Pharyngeal weakness can lead to episodes of aspiration, nasal regurgitation of liquids and nasal voice quality. The function of the extraocular muscles remains well preserved. Incontinence due to anal and urethral sphincter weakness is an uncommon and very late event.

Contractures most often involve the ankles (*see* Fig. 25.3 in CD), knees, hips, and elbows. *Scoliosis* is common. The thoracic deformity further compromises pulmonary capacity and compresses the heart.

Enlargement of the calves (pseudohypertrophy) and wasting of thigh muscles are characteristic features. The enlargement is caused by hypertrophy of some muscle fibers, infiltration of muscle by fat, and proliferation of collagen. After the calves, the next most common site of muscular hypertrophy is the tongue, followed by muscles of the forearm. Fasciculations of the tongue do not occur. The voluntary sphincter muscles are rarely involved.

The knee deep tendon reflexes may be present until about 6 yr, but are less brisk than the ankle jerks and are ultimately lost. Ankle deep tendon reflexes remain well preserved until terminal stages, unless ankle contractures are severe. In the upper extremities, brachioradialis reflex is usually stronger than the biceps or triceps brachii reflexes.

Cardiomyopathy, including persistent tachycardia and myocardial failure, is seen in 50–80% of patients with the disease.

Intellectual impairment occurs in all patients, although only 20–30% patients have an IQ < 70. The majority have learning disabilities, but still study in the regular classroom, with remedial help. A few patients are mentally retarded. Epilepsy is slightly more common than general population. Dystrophin is expressed in brain, retina, and striated and cardiac muscle, but the level is less in brain than in muscle. Abnormalities in cortical architecture and of dendritic arborization may be detected neuropathologically. Cerebral atrophy is demonstrated by MRI late in the clinical course of the disease. Myalgias and muscle spasms do not occur. Calcinosis of muscle is rare.

Death usually occurs at about 18–20 yr of age. The causes of death are respiratory failure in sleep, intractable heart failure, pneumonia, or occasionally aspiration and airway obstruction.

In *Becker muscular dystrophy*, boys remain ambulatory until late adolescence or early adult life. Calf pseudohypertrophy, cardiomyopathy, and elevated serum levels of creatine kinase (CK) are similar as seen inpatients with DMD. Learning disabilities are less common. The onset of weakness

occurs late in Becker than in DMD. Death often occurs in the mid to late 20s.

Diagnosis: The serum CK level is markedly elevated in DMD, even in presymptomatic stages, including at birth. The usual serum concentration is 15,000–35,000 (normal <160 IU/L). A normal serum CK level excludes the diagnosis of DMD. Other lysosomal enzymes present in muscle, such as aldolase and aspartate amiotransferase are increased, but they are less specific. Cardiac assessment by echocardiography, electrocardiography (ECG), and radiography of the chest is essential and should be repeated periodically. Electromyography (EMG) shows characteristic myopathic features but is not specific for DMD. No evidence of denervation is found. Motor and sensory nerve conduction velocities are normal.

Polymerse chain reaction (PCR) for the dystrophic gene mutation is the primary test, if the clinical features and serum CK are consistent with the diagnosis. If the blood PCR is diagnostic, muscle biopsy is deferred. The *muscle biopsy* is diagnostic and shows characteristic changes including endomysial connective tissue proliferation, scattered degenerating and regenerating myofibers, foci of mononuclear inflammatory cell infiltrates as a reaction to muscle fiber necrosis, mild architectural changes in still-functional muscle fibers and many dense fibers. These hypercontracted fibers probably result from segmental necrosis at another level, allowing calcium to enter the site of breakdown of the sarcolemmal membrane and trigger a contraction of the whole length of the muscle fiber. Calcifications within myofibers are correlated with secondary β-dystroglycan deficiency.

Treatment: There is neither a medical cure for the disease nor slowing its progression. Physiology delays but does not always prevent contractures. Preservation of a good nutritional state is important. Dietary restrictions are needed in children with obesity because a patient with myopathy even less functional because part of the limited reserve muscle strength is dissipated in lifting the weight of excess subcutaneous adipose tissue. Cardiac decompensation and pulmonary infections should be promptly treated.

2. Emery-Dreifuss Muscular Dystrophy

Emery-Dreifuss muscular dystrophy, also known as scapuloperoneal or scapulohumral muscular dystrophy is a rare dystrophy and is of two types: i). X-linked recessive dystrophy; the locus is on the long arm within the large Xq28 region. ii). Autosomal dominant trait and is located at 1q. This form can manifest quite late in adolescence or early adult life, although the muscular or cardiac symptoms and signs

---

Box 25.1: Characteristic features of
Emery-Dreifuss muscular dystrophy

1. Muscles do not hypertrophy
2. Contractures of elbows and ankles develop early
3. Muscle becomes wasted in a scapulohumeroperoneal distribution
4. Facial weakness does not occur
5. Myotonia is absent
6. Intellectual function is normal
7. Cardiomyopathy is severe*
8. Serum CK value is mildly elevated
9. Muscle biopsy—nonspecific myofiber necrosis and endomysial fibrosis

*Associated with conduction defects, ventricular fibrillation, and myocardial failure

---

are similar, and sudden death from ventricular fibrillation is a risk.

Clinical manifestations begin at between 5 and 15 yr of age. Many patients survive to late adult life because of its slow progression of its course. A rare severe infantile presentation also is documented. The characteristic features are listed in Box 25.1.

Treatment should be supportive, with special attention to cardiac conduction defects and can require medications or a pacemaker. The cause of death more commonly is from conduction defects and sudden ventricular fibrillation than from intractable myocardial failure.

3. Myotonic Muscular Dystrophy

Myotonic dystrophy (Steinert disease) is the second most common muscular dystrophy in North America, Europe, and Australia, having an incidence varying from 1:100,000 to 1:30,000 in the general population. Myotonic dystrophy is an example of a genetic defect causing dysfunction in *multiple organ systems*. The distal distribution of muscle wasting in myotonic dystrophy is an exception to the general rule of myopathies having proximal and neuropathies having distal distribution patterns. Myotonic muscular dystrophy is inherited as an autosomal dominant trait. Classic myotonic dystrophy (DM1) is located on chromosome 19q13.3, DM2 on chromosome 3q21, and a third, late form DM3 is identified, at locus 15q21–q24.

Clinical manifestations: In the usual clinical course, excluding the severe neonatal form, infants may appear normal at birth. The facial appearance is characteristic, consisting of an inverted V-shaped upper lip, thin cheeks, and scalloped, concave temporalis muscles. The head may be narrow, and the palate is high and arched. Progressive wasting of distal muscles becomes increasingly evident, particularly involving intrinsic muscles of the hands. The thenar and hypothenar muscles eminences are flattened and the affected dorsal interossei leave deep grooves between the fingers. The dorsal forearm muscles and anterior compartment muscles of the lower legs also become wasted. The tongue is thin and atrophic. Wasting of sternocleidomastoid gives the neck a long, thin, cylindrical contour. Proximal muscles also eventually undergo atrophy, and scapular winging appears. Difficulty with climbing stairs and Gowers sign are progressive. Tendon stretch reflexes are usually preserved. The muscular atrophy and weakness in myotonic dystrophy are slowly progressive throughout childhood and adolescence and continue into adulthood. Frontal baldness is also characteristic in males and often begins in adolescence.

Myotonia appears at about 5 yr of age and in exceptional patients develops as early as 3 yr. Myotonia is a very slow relaxation of muscle after contraction, whether the contraction was voluntary or was induced by a stretch reflex or electrical stimulation. Myotonia may be demonstrated by asking the patient to make tight fists and then to quickly open the hands. It may be induced by striking the thenar eminence with a rubber percussion hammer, and it may be detected by watching the involuntary drawing the thumb across the palm. Myotonia may also be demonstrated in the tongue by pressing the edge of a wooden tongue blade against its dorsal surface and by observing a deep furrow that disappears slowly. Myotonia is not a painful muscle spasm. Myalgias do not occur in myotonic dystrophy.

The speech of patients with myotonic dystrophy is often articulated poorly and is slurred because of the involvement of the muscles of the face, tongue, and pharynx. Difficulties with swallowing may sometimes occur. Aspiration pneumonia is a risk in severely involved children. Incomplete external ophthalmoplegia may sometimes result from extraocular muscle weakness.

Smooth muscle involvement of the *gastrointestinal tract* results in slow gastric emptying, poor peristalsis, and constipation. Some patients have encopresis associated with anal sphincter weakness. Women with myotonic dystrophy may have ineffective or abnormal uterine contractions during labor and delivery.

Cardiac involvement is usually manifested as heart block in the Purkinje conduction system and arrhythmias.

Endocrine abnormalities include hypothyroidism (rarely hyperthyroidism), and adrenocortical insufficiency, which may lead to an Addisonian crisis even in infancy. Diabetes mellitus is common. Onset of puberty may be precocious or, more, often delayed. Testicular atrophy and testosterone deficiency are common in adults and are responsible for a high incidence of male infertility. Ovarian atrophy is rare.

Immunologic deficiencies are common in myotonic dystrophy; the plasma IgG level is often low.

Cataracts occur frequently; they may be congenital or they may begin any time during childhood or adult life.

About half of the patients are *intellectually impaired*, but severe mental retardation is unusual. Epilepsy is not common.

A severe congenital form of myotonic dystrophy appears in minority of infants born to mothers with myotonic dystrophy. These infants have club foot deformities or more extensive contractures of many joints, generalized hypotonia and weakness at birth and facial wasting. Infants may require gavage feeding or ventilator support.

Diagnosis: The primary diagnostic test is a DNA analysis of the blood to demonstrate the abnormal expansion of the cytosine-thymine-guanine (CTG) repeat. Prenatal diagnosis is also feasible. The muscle biopsy specimen in older children shows many muscle fibers with central nuclei and selective atrophy of histochemical type 1 fibers, but degenerating fibers are usually a few and widely scattered, and there is a little or no fibrosis of muscle. The classic myotonic electromyogram is not found in infancy but may appear in toddlers or during the early school years. The level of serum CK and other serum enzymes from muscle may be normal or only mildly elevated. ECG should be performed annually in early childhood. Ultrasound imaging of the abdomen may be indicated in affected infants to determine diaphragmatic function. Radiographs of the chest and abdomen and contrast studies of the gastrointestinal motility may be needed. Endocrine assessment should be done to determine thyroid and adrenal cortical function and to verify carbohydrate metabolism (glucose tolerance test). Immunoglobulins should be examined.

Treatment: There is no specific medical treatment, but the cardiac, endocrine, gastrointestinal, and ocular complications can often be treated. Physiotherapy and orthopedic treatment of contractures in neonatal form of disease may be beneficial. Myotonia may be diminished, and function may be restored by drugs that raise the depolarization threshold of muscle membranes, such as phenytoin (3–9 mg/kg/24 hr bid), carbamazepine (10–30 mg/kg/24 hr tid), mexiletine, procainamide, and quinidine sulfate. Serum concentrations of 10–20 µg/ml for phenytoin and for 8–12 µg/ml carbamazepine should be maintained.

Other Myotonic Syndromes

***Myotonic chondrodystrophy* (Schwartz-Jampel disease):** Myotonic chondrodystrophy is characterized by generalized muscle hypertrophy and weakness, dysmorphic phenotypical features, dwarfism, joint abnormalities, and blepharophimosis. EMG reveals continuous electrical activity in muscle fibers closely resembling or identical to myotonia.

***Myotonia congenita* (Thomsen disease):** Myotonia congenita is characterized by weakness and generalized muscular hypertrophy so that affected children resemble body builders. Myotonia is prominent and may develop at age 2–3 yr, earlier than in myotonia dystrophy. The EMG demonstrates myotonia.

Paramyotonia: Paramyotonia is a temperature-related myotonia that is aggravated by cold and alleviated by warm external temperatures. Patients have difficulty when swimming in cold water or if they are dressed inadequately in cold weather.

4. Limb-girdle Muscular Dystrophies

Limb-girdle muscular dystrophies (LGMD) includes a group of progressive hereditary myopathies that mainly affect muscles of the hip and shoulder girdles. Distal muscles also eventually become atrophic and weak. Hypertrophy of the calves and ankle contractures develop in some forms causing potential confusion with Becker muscular dystrophy. Most cases of LGMD are of autosomal recessive inheritance, but some families express an autosomal dominant trait. The latter often follows a benign course with a little functional impairment.

The initial *clinical manifestations* rarely appear before middle or late childhood or may be delayed until early adult life. Low back pain may be a presenting complaint because of the lordotic posture resulting from gluteal muscle weakness. Patients are confined to wheelchair usually at about 30 yr of age. Weakness of neck muscles is present but facial, lingual and other bulbar innervated muscles are rarely involved. As weakness and muscle wasting progress, tendon stretch reflexes become diminished. Cardiac involvement is unusual. Intellectual function is generally normal.

Diagnosis and differential diagnosis: The differential diagnosis of LGMD includes juvenile spinal muscular atrophy (Kugelberg-Welander disease), myasthenia gravis, and metabolic myopathies. The EMG and muscle biopsy show confirmatory evidence of muscular dystrophy, but none of the findings is specific enough to make the definitive *diagnosis* without additional clinical criteria.

5. Facioscapulohumeral Muscular Dystrophy

Facioscapulohumeral muscular dystrophy also known as Landouzy-Dejerine disease is probably not a single disease entity but a group of diseases with similar clinical manifestations. The frequency is 1: 20,000. Autosomal dominant inheritance is the rule and the gene is in the subtelomeric region at the 4q35 locus. About 10% of families do not map to the 4q35 locus.

Clinical manifestations: Facioscapulohumeral muscular dystrophy shows the earliest and most severe weakness in facial and shoulder girdle muscles. The mouth in facioscapulohumeral muscular dystrophy is rounded and appears puckered because the lips protrude. Inability to close the eyes completely in sleep is indicative of upper facial weakness. Some patients have extraocular muscle weakness, although ophthalmoplegia is rarely complete. Mobius syndrome is associated in a few cases. Pharyngeal and tongue weakness may be absent and if present it is not as severe as the facial involvement. Hearing loss which may be subclinical and retinal vasculopathy (indistinguishable from Coats disease) are associated features, particularly occur in severe cases with early childhood illness.

Scapular winging is prominent, often even in infants. Flattening or even concavity of the deltoid contour is seen. Biceps and triceps brachii muscles are wasted and weak. Muscles of the hip girdle and thigh eventually loose strength and undergo atrophy, and Gowers sign and a Trendelenburg gait appear. Contractures of the extremities rarely occur. Finger and wrist weakness is occasionally the first symptom. Weakness of the anterior tibial and peroneal muscles leading to foot-drops usually occurs in advance cases. Lumbar lordosis and kyphoscoliosis are common complications of axial muscle involvement. Calf pseudohypertrophy is not a usual feature, but is rarely described.

Facioscapulohumeral muscular dystrophy can also be mild disease causing minimal disability. Clinical manifestations are not seen in childhood and are seen into middle adult life. Unlike most other muscular dystrophies asymmetry of weakness is common. About 30% of affected patients are asymptomatic or show only mild scapular winging and decreased tendon reflexes of which patients were unaware before neurologic examination was performed.

Diagnosis and differential diagnosis: Serum levels of CK and other enzymes vary normal or near normal to elevations of several thousands. ECG should be performed, although the findings are usually normal. EMG shows nonspecific myopathic muscle pattern.

Diagnostic molecular testing in individual cases and within families is indicated for prediction.

Muscle biopsy distinguishes more than one form of facioscapulohumeral muscular dystrophy, consistent with clinical evidence that several distinct diseases are included by the term *FISH dystrophy*. Muscle biopsy and EMG also distinguish the primary myopathy from a neurogenic disease with a similar distribution of muscular involvement. The histological findings of the muscle biopsy are extensive proliferation of connective tissue between muscle fibers, extreme variation in fiber size with many hypertrophic and atrophic myofibers and scattered degenerating and regenerating fibers. An "inflammatory" type of facioscapulohumeral muscular dystrophy is also distinguished, characterized by extensive lymphocytic infiltrates within muscle fascicles.

Treatment: Foot-drop and scoliosis may be treated by orthopedic measures. Cosmetic improvement of the facial muscles of expression may be achieved by reconstructive surgery. Physiotherapy is of no value in regaining strength or in retarding progressive weakness or muscle wasting.

6. Congenital Muscular Dystrophy

Congenital muscular dystrophy (CMD) encompasses several distinct diseases with a common characteristic of severe involvement at birth but that usually follows a benign clinical course and has an autosomal recessive mode of inheritance.

Clinical manifestations: infants often have contractures or arthrogryposis at birth and are diffusely hypotonic. The muscle mass is thin in the trunk and extremities. Head control is poor. Facial muscles may be mildly involved, but ophthalmoplegia, pharyngeal weakness, and weak sucking are not common. A minority of cases has severe dysphagia and requires gavage or gastrostomy. Tendon stretch reflexes may be hypoactive or absent. Congenital contractures of elbows have a high association with the Ullrich type of congenital muscular dystrophy owing to a defect in 1 or more of the 3 collagen VI genes, each at a different locus.

The Fukuyama type of congenital muscular dystrophy is the second most common muscular dystrophy in Japan (after DMD). It has been also reported in children in Dutch, German, Scandinavian, and Turkish ethnic backgrounds. In the Fukuyama variety, severe cardiomyopathy and malformations of the brain usually accompany the skeletal muscle involvement. Signs and symptoms related to these organs are present: cardiomegaly and heart failure, mental retardation, seizures, microcephaly and failure to thrive. The genetic defect in Fukuyama type has been identified at the 8q31–33 locus in Japanese patients.

Neurologic disease may accompany forms of congenital muscular dystrophy other than Fukuyama disease. Mental and neurologic are the most important features. An apparently normal brain and normal intelligence do not preclude the diagnosis if other manifestations indicate this myopathy. The cerebral manifestations that occur vary from cerebral dysplasia (holoprosencephaly, lissencephaly) to milder conditions (cerebral agenesis of the corpus callosum, focal heterotropia of the cerebral cortex and subcortical white matter, cerebellar hypoplasia).

Congenital muscular dystrophy is a consistent association with cerebral dysgenesis in the Walker-Warburg syndrome and in muscle-eye-brain disease of Santavuori. Another separate form of congenital muscular dystrophy is characterized by microcephaly and mental retardation.

Diagnosis: Serum CK is usually moderately elevated. EMG shows nonspecific myopathic features. Investigations should include cardiac assessment and an imaging study of the brain. Muscle biopsy is essential for the diagnosis and shows features of myopathy.

Treatment: Supportive therapy is only available in general. Cyclosporin A might correct the mitochondrial dysfunction and muscular apoptosis in collagen VI myopathy.

Allen CMC, Lueck CJ. Muscular dystrophy. In: Haslett C, Chilvers ER, Boon NA, Colledge NR, Hunter JAA (eds). *Davidson's Principles and Practice of Medicine.* 19th edn. Edinburgh: Churchill Livingstone, 2002; 1186–1187.

Kumar Sudhir. Muscular Dystrophies in Children and Adolescents. In: Mathur GP, Mathur Sarla (eds). *Current Trends in Pediatrics.* Vol 1. Delhi: Academa Publishers, 2005; 463-470.

Mukherjee M, Mittal B. Muscular dystrophies. *Indian J Pediatr* 2004; 71:161–168.

Sarnat HB. Neuromuscular disorders. In: Kliegman RM, Behrman RE, Jenson HB, Stanton BF (eds). *Nelson Textbook of Pediatrics.* 18th edn. Vol. 2. Philadelphia: Saunders, 2007; 2531–2567.

Sarnat HB. Muscular dystrophies. In: Kliegman RM, Stanton BF, St.Geme JW, NF Schor NF, Behrman RE. *Nelson Textbook of Pediatrics.* 19th edn. New Delhi: Elsevier, 2011; 2119–2129.

25.3 METABOLIC MYOPATHIES

Periodic Paralysis (Potassium-related)

Episodic, reversible weakness or paralysis known as periodic paralysis is associated with transient alterations in serum potassium levels, usually hypokalemia but occasionally hyperkalemia. The disorder is inherited as an autosomal dominant trait. The defective genes are at the 17q13.1-13.3 locus in *hyperkalemic periodic paralysis*, the same as in paramyotonia congenita, and at the 1q13-32 locus in *hypokalemic periodic paralysis*.

In childhood, periodic paralysis is often an episodic event; patients are unable to move after awakening and gradually recover muscle strength during the next few minutes or hours. Muscles that remain active in sleep, such as the diaphragm and cardiac muscle, are not affected. Patients are normal between attacks, but in adult life the attacks become more frequent, and the disorder causes progressive myopathy with permanent weakness even between attacks. The disorder is precipitated in some patients by a heavy carbohydrate meal, insulin, and epinephrine including that induced by emotional stress, hyperaldosteronism or hyperthyroidism, administration of amphotericin B or ingestion of licorice.

Alterations in serum potassium level occur only during acute episodes and are accompanied by T-wave changes in the electrocardiogram (ECG). Muscle biopsy findings are often normal between attacks, but during an attack a vacuolar myopathy is demonstrated.

Treatment: Paralytic attacks of hypokalemic periodic paralysis are treated by the oral administration of potassium or even fruit juices that contains potassium. A low sodium intake and the administration of acetazolamide (125–250 mg bid or tid) in school-age children often are effective in abolishing attacks or at least reducing their frequency and severity. Spironolactone (100–200 mg/day PO) may be effective in school-aged children as well.

Malignant Hyperthermia

This syndrome is usually inherited as an autosomal dominant trait. It occurs in all patients with central core disease but is not limited to that particular myopathy. The gene is at the 19q13.1 locus in both central core disease and malignant hyperthermia without this specific myopathy. It occurs rarely in Duchenne and other muscular dystrophies, in various other myopathies, and in an isolated syndrome not associated with other muscle disease. Affected children may have peculiar faces. All ages are affected, including premature infants whose mothers underwent general anesthesia for cesarean section.

Acute episodes are precipitated by exposure to general anesthetics and occasionally to local anesthetic drugs. Patients suddenly develop extreme fever, rigidity of muscles, and metabolic and respiratory acidosis; the serum CK level rises to as high as 35,000 IU/L. Myoglobinuria may result in tubular necrosis and acute renal failure. Apart from the genetic disorder some drugs, such as valproic acid may induce this process in children with mitochondrial cytopathies or with carnitine palmitoyltransferase deficiency. Muscle biopsy during an episode or shortly afterward shows widely scattered necrosis of muscle fibers known as rhabdomyolysis. Between attacks, the muscle biopsy is normal unless there is chronic myopathy.

It is important to identify patients at risk of malignant hyperthermia. Patients at risk such as siblings, are identified by the caffeine contracture test: A portion of fresh muscle biopsy tissue in a saline bath is attached to a strain gauge and exposed to caffeine and other drugs; an abnormal spasm is diagnostic. Attacks of malignant hyperthermia can be prevented by administering dantrolene sodium before an anesthetic is given.

Mitochondrial Myopathies

Several diseases involving muscle, brain, and other organs are associated with structural and functional abnormalities of mitochondria. Kearns-Sayre syndrome having a single large mtDNA deletion is characterized by the triad of progressive external ophthalmoplegia, pigmentary degeneration of the retina and onset before age 20 yr. Chronic progressive external ophthalmoplegia may be isolated or accompanied by limb muscle weakness, dysphagia, and dysarthria. The diseases associated with mitochondrial myopathies include MERRF syndrome, *MELAS* syndrome, *Leigh subacute necrotizing encephalopathy, Cerebro-hepatorenal (Zellweger) disease, Cytochrome-c-oxidase deficiency,* and *Oculopharyngeal muscular dystrophy.*

Investigations for mitochondrial cytopathies include serum and sometimes CSF lactate, cardiac evaluation, and molecular markers in blood for the common diseases with known mtDNA point mutations. The muscle biopsy provides best evidence for all mitochondrial myopathies.

There is no effective treatment of mitochondrial cytopathies, but various "cocktails" are often used empirically to try to overcome the metabolic deficits. These include oral carnitine supplements, riboflavin, coenzyme Q_{10}, vitamin C, vitamin E, and other antioxidants.

Kumar Sudhir. Endocrine and Metabolic Myopathies in Children and Adolescents. In: Mathur GP, Mathur Sarla (eds). *Current Trends in Pediatrics.* Vol 3. Delhi: Academa Publishers, 2007; 285–291.

Sarnat HB. Neuromuscular disorders. In: Kliegman RM, Behrman RE, Jenson HB, Stanton BF (eds). *Nelson Textbook of Pediatrics.* 18th edn. Vol. 2. Philadelphia: Saunders, 2007; P2531–2567.

Sarnat HB. Endocrine and toxic myopathies. In: Kliegman RM, Stanton BF, St.Geme JW, NF Schor NF, Behrman RE. *Nelson Textbook of Pediatrics.* 19th edn. New Delhi: Elsevier, 2011; 2129-2132.

25.4 MYASTHENIA GRAVIS

Myasthenia gravis, a chronic disease is characterized by rapid fatigability of striated muscle. The most frequent cause is an immune-mediated neuromuscular blockade. There are three causes.

1. Post-synaptic muscle membrane or motor end plate that is less responsive than normal to acetylcholine (ACh), but the release of ACh into the synaptic cleft by the axonal terminal is normal.

2. Decreased number of available Ach receptors that is due to circulating receptor binding antibodies present in most cases of acquired myasthenia.

3. Deficiency of motor end plate ACh, designated AChE.

Clinical manifestations: Three clinical varieties are distinguished in childhood: juvenile myasthenia gravis in late infancy and childhood, congenital myasthenia, and transient neonatal myasthenia. In the *juvenile form*, ptosis and some degree of extraocular muscle weakness are the earliest and most constant signs. Older children may complain of diplopia. The papillary response to light is normal. Young children may hold open their eyes with their fingers or thumbs if the ptosis is severe enough to obstruct vision. Dysphagia and facial weakness are also common. Feeding difficulties in early infancy and poor head control because of weakness of neck flexors are present. Involvement of bulbar-innervated muscles and weakness involving limb-girdle muscles and distal muscles of the hands in most cases occur. Fasciculations of muscle, myalgias, and sensory symptoms do not occur. Tendon stretch reflexes may be diminished but rarely are lost.

Rapid fatigue of muscles is a characteristic feature of myasthenia gravis that distinguishes it from most other neuromuscular diseases. Ptosis increases progressively as patients are asked to sustain an upward gaze for 30–90 sec. Holding the head up from the surface of the examining table while lying supine is very difficult, and gravity cannot be overcome for more than a few seconds. Repetitive opening and closing of the fists produces rapid fatigue of hand muscles. Patients cannot elevate their arms for more than 1–2 mm because of fatigue of deltoids. Patients are more symptomatic late in the day or when tired. Dysphagia may interfere with eating, and the muscles of the jaw soon tire when an affected child chews.

Congenital myasthenia gravis is not related to maternal myasthenia that is nearly always a permanent disorder without spontaneous remission.

Infants born to myasthenic mothers may have a *transient neonatal myasthenic syndrome* secondary to placentally transferred anti-ACh receptor antibodies, distinct from congenital myasthenia gravis. They may have respiratory insufficiency, inability to suck or swallow, and generalized hypotonia and weakness. They may show a little spontaneous motor activity for several days to weeks. Some require ventilatory support and feeding by gavage during this period. After the antibodies disappear from the blood and muscle tissue, the infants regain normal strength and are not at increased risk of developing myasthenia gravis in later childhood.

Myasthenia gravis is occasionally associated with hypothyroidism usually due to *Hashimoto thyroiditis*. Postinfectious myasthenia gravis in children is transitory and usually follows a *varicella-zoster infection* in 2–5 wk as an immune response.

Diagnosis: Electromyography (EMG) is a more specifically diagnostic. A decremental response is seen in response to repetitive nerve stimulation; the muscle potentials diminish rapidly in amplitude until the muscle becomes refractory to further stimulation. This EMG pattern is reversed after a cholinesterase inhibitor is administered. Motor nerve conduction velocity remains normal.

A clinical test for myasthenia gravis is administration of a short acting cholinesterase inhibitor, usually edrophonium chloride. Ptosis and ophthalmoplegia improve within a few seconds, and fatigability of other muscles decreases. Electrocardiographic monitoring during the test is recommended. In the case of infants younger than 2 yr of age prostigmine methylsulfate (Neostigmine) is administered intramuscularly at a dose of 0.04 mg/kg; if the results are negative or equivocal, another dose of 0.04 mg/kg may be administered 4 hr after the first dose (a typical dose is 0.5–1.5 mg). The peak effect is seen in 20–40 min.

The serum creatine kinase (CK) level is normal in myasthenia gravis. A thyroid profile should always be examined. A heart is not involved and the electrocardiographic findings remain normal. Radiographs of the chest often reveal an enlarged thymus, but the hypertrophy is not a thymoma. It may be further defined by tomography or by CT scanning. The role of conventional muscle biopsy is limited.

Treatment: Some patients with mild myasthenia gravis do not require any treatment. Cholinesterase-inhibiting drugs are the primary therapeutic agents. Neostigmine methylsulfate (0.04 mg/kg) may be given

intramuscularly every 4 to 6 hr, but most patients tolerate oral neostigmine bromide, 0.4 mg/kg every 4–6 hr (Neostigmine 0.5 mg/mL; Prostigmin and Tilstigmin 15 mg tablet). If dysphagia is a major problem, the drug should be given about 30 minute before meals to improve swallowing. Pyridostigmine is slightly longer acting than neostigmine. Overdoses of cholinesterase inhibitors produce cholinergic crisis; atropine blocks the muscarinic effects but does not block the nicotinic effects that produce additional skeletal muscle weakness. Because of the autoimmune basis of the disease long-term steroid treatment with prednisolone may be effective. Thymectomy should be considered and may provide a cure. Treatment of hypothyroidism usually abolishes an associated myasthenia without the use of cholinesterase inhibitors or steroids. Intravenous immunoglobulin (IVIG) and plasmapheresis are effective treatment in some children.

Neonates with transient maternally transmitted myasthenia gravis require cholinesterase inhibitors for only a few days or occasionally for a few weeks, especially to allow feeding.

Complications: Children with myasthenia gravis do not tolerate neuromuscular blocking drugs, such as succinylcholine and pancuronium and may be paralyzed for weeks after a single dose. Aminoglycosides (gentamicin and others) may potentiate myasthenia and should be avoided.

Prognosis: Some patients undergo spontaneous remission after a period of months or years. Others have a permanent disease extending into adult life. Immunosuppression, thymectomy, and treatment of associated hypothyroidism may provide a cure.

Andrews PL. Autoimmune myasthenia gravis in childhood. *Semin Neurol* 2004; 24: 101–110.

Harpar CM. Congenital myasthenic syndromes. *Semin Neurol* 2004; 24: 111–123.

Sarnat HB. Neuromuscular disorders. In: Kliegman RM, Behrman RE, Jenson HB, Stanton BF (eds). *Nelson Textbook of Pediatrics*. 18th edn. Vol. 2. Philadelphia: Saunders, 2007; 2531–2567.

25.5 NEUROPATHIES

Hereditary Motor-Sensory Neuropathies

Peroneal muscular atrophy (Charcot-Marie-Tooth Disease; HMSN Type I): Most patients are asymptomatic until late childhood or early adolescence, but in some the onset of symptoms may be delayed until after the 5th decade. Children with this disorder are clumsy, falling easily, or tripping over their own feet. The peroneal and tibial nerves are the earliest and most severely affected. Muscles of the anterior compartment of the lower legs become wasted, and the legs have a characteristic stork-like contour. The muscular atrophy is accompanied by progressive weakness of dorsiflexion of the ankle and eventual footdrop. The process is bilateral but may be asymmetric. Pes cavus deformities invariably develop due to denervation of intrinsic foot muscles. Atrophy of muscles of the forearms and hands is less severe than that of lower extremities, but in advanced cases contractures of the wrist and fingers produce a claw hand. Proximal muscle weakness occurs late and is mild. Axial muscles are not involved.

The sensory involvement mainly affects large myelinated nerve fibers that conveyed propiocentive information and vibratory sense, but the threshold for pain and temperature may also increase. Nerves often become palpably enlarged. Tendon stretch reflexes are lost distally. Cranial nerves are not affected. Sphincter control remains well preserved. Autonomic neuropathy does not affect the heart, gastrointestinal tract, or bladder. Intelligence is normal. *Davidenkow syndrome* is a variant of HMSN type 1 with a scapuloperoneal distribution.

Laboratory findings and diagnosis: Motor and sensory nerve conduction velocities are greatly reduced. In new cases without a family history both parents should be examined, and nerve conduction studies should be performed. EMG and muscle biopsy are usually not required for diagnosis, but they show many cycles of denervation and reinnervation. Serum creatine kinase is normal. CSF protein may be elevated, but no cells appear in the CSF.

Sural nerve biopsy is diagnostic. Large and medium-sized myelinated fibers are reduced in number and collagen is increased and characteristic onion bulb formations of proliferated Schwann cell cytoplasm surround axons. This pathologic finding is called interstitial hypertrophic neuropathy. Extensive segmental demyelation and remyelation also occur. The definitive molecular genetic diagnosis may be made in blood.

Treatment: Stabilization of the ankles is the primary concern. External short-leg braces may be required when footdrop becomes complete. Surgical fusion of the ankle may be considered in some cases. The leg should be protected from traumatic injury. During sleep compression neuropathy may be prevented by placing soft pillows beneath or between the lower legs. No treatment is available to arrest or slow the progression.

Roussy-Levy syndrome: This syndrome is defined as a combination of HMSN type 1 and cerebellar deficit resembling Friedreich ataxia, but there is no cardiomyopathy.

Box 25.2: Toxic and metabolic neuropathies

Metals: Arsenic (insecticide, herbicide); Lead (paint, batteries, pottery); Mercury (metallic vapor); Thallium (rodenticide)

Occupational industry: Acrelamide (grouting, flocculation); carbon disulfide (solvent); cyanide; Dichlorophenoxyacetate; Dimethylaminopropionitrile; Ethylene oxide (gas sterilization); Hexacarbons (glue, solvents); Organophosphates (insecticide, petroleum additive); Polychlorinated biphenyls; Tetrachlorbiphenyl; Trichloroethylene

Drugs: Amiodarone; Chloramphenicol; Chloroquine; Cisplatin; Colchicine; Dapsone; Ethambutol; Ethanol; Gold; Hydralazine; Isoniazid; Metronidazole; Nitrofurantoin; Nucleosides (antiretroviral agents ddC, ddI, d4T); Penicillamine; Pentamidine; Phenytoin; Pyridoxine (excessive); Stilbamidine; Suramin; Thalidomide; Vincristine

Metabolic disorders: Fabry disease; Krabbe disease; Leukodystrophies; Porphyria; Tangier disease; Tyrosinemia; Uremia

Refsum disease: See section 26.3.

Toxic Neuropathies

Many chemicals, toxins, and drugs are responsible for causing peripheral neuropathies (Box 25.2).

Gordon N. Giant axonal neuropathy. *Dev Med Child Neurol* 2004; 46: 717–719.

Houlden H, Blake J, Reilly MM. Hereditary sensory neuropathies. *Curr Opin Neurol* 2004; 17: 569–577.

Mendell JR, Sahenk, Z. Painful sensory neuropathy. *N Engl J Med* 2003; 348: 1243–1255.

Pleasure D. New treatments for denerving diseases. *J Child Neurol* 2005; 20: 258–262.

Sarnat HB. Neuromuscular disorders. In: Kliegman RM, Behrman RE, Jenson HB, Stanton BF (eds). *Nelson Textbook of Pediatrics.* 18th edn. Vol. 2. Philadelphia: Saunders, 2007; 2531–2567.

25.6 FAMILIAL DYSAUTONOMIA

Familial dysautonomia (Riley-Day syndrome) is an autosomal recessive disorder that is common in Eastern European Jews. The defective gene is at the 9q31–q33 locus. The familial dysautonomia gene is identified as IKBKAP. This disease is characterized pathologically by a reduced number of small unmyelinated nerve fibers that carry pain, temperature, and taste sensations and that mediate autonomic functions.

Clinical manifestations: Infants have poor sucking and swallowing. Aspiration pneumonia may occur. Vomiting crisis may occur. Excessive sweating and blotchy erythema of the skin are common, especially at mealtime or when the child is excited. Infants are vulnerable to heatstroke. Breath-holding spells followed by syncope are common in the first 5 yr. Insensitivity to pain becomes evident in older affected children and traumatic injuries are frequent. Corneal ulcerations are common. Walking is delayed or clumsy or appears ataxic because of poor sensory feedback from muscle spindles. The ataxia is probably related more to deficient muscle spindle feedback and to vestibular dysfunction than to cerebellar involvement. Tendon stretch reflexes are absent. Scoliosis is a common problem and is progressive. Overflow tearing with crying does not normally develop until 2–3 months of age but fails to develop after that time or is severely reduced in children with familial dysautonomia. There is an increased incidence of urinary incontinence. Bradycardia and other arrhythmias may occur. Seizures occur in about 40% of patients. Puberty is often delayed, especially in girls. Under stature may occur. Speech is often slurred or nasal.

Allgrove syndrome is a clinical variant, characterized by achalasia, autonomic dysfunction, with orthostatic hypotension and altered heart rate variability and sensorimotor polyneuropathy, usually presenting in adolescence. Cholinergic dysfunction may be demonstrated.

Diagnosis: ECG shows prolonged correcting QT intervals with lack of appropriate shortening with exercise. Chest radiographs show atelectasis and pulmonary changes similar to cystic fibrosis. Urinary vanillylmandelic acid level is decreased, and homovanillic acid level is increased. Plasma level of dopamine β-hydroxylase (the enzyme that converts dopamine to epinephrine) is diminished. Sural nerve biopsy shows a decreased number of unmyelinated fibers. EEG is useful in evaluating seizures.

Slow IV infusion of norepinephrine produces an exaggerated pressor response. Hypotensive response to infusion of methacholine is increased. Intradermal injection of 1:1000 histamine phosphate fails to produce a normal axon failure and local pain is absent or diminished. Instillation of 2.5% methacholine into the conjunctival sac produces miosis in patients with familial dysautonomia and no detectable effect on a normal pupil.

Treatment: Symptomatic treatment includes management of respiratory and gastrointestinal systems, methylcellulose eye drops or topical ocular lubricants to replace tears and prevent corneal ulceration, orthopedic treatment of scoliosis and joint problems, and appropriate anticonvulsants for epilepsy. Chlorpromazine is given to control vomiting and may be given as rectal suppositories during autonomic crisis. Dehydration and electrolyte disturbances should be anticipated. Bethanechol may be an alternative drug for cyclic vomiting, which is also useful for enuresis and augment tear production. Pacemaker may be required by some children. Blood pressure monitoring is important. Protection from injuries is important because of the lack of pain as a protective mechanism. Growth velocity can be accelerated by treatment with growth hormone.

Prognosis: Most patients die in childhood, usually of chronic pulmonary failure or aspiration.

Axelord FB. Familial dysautonomia. *Muscle Nerve* 2004; 29: 352–363.

Freeman R. Autonomic peripheral neuropathy. *Lancet* 2005; 365: 1259–1270.

Sarnat HB. Neuromuscular disorders. In: Kliegman RM, Behrman RE, Jenson HB, Stanton BF (eds). *Nelson Textbook of Pediatrics*. 18th edn. Vol. 2. Philadelphia: Saunders, 2007; 2531–2567.

25.7 GUILLAIN-BARRÉ SYNDROME

Guillain-Barré Syndrome (GBS) is a postinfectious polyneuropathy involving mainly motor but sometimes also sensory and autonomic nerves.

Clinical manifestations: The syndrome affects people of all ages. The paralysis usually follows a nonspecific viral infection by about 10 days. The original infection may have caused only gastrointestinal (especially *Campylobacter jejuni*, but also *Helicobacter pylori*) or respiratory tract (especially *Mycoplasma pneumoniae*) symptoms. GBS is reported following administration of vaccines against rabies, influenza, poliomyelitis (oral), and possibly the conjugated meningococcal vaccine.

Weakness begins usually in the lower extremities and progressively involves the trunk, the upper limbs, and finally the bulbar muscles, a pattern known as *Landry ascending paralysis*. Proximal and distal muscles are involved relatively symmetrically, but asymmetry is found in 9% of patients. The onset is gradual and progresses over days or weeks. In cases with abrupt onset, tenderness on palpation and pain in muscles is common in initial stages. Children are irritable. Weakness may progress to inability or refusal to walk and later to flaccid paralysis. Paresthesias occur in some cases. The differential diagnosis of acute flaccid paralysis is shown in Sections 14.8 and 24.1).

Bulbar involvement occurs in about half of cases. Respiratory insufficiency may occur. Dysphagia and facial weakness are often impending signs of respiratory failure. There are eating difficulties and increased risk of aspiration. Some young patients may show symptoms of viral meningitis or meningo-encephalitis. The facial nerves may be involved. Extraocular muscle involvement is uncommon variant, oculomotor and other cranial neuropathies are severe early in the course of disease. Urinary incontinence or retention of urine is a complication in about 20% of patients but is usually transient. Miller-Fisher syndrome (MFS) is characterized by triad of external ophthalmoplegia, ataxia and areflexia. Papilledema is found in some cases, although visual impairment is not clinically evident. Miller-Fisher syndrome overlaps with Bicker-staff brainstem encephalitis, which also shares many features with Guillain-Barré syndrome with lower motor neuron involvement and indeed be the same basic disease.

Tendon reflexes are lost, usually early in the course of disease, but may be preserved until later. The autonomic nervous system may also be involved in some cases. Cardiovascular involvement includes blood pressure and cardiac rate changes, postural hypotension, episodes of profound bradycardia, and occasional asystole. A few patients require insertion of a temporary venous cardiac pacemaker.

Chronic relapsing polyradiculoneuropathy (also known as chronic inflammatory demyelinating polyradiculoneuropathy) or chronic unremitting polyradiculoneuropathy are chronic varieties of Guillain-Barré syndrome that recur intermittently or do not improve for a period of months or years. About 7% of children with Guillain-Barré syndrome suffer an acute relapse. Patients are usually severely weak and may have a flaccid tetraplegia with or without bulbar and respiratory muscle involvement.

Congenital Guillain-Barré syndrome presents as generalized hypotonia, weakness, and areflexia in an affected neonate, fulfilling all electrophysiologic and cerebrospinal fluid (CSF) criteria, in the absence of maternal neuromuscular disease. Treatment may not be required. There is gradual improvement over the first few months and by one year of age complete recovery.

Laboratory findings and diagnosis: The diagnosis of GBS is based primarily on the clinical evaluation. Confirmatory laboratory studies by cerebrospinal fluid (CSF) examination, The CSF protein is elevated to more than twice the upper limit of normal, glucose level is normal, and there is no pleocytosis. Fewer than 10 white blood cells/mm^3 are found. The results of bacterial cultures are negative and viral cultures rarely isolate specific viruses. The dissociation between high CSF protein and a lack of cellular response (*cytoalbumin dissociation*) with an acute or subacute polyneuropathy is diagnostic of Guillain-Barré syndrome.

Motor nerve conduction velocities are greatly reduced, and sensory conduction time is often slow. Electromyography (EMG) demonstrates evidence of acute denervation of muscle. Serum creatine kinase (CK) level may be mildly elevated or normal. Antiganglioside antibodies, mainly against GM1 and GD1, are sometimes elevated in the serum in Guillain-Barré syndrome. Muscle biopsy specimens appear normal in early stages and show evidence of denervation atrophy in chronic stages. Sural nerve biopsy tissue shows segmental demyelination, focal inflammation, and wallerian degeneration. Muscle biopsy and sural nerve biopsy are not usually required for diagnosis. Serological testing for *Campylobacter* and *Helicobacter* infections helps establish the cause if results are positive but does not alter the course of treatment. MRIs are not routinely indicated in the evaluation of GBS.

Treatment: Patients in early stages should be admitted to the hospital for observation because the ascending paralysis may rapidly involve respiratory muscles during the next 24 hr. Patients with slow progression may simply be observed for stabilization and spontaneous remission without treatment. Rapidly progressive ascending paralysis is treated with intravenous immunoglobulin (IVIG 0.4 g/kg/day for 5 consecutive days). Plasmapheresis, and/or immunosuppressive drugs are alternatives, if IVIG is ineffective. Combined administration of immuno-globulin and interferon is effective in some patients. Supportive care, such as respiratory support, prevention of decubitus ulcers in children with flaccid quadriplegia, and treatment of cardiac rhythm disturbances and secondary bacterial infections is important. Treatment of *Campylocacter jejuni* infection if present is not necessary, because it is self limited, and the use of antibiotics does not alter the course of the polyneuropathy. For the treatment of chronic neuropathic pain following GBS, gabapentin is more effective than carbamazepine.

Chronic relapsing polyradioneuropathy or unremitting chronic neuropathy is also treated with IVIG. Plasma exchange sometimes required. Remission in these cases may be sustained, but relapses may occur within days, weeks or after months, which usually respond to another course of plasmapheresis.

Prognosis: The clinical course is usually benign, and spontaneous recovery begins within 2–3 wk. Most patients with GBS achieve a full and functional recovery although some are left with residual weakness. Improvement usually follows inverse to the direction of involvement, with recovery of bulbar function first and lower extremity weakness resolving last. Bulbar and respiratory muscle involvement may lead to death if the syndrome is not recognized and treated. The tendon reflexes are usually the last function to recover. Three clinical features are predictive of poor outcome with sequelae: cranial nerve involvement, intubation, and maximum disability at the time of presentation.

Jackson AH, Barquis GD, Shah BL. Congenital Guillain-Barré syndrome. *J Child Neurol* 1996; 11: 407–410.

Ramachandran R, Kuruvilla A. Guillain-Barré syndrome in children and adolescents: A retrospective analysis. *J Indian Med Assc* 2004; 102: 480–482.

Rees JH, Soudain SE, Gregson NA, Hughes RAC. Campylobacter jejuni infection and Guillain- Barré syndrome. *N Engl J Med* 1995;333:1374–1379.

Sarnat HB. Neuromuscular disorders. In: Kliegman RM, Behrman RE, Jenson HB, Stanton BF (eds). *Nelson Textbook of Pediatrics*. 18th edn. Vol. 2. Philadelphia: Saunders, 2007; 2531–2567.

Yildizdas Dincer. Guillain-Barré Syndrome. In: Mathur GP, Mathur Sarla (eds). *Current Trends in Pediatrics*. Vol 1. Delhi: Academa Publishers, 2005; 367–380.

25.8 BELL PALSY

Bell palsy is an acute unilateral facial nerve palsy that is not associated with other cranial nerve neuropathies or brain-stem dysfunction (*see* Fig. 25.4 in CD). It is a common disorder at all ages from infancy through adolescence. Bell palsy usually develops abruptly about 2 wk after a systemic viral infection (Box 25.3). Active or reactivation of herpes simplex or varicella-zoster virus may be the most common cause of Bell palsy.

Clinical manifestations: The upper and lower portions of the face are paretic, and the corner of the mouth droops. Patients are unable to close the eye on the involved side and may develop an exposure keratitis at night. Taste on the anterior ⅔ of the tongue is lost on the involved side, in about ½ of cases; it will establish the anatomic limits of the lesion as being proximal or distal to the chorda tympani branch of

---

Box 25.3: Causes of acute peripheral facial palsy

Common: Herpes simplex virus type 1; Varicella-zoster virus
Less common infections: Otitis media ±cholesteatoma; Lyme disease; Epstein-Barr virus; Cytomegalovirus; Mumps; Human herpes virus 6; Intranasal influenza vaccine; Mycoplasma
Other less common conditions: Trauma; Tumor; Hypertension; Guillain-Barré syndrome; Sarcoidosis; Ribavirin; Interferon-α therapy for hepatitis C.

---

the facial nerve. Numbness or parasthesias do not usually occur, but ipsilateral numbness of the face is reported in a few cases and probably is due to viral (especially herpes) or postviral immunologic impairment of the trigeminal and facial nerves.

Treatment: Oral prednisolone (1 mg/kg/day for 1 wk, then a 1 wk taper) started within the first 3–5 days results in improved outcome. Because of the recovery of the herpes simplex virus in the neural fluid of the 7th nerve, some also recommend adding acyclovir to the prednisolone therapy. Physiotherapy to the facial muscles is recommended in some chronic cases with poor recovery. Protection of the cornea with methylcellulose eye drops or an ocular lubricant is especially important at night.

Prognosis: The prognosis is excellent. More than 85% of cases recover spontaneously with no residual facial weakness; another 10% have mild focal weakness as a sequela; only 5% suffer from permanent facial weakness.

Facial palsy at birth: This is usually a compression neuropathy from forceps application during delivery and recovers spontaneously in a few days or weeks in most cases. Congenital absence of the depressor angularis oris muscle causes facial asymmetry, especially when an affected infant cries; it is a cosmetic defect that does not interfere with feeding. Infants with Möbius syndrome may have bilateral or, less commonly, unilateral facial palsy; this syndrome is usually caused by symmetric calcified infarcts in the tegmentum of the pons and medulla oblongata during mid-gestation or late fetal life.

Gilden DH. Bell's palsy. *N Engl J Med* 2004; 351: 1323–1331.

Salinas RA, Alvarez G, Ferreira J. Corticosteroids for Bell's palsy (idiopathic facial paralysis). *Cochrane Database Syst Rev* 2004; 4: CD001942.

Sarnat HB. Neuromuscular disorders. In: Kliegman RM, Behrman RE, Jenson HB, Stanton BF (eds). *Nelson Textbook of Pediatrics*. 18th edn. Vol. 2. Philadelphia: Saunders, 2007; 2531–2567.

25.9 MUSCULOSKELETAL PAIN SYNDROMES

Musculoskeletal pain affects the muscles, ligaments and tendons, along with the bones. It is common in children, affecting 10–20% of school children. The common symptoms are pain, body ache, fatigue and sleep disturbances. Pain may vary from a single extremity to generalize without tenderness. Pain cannot respond to the NSAID and analgesic agents. Physical findings are normal and no specific laboratory findings. The diagnosis of musculoskeletal pain syndromes can be made by exclusion the causes of pain by repeated physical examinations and laboratory testing. The differential diagnosis include autonomic dysfunction, inflammatory myositis, muscular dystrophies, or neurologic disease, costochondritis, pericarditis, osteoid osteoma, ankylosing spondyloarthropathy, physical and sexual abuse, benign hypermobility syndrome and "Growing pains". Growing pains is described as intermittent pains in both legs without inflammation mainly occur at night, last several hours, are self-limited. Complications include impaired physical fitness, decreased socialization, prolonged school absences, and depression.

Treatment include cognitive restructuring, thought stopping, distraction, relaxation, and self-reward in an approach that combines restoration of a normal sleep pattern and activities of daily living, rehabilitation strategies including exercise for fatigue, and judicious use of nonsteroidal anti-inflammatory or analgesic medications.

Anthony KK, Schanberg LE. Pediatric pain syndromes and management of pain in children and adolescents with rheumatic disease. *Pediatr Clin North Am* 2005; 52: 611–639.

Goodyear-Smith F, Arroll B. Growing pains. *BMJ* 2006; 333: 456–457.

Miller ML. Musculoskeletal pain syndromes. In: Kliegman RM, Behrman RE, Jenson HB, Stanton BF (eds). *Nelson Textbook of Pediatrics.* 18th edn. Vol. 1. Philadelphia: Saunders, 2007; 1049–1051.

Metabolic Disorders

26.1 AN APPROACH TO INBORN ERRORS OF METABOLISM

Many childhood conditions are caused by gene mutations that encode specific protein. These mutations can result in the alteration of primary protein structure or the amount of protein synthesized. The functional ability of protein, whether it is an enzyme, receptor, transport vehicle, membrane or structural element, may be relatively or seriously compromised. These hereditary biochemical disorders are collectively termed inborn errors of metabolism. An inborn error of metabolism should be considered in a child with one or more clinical manifestations:

1. Unexplained mental retardation, developmental delay or regression, motor deficits, or convulsions
2. Unusual odor, particularly during an acute illness (Table 26.1)
3. Intermittent episodes of unexplained vomiting, acidosis, mental deterioration, or coma
4. Hypoglycemia
5. Hypocalcemia
6. Hepatomegaly
7. Renal stones
8. Muscle weakness
9. Cardiomyopathy

Table 26.1: Inborn errors of amino acids metabolism associated with abnormal odor

Inborn error of metabolism	Urine odor
Glutaric acidemia (type II)	Sweaty feet, acrid
Hawkinsinuria	Swimming pool
Isovaleric acidemia	Sweaty feet, acrid
Maple syrup urine disease	Maple syrup
Hypermethioninemia	Boiled cabbage
Multiple carboxylase deficiency	Tomcat urine
Oasthouse urine disease	Hops-like
Phenylketonuria	Mousy or musty
Trimethylaminuria	Rotting fish
Tyrosinemia	Boiled cabbage, rancid butter

Neonatal period: Inborn errors of metabolism causing clinical features in the neonatal period are usually severe and if not treated properly often death occurs. Infants with metabolic disorders are usually normal at birth. An inborn error of metabolism should be considered in the differential diagnosis of a severely ill neonatal infant, and special studies should be undertaken if the index suspicion is high. Initial findings include or more of the findings such as poor feeding, vomiting, lethargy, convulsions (not responsive to intravenous glucose or calcium), and coma. Exclude first the infection and investigate for the diagnosis of metabolic disorder. Obtain blood ammonia, pH and CO_2. If blood ammonia level is high and blood pH and CO_2 is normal, it is due to urea cycle defects. In case blood ammonia level is normal and blood pH and CO_2 with normal anion gap, it is due to aminoacidopathies or galactosemia. If blood ammonia level is normal and blood pH and CO_2 with high anion gap, it is due to acidosis (organic acidemias). A specific diagnosis may be established by measurement of abnormal metabolites in body fluids, by assay of the specific enzyme activity, or by identification of the mutant gene. Specific diagnosis, even in an infant in whom death seems inevitable, is of great importance for genetic counseling of the family. Every effort should be made to determine the diagnosis while the infant is alive.

Children after the neonatal period: Most newborn infants exhibit mild clinical manifestations of inborn errors of metabolism and may be attributed to perinatal insults. These children may escape detection during the neonatal period, and the diagnosis may be delayed for months or even years. An inborn error of metabolism should be considered in a child with one or more clinical manifestations mentioned earlier. Occasionally, a peculiar odor may offer an invaluable aid to the diagnosis (Table 26.1).

Rezvani I. An approach to inborn errors of metabolism . In: Kliegman RM, Behrman RE, Jenson HB, Stanton BF (eds). *Nelson Textbook of Pediatrics.* 18th edn. Vol 1. Philadelphia: Saunders, 2007; 527-529.

26.2 DEFECTS IN METABOLISM OF AMINO ACIDS

Phenylalanine

Phenylalanine is an essential amino acid. Dietary phenylalanine not utilized for protein synthesis is normally degraded by way of the tyrosine pathway. The hyperphenylalaninemias are a group of disorders resulting from impaired conversion of phenylalanine to tyrosine. Normally, the major metabolic pathway of phenylalanine involves the enzyme phenylalanine hydroxylase, which is found in appreciable amount in the liver and kidneys. Deficiency of the enzyme phenyl hydroxylase or of its cofactor tetrahydrobiopterin causes accumulation of phenylalanine in body fluids and the central nervous system.

Classic phenylketonuria (PKU): Severe hyperphenylalaninemia (plasma phenylalanine levels >20 mg/dl or >1,200 µmole/L), if untreated, results in the development of signs and symptoms of classic PKU. The affected infant is normal at birth. Mental retardation may develop gradually and may not be evident for the 1st few months. Vomiting sometimes very severe may be an early symptom; other findings are seborrheic or eczematoid rash, unpleasant odor of phenylacetic acid, which has been described as musty or mousey. These children also have microcephaly, prominent maxilla with widely spaced teeth, enamel hypoplasia, growth retardation. Older untreated children become hyperactive, with purposeless movements, rhythmic rocking, or athetosis.

Milder forms of Hyperphenylalaninemia, Non-PKU Hyperphenylalaninemias: Infants in whom initial plasma concentrations of phenylalanine are above normal (2 mg/dl, 120 µmole/L) but <20 mg/dl (<1,200 µmole/L). Clinically, these infants may remain asymptomatic, but progressive brain damage may occur gradually with age. ***Diagnosis:*** Early diagnosis is only possible by mass screening of all newborn infants because of the gradual development of clinical manifestations of hyperphenylalaninemia. The diagnosis should be confirmed by quantitative measurement of plasma pheylalanine.

The **FeCl$_3$ test** is both qualitative and non-specific; however, it is useful for monitoring the effectiveness of dietary therapy of patients with PKU. This test should not be used for screening purposes. The color reaction is when 10% FeCl$_3$ solution is added to patients fresh urine sample, it results in an emerald green color, and it is not stable but color disappears in 20 minutes.

Neonatal Screening for Hyperphenylalaninemia: The bacterial inhibition assay of **Guthrie's test** has been replaced by more precise and quantitative methods (fluorometric and tandem mass spectrometry). All these methods require a few drops of blood, which are placed on a filter paper. Blood phenylalanine in affected infants with PKU may rise to diagnostic levels as early as 4 hr after birth even in the absence of protein feeding. Therefore, it is recommended that the blood for screening be obtained in the 1st 24–48 hr of life after feeding protein to reduce the possibility of false negative results, especially in the milder form of this condition.

Treatment: The goal of therapy is to reduce phenylalanine in the body; formulas low in or free of this amino acid are available commercially. The diet should be started as soon as diagnosis is established. It is generally accepted that infants with persistent plasma levels of phenylalanine > 6 mg/dl (> 600 µmole/L) should be treated with a phenylalanine-restricted diet similar to that for classic PKU. No dietary restriction is currently recommended for infants whose phenylalanine levels are between 2 and 6 mg/dl (<120–360 µmole/L). Plasma concentrations of phenylalanine in treated patients should be maintained as close to normal as possible [between 2 and 6 mg/dll (<120–360 µmole/L)] at least to the 1st 12 yr of life. The current recommendation is that all patients be kept on a phenylalanine-restricted diet for life. Overtreatment may lead to phenylalanine deficiency manifested by lethargy, failure to thrive, anorexia, anemia, rashes, diarrhea, and even death.

Hereditary progressive dystonia, autosomal dominant DOPA-Responsive dystonia, Segawa disease: This rare form of dystonia, 1st described in Japan, is caused by guanosine triphosphate (GTP) cyclohydrolase deficiency. It is inherited as an autosomal dominant trait and is more common in females than males (4:1). Clinical manifestations usually occur around 5–6 yr of age and are heralded by dystonia of the lower limbs, which may spread to all extremities within a few years. Early development is normal. Symptoms usually have diurnal variation, becoming worse by the end of the day and improving with sleep. Parkinsonian signs may also be present or develop subsequently with advancing age.

Diagnosis may be confirmed by reduced levels of BH_4 and neopterin in the spinal fluid, by measurement of the enzyme activity, and by identification of the gene defect in children without hyperphenylalaninemia. Clinically, the condition should be differentiated from other causes of dystonias and childhood Parkinsonism, especially tyrosine hydroxylase and aromatic amino acid decarboxylase deficiencies. The striking diurnal pattern of dystonia is an important clinical finding in favor of GTP cyclohydrolase deficiency.

Treatment with L-dopa in conjunction with a peripheral dopa decarboxylase inhibitor usually produces dramatic improvement.

Tyrosine

Tyrosine is obtained from ingested proteins and synthesized endogenously from phenylalanine, is used for protein synthesis and is a precursor of dopamine, norepinephrine, epinephrine, melanin and thyroxine. Excess tyrosine is metabolized to carbon dioxide and water.

Tyrosine hydroxylase deficiency (infantile parkin-sonism, autosomal recessive dopa responsive dystonia): This condition is inherited as an autosomal recessive trait. The gene for tyrosine hydroxylase is mapped to chromosome 11p. Tyrosine hydroxylase enzyme catalyzes the formation of L-dopa from tyrosine; deficiency of this enzyme results in dystonia and Parkinsonism in children. Diagnosis should be considered in any patient with dystonia and Parkinsonism. *Diagnosis* is established by the laboratory findings and gene study. Laboratory findings include reduced levels of dopamine and its metabolite homovanillic acid (HVA). *Treatment* with L-dopa results in a dramatic response.

Albinism is caused by defects in the biosynthesis and distribution of melanin. Melanin is synthesized by melanocytes from tyrosine by the enzyme **tyrosinase**. The end products are two pigments: *pheomelanin*, which is yellow-red pigment; and *eumelanin*, a brown-black pigment. Many clinical forms have been identified based on the distribution of albinism in the body and the types of gene mutation (*see* Section 30.3).

Methionine

Homocystinuria due to Cystathionine β-Synthase (CBS) Deficiency (Classic Homocystinuria) is inherited as an autosomal recessive trait. The gene for cystathionine β-synthase is located on chromosome 12q22.3. Infants are normal at birth. During infancy clinical manifestations are nonspecific and may include failure to thrive and developmental delay. The diagnosis is usually made after 3 yr of age, when subluxation of the ocular lens (ectopia lentis) occurs. This causes severe myopia and iridodonesis (quivering of the iris). Other clinical findings include progressive mental retardation, psychiatric and behavioral disorders, skeletal abnormalities resembling Marfan syndrome and thromboembolic episodes involving both large and small vessels especially those of the brain. The risk of thromboembolism increases after surgical procedures. The *diagnosis* may be established by assay of the enzyme in liver biopsy specimens, cultured fibroblasts, or phytohemagglutinin-stimulated lymphocytes or by DNA analysis. *Prenatal diagnosis* is feasible by performing an enzyme assay of cultured amniotic cells or chorionic villi or by DNA analysis. *Treatment* with high doses of vitamin B_6 (200–1,000 mg/24 hr) causes dramatic improvement in most patients who are responsive to this therapy. Some patients may not respond because of folate depletion; a patient should not be considered unresponsive to vitamin B_6 until folic acid (1–5 mg/24 hr) has been added to the treatment regimen.

Cysteine/Cystine

Cysteine is a sulfur-containing nonessential amino acid that is synthesized from methionine. In the presence of oxygen, two molecules of cysteine are oxidized to form cystine. The most common disorders of cysteine/cystine metabolism are cystinuria and cystinosis. *Cystinosis* is a systemic disease caused by a defect in the metabolism of cystine, which results in accumulation of cystine crystals in most of the major organs of the body, notably the kidneys, liver, eye, and brain. Three clinical patterns have been described.

1. *Infantile or nephrogenic stenosis* is the most severe form of the disease present in the 2 yr of life with severe tubular dysfunction and growth failure. If the disease is not treated, the children develop end stage renal disease by the end of their 1st decade.
2. A *milder adolescent form* is characterized by less severe tubular abnormalities and a slower progression to renal failure.
3. A *benign adult form* with no renal involvement exists.

Clinical manifestations: Patients with nephropathic cystinosis present with pronounced tubular dysfunction and Fanconi syndrome, including polyuria and polydipsia, growth failure, and rickets. Retinopthy and impaired visual acuity, hypothyroidism, hepatosplenomegaly and delayed sexual maturation occur. *Diagnosis* of cystinosis is suggested by the detection of cystine crystals in the cornea and confirmed by measurement of increased leukocyte cystine content. Prenatal diagnosis is available for at-risk families. *Treatment* should be directed at correcting the metabolic abnormalities associated with Fanconi syndrome or chronic renal failure. Cysteamine is the drug of choice, which binds to cystine and converts it to cysteine. Cysteamine eye-drops is required for ocular treatment. Early initiation of the drug may prevent or delay deterioration of renal function. Patients with growth failure that does not improve with cysteamine may benefit from growth hormone treatment.

Cystinuria is an autosomal recessive disorder and accounts for 1% of renal calculi (cystine calculi) in children, which is due to the low solubility of cystine. The patients usually have acidic urine, which is responsible for higher rate of precipitation. The sulfur content of cystine gives these stones faint radiopaque appearance. *Treatment* involves reducing the concentration of cystine, by taking large amount of water, and increasing the solubility of cystine by maintaining alkaline urine (urinary pH >7.5) with sodium bicarbonate or sodium citrate. D-penicilline is a chelating agent that binds to cysteine or homocystine, increasing the solubility of the product. It is effective in dissolving cystine stones, although poorly tolerated by many patients. N-acetylcysteine appears to have low toxicity and may be effective in controlling cystinuria. Captopril can be used.

Tryptophan is an essential amino acid and a precursor for nicotinic acid and serotonin. *Hartnup disorder* causes disturbance in tryptophan absorption. This is an autosomal recessive disorder, named after the 1st reported family. There is a defect in the transport of monoamino-monocarboxylic amino acids (neutral amino acids) by the intestinal mucosa and renal tubules. Most children with Hartnup defect remain asymptomatic. The major clinical manifestation in symptomatic patient is cutaneous photosensitivity. The skin becomes rough and red after moderate exposure to the sun, and with greater exposure, a pellagra-like rash may develop. Some patients may have intermittent ataxia which may last a few days and usually recovers spontaneously. Most children diagnosed with Hartnup disorder by neonatal screening have remained asymptomatic. *Diagnosis* is established by the characteristic intermittent nature of symptoms and urinary findings of aminoaciduria, which is restricted to neutral amino acids (alanine, serine, threonine, valine, leucine, isoleucine, phenylalanine, tyrosine, tryptophan, histidine). *Treatment* with nicotinic acid or nicotinamide (50–300 mg/24 hr) and a high protein diet results in a favorable response in symptomatic patients.

Valine, leucine, isoleucine, and related organic acidemias: These disorders commonly cause metabolic acidosis, which usually occurs in the 1st few days of life.

Maple syrup urine disease (MSUD): Decarboxylation of leucine, isoleucine and valine is accomplished by a complex enzyme system (branched-chain α-ketoacid dehydrogenase) using thiamine pyrophosphate (vitamin B_1) as a coenzyme. Deficiency of this enzyme system causes MSUD, named after the sweet odor of maple syrup found in body fluids, especially urine. Based on clinical findings and response to thiamine administration, five phenotypes of MSUD have been identified (classic, intermediate, mild, thiamine responsive, and due to a deficiency of E3 subunit [dihydrolipoyl dehydrogenase]). All forms of MSUD are inherited as an autosomal recessive trait. In the classic MSUD, the infants appear normal at birth but develop frequent vomiting and failure to thrive in the 1st wk of life; lethargy and coma may ensue within a few days. Periods of hypertonicity and muscular rigidity with severe opisthotonos may alternate with bouts of flaccidity. Cerebral edema may be present; convulsions occur in most infants. Hypoglycemia is common, but correction of the blood glucose concentration does not improve the clinical condition. Without treatment, death usually occurs in the 1st few weeks or months of life. *Diagnosis* is often suspected because of the peculiar odor of maple syrup found in urine, sweat, and cerumen. It is usually confirmed by amino acid analysis showing marked elevations in plasma levels of leucine, isoleucine, valine, and alloisoleucine (a strereoisomer of isoleucine not normally found in blood of normal persons, but is typically found in MSUD) and depression of alanine. Early detection of MSUD is feasible by mass screening of newborn infants. *Treatment* of acute attack is aimed at hydration and quick removal of the branched-chain amino acids and their metabolites from the tissues and body fluids. This is carried out effectively by peritoneal dialysis or hemodialysis. Providing sufficient calories and nutrients intravenously or orally should reverse the patient's catabolic state. Cerebral edema may need to be treated with mannitol, frusemide, or hypertonic saline. Infants should be fed on a diet low in branched chain amino acids. Synthetic formulas devoid of leucine, isoleucine and valine are available commercially. Because these amino acids cannot be synthesized endogenously, small amounts of them should be added to the diet. Patients with MSUD should remain on the diet for the rest of their lives. Mental and neurologic deficits are common sequelae. Some children (thiamine-responsive MSUD) with mild or intermediate forms of MSUD, who are treated with high doses of thiamine (10 mg/24 hr, while some as much as 200 mg/24 hr) for 3 days have dramatic clinical and biochemical improvement.

Multiple carboxylase deficiencies (Defects in utilization of Biotin): Biotin, a water-soluble vitamin, is a cofactor for all four carboxylase enzymes in humans: pyruvate carboxylase, acetyl CoA carboxylase, propionyl CoA carboxylase, and 3-methylcrotonyl CoA carboxylase. The latter two are involved in the metabolic pathways of leucine, isoleucine, and valine. Deficiencies in this enzyme or in biotinidase result in malfunction of all the carboxylases and in organic academia.

Multiple carboxylase deficiency due to dietary biotin deficiency: Acquired deficiency of biotin may occur in infants receiving total parenteral nutrition without added biotin in patients receiving prolonged anticonvulsant drugs (phenytoin, primidone, carbamazepine) or in children with short bowel syndrome or chronic diarrhea who are receiving formulas low in biotin. Excessive ingestion of raw eggs may also cause biotin deficiency because the protein avidin in egg white binds biotin and makes it unavailable for absorption. Infants with biotin deficiency develop dermatitis, alopecia, and candidal skin infections.

Biotinidase deficiency (multiple carboxylase deficiency-juvenile or late form): The absence of biotinidase results in biotin deficiency. The gene for biotinidase is located on chromosome 3p25 and many disease-causing mutations have been identified in different families. Clinical manifestations are similar to those seen in infants with holocarboxylase synthetase deficiency, but symptoms appear late. Laboratory findings and the pattern of organic acids in the body fluids resemble those associated with holocarboxylase synthetase deficiency. *Diagnosis* can be established by measurement of the enzyme activity in the serum. *Prenatal diagnosis* is possible by the measurement of the enzyme activity in the amniotic cells or by identification of the mutant gene. **Treatment** with biotin (5–20 mg/24 hr) results in a dramatic clinical and biochemical response.

Glutamic Acid

Glutathione (γ-glutamylcysteinylglycine) is the major product of glutamic acid in the body. This is synthesized and degraded through a complex cycle called the γ-glutamyl cycle. The common consequence of glutathione deficiency is hemolytic anemia. Glutathione also participates in amino acid transport across the cell membrane through the γ-glutamyl cycle.

Glutathione synthetase deficiency: Three forms (severe, moderate, and mild) of this condition have been reported. In all forms, patients have hemolytic anemia secondary to glutathione deficiency. All forms of the condition are inherited as an autosomal recessive trait. The gene for this enzyme is located on chromosome 20q11.2. *Treatment* of acute attack includes hydration, correction of acidosis (by infusion of sodium bicarbonate), and measures to correct anemia and hyperbilirubinemia. Chronic administration of alkali is usually needed indefinitely. Administration of large doses of vitamins C and E has been recommended. Drugs and oxidants that are known to cause hemolysis and stressful catabolic states should be avoided. Oral administration of glutathione analogs has been tried with variable success. In mild form treatment is that of hemolytic anemia and avoidance of drugs and oxidants that can trigger the hemolytic process.

Pyridoxine (vitamin B₆) dependency with seizures: This autosomal recessive condition is due to GABA deficiency in the brain, which is presumably caused by decreased activity of glutamic acid decarboxylase (GAD). Linkage studies have mapped the condition to the long arm of chromosome 5q31.2. The main *clinical manifestation* of this condition is seizures, which usually occur in the 1st few hours of life and are unresponsive to conventional anticonvulsant therapy. *Laboratory studies* have revealed increased glutamate and decreased GABA levels in the brain and in the spinal fluid (*see* Section 24.8).

Urea Cycle and Hyperammonemia

The catabolic pathway of amino acid leads to the production of free ammonia. Ammonia is as such very toxic to central nervous system. Ammonia is detoxified to urea through a series of reactions known as the Krebs-Henseleit or urea cycle. In addition to genetic defects of the urea cycle enzymes, a marked increase in plasma level of ammonia is observed in other inborn errors of metabolism.

Clinical manifestations of hyperammonemia: The affected *neonate* is normal at birth but becomes symptomatic within a few days of protein feeding. Refusal to eat and vomiting, tachypnea, and lethargy quickly progress to a deep coma. Convulsions are common. Physical examination may reveal hepatomegaly in addition to the neurologic signs of deep coma. In *infants and older children* acute hyperammonemia is manifested by vomiting and neurologic abnormalities such as ataxia, mental confusion, agitation, and irritability. These manifestations may alternate with periods of lethargy and somnolence that may progress to coma.

Routine *laboratory studies* show no specific findings when hyperammonemia is due to defects of the urea cycle enzymes. Blood urea nitrogen is usually low. Serum pH is usually normal or mildly elevated. In infants with organic acidemias, hyperammonemia is commonly associated with severe acidosis. Newborn infants with hyperammonemia are often misdiagnosed as having sepsis; they usually die without a correct diagnosis. CT may reveal cerebral edema. It is imperative to measure the plasma ammonia levels in any ill infant whose clinical manifestations cannot be explained by an obvious infection.

Diagnosis: The main criterion for diagnosis is hyperammonemia. The plasma ammonia concentration in the ill infant is usually >200 μmole/L (normal values <35 μmole/L). *Treatment of acute hyperammonemia:* Acute hyperammonemia should be treated promptly and vigorously. The goal of therapy is to remove ammonia from the body and to provide adequate calories and essential amino acids to stop further breakdown of endogenous proteins (Table 26.2). There may be considerable lag between the normalization of ammonia and an improvement in the neurologic status of the patient. Several days may be needed before the infant becomes fully alert.

Long-term therapy: Once the infant is alert, therapy should be tailored to the underlying cause of the

Table 26.2: Treatment of acute hyperammonemia in an infant

1. Provide adequate calories, fluid, and electrolytes intravenously (10% glucose and intravenous lipids 1 g/kg/24 hr). Add minimal amounts of protein preferably as a mixture of essential amino acids (0.25 g/kg/24 hr) during 1st 24 hr of therapy.
2. Give priming doses of the following compounds: To be added to 20 ml/kg of 10% glucose and infuse IV within 1–2 hr
   Sodium benzoate 250 mg/kg (5.5 g/nm^2)*
   Sodium phenylacetate 250 mg/kg (5.5 g/nm^2)*
   Arginine hydrochloride 200–600 mg/kg (4.0–12.0 g/nm^2) as a 10% solution
3. Continue infusion of sodium benzoate* (250–500 mg/kg/24 hr), sodium phenylacetate* (250–500 mg/kg/24 hr), and arginine (200–600 mg/kg/24 hr[1]) following the above priming dose. These compounds should be added to the daily intravenous fluid.
4. Initiate peritoneal dialysis or hemodialysis if above treatment fails to produce an appreciable decrease in plasma ammonia.

*These compounds are usually prepared as a 1–2% solution for intravenous use. Sodium from these drugs should be included as part of the daily sodium requirement.
[1]The higher dose is recommended in the treatment of patients with citrullinemia and argininosuccinic aciduria. Arginine is not recommended in patients with arginase deficiency and in those whose hyperammonemia is secondary to organic academia.

hyperammonemia. In general, all patients require some degree of protein restriction (1–2 g/kg/24 hr) regardless of the enzymatic defect. In patients with defects in the urea cycle, chronic administration of benzoate (250–500 mg/kg/24 hr), phenylacetate (250–500 mg/kg/24 hr), and arginine (200–400 mg/kg/24 hr), or citrulline (in patients with OTC deficiency, 200–400 mg/kg/24 hr) is effective in maintaining blood ammonia levels within the normal range. Phenylbuterate may be used in place of phenylacetate, because the patient and the family may not accept the latter owing to its offensive odor. Carnitine supplementation is recommended because benzoate and phenylacetate may cause carnitine depletion, but the clinical benefit of this compound is not yet proved. In a few patients skin lesions resembling acrodermatitis enteropathica have been noted with different types of urea cycle defects, presumably due to deficiency of essential amino acids, especially arginine. Catabolic states triggering hyperammonemia should be avoided.

Aspartic Acid (Canavan Disease)

N-acetylaspartic acid, a derivative of aspartic acid, is synthesized in the brain and is found in a high concentration. Its function is unknown, but excessive amounts of *N*-acetylaspartic acid in urine and deficiency of the enzyme aspartoacylase that cleaves the *N*-acetyl group from *N*-acetylaspartic acid is associated with Canavan disease. Canavan disease is an autosomal recessive disorder, characterized by spongy degeneration of the white matter of the brain that leads to a severe form of leukodystrophy. It is more prevalent in individuals of Ashkenazi Jewish descent than in other ethnic groups.

Clinical manifestations: Infants usually appear normal at birth and may not manifest symptoms of the disease until 3–6 mo of age, when they develop progressive macrocephaly, severe hypotonia, and persistent head lag. As the infant grows older, delayed milestones become evident. These children become hyperreflexic and hypertonic; joint stiffness may be encountered. As they grow older, seizures and optic atrophy develop. Feeding difficulties, poor weight gain, and gastroesophageal reflux may occur in the 1st yr of life; swallowing deteriorates in the 2nd and 3rd yr of life, and nasogastric feeding or permanent gastrostomy may be required. Most patients die in the 1st decade of life; with improved nursing care, they may survive through the 2nd decade.

Diagnosis: CT scans and MRI reveal diffuse white matter degeneration, primarily in the cerebral hemispheres, with less involvement in the cerebellum and brainstem. The differential diagnosis of Canavan disease should include Alexander disease, which is another leukodystrophy with macrocephaly. Progression is usually slow in Alexander disease; hypotonia is not as pronounced as it is in Canavan disease. Brain biopsy shows spongy degeneration of the myelin fibers, astrocytic swelling, and elongated mitochondria. Definitive diagnosis can be established by finding elevated amounts of *N*-acetylaspartic acid in the urine or blood. A deficiency of aspartoacylase can be found in cultured skin fibroblasts.

Treatment and prevention: There is no specific treatment available. Feeding problems and seizures should be treated on an individual basis. Genetic counseling, carrier testing, and prenatal diagnosis are the only methods of prevention.

Dell KM, Avner ED. Renal tubular acidosis. In: Kliegman RM, Behrman RE, Jenson HB, Stanton BF (eds). *Nelson Textbook of Pediatrics.* 18th edn. Vol 2. Philadelphia: Saunders, 2007; 2197–2200.

Elder JS. Urinary lithiasis. In: Kliegman RM, Behrman RE, Jenson HB, Stanton BF (eds). *Nelson Textbook of Pediatrics.* 18th edn. Vol 2. Philadelphia: Saunders, 2007;2267–71.

Grossse SD, Dezateux C. Newborn screening for inherited metabolic disease. *Lancet* 2007;369:5–6.

Matalon R. Aspartic Acid (Canavan disease). In: Kliegman RM, Behrman RE, Jenson HB, Stanton BF (eds). *Nelson Textbook of Pediatrics.* 18th edn. Vol 1. Philadelphia: Saunders, 2007;563–7.

Mitchell GA, Rezvani I. Tyrosine. In: Kliegman RM, Behrman RE, Jenson HB, Stanton BF (eds). *Nelson Textbook of Pediatrics.* 18th edn. Vol 1. Philadelphia: Saunders, 2007;532–6.

Njalsson R. Glutathione synthetase deficiency. *Cell Mol Life Sci* 2005;62:1939–45.

Phornphurkul C, Introne WJ, Perry MB, et al. Natural history of alkaptonuria. *N Engl J Med* 2002;347:2111–21.

Rezvani I. An approach to inborn errors of metabolism . In: Kliegman RM, Behrman RE, Jenson HB, Stanton BF (eds). *Nelson Textbook of Pediatrics.* 18th edn. Vol 1. Philadelphia: Saunders, 2007;527–9.

Rezvani I. Phenylalanine. In: Kliegman RM, Behrman RE, Jenson HB, Stanton BF (eds). *Nelson Textbook of Pediatrics.* 18th edn. Vol 1. Philadelphia: Saunders, 2007;529–32.

Rezvani I, Rosenlatt DS. Methionine. In: Kliegman RM, Behrman RE, Jenson HB, Stanton BF (eds). *Nelson Textbook of Pediatrics.* 18th edn. Vol 1. Philadelphia: Saunders, 2007;536–9.

Rezvani I. Cysteine/Cystine. In: Kliegman RM, Behrman RE, Jenson HB, Stanton BF (eds). *Nelson Textbook of Pediatrics.* 18th edn. Vol 1. Philadelphia: Saunders, 2007;539.

Rezvani I. Tryptophan. In: Kliegman RM, Behrman RE, Jenson HB, Stanton BF (eds). *Nelson Textbook of Pediatrics.* 18th edn. Vol 1. Philadelphia: Saunders, 2007;539–540.

Rezvani I, Rosenblatt DS. Valine, leucine, isoleucine, and related organic acidemias. In: Kliegman RM, Behrman RE, Jenson HB, Stanton BF (eds). *Nelson Textbook of Pediatrics.* 18th edn. Vol 1. Philadelphia: Saunders, 2007;540–9.

Rezvani I. Glutamic Acid. In: Kliegman RM, Behrman RE, Jenson HB, Stanton BF (eds). *Nelson Textbook of Pediatrics.* 18th edn. Vol 1. Philadelphia: Saunders, 2007;553–5.

Rezvani I. Urea cycle and hyperammonemia. In: Kliegman RM, Behrman RE, Jenson HB, Stanton BF (eds). *Nelson Textbook of Pediatrics.* 18th edn. Vol 1. Philadelphia: Saunders, 2007;555–61.

26.3 DISORDERS IN METABOLISM OF LIPIDS

Disorders of mitochondrial fatty acid β-oxidation: Mitochondrial β-oxidation of fatty acids is an essential energy-producing pathway helpful in starvation and when our body is switched to reduced calorie intake in gastrointestinal illness or increased energy expenditure during febrile illness. Characteristically involve tissues are liver, skeletal, and cardiac muscle. The most common presentation is an acute episode of life-threatening coma and hypoglycemia induced by a period of fasting due to defective hepatic ketogenesis. Other manifestations include chronic cardiomyopathy and muscle weakness or exercise-induced acute rhabdomyolysis. *Diagnosis:* During acute episodes, hypoglycemia is usually present. Plasma and urinary ketone bodies concentrations are inappropriately low (*hypoketotic hypoglycemia*). Elevated levels of liver enzymes (ALT, AST) along with elevated blood ammonia, and prolonged prothrombin (PT) and partial thromboplastin times (PTT). Liver biopsy at times of acute illness shows microvesicular or macrovesicular steatosis due to triglyceride accumulation. *Treatment:* Acute illnesses should be promptly treated with intravenous fluids containing 10% dextrose to treat or prevent hypoglycemia and to suppress lipolysis as rapidly as possible. The fasting must be avoided in patients. This usually requires simply adjusting the diet to ensure that overnight fasting periods are limited to < 10–12 hr.

Medium-chain acyl CoA dehydrogenase (MCAD) deficiency: MCAD deficiency usually requires simply adjusting the diet to ensure that overnight fasting periods are limited to < 10–12 hr. Affected patients usually present in the first three months to three years of life with episodes of acute illness triggered by prolonged fasting lasting longer than 12–16 hr. Signs and symptoms include vomiting and lethargy, which rapidly progress to coma or seizures and cardio-respiratory collapse. Sudden unexpected infant death may occur. The liver may be slightly enlarged with fat deposition. Attacks are rare until the infant is beyond the 1st few months of life, presumably due to more frequent feedings at a younger age. Affected older infants are at higher risk of illness as they begin to fast through the night or are exposed to fasting stress during an intercurrent childhood illness. Presentation in the 1st days of life has been reported in newborns that were fasted inadvertently before successful breastfeeding. Up to 25% of unrecognized patients may die during their 1st attack of illness. There is frequently a history of a previous sibling death due to unrecognized MCAD deficiency. Some patients may develop permanent brain injury during an attack of profound hypoglycemia. The prognosis for survivors without brain damage is excellent. Fasting tolerance improves with age and the risks of illness decreases. As many as 50% of affected patients have never had an episode; therefore, testing of siblings of affected patients is important to detect asymptomatic family members.

Primary carnitine deficiency: Primary carnitine deficiency is the only genetic defect in which carnitine deficiency is the cause. The most common presentation is progressive cardiomyopathy with or without skeletal muscle weakness beginning at 1–4 yr of age. A smaller number of patients may present with fasting hypoketotic hypoglycemia in the 1st yr of life before the cardiomyopathy becomes symptomatic. The underlying defect involves the plasma membrane sodium gradient-dependent carnitine transporter that is present in heart, muscle, and kidney. This transporter is responsible both for maintaining intracellular carnitine concentrations 20- to 50-fold higher than plasma concentrations and for renal conservation of carnitine. Patients have extremely reduced carnitine levels in plasma and muscle (1–2% of normal). Heterozygote parents have plasma carnitine levels ~50% of normal. *Treatment:* carnitine (100–200 mg/kg/dayPO) is highly effective in correcting the cardiomyopathy and muscle weakness as well as any impairment in fasting ketogenesis.

Zellweger syndrome (ZS): See Section 17.2.

Refsum disease: Patients with *infantile Refsum disease* are able to walk, although gait may be ataxic and broad based. All have sensory hearing loss and pigmentary degeneration of the retina. They have moderately dysmorphic features that may include epicanthal folds, a flat bridge of the nose, and low set ears. Early hypotonia and hepatomegaly with impaired function are common. Levels of plasma cholesterol and high- and low-density lipoproteins are often moderately reduced. The mode of inheritance is autosomal recessive. Patients have survived to the 2nd decade or longer.

Classic refsum disease: The defective enzyme (phytanoyl CoA oxidase) is localized to the peroxysome. The manifestations include impaired vision from retinitis pigmentosa, ichthyosis, peripheral neuropathy, ataxia, and occasionally, cardiac arrhythmias. In contrast to infantile Refsum disease, cognitive function is normal and there are no congenital malformations. Classic Refsum disease often does not manifest until young adulthood, but visual disturbances such as night blindness, ichthyosis, and peripheral neuropathy may already be present in childhood and adolescence. Early diagnosis is important because institution of phytanic acid-restricted diet can reverse the peripheral neuropathy and prevent the progression of visual and central nervous system manifestations.

Adrenoleukodystrophy (X-Linked): X-ALD is a genetically determined disorder associated with the accumulation of saturated very long chain fatty acids (VLCFA). Excess hexacosanoic acid (C26:0) is the most striking feature. The gene has been mapped to chromosome Xq28. The minimum incidence of X-ALD in males is 1/21,000, and the combined incidence of X-ALD males and heterozygous females in the general population is estimated to be 1/17,000. All races are affected. The various phenotypes often occur in members of the same kindred.

Clinical manifestations: X-ALD is a disorder characterized by a progressive dysfunction of the adrenal cortex and central and peripheral nervous system white matter. There are five relatively distinct phenotypes, three of which present in childhood with symptoms and signs. In all the phenotypes, development is usually normal in the 1st 3–4 yr. In the *childhood cerebral form of ALD*, symptoms are 1st noted between the ages of 4 and 8 yr. The clinical features include hyperactivity (most common initial manifestation), impaired auditory discrimination (tone perception is preserved), disturbances of vision, ataxia, poor handwriting, seizures, and strabismus. Impaired cortisol response to ACTH stimulation is present in 85% of patients, and mild hyperpigmentation is noted only after the condition is diagnosed because of the cerebral symptoms. *Cerebral childhood ALD* tends to progress rapidly with increasing spasticity and paralysis, visual and hearing loss, and loss of ability to speak or swallow. The mean interval between the 1st neurologic symptom and an apparently vegetative state is 1.9 yr. Patients may continue in this apparently vegetative state for 10 yr or more. *Adolescent ALD patients* experience neurologic symptoms between the ages of 10–21 yr. the manifestations resemble those of childhood cerebral ALD except that progression is slower. About 10% of patients present acutely with status epilepticus, adrenal crisis, acute encephalopathy, or coma. Adrenomyeloneuropathy first manifests in late adolescence or adulthood as a progressive paraparesis caused by long tract degeneration in the spinal cord. Approximately half of the patients also have involvement of the cerebral white matter. In *"Addison only"* phenotype male patients with Addison disease, 25% may have the biochemical defect of ALD. Many of these patients have intact neurologic symptoms, whereas others have subtle neurologic signs. Many acquire adrenomyeloneuropathy in adulthood.

Asymptomatic ALD persons have the biochemical defect of ALD but are free of neurologic or endocrine disturbances. Nearly all persons with gene defect eventually become neurologically symptomatic. A few have remained asymptomatic even in the 6th or 7th decade. Approximately 50% of female heterozygotes acquire a syndrome that resembles adrenomyelo-neuropathy but is milder and of later onset. Adrenal insufficiency is rare.

Diagnosis: There are abnormally high levels of VLCFA in plasma, red blood cells, or cultured skin fibroblasts. More than 85% of patients with the childhood form of ALD have elevated levels of ACTH in plasma and a subnormal rise of cortisol levels in plasma following intravenous injection of 250 μg of ACTH. Patients with childhood cerebral or adolescent ALD show cerebral white matter lesions that are characteristic with respect to location and attenuation patterns on MRI. In 80%

of patients, the lesions are symmetric and involve periventricular white matter in the posterior parietal and occipital lobes. About 50% show location of a garland of accumulated contrast material adjacent and anterior to the posterior hypodense lesions. This zone corresponds to the zones of intense perivascular lymphocytic infiltration where the blood–brain barrier breaks down. In 12% of patients, the initial lesions are frontal. Unilateral lesions that produce a mass effect suggestive of a brain tumor may occur.

Treatment: Corticosteroid replacement for adrenal insufficiency or adrenocortical hypofunction is effective, but does not alter the course of the neurologic disability. Bone marrow transplantation (BMT) benefits patients who show early evidence of the inflammatory neurologic disability in boys and adolescents with the cerebral X-ALD phenotype. The administration of Lorenzo's oil (4:1 mixture of glyceryl trioleate and glyceryl trierucate) combined with a dietary regimen in neurologically asymptomatic boys who have normal brain MRI and are younger than 8 yr, reduces the risk of developing the childhood cerebral phenotype by a factor of two or more. Lorenzo's oil has not been shown to alter disease progression in patients who already have cerebral involvement.

The progressive behavioral and neurologic disturbances associated with the childhood form of ALD are extremely difficult for the family. Counseling and communication with school authorities are of prime importance.

Genetic counseling and prevention: Family screening should be offered to all at risk relatives of symptomatic patients. The plasma assay permits reliable identification of affected males in whom plasma VLCFA levels are increased already on the day of birth. Identification of asymptomatic males permits institution of steroid replacement therapy when appropriate and prevents the occurrence of adrenal crisis, which may be fatal.

Prenatal diagnosis of affected male fetuses can be achieved by measurement of VLCFA levels in cultured amniocytes or chorionic villus cells and by mutation analysis.

Moser HW, Raymond GV, Dubey P. Adrenoleuko-dystrophy: New approaches to a neurodegenerative disease. JAMA 2005;294:3131–4.

Moser HW, Raymond GV, Lu SE, et al. Follow-up of 89 Lorenzo's Oil treated asymptomatic adrenoleukodystrophy patients Arch Neurol 2005;62:1073–80.

Moser HW. **Disorders of Very Long Chain Fatty Acids.** In: Kliegman RM, Behrman RE, Jenson HB, Stanton BF (eds). *Nelson Textbook of Pediatrics.* 18th edn. Vol 1. Philadelphia: Saunders, 2007;573–80.

Stanley CA, Bennett MJ. Disorders of mitochondrial fatty acid β-oxidation. In: Kliegman RM, Behrman RE, Jenson HB, Stanton BF (eds). *Nelson Textbook of Pediatrics.* 18th edn. Vol 1. Philadelphia: Saunders, 2007;567–73.

Wanders RJ, Jansen GA, Skjeldal OH. Refsum disease, peroxisomes and phytanic acid oxidation: A review. *J Neuropathol Exp Neurol* 2001;60:1021–31.

Lipidoses

The lysosomal storage diseases are due to an inherited deficiency of a lysosomal hydrolase leading to the lysosomal accumulation of the enzyme's particular substrate. Progressive lysosomal accumulation of glycosphingolipids in the central nervous system lead to neurodegeneration, whereas storage in visceral cells can lead to organomegaly, skeletal abnormalities, pulmonary infiltration, and other manifestations. Diagnostic assays for the identification of affected individuals rely on the measurement of the specific enzyme activity in isolated leukocytes or cultured fibroblasts. For most disorders carrier identification and prenatal diagnosis are available. Inheritance is autosomal recessive except for X-linked Fabry disease.

GM$_1$ gangliosidosis: GM$_1$ gangliosidosis, most frequently presents in early infancy (type 1 disease) but has been described in patients with a juvenile onset (type 2). Both are autosomal recessive traits; each results from the deficient activity of β-galactosidase, a lysosomal enzyme encoded by a gene on chromosome 3 (3p21.33). Although the disorder is characterized by pathologic accumulation of GM$_1$ gangliosides in the lysosomes of both neural and visceral cells, GM$_1$ ganglioside accumulation is most marked in the brain. In addition, keratan sulfate, a mucopolysaccharide, accumulates in liver and is excreted in the urine of patients with GM$_1$ gangliosidosis.

The clinical manifestations of the infantile form of GM$_1$ gangliosidosis (type 1 disease) are present in the newborn as hepatosplenomegaly, edema, and skin eruptions (*angiokeratomata*). It most frequently presents in the 1st 6 mo of life with developmental delay followed by progressive psychomotor retardation and the onset of tonic-clonic seizures. A typical facies is characterized by low set ears, frontal bossing, a depressed nasal bridge, and abnormally long philtrum. Up to 50% of patients have a macular cherry red spot. Hepatosplenomegaly and skeletal abnormalities including anterior beaking of the vertebrae, enlargement of the sella turcica, and thickening of the calvarium, are present. By the end of the 1st yr of life, most patients are blind and deaf, severe neurologic impairment characterized by decerebrate rigidity. Death usually occurs by 3–4 yr

of age. Affected patients of juvenile-onset form of GM$_1$ gangliosidosis (type 2) present primarily with neurologic symptoms including ataxia, dysarthria, mental retardation, and spasticity. Deterioration is slow; patients may survive through the 4th decade of life. There is no specific treatment for either form of GM$_1$ gangliosidosis.

The diagnosis of GM$_1$ gangliosidosis should be suspected in infants with typical clinical features and is confirmed by the demonstration of the deficiency of β-galactosidase activity in peripheral leukocytosis or cultured skin fibroblasts. Prenatal diagnosis is accomplished by determination of the enzymatic activity in cultured aminocytes or chorionic villi.

GM$_2$ gangliosidoses: The GM$_2$ gangliosidoses include Tay-Sachs disease and Sandhoff disease, each result from the deficiency of β-hexosaminidase activity and the lysosomal accumulation of GM$_2$ gangliosides, particularly in the central nervous system. Both disorders have been classified into infantile-, juvenile-, adult-onset forms based on the age at onset and clinical features. β-hexosaminidase results from mutations in the α-subunit and causes Tay-Sachs disease, whereas mutations in the β-subunit gene result in the deficiency of both β-hexosaminidases A and B and cause Sandhoff disease. Both are autosomal recessive traits, with Tay-Sachs disease having a prediction in the Ashkenazi Jewish population, where the carrier frequency is about 1/25.

Patients with the infantile form of *Tay-Sachs disease* have clinical manifestations in infancy of loss of motor skills, increased startle reaction, and macular pallor and retinal cherry red spots. Affected infants usually develop normally until 4–5 mo of age when decreased eye contact and an exaggerated startle response to noise (hyperacusis) are noted. Macrocephaly, not associated with hydrocephalus, may develop. In the 2nd yr of life, seizures requiring anticonvulsant therapy develop. Neurodegeneration is relentless, with death occurring by the age of 4 or 5 yr. The juvenile-onset form initially presents with ataxia and dysarthria and may not be associated with cherry red spot.

The clinical manifestations of *Sandhoff disease* are similar to those for Tay-Sachs disease. Infants with Sandhoff disease, however, have hepatosplenomegly, cardiac involvement, and bony abnormalities. The juvenile form of this disorder presents as ataxia, dysarthria, and mental deterioration, but without visceral enlargement or a macular cherry red spot.

No treatment is available for Tay-Sachs disease or Sandhoff disease.

The diagnosis of infantile Tay-Sachs disease and Sandhoff disease is usually suspected in an infant with neurologic features and a cherry red spot. Definitive diagnosis is by determination of the level of β-hexosaminidases A and B in isolated blood leukocytes. Future at-risk pregnancies for both disorders can be monitored by prenatal diagnosis by amniocentesis or chorionic villus sampling. Identification of carriers in families is also possible by β-hexosaminidases A and B determination. Newborn screening may be possible by measuring specific glycosphingolipid markers.

Gaucher disease: This disease is a multisystemic lipidosis autosomal recessive trait characterized by hematologic problems, organomegaly, and skeletal involvement, the latter usually manifesting as bone pain and pathologic fractures. Gaucher disease results from the deficient activity of the lysosomal hydrolase, acid β-glucosidase, which is encoded by a gene located on chromosome 1q21–q31. Clinical manifestations of *type 1 Gaucher disease* have variable age of onset, from early childhood to late adulthood, with most symptomatic patients presenting by adolescence. At presentation, patients may have bruising from thrombocytopena, chronic fatigue secondary to anemia, hepatomegaly with or without elevated liver function test results, splenomegaly, and bone pain. Occasionally patients have pulmonary involvement at the time of presentation. Most patients develop radiologic evidence of skeletal involvement, including an Erlenmeyer flask deformity of the distal femur (distal end of the femur is splayed). The pathologic hallmark of Gaucher disease is the Gaucher cell in the reticuloendothelial system, particularly in the bone marrow. These cells are 20–100 um in diameter, have a characteristic wrinkled paper appearance resulting from the presence of intracytoplasmic substrate inclusions. The cytoplasm of the Gaucher cell reacts strongly positively with the periodic acid-Schiff stain. The presence of this cell in bone marrow and tissue specimens is highly suggestive of Gaucher disease, although it also may be found in patients with granulocyte leukemia and myeloma. **Gaucher disease type 2** is characterized by a rapid neurodegenerative course with extensive visceral involvement and death within the 1st 2 yr of life. **Gaucher disease type 3** presents with neurologic involvement, which occurs later in childhood with decreased severity compared with type 2 disease and death occurs by age 10–15 yr.

Prenatal diagnosis is available by determination of enzyme activity in chorionic villi or cultured amniotic fluid cells. Treatment of patients with Gaucher disease type 1 includes enzyme replacement therapy, with recombinant acid β-glucosidase (imiglucerase).

Neimann-Pick disease (NPD): There are three subtypes of NPD. **Type A NPD** is a fatal disorder characterized by failure to thrive, hepatosplenomegaly, and a rapid progressive neurodegenerative course that leads to death by 2–3 yr of age. **Type B NPD** is a non-neuronopathic form observed in children and adults. Most are diagnosed in infancy or childhood when enlargement of the liver or spleen, or both, is detected during a routine physical examination. At diagnosis, Type B NPD patients **Type C NPD** is a neuronopathic form that results from defective cholesterol transport. All the subtypes are inherited as autosomal recessive traits. NPD types A and B result from the deficient activity of acid sphingomyelinase, a lysosomal enzyme encoded by a gene on chromosome 11 (11p15.1–p15.4). The enzymatic defect results in the pathologic accumulation of sphingomyelin, a ceramide phospholipid, and other lipids in the monocyte-macrophage system, which is the primary pathologic site. The progressive deposition of sphingomyelin in the central nervous system results in the neurodegenerative course seen in Type A NPD, and in non-neural tissue in the systemic disease manifestations of Type B NPD including progressive lung disease in some patients. **Type C NPD** patients often present with prolonged neonatal jaundice, appear normal for 1–2 yr, and then experience a slowly progressive and variable neurodegenerative course. There is no specific treatment for NPD.

Fabry disease: It is X-linked recessive trait that is manifested in affected males. Heterozygous females for the classic phenotypes can be asymptomatic or as severely affected as the males, the variability due to random X-inactivation. The disease results from the deficient activity of α-galactosidase A, a lysosomal enzyme encoded by a gene located on the long arm of the X chromosome (Xp22). The enzymatic defect leads to the systemic accumulation of neutral glycosphingolipids, particularly in the plasma and lysosomes of vascular endothelial and smooth muscle cells. The progressive vascular glycosphingolipid deposition in affected males results in ischemia and infarction, leading to the major disease manifestations.

Affected males with the classic phenotype have the skin lesions, acroparesthesias, hypohidrosis, and ocular changes, whereas males with the later onset phenotypes lack these findings and present with cardiac and/or renal disease in childhood. The classic **angiokeratomas** usually occur in childhood and may lead to early diagnosis. The lesions are punctate, dark red to blue-black, and flat or slightly raised. They do not blanch with pressure, and the larger ones show slight hyperkeratosis. Corneal opacities and lenticular lesions, observed under slit-lamp examination are present in affected males as well as in ~70% of asymptomatic heterozygotes. *Pain* is the most debilitating symptom in childhood and adolescence. *Treatment* of Fabry disease includes the use of phenytoin and/or carbamazepine to decrease the frequency and severity of the chronic acroparesthesias and the periodic crises of excruciating pain. Renal transplantation and long-term hemodialysis are life saving procedures for patients with renal failure. Recombinant α-galactosidase is a safe and effective enzyme replacement therapy for Fabry disease at a dose of 1 mg/kg every other week.

Fucosidosis: This is a rare autosomal recessive disorder caused by the deficient activity of α-fructosidase and the accumulation of fucose-containing glycosphingo-lipids, glycoproteins, and oligosaccharides in the lysosomes of the liver, brain and other organs. The α-fucosidase gene is on chromosome 1 (1p24). Although the disorder is panethic, most affected patients are from Italy and the United States. Severely affected patients present in the first year of life with developmental delay and somatic features including frontal bossing, hepatosplenomegaly, coarse facial features, and macroglossia. The central nervous system storage results in a relentless neurodegenerative course, with death in childhood. Patients with milder disease have angiokeratomas and longer survival. The disorder can be diagnosed by the demonstration of deficient α-fucosidase activity in peripheral leukocytes or cultured fibroblasts. Carrier identification studies and prenatal diagnosis are possible by determination of the enzymatic activity. No specific therapy is available for this disorder.

Schindler disease: It is an autosomal recessive neurodegenerative disorder that results from the deficient activity of α-*N*-acetylgalactosaminidase and the accumulation of sialylated and asialoglycopeptides and oligosaccharides. The gene for the enzyme is mapped to chromosome 22 (22q13.1–13.2). The disease is clinically identified in two major phenotypes. Type I disease is an infantile onset with normal development for the 1st 9–15 mo of life followed by a rapid neurodegenerative course that results in severe psychomotor retardation, cortical blindness, and frequent myoclonic seizures. Type II disease is characterized by a variable age at onset, mild retardation, and angiokeratomas. The diagnosis is confirmed by demonstration of the enzymatic deficiency in leukocytes or cultured skin fibroblasts. There is no specific therapy for this disorder.

Krabbe disease: This condition, also called globoid cell leukodystrophy, is an autosomal recessive fatal disorder of infancy. It results from the deficiency of the enzymatic activity of galactocerebrosidase and the white matter accumulation of galactosylceramide, which is normally found almost exclusively in the myelin sheath. The galactocerebrosidase gene is on chromosome 14 (14q31). The **infantile form** of Krabbe disease is rapidly progressive and patients present with irritability, seizures, hypertonia, optic atrophy, mental retardation and die before 3 yr of age. A second, **late infantile form** of Krabbe disease appears after the age of 2 yr and affected individuals have a disease course similar to that of the early infantile form. The diagnosis of Krabbe disease can be confirmed by demonstration of the specific enzymatic deficiency in white blood cells or cultured skin fibroblasts. Carrier identification and prenatal diagnosis are available.

Metachromatic leukodystrophy (MLD): It is an autosomal recessive white matter disease caused by a deficiency of arylsulfatase A (ASA), which is required for the hydrolysis of sulfated glycosphingolipids. Another form of MLD is caused by a deficiency of sphingolipid activator protein (SAPI), which is required for the formation of the substrate-enzyme complex. The deficiency of this enzymatic activity results in the white matter storage of sulfated glycosphingolipids, which leads to demyelination and a neurodegenerative course. The ASA gene is on chromosome 22 (22q13.31qter); specific mutations are known to fall into two groups that correlate with disease severity.

The *late infantile form* of MLD, which is most common, usually presents between 12 and 18 mo of age as irritability, inability to walk, and hyper-extension of the knee, causing genu recurvatum. Deep tendon reflexes are diminished or absent. Gradual muscle wasting, weakness, and hypotonia become evident and lead to a debilitated state. As the disease progresses, nystagmus, myoclonic seizures, optic atrophy, and quadripaesis appear, with death in the first decade of life. The *juvenile form* of MLD with onset as late as 20 yr of age is characterized by gait disturbances, mental deterioration, urinary incontinence, and emotional difficulties. The *adult form* of MLD, which presents after the 2nd decade, is similar to the juvenile form in its clinical manifestations, although emotional difficulties and psychosis are more prominent features. Dementia, seizures, diminished reflexes, and optic atrophy also occur in both the juvenile and adult forms. The characteristic pathologic finding is the deposition of metachromatic bodies, which stain strongly positive with periodic acid-Schiff and alcain blue in the white matter of the brain. Neuronal inclusions may be seen in the white matter of the brain. Neuronal inclusions may be seen in the midbain, pons, medulla, retina, and spinal cord;

demyelination occurs in the peripheral nervous system.

The *diagnosis* of MLD should be suspected in patients with the clinical features of leukodystrophy. Decreased nerve conduction velocities, increased cerebrospinal fluid protein, metachromatic deposits in sampled segments of sural nerve, and metachromatic granules in urinary sediment are all suggestive of MLD. Confirmation of the diagnosis is based on the demonstration of the reduced activity of ASA in leukocytes or cultured skin fibroblasts.

Supportive care is the main *treatment* of MLD. Bone marrow transplantation has resulted in normal enzymatic levels in peripheral blood but no clear evidence for clinical efficacy in terms of the neurologic course.

Multiple sulfatase deficiency: This is an autosomal recessive disorder that results from the deficiency of three enzymatic deficiencies: arylsulfatases A, B, and C. Sulfatides, mucoplysaccharides, steroid sulfates, and gangliosides accumulate in the cerebral cortex and visceral tissues, resulting in a clinical phenotype with features of leukodystrophy as well as of mucopoly-saccharidoses. Severe ichthyosis may also occur. Carrier testing and prenatal diagnosis can be performed by measurement of the enzymatic activity. There is no specific treatment for multiple sulfatase deficiency other than supportive care.

Farber disease: This is an autosomal recessive disorder that results from the deficiency of the lysosomal enzyme ceramidase and the accumulation of ceramide in various tissues, especially the joints. Symptoms can begin as early as the 1st yr of life with painful joint swelling and nodule formation. As the disease progresses, nodule or granulomatous formation on the vocal cords can lead to hoarseness and breathing difficulties. Failure to thrive is common. There is also central nervous system dysfunction and recurrent pneumonias. The diagnosis of Farber disease should be suspected in patients who have nodule formation over the joints but no other findings of rheumatoid arthritis. In such patients, ceramidase activity should be determined in cultured skin fibroblasts or white blood cells. Carrier detection and prenatal diagnosis are available.

Wolman disease and cholesterol ester storage disease (CESD): These are autosomal recessive lysosomal storage diseases that result from the deficiency of acid lipase and the accumulation of cholesterol esters and triglycerides in histiocytic foam cells of most visceral organs. The gene for lysosomal acid lipase is on chromosome 10 (10q24–q25).

Wolman disease is the more severe clinical phenotype and is a fatal disorder of infancy. The clinical features of the disease become apparent in the 1st wk of life and include failure to thrive, relentless vomiting, abdominal distension, steatorrhea, and hepatosplenomegaly. There is usually hyperlipidemia. Hepatic dysfunction and fibrosis may occur. Calcification of the adrenal glands is pathognomic for the disorder. Death usually occurs within 6 mo.

Cholesterol ester storage disease is less severe disorder that may not be diagnosed until adulthood. Hepatomegaly is the only detactable abnormality, but affected individuals are at significant risk for premature atherosclerosis. Adrenal calcification does not occur.

Diagnosis and carrier identification are based on measuring acid lipase activity in leukocytes or cultured skin fibroblasts. Prenatal diagnosis depends on measuring decreased enzyme levels in cultured chorionic villi or aminocytes.

There is no specific treatment for these disorders. Pharmacologic agents to suppress cholesterol synthesis, in combination with cholestyramine and diet modification, have been used in patients with cholesterol ester storage disease.

Clark JTR. Narrative review: Fabry disease. *Ann Intern Med* 2007; 146: 425–433.

McGovern MM, Desnick RJ. Lipidoses. In: Kliegman RM, Behrman RE, Jenson HB, Stanton BF (eds). *Nelson Textbook of Pediatrics*. 18th edn. Vol 1. Philadelphia: Saunders, 2007; 593–601.

Meikle PJ, Ranieri E, Simonsen H, et al. Newborn screening for lysosomal storage disorders: Clinical evaluation of a two tier strategy. *Pediatrics* 2004; 114: 909–916.

26.4 DEFECTS IN METABOLISM OF CARBOHYDRATES

Carbohydrate synthesis and degradation provide the energy required for most metabolic processes. The important carbohydrates include monosaccharides (glucose, galactose, and lactose) and a polysaccharide, glycogen. Most of these conditions are inherited as autosomal recessive traits.

Lactase Deficiency

Some infants may have deficiency of the enzyme lactase (congenital or acquired) and they show intolerance to lactose, the sugar of milk and symptoms include diarrhea, flatulence, abdominal cramps and distension. As lactose is not hydrolyzed due to deficiency of lactase in a single or all brush border oligosaccharides, the accumulation of lactose in the intestinal tract, which is "osmotically active" and holds water, producing diarrhea. Accumulated lactose is fermented by intestinal bacteria producing flatulence, distention and abdominal cramps. If symptoms of flatulence, abdominal discomfort, bloating, or diarrhea occur after consumption of one or two glass of milk or a large portion of ice cream or yogurt, lactose intolerance should be suspected.

Disorders of Galactose Metabolism

Milk and dairy products contain lactose, the major dietary source of galactose. The metabolism of galactose produces fuel for cellular metabolism through its conversion to glucose-1-phosphate. Galactose also plays an important role in the formation of galactosides, which include glycoproteins, glycolipids, and glycosaminoglycans. Galactose is an essential component of many nervous system structural proteins. Galactosemia denotes the elevated level of galactose in the blood and is due to deficiency of one of the 3 enzymes: galactose-1-phospahte uridyl transferase, galactokinase, and uridine diphosphate galactose-4-epimerase.

Galactose-1-Phospahte Uridyl Transferase Deficiency Galactosemia: Transferase deficiency galactosemia is an autosomal recessive disorder. Two forms of the deficiency exist: infants with complete or near complete deficiency of enzyme (classic galactosemia) and those with partial transferase deficiency. **Classic galactosemia** is a serious disease with onset of symptoms typically by the 2nd half of the 1st week of life. The incidence is 1/60,000. The newborn infant receives high amounts of lactose (up to 40% in breast milk and certain formulas) which consists of equal parts of glucose and galactose. Without the transferase enzyme, the infant is unable to metabolize galactose-1-phosphate, the accumulation of which results in injury to kidney, liver, and brain. This injury may begin prenatally in the affected fetus by transplacental galactose derived from the diet of the heterozygous mother or by endogenous production of galactose in the fetus. The diagnosis of uridyl transferase deficiency should be considered in newborn or young infants with any of the following features: jaundice, hepatomegaly, vomiting, hypoglycemia, convulsions, lethargy, irritability, feeding difficulties, poor weight gain or failure to regain birth weight, aminoaciduria, nuclear cataracts, vitreous hemorrhage, hepatic failure, liver cirrhosis, ascites, splenomegaly, or mental retardation. Symptoms are milder and improve when milk is temporarily withdrawn and replaced by intravenous or lactose-free nutrition.

Partial transferase deficiency is generally asymptomatic. It is more frequent than classic galactosemia and is diagnosed in newborn screening because of moderately elevated blood galactose and/or low transferase activity. Galactosemia should be considered for the newborn or young infant who is not thriving or who have any of the findings mentioned in the classic galactosemia.

Diagnosis: The preliminary diagnosis galactosemia is made by demonstrating a reducing substance in urine specimens by Clinitest (glucose, galactose, others) and can be identified by chromatography or by an enzymatic test specific for galactose. Direct enzyme assay using erythrocytes establishes the diagnosis. Carrier testing and prenatal diagnosis can be performed by direct enzyme analysis of aminocytes or chorionic villi; testing can also be DNA based.

Treatment and prognosis: Various milk substitutes are available (casein hydrolysates, soybean-based formula). Elimination of galactose from the diet reverses growth failure and renal and hepatic dysfunction. Cataract regress and most patients have no impairment of eye-sight. Early diagnosis and treatment have improved the prognosis of galactosemia; patients on long-term follow-up may manifest ovarian failure with primary or secondary amenorrhea, decreased bone mineral density, developmental delay, and learning disabilities that increase in severity with age. Most manifest speech disorders.

Disorders of Fructose Metabolism

1. *Deficiency of Fructokinase (Essential or Benign Fructosuria)* is not associated with any clinical manifestations, but it is an accidental finding when the asymptomatic patient's urine contains reducing substance, which can be identified as fructose by chromatography. No treatment is necessary and the prognosis is excellent.

2. *Deficiency of fructose-1, 6-Bisphosphate aldolase (Aldolase B, Hereditary Fructose Intolerance)* can be diagnosed by direct DNA analysis. Patients with hereditary fructose intolerance (HFI) are perfectly healthy and asymptomatic until fructose sucrose (table salt) is ingested (usually from fruit, fruit juice, or sweetened cereal). Symptoms may occur early in life, soon after birth if foods or formulas containing these sugars are introduced into the diet. Certain patients are very sensitive to fructose, where others can tolerate moderate intakes (up to 250 mg/kg/day). Early clinical manifestations resemble galactosemia and include jaundice, hepatomegaly, vomiting, lethargy irritability, and convulsions. Acute fructose ingestion produces symptomatic hypoglycemia and chronic ingestion results in failure to thrive and hepatic disease. If the intake of the fructose persists,

hypoglycemic episodes recur, and liver and kidney failure progress, eventually leading to death.

Laboratory findings include a prolonged clotting time, hypoalbuminemia, elevation of bilirubin and transminase levels, and proximal tubular dysfunction. Suspicion of the enzyme deficiency should be considered if a reducing substance is present in the urine during an episode. An intravenous fructose tolerance test is administered with great care. Definitive diagnosis can be made by assay of fructose aldolase B activity in the liver. Gene-based diagnosis is also available for most patients with this disease. *Treatment* consists of complete elimination of all sources of sucrose, fructose, and sorbitol from the diet. It may be difficult because these sugars are widely used additives, found also in most medical preparations. With treatment, liver and kidney dysfunction improves, and catch-up in growth is common. Intellectual function is usually unimpaired. As the patient matures, symptoms become milder even after fructose ingestion. The long-term prognosis is good. Affected patients have a few caries because of dietary avoidance of sucrose.

Defects in Intermediary Carbohydrate Metabolism Associated with Lactic Acidosis

Lactic acidosis occurs with defects of carbohydrate metabolism that interfere with the conversion of pyruvate to glucose via the pathway of gluconeogenesis or to carbon dioxide and water via the mitrochondrial enzymes of the citric acid cycle.

Deficiency of pyruvate carboxylase secondary to deficiency of holocarboxylase synthetase or biotinidase: HCS and biotinidase enzyme deficiencies are autosomal recessive traits and are located on chromosome 21q22 and 3p25, respectively. Deficiency of either holocarboxylase synthetase (HCS) or biotinidase, which are enzymes of biotin metabolism, result in multiple carboxylase deficiency and in clinical manifestations associated with rash, lactic acidosis, and alopecia. The course of HCS or biotinidase deficiency can be protracted, with intermittent exacerbation of chronic lactic acidosis, failure to thrive, seizures, and hypotonia leading to spasticity, lethargy, coma, and death. Late-onset milder forms have also been reported. Laboratory findings include metabolic acidosis and abnormal organic acids in urine. In HCS deficiency, biotin concentrations in plasma and urine are normal. *Diagnosis* can be made in skin fibroblasts or lymphocytes by assay for HCS activity, and in case of biotinidase, in the serum by a screening blood spot. *Treatment* consists of biotin supplementation (5–20 mg/day).

Leigh disease (subacute necrotizing encephalomyelopathy): Leigh disease is a heterogenous neurologic disease that remains a neuropathologic description characterized by demyelination, gliosis, necrosis, relative neuronal sparing and capillary proliferation in specific brain regions. In decreasing order of severity, the affected areas are the basal ganglia, brain stem, cerebellum, and cerebral cortex. The classic presentation in an infant who presents with central hypotonia, developmental regression or arrest, and signs of brainstem or basal ganglia involvement. Diagnosis is usually confirmed by radiologic or pathologic evidence of symmetric lesions affecting the basal ganglia, brainstem, and subthalamic nuclei.

Defects in Pentose Metabolism

About 90% of glucose metabolism in the body is via the glycolytic pathway with remaining 10% via the hexose monophosphate pathway. The hexose monophosphate shunt leads to formation of pentoses, as well as providing nicotinamide-adenine dinucleotide (NADH).

Essential pentosuria: Essential pentosuria is a benign disorder encountered principally in Ashkenazi Jews and is an autosomal recessive trait. The urine contains L-xylulose, which is excreted in increased amounts because of a block in the conversion of L-xylulose to xylitol due to xylitol dehydrogenase deficiency. The condition is usually discovered accidently in a urine test for reducing substances. No treatment is required.

Glycogen Storage Diseases

The disorders of glycogen metabolism, the glycogen storage diseases (GSDs) result from deficiencies of various enzymes or transport proteins in the pathway of glycogen metabolism are autosomal recessive disorders. The glycogen found in these disorders is abnormal in quantity, quality, or both. There are more than 12 forms of glycogenoses. Types I, II, III, and X are most common that typically present in early childhood; type V is the most common in adolescents and adults. They may primarily affect the liver or muscle. The frequency of all forms of GSD is ~1/20,000 live births. List of glycogen storage diseases (GSD Type I to GSD Type VII) is shown in Table 26.3.

Liver glycogenoses: The GSDs that principally affect the liver include types I, III, IV, VI, IX, glycogen synthetase deficiency (type 0), and glucose transporter-2 defect. Because hepatic carbohydrate metabolism is responsible for plasma glucose homeostasis, this group of disorders typically causes fasting hypoglycemia and hepatomegaly. Some (type III, type IV, type IX) can be associated with cirrhosis. Other organs can also be

Table 26.3: List of glycogen storage diseases

Type	Deficient enzyme	Eponym
GSD Type I	Glucose-6 phosphatase or translocase	von Gierke
GSD Type II	Acid α-1, 4-glucosidase (acid maltase)	Pompe
GSD Type III	Debrancher enzyme	-
GSD Type IV	Brancher enzyme	Andersen
GSD Type V	Muscle phosphorylase (PYGM)	McArdle
GSD Type VI	Liver phosphorylase	Hers
GSD Type VII	Muscle phospho-fructokinase	Tarui

involved and may manifest as renal dysfunction in type I and myopathy (skeletal and/or cardiomyopathy) in types III and IV, as well as some rare forms of phosphorylase kinase deficiency. Treatment for liver phosphorylase kinase deficiency includes a high carbohydrate diet and frequent feedings prevent hypoglycemia; most patients require no specific treatment. Prognosis for the X-linked and certain autosomal forms is good.

Muscle glycogenoses: The role of glycogen in muscle is to provide substrates for the generation of ATP for muscle contraction. The muscle GSDs are broadly divided into 2 groups. The 1st group is characterized by hypertrophic cardiomyopathy, progressive skeletal weakness and atrophy, or both, and is represented by type II GSD and LAMP2. The 2nd group comprises muscle energy disorder characterized by muscle pain, exercise intolerance, myoglobinuria, and susceptibility to fatigue. This group includes type V GSD and type VII GSD.

Kishnani PS, Chen YT. Defects in metabolism of carbohydrates. In: Kliegman RM, Behrman RE, Jenson HB, Stanton BF (eds). *Nelson Textbook of Pediatrics.* 18th edn. Vol 1. Philadelphia: Saunders, 2007; 601–620.

Kishnani PS, Chen YT. Defects in galactose metabolism. In: Kliegman RM, Behrman RE, Jenson HB, Stanton BF (eds). *Nelson Textbook of Pediatrics.* 18th edn. Vol 1. Philadelphia: Saunders, 2007; 609–610.

Kishnani PS, Chen YT. Defects in fructose metabolism. In: Kliegman RM, Behrman RE, Jenson HB, Stanton BF (eds). *Nelson Textbook of Pediatrics.* 18th edn. Vol 1. Philadelphia: Saunders, 2007; 611.

Kishnani PS, Chen YT. Defects in intermediary carbohydrate metabolism associated with lactic acidosis. In: Kliegman RM, Behrman RE, Jenson HB, Stanton BF (eds). *Nelson Textbook of Pediatrics.* 18th edn. Vol 1. Philadelphia: Saunders, 2007; 611–614.

Kishnani PS, Chen YT. Defects in pentose metabolism. In: Kliegman RM, Behrman RE, Jenson HB, Stanton BF (eds). *Nelson Textbook of Pediatrics.* 18th edn. Vol 1. Philadelphia: Saunders, 2007; 614–617.

Kishnani PS, Chen YT. Glycogen storage diseases. In: Kliegman RM, Behrman RE, Jenson HB, Stanton BF (eds). *Nelson Textbook of Pediatrics.* 18th edn. Vol 1. Philadelphia: Saunders, 2007; 601–609.

Zeviani M, Di Donato S. Mitochondrial disorders. *Brain* 2004; 127: 2153–2172.

Disorders of Glycoprotein Degradation and Structure

Sialidosis and galactosialidosis: Sialidosis is an autosomal recessive disorder that results from the primary deficiency of neuraminidase due to mutations in the gene that encodes this protein, which is located on chromosome 10. In contrast, galactosialidosis is due to deficiency of 2 lysosomal enzymes, neuraminidase and β-galactosidase.

The clinical phenotype associated with neuraminidase deficiency is variable and includes **type I sialidosis**, which usually present in the 2nd decade of life with myoclonus and the presence of a cherry red spot. In contrast, **type II sialidosis** occurs as congenital, infantile and juvenile forms. The congenital and infantile forms result from isolated neuraminidase deficiency, whereas the juvenile form results from both neuraminidase and β-galactosidase deficiency. The **congenital type II disease** is characterized by hydrops fetalis, neonatal ascites, hepatosplenomegaly, stippling of the epiphyses, periosteal cloaking, and stillbirth or death in infancy. The **type II infantile form** presents in the 1st yr of life with dysostosis multiplex, moderate mental retardation, visceromegaly, corneal clounding, cherry red spot and seizures. The **juvenile type II** form of sialidosis has a variable age of onset ranging from infancy to adulthood. In infancy the phenotype is similar to that of GM$_1$ gangliosidosis with edema, ascites, skeletal dysplasia, and cherry red spot. Patients with later-onset disease have dysostosis multiplex, visceromegaly, mental retardation, dysmorphism, corneal clouding, progressive neurologic deterioration, and bilateral cherry red spots. The diagnosis of sialidosis and galactosialidosis is confirmed by the demonstration of the specific enzyme deficiency. Prenatal diagnosis using cultured amniotic cells is also possible. No specific therapy is available for any form of disease.

Collins AE, Ferriero DM. The expanding spectrum of congenital disorders of glycosylation. *J Pediatr* 2005;147:728–30.

McGovern MM, Desnick RJ. Disorders of glycoprotein degradation and structure. In: Kliegman RM, Behrman RE, Jenson HB, Stanton BF (eds). *Nelson Textbook of Pediatrics.* 18th edn. Vol 1. Philadelphia: Saunders, 2007;617–20.

26.5 MUCOPOLYSACCHARIDOSES

Mucopolysaccharidoses (MPS) are hereditary, progressive diseases caused by mutations of the genes coding for lysosomal enzymes needed to degrade glycosaminoglycans (acid mucopolysaccharides). Mucopolysaccharidoses are autosomal recessive disorders, with the exception of Hunter disease, which is X-linked recessive. The most common subtype is MPS-III, followed by MPS-I and MPS-II.

MPS-I

Hurler disease: An infant with Hurler syndrome appears normal at birth, but inguinal hernias are often present. Diagnosis is usually made between 6 and 24 mo of age with evidence of hepatosplenomegaly, coarse facial features, corneal clouding, large tongue, prominent forehead, joint stiffness, short stature, and skeletal dysplasia. Valvular heart disease with incompetence, notably of the mitral and aortic valves and coronary artery narrowing regularly develops. Radiographs show a characteristic skeletal dysplasia known as dysostosis multiplex. The earliest radiographic signs are thick ribs and ovoid vertebral bodies. Obstructive airway disease, respiratory infection, and cardiac complications are the common causes of death, usually by 10 yr of age.

Hurler-Scheie disease is characterized by progressive somatic involvement, including dysostosis multiplex with a little or no intellectual dysfunction. Some patients have spondylolisthesis, which may cause cord compression. Cardiac involvement and upper airway obstruction contribute to clinical morbidity. The onset of symptoms is usually observed between 3 and 8 yr of age; survival to adulthood is common.

Scheie disease is a comparatively mild disorder characterized by joint stiffness, aortic valve disease, corneal clouding, and mild dysostosis multiplex. Patients with *Scheie disease* have normal intelligence and stature, but have significant joint and ocular involvement. Onset of symptoms is usually after age of 5 yr and diagnosis is usually made between 10 and 20 yr of age.

MPS-II: Hunter disease manifests almost exclusively in males; it has been reported in a few females. Patients with **severe MPS-II** have features similar to those of Hurler disease except for the lack of corneal clouding and the somewhat slower progression of somatic and CNS deterioration. Coarser facial features, short stature, dysostosis multiplex, joint stiffness, and mental retardation manifest between 2 and 4 yr of age. Grouped skin papules are present in some patients. Extensive Mongolion spots have been observed in African and Asian patients since birth and may be an earlier marker of the disease. Gastrointestinal storage may produce chronic diarrhea. Communicating hydrocephalus and spastic paraplegia may develop due to thickened meninges. In severely affected patients, extensive, slowly progressive neurologic involvement precedes death, which usually occurs between 10 and 15 yr of age. Patients with the **mild MPS-II** have a prolonged life span, minimal CNS involvement, and slow progression of somatic deterioration with preservation of intelligence in adult life. Adult height may exceed 150 cm. Airway involvement, valvular cardiac disease, hearing impairment, carpal tunnel syndrome, and joint stiffness are common and can result in significant loss of function in both the mild and severe forms.

MPS-III: Patients with Sanfilippo disease are characterized by slowly progressive, severe CNS involvement with mild somatic disease. Onset of clinical features usually occurs between 2 and 6 yr in a child who previously appeared normal. Presenting features include delayed development, hyperactivity with aggressive behavior, coarse hair, hirsutism sleep disorders, and mild hepatosplenomegaly. Severe neurologic deterioration occurs in most patients by 6–10 yr of age, accompanied by rapid deterioration of social and adaptive skills. Severe behavior problems such as sleep disturbance, uncontrolled hyperactivity, temper tantrums, destructive behavior, and physical aggression are common.

MPS-IV: Morquio disease are characterized by short-trunk dwarfism, fine corneal deposits, a skeletal dysplasia that is distinct from other mucopolysaccharidoses, and preservation of intelligence.

MPS-VI: Maroteaux-Lamy disease is characterized by severe to mild somatic involvement, as seen in MPS I, but with preservation of intelligence. The somatic involvement of the severe form of MPS VI is characterized by corneal clouding, coarse facial features, joint stiffness, valvular heart disease, communicating hydrocephalus, and dysostosis multiplex.

MPS-VII: Some severely affected newborns survive for some months and have or develop, signs of lysosomal storage including thick skin, visceromegaly, and dysostosis multiplex. Less severe forms of MPS-VII present in the 1st years of life with features of MPS-I but slower progression. Corneal clouding varies. Patients with manifestation after 4 yr of life have skeletal abnormalities of dysostosis multiplex but normal intelligence and usually clear corneae. They may be found incidently on the basis of a blood smear that demonstrates coarse granulocytic inclusions.

Treatment: Bone marrow transplantation from related or unrelated donors or cord blood transplantation results in significant clinical improvement of somatic disease in MPS I, II, and IV. *Enzyme replacement* using recombinant enzymes are approved for patients with MPS I, MPS II and MPS VI. It reduces organomegaly, ameliorates rate of growth and joint mobility, and reduces the number of episodes of sleep apnea and urinary GAG excretion. The combination of enzyme replacement therapy and stem cell transplantation may offer the best treatment.

Allen JL. Treatment of respiratory system (not just lung) abnormalities in mucoplysaccharidosis I. *J Pediatr* 2004;144: 561–2.

Fuller M, Rozaklis T, Ramsay SL, et al. Disease specific markers for the mucopolysaccharidoses. *Pediar Res* 2004;56: 733–8.

Spranger J. Mucopolysaccharidoses. In: Kliegman RM, Behrman RE, Jenson HB, Stanton BF (eds). *Nelson Textbook of Pediatrics.* 18th edn. Vol 1. Philadelphia: Saunders, 2007;620–6.

26.6 DISORDERS OF PURINE AND PYRIMIDINE METABOLISM

Lesch Nyhan disease (LND) is characterized by complete deficiency of hypoxanthine-guanine phosphoribosyltransferase (HPRT), the major enzyme of the purine salvage pathways. This sex-linked disorder is manifested clinically by mental retardation, dystonic movements and behavioral problems (self-mutilation of the mouth and fingers and aggressiveness). Biochemically this syndrome is manifested by hyperuricemia, hyperuricaciduria, and markedly decreased levels of HPRT in erythrocytes, fibroblasts, and other cells. Treatment focuses on prevention of renal failure by pharmacologic treatment of hyperuricemia with high fluid intake along with alkali and allopurinol. Self-mutilation is reduced through behavior management and the use of restraints, removal of teeth, or both. Diazepam may be helpful for anxiety symptoms, and carbamazepine or gabapentin for mood stabilization. Each of these medications may reduce self-injurious behavior by helping to reduce anxiety and stabilize mood.

Gout presents with hyperuricemia, uric acid nephrolithiasis and acute inflammatory arthritis. Gouty arthritis is due to monosodium urate crystal deposits that result in inflammation in joints and surrounding tissues. The presentation is most commonly monoarticular, typically in the metatarsophalangeal joint of the big toe. Tophi deposits of monosodium urate crystals may occur over points of insertion of tendons at the elbows, knees and feet or over the helix of the ears. Primary gout ordinarily occurs in middle-aged men. When hyperuricemia and gout occur in childhood, it is most often secondary gout, the result of another disorder in which there is rapid tissue breakdown or cellular turnover leading to increased production or decreased excretion of uric acid; during therapy for malignancy or with dehydration, lactic acidosis, ketoacidosis, starvation, diuretic therapy, and renal shutdown. Excessive purine, alcohol, or carbohydrate ingestion may increase uric acid levels. Treatment of hyperuricemia includes the combination of allopurinol (a xanthine oxidase inhibitor) to decrease uric acid production, probenecid to increase uric acid clearance in those with normal renal function, alkalinization of the urine to increase the solubility of uric acid, and increased fluid intake to reduce the concentration of uric acid. A low purine diet, weight reduction, and reduced alcohol intake are recommended.

Harris JC. Disorders of purine and pyrimidine metabolism. In: Kliegman RM, Behrman RE, Jenson HB, Stanton BF (eds). *Nelson Textbook of Pediatrics.* 18th edn. Vol 1. Philadelphia: Saunders, 2007;627–36.

26.7 PORPHYRIAS

Porphyrias are inherited and acquired metabolic disorders in which the activities of the enzymes of the heme biosynthetic pathway are either partially or almost completely deficient. It results in production of abnormally high levels of porphyrins and/or their precursors. These products accumulate in tissues and are excreted in urine and stool. Heme is composed of ferrous iron and protoporphyrin IX, and is an essential molecule for life as the prosthetic group of hemeproteins, such as hemoglobin, myoglobin, mitochondrial and microsomal cytochromes, catalase, peroxidases, and tryptophan pyrrolase. Pathophysiologic consequences of porphyrins and their precursors are photosensitivity and neurological disturbances. Porphyrias are classified into 8 types.

1. *δ-Aminolevulinic acid dehydratase deficiency (ADP)* is an autosomal recessive disorder. Patients with ADP show vomiting, pain in the arms and legs, and neuropathy exacerbated following stress, alcohol use, or decreased food intake. Treatment of acute attack is similar to the treatment of AIP.

2. *Acute intermittent porphyria (AIP)* is an autosomal dominant disorder that results from a partial deficiency of the enzyme porphobilinogen-deaminase (PBGD).

Abdominal pain and neuropathy are common features of AIP. *Treatment* of AIP, as well as that of ADP, HCP, and VP is essentially identical. Treatment between attacks consists of adequate nutritional intake, avoidance of drugs known to exacerbate porphyria, and prompt treatment of other intercurrent diseases or infections. Unresponsive severe cases should be treated with intravenous administration of dextrose (a minimum of 300 g). High doses of glucose (400 g/day) is given as a 10% solution; amounts up to 500 g daily may be more effective. Intravenous hematin (4 mg/kg q12 hr) is also effective in reducing the ALA and PBG excretion as well as in curtailing acute attacks. Bromides, gabapentin, and probably vagabatrin are safe drugs for treatment of seizures. Most classic anti-seizure medicines can lead to acute porphyria attacks.

3. *Congenital erythropoietic porphyria* (CEP) also termed Günther disease is an autosomal recessive disease due to a marked deficiency of the enzyme uroporphyrinogen III synthase (UROS). The diagnosis of CEP is suggested at birth by pink to dark brown staining of the diapers in infants, due to large amounts of porphyrins in urine. With sun exposure, severe blistering lesions appear on exposed areas of skin on the face and hands. Treatment includes protection from sunlight exposure and avoidance of trauma, and prompt treatment of any cutaneous infections. Sunscreen lotions and beta-carotene are sometimes beneficial.

4. *Porphyria cutanea tarda* (PCT) is due to a marked deficiency of hepatic UROD. It occurs in mid or late adult life, and is rare in children. PCT is characterized by skin lesions and liver abnormalities. PCT is recognized by blistering and crusted skin lesions on the backs of the hands, which are the most sun exposed areas of the body, and somewhat less commonly on the forearms, face, ears, neck, legs, and feet. The fluid-filled vesicles commonly rupture and become crusted or denuded areas heal slowly and are subject to infection. Facial hypertrichosis and hyperpigmentation are also common.

Treatment of PCT includes choice of 2 specific and effective forms of treatment, phlebotomy or low-dose hydroxychloroquine, and removal of susceptibility factors when possible.

5. *Hepatoerythropoietic porphyria* (HEP) is characterized by the childhood onset of severe photosensitivity and skin fragility. Avoidance of sunlight exposure and the use of topical sunscreens is most important in the management of HEP.

6. *Hereditary coproporphyria* (HCP) disease is similar to ADP or AIP, although it is usually milder; additionally, HCP may be associated with photosensitivity. Attacks are precipitated most commonly with phenobarbital. Pregnancy, menstrual cycle and

contraceptive steroids can also precipitate attacks. Treatment of acute attack is similar to the treatment of AIP.

7. *Variegate porphyria* (VP) is characterized by neurovisceral symptoms, photosensitivity, or both. The neurovisceral symptomatology is identical to that observed in ADP, AIP, and HCP. Barbiturates, dapsone, contraceptive steroids, pregnancy, and decreased carbohydrate intake all induce or exacerbate VP. Management of the case includes avoidance of precipitating factors, protective clothing and oral β-carotene and treatment of neurovisceral symptoms identical to that described for AIP.

8. *Erythropoietic protoporphyria* (EPP), an autosomal dominant disorder is characterized by the childhood onset of cutaneous photosensitivity in light-exposed areas. Exposure to sunlight should be avoided. Use of topical sun-screen agents may be helpful. Oral β-carotene (120–180 mg daily) leads to clinical improvement.

Anderson KE, Lee C, Desnick RJ. The porphyrias. In: Kliegman RM, Behrman RE, Jenson HB, Stanton BF (eds). *Nelson Textbook of Pediatrics*. 18th edn. Vol 1. Philadelphia: Saunders, 2007;637–55.

Badcock NR, O'Reilly DA, Zoanetti GD, et al: Childhood porphyrias: implications and treatments. *Clin Chem* 1993; 39(6): 1334–40.

Jensen JD, Resnick SD. Porphyria in childhood. *Semin Dermatol* 1995;14(1):33–39.

26.8 HYPOGLYCEMIA

Definition. Any value of blood glucose < 50 mg/dl in *neonates* be viewed with suspicion and vigorously treated. This is particularly applicable after the initial 2–3 hr of life, when glucose normally has reached its nadir; subsequently, blood glucose levels begin to rise and achieve values of 50 mg/dl or higher after 12–24 hr. In older *infants and children*, a whole blood glucose concentration of < 50 mg/dl (10–15% higher for serum or plasma) represents hypoglycemia.

Clinical manifestations: Clinical features generally fall into two categories. The 1st category includes symptoms associated with the activation of the autonomic nervous system and epinephrine release, usually seen with a rapid decline in blood glucose concentration (anxiety, perspiration, palpitation, pallor, tremulousness, weakness, hunger, nausea, vomiting and angina). The 2nd category includes symptoms due to decreased cerebral glucose utilization, usually associated with a slow decline in blood glucose level or prolonged hypoglycemia (headache, mental confusion, visual disturbances, personality changes, inability to concentrate, dysarthria, ataxia, seizure, coma, and decerebrate or decorticate posture).

Neonatal Transient Hypoglycemia

i. Small for gestational age and premature infants
ii. Infants born to diabetic mothers: *See* section 8.15
iii. Infants born with erythroblastosis fetalis may also have hyperinsulinemia and share many physical features, such as large body size, with infants born to diabetic mothers. The cause of hyperinsulinemia in infants with erythroblastosis is not clear.

Persistent or Recurrent Hypoglycemia in Infants and Children

Hyperinsulism: Hyperinsulism is the most common cause of persistent hypoglycemia in early infancy. There is no history or biochemical evidence of maternal diabetes. The onset is from birth to 18 mo of age, but occasionally it is 1st evident in older children. In affected infants, the plasma insulin concentrations at the time of hypoglycemia are commonly > 5–10 μU/ml. Some authorities consider any value of insulin > 2 μU/ml with hypoglycemia is abnormal. The insulin (U/ml): glucose (mg/dL) ratio is commonly > 0.4; plasma insulin-like growth factor binding protein-1 (IGFBP-1), ketones, and FFA levels are low. Macrosomic infants with hyperinsulinemia may present with hypoglycemia from the 1st days of life reflecting the anabolic effects of insulin in utero. Infants with lesser degrees of hyperinsulinemia may manifest hypoglycemia after the 1st few weeks to months, when the frequency of feedings has been decreased to permit the infant to sleep through the night. Increasing appetite and demands for feeding, jitteriness, and frank seizures are the most common presenting features. The differential diagnosis of endogenous hyperinsulism includes diffuse β-cell hyperplasia or focal β-cell microadenoma. The distinction between these two major entities is important because the former, if unresponsive to medical therapy, requires near total pancreatectomy, despite which hypoglycemia may persist or diabetes mellitus may ensue at some later time. By contrast, focal adenomas diagnosed preoperatively or intraoperatively permit localized curative resection with subsequent normal glucose metabolism. Insulin secreting macroadenomas are rare in childhood and may be diagnosed preoperatively via CT or MRI.

Persistent hyperinsulinemic hypoglycemia of infancy (PHHI) may be inherited or sporadic, is severe and is caused by mutations in the regulation of the potassium channel intimately involved in insulin secretion by the pancreatic β cell. The familial forms of PHHI are more common in certain populations, notably Arabic and Ashkenazi Jewish communities.

Hypoglycemia associated with hyperinsulinemia is also seen in ~50% of patients with the Beckwith-Wiedemann syndrome. This syndrome is characterized by omphalocele, gigantism, macroglossia, microcephaly, and visceromegaly. Distinctive lateral ear lobe fissures and facial nevus flammeus are present; hemihypertrophy occurs in many of these infants. Diffuse islet cell hyperplasia occurs in infants with hypoglycemia.

Hyperinsulinemic hypoglycemia in infancy is reported as a manifestation of one form of congenital disorder of glycosylation. Disorders of protein glycosylation usually present with neurologic symptoms but may also include liver dysfunction with hepatomegaly, intractable diarrhea, protein-losing enteropathy, and hypoglycemia.

Hyperinsulinemia due to islet cell adenoma should be considered in any child 5 yr or older presenting with hypoglycemia. Fasting for up to 24–36 hr usually provokes hypoglycemia; coexisting hyperinsulinemia confirms the diagnosis, provided that fictitious administration of insulin by the parents, a form of Munchausen syndrome of proxy, is excluded. Exogenously administered insulin can be distinguished from endogenous insulin by measurement of C-peptide concentration. If C-peptide levels are elevated, endogenous insulin secretion is responsible for the hypoglycemia; if C-peptide levels are low but insulin values are high, exogenous insulin has been administered, perhaps as a form of child abuse. Islet cell adenomas at this age are treated by surgical excision. Other possibilities such as familial multiple endocrine adenomatosis type I (Wermer syndrome), antibodies to insulin or the insulin receptor (insulin mimetic action), deliberate or accidental ingestion of drugs (sulfonylurea or related compound that stimulates insulin secretion) should be considered for hypoglycemia. In such cases, insulin and C-peptide concentrations in blood will be elevated.

A rare form of hyperinsulinemic hypoglycemia has been reported after exercise. Whereas glucose and insulin remain unchanged in most people after moderation, short-term exercise, and rare patients manifest severe hypoglycemia with hyperinsulinemia 15–50 minutes after the same standardized exercise. This form of exercise-induced hyperinsulism may be caused by an abnormal responsiveness of β-cell insulin release in response to pyruvate generated during exercise.

Endocrine deficiency: Hypoglycemia associated with endocrine deficiency is usually caused by adrenal insufficiency with or without associated growth hormone deficiency. In panhypopituitarism, isolated adrenocorticotrophic hormone (ACTH) or growth hormone deficiency, or combined ACTH deficiency plus growth hormone deficiency, the incidence is as high as 20%. In the newborn period, hypoglycemia may be the presenting feature of hypopituitarism; in males, a microphallus may provide a clue to a coexistent deficiency of gonadotropin. When adrenal disease is severe as in congenital adrenal hyperplasia disturbances in serum electrolytes with hyponatremia and hyperkalemia or ambiguous genitals may provide diagnostic clue. Hyperpigmentation may provide the clue to Addison disease.

Glucagon deficiency in infants or children may rarely be associated with hypoglycemia.

Substrate Limited

Ketotic hypoglycemia: This is the most common form of childhood hypoglycemia. This condition usually presents between the ages of 18 mo and 5 yr and remits spontaneously by the age of 8–9 yr. Hypoglycemic episodes typically occur during periods of intercurrent illness when food intake is limited. At the time of documented hypoglycemia, there is associated ketonuria and ketonemia; plasma insulin concentrations are appropriately low ≤ 5–10 μl/ml, thus excluding hyperinsulinemia. The etiology of ketotic hypoglycemia may be a defect in any of the complex steps involved in protein catabolism, oxidative deamination of amino acids, transamination, alanine synthesis, or alanine efflux from muscle. Children with ketotic hypoglycemia are frequently smaller than age-matched controls and often have a history of transient neonatal hypoglycemia. Although the defect may be present at birth, it may not be evident until the child is stressed by more prolonged periods of caloric restriction. Spontaneous remission observed in children at age 8–9 yr might be explained by the increase in muscle bulk with its resultant increase in supply of endogenous substrate and the relative decrease in glucose requirement per unit of body mass with increasing age. In addition to that impaired epinephrine secretion from immaturity of autonomic innervation contributes to ketotic hypoglycemia. In anticipation of spontaneous resolution of this syndrome, treatment of ketotic hypoglycemia consists of frequent feedings of a high-protein, high-carbohydrate diet. During intercurrent illness, parents should test the child's urine for the presence of ketones, the appearance of which precedes hypoglycemia by several hours. In the presence of ketonuria, liquids of high carbohydrate content should be offered to the child. If these cannot be tolerated, the child should be admitted to the hospital for intravenous glucose administration.

Branched Chain Ketonuria (Maple Syrup Urine Disease): The hypoglycemic episodes are due to the interference with the production of alanine and its availability as a gluconeogenic substrate during calorie deprivation is responsible for hypoglycemia.

Glycogen storage diseases associated with hypoglycemia include glucose-6-phosphatase deficiency (Type 1 glycogen storage disease), type III glycogen storage disease, type VI and glycogen synthetase deficiency. Hypoglycemia can be prevented by feeding diet containing carbohydrate providing 60–70% calories, protein 12–15% calories, and fat 15–25% calories.

Disorders of gluconeogenesis associated with hypoglycemia include fructose-1,6-diphosphatase deficiency, defects in fatty acid oxidation, acute alcohol intoxication, salicylate intoxication, phosphoenol pyruvate carboxykinase deficiency, and pyruvate carboxylase deficiency.

Other enzyme defects: Galactosemia (Galactose-1-Phosphate Uridyl Transferase Deficiency) and fructose intolerance (Fructose-1-Phosphate Aldolase Deficiency) are associated with hypoglycemia.

Defects in glucose transporters: Infants with GLUT-1 deficiency are associated with seizures. A ketogenic diet has been reported to reduce the severity. Children with hepatomegaly, galactose intolerance and renal tubular dysfunction (Fanconi- Bickel syndrome) have been shown to have a deficiency of the GLUT-2 deficiency.

Systemic disorders: Several systemic disorders are associated with hypoglycemia in infants and children. Neonatal sepsis is often associated with hypoglycemia, possibly as a result of diminished caloric intake with impaired gluconeogenesis. Similar mechanisms may apply to the hypoglycemia found in severely malnourished infants or in infants with severe malabsorption.

Hyperviscosity with a central hematocrit of > 65% is associated with hypoglycemia at least 10–15% of affected infants.

Falciparum malaria has been associated with hyperinsulinemia and hypoglycemia.

Heart and renal failure have also been associated with hypoglycemia, but the mechanism is obscure.

Infants and children with Nissen fundoplication, a relatively common procedure used to ameliorate gastroesophageal reflux, frequently have an associated "dumping" syndrome with hypoglycemia. Characteristic features include significant hyperglycemia of up to 500 mg/dl 30 min postprandially and severe hypoglycemia 1.5–3.0 hr later. The early hyperglycemia phase is associated with brisk and excessive insulin release that causes the rebound hypoglycemia.

Glucagon responses have been inappropriately low in some. Acarbose, an inhibitor of glucose absorption has been reported to be successful.

Diagnosis and differential diagnosis: A careful and detailed history is essential in every suspected or documented case of hypoglycemia. Specific points to be noted include age at onset, relation to meals or caloric deprivation, and a family history of prior infants known to have had hypoglycemia or of unexplained infant death. In the 1st wk of life, the majority of infants have the transient form of neonatal hypoglycemia either as a result of prematurity/intrauterine growth restriction (IUGR) or by virtue of being born to diabetic mothers. The absence of a history of maternal diabetes, but the presence of macrosomia and the characteristic large plethoric appearance of an "infant of a diabetic mother" should arouse suspicion of hyperinsulinemic hypoglycemia of infancy probably due to a K_{ATP} channel defect that is familial (autosomal recessive) or sporadic; plasma insulin concentrations $>10~\mu U/mL$, in the presence of documented hypoglycemia confirm this diagnosis. The presence of hepatomegaly should arouse suspicion of an enzyme deficiency; if non-glucose-reducing sugar is present in the urine, galactosemia is most likely. In males, the presence of a microphallus suggests the possibility of hypopituitarism, which also may be associated with jaundice in both sexes.

After the neonatal period, clues to the cause of persistent or recurrent hypoglycemia can be obtained through a careful history, physical examination and initial laboratory findings. The relation of the hypoglycemia to food intake may suggest that the defect is one of gluconeogenesis, if symptoms occur 6 hr or more after meals. If hypoglycemia occurs shortly after meals, galactosemia or fructose intolerance is most likely, and the presence of reducing substances in the urine rapidly distinguishes these possibilities. The autosomal dominant forms of hyperinsulinemic hypoglycemia need to be considered, with measurement of glucose, insulin, and ammonia, and careful history for other family members of any age. Measurement of insulin-like growth factor binding protein-1 (IGFBP-1) may be useful; it is low in hyperinsulinemia states and high in other forms of hypoglycemia. The presence of hepatomegaly suggests one of the enzyme deficiencies in glycogen breakdown or in gluconeogenesis. The absence of ketonemia or ketonuria at the time of initial presentation strongly suggests hyperinsulinemia or a defect in fatty acid oxidation. In most other causes hypoglycemia, with the exception of galactosemia and fructose intolerance, ketonemia and ketonuria are present at the time of fasting hypoglycemia. At the time of the hypoglycemia,

serum should be obtained for determination of hormones and substrates, followed by repeated measurement after an intramuscular or intravenous injection of glucagon. Hypoglycemia and ketonuria in children between ages 18 mo and 5 yr is most likely to be ketotic hypoglycemia, especially if hepatomegaly is absent. The ingestion of a toxin, including alcohol and salicylate, can usually be excluded rapidly by the history. Inadvertent or deliberate drug ingestion and errors in dispensing medicines should also be considered.

When the history is suggestive, but acute symptoms are not present, a 24–36 hr supervised fast can usually provoke hypoglycemia and resolve the question of hyperinsulinemia or other conditions. Such a fast is contraindicated if a fatty acid oxidation defect is suspected; other approaches such as mass tandem spectrometry or molecular diagnosis, or both, should be considered. Because adrenal insufficiency may mimic ketotic hypoglycemia, plasma cortisol levels should be determined at the time of documented hypoglycemia, increased buccal or skin pigmentation may provide the clue to primary adrenal insufficiency with elevated ACTH (melanocyte-stimulating hormone) activity. Short stature or a decrease in the growth rate may provide the clue to pituitary insufficiency involving growth hormone as well as ACTH. Definitive tests of pituitary-adrenal function such as the arginine-insulin stimulation test for growth hormone IGF-1, IGFBP-1, and cortisol release may be necessary.

In the presence of hepatomegaly and hypoglycemia, a presumptive diagnosis of the enzyme defect can often be made through the clinical manifestations, presence of hyperlipidemia, acidosis, hyperuricemia, response to glucagon in the fed and fasted states, and response to infusion of various appropriate precursors. A liver biopsy is required in making a definite diagnosis of glycogen storage disease.

Treatment: It is important to prevent hypoglycemia and its resultant effects on CNS development in the newborn period. Therefore, in neonates with hyperinsulinemia not associated with maternal diabetes, subtotal or focal pancreatectomy may be needed, unless hypoglycemia can be readily controlled with long-term diazoxide or somatostatin analogs.

Treatment of acute symptomatic neonatal or infant hypoglycemia includes intravenous administration of 2 ml/kg of $D_{10}W$, followed by a continuous infusion of glucose at 6–8 mg/kg/min, adjusting the rate to maintain blood glucose levels in the normal range. If hypoglycemic seizures are present, some recommend a 4 ml/kg bolus of D_{10} W.

The management of persistent neonatal or infantile hypoglycemia includes increasing the rate of intravenous glucose infusion to 10–15 mg/kg/min or more, if needed. This may require a central venous or umbilical venous catheter to administer a hypertonic 15–25% glucose solution. If hyperinsulinemia is present, it should be medically managed initially with diazoxide and then somatostatin analogs or calcium channel blockers. If hypoglycemia is unresponsive to intravenous glucose plus diazoxide (maximal doses up to 25 mg/kg/day) and somatostatin analogs, surgery via partial or near-total pancreatectomy should be considered.

Oral diazoxide, 10–25 mg/kg/24 hr given in divided doses every 6 hr, may reverse hyperinsuilinemic hypoglycemia but may also produce hirsutism, edema, nausea, hyperuricemia, electrolyte disturbances, advanced bone age, IgG deficiency, and, rarely hypotension with prolonged use. A long-acting somatostatin analog (octerotide) is sometimes effective in controlling hyperinsulinemic hypoglycemia in patients with islet cell disorders not caused by genetic mutations in K_{ATP} channel and islet cell adenoma. Octerotide is administered subcutaneously every 6–12 hr in doses of 20–50 µg in neonates and young infants. Complications include poor growth due to inhibition of growth hormone release, pain at the injection site, vomiting, diarrhea, and hepatic dysfunction (hepatitis, cholelithiasis). Octreotide is usually employed before subtotal pancreatectomy for K_{ATP} channel disorders. It may be particularly useful for the treatment of refractory hypoglycemia despite subtotal pancreatectomy. Continued prolonged medical therapy without pancreatic resection to control hypoglycemia is worthwhile because some children have spontaneous resolution of the hyperinsulinemic hypoglycemia.

Prognosis: The prognosis is good in asymptomatic neonates with hypoglycemia of short duration. Hypoglycemia recurs in 10–15% of infants after adequate treatment. Symptomatic infants with hypoglycemia, particularly low-birth weight infants, those with persistent hyperinsulinemic hypoglycemia, and infants of diabetic mothers, have a poorer prognosis for subsequent normal intellectual development. The major long-term sequelae of severe, prolonged hypoglycemia are mental retardation, recurrent seizure activity, or both. Transient isolated hypoglycemia of short duration does not appear to be associated these severe sequelae.

Dalgic N, Ergenekon E, Soysal S, et al. Transient neonatal hypoglycemia-Long-term effects on neurodevelopmental outcome. *J Pediatr Endocrinol Metab* 2002;15:319–24.

De Lonlay P, Giurgea I, Touati, et al. Neonatal hypo-glycemia: Aetiologies. *Semin Neonatol* 2004;9:49–58.

Mayefsky JH, Sarnaik AP, Postellon DC. Fictitious hypoglycemia. *Pediatrics* 1982;69:804–5.

Sperling MA. Hypoglycema. In: Kliegman RM, Behrman RE, Jenson HB, Stanton BF (eds). *Nelson Textbook of Pediatrics.* 18th edn. Vol 1. Philadelphia: Saunders, 2007;655–69.

Sperling MA, Menon RK. Differential diagnosis and management of neonatal hypoglycemia. *Pediatr Clin North Am* 2004;51:703–23.

Stanley CA. Advances in diagnosis and treatment of hyperinsulism in infants and children. *J Clin Endocrinol Metab* 2002;87:4857–9.

26.9 PROGERIA

Progeria is an autosomal dominant ageing disease which is caused by sporadic mutations in the LMNA-gene. Progeria of childhood characterized by premature aging that occurs at about 8 to 10 times the normal rate of aging. Because of this accelerated aging, a child of ten years will have similar respiratory, cardiovascular, and arthritic conditions that a 70-year-old would have. The condition is estimated to affect ~1/8,000,000. The children have a remarkably similar appearance, despite different ethnic background. Children with progeria usually appear normal in early infancy, but manifestations such as mid-facial cyanosis, "sculpted nose" and "sclerodema" may suggest the existence of the syndrome at birth. Profound growth failure occurs in the 1st yr of life. The clinical manifestations include short stature; weight distinctly low for height; diminished subcutaneous fat; head disproportionately large for face; micrognathia; prominent scalp veins; generalized alopecia; prominent eyes; delayed and abnormal dentition; pyriform thorax; short, dystrophic clavicles; "horse riding" stance; wide-based shuffling gait; coax valga; thin limbs and prominent, stiff joints; and failure to complete sexual maturation (do not become sexually mature). Other features frequently present are skin that is thin, taut, dry, wrinkled, and brown-spotted in various areas; sclerodermatous skin over the lower abdomen, proximal thighs, and buttocks, prominent superficial veins; loss of eyebrows and eyelashes; persistently patent anterior fontanel; sculpted, beaked nasal tip; faint nasolabial cyanosis; thin lips; protruding ears; absence of ear lobules; thin, high-pitched voice; dystrophic nails; and progressive radiolucency of the terminal phalanges and distal clavicles (acro-osteolysis). Children with progeria usually have severe atherosclerosis, and death occurs as a result of complications of cardiac or cerebrovascular disease, generally between age 5 and 20 yr, with a median lifespan of ~13 yr.

Brown WT, Gordon LB, Collis FS. Hutchinson-Gilford progeria syndrome. In Gene Reviews at Gene Tests: Medical Genetics Information Resource [data base outline]. Available at http://w.w.w, genetests.org/updated August 2006.

Brown WT. Progeria. In: Kliegman RM, Behrman RE, Jenson HB, Stanton BF (eds). *Nelson Textbook of Pediatrics.* 18th edn. Vol 1. Philadelphia: Saunders, 2007;836–7.

Pediatric Dentistry

27.1 INTRODUCTION

Humans have two sets of teeth: Primary teeth (deciduous/ milk teeth/baby teeth) and Permanent teeth (adult teeth) (Table 27.1).

Stages of Dentition

- *Primary dentition:* This dentition contains only primary or milk teeth. This dentition begins with the eruption of the first primary tooth and will last till the eruption of the first permanent tooth. Usually by the age of six months (6–8 months) the primary incisor tooth erupts. The first permanent tooth to erupt is lower first molar, i.e. by 6 years. So the primary dentition stage is from 6 months to 6 years.
- *Mixed dentition:* Six years onwards, the permanent teeth start erupting with simultaneous shedding of the primary teeth. This process of eruption and shedding is seen in mixed dentition which is unique in having both primary as well as permanent teeth. So mixed dentition stage is from 6 years up to 12 years.
- *Permanent dentition:* Usually by 12 years, shedding of all primary teeth is completed and hence only adult teeth are present.

Structure of Tooth

The **crown** is the part of the tooth that is visible above the **gum.** The **neck** is the region of the tooth that is at the gum line, between the root and the crown. The **root** is the region of the tooth that is below the gum. Some teeth have only one root, for example, incisors and canine teeth, whereas molar and premolar have 2 to 4 roots. The crown of each tooth has a coating of **enamel,** which protects the underlying dentine. Enamel is the hardest substance in the human body,

even harder than bone. It gains its hardness from tightly packed rows of calcium and phosphorus crystals within a protein matrix structure. This structure of enamel renders it brittle. On the cusps of molars and premolars it attains a maximum thickness of about 2 to 2.5 mm thinning down to almost a knife edge at the neck of the tooth. The specific gravity of enamel is 2.8. Its colour ranges from yellowish white to grayish. It mainly consists of inorganic material (96%) and only a small amount of organic substance and water (4%). Once the enamel has been formed during tooth development, there is a little turnover of its minerals during life. Mature enamel is not considered to be a 'living' tissue.

The major component of the inside of the tooth is **dentin.** It provides the bulk and general form of the tooth. This substance is slightly softer than enamel, with a structure more like bone. It is elastic and compressible in contrast to the brittle nature of enamel. Dentin is usually light yellowish in colour, becoming darker with age. It consists of 65% inorganic and 35% organic material. Dentin is sensitive. It contains tiny tubules throughout its structure that connect with the central nerve of the tooth within the pulp. Dentin is a 'live' tissue.

Below the gum, the dentin of the root is covered with a thin layer of **cementum,** rather than enamel. Its hardness is less than that of dentin, and is light yellow in color. It contains about 45–50% inorganic and 50–55% organic material and water. Cementum is a hard bone-like substance onto which the **periodontal membrane** attaches. This membrane bonds the root of the tooth to the **bone** of the jaw. It contains elastic fibres to allow some movement of the tooth within its bony socket. It is 'avascular'.

The **pulp** forms the central chamber of each tooth and consists of soft connective tissue. It contains **blood vessels** to supply nutrients to the tooth, and **nerves** to enable the tooth to sense heat and cold. It also contains small lymph vessels which carries white blood cells to the tooth to help fight bacteria. The total volume of all permanent teeth pulp organs is 0.38 cc, and the mean volume of a single adult human pulp organ is 0.02 cc (molar pulps are 3 to 4 times larger than incisor pulps).

The extension of the pulp within the root of the tooth is called the **root canal**. The root canal connects with the surrounding tissue via the **apical foramen** at the tip of the root. This is an opening in the cementum through which the tooth's nerve supply and blood supply enter the pulp from the surrounding tissue. The average size of the apical foramen of the maxillary teeth in the adult is 0.4 mm, and in mandibular teeth it is 0.3 mm in diameter.

Eruption and Shedding

- *Eruption:* Eruption is the axial or occlusal movement of the tooth from its developmental position within the gums to its functional position in the occlusal plane (Box 27.1).
- *Shedding:* The physiologic process resulting in elimination of the deciduous dentition due to progressive resorption of the roots of teeth and their supporting tissue.
- *Teething:* Teething is the common term used for eruption of primary dentition. This usually begins in the fifth or sixth months after birth. Appearance of teeth is an important milestone in a child's life and for the parents. In most of the cases, this process may remain uneventful causing no distress to the

> **Box 27.1:** Eruption hematoma and other than normal primary dentition
>
> *Natal teeth:* Teeth present at the time of birth.
> *Neonatal teeth:* Teeth which erupt within 30 days after birth.
> *Eruption hematoma:* A bluish purple, elevated area of tissue which occasionally develops a few weeks before the eruption of a primary or permanent tooth.

child but in some children it causes local symptoms. These "**teething troubles**" include signs of local irritation, drooling saliva, redness and swelling of the gums. The child wants to put fingers in the mouth or any object/toy in the mouth because of local itching. Some young children become restless and fretful during this time. Inflammation of gingival tissues subsides within a few days after the complete emergence of the crown of the erupting tooth. Some systemic symptoms are attributed to teething like fever, diarrhea, convulsions, bronchitis, etc. Eruption is a normal physiologic process. Attributing systemic disturbances to eruption is not justified, but is coincidental. Child putting his hands and objects frequently in the mouth may contribute to contamination and hence diarrhea and vomiting followed by fever.

Local massage to the gum pads relieves the discomfort. Topical anesthetic gel may also give temporary relief. Child may be allowed to chew on a piece of toast or biscuit or a clean teething object.

27.2 DENTAL CARIES

Dental Caries is defined as an infectious, microbial disease affecting the hard parts of the tooth, resulting

Table 27.1: Chronology of human dentition			
Primary dentition	*Eruption chronology*		*Shedding chronology*
Tooth	Mandibular	Maxillary	
Central incisor	6 months	7½ months	7–8 years
Lateral incisor	7 months	9 months	7–9 years
Canine	16 months	18 months	10–12 years
First molar	12 months	14 months	9–11 years
Second molar	20 months	24 months	11–12 years
Permanent dentition			
Central incisor	6–7 years	7–8 years	
Lateral incisor	7–8 years	8–9 years	
Canine	9–10 years	11–12 years	
First premolar	10–12 years	10–12 years	
Second premolar	11–12 years	10–12 years	
First molar	6–7 years	6–7 years	
Second molar	11–13 years	12–13 years	
Third molar	17–21 years	17–21 years	

in demineralization of the inorganic components and dissolution of the organic constituents of the tooth. It is a complex disease with a variety of factors involved resulting into the destruction of the tooth structure (Box 27.2).

Etiology of dental caries: It is a multifactorial disease. But the three primary factors are:
1. The host (Tooth)
2. Microflora (Bacteria)
3. Substrate (Fermentable)

Pathogenesis: The tooth surface is such that it provides excellent mechanical retention area for bacteria and food particles (especially if not cleaned well). The bacteria will form a biofilm (plaque) that adheres to the tooth surface. Over a period of time the food (substrate) serves as a nutrient for the bacteria to grow. Thus bacteria will produce acids that can demineralize the tooth causing dental caries. Fermentable, sticky carbohydrates are found to be the most adherent to the tooth surface, are difficult to be cleansed and most frequently attacked by the bacteria, producing acids. The microorganisms which are found most damaging for causing the disease are "**Mutans streptococci group**", especially the subspecies of this group, i.e. "*Streptococci mutans*".

Acids formed by the bacteria such as lactic acid, propionic acid, etc. can dissolve the tooth. Enamel is made of hydroxyapatite crystals containing calcium phosphate, hydroxyl ions and carbonate. Due to the dissolution of inorganic components, there occurs leaching of calcium and phosphorus causing "demineralization". Once the damaged enamel surface layer loses all support, cavitation takes place. Thus dental caries progresses and damages tooth until a change in the environment occurs. If therapeutic and preventive strategies are implemented, "Remineralisation" can occur up to a certain extent (Fig. 27.1).

Bacterial enzyme + Fermentable carbohydrates = Acid

Acid + Enamel = Dental caries

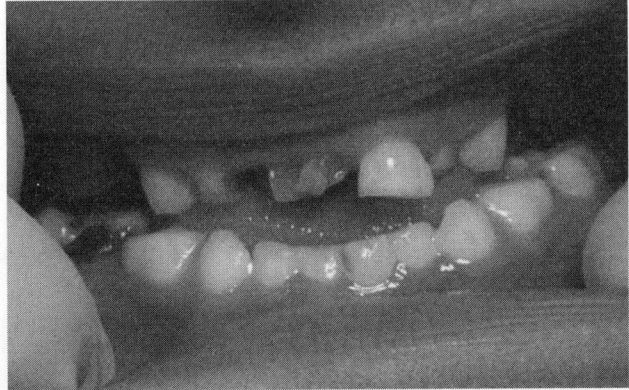

Fig. 27.1: Dental caries

Predisposing and Contributing Factors

A. Tooth
   1. Composition
   2. Anatomic characteristics
   3. Arch form
   4. Presence of restorations and /or appliance
B. Saliva
   1. Composition
   2. Flow rate
   3. pH
   4. Viscosity
   5. Antibacterial factors
C. Microflora
   1. Acidogenic: *Streptococcus mutans*, Actinomyces
   2. Aciduric: Lactobacilli
   3. Others: Those producing IgA-l proteases
   4. Plaque
D. Diet
   1. Type—cariogenicity
   2. Monosaccharides, disaccharides, polysaccharides
   3. Quantity consumed
   4. Form—refined or coarse
   5. Nature—sticky or easily cleared and cleansed
   6. Biochemical properties—fermentable or non-fermentable carbohydrates.
   7. Food retention—time factor
   8. Cooking and processing
   9. Frequency—snacking habit
   10. Trace elements and role of vitamins.
E. Socioeconomic status
F. Hereditary factors

Early childhood caries: Dental caries in infants and toddlers is specifically and broadly called early childhood caries. This can be rampant caries, nursing caries, nursing bottle caries, baby bottle decay, and milk bottle syndrome, etc.

Rampant caries: Massler defined it as "suddenly appearing, rapidly burrowing type of caries, resulting in early involvement of pulp and affecting those teeth which are usually regarded as immune to decay".

Rampant caries lesions have an acute onset and are widespread. These lesions involves teeth and areas

> **Box 27.2:** Important consideration in children contributing to dental caries
>
> 1. Liking for sweets
> 2. Snacking
> 3. Peer pressure, environment and media
> 4. Nursing habits and weaning
> 5. Oral cleansing habits
> 6. Introduction to dentistry—fear

that are usually not susceptible, e.g. facial and lingual surfaces of the incisors, interproximal surfaces of lower anterior teeth, etc.

Rampant caries is mainly attributed to inadequate maintenance of oral hygiene. Emotional disturbance is also a major contributing factor leading to craving for sweets and habit of snacking. This may further worsen the situation by salivary deficiency. Nutritional deficiencies also contribute to such lesions.

Nursing caries/nursing bottle caries: It is a type of rampant caries caused due to sleep time nursing habits. When the child sleeps immediately after being bottle fed, then the milk in the oral cavity supplies the required carbohydrate for the acidogenic bacteria and thus causes dental damage. Same result occurs if a child takes juice or sweetened pacifier at sleep time. Multiple caries lesions develop at a rapid speed. This is further supported by reduced salivary flow during sleep as swallowing reflex is absent. Opportunistic cariogenic bacteria can then cause great damage thus causing dental decay. Pattern of these lesions is significant, as lower incisors escape the damage due to protection by the tongue and their proximity to the salivary gland openings.

Management of dental caries: Treatment protocol both preventive and restorative management is presented in Table 27.2.

27.3 ORTHODONTICS—PREVENTIVE AND INTERCEPTIVE

1. Introduction

Orthodontics is that branch of dental sciences which studies the normal growth and development of the body generally and face, jaws and teeth particularly, their infinite variations and abnormalities and the prevention and treatment of the dento-facial abnormalities within certain biological limits.

Occlusion of the Teeth

The relationship which the teeth of one arch bear to the other arch when the jaws are closed into maximum cuspal relationship, is known as occlusion. In normal occlusion, each tooth occupies a reasonably definite position in the arch and bears a definite relationship with its neighbor of the same and the opposing arch. For the development of normal occlusion, the following status of teeth and jaws should persist:
1. The maxillary teeth should be in correct relationship to one another and to the maxillary basal bone.
2. And the mandibular teeth should be in correct relationship to one another and to the mandibular basal bone.
3. And the maxillary and mandibular bases should be in correct relationship with one another.

But this does not happen in all cases, so derangements in occlusion (malocclusion) may take place. These derangements may be aggravated or sometime masked by the morphology and behavior of soft tissues (lip, cheeks, tongue) and other environmental factors (e.g. habits).

2. Malocclusion

Malocclusion is defined as an irregularity of teeth beyond the accepted range of the normal. Malocclusion may be associated with one or more of the following conditions:
1. Malposition of individual teeth.
2. Malrelationship of the dental arches, unfavorable for the production of normal occlusion; and
3. Malrelationship of dental base, i.e. skeletal morphology unfavorable for the production of normal arch relationship and occlusion.

Table 27.2: Treatment protocol for dental management

Preventive	Restorative
A. Professional care	A. Incipient lesion
• Diet counseling	• Fluoride treatment
• Oral hygiene methods and education	• Pit and Fissure sealants
• Fluoride treatment	B. Carious enamel and dentin
• Pit and fissure sealants	• Preventive resin restoration
• Dental health education	• Glass ionomer restorations
B. Home care	• Composite filling for anterior and posterior teeth
• Diet modification	• Amalgam restoration
• Discontinuation of habits like bottle feed, feed at sleep time, pacifiers, etc.	• Cermet restoration
• Infant oral care	• Anterior and posterior crowns.
• Oral hygiene methods.	C. Carious lesions involving dental pulp.
• Fluoride toothpaste is to be used.	• Pulp therapy followed by crowns
• Regular dental checkups.	• Extraction and space management.

Malrelation of the dental arches: Variations from the normal relationship of the dental arches may take place in three planes of space:
a. Anteroposterior (sagittal plane)
b. Lateral plane
c. Vertical plane

3. Angle's Classification

In orthodontics, many classifications have been proposed, but the Angle's classification has received universal acceptance. Angle's classification in useful in determining the anteroposterior relationship of the maxillary and mandibular dental arches and these may also reflect the jaw relationship.

The 'key' teeth used in Angle's classification are the first permanent molars and relationship of these molars in the anteroposterior plane determines the different classes (class I, II, III) in this classification.

In normal occlusion, the mesiobuccal cusp of the upper first molar of both sides (6/6) occlude with the buccal groove of the lower first molars of both sides with all teeth well aligned and incisors with normal overjet and overbite. The normal overbite and overjet is produced as follows:
a. The palatal surface of upper incisors overlap the incisal third of the labial surface of lower incisors and this produces a normal overbite.
b. The palatal surface of upper incisors protrude 1–2 mm anteriorly to the labial surface of lower incisors and this produces a normal overjet.

Class I: Malocclusions in which the lower first permanent molars are correctly related to the upper first permanent molars, i.e. the mesiobuccal cusp of the upper first molar of both sides (6/6) occlude with the buccal groove of the lower first molars of both sides. This arch relationship is also 'neutro-occlusion'.

Class II: In these cases, the lower arch occludes at least half a cusp distal than normal in relation to the upper arch, judged by the first molar relationship. This arch relationship is also called 'disto-occlusion' or 'post-normal occlusion'. Class II is divided according to the inclination of the upper incisors into two divisions.

Division 1: The maxillary central incisors are proclined or of average inclination so that there is an increase in overjet.

Division 2: The maxillary central incisors are retroclined (less than 105 degree to the maxillary plane). The overjet is usually average, but may also be increased (in severe skeletal cases). The upper lateral incisors are usually proclined and rotated. Overbite is usually increased.

Class III: In this class, the lower dental arch occlude at least half a cusp forward than normal in relationship

to the upper dental arch, judged by the 1st permanent molar relationship. Frequently the lower incisors are in labial relationship to the upper incisors. This arch relationship is also called 'mesio-occlusion' or pre-normal occlusion.

4. Preventive Orthodontics

This includes actions taken to preserve the integrity of what appears normal for that age. It includes procedures undertaken prior to the onset of a malocclusion in anticipation of a developing malocclusion.

5. Interceptive Orthodontics

It is a procedure that is undertaken at an early age of malocclusion to eliminate or reduce the severity of the same. By undertaking appropriate interceptive procedures, it is possible to prevent the establishment of a full fledged malocclusion that may require long term orthodontic treatment at a later age.

Terms preventive and interceptive orthodontics are sometimes used synonymously. But it should be understood that preventive orthodontic procedures are undertaken when the dentition and occlusion are perfectly normal, while interceptive procedures are carried out when signs and symptoms of malocclusion have appeared.

6. Procedure Undertaken in Preventive Orthodontics

1. Parent education
2. Caries control
3. Care of deciduous dentition
4. Management of ankylosed tooth
5. Maintenance of quadrant wise tooth shedding time table
6. Check-up for oral habits and habit breaking appliances if necessary are given
7. Occlusal equilibration (if there are any occlusal prematurities)
8. Prevention of damage to occlusion, e.g. Milwaukee braces.
9. Extraction of supernumerary teeth
10. Space maintenance
11. Management of deeply locked first permanent molar
12. Management of abnormal frenal attachments

7. Procedure Undertaken in Interceptive Orthodontics

1. Planned extraction
2. Correction of developing cross bite
3. Control of abnormal habits
4. Space regaining
5. Muscle exercises

Table 27.3: Classification of habits

Obsessive (Deep rooted)		Nonobsessive (easily learned and dropped)	
Intentional or meaningful	Masochistic or self-inflicting injury	Unintentional	Functional
Examples: Nail biting; Digit sucking; Lip biting	Examples: Gingival stripping	Examples: Abnormal pillowing; Chin propping	Examples: Mouth breathing; Tongue thrusting; Bruxism

6. Interception of skeletal malrelations
7. Removal of soft tissues or bony barrier to enable eruption of teeth.

8. Habits

Habit can be defined as fixed or constant practice established by frequent repetition. Habits are acquired as a result of repetition. In the initial stages there is conscious effort to perform the act. Later the act becomes less conscious and if repeated often, enough may enter the realm of subconsciousness. Habits are classified into obsessive and nonobsessive types (Table 27.3). Dentists have to help patients overcome these habits not only by providing habit breaking appliance (mechanotherapy) but also by professional counseling (Table 27.4).

27.4 CLEFT LIP AND CLEFT PALATE

1. *Embryologically*, the clefts of lip and palate are due to failure of the maxillary and nasal processes to unite. The above union is usually completed between 5 and 6 weeks intrauterine life. Failure of this union due to lack of disintegration of epithelium or due to any other cause will produce total cleft of primary palate, while partial fusion will produce subtotal clefts. The secondary palate develops from a pair of palatal shelves (palatal processes) arising from the inner side of the maxillary processes, which unite with the nasal septum from before backwards and any arrest of union thus result in a defect that varies from a bifid uvula to a complete cleft of the secondary palate. The union between the palatal processes and nasal septum is at 8–10 weeks intrauterine life.

Table 27.4: Habit and habit breaking appliance

Habit	Appliance
Thumb sucking habit	Removable/fixed habit breaking appliance with palatal cribs
Tongue thrusting habit	Removable/fixed habit breaking appliance with palatal rakes
Mouth breathing	Oral screen
Bruxism	Occlusal splints
Lip biting/sucking	Lip bumper

2. *Etiology*
Genetic factors: Cleft lip associated with cleft palate is more common in males. Cleft palate is alone more common in female. This shows vague influence of heredity over occurrence of cleft. In about one-fifth of these patients, a positive family history can be elicited. In rare clefts, the heredity factors seem to be very unusual.

Gene-environment interactions: Many cleft lip and palate cases show a slight familial tendency but do not give rise to the Mendelian patterns of inheritance. In these cases, the interaction between multiple genes with small defects and environmental factors results in the defects. There is an increasing evidence that most clefts in human being appears due to multifactorial causes, i.e. due to combined effect of genetic influence and various environmental factors.

Environmental factors
- Various environmental factors like fever with rashes (e.g. Rubella), expose to radiation, drugs, trauma and complications of pregnancy (e.g. development of amniotic bands and oligohydramnious) during the first trimester of pregnancy can lead to development of various types of defects.
- Various drugs which can cause significant increases in the incidence of cleft and other congenital anomalies are thalidomide, antiepileptic drugs (diphenyl hydantoin), hormonal pills, LSD, quinine, antibiotic drugs.
- Consumption of alcohol, smoking and hypoxic condition in the mother are also considered to play an important role in development of clefts.
- Riboflavin deficiency (Riboflavin is necessary for organogenesis).
- Radiation may cause chromosomal aberration.
- Antimetabolite-block enzymes which interfere with DNA synthesis.
- Cortisone: Inhibits palatal shelf elevation; Reduces amniotic fluid; Reduces RNA synthesis
- Tolbutamide—decreases uptake of glucose.
- Oligohydramnious (reduced amniotic fluid)—causes hyperflexion of the head fold resulting in micrognathia. The small jaw pushes the tongue up between the palatal shelves.

Table 27.5: Type cleft lip and cleft palate

Type of cleft	Incidence (percent of all cleft cases)
Cleft lip alone	25%
Cleft palate alone	25%
Cleft lip and palate both	50%

3. *Incidence:* The overall incidence of cleft lip and palate varies from 0.5 to 3.63 per 1000 live births. Tog-Anderson (1942) has studied the distribution according to the type of cleft (Table 27.5).
4. *Sex:* Cleft lip is higher among males but cleft palate is common in females.
5. *Parental age:* Increase in frequency of cleft lip with or without cleft palate, with increasing parental age is seen.
6. *Associated malformation:* A number of studies have shown that in individuals born with cleft lip and/or palate, there is increased likelihood of other congenital malformation. 10–20 percent cases have congenital heart diseases.
7. *Syndromes associated with cleft palate are:*
    1. Cleidocranial dysostosis
    2. Craniofacial dysostosis
    3. Pierre Robin syndrome
    4. Marfan's syndrome
    5. Down's syndrome (Trisomy 21)
    6. Wardenburg's syndrome
    7. van der Woude's syndrome (lip pits)
    8. Klippel-Feil syndrome

8. *Treatment*

The treatment of this condition is usually shared between pediatrician, plastic surgeon, dental surgeon, orthodontist, speech therapist, otolaryngologist and sometimes other specialists. All should work together soon after the birth of the child. Their close co-operation during the treatment is very important. The aim of the treatment is to improve the appearance, speech and function (Tables 27.6 and 27.7).

Table 27.6: Total dental management of children with cleft lip and palate

Age	General dental and pediatric dental care	Orthodontic care	Surgical care
Birth	Initial contact and interview with parents. Case discussion with surgical and orthodontic teams.	Construction of presurgical orthopedic appliance if required.	Initial assessment
3–6 months	Introduce dental care plan. Study models at the time of lip repair.		Primary surgical repair of lip.
12 months to 2 years	Review.		Surgical repair of palate.
2–6 years	6 monthly reviews for assessment of growth and development, preventive advise. Topical fluoride applications and fissure sealing.		Possible revision of lip repair. Pharyngoplasty if required. Myringotomy and grommets by ENT
6–7 years	Fissure sealing of first permanent molars. Composite resin restoration of hypoplastic teeth adjacent to cleft. Preventive advice.		Myringotomy and grommets by ENT as required.
8–10 years	Case discussion with surgical and orthodontic teams for bone grafting. Possible extraction of supernumerary teeth. Interim bridge or partial denture.	Assessment for maxillary expansion prior to bone grafting. Skeletal age assessment.	Bone grafting at one-half to two-third root development of canine.
11–15 years	Retention of palatal expansion 6 monthly review. Fissure sealing of bicuspids and second molars.	Full fixed appliance therapy. Minor tooth irregularities may be corrected by removable appliance.	Review and possible surgical revision if required
16–17 years	Restoration of teeth in the cleft by crowns, bridges, implants, dentures, etc.	Retention, following orthodontic therapy.	Assessment of the need for orthognathic surgery.

Table 27.7: Management of cleft lip and palate patients

Experts involved	Role
Obstetrician	Refers the child to plastic surgeon and pediatrician for expert opinion counseling the parents.
Pediatrician or neonatologist	Provides medical care. Refers the child to the plastic surgeon
Plastic surgeon	Heads the team of cleft lip and palate case
	Discusses the case with members of the team in the conference held monthly or weekly
	Carries out initial lip repair and palate surgery
	Performs pharyngoplasty or reversionary lip and nose surgery.
Oromaxillofacial surgeon	Usually comes in the picture of bone grafting
	If any final orthopedic surgery is performed at later stage.
Neurosurgeon	If any Craniofacial syndrome is associated.
Pedodontist	A key member who sees the baby and the parent at the time of repair of the lip.
	Provided pre-surgical orthopedic treatment for the baby
	Pedodontist monitors the growth and development
	To maintain perfect oral health
	To guide the occlusion and facial growth
	Motivates the parent and the child to cooperate with the treatment.
Orthodontist	Provided pre-surgical dental orthopedic consultation at the initial state. Carries out definitive orthodontic treatment once the full permanent dentition is erupted.
Speech Pathologist	Monitors the speech development to normal Test for an adequate palatopharyngeal closure and guiding the surgeons about whether a pharyngeal flap may be necessary.
Audiologist	To test hearing in the infant, baby and the young child, providing essential information about hearing loss for both speech pathologist and otolaryngologist.
Otolaryngologist	Concerns with the health of nasopharyngeal tissues.

A. *Surgery:* Most clefts of lip are repaired between 3 and 6 months, while the clefts of the hard and soft palate are repaired at about 18 months of age. ***Pre-surgical orthopedic treatment:*** In unilateral and bilateral cleft of lip and palate, the fragmented segments are often malrelated to each other with wide separation or overlapping, tilting, etc. Therefore, some surgeons consider that, the result of lip and palate repair is better if the segments are aligned before surgery by presurgical orthopedic treatment. Such alignment of displaced segments is done by fitting a plate which is designed to mould the gum pads into better relationship. For better result, this treatment is undertaken soon after birth. One or more successive plate may be required to achieve the satisfactory alignment.

B. *Dental treatment:* This consists of: (i) Routine dental care; (ii) Orthodontic treatment; and (iii) Retention and prosthesis.

 i. *Routine dental care:* This consists of instructions and advises for the maintenance of good oral hygiene, and regular check-up of the patient for undertaking preventive measures such as application of topical fluoride, fissure sealants, etc.

 ii. *Orthodontic treatment:* Usually no orthodontic treatment is undertaken in the early mixed dentition stage. However, lingually placed permanent incisors can be moved over the bite and a supernumerary or malposed tooth can be removed surgically, if necessary. Expansion of the upper arch is not usually undertaken at this stage. Full orthodontic treatment is undertaken in the early permanent dentition stage. The child's sensitive general and dental health, cooperation expected, severity of the condition, and the limits set by the skeletal pattern and soft tissues, etc. must be adequately considered before planning and undertaking an elaborate orthodontic procedure. Where the arches are in reasonably good position, the treatment should confine to the correction of local dental irregularities followed by partial denture or bridge work to replace any missing tooth. A malformed tooth may also require a crown. Where the occlusion is not satisfactory due to collapse or displacement of the arches, the condition should be treated by rapid expansion of the arches using strong forces so as to move the fragments of bone, by stretching the scar tissue, rather than moving the teeth within the bone, in extreme cases, it may be desirable to accept some degree of cross bite.

Recently a new technique of bone grafting is being tried to fill up the bony gap after rapid expansion of the arches. It has been claimed that by inserting bone in the alveolar region, it is possible to move the adjacent teeth into the grafted area and that bone grafting obviates the need for permanent retention. Local teeth irregularities are then corrected following removal of poor teeth, in bilateral cases, every effort should be made to save and align at least the central incisors. In extreme cases, it may be necessary to remove the primary palate, although this adds considerably to the difficulty of denture construction.

iii. *Retention and prosthesis:* Following expansion of the arches and alignment of teeth, fitting of permanent retainer is necessary to hold the expanded arches. Such retainer may also carry the necessary pontic for any missing tooth. A cast partial denture or bridge prosthesis is usually fitted to serve both these purposes. An acrylic partial denture is not satisfactory long term prosthesis for the cleft palate patient, as it adds to the difficulties in speech and in maintaining satisfactory oral hygiene.

C. *Speech therapy:* Despite deformities of soft and hard palate and associated structures, a remarkably high proportion of cases, manage to produce satisfactory speech sounds. However, some patients may require the help of speech therapist to complete the treatment.

D. *Counseling:* Parents are usually not prepared to face this problem, hence supportive counseling sessions are required to have future treatment success.

27.5 PREVENTIVE DENTISTRY AND DENTAL HEALTH EDUCATION

WHO denotes prevention as procedure or course of action that prevents the onset of disease. This includes the efforts and procedures employed in practice of dentistry and community dental health which prevent the occurrence of oral diseases. The concept of prevention has also given birth to the concept of Minimal Intervention Dentistry (MID) or Minimal Invasive Dentistry which involve ultra-conservative treatment approach towards the oral tissues.

Three Levels of Prevention

Primary: Actions taken prior to the onset of disease which removes the possibility that a disease will ever occur.

Secondary: Treatment methods to terminate a disease process and to restore the tissues to as near normal as possible.

Tertiary: Treatment methods employed to replace lost tissues and to rehabilitate patients to the point that function is as near normal as possible thus preventing disease complications.

The broad concept of preventive dentistry places more emphasis on primary preventive care. Dental caries and periodontal disease are infections diseases caused by the microorganisms of dental plaque. All strategies to prevent and to arrest are directed towards 'plaque control'. In addition, there is attempt to improve the defense potential of the teeth and periodontal ligament tissues, with enhancement of their repair capability. Ten methods being used and developed are discussed.

1. *Dental health education:* This involves the various programs to increase the general public "awareness". Various dental public health activities are the organized efforts to improve the oral health of the public. This is much needed for the large percentage of the population that either doesn't seek or doesn't have geographic or economic access to timely preventive and/or therapeutic care. Firstly the population problem is identified. This can be achieved by epidemiologic surveys that collect the prevalence and/or incidence data. Then the public health programs are planned. Dental health education and prevention programs devoted to 'school children' have been very successful. For their effective functioning, these programs have to be well evaluated and monitored. Successful campaigns targeting children and adults need more dedication and enthusiastic people. Media plays a great role in dental health education as it reaches the masses more easily. Thus educating the masses about the dental disease occurrence, prevention and dental treatment will bring a further decrease in dental diseases (dental caries, periodontal diseases, oral cancers) than achieved till today.

2. *Advanced diagnostic methods:* These are important so as to detect dental diseases at an early stage and prevent at a younger age.

i. *Caries activity tests:* These are means of measuring the activity of bacteria causing dental caries which includes new carious lesions and enlargement of the existing cavities during a certain period of time. This will help in treatment planning, both therapeutic and preventive. The reliable test could be developed to signal the early stage of dental carious lesion. Some of these tests are:

a. Lactobacillus count/test: Counts the number of bacterial colonies using quebec counter.

b. Snyder test: Measures the rapidity of acid formation by bacteria.

c. Salivary reductase test: Measures the enzyme reductase in saliva.

ii. Saliva analysis

iii. Plaque discoloring agents

3. *Diet counseling:* Food that contributes in formation of the plaque will lead to the development of dental caries and periodontal diseases. If exogenous refined carbohydrates do not reach the plaque bacteria which thrive on them, excess plaque build up can be prevented. The defense system includes salivary peroxidase, lactoferrin, lysozymes, cells like osteocytes, fibroblasts, epithelial cells from the repair system along with essential components of the immunologic and humoral mechanisms. All theses all defense systems need adequate quantity and quality of foods to resist the challenging microorganisms. Thus "nutrition" has a great role in primary prevention against plaque diseases. It has been proved that "sucrose" aids in the implantation of *'Streptococcus mutans'* in animals. Fructose and glucose are also cariogenic but sucrose has highest cariogenic potential. Hence sweet intake in children has to be restricted and guided from the early childhood.

Healthy *'snacking'* habits should be installed early in life including restrictions of excess intake of sticky and fermentable carbohydrates. 'Self cleansing' foods should be incorporated in diet which include the detergent effect of fruits and vegetables like apple, carrot, celery. The vigorous mastication demanded by fibrous foods provides physical stimulation to periodontium, promotes keratinisation, increases salivary flow. Thus help in caries prevention. Balanced diet is to be taken with adequate vitamins and minerals.

Inquiring the dietary habit is an important component of history taking. Diet modification may be told to the patient while diet counseling which will include future ranges in the diet to prevent dental decay. Emphasis should also be given on baby bottle feeding and further diet weaning habits to prevent rampant caries.

General diet recommendations
1. Restricting the frequency of meals especially sweets and sticky carbohydrates.
2. Encourage healthy 'snacking' habits.
3. Restricting candies, toffees and chocolates in children.
4. Restricting intake of soft drinks (acid colas).
5. Restricting milk and other sweetened liquids at bedtimes for the small babies to prevent early childhood caries.
6. Advise an infant diet weaning.
7. Use of sugar substitutes.
8. Encourage maintaining 'Diet Chart'

4. *Plaque control methods:* Use of various oral hygiene aids to control plaque helps in dental disease prevention. The primary objective of using oral hygiene aids, being the removal of dental plaque, which causes caries and periodontal diseases. Various methods include:
   i. Use of toothbrushes
   ii. Dentifrices/toothpaste
   iii. Dental floss
   iv. Oral rinses/mouthwashes
   v. Use of interdental brushes
   vi. Professional tooth cleaning
   vii. Use of toothpicks
   viii. Use of tongue cleaner

5. *Sugar substitutes:* The term 'sugar' refers to the commonly used household stuff which is most commonly used sweetener. Fructose, maltose and lactose are also caloric sugars found in nature, but sucrose is the only one of many, used by man. Eating large amounts of sucrose can increase the dental caries incidence depending upon the physical form in which sucrose is eaten, other ingredients with which it is eaten, presence of acid producing microorganisms in dental plaque and frequency of ingestion. Several human studies have supported and clarified the role of sucrose in causing dental caries (Hopewood House study, Vipeholm study). Hence the need to develop sweeteners has been recognized. Sweeteners can be caloric or non-caloric.

Caloric sweeteners: These are sweeteners with same caloric content as sucrose. These include monosaccharides and disaccharides, corn syrup, polyols (sugar alcohols) like sorbitol, xylitol, and mannitol.

Non-caloric sweetener: These are concentrated sweeteners which are expensive. Their sweetness is much more than sucrose, e.g. saccharin, aspartame, acesulfame K.

Xylitol, sorbitol, mannitol are claimed to be non-cariogenic substantiated by clinical trials. They are often used in chewing gums, toothpaste, some candies, mouth rinses for their "tooth friendly" benefits. Safety parameters regarding the use of saccharin, aspartames, etc. are very controversial topics. From dental point of view, these sweeteners offer a considerable decrease in caries incidence.

6. *Use of fluorides:* Effectiveness of fluorides in reducing number of carious lesions is well documented related to smooth surfaces of the teeth.

7. *Pit and fissure sealants:* Deep pits and fissures on the occlusal surface of teeth are the areas where approximately two-thirds of all carious lesions occur. Pit and fissure on the occlusal surface demand special attention and care. Sealants were developed with the aim of blocking the pits and fissures. So that food lodgement is prevented and this further prevents caries. In 1972 Nuva-Seal was the first successful commercial material available to seal deep pit and fissures. Sealants are very easy to apply but they follow a very sensitive technique. No cutting of tooth structure is required, hence they are very useful in children. They can be placed by the dentist as soon as the molars erupt. Thus prevention can be achieved at the earliest. If followed along with the other preventive regimes, they are a boon to the preventive dentistry.

8. *Atraumatic restorative treatment (ART):* The atraumatic restorative treatment procedure is a non-invasive procedure in which caries removal is done with the hand instruments only followed by the restoration. Restorative material of choice is glass ionomer cement. This technique evolved due to the rising needs of community dentistry in remote areas where the dental needs were on rise but feasibility of taking the drilling equipment from place to place to cover large population, was limited. If applied carefully and properly, this is a painless procedure with remarkable results. The use of this method is great in preventive health programs but cannot be used in extensive carious lesions with pulp involvement, abscess, fistula, etc.

9. *Preventive resin restoration:* Preventive resin restoration (PPR) approach of treatment involves restorations of incipient caries using composite resins. It is a conservative approach of treatment wherein small incipient carious lesions are treated without extensive tooth cutting based on the extent and depth of carious lesion. Minimal cutting of tooth is done with the dental bur followed by the composite resin restoration. It is very useful in children especially in young permanent teeth. It is also used in suspicious pits and fissures where caries removal is limited in enamel only.

10. *Caries vaccine:* Efforts and research is being done to form a vaccine against Streptococcus mutans. Immunization studies are being carried all over the world on animals and humans. The feasibility is high as *S. mutans* are the identified causative agent. There are limitations too as dental caries is a multifactorial disease involving other microorganisms too. As caries is not a life threatening disease, careful clinical studies to determine possible adverse side reactions are under consideration.

Duggal MS. *Restorative techniques in Paediatric Dentistry.* 2nd edn. London: Martin Dunitz Ltd, 2002.

Graber, Vanarsdall, Vig. *Orthodontics—Current principles and techniques.* 4th edn. Philadelphia: Mosby, 2005.

Koch G, Poulsen S. *Pediatric Dentistry—A clinical approach.* 1st edn. Copenhagen: Munksgaard, 2001.

Litman Ronald S. *Pediatric anesthesia—The requisites in Anesthesiology.* 1st edn. Philadelphia: Mosby, 2004.

McDonald, Avery, Dean. *Dentistry for the child and adolescent.* 8th edn. St Louis, Missouri: Mosby, 2004.

Pinkham. *Pediatric Dentistry-Infancy through adolescence.* 3rd edn. Philadelphia: WB Saunders, 2001.

Shobha Tandon. *Textbook of Pedodontics.* 1st edn. Hyderabad: Paras Medical Publisher, 2001.

Soben Peter. *Essentials of Preventive and Community Dentistry.* 2nd edn. New Delhi: Arya (Medi) Publishing House, 2003.

Stewart Ray E. *Pediatric Dentistry—Scientific foundations and clinical practice.* St Louis, Missouri: Mosby. 1982.

White GE. Protocols for clinical Pediatric Dentistry. *J Clinical Pediatric Dentistry* Annual 1996, Vol 4.

28 ◆ Disorders of the Eye

28.1 EXAMINATION OF THE EYE

Examination of the eyes is a routine part of the periodic pediatric examination beginning in the newborn period.

External examination: External examination of eyes consists of inspection of the eyelids, surrounding tissues and palpebral fissure. Viewing the eyes and lids from above aids in detecting orbital asymmetry, lid masses, proptosis (exophthalmos). Palpation helps in detecting orbital and lid masses.

The lacrimal apparatus is assessed by looking for evidence of tear deficiency, overflow of tears (epiphora), erythema and swelling in the region of tear sac or gland. The sac is massaged when obstruction is suspected. The presence and position of the puncta is also checked.

The lids, conjunctivae and sclera are examined for local lesions, foreign bodies, and inflammatory signs. Also note loss and maldirection of lashes. When necessary, the lids can be everted in the following manner:

1. Instruct the patient to look down
2. Grasp the lashes of the patient's upper lid between the thumb and index finger of one hand
3. Place a probe, a cotton-tipped applicator, or the thumb of the other hand at the upper margin of the tarsal plate; and
4. Pull the lid down and outward, evert it over the probe, using the instrument as a fulcrum. Foreign bodies commonly lodge in the concavity just above the lid margin and are exposed only by fully everting the lid.

The anterior segment of the eye is then evaluated with oblique focal illumination, noting the lusture and clarity of the cornea, the depth and clarity of the anterior chamber, and the features of the iris. Transillumination of the anterior segment aids in detecting opacities and in demonstrating atrophy or hypopigmentation of the iris; these latter signs are important when ocular albinism suspected. Fluorescein dye can be used to aid in diagnosing abrasions, ulcerations, and foreign bodies.

Visual acuity: Visual acuity is the eye's ability to detect fine details and is the quantitative measure of the eye's ability to see an in-focus image at a certain distance. The standard definition of normal visual acuity (20/20 or 6/6 vision) is the ability to resolve a spatial pattern separated by a visual angle of one minute of arc. The E test, in which a child points in the direction of the letter, is the most widely used visual acuity test for preschool children. An adult-type Snellen chart can be used at about 5 or 6 yr of age if the child knows letters.

Visual field testing: To perform the test, the individual occludes one eye while fixated on the examiner's eye with the non-occluded eye. The patient is then asked to count the number of fingers that are briefly flashed in each of the four quadrants. In case of children, the child's bottle, a favorite toy, and lollipops are particularly effective attention getting items. Common problems of the visual field include scotoma (area of reduced vision), hemianopia (half of visual field lost), homonymous quadrantanopia (involving both eyes) and bitemporal hemianopia of a chiasmal lesion.

Color vision testing: Color vision testing is not frequently necessary in young children, but parents sometimes request it, particularly if their child seems to be slow in learning colors. A change in color discrimination can be a sign of optic nerve or retinal disease.

Pupillary function: An examination of pupillary function includes inspecting the pupils for equal size (1 mm or less of difference may be normal), regular shape, reactivity to light, and direct and consensual accommodation. These steps can be easily remembered with the mnemonic *PERRLA (D+C):* Pupils Equal and Round; Reactive to Light and Accommodation (Direct and Consensual). If there is a unilateral small pupil with normal reactivity to light, it is unlikely that a neuropathy is present. However, if accompanied by ptosis of the upper eyelid, this may indicate Horner's syndrome. If there is a small, irregular pupil that constricts poorly to light, but normally to accommodation, this is an Argyll Robertson pupil.

Ocular motility: Ocular motility should always be tested, especially when patients complain of double vision or physicians' suspect neurologic disease. Test the inferior, superior, lateral and medial rectus muscles of the eye, as well as the superior and inferior oblique muscles.

Binocular vision: A determination of the degree of binocular vision is commonly performed by an ophthalmologist. The Titmus test is probably the most frequently used test; a series of three-dimensional images are shown to the child while he or she wears a set of Polaroid glasses.

Ophthalmoscopy (fundus examination): Ophthalmoscopy allows the one to look directly at the retina and other tissue at the back of the eye. This is best done after the pupil has been dilated with eye drops. Tropicamde (Mydriacyl) 0.5–1% and phenylephrine (Neo-Synephrine) 2.5% are recommended as mydriatics of short duration. The appearance of the optic disc and retinal vasculature are the main focus of examination during ophthalmoscopy. Beginning with posterior landmarks, the disc and the macula, the four quadrants are symmetrically examined by following each of the major vessel groups to the periphery. More of the fundus can be seen if a child is directed to look up and down, and to the right and left. A red reflex can be seen when looking at a patient's pupil through a direct ophthalmoscope. This part of the examination is done from a distance of about 50 cm and is usually symmetrical between the two eyes. An opacity may indicate a cataract.

Slit-lamp examination (Biomicroscopy): Close inspection of the anterior eye structures and ocular adnexa are often done with a slit lamp machine.

Refraction: This determines the refractive state of the eye: the degree of nearsightedness, farsightedness, or astigmatism. Retinoscopy provides an objective determination of the amount of correction needed and can be performed at any age. In young children it is best done with cycloplegia.

Intraocular pressure: Intraocular pressure (IOP) can be measured by tonometry devices. A gross estimate of pressure can be made by palpating the globe with the index fingers placed side by side on the upper lid on the tarsal plate.

Isenberg SJ. Clinical application of the pupil examination in neonates. *J Pediatr* 1991; 118: 650–652.

Olitsky SE, Hug D, Smith LP. Examination of the eye. In: Kliegman RM, Behrman RE, Jenson HB, Stanton BF (eds). *Nelson Textbook of Pediatrics.* 18th edn. Vol 2. Philadelphia: Saunders, 2007; 2569–2572.

28.2 REFRACTIVE ABNORMALITIES IN CHILDREN

Refraction is an essential part of every complete ocular examination. Four types of refractive abnormalities reported in children include hyperopia, myopia, astigmatism, and anisometropia.

Hyperopia: Hyperopia results when the axial length of the eye is relatively short, when there is reduced refractive power of the cornea or lens, or from a combination of these factors. Low to moderate levels of hyperopia are commonly found in early childhood. Since young eyes possess large amplitudes of accommodation, and accommodative ability is well developed by the age of 4 months, the vast majority of hyperopic children are able to see clearly without a need for optical correction.

Myopia: Myopia occurs when the axial dimension of the eye is relatively long, when there is excessive refractive power in the cornea or lens, or with some combination of these factors. Mild to moderate degrees of uncorrected myopia in early childhood do not result in significant visual impairment, since most activities at this stage of life do not require sharp distance vision. The child quickly learns to bring objects of interest closer in order to obtain clear retinal images. High myopia in infancy or early childhood is uncommon and should alert the examiner to search for a possible cause.

Astigmatism: Astigmatism results when one or more of the refractive elements of the eye is toroidal rather than spherical. Uncorrected astigmatism in childhood may cause bilateral amblyopia that limits corrected visual acuity when glasses are initially prescribed. With continued wearing of glasses, vision often approaches the normal level over time.

Anisometropia: The high percentage of patients with anisometropia who also have strabismus has led to speculation that there may be an etiologic relationship in one direction or the other.

Accommodation: During accommodation, the ciliary muscle contracts, the suspensory fibres of the lens relax and the lens assumes a more rounded shape to bring rays of light into focus of the retina. The amplitude of the accommodation is greatest during childhood and gradually diminishes with age. The physiologic decrease in accommodative ability that occurs with age is called presbyopia. Premature presbyopia is occasionally seen in young children. Neurogenic causes of accommodative paralysis include lesions affecting the occulomotor nerve (3rd cranial nerve) in any part of its course. Differential diagnosis includes tumors, degenerative diseases, vascular lesions, trauma, and infectious diseases. Systemic disorders that may cause impairment of accommodation include botulism, diphtheria, Wilson disease, diabetes mellitus and syphilis.

Olitsky SE, Hug D, Smith LP. Abnormalities of refraction and accommodation. In: Kliegman RM, Behrman RE, Jenson HB, Stanton BF (eds), *Nelson Textbook of Pediatrics,* 18th edn Vol. 2. Philadelphia: Saunders, 2007; 2572–2573.

Safir A, Hyams L, Philpot J, et al. Studies in refraction. The precision of retinoscopy. *Arch Ophthalmol* 1970; 84:49.

Singhal S, Tomar A. Refractive abnormalities in children. In: Mathur GP, Mathur Sarla (eds). *Current Trends in Pediatrics.* Vol 1. Delhi: Academa Publishers, 2005; 321–326.

28.3 DISORDERS OF VISION

Severe visual impairment (corrected vision poorer than 6/60) and blindness in children may be due to multiple defects affecting any structure or function along the visual pathways.

Amblyopia: This is a decrease in visual acuity, unilateral or bilateral, that occurs in visually immature children as a result of a lack of a clear image falling on the retina. The development of visual acuity normally proceeds rapidly in infancy and early childhood. Anything that interferes with the formation of clear retinal image during this early developmental period can produce amblyopia. *Treatment* first consists of removing any media opacity or prescribing appropriate glasses, if needed, so that a well focused retinal image can be produced in each eye.

Diplopia or double vision is generally a result of a misalignment of the visual axes. The onset of diplopia in any child warrants prompt evaluation; it may signal the onset of a serious problem such as increased intracranial pressure, a brain tumor, or an orbital mass. Monocular diplopia results from dislocation of the lens, cataract, or some defect in the media or macula.

Suppression: In the presence of strabismus, diplopia occurs secondary to the same image falling on different regions of the retina in each eye. In a visually immature child, a process may occur in the cortex that eliminates the disability of seeing double. This is an active process and is termed suppression.

Amaurosis is partial or total loss of vision; the term is usually reserved for profound impairment, blindness, or near blindness. The first clue to amaurosis may be nystagmus or strabismus.

Nyctalopia or night blindness is vision that is defective in reduced illumination. It generally implies impairment in function of the rods, particularly in dark adaptation time and perceptual threshold. Children may have excessive problems going to sleep in a dark room, which may be mistaken for a behavioral problem. Progressive night blindness usually indicates primary or secondary retinal, choroidal, or viteroretinal degeneration. Nictalopia occurs also in vitamin A deficiency or as a result of retinotoxic drugs such as quinine.

Color blindness is an abnormal condition characterized by the inability to clearly distinguish different colors of the spectrum. Human color vision is normally trichomatic, i.e. the mixture of red, green and blue light. Most color vision defects are congenital and permanent. Red-green defects show the highest prevalence in the general population. Persons with defective color vision are at a disadvantage especially for employment purposes such as pilots, drivers, in defence services, and in technical fields, such as engineering and medical profession.

Psychogenic disturbances: Vision problems of psychogenic origin are common in school-aged children. Important clues to the diagnosis are inappropriate affect, excessive grimacing, inconsistency in performance, and suggestibility. A thorough ophthalmic examination is essential to differentiate organic from functional visual disorders.

Reassurance and positive suggestions help the children with psychogenic disturbances.

Dyslexia is the inability to develop the capability to read at expected level despite in otherwise normal intellect. Most dyslexic individuals also display poor writing ability. Dyslexia is a primary reading disorder and should be differentiated from secondary reading difficulties due to mental retardation, environmental or educational deprivation, and physical or organic diseases. Dyslexia is a language-based disorder and is not caused by any defect in the eye or visual acuity per se, nor is it attributable to a defect in ocular motility or binocular alignment. Ophthalmologic evaluation with reading problem is recommended to diagnose and correct any concurrent ocular problems such as a refractive error, amblyopia, or strabismus.

Holmes JM, Clarke MP. Amblyopia. *Lancet* 2006; 367:1343–1351.

Lyon GR, Shaywitz SE, Shaywitz BA. Dyslexia. In: Kliegman RM, Behrman RE, Jenson HB, Stanton BF (eds). *Nelson Textbook of Pediatrics.* 18th edn. Vol 1. Philadelphia: Saunders, 2007; 150–152.

Olitsky SE, Hug D, Smith LP. Disorders of vision. In: Kliegman RM, Behrman RE, Jenson HB, Stanton BF (eds). *Nelson Textbook of Pediatrics.* 18th edn. Vol 2. Philadelphia: Saunders, 2007; 2573–2576.

Olitsky SE, Nelson LB. Reading disorders in children. *Pediatr Clin North Am* 2003; 50: 213–224.

28.4 DISORDERS OF CONJUNCTIVA

Conjunctivitis

The conjunctiva reacts to infectious agents (bacterial and viral), allergens, irritants, toxins, and systemic diseases. Conjunctivitis is common illness in childhood and may be infectious and noninfectious.

Ophthalmia Neonatorum

This form of conjunctivitis occurs in infants within 4 weeks of birth, is the most common eye disease of newborns. Conjunctivitis during the neonatal period is usually acquired during vaginal delivery and reflects the sexually transmitted infections prevalent in the community. It can be aseptic or septic. Aseptic occurs due to instillation of silver nitrate and is a reaction to the solution. The onset of inflammation occurs within 6–12 hr after birth, with clearing by 24–48 hr. Not seen as frequently nowadays as erythromycin eye ointment is used for prophylaxis. Septic can be due to bacterial, chlamydial, or viral etiology. Bacterial infections include *N. gonorrhoeae, C. trachomatis, Staphylococcus aureus,* and *Pseudomonas aeruginosa.* The usual incubation period for conjunctivitis due to *N. gonorrhoeae* is 2–5 days, and for that due to *C. trachomatis* is 5–14 days. Herpes simplex keratoconjunctivitis usually presents in infants with generalized herpes simplex with corneal epithelial involvement or vesicles on the skin (which surround the eye). Serious systemic complications, such as encephalitis, may occur in these neonates due to their poor immunologic response. This is usually seen within 2 weeks after birth.

Clinical manifestations: Ophthalmia neonatorum is characterized by redness and chemosis (swelling) of the conjunctiva, edema of eyelids, and discharge, which may be purulent. They may also have associated systemic manifestations that require treatment.

Diagnosis: Conjunctivitis appearing after 48 hr should be evaluated for a possible infectious cause. Gram stain of the purulent discharge should be performed and the material cultured. If a viral cause is suspected, a swab should be submitted in tissue culture for virus isolation. In chlamydial conjunctivitis, the diagnosis is made by examining Giemsa-stained epithelial cells scrapped from the tarsal conjunctivae for the characteristic intracytoplasmic inclusions, by isolating the organisms from a conjunctival swab using special tissue culture techniques, by immunofluorescent staining of conjunctival scrapings for chlamydial inclusions, or by tests for chlamydial antigen or DNA.

Differential diagnosis: The differential diagnosis includes dacryocystitis caused by congenital lacrimal duct obstruction with lacrimal sac distension (dacryocystocele).

Treatment of infants in whom gonococcal ophthalmia is suspected and the Gram stain shows the characteristic intracellular gram-negative diplococci should be initiated immediately with ceftriaxone, 50 mg/kg/24 hr for one dose, not to exceed 125 mg. The eye should be irrigated initially with saline every 10–30 min, gradually increasing to 2-hr intervals until the purulent discharge is cleared. An alternative regimen includes cefotaxime (100 mg/kg/24 hr given IV or IM every 12 hr for 7 days, or 100 mg/kg as a single dose). Treatment is extended if sepsis or other extraocular sites are involved (meningitis, arthritis). Inclusion blennorrhea is treated with oral erythromycin (50 mg/kg/24 hr in 4 divided doses) for 2 wk. This cures conjunctivitis and may prevent subsequent chlamydial pneumonia. *Pseudomonas* neonatal conjunctivitis is treated with systemic antibiotics, including an aminoglycoside, plus local saline irrigation and gentamicin ophthalmic ointment. Staphylococcal conjunctivitis is treated with parenteral methicillin and local saline irrigation.

Prevention: Drops of 0.5% erythromycin or 1% silver nitrate are instilled directly into the open eyes at birth using plastic single dose containers. Silver nitrate is ineffective against active infection. Povidone-iodine may also be an effective prophylactic agent.

Identification of maternal gonococcal infection and appropriate treatment is a standard element of routine prenatal care. An infant born to a woman who has untreated gonococcal infection should receive a single dose of ceftriaxone, 50 mg/kg (maximum 125 mg) IV or IM, in addition to topical prophylaxis. The dose should be reduced for premature infants. If the mother's gonococcal isolate is known to be penicillin sensitive, her infant should be given penicillin (50,000 U).

Acute purulent conjunctivitis: Acute purulent conjunctivitis is characterized by generalized conjunctival hyperemia, edema, mucopurulent exudates, glued eyes (lids stuck together after sleeping), and various degrees of pain in the eye and discomfort. It is usually a result of bacterial infection. The most frequent causes are *Haemophilus influenzae*, pneumococci, staphylococci, and streptococci. *N. gonorrhoeae* and *Chlamydia* are relatively common causes of acute purulent conjunctivitis in children beyond the newborn period, especially in adolescents and require specific testing and treatment. Conjunctival smear and culture are helpful in differentiating specific types. These common forms of acute purulent conjunctivitis usually respond well to warm compresses and frequent topical instillation of antibiotic drops.

Viral conjunctivitis: This is generally characterized by a watery discharge. Follicular changes (small aggregates of lymphocytes) are often found in the palpebral conjunctiva. Conjunctivitis resulting from adenovirus infection is relatively common, sometimes with corneal involvement as well as pharyngitis or pneumonia. Conjunctivitis caused by enterovirus may be hemorrhagic. Conjunctivitis is commonly associated with such systemic viral infections as the childhood exanthems, particularly measles. Viral conjunctivitis is usually self-limited. Patients with AIDS may develop a transient nonspecific conjunctivitis, characterized by irritation, hyperemia, and tearing, that requires no specific treatment.

Epidemic keratoconjunctivitis: This is caused by adenovirus type 8 and is transmitted by direct contact. The initial presentation is a sensation of a foreign body beneath the lids, with itching and burning. Edema and photophobia develops, and large oval follicles appear within the conjunctiva. Preauricular adenopathy and a pseudomembrane on the conjunctival surface occur frequently. Subepithelial corneal infiltrates may develop and may cause blurring of vision; these usually disappear but may permanently reduce visual acuity. Children may have associated upper respiratory tract infection and pharyngitis. There is no specific medical treatment.

Membranous and pseudomembranous conjunctivitis: The classic membranous conjunctivitis is that of diphtheria accompanied by fibrin-rich exudates that forms on the conjunctival surface; the membrane is removed with difficulty and leaves raw bleeding areas. In pseudomembranous conjunctivitis, the layer of fibrin-rich exudates is superficial and can often be removed easily, leaving the surface smooth. This type occurs with many bacterial and viral infections, including staphylococcal, pneumococcal, streptococcal or chlamydial conjunctivitis, and in epidemic keratoconjunctivitis. It is also found in vernal conjunctivitis and in Stevens-Johnson disease.

Allergic conjunctivitis: See Section 11.9.

Vernal conjunctivitis: See Section 11.9.

Parinaud oculoglandular syndrome: This represents a form of cat-scratch disease caused by *Bartonella henselae*, which is transmitted to humans when they are scratched by an infected cat. The bacteria can then be deposited on the conjunctiva after rubbing one's eyes after handling the cat. The characteristic clinical features are lymphadenopathy and conjunctivitis including conjunctival granulomas. The course is generally self-limited, but antibiotics may be used in some cases.

Chemical conjunctivitis: See Section 28.17.

Other Conjunctival Disorders

Subconjunctival hemorrhage: This is manifested by bright or dark red patches in the bulbar conjunctiva and may result from injury or inflammation. It occurs spontaneously. It may occasionally result from severe sneezing or coughing. Rarely may it be a manifestation of a blood dyscrasia.

Pinguecula: It is a yellowish-white, slightly elevated mass on the bulbar conjunctiva, usually in the interpalpebral region. It represents elastic and hyaline degenerative changes of the conjunctivae. No treatment is required except for cosmetic reasons, in which case an excision is performed.

Pterygium: This is a fleshy, triangular conjunctival lesion that may encroach on the cornea. It typically occurs in the nasal interpalpebral region. The pathologic findings are similar to those of a pinguecula. Pterygium should be removed when it encroaches far onto the cornea. Recurrence is common after removal.

Dermoid cyst and dermolipoma: These are benign lesions, clinically similar in appearance. They are smooth, elevated, round to oval lesions of various sizes. The color varies from yellowish white to fleshy pink. The most frequent site is the upper outer quadrant of the globe; they also commonly occur near or straddling the limbus. Excision is performed for cosmetic reasons.

Conjunctival nevus: The conjunctival nevus is a small, slightly elevated lesion that may vary in pigmentation from pale salmon to dark brown. It is usually benign but progressive growth or a change is suggestive of malignancy.

Symblepharon: It is a cicatrical adhesion between the conjunctiva of the lid and the globe; the lower lid is usually affected. It follows operation or injuries, especially burns. It is a serious complication of Stevens-Johnson syndrome.

Maroba A. Ocular viral infections. *Pediatr Infect Dis* 1984; 3: 358–368.

O'Hara MA. Ophthalmia Neonatorum. *Pediatr Clin North Am* 1993; 40: 715.

Olitsky SE, Hug D, Smith LP. Disorders of the conjunctiva. In: Kliegman RM, Behrman RE, Jenson HB, Stanton BF (eds). *Nelson Textbook of Pediatrics.* 18th edn. Vol 2. Philadelphia: Saunders, 2007; 2588–2591.

Trachoma

Trachoma is caused by the bacterium *Chlamydia trachomatis*. Trachoma is responsible for 15 per cent of all blindness worldwide. It is the most important preventable cause of blindness in the world. A, B, Ba, and C serotypes of *C. trachomatis* are commonly involved. In India alone, an estimated 865,000 people have turned blind due to trachoma. The key factors in the geographical distribution of trachoma are a lack of adequate clean water supplies for washing and basic hygiene, plus inadequate health care resources. Flies are responsible for transmitting the disease from one eye to the other.

Clinical manifestations: The World Health Organization suggests that at least two of the following four criteria must be present for diagnosis of trachoma:
1. Lymphoid follicles on the upper tarsal conjunctivae
2. Typical conjunctival scarring
3. Vascular pannus, and
4. Limbal follicles. Children below 3 years had a much lower prevalence of scarring manifestations compared to older children.

The WHO grading system for field assessment of trachoma is as follows: *TF (Follicular Trachoma):* Presence of 5 or more follicles $\geq$ 0.5 mm diameter in the upper tarsal conjunctiva; *TI (Intense Trachomatous Inflammation):* 2/3 or more of the upper tarsal conjunctiva is inflamed and normal blood vessels in this region are obliterated; *TS (Trachomatous Scarring):* Scars are easily visible as white lines, bands or sheets in the tarsal conjunctiva; *TT (Trachoma Trichiasis):* At least one eyelash rubs against the eyeball. Evidence of recent removal of inturned eyelashes is also graded as Trichiasis; *CO (Corneal Opacity):* A visible whitish opacity covering the pupillary margin which thus appears blurred.

Diagnosis: It is confirmed by culture and appropriate staining techniques, performed during active stages of disease. Other diagnostic methods include direct immunofluorescence assay and polymerase chain reaction for *Chlamydia trachomatis* antigen, and antigen detection assay using a monoclonal antibody-based immunofluorescence assay.

Treatment: The key to the treatment of trachoma is the SAFE strategy developed by the WHO. "S" stands for trichiasis surgery. The antibiotics ("A"), facial cleanliness ("F"), and environmental improvement ("E") are components of this strategy. Surgery (S): Eyelid surgery (bilamellar tarsal rotation) to correct entropion and/or trichiasis may prevent blindness in individuals at immediate risk. It limits the progression of corneal scarring. Even after successful surgery, patients remain at risk for recurrence. Antibiotic (A): The WHO recommends 2 antibiotics for trachoma control: oral azithromycin and tetracycline eye ointment. The dose of oral azithromycin for children is 20 mg/kg (maximum 1 g) in a single dose. The second-line treatment is topical tetracycline eye ointment 1%. Topical tetracycline is applied to both eyes twice a day for 6 weeks. Treating individual and not treating infected family members leaves the individual at risk for repeat infection. All family members, including infants, should be treated. Facial cleanliness (F): Epidemiologic studies and community-randomized trials have shown that facial cleanliness in children reduces both the risk and the severity of active trachoma. Environmental (E): The environmental improvement activities are the promotion of improved water supplies and improved household sanitation, particularly methods for safe disposal of human feces and controlling fly populations by spraying insecticide.

Prevention: Poverty and lack of sanitation are important factors in the spread of trachoma. As socioeconomic conditions improve, the incidence of the disease decreases substantially. Endemic trachoma has been controlled in most instances by administrating topical tetracyclines (or rarely, erythromycin ointment) daily for periods of 6–10 wk or intermittently over a 6 mo period.

Hammerschlag MR. Chlamydial infections. In: Kliegman RM, Behrman RE, Jenson HB, Stanton B (eds). *Nelson Textbook of Pediatrics.* 18th edn. Vol. 1. Philadelphia: Saunders, 2007; 1283–1287.

28.5 DISEASES OF THE PEDIATRIC CORNEA

Congenital corneal disorders are important causes of childhood blindness. They can occur in isolation or in combination, or as part of a syndrome. Congenital hereditary endothelial dystrophy (CHED) presents as bilaterally symmetrical diffuse corneal opacification and edema of varying degree. The non-CHED congenital corneal opacities are frequently associated with glaucoma, dermoid, and metabolic diseases

Metabolic causes: Metabolic diseases are usually associated with clear corneas at birth followed by progressive opacification. Corneal clouding may be a part of many metabolic disorders including those involving aminoacids, lipids, carbohydrates, purines, etc. Systemic mucopolysaccharidosis (MPS) are lysosomal storage disorders that affect the glyco-saminoglycan catabolism and Hurler, Scheie, Morquio, Maroteaux-Lamy and Sly's are associated with variable amounts of corneal clouding.

Sclerocornea: Sclerocornea is a primary, nonprogressive anomaly in which scleralization of a peripheral part of the cornea, or the entire corneal tissue, occurs.

Birth trauma: Birth trauma caused by forceps blade placement across the orbit and globe during delivery can result in blunt trauma and rupture of Descemet's membrane. Diffuse stromal and epithelial edema in the immediate postpartum period due to birth trauma usually clears within weeks or months.

Aniridia: The most apparent clinical finding in aniridia is the absence of iris tissue but additional ocular structures are often affected. Corneal lesions in aniridia include peripheral pannus and epithelial abnormalities that may advance centrally (*see* Fig. 28.4 in CD).

Posterior polymorphous dystrophy (PPMD): PPMD an autosomal dominant disorder is usually a bilateral disease, typically occurs in the second or third decade of life. It may also be congenital or develop early in life. It may be seen in Alport's syndrome.

Keratoconus: Keratoconus is a noninflammatory ectatic disorder of cornea where cornea becomes cone shaped due to stromal thinning (*see* Fig. 28.5 in CD).

Acquired traumatic: Penetrating injuries cause acquired corneo-iridic scars, which are managed by keratoplasty.

Acquired non-traumatic: Acquired corneal scarring in the western nations before 6 years of age is herpes simplex keratitis, while in developing nations, infectious keratitis, corneal ulceration with perforation and post-infectious keratitis corneo-iridic scars. Keratomalacia due to vitamin A deficiency is an important cause of preventable corneal opacification.

Vitamin A deficiency disorders: The major cause of blindness in children worldwide is xerophthalmia caused by vitamin A deficiency. Vitamin A deficiency is the single most frequent cause of blindness among preschool children in developing countries. Clinical features include night blindness, Bitot's spot—triangular keratotic, foamy areas of interpalpebral bulbar conjunctiva, xerosis of the conjunctiva and cornea (xerophthalmia—dry lusterless poorly wettable surface), and corneal ulceration and necrosis of the cornea.

Pediatric keratitis: World Health Organization (WHO) has reported that of the 1.5 million blind children worldwide, 70,000 have active corneal involvement. Ocular trauma and corneal ulceration are significant causes of corneal blindness that are often underreported and may be responsible for 1.5–2.0 million new cases of monocular blindness every year. Infectious keratitis is one of the leading causes of preventable and treatable monocular blindness in developing world. Causes of childhood blindness (about 1.5 million worldwide with 5 million visually disabled) include xerophthalmia (350,000 cases annually), ophthalmia neonatorum, measles, and less frequently seen ocular diseases such as herpes simplex virus infections and vernal keratoconjunctivitis.

Infectious keratitis: Trauma is the most common predisposing factor. The other important predisposing factors are: associated systemic illness, previous ocular surgery (e.g. congenital glaucoma surgery), malnutrition. Beside this increased colonization during birth is another important factor. Recently contact lens wear has been found to be most common factor in adolescent age group. Infectious keratitis is caused by bacterial, viral, and fungal infectious agents. *Acanthamoeba keratitis* is rare among children. These are commonly found in fresh water sources, including bottled water, swimming pools, hot tubs, and bathroom tap water. Contact lens solutions are also source of these organisms. It can be seen in children using aphakic contact lens. But non-contact lens related keratitis is also seen. A ring infiltrate has been described as pathognomonic for *Acanthamoeba keratitis.*

Al-Ghamdi A, Al-Rajhi A, Wagoner MD. Primary pediatric keratoplasty: indications, graft survival, and visual outcome. *J AAPOS* 2007 Feb;11(1): 41–47.

M.Vanathi, Shalini Mohan, Rakhi Kusumesh. Disorders of pediatric cornea. In Z Chaudhuri, M Vanathi, *Postgraduate Ophthalmology.* New Delhi: Jaypee Highlights, 2011.

Vanathi M, Panda A, Vengayil S, Chaudhuri Z, Dada T. Pediatric keratoplasty. *Surv Ophthalmol* 2009 Mar-Apr; 54(2): 245–271.

28.6 ABNORMALITIES OF THE LENS

Cataracts

A cataract is an opacification of the lens. Congenital cataracts usually are diagnosed at birth. If a cataract goes undetected in an infant, permanent visual loss may ensue.

Signs and symptoms: As a cataract becomes more opaque, clear vision is compromised. A loss of visual acuity is noted. Contrast sensitivity is also lost, so that contours, shadows and color vision are less vivid. The affected eye will have an absent red reflex. A contrast sensitivity test should be performed and if a loss in contrast sensitivity is demonstrated, an eye specialist consultation is recommended. In the developed world, particularly in high-risk groups such as diabetics, it may be advisable to seek medical opinion if a 'halo' is observed around street lights at night, especially if this phenomenon appears to be confined to one eye only.

Treatment: When a cataract sufficiently interferes with vision, the treatment includes:

1. Surgical removal of the lens material to provide an optically clear visual axis
2. Correction of the resultant aphakic refractive error with spectacles, contact lenses, or intraocular lens implantation; and
3. Correction of any associated sensory deprivation amblyopia. Because the use of spectacles may not be possible in children after cataract removal, the use of contact lenses for visual rehabilitation is a medical necessity.

Ectopia Lentis

Normally the lens is suspended in place behind the iris diaphragm by the zonular fibers of the ciliary body. Abnormalities of the suspensory system resulting from a developmental defect, disease, or trauma may result in instability or displacement of the lens. Displacement of the lens is classified as luxation (dislocation-complete displacement of lens), or subluxation (partial displacement-shifting or tilting of the lens). Symptoms include blurring of vision because of refractory changes such as myopia, astigmatism, aphakic hyperopia, or diplopia. An important sign of displacement is iridodonesis, a tremulousness of the iris caused by the loss of its usual support. The anterior chamber may appear deeper than normal. Sometimes, the equatorial region ("edge") of the displaced lens may be visible in the pupillary aperture. On ophthalmoscopy, this may appear as a black crescent. Also, the difference between the phakic and aphakic portions can be appreciated when focusing on the fundus.

Causes of lens displacement: The lens displacement may occur as a result of trauma (commonest cause), uveitis, intraocular tumor, congenital glaucoma, high myopia, megalocornea, aniridia, or in association with cataract. Systemic disorders associated with displacement of the lens include Marfan syndrome, homocystinuria, Weill-Marchesani syndrome, sulfite oxidase deficiency, Ehlers-Danlos, Sturge-Weber, Crouzon, and Klippel-Feil syndromes; oxycephaly; and mandibulofacial dysostosis.

Treatment and prognosis: Displacement of the lens results often in optical problems, but in some cases more serious complications may develop such as glaucoma, uveitis, retinal detachment, or cataract. For many patients, optical correction by spectacles or contact lenses can be provided. In selected cases, the best treatment is surgical removal of the lens. Treatment of any associated amblyopia must be instituted early. Safety precautions must be taken for children with ectopia lentis to prevent injury to the eye.

Fallaha N, Lambert SR. Pediatric cataracts. *Ophthalmol Clin North Am* 2001; 14: 479–492.

Nelson LB, Maumenee IH. Ectopia lentis. *Surv Ophthalmol* 1982; 27: 143.

Olitsky SE, Hug D, Smith LP. Abnormalities of the lens. In: Kliegman RM, Behrman RE, Jenson HB, Stanton BF (eds). *Nelson Textbook of Pediatrics.* 18th edn. Vol 2. Philadelphia: Saunders, 2007; 2593–2597.

28.7 ABNORMALITIES OF PUPIL AND IRIS

Aniridia: The term aniridia is a misnomer, because iris tissue is usually present, although it is hypoplastic. The condition is bilateral in 98% of all patients. Aniridia is a panocular disorder, not an only isolated iris defect and is associated with ocular abnormalities:

1. Macular and optic nerve hypoplasias (commonly present) leading to decreased vision and sensory nystagmus;
2. Cornea may be small and a cellular infiltrate (pannus) occasionally develops, clinically appears as a gray opacification;
3. Lens abnormalities include cataract formation and partial or total lens dislocation; and
4. Glaucoma develops in about 75% cases. One fifth of aniridic sporadic cases may develop Wilms' tumor. Therefore, these children should be screened using renal ultrasonography every 3–6 mo until approximately 5 yr of age.

Coloboma of the iris: This developmental defect may present as a defect in a sector of the iris, a hole in the substance of the iris or a notch in the pupillary margin.

Microcoria (Congenital miosis): This appears as a small pupil that does not react to light or accommodation and that dilates poorly, if at all with medication. The eye may be otherwise normal or may be associated with other abnormalities of the anterior segment.

Congenital mydriasis: In this disorder, the pupils appear dilated, do not constrict significantly to light or near gaze, and respond minimally to miotic agents. Trauma, pharmacologic mydriasis, and neurologic disorders should be considered in the differential diagnosis.

Marcus Gunn pupil: This relative afferent pupillary defect indicates an asymmetric, prechiasmatic, afferent conduction defect. It is best demonstrated by the swinging flashlight test. With patients fixing on a distant target (to control accommodation), a bright focal light is directed alternately into each eye in turn. In the presence of an afferent lesion, both the direct response to light in the affected eye and the consensual response in the other eye are subnormal. Swinging the light in the better or normal eye causes both pupils to react (constrict) normally. Swinging the light back to the affected eye causes both pupils to redilate to some degree, reflecting the defective conduction. This is a very sensitive and useful test for detecting and confirming optic nerve and retinal disease.

Horner syndrome: The principal signs of oculosympathetic paresis (Horner syndrome) are homolateral miosis, mild ptosis and apparent enophthalmos with slight elevation of the lower lid. Patients may also have decreased facial sweating, increased amplitude of accommodation, and transient decrease in intraocular pressure. If paralysis of the ocular sympathetic fibers occurs before the age of 2 yr, heterochromia iridis with hypopigmentation of the iris may occur on the affected side.

Paradoxical pupil reaction: Some children exhibit paradoxical constriction of the pupils to darkness. An initial brisk constriction of the pupils occurs when the light is turned off, followed by slow redilation of the pupils. The response to direct light stimulation and the near response are normal. The mechanism is not clear, but paradoxical constriction of the pupils in reduced light can be a sign of retinal or optic nerve abnormalities. Paradoxical pupil reaction has been observed in children with congenital stationary night blindness, albinism, retinitis pigmentosa, Leber congenital retinal amaurosis, Best disease, optic nerve anomalies, optic neuritis, optic atrophy, and possibly amblyopia.

Heterochromia: In heterochromia, the two irides are of different color (heterochromia iridium) or a portion of an iris differs in color from the remainder (heterochromia iridis). Simple heterochromia may occur as an autosomal dominant trait. Congenital heterochromia is also a feature of Waardenburg syndrome, an autosomal dominant condition characterized by lateral displacement of the inner canthi and puncta, pigmentary disturbances (usually a median white forelock, and patches of hypopigmentation of the skin), and defective hearing. Changes in the color of the iris may occur as a result of trauma, hemorrhage, intraocular inflammation (iridocyclitis, uveitis), intraocular tumor (especially retinoblastoma), intraocular foreign body, glaucoma, iris atrophy, oculosympathetic palsy (Horner syndrome), melanosis oculi, previous intraocular surgery, and some glaucoma medicines.

Other iris lesions: Discrete nodules of the iris, referred to as Lisch nodules, are commonly seen in patients with neurofibromatosis. Lisch nodules represent melanocytic hamartomas of the iris and vary from slightly elevated pigmented areas to distinct ball-like excrescences. Lisch nodules are found in 92–100% of individuals older than 5 yr of age who have neurofibromatosis.

In leukemia, there may be infiltration of the iris, sometimes with hypopyon, an accumulation of white blood cells in the anterior chamber, which may herald relapse or involvement of the central nervous system.

The lesion of juvenile xanthogranuloma (nevoxanthoendothelioma) may occur in the eye as a yellowish fleshy mass or plaque of the iris. Spontaneous hyphema (blood in the anterior chamber), glaucoma, or a red eye with signs of uveitis may be associated. In many cases, the ocular lesion responds to topical corticosteroid therapy.

Leukocoria: This includes any white pupillary reflex, or so-called cat eye reflex. The primary consideration in any child with leukocorea is cataract, persistent hyperplastic primary vitreous, cicatrical retinopathy of prematurity, retinal detachment and retinoschisis, larval granulomatosis and retinoblastoma. Other conditions to be considered are endophthalmitis, organized vitreous hemorrhage, leukemic ophthalmopathy, exudative retinopathy (as in Coats' disease), and less common conditions such as medulloepithelioma, massive retinal gliosis, the retinal pseudotumor of Norrie (pseudoglioma of the Norrie disease).

The diagnosis can often be made by direct examination of the eye by ophthalmoscopy and biomicroscopy. Ultrasonographic and radiologic examinations are often helpful. In some cases the final diagnosis is made by pathologic examination.

Francois J. Differential diagnosis of leukokoria in children. *Ann Ophthalmol* 1978; 10: 1375–1378.

Olitsky SE, Hug D, Smith LP. Abnormalities of pupil and iris. In: Kliegman RM, Behrman RE, Jenson HB, Stanton BF (eds). *Nelson Textbook of Pediatrics*. 18th edn. Vol 2. Philadelphia: Saunders, 2007; 2576–2578.

Thompson HS. Segmental palsy of the iris sphincter in Adie's syndrome. *Arch Ophthalmol* 1978; 96: 1615–1620.

28.8 DISORDERS OF THE UVEAL TRACT

Uveitis (Iritis, Cyclitis, Choreoretinitis): The uveal tract is the inner vascular coat of the eye, consisting of the iris, ciliary body, and choroids. Inflammation occurs in a number of systemic diseases, both infectious and noninfectious, and in response to exogenous factors, including trauma and toxic agents. Inflammation may affect any one portion of the uveal tract or all parts together.

Panophthalmitis is inflammation involving all parts of the eye. It is frequently suppurative, most often as a result of a perforating injury or of septicemia. It produces severe pain, marked congestion of the eye, inflammation of the adjacent orbital tissues and eyelids, and loss of vision. The eye is lost in many cases despite intensive treatment of the infection and inflammation. Enucleation of the eye or evisceration of the orbit may be necessary.

Sympathetic ophthalmia is a rare type of inflammatory response that affects the uninjured eye after a perforating injury. Hypersensitivity phenomenon is the most probable cause. Loss of vision in the uninjured (sympathizing) eye may result weeks, months, or even years after the injury. Removal of the injured eye prevents the development sympathetic ophthalmia but does not stop the progression of the disease once it has occurred. Early enucleation should be considered if there is no hope of visual recovery after a severe injury.

Treatment: The various forms of intraocular inflammation are treated according to their causal factors. When infection is proved or suspected appropriate systemic antimicrobial or antiviral therapy should be used. In some cases, intravitreal injection is needed. Anterior inflammation may respond well to corticosteroid treatment. Posterior cases often require systemic therapy. The use of topical and systemic corticosteroids can lead to the development of glaucoma and cataracts. To reduce the need for corticosteroids, systemic immunosuppressive therapy (methotrexate, cyclosporine and tumor necrosis factor inhibitors) is often used in patients requiring long-term treatment. Cycloplegic agents, particularly atropine is also used to reduce inflammation and prevents adhesion of the iris to the lens (posterior synechiae), especially in anterior uveitis. Surgery is required in patients who develop glaucoma or cataract.

Chu DS, Foster CS. Sympathetic ophthalmia. *Int Ophthalmol Clin* 2002; 42: 176–185.

Kadayifecilar S, Eldem B, Tumer B. Uveitis in childhood. *J Pediatr Ophthalmol Strabismus* 2003; 40: 335–340.

Olitsky SE, Hug D, Smith LP. Disorders of the uveal tract. In: Kliegman RM, Behrman RE, Jenson HB, Stanton BF (eds). *Nelson Textbook of Pediatrics*. 18th edn. Vol 2. Philadelphia: Saunders, 2007; 2597–2598.

Patel H, Goldstein D. Pediatric uveitis. *Pediatr Clin North Am* 2003; 50; 125–138.

28.9 DISORDERS OF THE RETINA AND VITREOUS

Retinopathy of Prematurity (ROP)

ROP is a disease of the developing retinal vasculature in premature infants. Beginning at 16 wk of gestation, retinal angiogenesis normally proceeds from the optic disc to the periphery, reaching the outer rim of the retina (ora serrata) nasally at about 36 wk and extending temporally by approximately 40 wk. The basic pathogenesis is still unknown. The major risk factors associated with ROP are prematurity and the associated retinal immaturity at birth. The other contributory factors are oxygenation, respiratory distress, apnea, bradycardia, heart disease, infection, hypercarbia, acidosis, anemia and the need for transfusion. Generally, the lower the gestational age, the lower the birth weight, and the sicker the infant are, the greater the risk is for ROP.

Clinical manifestations and prognosis: In more than 90% of at-risk infants, the course is one of spontaneous arrest and regression, with a little or no residual effects or visual disability. Fewer than 10% of infants have progression toward severe disease, with significant extrarenal vasoproliferation, cicatrisation, detachment of the retina, and impairment of vision. Some children with arrested or regressed ROP show demarcation lines, undervascularization of the peripheral retina, or abnormal branching, tortuosity, or straightening of the retinal vessels, retinal pigmentary changes, dragging of the retina (so-called dragged disc), ectopia of the macula, retinal folds, or retinal breaks. Others proceed to total retinal detachment, which commonly assumes a funnel-like configuration. The clinical picture is often that of a retrolental membrane, producing leukocoria (a white reflex in the pupil). Some patients develop cataract, glaucoma, and signs of inflammation. The end stage is often a painful blind eye or a degenerated phthisical eye. The spectrum of ROP also includes myopia, which is often progressive and of significant degree in infancy. The incidence of anisometropia, strabismus, amblyopia, and nystagmus may also be increased.

Diagnosis: Systemic serial ophthalmoscopic examination of the infants at risk is recommended. Infants weighing less than 1,500 g at birth and those born before 31 wk of gestational age and infants born weighing more than 1,500 g who have an unstable clinical course should be examined for ROP. The initial examination should be performed at 4–6 wk of chronological age or at 31–33 wk postconceptional age. ROP is diagnosed most often at 32–44 wk after conception. The examination can be stressful to fragile preterm infants, and the dilating drops can have untoward side effects; thus, discretion must be used in timing the eye examination, and infants must be carefully monitored during and after the examination. Follow-up is based on the initial findings and risk factors but is usually 2 wk or less.

Treatment: In selected cases, cryotherapy or laser photocoagulation of the avascular retina reduces the more severe complications of progressive ROP.

Prevention of ROP ultimately depends on prevention of premature birth and its attendant problems.

Retinitis pigmentosa: The progressive retinal degeneration is characterized by pigmentary changes, arteriolar attenuation, some degree of optic atrophy, and progressive impairment of visual function. Other ocular findings include subcapsular cataract, glaucoma, and keratoconus. Impairment of night vision or dark adaptation is often the first clinical manifestation. Progressive loss of peripheral vision occurs. There may be loss of central vision manifestations commonly begin in childhood. The disorder may be autosomal recessive, autosomal dominant, or X linked. Only supportive treatment is available.

Cherry red spot: A cherry red spot is a bright to dull red spot at the center of the macula surrounded and accentuated by a grayish-white or yellowish halo. The halo is a result of a loss of transparency of the retinal ganglion cell layer secondary to edema, lipid accumulation, or both. The cherry red spot that characteristically occurs as a result of retinal ischemia secondary to vasospasm, ocular contusion, or occlusion of the central retinal artery must be differentiated from the cherry red spot of neurodegenerative diseases.

Phakomas: These are the herald lesions of the hamartomatous disorders. In Bourneville disease (tuberous sclerosis) the distinctive ocular lesion is a refractile, yellowish, multinodular cystic lesion arising from the disc or retina; the appearance is often compared with that of an unripe mulberry. Rarely similar retinal phakomas occur in von Recklinghausen disease, von Hippel-Lindau disease and Sturge-Weber syndrome.

Retinal detachment: A retinal detachment is a separation of the outer layers of the retina from the underlying retinal pigment epithelium (RPE). The detachment can occur as a congenital anomaly but more commonly arises secondary to other ocular abnormalities or trauma. The presenting sign of retinal detachment in an infant or child may be loss of vision, secondary strabismus, or nystagmus, or leukocoria (white papillary reflex). Prompt treatment is essential in restoring the vision.

Hypertensive retinopathy: In the early stages of hypertension, no retinal changes occur. Generalized constriction and irregular narrowing of the arterioles are usually the first signs in the fundus. Other findings include retinal edema, flame-shaped hemorrhages, cotton-wool spots (retinal nerve fiber layer infarcts), and papilledema. These changes are reversible if the hypertension can be controlled in the early stages, but in long-standing hypertension, irreversible changes may occur. Thickening of the vessel wall may produce a silver- or copper-wire appearance. Hypertensive retinal changes in a child should alert the physician to renal disease, pheochromocytoma, collagen disease, and cardiovascular disorders, particularly coarctation of the aorta.

Diabetic retinopathy: The retinal changes of diabetes mellitus are classified as nonproliferative or proliferative. Nonproliferative diabetic retinopathy is characterized by retinal microaneurysms, venous dilatation, retinal hemorrhages, and exudates. The microaneurysms appear as tiny red dots. The hemorrhages may be of both the dot and blot type, representing deep intraretinal bleeding, and the splinter or flame-shaped type, involving the superficial nerve fiber layer. The exudates are deep and appear waxy. There may also be superficial nerve fiber infarcts called cytoid bodies or cotton-wool spots, as well as retinal edema. These signs may wax and wane. They are seen primarily in the posterior pole, around the disc and macula. Involvement of the macula may lead to decreased vision.

Proliferative retinopathy, the more serious form is characterized by neovascularization and proliferation of fibrovascular tissue on the retina, extending into vitreous. The vision-threatening complications of the proliferative diabetic retinopathy are retinal and vitreous hemorrhages, cicatrisation traction, and retinal detachment. Neovascularization of the iris may lead to secondary glaucoma, if not treated promptly.

Treatment: Photocoagulation may be used to decrease the risk of continued vision loss in patients with macular edema. Patients with proliferative retinopathy should undergo panretinal photocoagulation to preserve their central vision. Neovascularization of the iris is also treated with panretinal photocoagulation to stop the development of neovascular glaucoma. Vitrectomy and other intraocular surgery may be necessary in patients with nonresolving vitreous hemorrhage or traction retinal detachment.

Subacute bacterial endocarditis: At sometime during the course of the disease, retinopathy is present in approximately 40% of cases of subacute bacterial endocarditis. The lesions include hemorrhages, hemorrhages with white centers (Roth spots), papilledema, and, rarely, embolic occlusion of the central retinal artery.

Blood disorders: In primary and secondary anemias, retinopathy in the form of hemorrhages and cotton-wool patches may occur. Vision can be affected if hemorrhage occurs in the macular area. The hemorrhages may be light and feathery or dense and preretinal. In polycythemia vera, the retinal veins are dark, dilated, and tortuous. Retinal hemorrhages, retinal edema, and papilledema may be observed. In leukemia, the veins are characteristically dilated, with sausage-shaped constrictions; hemorrhages, particularly white-centered hemorrhages and exudates are common during the acute stage. In the sickling disorders, fundus changes include vascular tortuosity, arterial and venous occlusions, "salmon patches," refractile deposits, pigmented lesions, arteriolar-venous anastomosis, and neovascularization (with "sea-fan" formations), sometimes leading to vitreous hemorrhage and retinal detachment.

Trauma-related retinopathy: Retinal changes may occur in patients who suffer trauma to other parts of the body. Retinal hemorrhages occur in infants who have been physically abused. Retinal, subretinal, subhyaloid, and vitreous hemorrhages have been described in infants and young children with inflicted neurotrauma. Often there are no signs of direct trauma to the eye, periocular region, or head. Such cases may result from violent shaking of an infant, and permanent retinal damage may result. In patients with severe head or chest compressive trauma, a traumatic retinal angiopathy can occur.

Retinoblastoma (Rb)

See Section 34.8.

Hartong DT, Berson EL, Dryia TP. Retinitis pigmentosa. *Lancet* 2006; 368: 1795–1809.

Olitsky SE, Hug D, Smith LP. Disorders of the retina and vitreous. In: Kliegman RM, Behrman RE, Jenson HB, Stanton BF (eds). *Nelson Textbook of Pediatrics*. 18th edn. Vol 2. Philadelphia: Saunders, 2007; 2598–2605.

Optic nerve aplasia: Optic nerve aplasia, a rare congenital anomaly is typically unilateral. The optic nerve, retinal ganglion cells, and retinal blood vessels are absent. A vestigial dural sheath usually connects with the sclera in a normal position, but no neural tissue is present within this sheath.

Optic nerve hypoplasia: Hypoplasia of the optic nerve (unilateral or bilateral), a nonprogressive condition is characterized by a subnormal number of optic nerve axons with normal mesodermal elements and glial supporting tissue. In typical cases, the nerve head is small and pale, with a pale or pigmented peripapillary halo or double-ring sign.

Patients should be tested for early diagnosis of diabetes mellitus and in detecting abnormal endocrine function.

Papilledema: The term papilledema is reserved to describe swelling of the nerve head secondary to increased intracranial pressure (ICP). *Clinical manifestations* of papilledema include edematous blurring of the disc margins, fullness or elevation of the nerve head, partial or complete obliteration of the disc cup, capillary congestion and hyperemia of the nerve head, generalized engorgement of the veins, loss of spontaneous venous pulsation, nerve fiber layer hemorrhages around the disc and peripapillary exudates. In some cases, edema extending into the macula may produce a fan- or star-shaped figure. In addition, concentric peripapillary retinal wrinkling (Paton lines) may be noted. Transient observation of vision may occur, lasting seconds and associated with postural changes. Vision is usually normal in acute papilledema. Normally, when the ICP is relieved, the papilledema resolves and the disc returns to a normal or nearly normal appearance within 6–8 wk. sustained chronic papilledema or long-standing unrelieved increased ICP may lead to permanent nerve fiber damage, atrophic changes of the disc, macular scarring, and impairment of vision. Papilledema is a neurologic emergency. It may be associated with other signs of increased ICP, including headaches, nausea, and vomiting.

Optic neuritis: This is an inflammation or demyelinization of the optic nerve leading to impairment of function. The process is usually acute, with rapidly progressive loss of vision. It may be unilateral or bilateral. Pain on movement of the globe or pain on palpation of the globe may precede or accompany the onset of visual symptoms. There is decreased visual activity, decreased color vision and contrast sensitivity, a relative afferent pupillary defect, and a normal macular and peripheral retina.

When the retrobulbar portion of the nerve is affected without ophthalmoscopically visible signs of inflammation at the disc, the term retrobulbar optic neuritis is applied. When ophthalmoscopically visible evidence of inflammation of the nerve head is present, the term papillitis or intraocular optic neuritis is used. When there is involvement of both retina and papilla, the term optic neuroretinitis is used.

In most cases of acute optic neuritis, some improvement in vision begin within 1–4 wk after onset, and vision may improve to normal or near normal within weeks or months, depending on the cause. The central vision may fully recover, but permanent defects in other areas of visual function (contrast sensitivity, color, brightness sense, and motion perception) have been reported.

Optic atrophy: The term optic atrophy denotes degeneration of optic nerve axons with loss of unction. The ophthalmoscopic signs of optic atrophy are pallor of the disc and loss of substance of the nerve head, sometimes with enlargement of the disc cup. The cause may be traumatic, inflammatory, degenerative, neoplastic or vascular intracranial tumors and hydrocephalus, and autosomal recessive inherited congenital atrophy.

Optic nerve glioma: It is the most frequent tumor of the optic nerve in childhood that may develop in the intraorbital, intracanalicular, or intracranial portion of the nerve; the optic chiasma is often involved. Surgical removal may be appropriate when the tumor is confined to the intraorbital, intracanalicular, or prechiasmal portion of the nerve. When the optic chiasma is involved, resection is usually not indicated and radiation and chemotherapy may be necessary.

Traumatic optic neuropathies: Injury to the optic nerve may result from direct and indirect trauma. The treatment includes high-dose corticosteroids or optic canal decompression.

Balcer LJ. Optic neuritis. *N Engl J Med* 2006; 354:1273–1280.

Olitsky SE, Hug D, Smith LP. Abnormalities of the optic nerve. In: Kliegman RM, Behrman RE, Jenson HB, Stanton BF (eds). *Nelson Textbook of Pediatrics*. 18th edn. Vol 2. Philadelphia: Saunders, 2007; 2605–2608.

Repka MX, Miller NR. Optic atrophy in children. *Am J Ophthalmol* 1988; 106: 191–193.

Weiss AH, Beck RW. Neuroretinitis in childhood. *J Pediatr Ophthalmol Strabismus* 1989; 26: 198–203.

28.11 STRABISMUS

Strabismus, or misalignment of the eyes, is one of the most common eye problems encountered in children. Strabismus can result in vision loss (amblyopia) and significant psychologic effects. Restoration of proper alignment of the visual axis must occur at an early stage of vision development so that these children have a chance to develop normal binocular vision. The word *strabismus* means "to squint or to look obliquely."

Diagnosis: In a child with strabismus or any other ocular disorder, assessment of visual acuity is mandatory. Two tests (corneal light-reflex tests and cover tests) are used to diagnose strabismus.

Corneal light-reflex tests are particularly useful in children who are uncooperative and in those who have poor ocular fixation. To perform the Hirschberg corneal reflex test, the examiner projects a light source onto the cornea of both eyes simultaneously as a child looks directly to the light. Comparison should then be made of the placement of the corneal light reflex in each eye. In straight eyes, the light reflection appears symmetric and, because of the relationship between the cornea and the macula, slightly nasal to the center of each pupil. If strabismus present, reflected light is asymmetric, and appears displaced in one eye. The Krimsky method of the corneal reflex test uses prisms placed over one or both eyes to align the light reflections. The amount of prism needed to align the reflections is used to measure the degree of deviation. Corneal reflex tests may not detect a small angle or an intermittent strabismus.

Cover tests for strabismus require a child's attention and cooperation, good eye movement capability, and reasonably good vision in each eye. The results of cover tests might not be valid, if any of these are lacking. These tests consist of the cover-uncover test and the alternate cover test. In the cover-uncover test, a child looks at an object in the distance, preferably 6 meter away. If the child has an ocular deviation, the eye rapidly moves as the cover is shifted to the other eye. Both the cover-uncover test and the alternate cover test should be performed at both distance and near fixation. The cover-uncover tests differentiates tropias, or manifest deviations, from latent deviations, or phorias.

Clinical manifestations: There are nonparalytic and paralytic forms of strabismus.

1. *Nonparalytic strabismus:* It is the most common type of strabismus. The individual extraocular muscles usually have no defect. The amount of deviation is constant, or relatively constant, in various directions of gaze. Nonparlytic strabismus may rarely be congenital. Congenital exotropia may be associated with neurologic disease or abnormalities of bony orbit, as in Crouzon syndrome.

Pseudostrabismus (pseudoesotropia): This condition is characterized by the false appreciation of strabismus when the visual axes are aligned accurately. This appearance may be caused by a flat, broad nasal bridge, prominent epicanthal folds, or a narrow interpupillary distance. The observer might see less white sclera nasally than would be expected and the impression is that the eye is turned in toward the nose; especially when the child gazes to either side. Parents say that when the child looks to the side, the eye almost disappears from the view. Pseudoesotropia can be differentiated from a true misalignment of the eyes when the corneal light reflex is centered in both eyes and when the cover-uncover test shows no refixation movement. Once pseudoesotropia has been confirmed, parents can be reassured that the child will outgrow the appearance of esotropia.

2. *Paralytic strabismus:* When an eye muscle is paretic, palsied, or restricted, muscle imbalance occurs in which the deviation of the eye varies according to the direction of gaze. The symptom of recent onset of paresis is double vision that increases in one direction. It is important to differentiate a noncomitant strabismus from a comitant deviation because noncomitant forms of strabismus are often associated with trauma, systemic disorders, or neurologic abnormalities.

Third nerve palsy: It may be congenital or acquired. The congenital form is often associated with a developmental anomaly or birth trauma. The acquired causes include inflammatory or infectious lesions, head trauma, postviral syndromes, migraine, or an intracranial neoplasm or aneurism. A 3rd nerve palsy, whether congenital or acquired, usually results in an exotropia and a hypotropia, or downward deviation of the affected eye, as well as complete or partial ptosis of the upper lid. The strabismus results from the action of the normal, unopposed muscles, the lateral rectus muscle and superior oblique muscle. If the internal branch of the 3rd nerve is involved, papillary dilation may be noted as well. Eye movements are usually limited nasally in elevation and in depression.

Fourth nerve palsy: Fourth nerve palsies more commonly congenital than traumatic. A palsied 4th nerve results in weakness in the superior oblique muscle, which causes an upward elevation of the eye, a hypertropia. Because the antagonist muscle, the inferior oblique, is relatively unopposed, the affected eye demonstrates an upshoot when looking toward the nose. Children typically present with a head tilt to the shoulder opposite the affected eye, their chin down, and their face turned away from the affected side. This head position places the eye away from the area of greatest action of the affected muscle and therefore, minimizes the deviation and the associated double vision.

Sixth nerve palsy: Sixth nerve palsies produce markedly crossed eyes with limited ability to move the affected eye laterally. Children often present with their head turned toward the palsied muscle, a position that helps preserve binocular vision.

Elder J. Pediatric Ophthalmology and strabismus. J Pediatr Child Health 2003; 39: 724.

Kraft SP. Selected exotropia entities and principles of management. In: Rosenbaum AL, Santiago AP (eds). *Clinical Strabismus Management. Principles and Surgical Techniques.* Philadelphia: WB Saunders Co, 1999.

Olitsky SE, Hug D, Plummer LS, Stass-Isern M. Disorders of eye movement and alignment. In: Kliegman RM, Stanton BF, St.Geme JW, Schor NF, Behrman RE. *Nelson Textbook of Pediatrics.* 19th edn. New Delhi: Elsevier, 2011; 157–2162.

Singh K. Squint in Children. In: Mathur GP, Mathur Sarla (eds). *Current Trends in Pediatrics.* Vol 3. Delhi: Academa Publishers, 2007; 349–361.

28.12 ABNORMAL EYE MOVEMENTS

Nystagmus: Nystagmus (Greek word; to nod) is defined as involuntary, rhythmic oscillations of one or both eyes. The condition is almost always bilateral. Nystagmus may be characterized by rate (rapid or slow), amplitude (coarse or fine), direction (horizontal, vertical or rotational), and type of movement (pendular jerk). Acquired nystagmus requires prompt and thorough evaluation. The pathologic types are the gaze-paretic or gaze-evoked oscillations of cerebellar, brainstem, or cerebral disease. Spasmus nutans is an acquired nystagmus and is characterized by the triad of pendular nystagmus, head nodding, and torticollis. The nystagmus is characteristically very fine, very rapid, horizontal and pendular; it is often asymmetric, sometimes unilateral. Signs usually develop within the 1st yr or 2 of life. In many cases the condition is benign and self-limited, usually lasting a few months sometimes years. Those resolve spontaneously, the cause is unknown. Some children have underling brain tumors, particularly hypothalamic and chiasmal optic gliomas.

Opsoclonus: Opsoclonus and ataxic conjugate movements are spontaneous, nonrhythmic, multidirectional, chaotic movements of the eyes. The eyes appear to be in agitation, with bursts of conjugate movement of varying amplitude in varying directions. Opsoclonus is most often associated with encephalitis and may be the first sign of neuroblastoma.

Ocular motor dysmetria: It is characterized by an overshoot (or undershoot) of the eyes with several corrective to and fro oscillations on looking from one point to another. Ocular motor dysmetria is a sign of cerebellar or cerebellar pathway disease.

Flutter like oscillations: These intermittent to-and-fro horizontal oscillations of the eyes may occur spontaneously or on change of fixation. They are characteristic of cerebellar disease.

Leigh RJ, Zee DS. Diagnosis of central disorders of ocular motility. In: *The Neurology of eye movements.* 3rd edn. New York: Oxford University press, 1999;405–610.

Miller SJH. Nystagmus. In: *Parson's Diseases of the Eye.* 18th edn. Edinburgh: Churchill Livingstone, 1990;334–7.

Olitsky SE, Hug D, Smith LP. Disorders of eye movement and alignment. In: Kliegman RM, Behrman RE, Jenson HB, Stanton BF (eds). *Nelson Textbook of Pediatrics.* 18th edn. Vol 2. Philadelphia: Saunders, 2007;2578–84.

Prasad VN. Nystagmus and Abnormal Ocular Movements. In: Mathur GP, Mathur Sarla (eds). *Movement Disorders in Children & Adolescents.* New Delhi: Jaypee Brothers Medical Publishers (P) Ltd., 2003;104–10.

28.13 CHILDHOOD GLAUCOMA

Congenital glaucoma is a potentially blinding condition that afflicts infants and young children, either immediately at birth or within first few months or years of life. The classical tried of symptoms of congenital glaucomas comprises epiphora, photophobia and blephrospasm. Enlargement of eye, particularly cornea is seen early in life before 3 years of life. Progressive myopia develops due to enlargement of eyeball, due to elevated IOP. Disc cupping, which is reversible after successful control of IOP in early childhood, is also seen. Visual field defects may be documented in older children. Anisometropic ambylopia may occur as a consequence of progressive, uncorrected undetected myopia in a patient with late onset congenital glaucoma. Lens subluxation may occur due to stretching of zonules. Blunt trauma in these enlarged eyes may easily lead to hyphema and rupture of the globe.

Depending on the patient's age and degree of cooperation the examination may be carried out as an office procedure but with patience, or under sedation (Chloral hydrate 25–50 mg/kg body weight) or under general anesthesia. Important parameters to be noted on examination are adequacy of lacrimal drainage system, corneal diameter measurement with calipers, corneal clarity, intraocular pressure (IOP) and other intraocular abnormalities. Tonometry may be performed with noncontact tonometer or with Storz tonometer.

Ophthalmoscopy: It is best done through a semidiated pupil using Koeppe contact lens, which neutralizes irregular corneal reflexes. A cup disc ratio of greater than 0.3 or an asymmetry of more than 0.2 is highly suspicious of glaucoma. The cup enlargement is reversible with lowering of IOP, early enough. Cup enlargement may occur due to the enlargement of scleral canal though there may not be any neuronal loss.

Treatment: The treatment of congenital glaucoma includes medical and surgical management.

Medical management: Acetazolamide may be used immediately before or after surgery (as an oral suspension, 5–10 mm/kg body weight, every 6–8 hours).

Surgical management: Procedures to treat glaucoma in children include surgery to establish a normal anterior chamber angle (include goniotomy and trabeculotomy), to create a site for aqueous fluid to exit the eye (trabeculectomy and Saton surgery), or to reduce aqueous fluid production (cyclocryotherapy and cyclophosphocoagulation). Although vision may be reduced secondary to glaucomatous optic nerve damage or corneal scarring, amblyopia is the most common cause of loss of vision in these children.

Visual rehabilitation: It is as important in the management of the disease, as is the IOP control. This involves correction of refractive errors, correction of opacities in the media such as corneal scarring and cataract and orthoptic treatment to stimulate the development of binocular stereoscopic vision. Anisometropic ambylopia must be treated aggressively. These measures should be undertaken as early as possible.

Dickens CJ, Hoskens HD. Epidemiology and pathophysiology of congenital glaucoma. In: Ritch R, Sheelds MB, Krupin T (eds). *The glaucomas.* 2nd edn. Edinburgh: Mosby, 1996;729–38.

Kepp MA. Childhood glaucoma. *Pediatr Clinic N Am* 2003, 50:89–104.

Miller SJH (Ed). Glaucoma. In: *Parsons' Diseases of the Eye.* 18th edn. Oxford: Butterworth-Heinemann, 1998;213–28.

Olitsky SE, Hug D, Smith LP. Chidhood Glaucoma. In: Kliegman RM, Behrman RE, Jenson HB, Stanton BF (eds). *Nelson Textbook of Pediatrics.* 18th edn. Vol. 2. Philadelphia: Saunders, 2007;2608–10.

Rubin SE, Marcus CH. Glaucoma in childhood. *Ophthalmol Clin North Am* 1996;2:215.

28.14 ABNORMALITIES OF THE LIDS

Congenital Anomalies of the Lids

Congenital ptosis: It is also known as blepharoptosis. It can be simple ptosis existing as an isolated anomaly, or can be complicated when associated with other anomalies as superior rectus palsy, etc.

Congenital ectropion is usually associated with blepharophimosis syndrome and ichthyosis. It is caused by vertical insufficiency of anterior lamella of the lids. It can give rise to exposure keratitis and epiphora in severe cases.

Epicanthus is a medial canthal fold and is usually bilateral. It can result in pseudostrabismus due to decreased scleral exposure nasally resulting in false sense of esotropia.

Epiblepharon: The lower eyelid pretarsal muscle and skin override the lower lid margin so that the eyelid cilia are directed vertically. The lid margin is in normal position.

Congenital entropion: In this lid margin inversion is presents compared to epiblepharon.

Lid hemangiomas: Usually capillary hemangioma is present in the lid, which manifest at first week or month of life, increase in size till one year of age and then decreases over next 4–5 years. Treatment is required in cases causing amblyopia if involving the visual axis, strabismus or cosmetic disfigurement. Intralesional steroid injection can be tried. Alternatively well circumscribed lesions can be surgically excised.

Acquired Eyelid Lesions

Chalazion results from obstruction of the meibomian gland which is located in the tarsal plate and open posterior to the grey line. Treatment consists of warm compresses and topical antibiotic or anti-inflammatory medication in acute stage and incision and curettage in chronic lesions. The incision in posterior aspect of the lid is oriented vertically to avoid injury to vertically arranged meibomian glands. The incision on skin side should be horizontal to prevent scarring. An infected chalazion can result in internal hordeolum.

Stye (external hordeolum). An acute infection of gland of Zeis is known as stye. The infection appears to center around the lash follicle and the lash can be plucked to promote drainage.

Eyelid Neoplasms

Eyelid tumors, benign (papillomas; dermal melanocytosis) and malignant can arise from various layers in periocular skin, i.e. epidermis, dermis or eyelid adnexa. Usually 15–20% of eyelid lesions are malignant. These are more common in adults.

Doxanas MT, Andersons RL. Oriental eyelids. An anatomic study. *Arch Ophthalmol* 1984; 102: 1232–1235.

Stewart WB. *Surgery of the Eyelid, Orbit and Lacrimal system.* Ophthalmology Monograph 8. Vol 2. San Francisco: American Academy of Ophthalmology, 1994; 85.

28.15 DISORDERS OF THE LACRIMAL APPARATUS

Congenital nasolacrimal obstruction: Congenital NLDO usually caused by membranous block of valve of Hasher, occurs in 50% of the newborn infants. These open in 90% of cases in first year of life. Conservative management with topical antibiotics and properly done nasolacrimal massage resolves most of the cases and this conservative management is followed till the age of 6–9 months according to various studies.

Usually after 9 months syringing and probing under general anesthesia is performed for congenital nasolacrimal duct obstruction. Silicone intubation is performed for children with recurrent epiphora following probing syringing and probing or in older children where stenosis or scarring is found on initial syringing and probing. Balloon dacryoplasty is recently being used in management of congenital NLDO in which a collapsed balloon catheter is placed in the nasolacrimal duct and inflated at various places to relieve the obstruction. After the age of 3 years external dacryocystorhinostomy (DCR) is performed in which an opening from lacrimal sac is made in the nasal cavity opening below the middle turbinate for drainage.

Dacryocystocele: A dilated lacrimal sac at birth presenting in absence of inflammatory signs may indicate a congenital dacryocystocele or mucocele. It occurs due to obstruction of nasolacrimal duct and accumulation of amniotic fluid and mucus (secreted from goblet cells of the lacrimal sac) into the lacrimal sac. A congenital dacryocystocele can even extend inferiorly under the inferior turbinate. In initial phase when it is sterile congenital dacryocystocele can be managed conservatively by topical antibiotics and massage; in cases of non response and infection probing of the tear system is indicated. Urgent treatment is requires in cases of bilateral prolapse of dacryocystocele into the nasal cavity causing difficulty in breathing.

Punctal agenesis and dysgenesis: The punctum can sometimes be absent or the opening can be covered by a thin membrane. The membrane can be cut with sharp probe or dilator in these cases. Usually an absent punctum can be associated with absence of underlying canalicular tissue. Complete absence of punctum and canalicular system requires a conjunctivodacryo-cystorhinstomy.

Katowitz JA, Welsh MG. Timing of initial probing and irrigation in congenital nasolacrimal duct obstruction. *Ophthalmology* 1987; 94: 698–705.

Kushner BJ. Congenital nasolarimal system obstruction. *Arch Ophthalmol* 1982; 100: 597–600.

Mansour AM, Cheng KP, Mumma JV, et al. Congenital dacryocele: A collaborative review. *Ophthalmology* 1991; 98: 1744–1751.

28.16 ORBITAL ABNORMALITIES

Orbital malformations: Orbital malformations can be a part of syndrome or can present as isolated condition. Measurements of orbit can be made by using a transparent ruler and compared to normal reference values according to data available keeping in account the racial variations.

Hypotelorism: It is the reduced distance between the medial walls of the orbits with reduced inner and outer canthal distances. It can be a result of skull malformation or failure in brain development. It is a part of various syndromes seen in children such as Down syndrome, Goldenhar syndrome, oculodento-digital syndrome.

Hypertelorism is an increase in both inner and outer intercanthal distance. It occurs due to early ossification of lesser wing of the sphenoid bone which fixes the orbit in fetal position, can be due to protusion of primitive brain as in frontal encephalocele, or maldevelopment of skull base as in craniosynostosis. It is seen in various syndromes as Apert syndrome, Noonan syndrome.

Telecanthus: It is characterized by increased distance between the inner canthus. It is seen in blepharophimosis syndrome, fetal alcohol syndrome.

Dystopia canthorum: It is defined as lateral displacement of both inner canthi and the lacrimal puncta such that imaginary vertical line drawn connecting the upper and lower puncta crosses the cornea.

Enophthalmos: True congenital enophthalmos is a rare entity. It occurs when the primary optic vesicle fails to grow out from the cerebral vesicle during embryonic development. The impure variant consists of unilateral small orbit and no visible eye and a small microphthalmic globe is present in the orbital soft tissues.

Microphthalmos is a developmental defect that causes reduction in size of the eye. Microphthalmos with orbital cyst results failure of closure of choroidal fissure in the embryo.

Craniosynostosis: It is premature closure of one or more sutures in bones of the skull, resulting in skeletal malformations. Various craniosynostosis syndromes such as Crouzon syndrome and Apert syndrome have hypertelorism and proptosis as a common manifestation.

Orbital Infections

Infections of the orbit can arise from three sources namely direct spread from adjacent sinuses, direct inoculation from trauma or skin infection or bacterial spread from a distant focus, i.e. caries tooth, otitis media. Periorbital infections can be classified into preseptal or orbital cellulitis.

Preseptal cellulitis: It is defined as inflammation and infection confined to the eyelids and periorbital structures anterior to the orbital septum. In children the most common cause is extension of the infection from surrounding sinuses. The globe is usually uninvolved. The manifestations are eyelid edema, erythema and inflammation. Pupillary reaction, visual acuity and ocular motility are not involved. CT scan of paranasal sinuses can delineate underlying sinusitis. In children infection is usually treated by intravenous antibiotics.

Orbital cellulitis: Active infection of the orbital soft tissue is present posterior to the orbital septum. The clinical findings are fever, proptosis, chemosis, restriction of ocular motility and pain on movement of the globe. Decrease in visual acuity and pupillary abnormalities indicate involvement of the orbital apex.

Involvement of the lateral rectus of the other eye indicates spread of infection to cavernous sinus. In more than 90% of cases sinusitis is the underlying cause. An intravenous antibiotics are used in treatment with surgical drainage any localized subperiosteal abscess develops. Monitoring for involvement of orbital apex and cavernous sinus should be done.

Necrotizing fasciitis: It is severe bacterial involvement of the underlying subcutaneous tissue, particularly superficial and deep fascia. Usually occurs in patients with history of trauma or relatively immunocompromised status, e.g. diabetes. It is associated with swelling, erythema and pain and tends to track along the avascular planes, and can be associated with disproportinate complaint of pain and typical change in skin color progressing from rose discoloration to bluish grey and skin necrosis. Rapid deterioration can be noticed, resulting in hypotension, renal failure and respiratory distress.

Phycomycosis: It is fungal infection of the orbit usually caused by Mucor and Rhizopus fungus, more common in immunocompromised adults.

Orbital tuberculosis: It usually affects the orbit as a chronic inflammatory process, such as periostitis, commonly known as cold abscess. It usually spreads to orbit hematogenously from underlying pulmonary focus or can be associated with adjacent tubercular sinusitis. Proptosis, motility dysfunction, bone destruction, and chronic draining fistulas can be the presenting manifestations. Fine needle aspiration cytology with culture can help in establishment of the diagnosis. Antitubercular therapy is usually curative.

Orbital Tumours

Hamartoma is characterized by anomalous growth of tissue present normally at the site, e.g. capillary hemangioma and neurofibromatosis. Choristomas consist of tissue not normally found at the involved site, e.g. dermoid cyst, teratoma, etc.

Dermoid cyst: It is among the most common orbital tumour in children. It consists of keratinized epidermis with dermal appendages such as sebaceous glands and hair follicles. These are usually located adjacent to lateral brow and may have dumbbell extension posteriorly. Therefore a CT scan is usually needed to rule out posterior extension. Treatment is surgical removal of the cyst in total; rupture of cyst during removal can lead to acute inflammatory process.

Capillary hemangiomas are common primary benign tumours of the orbit in children. Capillary hemangiomas are seen primarily in children in first year of life, appearing in first week or two after birth and enlarge dramatically over 6 months to one year. After first year they start decreasing in size. Superficially located capillary hemangiomas can strawberry to bluish discoloration of skin depending on depth, while more deeply located tumours can present as progressively enlarging mass, proptosis. Capillary hemangiomas of eyelid and orbit can cause anisometropia, strabismus or deprivation amblyopia which is usually indications of treatment. Initial treatment consists of local steroid injection but can lead to subcutaneous fat atrophy, embolic visual loss. Smaller lesions refractory to steroid injection can be surgically excised.

Lymphangiomas: Ocular involvement includes conjunctiva, eyelids and orbit. Spontaneous hemorrhage within the lesion can lead to enlargement of the lesion. These are diffusely infiltrative lesions with ill defined margins making complete resection difficult.

Neurofibromas: Neurofibromas of orbit can present as S-shaped lid deformity presenting as lid neurofibromas, dysplasia of the orbital walls presenting as pulsating proptosis and optic nerve gliomas.

Optic nerve gliomas: Section 28.10.

Rhabdomyosarcomas: See Section 34.10.

Dutton JJ. *Atlas of clinical and surgical Orbital anatomy.* Philadelphia: Saunders, 1994.

Dutton JJ. Gliomas of the anterior visual pathway. *Surv Ophthalmol* 1994; 38: 427–452.

Sheilds JA, Kaden IH, Eagle RC et al. Orbital dermoid cysts: clinicopathological correlations, classification, and management. *Ophthal Plast Reconstr Surg* 1997; 13: 265–276.

Wright JE, Sullivan TJ, Garner A, et al. Orbital venous anomalies. *Ophthalmology* 1997; 104: 905–913.

28.17 INJURIES TO THE EYES

Trauma is the most important cause of blindness in children. About 1/3 of blindness in children is as a results from trauma. Boys 11–15 yr of age are the most vulnerable; injuries outnumber in boys than those in girls by a ratio of 4:1. The majority of injuries are related to sports, toy darts, other projectiles, sticks, stones, fireworks, paint balls, and air-powdered BB guns. Any part of the orbit or globe may be affected.

Ecchymoses and swelling of the eyelids: These are common after blunt trauma. Hemorrhage into the lids and periorbital region ("black eye" or "shiner") is usually of no consequence and absorbs spontaneously, but it should prompt careful examination of the eye for deeper, more serious injury, such as a blowout fracture of the orbit, an intraocular hemorrhage, or rupture of the globe.

Lacerations of the eyelids: In all cases of lid laceration, examination of the globe for perforating injury is mandatory. Proper primary repair often achieves a superior outcome to secondary repair at a later date.

Superficial abrasions of the cornea: This is accompanied by pain, tearing, photophobia, and decreased vision. Corneal abrasions are detected by instilling fluorescein dye and inspecting the cornea using a blue-filtered light. A slit lamp is ideal for this examination.

Treatment of a corneal abrasion is directed at promoting healing and relieving pain. Abrasions are treated with frequent applications of a topical antibiotic ointment until the epithelium is completely healed. A topical cycloplegic agent (cyclopentolate hydrochloride 1%) can relieve the pain from ciliary spasm in patients with large abrasions.

Foreign body on or in the cornea or conjunctiva: This usually produces acute discomfort, lacrimation, and inflammation. Most foreign bodies can be detected by examination in good light with the aid of magnification or a direct ophthalmoscope set on a high plus lens (+10 or +12). In many cases, especially if the particle is deep or metallic, slit-lamp examination is required. Some conjunctival foreign bodies tend to lodge under the upper eyelid, causing the sensation of corneal foreign body as they come into contact with the globe on eyelid movement; they may also produce vertically oriented linear corneal abrasions. If these abrasions are present, eversion of the lid may be necessary. If a foreign body is suspected but not found, further examination is indicated. If there is history of injury with a high-velocity particle, radiologic examination of the eye may be needed to explore the possibility of an intraocular foreign body.

Removal of a foreign body can be facilitated by instillation of a drop of topical anesthetic. Many foreign bodies can be removed by irrigating or by gently wiping them away with a moistened cotton-tipped applicator. Embedded foreign bodies should be treated by an ophthalmologist. Removal of corneal foreign bodies may leave epithelial defects, which are treated as corneal abrasions. Metallic foreign bodies may cause rust to form in the corneal tissues; examination by an ophthalmologist 1 or 2 days after removal of a foreign body is recommended because a rust ring might require further treatment (curettage).

Hyphema: Presence of blood in the anterior chamber of the eye is known as hyphema. It may occur with either a blunt or perforating injury. Hyphema appears as a bright or dark red fluid level between the cornea and iris or as a diffuse murkiness of the aqueous humor. Children complaints of pain and may be somnolent. The treatment of hyphema includes bed rest, with head elevated 30–45 degrees to promote settling and resorption of the blood. Hospitalization and sedation may be necessary to ensure compliance in some children. In most cases, topical mydriatics, topical or oral corticosteroids, or oral aminocaproic acid are used to prevent rebleeding. Secondary bleeding typically occurs 3–5 days, after the initial hemorrhage, increasing the risk of sequelae. The blood in the anterior chamber may produce elevation of intraocular pressure and blood staining of the cornea. These complications may affect vision. In such cases, surgical evacuation of the clot and irrigation of the anterior chamber may be necessary.

Lacerations and perforating wounds of the cornea or sclera: Important clues to perforating injury of the eye are collapse of the anterior chamber, distortion and displacement of the pupil, and protusion of dark tissue (uvea) into the wound. These require immediate referral to an ophthalmologist and prompt surgical care. Emergency treatment consists of protecting the injured eye from further damage by applying a sterile bandage and a rigid eye shield. If these medical supplies are not on hand, an adequate eye shield can be fashioned from a plastic or from a piece of cardboard bent into a box or cone shape. Manipulation should be kept to minimum. No medication should be instilled except under the direction of ophthalmologist.

Ruptured globe: If the globe is compressed along its anteroposterior diameter with enough force, it will rupture at its weakest point. These weak points generally include the area where the sclera and cornea meet (limbus), near the insertions of the rectus muscles and at the site of previous intraocular surgery. Prognosis in these injuries is poor.

Optic nerve trauma: Injury to the globe may produce a traumatic optic neuropathy. Indirect damage to the optic nerve may occur after blunt trauma to the forehead secondary to shock waves that pass through the optic canal. Patients may complain of reduced vision. More frequently, these patients are unconscious and the only clue to the injury may be the presence of an afferent papillary defect. In such cases, the imaging studies should be performed to look for the presence of a fracture or hematoma.

Chemical injuries: Chemical injuries are caused by alkali or acid burns. Alkali burns are usually more destructive than acid burns because they react with fats to form soaps, which damage cell membranes, allowing further penetration of the alkali into the eye. Acids generally cause less severe, more localized tissue damage. Most stronger acids precipitate tissue proteins, creating a physical barrier against their further penetration. The corneal epithelium offers moderate protection against weak acids, and a little damage occurs unless the pH is 2.5 or less.

Mild acid or alkali burns are characterized by conjunctival injection and swelling and mild corneal epithelial erosions. The corneal stroma may be mildly edematous, and the anterior chamber may have mild to moderate cell and flare reaction. With strong acids, the cornea and conjunctiva rapidly become white and opaque. The corneal epithelium may slough, leaving a relatively clear stroma; this appearance may initially mask the severity of the burn. Severe alkali burns are characterized by corneal opacification.

Chemical burns of the cornea and adnexal tissue are among the most urgent of the ocular emergencies. Emergency treatment of a chemical burn begins with copious immediate irrigation with water or saline. Local debridement and removal of foreign particles should be performed while still irrigating. If the nature of chemical injury is unknown, the use of pH test paper is helpful in determining whether the agent was basic or acidic. Irrigation should continue for at least 30 minutes or until 2 L of irrigant has been instilled in mild cases and for 2–4 hr or until 10 L of irrigant has been instilled in severe cases. At the end of irrigation, the pH should be checked again approximately 30 min after irrigation to ensure that it has not changed.

Fractures: Floor fractures are common when objects larger than the orbital opening, such as a ball, fist, or the dash board of an automobile, strike the orbit, particularly the inferior lateral orbit. A direct orbital floor fracture is a floor fracture associated with an orbital rim fracture. An indirect orbital floor fracture is an isolated floor fracture and is more commonly known as a "blowout fracture."

The characteristic clinical sign of an orbital floor fracture is limitation of upward gaze. Other signs include lower eyelid ecchymosis, nosebleed, orbital emphysema, and hypesthesia of the ipsilateral cheek and upper lip. The last sign results from disruption of the infraorbital nerve as it traverses the orbital floor. Radiographic studies (plain film radiography and CT) will help in visualizing the orbital fractures.

Treatment for children with acute orbital fractures includes antibiotic prophylaxis, nasal decongestants, and ice packs. Surgical repair is necessary.

Penetrating wounds of the orbit: Careful evaluation for possible damage to the eye, the optic nerve, or the brain and investigation for retained foreign body is required. Orbital hemorrhage and infection are common with penetrating wounds of the orbit; such injuries must be treated as emergencies.

Child abuse: This is a major cause of injuries to the eye and orbital region. The possibility of nonaccidental trauma must be considered in any child with ecchymosis or laceration of the lids, hemorrhage in or about the eye, cataract or dislocated lens, retinal detachment, or fracture of the orbit. Inflicted childhood neurotrauma (shaken baby syndrome) occurs secondary to violent, nonaccidental, repetitive, unrestrained acceleration-deceleration head and neck movements, with or without blunt head trauma in children typically younger than 3 yr. Retinal hemorrhage is the most common ophthalmic finding and occurs at all levels of the retina. Detection of abuse is not only important in order to treat but also to prevent further abuse or even death.

Fireworks related injuries: Injuries related to the use of fireworks can be most devastating of all ocular traumas that occur in children. It is reported that 1/5th of the emergency department visits for fireworks-related injuries are for ocular trauma.

Sports-related ocular injuries and their prevention: Sports injuries occur in all age groups. Children and adolescents especially participate in high-risk sports than do adults suffer more injuries. The sports with the highest risk of eye injury are those in which no eye protection can be worn, including boxing, wrestling, and martial arts. High-risk sports include those that use a rapidly moving ball or puck, bat, stick, racquet, or arrow (baseball, hockey, lacrosse, racquet sports, and archery) or involve aggressive body contact (football and basketball). Related to both risk and frequency, of participation, the highest percentage of eye injuries are in basketball and baseball. Protective eyewear designed for a specific activity is available for most sports.

American Academy of Pediatrics Committee on Sports Medicine and Fitness, American Academy of Ophthalmology Committee on Eye Safety and Sports Ophthalmology: Protective eyewear for young athletes. *Pediatrics* 1996; 98:311–313.

Khaw PT, Shah P, Elkington AR. Injury to the eye. *Br Med J* 2004; 328: 36–38.

Kivlin JD, Simons KB, Lazoritz S, et al. Shaken baby syndrome. *Ophthalmology* 2000; 107:1246–1254.

Olitsky SE, Hug D, Smith LP. Disorders of vision. In: Kliegman RM, Behrman RE, Jenson HB, Stanton BF (eds). *Nelson Textbook of Pediatrics.* 18th edn. Vol 2. Philadelphia: Saunders, 2007; 2612–2615.

29 Disorders of the Ear, Nose, Throat, Head and Neck

29.1 EXAMINATION OF EAR, NOSE, THROAT, AND NECK

Examination of ear, nose, throat, and neck is a routine part of periodic assessment. Hearing loss must be detected early. Examination of cranial nerves particularly olfactory nerve (1), facial nerve (7) and auditory nerve (8) should also be performed. Enquire history of atopy and allergy in children and family members.

Eight prominent signs and symptoms associated with diseases of the ear and temporal bone includes: 1. Hearing loss, 2. Tinnitus, 3. Discharge (Otorrhoea), 4. Pain (Otlagia), 5. Vertigo, 6. Swelling around the ear, 7. Nystagmus, 8. Facial paralysis

Basic tests of hearing: A patient with normal hearing should hear equally as well in both ears. To make a basic assessment of a patients hearing, you need to mask the non test ear, say by inserting your finger into it, and then ask them to repeat random numbers (e.g. 31, 45, 17, 64, etc.) that you speak into the test ear. Start with a quiet whisper, then a 'stage' whisper, then quiet speech, loud speech and finally a shout, stop at the level at which the patient can accurately repeat the numbers you are giving them. It is important that the patient cannot see your face as many deaf patients can lip read. Repeat this on the other side and you can get a rough measure of their hearing. Hearing levels are objectively and accurately assessed by pure tone audiometery.

Tuning fork tests: These test hearing in both ears and can help distinguish between a sensorineural and conductive hearing loss. Ideally you should use a 512Hz tuning fork. If unavailable a 265Hz will suffice. Strike the tuning fork against your elbow or knee to make it vibrate. Striking it against a metal object can introduce unwanted harmonic vibrations into the sound signal.

Weber test. Place the fork in the middle of the head (vertex). Ask the patient if he can hear the sound equally in both ears, or if it is louder on one side. A patient with normal hearing should hear the sound equally in both ears. If a patient has a unilateral conductive loss, the Weber test will localise to the affected ear.

Rinne test. Place the fork behind the ear, pressing on the mastoid process (firmly) and then hold the fork about three inches away from the ear. In a normal ear, the patient should hear the tuning fork louder in front (air conduction) and quieter behind (bone conduction). This is called a positive Rinne test. If a patient has a conductive hearing loss (usually of around 20 dB or greater), then they will hear the bone conduction (behind the ear) louder than the air conduction and this is called a negative Rinne test. If a patient has a non-hearing ear on one side ('dead' ear), then they will still hear the bone conduction louder, because the sound will be transmitted around the skull and heard by the other cochlea. This is called a false negative Rinne test.

Vestibular function can be evaluated by the caloric test. Approximately 5 ml of ice water is delivered by syringe into the external auditory canal with patient's head elevated 30 degrees from the horizontal position. In obtunded or comatose patients with an intact brainstem, there is prompt deviation of the eyes to the side of the stimulus. A much smaller quantity of ice water (0.5 ml) is used in alert, awake subjects. In normal subjects, introduction of ice water produces nystagmus with the quick component in the opposite direction to the stimulated labyrinth. No response implies severe dysfunction of the brainstem and medial longitudinal fasciculus. If the otoscopic examination reveals a ruptured tympanic membrane, the test should not be performed in that ear.

Examination of the nose: Examination of the nose also involves assessment of function: Airway resistance and occasionally sense of smell. Examination of the nose is incomplete without looking into the mouth and pharynx. The main symptoms of nasal disease are:
1. Airway obstruction
2. Runny nose (rhinorrhea)
3. Sneezing
4. Loss of smell (anosmia)
5. Facial pain due to sinusitis
6. Snoring associated with nasal obstruction.

Throat examination: The throat examination includes a thorough examination of the oral cavity including tongue, tonsils, uvula, soft palate, hard palate, teeth, buccal region and the gingivolabial/gingivobuccal sulcus—the space between the cheek and the gums, floor of the mouth. Examination of the nasopharynx and larynx are done by using mirrors or flexible fibre—optic nasendoscopes.

Neck examination: The neck should be examined in a systematic manner. Examine the following areas: parotid region; midline from chin to sternal notch; anterior triangle including submandibular triangle; anterior jugular chain of lymph nodes; posterior triangle.

Facial nerve (7th cranial nerve): Decreased voluntary movement of the lower face with flattening of the nasolabial angle on the ipsilateral side indicates an upper motor neuron or supra nuclear corticospinal lesion. A lower motor neuron tends to involve upper and lower facial muscles equally. Taste for anterior two-thirds of the tongue may be tested in a cooperative child by placing a solution of saline or glucose on either side of the extended tongue. Normal children can identify the substance with a little difficulty.

Haddad J Jr. General consideration and evaluation. In: Kliegman RM, Behrman RE, Jenson HB, Stanton BF (eds). *Nelson Textbook of Pediatrics.* 18th edn. Vol 2. Philadelphia: Saunders, 2007;2617–19.

Haddad J Jr. Congenital malformations. In: Kliegman RM, Behrman RE, Jenson HB, Stanton BF (eds). *Nelson Textbook of Pediatrics.* 18th edn. Vol 2. Philadelphia: Saunders, 2007;2628–29.

Haslam RHA. Neurologic evaluation. In: Kliegman RM, Behrman RE, Jenson HB, Stanton BF (eds). *Nelson Textbook of Pediatrics.* 18th edn. Vol 2. Philadelphia: Saunders, 2007;2433–43.

29.2 HEARING LOSS

The estimates vary because of differences in criteria for defining hearing impairment, the age group surveyed, and the testing methods used. Approximately 1–2 newborns/1,000 live births have moderate (30–50 dB), severe (50–70 dB), or profound (>70 dB) bilateral neural hearing loss, including 0.5–1/1,000 with bilateral hearing loss >75 dB. An additional 1–2/1,000 may have milder or unilateral impairments; by 19 yr of age.

Types of hearing loss: Hearing loss can be *peripheral* or *central* in origin. Peripheral hearing loss can be conductive hearing loss (CHL), sensorineural hearing loss (SNHL) or mixed. CHL is commonly caused by dysfunction in the transmission of sound through the external or middle ear or by abnormal transduction of sound energy into neural activity in the inner ear and the 8th nerve. CHL is the most common type of hearing loss in children and occurs when sound transmission is physically impeded in the external and/or middle ear. Common causes of CHL in the ear canal include atresia or stenosis, impacted cerumen, or foreign bodies. In the middle ear, perforation of the tympanic membrane (TM), discontinuity or fixation of the ossicular chain, otitis media (OM) with effusion, otosclerosis, and cholesteatoma can cause CHL.

Damage to or maldevelopment of structures in the inner ear can cause SNHL. Causes include hair cell destruction from noise, disease, or ototoxic agents; cochlear malformation; perilymphatic fistula of the round or oval window membrane; and lesions of the acoustic division of the 8th nerve. A combination of CHL and SNHL is considered a mixed hearing loss.

Effects of hearing impairment: The effects of hearing impairment depend on the nature and degree of the hearing loss and on the individual characteristics of the child. Hearing loss may be unilateral or bilateral, conductive, sensorineural or mixed; mild, moderate, severe, or profound; of sudden or gradual onset; stable, progressive, or fluctuating; and affecting a part, or all, of the audible spectrum. Other factors, such as intelligence, medical or physical condition (including accompanying syndromes), family support, age at onset, age at time of identification, and promptness of intervention, also affect the impact of hearing loss on a child.

Hearing screening: Hearing impairment can have a major impact on a child's development. Early identification and prompt intervention improves prognosis. The recommended hearing screening techniques are either otoacoustic emissions (OAE) testing or auditory brainstem evoked responses (ABR). The ABR test, an auditory evoked electrophysiologic response that correlates highly with hearing, is cost effective to screen newborns and to identify further the degree and type of hearing loss. OAE tests are quick, easy to administer, and inexpensive, and provide a sensitive indication of the presence of hearing loss. Results are relatively easy to interpret. OAE tests elicit no response if hearing is worse than 30–40 dB, no matter what the cause. Those children who fail OAE tests undergo an ABR for a more definitive evaluation.

Identification of hearing impairment: Parental concern about hearing and any delayed development of speech and language should alert the pediatrician, because parental concern usually precedes formal identification and diagnosis of hearing impairment by 6 mo to 1 yr of age. Any child with a known risk factor for hearing loss should be evaluated in the 1st 6 mo of life. Children suspected of hearing loss should be referred for hearing assessment. Children with speech delay should be referred for audiologic assessment. Children with normal hearing develop an extensive language by 3–4 yr of age.

Clinical audiologic evaluation: When hearing impairment is suspected in a young child, reliable and valid estimates of auditory function can be obtained.

Treatment. Once a hearing loss is identified, a full developmental and speech and language evaluation is needed. Parental counseling and involvement are required in all stages of the evaluation and treatment or rehabilitation. Infants and young children with profound congenital or prelingual onset of deafness have benefited from multichannel cochlear implants.

Genetic counseling: Families of children with the diagnosis of SNHL, or a syndrome associated with SNHL and/or CHL should consider genetic counseling, which will allow for a discussion of the likelihood of similar diagnoses in future pregnancies.

Grote JJ. Neonatal screening for hearing impairment. *Lancet* 2000; 355: 513–514.

Haddad J Jr. Hearing loss. In: Kliegman RM, Behrman RE, Jenson HB, Stanton BF (eds). *Nelson Textbook of Pediatrics.* 18th edn. Vol. 2. Philadelphia: Saunders, 2007; 2620–2628.

Smith RJH. Deafness from bedside to bench and back. *Lancet* 2002; 260: 656–657.

Smith RJH, Bale JF Jr, White KR. Sensorineural hearing loss in children. *Lancet* 2005; 265: 879–890.

Williams PJ. Genetic causes of hearing loss. *N Engl J Med* 2000; 342: 1101.

Deaf Mutism and Cochlear Implant

Deaf mutism is a very agonizing health condition which can greatly undermine the potentials of those affected. Cochlear implant has established itself as a means of optimizing the potentials of such children. Deafness is severe hearing loss with a little or no residual hearing. Such a person's hearing is non-functional for ordinary purposes of life. The degree of hearing impairment in decibels in children is graded as normal (0–15); mild (16–40); moderate (41–55); moderately severe (56–70); severe (71–90) and profound (91–110).

Normal hearing is, essential in early life to ensure speech and language development especially in the first 2–3 years of life. This auditory linked acquisition of language in humans is a time linked function related to early maturational processes in an infant's life. Reception of speech and language inputs from early infancy (even earlier, since the baby is born with fully developed functioning cochlea) is gradually converted to expression in first life and into the second year of life. After the age of two years it becomes progressively more difficult, and by the age of two in the average normal hearing child a good vocabulary and the capacity to string words together into simple sentences has already been acquired.

It is certain, however, that if a child is to begin to speak at the normal average age of 9–15 months, deafness must be diagnosed and an aid given by the age of six months. That aid may be in the form of cochlear implant. A cochlear implant (CI) is a surgically implanted electronic device that provides a sense of sound to a person who is profoundly deaf or severely hard of hearing. The cochlear implant unlike the hearing aid does not amplify sound, but works by directly stimulating any functioning auditory nerves inside the cochlear with electrical impulses.

Hearing impairment is the most prevalent sensory deficit in the human population with about 1 in 800 children born with serious hearing impairment. Cochlear implant has improved the hearing of many children.

Deaf mutism: Deaf mutism is inability to acquire speech as a result of severe deafness. Deafness can be conductive or sensorineural type. For hearing loss to be severe enough to lead to mutism, it has to be bilateral. The causes of deafness may be congenital or acquired (Boxes 29.1 and 29.2).

Management of deaf mutism: Early detection is the hallmark of management. This is important so that early auditory rehabilitation is instituted which will ensure optimal speech development, educational development, social interactions and psychological

---

Box 29.1: Causes of congenital deafness

Congenital conductive deafness: Atresia of the external auditory meatus; Ossicular anomalies: Congenital absence of oval window

Congenital sensorineural deafness:

a. Syndromic (when sensorineural hearing loss occurs in addition to other conditions): Waardenburg's syndrome (congenital perceptive deafness, hypertelorism, heterochromia iridiae frontal bossing and white forlock); Albinism; Usher's syndrome (deafness and night blindness); Pendred's syndrome (deafness and goiter in non-endemic area).

b. Non-syndromic: Michel's aplasia (complete failure of development of the inner ear); Mondini (incomplete development of bony and membraneous labyrinth); Scheribe (membraneous cochlear and sacular aplasia); Chromosomal abnormalities – Trisomy 13, 18, 12; Connexin 26 R143N mutation.

Intrauterine infections (usually first infections where there is lack of maternal immunity): Congenital rubella; Congenital syphilis; Congenital Toxoplasmosis; Congenital Cytomegalovirus (CMV); Varicella infection (rare)

Maternal infections other than rubella occurring within the first trimester: Mumps; Measles; Scarlet fever

Maternal drug ingestion (first trimester): Thalidomide

Miscellaneous maternal factors (may affect fetus): Toxaemia of pregnancy; diabetes mellitus: thyrotoxicosis: abdominal radiography in pregnancy

---

Box 29.2: Causes of acquired deafness

1. Kernicterus from Rhesus iso-immunization, ABO incompatibility, G-6PD deficiency
2. Severe birth asphyxia HIE
3. Neonatal meningitis, neonatal seizures, neonatal tetanus
4. Administration of ototoxic drugs in the neonatal period, e.g. furosemide
5. Prematurity has been associated with deafness

---

adjustments which hitherto may be adversely affected by hearing impairment. For this reason, all infants should be screened while still in the hospital or within the first month of life. Recently Otoacoustic emissions (OAE) have been suggested as a procedure by which significant sensorineural hearing loss may be identified in the newborn.

Normally a newborn responds to loud sound by moving its head, legs and arms—Startle reflex. Also a loud sound made near a healthy infant causes blinking of its eyes—Cochleopalpebral reflex. Absence of these reflexes could call attention of parents or care giver to the fact that all may not be well with the baby's hearing. Detailed history from the mother on the pregnancy, birth, and developmental milestones as well as behavioral assessment are vital in detecting the "at risk group". The "at risk babies" form about 20% of the infant population and among this group deafness is 14 times more common than the remaining 80%. First test is done at 6–9 months, second repeated at 18 months–2 years and thirdly just before entering school. At any time abnormality is detected the child is subjected to more in-depth assessment in the audiology clinic and intervention initiated accordingly medically or surgically. Profound deafness in children can be very disastrous whether it is congenital or acquired. In the case of congenital deafness, the child may fail to develop any spoken language and will be denied access to the world of hearing even with the most powerful conventional hearing aid. In these cases both congenital and acquired cochlear implantation could be very useful.

Cochlear implant: Cochlear implant (CI) is essentially an alternative form of hearing device applicable to some people who, because of bilateral sensorineural hearing loss due to cochlear failure are unable to benefit from even the most powerful conventional hearing aid. Cochlear implant is a surgically implanted electronic device that provides a sense of sound to a person who is profoundly deaf or severely hard of hearing. Unlike the hearing aids the CI does not amplify sound but works by directly stimulating any functioning auditory nerve inside the cochlear with electrical impulses.

Cochlear implant consists of a small electronic device that is surgically implanted under the skin behind the ear and an external speech processor which is usually worn on a belt or in a pocket. A microphone is also worn outside the body as a head piece behind the ear to capture incoming sound. The speech processor translates the sound into distinctive electrical signals. These signals travel up a thin cable to the headpiece and are transmitted across the skin via radio waves to the implanted electrodes in the cochlea. The electrodes' signals stimulate the auditory nerve fibers to send information to the brain where it is interpreted as meaningful sound. The indications for cochlear implant are listed in Box 29.3.

Benefits of cochlear implants: Cochlear implants do not restore normal hearing, and benefits vary individually. Most users find that the implants help them communicate better through improved lip reading.

- Help discriminate speech without visual cues.
- Hearing ranges from near normal ability to understand speech to no hearing benefit at all.
- Adults often benefit immediately and continue to improve for about 3 months after the initial tuning session.
- Then, although performance continues to improve, improvements are slower. Cochlear implant users' performances may continue to improve for several years.
- Children may improve at a slower pace. A lot of training is needed after implantation to help the child use the new 'hearing' he or she now experiences.
- Most perceive loud, medium and soft sounds. People report that they can perceive different types of sounds, such as footstep, slamming of doors, sounds of engines, ringing of the telephone, barking of dogs, whistling of the tea kettle, rustling of leaves, the sound of a light switch being switched on and off, and so on.
- Many understand speech without lip reading. However, even if this is not possible using the implant helps in lip-reading.
- Many can make telephone calls and understand familiar voices over the telephone. Some good performances can make normal telephone call and even understand an unfamiliar speaker. However, not all people who have implants are enabled to use the phone.
- Many can watch TV more easily, especially when they also see the speaker's face. However, listening to the radio, is often more difficult as there are no visual cues available.
- Some can enjoy music. Some enjoy the sound of certain instruments (piano or guitar, for example) and certain voices. Others do not hear well enough to enjoy music.

Box 29.3: Indications for CI implantation

- Patient must have profound severe hearing loss in both ears
- Patient derives no benefit from the most powerful hearing aid
- Family willing to work towards speech and language skills and therapy
- No medical contraindication to surgery
- Realistic expectation as to the benefits of implantation
- Availability of adequate post surgical aural rehabilitation services (speech language pathologist, deaf educator or auditory verbal therapist)

Complications of cochlear implant: The complications that could arise from cochlear implant surgery include:

1. Injury to the facial nerve
2. Meningitis
3. Leakage of cerebrospinal fluid
4. Perilymph fluid leak from the cochlear
5. Skin infection
6. Tinnitus
7. Taste disturbances
8. Numbness
9. Reparative granuloma
10. Destruction of any residual hearing
11. Device failure. People with cochlear implant may hear sounds differently initially and may loose residual hearing.

Brobby GW, Muller-Myshok B, Horsfman RD. Connexin 26 R 143 Mutation associated with non-syndromic sensori-neural deafness in Africa. *N Engl J Med* 1988;8:548–50.

Downs MP, Sterritt GM. Identification audiometry for neonates: A preliminary report. *J Aud Res* 1964;4:69–80.

Joint Committee on Infant Hearing: Position statement. *Pediatrics* 1982;70:496–7.

Gibbon KP. Cochlear implantation in children Scott Brown. In: Adams DA, Cinnamond MJ (eds). *Scott Brown's otolaryngology.* vol 6. Paediatrics otolaryngology Reed Educational and Professional Publishing Ltd., 1997; 6/11/1–11/4.

Lysons K. *Understanding Hearing loss.* Pennsylvania: Jessica Kingsley Publishers, 1996;108–119.

Magbol M. *Text book of Ear, Nose and Throat Diseases.* 10th edn. New Delhi: Jaypee Brothers Medical Publishers (P) Ltd., 2003;86–98.

Makhdoum MJ, Snik AFM, Broek PVD. Cochlear implantation: a review of the literature and the Nijinegen results. *J Laryn Otology* 1999; III: 1008–1017.

Manson SR. *Diseases of the Ear.* 3rd edn. Edward Arnold 1974;123–70.

Morgan DE, Canalis RF. Auditory screening of infants. *Otolaryn Clin North Am* 1991;24(2):277–84.

Steel KP. New interventions in hearing impairment. *Brit Med J* 2000;320:622–5.

29.3 EXTERNAL OTITIS (OTITIS EXTERNA)

External otitis, also known as swimmer's ear, although it can occur without swimming, is caused most commonly by *P. aeruginosa*, but *S. aureus*, *Enterobacter aerogenes*, *Proteus mirabilis*, *Klebsiella pneumoniae*, streptococci, cogulase-negative staphylococci, diphtheroids, and fungi such as *Candida* and *Aspergillus* also may be isolated. Diseases of the external ear include furunculosis, acute cellulitis, perichondritis, and chondritis, dermatosis (seborrheic, contact, infectious, eczematoid, or neurodermatoid), and herpes virus infection including Ramsay Hunt syndrome, bullous myringitis, exostosis and osteoma. Ramsay Hunt syndrome (herpes zoster oticus) may present with herpes vesicles in the ear canal and on the pinna and with facial paralysis and pain, 8th nerve may be involved.

Clinical manifestations: The predominant symptom is acute ear pain, accentuated by manipulation of the pinna or pressure on the tragus. Itching often is a precursor of pain and usually is characteristic of chronic inflammation of the canal or resolving acute otitis externa. Conductive hearing loss may result from edema of the skin and tympanic membrane (TM), serous or purulent secretions, or the canal of skin thickening associated with chronic external otitis. The signs of acute disease are edema of the ear canal, erythema, and thick, clumpy otorrhea; cerumen usually is white and soft in consistency as opposed to its usual yellow and firmer consistency. Complete otoscopic examination may be delayed until the acute swelling subsides. If the TM can be visualized, it may appear either normal or opaque. TM mobility may be normal or, if thickened, reduced in response to positive and negative pressure. Other physical findings may include palpable and tender lymph nodes in the periauricular region, and erythema and swelling of the pinna and periauricular skin.

Rarely, facial paralysis, other cranial nerve abnormalities, vertigo, and/or sensorineural hearing loss are present, indicating invasive infection of the temporal bone and skull base and the occurrence of *necrotizing (malignant) otitis externa.* This requires immediate culture, intravenous antibiotics, and imaging studies to evaluate the extent of the disease. Surgical intervention to obtain cultures or debride devitalized tissue may be necessary. *P. aeruginosa* is the most common causative organism of necrotizing otitis externa. This disease is rare in children and is seen only in association with immunocompromise or severe malnourishment.

Diagnosis: External otitis externa may be confused with furunculosis, otitis media (OM) and mastoiditis.

Treatment: Topical otic preparations containing neomycin with either colistin or polymyxin and corticosteroids are highly effective in treating most forms of acute external otitis. If canal edema is marked, the patient may need cleaning and possible wick placement. A wick can be inserted into the ear canal and topical antibiotics applied to the wick 3 times a day for 24–48 hr. The wick can be removed after 2–3 days, at which time the edema of the ear canal usually is markedly improved, and the ear canal and TM are better seen. Topical antibiotics are then continued by direct instillation. When the pain is severe, oral analgesics (e.g., ibuprofen, codeine) may be necessary for a few days. Removal of all jewelry is mandatory in the presence of infection.

As the inflammatory process subsides, cleaning the canal with a suction or cotton-tipped applicator to remove the debris enhance the effectiveness of the topical medications. In subacute and chronic infections, periodic cleansing of the canal is essential. In severe, acute external otitis associated with fever and lymphadenitis, oral or parenteral antibiotics may be indicated. An ear canal culture should be done, and empiric antibiotic treatment can then be modified if necessary, based on susceptibility of the organism cultured. A fungal infection of the external auditory canal (otomycosis) is characterized by fluffy white debris, and sometimes with black spores seen; treatment includes cleaning and application of antifungal solutions such as clotrimazole or nystatin.

Prevention: In individuals, who are susceptible to recurrences, especially children who swim preventing external otitis may be necessary. The most effective prophylaxis is instillation of dilute alcohol or acetic acid (2%) immediately after swimming or bathing. During an acute episode of otitis externa, patients should not swim and the ears should be protected from excessive water during bathing.

29.4 OTITIS MEDIA

Otitis media (OM) is a common condition and has two main components: acute infection, which is termed *suppurative or acute otitis media* (AOM); and inflammation accompanied by effusion, termed nonsuppurative or secretory otitis media, or otitis media with effusion (OME). Middle-ear-effusion (MEE) is a feature of both AOM and OME. MEE results in the conductive hearing loss associated with OM. Hearing losses of 21–30 dB HL are usual.

Epidemiology: Factors which affect the occurrence of OM include age, gender, race, genetic background, socioeconomic status, type of milk (breastfeed) or formula used in infant feeding, tobacco smoke exposure, degree of exposure to other children, presence or absence of respiratory allergy, season of the year, congenital anomalies and pneumococcal vaccination status.

Etiology
Acute otitis media (AOM): Pathogenic bacteria are isolated in 65–75% cases and include: *S. pneumoniae* (40%); nontypable *Haemophilus influenzae* (25–30%); *Moraxella catarrhalis* (10–15%); and other pathogens-group A streptococcus, *Staphylococcus aureus*, and gram-negative organisms (5%). Respiratory viruses may be found in middle-ear exudates either alone or, more commonly, in association with pathogenic bacteria, includes rhinovirus and respiratory syncytial

virus (RSV). AOM is a known complication of bronchiolitis.

Otitis media with effusion (OME): The pathogens typically found in AOM can be recovered in approximately in 30% of children with OME.

Clinical manifestations: Ear pain, often manifested by irritability, a change in sleeping or eating habits, and, occasionally, holding or tugging at the ear. Fever also may be present and, rarely, rupture of the tympanic membrane with purulent otorrhea. Systemic symptoms and symptoms associated with upper respiratory tract infections also occur. Older children may complain of mild discomfort or a sense of fullness in the ear.

Conjunctivitis otitis media syndrome: Simultaneous appearance of purulent and erythematous conjunctivitis with OM in most children is due to non-typable *Haemophilus influenzae*. The disease often is present in multiple family members and affects young children and infants.

Diagnosis: The diagnosis of OM is based on all the following findings:
1. Recent and usually acute onset of illness
2. Presence of MEE; and
3. Signs and symptoms of middle-ear inflammation, including erythema of the tympanic membrane or otalgia.

A diagnosis of AOM is established, when, in addition to having MEE, a child gives evidence of recent ear pain, or the tympanic membrane shows marked redness or distinct fullness or bulging. The diagnosis between AOM and OME is important. In OME, bulging of the tympanic membrane is absent or slight, or the membrane may be retracted; erythema also is absent or slight, but may increase with crying or with superficial trauma to the external auditory canal incurred in clearing the canal of cerumen. In children with MEE but without tympanic membrane fullness or bulging, the presence of unequivocal ear pain usually is indicative of AOM.

Treatment

Management of acute otitis media: Prompt and adequate antimicrobial treatment may prevent the development of suppurative complications. Patient should be provided with adequate analgesic medications—acetaminophen or ibuprofen-during period of observation. Topical otic agents (containing benzocaine and lignocaine preparation) also may be effective for pain relief. The duration of treatment of AOM is 10 days. Treatment for >10 days may be required for children who are very young or are having severe episodes or whose previous experience with OM has been problematic. Follow-up of cases is essential to assess the outcome of treatment and to differentiate between inadequate response to treatment and early recurrence. Follow-up within 2 wk is appropriate for the infant or young child who apparently has been having frequent recurrences. In the child with only a sporadic episode of AOM and prompt symptomatic treatment, follow-up 1 mo after initial examination is necessary; in older children, no follow-up may be necessary.

Second-line treatment: When treatment of AOM with a first-line antimicrobial drug has proven inadequate, a number of second-line alternatives are available. Drugs chosen for second-line treatment should be effective against β-lactamase-producing strains of *H. influenzae* and *M. catarrhalis* and against susceptible and most nonsusceptible strains of *S. pneumoniae*. Only 3 drugs have been shown to meet the requirement: amoxicillin-clavulanate, cefuroxime axetil, and intramuscular ceftriaxone. Clindamycin is active against most strains of *S. pneumoniae*, including resistant strains, but is not active against *H. influenzae* and *M. catarrhalis*. It should, therefore, be reserved for patients known to have infection caused by penicillin—nonsusceptible *S. pneumoniae*.

Myringotomy and tympanocentesis: Indications for myringotomy in children with AOM include severe, refractory pain; hyperpyrexia; complications of AOM such as facial paralysis, mastoiditis, labyrinthitis, or central nervous system infection; and immunologic compromise. Myringotomy should be considered as third-line therapy in patients who have failed 2 courses of antibiotics for an episode of AOM. In children with AOM in whom second-line treatment has been unsatisfactory, either diagnostic tympanocetesis or myringotomy is indicated to enable identification of the offending organism and its sensitivity profile.

Management of Otitis Media with Effusion (OME)

To determine the course of an episode of OME, and to distinguish between persistence and recurrence, examination should be conducted monthly until resolution, and hearing should be assessed if effusion has been present for >3 mo. Most cases of OME resolve without treatment within 3 mo. Antimicrobials have definite but limited efficacy in resolving OME, presumably because they help eradicate nasopharyngeal infection or inapparent middle-ear infection, or both. Treatment with antimicrobials should be limited to cases in which there is evidence of associated bacterial upper respiratory tract infection or untreated middle ear infection. For this purpose, the most broadly effective drug available should be used, as recommended for AOM.

When OME persists despite an ample period of watchful waiting, usually 3–6 mo or perhaps longer in children with unilateral effusion, myringotomy alone, without tympanostomy tube insertion, permits evacuation of middle-ear effusion and sometimes is not effective; often, because the incision heals before the middle ear mucosa returns to normal, the effusion soon reaccumulates. However, placement of tympanostomy tubes usually is quite effective in providing resolution of OME in children.

Prevention: The general measures to prevent OM consist of breast-milk feeding, avoidance, insofar as possible, of exposure to individuals with respiratory infection; avoidance of a environmental tobacco smoke; and pneumococcal vaccination (heptavalent pneumococcal conjugate vaccine).

29.5 INNER EAR AND DISEASES OF THE BONY LABYRINTH

The inner ear and diseases of the bony labyrinth include conductive and sensorineural hearing loss (SNHL) as well as vestibular dysfunction. Genetic factors may affect the anatomy and function of the inner ear. Infectious agents may cause abnormal function, most commonly as sequelae of congenital infection or bacterial meningitis. Tumors of the ear and temporal bone produce hearing loss.

Sensorineural hearing loss (SNHL): Viruses causing sensorineural hearing loss (SNHL) are congenital cytomegalovirus (CMV), congenital rubella as well as acquired measles, mumps, rubella, parvovirus B19. Toxoplasmosis may cause congenital SNHL. SNHL has been reported in children suffering bacterial meningitis (*Haemophilus influenzae* type b, *Streptococcus pneumoniae* and *Neisseria meningitidis*). Congenital syphilis may cause SNHL in affected children. When the condition is identified, treatment with antibiotics and corticosteroids may improve the hearing loss.

Other diseases of the inner ear include labyrinthitis, otosclerosis, osteogenesis imperfecta, and osteopetrosis.

Tumors of the ear and temporal bone: Tumors include osteomas and fibrous dysplasia, eosinophilic granuloma, rhabdomyosarcoma, non-Hodgkin lymphoma and leukemia. Primary neoplasms of the middle ear, such as adenoid cystic carcinoma, adenocarcinoma, and squamous cell carcinoma are uncommon in children.

American Academy of Family Physicians; American Academy of Otolaryngology-Head and Neck Surgery; American Academy of Pediatrics Subcommittee on Otitis Media With Effusion: Otitis media with effusion. *Pediatrics* 2004;113:1412–29.

American Academy of Pediatrics Subcommittee on Management of Acute Otitis Media: Diagnosis and management of acute otitis media. *Pediatrics* 2004;113:1451–65.

Bodor FF. Systemic antibiotics for treatment of the conjunctivitis-otitis-media syndrome. *Pediatr Infect Dis J* 1989; 8:287–90.

Haddad J Jr. External otitis (Otitis externa). In: Kliegman RM, Behrman RE, Jenson HB, Stanton BF (eds). *Nelson Textbook of Pediatrics.* 18th edn. Vol 2. Philadelphia: Saunders, 2007; 2629–32.

Haddad J Jr. The inner ear and diseases of the bony labyrinth. In: Kliegman RM, Behrman RE, Jenson HB, Stanton BF (eds). *Nelson Textbook of Pediatrics.* 18th edn. Vol 2. Philadelphia: Saunders, 2007;2646–7.

Kerschner JE. Otitis media. In: Kliegman RM, Behrman RE, Jenson HB, Stanton BF (eds). *Nelson Textbook of Pediatrics.* 18th edn. Vol 2. Philadelphia: Saunders, 2007;2632–46.

29.6 MASTOID DISEASE IN CHILDREN

The term " Mastoiditis" includes any inflammatory processes of the mastoid air cells of the temporal bone. Since mastoid is a part of middle ear cleft, virtually every child or adult with acute otitis media (AOM) or chronic middle ear inflammatory disease has mastoiditis. In most cases, the symptomatology of the middle ear disease predominates (e.g. fever, pain, conductive hearing loss), and the disease within the mastoid is overlooked.

Epidemiology: Actual incidence is unknown. Acute mastoiditis is rarely seen today. The incidence has dropped significantly with the advent of antibiotics.

Bacteriolgy: The most common etiologic agent causing surgical mastoiditis is *Streptococcus pneumoniae* followed by *Haemophilus influenzae* and group A *Streptococcus pyogenes* (GAS). More than half of the *S. pneumoniae* recovered are of serotype 19, followed by serotypes 23 and 3. Other etiologic organisms include coagulase-positive staphylococci, *Pseudomonas* species, *S. aureus. E. coli*, and *Proteus.*

Pathophysiology: As with most infectious processes, one must consider host and microbial factors when evaluating surgical mastoiditis. Host factors include mucosal immunology, temporal bone anatomy, and systemic immunity. Microbial factors include protective coating, antimicrobial resistance, and ability to penetrate local tissue or vessels (i.e. invasive strains).

Evaluation of the patient: Evaluation of the patient with acute mastoiditis begins with the history and physical examination. The majority of the diagnosis is based on clinical judgment. Laboratory evaluation reveals a leukocytosis and elevated erythrocyte sedimentation rate (ESR). Mastoid radiographs are characteristic and will show cloudiness of the mastoid air cells associated with fuzziness of the bony partitions. Although helpful in the diagnosis, most agree that mastoid X-rays are not helpful in determining whether mastoid surgery is necessary. CT scan of the temporal bones is helpful in evaluation of concomitant intracranial complications as well as discerning any anatomical variations preoperatively. Chest x-ray is useful to rule out infiltrates in patients with septicemia and possible embolic phenomena secondary to lateral sinus thrombosis.

Disease progression: Mastoiditis progresses in 5 stages and may be arrested at any point:

1. Hyperemia of the mucosal lining of the mastoid air cells
2. Transudation and exudation of fluid and/or pus within the cells
3. Necrosis of bone by loss of vascularity of the septa
4. Cell wall loss with coalescence into abscess cavities
5. Extension of inflammatory process to contiguous areas

Clinical features: The signs and symptoms of acute mastoiditis mimic severe acute suppurative otitis media; the disease entities are distinguished by the duration of symptoms. When the symptoms persist or recur after several weeks of acute otitis media, they point toward development of a coalescent process within the mastoid. The most common symptoms are otorrhea and otalgia. Subperiosteal abscess is noted by a fluctuant mass with overlying edema and erythema. This process produces displacement of the ear thickening of the periosteum overlying the bone in the area of the antrum. Neurologic changes may be seen with intracranial complications. Perforation of the mastoid tip along the medial aspect of the SCM through the incisura mastoidea produces a deep abscess in the neck known as a Bezold's abscess.

Signs: Otitis media is revealed on otoscopy, often with one of the following additional features:

1. Sagging of the posterosuperior canal wall (possibly a sign of ASM)
2. The tympanic membrane can simply appear normal, thickened or can demonstrate a small central perforation; nipple like protrusion of the middle ear mucosa through a small central perforation of the tympanic membrane, usually oozing pus.

Findings consistent with complications are extension beyond the mastoid process and its covering periosteum or another intratemporal complication such as facial palsy. Tenderness and inflammation over the mastoid process is the most consistent sign of ASM. Periosteal thickening requires comparison to the other side, and some lateral displacement of the auricle may be present. Subperiosteal abscess displaces the auricle

---

Box 29.4: Complications of mastoiditis

1. Posterior extension to the sigmoid sinus (causing thrombosis)
2. Posterior extension to the occipital bone to create an osteomyelitis of calvarium
3. Superior extension to posterior cranial fossa, subdural space, and meninges
4. Anterior extension to the zygomatic root
5. Anterior extension into posterior canal wall forming Luc's abscess
6. Antero-inferior extension into posterior belly of digastric—Citelli's abscess
7. Lateral extension to form a subperiosteal abscess
8. Inferior extension to form a Bezold abscess
9. Medial extension to the petrous apex
10. Intratemporal involvement of facial nerve and/or labyrinth

---

laterally and obliterates the postauricular skin crease. If the crease remains, the process is lateral to the periosteum. *Complications* of mastoiditis are further extensions of the infectious process within or beyond the mastoid itself (Box 29.4).

Investigations: A culture from the middle ear fluid should be obtained prior to beginning antimicrobial therapy to find out the cusative micro-organism. While this is facilitated with the use of an operating microscope and specifically designed suction traps, an otoscope, spinal needle, and syringe are equally efficient in obtaining specimens from the middle ear. Sterilize the canal with an antiseptic, and, with the child restrained, aspirate from the anterior half of the tympanic membrane. CBC and sedimentation rate are obtained for baseline studies used to evaluate efficacy of therapy. Obtain and evaluate spinal fluid if any suggestion exists of intracranial extension of the process.

Imaging studies: CT scanning of the temporal bone, the standard for evaluation of mastoiditis shows:

1. Clouding or haziness of the mastoid air cells and middle ear by inflammatory swelling of mucosa and by collection of fluid
2. Loss of sharpness or visibility of mastoid cell walls due to demineralization, atrophy, or necrosis of bony septa
3. Haziness or distortion of mastoid outline, possibly with visible defects of the tegmen or mastoid cortex
4. Enhancement of areas of abscess formation
5. Elevation of periosteum of mastoid process or posterior cranial fossa; and
6. Osteoblastic activity in chronic mastoiditis. MRI is not typically the radiographic study of choice; however, it is helpful in showing inflammatory processes and differentiating certain tumors. Do not

use MRI as a method of evaluating the mastoid, although it is the standard for evaluation of contiguous soft tissue, particularly the intracranial structures. Plain radiographs of the mastoids demonstrate clouding of the air cells with bone destruction in ASM, but lack the sensitivity to differentiate the stages of the disease and fail to show the petrous apex in any great detail.

Other tests: Audiometry is seldom appropriate or useful in children with ASM, but it must be performed after convalescence from the acute phase and in children with chronic mastoiditis. In the at-risk population (children <2 yr), thresholds for air and bone conduction under headphones are obtained only rarely.

Treatment

Medical therapy: Antibiotics are the principal medications used in ASM. Culture results and the sensitivity of the organism ultimately govern selection of medications. Until microbiology information is available, the following principles guide the selection:

1. The antimicrobial must be appropriate to cover the invasive strains of bacteria most common for AOM
2. The selected antibiotic should cross the blood–brain barrier, and
3. The selected therapeutic spectrum should include consideration of those MDRSP prevalent in the individual community.

Specific microbiologic diagnoses should be treated with appropriate antibiotics. Antibiotic therapy is guided by the patients' history. If the history is otherwise uncomplicated by ear disease or protracted episode of otitis media, the infecting organism is probably *S. pneumoniae* or *S. pyogenes* which is best treated by ampicillin. If the patient has a protracted course of otitis media, then coverage for *S. aureus* and gram negative organisms is necessary with a penicillinase resistant penicillin and an aminoglycoside or single antibiotic coverage with a cephalosporin. Anaerobic coverage should be added to the above therapy when suspected. If open mastoid surgery is not undertaken, use of single, high-dose intravenous steroids is warranted to decrease mucosal swelling and to promote natural drainage through the aditus and antrum into the middle ear. Other medications used include analgesics, antipyretics, and topical antibiotic/steroid combinations. After placement of a tympanostomy tube with or without mastoidectomy, a pH-balanced solution or suspension of an antibiotic and steroid is useful to decrease mucosal swelling and to deliver topical antibiotics to the middle ear and mastoid. Continue the drops until otorrhea ceases and the view through the tube shows healing mucosa

without swelling or obstruction. Multiple combinations are available, the best being those thin enough to rub through the tube into the middle ear. Early consultation with an otolaryngologist is appropriate and necessary if the condition does not improve and patient requires tympanocentesis or surgical intervention.

Surgical therapy: Surgical therapy confined to the ear takes one of the following forms:

1. Myringotomy/tympanocentesis
2. Tympanostomy tube placement
3. Mastoidectomy.

Indications for surgery include acute mastoiditis with subperiosteal abscess, acute mastoiditis not responsive after 24 to 48 hours of intravenous antibiotics and myringotomy, and intracranial complications with evidence of mastoid coalescence.

Medicolegal pitfalls relate almost entirely either delay of diagnosis or iatrogenic injury during therapy. A high index of suspicion and judicious use of diagnostic modalities and close follow-up care are recommended to make a diagnosis in a timely manner. Although facial nerve monitoring is a useful adjunct, nothing substitutes for experience and attention to detail when preserving the facial nerve. Experienced otologists are unlikely to injure the ossicular chain during mastoid surgery.

Prognosis: Patients with ASM to recover completely provided the facial nerve, vestibule, or intracranial structures are not involved. Cosmetic deformity of the operated ear usually can be prevented with judicious placement of the incision and the development of flaps to pull the ears posteriorly when replaced. Conductive hearing loss should resolve provided the ossicular chain remains intact.

Gupta P, Varshney S, Chaterjee B, Saxena RK. Mastoid abscess caused by Nocardia in a child with visceral Leishmaniasis. *Tropical Doctor* 2005;35:45–46.

Ginsburg CM, Rudoy R, Nelson JD. Acute mastoiditis in infants and children. *Clin Pediatr* 1980;19:549–53.

Kvestad E, Kvaerner KJ, Mair IW: Acute mastoiditis: predictors for surgery. *Int J Pediatr Otorhinolaryngol* 2000 Apr 15;52(2):149–55.

Varshney S, The charge of Chronic Ear Discharge. *Physician's Digest* 1998;6:11–19.

Varshney S, Gupta P. Bacteriological study of CSOM. *Indian Journal of Otology* 1999;5:87–91.

Varshney S. Mastoid Disease in Children. In: Mathur GP, Mathur Sarla (eds). *Current Trends in Pediatrics*. Vol 2. Delhi: Academa Publishers, 2006;275–83.

29.7 NOSE AND DISORDERS OF NOSE

The nose is the main gate to the respiratory system, body's system for breathing. After the air is inhaled through nostrils, the air enters the nasal passages and travels into nasal cavity. The air then passes down the back of the throat into the trachea on its way to the lungs. Nose is also a two-way passage. When you exhale the old air from the lungs, the nose is the main way for the air to leave the body. But nose is more than a passage-way for air. The nose also warms, moistens (humidification), and filters the inspired air before it goes to the lungs. Nose lets you smell and you cannot taste anything without some help from the nose. The ability to smell and taste go together because odors from foods allow us to taste more fully. Nose is an organ to beautify face. Because of the special nature of the blood supply to the human nose and surrounding area, it is possible for retrograde infections from the nasal area to spread to the brain. For this reason, the area from the corners of the mouth to the bridge of the nose, including the nose and maxilla, is known as the *dangerous area of the face*.

Disorders of the Nose

1. *Choanal atresia:* This is the most common congenital anomaly of the nose and is approximately present in 1/7,000 live births. It consists of a unilateral or bilateral bony (90%) or membranous (10%) septum between the nose and the pharynx; most cases are a combination of bony and membranous atresia. Nearly 50% of affected infants have other congenital abnormalities, more frequently in bilateral cases. The CHARGE syndrome—Coloboma; *H*eart disease; *A*tresia choanae; *R*etarded growth and development or CNS anomalies or both; *G*enital anomalies or hypogonadism or both; and *E*ar anomalies or deafness or both—is one of the more common anomalies associated with choanal atresia.

Diagnosis: When unilateral often the diagnosis is suggested by nasal discharge or persistent nasal obstruction after first respiratory infection. Infants with bilateral choanal atresia, who have difficulty with mouth breathing make vigorous attempts to inspire, often suck in their lips, and develop cyanosis. Diagnosis is established by the inability to pass a firm catheter through each nostril 3–4 cm into the nasopharynx. The atretic plate may be seen directly with fiberoptic rhinoscopy. The anatomy is best evaluated by using high-resolution CT.

Treatment: Initially, this consists of prompt placement of an oral airway, maintaining the mouth in an open position, or intubation. Once an oral airway is established, the infant can be fed by gavage until breathing and eating without the assisted airway is possible. In bilateral cases, intubation or tracheotomy may be indicated. If the child is free of other serious medical problems, operative intervention is considered in neonate, and tracheotomy should be considered in bilateral atresia with potentially life threatening problems and in whom early repair may not be appropriate or feasible. Transnasal repair is now more common. Stents are usually left in place for weeks after repair to prevent closure or stenosis. Operative correction of unilateral obstruction may be deferred for several years. In both unilateral and bilateral cases, re-stenosis necessitating dilation or reoperation or both, is common. Mitomycin-C has been used to help prevent the development of granulation tissue and stenosis.

2. *Congenital defects of the nasal septum:* Congenital defects of the nasal septum such as perforation or deviation are rare. Perforation is more commonly acquired after birth secondary to infection, such as syphilis, tuberculosis or trauma (e.g., continuous positive airway pressure cannula). Trauma from delivery is the most common cause of septal deviation noted at birth. When recognized early, it may be corrected with immediate realignment using blunt probes, cotton applicators, and topical anesthesia.

3. *Pyriform aperture stenosis* is a bony abnormality of the anterior nasal aperture. These infants present with severe nasal obstruction at birth or shortly thereafter. Diagnosis is made by CT of the nose; surgical repair by means of an anterior, sublabial approach may be needed if the child cannot feed or breathe without difficulty.

4. *Nasal masses:* Congenital midline nasal masses include dermoids, gliomas, and encephaloceles in descending order of frequency. They present intranasally or extranasally and may have intracranial connections. Other nasal masses include hemangiomas, congenital nasolacrimal duct obstruction, nasal polyps, tumors such as rhabdomyosarcoma.

5. *Nasal sinuses:* Poor development of paranasal sinuses and a narrow nasal airway are associated with recurrent or chronic upper airway infection in Down syndrome.

6. *Foreign body:* Food, crayons, small toys, erasers, paper wads, beads, beans, stones, pieces of sponge, and other foreign bodies are frequently introduced into the nose of children. Initial symptoms are local obstruction, sneezing, relatively mild discomfort, and, rarely pain. Irritation results in mucosal swelling, and, because some foreign bodies are hygroscopic and increase in size as water is absorbed, signs of local obstruction and discomfort may increase with time. Infection usually follows and gives rise to a purulent, malodorous, or bloody

discharge. The patient may also present with a generalized body odor known as bromhidrosis. Disk batteries are dangerous when placed in the nose; they leach base, which causes pain and local tissue destruction within a few hours. Tetanus may rarely occur in nonimmunized children. Toxic shock syndrome is also rare and most commonly occurs from nasal surgical packing.

Diagnosis: Unilateral nasal discharge and obstruction should suggest the presence of a foreign body, which can often be seen on examination with a nasal speculum. When of long standing, a foreign body may become embedded in granulation tissue or mucosa and appear as a nasal mass. A lateral skull radiograph assists in diagnosis if the foreign body is metallic or radiopaque.

Treatment: The foreign body should be carried out promptly to minimize the danger of aspiration and to prevent local tissue necrosis. This can usually be performed with topical anesthesia, using either forceps or nasal suction. If there is marked swelling, bleeding, or tissue overgrowth, general anesthesia may be needed to remove the object. Infection usually clears promptly after the removal of the object, and generally no further therapy is necessary.

7. *Epistaxis:* Epistaxis is one of the most frequent causes of bleeding. Nosebleeds are rare in infancy, common in childhood; their incidence decreases after puberty. In the majority of the cases, bleeding is in small quantities and self-limited, but sometimes it can be very intense and life threatening. That's why epistaxis should never be treated as a harmless event either from the diagnostic or therapeutic point of view. The blood supply of the nasal cavity is provided by both the internal and external carotid artery and their accompanying veins. Bleeding from Kiesselbach's plexus, a vascular plexus on the anterior nasal septum, is by far, the most common type of epistaxis. The mucosa in this area is very fragile and is tightly adherent to the underlying cartilage and thus offers a little resistance to mechanical or functional stress. Little's area is situated in the anterior inferior part of nasal septum, just above the vestibule. Four arteries—anterior ethmoidal, septal branch of superior labial, septal branch of sphenopalatine and the greater palatine, anastomose here to form a vascular plexus called *"Kiesselbach's plexus"*. This area is exposed to the drying effect of inspiratory current and to finger-nail trauma, and is the commonest site for epistaxis in children and young adults.

Etiology: The causes of epistaxis are divided into local, general and idiopathic.

1. *Local causes:* Nose:
   i. Nasal trauma (nose picking, foreign bodies, forceful nose blowing, violent sneeze, injuries of nose, fractures of middle third of face and base of skull)
   ii. Rhinitis
   iii. Maggots
   iv. Drying of the nasal mucosa from low humidity
   v. Deviation of nasal septum
   vi. Bleeding polyp of the septum
   vii. Tumors, particularly malignant tumor of the nose or paranasal sinuses

Nasopharynx:
   i. Adenoiditis
   ii. Tumors of the nasopharynx (juvenile angiofibroma, malignant tumors)

2. *General causes:*
   i. Cardiovascular system (hypertension, mitral stenosis)
   ii. Blood diseases (leukemia)
   iii. Bleeding disorders [thrombocytopenic purpura, idiopathic thrombocytopenic purpura (ITP)]
   iv. Coagulation disorders (hemophilia, over dosage with anticoagulants, deficiency of vitamin K)
   v. Endocrine causes (epistaxis during pregnancy, and pheochromocytoma which causes hypertensive crisis due to circulating catecholamine)
   vi. Hereditary hemorrhagic telangiectasia with typical mucosa lesions—Osler-Weber-Rendu syndrome - which causes recurrent mild to modest, and often multifocal bleeding

3. *Idiopathic:* Many times the cause of epistaxis can not be ascertained, such cases are included in the idiopathic group.

Sites of epistaxis: There are six sites from where bleeding takes place.

1. Little's area. In 90% cases of epistaxis bleeding occurs from the Little's area.
2. Above the level of middle turbinate. Bleeding from above the middle turbinate and corresponding area on the septum is often from the anterior and posterior ethmoidal vessels (internal carotid system).
3. Below the level of middle turbinate. Bleeding from the branches of sphenopalatine artery.
4. Posterior part of nasal cavity. Here blood flows directly into the pharynx.
5. Diffuse. Bleeding occurs both from septum and lateral nasal wall. This is generally seen in general systemic disorders.
6. Nasopharynx.

Classification of epistaxis: Epistaxis is classified on the basis of blood flow into anterior or posterior epistaxis. *Anterior epistaxis:* The blood flows out from the front of the nose with the patient in sitting position. *Posterior epistaxis:* The blood mainly flows back into the throat. The patient may swallow it and later, have a "coffee colored" vomitus. This may be erroneously diagnosed as hematemesis.

Diagnostic steps: In order to correctly diagnosing a case of epistaxis regarding the location and cause, a detailed history, physical examination, laboratory tests and radiologic examination is required. Profuse unilateral epistaxis associated with a nasal mass in an adolescent boy near puberty may signal a juvenile nasopharyngeal angiofibroma. This unusual tumor has also been reported in a 2 yr old and in 30–40 yr old, but the incidence peaks in adolescence and preadolescent boys. CT with contrast medium enhancement and MRI are part of the initial evaluation; arteriography, embolization, and extensive surgery may be needed.

- History—In this case ask for previous bleeding, hypertension, hepatic diseases, use of anti-coagulants, nasal trauma, family history of bleeding, etc.
- Localize the source of the bleedings and determine its cause.
- Measurement of the blood pressure.
- Laboratory tests—platelet count, bleeding time (BT), activated partial thromboplastin time (APTT), prothrombin time (PT), coagulation time (CT).
- Radiographs of the skull, nose and sinuses and possibly tomograms.
- Exclude generalized causes.

Differential diagnosis: It includes bleeding which doesn't arise in the nose but in which the blood escapes through the nose, for instance, hemoptysis, bleeding esophageal varices, bleeding due to injury to the vessel around the base of the skull escaping via the sphenoid sinus or the eustachian tube.

Treatment: The treatment of a case of epistaxis depends on the location and cause. In the majority of the cases, bleeding is in small quantities and self-limited, but sometimes it can be very intense and life threatening. Surgical intervention is needed in patients with juvenile nasopharyngeal angiofibroma and uncontrolled bleeding from the internal maxillary artery or other vessels that can cause bleeding in the posterior nasal cavity.

First aid: Most of the time, bleeding occurs from Little's area and can be easily controlled by pinching the nose with thumb and index finger for about 5 minutes. This compresses the vessels of the Little's area. Cold compresses should be applied to the nose to cause reflex vasoconstriction.

General symptomatic treatment includes:
- Calming the patient (if necessary with medication).
- The patient should sit with the upper part of the body tilted forward and the mouth open so that he can spit out the blood and don't have to swallow it.
- Cold compresses are applied to the nape of the neck and also to the dorsum of the nose.
- Keep check on pulse, blood pressure (BP), and respiration.
- Lowering of blood pressure in hypertension.
- Discontinuation of anticoagulants.
- Antibiotics may be given to prevent sinusitis, if pack is to be kept beyond 24 hours.
- Intermittent oxygen may be required in-patients with bilateral packs because of increased pulmonary resistance from nasopulmonary reflex.
- Administration of fluid expanders in severe bleeding; blood transfusion may be required.
- Investigate and treat the patient for any underlying local or general cause.

Local measures required to control bleeding include:
- Digital compression for several minutes.
- Those that continue to bleed after 3 or 4 minutes can be controlled by one of the two approaches. The easiest is applying pressure to the bleeding site with anterior nasal packing. A second approach is to stop the bleeding with vasoconstrictors such as topical oxymetazoline hydrochloride 0.1% (Nasivion), xylometazoline hydrochloride 0.1% (Otrivin) or epinephrine 1:100,000, and then to cauterize the bleeding site.
- Cautery of the hemorrhagic point. When visible the bleeding site may be cauterized with silver nitrate or electrocautery.
- Anterior nasal packing: Sometimes it is required to achieve hemostasis in more intense bleeding.
- Posterior nasal packing: It is used when the bleeding is intense and from the posterior part of nasal cavity. When we use nasal packing, we should use antibiotics to avoid sinuses infection.
- Vascular ligation: This procedure is used for uncontrolled life-threatening epistaxis if the methods described before have not been effective.
- After control of epistaxis: The patient is advised to avoid vigorous exercise for several days. Avoidance of hot or spicy food and tobacco is also advisable as they may cause vasodilatation. Avoiding nasal trauma, including digital self-trauma is an obvious necessity.

Prevention: Children should be discouraged not to do nose picking. Proper humidification during dry weather of the bedroom helps to prevent many nosebleeds. Prompt attention to nasal infections and allergies is beneficial to nasal hygiene. Prompt cessation of nasal steroid sprays prevents ongoing bleeding.

8. *Nasal polyps:* Nasal polyps are benign peduncu-lated tumors formed from edematous, usually chronically inflamed nasal mucosa. They commonly originate from the ethmoidal sinus and present in the middle meatus, and occasionally, within the maxillary antrum and extend to the nasopharynx (antrochoanal polyp). Large or multiple polyps may completely obstruct the nasal passage. The polyps originating from the ethmoidal sinus are usually smaller and multiple, as compared with the large and usually single antral choanal polyp. Nasal polyposis is associated with cystic fibrosis (commonest cause especially in children less than 12 yr), chronic sinusitis, and allergic sinusitis.

Diagnosis: Obstruction of nasal passages is prominent, associated with hyponasal speech and mouth breathing. Profuse mucoid or mucopurulent rhinorrhea may also be present. An examination of the nasal passages shows glistening, gray, grape-like masses squeezed between the nasal turbinates and the septum. Ethmoidal polyps can be readily distinguished from the well-vascularized turbinate tissue, which pink or red; antrochoanal polyps may have a more fleshy appearance. Prolonged presence of ethmoidal polyps in a child may widen the bridge of the nose and erode adjacent osseous structures.

Treatment: Polyps should be removed surgically if complete obstruction, uncontrolled rhinorrhea or deformity of the nose appears. Local or systemic decongestants are not usually effective in shrinking the polyps, although they may provide symptomatic relief from the associated mucosal edema. Intranasal steroid sprays, and sometimes systemic steroids, may provide some shrinkage of nasal polyps with symptomatic relief and is useful in children with cystic fibrosis.

9. *Rhinosinusitis (Common cold):* The common cold is a viral disease in which the symptoms of rhinorrhea and nasal obstruction are prominent and systemic symptoms such as myalgia and fever are absent or mild and there is also involvement of sinus mucosa and is more correctly termed rhinosinusitis. Colds occur year round, but the incidence is greatest in April–May and August–October. The most common pathogens associated with the common cold are the rhinoviruses (frequent) and coronaviruses (occasional). But the agents primarily associated with other clinical syndromes that also cause common cold symptoms include respiratory syncytial virus (RSV), influenza viruses, parainfluenza viruses, adenoviruses, and enteroviruses.

The most common complication of rhinosinusitis (common cold) is otitis media; other complications are: sinusitis and exacerbation of asthma.

Diagnosis: The onset of common cold symptoms such as rhinorrhea and nasal obstruction typically occurs 1–3 days after viral infection. The physical findings of the rhinosinusitis (common cold) are limited to the upper respiratory tract. The usual common cold symptoms persist about a week, but in approximately 10% cases it may last for 2 weeks. The differential diagnosis of common cold includes noninfectious disorders and other upper respiratory infections such as allergic rhinitis, foreign body, sinusitis, streptococcal nasopharyngitis, pertussis, and congenital syphilis.

A nasal smear for eosinophils may be useful if allergic rhinitis is suspected. A predominance of polymorphonuclear leukocytes in the nasal secretions is characteristic of uncomplicated rhinosinusitis and does not indicate bacterial superinfection. Bacterial cultures or antigen detection are useful only when group A *Streptococcus, Bordetella pertussis*, or nasal diphtheria is suspected. The viral pathogens associated with the common cold may be detected by culture, antigen detection, or serologic methods; but are indicated only when treatment with an antiviral agent is contemplated and not generally for making a specific etiologic diagnosis.

Treatment: The management of common cold consists primarily of symptomatic treatment. Nasal obstruction can be relieved by topical adrenergic agents (nasal decongestants), such as xylometazoline, oxymeta-zoline, or phenyephrine as either intranasal drops or nasal spray. Prolonged use of topical adrenergic agents should be avoided to prevent the development of *rhinitis medicamentosa*, an apparent rebound effect that causes the sensation of nasal obstruction when the drug is discontinued. Rhinorrhea may be treated with the first degree antihistamines and ipratropium bromide (a topical anticholinergic agent). The side effect of antihistamine is sedation and that of ipratropium bromide are nasal irritation and bleeding. Sore throat is generally not severe, but if associated with myalgia or headache, paracetamol is indicated. Aspirin should not be given because of the risk of Reye syndrome in children. For fever which is infrequently associated with uncomplicated rhinosinusitis, antipyretic is generally not indicated. Cough suppression is generally not necessary, but in some patients appears to be due to upper respiratory tract irritation associated with postnasal drip; in these patients treatment with first degree antihistaminic may be helpful. In other patients, cough may be a result of virus-induced reactive airway disease. These patients have cough that persists for days to weeks after the acute illness and may benefit from bronchodilator therapy.

At present many common cold remedies such as Vitamin-C, zinc, guaifenesin, codeine, dextromethorphan hydrobromide, and inhalation of warm, humidified air have all been found to be ineffective treatments than placebo for the symptomatic treatment of colds.

10. *Sinusitis:* Sinusitis is a common illness of childhood and adolescence, which is associated with significant morbidity and may be with serious complications. Sinusitis is acute and chronic type. Acute sinusitis is due to viral and bacterial infections. The common cold produces a viral, self-limited rhinosinusitis; one-half to 2% of viral upper respiratory tract infections are complicated by acute bacterial sinusitis in children and adolescents. Some children with the underlying predisposing conditions may have chronic sinus disease. The common bacterial pathogens causing acute bacterial sinusitis in children and adolescents include *Streptococcal pneumoniae*, *Haemophilus influenzae* and *Moraxella catarrhalis*. *Staphylococcus aureus*, other streptococci, and anaerobes are uncommon causes of acute bacterial sinusitis. Predisposing conditions include viral upper respiratory tract infections, allergic rhinitis, and cigarette smoke exposure. Children with immune deficiencies, cystic fibrosis, ciliary dysfunction, abnormalities of phagocytic function, gastroesophageal reflux, anatomic defects (e.g. cleft palate), nasal polyps, and nasal foreign bodies (including nasogastric tubes) may develop chronic sinus disease.

Because of the close proximity of the paranasal sinuses to the brain and eyes, serious orbital and/or intracranial complications may result from acute bacterial sinusitis and progress rapidly. Orbital complications include periorbital cellulitis and orbital cellulitis. Intracranial complications may include meningitis, cavernous sinus thrombosis, subdural empyema, epidural abscess and brain abscess. Other complications include osteomyelitis of the frontal bone (Pott puffy tumor), and mucoceles.

The paranasal sinuses continue to develop throughout childhood. Both the ethmoidal and maxillary sinuses are present at birth, but only the ethmoidal sinuses are pneumatized. The maxillary sinuses are not pneumatized until 4 yr of age. The sphenoidal sinuses are present by 5 yr of age, whereas the frontal sinuses begin development at the age of 7 to 8 yr and are not completely developed until adolescence. The ostea draining the sinuses are narrows (1–3 mm) and drain into the ostiomeatal complex in the middle meatus. The paranasal sinuses are normally sterile, maintained by the mucociliary clearance system.

Diagnosis: Children and adolescents with sinusitis may present with nonspecific complaints, including nasal congestion, nasal discharge (unilateral or bilateral), fever and cough. Less common symptoms include bad breath (halitosis), a decreased sense of smell, periorbital edema, headache and facial pain in children. Physical examination may reveal mild erythema and swelling of the nasal mucosa with nasal discharge and sinus tenderness.

Persistent symptoms of upper respiratory tract infection, including nasal discharge and cough, for longer than 10–14 days without improvement, or severe respiratory symptoms, including temperature of at least 102°F (39°C) and purulent nasal discharge for 3–4 consecutive days, are suggestive of a complicating *acute bacterial sinusitis*. Children with *chronic sinusitis* have a history of persistent respiratory symptoms, including cough, nasal discharge, or nasal congestion, lasting more than 90 days.

Sinus aspirate culture is the only accurate method of diagnosis. Transillumination of the sinus cavities may demonstrate the presence of fluid. Radiographic studies (e.g. sinus plain films, and CT scans) will show opacification, mucosal thickening, or presence of an air-fluid level; but such findings cannot differentiate, viral, bacterial, or allergic causes of inflammation.

Differential diagnostic considerations include viral upper respiratory tract infection, allergic rhinitis, non-allergic rhinitis, and nasal foreign body. Viral upper respiratory tract infections are characterized by nasal discharge, cough, and initial fever; symptoms usually do not persist beyond 10–14 days. Allergic rhinitis may be seasonal; examination of nasal secretions should reveal significant eosinophils.

Treatment: Acute bacterial sinusitis should be treated with antimicrobial agents to promote resolution of symptoms and prevent suppurative complications. Children with uncomplicated acute bacterial sinusitis should be treated with amoxicillin (45 mg/kg/day). Treatments for the penicillin-allergic patients include cefuroxime axetil, cefpodoxime, clarithromycin, or azithromycin. For children with risk factors (i.e. antibiotic treatment in the preceding 1–3 months, day care attendance, or age younger than 2 years) for the presence of resistant bacterial species and for children who fail to respond to initial therapy with amoxicillin within 72 hr, treatment with "high dose" amoxicillin-clavulanate (80–90 mg/kg/day of amoxicillin and 6.4 mg/kg/day of clavulanate) should be initiated. Treatment of sinusitis should be for 7 days after resolution of symptoms. Maxillary sinus aspiration for culture and susceptibility testing may be necessary. Abscesses may require surgical drainage.

11. *Acute pharyngitis:* Acute pharyngitis is caused by viruses (adenoviruses, coronaviruses, enteroviruses, rhinoviruses, respiratory syncytial virus, Epstein-Barr virus, herpes simplex virus, metapneumovirus) and group A β-hemolytic *Streptococcus, Mycoplasma pneumoniae, Neisseria gonorrhoeae,* and *Corynebacterium diphtheriae.*

Clinical manifestations: The onset of streptococcal pharyngitis is often rapid with prominent sore throat, absence of cough, and fever. Headache and gastrointestinal symptoms (abdominal pain, vomiting) are frequent. The pharynx is red, and the tonsils are enlarged and classically covered with a yellow, blood-tinged exudate. There may be petechiae on the soft palate and posterior pharynx, and the uvula may be red, stippled, and swollen. The anterior cervical lymph nodes are enlarged and tender. The incubation period is 2–3 days. Some patients demonstrate the additional stigmata of scarlet fever, circumoral pallor, strawberry tongue, and a red, finely popular rash that feels like sandpaper and resembles sunburn with goose pimples.

Treatment: Penicillin V is given bid or tid for 10 days: 250 mg/dose for children and 500/dose for adolescents and adults; or a shorter, 6 day course of oral amoxicillin (50 mg/kg/day divided bid; adult dose 1 gm bid).

12. *Retropharyngeal and lateral pharyngeal abscess:* Retropharyngeal abscess occurs most commonly in children < 3–4 yr of age, with boys affected more often than girls. Infection is often polymicrobial; the usual pathogens include group A streptococcus, oropharyngeal anaerobic bacteria, and *Staphylococcus aureus.* The *clinical manifestations* include fever, irritability, decreased oral intake, and drooling. Neck stiffness, torticollis, and refusal to move the neck may also be present. Other signs may include muffled voice, stridor, respiratory distress, bulging of the pharyngeal wall, and cervical lymphadenopathy. The *differential diagnosis* includes acute epiglottitis and foreign body aspiration. *Treatment options* include intravenous antibiotics with or without surgical drainage. A 3rd-generation cephalosporin combined with ampicillin-sulbactam or clindamycin to provide anaerobic coverage is effective. The optimal duration of treatment is for several days with IV antibiotics until the patient has begun to improve followed by a course of oral antibiotic is typically utilized. Drainage is necessary in the patient with respiratory distress or failure to improve with IV antibiotic therapy.

13. *Peritonsillar cellulitis/abscess:* Peritonsillar cellulitis/abscess is caused by bacterial invasion through the capsule of the tonsil, leading to cellulitis and/or abscess formation in the surrounding tissues. *Clinical manifestations* include sore throat, fever, trismus, and dysphagia. *Physical examination* reveals an asymmetric tonsillar bulge with displacement of the uvula, which is diagnostic. CT is helpful in revealing the abscess. Group A streptococci and mixed oropharyngeal anaerobes are the most common pathogens, with more than 4 bacterial isolates per abscess typically recovered by needle aspiration. *Treatment* includes surgical drainage and antibiotic therapy effective against group A streptococci and anaerobes. Surgical drainage may be accomplished through needle aspiration, incision and drainage, or tonsillectomy.

14. *Obstructive sleep apnea and hypoventilation:* Obstructive sleep apnea and hypoventilation (OSA/H) is a disorder of breathing during sleep characterized by prolonged partial upper airway obstruction and/or intermittent complete obstruction (obstructive apnea) that disrupts normal ventilation during sleep and normal sleep patterns. If unrecognized and untreated, it can lead to impaired day time functioning as well more serious complications, such as heart failure, developmental delay, poor growth, and death. The most common predisposing condition is adeno-tonsillar hypertrophy. Conditions that predispose to obstructive sleep apnea and hypoventilation include:

a. *Nasal disorders* (anterior and chronic nasal stenosis, deviated nasal septum, seasonal or perennial rhinitis, nasal polyps, foreign body, hamartoma, mass lesion)
b. *Nose:* Anterior and chronic nasal stenosis, deviated nasal septum, seasonal or perennial rhinitis, nasal polyps, foreign body, hamartoma, mass lesion
c. *Nasopharyngeal and oropharyngeal:* Adenotonsillar hypertrophy, macroglossia
d. Cystic hygroma
e. Velopharyngeal flap repair
f. Cleft palate repair
g. Pharyngeal mass lesion
h. *Craniofacial:* Micrognathia/retrognathia, mid-face hypoplasia (trisomy 21, Crouzon, Apert syndrome)
i. Mandibular hypoplasia (Pierre Robin sequence, Treacher Collins, Cornelia de Lange)
j. Craniofacial trauma
k. Achondroplasia
l. *Skeletal and storage diseases:* Glycogen storage disease (Hunter, Hurler syndrome, etc.)
m. Obesity.

Diagnosis: Common clinical manifestations of OSA/H include chronic mouth breathing, snoring, and restlessness during sleep with or without frequent awakenings. Children with more severe presentation also have noisy, mildly labored awake breathing that clearly worsens during sleep.

Although obesity is a risk factor for OSA/H in children, most children with OSA/H are not obese. Some children, especially children younger than 3 yr of age, are underweight or present with failure to thrive.

Clinical examination features include dysmorphic facies, mouth breathing, hyponasal speech, macroglossia, cleft palate, or enlarged tonsils. Specific craniofacial anomalies may be apparent. Pectus excavatum deformity can develop in long standing upper airway obstruction.

Polycythemia and respiratory acidosis with a metabolic alkalosis support the diagnosis of OSA/H when present but are absent in the majority of pediatric patients. Right ventricular hypertrophy on electro-cardiography and dysfunction on echocardiography are seen only in severe OSA/H. A lateral soft tissue radiograph of the neck can identify adenoidal tissue.

Treatment: Adenotonsillectomy is the most common therapy for OSA/H in children. However, the treatment of a particular child will depend on the underlying abnormalities, the site of obstruction, and the presence or absence of contributing neurologic or functional abnormalities. *Medical therapies* include nasopharyngeal airway, continuous positive airway pressure via nasal mask, supplemental oxygen to minimize hypoxemia, drug administration (topical nasal steroids, antibiotics, nasal decongestants for short term only), and weight loss in children with obesity. *Surgical therapies* include adenotonsillectomy, correction of deviated septum, nasal polypectomy, stenting procedures for nasal stenosis/atresia, uvulopalatopharyngoplasty, cleft palate revision procedures, mandibular/maxillary plastic surgical procedures, mandibular distraction osteogenesis, tracheostomy. Pharmacologic management has only a limited role in pediatric patients. If severe airway obstruction is present in wakefulness and sleep, then tracheostomy is the treatment of choice, particularly when vocal cord dysfunction, impaired swallowing, or absent laryngeal reflexes exists. When procedures require sedation or anesthesia, extreme caution is required, as such medications have profound effects on upper airway muscle tone, and respiratory decompensation can occur in these children.

Prevention: Because obesity is a risk factor for the increased severity of OSA/H in children with adenotonsillar hypertrophy persistence of OSA/H after adenotonsillectomy, and the development of OSA/H in adulthood, weight management should be a long-term goal in a child at risk or diagnosed with OSA/H.

15. *Nasopharyngeal carcinoma* though rare but is one of the most common nasopharyngeal tumors to occur in pediatric patients. It occurs in males twice as often as in females. It is associated with Epstein-Barr-virus. Cervical lymphadenopathy, epistaxis, trismus, and cervical nerve deficits may be present. The diagnosis is established from biopsy of the nasopharynx or cervical lymph nodes. Evaluation of head and neck with CT or MRI is performed to determine the extent of locoregional disease. Chest radiography, CT, bone scan, and liver scan are used to evaluate for metastatic disease. Treatment is a combination of cisplatin-based chemotherapy given before or concurrent with irradiation. The outcome depends on the extent of disease; those with distant metastasis have a very poor prognosis. Late effects as a result of radiation therapy are common, including hormonal dysfunction, dental caries, fibrosis, and second malignancies.

Dhingra PL. Epistaxis. In: Dhingra PL (Ed). *Diseases of Ear, Nose and Throat.* 3rd edn. New Delhi: Elsevier, 2004;165–256.

Dhingra PL. Anatomy of Nose. In: Dhingra PL (Ed). *Diseases of Ear, Nose and Throat.* 3rd edn. New Delhi: Elsevier, 2004;165–70.

Haddad J Jr. Epistaxis. In: Kliegman RM, Behrman RE, Jenson HB, Stanton BF (eds). *Nelson Textbook of Pediatrics.* 18th edn. Vol 2. Philadelphia: Saunders, 2007;1745–6.

Haddad J Jr. Congenital Disorders of Nose. In: Kliegman RM, Behrman RE, Jenson HB, Stanton BF (eds). *Nelson Textbook of Pediatrics.* 18th edn. Vol 2. Philadelphia: Saunders, 2007; 1742–1744.

Haddad J Jr. Acquired Disorders of Nose. In: Kliegman RM, Behrman RE, Jenson HB, Stanton BF (eds). *Nelson Textbook of Pediatrics.* 18th edn. Vol 2. Philadelphia: Saunders, 2007; 1744–6.

Haddad J Jr. Nasal polyps. In: Kliegman RM, Behrman RE, Jenson HB, Stanton BF (eds). *Nelson Textbook of Pediatrics.* 18th edn. Vol 2. Philadelphia: Saunders, 2007;1746–7.

Mathur Sumit. Epistaxis. In: Mathur GP, Mathur Sarla (eds). *Current Trends in Pediatrics.* Vol 1. Delhi: Academa Publishers, 2005;315–320.

Mathur Sumit. Nose and disorders of Nose. In: Mathur GP, Mathur Sarla (eds). *Current Trends in Pediatrics.* Vol 3. Delhi: Academa Publishers, 2007;370–87.

Pappas DE, Hendley JO. Sinusitis. In: Kliegman RM, Behrman RE, Jenson HB, Stanton BF (eds). *Nelson Textbook of Pediatrics.* 18th edn. Vol 2. Philadelphia: Saunders, 2007;1749–52.

Rose CL, Kass LJ, Haddad GG. Obstructive Sleep Apnea and Hypoventilation. In: Behrman RE, Kliegman RM, Jenson HB (eds). *Nelson Textbook of Pediatrics.* 17th edn. Philadelphia: Saunders, 2004;1397–1401.

Turner RB, Hayden GF. The Common Cold. In: Kliegman RM, Behrman RE, Jenson HB, Stanton BF (eds). *Nelson Textbook of Pediatrics.* 18th edn. Vol 2. Philadelphia: Saunders, 2007; 1747–9.

29.8 TONSILS AND ADENOIDS

Adenoids and tonsils both work to help the body stay healthy. In children infection and airway obstruction is the most important cause and rarely neoplastic disease occurs. Lymphoid tissues develop rapidly, reaching adult size by age 6 yr and continuing to hypertrophy throughout childhood and early adolescence (10–13 yr) before receding to adult size. Before deciding to perform tonsillectomy, adenoidectomy or both, one should keep in mind the normal growth and development of lymphoid tissue and immunologic role of tonsils and adenoids.

Waldeyer ring: Waldeyer ring consists of lymphoid tissue that surrounds the opening of the oral and nasal cavities into the pharynx and includes the palatine tonsils—located on both sides of the back of the throat, pharyngeal tonsils, or adenoids—located high in the throat, behind the nose, lymphoid tissue surrounding the eustachian tube orifice in the lateral walls of the nasopharynx, the lingual tonsils—located at the base of the tongue, and scattered lymphoid tissue throughout the remainder of the pharynx but especially behind the posterior pharyngeal pillars and along the posterior pharyngeal wall.

Lymphoid tissue located between the palatoglossal fold (anterior tonsillar pillar and the palatopharyngeal fold (posterior tonsillar pillar) forms the palatine tonsil. This lymphoid tissue is separated from the surrounding pharyngeal musculature by a thick fibrous capsule. The adenoid is a single aggregation of lymphoid tissue that occupies the space between the nasal septum and the posterior pharyngeal wall. A thin fibrous capsule separates it from the underlying structures; the adenoid does not contain the complex crypts that are found in the palatine tonsils but rather more simple crypts. Lymphoid tissue at the base of the tongue forms the lingual tonsil that also contains simple tonsillar crypts.

Normal function: Waldeyer ring of lymphoid tissue surrounds the entrance to the air-food inlet and thus provides initial contact with incoming organisms. The crypts and folds of the adenoids and tonsils serve to collect antigens for immune processing. Sensitized B-lymphocytes produce IgA locally (and at other sites) whilst T-lymphocytes are part of the immune system against certain viruses. Approximately two thirds of the lymphocytes that make up the lymphoid tissue of Waldeyer ring are B-lymphocytes, the remainder being either T-lymphocytes or plasma cells. The immunologic role of the tonsils and adenoids is to induce secretory immunity and secretory immunity and to regulate the production of the secretory immunoglobulins. This function is thought to be important when people are very young and their immune systems are still developing. Lymphoid tissue of Waldeyer ring is most immunologically active between 4–10 yr of age with a decrease after puberty.

Pathology: Acute and chronic infections commonly involve the tonsils and adenoids and neoplasms rarely. The infective agents of acute infection include viral, bacterial and fungal agents. Most episodes of acute pharyngotonsillitis are due to viral infection. Group A β-hemolytic *Streptococcus* (GABHS) is the most common cause of bacterial infection in the pharynx. Other bacterial organisms may include other β-hemolytic streptococcal species (i.e. group C), *Staphylococcus aureus*, gram-negative organisms, *Mycoplasma pneumoniae*, and, rarely, *Neisseria gonorrhoeae* and *Corynebacterium diphtheriae*. Oral candidiasis may occur in immunocompromised patients or children who have been treated chronically with antibiotics. *Candida albicans* accounts for the most human infections. Oral thrush, or oral pseudo-membranous candidiasis, is a superficial membrane infection which may be found on the lips, buccal mucosa, tongue, and palate. Removal of plaques from these surfaces may cause mild punctate areas of bleeding, which helps to confirm the diagnosis.

The tonsils and adenoids may be infected chronically in a polymicrobial manner that may include a high incidence of β-lactase-producing organisms. Both aerobic species, such as streptococci and *Haemophilus influenzae*, and anaerobic species, such as *Peptostreptococcus*, *Prevotella*, and *Fusobacterium*, predominate.

Clinical manifestations: The clinical features of tonsillitis include redder than normal tonsils, white or yellow coating on the tonsils, slight voice change due to swelling, sore throat, uncomfortable or painful swallowing, swollen lymph nodes in the neck, fever, and bad breath. Enlarged adenoids and their symptoms include breathing through the mouth instead of the nose most of the time, nose sounds "blocked" when the person speaks, noisy breathing during the day, recurrent ear infections, snoring at night, breathing stops for a few seconds at night during snoring or loud breathing (sleep apnea).

The goal of specific diagnosis is to identify GABHS infection. It can cause secondary damage to the heart valves (rheumatic fever) and kidneys (glomerulonephritis). It can also lead to a skin rash (scarlet fever), sinusitis, pneumonia, and ear infections. The clinical presentations of streptococcal and viral pharyngitis show considerable overlap. Antistreptolysin O (ASO) is measured to detect the GABHS infection (upper limit of normal: 2–5 yr 120–160 Todd units, 6–8 yr 240 Todd units, 10–12 yr 320 Todd unit). Throat swab culture is advised if the test is negative. A complete blood cell count (CBC) showing many atypical lymphocytes and a positive slide agglutination test can help to confirm a clinical diagnosis of EBV infectious mononucleosis.

Viral infections occur most commonly in winter and spring and are spread by close contact. The onset of viral pharyngitis may be more gradual, and symptoms more often include rhinorrhea, cough and diarrhea. Adenovirus pharyngitis may feature concurrent conjunctivitis and fever (pharyngoconjuctival fever). Coxsackievirus pharyngitis may produce small (1–2 mm) grayish vesicles and ulcers in the posterior pharynx or small (3–6 mm), yellowish white nodules in the posterior pharynx. In Epstein-Barr virus (EBV) pharyngitis, there may be prominent tonsillar enlargement with exudates, cervical lymphadenitis, hepatosplenomegaly, and rash. Primary herpes simplex virus infections often present in young children as high fever and gingivostomatitis.

Airway obstruction: Both the tonsils and adenoid are a major cause of upper airway obstruction in children. Airway obstruction is typically manifested in sleep-disordered breathing, including obstructive sleep apnea, obstructive sleep hypopnea, and upper airway resistance syndrome. The diagnosis of airway obstruction may be made by history and physical examination.

Tonsillar neoplasm: The rapid unilateral enlargement of a tonsil, especially if accompanied by systemic signs of fever, weight loss, and lymphadenopathy is highly suggestive of a tonsillar malignancy typically lymphoma in children.

Investigations before tonsillectomy and adenoidectomy: The list of investigations is blood for total and differential white blood cell (WBC) count and hemoglobin (Hb%) blood grouping, bleeding Time (BT) and coagulation time (CT), and X-ray skull-(lateral view in case of adenoidectomy).

Treatment

Medical management: The treatment of acute pharyngotonsillitis is with oral penicillin (Pentids 400 mg bid-tid) for 10 days or a single intramuscular injection of benzathine penicillin G (Penidure LA 6. 600,000 IU for ≤ 30 kg, Penidure LA 12. 1.2 million IU for >30 kg). Erythromycin (erythromycin estolate 20–40 mg/kg/24 hr divided bid-qid PO or erythromycin ethylsuccinate 40 mg/kg/24 hr divided bid or qid PO) is given for 10 days for patients allergic to penicillin. Cephalosporin or clindamycin may be more efficacious in the treatment of chronic throat infections caused by staphylococci or anaerobes producing

---

> **Box 29.5:** Criteria for tonsillectomy
>
> - Seven or more throat infections treated with antibiotics in the preceding year or
> - Five or more throat infections treated in each of the preceding 2 yr or
> - Three or more throat infections treated by antibiotics in each of the preceding 3 yr.

β-lactamase that may inactivate penicillin. Children with cryptic tonsillitis may be able to manually express tonsillolith or debris with either a cotton-tipped applicator or a dental water jet device.

Surgical management: Tonsillectomy alone is usually performed for recurrent or chronic pharyngotonsillitis. Although there is no strict criteria for number of infections but the criteria developed for the Children's Hospital of Pittsburgh study should be considered as the basis of performing tonsillectomy (Box 29.5).

Criteria for adenoidectomy: Adenoidectomy alone may be indicated for the treatment of chronic nasal obstruction (chronic adenoiditis), chronic sinus infections that have failed medical treatment, and recurrent bouts of acute otitis media, including those in children with tympanostomy tubes who suffer from recurrent otorrhea, chronic or recurrent otitis media with effusion.

Criteria for tonsillectomy and adenoidectomy: The criteria for both tonsillectomy and adenoidectomy for recurrent infection are the same as mentioned for tonsillectomy alone. The other indication for performing both procedures together is upper airway obstruction secondary to adenotonsillar hypertrophy that results in sleep-disordered breathing, failure to thrive, craniofacial or occlusive developmental abnormalities, speech abnormalities, or, rarely cor-pulmonale.

Complications of tonsillectomy and adenoidectomy: Bleeding may occur in immediate postoperative period or may be delayed after separation of the eschar. Swelling of the tongue and soft palate may lead to acute airway obstruction in the first few hours of surgery. Children with hypotonia or having cranial facial anomalies are at greater risk to suffer this complication. Dehydration may occur from odynophagia during the first postoperative week. Rare complications include velopharyngeal insufficiency, nasopharyngeal or oropharyngeal stenosis, and psychological problems.

Dhingra PL. *Diseases of Ear, Nose and Throat.* 3rd edn. New Delhi: Elsevier, 2004;289–331:489–94.

Mathur Sumit. Tonsils and Adenoids: When to operate. In: Mathur GP, Mathur Sarla (eds). *Current Trends in Pediatrics.* Vol 2. Delhi: Academa Publishers, 2006;284–90.

Owens JA. Sleep Medicine. In: Kliegman RM, Behrman RE, Jenson HB, Stanton BF (eds). *Nelson Textbook of Pediatrics*. 18th edn. Vol 1. Philadelphia: Saunders, 2007;91-100.

Paradise JL. Tonsillectomy and adenoidectomy. In: Bluestone CD, Stool SE, Alper CM, et al (eds). *Pediatric Otolaryngology*. 4th edn. Philadelphia: WB Saunders, 2002; 1210–22.

Wetmore RF. Tonsils and Adenoids. In: Kliegman RM, Behrman RE, Jenson HB, Stanton BF (eds). *Nelson Textbook of Pediatrics*. 18th edn. Vol 2. Philadelphia: Saunders, 2007;1756–8.

29.9 EAR, NOSE AND THROAT EMERGENCIES

Emergencies involving the ears, nose, and throat (ENT) are a source of much consternation for the emergency clinician. ENT emergencies range from minor ones to life threatening ones.

Ear Emergencies

Perichondritis: Perichondritis of the pinna can result secondary to an infection in the external auditory canal (EAC) or as a result of trauma to the pinna. Treatment consists of antibiotics with pressure dressing of the affected area. If there is abscess formation, it should be drained.

Hematoma of auricle: Blunt trauma can result in accumulation of blood between perichondrium and cartilage. Treatment consists of repeated aspiration under sterile conditions and pressure dressings.

Laceration of pinna: It is usually traumatic. Simple laceration requires thorough cleaning of wound, conservative debridement of necrotic skin edges and cartilage and closure of skin. Prophylactic antibiotics should be given. Complicated laceration requires staging with use of grafts or reconstructive flaps. In case of avulsion, microvascular reconstruction is required.

Impacted wax: Impacted wax can present as otalgia. Treatment is by removal of wax. If wax is very hard, then commercially available ear drops like paradichlorobenzene can be used and after a few days one can attempt again.

Otitis externa (Swimmer's ear): Otitis externa can be acute or chronic. Usual causative organisms are staphylococcus, pseudomonas or fungal infection (Otomycosis). Infection usually follows exposure to water. The ear canal will be exquisitely tender, and pressure on the tragus in front of the ear will exacerbate the pain *(Tragus sign)*. Treatment consists of topical antibiotic and antiseptic drops with combination of steroids. In case the ear canal is completely occluded, aural toilet and insertion of an antiseptic wick may be required.

Malignant otitis externa: This is a severe infection of the external auditory canal usually caused by *Pseudomonas*. This disease occurs most commonly in diabetics and immunocompromised patients. This infection spreads to the temporal bone and can lead to osteomyelitis of the temporal bone and eventually the skull base if not adequately treated. Main stay of treatment is intravenous anti pseudomonal antibiotics, e.g. ceftazidime, cefipime along with aminoglycosides if the renal parameters are not altered. Debridement may be required in selected cases. Treatment usually lasts for three to six months.

Foreign bodies in the ear: This condition is usually seen in children. It is characterized by pain with heaviness in the ear. Foreign body in the ear can be usually removed under local anesthesia. In case of impacted foreign body or uncooperative child general anesthesia may be required. Live insects should be suffocated with oil, 2% xylocaine or ether and removed with large metal suction tip.

Traumatic perforation of tympanic membrane: Various causes are injury from sharp objects, pressure from slap, blast injury, scuba diving or fracture of skull base. Patient usually complains of pain, deafness and bleeding from the ear. Inner ear trauma should be suspected if there is complete hearing loss or severe vertigo. Antibiotics are usually not required for traumatic perforation of tympanic membrane unless there are any signs of infection. Patient is instructed to keep water out of the ear. Most of the traumatic perforations tend to heal on its own, otherwise reconstructive surgery of tympanic membrane (Myringoplasty/tympanoplasty) is required.

Acute suppurative otitis media (ASOM): Common causative organisms are pneumococcus or *Haemophilus influenzae*. Infection can travel through eustachian tube and reach middle ear. Patient usually complains of pain. Treatment consists of antibiotics, analgesics and nasal decongestants. Occasionally there can be perforation in the tympanic membrane which results in discharge from the ear. The complication of acute otitis media is acute mastoiditis. Infection can spread further through the thin layer of bone separating the mastoid air cells from the cranial cavity, resulting in meningitis or intracranial abscesses. Other complications can be facial nerve paralysis or labyrinthitis.

Facial nerve paralysis: Facial nerve paralysis is usually lower motor neuron type of paralysis. The various reasons can be Bell's palsy, temporal bone trauma or facial laceration in parotid area, tumors (e.g. acoustic neuroma or parotid), infection (e.g. acute or chronic otitis media, Ramsay Hunt syndrome), Guillain-Barré syndrome, sarcoidosis, diabetes, etc. In all such patients' complete assessment of the external auditory canal, eardrum, parotid region and full CNS examination should be done. Treatment depends upon the pathology.

Sudden sensorineural hearing loss (SSNHL): The causative factors for sudden sensorineural hearing loss/deafness are not completely understood. In most of the cases it appears to be due to a vascular compromise. Other cause can be viral infection, post meningitis, cerebropontine angle lesions, or idiopathic. Treatment of this condition also remains unsatisfactory. The proposed treatment is oral steroids with vasodilating agents.

Vertigo: Vertigo can be central or peripheral. Vertigo secondary to ear pathology is usually peripheral. Various causes are vestibular neuritis, Meniere's disease, benign positional paroxysmal vertigo, acoustic neuroma, otosclerosis, cholesteatoma and ototoxic drugs. Treatment again depends upon the causative factors. Commonly used labyrinthine sedatives are cinnarizine and betahistine.

Nose Emergencies

Foreign body: It may be asymptomatic or can lead to offensive, unilateral nasal discharge, if it goes undetected for a long time. If foreign body can be visualized in anterior part of nose, it can be removed with a bent hook or pair of forceps. But if removal is difficult or child is uncooperative especially in a posteriorly located foreign body general anesthesia (GA) is preferred. Sudden posterior dislodgment with inhalation of the foreign body can be very dangerous (*see* Section 29.7).

Acute rhinosinusitis: It is one of the common ENT emergencies. In this condition there is inflammation of one or more paranasal sinuses. Maxillary sinus is the commonest to get affected. It can be viral, bacterial or fungal. Main bacteria responsible are streptococcus, staphylococcus and *Haemophilus influenzae*. Patient presents with nasal blockage, nasal discharge, headache and fever. On examination the affected paranasal sinus may show tenderness. On anterior rhinoscopy one can see the mucopurulent discharge in the middle meatus. Treatment consists of antibiotics, nasal decongestants, analgesics and steam inhalation. In the case of fungal sinusitis mucormycosis is the main causative factor. It mainly affects the immuno-compromised patients, e.g. diabetics, patients on dialysis, patients with multiple system failure. The fungus grows in the blood vessels causing thrombosis and distal ischemia. It can cause frank necrosis of the tissue (which has been infarcted). Usually the infection starts in the sinuses but rapidly spreads to the nose,

eye, palate, and up to the optic nerve of the brain. Treatment is immediate correction of the acidosis and metabolic stabilization and wide debridement usually consisting of a maxillectomy along with amphotericin B.

Epistaxis: In children it is often in Little's (Kiesselbach plexus) area, located anteriorly on nasal septum where as in hypertensive patients it is more posteriorly situated. When the patient presents with nasal bleed first thing which should be looked for is signs of shock, i.e. low blood pressure, weak pulse, cool, pale skin, etc. Firm compression of the lower half of the nose will stop bleeds by direct compression of the bleeding point, which is often in Little's area. Ice compression can also be given. If a bleeding vessel is visualized, it can be cauterized using silver nitrate ($AgNO_3$) or trichloroacetic acid. Anterior nasal pack will be required if the bleeding continues. It can be done by the ribbon gauze or by merocel nasal pack. Most of the times bleeding will stop with these measures but if posterior bleed persists even after anterior pack then posterior nasal packing is required. It may be done by balloon or Foley urethral catheter inserted back along floor of nose, or by traditional posterior nasal pack using gauze. If still the bleeding does not stop, ligation of the arteries can be done, usually the last resort in control of intractable epistaxis. It can be anterior or posterior ethmoidal artery, maxillary artery or the external carotid artery (*see* Section 29.7).

Nasal bone fractures: Nasal bone fractures can be isolated or it can be associated with other facial fractures. Various deformities which can be resulted are hump, a wide nasal dorsum, depression of the nasal dorsum, depression of the cartilaginous tip, deviation of the nose, splaying of the tip, saddle deformity, columella retraction, septal deflections, spurs, and complex angulations. Septal hematoma can be resulted which, causes persistent nasal pain and excessive swelling of the septum. Hematoma must be evacuated through external or internal incisions. If not treated timely it can result in septal abscess which can cause depression of the nose.

CSF rhinorrhoea: It is defined as leakage of CSF from the nasal cavity. Etiology is traumatic in most of the cases. Other etiological factors are tumors, congenital skull base defect. Patient complains of clear watery discharge from nasal cavity usually after bending or straining. Diagnosis can be made by CT scan or by injecting the fluorescein dye intrathecally and examining its presence in nasal cavity. In traumatic cases initial treatment is conservative. For persistent leaks, surgical closure should be done.

Nasal myiasis (Maggots): Maggots are larval forms of flies. They can infest nose and paranasal sinuses in old and debilitated people and can cause destruction of tissue. If not treated, it can be fatal. Treatment consists of removal of maggots. Chloroform oil can be used to kill them.

Throat Emergencies

Acute tonsillitis: It can be viral or bacterial. Main bacteria responsible for this are group A beta hemolytic Streptococcus. Patient presents with fever and odynophagia. Occasionally there may be formation of a membrane over the tonsil. In such cases other causes of the membrane over the tonsil like diphtheria, glandular fever, etc. should be ruled out. Treatment generally consists of broad spectrum antibiotics, and analgesics.

Peritonsillar abscess: Patient presents with spiking temperatures, muffled voice, dysphagia, referred earache and trismus. Examination shows unilateral swelling of soft palate, displacement of the tonsil down and medially. All the patients of peritonsillar abscess should be hospitalized. In early stage where there is more cellulitis, the treatment consists of broad spectrum antibiotics and analgesics. But once the abscess is formed, it should be drained.

Ludwig's angina: Ludwig's angina is rapidly progressive cellulitis involving the submandibular space. Main organisms involved are Streptococcus, Staphylococcus, *Bacillus fragilis* and anaerobes. Most common etiological factor is tooth infection. Roots of the second and third molars are behind and below the mylohyoid line. Therefore, if these teeth are abscessed, the pus will go into the submandibular space. From here it can spread to parapharyngeal space and other deep spaces of neck. Swelling of the neck appears woody or brawny. There may be tenderness or stiffness in the neck. Due to involvement of floor of mouth, the tongue may be pushed up and back and can obstruct the patient's airway. Trismus may be present especially if the abscess has involved the parapharyngeal space. Antibiotics should be started initially. Antibiotic coverage should include oral cavity anaerobes also. If abscess is formed then the treatment is incision and drainage. Incision is given from one angle of mandible to the other. Tracheostomy may also be required in case of obstructed airway. Complications of Ludwig's angina include aspiration, mediastinitis, septicemia, involvement of parapharyngeal space, etc. All these complications can be potentially fatal.

Retropharyngeal abscess: Retropharyngeal space is situated between the prevertebral fascia and buccopharyngeal fascia. It contains loose areolar tissue and a group of lymph nodes. It can get involved in acute bacterial infections of head and neck especially in children, injuries by foreign bodies and less commonly by tubercular infection. Retropharyngeal abscess caused by acute bacterial infections or by foreign bodies is termed acute retropharyngeal abscess whereas infection caused by tubercular bacilli is called chronic retropharyngeal abscess. Acute retropharyngeal abscess can cause laryngeal edema leading on to respiratory distress which may require tracheostomy. Treatment of acute retropharyngeal abscess is by drainage and a broad spectrum antibiotic whereas in cases of chronic retropharyngeal abscess, anti-tubercular treatment is used.

Parapharyngeal abscess: Parapharyngeal space is a pyramidal shaped space, its base being situated at the base of the skull and its apex at the level of hyoid bone. Parapharyngeal space abscesses are usually secondary to the infection in the pharynx, mainly the tonsils or dental infections. Patient presents with severe pain in throat with trismus and a swelling over the neck. On examination a bulge can also be seen in the oropharynx along with external swelling. Treatment consists of drainage of the pus via external incision. If untreated, it can lead on to laryngeal edema, thrombosis of internal jugular vein, mediastinitis, septicemia, etc.

Acute epiglottitis: It is the acute inflammation of the epiglottis seen mostly in children caused by *H. influenzae*. It presents as a sudden onset of high grade fever and rapidly progressive stridor. On examination the child appears sick. There is drooling of saliva as the child is unable to swallow because of excessive pain. Indirect laryngoscopy shows an edematous and congested epiglottis. But one should be careful while doing indirect laryngoscopy as it can occasionally cause fatal laryngeal spasm. X-ray neck shows edematous epiglottis which is referred to as *"thumb sign"*. Treatment includes broad spectrum antibiotics with humidified air. Because of respiratory distress child may require tracheostomy.

Foreign bodies of the upper aerodigestive tract: The various areas where the foreign body can get stuck in upper aerodigestive tract are base of tongue, tonsillar pillars and tonsils posterior pharyngeal wall, pyriform fossae, cricopharyngeal sphincter, upper part of esophagus, larynx, trachea and bronchus. Commonly encountered foreign bodies are peanuts, coins, fish or chicken bone and dentures.

Foreign body in the tonsils, tonsillar pillars, base of tongue and posterior pharyngeal wall can be removed in OPD settings most of the times unless the patient is not cooperative. For rest of the foreign bodies, general anesthesia is needed for most of the cases. If the foreign body is in pyriform fossa or cricopharynx, it can be removed by direct laryngoscopy. In case of esophageal foreign bodies, removal is done by rigid esophagoscope. Foreign bodies in the airway are managed by bronchoscopy. Occasionally tracheostomy may be required for airway foreign body. Occasionally the foreign body can completely obstruct the upper airway. This can be dislodged by suddenly increasing the intrathoracic pressure. This is done by using Heimlich maneuver: stand behind the patient and grasp him or her around the upper abdomen; an upward thrust in the epigastric region may dislodge the offending article.

Bilateral abductor vocal cord palsy: It can be congenital (rare) or acquired. These days the commonest acquired cause is thyroid surgery. Because of bilateral abductor vocal cord palsy the vocal cords come in paramedian position. A minimal insult to the larynx then can cause significant airway obstruction. Emergency tracheostomy is required. Various definite treatment options are arytenoidectomy, vocal cord lateralization and nerve muscle implant.

Laryngeal tumors causing obstruction: Patients with laryngeal tumors can present to casualty with breathing difficulty or stridor. The tumor can be benign or malignant. Benign tumors can be laryngeal papillomatosis, amyloidosis, chondroma, neurogenic tumors, etc. Laryngeal papillomatosis is actually a viral infection caused by human papilloma virus. It can be juvenile or adult papillomatosis. Juvenile papillomas are multiple. They present with breathing difficulty and are notorious for recurrence after removal. In malignant tumors the commonest tumor is squamous cell carcinoma. Other malignant tumors can be chondrosarcoma, malignant salivary gland tumors, etc. Various treatment options for malignant tumors are surgery, radiotherapy or chemotherapy. Surgery can be partial or total laryngectomy with or without neck dissection depending upon extent of the disease.

Laryngotracheal trauma: Most of the cases of laryngotracheal trauma are suicidal, assault or road traffic accidents. Early diagnosis is the key to successful management. Various injuries which can occur are Hyoid bone fracture, laryngeal fracture, tracheal fracture, penetrating injuries, supraglottic hematoma, arytenoid dislocation, cricotracheal separation and recurrent laryngeal nerve paralysis.

Majority of the patients present with pain, hoarseness, hemoptysis and breathing difficulty. Breathing difficulty can develop even several hours after the injury. On examination, there may be subcutaneous emphysema with loss of surface land marks. Crepitus may be felt in larynx or trachea. Diagnosis can be made on the basis of X-ray neck (soft tissue) or a CT scan. Chest X-ray should also be done to rule out concomitant chest injury. In case of breathing difficulty it is always safer to do a tracheostomy rather than intubation as the anatomical landmarks for intubation might have been lost. Open reduction of fractures and careful suturing of lacerations should be done, as soon as possible after injury.

Corrosive injuries: It can be suicidal or accidental. Corrosive injuries can be caused by acids or alkalis. Burns caused by alkaline materials are more dangerous and can cause severe mucosal injuries. In upper aerodigestive tract, there can be oral ulcerations. More dangerous is the involvement of the larynx by the burns which can cause breathing difficulty or stridor. In such cases emergency tracheostomy is required.

Angioneurotic edema: It can present as severe laryngeal edema of sudden onset and can be fatal if not diagnosed and treated timely. Patient may require emergency intubation or tracheostomy. Systemic steroids can be given to reduce edema.

Bansal A, Miskoff J, Lis RJ. "Otolaryngeal critical care." *Crit Care Clin* 2003 January; 19 (1):55–72.

Flynn TR. "The Swollen Face: Severe Odontogenic Infections." *Emerg Med Clin North Am* 2000 August; 10 (3). 101 519.

Garantziotis S, Kyrmizakis DE, Liolios AD. "Critical care of the head and neck patient." *Crit Care Clin* 2003 January; 19 (1):73–90.

Gradon JD. "Infectious Disease Emergencies: Space-occupying and Life-Threatening Infections of the head, Neck, and Thorax." *Inf Dis Clin North Am* 1996 December; 10(4):857–78.

Howes DS, Dowling PJ. "Oral-Facial Emergencies: Triage and Initial Evaluation of the Oral Facial Emergency." *Emerg Med Clin North Am* 2000 August; 18(3):371–378.

Murphy SC. "The person behind the eponym: Wilhelm Frederick von Ludwig (1790–1865)." *J Oral Pathol Med* 1996; 25 (9):513–5.

Padgham N. Epistaxis: anatomical and clinical correlates. *J Laryngol Otol* 1990;104(4):308–11.

Verghese S T, Hannallah R S. Pediatric otolaryngolic emergencies. *Anesthesiol Clin North Am* 2001;19:237–56.

30 ◆ Pediatric Dermatology

30.1 ANATOMY OF SKIN

Human skin is a complex multi-layered structure, consisting of a stratified cellular epidermis and an underlying dermis. The dermal-epidermal junction is undulating in section; ridges of the epidermis (known as rete ridges) project into the dermis, while dermis projects as dermal papillae. The junction provides mechanical support for the epidermis and acts as a selective barrier against exchange of cells and large molecules. Below the dermis is a fatty layer, the panniculus adiposus usually designated as 'subcutis' or 'hypodermis'.

Regional variation: Human skin shows marked regional variations in terms of thickness, structure and presence of appendages. The thickness varies between 06.mm (e.g. eyelids) and 3 mm (e.g. palms and soles). Skin over palms and soles is 'glabrous' or non-hairy, and it is grooved on the surface by alternating ridges and sulci, in individually unique configurations known as dermatoglyphics. Hair-bearing skin, present elsewhere over the body, is characterised by the presence of hair follicles and sebaceous glands. The axilla and anogenital region are notable due to the presence of apocrine glands in addition to eccrine sweat glands, which are found throughout the body.

Normal Microanatomy of Skin

The epidermis is a stratified multilayered structure, which renews itself continuously by cell division in germinative layer. The principal cell of epidermis is the ectoderm-derived *keratinocyte* that constitutes at least 80% of the epidermal cells. Other epidermal cells include melanocytes, Langerhans cells, and Merkel cells. From below upwards, the layers of the skin are as follows: stratum basale (stratum germinativum), stratum spinosum, stratum granulosum. As the cells of granular layer move up, they become more flattened, lose their nuclei and other organelles and end up as enucleate dead cells (or corneocytes) of stratum corneum or horny layer. The epidermal turnover time or transit time has been used to represent the time taken for a cell to pass from basal layer to the surface of the skin. In normal skin, the total time varied from 52–75 days, but this is greatly reduced in psoriatic epidermis.

Other Cells of the Epidermis

i. **Melanocytes** are melanin pigment producing cells located in the basal layer of epidermis. They are also present in hair follicles, eye, inner ear, peripheral nerves, and leptomeninges of brain. These cells synthesize melanin pigment in oval or round bodies called melanosomes, which are then transferred to adjacent keratinocytes. A single melanocyte supplies melanosomes to a group of about 36 keratinocytes, and this constitutes the epidermal melanin unit. Density of *epidermal melanocytes* in different parts of the body varies, being greatest in facial skin and male genitalia. The colour difference between white, oriental and black skin is due to the amount and arrangement of melanosomes. Melanin contributes to the colour of human skin and provides protection from the harmful effects of ultraviolet radiation.

ii. **Langerhans cells** are derived from the bone marrow, these cells are located in mid-portion of stratum spinosum and possess dendritic processes. On electron microscopy, characteristic tennis racquet shaped granules called Birbeck granules are seen in cytoplasm of Langerhans cells. These cells are functionally related to the monocyte-macrophage-histiocyte series, and behave as epidermal antigen processing cells. Thus, they play a crucial role in contact sensitization and in immunosurveillance against viral infections and neoplasms of the skin.

iii. **Merkel cells** are present in basal layer, scarce and irregularly distributed. They function as specialized touch receptors.

Epidermal Appendages

The epidermal appendages include hair, nails, eccrine and apocrine sweat glands, and sebaceous glands.

Hair: Hair are found all over the skin except on the palms, soles, glans penis, and vaginal introitus (glabrous skin). Hair and sebaceous gland together constitute the pilosebaceous unit. There are 3 types of hair. 1. Lanugo hair—found in the foetus and usually shed in-utero in eighth to ninth month gestation. 2. Vellus hair—short, soft, occasionally pigmented hair present all over the body. 3. Terminal hair—long, coarse and darkly pigmented hair. They are limited to scalp, eyebrows and eyelashes before puberty. After puberty, secondary sexual terminal hair develop from vellus hair in response to androgens.

Nail: Nails form an essential covering over distal phalanges of fingers and toes. Hardness of nails is due to the presence of hard keratin. The rectangular nail plate is the major structure that rests on and is firmly attached to the underlying nail bed. Approximately one-quarter of the nail is covered by the proximal nail fold, and a narrow margin of the sides of the nail plate is occluded by lateral nail folds. Fingernails grow approximately 0.1 mm/day or 0.3 cm every month and toenails at one-third of this rate.

Eccrine sweat glands: Two to three million sweat glands are present all over the body, being most numerous on the palms, soles and axillae. Each gland consists of a secretory coil present deep in the dermis and subcutaneous tissue, and a duct which passes through the dermis and epidermis and conveys the secreted sweat to the skin surface. Sweat contains water, sodium, potassium, chloride, urea, ammonia, lactate, and few other organic as well as inorganic substances. In cystic fibrosis, abnormalities in a membrane chloride channel results in elevated sodium and chloride levels in the sweat, which can be diagnosed by quantitative pilocarpine iontophoresis sweat test. The functions of eccrine glands are 1) evaporation of sweat resulting in cooling of the body, 2) moistening the skin of palms and soles resulting in improved grip, and 3) excretion of drugs like griseofulvin and ketoconazole.

Apocrine sweat glands: The structure of these specialized sweat glands is similar to that of eccrine sweat glands, consisting of a convoluted secretory coil (present deep in the dermis or subcutis) and an apocrine duct. They are present in the axillae, groins, perianal region, and areolae of breasts. They are poorly developed in childhood, and begin to enlarge at puberty under the influence of androgens. They secrete very small quantities of an oily fluid, which gives a characteristic odour after reaching the surface due to bacterial decomposition. Apocrine glands are responsible for producing body odour and may play some part in human olfactory communication.

Sebaceous glands: Sebaceous glands are found on all areas of the skin except for palms and soles and only scarcely present over dorsa of hands and feet. They are associated with hair follicles over most areas of the body forming the pilosebaceous unit. However, they may open directly to the surface of skin and this includes Meibomian glands of eyelids, Tyson's glands of prepuce, free glands in areolae of nipples, female genitalia, as well as over margin of upper lip and buccal mucosa appearing as minute pale-yellow specks called Fordyce's spots. The gland is multilobed and contains lipid-rich cells that completely disintegrate to form the sebaceous secretion (holocrine secretion). The lobular ducts converge to the main sebaceous duct which opens into the upper part of the hair follicle. Sebum is a complex mixture of lipids and consists of triglycerides, squalene, cholesterol and related esters. It also contains free fatty acids which are produced by lipolysis of triglycerides by a skin surface bacterium called *Propionibacterium acnes*.

McGrath JA, Uitto J. Anatomy and Organization of Human Skin. In: Burns T, Breathnach S, Cox N, Griffiths C (eds) . *Rook's Textbook of Dermatology*. 8th edn. London: Blackwell science, 2010; 3.1–3.53.

Moschella SL, Hurleh HJ (eds). Structure and Function of Skin. *Dermatology*. Philaelphia: W B Saunders, 1992; 1–53.

Wolff K, Goldsmith LA, Katz SI, Gilchrest BA, Paller AS, Leffell DJ (eds). Overview of biology, development, and structure of Skin. *Fitzparick's Dermatology in General Medicine*. 7th edn. New York: McGraw Hill, 2008: 57–87.

30.2 EVALUATION OF THE DERMATOLOGIC PATIENT

Disorders of the skin in infants and young children vary in many respects from occurrence of the same diseases in older children and adults. The diagnosis and treatment of skin diseases in children differ because of more sensitive reaction patterns, tendency towards easier blister formation, and therapeutic dosages and regimes that frequently differ from those of adults.

History: In obtaining history, careful questioning by the examiner is necessary to elucidate the relationship of the onset of the initial eruption or of recurrences to: previous treatment—prescribed by physician or self-administered exposure to sunlight, seasonal variations, immediate environment, e.g. contact with plants, animals, chemicals, metals, etc. specific foods or additives, and immunization. The family history may suggest a hereditary or contagious process and the clinician may need to examine other members of the family.

Examination: Examination of the entire skin should be done routinely including the scalp, hair, palms and soles, nails, and mucosae (oral, ocular, nasal, and ano-genital). Identification of the primary lesion is the key to accurate interpretation and description of cutaneous disease. Secondary lesions evolve from the primary lesions or result from scratching of primary lesion by the patient.

Primary lesions include: *Macule* is a flat, non-palpable lesion with color or subtle texture change only, without elevation above the skin surface. *Papule* is a small (up to 5 mm), solid, superficial, circumscribed, palpable lesion elevated above the skin surface. *Plaque* is a palpable lesion elevated above the skin surface 5 mm or more in diameter. *Nodule* is a solid mass in the skin, more than 5 mm in diameter, can be seen as an elevation or can be palpated. *Vesicle* is an elevated, circumscribed lesion up to 5 mm in diameter that contains clear fluid. *Bulla* is a fluid-filled lesion with diameter greater than 5 mm. *Pustule* is a superficial elevated lesion that contains pus or purulent exudates. *Petechiae* are punctate hemorrhagic spot of size up to 4 mm. These are known as *purpura* if size is upto 1 cm. *Ecchymoses* are larger bruise like purpuric lesions of size more than 1 cm. *Telangiectasia* are permanent dilatations of capillaries that may or may not disappear with application of pressure. *Comedone* is a plug of keratin and sebum in dilated pilosebaceous orifice typically seen in acne and acneiform eruptions. *Burrow* is a small tunnel in the skin that houses the female scabies mite. *Wheal* is a white or pale red, compressible transient or evanescent, rounded or flat topped area of dermal or dermal and hypodermal edema. It is characteristic lesion of urticaria.

Secondary lesions include: *Scale* refers to abnormal shedding or accumulation of stratum corneum in perceptible flakes. *Excoriation* refers to superficial excavations of the epidermis that may be linear or punctate and result from scratching. *Erosion* is a moist, circumscribed, usually depressed lesion that results from loss of all or a portion of the viable epidermis and up to one third of dermis and heals without scarring. *Ulcer* is an erosion in which there is destruction of epidermis and more than one third of dermis. *Fissure* is a linear cleavage or crack in the skin. *Atrophy* can be epidermal or dermal or both. Epidermal atrophy refers to thinning of the epidermis. Dermal atrophy results from a decrease in the papillary or reticular dermal connective tissue and is usually manifests as a depression of the skin. *Scar* results from replacement by fibrous tissue of another tissue that has been destroyed by injury or disease. *Lichenification* is thickening of the skin with hyperpigmentation and accentuation of skin markings in response to prolonged rubbing. *Sclerosis* refers to a circumscribed or diffuse hardening or induration in the skin. It may also involve the dermis when the overlying epidermis may be atrophic. *Alopecia* refers to absence of hair from a normally hairy area. *Callus* is a localised hyperplasia of stratum corneum. *Sinus* is a cavity or tract with a blind ending. *Cyst* is a closed cavity or sac with an epithelial, endothelial or membranous lining and containing fluid or semisolid material. *Fistula* is an abnormal passage from a deep structure to skin surface or between two structures, often lined with squamous epithelium. *Milium* a tiny white cyst containing lamellated keratin. *Poikiloderma* is the association of cutaneous pigmentation, atrophy and telangiectasia.

Koebner phenomenon is the development in a patient with preexisting dermatoses of new lesions of similar morphology in otherwise normal skin following trauma. This reaction occurs in traumatized normal skin is vitiligo, psoriasis and lichen planus. It may occur in recent scars or at pressure points.

Bedside tests and procedures: **Magnification**—A hand lens magnifier allows critical examination of skin surface and detection of fine morphologic details of skin lesions. Addition of a drop of mineral oil to the lesions produces an even better image.

Diascopy/vitropression: Diascopy consists of firmly pressing a transparent, hard, flat object (such as glass slide or colourless tongue depressor) over the surface of a skin lesion. This causes exclusion of blood out of small vessels to allow evaluation of other colours. This may aid in differentiating a macule or papule due to capillary dilatation (erythema) from extravasation of blood (purpura). It is of particular value in detecting granulomatous nodules, which have a translucent brownish colour known as apple jelly nodules (in lupus vulgaris). It may also help in differentiating nevus anemicus (a localized area of vasoconstriction) from a nevus hypochromicus where there is a deficiency of melanin pigment.

Nikolsky's sign refers to the sheet like removal of epidermis by gentle traction. It is seen in pemphigus vulgaris and toxic epidermal necrolysis. Marginal Nikolsky sign, elicited in the vicinity of an active lesion is more sensitive but less specific than direct Nikolsky for the diagnosis of pemphigus. The latter involves similar removal of epidermis in normal looking skin distant from the lesions and indicates active disease.

Auspitz sign for psoriasis is elicited by the Grattage test which has three components. Gentle scraping of scale from psoriatic plaque produces an initial increase in scaling. Continuing further scrapping produces the skin supra-papillary membrane known as the Berkeley's membrane. Appearance of pin-point dots of blood at the tops of ruptured capillaries on removal of this membrane is known as the Auspitz sign.

Wood's lamp examination: Some important uses of this technique include pigmentary disorders, infections, and porphyrias.

Microscopy: Skin scrapings may be examined under potassium hydroxide (KOH 10%) for diagnosis of fungal infections, or stained with specific stains for viral or bacterial infections. **Tzanck smear** is an important diagnostic tool in the evaluation of blistering diseases. It involves obtaining material from the base of a vesicle by gentle curettage, smearing it on a glass slide and staining with Giemsa's or Wright's stain. These are then examined under a microscope to look for multinucleate giant epithelial cells (seen in herpes simplex/zoster and varicella) or acantholytic cells (seen in pemphigus). Gram stain should be made in lesions suspected of being of bacterial origin. Sterile pustules of pustular psoriasis may reveal multiple polymorphonuclear leucocytes in the absence of any organisms.

Skin biopsy: A commonly technique for skin biopsy using local anesthesia employs a 5 mm punch—a small tubular knife. Nodules and tumors may require a larger wedge shaped scalpel biopsy including the subcutaneous tissue. Specimens for light microscopy should be fixed immediately in 10% aqueous formalin. Formalin should not be used in collection of skin biopsy specimens for bacterial, mycobacterial and mycotic tissue cultures. Normal saline or appropriate culture media should be used in such cases, ideally in consultation with the microbiology or pathology laboratory.

Cox NH, Coulson IH. Diagnosis of Skin Disease. In: Burns T, Breathnach S, Cox N, Griffiths C (eds). *Rook's Textbook of Dermatology.* 7th edn. Vol 1.Oxford: Blackwell Science. 2004; 5.1–5.20.

Levy ML. Principles of diagnosis. In: Schachner LA, Hansen RC (eds). *Pediatric Dermatology.* 2nd edition. Vol 1. New York: Churchill Livingstone, 1995; 139–163

Paller AS, Mancini AJ (eds). *Hurwitz Clinical Pediatric Dermatology: A Textbook of Skin Disorders of Childhood and Adolesecence.* 3rd edn. Philadelphia: Elsevier, 2006; 1–15.

30.3 VITILIGO AND ALBINISM

Normal skin color in humans ranges from pale white to black. Melanin, formed in melanocytes, is the major component imparting color to the skin. Others responsible for skin color are oxyhemoglobin, deoxygenated hemoglobin and carotenoids. Disorders of melanin pigmentation can be divided on morphological grounds into two types. The first is *hypermelanosis* where there is an increased amount of melanin in the skin. The second type is *hypomelanosis* where there is a lack of pigment in the skin, which appears white or lighter than the normal colour. Amelanosis is when there is total lack of melanin in the skin. The term depigmentation is used to describe a loss of pre-existing pigment from the skin.

Vitiligo

Vitiligo is a common, idiopathic, acquired disorder of pigmentation, characterized by depigmentation of skin and hair. There is absence of melanin and melanocytes in the epidermis. The etiology of vitiligo is complex. There appears to be a certain genetic predisposition. Between 30 and 40% of patients have a positive family history. It has been reported in monozygotic twins. Inheritance may be polygenic or determined by an autosomal dominant gene of variable penetrance. HLA association is variable and has shown inconsistent results. Some antigens and alleles found with increased frequency are HLA-A2, HLA-DR4 and HLA-DR7. Various theories, all centered on the mechanisms for the destruction of melanocytes have been suggested such as: autoimmune hypothesis, neurogenic hypothesis, and self destruct theory of Lerner.

Clinical manifestations: Onset of vitiligo can occur at any age and has been reported from birth to 81 yrs of age. Congenital vitiligo is very rare. The peak age of onset in all series is between 10 and 30 years and in 50% of cases, it develops before the age of 20 years.

Among 50% of the pediatric cases, onset of lesion is between 4 and 8 years of age. Lesions may develop either spontaneously or sometimes attributed to a severe physical or emotional stress. In some cases, physical damage to previously normal skin like a cut, abrasion or burn may result in depigmentation known as isomorphic or Koebner phenomenon and is seen in up to 30% of patients. In these patients sites subjected to repeated friction and trauma like dorsa of knuckles, elbows, feet, ankles, knees and other bony prominences and areas frequently rubbed by clothing-shoulder strap, waistband and collar areas are particularly prone to develop vitiligo.

Typical vitiligo lesion is a round to oval milky white macule measuring a few millimeters to centimeters in size. The lesions are usually progressive and the advancing interface between normal and vitiligo skin has a convex outline resulting in a scalloped margin indicating active disease process. The pigment loss is usually complete but may be partial at interface between the normal and vitiligo skin, giving rise to a narrow band of tan coloration called trichrome vitiligo. In some cases of repigmenting vitiligo, a fourth color of perifollicular or marginal hyperpigmentation may be seen referred to as quadrichrome. When the border of lesions is raised and erythematous, it is termed inflammatory vitiligo. A few or all the hairs in vitiligo macules may become depigmented (leucotrichia) and it has been reported in 9 to 45% patients. Leucotrichia adversely affects the rate and degree of repigmentation but it helps to differentiate vitiligo from other hypopigmented disorders described in differential diagnosis. Vogt-Koyanagi syndrome presents with vitiligo, uveitis, and premature graying of hair along with involvement of central nervous system.

Diagnosis: The distribution of lesions, age of onset and characteristic margin of progressing lesions aid in making a diagnosis. Sometimes, Wood's lamp examination may be required in patients with lighter skin types to assess the true extent of the disease. Clinically inapparent lesions stand out prominently through Wood's lamp examination.

Differential diagnosis: Vitiligo needs to be differentiated from the hypo/depigmented lesions from a number of diseases, such as piebaldism, nevus depigmentosus, hypomelanosis of Ito, pityriasis alba, tinea versicolor, lichen sclerosus, scleroderma, leprosy, tuberous sclerosis, Waardenburg syndrome, chemical leukoderma (previous history of exposure to phenolic compounds), and post inflammatory hypopigmentation.

Course and prognosis: Lesions start abruptly and continue to progress for a while and then might become static. Repigmentation of some lesions and simultaneous extension of others or appearance of new lesions also occur. The face, arms, trunk, and legs respond best.

Treatment: Currently there is no universally effective therapeutic modality for vitiligo; however, there are a number of active medical and surgical approaches, which have shown variable efficacy. In addition to attempts at repigmentation, sunscreens, cosmetic camouflage and behavioral therapy constitute important adjunctive therapies.

Medical treatment: A number of options are available such as (i) Corticosteroids (topical and systemic), (ii) Photochemotherapy (PUVA) [a combination of Psoralen (P) and ultraviolet A radiation (UVA)], (iii) Narrow band UVB, (iv) Tacrolimus, (v) Calcipotriol [synthetic analogue of vitamin D_3], (vi) 308 nm excimer laser, (vii) Levamisole (antihelminthic drug).

Surgical treatment: In those patients who fail medical therapy, various surgical techniques are available. However, best results have been achieved in segmental vitiligo. Various surgical modalities include: 1. autologous thin epidermal graft (Thiersch) from normally pigmented skin; 2. grafting of suction blister epidermis; 3. minigrafting of small punch biopsies; and 4. autologous grafting of cultured melanocytes. Combination of grafting and PUVA has resulted in increased success rates.

Tattoing: To achieve the best cosmetic results, appropriate proportion of various tattoo pigments are mixed depending on the color of normally pigmented skin, residual pigment in affected skin and quantity of blood flow through the affected skin.

Cosmetic camouflage: It includes makeup and color matched dyes for a cosmetic camouflage for lesions on exposed skin. Although it causes neither repigmentation, nor regression of the disease, it is a practical solution for treatment resistant cosmetically disabling lesions.

Bleaching: In patients with extensive vitiligo and a few residual areas of normal pigmentation, removal of the remaining pigment to give a uniform white appearance may be more desirable cosmetically. Depigmentation may be achieved by daily night time use of 20% cream of monobenzyl ether of hydroquinone for 6–9 months.

Behavioral therapy: Reassurance, explanation of prognosis and psychological counseling are essential components of all treatment protocols.

Albinism

Albinism a genetically determined condition characterized by reduced melanin in the skin, hair and eyes. Melanocytes are present in normal distribution but fail to synthesize melanin adequately. Hypopigmentation primarily involving the retinal pigment epithelium of the eyes is termed ocular albinism (OA), while involvement of skin, hair and eyes is termed oculocutaneous albinism (OCA). The characteristic ocular abnormalities common to all types of OCA and OA include photophobia, nystagmus, reduced melanin in the retinal pigment epithelium, foveal hypoplasia, reduced visual acuity, refractory errors and misrouting of the optic nerves at the chiasma.

Oculocutaneous albinism: It is seen at a frequency of 1:20,000 in general population. There are several variants divided on the basis of genetic locus involved and all of them have an autosomal recessive inheritance except a poorly defined rare type with an apparent autosomal dominant inheritance that is now thought to be due to quasi-dominant pedigree patterns. No treatment is possible except: 1. physical photoprotection in the form of full sleeved clothes and appropriate headgear and meticulous regular use of broad spectrum sunscreen; 2. regular examination for early detection and treatment of premalignant and malignant conditions of the skin; 3. and annual ophthalmologic examination for correction of refractory errors.

Chédiak-Higashi syndrome: It is a rare autosomal recessive disorder characterized by hypopigmentation of skin and hair, severe immunological defects, progressive neurological dysfunction and the presence of giant peroxidase positive lysosomal granules in peripheral blood granulocytes. Patients have a marked tendency to infections—bacterial, viral, intractable respiratory and cutaneous infections, and usually prove fatal before the age of 10 years.

Halder RM, Grimes PE, Cowan CA, Enterline JA, Chakrabarti SG, Kenney JA Jr. Childhood vitiligo. *J Am Acad Dermatol* 1987;16:948–54

Handa S, Dogra S. Epidemiology of childhood vitiligo, a study of 625 patients from North India. *Pediatr Dermatol* 2003; 20:207–10.

Kanwar AJ, Dogra S. Narrow-band UVB for the treatment of generalized vitiligo in children. *Clin Exp Dermatol* 2005; 30:332–6.

Savant SS. Tattooing. In: Savant SS (Ed). *Textbook of dermatosurgery & cosmetology*. 2nd edn. Mumbai: ASCAD, 2005; 338–44.

Singal Archana, Aggarwal Puneet. Vitiligo and Albinism. In: Mathur GP, Mathur Sarla (eds). *Current Trends in Pediatrics*. Vol 3. Delhi: Academa Publishers, 2007;327–36.

30.4 IMMUNE MEDIATED BLISTERING DISEASES OF CHILDHOOD

Pemphigus vulgaris: This disorder usually affects middle aged individuals and rarely occurs in children. Oral erosions are the presenting sign in most of the children with pemphigus vulgaris. Both mucosae as well as the skin are affected in the course of the disease in up to 80% of children. The blisters are flaccid, appear on normal skin and are filled with clear or slightly hemorrhagic fluid. Face, scalp, neck, chest, axillae and groin are the frequently involved sites. Lesions may be asymptomatic or may be associated with itching or burning sensation. Lateral pressure applied to the normal appearing skin at the periphery of the lesions results in shearing of the skin—*Nikolsky sign*. Lateral or vertical pressure over an intact bulla may also produce peripheral extension of the lesion (*bulla spread sign*). Histopathological examination of the blister shows suprabasal cleft and basal cells attached to basement membrane, giving the basal layer, a characteristic *row of tombstone* appearance. Direct immunofluorescence (DIF) tests on biopsied samples show IgG bound to intercellular areas of the epidermis. Indirect immunofluoroscent (IIF) studies of the serum of patients show IgG antibodies to Dsg-3 (mainly) and 1.

Treatment: In mild and localized forms of pemphigus, topical corticosteroids may be sufficient. However, in majority of cases, systemic corticosteroids in doses of 0.5–5 mg/kg per day are required initially to suppress the disease activity which can be later tapered slowly. Intravenous steroids in the form of pulse therapy (0.5–1 g methylprednisolone or 50–100 mg dexamethasone in 5% dextrose intravenously over 1–3 hours on 3 consecutive days per month) can be given in patients with extensive disease to achieve early control and to reduce long term side effects of daily steroids. Other immunosuppressants like azathioprine, cyclophosphamide and methotrexate can be used as steroid sparing agents. Pemphigus vulgaris is a severe chronic disease in children, which can be fatal at times.

Pemphigus neonatorum: Pemphigus neonatorum is due to transplacental passage of autoantibodies against intercellular substance from the mother. It must be distinguished from primary pemphigus vulgaris in a neonate. Pemphigus seen in neonates is usually pemphigus vulgaris and very rarely pemphigus foliaceus. Pemphigus foliaceus is characterized by intraepidermal blistering; the site of cleavage is high in the epidermis rather than suprabasal as in pemphigus vulgaris. The prognosis in neonatal pemphigus is good. Healing of the lesions occurs within 3 weeks, and is most probably related to the decrease in maternal antibodies. As spontaneous recovery occurs, no treatment is necessary.

Drug-induced pemphigus: The most commonly implicated agents are penicillamine and captopril. Other implicated agents are penicillin, rifampicin, progesterone, ceftazidime, etc. Drug-induced pemphigus usually presents as pemphigus foliaceous and rarely as pemphigus vulgaris. Mucosal involvement is rare. Drug-induced pemphigus usually clears with treatment of pemphigus and withdrawal of the offending agent.

Pemphigoid gestations: It is the subepidermal blistering disorder occurring during second or third trimester of pregnancy or in immediate postpartum period. Cutaneous involvement of the newborn occurs in about 10% of infants born to mothers with this disorder as a result of passively transferred antibodies. With the decline in transferred antibody levels, the lesions remit spontaneously within several weeks and thus, do not require any therapy.

Chronic bullous disease of childhood (syn. linear IgA bullous dermatosis): Chronic bullous disease of childhood (CBDC) is a benign chronic subepidermal blistering disease of childhood characterized by deposition of IgA in basement membrane zone in immunofluoroscent studies. It is more common in children from developing communities like China and India. The mean age of onset is under 5 years. Large, tense, clear or hemorrhagic bullae appear on a normal or erythematous base over perioral area, scalp, genitalia, buttocks, inner thighs, legs, and dorsal aspect of feet. The bullae may form characteristic annular or rosette like lesions composed of vesicles surrounding a central crust, the *"string of pearls"* sign. Involvement of mucous membranes is common. Histologically, it is characterized by subepidermal bullae with a dermal infiltrate of neutrophils, eosinophils, and mononuclear cells. Dapsone is the drug of choice in linear IgA disease, but patients have also responded to erythromycin and flucloxacillin. Systemic corticosteroids, azathioprine and mycophenolate mofetil are alternative therapies.

Wojnarowska F, Venning VA. Immunobullous diseases. In: Burns T, Breathnach S, Cox N, Griffiths C (eds). *Rook's Textbook of Dermatology*, 8th edn. Vol 2. London: Blackwell Science, 2010; 40.1– 40.62.

30.5 ECZEMA IN PEDIATRIC AGE GROUP

Eczema is a generic designation for a particular type of reaction pattern in the skin, which includes exudation, lichenification, and pruritus. Acute eczematous lesions are characterized by erythema, weeping, oozing, and the formation of microvesicles within the epidermis. Chronic lesions are generally thickened, dry and scaly with coarse skin markings (lichenification) and altered pigmentation. Many types of eczema occur in children; the most common is atopic dermatitis (*see* Chapter 11).

Infantile seborrheic dermatitis: The eruption usually appears between the third and the eighth week of life. Most often, it starts in the napkin area and tends to spread rapidly to involve the scalp, face neck and axillae. The vertex and the frontal areas are the sites of predilection on the scalp. On the face, eyebrows, eyelashes and nasolabial folds are worst affected. The classical asymptomatic erythemo-squamous eruption may be discrete to coalescent with adherent yellow brown scales which are large and greasy on the scalp known as 'cradle cap' but smaller, whiter and drier elsewhere. When considering differential diagnose of seborrhoeic dermatitis, all scaling eruptions should be considered particularly psoriasis and disseminated irritant napkin dermatitis. The condition is usually self limiting. After bathing, treatment with anti-yeast agents like 1 % clotrimazole or 2 % miconazole with or without 1 % hydrocortisone, for 10–14 days is sufficient in most cases.

Contact dermatitis in childhood: Contact dermatitis in the pediatric age group is mostly transient. Factors that contribute to the high incidence of irritant dermatitis in this age group especially infancy include inappropriate widespread application of antiseptics, prolonged skin contact with urine and feces and frequent presence of occlusive conditions. The usual clinical pattern of primary irritant dermatitis in infancy is perianal dermatitis and napkin dermatitis. True allergic contact dermatitis has been uncommonly described in childhood. However, dermatitis from nickel (ear-rings), epoxy resins (plastic items) and components of various topical applications has been described.

Diaper dermatitis (Syn. primary irritant napkin dermatitis): Diaper dermatitis includes all inflammatory eruptions that occur in the diaper area. Prolonged contact with water can cause maceration of the stratum corneum due to frictional damage and subsequently impair the barrier function, thereby, increasing the transepidermal permeability to irritants. Friction between the skin and the napkin fabric has been implicates in its etiology. The irritant potential of fecal enzymes like proteases and lipases in combination with increased urinary pH and impaired epidermal barrier, may contribute to the diaper dermatitis. Secondary invasion by *Candida albicans* appears to be a risk in cases where it has been isolated from the faces.

Primary irritant napkin dermatitis has peak prevalence between the 7th and 12th months. Primary irritant contact dermatitis usually causes confluent erythema of the buttocks, the genitalia, lower abdomen and pubic area, i.e. the areas in close contact with the napkins, sparing the intertriginous areas. Postinflammatory depigmentation may be a striking feature in racially pigmented infants. Among the distinctive variants, confluent erythema of the perianal area with elevated margins and the satellite pustular lesions associated with proliferation of Candida albicans has been observed. Psoriasiform, herpetiform, granutomatous infantile gluteal granuloma and disseminated eruptions are encountered rarely.

A variety of conditions need to be differentiated include infections (congenital syphilis, herpes simplex of the genital area), zinc deficiency and Langerhans cell histiocytes, which may be present with similar skin lesions during infancy.

Recognition of relevant causative factors and adequate local cleansing with water and nonirritant soaps and detergents forms the mainstay of treatment. Mild topical corticosteroid alone or in combination with anti-Candida agents is usually effective in most cases. The use of good quality disposable napkins containing absorbent gelling material and increased frequency of napkin change following soiling with urine or feces, is associated with a lower incidence of napkin dermatitis.

Pityriasis alba: This is a common endogenous, eczematous disorder characterized by hypopigmented, slightly raised, fine, scaly plaques with indistinct borders. It usually affects face (midforhead and malar areas), lateral upper arms and rarely thighs. Macules are about 2–3 in number usually and vary in size from 0.5 to 3 cm. The lesions appear in young children, commonly in 6–12 years age group and disappear by early adulthood. This disease is to be differentiated from tinea versicolor and vitligo. The condition is usually self limiting and hypopigmentation fades with time. Short course PUVA has been found to be helpful in extensive pityriasis alba.

Holden CA, Parish WE. Atopic Dermatitis. In: Champion RH, Burton JL, Burns DA, Breathnach SM (eds). *Rooks Textbook of Dermatology.* 6th edn, Vol 1. Oxford: Blackwell publications, 1998; 681–708.

Krafenik BR. Eczematous Dermatitis. In: Schachner LA, Hansen RC (eds). *Pediatric Dermatology.* 2nd edn. Vol 1. New York: Churchill Livingstone publications, 1995; 685–702.

Singal Archana, Mehta Shilpa. Eczema in Pediatric Age Group. In: Mathur GP, Mathur Sarla (eds). *Current Trends in Pediatrics.* Vol 2. Delhi: Academa Publishers, 2006; 296–306.

30.6 PSORIASIS

Etiopathogenesis: Psoriasis has a multifactorial etiology encompassing genetic, immunological and environmental determinants. Recent streptococcal infection has been especially implicated in the development of guttate psoriasis in children. *Koebner's phenomena* or the appearance of skin lesions following

trauma has been described in 30–50% of psoriatic patients. Several other risk factors like HIV infection, smoking, alcohol consumption, drugs (lithium, beta blockers and antimalarials), stress and withdrawal of corticosteroids have been accepted in provoking a new episode of psoriasis or in exacerbating pre-existing disease. The prevalence of the disease is 1–3%. Incidence of psoriasis is equal in both the sexes; however, females tend to develop psoriasis earlier than males. There are two peaks of age of onset of disease: first one at 15–22 years and the second one at 57–60 years. However, about 15% of the patients have their first episode before the age of 15 years.

Clinical Manifestations

Psoriasis vulgaris (chronic plaque psoriasis) is the most frequent clinical form of psoriasis observed in about 60–70% of pediatric patients and characterized by the insidious development of erythematous, sharply demarcated, plaques with a silvery, adherent scale. The successive removal of the psoriatic scale usually reveals a underlying smooth, glossy red membrane with multiple bleeding points where thin suprapapillary epithelium is torn off (*Auspitz's sign*). When the scaling is not evident, it can induce by light tangential scratching with the edge of glass slide (*Grattage sign*). Koebner's phenomenon has been observed. Scalp is the most frequently affected site of involvement in pediatric psoriasis, followed by the appearance of lesions on the extensor surfaces of the extremities and trunk. Although not common in adult psoriasis, the face, ears and anogenital areas are often involved. The so-called *napkin psoriasis* is the usual early expression of the disease in infants. It is characterized by slightly itchy, erythematous papules and plaques with discrete scaling spread over napkin area starting from age three months.

Guttate psoriasis describes the shower of small lesions appearing more or less generally over the body particularly in children and young adults after an acute streptococcal infection. The lesions are from 2–3 mm to 1 cm in diameter round or slightly oval. They are scattered particularly over the trunk and proximal parts of extremities, sometimes on the face, scalp and the ear. Guttate psoriasis resolve spontaneously in weeks or months; responds more readily than plaque psoriasis.

Generalized pustular psoriasis (von Zumbusch psoriasis) is a rare and serious form of psoriasis. Numerous tiny pustules evolve from an erythematous base and coalesce to form lake of pus on the trunk, flexures and other glabrous areas of the body. These pustules readily rupture and dry up. The patient is toxic, febrile and has leukocytosis. Topical medications such as tar and anthraline, and sudden withdrawal of topical or systemic steroids may precipitate episode in patients with unstable psoriasis.

Erythrodermic psoriasis (exfoliative erythroderma) is an acute condition that usually results from a progressive worsening of psoriasis in an acute or chronic fashion. The skin becomes diffusely and intensely red, edematous and profoundly scaly and effects 75 % or greater of body surface area. It frequently arises in patients with unstable psoriasis vulgaris. There is usually associated pruritus. Constitutional symptoms, such as fever, myalgias are often present. The etiological agents of erythroderma in psoriasis have been ascribed to intercurrent infections, harsh topical treatments and withdrawal of systemic steroids.

Nail psoriasis occurs in 7% to 40% of children. Nail pitting, ridges and grooves are due to psoriasis in the nail matrix, whereas onycholysis and subungual hyperkeratosis are due to defects in the proximal portion of the matrix. It is frequently seen in combination with psoriatic arthropathy. Psoriasis is probably the disease most often associated with nail pathology.

Psoriatic arthritis is classified as a seronegative spondyloarthropathy, a loosely organized group of disorders that also includes ankylosing spondylitis, enteropathic arthritis and Reiter's syndrome. The frequency of psoriatic arthritis is in the range of 5% to 8% among the psoriatic.

Juvenile psoriatic arthritis shows a peak incidence between the ages of 2 and 4 in females and a second peak between 11 and 12 in both sexes with a slight male predominance. The characteristic features include the distinctive asymmetric pattern of joint involvement, the simultaneous presence of ankylosis, periosteal new bone formation, erosions and osteolysis in various joints and the pathognomonic distal interphalangeal joint involvement. The most common presentation of pediatric psoriatic arthritis is monoarticular, often acute arthritis of the knee. However, the long term course is typically polyarticular with asymmetric involvement of both upper and lower extremities.

Spinal column involvement is much less frequent in juvenile psoriatic arthritis, but when found, is associated with an increased incidence of HLA B27. Another feature shared by the spondyloarthropathies is involvement of the periarticular structures in a distinctive inflammatory process that affects tendons and ligaments at their insertions, resulting in tendinitis, dactylitis and fascitis. The diagnosis of psoriatic arthritis in childhood is often delayed since arthritis precedes psoriasis in many patients. In the absence of skin lesions, typical nail changes and a family history of psoriasis could suggest the diagnosis, especially in patients with an asymmetric arthritis and dactylitis.

Histopathology: A biopsy from the suspected lesions is required to confirm the diagnosis. Histopathological criteria for the diagnosis of psoriasis considered are: epidermal hyperplasia from sight to prominent, parakeratosis, focal or confluent, neutrophils in the cornified layer also called the *Munromicro* abscess, neutrophilic infiltrate in the granular layer or the *Kogoj's* abscess, diminution or disappearance of the granular layer, at least focally suprapapillary thinning, dilated and tortuous blood vessels that spiral up within dermal papillae, and superficial perivascular lymphohistiocytic infiltrate.

Treatment: Management of pediatric psoriasis involves: 1. Education of the child and parents concerning the relapsing and remitting nature of psoriasis and the effects of treatment; 2. Genetic counseling may be provided if needed based on population data; and 3. Environmental triggers of psoriasis should be sought particularly infection.

Psoriasis can usually be treated effectively in children with topical agents including emollients, coal tar, corticosteroids, dithranol and calcipotriol according to age and the sites affected. Phototherapy (*UVB therapy*) is initiated only in the presence of extensive and widespread disease. Resistance to topical treatment is another indication for phototherapy. Methotrexate (MTX) has been used in children suffering from recalcitrant plaque, pustular, erythrodermic and severe psoriatic arthritis. The usual dose of MTX is about 0.3 mg/kg given in orally or parenterally once a week. Acitretin (systemic retinoids) is only used in severe forms of the disease such as erythrodermic, pustular and arthritic psoriasis.

Benoit S, Hamm H. Childhood psoriasis. *Clin Dermatol* 2007; 25(6): 555–562.

Habif TP. Psoriasis and other papulo-squamous diseases. In: Habif TP (Ed). *Clinical dermatology: A color guide to diagnosis and therapy.* 4th edn. Pennysylvania, USA: Mosby, 2004: 209–238.

Paller AS and Mancini AJ. Papulo-squamous and related disorders. In: Paller AS, Mancini AJ (eds). *Hurwitz clinical and pediatric dermatology.* 3rd edn. Elsevier: Saunders, 2006; 85–107.

30.7 ACNE IN CHILDREN

Acne is a chronic inflammatory disease of the pilosebaceous unit. Acne can be seen in the first year of life, early childhood, prepubertal age, and puberty. However, in mid-childhood, between 1 and 7 years, acne is uncommon, and when it is encountered, it should be evaluated for hyperandrogenism. Approximately 40% of adolescents below the age of 15 years will develop physiological acne and in 15% of these patients, the acne is sufficiently troublesome to merit a visit to their physician. Although not a serious disease, severe acne and acne scarring can be a cause of emotional distress and concern for the parents. Studies on quality of life (QOL) have revealed that in acne patients QOL is markedly impaired thus ensuring that treatment is required not just for the cosmetic reasons but also for improving QOL and psychosocial well-being of the patient.

Etiopathogenesis: Acne vulgaris (AV) has a familial trend with probable autosomal dominant inheritance. Four key pathogenic factors have been recognized for acne: follicular epithelial hyper-proliferation and resultant follicular plugging, androgen stimulation, presence and activity of *Propionibacterium acnes* (*P. acnes*), inflammation. Stress appears to be a trigger factor for development of acne as it stimulates hypothalamic-pituitary-adrenal axis and the resultant increase in androgen production. Role of diet in pathogenesis of acne is controversial. Recently, the toll-like receptor 2 (TLR-2) has been implicated in the pathogenesis of acne. TLR-2 is a pattern recognition receptor that is activated by *P. acnes*. When bound, TLR-2 activates a transcription factor that up-regulates production and the release of pro-inflammatory cytokines like IL-12 and IL-8 from monocytes. TLR-2 is expressed on infiltrating inflammatory cells around the pilosebaceous follicle in those with acne and its expression increases as the acne lesion ages and becomes more inflamed.

Clinical manifestations: Acne is a polymorphic disease occurring predominantly over the areas with greatest concentrations of sebaceous glands, i.e. face (particularly cheeks and forehead) and frequently spread to involve all parts of the face, as well as the neck and trunk. Occasionally a patient is seen with little or no facial acne but considerable truncal acne.

Physical signs: Seborrhoea non-inflamed lesions, i.e. comedones—open comedone (black head), and closed comedone (white head), superficial inflamed lesions (papules, superficial pustules), deep inflamed lesions (nodules), scarring can occur at any age including as

early as 9 or 10 years. Scarring associated with increased collagen is less frequent and include hypertrophic scars and keloids.

The American Academy of Dermatology (AAD) developed a classification scheme for primary acne vulgaris. This grading scale delineates three levels of acne: i. *Mild acne:* A few to several papules and pustules, but no nodules; ii. *Moderate acne:* Several to many papules and pustules, along with a few to several nodules; iii. *Severe acne:* Numerous or extensive papules and pustules, as well as many nodules.

Treatment: The pathophysiologic features of acne suggest that combination therapy should be utilized as early as possible (except in patients requiring oral isotretinoin), preferably at the initiation of therapy, to simultaneously attack two or three pathogenic factors. Treatment guidelines for acne vulgaris are summarized in Table 30.1.

Antoniou C, Dessinioti C, Stratigos AJ, Katsambas AD. Clinical and therapeutic approach to childhood acne: an update. *Pediatr Dermatol* 2009; Jul-Aug 26(4): 373–80.

Cohen BA, Schachner LA. Acne. In: Schachner LA, Schchner RC editors. *Pediatric dermatology*. 2nd edn, Churchill Livingstone; 1995:661–83.

Paller AS, Mancini AJ. Disorders of the sebaceous and sweat glands. In: Paller AS, Mancini AJ (eds). *Hurwitz clinical pediatric dermatology: a textbook of skin disorders of childhood and adolescence*. 4th edn, Philadelphia: Elsevier, 2011: 167–183.

30.8 SEXUALLY TRANSMITTED DISEASES

The term sexually transmitted disease (STD) is used for all infections that are transmitted mainly through sexual contact, during unprotected vaginal, anal or oral intercourse. Some are also transmitted from mother to child before or during birth and through unsafe blood, donated organs or contaminated needles. According to World Health Organization estimates 333 million curable STDs occur globally in a year. In addition to classical venereal diseases like syphilis, chancroid, gonorrhea, granuloma inguinale and lymphogranuloma venereum, the spectrum of STDs that may be observed in the pediatric age group include: *human immunodeficiency virus (HIV), hepatitis B, hepatitis C*, genital types of *herpes simplex* and

Table 30.1: Acne treatment plan			
Comedonal acne	*Mild to moderate papulo-pustular acne*	*Severe inflammatory acne*	*Severe nodulo-cystic acne*
Topical retinoids, Comedone Extraction	Topical retinoids + benzoyl peroxide/topical antibiotic (clindamycin, erythromycin)	Oral antibiotics, i.e. doxycycline/ tetracycline/minocycline/ erythromycin + topical retinoids	Oral isotretinoin, intralesional steroid

Trichomoniasis. The mode of acquiring STDs in an adolescent may be consensual sexual activity or sexual abuse. In prepubertal children the cause is often sexual abuse. Infections like gonorrhea and chancroid are highly suggestive of abuse. Trans-placental or intrapartum exposure may cause congenital syphilis, neonatal herpes infections, genital warts or HIV in childhood.

Syphilis

It is caused by *Treponema pallidum*. It is a chronic, systemic infection capable of involving every organ in the body and it can persist as latent disease for years. The disease is divided into early syphilis which includes primary and secondary stage, and the tertiary or late stage. Most infections are transmitted in early syphilis, including early latent syphilis (up to 1 year).

Epidemiology: The distribution of syphilis is worldwide and resurgence has been documented with the HIV epidemic. However, a reduction in tertiary syphilis and congenital syphilis has been noted. Acquired syphilis in children is almost always associated with abuse. Uncommon modes of infection include non-sexual in health care workers or children (by breast feeding) and by transfusion of fresh blood components.

Clinical Manifestations

Primary: After an incubation period of 10 to 90 days, primary chancre appears at the site of inoculation. Starting as a papule, the chancre ulcerates to form a single, painless, button like indurated, round to oval, clearly defined ulcer. The sites of predilection include prepuce, coronary sulcus, frenulum or glans in males and labia in females. Special attention should be given to anal chancres, and extragenital sites like lips, tongue, nipples or hands. Kissing ulcers occur in the urethral meatus and coronal sulcus. In children, the chancres are said to be smaller and thus easily missed. The syphilitic ulcer may be atypical due to coexistence with the lesions of herpes simplex, chancroid or other STDs. The ulcer is accompanied by firm, nontender, regional lymphadenopathy. Spontaneous resolution of the chancre and lymphadenopathy usually occurs within 4 to 6 weeks leaving a depressed scar at site of ulcer in some patients.

Secondary syphilis: After a period ranging from 6 weeks to 6 months after healing of chancre, 40% of infected individuals develop secondary syphilis. An overlap between the two stages may also be seen. The patients may develop a flu-like prodrome with fever, malaise, myalgia, arthralgia, and rhinorrhoea. The lymphadenopathy is generalized, nontender, and can involve the cervical, axillary or epitrochlear chains. The initial eruption is faint pink, macular over the trunk, lasting for up to 3 weeks. This is followed by a copper coloured, maculopapular or papulosquamous eruption in about 50% of the patients over trunk, flexors of upper extremities and palms and soles, which may mimic psoriasis, lichen planus or pityriasis rosea. The corresponding lesions in the warm and moist areas are large, moist and referred to as condyloma lata and are highly infectious. Papules along the hair line are arranged in a crown like pattern (corona veneris). Scalp lesions are associated with moth eaten alopecia. Pressure with blunt side of pin over a papule will elicit deep dermal tenderness (Buschke Ollendorf sign). Mucous patches are intraoral plaques with slightly raised grayish-white margins and frequent ulceration. Snail track ulcers may present on oral and genital mucosa. Systemic features can include mild hepatitis, iritis, uveitis, arthritis, parotitis, and glomerulonephritis. Untreated syphilis may develop clinical relapse with secondary features in approximately 25%.

Latent syphilis: It is defined as reactive serology with positive specific tests in the absence of clinical signs and symptoms, CSF abnormality or adequate treatment.

Tertiary syphilis: Progression to tertiary syphilis is seen in one third of cases of late latent syphilis. Among these patients, half develop gummatous syphilis, 25% each cardiovascular and neurosyphilis. It is extremely rare in the pediatric age group.

Syphilis and HIV: Syphilitic ulcer increases transmission of HIV. In the presence of HIV infection, syphilis may present with multiple and atypical chancres, early progression to neurosyphilis, pustular or malignant syphilis, multi-organ involvement in secondary stage and misleading serological tests (including false negative results).

Congenital syphilis: It represents a failure of appropriate case detection and treatment in the antepartum period. World Health Organization estimates that maternal syphilis causes 460,000 abortions or stillbirth, 270,000 cases of congenital syphilis and 270,000 premature babies. Maternal treatment for syphilis can successfully prevent congenital syphilis in 83% fetuses. *Congenital syphilis* can be divided into early, late, and stigmata.

Early congenital syphilis: The division is arbitrarily at 2 years. The lesions are infectious and resemble acquired secondary syphilis. The onset of clinical signs is at birth in 32% and by 4 weeks in 64% of neonates. The infant tends to be irritable, low birth weight and has a feeble cry. Generalized lymphadenopathy, hepatosplenomegaly, lacrimation, rhinitis (snuffles) and mucosal ulceration may be present. The common skin lesions are macular, papular, coppery red, scaly, predominantly present on palms, soles and diaper area. Radiating fissures at the angle of the mouth, nares and anus may heal leaving linear scars (rhagades). Involvement of the long bones in the form of osteochondritis in the first six month is a characteristic finding. Syphilitic epiphysitis may cause local pain and tenderness and the limb is held immobile (pseudoparalysis of Parrot). Another characteristic sign is the Wimberger's sign (loss of density on the medial side of the upper end of tibia). The signs of osteochondritis disappear after 6 months, but periosteum lesions persist, presenting in radiographs as 'onion peel' periosteum. Osteitis of the proximal phalanges may produce dactylitis in the second year of life. Involvement of nervous system in the form of abnormal CSF findings is seen in 40–60% of infected infants. Symptomatic infants with leptomeningitis or encephalitis present with seizures, bulging fontanelles, neck rigidity and hydrocephalus. Choroiditis is common in early months of life and glaucoma and uveitis can rarely be seen.

Late congenital syphilis: The early stage may go unnoticed in about 80% of the cases. Late syphilis presents after 2 years and is rare after 30 years of age. These patients are usually non-infectious. Subcutaneous or submucous gummata soft tissue appear from 5 years of age. These can result in ulceration of soft palate and nasopharynx. Hutchinson's triad is pathognomonic and comprises interstitial keratitis, Hutchinson's teeth and eighth nerve deafness. Hutchinson's teeth are barrel or peg shaped, notched, permanent upper central incisors that form due to defective enamel formation. Mulberry or moon molars teeth affect the lower first molar most commonly and have four defective dwarfed cusps. Bone involvement mostly is in the form of sclerosis and new bone formation. Tibia is most frequently involved in the middle third (saber tibia) and also the inner end of clavicle (Higoumenaki's). Osteoperiostitis of bones of the skull vault leads to rounded bony swelling, called Parrot's nodes. Both the knee joints may show symptomless effusion (Clutton joints). Neurosyphilis may be symptomatic. Juvenile paresis has been observed more frequently than juvenile tabes dorsalis. Cardiovascular syphilis is very rare and only a few cases of aneurysm and aortic incompetence have been reported.

Stigmata of congenital syphilis: Stigmata are scars from early or late congenital syphilis and represent permanent evidence of the infection. These include saddle nose, frontal bossing of Parrot, short maxillae,

bull dog jaws, high arched palate, Hutchinson's teeth, moon molars, saber tibia, Higoumenaki's sign, scaphoid scapula, Clutton's joint, corneal opacities, optic atrophy, deafness, hydrocephalus and rhagades.

Diagnosis: The diagnosis of syphilis can be confirmed by one of the following methods: demonstration of *Treponema pallidum* by dark field examination is approximately 80%. Care should be taken to distinguish commensal spirochaetes. Direct fluorescent antibody test from exudates for *T. pallidum* differentiates pathogenic from non-pathogenic strains and increases the sensitivity. Polymerase chain reaction (PCR) may be helpful in cases of congenital syphilis, neurosyphilis and in early primary syphilis. Serology (nontreponemal tests): Venereal disease research laboratory (VDRL) and Rapid Plasma Reagin. These correlate well with disease activity and can be used to assess response to treatment. False positive results may be seen in children following immunization, or *mycoplama* or *pneumococcal* pneumonia, measles, mumps, varicella, leprosy, malaria, *hepatitis B* and rheumatic diseases. Specific treponemal tests: Fluorescent treponemal antibody absorbed (FTA-Abs) and Microhemagglutination assay for antibody (MHA-TP). Treponemal tests may stay reactive for a lifetime and cannot be used to monitor the disease activity. Detection of treponemal IgM antibodies: IgM capture ELISA, IgM FTA-Abs, 19S-IgM-FTA Abs or Western blot is especially useful and indicated in congenital syphilis and neurosyphilis. All patients with sexually transmitted diseases or sexually abused children should be subjected to a screening VDRL for syphilis.

Treatment: Early (primary, secondary, early latent): Adult: Benzathine penicillin G 2.4 million units IM in a single dose; Children: 50,000 units/kg IM up to adult dosage; Penicillin allergy: Doxycycline 100 mg every 12 hours for 14 days. *Late syphilis:* Benzathine penicillin G 7.2 million units, as 3 doses of 2.4 million units IM at 1 week interval; Children 150,000 units/kg divided in three weekly doses. Neurosyphilis: Aqueous crystalline penicillin G 18–24 million units every 4–6 hours for 10–14 days. *Early congenital syphilis:* Aqueous crystalline penicillin G 100,000–150,000 units/kg/day given as 50,000 units/kg/dose IV every 12 hours during the first 7 days of life and every 8 hours thereafter for total of 10 days. *Late congenital syphilis:* With a normal CSF give Benzathine penicillin G, 50,000 U/kg IM in 3 weekly doses. *The Jarisch-Herxheimer reaction* is an acute hypersensitivity reaction presenting as fever, headache, myalgia within 24 hrs of effective therapy for syphilis. Partner notification and treatment, if possible, should be promoted.

Chancroid

It is an acute, autoinoculable, ulcerative disease caused by the bacterium *Haemophilus ducreyi.* It is rare in the pediatric age group but may occur in sexually active teens or following child abuse. After an incubation period varying from 1 to 10 days, a small erythematous papule appears which progresses to a pustule and ulcerates. Subsequently, multiple, painful non-indurated ulcers varying in size from 3 mm to 2 cm with ragged undermined edge appear. The floor is covered with yellow necrotic exudates and vascular granulation tissue which bleeds on gentle manipulation. They may present anywhere on the anogenital skin and rarely extragenital sites including breast, lips, tongue and oropharynx.

Diagnosis: Smears stained with Gram stain show "school of fish" appearance; that is gram negative coccobacilli arranged in short parallel chains. The gold standard for diagnosis is culture of the organism. Multiplex test combining PCR for *H. ducreyi, T. pallidum* and *herpes simplex* virus is available.

Treatment: Azithromycin 1 gm orally, or ceftriaxone 250 mg intramuscular for 3 days, or erythromycin base 500 mg tab for 7 days. Worldwide, resistance to ciprofloxacin and erythromycin is reported. The fluctuant bubo should be aspirated from non-dependent part. Treatment failure is said to be predictive of associated HIV.

Gonorrhea

It is one of the commonest sexually transmitted disease, caused by *Neisseria gonorrhoeae.* In the prepubertal child it is diagnostic of abuse with very rare exceptions. Reported rates of infection in abused children vary from 3 to 20%. In pubertal children, the features are similar to that seen in adults. After an incubation period of 2 to 7 days, the presentation is with purulent urethral discharge, dysuria in males and with cervicitis, vaginal discharge, dysuria, menstrual abnormalities and abdominal pain in females. Complications in males include epididymitis, prostatitis, periurethral abscess, penile lymphangitis and urethral stricture. In females spread can lead to salpingitis, tubo-ovarian abscess and pelvic peritonitis. Up to 44% teens may be asymptomatic, which increases the probability of complications. Prepubertal children are mostly symptomatic. Females present with signs of vaginitis like vulvar erythema, purulent discharge, pruritus, and dysuria. Ascending infections are less common and cervicitis is absent. In both sexes pharyngitis and proctitis may be seen. Though, mostly asymptomatic, pharyngeal gonorrhoea can present as sore throat or cervical adenitis and anorectal disease as anal pruritus, proctitis, tenesmus, bleeding and purulent discharge per anum. Rarely conjunctivitis is documented in older children. Disseminated gonococcal infection occurs infrequently in children.

Neonatal gonorrhea: Perinatal transmission can result in conjunctivitis, asymptomatic pyuria, urethritis, vaginitis, proctitis, pharyngitis, rhinitis, scalp abscess, arthritis, meningitis, septicemia and pelvic inflammatory disease.

Ophthalmia neonatorum: Any inflammation accompanied by discharge that occurs in the eye of an infant within 21 days of birth. The causes of purulent conjunctivitis include gonococcal or chlamydial infection and organisms like Streptococcus, Staphylococcus, diphtheria and chemical irritation. The risk of acquiring gonococcal ophthalmia neonatorum from infected mother is 10%. The signs of infection appear on 3rd day. There is profuse mucopurulent discharge, conjunctival congestion and edema. Corneal perforation leading to blindness can occur (*see* Chapter 14).

Diagnosis: Microscopy: Specimen should be collected using rayon or polyester swabs. A Gram stain of the smear will demonstrate intracellular gram-negative diplococci. The specificity is 95% in male urethra but only 40–60% in endocervical smears. It is not recommended in prepubescent age group. Culture is the gold standard test and indicated in all females, prepubescent children, and for pharyngeal and rectal infection. Samples are taken from vagina, urethra, pharynx and rectum. Multiplex PCR for both *Neisseria gonorrhoeae* and *Chlamydia trachomatis* is available.

Treatment: Uncomplicated: Ceftriaxone 125 mg IM or cefixime 400 mg orally or ciprofloxacin 500 mg orally single dose or spectinomycin 2 gm IM single dose or Levofloxacin 250 mg orally. Worldwide quinolone resistance is reported and ceftriaxone 250 mg dose is recommended by National AIDS Control Organization. Concomitant *C. trachomatis* treatment should be given if screening is not carried out. *Complicated infection* ceftriaxone 1 gm IM or IV every 24 hours or cefotaxime 1 gm IV 8 hourly or levofloxacin 250 mg IV daily or Spectinomycin 2 g IM every 12 hours. After 48 hours of clinical improvement, oral cefixime 400 mg every 12 hours should be administered to complete 7 days. Infants: Ceftriaxone 25–50 mg/kg, IV or IM in single dose, not to exceed 125 mg. In complication give ceftriaxone for 7 to 14 days. *Ophthalmia neonatorum* prophylaxis is carried out by the instillation of a prophylactic agent like silver nitrate 1% solution, erythromycin 0.5% ointment or tetracycline 1% ophthalmic ointment in a single dose into the eyes of all newborns. The efficacy against chlamydial eye disease is unknown and colonization at other sites is not treated but it is recommended in populations with inadequate prenatal care.

Lymphogranuloma Venereum

LGV is caused by *C. trachomatis* serotypes L1, L2, and L3. LGV is prevalent in less developed countries and is rarely reported in children or early adolescence. The age group affected is 15–40 years. The clinical course of LGV is divided into primary, secondary and tertiary stages. *Primary:* After an incubation period of 5 to 21 days, a small painless papule associated with urethritis or cervicitis develops. The lesion heals without scarring within a week. *Secondary:* Inguinal syndrome This occurs 1 to 6 weeks after healing of primary lesion. There is painful, suppurative inguinal lymphadeno-pathy accompanied by fever, malaise and arthralgia. These fluctuant, tender glands (buboes) may ulcerate and lead to sequel. *Tertiary:* The complications can include perirectal abscess, fistula, strictures and stenosis of the rectum, chronic ulcerations, elephantiasis and gross distortion of the penis (saxophone penis) and esthiomene in females.

Treatment: Lymphogranuloma venereum: Doxycycline 100 mg twice a day for 21 days or erythromycin base 500 mg four times a day for 21 days. The buboes may require aspiration through intact skin. *Urethritis and cervicitis: Regimen for adults and children ≥ 8 years:* Azithromycin 1 g single dose or doxycycline 100 mg twice a day for 7 days or erythromycin base 500 mg orally four times a day for 7 days or levofloxacin 500 mg once a day for 7 days. *Infants:* Erythromycin base 50 mg/kg/day orally divided into 4 doses daily for 14 days.

Herpes Simplex Virus (*See* Section 14.8)

Anogenital Warts (Condyloma Acuminatum)

There are over 100 different HPV genotypes isolated till date, and more than 40 infect the epithelial and mucosa lining (*see* Section 14.8). HPV strains can be classified into low risk (HPV 6 and 11) and high risk (HPV 16 and 18) for causing malignancy. HPV types are known to cause carcinoma of cervix, vulva, anus, penis and oropharynx. Ninety percent of external genital warts are caused by HPV 6 and 11. Most children present with asymptomatic, clusters of flat, papillomatous or pedunculated lesions and occasionally cauliflower type masses. The perianal site is most commonly involved occurring in 37% girls and 57% boys. Other sites of involvement include labia and hymen or vestibular fossa in females and penis and scrotum in males. HPV 6 and 11 are detected in 40–90% lesions. Some children may complain of itching, pain and bleeding. Laryngeal papilloma is the most common tumor of the larynx in childhood. The mean age of diagnosis is 4 years and it manifests as progressive hoarseness, stridor and cough. The predominant HPV type is HPV 6 and 11. Multiple surgeries may be required for treatment. Spontaneous resolution of pediatric condyloma occurs in more than half of cases in 5 years. The treatment options are summarized in Table 30.2. HPV vaccine is used as a preventive measure, *see* Section 40.11. The lesions (genital warts and HIV) are larger, respond poorly to therapy, recur frequently and have higher progression to dysplasia and squamous cell carcinoma.

Trichomoniasis

Trichomoniasis is caused by *Trichomonas vaginalis*, a flagellate protozoan. The incubation period is 4 to 28 days. About 50% of women are asymptomatic. Symptomatic women present with vulvovaginitis; an itchy, copious, homogenous, maldourous, yellow green discharge. Strawberry cervix is present due to punctuate hemorrhages. There may be associated abdominal pain, regional lymphadenitis, endometritis or salpingitis. Reproductive complications include premature rupture of membranes, preterm labor and puerperal infection. Infection is rare before puberty due to the absence of glycogen and the alkaline vaginal pH. In men the infection may be asymptomatic or present with urethritis and urethral discharge. It is

Table 30.2: Treatment of HPV lesions		
Surgery	Scalpel, curette, scissors (snip)	Pedunculated warts
	Electrosurgical	
	Laser therapy	Laryngeal papilloma
Destructive	Cryotherapy	Mucosal and genital warts
	Photodynamic therapy	Laryngeal papilloma
Anti-proliferative agents	Podophyllotoxin 0.5%, Podophyllin 20%	Warts
Antiviral	Cidofovir	Anogenital, mucosal, laryngeal papilloma
Immunotherapies	Imiquimod 5%	
Interferon	Anogenital	
laryngeal papilloma		

reported to cause 1–17% of cases of non-chlamydial non-gonococcal urethritis. The complications can include balanoposthitis, urethral stricture, epididymitis and infertility. It increases risk of HIV transmission.

Diagnosis: Direct wet mount microscopic examination of smears from vaginal and urethral discharge or urine has subjective interpretation and a sensitivity range of 42 to 92%. Culture is the gold standard test. PCR has a sensitivity of 84% and 94% specificity. It is especially useful if urine is used as specimen. A nucleic acid probe test that evaluates for *T. vaginalis*, *G. vaginalis* and *C. albicans* is available.

Treatment: Metronidazole 2 g orally, single dose or Tinidazole 2 g orally, single dose, or metronidazole 500 mg orally twice a day for 7 days. In Children metronidazole is given 30 mg/kg/day in 3 doses for 7 days. Sex partners, if available, should be treated.

Hadlich SF, Kohl PK. Sexually transmitted diseases in children: A practical approach. *Dermatol Clin* 1998;16:859–61.

Joyee AG, Thyagarajan SP, Sowmya B, Venkatesan C, Ganapathy M. Need for specific and routine strategy for the diagnosis of genital chlamydial infection among patients with sexually transmitted diseases in India. *Indian J Med Res* 2003; 118:152–7.

Krause W, Happle R. Sexually transmitted diseases. In: Schachner LA, Hansen RC (eds). *Pediatric Dermatology*. 2nd edn. New York: Churchill Livingstone, 1995;1393–1443.

Murugan S. Sexually transmitted disease in children. In: Sharma VK (Ed). *Sexually Transmitted Diseases and AIDS*. 1st edn. New Delhi: Viva Books Pvt. Ltd., 2003;353–60.

Sharma RC. Sexually transmitted infections in neonates and infants. In: Kumar B, Gupta S (eds). *Sexually Transmitted Infections*. 1st edn. New Delhi: Elsevier, 2005;897–908.

30.9 NEVI, VASCULAR DISORDERS

NEVI

A nevus can be defined as a circumscribed lesion of skin and/or neighboring mucosae, which is permanent or at least very long lasting and which is not neoplastic. Nevi generally are a result of genetic mosaicism. They can be classified according to their origin from epidermal or dermal structures.

Epidermal nevi are hamartomatous lesions arising from the embryonic ectoderm. They generally present as linear streaks and swirls over body as they are a result of genetic mosaicism. This characteristic pattern is known as lines of Blaschko. They may be keratinocyte nevi, follicular nevi, sebaceous nevi, apocrine nevi or eccrine nevi. *Becker's nevus* is of fairly common occurrence, seen more in males, first becoming apparent at puberty. It generally starts of as an irregular pigmented area over shoulder, chest or scapular region, which goes on to develop thickening and increased hair growth. Once present, the nevus tends to persist indefinitely.

Dermal and subcutaneous nevi are classified on the basis of their predominant constituents, into connective tissue nevi, smooth muscle nevi, fat nevi or vascular nevi.

Vascular Nevi may be of two main types, hemangiomas or vascular malformations.

Infantile Hemangiomas

Infantile hemangiomas are benign, proliferative vascular tumors that appear during the first months of life. Infantile hemangiomas are the commonest tumors of infancy with 90% becoming visible within first month of life and 100% by nine months. *Superficial hemangiomas* are commonly first seen as a macular area of hyperemia or pallor which goes on to develop soft, domed, lobed swellings of scarlet red color. *Deep infantile* hemangiomas are seen as soft, warm, round bluish masses which give the feeling of bag of worms. *Mixed hemangiomas* are the ones having both a superficial and deep component. Virtually 100% of infantile hemangiomas undergo spontaneous regression with age. An early onset of resolution is associated with more rapid disappearance and superior cosmetic result. Resolution is heralded by softening of the lesion and appearance of pinkish grey areas in the centre which gradually coalesce. In larger lesions, areas of atrophy or telangiectasia may remain even after complete resolution. Still larger lesions may leave areas of loose, redundant skin.

Treatment: For infantile hemangiomas the best treatment policy is that of 'wait and watch', especially for the lesions where a good cosmetic result can be predicted and complications are unlikely to happen. However, all actively growing lesions need periodic and close supervision. Various indications for treatment include: 1. Hemangioma causing or threatening tissue loss secondary to ulceration, 2. Airway or feeding obstruction, 3. Interference with important structures like eye, and 4. Significant cosmetic handicap.

1. *Systemic corticosteroids:* Oral prednisolone, given in a daily dose of 2–5 mg/kg for 4–8 weeks is the treatment of choice for most cases. However, it is effective only during the proliferative phase of the hemangioma. The dose is gradually reduced over a period of several weeks. If no response is seen over 3–4 weeks, this approach may be abandoned. **2.** *Intralesional corticosteroids:* Rapid shrinkage, especially in eyelid lesions can be produced by 2–3 treatments with intralesional corticosteroids, given at 6 weeks interval. 3. *Laser therapy.* 4. *Compression* *therapy:* It can be used to provide temporary reduction of bulk or for accessible cutaneous lesions. **5. *Surgical excision:*** Most common indication for surgical excision is redundant folds of skin after the resolution of hemangioma. **6. *Embolization:*** Hepatic hemangiomas or those with high output cardiac failure can be dealt with embolization of the feeder vessel. **7. *Sclerosant injection:*** The use of sodium citrate 30%, monoethanolamine oleate 5%, glucose 30%, metallic magnesium, polidocanol 3% and other such sclerosing agents is particularly of value in treating lesions which are not regressing any further or are very large and deep. **8. *Interferon α-2a:*** They are effective only during the proliferative phase and the cost of therapy is prohibitive.

Vascular Malformations

1. ***Salmon patch:*** Lesions are in the form of irregular dull areas over nape of neck and other facial areas. They fade rapidly over the first year, though nuchal and lumbosacral lesions may persist.

2. ***Port wine stain (Nevus flammeus):*** This is a capillary vascular malformation. Face is the most common site but lesions may be present on other parts as well. Leptomeningeal vascular abnormality is clinically manifest in the form of seizures, hemiplegia and progressive neurological deterioration. Portwine stains particularly those on the face have cosmetic significance and hence a profound psychological impact.

3. ***Cutis marmorata telangiectatica congenita:*** It is a combined capillary and venous vascular malformation. Generally presents as a flat or depressed area of reticulate erythema of variable extent, producing a marbled effect. Atrophy of subcutaneous fat is seen in many lesions. A wide variety of other congenital anomalies may be associated, e.g. limb defects, developmental delay, spina bifida, patent ductus arteriosus.

4. ***Blue rubber bleb nevus syndrome:*** It is a venous vascular malformation of skin, gastrointestinal tract and other sites. Cutaneous lesions are multiple compressible, blue or purple, soft rubbery nodules with a wrinkled surface. They may occur virtually anywhere on skin and are often spontaneously painful, particularly at night. They may be present at birth or may appear progressively during early childhood. Analogous lesions affect the gastrointestinal mucosa where they may bleed or cause obstruction. They may affect virtually any other organ of body or tend to remain the same throughout life. Treatment involves symptomatic treatment of complications like anemia. Resection of heavily involved lengths of bowel or endoscopic cauterization may also be done.

Habif TP. Vascular tumors and malformations. In: Habif TP (Ed). *Clinical Dermatology: A color guide to diagnosis and therapy.* 4th edn. Pennsylvania, USA: Mosby, 2004; 814–824.

Paller AS and Mancini AJ. Cutaneous tumors and tumors syndrome. In: Paller AS, Mancini AJ (eds). *Hurwitz clinical and pediatric dermatology.* 3rd edn. Elsevier: Saunders, 2006; 205–245.

30.10 DISEASES OF THE SKIN APPENDAGES

Appendages like *hair, nails* and *sweat glands* are an integral part of the skin. The appendages may be involved in a variety of diseases that affect the skin, and may be involved in systemic diseases as well.

Disorders of Hair

Ectodermal dysplasia: (a) *Hypohidrotic/anhidrotic ectodermal dysplasia* can be both sex-linked and autosomal dominant. It is seen in male patients. Children affected by this disorder have hypotrichosis, with sparse, fine and twisted terminal hair. Dentition is absent or abnormal with absent sweat glands. (b) *Hidrotic ectodermal dysplasia* is autosomal dominant in nature. There is generalized hypotrichosis with sparse, fine, blonde, and brittle hair. Teeth and sweat glands are normal. There may be hyperkeratosis of palms and soles.

Alopecia areata: This common disorder is believed to be autoimmune and characterized by well defined, oval, or rounded patches of hair loss. Disease may be associated with other autoimmune diseases like thyroid disease, vitiligo and inflammatory bowel disease. Atopic dermatitis may be associated with many cases of alopecia areata. Clinically the lesions are round or oval bald patches with normal skin in the patch. Depending upon the clinical pattern may have three variants: Alopecia areata—characterized by patchy hair loss, Alopecia totalis—hair loss involves the entire scalp, Alopecia universalis—involves the whole body. In oophiasis pattern hair loss occurs along the nape of the neck and scalp margins. Nail changes in the form of fine pitting and trachyonychia may be present. Early age of onset, oophiasis pattern, positive family history, association with other autoimmune diseases are bad prognostic signs for this disease.

Treatment: Intralesional therapy is particularly useful for localized disease with a few patches. Injection triamcinolone acetomide is administered with 30 gauge needle in concentration of 2.5–5/mg, 1–2 mm apart repeated after 4–6 weeks. Improvement can be seen after 4–6 weeks. Topical steroids (mid to super potent) creams are applied twice a day for 6–12 weeks. Topical sensitizers like squaric acid dibutyl ester (SADE) or diphenyl cyclopropenone (DPCP) should be used in children above 10 years of age with minimum 50% involvement of scalp. Topical anthralin has been used in varying concentrations either as short contact therapy or for overnight treatment. Topical minoxidil 2–5% is also used. PUVA therapy has also been found to be useful in some cases of alopecia areata, though it cannot be used in children below 10 years of age. Systemic steroids are recommended for extensive cases with rapid onset, this modality is associated with high relapse rate on withdrawal of steroids.

Trichotillomania: It is due to probably some underlying psychiatric problem that manifests, as compulsive habit of pulling hair. In young children 2–6 years, the condition develops as harmless hair pulling tic and tends to occur when child is studying, watching TV or before he goes to sleep. In adolescents or adults it is an obsessive compulsive disorder. It is compulsive desire to pluck hair in the frontal or fronto temporal region resulting in patchy hair loss in bizarre pattern. Females outnumber males. A hair ball (trichobezoar) may be rare accompaniment of trichotillomania in those who eat plucked hair. The condition is self limiting. Young children does not require any treatment. Trichotillomania in adolescents is a difficult condition to treat. Help of a psychologist or psychiatrist should be sought for behavioral problem. Drugs like clomipranine and neuroleptic agents are helpful in some cases.

Nail Disorders

Paronychia is infection of periungual tissues particularly the nail folds. Paronychia can be acute or chronic. Acute paronychia is usually due to Staphylococcus, can also occur as a complication of chronic paronychia. Chronic paronychia is usually seen in individuals whose profession demands prolonged wetting of hands. It can also be seen in children and most cases in children are due to finger or thumb sucking. Any finger may be involved, most often index and middle fingers of right hand and the middle finger of left hand are involved. Common organisms responsible for chronic paronychia are Staphylococcus, Streptococcus and Candida. The condition is characterized by painful, erythmatous induration of proximal and lateral nail folds. Inflammation adjacent to nail matrix, disturbs nail growth that results in surface irregularities of nail plate. Treatment consists of removal of predisposing factors, i.e. to keep hands dry and avoid repeated wetting. Topical application of combination of steroid and antifungal agents is helpful.

Ingrowing toe nail is common problem in infancy, childhood and teens. In this condition the edge of the nail plate penetrates into lateral nail fold resulting in pain, sepsis and there may be formation of granulation tissue. Great toes are commonly affected. The deformity results mainly from the compression of the toe due to ill fitting shoe wear. Cutting of toe nail in half circle instead of straight line may be contributing factor. Rarely the condition may be congenital. Complications of ingrowing toe nail include secondary infection often with pseudomonas and resulting paronychia. Treatment of ingrowing toe nail may be difficult and prolonged. In uncomplicated cases packing with sterile cotton will do the needful. If there is presence of granulation tissue, silver nitrate cauterization is to be done. Patient should be instructed to cut nail in a straight line instead of semicircle, should wear wide shoes. Cases of severe superadded infection are treated with appropriate antibiotics. If conservative measures fail, operative intervention in the form of removal of nail plate with phenolization of the relevant part of nail matrix may be required. Rarely total nail avulsion is needed.

Onychogryposis is due to hypertrophy on the nails, which may result from trauma, infection or peripheral vascular disorders. The nail plate is thickened and may resemble claws.

Diseases of the Sweat Glands

Out of various diseases of sweat glands like hypohydrosis, hyperhidrosis, chromhidrosis and bromhidrosis and miliaria; miliaria is most commonly seen in infancy and childhood.

Miliaria: Miliaria occurs due to occlusion of eccrine sweat ducts and is common in hot and humid climate. Due to occlusion, normal secretion of sweat is prevented and due to back pressure sweat gland or duct ruptures. Depending upon level of obstruction of sweat glands, 3 different types of miliaria are recognized.

Miliaria crystallina: It is characterized by small, clear and very superficial vesicles with no surrounding erythema or inflammation. Condition is accentuated in folds. It can be congenital or develop in first few weeks of life; it can also follow sun burn. In this case level of obstruction is subcorneal or intracorneal. Lesions are self limiting. Generally no treatment is required for miliaria crystallina.

Miliaria rubra (prickly heat): This condition is common in febrile, overheated infants or in hot weather. Lesions are discrete, generally extremely pruritic 1–3 mm non follicular papules, vesicles, or papules with an erythmatous base. Condition is accentuated in intertrignous areas. In this case obstruction is intraepidermal. Treatment is avoidance of excessive heat and occlusion. Light clothing is recommended. Cool bath and air conditioning are useful. Topical calamine lotion is soothing.

Miliaria profunda: This is characterized by skin colored, erythmatous papules or pustules. It can prevent adequate sweating leading to hyperthermia in older children. Obstruction is at dermo epidermal junction.

Miliaria pustulosa: This special variant of miliaria is due to preceding dermatitis that has produced injury, destruction or blockade of the sweat glands. Lesions in this case are distinct, superficial, non pururitic pustules in the flexors, and in intertrignous areas. Usually the lesions are sterile but may contain non pathogenic cocci.

Mallory SB, Bree A, Chern P (eds). *Illustrated Manual of Pediatric dermatology: Diagnosis and management.* 2nd edn. New York: Taylor and Francis Group: 2005; 1–220.

Paller AS, Mancini AJ. Disorders of hair and nails. In: Paller AS, Mancini AJ (eds). *Hurwitz Clinical Pediatric Dermatology: A Textbook of Skin Disorders of Childhood and Adolesecence.* 3rd edn. Philadelphia: Elsevier, 2006; 145–205.

Silverman R. Nail and appendageal abnormalities. In: Schachner LA, Hansen RC (eds). *Pediatric Dermatology.* 2nd edn. Vol 1. New York: Churchill Livingstone, 1995; 615–660.

30.11 BACTERIAL INFECTIONS

Impetigo is a common superficial, contagious, pyogenic infection affecting pre-school and school going children. Impetigo may occur primarily on normal skin or may complicate wounds, insect bites, or other dermatosis like scabies, pediculosis, varicella and atopic dermatitis. Bullous impetigo and non-bullous impetigo are two different clinical presentations. Bullous impetigo (Impetigo bullosa) is caused by *coagulase positive Staphylococcus aureus (most common group II phage 71), rarely by S. pyogenes.* Non-bullous impetigo (impetigo contagiosa), common clinical form, caused by Streptococcal, *Staphylococcus,* or by both. *S. aureus* may be a secondary invader in *Streptococcal* impetigo. Face and extremities are most commonly affected. *Treatment:* Adequate cleaning of the lesion along with gentle removal of crust is important. Topical antibiotic—Mupirocin (1%) or fusidic acid (2%) has been shown to be as effective as systemic antibiotic. Systemic antibiotic is administered for widespread infection—dicloxacillin (25–50 mg/kg/day) in four divided doses, cephalexin (25–50 mg/kg/day), azithromycin (5–10 mg/kg/day) or erythromycin (30–50 mg/kg/day). Treatment of impetigo does not alter risk for acute glomerulonephritis. Nasal carriage may lead to recurrence which can be reduced by applying mupirocin in the nares.

Ecthyma is characterized by deep ulcerative infection with a thick overlying crust. Ecthyma is a distinct ulcerative infection caused mainly by *Group A beta hemolytic Streptococcus. S. aureus* has also been isolated. The infection affects both the epidermis and the dermis. It begins as a vesicle that evolves into a vesico-pustule. It later forms a thick crust the removal of which reveals a deep, punched out, pus filled ulcer. Lesions are painful and often associated with lymphadenopathy; surrounding cellulitis may also be seen. The lesions heal with scarring. Shins and the dorsa of feet are most common sites to be affected. *Treatment:* Oral penicillin in dose of 50 mg/kg/day in four divided doses given for 10–14 days. Other antibiotics which may be administered include long acting benzathine penicillin, oral erythromycin, clindamycin and cephalosporins. Local cleansing and application of topical mupirocin may speed reepithelization.

Erysipelas is a form of superficial cellulitis involving the dermis and the superficial subcutaneous tissue. The superficial lymphatics may be involved. Causative organisms include *Group A beta hemolytic Streptococcus, Streptococcus pneumoniae, H. influenzae* and rarely *Staphylococcus, Aeromonas* and *Pseudomonas.* Characteristic lesion is a well demarcated, raised plaque with rapidly advancing margins. Hallmark sign is a well defined, raised edge. Local edema, tenderness, sometimes with a peau' de orange and superficial bulla formation may be present. Constitutional symptoms like high grade fever, chills, headache, arthralgia, myalgia may occur. Site may be surgical wound, umbilicus in neonate, face and lower limbs are the most commonly affected. *Treatment:* Cultures (blood and pus) are advised for finding the causative organism and then directing appropriate antibiotic therapy. Mild and limited disease: Oral broad spectrum antibiotics like penicillin, cephalosporins and erythromycin. In extensive disease: Hospitalization and intravenous antibiotic are advised. Intravenous ciprofloxacin (20–30 mg/kg/day), ticarcillin (200–300 mg/kg/day), teicoplanin, or imipenem/cilastatin (60–100 mg/kg/day) should be considered. Bed rest, limb elevation, and warm compresses add to patient comfort and speed of resolution.

Cellulitis is deeper inflammation of the dermis and the subcutaneous tissue. It is characterized with ill defined margins. It may involve intact skin or may occur secondary to surgical wounds, trauma, tinea infections or ulcerations. Most common implicated organisms *Group A beta hemolytic Streptococcus, S. aureus, H. influenzae, S. pneumoniae.* Other organisms include *E.coli, Proteus, Enterobacter aerogenes, Pasturella,*

Pseudomonas and *Clostridium*. Cellulitis is an acute, subacute or chronic painful, erythematosus inflammation of the dermis and the subcutaneous tissue. Clinically characterized by increased temperature, erythema, edema and advancing borders. Legs, digits, face, feet, hand, buttocks are commonly involved. Cellulitis may extend superficially and erysipelas deeper, so that the two conditions may coexist. Constitutional symptoms are present and the total leukocyte count is elevated. *Treatment:* Empirical therapy with penicillinase resistant penicillin, first generation cephalosporin, amoxicillin-clavulanate, fluoroquinolone and macrolide are appropriate. Benzyl penicillin 450,000–500,000 U/kg/day is given for at least 10 days. In immunocompromised patients, known diabetics, patients not responding to conventional antibiotics second generation cephalosporins (along with aminoglycoside) are considered. *Adjunctive therapy* includes cold compresses, analgesics for associated pain, and immobilization and elevation of the affected extremity. Limited disease may respond to oral antibiotics but, in case of extensive involvement intravenous antibiotic should be administered.

Folliculitis refers to inflammation around the pilo-sebaceous unit. It is classified according to depth of involvement and origin into superficial and deep folliculitis. Inflammation may result from Gram positive organisms (predominantly *Staphylococcal*), and Gram negative bacteria. It may occur secondarily due to irritation or injury. Common sites include scalp, back and extremities. Non-infective folliculitis occurs as a complication of occlusive therapy after use of emollients, plastic occlusion or wet dressings. It may also be as a result of injury, abrasion, waxing, and exposure to chemicals, mineral oil, tars or complication of occlusive therapy. Beard and neck are the most common sites to get involved. *Treatment:* Removal of the inciting factors. Good hygiene and topical antibacterials like mupirocin are usually successful. Oral anti staphylococcal antibiotics are indicated for recurrent lesions and cases not responding to topical therapy.

Sycosis barbae is a subacute or chronic pyogenic infection involving the entire hair follicle usually associated with scarring. Males in the third to fourth decade are commonly affected. Occurs mainly in the shaved beard or scalp. *S. aureus* and *dermatophytide* have both been isolated. Follicle is packed with neutrophils, which also infiltrate the wall. A chronic granulomatous infiltrate in which lymphocyte, plasma cells, histiocytes and foreign body giant cells are present. *Treatment:* Subacute forms are clinically controlled by topical antibiotics, but tend to relapse when the topical antibiotics are stopped. If the nasal swab is positive, the antibiotic is to be applied to the nares. In chronic forms, the response may be enhanced by using antibiotic steroid combination. In resistant cases, systemic antibiotics given for 10–14 days may be tried.

Furuncle is a deeper infection of the hair follicle caused by *coagulase positive S. aureus*. Predisposing factors include maceration caused by friction and sweating, cutaneous injury and abrasions. It may result in firm, painful, fluctuant mass walled off with purulent material. Begins as tender, follicular nodule, which is firm initially, later develops suppuration and becomes fluctuant. Central necrosis develops and the lesions drains to leave a violaceous macule followed by a scar. Lesions may be solitary or multiple. Face, neck, arms, wrists, buttocks, anogenital region and fingers are the most commonly affected sites.

Carbuncle: Coalescence of closely spaced furuncles may result in a broad, erythematous, swollen, tender mass termed carbuncle. It is associated with intense inflammatory changes in the underlying connective tissue, including the subcutaneous fat. Predisposing conditions include diabetes mellitus, skin occlusion, mechanical damage, HIV, atopy and scabies. Gram stain reveals gram positive cocci and cultures reveal *S. aureus*. *Treatment:* Warm compresses. Systemic anti-staphylococcal antibiotics include penicillinase resistant penicillin like cloxacillin (50–100 mg/kg/day), first generation cephalosporins given in three to four divided doses. Topical antibiotics have an adjuvant role with systemic therapy. Diabetes and other underlying conditions should be ruled out.

Staphylococcal scalded skin syndrome (SSSS) is a generalized blistering and peeling skin condition caused by **exfoliation** toxin producing *S. aureus*. Mostly seen in children less than 5 years of age, rarely in adults. At the onset of the disease, a history/clinical evidence of purulent pharyngitis, conjunctivitis, rhinitis, wound infection is usually present. A macular erythema is noticed around the lips and nose; the eruption later becomes generalized developing a sandpaper quality. Flexures are more involved. The skin develops a wrinkled appearance and peels off in large sheets. Mucosa is usually uninvolved. Over 2–3 days the skin that peels dries and crusts. Complete recovery takes 2–3 weeks. Now that the condition is well recognized and can be easily treated, the mortality is low. SSSS should be differentiated from staphylococcal scalded fever, Kawasaki disease, and TSS (toxic shock syndrome). *Treatment:* Supportive measures—sterile sheets, use of cradle, analgesia, intravenous fluids. Minimal handling is advised because of the extreme skin tenderness. Penicillinase resistant antibiotics reduce the risk of septic complications and spread to other children. Though, it does not significantly alter the course of the disease when started late. Systemic steroids are contraindicated.

Streptococcal toxic shock syndrome: Fever, myalgia and flu like symptoms are associated with pain in the legs and the extremities. A rash followed by desquamation, circulatory shock and multi-system disease characterize this syndrome. *Group A Streptococcus* producing pyrogenic exotoxin characterizes this syndrome. The condition is similar to Staphylococcus toxic skin syndrome, except that it has a high mortality. Surgical wounds, throat infections, wound infections due to *Group A Streptococcus* may be followed by Streptococcus toxic shock syndrome. ***Diagnosis:*** Swabs from site of infection are positive for Streptococcus; cultures are also frequently positive. Treatment: Systemic penicillin, erythromycin, clindamycin may be administered. Debridement may be required in necrotizing infections.

Hay RJ, Adrians BM. Bacterial infections. In: Burns T, Breathnach S, Cox N, Griffiths C (eds). Rook's Textbook of Dermatology, 7th Edition. Vol 2. London: Blackwell Science, 2004; 27.1–27.85.

30.12 FUNGAL INFECTIONS

Dermatophytosis: Superficial fungal infections in children are usually caused by dermatophytes; *Trichophyton, Microsporu* and *Epidermophyton.* Dermatophytic infections are commonly referred to as ringworm, or tinea.

Tinea capitis (synonyms: ringworm of the scalp) is a form of superficial mycosis affecting the skin of the scalp, eyebrows, and eyelashes. Mode of spread is from person-to-person transmission (through combs, brushes, couches, and sheets).

Clinical manifestations: T. capitis has different clinical presentations:

i. **Grey patch**—characterized by well defined round/oval patch of partial alopecia. It is commonly caused by *Microsporum* and produces yellow-green fluorescence under Wood's light examination.

ii. **Black dot**—when the hairs are black, this result in the appearance of black dots. *T. tonsurans* is the commonest pathogen.

iii. **Inflammatory type**—the lesions range from pustular folliculitis to kerion. **Kerion** begins as small furuncles, which enlarge and becomes inflamed giving rise to boggy swelling. Follicular abscesses develop and pus may exude from multiple sites. The active inflammation generally lasts from 5 weeks to 5 months. Occasionally there is residual scarring alopecia. Systemic manifestations include adenopathy, fever, and malaise.

Favus is another type of inflammatory type caused by *T. schoenleinii* and is characterized by the formation of scutula. These cup-shaped, yellow crusts form within the hair follicles and are composed of hyphae, epidermal cells and neutrophils.

Differential diagnosis: Tinea capitis infection is to be differentiated from alopecia areata, folliculitis decalvans, discoid lupus erythematosus, psoriasis, seborrheic dermatitis.

Treatment: Systemic treatment is required. Oral griseofulvin (15–25 mg/kg/day) for 6–12 weeks is the gold standard treatment and only FDA approved for the condition. Alternative systemic drugs are oral terbinafine (5 mg/kg/d) for 2–4 wks, fluconazole (6 mg/kg/d), itraconazole (5 mg/kg/d) for 2–4 weeks. Adjunctive therapy—periodic use of ketoconazole shampoo to help reduce shedding of infected hair and prevent its spread.

Tinea corporis is a superficial dermatophyte infection characterized by inflammatory or noninflammatory lesions on the glabrous skin, i.e. skin regions except the scalp, groin, palms, and soles. Three genera cause dermatophytoses: *Trichophyton, Microsporum,* and *Epidermophyton.* The lesion begins as an erythematous, scaly plaque that may rapidly worsen and enlarge. Following central resolution, the lesion may become annular in shape. Scale, crust, vesicles, and papules often develop, especially in the advancing border. ***Treatment:*** It comprises topical and systemic therapy. *Topical therapy* is recommended for a localized infection. The topical azoles (fungistatic), e.g. econazole, ketoconazole, clotrimazole, miconazole, oxiconazole, sulconazole, sertaconazole and topical allylamines (e.g. naftifine, terbinafine) may be used. *Systemic therapy* is indicated for extensive infection, in immunocompromised patients, or is patients refractory to topical therapy. Systemic therapy includes Griseofulvin in dose of 10 mg/kg/day for 4–8 weeks; systemic azoles—fluconazole (50–100 mg/day or 150 mg once weekly for 2–4 weeks), itraconazole (100 mg/day for 2 weeks, 200 mg/d for 1 week); oral terbinafine (250 mg/day for 2–4 weeks).

Tinea cruris is a pruritic superficial fungal infection of the groin and adjacent skin. *T rubrum* (most common), *E. floccosum, T. verrucosum* and *T. mentagrophytes* are commonly identified. Contagious infection is transmitted by fomites or by autoinoculation from a reservoir on the hands or feet. Clinically it is characterized by large patches of erythema with central clearing; sharply marginated scale centered on the inguinal creases and extends distally down the medial aspects of the thighs and proximally to the lower abdomen and pubic area. In acute infections, the rash may be moist and exudative. Chronic infections typically are dry with a popular, annular or arciform border and barely perceptible scale at the margin. Central areas typically are hyperpigmented and contain a scattering of erythematous papules and a little scale. Secondary changes of excoriation, lichenification, and impetiginization may be present as a result of pruritus. Chronic infections modified by the application of topical corticosteroids are more erythematous, less scaly, and may have follicular pustules. *Treatment:* In uncomplicated infection— topical antifungal agents such as imidazoles or allylamines are effective. For extensive or recalcitrant infection, systemic antifungal are required.

Tinea pedis, ringworm of the foot is common in tropical climates and in the summer. The infection is mostly bilateral and recurrences are common. The fungus is usually acquired from infected socks, shoes, games-kit or towels, and is easily picked up from wet floor-boards. Causative organisms are *T. interdigitale*, *T. rubrum* and *E. floccosum*.

Three clinical types are known: i. *Interdigital type* (commonest). The skin between the toes (particularly, the fourth and fifth) is sodden, white and macerated; ii. *Vesicular type*—affects the sides of the toes and the backs of the feet; and iii. *Hyperkeratotic type*—thickened and scaly lesions on the sides of the feet and the heel. Treatment: Reduction of moisture is essential—(careful drying after bath, frequent changing of cotton socks, use of ventilated footwear) are recommended. Topical antifungal creams and powders help in controlling the infection. Recurrence is diminished by courses of oral antifungals for 4–6 weeks. Long-standing cases may need oral antifungals for 2–3 months. In hyperkeratotic type, antifungal applications should be combined with keratolytic preparations (e.g. salicylic acid).

Tinea mannum is a dermatophyte infection of the hand. The infection often is unilateral and is virtually always associated with bilateral involvement of the feet. Tinea mannum also may involve the fingernails. The clinical presentation is similar to vesicular and hyperkeratotic types of tinea pedis. Treatment includes similar general measures, topical and systemic treatment as administered for tinea pedis.

Tinea faciei is a superficial dermatophyte infection limited to the glabrous skin of the face. In pediatric and female patients, the infection is seen on any surface of the face, including the upper lip and chin. In men, the condition is known as tinea barbae when infection of bearded areas occurs. Tinea faciei is caused by zoophilic dermatophytes—*T. mentagrophytes* var. *granulosum* and *T. verrucosum* clinically present as inflammatory kerion-like plaques. Inflammatory type which present as an inflamed nodule/ nodules with multiple pustules and draining sinuses on its surface and loose or broken hairs. Non-inflammatory type caused by antropophilic dermatophytes present as erythematous patches with a raised border studded with papules, pustules or crusts and broken hairs. Tinea faciei must be differentiated from bacterial folliculitis, atopic dermatitis, contact dermatitis, seborrheic dermatitis. *Treatment:* Topical antifungal agents alone or in combination with systemic therapy (for chronic and/or multiple lesions) is recommended.

Tinea versicolor is a common, benign, superficial cutaneous fungal infection usually characterized by hypopigmented or hyperpigmented macules and patches on the chest and the back. Tinea versicolor is caused by the dimorphic, lipophilic organism, *Malassezia furfur*. Tinea versicolor can present in three forms: classical, inverse, and follicular. *Classical*— numerous, well-marginated, finely scaly, oval-to-round macules scattered over the trunk, chest, with occasional extension to the abdomen, neck, and proximal extremities. The macules tend to coalesce, forming irregularly shaped patches with pigmentary alteration. As the name versicolor implies, the disease characteristically reveals a variance in skin hue. The involved areas can be either darker or lighter than the surrounding skin. *Inverse*—affects the flexures (face, or isolated areas of the extremities), more often seen in immunocompromised patients. **Follicular**—affects hair follicle, lesions are typically localized to the back, the chest, and the extremities. *Treatment:* The treatment consists of application of *topical agents*— selenium sulfide, sodium sulfacetamide, ciclopiroxolamine, as well as azole and allylamine antifungals, and *oral therapy*—ketoconazole (400 mg weekly for 2 weeks), fluconazole (300 mg weekly), and itraconazole (200 mg daily for 5–7 days).

Onychomycosis refers to a fungal infection that affects the toenails or the fingernails. It may involve any component of the nail unit, including the nail matrix, the nail bed, or the nail plate. *T. rubrum* accounts for 70% and *T. mentagrophytes* accounts for 20% of all cases. Yeasts and nondermatophyte molds account for 8% and 2% of the cases, respectively. *Candida albicans* primarily causes chronic mucocutaneous candidiasis of the nail. Clinical types are i. Distal lateral subungual onychomycosis (DLSO); ii. Endonyx (EO); iii. White superficial onychomycosis (WSO); iv. Proximal subungual onychomycosis (PSO); v. Candidal nail infection; and vi. Total dystrophic onychomycosis (TDO). *Treatment:* Factors that influence the choice of therapy include clinical presentation and severity, current medications and previous therapies for onychomycosis and their response. *Systemic antifungals* are required. Oral griseofulvin for 9–12 months, terbinafine for 6–12 weeks. *Transungual delivery systems* such as amorolfine 5% nail lacquer and ciclopirox olamine 8% nail lacquer are also used.

Candidiasis: Candida is both normal flora and an invasive pathogen. It is a unicellular yeast whose cells reproduce by budding. This organism can flourish in most environments. It frequently colonizes the oropharynx, skin, mucous membranes, and lower respiratory, and gastrointestinal and genitourinary tracts.

Etiology: C. albicans is the most common pathogenic species identified. Other species that are commonly found include *C. glabrata, C. parapsilosis, C. tropicalis,* and *C. krusei.* Risk factors for oral infection include antibiotic use, immunodeficiency, xerostomia, inhaled corticosteroids, and denture use.

Clinical manifestations: Oral candidiasis (thrush) is characterized by creamy curd-like patches on the tongue and oral mucosa. These patches are a pseudomembrane of *Candida,* desquamated epithelial cells, keratin, leukocytes, bacteria, necrotic tissue, and food debris. Symptoms include dry mouth, loss of taste, and occasionally, pain with eating. Chronic atrophic candidiasis, or denture sore mouth, is a chronic inflammatory reaction with epithelial thinning under dental plates. Candidal leukoplakia is firm, white plaques affecting the cheeks, lips, and tongue, which frequently have a protracted course and can be precancerous. Angular cheilitis is characterized as erythema and fissuring at the corners of the mouth.

Cutaneous candidiasis syndromes: 1. **Intertrigo** develops in sites where skin surfaces are apposed. Lesions begin as vesico-pustules that enlarge, rupture, and develop maceration and fissuring. Satellite lesions may be present. 2. **Generalized cutaneous candidiasis** is characterized by widespread eruptions with increased severity in the genitocrural folds, anal region, axillae, and hands and feet. 3. **Candidal paronychia** infection of the nail folds. 4. **Diaper rash.** Skin irritation is exacerbated by wet diapers. 5. **Perianal candidiasis.** Skin maceration and pruritus are frequent with frequent extension to the perineum. 6. **Neonatal invasive candidiasis** occurs with an incidence inversely proportional to birth weight. Candida colonization is found in approximately 30% of infants weighing less than 1500 grams at birth weight. Sources of invasive infection include blood (70%), urine (15%), cerebrospinal fluid (10%), and peritoneal fluid (5%). *C. albicans* and *C. parapsilosis* are the most common species found in neonates. 7. **Candida amnionitis** may occur after prolonged rupture of the membranes in mothers given parenteral

antibiotics. A neonate's skin may have pustules, vesicles, or diffuse erythema. *Treatment:* Mucocutaneous infection typically responds to topical therapy such as nystatin and clotrimazole. Addition of a topical steroid may be required for diaper rash. Intertrigo and diaper rash respond to decreased moisture around the skin.

Hay RJ, Moore MK. Mycology. In: Burns T, Breathnach S, Cox N, Griffiths (eds). *Rook's Textbook of Dermatology.* 7th edn. Vol 2. London: Blackwell Science, 2004;31.1–31.101.

Paller AS, Mancini AJ. Skin disorders due to fungi. In: Paller AS, Mancini AJ (eds). *Hurwitz Clinical Pediatric Dermatology: A Textbook of Skin Disorders of Childhood and Adolesecence.* 3rd edn. Philadelphia: Elsevier, 2006;365–96.

Stein DH. Fungal infections. In: Schachner LA, Hansen RC (eds). *Pediatric Dermatology.* 2nd edn. Vol 2. New York: Churchill Livingstone, 1995;1295–1329.

30.13 VIRAL INFECTIONS OF THE SKIN

Common viral infections mainly involving skin in children are warts, molluscum contagiosum, herpes simplex, varicella, herpes zoster (*see* Chapter 14).

Warts

Warts are caused by human papillomavirus (HPV). HPV is a small DNA virus. The incubation period varies from weeks to over a year. Infection is transmitted from person to person by direct contact through areas of trauma to skin. Anogenital warts are transmitted by sexual contact, though may be acquired at the time of delivery from mother.

Clinical manifestations: Warts can occur at any age, but are unusual in infancy and early childhood. Most commonly occur in school going children. Warts are more common and widespread in patients receiving immunosuppressive drugs and in those with immune deficiency states including lymphoma, chronic lymphocytic leukemia, Hodgkin's disease and human immunodeficiency virus (HIV) infection.

Clinical Types

Common warts (verruca vulgaris): Most commonly caused by HPV type 2, commonly in ages of 12–16 years. Commonest site of involvement is dorsa of fingers and hands but may occur anywhere on the body. Common warts are small, skin colored, hyperkeratotic papules that of size less than 1 mm to 1 cm. Kobner's phenomenon, i.e. appearance of lesions at the site of trauma may be seen. Differential diagnosis: Molluscum contagiosum and hypertrophic lichen planus.

Filiform warts: These are soft, slender, finger like projections mostly seen on the face, scalp and neck.

Plane warts (Verruca plana): Plane warts are mainly caused by HPV 3 and 10, are flesh colored, discrete papules most frequently appearing on the face, neck, external aspect of forearms and hands. There number may vary from 2–3 to many hundreds.

Differential diagnosis: Lichen planus, lichen nitidus, seborrhoeic keratosis, epidermal naevus

Plantar warts: Plantar warts are caused by HPV 1, 2, 4 and 5 to 7. They are hyperkeratotic, firm, flat or elevated lesions. Mostly seen on the pressure points. They can be painful and disrupt the natural lines of skin. Multiple black or red spots can be seen on paring on the surface of warts due to thrombosed capillaries. Confluence of multiple, hyperkeratotic lesions into one group give rise to mosaic appearance. They need to be differentiated from corns and callosities.

Anogenital or venereal warts (Condylomata accuminata): These warts are caused by HPV 6, 11, 16, 18. They can range from asymptomatic lesions to cauliflower like growth on shaft of penis, urethral meatus, preputial opening, scrotal and perineum in males. In females anogenital warts can be situated on labia, vagina or cervix. If anogenital warts are present in prepubertal children, the possibility of sexual abuse must be entertained. Laryngeal papilloma in children less than 3 years of age can be due to HPV infection from the mother during passage through infected birth canal.

Diagnosis is mainly clinical. Histology shows vacuolated epidermal cells (Koilocytes) with hypergranulomatosis and presence of eosinophilic inclusions. PCR (Polymerase chain reaction) and FISH (Fluorescent *in situ* hybridization) are also useful investigations. The use of a colposcope is invaluable in assessing vaginal and cervical lesions. Papanicolaou (Pap) smears prepared from cervical or anal scrapings often show cytologic evidence of HPV infection.

Differential diagnosis: Warts must be distinguished from condylomata lata, a manifestation of secondary syphilis.

Treatment: Choice of treatment depends upon number, size, location of lesions, physician's or patient's preference, convenience, cost, etc.

Common warts: Destruction by light electrodessication and curettage, cryotherapy with liquid N_2. CO_2 laser and pulse dye laser can be used for recalcitrant warts

Plane warts: Wart paint (5–20 % salicylic acid and 5–20% lactic acid in flexible collodion) and tretinoin 0.25% to 0.05% may be particularly useful in plane warts.

Plantar warts: Can be treated with cryosurgery with liquid nitrogen and/or wart paint.

Condylomata accuminata: Various therapeutic modalities have been used such as application of 25% podophyllin in tincture benzoin, TCA, podophyllotoxin, imiquimod and cryosurgery.

Prognosis: With all forms of therapy genital warts commonly recur, and approximately half of children and adolescents require a 2nd or 3rd treatment. Prognosis of cervical disease is better, with 85–90% cure rates after a single treatment.

Prevention: Gradasil, the human papillomavirus vaccine [Quadrivalent human papillomavirus (Types 6, 11, 16, 18); recombinant vaccine] is 98% effective against cervical cancer caused by HPV types 16 and 18. HPV types 16 and 18 cause ~70% of cervical cancers. Three doses of HPV are administered IM on day 1, 2 mo, and 6 mo in women 15 yr to 26 yr.

Molluscum Contagiosum

Molluscum contagiosum is caused by DNA virus; largest known pox virus. Disease is largely confined to human beings though it has also been reported in monkeys. The incubation period varies from 2 weeks to 6 months. Disease is contracted from other people by direct contact or through fomites, and by autoinoculation. Swimming pool outbreaks occur frequently. Atopic children are infected more commonly.

Clinical manifestations: In children face, trunk and extremities are the common sites of involvement. In adults the lesions are mainly seen on lower abdomen and pubic area and may be sexually transmitted. Disease is common in patients with AIDS as an opportunistic infection. Most lesions are asymptomatic. Individual lesions are shiny, pearly white, hemispherical papules with central umbilication. Lesions enlarge slowly and may reach a diameter of 5–10 mm. A minority of patients may have surrounding erythmatous and scaly dermatitis. The lesions in HIV patients are widespread, refractory and may become giant nodules up to 1.5 cm in size, suggesting that cell mediated immunity helps in eliminating the virus. Disease is self limiting with majority of the cases showing spontaneous resolution within span of 9 months, however in some cases lesions may persist for years together.

Diagnosis is mainly clinical. Extraction of keratinous material from a papule and inspection under microscope with Wright's stain or KOH will show characteristic pear shaped molluscum bodies. Differential diagnosis: This includes warts, closed comedons, milia, pyogenic granuloma, and keratoacanthoma.

Treatment: Patients should be advised to avoid swimming pools, communal baths, shared towels, etc. till they are cured of the disease to prevent spread of infection in the community. Treatment modalities like mechanical removal by squeezing out the lesions with forceps, piercing the lesions with orange stick and curettage are very effective but young children dislike them. Topical preparations like TCA 25–50%, silver nitrate 40%, phenol 20% are effective in the treatment of mollusca but should be used under medical supervision. Topical .05 –.1% tretinoin cream, KOH 10–20%, wart paint can be used in children. Topical cidofovir, 5 FU have all been effective in the treatment of recalcitrant molluscum contagiosum. Cryotherapy with liquid nitrogen by spray is very effective and popular modality of treatment. Pulsed dye laser have been reported to be effective for recalcitrant molluscum contagiosum in immunocompromised patients.

HERPES SIMPLEX (*see* Section 14.8)

Frieden IJ, Penneys NS. Viral infections. In: Schachner LA, Hansen RC (eds). *Pediatric Dermatology*. 2nd edn. Vol 2. New York: Churchill Livingstone, 1995;1257–94.

Morelli JG. Cutaneous viral infections. In: Kliegman RM, Behrman RE, Jenson HB, Stanton BF (eds). *Nelson Textbook of Pediatrics*. 18th edn. Vol. 2. Philadelphia: Saunders, 2007; 2751–54.

Moscicki AB. Human papillomaviruses. In: Kliegman RM, Behrman RE, Jenson HB, Stanton BF (eds). *Nelson Textbook of Pediatrics*. 18th edn. Vol. 1. Philadelphia: Saunders, 2007;1402–06.

Sterling JC. Immunobullous diseases. In: Burns T, Breathnach S, Cox N, Griffiths C (eds). *Rook's Textbook of Dermatology*, 8th edn. Vol. 2. London: Blackwell Science, 2010; 33.1– 33.78.

30.14 LEPROSY

Etiology: Leprosy is a chronic granulomatous infection of the skin and peripheral nerves cause by intracellular bacterium Mycobacterium leprae.

Epidemiology: In India the prevalence is less than 1:10000 and the most common type is the pauciba-cillary or PB type. Risk of transmission of leprosy from a marriage partner is only 5% (Conjugal leprosy). Risk of children acquiring infection from infected adults in the family is 60%.

Route of transmission: Main mode of exit is nasal mucosa of untreated cases. Although mode of transmission is still uncertain it seems most likely that *M. leprae* are transmitted via respiratory route. Infection may occur through skin-to-skin (abraded skin) contact with leprosy patients, particularly those at the lepromatous end. Incubation period is 2–7 years (average 3–5 years).

Host response: Most persons exposed to *M. leprae* will not develop leprosy. In susceptible individuals an indeterminate lesion may form. Indeterminate leprosy often spontaneously heals, but it may progress into the leprosy spectrum. The varying clinical forms of leprosy are determined by the underlying immuno-logical response of the host to *M. leprae.*

At one pole, patients with *tuberculoid leprosy* **(TT)** have a high cellular immune response to the mycobacterium, which limits the disease to a few well-defined skin patches or nerve trunks. At the other pole, *lepromatous leprosy* **(LL)** is characterised by the absence of specific cellular immunity but intact immunity to the related *M. tuberculosis*. There is therefore uncontrolled proliferation of leprosy bacilli with many lesions and extensive infiltration of the skin and nerves. Most patients have the intermediate forms of borderline tuberculoid **(BT)**, mid-borderline **(BB)**, and borderline lepromatous **(BL)** leprosy. The *borderline forms* are clinically unstable, and patients either show slow change towards the lepromatous pole or experience sudden type I or reversal reactions.

Clinical Manifestations

Skin involvement: The most common skin lesions are macules or plaques; more rarely papules and nodules are seen. Lesions are hypopigmented in borderline tuberculoid and tuberculoid leprosy, and infiltrated with a raised edge. On pale skins, lesions can appear erythematous. In lepromatous leprosy, diffuse infiltration of the skin commonly occurs. Patients with tuberculoid disease have a few, hypopigmented lesions with reduced sensation, whereas those with lepromatous forms have many lesions, confluent in some cases, and many of them are not hypoaesthetic.

Nerve damage: Damage to the nerves occurs in two settings—peripheral nerve trunks and small dermal nerves. Peripheral nerves are affected in fibro-osseous tunnels near the surface of the skin, including the great auricular nerve (neck), ulnar nerve (elbow), radial-cutaneous nerve (wrist), median nerve (wrist), lateral popliteal nerve (neck of the fibula), and posterior tibial nerve (medial malleolus). The ulnar nerve is the most commonly affected, followed by the median, lateral popliteal and facial nerves. The earliest sensation to be lost is the cold followed by warm sensation, touch and pain. Small dermal sensory and autonomic nerves are affected producing hypoaesthesia and anhidrosis within borderline-tuberculoid and tuberculoid lesions, and glove and stocking sensory loss in lepromatous disease resulting in anesthetic hands and feet. Pure neuritic leprosy presents with asymmetrical involve-ment of peripheral nerve trunks and no visible skin lesions.

Bone involvement: Bone changes occur as a consequence of leprosy neglected over many years, therefore seen rarely in children. In majority bone damage is confined to hands, feet and skull. In hands phalanges undergo slow atrophy and absorption, and the finger shorten, but metacarpals and carpal bones are spared. In the feet the atrophic changes occur in phalanges, metatarsals and tarsal bones. In both hands and feet, the affected bones become thin and pointed as a result of concentric bone atrophy. Various factors responsible for these changes are; repeated trauma to anesthetic hands and feet, disuse osteoporosis, impaired blood and nerve supply and secondary osteomyelitis complicating chronic ulceration of the overlying skin. In the skull, two pathognomonic changes take place; atrophy of a. anterior nasal spine leading to nasal collapse and b. of maxillary alveolar process causing loss of upper central incisor teeth.

Eye involvement: Eye damage results from both nerve damage and direct bacillary invasion. Lagophthalmos results from paresis of the orbicularis oculi caused by involvement of the zygomatic and temporal branches of the facial (VIIth) nerve. Corneal ulceration is a dreaded sequel of unattended ocular leprosy and is better prevented than treated.

Systemic features: These features are seen mainly in lepromatous patients and are due to bacillary infiltration affecting nasal mucosa, bones, and testes. Testicular atrophy results from diffuse infiltration and the acute orchiitis that occurs with ENL reactions. The consequent loss of testosterone leads to azoospermia and gynaecomastia. Renal involvement and amyloidosis are now rarely seen with effective MDT.

Leprosy in children: Most studies have found that 63% are of PB and 37% of MB type in children. The clinicopathological correlation in childhood leprosy is low, at 45–63%. Exposed parts were the most common sites. Nerve involvement is seen in 55% to 70 % of cases.

Diagnosis

Cardinal signs of leprosy. Leprosy is diagnosed by finding at *least one* of the following cardinal signs:

1. Definite loss of sensation in a pale (hypopigmented) or reddish skin patch.
2. A thickened or enlarged peripheral nerve, with loss of sensation and/or weakness of the muscles supplied by that nerve.
3. The presence of acid-fast bacilli in slit skin smears.

Skin smear: Skin slit smears are made from eyebrow, ear lobule, skin lesion if any and from dorsum of finger, stained with Ziehl-Neelsen staining method and interpreted in terms of

- *Bacteriological index:* **BI** denotes density of bacilli in slit skin smears and includes both live and dead bacilli. BI is represented on a scale of 1+ to 6+ and falls by 1 log/year following MDT.
- *Morphological index:* **MI** is the percentage of solid-stained bacilli, calculated after examining 200 red staining elements lying singly. MI is an important indicator to monitor response to therapy and steadily fall to zero in 6 weeks of therapy.

Serology and PCR for diagnosis: A simple diagnostic test to support the diagnosis of paucibacillary leprosy would be useful. Neither serology nor PCR has a role for this at present. Antibodies to the *M. leprae* specific PGL-I are present in 90% of patients with untreated lepromatous disease, but only 40–50% of patients with paucibacillary disease, and 1–5% of healthy controls. PCR for detection of *M. leprae* DNA encoding specific genes or repeat sequences is potentially highly sensitive and specific, since it detects *M. leprae* DNA in 95% of multibacillary and 55% of paucibacillary patients. Currently PCR is not used in clinical practice.

Classification

1. **Ridley-Jopling classification:** It combines clinical, histopathological, and immunological criteria to identify five forms of leprosy: tuberculoid (TT), borderline tuberculoid (BT), mid-borderline (BB), borderline lepromatous (BL), and lepromatous (LL) leprosy.
2. **World Health Organization classification:** was designed for distinct multidrug therapy regimens. It includes two broad categories:
   Paucibacillary (PB): includes TT and BT,
   Multibacillary (MB): includes BB, BL and LL.
3. **Indian-Indeterminate and Neuritic (+RJ types).**
4. **Classification by NLEP (National Leprosy Eradication Programme)**

Lesion Count: PB-1–5 skin lesions, MB-5 lesions, Polyneuritic-1 nerve trunk involvement, SSL (single skin lesions), with sensory loss but no nerve enlargement, infiltration.

If a skin smear is positive, the patient must be classified as MB whatever is the number of skin lesions.

Salient Clinical Features of Ridley-Jopling Types

1. **Tuberculoid (TT)**
   i. Single or a few, asymmetrical, well-defined, hypopigmented, erythematous or copper-colored palques.

ii. Hypopigmented patches not raised above the level of the surrounding skin.

iii. Psoriasiform rarely.

Initially a single peripheral nerve trunk related to the lesion is enlarged; nerve abscess may be formed. Foci of lymphocytes, epitheloid cells and Langhans giant cells are seen in the dermis. Nerves are densely infiltrated and often destroyed by the granuloma.

2. Borderline Tuberculoid (BT)

i. A few asymmetrical lesions, usually well-demarcated, somewhat dry.

ii. May be annular with *clearly-defined, outer* border with satellite lesions.

iii. Asymmetric nerve enlargement.

3. Borderline-Borderline (BB)

i. Mixture of lesions of TT and LL type. Asymmetrical less well-demarcated, somewhat shiny lesions.

ii. Often annular lesions with characteristic, punched-out or swiss cheese appearance (the outer border is vague, *inner border is clearly defined*).

iii. Widespread and asymmetrical nerve enlargement.

4. Borderline-Lepromatous (BL)

i. Many roughly symmetrical lesions. Shiny macules, papules, nodules and plaques with sloping edges.

ii. Lesions are raised in the center and *sloping towards the periphery* "inverted saucer" appearance.

5. Lepromatous (LL)

Very numerous symmetrically distributed erythematous or copper-colored, **shiny**, macules, papules and nodules; the papules lie over infiltrated skin; **macules are ill-defined;** patient may have **leonine face,** loss of eyebrows and eyelashes, with infiltration of the ear lobes.

Salient Features of other Types (Indian Classification) Indeterminate Leprosy

Most common type in India. It has been observed that the large majority of the single leprosy lesions were in posterior aspect of the upper extremity and anterior aspect of the lower extremities, which are injury and abrasion prone areas facilitating entry of bacilli.

- Patient is usually a child.
- One or more hypopigmented faintly erythematous macules
- No sensory loss, no nerve enlarged.
   Lepromin Test: (+/−).
   Slit smear for AFB (−).

Biopsy: Mild periappendegeal and perivascular infiltrate.

- Usually heals spontaneously; about 30% progress to determinate.

Lucio Leprosy

The Lucio leprosy is described in Mexico.

Clinical features: Diffuse non-nodular; Shiny thickened skin, loss of body and facial hair, puffy hands, chronic edema and ulceration of legs, widespread sensory loss; Eyes have shiny, thickened upper eyelids with a sleepy look; Ulceration of nasal mucosa presents with epistaxis; Laryngeal involvement presents as a hoarse voice; Develop peculiar form of lepra reaction, Lucio phenomenon.

HISTOID LEPROSY—VARIANT OF LL

The Term is introduced by Wade

- Type of lepromatous leprosy but with better C.M.I.
- Usually seen in patients whose disease is relapsing due to:
   i. Stoppage of treatment.
   ii. Drug resistance.
- Skin lesions: Firm, erythematous, round to oval, shiny, succulent **nodules**.
- AFB seen of slit smear: Longer, lying singly or in parallel bundles.

Reaction in Leprosy

Reactions are acute episodes of hypersensitivity reactions due to fluctuations in the immune status of a leprosy patient. In children reactions are relatively uncommon.

There are two main types of reactions:

- Type 1 reaction
- Type 2 reaction (erythema nodosum leprosum)

Signs of a reaction

In the skin	— Inflamed skin patches
In the nerves	— Pain or tenderness in a nerve
	— New loss of sensation
	— New muscle weakness
In the eye	— Pain and redness in the eye
	— New loss of vision
	— New weakness in eye closure

Type 1 reaction: It is Type IV hypersensitivity reaction (Coombs' and Gell type) and is associated with alteration in cell mediated immunity (CMI); *upgrading* or *reversal reactions* are due to sudden increase in CMI; *downgrading reactions* are due to decrease in CMI. About 25% of all leprosy patients, both with PB and MB disease are likely to get a Type 1 reaction. Mostly occurs in patients with borderline disease (BB, BT, BL);

may occur in sub polar lepromatous (LLs) and in tuberculoid leprosy patients under treatment.

Time: Upgrading (reversal) reaction usually occurs during the *first six months* of therapy in BT and BB patients, but longer intervals have been observed in BL patients. Downgrading reaction occurs spontaneously in untreated patients and reaction is often the first sign of the disease for which patient seeks medical help or in patients whose treatment has been interrupted. On restarting treatment, they may show reversal reaction.

On rare occasions, a Type 1 reaction can occur up to five years after treatment. Reactions occurring after treatment are sometimes mistaken for a leprosy relapse: that is, a return of the disease itself.

Clinical Manifestations

Upgrading reaction: Some or all the existing leprosy lesions show signs of acute inflammation (pain, tenderness, erythema and edema). Necrosis and ulceration occur in severe cases. Lesions desquamate as they subside. *New lesions* might appear occasionally in upgrading reactions. As the edema is profound the existing lesion (swiss cheese appearance) becomes more profound. Rapid swelling of one or *more nerves with pain* and tenderness at the site of nerve swelling; edema of hands, feet or face may be present; *nerve abscesses* may form.

Downgrading reaction: Lesions worsen and progress towards the lepromatous pole and new skin lesions may appear, each typically lepromatous in appearance.

Very severe reaction with necrosis and ulceration is also called "Lazarine Leprosy".

Type 2 reaction: It is also known as erythema nodosum leprosum (ENL). It is a Type III hypersensitivity reaction, immune complex syndrome and occurs in BL, LL leprosy usually after 6 months of therapy and rarely de novo. It occurs when large numbers of leprosy bacilli are killed. Proteins from the dead bacilli provoke an allergic reaction, causing generalized symptoms. Because it takes the body a long time to clear the dead bacilli, patients may develop episodes of type 2 reaction years after stopping treatment.

Clinical Manifestations

- ENL is triggered by infection, vaccination, drugs and stress.
- Marked constitutional symptoms are present.
- Characterized by tender, erythematous, evanescent nodules that come in crops, called erythema nodosum leprosum (ENL).

- ENL occurs over the face, arms and thigh in a bilateral and symmetrical fashion.
- ENL resolve with residual bluish hyperpigmentation.

Systemic

- May have systemic involvement in the form of conjunctivitis, keratitis, iritis, iridocyclitis, orchitis, hepatomegaly and lymphadenopathy.
- Most common cause of death in lepromatous leprosy is renal failure.
- Type of anaemia seen in leprosy is dimorphic anaemia.
- Cause of blindness in lepromatous variety is due to iridiocyclitis.

Treatment

Various important antileprosy drugs are discussed.

1. **Rifampicin** is the most rapidly acting bactericidal drug against *M. leprae*. It inhibits bacterial DNA-dependent RNA polymerase. It is administered as a single monthly dose in leprosy. Minor side effects of rifampicin include red discolouration of urine, abdominal pain and other gastrointestinal symptoms and skin rash. Fl-like syndrome is seen with intermittent administration. Serious side-effects are uncommon, and include hepatitis, psychosis, thrombocytopenia, osteomalacia, and severe hypersensitivity reactions like Stevens Johnson syndrome, porphyria cutanea tarda and pemphigus vulgaris.

2. **Dapsone** is a bacteriostatic drug and an essential component of anti-leprosy regimes. It inhibits dihydropteroate synthase enzyme, thereby interfering with bacterial folate biosynthesis. The drug has a half-life of 24 hours and used as once daily dose.

   Side effect of dapsone is hemolysis (individuals deficient in G6PD are more prone). Other side effects include: methaemoglobinaemia, agranulocytosis, mild thrombocytopenia, hepatitis, polyneuropathy, insomnia, irritability and psychosis. Cutaneous side effects include exanthematous rash, exfoliative dermatitis, toxic epidermal necrolysis, Stevens-Johnson syndrome and fixed drug eruptions. Dapsone syndrome (DDS syndrome) is an uncommon but dangerous hypersensitivity reaction manifesting as fever, lymphadenopathy, liver involvement and hematological abnormailites.

3. **Clofazimine** is an iminophenazine dye. It has dual effect in leprosy. The drug is bacteriostatic against *M. leprae* and has additional anti-inflammatory effects helpful in lepra reaction. Side effects are: gastrointestinal disturbances like diarrhea, skin and

conjunctival pigmentation (red brown discoloration), red discoloration of body fluids and icthysosis (particularly over forearms and legs).

The drug schedule and dosages for adults and children till 10 years of age are summarized in Table 30.3.

The appropriate dose for children under 10 years of age can be decided on the basis of body weight [Rifampicin: 10 mg per kilogram body weight, clofazimine: 1 mg per kilogram per body weight daily and 6 mg per kilogram monthly, dapsone: 2 mg per kilogram body weight daily].

First dose containing rifampicin, clofazimine and dapsone for MB leprosy and rifampicin and dapsone for PB leprosy is given once in a month (Day 1of every blister pack) under direct supervision of health care worker of physician. Following this daily dose of dapsone and clofazimine for MB and only dapsone for PB leprosy, that is taken by the patient at home.

Patient categories: Candidates for MDT belong to either of the following category

New Cases: Leprosy patient who have never received treatment before.

Relapse cases: Persons who have developed new lesion at any time after the completion of a full course of treatment. Such cases receive exactly the same treatment as new cases (either PB or MB).

Default cases: Persons who fail to complete the treatment within maximally allowed time framework (either PB or MB). They receive exactly the same treatment as new cases (either PB or MB).

Accompanied-MDT (A-MDT)—Give the full course on the first visit.

Uniform MDT (U-MDT)—6 months to all patients irrespective of classification.

Fixed Drug Therapy (FDT): As per the latest guidelines the therapy is called FDT, i.e. at the end of duration irrespective of the activity of disease the medicine is stopped.

Newer antileprosy drugs. Various regimens have been proposed with the following drugs for shorter duration therapy and in patients with multi-drug resistance to MDT drugs:
1. Quinolones—Perfloxacin, ofloxacin, ciprofloxacin, sparfloxacin
2. Tetracyclines—Minocycline
3. Macrolides—Clarithromycin, Roxithromycin
4. Dapsone analogs
5. Clofazimine derivatives.
6. Ansamycins—Rifamycin, Rifapentine, Rifabutine.
7. Amoxycillin + Clavulanic acid

Treatment of Reactions

Type I reaction: Most type 1 reactions settle down within six months, but without treatment, nerve involvement may lead to permanent loss of function. The drug of choice remains **Prednisolone.** Other drugs like aspirin, NSAIDS and chloroquine are used as adjuvants. Prednisolone is given orally in a decreasing dosage over several months. Patients with PB leprosy receive different dosages of steroids than multibacillary (MB) in addition to MDT. Patients who have completed their course of MDT do not need antileprosy treatment while on steroids. For **PB patients** the standard treatment of prednisolone therapy is given for a total duration of twelve weeks (1–2 wk 40 mg, 3–4 wk 30 mg, 5–6 wk 20 mg, 7–8 wk 15 mg, 9–10 wk 10 mg, 11–12 wk 5 mg).

For **MB patients** the standard treatment of prednisolone therapy is given for a total duration of 24 weeks, exactly double the PB course (1–4 wk 40 mg,

Type of leprosy	Drugs used	Frequency of Administration Adults (children in bracket)	Dosage (adult) 15 years and above	Dosage (Children 10–14 years)	Dosage (Children below 10 years)	Criteria for RFT
MB leprosy	Rifampicin	Once monthly	600 mg	450 mg	300 mg	Completion of
	Clofazimine	monthly	300 mg	150 mg	100 mg	12 monthly pulses
	Dapsone	Daily Once	100 mg	50 mg	25 mg	pulses in 18
	Clofazimine	Daily for adults (every other day for children)				consecutive months
			50 mg	50 mg (alternate day, not daily)	50 mg (weekly twice)	
PB leprosy	Rifampicin	Once monthly	600 mg	450 mg	300 mg	Completion of
	Dapsone	Daily	100 mg	50 mg	25 mg daily or 50 mg alternate day	6 monthly pulses in 9 consecutive months

Table 30.3: MDT regimen

5–8 wk 30 mg, 9–12 wk 20 mg, 13–16 wk 15 mg, 17–20 wk 10 mg, 21–24 wk 5 mg).

Splinting of the limb in case of neuritis is advisable and drainage of nerve abscess is not advisable as this would cause permanent disability as the nerve involved are motor nerves, the systemic steroid is the treatment of choice for abscess.

Newer Drugs: Azathioprine, Cyclosporine.

Type 2 reaction: Mild—aspirin, chloroquine, clofaza-mine; Severe-thalidomide, Steroids—prednisolone. Prescribe prednisolone in the doses over a short course of six weeks (1 wk 40 mg, 2 wk 30 mg, 3 wk 20 mg, 4 wk 15 mg, 5 wk 10 mg, 6 wk 5 mg).

Prescribing treatment for severe type 2 reactions: Type 2 reactions can often last for months or even years, and so there is a risk of people becoming dependent on steroids. This makes the reactions very hard to manage, with the result that it can become difficult to reduce and eventually terminate the treatment.

Clofazimine is given in decreasing doses as follows: 300 mg daily for 1 month, 200 mg daily for 3–6 months, 100 mg daily for as long as symptoms remain. It is a normal component of MDT, and the usual adult dose is 50 mg per day; however, the higher doses are needed to suppress the ENL reaction. Clofazimine takes some time to have an effect, but by the time the steroid dose is reduced to a low level it should be working well, allowing the steroids to be stopped completely.

Thalidomide is an effective drug for treating type 2 reactions, but because of its side-effects one must monitor it very carefully. It should only be considered for patients whose type 2 reaction cannot be controlled by the first two drugs mentioned above.

The usual dosage is 200–400 mg daily, in divided doses.

Dayal R, Sanghi S. Leprosy in children. In: Kar HK, Kumar B (eds). *IAL Textbook of Leprosy*. Delhi: Jaypee Brothers Medical Publishers, 2010; 325–335.

Jopling WH, McDougall AC. *Handbook of Leprosy*. 5th edn. Delhi: CBS Publishers and Distributors, 1996; 120–140.

Mahajan S, Sardana K, Bhushan P, Koranne RV, Mendiratta V. A study of leprosy in children, from a tertiary pediatric hospital in India. *Lepr Rev* 2006; 77(2): 160–162.

Report of the Tenth Meeting of the WHO Technical Advisory Group on Leprosy Control New Delhi, India, 23 April 2009 SEA–GLP–2009.5 Distribution: General © World Health Organization 2009.

Walker SL, Lockwood DN. Leprosy. *Clin Dermatol* 2007; 25(2): 165–172.

30.15 ARTHROPOD BITES AND INFESTATIONS

Arthropods of dermatologic significance are the eight-legged arachnids (mites, ticks, spiders and scorpions) and the six-legged insects (lice, flies, mosquitoes, flee, bug, bees, wasps, ants, and beetles).

Scabies

Scabies is caused mite *Sarcoptes scabiei var hominis*. The mite is an obligate parasite that completes its entire life cycle on humans. The adult female mite has a rounded body measures 0.4 mm long by 0.3 mm broad and has four pair of legs, the hind two containing bristles. The male is about one third of the size of the female. Usually a female mite can live away from the host for 24 to 36 hrs and remain capable of infestation and epidermal burrowing. The female mite after being fertilized on the skin surface excavates a sloping burrow in the stratum corneum to the boundary of stratum granulosum. Along a path that may be up to 1 cm long, the female mite leaves a trail of eggs and feces behind in the burrow. The female mite has a life span of around 15 to 30 days and lays 1 to 4 eggs per day. After hatching, the immature forms leave the burrow and take shelter in the hair follicles. The larvae mature into adult mites in 10 to 14 days and the duration of the whole life cycle is 30–60 days.

The disease is worldwide in all races and in all age groups. It is transmitted sexually as well as by non-sexual close skin to skin contact especially within the family and school. Infected bedding and clothing can sometimes transmit the disease, especially from patients with crusted scabies. The more parasites present in a person, the greater is the likelihood of transmission—either direct or indirect.

Predisposing factors: The burden of disease is highest in crowded living conditions in tropical countries where scabies is endemic. Scabies disproportionately affects women and children as well as individuals with immunodeficiency, mental or physical handicap or HIV infection. The prevalence of scabies is highest in infants younger than 2 years of age. The average number of adult female mites per infested patient is 11.

Incubation period: It is 3–6 weeks for primary infestation, the time required for sensitization to acarine products. Reinfestation may result in symptoms within 24 hours.

Clinical manifestations: The hallmark of scabies is nocturnal itching often disturbing sleep and evident well before the clinical signs become apparent. The pathognomonic lesion is an intact or excoriated burrow—a short wavy, dirty gray, elevated scaly line measuring 1–2 mm on the skin surface. The terminal end of the burrow is often capped with a small vesicle. These are more easily found on in the finger web space, on the wrist and on genitals in males. They are often present on the palms and soles of young children.

Numerous erythematous intact as well as excoriated papules may be seen around the axillae, periareolar regions and abdomen especially around the umbilicus, buttocks and thighs. These develop as a result of hypersensitivity to the mite or its products. In young children and infants, the hands, palms, wrist, feet, retroauricular area and periumbilical region and skin folds are most commonly involved. In infants, particularly in warm weather, lesions may occur on scalp and face also.

Infants and young children may also experience irritability, fussiness and poor feeding due to interference with sleep resulting from constant irritation.

Complications: Non-specific secondary lesions including excoriations, eczematization and secondary infections by group 'A' *Streptococcus* and *Staphlycoccus aureus* are common in children, particularly affecting the hands and feet.

Diagnosis: The diagnosis is chiefly clinical and is suggested in the child with nocturnal pruritus with a positive family history, a papular or papulovesicular eruption with burrows and the characteristic distribution pattern. A definite diagnosis is made by demonstration of mite, eggs, egg shell fragments or mite pellets. This can be done by mineral oil examination of the scrapings from burrow. Visualization of the mite or its eggs or scybala is confirmatory. However, failure to find mites is common and does not rule out scabies.

Differential diagnosis: Impetigo contagiosa, papular urticaria, animal scabies, atopic eczema should be considered in the differential diagnosis of scabies.

Treatment: Management involves treatment of symptoms, secondary infection and destruction of mite.

Principles of treatment: 1. Treatment is best done at night before going to bed; 2. The medication provided should be rubbed into the skin. All parts of the body from chin downwards, whether involved or uninvolved should be treated with special attention to groins, axillae, web spaces and nails, intertriginous and retroauricular areas; 3. Avoid touching your mouth or eyes with your hands; 4. Medication should be thoroughly washed off after the recommended time; 5. Change of clothes and bed linen next day and launder them; 6. Itching and eczematization might persist for a week or more, but usually do not require treatment to be repeated; 6. Close physical contacts of infected persons should be treated at the same time.

Topical treatment: Permethrin and lindane are the two most studied drugs. Permethrin (5% cream or lotion) is applied for 8–12 hours usually at night. High cure rates are achieved with a single application, though many physicians prefer to use a second one 5–7 days later. It is available as to be. Permethrin should not be used in infants younger than 2 months of age or in pregnant or nursing women. Adverse reactions are mild and transient; burning, stinging or exacerbation or recurrence of pruritus or rarely contact dermatitis. *Lindane or gamma benzene hexachloride* acts on central nervous system of mite and leads to increased excitability, convulsions and death. A single 6–8 hours application is effective in the treatment of scabies. Adverse effects are particularly significant in children or infants with overexposure or an altered skin barrier. The clinical signs of CNS toxicity include headache, nausea, dizziness, vomiting, restlessness, tremors, disorientation, and weakness, twitching of eyelids, convulsions, respiratory failure, coma and death. It may also cause aplastic anemia, thrombocytopenia and pancytopenia. Application should be on dry skin to limit the percutaneous absorption. It should not be used in infants, young children or pregnant or nursing mothers or in patients with seizure disorders or other neurological diseases.

Crotamiton: An alternative scabicide is crotamiton which also has an antipruritic effect. Formulated in a 10% lotion and cream, crotamiton requires two applications applied at 24 hours interval. Side effects are minimal. Crotamiton is irritating to denuded skin as well as capable of inducing an allergic reaction.

Five to 10% precipitated sulphur in a petroleum base is the oldest anti-scabitic in use. It is to be applied on three successive nights usually as 6% ointment and washed off 24 hrs after the last application. Although the preparation is messy, malodorous and tends to stain the skin and can produce an irritant dermatitis, it is cheap and considered safe, especially in pregnant and lactating women and infants less than 2 months of age.

Papular Urticaria

Etiology: Papular urticaria represents delayed hypersensitivity reactions to a variety of biting or stinging arthropods.

Clinical manifestations: Papular urticaria is characterized by the presence of small 3–10 mm in diameter, pruritic erythematous papules, sometimes surmounted by a vesicle. These are arranged in clusters over the extensor surfaces of arms and legs, shoulders, buttocks. Individual papules have a tiny central punctum and are more persistent than typical urticaria and may last from weeks to months. These usually appear in recurrent crops each lasting 2–10 days. Excruciating pruritus leads to excoriations with secondary eczematization. Lesions may result in temporary hyperpigmentation once they resolve. Papular urticaria occurs predominantly between the ages of 18 months and 7 years. The genital, perianal and axillary regions are usually uninvolved. Characteristically the affected child is the only member of the household involved. The problem may persist for many years and most often begins in spring or summer.

Differential diagnosis: Atopic dermatitis, papular drug reaction, id eruption, miliaria rubra, allergic contact dermatitis, and paulovesicular polymorphous light eruption should be considered in the differential diagnosis of papular urticaria. Scabies, prurigo simplex and delusions of parasitoses may also be confused with papular urticaria.

Treatment: The ideal treatment for popular urticaria is identification and removal of cause. Dogs or cats should be treated for fleas and mites and household fumigation may be necessary. Protective clothing such as long sleeves may be useful. Mosquito nets and mats may also be helpful. Use of insect repellants may make the child less attractive to the insect. Fleas or mites living in carpets or furniture may be eliminated by treatment with a commercial insecticide. Window casings should be treated in the case of bird mites. The extreme sensitivity of the affected person should be explained. Use of mild to moderate potency topical steroids and systemic antihistamines is advocated for control of pruritus. Long standing neglected cases may develop secondary infection and require systemic antibiotics.

Pediculosis

Infestation with lice is called pediculosis. Lice are six-legged obligate human parasite that can survive off their host from 10 days to 3 weeks. Three kinds of lice infest humans: *Pediculus humanus* var. *capitis* (Head louse); *Pediculus humanus* var. *corporis* (Body louse); Pthirus pubis (Pubic or crab louse). All three have similar anatomic characteristics. The body louse is the largest and the crab louse is the smallest with a short oval body and prominent claws. The female lice lay approximately 6 eggs or nits up to one month and then die.

Pediculosis capitis: Lice are transmitted by close personal contact with an infested person but fomite transmission with hats, brushes, combs, bedding is also common. Lice infestation of the scalp is most common in children, especially girls. Though any part of the scalp may be infested, head lice are most commonly seen on the back of the head and neck,

and behind the ears. Scratching causes inflammation and secondary infection with cervical lymphadenopathy. Eyelashes may be involved causing redness and swelling. Nits are cemented in the hair and can be taken out along the hair shaft with difficulty, whereas dandruff scale can easily be removed.

Pediculosis corporis: Infestation by body lice is uncommon in children. It is a disease of people with poor hygiene in underdeveloped countries. Body lice live and lay their eggs in the seams of clothing and come to skin only to feed. Body lice induce pruritus which leads to scratching and secondary infection.

Pediculosis pubis: Not often seen in infants and young children. May occur in adolescence through sexual transmission. Patient may present with grey blue macules (maculae ceruleae) in the groin that may represent altered blood pigment.

Eyelash infestation: Seen almost exclusively in children. The lice are acquired from other children or infested adults with pediculosis pubis. It induces blepharitis with lid itching, scaling, crusting, and discharge. Eyelash infestation is an indicator of child abuse.

Diagnosis: Lice are suspected when a patient complains of itching in a localized area without an apparent rash. Scalp and pubic lice can be seen on careful examination.

Treatment: Permethrin cream rinse 1% is applied to the scalp and hair thoroughly after the hair is shampooed and dried. The medication is rinsed out with water after 10 minutes. It is not 100% ovicidal but a higher cure rate can be achieved by second application one week after the first treatment. Ivermectin causes paralysis and death of lice. The drug has selective activity against parasites without systemic effects. A single oral dose of ivermectin 200 µg/kg repeated in 10 days is effective. The medical therapy should be combined with combing the hair with a fine toothed comb. The close contacts should be screened and treated as necessary.

Burns DA. Diseases caused by arthropods and other noxious animals. In: Burns T, Breathnach S, Cox N, Griffiths C (eds). *Rook's Textbook of Dermatology.* 7th edn. Vol 2. Oxford: Blackwell Science. 2004; 33.1 –33.63.

Stone SP. Scabies and pediculosis. In: Freedberg IM, Eisen AZ, Wolff K, Austen KF, Goldsmith LA, Katz SI (eds). *Fitzpatrick's Dermatology in General Medicine.* 6th edn. Vol 2. New York: McGraw Hill, 2003; 2283–2286.

30.16 PHOTOSENSITIVITY IN PEDIATRIC AGE GROUP

Photosensitive disorders are those in which abnormal cutaneous response occurs after exposure to non-ionizing ultraviolet (UV) radiations. Many photo-sensitivity disorders present in childhood. Prompt diagnosis of these disorders becomes difficult at times because of overlapping clinical pictures. Apart from classic photo distribution of lesions, many genodermatoses and metabolic disorders may have systemic involvement, thereby making a coordinated approach by a dermatologist and pediatrician necessary in the diagnosis and management. Causes of photosensitivity in children have been listed in Table 30.4.

Photosensitization disorders: These are i. drug induced photosensitivity and ii. phytophotodermatitis.

i. *Drug induced photosensitivity:* Symptoms may range from prickling or burning sensation to erythema, edema, and skin fragility over sunexposed sites such as forehead, cheeks, chin, ear lobules, 'V' of the neck and dorsa of hands. Drugs responsible for photosensitivity are reported as follows:

1. Antibiotics: Tetracyclines; Sulphonamides; Fluoroquinolones; Nalidixic acid; **2. Antifungals:** Griseofulvin; **3. Diuretics, antihypertensives:** Thiazides; Frusemide; Amiodarone; Nifedipine; Quinidine; **4. NSAIDS:** Naproxen; Piroxicam; Ibuprofen; Tiaprofenic acid; **5. Retinoids:** Isotretinoin; Acitretin; **6. Psychoactive drugs:** Phenothiazines; Protriptyline; **7. Psoralens;** **8. Photodynamic therapy agents:** Foscan.

ii. *Phytophotodermatitis:* Phytophotodermatisis results from contact with plant extracts containing furocoumarins (*psoralens*) and subsequent activation of these chromophores by ultra violet radiation. Citrus fruits specially lemons, limes, mangoes and many common weeds contain these tropically photosensitizing chemicals. Lime juice which contain ten times the oil of bergamot as other citrous fruits, is the commonest offending agent. Handling flowers of the composite group of plants (e.g. chrysanthemum, marigold, dahlia and sunflower), which contain oleoresins may give rise to photosensitivity. Topical antimicrobials included in soaps, cosmetics and medicaments like halogenated salicylanilides, clioquinol, and sulfonamides are common photosensitizers and may go unnoticed unless a detailed history is evaluated. The clinical presentation include dramatic erythema and hyper pigmentation over upper lip from drinking citrus beverages, the hands from handling culprit weeds and the legs from contact with certain grasses. Bizarre streaks may appear secondary to dripping liquid or it may present as linear vesicle formation and subsequent hyper pigmentation over exposed limbs.

Management: Reduction of light exposure is paramount in the management of all photosensitivity disorders. Psychological and socioeconomic factors make complete avoidance of sunlight difficult; however, a three-fold strategy is recommended to decrease the amount of unnecessary irradiations that include: i. Sun avoidance including behavioral change; ii. Photo protective clothing; iii. Sunscreens; iv. Avoidance of photosensitizing drugs.

Harber LC, Bickers DB, Photosensitive diseases. *Principles of Diagnosis and Treatment.* Toronto, BC Decker, 1998, 241, 263–276.

30.17 DERMATOLOGIC THERAPEUTICS IN PEDIATRIC POPULATION

Topical medications and therapies are necessary for the proper management of skin diseases in children; however, physicians must be aware of the differences

Table 30.4: Causes of photosensitivity in children	
1. Genetic Disorders	Xeroderma pigmentosum; Cockayne's syndrome; Bloom's syndrome; Rothmund-Thomson syndrome; Trichothiodystrophy
2. Metabolic and Nutritional Disorders	• Disorders of tryptophan metabolism: Hartnup disease, Pellagra • Porphyrias: Erythropoietic Protoporphyria (EPP); Porphyria Cutanea Tarda (PCT); Variegate Porphyria (VP); Congenital Erythropoietic Porphyria (CEP)
3. Melanin Deficiency Syndromes	Albinism; Phenyl ketonuria; Vitiligo
4. Idiopathic, Acquired photodermatoses	Polymorphous light eruption; Actinic prurigo; Hydroa vacciniforme; Juvenile spring eruption; Solar urticaria
5. Photoaggravated Dermatosis	Neonatal Lupus Erythematosus; Childhood Systemic Lupus Erythematosus; Juvenile Dermatomyositis; Others
6. Photosensitization	Phototoxicity (Drug induced photosensitivity, phytophotodermatitis); Photoallergy (Eczematous reaction)

Box 30.1: Potency ranking of some commonly used topical glucocorticoids

Class I (Superpotent): Clobetasone propionate cream/ointment (0.05 %); Betamethasone dipropionate ointment (optimized vehicle) (0.05 %)

Class 2 (potent): Betamethasone dipropionate ointment (0.05 %); Betamethasone dipropionate cream (optimized vehicle) (0.05%); Mometasone furoata ointment (0.1 %); Flucinonide cream / ointment (0.05%)

Class 3 (potent): Triamcinolone acetonide ointment (0.1%); Fluticasone propionate ointment (0.005%); Betamethasone dipropionate cream (0.05%)

Class 4 (mid-strength): Mometasone furoate cream (0.1%); Betamethasone valerate foam (0.12%); Fluocinonide ointment (0.025%)

Class 5 (mid-strength): Fluticasone propionate cream (0.05%); Betamethasone dipropionate lotion (0.05%); Betamethasone valerate cream (0.1%); Hydrocortisone butyrate cream 0.1%)

Class 6 (mild): Desonide cream (0.05%); Betamethasone valerate lotion (0.1%)

Class 7 (mild): Hydrocortisone acetate (0.5%, 1%, 2.5%)

---

while prescribing topical steroids in children when compared to adults. The success of topical therapy depends on the vehicle, ease of application and cost.

FTU (finger tip unit): It is useful for measurement of topical corticosteroid. Weight of a strip of cream or ointment squeezed from a tube and extending from the tip of the finger to the crease at the distal interphalangeal joint in an adult is 0.5 g.

Rule of hand 4 adult flat hand = 2 FTU = 1 gm cream/ointment. Means 1 gm of topical corticosteroid is adequate for skin surface of 4 adult flat hands.

Principle of topical therapy in dermatology: If lesion is wet, dry it or if lesion is dry, wet it.

Information to be given to Parents

Liberal amounts of a lubricant/emollient cream should be applied to the skin immediately after bathing. Emollients should be applied once or twice daily to prevent skin dryness and irritation.

Patients generally prefer emollient creams over ointments for daytime use because emollients have a nongreasy, cosmetic appearance. Lubricating ointments may be preferred for night time use because of their superior hydrating properties.

1. Advise to use the drug in as small amount as possible, to cover diseased area with thin layer of medicine.
2. Treated area should not be bandaged or wrapped.
3. Avoid the use of plastic or disposable diapers.
4. Avoid contact with eyes.

Steroid Therapy in Children

Corticosteroids (CS) are mainstay of therapy in dermatology because of their antiproliferative, anti-inflammatory, immunosuppressive and vasoconstrictive action.

Indications of systemic corticosteroids: Bullous dermatosis, papulo-squamous dermatosis, atopic dermatitis and contact dermatitis, autoimmune connective tissue disease.

Indication of topical corticosteroids: Papulosquamous dermatoses, atopic dermatitis, diaper dermatitis, dyshidrotic eczema, lichen planus, alopecia areata, vitiligo, etc. Potency ranking of some commonly used topical glucocorticoids are listed Box 30.1.

Contraindication of topical corticosteroids (TCS): Absolute—hypersensitivity to topical corticosteroids (TCS); Relative—infection at site of application, infestation, ulceration or other wound.

Contraindication of systemic corticosteroids: **Absolute:** Systemic fungal infection, herpes simplex keratitis; **Relative:** Psychosis, severe depression, glaucoma, cataract, osteoporosis, diabetes mellitus, active TB or positive tuberculin test.

Adverse effects of corticosteroids (CS) (*see* Box 11.7)

Metry DW, Hebert AA. Topical therapies and medications in the pediatric patient. *Pediatr Clin North Am* 2000; 47: 867–876.

Pasic A, Ceovic R, Lipozenci? J, Phototherapy in pediatric patients. *Pediatr Dermatol* 2003;20:71–77.

Orthopedic Problems

31.1 GROWTH AND DEVELOPMENT

Each of the individual components of the skeletal system grows by different mechanisms. The long bones of the extremities (humerus, radius-ulna, femur, and tibia-fibula) have growth plates or physes at each end. Each contributes a varying proportion to the longitudinal growth of the individual bone as well as the extremity through a process termed enchondral ossification. The ends of each long bone are composed of the epiphyses. These are covered by articular cartilage and form the associated joints. Initially, the epiphyses are almost entirely cartilaginous and become progressively more ossified during growth. The articular cartilage also has growth potential, which contributes to the growth of the epiphysis. The perichondrial ring around physes, the perichondrium around the epiphyses and the periosteum, which surrounds the metaphysis and diaphyseal regions of the bone, contributes to appositional or circumferential growth.

Bones without physes, such as the pelvis, scapulae, carpals, and tarsals, grow by appositional bone growth from their surrounding perichondrium and periosteum. Other bones, such as the metacarpals, metatarsals, phalanges and spine, grow by a combination of both appositional and endochondral ossification.

31.2 EVALUATION OF THE CHILD

The key to an accurate diagnosis is a careful history, a thorough physical examination, appropriate radiographic imaging, and occasionally, laboratory testing. The history of the presenting symptom is often the most important part of the evaluation. This is usually obtained from the parents or guardian, but the child, if old enough and cooperative, can also give useful information. The chief complaint is established first. In children with chronic symptoms, the past medical history is also important. The prenatal or pregnancy history should be obtained. The condition of the child during the neonatal period is important. In older infants and young children, evaluation of the presence and delay of developmental milestones for posture, locomotion, dexterity, social activities, and speech is important. Pediatric orthopedics disorders may be associated with pain, deformity, neurologic changes, or a combination of these factors.

Physical examination: The physical examination of a child with a musculoskeletal disorder includes careful evaluation of the musculoskeletal and neurologic systems as well as an appropriate general physical examination. The examination of the musculoskeletal system includes four parts: observation, palpation, assessment of joint range of motion, and gait assessment in ambulatory children.

Gait assessment: Gait disturbances are one of the most important parental concerns in children. It is, therefore, important to have a thorough understanding of the development of normal gait. Human gait is dynamic, complex, and repetitive. The gait cycle is the time between right heel strike followed by left toe-off, left

Table 31.1: Common causes of limping according to age

Age	Antalgic	Trendenlenburg	Leg-lengthening discrepancy
Toddler (1–3 yr)	(i) Infection: Septic arthritis (hip, knee); Osteomyelitis; Diskitis (ii) Occult trauma: Toddler's fracture (iii) Neoplasia	(i) Hip dislocation (DDH) (ii) Neuromuscular disease (Cerebral palsy; Poliomyelitis)	Absent
Childhood (4–10 yr)	(i) Infection: Septic arthritis (hip, knee); Osteomyelitis; Diskitis; Transient synovitis, hip (cerebral palsy; poliomyelitis) (ii) LCPD (iii) Tarsal coalition (iv) JRA (v) Trauma (vi) Neoplasia	(i) Hip dislocation (DDH) (ii) Neuromuscular disease	Present
Adolescence (11+ yr)	(i) SCFE (ii) JRA (iii) Trauma (Fracture; Overuse) (iv) Tarsal coalition (v) Neoplasia	—	Present

DDH, developmental dysplasia of hip; JRA, juvenile rheumatoid arthritis; LCPD, Legg- Calvé- Perthes Disease; SCFE, slipped capital femoral epiphysis.

heel strike, and right toe-off and ends with right heel strike. The five events describe one gait cycle and include two phases: stance and swing. The stance phase is the period of time during which one of the two feet is on the ground. The swing phase is the portion of the gait cycle during which a limb is being advanced forward without ground contact.

Limping is categorized into either painful (antalgic) or nonpainful (Trendelenburg gait) on the basis of the length of the stance phase (Table 31.1). In a painful gait, the stance phase is shortened as the child decreases the time spent on the painful extremity. In a nonpainful gait, which is indicative of underlying proximal muscle weakness or hip instability, the stance phase is equal between the involved and uninvolved sides, but the child will lean or shift the centre of gravity over the involved extremity for balance. If the disorder is bilateral, it produces a waddling gait.

Neurologic evaluation: A careful neurologic evaluation must be performed and includes muscle strength testing, sensory assessment and evaluation of deep tendon and pathologic reflexes like Babinski reflex.

Radiographic assessment: Radiography is the principle method of evaluation of paediatric musculoskeletal system. This includes routine radiographs as well as ultrasonography, CT, MRI and bone scans.

Beebe AC, Kerpsac JM. Pediatric musculoskeletal examination. In: Dormans JP (Ed). *Pediatrics Orthopedics: Core Knowledge in Orthopedics.* Philadelphia: Mosby, 2005; 15–35.

Herring JA. The orthopaedic examination. A comprehensive overview. In: Herring JA (Ed). *Tachdjian's Pediatric Orthopaedics.* 3rd edn. Philadelphia: WB Saunders, 2002; 25–61.

Hosalkar HS, Wells L. Growth and development. In: Kliegman RM, Behrman RE, Jenson HB, Stanton BF (eds). *Nelson Textbook of Pediatrics.* 18th edn. Vol. 2. Philadelphia: Saunders, 2007; 2771–2773.

Hosalkar HS, Wells L. Evaluation of the child. In: Kliegman RM, Behrman RE, Jenson HB, Stanton BF (eds). *Nelson Textbook of Pediatrics.* 18th edn. Vol. 2. Philadelphia: Saunders, 2007; 2773–2776.

31.3 THE FOOT AND TOES

The foot and toes are important in stance and locomotion. Abnormalities affecting the foot can produce pain and abnormal shoe wear and can adversely affect limb function. The foot is divided into three regions: hind foot, midfoot, and fore foot. The hind foot is composed of the talus and calcaneus. The midfoot is composed of the navicular, cuboid, and three cuneiform bones. The forefoot is composed of the metatarsals and toes.

Calcaneovalgus feet: The calcaneovalgus foot is a relatively common finding in the newborn and is secondary to in utero positioning. A hyperdorsiflexed foot with forefoot abduction and increased heel valgus manifests this condition. It is usually associated with external tibial torsion. It is often unilateral but may be bilateral. Anteroposterior and lateral simulated weight-bearing radiographs of the feet may be necessary to differentiate between the calcaneovalgus foot and a congenital vertical talus. The typical calcaneovalgus foot requires no treatment. The hyperdorsiflexion of the foot resolves during the first 6 months of life. The external tibial torsion, however, persists. Spontaneous improvement does not occur until the child begins to stand and walk independently.

Metatarsus adductus: It is the medial deviation of the forefoot at the level of the midtarsal joints of the foot. Metatarsus adductus is the most common congenital foot deformity, present in 1 of 1000 live births. The etiology is not completely understood, but the disorder is theorized to result from intrauterine mechanical forces applied to the foot. The purpose of the foot examination is to judge the extent of deformity and the level of flexibility. The foot with metatarsus adducts is described as "bean shaped" (kidney bean). The foot has a deep medial crease along the instep and a convex lateral border (*see* Fig. 31.3.1 in CD). Radiographs are usually unnecessary in the initial evaluation of metatarsus adductus. It has been suggested that a foot that corrects beyond the midline when its lateral border is stroked does not require treatment. Serial casting may then be applied, with a new cast every 1 or 2 weeks. The indication for surgery is the inability to achieve treatment goals through nonoperative means. Surgery is not considered before a child is 4 years old. The use of multiple metatarsal osteotomies through the bases of the metatarsals is a more reasonable operation.

Club foot: The term is commonly used to describe a foot deformed in hind foot equinus, midfoot varus and forefoot adductus or talipes equinovarus. The deformity has been further divided into congenital and acquired. Acquired clubfoot is associated with neuromuscular diseases, such as cerebral palsy, myelomeningocele, and polio or external forces such as amniotic band syndrome. Males are affected twice as often as females. Congenital talipes equinovarus feet are positioned in hind foot equinus, hindfoot varus, midfoot adduction and, often, cavus. However, they vary greatly in stiffness, bone deformity; muscle involvement, and response to treatment. It is important to examine for associated anomalies of the upper extremities, back, legs, abnormal reflexes, and so on, as they can provide information about etiology as well as the likelihood of successful treatment. Radiographic evaluation is useful in documenting the deformity just before surgical correction or to confirm adequate correction by any method. In the older patient with clubfoot, radiographic evaluation can help identify deformity, degenerative changes, stress changes and fractures. During the last decade, the Ponseti method of combined manipulation and Achilles tenotomy has become very popular. Treatment is begun as soon as is practical after birth, consist of weekly casting for 4 to 8 weeks or until the foot has been abducted 60 degrees. Achilles tenotomy is then performed with the use of local or general anaesthesia, followed by continued casting for 1 month. After Ponseti manipulation and tenotomy, the child must wear Denis Browne-style bar-and-shoes. Older children and those who do not respond to conservative treatment may require soft tissue releases or bony corrective procedures.

Flat foot (Planovalgus) is a common deformity consisting of hind foot valgus compensatory midfoot supination and abduction. Foot flexibility and pain are the central issues to consider when one is evaluating the child with planovalgus feet. Flexible flat feet without pain require no treatment. Conversely, stiff feet even in the absence of pain are cause for concern and require investigation.

Congenital vertical talus (CVT) is an anomaly characterized by a stiff rocker-bottom foot. The appearance is secondary to a dorsal dislocation of the navicular bone onto the head of the talus. CVT may occur without a predisposing condition (idiopathic), although more commonly it is associated with arthrogryposis multiplex congenita (AMC), myelomeningocele, congenital myopathy, and intraspinal lesions (i.e. syringomyelia). Examination of the foot reveals an equinus hind foot and a dorsiflexed and abducted midfoot. The talar head is palpable along the plantar surface of the foot. Diagnosis of CVT is confirmed with radiographs. Manipulation and casting techniques stretch the skin, making wound closure easier at the time of surgery, but cannot reduce the dislocation. The only corrective treatment for CVT is surgery, with best results in children who undergo operative intervention before they are 2 years old.

Tarsal coalition: Tarsal coalition is a failure of segmentation between adjoining tarsal bones so that a normal mobile joint does not form. The coalitions are composed of fibrous tissue (syndesmosis), cartilaginous tissue (synchondrosis), or osseous tissue (synostosis). Intertarsal motion in presence of coalition produces pain in some patients. Coalitions may exist between any two of the tarsal bones, but talocalcaneal (TCC) and calcaneonavicular (CNC) coalitions are the most common. Subtalar motion is limited or absent. The presence of a tarsal coalition is confirmed on standing weight-bearing AP, lateral, and oblique radiographs. CT is helpful in assessing the location and percentage of joint surface occupied by the coalition. Initial treatment consists of 1 month of immobilization in a short-leg walking cast. Patients with a small TCC (less than 50% of the subtalar joint) or CNC usually require surgical coalition resection with fat, muscle, or tendon interposition. Extensive or multiple coalitions are treated with an arthrodesis.

Cavus feet: A cavus foot has a "high arch" with no contact between the floor and the instep (*see* Fig. 31.3.2 in CD). Elevation of the arch is due to plantar-flexion of the medial metatarsals. Ambulation on the lateral border of the foot leads to fifth metatarsal pain and pre-disposes to inversion injuries. The subtalar joint is initially mobile and passively correctable, with time however, heel varus becomes fixed. Cavus is the result of a peripheral neuropathy that affects intrinsic foot muscles and peroneal muscles, especially the peroneal longus. Intrinsic weakness can also lead to clawing of the toes. Conditions that lead to a cavus foot may be idiopathic or due to Charcot-Marie-Tooth (CMT) disease, myelomeningocele, Friedreich ataxia, or a spinal cord lesion (i.e. syringomyelia and tumor). A triple arthrodesis (calcaneocuboid, talonavicular, and subtalar) may be required for severe feet (or recurrent deformities) in older patients. Foot surgery is indicated in progressive or painful deformities. Tendon transfers, plantar releases, and first metatarsal dorsiflexion osteotomies may be required.

Foot pain: Several conditions cause foot pain in the absence of a deformity (i.e. cavus and planovalgus). The causes of non mechanical foot pain are divided into inflammatory, infectious, vascular, neoplastic, and traumatic. Köhler disease, Freiberg infarction, and Sever disease are examples of osteochondrosis of unknown etiology. Köhler disease involves the navicular bone, Freiberg infarction the metatarsal head, and Sever disease the calcaneal apophysis.

Juvenile hallux valgus (Bunion): Hallux valgus is a deformity of the first ray characterized by abduction of the first metatarsal, with adduction and pronation of the great toe (*see* Fig. 31.3.3 in CD). The prominence formed by the medial aspect of the first metatarsal is known as a bunion. Both extrinsic and intrinsic factors lead to the development of hallux valgus. Extrinsic factors include shoes with a narrow toe box, an elevated heel, or both. Intrinsic factors include hereditary tendency and planovalgus foot. Although bunions can be painful, most are not. Some patients are merely unhappy with their foot's aesthetic but do not have functional problems. Treatment begins with shoe modifications. Patients should wear a shoe with a wide toe box. The goal of surgery is a painless,

shoeable foot. The surgical treatment of juvenile bunion has a high recurrence rate.

Deformities of the lesser toes: Curly toe is a nonprogressive deformity of a lesser toe. Most cases are idiopathic. Curly toe is to be distinguished from claw toe, or dorsiflexed metatarsophalangeal joint with plantarflexed interphalangeal joints. Claw toe is a progressive deformity associated with spinal cord disease (e.g. myelomeningocele, syringomyelia) or a hereditary motor sensory neuropathy such as Charcot-Marie-Tooth disease. Curly toes occur most frequently with fourth and fifth toes. The deformity is initially flexible and painless. Pain does not appear until the child begins to wear shoes. Observation is the initial treatment. For most children, the condition either resolves spontaneously or remains asymptomatic. Persistent pain and difficulty with shoe wear are the indications for surgery. Syndactyly is a failure of segmentation of digits. Toe syndactyly can be either partial (a portion of the toe) or complete (entire toe) and either simple (skin only) or complex (involves osseous connections). Polydactyly is an error of duplication, resulting in an extra digit. The extra digit can be pre-axial (medial to the first toe) (*see* Fig. 31.3.4 in CD), postaxial (lateral to the fifth toe) or central. Patients with foot polydactyly may have extra digits on their hands as well. The extra toe may be rudimentary (lacking osseous structures) or may be a complete digit with its own metatarsal. The indications for amputation are cosmesis, difficulties with shoe wear, and foot pain.

31.4 TORSIONAL AND ANGULAR DEFORMITIES

The most common torsion and angular changes of the lower extremity are related to normal in utero positioning or acquired disorders. In the typical in utero position, the hips are flexed, abducted, and externally rotated; the knees are flexed and lower legs are internally rotated; and the feet are in slight equines, supinated, and in contact with the posterolateral aspect of the opposite thigh. The combination of the external rotation of the hip and the internal rotation of the lower leg produces a bowed appearance of the lower extremities when the child begins to ambulate. *Physiologic genu varum* or bow legs resolves with 6–12 months of independent ambulation. *Physiologic genu valgum* or knock knees is seen between 3 and 4 yr of age. This is true genu valgum and not the result of a rotational combination, and also resolves with growth, with the normal adult knee alignment obtained between 5 and 8 yr of age. The mean tibiofemoral angle at birth is 15 degrees of varus. This decreases to approximately 10 degrees by 1 yr of age. Neutral alignment occurs between 18 and 20 months of age.

maximal valgus of 12 degrees occurs at 3 to 4 yr of age. The values are similar for boys and girls. By 7 yr the valgus alignment corrects to that of a normal adult (8 degrees in women; 7 degrees in men). Approximately 95% of physiologic genu varum and genu valgum cases resolve with growth.

Coronal limb abnormalities: Genu varum (bow legs) and genu valgum (knock knees) are the two most common deformities found in the coronal plane. The infant is born with knees in varus. Varus persists until 2 years of age, when the legs straighten. The limbs then overcorrect and become maximally valgus between 3 and 4 years of age. In a child 6 to 7 years old, a mature knee alignment is achieved, with 5 to 7 degrees of valgus. Physiologic genu varus and genu valgus, which are characterized by spontaneous resolution, must be distinguished from pathologic conditions that will persist without treatment.

The genu varum (bow legs) is classified:
1. Physiologic
2. Asymmetric growth (tibia valga; trauma to proximal tibial metaphysis and physis; infection; tumor)
3. Metabolic disorders (vitamin D deficiency [nutritional rickets]; vitamin D resistant rickets; renal osteodystrophy)
4. Skeletal dysplasias
5. Congenital abnormalities (congenital dislocation of the patella)
6. Neuromuscular disorders (cerebral palsy, poliomyelitis, myelodysplasia).

The genu valgum (knock knees) is classified:
1. Physiologic (*see* Fig. 3.17 in CD)
2. Asymmetric growth (tibia vara (Blount disease) (infantile, juvenile, adolescent); focal fibro-cartilaginous dysplasia (trauma including physeal injury, infection, tumor)
3. *Metabolic disorders:* Vitamin D deficiency (nutritional rickets), vitamin D resistant rickets, hypophosphatasia
4. *Skeletal dysplasia:* (metaphyseal dysplasia, achondroplasia, enchondromatosis).

The diagnosis of idiopathic genu valgum is one of exclusion. When the disorder is severe, patients complain of knee instability or pain. The angular deformity is apparent on physical examination. The degree of knee deformity is measured on plain radiograph or computed tomography. Treatment is surgical, and a medial hemiepiphysiodesis is performed if adequate growth remains for the lateral physis to catch up. In the mature patient or the child in whom inadequate growth remains in the lateral physis for correction, a realignment osteotomy is performed.

Blount disease: Blount disease is an idiopathic, nonphysiologic form of genu varum. Classification is based on age at presentation. The infantile (presentation from birth to 4 years) and juvenile (5 to 10 years) forms of Blount disease are grouped together as early onset, and the adolescent form (presentation from 11 years to maturity) is categorized as late onset. Risk factors for infantile Blount disease are early ambulation and weight more than the 95% for age. Distinguishing physiologic genu varum from Blount disease is a difficult task in patients younger than 2 years. The child with infantile Blount disease has an angular deformity limited to the proximal tibia (no femoral involvement), and a lateral thrust is typically present. The radiographic changes associated with infantile Blount disease were described and divided into six stages by Langenskiold. These stages are characterized by progressive medial physeal inclination of the proximal tibia.

Observation is the mainstay of treatment for infantile Blount disease in children younger than 3 years. A brace is prescribed before 3 years of age for a child with a lateral thrust. Surgery is recommended after brace failure or once a child is older than 4 years. Surgery consists of a proximal tibial realignment osteotomy.

Tibial bowing: Congenital pseudoarthrosis of the tibia is a structural defect within the tibia that is susceptible to fracture and resistant to healing. Typically, the lesion is diaphyseal, located at the junction of the middle and distal thirds. Neurofibromatosis is the most common associated condition. Radiographs show a narrowing and sclerosis of the diaphysis. Early treatment, before the occurrence of fracture and significant angular deformity consists of bracing. Fracture or progressive bowing is an indication for surgical intervention.

Fibula hemimelia is a longitudinal deficiency in the lateral portion of the lower limb in which part or all of fibula may be missing. The foot commonly is missing its lateral rays and may be in severe valgus.

31.5 LEG-LENGTH DISCREPANCY

Approximately 65% of the growth of the entire lower extremity comes from the distal femoral (37%) and proximal tibial (28%) physes. Thus, growth disturbances around the knee can have the most adverse effect on leg length. Common causes of lower extremity length discrepancies include:
1. *Congenital:* Proximal femoral focal deficiency, coxa vara, developmental dysplasia of the hip
2. *Developmental:* Legg-Calvé-Perthes disease
3. *Neuromuscular:* Poliomyelitis, cerebral palsy (hemiplegia)

4. *Infectious:* Pyogenic osteomyelitis with physeal damage

5. *Trauma:* Physeal injury with premature closure, overgrowth, malunion (shortening)

6. *Tumor:* Physeal destruction, radiation induced physeal injury, overgrowth.

Radiographic evaluations are the most accurate methods of assessing leg length. Four different types of radiographic techniques are available including teleroentgenogram, orthoroentgenogram, scanogram and CT.

Discrepancies of greater than 2 cm at skeletal maturity usually require treatment because these often cause the patient to limp. Equalization can be achieved by non-surgical and surgical methods—extremity shortening or lengthening procedures. Extremity shortening procedures include epiphysiodesis, epiphyseal stapling and bone resection.

The advantages of lengthening are equalization of significant leg-length discrepancies, maintenance of ultimate adult height, preservation of normal body proportions, surgery on the affected limb, correction of existing angular deformities, and elimination of orthoses. The procedures include transiliac or pelvic lengthening and callotaxis technique by Ilizarov methodology.

31.6 KNEE

The tibiofemoral articulation is constrained only by soft tissues. The distal femur is cam-shaped, allowing it to have a gliding, hinged motion. The major constraints of the knee are the medial and lateral collateral ligaments, the anterior and posterior cruciate ligaments, and the medial and lateral menisci. Weight is transmitted through both the articular cartilage and the menisci. Patellofemoral joint is the common site of problems especially during adolescence. Pain around the knee is a common complaint in older children and adolescents. This may be insidious in onset or the result of trauma. Accumulation of fluid (effusion) in the knee occurs with arthritis (septic, viral, postinfectious, juvenile rheumatoid arthritis, systemic lupus erythematosus), hemorrhage secondary to hemophilia, overactivity and trauma. This fluid is aspirated to relieve discomfort and to make the diagnosis.

Discoid lateral meniscus (*see* Chapter 32)

Popliteal cyst: The popliteal cyst (Baker cyst) is commonly seen during the middle childhood years. There is distension of the gastrocnemius and semimembranous bursa along with the posterior aspect of the knee by synovial fluid from a tendon sheath or the knee joint. It is not due to intra-articular pathologic conditions. The diagnosis is confirmed by ultrasonography or aspiration. The resolution over several years usually occurs, especially in children 10 yr of age and younger. The only indications for surgical excision are the presence of symptoms or progressive enlargement.

Anderson M, Green WT, Messner MB. Growth and predictions of growth in the lower extremities. *J Bone Joint Surg Am* 1963; 45-A: 1–14.

Drennan JC. Congenital vertical talus. *Instr Course Lect* 1996; 45:315–22.

Hosalkar HS, Spiegel DA, Davidson, RS. The foot and toes. In: Kliegman RM, Behrman RE, Jenson HB, Stanton BF (eds). *Nelson Textbook of Pediatrics.* 18th edn. Vol. 2. Philadelphia: Saunders, 2007;2776–84.

Hosalkar HS, Wells L. Torsional and angular deformities. In: Kliegman RM, Behrman RE, Jenson HB, Stanton BF (eds). *Nelson Textbook of Pediatrics.* 18th edn. Vol. 2. Philadelphia: Saunders, 2007;2784–91.

Hosalkar HS, Gholve PA, Spiegel DA. Leg-length discrepancies. In: Kliegman RM, Behrman RE, Jenson HB, Stanton BF (eds). *Nelson Textbook of Pediatrics.* 18th edn. Vol. 2. Philadelphia: Saunders, 2007;2791–96.

Hosalkar HS, Wells L. The knee. In: Kliegman RM, Behrman RE, Jenson HB, Stanton BF (eds). *Nelson Textbook of Pediatrics.* 18th edn. Vol. 2. Philadelphia: Saunders, 2007;2796–2800.

Staheli LT. Rotational problems in children. *Instr Course Lect* 1994;43:199–209.

Staheli LT, Corbett M, Wyss C, King H. Lower-extremity rotational problems in children. Normal values to guide management. *J Bone Joint Surg Am* 1985;67(1):39–47.

31.7 HIP

Developmental dysplasia of the hip: About 2.5 to 6.5 cases per 1000 live births develop hip dysplasia, and a significant percentage of these cases are not evident on neonatal screening examinations (*see* Section 8.2). DDH encompasses the entire spectrum of abnormalities involving the growing hip, ranging from simple dysplasia to dysplasia plus subluxation or dislocation of the hip joint. The condition has the following three characteristic components:

1. Varying levels of abnormality in the slope of the acetabulum

2. Excessive laxity of the hip joint that allows the femoral head to slide upward and laterally out of its normal relationship with the acetabulum, and

3. Abnormal rotation of the upper end of the shaft leading to a malalignment of the femoral head and the acetabulum.

Although some studies suggest that a high percentage of newborns with DDH may spontaneously improve without treatment, many untreated cases of unilateral DDH progress, with development of a leg length discrepancy and a painless Trendelenburg gait (limp) in childhood or young adulthood. Osteoarthritis may occur in later life. About 1% of infants have dislocated, dislocatable, or subluxatable hips. Risk factors for DDH include female gender, breech presentation, positive family history, and reduced space in utero. Seventy percent of hip dislocations occur in girls. A child with DDH should be examined for other "molding" or "packing" deformities, such as congenital muscular torticollis, plagiocephaly (flat portion of head), metatarsus adductus, and congenital hyperextension of the knee. The most reliable clinical methods of DDH detection in the newborn are the Ortolani and Barlow (provocative) maneuvers. Asymmetry of thigh and gluteal skin folds may be present in 10% of normal infants but is suggestive of DDH. In infants younger than 6 months, the acetabulum and proximal femur are predominantiy cartilaginous and thus not visible on plain radiographs. In this age, these structures are best visualized with ultrasound. Radiographs are recommended for an infant once the proximal femoral epiphysis ossifies, usually by 4 to 6 months.

The goal in management of DDH is to achieve and maintain a concentric reduction of the femoral head within the acetabulum in order to provide the optimal environment for normal development of both the femoral head and acetabulum. Pavlik harness is the most commonly used device for the treatment of DDH. Use of the Pavlik harness should be discontinued if no reduction of the hip can be documented after 3 to 4 weeks of use. If Pavlik harness treatment fails, the child can be taken for an examination under anaesthesia, an attempt at closed reduction, and spica casting. Failure of closed reduction and immobilization necessitates an open reduction. Surgical options vary as per age of the patient at presentation.

Legg-Calvé-Perthes disease: LCPD is a disorder of the femoral head of unclear etiology. It involves temporary interruption of the blood supply to the bony nucleus of the proximal femoral epiphysis that leads to impairment of epiphyseal growth and an increase in bone density. The dense bone is subsequently replaced by new bone, resulting in flattened and enlarged femoral head. Once new bone is in place, the femoral head slowly remodels until skeletal maturity. LCPD generally affects children 4 to 12 years old. Boys are more commonly affected than girls. The incidence of bilateralism is 10% to 12%. LCPD may be an avascular phenomenon of the femoral head.

The clinical course of LCPD can be broken down into four pathologic phases:

1. The incipient, or synovitis phase
2. The osteonecrosis phase
3. The fragmentation phase, and
4. Regeneration and revascularization (healing) phase.

Children with LCPD usually present with a limp accompanied by hip pain or pain referred to the thigh or knee. In the early phase of LCPD, spasm may be the cause of restriction in motion. As the disease progresses, the range of motion of the affected hip becomes progressively limited, particularly in abduction and medial rotation. Treatment involves initial rest and traction followed by bracing/casting or operative containment (femoral or pelvis osteotomy) and salvage procedures in advanced cases.

Slipped capital femoral epiphysis (SCFE) affects adolescents, most often between ages 12 and 15. It involves displacement of the capital femoral epiphysis from the metaphysis through zone of the hypertrophy layer of the physeal plate. Obesity is the most closely associated factor in the development of SCFE. The higher prevalence of SCFE in children who are receiving growth hormone supplementation and who have hypothyroidism, hyperthyroidism, hypogonadism, hypopituitarism, or renal osteodystrophy also suggests an association between this disorder and an endocrine derangement. Two main concerns are:

1. Progression of the slip and
2. The development of degenerative joint disease. Child with SCFE often complains of knee or distal thigh pain (referred pain from hip). The gait is usually antalgic or trendelenburg. The slip may be acute, chronic or acute on chronic. The clinical classification for SCFE depends on the patient's ability to walk. SCFE is considered "stable" if the child is able to walk with or without crutches. A child with "unstable" SCFE is unable to walk, with or without crutches. The opposite hip may be susceptible to a slip simultaneously or later and should be watched for. Initial management includes a period of rest followed by in situ operative fixation to prevent progression of slip or corrective osteotomies for deformities. Complications include osteonecrosis and chondrolysis that are seriously disabling.

Bloom ML, Crawford AH. Slipped capital femoral epiphysis. An assessment of treatment modalities. *Orthopedics* 1985;8:36–40.

Haynes RJ. Developmental dysplasia of the hip: etiology, pathogenesis, and examination and physical findings in the newborn. *Instr Course Lect* 2001;50:535–40.

Herring JA. Legg-Calve-Perthes disease. In: Herring JA (Ed). *Tachdjian's Pediatric Orthopaedics*. 3rd edn. Philadelphia: WB Saunders; 2002:655–709.

Hosalkar HS, Horn D, Friedman JE, Dormans JP. The hip. In: Kliegman RM, Behrman RE, Jenson HB, Stanton BF (eds). *Nelson Textbook of Pediatrics*. 18th edn. Vol. 2. Philadelphia: Saunders, 2007;2800–11.

31.8 SPINE

Back pain is less common in childhood and adolescence than in adulthood but is more likely to have an identifiable cause. In the evaluation of a child with back pain, the patient's history is extremely important. Overuse injuries, although less common than in adults, can cause backaches in children. Activity pain usually resolves after a few days of rest. Children and adolescents can sustain fractures, disk herniations, and ligamentous injuries to their spinal columns. The pediatric spine, however, has greater elasticity than the mature spine. Because the bones and ligaments of the paediatric spine can tolerate more stretch than the spinal cord, children are at risk of having neurologic injuries even if radiographic findings are normal; this pattern of injury is referred to as spinal cord injury without radiographic abnormality (SCIWORA). Infections of the pediatric spine may involve the disk space (diskitis) or the vertebral body (osteomyelitis). Frequently, however, it is difficult to determine where the initial bacterial seeding began, and an entire vertebra-disk-vertebra unit becomes involved (spondylitis) subsequently. Tumors also may manifest as back pain, which often occurs at night. If the patient also has constitutional symptoms, such as fever and malaise, malignancy must be considered.

Idiopathic scoliosis is defined as scoliosis not associated with any other condition. On a standing radiograph, the lateral curvature of the spine should measure at least 10 degrees using the Cobb technique before being labelled true scoliosis. Long, gentle, flexible curves that disappear with forward bending and are not associated with a rib hump or rotational changes may be due to postural changes rather than true scoliosis. A curve should be classified as idiopathic only after other causes have been excluded. Idiopathic scoliosis can be classified according to the age of onset. The subtypes are infantile (onset between birth and 3 years), juvenile (onset between 3 and 10 years), and adolescent (onset after age 10, or post pubescent onset). It was noted that progression of curves after skeletal maturity was greatest for curves larger than 50 degrees, especially in the thoracic spine. Conversely, curves smaller than 30 degrees tended to be stable. Large curves have been implicated in pulmonary dysfunction and a higher incidence of back pain in adulthood.

Congenital scoliosis refers to a lateral curvature of the spine that is due to vertebral anomalies that develop in the embryonic period. Sagittal plane deformities, such as congenital kyphosis and lordosis, may also occur. Congenital anomalies are classified into two groups, those caused by failures of formation and those caused by failures of segmentation. A failure of formation results in incomplete formation of a vertebra. Depending on how much of the vertebra is lacking, various degrees of deformity may occur. A failure of segmentation may be unilateral or bilateral and may involve two or more vertebrae. If only one side is affected, a unilateral unsegmented bar arises that forms a bony bridge, and the other side may continue to grow and create a convexity. If, however, both sides fail to segment, a block vertebra forms, resulting in a shortened segment. The unilateral unsegmented bar with a contralateral, fully segmented hemivertebra has the worst prognosis and should be treated surgically once recognized. Curves due to nonsegmented hemivertebrae, incarcerated hemivertebrae, and block vertebrae may progress slowly or not at all and can usually be observed. Bracing is ineffective for controlling congenital curves. It has been found that some patients with congenital spinal deformities have an associated intraspinal defect, such as tethered cord, diastematomyelia, a low-lying conus, teratoma, or syringomyelia. MRI may not be necessary for every patient with congenital scoliosis; however, the modality may be performed for any suspicious clinical or radiologic findings or in a patient about to undergo surgery to correct the deformity.

Spondylolysis and spondylolisthesis: Spondylolysis refers to a defect in the pars interarticularis that may be unilateral or bilateral. Spondylolisthesis refers to the forward slippage of one vertebra on another. Patients may be asymptomatic or may manifest as pain. Patients frequently have tight hamstrings and walk with a bent knee, flexed-hip gait. Nerve root impingement usually of the L5 root, can occur. For patients experiencing pain, full time weaning of a brace for 3 to 6 months, followed by gradual wearing may relieve symptoms. Physical therapy that emphasizes abdominal strengthening and stretching of the lumbosacral fascia and hamstrings is also recommended. Surgery should be considered for patients suffering from spondylolisthesis with refractory pain, rapid slip progression, more than 50% slippage, or neurologic changes.

Scheuermann kyphosis: Excessive rounding of the back can be caused by postural changes or structural abnormalities. One can distinguish postural round back from true Scheuermann kyphosis by assessing the flexibility of the curve and looking for vertebral changes. Postural round back is corrected with hyperextension, demonstrates no structural changes in the vertebral bodies or intervertebral disks, and tends to improve with hyperextension exercise programs. Scheuermann kyphosis, however, is a more rigid condition. Scheuermann kyphosis has an incidence of 0.4% to 8% and appears to have a male preponderance. Patients tend to present during adolescence. Clinical findings consist of observation of a cosmetic deformity by the patient or other observer, and a complaint of back pain, especially toward the end of the adolescent growth. Scheuermann kyphosis usually occurs in the thoracic region, with an apex localized between T7 and T9. Mild scoliosis may be associated with the deformity. A thoracolumbar form, with an apex between T10 and T12, also occurs. For patients with stable curves smaller than 60 degrees, the natural history of Scheuermann kyphosis tends to be rather benign. Adolescents with curves smaller than 50 degrees rarely need any treatment other than observation. Treatment, either nonoperative or surgical, is reserved for patients with rapidly progressing kyphosis or vertebral wedging, unrelenting pain, and respiratory dysfunction due to deformity. Bracing is the most common treatment for Scheuermann kyphosis. Surgery may be indicated for a curve that is larger than 75 degrees or that rapidly progresses despite bracing.

Neuromuscular diseases: Spinal deformities are commonly associated with neuromuscular disorders. Cerebral palsy and myelodysplasia are the most common, but conditions such as muscular dystrophies, spinal muscular atrophy, Friedreich ataxia, and neurofibromatosis also occur and cause spinal changes. Any condition that interrupts or interferes with control of distal motor units by the central nervous system can affect neuromuscular balance, thus causing weakness, contractures, or deformity.

Disk space infection: Intervertebral diskitis is the term used for the association of back pain, progressive loss of intervertebral disk height, and erosion of adjacent vertebral end-plates usually in the lumbar regions. Rarely patients have severe back pain, high fever, and signs of bacteremia consistent with acute osteomyelitis. In most, the inflammatory process is much less severe. Toddlers may cease walking. Older children and adolescents complain of back, abdominal or pelvic pain. The physical findings in a child with a disk space infection are usually characteristic. The child maintains the spine in a straight, stiff, or splinted position and refuses to flex the lumbar spine. The normal lumbar lordosis is reversed, and there may be paravertebral muscle spasm. Radiographic signs lag behind clinical symptoms. Bone scans and MRI scans become abnormal early in the disease. MRI is most helpful in distinguishing diskitis from vertebral osteomyelitis. In patients with constitutional symptoms and signs suggestive of a bacterial cause,

initial treatment should include a combination of immobilization and antibiotics. Surgical drainage is usually reserved for patients who do not respond to initial therapy or who have MRI evidence of abscess formation in the paravertebral area.

Brown R, Hussain M, McHugh K, Novelli V, Jones D. Discitis in young children. *J Bone Joint Surg Br* 2001; 83: 106–111.

Jones GT, Macfarlane GJ. Epidemiology of low back pain in children and adolescents. *Arch Dis Child* 2005; 90: 312–316.

Spiegel DA, Hosalkar HS, Dormans JP. The spine. In: Kliegman RM, Behrman RE, Jenson HB, Stanton BF (eds). *Nelson Textbook of Pediatrics*. 18th edn. Vol. 2. Philadelphia: Saunders, 2007; 2811–2822.

31.9 NECK

Torticollis: Torticollis (*torqueo*, "to twist" + *collum*, "neck") is the term applied to the clinical finding of a twisted neck. In most instances, the head is tipped toward one side and the chin rotated toward the other. Torticollis that is present at birth may be the result of in utero positional (postural) effects or traumatic lesions of the sternomastoid muscle or of congenital abnormalities of the cervical spine. Torticollis in later childhood may be the result of trauma, inflammatory processes, spinal or central nervous system neoplasia. Muscular torticollis is the most common variety and is presumed to result from injury to the sternocleidomastoid muscle during delivery. In affected infants, rotation of the neck during delivery produces bleeding within the substance of the sternocleidomastoid muscle (tumor) and a localized increase in pressure within the muscular compartment contained by the sternocleidomastoid fascia. Increased pressure produces focal ischemia and secondary fibrosis. Significant correction usually occurs within the first few months of life. Surgical release of the sternocleidomastoid muscle is occasionally required in patients before the development of facial asymmetry (plagiocephaly).

Klippel-Feil syndrome: The clinical triad of short neck, low hairline, and restriction of neck motion in a patient with multiple coalitions of the cervical vertebrae defines this syndrome. There is an association of the Klippel-Feil triad with congenital abnormalities of the genitourinary trait, auditory system, spinal cord, arid cardiovascular system, as well as with other abnormalities of the musculoskeletal system. Sprengel anomaly (congenital elevation of the scapula is a common associated finding. Affected children characteristically have low hairlines and short, sometimes webbed necks. Decreased active and passive motion of the cervical spine is usually present.

Initial evaluation should include anteroposterior, lateral, and oblique views of the cervical spine.

Atlantoaxial instability: Instability of the upper cervical spine in children is uncommon but potentially devastating. Developmental, traumatic inflammatory or metabolic lesions that affect the stability of the occiput-C1 or C1-2 joint have serious implications. Progressive myelopathy may develop in patients with chronic instability; acute impingement and death are possible in patients with severe instability. Hypoplasia and absence of the odontoid process—rudimentary formation or absence of the odontoid process is well documented in disorders such as Morquio syndrome. Symptoms vary depending on the degree of C1-2 instability. MRI is indicated. In normal asymptomatic patients without radiographic evidence of instability, restriction of contact sports and close observation is appropriate. In patients with Morquio syndrome, cervical stabilization should be considered even when such patients are asymptomatic and have little instability. In patients with cervical instability or abnormal neurologic findings, stabilization of the cervical spine is essential.

Down syndrome: Down syndrome cases are associated with instability of the upper cervical spine in the range of 10–25%. Reported abnormalities include occipitoatlantal instability, atlantoaxial instability and occipitalization of the atlas.

Brockmeyer D. Down syndrome and craniovertebral instability. Topic review and treatment recommendations. *Pediatr Neurosurg* 1999; 31: 71–7.

Herman MJ, Pizzutillo PD. Cervical spine disorders in children. *Orthop Clin North Am.* 1999; 30: 457–66.

Spiegel DA, Hosalkar HS, Dormans JP, Drommond DS. The Neck. In: Kliegman RM, Behrman RE, Jenson HB, Stanton BF (eds). *Nelson Textbook of Pediatrics.* 18th edn. Vol. 2. Philadelphia: Saunders, 2007; 2822–2826.

31.10 UPPER LIMB

Sprengel deformity: Failure of the scapula to descend to its normal location is termed Sprengel deformity. The scapula is located at an abnormally high position with respect to the child's neck and thorax. This uncommon abnormality occurs with varying degrees of severity. Webbing of the skin between the neck and scapula and a low posterior hairline may be associated findings. In the severe form, a bone (omovertebral) may connect the scapula with the cervical spine and prevent scapulothoracic movement. A Klippel-Feil anomaly (congenital fusion of one or more of the cervical spine vertebra) may also occur with Sprengel deformity. The best outcome in severe Sprengel deformity is achieved by surgically repositioning or, occasionally, partially resecting the scapula. This improves the cosmetic appearance. Mild cases when operated may yield a cosmetically better appearance but no function is gained.

Nursemaid's elbow (pulled elbow): When longitudinal traction is applied to the upper extremity with the elbow in extension, the annular ligament can slide over the radial head and become partially entrapped in the radiohumeral joint. This leads to pulled elbow. The subluxation of the annular ligament is initiated by either a jerk on the arm when the child falls while the hand is being held by a parent or when the child is forcibly lifted by the hand. The hand typically is held in a pronated position, and the child may refuse to use the hand and may cry when the elbow is moved. Treatment involves rotating the hand and forearm to a supinated position with pressure over the radial head.

Syndactyly is the most common hand congenital deformity after polydactyly. Half of cases are bilaterally symmetrical. The rays most commonly involved are the middle and ring fingers (third web space). Simple syndactyly involves only soft tissues and complex syndactyly involves the bones as well. The timing of syndactyly correction depends on the type and cosmetic deformation. For simple and incomplete syndactyly, the best surgical result can be achieved when the child is older, but usually before school starts. However, early separation during the first year of age is indicated in cases of complex syndactyly associated with Apert syndrome.

Polydactyly is the most common congenital hand deformity. Postdactyly most commonly affects the border digits and is extremely rare in the central digits. Thumb (radial) polydactyly can occur in isolation or as part of a syndrome. Surgical correction, which can be carried out when the child is between 1 and 3 years old, usually involves deletion of the smaller thumb.

Ulnar polydactyly usually occurs in isolation. Those attached by a wider base or by bone should be excised in the operating room after the patient's first birthday, when general anesthesia is safer.

Chan O, Hughes T. Hand. *Br Med J* 2005; 330: 1073–1075.

Cornwall Roger. Upper limb. In: Kliegman RM, Behrman RE, Jenson HB, Stanton BF (eds). *Nelson Textbook of Pediatrics.* 18th edn. Vol. 2. Philadelphia: Saunders, 2007; 2826–2829.

Knight SL, Kay SPJ. Classification of congenital anomalies. In: Gupta A, Kay SPK, Scheker LR (eds). *The Growing Hand: Diagnosis and Management of the Upper Extremity in Children.* London: Mosby, 2000.

31.11 SKELETAL DYSPLASIAS

The skeletal dysplasias, also known as osteochondrodysplasias, are a group of genetic disorders characterized by generalized disorders of growth and development of bone and cartilage.

Pseudochondroplasia: Newborns with pseudo-chondroplasia are average in size and appearance. Gait abnormalities and short stature mainly affect the limbs and become apparent in late infancy. The hands are short, broad and deviation an ulna direction; the forearms are bowed. Developmental milestone and intelligence are usually normal. Lumbar lordosis and deformities in the knee develop during childhood; the latter frequently requires surgical correction. Pain is common in weight bearing joints during childhood and adolescence, leading to osteoarthritis in late 2nd decade of life. Skeletal radiographs of thoracolumbar spine shows central protrusion (tonguing) of the anterior aspect of the upper lumbar and lower thoracic vertebrae and reduced vertebral body heights (platyspondyly) and secondary lordosis. Lower extremity radiograph shows large metaphyses, poorly formed epiphyses, and marked bowing of long bones.

Multiple epiphyseal dysplasia (MED): MED, one of the most common skeletal dysplasias, is characterized by delayed epiphyseal ossification and limb deformities. MED is transmitted as an autosomal dominant condition. Children with MED are usually referred to orthopaedic surgeons, later in childhood, for joint pain in the lower limbs, decreased range of motion of the hips and knees, or gait disturbance. Angular deformities of the lower limbs, including coxa vara, genu varum, and genu valgum, are common.

Radiographs reveal delayed epiphyseal ossification with subsequent irregular ossification and joint surface deformation. Upper extremity involvement is mild. Treatment involves corrective osteotomies for limb deformities when the child nears maturity.

Achondroplasia is the most common form of short limb dwarfism. It is an autosomal dominant condition, although two thirds of cases arise from spontaneous new mutations. The mutation of achondroplasia is in the gene encoding fibroblast growth factor receptor 3 (*FGFR3*). The achondroplasia group consists of thanatophoric dysplasia, achondroplasia and hypochondroplasia; all three have mutations in a small number of locations in the *FGFR3* gene and there is a strong correlation between the mutations and the clinical phenotype. Thanatophoric dysplasia (TD) is the most common lethal chondrodysplasia with an incidence of 1/35,000, achondroplasia is the most nonlethal chondrodysplasia with an incidence of 1/15,000 to 1/40,000 births and hypochondroplasia resembles achondroplasia but is milder. Achondro-plasia is recognizable at birth with short limbs, a long narrow trunk, and a large head with midfacial hypoplasia and prominent forehead. The limb shortening is greatest in the proximal segments, and digits of the hand have extra space between the third and fourth, so the digits are separated into three groups—the 'trident hand'. Most joints are hyper extensible, but extension is restricted at the elbow. A thoracolumbar gibbus is often found. Usually birth length is slightly less than normal. Developmental motor milestones are frequently delayed. Intelligence is normal unless central nervous system develops. Frontal bossing, flattening of the nasal bridge, and mid-face hypoplasia are typical facial features of children with achondroplasia. Other problems include obesity, frequent ear infections, compromised pulmonary function and varied neurologic signs due to foramen magnum stenosis and thoracolumbar spinal stenosis. Foramen magnum stenosis is measured most accurately on computed tomography (CT) or magnetic resonance imaging (MRI). Skeletal radiographs confirm the diagnosis. The calvarial bones are large, whereas the cranial base and facial bones are small. The vertebral pedicles are short throughout the spine on a lateral radiograph and the interpedicular distance, which normally increases from the 1st to the 5th lumbar vertebra decreases in achondroplasia. The iliac bones are short and round and the acetabular roofs are flat. The tubular bones are short with mildly irregular and flared metaphyses. The fibula is disproportionately long compared to tibia. Initial treatment consists of spinal bracing, failing which posterior spinal fusion may be required. Limb deformities may require operative correction.

Jansen metaphyseal chondrodysplasia is a rare dominantly inherited chondrodysplasia characterized by severe shortening of limbs associated with an unusual facial appearance. Sometimes it is accompanied by clubfoot and hypercalcemia. It is caused by activating mutations of PTHR1.

Osteogenesis imperfecta (OI) is an autosomal dominant disorder. OI is due to the presence of abnormal type I collagen fibrils and relatively increased levels of types III and V collagen. OI has a triad of fragile bones, blue sclerae, and early deafness.

It is seen with varying levels of severity, from multiple fractures in an infant to only a few fractures before maturity in a child. Due to repeated fractures and deformity children are short stature. Sillence classification system is most commonly used which divides OI into four types based on clinical and radiographic criteria. Additional types (types V, VI, VII) have been proposed based on histologic distinctions. Type 1 is the most common and mild while type 2 is lethal. Type III is the most severe nonlethal form of OI, whereas type IV is moderately severe form. The morbidity and mortality of OI are cardiopulmonary. Recurrent pneumonias and declining pulmonary function occur in childhood. Neurologic complications include basilar invagination (best detected with spiral CT of the craniocervical junction), brain stem compression, hydrocephalus, and syringohydromyelia. Radiographs reveal generalized osteopenia and deformities owing to repeated microfractures and fractures. A characteristic deformity is the 'Shepherd Crook' deformity in the proximal femur. There is no cure for OI. Adolescents with OI may require psychologic support with body image issues. Treatments with calcium, fluoride supplements or calcitonin do not improve OI. Growth hormone improves bone histology in growth responsive children (usually types I and IV). A short course of treatment with bisphosphonates confers some benefit. Orthopedic management is aimed at fracture management and correction of deformity to enable function. Fractures and deformities are amenable to either closed or operative correction or fixation. Callus formation is normal but is plastic and easily deformed.

Marfan syndrome: Marfan syndrome is an autosomal dominantly inherited connective tissue disorder. The incidence of this disorder is about 1 per 5,000–10,000 births. The pathogenesis is related to abnormal biosynthesis of fibrillin-1 (FBN-1). The locus of FBN-1 resides within the long arm of chromosome 15 (15q21). The diagnosis of Marfan syndrome is based on the clinical findings consisting of tall stature (present at birth and persist to adulthood), diminished subcutaneous fat, hypotonia, ligamentous laxity and musculoskeletal, cardiovascular, and ocular abnormalities.

Marfan syndrome individuals are *tall stature* and a *long, thin face* with narrowness of the maxilla and *dental crowding. Ocular abnormalities* include blue sclerae, myopia affecting in 60% of affected individuals, increased intraocular pressure, retinal detachment, and lens dislocation. *Musculoskeletal system* abnormalities include dolichostenomelia (long, thin limbs), and the arm span exceeds the height (>1.05 times higher). The lower segment (distance from pubis to heel) is increased in comparison to the upper segment (height minus lower segment) and contributes to a diminished upper segment: lower segment ratio (U/L). Hand findings include long thin fingers (arachnodactyly) that are hyperextensible. The thumb may be adducted across the narrow palm (Steinberg sign). When the hand is clenched without assistance, the entire thumb nail projects beyond the border of the hand (Thumb sign). When the wrist is grasped by the contralateral hand the thumb may appreciably overlap the 5th finger (Wrist sign). Long gracile ribs may contribute to various sternal anomalies including pectus excavatum (funnel chest) or pectus carinatum (pigeon breast). *Cardiovascular defects* include aortic root dilatation and mitral valve prolapse (MVP). There is increased risk of spontaneous pneumothorax and dural ectasia because of increases distension of lung parenchyma and dura respectively.

The differential diagnosis includes homocystinuria, Loeys Dietz aneurysm syndrome, familial aortic dissection, familial ectopia lentis, and MASS (myopia, mitral valve prolapse, mitral aortic dilation, skin striae, skeletal features like Marfan syndrome) syndrome.

Therapy focuses on prevention of complications and genetic counselling.

Beighton P, Giedion ZA, Gorlin R, Hall J, Horton B, Kozlowski K, Lachman R, Langer LO, Maroteaux P, Poznanski A, et al. International classification of osteochondrodysplasias. International Working Group on Constitutional Diseases of Bone. *Am J Med Genet* 1992; 44: 223–229.

Horton WA, Hecht JT. General considerations, the skeletal dysplasia. In: Kliegman RM, Behrman RE, Jenson HB, Stanton BF (eds). *Nelson Textbook of Pediatrics.* 18th edn. Vol. 2. Philadelphia: Saunders, 2007; 2869–2873.

Marini JC. Osteogenesis imperfecta. In: Kliegman RM, Behrman RE, Jenson HB, Stanton BF (eds). *Nelson Textbook of Pediatrics.* 18th edn. Vol. 2. Philadelphia: Saunders, 2007; 2887–2890.

Roninson LK, Fitzpatrick E. Marfan syndrome. In: Kliegman RM, Behrman RE, Jenson HB, Stanton BF (eds). *Nelson Textbook of Pediatrics.* 18th edn. Vol. 2. Philadelphia: Saunders, 2007; 2890–2893.

31.12 METABOLIC BONE DISEASE

Rickets: Lack of calcium and phosphorus may be due to inadequate intake of calcium and vitamin D, impaired absorption of phosphorus or vitamin D, decreased conversion of vitamin D to its active form, end-organ insensitivity to vitamin D, impaired release of calcium from bone, and phosphate wasting.

The causes of rickets are classified into 3 groups: Deficiency diseases: Vitamin D-deficient rickets (inadequate intake of vitamin D ± no sunlight), chelators in the diet (i.e. phytates, oxylates), phosphorus deficiency, gastrointestinal disorder, hepatobiliary rickets (free fatty acids in gut binding calcium).

Vitamin D-resistant rickets: Hypophoshatemic rickets (decreased tubular reabsorption of phosphate), decrease in 1, 25-dihydroxyvitamin D production, end-organ insensitivity to autogenous 1,25-dihydroxy vitamin D, renal tubular acidosis. It is commonly transmitted as an X-linked dominant disorder.

Unusual forms of rickets: Rickets in association with soft tissue and bone tumors, rickets in association with fibrous dysplasia, rickets in association with neurofibromatosis, rickets in association with anticonvulsant medications, renal osteodystrophy.

Children with rickets usually have short stature, often less than the third percentile. Muscle weakness of the abdomen and extremities may be seen. Frontal bossing and enlargement of the suture lines (e.g. caput quadratum) are common. Delayed dentition, enamel, defects, and extensive caries are common dental anomalies. Examination of the chest is likely to show enlargement of the costal cartilage (rachitic rosary), indentation of the lower ribs where the diaphragm inserts (Harrison groove), and, occasionally, pectus carinatum. The spine is commonly affected most characteristically with a long thoracic kyphosis. Lower limb deformities—genu varum and valgum are common and depend on the age of onset of the disease.

Radiographic findings include osteopenia, thin cortices, and small trabeculae with an overall decrease in bone mass. The appearance of the growth plates, including irregular widening or cupping, splaying, fraying is the most classic finding. Looser lines or incomplete fractures may also be seen.

The main diagnostic laboratory tests are measurements of serum calcium, phosphate, and alkaline phosphatase levels. Also helpful are determinations of serum 25-hydroxyl vitamin D, 1, 25-dihydroxyvitamin D and PTH levels and of urine calcium and phosphate levels. Children with classic or vitamin D-deficient rickets usually have low to low-normal levels of serum calcium, low levels of serum phosphorus, elevated levels of serum alkaline phosphatase and PTH, low concentrations of vitamin D.

Treatment is medical in the form of high doses of vitamin D and calcium with emphasis on adequate diet and periods of sunlight exposure. Limb deformities, if do not resolve spontaneously, may require corrective surgeries.

Renal osteodystrophy includes bone diseases that occur as a result of renal failure. In renal osteodystrophy, glomerular damage leads to phosphate retention, and tubular injury causes decreased production of 1,25-dihydroxyvitamin D, the active form of vitamin D. These two factors severely inhibit the gut's ability to absorb calcium. The resultant hypocalcemia triggers severe secondary hyperparathyroidism, which remains ineffective in increasing intestinal absorption of calcium. Therefore, the body's only means of raising serum calcium levels is through bone resorption. Patients with chronic renal disease are hyperphosphatemic, and even when pH is reduced, shifting the solubility product, they depend on a decreased serum calcium level to avoid precipitation of the relatively insoluble $CaHPO_4$. If for

any reason (e.g. dietary indiscretion, spontaneous improvement, or dialysis) calcium increases to near-normal levels, calcium salts may be precipitated at a variety of ectopic sites. Patients with renal osteodystrophy may have all the features of rickets. But generally they have a more 'sick' look. The presence of calcification in the conjunctivae and skin can produce significant irritation and itching. The periarticular calcification and ossification can cause severe limitation and pain in one or more joints. Slipped epiphysis especially in the proximal femur is common. Radiographic changes seen in renal osteodystrophy are unique, consisting of "salt-and-pepper" skull, subperiosteal resorption of the ulnas, terminal tufts of distal phalanges, clavicle, and medial proximal tibias. Brown tumors may also be seen as lytic areas. Management involves medical treatment of the underlying metabolic disturbance as the first step. This may involve oral or injectable vitamin D preparations, calcium and phosphate supplements and alkalinizing solutions. Fractures and deformities may require closed or surgical correction after metabolic stabilization. There is a high recurrence rate of deformities even after surgical correction.

Metaphyseal dysplasia (primary chondrodystrophy): This autosomal dominant condition is characterized by bowing of the legs, short stature, and a waddling gait in the absence of abnormalities of serum levels of calcium and phosphate, alkaline phosphatase activity, or vitamin D metabolites. Metaphyseal dysostosis results from defects in endochondral bone formation and metaphyseal modelling. Allogeneic bone marrow transplantation has been used as a therapeutic approach.

Hypophosphatasia is an autosomal recessive disorder that radiographically resembles rickets but has low serum alkaline phosphatase activity. The tissue-nonspecific (liver/bone/kidney) alkaline phosphatase isoenzyme (TNSALP) is deficient. Patients with mild disease may present with bowing of the legs and variable statural shortening. Hypercalcemia is common in the neonatal and infantile forms. Bone marrow transplantation has been successful using donors with normal TNSALP values.

Hyperphosphatasia is an autosomal recessive disorder with normal serum calcium and phosphate levels and elevated serum alkaline phosphatase activity. The onset of disease is usually by 2–3 yr of age when painful deformity develops in the extremities leading to abnormal gait and sometimes fractures. The clinical findings include bowing and thickening of diaphyses, pes craniatum, kyphoscoliosis, rib fraying, large skull and hearing loss. Transient hyperphosphatasia occurs between 2 mo to 2 yr of age with some mild gastrointestinal symptoms; both liver and bone isoenzymes are elevated. Resolution usually occurs within 4–6 months.

Osteoporosis is the most common bone disorder in adults but uncommon in children. In osteoporosis there is reduced amount of bone tissue (osteopenia), which is associated with atraumatic (pathological) fractures. Osteoporosis in children may be primary or secondary. The primary forms of osteoporosis include osteogenesis imperfect, Bruck syndrome, osteoporosis-pseudoglioma syndrome, Ehlers-Danlos syndrome, Marfan syndrome, homocystinuria, and idiopathic juvenile osteoporosis. Secondary forms of osteoporosis include various neuromuscular disorders, chronic illness, endocrine disorders, inborn errors of metabolism, including lysinuric protein intolerance and Gaucher disease, and drug-induced (alcohol, glucocorticoids, thyroxine, anticonvulsants, heparin, gonadotropin-releasing hormone agonist, cyclosporine, chemotherapy, cigarettes). Idiopathic juvenile osteoporosis should be considered, especially following clinical features are present: onset prior to puberty, long bone and lower back pain, vertebral fractures, a washed out appearance of the spine and appendicular skeleton, and improvement after puberty. Blood values of minerals, vitamin D metabolites, alkaline phosphatase, and parathyroid hormone are normal. Bone mineral content and bone density by dual-energy X-ray absorptiometry or less often quantitative CT shows markedly reduced values. Therapy including oral calcium supplements, calcitriol, bisphosphonates and calcitonin has been used with some success in individual cases. Spontaneous recovery has been reported in more than 75% cases after the onset of adolescence.

Chesney RW. Metabolic bone disease. In: Kliegman RM, Behrman RE, Jenson HB, Stanton BF (eds). *Nelson Textbook of Pediatrics*. 18th edn. Vol. 2. Philadelphia: Saunders, 2007; 2893–2898.

Cundy T, Wheadon L, King A. Treatment of idiopathic hyperphospatasia with intensive bisphosphonate therapy. *J Bone Miner Res* 2004; 19: 703–711.

Fewtrell MS. Bone densitometry in children assessed by dual X-ray absorptiometry: Uses and pitfalls. *Arch Dis Child* 2003; 88: 795–798.

Mankin HJ. Rickets, osteomalacia, and renal osteodystrophy. An update. *Orthop Clin North Am* 1990; 21: 81–96.

Solomon CG. Bisphosphonates and osteoporosis. *N Engl J Med* 2002; 346: 642.

31.13 ARTHROGRYPOSIS

Arthrogryposis is a congenital neuromuscular disorder involving both upper and lower extremities.

It is characterized by multiple joint contractures and decrease in muscle bulk and number. Arthrogryposis multiplex congenita signifies numerous congenital contractures. The upper extremities in arthrogryposis have fixed joint contractures with internal rotation of the shoulder, extension of the elbow, flexion and ulnar deviation of the wrist, flexed digits, and thumb-in-palm deformity. Most children with arthrogryposis are of above-average intelligence. There are no associated visceral abnormalities, and life expectancy is normal. The consistent goal of any treatment should be to enhance the quality of life and facilitate functional independence. Treatment usually starts with splinting and occupational therapy. The goal of the surgery is to allow for full flexion at the elbow and 40 degrees of extension at the wrist. Although this is not a progressive disease, the joint contracture commonly recurs after surgery without long-term splinting and therapy.

Hosalkar HS, Drummond DS. Arthrogryposis. In: Kliegman RM, Behrman RE, Jenson HB, Stanton BF (eds). *Nelson Textbook of Pediatrics*. 18th edn. Vol. 2. Philadelphia: Saunders, 2007; 2829–2834.

31.14 OSTEOMYELITIS AND SUPPURATIVE ARTHRITIS

Osteomyelitis and suppurative arthritis are most common in young children. This is particularly true of arthritis, in which half of all cases occur by 2 years of age and three fourths of all cases occur by 5 years of age, compared with about one third and one half respectively, for osteomyelitis among these age groups. Osteomyelitis is more common in boys than girls. The majority of infections in otherwise healthy children are of hematogenous origin. Minor, closed trauma is a common preceding event in cases of osteomyelitis, occurring in about one third of patients.

Bacteria are the most common pathogens in acute skeletal infections. In osteomyelitis, *Staphylococcus aureus* is the most common infecting organism in all age groups, including newborns. Group B Streptococcus and gram-negative enteric bacilli are also prominent pathogens in neonates. Cases of Pseudomonas are related almost exclusively to puncture wounds of the foot. Other organisms include *Haemophilus influenzae*, *Salmonella*, group A Streptococcus and *Streptococcus pneumoniae*.

Neonates may exhibit pseudo-paralysis or pain with movement of the affected extremity. Half of neonates do not have fever and may not appear ill. Older infants and children are more likely to have fever, pain, and localizing signs such as edema, erythema, and warmth. With involvement of the lower extremities, limp or refusal to walk is seen in approximately half of patients.

Long bones are principally involved in osteomyelitis. The femur and tibia are equally affected and together constitute almost half of all cases. The bones of the upper extremities account one fourth of all cases. Flat bones are less commonly affected. There is usually only a single site of bone or joint involvement. Several bones or joints are infected in fewer than 10% of cases; notable exceptions are gonococcal infections and osteomyelitis in neonates, in whom two or more bones are involved in almost half of the cases.

Aspiration of the infected site for Gram stain and culture when history and physical findings indicate a strong likelihood of osteomyelitis or suppurative arthritis remains the definitive diagnostic technique and provides the optimal specimen for culture to confirm the diagnosis.

Tests such as white blood cell count and differential, erythrocyte sedimentation rate (ESR), and C-reactive protein (CRP) are very sensitive for bone and joint infections but are non specific and not helpful in distinguishing between skeletal infection and other inflammatory processes.

Conventional radiographs, ultrasound, CT, MRI and radionuclide studies may all contribute to establishing the diagnosis. Lytic bone changes are not visible on radiographs until 30–50% of the bone matrix is destroyed, which is usually 7–14 days after onset of infection.

The initial empirical antibiotic therapy is based on knowledge of likely bacterial pathogens at various ages, the results of the Gram stain of aspirated material, and additional considerations. In neonates, an antistaphylococcal penicillin, such as oxacillin (150–200 mg/kg/24 hr divided q 6 h IV), and a broad-spectrum cephalosporin, such as cefotaxime (l50–200 mg/kg/24 hr divided q 8 h IV), provide coverage for the *S. aureus*, group B Streptococcus, and gram-negative bacilli. When the pathogen is identified appropriate adjustments in antibiotics are made if necessary. If a pathogen is not identified and the patient condition is improving, therapy is continued with the initially selected antibiotics. Duration of antibiotic therapy is individualized depending on the organism isolated and clinical course. Changing antibiotics from the intravenous route to oral administration when a patient's condition has stabilized, generally after 1 week of intravenous therapy may be considered. When frank pus is obtained from subperiosteal or metaphyseal aspiration, a surgical drainage is usually indicated. Infection of the hip joint is considered a surgical emergency because of the vulnerability of the blood supply to the head of femur.

Treatment of chronic osteomyelitis consists of surgical removal of sinus tracts and sequestrum. Antibiotic therapy is continued for several months or longer until clinical and radiologic findings suggest that healing has occurred.

Huber AM, Lam PY, Duffy CM, et al. Chronic recurrent multifocal osteomyelitis: Clinical outcomes after more than five years of follow-up. *J Pediatr* 2002;141:198–203.

Lampe RM. Osteomyelitis. In: Kliegman RM, Behrman RE, Jenson HB, Stanton BF (eds). *Nelson Textbook of Pediatrics.* 18th edn. Vol. 2. Philadelphia: Saunders, 2007; 2841–45.

Lampe RM. Suppurative arthritis. In: Kliegman RM, Behrman RE, Jenson HB, Stanton BF (eds). *Nelson Textbook of Pediatrics.* 18th edn. Vol. 2. Philadelphia: Saunders, 2007;2845–47.

Lew DP, Waldvogel FA. Osteomyelitis. *Semin Musculoskelt Radiol* 2004;8:243–53.

Nelson JD. Bugs, drugs, and bones: a pediatric infectious disease specialist reflects on management of musculoskeletal infections. *J Pediatr Orthop* 1999;19:141–2.

31.15 FRACTURES IN CHILDREN

Sites and patterns of fractures and their healing in children are grossly different from adults. Bones of children have a tremendous remodeling capacity enabling majority of pediatric fractures to be treated conservatively. But fractures near physis need to be followed up for longer periods to watch for late complications and treatment thereof. In addition to the complete fractures as seen in adults, bones of child present specific fracture patterns.

Greenstick fractures are caused by angulation forces on a long bone when the force is insufficient to cause a complete fracture but sufficient to cause plastic deformation of the bone. It causes a break in the tension side and a buckling at the compression side of the long bone.

Torus fractures are metaphyseal compression fractures in young children; frequent sites being distal radius and tibia. These are stable injuries and require no specialized treatment except relative immobilization.

Bend fractures are caused by plastic deformation of bone due to angulation producing forces that are insufficient to produce a complete fracture. These are different from greenstick fractures as there is no break in cortex and are commonly seen in ulna and fibula.

Epiphyseal injuries: Salter and Harris classified epiphyseal injuries depending upon the involvement of the physis, epiphysis, and the joint (*see* Fig. 31.23 in CD).

Open fractures: An open fracture should be treated as contaminated. Open fracture wounds need to be enlarged, irrigated and debrided in a sterile operating suite with the patient under general or regional block anesthesia and the patient should be treated with intravenous antibiotics. External fixation is the method of choice but transfixing pins should be avoided in physes and adequate incisions should be used for pin insertion to prevent skin necrosis and infection (*see* Fig. 31.24 in CD). Delayed union and nonunion, though not so common in pediatric fractures, may be seen in open injuries.

Pathological fractures: Children with pathological fractures such as in pseudoarthrosis of tibia due to neurofibromatosis, fractures through cystic areas in unicameral bone cysts and multiple fractures of long bones as in myelomeningocele or osteogenesis imperfecta are difficult to treat. Bones of children have a tremendous remodeling capacity enabling majority of pediatric fractures to be treated conservatively (*see* Fig. 31.25 in CD). These children usually require open reduction and internal fixation and occasionally bridging of large bone defects by bone grafting.

Fractures at birth: These fractures commonly occur in the clavicle, humerus, hip and femur due to trauma during delivery especially in difficult, prolonged labor and narrow birth canal.

Fractures an indication of child abuse: The highest percentage of child abuse occurs between birth and 2 years of age. In any child under 2 years old with a significant fracture and a questionable history of its occurrence, child abuse should be suspected. A bone scan or skeletal survey generally is indicated to investigate a suspected battered child. Multiple fractures in different stages of healing are almost always indicative of child abuse. Multiple areas of large ecchymoses in different stages of resolution are also pathognomonic of child abuse. Epiphyseal-metaphyseal fractures (Corner fractures) are caused by pulling and twisting forces that are rarely accidental. These are another pointer towards child abuse. Other suspicious fractures could be posterior rib fractures, scapular fractures, spinous process fractures and sternal fractures. Epiphyseal separations, vertebral body fractures, complex skull fracture, digit fractures, and spiral fractures in non-ambulatory infants are also highly suggestive of non accidental trauma.

Canale ST. Fractures and dislocations in children. In: Canale ST (Ed). *Campbell's Operative Orthopaedics*. Philadelphia: Mosby, 2003; 1391–1568.

Cheng JC, Shen WY. Limb fracture pattern in different pediatric age groups: a study of 3350 children. *J Orthop Trauma* 1993; 7: 15–22.

Gholve PA, Hosalkar HS, Dormans JP, Wells L. Common fractures. In: Kliegman RM, Behrman RE, Jenson HB, Stanton BF (eds). *Nelson Textbook of Pediatrics*. 18th edn. Vol. 2. Philadelphia: Saunders, 2007; 2834–2841.

Overly F, Steele DW. Common pediatric fractures and dislocations. *Clin Pediatr Surg Med* 2002; 3: 106–117.

Salter RB, Harris WR. Injuries involving the epiphyseal plate. *J Bone Joint Surg Am* 1963; 45: 587–622.

Silber JS, Flynn JM, Koffler KM. Analysis of the cause, classification, and associated injuries of 166 consecutive pelvic fractures. *J Pediatr Orthop* 2001; 21: 446–450.

32 ◆ Sports Medicine

32.1 INTRODUCTION

Sports injuries account for nearly a quarter of all injuries in children and adolescents. So, those caring for young athletes must be aware of the special characteristics of injuries incurred on the field of play. Physicians, thus, have an important role in sports injuries as a caregiver. They have the responsibility of providing medical clearance for participation in physical activity and sports and for diagnosis, treatment and rehabilitation of sports injuries. In case of injury or non-compliance to the sport, he is called upon to rule out an organic etiology, review the training schedule, and accordingly suggest adjustments in physical activity or reduction in training. Though, many potential acute and overuse injuries that can occur to skeletally immature athlete, the beneficial aspects of recreational and organized sports far outweigh the hazards. Most important of all the benefits is the development of an active and healthy lifestyle that facilitates weight control, helps strengthen bones, and can improve cardiovascular risk factors. This lays the groundwork for a lifetime of fitness. Physicians can play a key role in helping young patients find and maintain activities they enjoy while keeping the risk of injury to a minimum.

32.2 INJURY PREVENTION

A pre-participation sports examination is the key to injury prevention in athletes. An assessment of general health, physical fitness, strength, flexibility, and joint stability and alignment should be performed. The purpose of this examination and thorough history taking includes detecting medical conditions that delay or disqualify athletic participation owing to a risk of injury or death; detecting previously undiagnosed medical conditions; detecting medical conditions that need further evaluation or rehabilitation before participation; providing guidance for sports participation for patients with health conditions; and meeting legal and insurance obligations. This should be combined with a comprehensive annual checkup with emphasis on preventive health care. Recognizing mechanisms of injury and enforcing rules that reduce the likelihood of that mechanism of injury, including penalizing dangerous play, using protective gear, nursing appropriate field and weather conditions can reduce injury rates. Strength training is beneficial for development and maintenance of muscular strength and for enhancement of endurance, flexibility, and prevention of injury. Adolescents participating in sports and athletics should be subjected to resistance and endurance training as part of a well-balanced fitness program. Weight training may cause damage to physes or joints; hence lightweight exercises with high repetitions are most beneficial and safest for athletes of this age group.

32.3 PRINCIPLES OF REHABILITATION

Rehabilitation is a process in which a series of structured activities enables an athlete to return to normal activity or function. The rehabilitation program requires expert supervision to determine when joint functions, muscle strength, and sport-specific functions have been restored back after an injury. The phases of rehabilitation include the initial period of acute care when pain and inflammation are controlled and the limb is put to relative rest. The next phase, or intermediate phase, is aimed at resolution of pain and restoration of joint motion, flexibility and strength. Later care involves progressive strengthening, functional and sport-specific drills, as well as proprioceptive training. Finally, a maintenance program to prevent further injury is instituted.

Widespread publicity about performance-enhancing drugs like anabolic steroids and the perception of societal reward for exceptional athletic performance drives young athletes to consider the use of these substances. If used in conjunction with a strength-training program and proper diet, anabolic steroids have been shown to increase muscle size and strength for short durations; but there is a little evidence that their continued use results in increased aerobic capacity or improved athletic performance. The adverse effects far outnumber the doubtful gains that these substances claim to achieve.

Sports injuries may be acute affections or chronic and overuse injuries. Acute affections include soft tissue injuries and bony injuries. Studies in developed countries indicate that the majority of musculoskeletal injuries are soft tissue affections including contusions, sprains and strains, while only five percent of pediatric sports injuries are fractures (twenty-five percent of these fractures involve the epiphysis). The distribution of injuries by body part reveals that more than 50% of all reported injuries were to the lower extremity with knee and ankle the most affected. Injuries to the upper extremity accounted for 18.3% of sports injuries (Table 32.1). In general, injuries to the upper extremity occur more frequently in younger children, due to falls, whereas lower extremity injuries occur more frequently in older children and adolescents. Football is the highest contributor to injuries among all sports in western world and girls have accounted for higher injury rates in sports they participate in. Chronic and overuse injuries are caused by prolonged participation in sports and athletic activities.

Table 32.1: Distribution of sports injuries in body parts	
Body parts	*Injuries in percentage (%)*
Lower extremity	54
Upper extremity	18
Trunk/Back	13
Head/Neck	10
Other systems	5

Source: Hootman JM, Dick R, Agel J Epidemiology of collegiate injuries for 15 sports: summary and recommendations for injury prevention initiatives. *J Athl Train* 007; 42(2): 311–319.

32.4 ACUTE INJURIES

Soft Tissue Injury

Contusions involve direct impact to soft tissues causing bleeding and crushing of tissues without breaking the skin. Young patients are more susceptible to severe contusion and hematoma formation due to increased vasculature in their muscles.

Sprains: These occur when forces directed on a ligament or joint capsule cause them to stretch or rupture. The quantum of injury depends on the amount and rate of force applied and position of the limb at the time of injury. These may involve tearing of some fibers of the ligament (grade I), tearing of considerable number of fibers with pathological laxity and loss of motion (grade II) or complete tear of ligament and resulting instability (grade III). Grade III injuries are uncommon in children and adolescents as the force involved usually causes physeal injuries earlier than ligament rupture.

Strains involve injuries to the muscle-tendon unit as a result of muscle contraction. Specifically, eccentric contraction, which stretches a preloaded muscle, is the causative factor in most cases. The musculotendinous junction is the most common site for muscular strains. Moreover, muscles with a high content of type II fibers (fast twitch) and muscles that cross two joints (like hamstrings) are most susceptible to strains. Strain may be associated with mild tenderness on stretching (grade I), muscle spasms (grade II) or a palpable defect indicating complete tear of muscle (grade III).

Management of soft tissue injury involves *r*est, *i*ce, *c*ompression, and *e*levation (RICE). This initial management should be given within the first 48–72 hours after injury. Resting protects the soft tissue structures from re-injury and minimizes swelling. Ice causes local vasoconstriction decreasing bleeding and inflammation, helping to reduce edema and pain. Compression limits compartment volume, increases interstitial pressure and reduces transudation of fluid from the capillaries. Elevation (above the level of heart) assists in controlling edema by improving lymphatic and venous return from the injury site. Once the injured soft tissues respond to the initial management, the patient is rehabilitated with graduated mobilization and subsequent endurance and agility training when range of motion and strength recover.

Shoulder injuries: Besides fractures of the clavicle and proximal humerus, shoulder dislocation and acromioclavicular injuries are the most common injuries around the shoulder region. The shoulder joint is a highly mobile but equally unstable joint due to the bony configurations involved wherein a large humeral head articulates with a small, shallow glenoid fossa. Static and dynamic soft tissue stabilizers play an important role in the stability of the shoulder joint.

In *traumatic shoulder dislocation*, the arm and shoulder are forced into an abducted and externally rotated position as the humeral head is levered over the glenoid anteriorly. This usually occurs after a fall on an outstretched hand and forced abduction and external rotation injuries in contact sports. Posterior dislocations are far less common. The patient presents with pain and swelling around the shoulder. The glenoid fossa is found to be hollow and the head is palpable anteriorly. The contour of shoulder is lost. Axillary nerve is susceptible to injury in shoulder dislocations. The injury is usually a neuropraxia and leads to deltoid muscle weakness and hypoesthesia over the upper outer aspect of arm.

Anteroposterior radiographs and special views are indicated to look for any associated fracture. Radiographic features suggestive of recurrent dislocation of shoulder may also be appreciated. Closed reduction of the dislocation is performed as early as possible by any of the standard maneuvers under anesthesia. Abduction and extreme external rotation of the shoulder should be restricted following reduction. The patient is gradually mobilized after 3 weeks and subjected to rotator cuff strengthening exercises.

The *acromioclavicular joint* is usually injured during a violent fall. Patients have discrete tenderness over the acromioclavicular joint with a palpable step between the lateral end of clavicle and acromion process. The injury needs to be distinguished from a Salter-Harris physeal injury of the lateral end of clavicle by radiographs. Stress radiographs of the acromioclavicular joint may demonstrate subtle injuries. Most of these injuries are treated conservatively supporting the arm in a sling. Severe disruptions may need surgical intervention. The patient is gradually started on range of motion exercises after initial symptoms subside. Subsequently strengthening of rotator cuff, deltoid and trapezius muscles is initiated.

Elbow injuries: Besides fractures of the distal humerus and proximal radius and ulna, elbow dislocations are common occurrence during sports activities. *Elbow dislocation* is usually posterior and is caused by a fall on an outstretched arm with the elbow extended. The injury is extremely painful and is usually obvious by the deformity at the elbow. Thorough neurovascular assessment of the distal extremity is necessary as the dislocation compromises the brachial artery and median nerve in some cases. Rich collateral circulation around the elbow maintains viability of the distal limb.

Radiographs of the elbow-anteroposterior and lateral are mandatory to look for associated fractures. Reduction of the elbow is usually easily achieved if not complicated by fractures by longitudinal traction on the forearm and subsequent flexion. It requires immobilization to aid soft tissue healing and subsequent gradual rehabilitation. High incidence of myositis ossificans is associated with this injury.

Hand, wrist and forearm injuries: Salter-Harris injuries of the distal radius and ulna are the most common injuries in this region. Fractures of shafts of forearm bones, torus fractures, fractures of metacarpals and phalanges may all be associated with sports related trauma.

Pelvic avulsion fractures: Avulsion fractures are caused by sudden powerful contractions of a muscle pulling on a developing apophysis. Large muscles contract and create force greater than the strength of attachment of the muscle to the apophysis causing the injury. Common sites include sartorius origin at anterior superior iliac spine; origin of rectus femoris from anterior inferior iliac spine; hamstrings and adductors from ischial tuberosity (*see* Fig. 32.1 in CD) and ilio-psoas insertion at lesser trochanter. Anterior superior iliac spine and ischial avulsions are the most common. Physical examination elicits pain and localized swelling around the injured apophysis. Anteroposterior, oblique, inlet and outlet views of the pelvis are indicated.

The usual treatment is a period of rest or protected weight bearing. Failure of conservative management or large displaced fragments may require surgery.

Knee injuries: Acute knee injuries that cause immediate disability are fractures, patellar dislocations and internal derangement of knee. Internal derangement of knee includes injuries to the cruciate and collateral ligaments, menisci and chondral lesions.

Patellar dislocations are relatively common in children and are more common in girls. It is usually a no contact injury and occurs when the quadriceps muscle forcefully contract to extend the knee while the lower leg is externally rotated. The injury is predisposed by the eccentric pull of quadriceps. Patella almost always dislocates laterally (*see* Fig. 32.2 in CD). The knee may be swollen due to a hemarthrosis and tenderness is elicited over the medial retinaculum. Radiographs should be obtained to rule out osteochondral fractures and possibility of loose bodies in the knee joint. These include anteroposterior, lateral and skyline views (*see* Fig. 32.3 in CD). A dislocated patella usually relocates in extension of knee. An irreducible dislocation should be reduced under anesthesia. Failure of closed reduction and old dislocations may require operative reduction and appropriate soft tissue repair and reconstructions. Recurrent dislocations require specialized operative procedures. Rehabilitation includes strengthening of vastus medialis obliquos in particular.

Anterior cruciate ligament (ACL) tears are quite common in children and adolescents indulging in sports activities. The mechanisms of ACL injury in children and adults are similar; resulting from twisting of knee while the foot is planted on the ground. Usually a 'pop' or 'give way' is felt. Knee hemarthrosis occurs and there is a feeling of knee instability and inability to bear weight on the affected extremity. Physical examination includes specific tests aimed at eliciting instability including anterior drawer test and Lachman test. Radiographs of the knee are required to rule out bony injury and osteochondral fragments. An MRI is frequently required to visualize the tear that may be partial or complete. Initial management includes knee immobilization, ice and rest. Initially, all patients undergo rehabilitation program designed to restore the patient's range of motion and muscle strength. But results of non-operative treatment have been disappointing. On the other hand, operative treatment may jeopardize the physis; hence timing of surgery is to be coordinated with the growth potential left in the physis. Operative treatment includes use of auto or allograft for ligament reconstruction.

Posterior cruciate ligament sprains occur from a direct blow to the region of the proximal tibia. Medial collateral ligament injury occurs due to a valgus blow at the knee. Lateral collateral ligament injury is rare in children.

Meniscal tears are less common in children than in adults. The mechanism of injury is rotation as the flexed knee is being extended. The knee effusion is usually delayed in appearance in case of isolated meniscal injuries; findings include joint line tenderness and a click with knee flexion. MRI is the key to diagnosis. Management varies from simple immobilization in small peripheral tears to operative repair or partial excision of meniscus in large tears that cannot be repaired.

Tibial spine fractures occur in the region of insertion of ACL as bone fails before ligaments under tensile or shear stresses in children. The mechanism involved is usually a hyperextension or hyperflexion force, with or without the combination of varus or valgus, and a rotational moment about the knee. The fracture may be undisplaced, hinged or displaced and are usually associated with meniscal and collateral ligament injuries. Aim of treatment is anatomical reduction and open reduction and internal fixation is often required if reduction of fragment is not achieved by full extension of the knee.

Knee osteochondral fractures typically involve the medial and lateral femoral condyles or patella. The mechanism of injury is typically flexion rotation twist of the knee. Hemarthrosis is usually present and tenderness may be elicited in the involved area. Anteroposterior, lateral and tunnel views are required. Some fractures may not be visible on plain radiographs; for these, CT scan may be advisable. Treatment includes immobilization for small lesions in non-weight bearing areas of the condyle and debridement or operative fixation of large fragments.

Ankle injuries: Ankle injuries are the most common acute athletic injury amongst all age groups. Eighty-five percent of ankle injuries are sprains and a further 85% of those are inversion injuries.

In adolescents, **physeal injuries** in the ankle is also the most common site . The amount and location of injury depends on the direction of the deforming force and the position of the foot at the time of trauma. There may be deformity, swelling and inability to bear weight on the affected extremity. The bony landmarks should be palpated to decipher the anatomical structure involved. Inversion and eversion stress tests and anterior drawer test should be performed to assess the competence of anterior talofibular ligament, which is the ligament that is commonly injured. The ligamentous injuries need to be distinguished from Salter-Harris injuries of the lower ends of tibia and fibula.

Radiographs are indicated if the patient has pain in the malleolar area, is unable to bear weight or has bony tenderness (Ottawa rules). Radiographs include anteroposterior, lateral and mortise views. Treatment is usually conservative. Initial management includes RICE and immobilization in short leg cast followed by gradual mobilization as pain and swelling subside. These injuries are notorious for recurrence due to inadequate rehabilitation of a previous injury. Physeal injuries require anatomical reduction of the fracture either closed or open.

Tillaux and triplane fractures are seen in adolescents with partially closed physis due to violent pull of distal anterior tibiofibular ligament. Treatment includes closed/open reduction and immobilization.

Fractures of the fifth metatarsal are common in young athletes. These may be within the metatarsal shaft or the tuberosity. The tuberosity fracture is usually an apophyseal separation due to violent pull of peroneus brevis in inversion injuries. Conservative treatment in the form of immobilization in a short leg cast is usually sufficient but fractures of the shaft of fifth metatarsal are prone to go into nonunion and require prolonged immobilization.

32.5 CHRONIC AND OVERUSE INJURIES

Overuse injuries are caused by repetitive micro-trauma that exceeds the body's rate of repair. Although stress is normal for connective tissue development, excessive stress without intervening periods of rest can cause soft tissue as well as chondral and bone injuries. Overuse injuries can occur not only in an unconditioned athlete with poor biomechanics or technique but also in the highly conditioned athlete whose training regimen exceeds the limits of the musculoskeletal system.

Chronic Shoulder Injuries

Proximal humeral stress fracture or epiphysiolysis (thrower's shoulder) is usually an overuse injury of the proximal humeral physis. Symptoms are usually nonspecific characteristically with pain with throwing. Radiographs of the shoulder reveal a widening of the proximal humerus physis indicating a fatigue fracture. Treatment is usually conservative with avoidance of throwing activities and relative rest to the involved shoulder. A program of progressive strengthening and gradual return to interval throwing is recommended.

Glenohumeral instability may occur after an episode of acute traumatic shoulder dislocation or as a sequel of repetitive stress (*see* Fig. 32.4 in CD). This causes inflammation of the rotator cuff muscles and surrounding soft tissues producing restriction of pain-free motion and positive impingement sign. Relative rest, use of non-steroidal ant-inflammatory drugs (NSAIDs) and gradual strengthening of the rotator cuff usually are enough. Non-responders may require surgical decompression—either arthroscopic or as an open procedure.

Chronic Elbow Injuries

Thrower's elbow (Little League elbow) encompasses a number of conditions consisting of overstress of the medial elbow stabilizing structures and repetitive compression injuries to the radiocapitellar articulation. These include traction apophysitis of the medial epicondyle, avulsion of the medial epicondyle and capitellar osteochondritis dissecans.

Medial epicondyle apophysitis is usually precipitated by repetitive throwing motions putting undue stress on the elbow joint. Ulnar collateral ligament is also vulnerable to microtrauma due to overuse; both of these conditions presenting as pain localized to the medial aspect of the elbow with point tenderness over the medial epicondyle. Radiographs are usually inconclusive but occasionally may show widening of apophysis. Treatment consists of rest and avoidance

of the offending activity. Severe affections may require cast immobilization and displaced avulsions may require operative fixation.

Osteochondritis dissecans of capitellum occurs due to excessive compressive forces on the lateral side of the joint, resulting in microfractures, edema, avascular necrosis and potential loose body formation. Pain on the lateral aspect of elbow and tenderness of the radio-capitellar joint call for radiographs of the elbow that may reveal increased density of capitellum and occasional loose bodies. There may be mechanical symptoms like popping and locking of the joint. Treatment consists of rest and initial immobilization. The healing of this lesion is delayed and warrants prolonged absenteeism from the sport. Large fragments and loose bodies may require surgical debridement or fixation.

Lateral epicondylitis (tennis elbow) is usually inflammation of the origin of the extensor muscles at the lateral epicondyle. Lateral epicondyle is tender on palpation and tenderness is exacerbated by passive wrist flexion or resisted extension. Radiographs are usually normal. Treatment varies from simple rest to immobilization, local heat, local steroid injections, extensor strengthening exercises and surgical exploration. Resolution is slow and rehabilitation is prolonged.

Chronic wrist injuries: Chronic repetitive mechanical loading of the distal radius as seen in gymnasts (*Gymnast's wrist*) leads to symptoms ranging from mild discomfort without radiographic changes to disabling pain and mechanical symptoms secondary to alteration in anatomy and subsequent biochemical changes in the wrist. Treatment includes early recognition, modification of activity and immobilization.

Chronic Pelvic and Hip Injuries

Osteitis pubis is an inflammation at the pubic symphysis caused by excessive rocking motion of the pelvis in certain sports as hockey and roller-blading. Radiographs of pelvis reveal irregularity, sclerosis and widening of the symphysis 6–8 weeks after onset of symptoms. Treatment includes relative rest and anti-inflammatory medication.

Piriformis syndrome usually manifests as radiating pain in the lower limb due to injury to the piriformis muscle secondarily involving the sciatic nerve passing through it. Straight leg raising test and the 'figure of four' test are usually positive. Treatment is by relative rest, anti-inflammatory medication and local warmth.

Trochanteric bursitis is invariably associated with iliotibial tendonitis or snapping hip syndrome in skeletally immature athletes. Pain in the trochanteric region accentuated by adduction and external rotation of hip and a reproducible snap are highly indicative. Treatment may be conservative in the form of rest, NSAIDs and iliotibial stretching or may require local steroid injections or surgical release in non-responders.

Chronic knee injuries: Anterior knee pain is a common entity seen in the adolescence, particularly in athletes. The musculoskeletal conditions that may be implicated include Osgood-Schlatter syndrome, Sinding-Larsen-Johansson syndrome, idiopathic knee pain, and osteochondritis dissecans.

Osgood-Schlatter syndrome is a traction apophysitis of the tibial tubercle commonly seen in pre-teen rapidly growing boys and with some frequency in girls as well (*see* Fig. 32.5 in CD). The patient is usually a high-impact runner or jumper though kneeling and excessive stair climbing may also lead to the apophysitis. There is a painful prominence at the anterior proximal tibia and radiographs demonstrate fragmentation and occasional separation of the anterior tibial tubercle. Treatment is mostly conservative involving quadriceps and hamstring stretching program, relative rest and local warmth. The disease is self-limiting on closure of growth plate.

Sinding-Larsen-Johansson syndrome is an apophysitis of the inferior pole of patella with similar presentation and treatment as in Osgood-Schlatter syndrome. Radiographs show fragmentation in a small ossicle at the inferior pole of patella. Management is conservative.

Idiopathic knee syndrome is labeled when anterior knee pain exists in the absence of positive clinical findings. The pain is usually diffuse, bilateral and exacerbated by activity or prolonged knee flexion. Malalignment of the knee including genu valgum, femoral or tibial torsion, patellar maltracking, pes planus should all be looked for. Radiographs are mostly normal. Treatment consists of quadriceps and hamstring stretching and strengthening exercises, activity modification and local warmth or ice.

Osteochondritis dissecans is an osteochondral lesion that affects the subchondral bone and overlying articular cartilage. The knee is the most common site involved followed by elbow and ankle. The lesion may be asymptomatic or present with generalized knee pain that worsens with strenuous activity. Radiographs may demonstrate an osteochondral fragment that may be undisplaced, hinged or loose body in the joint. MRI is useful to determine the health of articular cartilage. Treatment involves non-weight bearing and immobilization for early lesions and debridement and grafting for large lesions.

Discoid meniscus is one of the causes of 'snapping' sensation in the knee and almost always involves the lateral meniscus. The anomaly in shape is usually congenital. These menisci are more prone to tears because of increased mechanical stress transmitted to their larger surface area, and because of hypermobility. The snapping is audible when the knee is brought to extension from a flexed position and is usually painless and palpable. Injury causes joint pain, tenderness, effusion, and a feeling of locking, catching or giving way. MRI is the most useful investigation. Treatment is required if the meniscus injury is symptomatic and involves arthroscopic partial meniscectomy.

Chronic Leg and Ankle Injuries

Shin splints denote tibial pain due to overuse of the lower leg as in prolonged running or hiking. The condition is limited to musculotendinous inflammation and diagnosis should exclude stress fractures of tibia. The patient experiences pain along the posteromedial border of tibia with tenderness elicited over the tibialis posterior muscle belly and exacerbated by active resisted plantar flexion. Radiographs are usually normal but are necessary to exclude stress fracture. Treatment consists of relative rest and local ice. Severe cases may require immobilization. Lower limb misalignment, if any, should be corrected.

Stress fractures result from repetitive physical stress that disrupts the normal bone-remodeling mechanism, the stress being below the threshold needed to cause an acute fracture and rate of bone resorption exceeding that of osteoblastic activity. The most common site for stress fracture in children is the proximal tibia, followed by distal fibula and metatarsals. Sprints, hurdles and jumps account for a significant number of such injuries. Patients experience pain that is related to activity. Radiographs may not be conclusive in early stages and demonstrate a radiolucent line and periosteal reaction usually after 3 weeks. Bone scan is beneficial in confirming the diagnosis. Treatment includes immobilization in cast and gradual return to activity but it may warrant activity modification.

Chronic exertional compartment syndrome is characterized by increased intracompartmental pressure (usually anterior and deep posterior) that is sufficient to cause pain in the leg, is precipitated by running and usually persists after training has ended. Physical examination and radiographs are often normal and call for compartment pressure measurements. Conservative treatment methods have been unsuccessful and fasciotomy of the involved compartment is required.

Sever disease (Calcaneal apophysitis) is an inflammation of the apophysis at the posterior aspect of calcaneum predisposed by a tight gastro-soleal complex and tight plantar fascia (*see* Fig. 32.6 in CD). It is usually seen in high impact running and jumping sports. Swelling and tenderness are present at the insertion of Achilles tendon and are exacerbated by activity. Radiographs may reveal fragmentation and separation of calcaneal apophysis. The disease is usually self-limiting and treatment includes relative rest, ice, stretching and strengthening of Achilles tendon, heel lifts and correction of abnormal foot morphology.

32.6 BACK INJURIES

Spondylolysis denotes a stress fracture of the pars interarticularis. This can be due to direct spinal trauma or a stress injury due to repetitive extension loading of the lower spinal column as seen in weight lifters and gymnasts. The patient has pain in activities involving spinal extension. The diagnosis is usually delayed and established by oblique radiographs of the lumbosacral spine or CT scan. Treatment is mostly conservative and involves restriction of spinal extension by activity modification or suitable bracing. Highly unstable traumatic defects and significant spondylolisthesis may require spinal decompression and stabilization.

Facet syndrome is caused by instability in the facet joint posterior to pars interarticularis. The management is conservative similar to spondylolysis.

Lumbar disc herniation is rare in young athletes but not in older adolescents. The acute event is usually precipitated by a sudden jerk or back strain. The typical symptom is sciatica with pain radiating to lower limbs along the distribution of sciatic nerve often below the knee with or without sensory symptoms. Straight leg raising test is positive and sciatica worsens on forward bending. Radiographs are inconclusive and MRI aids in diagnosis. Management is mostly conservative including analgesia, brief periods of rest and physical therapy, as tolerated.

32.7 HEAD AND NECK INJURIES

Head and neck injuries are the leading cause of permanent disability resulting from sports participation. But their incidence is on a steady decline owing to improved equipment standards and stricter norms in sports. The most common sequel of mild head injury is concussion, a traumatically induced alteration of mental status not necessarily resulting in loss of consciousness. There may be disturbance of vision, equilibrium and cognitive function besides headache. Repeated concussions may cause impaired memory, attention and cognitive dysfunction. This requires absenteeism from contact sports for a duration that depends on the number and severity of concussions.

Epidural hematoma is a rapidly accumulating hematoma between the dura and cranium usually associated with skull fracture and laceration of middle meningeal artery. There is loss of consciousness followed by lucid interval associated with a severe headache. Patients respond excellently to surgical evacuation.

Subdural hematoma occurs due to tear of a bridging vessel between dura and brain parenchyma. It is the most common cause of death in sports-related head injuries. Patients may lose consciousness at the time of injury but gradually recover. Massive collections of blood may need surgical drainage.

Cerebral contusion indicates bruising of brain parenchyma and can present as coup and countercoup injuries. It is characterized by loss of consciousness, severe headache and focal symptoms. Treatment is usually conservative.

Cervical fracture with or without dislocation is suspected in an athlete with head or neck injury when there is loss of consciousness, midline cervical tenderness, painful cervical motion or peripheral neurologic signs. ATLS protocol should be followed for initial management; patients should be strictly immobilized and subjected to radiological evaluation. CT and MRI should be done, as indicated. Further treatment is individualized as per the site and quantum of injury.

Brachial plexus injuries in sports are usually stretch injuries due to undue traction on nerve trunks. The symptomatology depends on the segment of plexus involved ranging from mild pain and paresthesias in arm, focal muscle weakness to complete paralysis of one or both upper limbs. An MRI is usually indicated to assess the plexus and management decided on the type of nerve injury (neuropraxia, neurotmesis or axonotmesis) that may include splintage and watchful expectancy or surgical exploration and repair.

32.8 HEAT INJURIES

Children's ability to tolerate heat stress is not as effective as that of adults. Children have a lower sweat rate and slower acclimatization process, absorb greater ambient heat secondary to their higher surface area to body mass ratio, and produce more metabolic heat per mass unit. Heat illness is a continuum of clinical signs and symptoms that can be mild to fatal.

Heat cramps are the most common heat injury mainly affecting the calf and hamstring muscles and respond to oral rehydration and stretching. Heat syncope is attributed to poor vasomotor tone and depletion of intravascular volume on prolonged exercise. Management includes supine positioning and fluid repletion.

Heat exhaustion or moderate heat injury is manifested as headache, nausea, vomiting, dizziness and possibly syncope. Treatment includes cooling the environment, ice application and rehydration, oral or intravenous.

Heat stroke is a medical emergency and indicates severe dehydration. Airway, breathing and circulation are maintained and aggressive cooling methods are used. Rapid intravenous fluid replenishment is done.

The most important aspect of heat injury is that it is preventable. Identification of medical conditions or drug intake that decreases heat tolerance should be identified before active indulgence in sports. Acclimatization to the playing conditions and prevention of dehydration by adequate fluid intake is of paramount importance.

32.9 FEMALE ATHLETE AND SPORTS

Special concerns are related to overtraining in young women and its effect on reproductive function and bone mineral status. In general, exercise promotes bone mineralization in the majority of young women and is to be encouraged. But females with eating disorders and those who follow a training schedule to achieve extreme weight loss having oligo or amenorrhea may end up with *osteopenia* due to exercise. These are more prone to stress fractures compared to their peers. Menstrual dysfunction can occur in young women participating in sports and athletics. These women should be investigated as for any other case of amenorrhea or oligomenorrhea. In the absence of any cause, hypothalamic amenorrhea is established by exclusion. Treatment includes lifestyle changes aimed at reduced energy expenditure and increased energy intake and gradual return to training if weight gain is evident. Calcium intake is promoted. Some patients with prolonged amenorrhea may require estrogen/progesterone therapy but this must be counterbalanced with the risk of early epiphyseal closure.

American Academy of Pediatrics: American Academy of Pediatrics policy statement: Use of performance enhancing substances. *Pediatrics* 2005; 115: 1103–1106

American Academy of Pediatrics Committee on Sports Medicine and Fitness Adolescents and anabolic steroids: a subject review. *Pediatrics* 1997; 99: 904–908.

Committee on Sports Medicine and Fitness. Medical conditions affecting sports participation. *Pediatrics* 2001; 107: 1205–1209.

Committee on Sports Medicine and Fitness. Climatic heat stress and exercising child and adolescent. *Pediatrics* 2000; 106: 158–159.

Committee on Sports Medicine and Fitness. Medical concerns in the female athlete. *Pediatrics* 2000; 106: 610–613.

Hergenroeder AC, Chorley JN. Sports Medicine. In: Behrman RE, Kliegman RM, Jenson HB (eds). *Nelson Textbook of Pediatrics*. 17th edn. Philadelphia: Saunders, 2004; 2302–2320.

33 Gynecologic Problems of Childhood

33.1 CLINICAL EXAMINATION AND GYNECOLOGIC IMAGING

Clinical Examination

Neonatal infant: All newborn infants should have first thorough physical examination. The initial gynecologic assessment of newborn infants begins with the breast examination. Commonly as a result of maternal endogenous estrogen production, breast tissue enlarges transiently in neonates; a milk-like nipple discharge may be noted. Persistent enlargement with tenderness and fever should suggest mastitis or rarely, a breast abscess. The abdomen is gently palpated for evidence of organomegaly. The external genitalia are assessed for any ambiguity. The labia should be gently separated, allowing inspection of the introitus-hymenal area. Abducting the hips with the labia gently retracted frequently facilitates inspection of the introital area. A normal protuberant hymen with associated thin white mucoid discharge from the vagina is often perceptible. In the first few weeks of life, a small amount of vaginal bleeding may occur, reflecting the decline of circulating levels of maternal estrogens. On completion of the inspection segment of examination, a rectal examination is performed. A midline structure, indicative of the uterus, is usually palpable, but the adnexa should not be palpable at this time.

Prepubertal child: The gynecologic examination in a pediatric or adolescent patient should be very comfortable. If the examination is painful or uncomfortable or if there is significant lack of rapport between the patient and examiner, the child may suffer lasting psychologic consequences. The history is

obtained primarily from the parent (s), who should be integrally involved in the physical examination of a child in this age group. Much information can be obtained by inspection of the vulvovaginal area. Ideally the patient is placed in a frog-leg position. This is followed by the knee-chest position with a Valsalva maneuver allowing adequate assessment of the intercoital lower third vaginal area. Magnification often can be accomplished with use of a colposcope or hand-held magnifying glass; appropriate documentation is also important. Visualizing the vestibule permits assessment of any discharge. Aspiration of any fluid in the vagina and lavage should be carried out with aseptic technique. An intravenous tube (butterfly) is passed into a soft number 12 catheter, all of which is then attached to a 1 ml tuberculin syringe. Wet mounts can be obtained and evaluated as indicated. Cultures should be taken for evaluation of vulvovaginitis. Gentle traction on the labia upward and outward further exposes the vaginal intercoitus for assessment. Note whether a patient has an imperforate, microperforate, or septate hymen. If an inadequate examination is accomplished, then sedation or examination under anesthesia should be considered.

Adolescent: A history in this age group may initially be taken in the presence of the patient's parents. However, an adolescent should be made aware of the concept of confidentiality and be given the opportunity to provide her own history in the absence of parents. This can be accomplished in the examination room before the physical examination. Explore her concern for the presence of vaginal discharge, sexually transmitted infections, pregnancy, or menstrual aberration. Indications for the first pelvic examination in adolescents include: Age 18 yr; Sexually active; Past or current (menstrual irregularities, severe dysmenorrheal, unexplained abdominal pain, unexplained dysuria, abnormal vaginal discharge).

Gynecologic imaging: A transabdominal ultrasonography is the most important diagnostic tool. A distended urinary bladder serves as an imaging window and facilitates identification of uterus and the ovaries; bladder distension with urine displaces gas-filled bowel loops out of the pelvis and enhances imaging. Ultrasonography makes appropriate diagnosis in patients presenting with ambiguous genitalia, ovarian or uterine masses, primary amenorrhea and abdominal or pelvic pain.

Pelvic masses can be identified at any age. Ovarian cysts and hydrocolpos or hydrometrocolpos are the most common abnormalities noted in neonates. Hydrocolpos is defined as dilatation of the vagina, which is usually associated with accumulation of serous fluid or urine (if there is urogenital sinus). Hydrometrocolpos causes dilatation of both the uterus and the vagina. It may also be associated with vaginal or cervical atresia, stenosis, or an imperfonate hymen. A solid mass requires histological diagnosis.

MRI is useful in evaluating müllerian duct anomalies. It should be used in conjunction with ultrasound assessment and, if necessary, such techniques as genitography. The three-dimensional Doppler studies more clearly differentiate benign from malignant ovarian lesions and reduce the false-positive findings with ultrasonography.

Porcu E. Imaging in pediatric and adolescent gynecology. *Endocr Dev* 2004; 7: 9–22.

Sanfilippo JS. History and physical examination. In: Kliegman RM, Behrman RE, Jenson HB, Stanton BF (eds). *Nelson Textbook of Pediatrics.* 18th edn. Vol. 2. Philadelphia: Saunders, 2007; 2273–2274.

Sanfilippo JS. Special gynecologic needs. In: Kliegman RM, Behrman RE, Jenson HB, Stanton BF (eds). *Nelson Textbook of Pediatrics.* 18th edn. Vol. 2. Philadelphia: Saunders, 2007; 2290.

Sanfilippo JS. Gynecologic imaging. In: Kliegman RM, Behrman RE, Jenson HB, Stanton BF (eds). *Nelson Textbook of Pediatrics.* 18th edn. Vol. 2. Philadelphia: Saunders, 2007; 2290.

33.2 VULVOVAGINAL AND MÜLLERIAN ANOMALIES

The diagnosis and management of young girls with mullerian anomalies requires not only knowledge of embryonic development of female reproductive tract, but also an awareness of their known association with other congenital anomalies.

Congenital hymenal abnormalities: The newborn may have bulging, translucent, yellow-gray mass at the vaginal introitus. Most of them are asymptomatic and resolve as the mucous is reabsorbed and estrogen levels decrease. However, large hydro/mucocolpos may obstruct the ureters, resulting in hydronephrosis or even respiratory distress.

The most common presentation of imperforate hymen is in a pubertal girl with cyclical or persistent pelvic pain and an abdominal mass bulging with a translucent bluish-tinged hymen secondary to significant hematocolpos and in severe cases, additional hematometra. Definitive surgery should take place after appropriate evaluation and abdomino-pelvic USG. Treatment is hymenotomy/hymenectomy to allow the menstrual flow and eventually comfortable sexual intercourse (*see* Fig. 33.1 in CD).

Anomalies of the Vagina

Transverse vaginal septum: Approximately 46% septa occur in upper vagina, 40% in the middle vagina and 14% in the lower vagina. On examination, the vagina is seen foreshortened ending in a blind pouch. A recto-abdominal bimanual examination may elicit a mass. Transverse vaginal septa commonly have a small central or eccentric opening. Ultrasound or MRI may define the septum and its thickness preoperatively. Management varies as cervical agenesis will require hysterectomy.

Longitudinal vaginal septum: It may be associated with one of the several uterine anomalies including a complete septate uterus, uterine didelphi and rarely, bicornuate uterine. Longitudinal vaginal, septa have also been reported to occur in association with anorectal malformations, including imperforate anus with rectovestibular fistula and cloaca. Treatment is by surgical resection. The septum should be completely removed while taking care to avoid damaging the cervix, where it is inserted.

OHVIRA: It is an acronym for obstructed hemivagina and ipsilateral renal agenesis. Treatment is resection of the obstructing septum (the common wall of the hemivagina) to create a single vaginal vault.

Vaginal atresia/distal vaginal agenesis/segmental vaginal agenesis: These anomalies occur when the urogenital sinus fails to contribute to the lower portion of the vagina. The uterus, cervix and upper vagina develop normally and the absent mid to lower section of the vagina is replaced by fibrous tissue. The most common presenting symptom is primary amenorrhea. Surgical correction is the treatment.

Vaginal agenesis (müllerian aplasia): Most patients present with primary amenorrhea around 15 years age, with normal secondary sexual characters. Müllerian aplasia is the second most common cause of primary amenorrhea after gonadal dysgenesis. On examination, there is a vaginal dimple or very foreshortened, blind-ending vagina. The hymenal fringe is usually present. A pelvic mass is usually absent. Transabdominal, pelvic and renal ultrasound may aid in diagnosis. An MRI is more accurate. Laparoscopy may be necessary if non-invasive imaging fails to make an accurate diagnosis and it allows for the removal of obstructed uterine structures. Furthermore, a karyotype will definitely differentiate androgen insensitivity from müllerian aplasia, if necessary.

Treatment: The patient's co-operation and positive attitude are vital to the ultimate success of the creation of a functional vagina. Creation of neovagina can be by both nonsurgical and surgical approaches. The non-operative method should be offered as first line therapy for this condition. Frank technique involves the use of hard graduated dilators to press against the vaginal dimple and create neovagina. Surgical correction can be offered to patients who fail nonoperative method or who choose surgery as the option. The modified Abbe-McIndoe is the most commonly performed surgical technique.

Rudimentary uterine horn: Since 7–10% of patients with vaginal agenesis may have a rudimentary uterus with some functional endometrium and no outflow tract, it is important to maintain a high index of an obstructed rudimentary horn as a cause of recurrent pain in patients with this diagnosis. Ultrasound and/or MRI can be useful and determine whether functional endometrium is present. Laparoscopy may be necessary to diagnose and remove the obstructed rudimentary horn.

Cervical atresia: It is a rare condition. MRI allows superior identification of the presence and integrity of the cervix. The classic management recommended for this condition is hysterectomy.

Disorders of the Uterus

a. *Complete uterine septum:* Most patients who are evaluated for repeated abortion are found to have a uterine anomaly—a septate uterus. If patient experiences pain, recurrent miscarriage, infertility or premature labour, the abnormality should be repaired by hysteroscopic resection.

b. *Bicornuate uterus:* The uterine fundus is deeply indented, often heart-shaped. In most cases, there is single cervix. Metroplasty has been recommended only in patients with bad obstetric history.

c. *Unicornuate uterus:* There is a single uterine horn that has only a single round ligament and fallopian tube (hemiuterus). The opposite horn may be absent or underdeveloped. Associated renal anomalies are common. Patients are at increased risk of premature labor and breech presentation.

Pregnancy outcome in women with müllerian duct anomalies: Women with müllerian anomalies seem to have an increased rate of unexplained infertility, endometriosis, spontaneous abortion, breech presentation and premature delivery. Those who have had segmental vaginal atresia corrected by creation of a neovagina are able to become pregnant and maintain a pregnancy, if a well-developed cervix and uterus are present. Patients with vaginal agenesis should always be counseled for adoption and surrogacy. The wider use of assisted reproductive technologies will surely enhance the reproductive capacity of women with congenital abnormalities of the reproductive tract.

Key Points

1. Each müllerian anomaly is distinct and an appropriate preoperative evaluation of reproductive and pelvic anatomy remains a crucial step before a patient is taken to operating room for surgical treatment.
2. The gynecologist should allay patient's anxiety by adequately counseling about the sexual and reproductive implications of her particular anomaly.
3. In patients with vaginal aplasia, non-surgical method of vaginal creation may be tried first as it is associated with high success rate.
4. In patients with müllerian agenesis, removal of uterine anlagen that contains endometrium and have the potential to cause obstruction and pelvic pain should be considered.
5. Hysteroscopic metroplasty is successful, minimally invasive technique for removal of uterine septum with improved pregnancy rate in patients of recurrent pregnancy loss.

American Fertility Society classification of müllerian anomalies. *Fertil Steril* 1988; 49: 952.

Buss JG, Lee RA. McIndoe procedure for vaginal agenesis: results and complications. *Mayo Clin Proc* 1989; 64: 758–761.

Sanfilippo JS. Vulvovaginal and Müllerian anomalies. In: Kliegman RM, Behrman RE, Jenson HB, Stanton BF (eds). *Nelson Textbook of Pediatrics*. 18th edn. Vol 2. Philadelphia: Saunders, 2007; 2287–2289.

The American Fertility Society classifications of adnexal adhesions, distal tubal occlusion, tubal occlusion secondary to tubal ligation, tubal pregnancies, müllerian anomalies and intrauterine adhesions. *Fertil Steril* 1988; 49: 944–955.

33.3 VULVOVAGINITIS

Vulvovaginitis is an inflammation of the vagina and vulva, most often nonspecific in childhood. Yet, it is the commonest gynecologic problem affecting prepubertal girls.

Vulvovaginitis in the young infant and toddler is usually diagnosed as "diaper dermatitis". Most commonly, these infants suffer from vulvitis due to local irritation from moisture, either urine or stool, which is part of a broader diaper dermatitis. Diapered infants can also suffer from specific infections like *Candida* dermatitis.

Nonspecific vulvovaginitis often occurs in the months prior to menarche and represents a physiologic response to increasing estrogen levels. Vulvovaginitis should be differentiated from this condition to avoid unnecessary anxiety to the child. Children with a visible discharge are significantly more likely to have a specific diagnosis than children who do not have a discharge at the time of examination.

Specific vulvovaginitis: Group A beta-hemolytic Streptococcus (GABHS) is another common cause of vulvovaginitis. It is often accompanied by an anal streptoccocal proctitis (which presents as a beefy, red, well demarcated ring, the size of a quarter around the anal area). GABHS vulvovaginitis presents with a purulent vaginal discharge which may manifest as soiling on the child's panties. Prepubertal girls may also have specific infections from sexually acquired organisms like *Gardnerella vaginalis*, *Trichomonas*, *C. trachomatis*, *Herpes simplex* and *Condyloma accuminata* as a result of sexual abuse.

Candidal vulvovaginitis is extremely uncommon in the prepubertal child who is no longer wearing diapers. However, some of these children do wear diapers at night only (nocturnal enuresis) until they are well beyond 5 years of age and they may be susceptible to a *Candidal* vulvovaginitis. *Candidal* vulvovaginitis may develop into chronic or recurrent *Candidal* infection in cases with diabetes mellitus, prolonged antibiotic use and immunodeficiency.

Prevention and Treatment

Nonspecific vulvovaginitis: A period of supervised defecation may be helpful, stressing the need to cleanse thoroughly and in right direction from anteriorly to posteriorly. Teach your child to urinate with her knees spread apart, so that the urine does not collect on the skin around or in the vagina. Good hand-washing after using the bathroom and before bed at night can also reduce the chances that bacteria will transfer from the girl's hand to her vaginal area, as she explores her body.

Avoid vaginal irritants such as bubble baths and creams. Use a nonperfumed, mild soap during baths, use warm water (not hot water) and keep baths brief (less than 10–15 minutes). Avoid using soap, or use just a little soap to clean the skin around the vagina before puberty and no scrubbing. Rinse the vaginal area well with clear water and a hand held sprayer when a bath is finished. Dry the vaginal area by gently patting with a towel (no rubbing) and consider using a hair dryer or just air dry it with her legs spread apart. Stress the importance of wearing loose-fitting, cotton

undergarments and change them frequently. Also wear loose fitting clothing (such as skirts, loose pants or shorts), and consider allowing her to sleep without underpants. Avoid prolonged wearing of tight clothing, especially wet swim suits, gymnastics outfits, and/or synthetic clothing. Also avoid sleeper pajamas. Having fabric, like underpants, over the vulva 24 hours a day can lead to chronic dampness and skin irritation. In a symptomatic child, sitz baths (warm water baths) in clear water 2–4 times a day may help provide relief. Apply bland ointment on the vulval skin that is irritated for symptomatic relief. 1/2% or 1% hydrocortisone cream 3–4 times a day helps to relieve severe burning and itching (stronger steroid creams in the vaginal area are not advisable). Severe itching can be relieved by oral diphenhydramine. If these methods are unsuccessful, do perform a vaginal culture. If a bacterial etiology seems likely, consider a course of broad-spectrum antibiotics. Streptococcal infections respond to penicillin or erythromycin. Treatment of the case and the entire family to eradicate pinworms with mebendazole or pyrantel pamoate may be done in suspected cases. Very rarely, an estrogen cream may be applied topically each night to the skin around the vaginal area to thicken and strengthen the skin and make it more resistant to irritation for a short time (2–4 weeks).

Specific vulvovaginitis: Medical treatment should be tailored to the suspected pathogen.

- Suspected child sexual abuse like sexually acquired infections such as *N. gonorrhoea* must be reported to the police. Further counseling with social worker and child welfare agency may be required. Treat STDs appropriately using pediatric doses. All STDs should prompt an evaluation for sexual abuse.
- Where a specific infection such as GABHS is cultured, appropriate oral antibiotics should be used.
- The rare occurrence of candidal vaginitis in the older child still in diapers should be treated with topical medications such as mycostatin or clotrimazole.

Key Points
1. The commonest cause of vulvovaginitis in prepubertal children is a "non-specific" irritation or inflammation.
2. Proper perineal hygiene and avoidance of known irritants remains the mainstay of prevention and treatment.

Kokotos F. Vulvovaginitis. *Pediatr Rev* 2006; 27: 116–117.
Owen MK, Clenney TL. Management of vaginitis. *Am Fam Physician* 2004; 70: 2125–2132.
Schroeder B. Vulvar disorders in adolescents. *Obstet Gynecol Clin North Am* 2000; 27: 235–251.
Stricker T, Navratil F, Sennhauser FH. Vulvovaginitis in prepubertal girls. *Arch Dis Child* 2003; 88: 324–326.

33.4 VAGINAL BLEEDING

Vaginal bleeding, before menarche requires evaluation. Menarche typically occurs at Tanner stage 3–4 of breast development. During neonatal period slight vaginal bleeding can occur within first few days of life due to withdrawal from exposure of high levels of maternal estrogen. Any bleeding after this early neonatal period but before breast budding (and in the absence of secondary sexual characteristics) should be evaluated carefully.

Vaginal Bleeding in Prepubertal Girls

Vulvar lesions: Vulvar excoriations can lead to bleeding. Urethral prolapse can present as a tender friable mass symmetrically surrounding the urethra that may bleed slightly. Condylomas appearing during first 3 years of life are usually perinatally acquired from maternal infection from human papilloma virus, but possibility of abuse should be considered. Prepubertal vulvar lichen sclerosus can lead to excoriations and hemorrhage.

Foreign body: Children have tendency to place small objects (toys or pieces of paper) inside their vagina. A foreign body may cause purulent or bloody vaginal discharge. Possibility of abuse should be considered in the presence of vaginal foreign bodies.

Precocious puberty: Precocious puberty may cause vaginal bleeding in the absence of secondary sexual characteristics, though there may be onset of breast budding and pubic hair before vaginal bleeding. Evaluation of precocious puberty is recommended for girls with pubertal development (either breast development or pubic hair) younger than 7 years of age (and younger than 6 years of age in case of African American girls).

Trauma: Trauma causing bleeding requires detailed inquiry of how the injury occurred. Detailed history should be obtained from the parents preferably both as well as the child herself to evaluate the possibility of trauma caused by sexual abuse. If physical findings are inconsistent with history possibility of sexual abuse should be strongly considered. Straddle injuries involve the anterior and lateral vulva, whereas penetrating injuries (least likely to occur as a result of accidental trauma) involve the fourchette and extend through the hymenal ring.

Abuse: Children with sexual abuse rarely present with acute injury, rather present with non-specific genital findings or no findings at all.

Vaginal tumors: The most common cause in prepubertal age group is rhabdomyosarcoma (sarcoma botryoides) presenting like a grape like mass. Other vaginal tumors though rare, should be ruled out.

Ovarian tumors which are hormonally active can lead to endometrial proliferation and bleeding.

Topical use of estrogens: If prescribed for labial adhesions or vulvovaginitis can cause bleeding.

Diagnosis

Examination: Genital bleeding in children demands a careful examination. If no obvious cause of bleeding is visible externally, an examination under anesthesia, using an endoscope should be done to visualize the cervix and vagina.

Imaging: Ultrasonography of the perineum and pelvis should be the first imaging study. The appearance of the ovaries (normal prepubertal) and prepubertal uterus (equal proportion of the cervix and the uterus and size in the range of 2 to 3.5 cm in length and 0.5 to 1 cm in width) can be noted.

Management is according to the cause of bleeding. Skin lesions like lichen sclerosus can be managed with the use of high potency topical steroids. If the child continues to have bloody discharge due to nonspecific vulvovaginitis, the presence of foreign body should be ruled out. Urethral prolapse can be managed medically with topical estrogen. Vaginal and ovarian tumors need specific evaluation and management.

Abnormal Bleeding in Adolescent Age Group

Anovulation

During first two years after menopause cycles are anovulatory. The transition to ovulatory cycles, by maturation of hypothalamic-pituitary-ovarian-axis usually occurs in first two years post menarche. Cycles that are longer than 42 days or shorter than 21 days and bleeding for more than 7 days are considered abnormal especially occurring after first two years after menarche. During adolescence greater irregularity is acceptable, if cycles are unassociated with anemia or hemorrhage.

To assess vaginal bleeding during adolescence, it is necessary to have an understanding of the range of normal menstrual cycles. In adolescent mean duration of menses is 4–7 days, cycle 21–40 days and average blood loss is 35 ml. Hypermenorrhea is blood loss > 80 ml/cycle. During the first two years after menarche, most cycles are anovulatory. The transition from anovulatory to ovulatory cycles results from "maturation of HPO axis" characterized by positive feedback mechanisms in which rising estrogen level triggers a surge of LH hormones and ovulation.

Anovulation causes usually heavy, prolonged and irregular bleeding. Anovulation results in continued estrogen secretion, causing endometrial proliferation with incomplete shedding. Ovulation is established usually in first 2 years post menarche. The younger the age at menarche the earlier ovulatory cycles are established.

Causes: 1.Polycystic ovary syndrome (PCO) and androgen disorders; 2.Thyroid dysfunction and hyperprolactinemias; 3. Pregnancy (whether abortion, ectopic or molar, or other pregnancy related complications); 4. Hematological abnormality (any hematological abnormality in its mildest form may have menorrhagia, most commonly diagnosed hematological abnormalities being idiopathic thrombocytopenic purpura and von Willebrand's disease); 5. Exogenous hormone (oral contraceptive pills, missed pills, other forms of hormonal contraceptives like injectables, implants); 6. Infections (sexually active adolescents have the highest incidence of Chlamydia and pelvic inflammatory disease); 7. Anatomic causes (partially obstructive or obstructive genital tract anomalies).

Diagnosis: A detailed physical examination to look for signs of androgen excess, hirsutism, or acanthosis nigricans, pelvic examination may be done in sexually active adolescents. Sensitive pregnancy test, complete blood count, and screening for coagulopathies and platelet dysfunction, thyroid function test need to be done. Testing for STD may be done in sexually active adolescents. If pelvic ultrasonography (transvaginal sonography may not be done), does not yield sufficient information MRI or rarely laparoscopy needs to be done to identify genital anatomic abnormality.

Management: Management depends on the cause. Pregnancy, thyroid, hepatic, or coagulation dysfunction or androgen excess syndromes should be managed by treating the underlying condition. NSAID's (mefenamic acid) and antifibrinolytic agent, tranexamic acid (more effective than NSAID's) can be used to decrease blood flow.

Mild bleeding as defined by adequate hemoglobin levels and minimal disruption of activity can be best managed by reassurance, menstrual charting close follow up, supplemental iron or a combination low dose OCs (oral contraceptives) prescribed in the manner in which it is used for contraception. Medroxyprogesterone acetate, 5–10 mg/day for last 10–13 days for 2–3 months may prevent excessive endometrial buildup and irregular shedding caused by unopposed estrogen, where OCPs (contraceptive pills) are unacceptable to the child or her parents.

Moderate bleeding: Patients who are bleeding acutely but in a stable condition, not requiring hospitalization will need use of combination monophasic OCs (every 6 hours for 4–7 days). After that dose is lapsed or stopped to allow withdrawal flow. Continue low dose OCs for 3–6 cycles, the pill may be discontinued and the menstrual cycle may be reassessed.

Acute bleeding: The need for hospitalization depends on existing severity of anemia and severity of bleeding. Generally there is no need for transfusion unless the patient is hemodynamically unstable. First stabilize the patient. After stabilization conjugated estrogens 25–40 mg /12 every 6 hours or 2.5 mg orally every 6 hours will be effective. Oral progestin therapy is administered for several days, to stabilize the endometrium after estrogens have controlled the bleeding.

Long-term menstrual suppression: This may be required for suppression in cases of coagulopathy or malignancy,
*   Progestins on a continuous basis
*   Continuous OCs without a withdrawal bleeding
*   Depot progestins (DMPA), with or without estrogens
*   GnRH analogues along with estrogen therapy

Although goal of long term suppression is amenorrhea all of these regimens may be accompanied by breakthrough bleeding.

Hypermenorrhagia

Diagnosis: Any adolescent with abnormal bleeding should undergo sensitive pregnancy testing. In addition to this other tests include complete blood count, coagulation studies, culture for gonorrhoea, tests for chlamydial infection, and thyroid tests. USG is helpful in ascertaining details of pelvic anatomy, ruling out pregnancy. MRI or CT can also be used.

Management: Base therapy on appropriate diagnosis. Thus management of bleeding abnormalities related to pregnancy, thyroid dysfunction, hepatic, hematologic abnormalities, or androgen excess should be directed to treat the underlying condition.

Polymenorrhagia

Cyclical bleeding which is both excessive and too frequent. It implies a disturbance in HPO axis and the endometrium. Here the ovary goes through its normal cycle but does so more quickly. The acceleration affects the follicular rather than the luteal phase. Endometrium goes through the usual phases but its proliferation increases and menstruation takes place every 2–3 weeks.

Causes: 1. Following menarche: occasionally seen during the few years; 2. Pelvic infection: chronic congestion of ovaries causes alteration in rhythm; 3. Stress induced: due to either a higher cortical effect on hypothalamic releasing factors or effect of neurohormonal substances from CNS directly on uterine vasculature; 4. Ovarian endometriosis.

Diagnosis: Any adolescent with abnormal bleeding should undergo pregnancy test. In addition to it other tests include complete blood count, USG, (CT and MRI are optional), culture for gonorrhoea and chlamydia test.

Treatment: Reassurance, when no organic cause is found; treatment aims at controlling symptoms cure being nearly always spontaneous. Non hormonal methods include PG synthetase inhibitors, antifibrinolytic agents.

Hormones: For moderately severe bleeding treatment can be initiated with up to 3–4 tablets/day of oral contraceptives and then gradually decreased to 1 tablet daily once bleeding stops. This dose is continued for 3 weeks.

Amenorrhoea

Definition: Refers to the absence of menstruation for 3 cycle length, 6 months after establishment of regular menses or by 18 months after menarche.

Causes: 1. Ovarian failure; 2. Pituitary/Hypothalamic lesions; 3. Altered GnRH secretion: 4. General disorders: Asherman's syndrome can be caused by infections such as tuberculosis and schistosomiasis.

Investigations: Exclude pregnancy and hypothyroidism and hyperprolactinemia.

Treatment: It varies according to the cause. The underlying disorder should be treated whenever possible for thyroid and hyperprolactinemia. Surgical removal, radiation therapy or both is advocated for CNS tumors other than prolactinomas.

Obesity/malnutrition/chronic disease, Cushing's syndrome, acromegaly should be specifically treated. Anorexia and stress induced amenorrhoea respond to psychotherapy.

When chronic anovulation caused by CAH corticosteroid administration is successful.

Anveden-Hertzberg L, Gauderer MW, Elder JS. Urethral prolapsed: An often misdiagnosed cause of urogenital bleeding in girls. *Pediatr Emerg Care* 1995; 11; 212–214.

Classens E, Cowell CA, Acute adolescent menorrhagia. *Am. J Obstet Gynecol* 1981; 139: 227–280.

Harlan WR. Secondary sex characteristics of girls 12 to 17 years of age. *J Pediatr* 1980; 96;1074–1078.

Marshall WA. Variations in pattern of pubertal changes in girls. *Arch Dis Child* 1969; 44: 291–303.

Merrit DF. Evaluation of vaginal bleeding in preadolescent child. *Semin Pediatr Surg* 1998;7: 35–42.

Phillip CS, Faiz A, Dowling N, et al. Age and prevalence of bleeding disorder in women with menorrhagia. *Obstet Gynecol* 2005: 105: 61–66.

33.5 BREAST DISORDERS

The breast is a modified sweat gland enveloped by superficial thoracic fascial layers and suspended from the chest wall by Cooper's ligaments (fibrous septae), extending from the pectoralis fascia to the dermis.

Congenital anomalies: Nipple anomalies: Polythelia, or extra nipples, is described in 1% to 2% of the general population and may be associated with other anomalies, such as genitourinary or cardiovascular defects. These accessory nipples can be located anywhere along the milk lines, from the axilla to the groin, other sites have been noted as well, such as over the back or buttock. The nipple and areola of the accessory tissue are usually smaller than a normal nipple and may be mistaken for a mole, melanoma, or hemangioma. An *inverted nipple* is one that does not project beyond the breast surface and is noted at birth; it is typically bilateral and usually reverts to normal in a few weeks. If it persists into the adolescent years, cosmetic and lactation concerns often arise. The infra-areolar breast tissue can be compressed and may lead to nipple protrusion. Infection can develop in an inverted nipple unless hygiene is excellent at all times and can lead to chronic areolar abscesses with swelling, erythema, pain, and discharge of the involved nipples. Management includes local heat application, antibiotics, and surgery to divide the breast ducts and raise the nipple; however, breastfeeding potential is then typically compromised. Acute onset of inversion in adolescence or adulthood suggests such problems as duct ectasia or malignancy and commonly presents as unilateral nipple inversion. *Athelia* is a very rare condition and can be unilateral and bilateral. This condition may occur due to androgen intake by mother during pregnancy. Others anomalies of nipple like *bifid nipple* need surgical correction. *Amastia* is rare and can be associated with Poland syndrome (various combinations of anomalies, such as amastia, pectoralis muscle aplasia, rib deformities, and upper limb defects) Work-up for ovarian failure is required in lack of breast development with delayed puberty. *Polymastia* is extra breast tissue seen along the milk line. It becomes apparent at puberty and requires referral for diagnostic and cosmetic purposes. Other nipple anomalies include a *bifid nipple* and a depressed nipple; the latter involves lactiferous ducts that directly open into a depressed areolar center; if severe, breastfeeding is prevented. Polythelia excision of the extra nipples is the typical management. If the patient requests cosmetic removal is with surgical correction as with the inverted nipple. The absence of a nipple, *athelia*, is a rare condition and may also be seen as a unilateral, bilateral, or familial condition; it may occur with exposure to exogenous androgen taken during pregnancy.

Developmental disorders of breast: Thelarche begins with the onset of puberty; average age of thelarche is 11 to 11.5 yrs. According to some research thelarche begins as early as the age of 6 years in African

American children. 48% of African America girls have thelarche between 8–9 yrs vs 15% in white girls.

Premature thelarche: Premature thelarche is defined by the isolated appearance of the breast in the female child to less than 6 – 8 yrs of age without other evidence of puberty. The causes are genetic, hormonal (primary hypothyroidism, raised FSH levels) and estrogen related (OCP, estrogen cream). Its management depends upon underlying etiology.

Infections of breast and nipple: Breast infections accounts for about 4% of all childhood breast conditions. Causes are infections, epidermoid cysts, foreign bodies in nipple, piercing, folliculitis and trauma. Presentation of infection can be induration, localized tenderness, erythema and even fluctuant mass locally. The most common organisms causing breast infections are *Staphylococcus aureus, Streptococcus pyogenes, E. coli, Pseudomonas aeruginosa*. Treatment involves antibiotics and/or surgical drainage. Antibiotic coverage should include methicillin resistant *S. aureus* until culture and sensitivity results are available.

Benign breast disorders: **Fibroadenoma:** It is most common mass encountered in the adolescent. This can be lobular, bilateral or multiple. Its feel may be rubbery, discrete and tenderness may not be there. Size is usually 2–3 cm, but solitary fibroadenoma can be as large as 10–15 cm (giant fibrodenoma—a slow growing tumor). Giant fibroadenoma is more commonly seen in African American girls. The lesion can be anywhere in breast tissue but upper lateral quadrant is most common site. Fibroadenoma are the estrogen sensitive tumor that can develop from breast tissue and shown at any age. There are many differential for breast mass but the diagnosis of fibrodenoma is made by its typical presentations. Malignant changes in fibroadenoma are very rare.

Treatment of fibroadenoma is surgical excision of mass. If the mass is close to areola, then circumareolar incision otherwise direct incision over the mass. Some fibroadenoma grow very fast should be distinguished from virginal hyperplasia, giant fibroadenoma, and cystosarcoma phyllodes. The giant fibroadenoma (juvenile cellular fibroadenoma) is an uncommon variant of fibroadenoma characterized by rapid growth. A giant or juvenile fibroadenoma is larger than 5 cm in diameter and sometimes doubles in size within 3 to 6 months, up to 15 or 20 cm; it may compress or replace normal breast tissue. Giant fibroadenomas should be excised because they cannot readily be distinguished from cystosarcoma phyllodes using physical examination, radiographic studies or fine needle aspiration.

Malignant breast disorders: Very few primary breast cancers occur in children and adolescents. Malignant breast masses in children more commonly result from metastases than from primary lesions; secondaries from rhabdomyosarcoma, Hodgkin and non-Hodgkin lymphoma, melanoma, and neuroblastoma. Two critical genes responsible for 7 –9% of all breast cancers in girls with an inherited predisposition to breast cancer are BRCA1 on chromosome 17 and BRCA2 on chromosome 13. Monthly self-examinations are recommended beginning between ages 18 and 21, and mammography at age 25 –35 years.

Nipple discharge: Nipple discharge must be carefully evaluated and a distinction made between the presence of galactorrhea (spontaneous flow of milk), blood or other discharge. Galactorrhea refers to breast milk secretion apart from birth or abortion, and the fluid may be white (milky) or clear, green, or yellow. For the confirmation of discharge of true galactorrhea, milk secretion should be sent for fat staining. Laboratory studies should include serum prolactin, follicular stimulating hormone, luteinizing hormone, and thyroid function studies. To resolve the galactorrhea the underlying disorder needs evaluation and treatment.

Causes of Nipple Discharge

1. **Milky discharge:** Lactation; Breast cancer; Drug intake; Pituitary microadenoma; Hypothyroidism; Acromegaly

2. **Bloody discharge:** Cystic ductal hyperplasia; Intraductal papilloma; Cystosarcoma phyllodes

3. **Brownish discharge:** Montgomery's gland secretion; Intraductal papilloma

4. **Serous:** Physiologic breast cyst

Draznin MB. Endocrine disorders. In: Greydanus DE, Patel DR, Pratt HD (eds). *Essentials of Adolescent Medicine*. New York: McGraw-Hill Medical Publishers, 2006; 299–327.

Jenkins RR. The breast. In: Behrman RE, Kliegman RM, Jenson HB (eds) *Nelson Textbook of Pediatrics*. Philadelphia: WB Saunders-Elsevier, 2004; 662–663.

Kaul P, Beach RK. Breast disorders. In: Greydanus DE, Patel DR, Pratt HD (eds). *Essentials of Adolescent Medicine*. New York: McGraw-Hill Medical Publishers, 2006; 569–590.

Mary E. Fallat M E, Ignacio R C. Breast Disorders in Children and Adolescents. *J Pediatr Adolesc Gynecol* 2008; 21:311–316.

33.6 POLYCYSTIC OVARIAN SYNDROME

Polycystic ovarian syndrome (PCOS) is the single most common endocrine abnormality of women of reproductive age group, occurring in about 1 in 15 women. PCOS is traditionally thought of as a triad of oligomenorrhea, hirsutism and obesity is now recognized as a heterogeneous disorder that results in overproduction of androgens, primarily from the ovary and is associated with insulin resistance. Most women with PCOS commonly date the onset of symptoms to the peripubertal or during early adolescence .Because the symptoms of PCOS emerge insidiously coincident with changes that accompany normal pubertal development, subtle features may not be realized in the early stages that may account for the failure to identify the disorder in young girls resulting in delayed treatment.

Definition: To maintain uniformity and lessen ambiguity, two major diagnostic criteria for PCOS have been proposed (Box 33.1).

Clinical manifestations: The developmental events of normal puberty include acceleration of growth in height, breast budding and enlargement, appearance of sexual hair and menstrual bleeding. PCOS is related to an abnormal expression of or response to these factors which initiate and regulate the process of puberty.

Menstrual dysfunction: Menstrual dysfunction in adolescents with PCOS may range from amenorrhea to oligomenorrhea to episodic menometrorrhagia. Rarely, an adolescent with PCOS can present with primary amenorrhea as the first manifestation. This group of adolescents exhibit more features of the metabolic syndrome and has higher androstenedione levels and may represent a more severe spectrum of the disease.

PCOS can also present before menarche in the form of androgen excess with premature pubarche and adrenarche.

Hyperandrogenism: This is typically manifested clinically by hirsutism, acne and/or androgenic alopecia. In contrast, signs of virilization (such as increased muscle mass, deepening of voice,

clitoromegaly) are not typical of PCOS. The most characteristic clinical feature of PCOS women is excessive hair growth (hirsutism). Usually increased facial hair is noted at or soon after puberty and the rate of growth is gradual in contrast to rapid appearance of severe hair growth, which suggests a neoplastic source of androgen production.

Acne vulgaris is a frequent clinical finding in adolescents. However, acne that is particularly persistent or late onset should suggest PCOS.

Obesity: The prevalence of obesity in PCOS women has been reported to be around 50%. Although obesity is common in adolescents who have PCOS, it is not necessary to make the diagnosis; the presence of obesity does however, amplifies the severity of PCOS and increases the risk for metabolic dysfunction. These girls generally have android or central pattern of obesity and increased waist to hip ratio. In addition to health consequences of obesity later in life, obesity in adolescents is correlated inversely with obstructive sleep apnea, fatty liver, orthopedic disorders and decreased quality of life.

Obstructive sleep apnea: It is more common in adolescents with PCOS and most likely related to central obesity and insulin resistance.

Insulin resistance: It has been well documented that most women with PCOS exhibit insulin resistance with compensatory hyperinsulinemia. The prevalence of insulin resistance in PCOS ranges from 20 to 40%. The risk for diabetes has been shown to be higher in women and adolescents who have PCOS. The 2 hour GTT is the most sensitive way to detect impaired glucose tolerance in such adolescents and is better than the fasting glucose levels.

Metabolic syndrome (MS): This syndrome is characterized by insulin resistance, obesity, atherogenic dyslipidemia, and hypertension. It is associated with an increased risk of cardiovascular disease and type 2 diabetes.

Endometrial hyperplasia: It is also present in PCOS.

Evaluation: The early recognition of PCOS in adolescent girls is predicted on clinical features, the most noticeable being evidence of hyperandrogenism.

Hormonal assays

- S. testosterone/DHEAS levels: Threshold values beyond which a neoplasm should be considered are 200 ng/dl and 7000 ng/dl for testosterone and DHEAS respectively. If circulating levels exceed these, then USG and MRI are done to locate the lesion. In PCOS, total testosterone is normal or slightly elevated but free testosterone is a more

---

Box 33.1: Criteria for defining PCOS

ESHRE/ASRM (Rotterdam) 2003
To include 2 of the following:
  i. Hyperandrogenism and/or hyperandrogenemia
 ii. Chronic anovulation
iii. Exclusion of related disorders

AFS 2006 criteria
To include all of the following:
  i. Hyperandrogenism (hirsutism and/or hyperandrogenemia)
 ii. Ovarian dysfunction (oligo-anovulation and/or polycystic ovaries)
iii. Exclusion of related disorders

sensitive test with levels > 10 pg/ml seen in 60–80% of patients with PCOS.

- LH/FSH ratio: It is important to check FSH and estradiol levels to exclude premature ovarian failure. Multiple studies have shown that an elevation of LH/LSH ratio > 2 is not required for diagnosis of PCOS.
- 17-Hydroxyprogesterone: It is a screening test to detect nonclassic adrenal hyperplasia (NCAH). Blood samples are drawn early morning (when adrenal secretion is highest). A follicular phase value of > 2 ng/ml should be followed by a corticotrophin stimulation test to rule out NCAH. Girls with Cushing syndrome may also present with a clinical picture consistent with PCOS. Optimal screening test is a 24 hours urinary free cortisol. Values that exceed the upper normal limit by 3 to 4 fold are highly suggestive of diagnosis.
- Oral glucose tolerance test: Adolescents who are obese should undergo a 2-hour 75 mg OGTT. This is a more sensitive test than fasting glucose levels to detect diabetes.
- Serum insulin: There is no accurate way to measure insulin resistance. A fasting glucose/insulin ratio < 4.5 suggests insulin resistance in an obese adult woman whereas a ratio < 7 is significant in adolescents.

Ultrasonography: The ultrasound definition of polycystic ovary is ≥ 12 follicles with a 2–9 mm diameter or ovarian volume >10 ml. Only 1 ovary consistent with such morphology is sufficient for diagnosis. In the adolescents as the ultrasound is performed transabdominally, it underestimates the prevalence of polycystic ovaries. But the diagnosis of PCOS in adolescents does not require imaging of the ovary and presence of hyperandrogenism and chronic anovulation is reason enough to initiate treatment provided other causes of androgen excess have been excluded.

Treatment: Treatment of the adolescent should be instituted early. Early interaction helps in treatment-of distressing symptoms such as hirsutism, acne and weight gain which in turn helps in improving self esteem and quality of life. It also helps in prevention of long term sequels of PCOS. Treatment options for PCOS in the adolescent include: 1. Weight loss for obese girls; 2. Symptom directed therapy; and 3. Metabolic correction of the underlying insulin resistance.

1. Weight Loss

It should be the first line treatment for all overweight and obese adolescents with PCOS. Weight loss has several metabolic effects upon clinical, endocrino-logical and metabolic features. Weight loss of approximately 5 to 10% leads to reduction in testosterone, increase in SHBG and resumption of menses.

Lifestyle modification: The emphasis on weight loss should be on lifestyle modification, with a program encompassing calorie restriction and an increase in formal exercise. Regular physical exercise is essential for weight loss and a minimum of 30 minutes of moderately intense exercise at least 3 days per week is recommended. Dietary interactions should focus on restricting calories and increasing energy expenditure. Decreases in insulin and total cholesterol are seen with weight loss.

2. Symptom Directed Therapy

Hirsutism: Hirsutism is a significant issue for the adolescent although in young children or adolescents the degree of hair growth may not be as severe as that encountered in adult women; but hirsutism is progressive and so sooner it is treated, the better is the success.

Cosmetic techniques of hair removal: The first line treatment for excess body or facial hair is hair removal techniques. It is best to encourage the patient to shave because this causes least trauma to the skin. Plucking or waxing should be discouraged because they may stimulate the growth of surrounding follicles and lead to folliculitis with subsequent development of ingrown hairs. Electrolysis/laser are the methods used for irreversible destruction of hair follicles. These are limited for their cost and the skills of the operating surgeons.

Hormonal therapy: Oral contraceptive (OC) pills: Use of oral contraceptive pills remain the predominant treatment for hirsutism, acne and cycle regulation in adolescent PCOS. Effects of OCP on acne can generally be observed by 2 months. In contrast, the effect on hair growth may not be evident for up to 6 months and the maximal effect is generally seen by 1 year due to the length of hair growth cycle.

GnRH agonists (e.g. leuprolide acetate depot 3.7 mg) and antiandrogens are not used because of side effects. Spironolactone, flutamide and finasteride are all equally effective in the treatment of hirsutism. None of these medications are approved by the US FDA for treatment of hirsutism. They are potential teratogens.

Abnormal bleeding: The goals of treating abnormal bleeding are to regulate menstrual cycle bleeding, thereby preventing anemia and also to prevent the long-term risk for endometrial hyperplasia.

a. Combined hormonal contraceptives: These offer excellent cycle control and also decrease menstrual flow.

b. Progestins: They can be administered on a cyclic or continuous schedule. Cyclic progestins are given for 10–14 days in a month. Drugs used are medroxyprogesterone acetate 5 to 10 mg, norethidrone acetate 5 mg or oral micronized progesterone 100 to 200 mg. Progestin only pill containing norethindrone in a dose of 0.35 µg/day can be used but incidence of abnormal spotting is higher.

3. Metabolic Correction

Metformin is the drug used for metabolic correction.

Chang JR, Coffler MS. Polycystic ovary syndrome: early detection in the adolescent. *Clin Obstet Gynecol* 2007; 50: 78–87.

Ehrmann DA, Barnes RB, Rosenfield RL et al. Prevalence of impaired glucose tolerance and diabetes in patients with polycystic ovary syndrome. *Diabetes Care* 1999; 22: 141–146.

Frank S. Polycystic syndrome in adolescents. *Int J Obes (London)* 2008; 32: 1032–1041.

The Rotterdam Eshre/ASRM sponsored PCOS consensus workshop group. Revised 2003 consensus on diagnostic criteria and long term health risks related to polycystic ovary syndrome. *Fertil Steril* 2004; 81: 19–25.

33.7 GENITAL TRACT TUMORS OF CHILDHOOD AND ABNORMAL PAP SMEAR MANAGEMENT

Gynecological tumors contribute to 1.5–2% of all malignancies in childhood and adolescence. Malignancies of the external genitalia are rare. Vaginal malignancies are common while cervical tumors are infrequent in childhood. Uterine tumors are rare but ovarian tumors represent up to 60–70% of childhood gynecological tumors. 1. *Cervical* and *vaginal tumors:* rhabdomyosarcomas, vaginal adenocarcinomas, embryogenic and yolk sac tumors. 2. *Ovarian tumors:* teratoma, germ cell tumors, sex cord-stromal tumors and epithelial cell tumors, both benign and malignant.

Fertility preservation in children and adolescents: Methods include substitution of alkylating agents, cyclical regimes, ovarian transposition during surgery and cryopreservation of ovarian tissue and oocytes.

Abnormal cervical cancer screening in adolescence: The overall rationale for management of abnormal cytology in adolescents is based on the following: (1) Adolescents have high rates of HPV and its associated LSIL; (2) Most of these spontaneously regress; (3) Adolescents frequently have multiple partners or serial monogamy, resulting in frequent new infections; (4) Rare CIN 3 that does occur is unlikely to progress to cancer during this age period.

HPV vaccine: *See* Section 40.11.

Billmire D, Vinocur C, Rescorla F et al. Children's Oncology Group (COG), Outcome and staging evaluation in malignant germ cell tumors of the ovary in children and adolescents: an intergroup study. *J Ped Surg* 2004; 39: 424–429.

Brandt ML, Helmrath MA. Ovarian cysts in infants and children. Sem Pediatr Surg 2005; 14(2): 78–85.

Hanprasertpong J, Chandeying V. Gynecologic tumors during childhood and adolescence. *J Med Assoc Thai* 2006; 89 Supp l4: S192–S198.

Widdice LE, Moscicki AB. Updated Guidelines for Papanicolaou Tests, Colposcopy, and Human Papillomavirus Testing in Adolescents. *J Adol Health* 2008; 43(4): S41–S51.

34 ◆ Cancer and Benign Tumors

34.1 LEUKEMIAS

The leukemias are the most common malignant neoplasms in childhood, and account for about 41% of all malignancies that occur in children younger than 15 yr of age. The leukemias may be defined as a group of malignant diseases in which genetic abnormalities in a hematopoietic cell give rise to a clonal proliferation of cells. The progeny of these cells have a growth advantage over normal cellular elements owing to an increased rate of proliferation, a decreased rate of spontaneous apoptosis, or both. This results in a disruption of normal marrow function and, ultimately, marrow failure.

Depending on the type of the cell of origin the disease can be a lymphoid or myeloid type of leukemia and the rapidity of the course of the disease determines whether it is acute or chronic. The clinical manifestations, laboratory findings, and responses to therapy vary depending on the type of leukemia. Acute lymphoblastic leukemia (ALL) accounts for about 77% of cases of childhood leukemia, acute myelogenous leukemia (AML) for about 11%, chronic myelogenous leukemia (CML) for 2–3%, and juvenile chronic myelogenous leukemia (JCML) for 1–2%. The remaining cases consist of a variety of acute and chronic leukemias that do not fit classic definitions for ALL, AML, CML, or JCML.

Acute Lymphoblastic Leukemia

Epidemiology: Acute lymphoblastic leukemia (ALL) accounts for about 77% of cases of childhood leukemia.

Childhood ALL peak incidence is between 2 and 6 yr of age and occurs more frequently in boys than in girls. The disease is more common in certain chromosomal abnormalities (Box 34.1). Among identical twins, the risk to the second twin if one develops leukemia is greater than that in the general population. The risk may be as high as 100% if the first twin is diagnosed during the first year of life and the twins shared the same (monochorionic) placenta. If the first twin develops ALL by 5–7 yr of age, the risk to the second twin is at least twice that in general population, regardless of zygosity.

Etiology: The etiology of ALL is unknown, although several genetic and environmental factors are associated with childhood leukemia (Box 34.1). There is an association between B-cell ALL and Epstein-Barr viral infections in certain developing countries.

Pathogenesis: The classification of ALL depends on characterizing the malignant cells in the bone marrow to determine the morphology, phenotypic characteristics as measured by cell membrane markers, and cytogenetic and molecular genetic features. The most important distinguishing morphologic features is the French–American-British (FAB) L3 subtype (also known as Burkitt leukemia), which is evidence of a mature B-cell leukemia. Phenotypically, surface markers show that about 85% of cases of ALL are derived from progenitors of B cells, about 15% are derived from T cells, and about 1% is derived from B cells. A small percentage of children have surface markers of both lymphoid and myeloid derivation.

Chromosomal abnormalities are found in most patients with ALL. The abnormalities, which may be related to chromosomal number, translocations or deletions, provide important prognostic information. Infants with ALL, who have chromosomal abnormalities such as t(9;22) or t(4;11), have even higher risk of relapse despite intensive therapy. Specific chromosomal findings, such as the t(9;22) translocation suggest a need for additional, molecular genetic studies.

Clinical manifestations: The clinical symptoms and signs are vague and non-specific initially. There may be anorexia, fatigue, irregular rise in temperature, and bone or joint pain, particularly may be present in the lower extremities. As the disease progresses, signs and symptoms of bone marrow failure become more obvious with the occurrence of pallor and petechial rashes on the mucus membranes and skin, and bruises and echymotic patches on the skin as well as fever which may be caused by infection. Nasal bleeding may occur. Sometimes hematuria and blood in stool may be seen. Unusually the patient may present with signs of increased intracranial pressure due to central nervous system infiltration by the leukemic cells, such as papilledema, retinal hemorrhages, and cranial nerve palsies. Respiratory distress may occur in patients with an obstructive airway problem due to mediastinal lymph node enlargement, which is most typically seen in adolescent boys with T-cell ALL (*see* Fig. 34.1 in CD).

Diagnosis: The increasing pallor with mild fever, purpuric rashes along with enlarged lymph nodes and hepatosplenomegaly with a history of illness starting around one month to six weeks suggests the disease and peripheral blood findings indicative of bone marrow failure. Anemia and thrombocytopenia are seen in most cases, but leukemic cells are often not seen in the peripheral blood in routine laboratory examinations. Most patients with acute lymphoblastic leukemia will have a total leukocyte count between 10,000 and 20,000/mm^3 (some patients have less than 10,000/mm^3), with predominant lymphocytes, some of which look abnormal (atypical lymphocytes). Bone marrow examination establishes the diagnosis. Bone marrow aspiration alone is usually sufficient, but sometimes a bone marrow biopsy is needed to provide adequate tissue for study or to exclude other possible causes of bone marrow failure. ALL is diagnosed when more than 25% of bone marrow cells are lymphoblasts and the figure may reach even 90%.

Differential diagnosis: ALL must be differentiated from AML; other malignant diseases that may invade the bone marrow and cause marrow failure such as neuroblastoma, rhabdomyosarcoma, Ewing's sarcoma, and retinoblastoma; and causes of primary bone marrow failure, such as aplastic anemia (either congenital or acquired) and myelofibrosis. Sometimes, failure of a single cell line, as in transient erythroblastic anemia, immune thrombocytopenia, and congenital or acquired neutropenia produces a clinical picture that is difficult to distinguish from ALL and they may require bone marrow examination. Any diseases, including infections like infectious mononucleosis, autoimmune diseases—like idiopathic thrombocytopaenic purpura, and collagen diseases—like rheumatoid arthritis may be considered in the differential diagnosis and for establishing the diagnosis peripheral blood smear examination and sometimes bone marrow examination is required.

Treatment: Three most important predictive factors are the age of the patient at the time of diagnosis, the initial leukocyte count and the speed of response to treatment (i.e. how rapidly the blast cells can be cleared from the marrow or peripheral blood). A patient between 1 and 10 yr of age and with a leukocyte count of less than 50,000/μl is used to define average risk. Patients considered being at higher risk who are older than 10 yr of age or who have an initial leukocyte count of more than 50,000/μl. Infants with ALL, who have chromosomal abnormalities such as t(9;22) or t(4;11), have even higher risk of relapse despite intensive therapy. The prognosis for patients with a slower response to initial therapy may be improved by therapy that is more intensive than the therapy considered necessary for patients who respond rapidly. The therapy is broadly divided into remission induction, CNS therapy to prevent CNS relapses, and maintenance therapy.

The *initial therapy* is designed to eradicate the leukemic cells from the bone marrow and is known as *remission induction.* During this phase, therapy is usually given for 4 weeks and consists of vincristine weekly, corticosteroid such as prednisone/ prednisolone or dexamethasone, and either repeated doses of L-asparaginase or a single dose of a long-acting asparaginase preparation. Intrathecal cytarabine or methotrexate, or both, may also be given. Intrathecal chemotherapy is usually given at the time of diagnosis and once more during induction. Patients at higher risk also receive daunomycin at weekly intervals. With this approach, 98% patients are in remission, as defined by 5% blasts in the marrow and to near-normal levels of neutrophil and platelet counts after 4–5 wk of treatment.

The *second phase of treatment* focuses on *CNS therapy* in an effort to prevent later CNS relapses. Intrathecal therapy is give repeatedly by lumbar puncture in conjunction with intensive systemic chemotherapy. The later CNS relapse is reduced to less than 5%. A small number of patients with features that predict a high risk of CNS relapse, such as those who have lymphoblasts in the CSF and elevated CSF leukocyte count at the time of diagnosis receive irradiation to the brain and spinal cord.

After *remission induction,* many regimens provide 14–28 wk of multiagent therapy, with the drugs and schedules used varying depending on the risk group of the patient. Finally, patients are given daily methotrexate, usually with intermittent doses of vincristine and a corticosteroid. This period, is known as the *maintenance phase of therapy,* lasts for 2–3 yr, depending upon the protocol used. A small number of patients with poor prognostic features, principally those with the t(9;22) translocation known as the Philadelphia chromosome, may undergo bone marrow transplantation during the first remission. In ALL, this chromosome is similar but not identical to the Philadelphia chromosome of chronic myelogenous leukemia (CML).

The major impediment to a successful outcome is relapse of disease. Bone marrow relapse occurs in 15–20% of patients with ALL and carries the most serious implications, especially if it occurs during or shortly after completion of therapy. Intensive therapy followed by allogeneic stem cell transplantation can result in long-term survival for a few patients with bone marrow relapse.

Patients with CNS relapse usually present with signs and symptoms of increased intracranial pressure and may present with isolated cranial nerve palsies. The diagnosis is confirmed by demonstration of leukemic cells in the CSF, rarely by imaging studies. The treatment includes intrathecal medication and craniospinal irradiation along with systemic chemotherapy because these patients are at high risk for subsequent bone marrow relapse. Most patients with leukemic relapse confined to the CNS do well, in whom the CNS relapse occurs after chemotherapy has been completed or during the latter phase of chemotherapy.

Testicular relapse occurs in 1–2% of boys with ALL, usually after completion of therapy. Patients present as painless swelling of one or both testes. The diagnosis is confirmed by biopsy of affected testis. Treatment includes systemic chemotherapy and local irradiation. Majority of boys with a testicular relapse can be successfully re-treated, and the survival rate of these patients is good.

Supportive care: Medical supportive care is essential in successively administrating aggressive therapeutic programs. Patients may require erythrocyte and platelet transfusion, and aggressive empirical antimicrobial therapy for sepsis in febrile children with neutropenia. Patients need to receive prophylactic treatment of *Pneumocystis carinii* pneumonia during chemotherapy and for several months after completing treatment.

Prognosis: Most children with ALL have long-term survival, with the rate greater than 80% after 5 yr. Adversely affect outcome include an age younger than 1 yr or older than 10 yr at diagnosis, a leukocyte count of more than 100,000/mL at diagnosis, or a slow response to initial therapy. Chromosomal abnormalities, including hypodiploidy, the Philadelphia chromosome, and t(4;11), portend a poorer outcome. More favorable characteristics include a rapid response to therapy, hyperdiploidy, and rearrangements of the TEL/AMLI gene.

Acute Myelogenous Leukemia

Epidemiology: Acute myelogenous leukemia (AML) accounts for about 11% cases of leukemia in childhood. One subtype, acute promyelocytic leukemia (APL) is more common in certain regions of the world, but the incidence of the other subtypes is generally uniform. Several chromosomal abnormalities associated with AML are identified, but no predisposing, genetic or environmental factors can be identified in most patients.

Pathogenesis: The characteristic feature of AML is more than 30% of bone marrow cells on bone marrow aspiration or biopsy constitute a homogeneous population of blast cells with features similar to those that characterize early differentiation states of the myeloid-monocyte-megakaryocyte series of blood cells. The most common classification of the subtypes of AML is the FAB system.

Clinical manifestations: Patients with AML may present with any or all of the findings associated with marrow failure in ALL. In addition, patients with AML present with signs and symptoms that infrequently occur with ALL, including subcutaneous nodules or "blueberry muffin" lesions, infiltration of the gingival, signs and laboratory findings of disseminated intravascular coagulation (especially indicative of acute promyelocytic leukemia), and discrete masses, known as **chloromas** or **granulocytic sarcomas**. These masses may occur in the absence of apparent bone marrow involvement and are typically associated with the M2 (acute myeloblastic leukemia with maturation) subcategory of AML with a t(8;21) translocation.

Diagnosis: Bone marrow aspiration and biopsy specimens of patients with AML examination typically reveals the features of a hypercellular marrow consisting of cells with features that permit FAB subclassification of disease. Special stains assist in identification of myeloperoxidase containing cells, thus confirming both the myelogenous origin of the leukemia and the diagnosis of AML. Some chromosomal abnormalities and molecular genetic markers are characteristic of specific subtypes of disease.

Treatment: Aggressive multiagent chemotherapy is required in successfully inducing remission in about 80% of patients. Up to 10% of patients die of either infection or bleeding before a remission can be achieved. Matched-sibling bone marrow or stem cell transplantation after remission has been shown to achieve long-term disease-free survival in 60–70% patients. Continued chemotherapy for patients who do not have a matched donor is less effective than marrow transplantation but is curative in some patients. Acute promyelocytic leukemia is very responsive to retinoic acid combined with anthracyclines. The supportive care needs of patients with AML are basically the same as those given for ALL.

Down syndrome and acute leukemia and myeloproliferation: Acute leukemia occurs about 14 times more frequently in children with Down syndrome than in general population. The ratio of ALL to AML in patients with Down syndrome is the same as that in general population. In ALL the expected outcome in children with Down syndrome is the same that for other children. But patients with Down syndrome are more sensitive to methotrexate and other antimetabolites, which can result in substantial

toxicity if standard doses are administered. In AML patients with Down syndrome have much better outcomes, with more than 80% survival rate, than is noted in the non-Down syndrome population. After induction therapy these patients require less intensive therapy to achieve the better results.

Chronic Myelogenous Leukemia

Epidemiology: Chronic myelogenous leukemia (CML) is a clonal disorder of the hematopoietic tissue that comprises 2–3% of all cases of childhood leukemia. About 99% of the cases are associated with a specific translocation, t(9;22)(q34;q11), known as the **Philadelphia chromosome**. The disease has been associated with exposure to ionizing radiation but in very few children history of such exposure is available.

Clinical manifestations: Typically, the disease exist in chronic phase, which terminates 3–4 yr after onset when the CML moves into the accelerated or "blast crisis" phase.

The presenting symptoms during chronic phase are entirely nonspecific and may include fever, weight loss, fatigue, and anorexia. Splenomegaly may also be present and often resulting in pain in the left upper quadrant of the abdomen. Additional manifestations may occur, including hyperuricemia and neurologic symptoms, which are related to increased blood viscosity with decreased CNS perfusion.

Diagnosis: The diagnosis is suggested in the chronic phase by an elevated leukocyte count with a predominance of mature forms but with increased numbers of immature granulocytes in the peripheral blood and bone marrow, and is confirmed by cytogenetic studies that demonstrate the presence of the characteristic Philadelphia chromosome. During the accelerated or "blast crisis" phase the blood counts are markedly elevated.

Treatment: The patients are treated with hydroxyurea in the chronic phase to control the signs and symptoms, which will gradually return the leukocyte to normal. However, this treatment is not definitive and does not eliminate the abnormal clone or prevent progression of disease. The elevated blood cell counts during the accelerated or "blast crisis" phase cannot be controlled by hydroxyurea. Therapy with interferon-α produces hematologic remission in up to 70% patients and cytogenetic remission in about 20% of patients. Combination chemotherapy has been successful in achieving remission in a small proportion of patients with CML. The optimum therapy is allogenic bone marrow or stem cell transplantation from an HLA-matched sibling, which is curative in up to 80% of children. **Imatinib mesylate**, which inhibits the *BCR-ABL* tyrosine kinase (specifically targeting the genetic abnormality of the malignant clone of cells), is very effective in adults, and trial of this drug in children should be carried out. Imatinib mesylate is administered orally; doses < 300 mg/day seem ineffective and may lead to development of resistance in adults. The side effects include fluid retention, nausea, muscle cramps, diarrhea, and skin rashes.

Juvenile Chronic Myelogenous Leukemia

Juvenile chronic myelogenous leukemia (JCML) also known as juvenile myelomonocytic leukemia is a clonal proliferation of hematopoietic stem cells that typically affects children younger than 2 yr of age, contributing less than 2% of all cases of childhood leukemia. Patients with JCML do not have the Philadelphia chromosome. Patients with neurofibromatosis have a predilection for JCML. Patients with JCML present with rashes, lymphadenopathy, and splenomegaly. Peripheral blood examination often shows an elevated leukocyte count, and may also show thrombocytopenia and erythroblasts. The bone marrow shows a myelodysplastic pattern with blast accounting for less than 30% of cells. The treatment is the same as mentioned in CML. The cure rate with stem cell transplantation is the best, but is much less than reported for classic CML.

Infant Leukemia

Leukemia during childhood occurs only in about 2% of cases before the age of 1 yr. Infants with ALL demonstrate rearrangements of the *MLL* gene in more than two-thirds of the cases, classically a translocation involving the q23 band of chromosome 11, with a very high relapse rate and poor prognosis. These patients often present with hyperleukocytosis and extensive tissue invasion, including CNS disease. Subcutaneous nodules **(leukemia cutis)** and tachypnea due to diffuse pulmonary infiltration by leukemic cells are more frequently seen in infants. The leukemic cell morphology is usually that of large irregular lymphoblasts. The treatment may be the same as that for older children with AML, but these patients need more supportive care and aggressive therapy.

Arico M, Valsecchi MG, Camitta B, et al. Outcome of treatment in children with Philadelphia chromosome-positive acute lymphoblastic leukemia. *N Engl J Med* 2000; 342: 998–1006.

Clark JJ, Smith FO, Arceci RJ. Update in childhood acute myeloid leukemia: Recent developments I the molecular basis of disease and novel therapies. *Curr Opin Hematol* 2003; 10: 31–39.

Pizzo PA, Poplack DG (eds). *Principles and Practice of Pediatric Oncology*. 5th edn. Philadelphia: Lippincort Williams & Wilkins, 2005.

Powel BL. Acute progranulocytic leukemia. *Curr Opin Oncol* 2001; 13: 8–13.

Puri CH, Evans WE. Treatment of acute lymphoblastic leukemia. *N Engl J Med* 2006; 354: 166–178.

Pui CH, Relling MV, Downing JR. Acute lymphoblastic leukemia. *N Engl J Med* 2004; 350: 1535–1548.

Sande LE, Arcecci RJ, Lampkin BC. Congenital and neonatal leukemia. *Semin Perinatol* 1999; 23: 274–285.

Shrestha AD. The Leukemias in Children. In: Mathur GP, Mathur Sarla (eds). *Current Trends in Pediatrics*. Vol 1. Delhi: Academa Publishers, 2005; 150–157.

Smith FO, Sanders JE. Juvenile myelomonocytic leukemia: What we don't know. *J Pediatr Hematol Oncol* 1999; 21: 461–463.

Tubergen DG, Bleyer A. The Leukemias. In: Kliegman RM, Behrman RE, Jenson HB, Stanton BF (eds). *Nelson Textbook of Pediatrics*. 18th edn. Vol. 2. Philadelphia: Saunders, 2007; 2116–2123.

34.2 LYMPHOMA

Lymphoma is the third most common cancer in childhood. There are two broad categories of lymphoma, Hodgkin disease and non-Hodgkin lymphoma (NHL), because of different clinical manifestations and treatments.

Hodgkin Disease

Epidemiology: Hodgkin disease (HD) accounts for about 5% of cancers in persons younger than 15 yr of age and for about 15% in persons 15–19 yr of age in industrialized countries, in contrast to developing countries, where the highest rate is in younger children. Three forms of Hodgkin disease have been identified in epidemiologic studies: a childhood form (≤ 14 yr), a young adult form (15–34 yr of age), and an older adult form (55–74 yr of age). Males predominate in patients younger than 10 yr of age at diagnosis, but the male female ratio is equal in adolescence. Risk factors include infection due to Epstein-Barr virus (EBV) and immunodeficiencies (congenital or acquired).

Etiology: The Reed-Sternberg cell, a large cell (15–45 μm in diameter) with multiple and multilobular nuclei, is considered the hallmark of Hodgkin disease, although similar cells are seen in infectious mononucleosis, NHL, and other conditions. The Reed-Sternberg cells arises from germinal center B-cells in most cases. An infiltrate of apparently normal lymphocytes, plasma cells, and eosinophils, various degrees of fibrosis and the presence of collagen bands, necrosis, or malignant reticular cells, helps to distinguish four major histologic subtypes: lymphocyte predominant, nodular sclerosing, mixed cellularity, and lymphocyte depleted.

Hodgkin disease appears to arise in lymphoid tissue and spreads to adjacent lymph node areas in a relatively fashion. Hematogenous spread also occurs, leading to involvement of the liver, spleen, bone, bone marrow, or brain, and is usually associated with systemic symptoms. Levels of various cytokines are elevated, which are responsible for the systemic symptoms of fever and night sweats (interleukin 1 or 2) and weight loss [tissue necrosis factor (TNF)], in addition to influencing the proliferation of Reed-Sternberg cells and including immunosuppression (transforming growth factor-β).

Clinical manifestations: The most common presenting sign is the painless, firm, cervical or supraclavicular lymphadenopathy. Inguinal or axillary lymphnodes are rarely involved. An anterior mediastinal mass is often present and rapidly disappear with therapy. Clinically hepatosplenomegaly is rarely detected. Depending on the extent and location of nodal and extranodal disease, patient might present with symptoms and signs of airway obstruction, pleural or pericardial effusion, hepatocellular dysfunction or bone marrow infiltration (anemia, neutropenia, or thrombocytopenia). Nephrotic syndrome is a rare presenting manifestation of Hodgkin disease.

Systemic symptoms classified as **B** symptoms that are considered important in staging are unexplained fever > 39°C, weight loss >10% total body weight over 3 months, or drenching night sweats. Some present as a fever of unknown origin. Less common symptoms not considered of prognostic significance are pruritus, lethargy, anorexia or pain that worsens after ingestion of alcohol.

Tuberculosis, fungal or varicella-zoster infection may complicate Hodgkin disease and predispose to complications during immunosuppressive therapy, because of the impaired humoral immunity.

Diagnosis: Any patient with persistent, unexplained lymphadenopathy unassociated with an obvious underlying inflammation or infectious process should have a chest radiograph to identify the presence of a mediastinal mass before undergoing node biopsy. Patients with persistently enlarged lymph nodes, even after serologically proven infectious mononucleosis, should also be considered for biopsy. Excisional biopsy is preferred over needle biopsy to ensure that adequate tissue is obtained, both for light microscopy and for appropriate immunocytochemical and molecular studies, culture, and cytogenetic analysis if routine studies fail to provide a firm diagnosis. A portion of the biopsy specimen should be frozen and stored to

---

Box 34.2: Modified Ann Arbor staging system for Hodgkin disease*

Stage I
Involvement of a single lymph node region or of a single extralymphatic organ or site

Stage II
Involvement of two or more lymphoid regions on the same side of the diaphragm or localized involvement of an extralymphatic organ or site and of one or more lymph node regions on the same side of the diaphragm

Stage III
Involvement of lymph node regions on both sides of the diaphragm, which may be accompanied by localized involvement of an extralymphatic organ or site or by splenic involvement

Stage IV
Diffuse or disseminated involvement of one or more extralymphatic organs or tissues, with or without associated lymph node enlargement

*Stages are further categorized as:
A or B, based on the absence or presence, respectively, of systemic symptoms of fever and/or weight loss
Bulky disease, based on mediastinal mass larger than one third thoracic diameter; lymph node masses ≥10 cm in diameter and/or four or more nodal regions involved.

Source: Lister TA, Crowther D, Sutcliffe SB, et al. Report of a committee convened to discuss the evaluation and staging of patients with Hodgkin's disease: Cotswolds meeting. *J Clin Oncol* 1989; 7: 1630–1636.

---

allow for additional studies. Once the diagnosis of Hodgkin disease is established, extent of disease (i.e., stage) should be determined (Boxes 34.2 and 34.3).

A complete blood cell count (CBC) identifies abnormalities that might suggest bone marrow involvement. Erythrocyte sedimentation rate (ESR), serum ferritin, serum copper levels are of some

---

Box 34.3: Clinical staging of Hodgkin disease

Measurement of palpable lymph nodes, liver, and spleen
Complete blood cell count
Erythrocyte sedimentation rate (ESR), serum ferritin, serum copper
Liver function tests
Chest radiograph with measurement of mediastinal ratio
Chest CT with contrast medium enhancement
Neck CT if high cervical lymph nodes palpable
Abdominal CT or MRI
Gallium scan
Bone marrow biopsy with advanced disease or "B" symptoms
Bone scan with elevated serum alkaline phosphatase level and/or bone pain

prognostic significance, and if abnormal at diagnosis, serve as a baseline to evaluate the effects of treatment. Liver function tests, although not particularly sensitive to the presence of liver involvement, can influence treatment and treatment complications. Chest radiograph is done to measure the size of the mediastinal mass in relation to the maximal diameter of the thorax. Chest CT more clearly defines the extent of a medastinal mass if present and identifies hilar nodes and pulmonary parenchymal involvement, which may not be evident on chest radiographs. Abdominal CT or MRI can identify gross subdiaphragmatic involvement of nodes together with enlargement and defects in the liver and spleen. Gallium-67 scan is particularly helpful in identifying areas of increased uptake, which can then be re-evaluated at the end of treatment, especially in patients with mediastinal masses that do not completely resolve on chest radiographs or CT. Lymphangiography is rarely performed in pediatric practice, although it can demonstrate the intrinsic abnormalities of lymph nodes, except upper para-aortic nodes. Bone marrow biopsy is necessary in only those patients with advanced (stage III or IV) disease or with "B" symptoms. Surgical staging should be considered only if findings will significantly influence therapy.

Treatment: Chemotherapy and radiation therapy are effective in the treatment of HD. It is determined by disease stage, patient's age at diagnosis, and presence or absence of "B" symptoms, and the presence of hilar lymphadenopathy and/or bulky nodal disease. Three risk groups have been identified. Favorable presentations include stage I and IIA. Intermediate presentations include stage I, IIB (with symptoms, bulky disease, or hilar lymphadenopathy), and stage IIIA. Unfavorable presentations include stages IIIB and IV.

Chemotherapy agents commonly used to treat children and adolescents with HD include cyclophosphamide, procarbazine, vincristine or vinblastine, prednisolone, or dexamethasone, doxorubicin, bleomycin, dacarbazine, etoposide, methotrexate, and cytosine arabinoside. The combination chemotherapy regime in current use are based on **COPP** (cyclophosphamide, vincristine [Oncovin], procarbazine, and prednisolone), or **ABVD** (doxorubicin [Adriamycin], bleomycin, vinblastine, and dacarbazine), with **BEACOPP** (bleomycin, etoposide, doxorubicin, cyclophosphamide,, vincristine, procarbazine, prednisolone) used typically in patients with advanced stage disease. The **COPP/ABV** ((cyclophosphamide, vincristine [Oncovin], procarbazine, and prednisolone doxorubicin [Adriamycin], bleomycin and vinblastine) is an

example to reduce potential toxicities. Originally, a minimum of six cycles of chemotherapy is given, with significant cumulative toxicity, including second malignancies, sterility, and cardiac and pulmonary dysfunction. "Risk-adapted" protocols are based on staging criteria as well as rapidity of response to initial chemotherapy, the aim is to reduce total drug doses and treatment duration and even eliminate radiation therapy.

Relapse: Most relapses occur within the first 3 yrs from diagnosis but relapses as late as 10 yr have been reported. Those patients who never achieve remission or who suffer relapse after initial remission of less than 12 months after chemotherapy or combined modality therapy have a poorer prognosis and are candidates for myeloablative chemotherapy and autologous stem cell or bone marrow rescue.

Prognosis: Most treatment programs result in disease-free survival rates of more than 60%, with overall cure rates greater than 90% in those with early stage disease and more than 70% in more advanced cases. All diagnosed cases in children and adolescents should be treated with combined modality therapy, choice of regimen is selected on the basis of risk category and observed or anticipated long-term complications.

Non-Hodgkin Lymphoma

Non-Hodgkin Lymphoma (NHL) accounts for approximately 60% of all lymphomas in children and adolescents. Most children, who develop NHL, have no obvious or environmental etiology.

Pathogenesis: The four major pathological subtypes of childhood and adolescent NHL are 1 Burkitt lymphoma (BL) 40%, 2 Lymphoblastic lymphoma (LL) 30%, 3 Diffuse large B-cell lymphoma (DLBCL) 20%, and 4 Anaplastic large cell lymphoma (ALCL) 10%. Most childhood and adolescent NHLs are high-grade tumors with an aggressive clinical behavior compared to those of adult NHL, which are low to intermediate-grade indolent tumors. Almost all childhood and adolescent NHL is derived from germinal center aberrations. Almost all forms of BL and DLBCL are of B cell origin; cases of LL are 80% T cell and 20% B cell and cases of ALCL are 70% T cell, 20% null cell, and 10% B cell origin.

Clinical manifestations: The presenting signs and symptoms of childhood and adolescent NHL depend primarily on pathological subtype and primary and secondary sites of involvement. NHLs are rapidly growing tumors and can cause symptoms based on size and location. Approximately 70% present with advanced disease of stages III or IV (Box 34.4), including extranodal disease manifests as gastrointestinal, bone marrow, and central nervous system (CNS) involvement. BL commonly presents with abdominal (sporadic type) or head and neck (endemic type) disease with involvement of the bone marrow or CNS. LL commonly presents with an intrathoracic or mediastinal supradiaphragmatic mass, and has a predilection for spreading to the bone marrow and CNS. DLBCL commonly presents with either an abdominal or mediastinal primary and, rarely, dissemination to the bone marrow or CNS. ALCL presents either with a primary cutaneous manifestation (10%) or with systemic disease (fever, weight loss) with dissemination to liver, spleen, lung, mediastinum, or skin; spread to bone marrow is rare.

Site-specific manifestations include:

i. Painless, rapid lymph node enlargement
ii. Cough, superior vena cava (SVC) syndrome, dyspnea with thoracic enlargement
iii. Abdominal (massive and rapidly enlarging) mass, intestinal obstruction, intussusceptions-like symptoms, ascites with abdominal enlargement
iv. Nasal stuffiness, earache, hearing loss, tonsil enlargement with Waldeyer ring enlargement and
v. Local bone pain (primary or metastatic).

Three clinical manifestations that require special alternative treatment strategies are:

i. SVC syndrome secondary to a large mediastinal mass obstructing various blood flow or respiratory airways
ii. Acute paraplegias secondary to spinal cord or central nervous system compression from neighboring localized NHL; and
iii. Tumor lysis syndrome (TLS) secondary to severe metabolic abnormalities, including hyperuricemia, hyperphosphatemia, hyperkalemia, and hypocalcemia from massive tumor cell lysis.

Diagnosis: Prompt tissue diagnosis and staging is important. To ensure adequate tissue for accurate diagnosis and subtyping, multiple needle biopsy specimens or a large wedge of tumor should be obtained. Pretreatment investigations are necessary to accurately stage the disease and provide baseline measurements of organ function before treatment is instituted (Box 34.5). The St. Jude staging system defines tumor extent, which is important for designing treatment (Box 34.4). Stage I applies to localized disease, stage II to regional disease (except for mediastinal tumors, which are designated as stage III, stage III to extensive disease, and stage IV to disseminated (CNS and/or bone marrow) disease. Elevated levels of serum lactic dehydrogenase (> 500 U/L) correlate with tumor mass and have proved useful for stratifying therapy intensity. A

Box 34.4: St Jude staging system for childhood non-Hodgkin lymphoma

Stage I
A single tumor (extranodal) or single anatomic area (nodal), with the exclusion of mediastinum or abdomen

Stage II
A single tumor (extranodal), with regional node involvement
Two or more nodal areas on the same side of the diaphragm
Two single (extranodal) tumors with or without regional node involvement on the same side of the diaphragm
A primary gastrointestinal tract tumor, usually in the ileocecal area, with or without involvement of associates mesenteric nodes only, which must be grossly (>90%) resected

Stage III
Two single tumors (extranodal) on opposite side of the diaphragm
Two or more nodal areas above or below the diaphragm
Any primary intrathoracic tumor (mediastinal, pleural, or thymic)
An extensive primary intra-abdominal disease

Stage IV
Any of the above, with initial involvement of central nervous system and/or bone marrow at time of diagnosis

Source: Murphy SB. Classification, staging and end results of treatment of childhood non-Hodgkin's lymphomas: Dissimilarities from lymphomas in adults. *Semin Oncol* 1980; 7: 332–399.

---

normal CBC does not preclude marrow involvement. CT or MRI of the chest or abdomen or both provides information regarding the extent of the disease.

Differential diagnosis: Head and neck lymphadenopathy should be differentiated from infectious lymphnode etiologies; mediastinal masses from HD and germ cell tumors; abdominal enlargement from other abdominal malignant masses such as Wilms' tumor, neuroblastoma, rhabdomyosarcoma; and bone

---

Box 34.5: Pretreatment studies for staging pediatric non-Hodgkin lymphoma

Complete blood cell count
Serum electrolytes, uric acid, lactate dehydrogenase, creatinine, calcium, phosphorus
Liver function tests (ALT, AST)
Chest radiographs and chest CT if abnormal
Neck, abdominal and pelvic ultrasonography and /or CT
Positive emission tomography scan
Bilateral bone marrow aspirate and biopsy
Cerebrospinal fluid cytology, cell count, protein
ALT, alanine aminotransferase; AST, aspartate aminotransferase

marrow involvement from precursor B (Pre-B) acute lymphoblastic leukemia.

Treatment: The primary modality of treatment for children and adolescent NHL is malignant systemic chemotherapy and intrathecal chemotherapy. Surgery is used mainly for diagnostic and/or biologic specimens and staging and is rarely used for removing large size masses. Radiation therapy is used in special circumstances such as CNS involvement in LL or occasionally BL, acute SVC, and acute paraplegias. Patients at diagnosis and at risk of TLS , especially advanced/bulky BL or LL, require vigorous hydration and either a xanthine oxidase inhibitor (allopurinol, 10 mg/kg/day PO divided tid) or, more often, recombinant urate oxidase (rasburicase, 0.2 mg/kg/day PO once daily for 1–3 days).

Specific treatment for localized and advanced disease is similar for BL and DLBCL. Localized BL and DLBCL require 6 wk to 6 mo of malignant chemotherapy. Common regimens include COPAD (cyclophosphamide, vincristine, prednisone and doxorubicin), or COMP (cyclophosphamide, vincristine [Oncovin], methotrexate, 6-mercaptopurine and prednisone). Advanced disease usually is treated by 4–6 mo of multiagent chemotherapy.

Localized and advanced LL usually requires almost 24 mo of therapy. The best results in advanced LL have been obtained by an induction cycle of chemotherapy by using therapeutic approaches similar to those for childhood acute leukemia, which includes an induction cycle of chemotherapy, consolidation phase, interim maintenance phase, reinduction phase (advanced disease only), and a year of maintenance therapy with 6-mercaptopurine and methotrexate.

Localized ALCL may require only cutaneous excision or more aggressive therapy similar to that for advanced ALCL. Advanced ALCL is treated similar to advanced LL or with a COG protocol of APO (doxorubicin, prednisone, and vincristine) with additional VP-16, Ara-C, or vinblastine.

Intrathecal chemotherapy is administered to moderate to advanced disease in all subtypes of childhood and adolescent NHL and may include intrathecal methotrexate, hydrocortisone, or Ara-C.

Patients with NHL who develop progressive or relapsed disease require reinduction chemotherapy and either allogeneic or autologous stem cell transplantation.

Supportive care: Indwelling central venous catheters routinely should be placed to facilitate frequent blood draws, chemotherapy and transfusion administration, and parenteral nutrition to prevent weight loss and nutritional debilitation.

Complications: Patients receiving multiagent chemotherapy for advanced disease are at acute risk for serious mucositis, infections, cytopenias (requiring RBC and platelets transfusions), electrolyte imbalance and poor nutrition. Long-term complications may include growth retardation, cardiac toxicity, gonadal toxicity with infertility and secondary malignancies.

Prognosis: The prognosis is excellent for most forms of childhood and adolescents NHL. Patients with localized disease have a 90–100% chance of survival, and patients with advanced disease have a 60–95% chance of survival.

Cairo MS, Brigid Bradley M. Lymphoma. In: Kliegman RM, Behrman RE, Jenson HB, Stanton BF (eds). *Nelson Textbook of Pediatrics.* 18th edn. Vol. 2. Philadelphia: Saunders, 2007; 2123–2128.

Flavell KG, Murray PG. Hodgkin's disease and Epstein-Barr virus. *Mol Pathol* 2000; 53:262-269.

Hudson MM, Donaldson SS. Treatment of pediatric Hodgkin's disease. *Semin Hematol* 1999; 36: 313–323.

Pinkerton CR. The continuing challenge of treatment for non-Hodgkin's lymphomas. *Br J Haematol* 1999; 107: 220–234.

Yung L, Linch D. Hodgkin's lymphoma. *Lancet* 2003; 361: 943–950.

34.3 CENTRAL NERVOUS SYSTEM TUMORS

See Section 24.12 and 24.14.

34.4 NEUROBLASTOMA

Neuroblastoma occurs with nearly the same frequency as Wilms tumor. Mean age at presentation is 24 months (range 1 to 4 yrs). The tumor may arise anywhere along the sympathetic chain. The most common site is suprarenal. Other sites include retroperitoneal, pelvic, posterior mediastinum and cervical. Neuroblastoma metastasizes early and may spread to bone, liver, skin, bone marrow or orbit at the time of presentation. Clinical presentation is often due to compression neuropathy and paraparesis; or due to paraneoplastic syndrome as a result of catecholamine production by the tumor. This includes episodes of flushing, sweating, headache, tachycardia and hypertension. There may be refractory diarrhea due to production of vasoactive intestinal peptide (VIP) by the tumor. Ataxia or opsomyoclonus ("dancing eyes and dancing feet") is also seen in neuroblastoma.

Plain radiograph often shows speckled calcification. The tumor frequently crosses the midline. Ultrasonography may help in defining the organ of origin, i.e. renal or extra renal. CT scan is the most helpful imaging modality as it also defines tumor extension and involvement of lymph nodes. Technetium 99m labeled radionuclide scan helps in detecting skeletal metastasis. MIBG scan also picks up tumor activity due to its catecholamine production.

Treatment options are combinations of surgery, chemotherapy and radiation. The tumor is often not resectable at diagnosis as it engulfs the great vessels (e.g. aorta and inferior vena cava in the abdomen). Hence neo-adjuvant chemotherapy is useful in shrinking the tumor preoperatively. Overall prognosis is much poorer when compared to Wilms' tumor. Stage 4S disease seen in infants has been shown to have spontaneous regression despite metastasis.

Ater JL. Neuroblastoma. In: Behrman RE, Kliegman RM, Jenson HB (eds). *Nelson Textbook of Pediatrics*. 17th edn. Philadelphia: Saunders, 2004;1709–11.

Moppett J, Haddadin I, Foot ABM. Neonatal neuroblastoma. *Arch Dis Fetal Neonatal Ed* 1999; 81: F134–37.

34.5 HEPATOBLASTOMA

Hepatoblastoma is the most common malignant hepatic tumor in children. Majority of the children are less than 3 yrs of age. Clinical features include upper abdominal mass, anorexia and weight loss. Extramedullary hematopoiesis and thrombocytosis are often associated. Tumor markers like alpha-feto-protein (AFP) and beta-human-chorionic-gonado-tropin (B-HCG) are elevated. Precocious puberty can be present due to secretion of B-HCG by the tumor. Ultrasonography and CT scan help to define the morphology and respectability of the tumor. Celiac arteriography is rarely required in the present era. Treatment is by combination of surgery and chemotherapy. These children have a fair prognosis if the tumor is completely resected and tumor marker levels come down to normal. Hepatocellular carcinoma is seen in older children often with underlying hepatic pathology like cirrhosis. The prognosis is poorer than hepatoblastoma.

Caty MG, Shamberger RC. Abdominal tumors in infancy and childhood. *Pediatr Clin North Am* 1993; 40(6):1253–1271.

34.6 WILMS' TUMOR (WT)

Introduction: WT was first described by Thomas F. Rance in 1814, but later in 1899 was given this name by Max Wilms. Wilms' tumor (WT) is one of the success stories of paediatric oncology with long term survival approaching 90% in localised disease and over 70% for metastatic disease quoted in the developed world. The prognosis is related not only to the stage of disease at diagnosis, the histopathologic features of the tumor, patient age, and tumor size, but also to the team approach to each patient by the pediatric surgeon, radiation oncologist, and pediatric oncologist. The success in management of WT encourages the outlook towards the management of pediatric malignant tumors in general.

Incidence: WT is the commonest renal tumors and accounts for 5–10% of all tumors in the western literature; the Indian literature states a similar incidence. Asian children have a lower incidence as compared to their Western counterparts and that the tumors in Asian children were encountered at younger age. Half of the tumors occur before the age of 3 yrs and 90% before the age of 6, and is equally common in boys and girls.

Molecular biology and associations: Chromosomal regions implicated in the development of WT include the short arm of chromosome 11 (likely contains two regions involved in WT), the long arm of chromosome 16 and the short arm of chromosome 1.

Of all the children affected by WT, 90% occur in children otherwise healthy and 10% of cases occur in those with recognized malformations. **Syndromic WT** (WAGR syndrome, Denys-Drash syndrome, Beckwith-Wiedemann syndrome, hemihypertrophy, etc.) occurs in approximately 10% of patients with WT. These syndromes have provided clues to the genetic basis of the disease. The phenotypic syndromes have been divided into overgrowth and non-overgrowth categories.

Diagnosis: Apart from the most common form of presentation of lump in abdomen (80%), abdominal pain and hematuria (25% each), hypertension, fever, anaemia and gross hematuria occurs in 5–30% of patients. Large tumors with lung metastases may present with tachypnoea/respiratory distress. A thorough clinical examination for the abdominal mass as well as for associated congenital malformations and syndromes.

Rare presentations of WT include varicocele, hernia, enlarged testis, congestive cardiac failure, acute renal failure, nephrotic syndrome, polycythemia, Cushing syndrome, cervical polyp (extra-renal WT), acquired von Willebrand disease, intestinal obstruction, hydrocephalus (metastases), acute anemia (intra-capsular hemorrhage), hemoptysis (metastases), acute abdominal pain mimicking appendicitis. Antenatal detection of WT has been also reported.

Ultrasonography of the abdomen remains the gold standard investigative modality. X-ray chest is essential for detecting metastases to the lungs. A contrast enhanced CT scan or a MRI could also be done for better delineation of the mass and its effects.

Staging: Since the Wilms' tumor is managed by 2 different approaches, 2 staging systems exist—the NWTS and the SIOP.

Management

Treatment of WT is one of the remarkable success stories in childhood cancer. Before the advent of modern therapy, 2-yr survival rates were 50% or less. However, the combined use of surgery, radiation therapy and chemotherapy (multimodal treatment approach) permits most patients treated today to be able to reach adulthood. All patients receive chemotherapy and surgery, while those with more extensive disease or those with adverse prognostic features receive additional radiotherapy. In North America, most children are registered on and subsequently treated according to a NWTSG clinical trial, while in Europe most children are managed based on studies designed by the International Society of Paediatric Oncology (SIOP).

NWTS advocates upfront nephrectomy followed by tumor staging and further therapy, chemotherapy and occasionally, radiotherapy. The rationale for the NWTSG approach is that accurate assessment of the extent of disease at diagnosis allows safe administration of the intensity of treatment for each individual. SIOP advocates upfront chemotherapy without tissue diagnosis.

Chemotherapy: The drugs used in the treatment of WT include vincristine and actinomycin D, given to all patients. Doxorubicin is added for those with more extensive disease or those with adverse prognostic features.

Radiation therapy: There is a very limited role of radiation therapy in the treatment of WT, and is restricted largely to treating symptoms caused by widespread disease, i.e., Stages III and IV disease, (i.e., palliation of metastatic disease). In the past two decades, researchers have identified which patients can be cured without the addition of radiation therapy. In addition, they have been able to show that the radiation dose initially recommended for children with Wilms tumor could be reduced significantly. Currently patients in North America receive 1080 cGy and those in Europe 1500 cGy, both given in combination with chemotherapy.

Bhatnagar S. Management of Wilms' tumor: NWTS vs SIOP. J Indian *Assoc Pediatr Surg* 2009; 14: 6–14.

Jaffe N, Huff V. Neoplasms of the kidney. In: Behrman RE, Kliegman RM, Jenson HB (eds). *Nelson Textbook of Pediatrics.* 17th edn. Philadelphia: Saunders, 2004; 1711–1714.

Huff V. Wilms' tumor genetics. *Am J Med Genet* 1998; 79: 260–267.

National Wilms' Study Committee: Wilms' tumor: Status report, 1990. *J Clin Oncol* 1991; 9: 877–887.

Paulino AC. Current issues in the diagnosis and management of Wilms' tumor. *Oncology* 1996; 10:1553–1571.

34.7 NEOPLASMS OF BONE

Malignant Tumors of Bone

Osteosarcoma

Osteosarcoma is the most common primary malignant bone tumor in children and adolescents, followed by Ewing sarcoma. Both tumor types occur most frequently in the second decade of life.

Epidemiology: The highest risk period for development of osteosarcoma is during the adolescent growth spurt, which suggests an association between rapid bone growth and malignant transformation. Patients with osteosarcoma are taller than their peers of similar age. The predisposing factors include retinoblastoma, Li-Fraumeni syndrome, Paget disease, and radiotherapy.

Clinical manifestations: Pain and swelling are the most common clinical manifestations. Additional clinical findings may include limitation of motion, joint effusion, tenderness, and warmth. The common site is metaphyses of long bones. Metastasis occurs in lungs and bones.

Diagnosis: Any bone or joint pain not responding to conservative therapy for sports injury or sprain within a reasonable amount of time should be thoroughly investigated. Results of routine laboratory tests, such as complete blood cell count and chemistry panel are usually normal except alkaline phosphatase or lactic dehydrogenase levels, which may be elevated. The diagnosis of a bone tumor should be suspected in a patient who presents with deep bone pain, often causing night time awakening, a palpable mass, and a radiograph demonstrating a lesion. The lesion may be mixed lytic and blastic in appearance, but new bone formation is usually visible. The classic radiographic appearance of osteosarcoma is the **sun-burst** pattern (*see* Fig. 34.2 in CD). The biopsy should be performed by the surgeon who will ultimately perform the definitive surgery so that the incisional biopsy site can be placed in a manner that will not compromise the ultimate limb salvage procedure. Tissue is usually obtained for molecular and biological studies at the time of the initial biopsy (spindle cell-producing osteoid). Before biopsy, MRI of the primary lesion and the entire bone should be performed to evaluate the tumor for its proximity to nerves and blood vessels and soft tissue and joint extension as well as for skip lesions. The metastatic work-up should also be performed before biopsy and includes CT of the chest and radionuclide of bone scan to evaluate for lung and bone metastases respectively. The differential diagnosis of a lytic bone lesion includes histiocytosis, Ewing sarcoma, lymphoma, and bone cyst.

Treatment: The current approach is to treat patients with preoperative chemotherapy in an attempt to facilitate limb salvage operations and to immediately treat micrometastatic disease. Up to 80% of patients are able to undergo limb salvage operations after initial chemotherapy. It is important to resume chemotherapy as soon as possible after surgery. Lung metastases present at diagnosis should be resected by thoracostomies at some time during the course of treatment. The multidrug therapy regimens include doxorubicin, methotrexate, cisplatin, and ifosfamide. After limb salvage surgery, intensive rehabilitation and physical therapy is necessary to ensure maximal functional outcome. For patients who require amputation, early prosthetic fitting and gait training is essential to enable them to resume normal activities as early as possible. Before definitive surgery, patients with tumors on weight-bearing bones should be instructed to use crutches to avoid stressing the weakened bone and causing a pathologic fracture. The role of chemotherapy in periosteal and perosteal osteosarcoma is not well defined.

Prognosis: Complete surgical resection of the tumor is important for cure. Surgical resection alone is curative only for patients with perosteal osteosarcoma. Conventional osteosarcoma requires multiagent chemotherapy. Up to 75% of patients with nonmetastatic extremity osteosarcoma are cured with multiagent treatment protocols. Patients with pelvic tumors do not have as favorable prognosis as those with extremity osteosarcoma. Cure rate is only 20–30% in patients who have limited numbers of pulmonary metastases with aggressive chemotherapy and resection of lung nodules, but patients with bone metastases and those with widespread lung metastases have an extremely poor prognosis. Patients who develop late isolated lung metastases may be cured with surgical resection alone. Late effects of chemotherapy such as cardiotoxicity from anthracycline should be monitored during follow up study.

Ewing Sarcoma

Epidemiology: Ewing sarcoma, an undifferentiated sarcoma of bone, may also arise from soft tissue. The term **Ewing sarcoma family of tumors** refers to a group of small round cell undifferentiated tumors thought to be of neural crest origin that generally carry the same chromosomal translocation. This family of tumors includes Ewing sarcoma of bone and soft tissue and **peripheral primitive neuroectodermal tumor (PPNET)**. Primary tumors arising in bone are evenly distributed between the extremities and central axis (pelvis, spine, and chest wall). Primary tumors arising in the chest wall are often referred to as **Askin tumors.**

Clinical manifestations: Pain, swelling, limitation of motion and tenderness over involved bone or soft tissue are the common presenting symptoms, similar to those observed in osteosarcoma. Patients with huge chest wall primary tumors, my present with respiratory distress. In case of paraspinal or vertebral primary tumors may present with symptoms of cord compression. Metastasis occurs in lungs and bones.

Diagnosis: The diagnosis of Ewing sarcoma should be suspected in a patient who presents with pain and swelling, with or without systemic symptoms such as fever or weight loss and with a radiographic appearance of a primarily lytic bone lesion with periosteal reaction, the characteristic **onion-skinning** (*see* Fig. 34.3 in CD). A large associated soft tissue mass is often visualized on MRI or CT. Thorough evaluation for metastatic disease includes CT of the chest, radionuclide bone scan, and bone marrow aspirate and biopsy specimens from at least two sites. MRI of the tumor and the entire length of involved bone should be performed to determine the exact extension of the soft tissue and bony mass and the proximity of tumor to neurovascular structures. The biopsy should be performed by the surgeon who will ultimately perform the definitive surgery so that the incisional biopsy site can be placed in a manner that will not compromise the ultimate limb salvage procedure. CT-guided biopsy of the lesion often provides diagnostic tissue. Histological findings will reveal undifferentiated small round cell, probably of neural origin. It is important to obtain adequate tissue for special stains, cytogenetics, and molecular studies. The differential diagnosis includes osteosarcoma, osteomyelitis, Langerhans cell histiocytosis, and primary lymphoma of bone; metastatic neuroblastoma or rhabdomyosarcoma in the case of a pure soft tissue lesion.

Treatment: Ewing sarcoma family of tumors is best treated with a multidisciplinary approach including multiagent chemotherapy, surgery and radiation. Chemotherapy causes shrinkage of the soft tissue mass and rapid of pain. The multidrug therapy regimens include vincristine, doxorubicin, cyclophosphamide, ifosfamide and etoposide. Ewing sarcoma is sensitive to radiotherapy and local control may be achieved with radiation or surgical resection. Radiation therapy is associated with a risk of radiation-induced second malignancies, especially osteosarcoma, as well as failure of bone growth in skeletally immature patients. Before definitive local control (radiation or surgery), patients with tumors on weight-bearing bones should be instructed to use crutches to avoid stressing the weakened bone and causing a pathologic fracture. Chemotherapy should be resumed as soon as possible after surgery.

Prognosis: Patients with small, nonmetastatic, distally located extremity tumors have the best prognosis with a cure rate up to 75%. Patients with pelvic tumors do not have a favorable prognosis as those with extremity Ewing sarcoma. Patients with metastatic disease at diagnosis especially bone or bone marrow metastases have a poor prognosis with less than 30% survival. Late effects of chemotherapy such as cardiotoxicity from anthracycline, second malignancies, especially in the radiation field, and late relapses even 10 yr after initial diagnosis should be monitored during follow up study.

Benign Tumors

Osteochondroma (exostosis) is one of the most common benign bone tumors in children. Most osteochondromas develop in childhood, arising from the metaphysic of long bones, particularly the distal femur, proximal humerus, and proximal tibia. The lesion enlarges with the child until skeletal maturity. Most are discovered from 5 to 15 yr of age when the child or parent notices a bony, non-painful mass. Osteochondrosarcoma appear radiographically as stalks or broad-based projections from the surface of the bone, usually in a direction away from the adjacent joint. Invariably, the lesion is radiographically smaller than suggested by palpation because the cartilage, "cap" covering the lesion is not seen. This cartilage cap may be up to 1 cm thick. Both the cortex of the bone and the marrow space of the involved bone are continuous with the lesion. Malignant degeneration to a chondrosarcoma may occur in as many as 1% of adults. Routine removal is not performed unless the lesion is large enough to cause symptoms or if rapid growth occurs. **Multiple hereditary exostoses** are characterized by the presence of multiple osteochondromas and involved children may have short stature, limb-length inequality, and deformity of both the upper and lower extremities.

Chondroblastoma is a rare lesion usually found in the epiphysis of long bones; common sites include the hip, shoulder, and knee. Most patients present in the second decade with complaints of mild to moderate pain in the adjacent joint, local tenderness and muscle atrophy. Radiographically, the lesion appears as a sharply marginated radiolucency within the epiphysis. Recognition is important because most lesions can be cured with curettage and bone grafting before joint destruction occurs.

Osteoid osteoma is a small benign bone tumor, mostly diagnosed between 5 and 20 yr of age. Males are affected more than females. The clinical pattern is characteristic, consisting of unremitting and gradually occurring pain that is often worst at night and relieved by aspirin. Any bone can be involved, but the most common sites are the proximal femur and tibia. Vertebral lesions may cause scoliosis or symptoms that mimic a neurologic disorder. Radiographs show a round or oval metaphyseal or diaphyseal lucency (0.5–1 cm diameter) surrounded by sclerotic bone. The central lucency or nidus shows intense uptake on bone scan. Osteoid osteoma not visualized on plain radiographs can be identified by CT. Treatment consists of en-bloc excision, curettage, or percutaneous CT-guided ablation. Patients with mild pain may be treated with aspirin. Some lesions spontaneously resolve after skeletal maturity.

Fibromas (nonossifying fibroma, fibrous cortical defect, metaphyseal fibrous defect) are fibrous lesions of bone that occur in 40% of children older than 2 yr of age. These lesions are usually asymptomatic. Radiographs show a sharply marginated eccentric lucency in the metaphyseal cortex. Lesions may be multilocular and expansile, with extension from the cortex into the medullary bone. The long axis of the lesion is parallel with that of the bone. Approximately 50% are bilateral or multiple. Spontaneous regression can occur. Curettage and bone grafting is recommended for lesions occupying more than 50% of the bone diameter because of the risk of pathologic fracture.

Fibrous dysplasia is characterized by fibrous replacement of cancellous bone. Lesions may be solitary or multifocal (polyostotic), relatively stable, or progressively more severe. Most children are asymptomatic. Children with skull involvement may have swelling or exophthalmos; pain and limp with proximal femoral involvement; limb-length discrepancy, bowing of the tibia or femur, and pathologic fractures. The triad of polyostotic disease, precocious puberty, and cutaneous pigmentation is known as **Albright syndrome**. Radiographs show a lytic or ground glass expansile lesion of the metaphysis or diaphysis and the lesion is sharply marginated and surrounded by a thick rim of sclerotic bone. Treatment usually involves observation. Surgery is indicated for patients with progressive deformity.

Eosinophilic granuloma usually occurs during the first 3 decades of life and is most common in boys 5–10 yr of age. The skull is most commonly affected, but any bone can be involved. Patients usually present with local pain, swelling, marked tenderness and warmth in the affected area of the involved bone. Spinal lesions may cause pain, stiffness, and occasional neurologic symptoms. Eosinophilic granuloma is a monostotic or polyostotic disease with no extra skeletal involvement.

This latter finding distinguishes eosinophilic granuloma from other forms of Langerhans histiocytosis. The radiographic findings include radiolucent lesions, which have well-defined or irregular margins with expansion of the involved bone and periosteal new bone formation. Biopsy is often necessary to confirm the diagnosis because of the broad radiographic differential diagnosis. Treatment includes curettage and bone grafting, low dose radiation therapy, or steroid injection. Observation for symptomatic lesions is necessary because most skeletal lesions heal spontaneously and do not recur.

Arndt CAS. Neoplasms of bone. In: Behrman RE, Kliegman RM, Jenson HB (eds). *Nelson Textbook of Pediatrics*. 17th edn. Philadelphia: Saunders, 2004;1717–1722.

Arndit CAS, Crist WM. Common musculoskeletal tumors of childhood and adolescence. *N Engl J Med* 1999; 341: 342–352.

34.8 RETINOBLASTOMA

Retinoblastoma (RB) is the most common primary malignant intraocular of childhood. It occurs in approximately 1/15,000 live births. There are two forms of the disease: hereditary and a non-hereditary. The hereditary form is usually bilateral and multifocal, whereas the nonhereditary form is generally unilateral and unifocal. Fifteen percent of unilateral cases are hereditary. The retinoblastoma gene is a recessive suppressor gene located on chromosome13 at the 13q14 region. Bilateral cases often present earlier than unilateral cases. Unilateral tumors are often large by the time they are recognized. The average age at diagnosis is 15 months for bilateral cases, compared with 25 mo for unilateral cases. Rarely, the tumor is discovered at birth, during adolescence, or even in early adulthood.

Clinical manifestations: The most common and obvious sign of retinoblastoma is a white pupillary reflex, leukocoria (*see* Figs 34.4 and 34.5 in CD). The second most frequent sign of retinoblastoma is strabismus. Other less common and less specific signs and symptoms are: pseudohypopyon (tumor cells layered inferiorly in front of the iris) caused by tumor seeding in the anterior chamber of the eye, hyphema (blood layered in front of the iris) secondary to iris neovascularization, vitreous hemorrhage and signs of orbital cellulitis. On examination, the tumor appears as a white mass. Vitreous haze or tumor seeding may be evident.

Diagnosis: The diagnosis is established by the characteristic ophthalmoscopic findings. Orbital ultrasonography, CT or MRI are used to evaluate the extent of intraocular disease and extraocular spread and also demonstrate calcification within the mass.

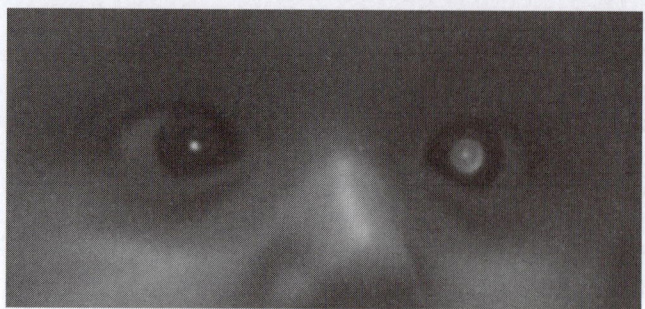

Fig. 34.4: Leukocoria in the left eye in a child with retinoblastoma

Occasionally, a pineal area tumor is detected, a phenomenon known as **trilateral retinoblastoma**. MRI allows for better evaluation of optic nerve involvement. A definitive diagnosis occasionally can not be made and removal of a blind eye in which the diagnosis of retinoblastoma is likely may be appropriate; biopsy is contraindicated. Histologically, retinoblastoma appears as a small round blue cell tumor with rosette formation. It may arise in any of the nucleated layers of the retina, exhibits various degrees of differentiation, and tends to outgrow its blood supply, resulting in necrosis and calcification.

The *differential diagnosis* includes hyperplastic primary vitreous, Coats disease, cataract, visceral larva migrans, choroidal coloboma, and retinopathy of prematurity.

Treatment: The position and size of the tumor as well as whether it is unilateral or bilateral are considered when choosing the type of treatment for the disease. In case of a solitary, large tumor, enucleation is performed if there is no potential for useful vision. With bilateral disease, chemoreduction in combination with focal therapy (laser photocoagulation or cryotherapy) of the more severely affected eye (no enucleation) and irradiation of the remaining eye. Small tumors can be treated with focal therapy with careful follow-up for evidence of recurrence or new tumor growth. Larger tumors often respond to multiagent chemotherapy including carboplatin, vincristine, and etoposide. If this approach fails, external-beam irradiation should be considered, but is associated with significant orbital deformity and increased incidence of second malignancies in patients with germ line mutations. Brachytherapy or episcleral plaque radiotherapy is an alternative with less morbidity. Enucleation may be required for unresponsive or recurrent tumors. Children of affected patients should be referred to an ophthalmologist when the peripheral retina examination.

Prognosis for children with retinoblastoma depends on the size and extension of the tumor. When confined to one eye, most tumors can be cured. The prognosis for long-term survival is poor when the tumor has extended into the orbit or along the optic nerve.

Chintagumpala M, Chevez-Barrios P, Paysse EA, Plon SE, Hurwitz R. "Retinoblastoma: review of current management." *Oncologist* 2007; 12 (10): 1237–1246.

Melamud A, Palekar R, Singh A. "Retinoblastoma." *Am Fam Physician* 2006; 73 (6): 1039–1044.

Herzog CE. Retinoblastoma. In: Kliegman RM, Behrman RE, Jenson HB, Stanton BF (eds). *Nelson Textbook of Pediatrics.* 18th edn. Vol. 2. Philadelphia: Saunders, 2007; 2151–2153.

Shields CL, Shields JA. Diagnosis and management of retinoblastoma. *Cancer Control* 2004; 11 (5): 317–327.

34.9 HISTIOCYTOSIS SYNDROMES OF CHILDHOOD

The childhood histiocytoses constitute a diverse group of disorders and are divided into three classes based on histopathologic findings.

Class I Histiocytoses

Langerhan's cell histiocytosis is applied to class 1 histiocytosis and includes clinical entities of eosinophilic granuloma, Hand-Schüller-Christian disease and Letterer-Siwe disease. No extraskeletal involvement occurs in patients with eosinophilic granuloma.

Clinical manifestations: Langerhans' cell histiocytosis (LCH) has an extremely variable presentation. The skeleton is involved in 80% of patients and may be the only affected site, especially in children older than 5 yr of age. Bone lesions may be single or numerous and are seen most commonly in the skull. They may be asymptomatic or associated with pain and local swelling. The other bones involved are vertebral body, flat and long bones. Lesions that involve weight-bearing long bones may result in pathologic fractures. Chronically draining infected ears are commonly associated with destruction in the mastoid area. Bone destruction in the mandible and maxilla may result in loose teeth.

Extra-skeletal involvement includes skin (seborrheic dermatitis, exanthema), lymphadenopathy, hepatosplenomegaly, retro-orbital area (leading to exophthalmos), gingival mucus membranes, pituitary, hypothalamus, and thyroid. Patients who are more severely involved may have systemic manifestations, including fever, weight loss, malaise, irritability, and failure to thrive. Bone marrow involvement may cause anemia and thrombocytopenia. Two uncommon but serious and unusual manifestations of LCH are hepatic involvement (leading to cirrhosis) and a peculiar central nervous system (CNS) involvement characterized by ataxia, dysarthria, and other neurologic symptoms.

Diagnosis: A thorough clinical and laboratory evaluation should be undertaken in addition to tissue biopsy (skin or bone lesions). This should include complete blood cell count, liver function tests, coagulation studies, skeletal survey, chest radiograph, and measurement of urine osmolality. Cellular characteristics of lesions are Langerhans' cells (CD 1a positive) with Birbeck granules. Birbeck granules, a tennis racket-shaped bilamellar granule, which when seen in the cytoplasm of lesional cells in LCH is diagnostic of the disease.

Treatment and prognosis: The clinical course of single-system disease (usually bone, lymph node, or skin) is generally benign, with a high chance of spontaneous remission. The aim should be minimal treatment and arresting the progression of a lesion (e.g., bone lesion) by curettage or low-dose local radiation therapy (5–6 Gy). Multisystem disease should be treated with systemic multiagent chemotherapy, which should include either vinblastine or etoposide, to reduce reactivation of disease and long-term consequences. Experimental therapies should be undertaken only for unresponsive disease, including immunosuppressive therapy with cyclosporine/antithymocyte globulin and possibly certain new agents and modalities such as 2-chlorodeoxyadenosine and stem cell transplantation.

Class II Histiocytosis: Hemophagocytic Lymphohistiocytosis

In Class II histiocytosis familial erythrophagocytic lymphohistiocytosis [also called familial hemophagocytic lymphohistiocytosis (FHLH)] and infection-associated hemophagocytic syndrome [also called secondary hemophagocytic lymphohistiocytosis (secondary HLH)] are included.

Clinical manifestations: The major forms of hemophagocytic lymphohistiocytosis (HLH), familial hemophagocytic lymphohistiocytosis (FHLH), and secondary HLH have similar manifestation, consisting of a generalized disease process, most often with fever, maculopapular and/or petechial rash, weight loss, and irritability. FHLH is also characterized by immunodeficiency. Children with FHLH are always younger than 4 yr of age, whereas children with secondary HLH my present at an older age. Physical examination frequently reveals hepatosplenomegaly, lymphadenopathy, respiratory distress and symptoms of CNS involvement, unlike that of aseptic meningitis in which the CSF cells are the same phagocytic macrophages as found in the peripheral blood or bone marrow. The diagnosis is based on the pathologic findings in skin or bone marrow biopsy. Associated laboratory findings in both forms of HLH include hyperlipidemia, hypofibrinogenemia, elevated levels of hepatic enzymes, extremely elevated levels of serum ferritin (often > 10,000), and cytopenias (especially pancytopenia from hemophagocytosis in the marrow). No absolute clinical or laboratory distinction can be made between FHLH and secondary HLH, although genetic markers for FHLH can complement a positive history for other affected children.

Treatment and prognosis: When FEL is diagnosed or suspected without documented infection, therapy includes etoposide and immunosuppressive therapy. Allogeneic bone marrow transplantation may be effective in curing a few patients with FEL. Treatment of infection along with supportive care should be done in the patients with infection. In IAHS, when an infection can be documented and effectively treated the prognosis is good without any other specific treatment. When a treatable infection cannot be documented in IAHS, the prognosis is as poor as that of FEL. In contrast, in secondary HLH, when an infection can be documented and effectively treated

Class III Histiocytosis

In the class III histiocytosis, acute monocytic leukemia (*see* acute myelogenous leukemia) and true malignant histiocytosis are included. Cellular characteristics of lesions include neoplastic proliferation of cells with characteristics of monocytes/macrophages or their precursors. Treatment includes antineoplastic chemotherapy, including anthracyclines

Ladisch G. Histiocytosis syndromes of childhood. In: Behrman RE, Kliegman RM, Jenson HB (eds). *Nelson Textbook of Pediatrics.* 17th edn. Vol.2. Philadelphia: Saunders, 2008; 2159–2162.

Writing Group of the Histiocyte Society: Histiocytosis syndromes of childhood. *Lancet* 1987; 1: 208–209.

34.10 RHABDOMYOSARCOMA

Rhabdomyosarcoma (RMS) is the most commonly occurring soft tissue sarcoma of all the sarcomas that occur in children. It is the only tumor that occurs in almost unlimited number of primary sites. RMS is a highly malignant, rapidly progressing, aggressive tumor that arises from the primitive embryonal mesenchymal cells that initiate striated and skeletal muscle differentiation. The hallmarks of this tumor are early local infiltration and metastatic dissemination if left untreated. One-fourth of all RMSs are genitourinary in origin. The genetic conditions and syndromes associated with RMS are unusual and include Li- Fraumeni cancer susceptibility syndrome, neurofibromatosis type I, Beckwith-Wiedemann

syndrome, Rubinstein-Taybi syndrome, Gorlin basal cell nevus syndrome, Costello syndrome.

Incidence: The estimated annual incidence of genitourinary rhabdomyosarcoma in the United States is 0.5 to 0.7 cases per 1 million children less than 15 yrs old. It occurs at 2 yrs age, peaks—the early peak in 2–6 yrs old children and late peak during adolescence between ages 15–19 yrs with a male preponderance of 3:1.

Clinical manifestations: The genitourinary especially bladder and prostatic RMS, can present in various forms depending on the site and extent of the tumor. Usually *bladder tumors* grow intra-luminally and cause obstructive urinary symptoms and bladder outlet obstruction which may lead to urinary retention, incontinence and infection, hematuria, and backpressure changes of the upper urinary tract. With breach of the overlying mucosa the tumor tissue can disrupt and be seen as tissue fragments in the urine. Mass prolapsing per urethra may be seen in a female patient. Lump in abdomen is another presenting feature found in exophytic bladder tumors as well as prostatic tumors. The **prostatic tumor** present as large pelvic masses with urinary retention, dysuria, strangury, and or constipation.

Diagnosis: RMS of the bladder and the prostate will clinically present according to the site of origin and the size of the tumor. The first and foremost mode of investigating the child is by ultrasonography of the abdomen and pelvis followed by a CT scan to confirm the ultrasound findings as well as to give a detailed tumor anatomy. A micturating cystourethrogram is the basic investigation to assess the involvement of the bladder and the status of the bladder outlet. MRI has been reported to be better than CT scan for diagnosis as well as follow-up as it gives a more accurate delineation of residual disease. A whole body MRI with STIR (Short tau inversion recovery) sequence has been proved to be as useful as bone-scan to detect skeletal metastases and even other sites of metastases. 18F-Deoxyglucose Positron Emission Tomography (PET) has been evaluated over recent yrs and has been found to be a useful adjunct in the staging of RMS. Though bone scintigraphy, whole body MRI and PET scan can be done for skeletal metastases, it has been found that the FDG - PET is more specific as compared to whole body MRI or bone scintigraphy. Immunoscans have also been reported in literature with the Fab-fragment of the monoclonal R11D10 labeled with 111Indium which show significant increased uptake in rhabdomyosarcoma and some other tumors. Urine cytology, a non-invasive investigation should be done as a preliminary test for round cells which clinch the diagnosis of RMS. Fine-needle aspiration cytology is a valuable investigation for early histopathological diagnosis, and gives the opportunity to study specific chromosomal abnormalities using the FISH probe. The final confirmative diagnosis is always on histopathology of the tumor tissue taken either via cystoscope, a trucut biopsy needle or via operative biopsy.

Management

According to the clinical groups, the survival rate has been found to be 93% in stage I, 81% in stage II, 73% in stage III, and as low as 30% in stage IV. There has been steady improvement in the results of treatment reflected in the IRS trials I–IV.

Management of the bladder and prostate RMS involves complete surgical excision of the primary non-metastatic lesion of the bladder/prostate followed by multi-agent chemotherapy and radiotherapy. Surgery plays a vital role in the therapeutic modalities of the management of RMS.

The surgical options for the bladder RMS would be partial, subtotal or total cystectomy with reconstruction of the bladder. The prostatic RMS can be approached through the bladder or via transpubic approach. Inadequate local control of the tumor by either of the modalities is a major cause for treatment failure. The incidence of relapse ultimately leading to death in RMS has been reported to be as high as 30%, in spite of the advances in treatment. Also, those who survived the first five years post therapy did have a good prognosis on the long term.

Chemotherapy: Vincristine, Actinomycin and Cyclophosphamide (VAC) constitute the standard chemotherapy regime in a majority of cases. Ifosfamide and doxorubicin have been used in the IRS study group for metastatic RMS.

Radiotherapy: In RMS, radiotherapy plays a major role in local tumor control as complete surgical resection of the tumor is not always feasible considering the complications and long term morbidity of these patients. The standard regime for conventional radiation was 45 Gy given by single daily fractions of 1.5 to 2.0 Gy.

Arndt CAS. Soft tissue sarcomas. In: Behrman RE, Kliegman RM, Jenson HB (eds). *Nelson Textbook of Pediatrics.* 17th edn. Philadelphia: Saunders, 2004; 1714–1717.

Arndit CAS, Crist WM. Medical progress: Common musculoskeletal tumors of childhood and adolescence. *N Engl J Med* 1999; 341: 342–352.

Kaefer M, Rink RC. Genitourinary rhabdomyosarcoma treatment options. *Urol Clin North Am* 2000; 27: 471–487.

Palumbo JS, Zwerdling J. Soft tissue sarcomas of infancy. *Semin Perinatol* 1999; 23: 299–309.

34.11 ONCOLOGIC EMERGENCIES

The overall survival of children with malignancy has increased as a result of advances in diagnosis and newer therapies including hematopoietic cell transplantation and use of growth factors. Oncologic emergencies may come as initial presentation of the malignancy, during course of disease or as a consequence of therapy. Early diagnosis and urgent management will save the life of the child and allow for treatment of the underlying malignancy. Six common emergencies likely to be encountered.

1. *Tumor lysis syndrome* is the set of metabolic abnormalities that results from acute destruction of neoplastic cells and release of their intracellular products into the circulation. The high rate of cell turnover overwhelms the body's normal homeostatic mechanisms for handling potassium, calcium, phosphorus, and uric acid, leading to hyperuricemia, hyperkalemia, hyperphosphatemia, hypocalcemia and uremia. These may be seen alone or in combination with one another. Tumor lysis syndrome occurs with a variety of tumors, most commonly the hematologic malignancies. Burkitt's lymphoma and T-cell lymphoblastic lymphomas are the most common causes.

   Prophylaxis is the first step in treatment. If a patient is found to be at high risk for tumor lysis syndrome, he or she should promptly be started on both intravenous fluid and allopurinol (300 mg/m^2 per day, orally) if there is no contraindication to it. Close observation during therapy is essential as transient urgent hemodialysis may reverse the toxicity.

2. *Hypercalcemia of malignancy* most commonly occurs in children with lymphoma. It is treated with hydration and bisphosphonates (pamidronate). Dieresis with furosemide should be started only after the patient is adequately hydrated.

3. *Superior vena cava syndrome* results from an increase in central venous pressure caused by vena caval obstruction. Typically this produces cough, dyspnea, and dysphagia combined with swelling and discoloration of the neck, face or upper extremities. Depending on the site of disease, both vocal cord paralysis and Horner syndrome can occur. Malignancies implicated include non-Hodgkin lymphoma, Hodgkin lymphoma, acute lymphoblastic leukemia, neuroblastoma and germ cell tumors.

   The treatment consists of elevating of the bed and giving diuretics and corticosteroids or chemotherapy; occasionally radiation therapy may be required.

4. *Spinal cord compression* is not immediately life-threatening unless it involves level cervical 3 (C3) or above, but it may lead to profound, permanent morbidity. Paraplegia or loss of sphincter control or both not only diminishes a patient's quality of life but also predisposes to further complications such as venous thrombosis, decubitus ulcers, and urinary obstruction.

Pain is the primary symptom. Other signs and symptoms are weakness, sensory deficits, and autonomic dysfunction. Magnetic resonance imaging with gadolinium is the investigation of choice. Prompt treatment with corticosteroids and radiation therapy may preserve the patient's ability to walk. Occasionally surgical intervention may be required.

5. *Strokes and seizures* are common in cancer patients. Initial treatment of strokes and seizures in cancer patient is the same as in patients without cancer. After initial stabilization, specific treatment of the tumor should be started.

6. *Treatment related emergencies.* Extravasation-leakage of chemotherapeutic drugs into the skin-results in pain, redness, swelling and even necrosis. Extravasation is important because large areas of skin may break down, leading to poor cosmetic results, secondary infection and contractures if the injury is over a joint. The most common culprits are vesicants, which cause blisters when they contact skin. Anthracyclines (e.g., doxorubicin and idarubicin) and vinca alkaloids (e.g., vincristine and vinorelbine) are the most common vesicants used in clinical practice.

If a patient is complaining of pain or problems during vesicant infusion, the infusion should be stopped, the line aspirated to remove residual drug and an antidote (if available) instilled through the line. Compression of the site should be avoided as this may spread the remaining drug further out from the injection site.

Neutropenic fever is common. Infectious complications are the most common emergencies seen in children with cancer. Neutropenia occurs due to disease and as a consequence of treatment with chemotherapy and/or radiation. Neutropenia is defined as a neutrophil count lower than 0.5×10^9/L (500/mm^3) or less than 1×10^9/L and expected to decline below 0.5 soon. A fever is defined as a single temperature of 38.3°C (101.0°F) or higher, or a temperature of 38.0°C (100.4°F) or higher lasting over 1 hr.

Blood cultures and cultures from specific sites of infection must be sent. All patients should receive a broad-spectrum antipseudomonal drug such as ceftazidime. They also should receive vancomycin to cover resistant gram-positive organisms if any of the following is present: severe mucositis, catheter infection, current quinolone prophylaxis, hypotension, or known colonization with gram-positive organisms. Often, despite a comprehensive search, the cause is never found; however, it is essential to start antibiotics immediately upon noting neutropenic fever. Antibiotics should be continued until the absolute neutrophil count exceeds 0.5×10^9/L and the patient is afebrile.

It is important for the patient and all of his or her contacts to routinely wash their hands.

Dehydration is a serious risk and is very common in cancer patients (often overlooked) because of cachexia caused by the disease or its treatment. Common treatment-related causes include emesis, diarrhea, and mucositis.

Hemorrhagic cystitis: Some chemotherapeutic drugs have toxic metabolites that are excreted by the kidney and can cause severe bladder hemorrhage. A common example is acrolein, which is formed by the metabolism of cyclophosphamide and ifosfamide. Hydrating the patient before chemotherapy is important, because hemorrhagic cystitis is more common when urinary output is low. Low urinary output increases the concentration of acrolein in the urine and the duration that the bladder mucosa is exposed to it.

Krimsky WS, Behrens RJ, Kerkvliet GJ. Oncologic emergencies for the internist. *Cleveland clinic Journal of Medicine* 2002;69(3):209–222.

Schiff D, Batchelor T, Wen PV. Neurologic emergencies in cancer patients. *Neurol Clin* 1998;16:449–283.

35 Environmental Health Hazards

35.1 PEDIATRIC RADIATION INJURIES

Radiation exposure may be natural or environmental (man-made). Medical procedures account for the largest component of environmental radiation. Some imaging procedures listed in Table 35.1.

Unnecessary diagnostic radiation: Selecting the correct examination is the responsibility of the ordering physician and may involve consultation with the pediatric radiologist. CT does not detect as many abnormalities as MRI, but CT involves radiation. MRI detects the subtle changes of congenital or acquired anomalies much more easily. Therefore, it is appropriate except in an emergent situation to obtain an MRI within a reasonable time frame instead doing two tests (CT followed by an MRI).

All radiologic procedures carry a risk. The risk incurred must be balanced against the benefit to the patient from the information obtained. The risk factors from contrast media in pediatric population are similar to those in adults. Factors that increase the risk to the patient can be considered in three headings: 1 due to radiation, 2 due to contrast media, and 3 due to technique.

Whole body irradiation: A large single exposure of penetrating radiation can result in acute radiation syndrome. The signs and symptoms of this syndrome result from damage to major organ systems that have different levels of radiation sensitivity, modulated by the rate at which the radiation exposure occurred. For example 100 rads delivered in 1 min would be symptomatic. But 1 rad/day for 100 days would not be symptomatic.

The *hematopoietic syndrome* results from acute whole body doses above 200 rads. A prodromal phase consists of nausea and vomiting within the first 12 hr, with symptoms usually lasting up to 48 hr. A latent period of 2–3 wk during which patients may feel quite well follows. Although patients are asymptomatic, bone marrow impairment has occurred. The most obvious laboratory finding is lymphocyte depression. Maximal bone marrow depression occurs approximately

Table 35.1: Imaging modalities	
Modality	*Source*
Plain film	Radiation (X-ray)
Ultrasound	Sound beams
Computed tomography (CT)	Radiation (X-ray)
Magnetic resonance imaging (MRI)	Magnetic field
Nuclear medicine	Radiation (injected isotope)
Positron emission tomography (PET)	Radiation (injected isotope)

30 days after exposure, when hemorrhage and infection can be major problems. If the bone marrow was not completely eradicated, a recovery phase then ensues. This radiation effect is similar to what occurs when whole body irradiation (given as 1,200 rads in 2 treatments) is used to obliterate the bone marrow in children with leukemia before bone marrow transplantation.

The *gastrointestinal syndrome* occurs from acute whole body doses above 800 rads. Prompt onset of nausea, vomiting and diarrhea follows. There is a latent period of approximately one week followed by recurrence of gastrointestinal symptoms, sepsis, and electrolyte imbalance, which may result in death.

The *cardiovascular/central nervous system syndrome* predominates at dose levels over 3,000 rad. Nausea, vomiting, prostration, hypotension, ataxia, and convulsions are almost immediate. Death usually occurs promptly.

Treatment: For the hematopoietic and gastrointestinal syndromes, treatment is supportive, involving transfusions, fluids, antibiotics, and antiviral agents.

Localized irradiation: Localized exposure involves a small amount of tissue, the systemic manifestations may be less severe, and patients may survive even if local absorbed doses are very high. The hand is the most common site for accidental localized irradiation injuries, usually as a result of picking up or playing with lost radiation sources. The second most common accidental site is the thigh and buttocks, predominantly from placing unsuspected highly radioactive sources in the pockets. The effects of a thermal burn are present almost immediately and patients invariably what burned them. If patients present with burn-like symptoms but no known cause, radiation should be suspected.

The permeability of the radiation is an important factor in the outcome of local radiation injury. In cases of low-energy irradiation, recovery and skin grafting are possibilities, even after high absorbed skin doses. Gamma and X-rays penetrate substantially and cause progressive obliterative endarteritis that may result in necrosis and gangrene. A few symptoms occur in the first 12 hr unless the dose has been extremely high. Patients may complain of hypersensitivity, tingling, or pain. Erythema is similar to that seen with a first degree burn. If erythema is seen within the first 48 hr, ulceration probably will occur. The erythema may present, disappear, and return days or 1–3 wk later. Transepidermal injury is similar to a second degree thermal burn. Blister formation may occur at 1–2 wk with doses in the range of 10,000 rads.

Some tissues that may receive localized radiation exposure are relatively radiosensitive. Cataract formation may occur with single gamma ray exposures in the range of 200–600 rads. Such cataracts usually take from 2 mo to several years to develop. *Oligospermea* may take up to 2 mo to develop. Transient infertility in men may result from doses as low as 15 rads, and permanent sterility may occur in men at dose levels between 300 and 600 rads.

Treatment: Skin therapy is directed at prevention of infections. Treatment of localized injuries usually involves plastic surgery and grafting, if the radiation exposure was not very penetrating. The full expression of radiation injury often is not apparent for 1–2 yr, owing to slow arteriolar narrowing that can cause delayed necrosis. After penetrating radiation, amputation may be necessary because of obliterative changes in small vessels.

Radiation therapy: Radiation therapy uses high doses to kill malignant cells. The sensitivity of normal cells is quite close to that of malignant cells. In order to achieve significant cure rates serious complications (5–10%) are noted. Most regimens use about 50 Gy (5,000 rads) given in about 25 fractions over 5 wk. A treatment scheme that uses doses much more than 10% higher than this or uses this dose with significantly fewer fractions poses a high incidence of severe complications. Childhood cancer affects 70–160 per million children annually between the ages of 0 and 14 yr. More than 70% of children are long-term survivors. At times it is difficult to separate the results of chemotherapy, radiation, or combined chemotherapy radiation. The kinds of effects depend on the age at radiation (amount of growth remaining, pubertal status). Radiation therapy increases the risk of second cancers in a dose-dependent manner for non-genetic neoplasms. Second cancers may account for 6–10% of all cancers in children or adults. Among childhood cancer survivors there is a 3– to 6-fold risk of a second cancer. 12% of children treated for one neoplasm will develop a second malignancy by the age of 25 yr. Almost 70% of the second neoplasms are in the field of the original radiation. Second cancers may account for 6–10% of all cancers in children or adults. The exact complications depend on the location of the treatment field. In children, because of the location of many childhood tumors, the central nervous system (CNS) commonly in the treatment field suffers from complications. More than half of the children who received 2,000–6,000 rads suffer from cortical atrophy; 26% have white matter changes (leukoencephalopathy), and 8% have calcifications and some also develop mineralizing microangiopathy. Radiation induced changes in the brain are potentiated by methotrexate administered before, during, or after radiation therapy. The younger the child is at the time of irradiation, the greatest is the atrophy.

Cerebral necrosis is a serious complication of radiation-induced vascular disease, which is usually diagnosed 1–5 yr after irradiation but can occur up to a decade later. Brain necrosis occurs when radiation therapy schemes exceed 4,000 rads in 10 fractions, 5,000 rads in 20 fractions, or 6,000 rads in 30 fractions, or when individual fractions exceed 300 rads. Brain necrosis may be manifested by headache, increased intracranial pressure, seizures, sensory deficits, and psychotic changes.

Spinal cord irradiation may result in *radiation myelitis*, which may be either transient or permanent. Acute transient myelitis often appears 2–4 mo after radiation. Patients with myelitis usually present with *Lhermitte sign*, a sensation of a little electrical shocks in the arms and legs occurring with neck flexion or other movements that stretch the spinal cord. Reversal myelopathy usually occurs between 8 and 40 wk and does not necessarily progress to delayed necrosis.

Delayed myelopathy occurs after a mean latent period of 20 mo, but it can occur earlier if the total dose or dose per fraction is high. This usually is manifested by discontinuous deterioration, which is irreversible. In the cervical and thoracic regions, sensory dissociation develops, followed by spastic, and then flaccid paresis. In the lumbar cord, flaccid paresis is dominant. The mortality for high thoracic and cervical lesions reaches 70%, with death due to pneumonia and urinary tract infections.

Other specific effects: The effect on growth is most pronounced when children are younger than 6 yr or during their adolescent growth spurt. Scoliosis and hypoplasia of bones may occur if fractionated treatment schemes exceed 4,000 rads. Fractional doses > 2,500 rads can result in slipped capital femoral epiphyses. An increase in the incidence of benign osteochondromas also has been reported after irradiation in children. Chest wall irradiation of girls with 1,500–2,000 rads over 1 wk impairs breast development and fractionated doses of 3,000–4,000 rads cause fibrosis and atrophy of breast tissue.

Karki D B, Tuladhar AS, Ghimire RK. Risk factors and adverse reactions in radiologic and medical imaging procedures. In: Mathur GP, Mathur Sarla (eds). *Current Trends in Pediatrics*. Vol 2. Delhi: Academa Publishers, 2006; 61–66.

Slovis TL. Biologic effects of radiation on children. In: Kliegman RM, Behrman RE, Jenson HB, Stanton BF (eds). *Nelson Textbook of Pediatrics*. 18th edn. Vol 2. Philadelphia: Saunders, 2007; 2899–2906.

35.2 CHEMICAL POLLUTANTS

Children are at increased risk of exposure to more than 80,000 chemicals, most of which have been developed since World War II. Effects of selected chemical pollutants on infants and children are listed in Table 35.2.

Etzel RA, Balk SJ (eds). *Handbook of Environmental Health for Children*. 2nd edn. Elik Grove Village, IL, American Academy of Pediatrics, 2003.

Frumkin H (Ed). *Environmental Health: From Global to Local*. San Franscisco, John Wiley and Sons, 2005.

Landrigan PJ, Forman JA. Chemical pollutants. In: Kliegman RM, Behrman RE, Jenson HB, Stanton BF (eds). *Nelson Textbook of Pediatrics*. 18th edn. Vol 2. Philadelphia: Saunders, 2007; 2906–2909.

35.3 HEAVY METAL INTOXICATION

The main threats to humans from heavy metals are associated with exposure to lead, cadmium, mercury, and arsenic. The most common cause of heavy metal toxicity is lead.

Arsenic

Arsenic exposure can occur from contaminated food or water. *Arsine gas* is the most toxic form of arsenic. Occupational exposure may occur in industries such as glass manufacturing, pottery, electronic components, semiconductors, lasers, mining, smelting, and refining.

Table 35.2: Effects of selected chemical pollutants on infants and children	
Chemical Exposure	*Effect*
Diethylstilbestrol	Adenocarcinoma of the vagina after intrauterine exposure
Thalidomide	Phocomelia after intrauterine exposure
Trichloroethylene	Increased risk of leukemia after intrauterine exposure
Alcohol	Fetal alcohol syndrome after intrauterine exposure
Lead	Neurobehavioral toxicity from low dose exposure
Nitrosamine, vinyl chloride, ionizing radiation	Increased risk of cancer after intrauterine exposure
Organophosphate insecticide	Developmental neurotoxicity
Environmental tobacco smoke	Increased risk of sudden infant death syndrome and asthma

Clinical manifestations: 10 ppb is the lower limit of safety. Arsine gas after a latent period of 2–24 hr produces hemolysis along with malaise, headache, weakness, dyspnea, nausea, vomiting, abdominal pain, hepatomegaly, pallor, jaundice, hemoglobinuria, and renal failure. Acute ingestion of arsenic produces gastrointestinal toxicity within minutes to hours (manifested by nausea, vomiting, abdominal pain, and diarrhea), hemorrhagic gastroenteritis, hypovolemic shock, cardiovascular toxicity (QT interval prolongation, ventricular tachycardia, congestive cardiomyopathy, pulmonary edema, and cardiogenic shock), and acute neurologic toxicity (delirium, seizures, cerebral edema, encephalopathy, and coma). Lethal doses of arsenates are 5–50 mg/kg; lethal doses of arsenites are < 5 mg/kg.

Late sequelae include hematuria, acute tubular necrosis, encephalopathy, sensorimotor peripheral neuropathy, gastroenteritis, alopecia, oral ulceration, peripheral edema, pruritic macular rash, and desquamation.

Chronic exposure to low levels of arsenic usually is from environmental or occupational sources. Over the course of years, dermatologic lesions develop, including hyperpigmentation, hypopigmentation, hyperkeratosis (especially on the palms and soles), squamous and basal cell carcinoma, and *Bowen disease* (cutaneous squamous cell carcinoma in situ). Encephalopathy and peripheral neuropathy may be present. Hepatomegaly, hypersplenism, noncirrhotic portal fibrosis, and portal hypertension occur. *Blackfoot disease* is an obliterative arterial disease of the lower extremities associated with chronic arsenic exposure that has been described in Taiwan. Carcinogenicity of chronic arsenic exposure is reflected in increased rates of cancers of the skin, lung, liver, bladder, and kidney, and of angiosarcomas.

Diagnosis: The diagnosis of arsenic intoxication is based on characteristic clinical findings, a history of exposure, and elevated urinary arsenic levels, which confirm the exposure. Concentrations greater than 50 µg/L in a 24-hr urine collection are consistent with arsenic intoxication. Abdominal radiographs may demonstrate ingested radiopaque arsenic.

Mercury

After absorption, mercury is distributed to all tissues, particularly the CNS and kidneys. Mercury reacts with sulfhydryl, phosphoryl, carboxyl, and amide groups, resulting in disruption of enzymes, transport mechanisms, membranes and structural proteins. Widespread dysfunction or necrosis results in the multiorgan toxicity, which is the characteristic feature of mercury poisoning.

Clinical manifestations: Five syndromes have been described. **1.** *Acute inhalation of elemental mercury vapor* results in rapid onset of cough, dyspnea, chest pain, fever, chills, headaches, and visual disturbances and gastrointestinal findings including metallic taste, salivation, nausea, vomiting, and diarrhea. **2.** *Acute ingestion of inorganic mercury salts* can present in a few hours with corrosive gastroenteritis manifested by metallic taste, oropharyngeal burns, nausea, hematemesis, severe abdominal pain, hematochezia, acute tubular necrosis, cardiovascular collapse, and death. **3.** *Chronic inorganic mercury intoxication* produces the classic triad of tremor, neuropsychiatric disturbances, and gingivostomatitis. Renal dysfunction ranges from asymptomatic proteinuria to nephrotic syndrome. **4.** *Acrodynia, or pink disease* is a rare idiosyncratic hypersensitivity reaction to mercury that occurs predominantly in children exposed to mercurous powders. The symptom complex includes generalized pain, paresthesias, and an acral (hands, feet) rash that may spread to involve the face. It typically is red-pink, popular, pruritic, and painful; it may progress to desquamation and ulceration. **5.** *Methyl mercury intoxication* also is referred to as *Minamata disease* after widespread mercury poisoning that occurred at Minamata Bay in Japan in people who had ingested contaminated fish. Methyl mercury poisoning presents as delayed neurotoxicity after a latent period of weeks to months, characterized by ataxia; dysarthria; paresthesias; tremors; movement disorders; impairment of vision, hearing, smell, and taste, memory loss; progressive dementia; and death. Infants exposed in utero are the most severely affected, with low birth weight, microcephaly, profound developmental delay, cerebral palsy, deafness, blindness, and seizures.

Diagnosis: The diagnosis of mercury intoxication is based on characteristic clinical findings, a history of exposure, and elevation of whole blood or urine mercury levels, which confirms the exposure. Levels < 10 µg/L in whole blood and < 20 µg/L in a 24-hr urine collection are considered normal. Thin-layer and gas chromatographic techniques can be used to distinguish organic from inorganic mercury. Abdominal radiographs may demonstrate ingested radiopaque mercury. Early neurotoxicity may be detected with neuropsychiatric testing and nerve conduction studies, whereas severe CNS toxicity is apparent on CT or MRI scans.

Treatment of arsenic and mercury intoxication: The principles of management for arsenic and mercury intoxication include prompt removal from the source of poisoning, aggressive stabilization and supportive care, decontamination, and chelation therapy when appropriate.

Supportive care for patients exposed to *arsine gas* requires close monitoring for signs of hemolysis, including evaluation of the peripheral blood smear and urinalysis. Transfusion of packed red blood cells may be necessary, as well as administration of intravenous fluids, sodium bicarbonate, and mannitol to prevent renal failure secondary to the deposition of hemoglobin in the kidneys. After inhalation of *elemental mercury vapor*, patients require monitoring of respiratory status, which may include pulse oximetry, arterial blood gas analysis, and chest radiography. Supportive care includes administration of supplemental oxygen and, in severe cases, intubation and mechanical ventilation. *Acute ingestion of inorganic arsenic and mercury salts* results in hemorrhagic gastroenteritis, cardiovascular collapse, and multiorgan dysfunction. Fluid resuscitation, pressor agents, and transfusion of blood products may be required for management of cardiovascular instability. Severe respiratory distress, coma with loss of airway reflexes, intractable seizures, and respiratory paralysis are indications for intubation and mechanical ventilation. Renal function must be monitored for signs of renal failure and the need for hemodialysis.

Gastrointestinal decontamination: Whole bowel irrigation is used to remove any radiopaque material remaining in the gastrointestinal tract. Because of the corrosive effects of inorganic arsenic and mercury salts induce emesis is not recommended.

Chelation for acute arsenic and mercury poisoning is most effective when administered as soon as possible after the exposure. Chelation should be continued until 24-hr urinary arsenic or mercury levels return to normal (< 50 µg/L for arsenic and < 20 µg/L for mercury), the patient is symptom-free, or the remaining toxic effects are believed to be irreversible. Dimercaprol [2, 3-dimercaptopropanol or British antilewisite (BAL)], is the chelator of choice if a patient cannot tolerate oral therapy. BAL is available suspended in peanut oil and benzyl benzoate in 3 ml ampoules at a concentration of 100 mg/ml for deep intramuscular (IM) injection. For **arsenic poisoning,** the recommended regimen of BAL is 2.5 mg/kg IM q6hr for the first 2 days, 2.5 mg/kg IM q12 hr on the third day, then 2.5 mg/kg/day IM for 10 days. For severe arsenic poisoning, the dose of BAL is increased to 3 mg/kg IM q4 hr for 2 days, 3 mg/kg IM q6hr on day 3, then 3 mg/kg IM q12 hr for 10 days. The dose of BAL for **inorganic mercury poisoning** is 5 mg/kg IM on the first day, then 2.5 mg/kg IM q12–24 hr for 10 days. The BAL-heavy metal complex is excreted in the urine and bile. A period of 5 days between courses of chelation is recommended. Adverse effects of BAL include pain at the injection site, hypertension,

tachycardia, diaphoresis, nausea, vomiting, abdominal pain, a burning sensation in the oropharynx, and a feeling of constriction in the chest. BAL may cause hemolysis in glucose-6-phosphate dehydrogenase (G6PD)-deficient individuals. BAL is contraindicated for chelation of methyl mercury because BAL redistributes methyl mercury to the brain from the other tissue sites, resulting in increased neurotoxicity.

Succimer, also known as 2,3-dimercaptosuccinic acid (DMSA) is an orally administered water-soluble derivative of BAL. DMSA is available in 100 mg capsules. The recommended regimen of DMSA is 1,050 mg/m^2/24 hr (or 30 mg/kg 24 hr) orally in three divided doses for 5 days, then 700 mg/m^2/24 hr (or 20 mg/kg/24 hr) orally in two divided doses for 14 days. The DMSA-heavy metal complex is excreted in the urine and bile. A period of 2 wks between courses of chelation is recommended. Mild adverse effects include nausea, vomiting, diarrhea, loss of appetite, and transient elevations in liver enzyme levels. DMSA also may cause hemolysis in G6PD-deficient patients. D-penicillamine, an orally administered chelator is not recommended due to the potential for significant leucopenia. Therapeutic abortion may be considered in pregnant patients due to the teratogenic effect of mercury.

Lead

Blood lead levels as low as 5 µg/dL in children have been associated with a variety of neurocognitive deficits, including decreased intelligence, shortened attention span, and increased risk of asocial behavior. A blood lead level (BLL) of 10 µg/dl or greater indicates a need for risk management.

Clinical manifestations: Gastrointestinal symptoms include anorexia, abdominal pain, vomiting, and constipation, often occurring and reoccurring over a period of weeks. *Lead encephalopathy* is more likely to be observed in children with BLLs > 100 µg/dl. CNS symptoms are related to increasing cerebral edema and increased intracranial pressure. Chronic lead exposure also may *delay puberty.* At higher levels (> 100 µg/dl), renal tubular dysfunction is observed. Lead also may induce a reversible Fanconi syndrome. At high BLLs *red cell survival* is shortened and may contribute to a hemolytic anemia, though most cases of anemia in lead-poisoned children are due to other factors such as iron deficiency and hemoglobinopathies. Older patients may develop a peripheral neuropathy.

Treatment: Lead when present in bone is released only slowly and is difficult to remove even with chelating agents. The cognitive/behavioral effects from lead may be irreversible. The main effort in treating lead poisoning is to prevent it from occurring and to prevent further ingestion by already poisoned children. The drug treatment is available for children with more severe lead poisoning that enhances lead excretion.

1. Identification and elimination of environmental sources of lead exposure. During repairs, repeated washes of surfaces and the use of vacuum cleaners will help reduce exposure to lead containing dust.
2. Behavioral modification to reduce non-nutritive hand-to-mouth activity. Hand-washing is best limited to the period immediately before nutritive hand-to-mouth activity occurs.
3. Dietary counseling to ensure sufficient intake of the essential elements calcium and iron. Because there is competition between lead and essential minerals, it is essential to promote a healthy diet that is sufficient in calcium and iron. For children 1 yr of age and up a calcium intake of about 1 g per day is sufficient (roughly the calcium content of a quart of milk is 1,200 mg/qt). A multivitamin containing vitamin D may be prescribed for children who do not drink sufficient milk or who have inadequate sunlight exposure. Iron requirements also vary with age, ranging from 6 mg/day, for infants to 12 mg/day for adolescents. For children identified biochemically as being iron-deficient, therapeutic iron at a daily dose of 5–6 mg/kg for 3 mo is appropriate. Iron absorption is enhanced when ingested with ascorbic acid (citrus juices).
4. Drug treatment that enhances lead excretion. A child with a venous BLL ≥ 45 μg/dl should be treated with DMSA. Repeat chelation is indicated if the BLL rebounds to ≥ 45 μg/dl. Children with initial BLLs > 70 μg/dl are likely to require more than one course. A minimum of 3 days between courses is recommended to prevent treatment-related toxicities, especially in the kidney.

With successful intervention, BLLs decline, with the greatest fall in BLL occurring in the first 2 mo after therapy is initiated. Subsequently the rate of change in BLL declines slowly so that by 6–12 mo after identification, the BLL of the average child with moderate lead poisoning (BLL >20 μg/dL) will be 50% lower.

Kondo K. Congenital Minamata disease: Warnings from Japan's experience. *J Child Neurol* 2000; 15: 458–464.

Mahajan PV. Heavy metal intoxication. In: Kliegman RM, Behrman RE, Jenson HB, Stanton BF (eds). *Nelson Textbook of Pediatrics*. 18th edn. Vol 2. Philadelphia: Saunders, 2007; 2909–2913.

Markowitz M. Lead poisoning. In: Kliegman RM, Behrman RE, Jenson HB, Stanton BF (eds). *Nelson Textbook of Pediatrics*. 18th edn. Vol 2. Philadelphia: Saunders, 2007; 2913–2918.

McLellan F. Arsenic contamination affects millions in Bangladesh. *Lancet* 2002; 359: 1127.

35.4 TEAR GAS AND MEDICAL PROBLEMS

Tear gas has gained widespread popularity in recent years as a means of controlling civilian crowds, for riot control, during hostage and siege situations and subduing barricaded criminals in several countries including India. It is used to help control individuals or groups without the need for lethal force. Three chemicals have been used worldwide as tear gas agents, including chloroacetophenone (CN), dibenzo-xazepine (CR), and chlorobenzylidene malononitrile (CS).

Clinical manifestations: The onset of symptoms occurs within 20 to 60 seconds, and if the exposed individual is placed in fresh air these findings generally cease in 10 to 30 minutes. Most organ systems of the body are affected; the eye being the most commonly affected organ causing epiphora, blepharospasm, a burning sensation, and visual problems even temporary blindness. Irritation of the mucus membranes of the nose, trachea, or lungs has been reported causing coughing, increased salivation, severe headaches, shortness of breath, tightness of chest, dizziness with induction of vomiting and possibly diarrhea. People coming in close contact with exploding tear gas fragments have been known to sustain traumatic penetrating injuries and blistering skin burns. Persons with pre-existing lung disease such as asthma or emphysema should be observed for exacerbation of their condition.

Treatment: Management is conservative, beginning with aeration and disposal of all contaminated clothing in plastic bags. Skin should be washed; although contact with water can briefly exacerbate skin symptoms from CS exposure, and a mild alkaline solution (6% sodium bicarbonate, 3% sodium carbonate, and 1% bezalkonium chloride) has been recommended. Persistent eye irritation can be relieved with application of a local anesthetic preparation and a patch. Contact dermatitis may respond to corticosteroid creams and antipruritics. Patients who present with signs of pulmonary edema should be kept under close observation and treated with humidified oxygen, bronchodilators and ventilator therapy as necessary. Prophylactic antibiotics have been suggested. Thiocyanate assay should be considered in cases of ingestion or extremely high exposure.

Based on the current knowledge, if CS tear gas is used by properly trained law enforcement officers and exposed combatants leave the area rapidly, few, if any, significant or long-term human disabling effects should occur.

Bennett PN, Brown MJ (eds). Incapacitating agents. In: *Clinical pharmacology.* 9th edn. Edinburgh: Churchill Livingstone, 2003; 162–163.

Fraunfelder FT. Is CS gas dangerous? *BMJ* 2000; 320:458–459.

Mathur GP, Mathur Sumit, Mathur Sarla. The use of tear gas and medical problems. In: Mathur GP, Mathur Sarla (eds). *Current Trends in Pediatrics.* Vol 3. Delhi: Academa Publishers, 2007; 462–463.

Yih JP. CS gas injury to the eye. *BMJ* 1995; 311:276.

35.5 BIOLOGIC AND CHEMICAL TERRORISM

Biologic and chemical agents used by terrorists are listed in Tables 35.3 to 35.5. Each potential agent of terrorism although produces its own unique clinical manifestations, it is useful to consider their effects in terms of a limited number of distinct clinical syndromes (Table 35.3). This will help clinicians to make prompt, rational decisions regarding empirical therapy.

Cieslak TJ, Henretig FM. Biologic and chemical terrorism. In: Kliegman RM, Behrman RE, Jenson HB, Stanton BF (eds). *Nelson Textbook of Pediatrics.* 18th edn. Vol 2. Philadelphia: Saunders, 2007; 2921–2927.

Markenson D, Reynolds S. American Academy of Pediatrics Committee on Pediatric Emergency Medicine, Task Force on Terrorism: The Pediatrician and disaster preparedness. Pediatrics 2006; 117:340–362.

Patt HA, Feigin RD. Diagnosis and management of suspected cases of bioterrorism: A pediatric perspective. Pediatrics 2002; 109: 685–692.

35.6 NONBACTERIAL FOOD POISONING

Mushroom Poisoning

Poisoning by species of *Amanita* and *Galerina* account for 95% of the fatalities due to mushroom intoxication. *Amanita* poisoning causes cellular necrosis of the gastrointestinal tract, acute yellow atrophy of liver and necrosis of the proximal renal tubules.

The clinical course produced by poisoning with *Amanita* or *Galerina* species is biphasic; after an initial 6–12 hr asymptomatic latent period. Nausea, vomiting, and severe abdominal pain ensue 6–24 hr after ingestion. Profuse watery diarrhea follows shortly thereafter and may last for 12–24 hr. During this time, as much as 9 L of fluid may be lost. From 24–48 hr after poisoning, jaundice, elevated transaminase levels (peaking at 72–96 hr), renal failure and coma occur. Death occurs 4–7 days after the ingestion. A prothrombin time less than 10% of control is a poor prognostic factor.

Treatment: Oral activated charcoal and lactulose combined with fluid and electrolyte replacement is administered as part of initial treatment. Forced diuresis should be avoided, because this increases renal exposure. Intravenous penicillin G (250 mg/kg/24 hr) administered as a continuous infusion combined with silibinin (intravenous dose of 20–50 mg/kg/24 hr) acts synergistically to inhibit binding of both toxins and to interrupt enterohepatic recirculation of amanito-toxin. Hemodialysis and hemoperfusion are also recommended as part of the initial treatment for intoxicated children. Orthotopic liver transplantation is recommended for children in whom severe hepatic failure develops.

Solanine Poisoning

Solanine is a mixture of several toxins found in "greened" or sprouted potatoes. Solanine alkaloids bind to serum cholinesterase. Clinical manifestations of solanine intoxication occur within 7–19 hr after ingestion. Common symptoms are vomiting and diarrhea, and in more severe instances of poisoning, fever, abdominal pain, coma and hypovolemic shock occur. Treatment of solanine poisoning is supportive. In the most severe cases, symptoms resolve within 11 days.

Seafood Poisoning

Seafood Poisoning is caused by i. *Ciguatera fish poisoning* (ciguatera, dolphin, eel, kingfish, and salmon); ii. *Scombroid (Pseudoallergic) fish poisoning* (tuna, bonita, and kingfish and nonscombroid fish and marine mammals, such as dolphin and blue fish); iii. *Paralytic shellfish poisoning* (mussels, scallops, clams, crustacean and fish); iv. *Diarrhetic shellfish poisoning* (mussels, cockles, and other shellfish containing okadaic acid); v. Azaspiracid poisoning: (contaminated shellfish, especially mussels).

Hughes JM, Potter ME. Scombroid fish poisoning: From pathogenesis toff SC. Nonbacterial food poisoning. In: Behrman RE, Kliegman RM, Jenson HB (eds) *Nelson Textbook of Pediatrics.* 17th edn. Philadelphia: Saunders, 2004; 2375–2378.

Whittle K, Gallachter S. Marine toxins. *BMJ* 2000; 56:236.

Table 35.3: Diseases caused by agents of chemical and biologic terrorism, classified by syndromes

	Neuromuscular symptoms prominent	*Respiratory symptoms prominent*	*Dermatologic findings prominent*
Sudden onset	Nerve agents	Chlorine; Phosgene; Cyanide	Mustard; Lewisite
Delayed onset	Botulism	Anthrax; Plague; Tularemia	Smallpox

Table 35.4: Critical biologic agents of terrorism

Disease	Initial Treatment	Prophylaxis
Anthrax (inhalational)* Incubation period- 1–5 days Isolation precautions:Standard Clinical findings:Febrile prodrome with rapid progression to mediastinal lymphadenitis and mediastinitis, sepsis, shock, meningitis	Ciprofloxacin[1] 10–15 mg/kg IV q 12 hr OR Doxycycline 2.2 mg/kg IV q 12 hr AND Clindamycin[2] 10–15 mg/kg IV q8 hr AND Penicillin G[3] 400–600 K U/kg/day IV divided q 4 hr	Ciprofloxacin 10–15 mg/kg PO q12 hr OR Doxycycline 2.2 mg/kg PO q12 hr
Plague (pneumonia) Incubation period: 2–3 days Isolation precautions: Droplet (for first 3 days of therapy) Clinical findings: Febrile prodrome with rapid progression to fulminant pneumonia, hemoptysis, sepsis, DIC	Gentamicin 2.5 mg/kg IV q 8 hr OR Doxycycline 2.2 mg/kg IV q 12 hr OR Ciprofloxacin 15 mg/kg IV q12 hr	Doxycycline 2.2 mg/kg PO q12 hr OR Ciprofloxacin 20 mg/kg PO q12 hr
Tularemia Incubation period: 2–10 days Isolation precautions: Standard Clinical findings: Pneumonic: Abrupt onset of fever with fulminant pneumonia Typhoidal fever, malaise, abdominal pain	Same as for plague	Same as for plague
Smallpox Incubation period: 7–17 days Isolation precautions: Airborne (+contact) Clinical findings: Febrile prodrome with synchronous, centrifugal, vesicopustular exanthema	Supportive care	Vaccination may be effective if given within the first several days after exposure
Botulism Incubation period: 1–5 days Isolation precautions: Standard Clinical findings: Afebrile descending symmetrical flaccid paralysis with cranial nerve palsies	Supportive care; antitoxin may halt the progression of symptoms but is unlikely to reverse them	None
Viral hemorrhagic fevers Incubation period: 4–21 days Isolation precautions: Contact (consider airborne in cases of massive hemorrhage) Clinical findings: Febrile prodrome with rapid progression in shock, purpura, and bleeding diatheses	Supportive care; ribavirin may be beneficial in select cases	None

*In a mass casualty setting where resources are severely constrained, it may be necessary to substitute oral therapy for the preferred parenteral option.
[1]Levofloxacin or ofloxacin may be acceptable alternatives to ciprofloxacin.
[2]Rifampin or clarithromycin may be acceptable alternative to clindamycin as drugs that target bacterial protein synthesis if ciprofloxacin or another quinolone is employed, doxycycline may be used as a second agent, because it also targets protein synthesis.
[3]Ampicillin, imipenem, meropenem or chloremphenicol may be acceptable alternative to penicillin as drugs with good central nervous system penetration.
DIC, disseminated intravascular coagulation.

Table 35.5: Critical chemical agents of terrorism

Agent	*Contamination**	*Management*
Nerve agents (Tabuin, Sarin, Soman, VX) Toxicity: Anticholinesterase: muscarinic, nicotinic CNS effects Onset: Seconds: Vapor; Minutes-hours: Liquids Clinical findings: Vapor: miosis, rhinorrhea, dyspnea Liquid: Diaphoresis, vomiting Both: Coma, paralysis, seizures, apnea	Vapor: Fresh air, remove clothes, wash hair Liquid: Remove clothes; wash skin, hair with copious soap and water; ocular irrigation	ABCs [1]Atropine: 0.05 mg/kg IV, IM (min 0.1 mg, max 5 mg), repeat q2–5 min pm for marked secretions, bronchospasm [2]Pralidoxime: 25 mg/kg IV, IM (max 1g IV; 2 g IM), may repeat within 30–60 min pm, then again q1hr for one or two doses pm for persistent weakness, high atropine requirement Diazepam: 0.3 mg/kg (max 10 mg) IV; lorazepam: 0.1 mg/kg IV, IM (max 4 mg); midazolam: 0.2 mg/kg (max 10 mg) IM pm for seizures or severe exposure
Vesicant-Mustard Toxicity: Alkylation Onset: Hours Clinical findings: Skin: Erythema, vesicles Eye: Inflammation Respiratory tract: Inflammation	Skin: soap and water Eyes: water (effective only if done within minutes of exposure)	Symptomatic care
Vesicant-Lewisite Toxicity: Arsenical Onset: Immediate pain	Skin: soap and water Eyes: water (effective only if done within minutes of exposure)	Possibly BAL 3 mg/kg IM q4–6hr for systemic effects of Lewisite in severe cases
Pulmonary agents (Chlorine; Phosgene) Toxicity: Liberate Hcl, alkylation Onset: Minutes: Eyes, nose, throat irritation; bronchospasm; Hours: Pulmonary edema Clinical findings: Eyes, nose, throat irritation (especially chlorine) Respiratory: Bronchospasm, pulmonary edema (especially phosgene)	Fresh air Skin: water	Symptomatic care
Cyanide Toxicity: Cytochrome oxidase inhibition: Cellular anoxia, lactic acidosis Onset: Seconds Clinical findings: Tachypnea, coma, seizures, apnea	Fresh air Skin: Soap and water	ABCs, 100% oxygen Na bicarbonate pm metabolic acidosis Na nitrate 3%; Dose (ml/kg) / Estimated Hgb (g/dl) 0.27 — 10 0.33 — 12 0.39 — 14 (max 10 ml) Na thiosulfate (25%): 1.65 ml/kg (max 50 ml)

*Decontamination, especially for patients with significant nerve agent or vesicant exposure.

[1]Atropine might have some benefit via endotracheal tube or inhalation, as might aerosolized ipratropium.

[2]Pralidoxime is reconstituted to 50 mg/ml (1 g in 20 ml water) for IV administration, and the total dose infused over 30 min, or may be given by continuous infusion (loading dose 25 mg/kg over 30 min, then 10 mg/kg/hr). For IM use it might be diluted to a concentration of 300 mg/ml (1 g added to 3 ml of water).

From Henreting FH, Cieslak TJ, Eitzen EM. Biological and chemical terrorism. *J Pediatr* 2002;14:311–326.

ABCs, airway, breathing and circulatory support; BAL, British antilewisite; CNS, central nervous system; HCl, hydrochloric acid; Hgb, hemoglobin concentration; max, maximum; min, minimum; pm, as needed.

35.7 ANIMAL AND HUMAN BITES

Dog, cats, rats and other rodents (rabbit, squirrel), and human bites are responsible for injuries. Dog bite-related injuries can be divided into three, almost equal categories: abrasions puncture wounds and lacerations, with or without an associated avulsion of tissue. Dog bites may be crush injuries. The most common type of injury from cat and rat bites is a puncture wounds. Human bite injuries are of two types: an occlusion injury that is incurred when the upper and lower teeth come together on a body part and, in older children and young adults, a clenched-fist injury that occurs when the injured fist, usually on the dominant hand, comes in contact with the tooth of another individual. In adolescents, fist-to-mouth (tooth) injuries are associated with fights. Preschool- and early school-aged children appear to be at greatest risk of sustaining from a bite by a human. Reduction of human bite injuries, particularly in day care centers and schools, can be achieved by a good surveillance of the children and adequate supervisory personal-to-child ratios.

Diagnosis: The diagnosis is based on history and physical examination of the bite victim. Careful attention should be paid to the circumstances surrounding the bite (e.g. type of animal, domestic or sylvatic, provoked or unprovoked, location of the attack); a history of drug allergies; and the immunization status of the child (tetanus) and animal (rabies). During physical examination, attention should be paid to the type, size, and depth of the injury; the presence of foreign material in the wound; the status of underlying structures; and in instances where the bite is on an extremity, the range of motion of the affected area. A diagram of the injury (s) should be recorded in the patient's medical record. A radiograph of the affected part should be obtained if there is likelihood that a bone or joint could have been penetrated or fractured or if foreign material is present. The possibility of a fracture or penetrating injury of the skull should be considered in individuals, particularly infants, who have sustained dog bite injuries to the face and head.

Complications: Infection is the most common complication of bite injuries, regardless of the species of biting animal. It is prudent to obtain material for culture from all animal bite wounds that are not brought to medical attention within 8 hr, regardless of species of the biting animal. All *human bite* wounds, regardless of the mechanism of injury, should be regarded as carrying high risk for infection and cultured. Because of the large incidence of anaerobic infection after bite wounds, it is important to obtain material for anaerobic and aerobic cultures.

Treatment: After the appropriate material has been obtained for culture, the wound should be anesthetized, cleaned, and vigorously irrigated with copious amounts of normal saline. Irrigation with antibiotic-containing solutions provides no advantage over irrigation with saline alone and may cause local irritation of the tissues. Puncture wounds should be thoroughly cleansed and gently irrigated with a catheter or blunt-tipped needle; high pressure irrigation should not be employed. Avulsed or devitalized tissue should be debrided and any fluctuant areas incised and drained.

There is general consensus that antibiotics should be administered to all victims of human bites and all but the most trivial of dog, cat, and rat bite injuries, regardless of whether there is evidence of infection. The bacteriology of bite wound infections is primarily a reflection of the oral flora of the biting animal and, to a lesser extent, a reflection of the skin flora of the victim. Because each of the multitudes of aerobic and anaerobic bacterial species that colonize the oral cavity of the biting animal has the potential to invade local tissue, multiply, and cause tissue destruction, most bite wound infections are polymicrobial.

The choice between an oral and parenteral antimicrobial agent should be based on the severity of the wound, the presence and degree of overt infection, signs of systemic toxicity, and the patient's immune status. Amoxicillin-clavulanate is the drug of choice for empirical oral therapy for human and animal bite wounds because of its activity against most of the strains of bacteria that have been isolated from infected bite injuries. Similarly, ticarcillin-clavulanate or ampicillin and sulbactam are preferred for patients who require empirical parenteral therapy. Azithromycin may be considered the therapeutic alternative for penicillin-allergic patients, because it has activity against aerobic and anaerobic bacteria that are present in infected bite wounds. Procaine penicillin remains the drug of choice for prophylaxis and treatment of rat-inflicted injuries. Tetracycline is the drug of choice for penicillin-allergic patients who have sustained rat bite injuries.

It is important to obtain an immunization history and to provide tetanus toxoid (TT) to all patients who are incompletely immunized or those in whom it has been longer than 10 yr since their last immunization. The need for postexposure rabies vaccine in victims of dog and cat bites on whether the biting animal is known to have been vaccinated. Postexposure prophylaxis for hepatitis B should be considered in rare instances in which an individual who is at high risk for hepatitis B. All but the most trivial bite wounds of the hand should be immobilized in position of function for 3–5 days, and patients with bite wounds of an extremity should be instructed to keep the affected extremity elevated for 24–36 hr or until the edema has resolved. All bite wound victims should be revaluated within 24–36 hr after the injury.

Centers for Disease Control and Prevention: Nonfatal dog bite-related injuries treated in hospital emergency departments—United States, 2001. *MMWR* 2003; 52: 605.

Centers for Disease Control and Prevention: Dog bite-related fatalities—United States, 1995–1996. *MMWR* 1997; 46: 463–467.

Ginsburg CM. Animal and human bites. In: Kliegman RM, Behrman RE, Jenson HB, Stanton BF (eds). *Nelson Textbook of Pediatrics*. 18th edn. Vol 2. Philadelphia: Saunders, 2007; 2928–2932.

35.8 SNAKEBITES AND MANAGEMENT OF SNAKEBITE

Snakebite is one of the most ancient medical problems of mankind. Epidemiological studies have revealed that the highest mortality rates of bites in Philippines, Thailand, Burma, Sri Lanka, India and Nepal were by cobras, kraits and Russell's vipers (*see* Figs 35.1 to 35.3 in CD).

Venom properties: Snake venom is the most complex of biochemical composition of all the known venoms. It consists of multiple enzymes and non-enzymatic components. The lethal dose of the venom ranges from 0.06 gm in krait to 0.15 gm in Russell's viper. The constituents can be broadly divided into enzymes and non-enzymatic proteins. The common enzymes are *Proteinases*, hyaluronidase, phospholipase A, *cholinesterase*, and phosphatase, while the non-enzymatic components are hemorrhagins, neurotoxins and cardiotoxins. Single venom contains 5–15 enzymes and 3–12 non-enzymatic proteins and peptides. The clinical manifestations of venom is a collective effect of all its constituents and almost every organ system is affected, the most important actions being on the neuromuscular, cardiovascular, hematopoietic and renal systems.

Clinical manifestations: Not all patients bitten by venomous snake, even with fang marks, will develop features of envenoming. The bites of venomous species are often "dry", i.e. no venom is injected. The majority of the snakebites are by non-venomous species. Fear, particularly the fear of death, may produce adrenergic symptoms and may mimic neuroparalytic syndrome. Use of a tourniquet may lead to a swollen and gangrenous limb. Clinical manifestations depend on the snake species. Elapid bite manifests predominantly with neuroparalytic features and mild to moderate local signs. Neuroparalytic symptoms manifest as ptosis and external ophthalmoplegia that are first to

appear. Cardiotoxicity in the form of myocarditis, sudden cardiac death and arrhythmias has been observed in a few elapid victims.

Viper bite is predominantly manifested by bleeding with severe local signs and symptoms. Bleeding from gingival sulci is usually the earliest sign of systemic envenoming. Intravascular hemolysis leading to hemoglobinaemia and hemoglobinuria has been reported. Such patients develop progressive anemia and renal failure. Circulatory shock is frequent in viperidae envenomation. Renal failure is observed among patients bitten by Russell's viper and tropical rattlesnakes. Viperidae may produce neurotoxic manifestations but these are less severe than that of elapids.

Management: Snakebite is a medical emergency and survival of the victim depends much on the appropriate first aid measures and immediate transportation to the nearest health canter. Management of envenoming comprises first aid measures and hospital-based treatment with anti snake venom serum (ASVS) and supportive care.

First Aid

DO'S. First aid can be carried out by the person who is bitten or by others who happen to be nearby at the time of bite, using materials that are readily available and close at hand. The aim of first aid measures is 1 retardation of systemic absorption of venom; 2 control of distressing and dangerous early symptoms of envenoming; and 3 preserve life and prevent complications before patient can receive medical-care. The recommended first aid measures are:

1. Reassurances, as most of the victims are terrified and apprehensive. Immobilization of the bitten limb is the most important and effective first aid measure. This can be achieved by pressure immobilization method. Pressure immobilization involves wrapping the bitten limb from distal to proximal with a firm crepe bandage (or other material available) at sufficient pressure only to block lymphatic spread but not to impede circulation. Then a splint is applied. This method is recommended for bites by neurotoxic elapid snakes, including sea snakes, but should not be used for viper bites because of danger of increasing the local effects of the necrotic venom.
2. Immediate transportation of the victim to the nearest health centers where anti-snake venom serum (ASVS) is available.

Since species diagnosis can help in the decision regarding ASV therapy, *the snake should be carried along to the hospital if it has already been killed.* However, if the snake is still at large, one should not risk further bites and waste time by searching for it. Even snakes that appear to be dead should not be handled with bare hands but carried in a bag or dangling across a stick. In some species (e.g. Hemachatus hemachatus) severed head can inject venom by reflex action up to 1 hr.

DON'TS. Traditional practices that inflict further trauma are potentially harmful with no proven benefit, should be abandoned and strongly denounced. (a) Certain common practices that need to be avoided include incision, excision, cauterization and amputation of the bitten digit. (b) Suction of the wound can cause tissue necrosis. (c) Instillation of chemical compounds, herbs, cryotherapy and electric shock can potentiate local tissue necrosis. (d) The offending snake must not be provoked further by attempt to capture it. However, if the snake is already killed, the snake should be carried along with the patient to the treatment centre.

Management at the Health Centre

Rapid clinical assessment, resuscitation and immediate infusion of ASV with other supportive care are the key to survival of the victim and must be provided immediately on arrival of the patient.

A. *Immediate management:* Assessment of vital signs and appropriate resuscitation should be the first step in the management of a snakebite victim. An IV line should be immediately secured and ASV should be made available. Patient should then be evaluated for the presence of local or systemic signs or symptoms of envenoming. Even if there are no features of envenoming, then the patient should be admitted and observed for a minimum period of 24 hrs. During the period of observation, the patient should be monitored hourly for local swelling, ptosis, diploplia, respiratory rate and effort, gingival bleed, bleeding from other sites, pulse rate and rhythm, blood pressure, urine output, cola colored urine, level of consciousness and any other signs of envenoming. Certain clinical situations demands urgent resuscitation, e.g. presence of profound hypotension and shock, respiratory failure, sudden deterioration or rapid development of severe systemic envenomation following release of tourniquet, cardiac arrest, acute renal failure and sepsis.

B. *Anti-snake venom serum (ASVS) therapy is available in two forms. Monovalent ASVS:* If the biting species is known or can reliably be deduced, the appropriate monovalent anti-snake venom serum should be used. *Polyvalent ASVS:* It contains specific antibodies against snake venom of two or more snake species. Lyophilized polyvalent anti snake venom serum (enzyme refined) Haffkine contains equivalent of 10 ml of purified globulin; 1 ml of reconstituted

serum neutralises 0.5 mg of dried cobra venom, 0.45 mg of dried common krait venom, 0.6 mg of dried Russels viper venom, 0.45 mg of dried saw scaled viper venom—Vial 10 ml.

C. *Indications of ASVS therapy*

 i. *Systemic envenoming*
 1. Neurotoxicity: Bilateral ptosis, external opthalmoplegia, respiratory paralysis. Cardiovascular abnormalities: Hypotension, shock, arrhythmias, cardiac failure, pulmonary edema.
 2. Hemostatic abnormalities: Spontaneous systemic bleeding, incoagulable blood, prolonged clotting time, elevated FDPs, decreased fibrinogen-level, thrombocytopenia.
 3. Generalized rhabdomyolysis
 4. Other significant indications include: hemoconcentration, severe anemia, neutrophil leucocytosis, elevated serum enzymes such as creatine phosphokinase and aminotransferases, uremia, myoglobinuria, hemoglobinuria, methemoglobinuria, oliguria, hypoxaemia, acidosis and vomiting in the absence of history of ingesting-emetic-agents.
 ii. *Severe local envenoming*
 1. Local swelling involving more than half the bitten limb, in absence of application of arterial tourniquet
 2. Swelling after bite on digit, especially finger
 3. Rapid extension of swelling, within a few hours
 4. Development of enlarge tender lymph nodes draining the bitten limb.

D. *Time of administration:* Anti-snake venom should be given as soon as indicated. However, it is never too late to give it as long as signs of systemic envenoming persist (e.g. up to 2 days after a sea snakebite and many days or even weeks for prolonged defibrination following bites by Viperidae). In contrast, local effects of venom may not be reversed if antivenom is delayed by more than 1–2 hrs after the bite.

E. *Dose of ASVS:* The average dose requirement for the krait envenoming in various studies were reported to range from 90 to 430 ml. Since there could be recurrence of bleeding after initial clearance, it is advisable to repeat the dose of ASV when coagulation defect recurs.

F. *Routes of administration:* The intravenous route is the most effective and the preferred one for ASV administration by either intravenous 'push' injection or by continuous intravenous infusion. In the absence of adequate expertise to administer the intravenous

ASV, it may be given by deep intramuscular route, in the anterior and lateral aspects of thigh, followed by message to promote absorption. It should not be given in the gluteal region. Absorption from intramuscular site is very slow.

G. *Response to ASVS:* Neurotoxic signs respond slowly. Blood coagulability, however, is usually restored in 3 to 9 hr.

H. *Criteria for repeating the dose of ASVS:* i. Persistent or recurrence of blood incoagulability after 6 hrs or bleeding after 1 to 2 hrs; ii. Deteriorating neurotoxic or cardiovascular signs after 1 to 2 hrs.

I. *Reactions to ASVS:* Three types of reactions may complicate ASV administration:
   i. Early (anaphylactic) reactions;
   ii. Pyrogenic reactions;
   iii. Late reactions
   i. ***Early (anaphylactic) reactions:*** The reactions usually develop within 10–20 min (IV bolus) or 30 min-3 hrs (IV infusions) of starting the ASV. The symptoms are initially in the form of restlessness, cough, itching, nausea, vomiting, feeling of heat, tachycardia and later urticaria, generalized pruritis, fever, tachycardia, autonomic symptoms, hypotension, airflow obstruction, angio-edema predominate the picture. Early reactions respond readily to adrenaline given by an intra-muscular route (into the deltoid muscle or the upper lateral thigh) in an initial dose of 0.5 mg for adults, 0.01 mg/kg body weight for children at the first sign of reaction. The dose can be repeated every 5 to 10 minutes if the patient's condition does not respond. Anti-H1 anti-histaminics such as chlopheniramine maleate (adults 10 mg, children 0.2 mg/kg by intravenous injection over a few minutes) should be given followed by intravenous hydrocortisone (adults 100 mg, children 2 mg/kg body weight). The corticosteroid may prevent recurrent anaphylaxis.
   ii. ***Pyrogenic reactions:*** It results from contamination of the anti-venom by endotoxin like compounds. High fever develops 1–2 hrs after treatment and is associated with rigors, followed by vasodilatation and a fall in blood pressure. Febrile convulsions may occur in children. It is treated with hydrotherapy and antipyretic drugs such as paracetamol.
   iii. ***Late reactions.*** It develops 1 to 12 (mean 7) days after treatment. The higher the dose of anti-venom the higher the incidence of these reactions and the speed of their development. Symptoms include fever, urticaria, subcutaneous and peri-articular swelling, polyarthritis, lymphadeno-pathy, mononeuritis multiplex, albuminuria and rarely encephalopathy. This is an immune complex disease, which responds to anti-histaminics in mild cases while corticosteroids (prednisolone 5 mg four times a day for 5 days) would be required in severe cases.

J. *Supportive measures*
1. *Role of anti-cholinesterase in neurotoxic snakebite:* Intravenous neostigmine, 0.5 mg is given at half hourly interval for five injections. This is followed by repeating the same dose at increasing intervals of 2 to 12 hrs according to the state of neurological recovery. Each dose of neostigmine is preceded by an intravenous injection of 0.6 mg atropine sulfate to ensure a rise in the pulse rate by 20 beats per minute. Patients who are able to swallow tablets may be maintained on atropine 0.6 mg twice each day, neostigmine 15 mg four times each day. Neostigmine-atropine in the recommended dosage schedule has been found to be completely free from any untoward effect and is considered fully safe. The encouraging results with the treatment suggest this treatment should be employed as a routine supplementary treatment to anti-venom therapy in all cases of neurotoxic snakebite.
2. *Artificial ventilation:* Neuroparalytic effects are reversible but may take long time and venom bind to pre-synaptic receptor is not neutralized by ASV. Once there is loss of gag reflex, pooling of secretions and loss of cough reflexes artificial ventilation with endotracheal intubation or tracheostomy, using cuffed tubes, is needed. The patient can be ventilated manually with an anaesthetic or Ambu bag or, preferably, with a mechanical ventilator.
3. Once specific anti-venom has been given to neutralize venom pro-coagulants, usually coagulability and platelet function is restored. However, patients may still need fresh whole blood, fresh frozen plasma, cryoprecipitates containing fibrinogen, factor VIII, fibronectin, and some factors V and XIII or platelet concentrates.
4. Hypotension and shock should be treated by infusing a plasma expander, preferably fresh whole blood or, failing that, fresh frozen plasma.
5. Infection at the site of the bite should be prevented with penicillin or erythromycin. It is important to obtain an immunization history and to provide tetanus toxoid (TT) to all patients who are incompletely immunized or those in whom it has been longer than 10 yr since their last immunization.
6. Development of acute renal failure (ARF) is a serious and significant complication and majority of cases of ARF result from viperidae envenomation. Early administration of ASVS is vital therapeutic measure that may prevent development of ARF.

Bawaskar HS. Snake Venom and Anti Venoms: Critical supply issues. *J Assoc Phys India* 2004; 52: 11–13.

Kakrani AL. Rationale Antisnake Venom Therapy: Randomized Controlled Trail or Clinical Judgement. *J Assoc Phys India* 1999; 47(4): 367–368.

Sawai Y. Epidemiology of snakebite in South East Asia Region. *Proceedings of the Inter-country Consultative Meeting on Snakebite Management.* WHO/SEARO, New Delhi, 12–14 November 1981.

Sellahewa KH. Snakebite in Sri Lanka. *Proceedings of 4th All Nepal Medical Conference.* Birganj, 6–9 Jan 1999; P91–93.

Sharma SK, Chappuis F, Jha N, Bovier PA, Loutan L, and Koirala S. Impact of snakebites and determinants of fatal outcomes in southeastern Nepal. *Am J Trop Med Hyg* 2004 Aug; 71(2): 234–8.

Sharma SK, Khanal B, Pokhrel P, Khan A, Koirala S. Snakebite-reappraisal of the situation in Eastern Nepal. *Toxicon* 2003; 41: 285–289.

Sharma SK, Koirala S, Dahal G. Krait bites requiring high dose antivenom: a case report. *Southeast Asian J Trop Med Public Health* 2002 Mar; 33(1): 170–171.

Sharma SK. Snakes, Snakebites and Management of Snakebite. In: Mathur GP, Mathur Sarla (eds). *Current Trends in Pediatrics.* Vol 1. Delhi: Academa Publishers, 2005; 208–220.

Whitaker R (Ed). *Common Indian Snakes: A field guide.* New Delhi: Macmillan, 1978.

35.9 SCORPION STING ENVENOMATION IN CHILDREN

Scorpions have been around for a long time. Scorpions live on every continent except Antarctica and are found in almost every kind of habitat. Most scorpions live in deserts. Some live in rain forests. Others live in grassy prairies, and still others live only beneath the bark of palm trees. Of the 1,500 known scorpion species, only 25 have a sting potent enough to be considered potentially dangerous to humans. Of the 86 species of scorpions known from India, only two species Hottentotta tamulus (formerly, Mesobuthus tamulus), the common red scorpion, and Palamneus swammerdami, are potentially lethal.

Scorpion venom: Venom in general serves two purposes—to acquire food and for self-defense. Scorpion venin is species-specific complex mixtures of short neurotoxic proteins (31–64 amino acid sequences). The toxin acts by opening sodium channel at presynaptic nerve terminals and inhibiting calcium dependent potassium channels. After a sting the venom enters the circulation very rapidly, with a tissue distribution half life of 5–6 minutes and peak tissue concentration is reached in 37 minutes. The excretion half-life of scorpion toxin is approximately 30 minutes.

Clinical manifestations: Species differences, venom dose/weight relationship determine the toxicity and clinical picture. Changes in body temperature may increase the sensitivity of venom and influence the course of toxicity. In India, Israel, Brazil and Mexico cardiac manifestations are common; in Iran tissue necrosis and hemolysis; in South Africa and USA neurological features and in Trinidad acute pancreatitis dominate the clinical picture. Symptoms after scorpion sting progress to a maximal severity in about five hours and subside within a day or two (Box 35.1).

Pain: Screaming within seconds to minutes due to pain after the sting, children appear irritable, at times excitable. There is a little or no skin reaction at sting site. Whenever local pain was severe, there was often no further progression of symptoms. Older children report paresthesia near the sting site. Reappearance of pain during recovery carries good prognosis. Serotonin found in scorpion venom is thought to contribute to pain associated with scorpion sting.

Autonomic storm: Features of cholinergic stimulation merge imperceptibly into those of adrenergic stimulation. Vomiting, salivation, sweating, priapism and bradycardia are early diagnostic signs. Sweating and salivation persist for 6–13 hrs. Increased oral secretions and bronchorrhea in the early cholinergic phase can worsen respiratory compromise.

Tachycardia seen within 4 hrs persists for 24–72 hrs. Tachycardia, hypertension, myocardial dysfunction, pulmonary edema and shock are part of spectrum of a single process, viz. autonomic storm. Vomiting and palmoplantar sweating precede development of myocardial injury. Marked tachycardia, S3 gallop and ice-cold extremities are seen in these children.

Hypertension lasts for 4–8 hrs in many due to outpouring of catecholamines from adrenal stimulation; it is prolonged in some due to direct stimulation of sympathetic centers in medulla. Hypertensive stress on myocardium, direct myocyte toxicity and catecholamines induced injury contribute to rhythm disturbances and left ventricular (LV) failure in a significant proportion of children.

Hypotension and bradycardia can be encountered within 1–2 hrs of sting due to cholinergic stimulation; hypotension and tachycardia later (4–48 hr) indicate severe LV dysfunction. During recovery stage (48–72 hr) hypotension can be seen; but the extremities are warm with good volume pulse and child is otherwise well. This state, due to an exhausted catecholamine stores awaiting replenishment, requires no intervention with dopamine agonists.

Fluid loss due to vomiting, salivation and perspiration complicate the clinical course and hemodynamic abnormalities in many children.

Pulmonary edema may develop within 30 minutes to three hours after a sting due to myocardial dysfunction. Development of symptoms associated with pulmonary edema is variable but may be rapid. Tachypnea or intractable cough at admission could mean pulmonary edema in evolution. Close monitoring is indeed vital to detect and treat pulmonary edema. Children appear pale with cold, clammy skin and have tachycardia with elevated blood pressure, retractions, nasal flaring and grunting. Some children land into acute pulmonary edema while showing apparent signs of recovery. Death within 30 minutes in some of these children is due to ventricular arrhythmias. Non-cardiac pulmonary edema due to ARDS is commonly reported from Brazil (Tityus serrulatus scorpion).

CNS manifestations: Neurological manifestations are often observed in severe scorpion-envenomed patients and they correlated with poor outcome. Encephalopathy, seizures, hemiplegia and motor aphasia have been documented. MRI findings may suggest brain infarcts. The cause of the infarct may be hypotension, shock or depressed left ventricular function, all of which are frequent in severe poisoning by scorpion sting.

Differential diagnosis: Scorpion sting envenomation in children is mostly a clinical diagnosis and very rarely a differential diagnosis like methamphetamine poisoning is considered. However, in adults and in regions where scorpion sting is not so common, the following differential diagnosis may be considered: spider bite by Latrodectus mactans (black widow), overdoses of neuroleptics, anticholinergics or tricyclic antidepressants, organophosphate poisoning, tetanus, botulism, diphtheria, meningitis, encephalitis, neurotoxic snakebite, thyroid storm, carcinoid or pheochromocytoma.

Investigations: Mild envenomation may not require any investigation. But an electrocardiogram (ECG) and chest X-ray will be helpful in cases of myocarditis and pulmonary edema. Hyper-acute tented T waves,

---

Box 35.1: Useful clinical dictum—scorpion sting envenomation

- Any male child presenting with cold peripheries and priapism—suspect scorpion sting.
- Tachypnea is the earliest and reliable indicator for onset of pulmonary edema
- Profuse diaphoresis may cause hypovolemia and requires judicious correction.
- The time interval between the sting and administration of prazosin for autonomic storm determines the outcome.
- It is prudent to monitor all children with scorpion sting for a minimum of 24 hours.

---

bradycardia, first degree heart block, transient ventricular and atrial ectopics, sinus tachycardia with ST segments depression, left anterior hemi-block, bundle branch block and prolonged QTc interval may be noted. ECG changes in scorpion envenomation have resembled those seen in Brugada syndrome (Genetic disease with sodium channel gene abnormality and sudden cardiac arrest) with a peculiar pattern of pseudo-RBBB and persistent elevation of ST segment in V1–V3. Chest X-ray may show bilateral batwing, patchy or interstitial pulmonary edema. Cardiac enzymes (both cTnI and IL-8) are useful to forecast the fatal outcome in scorpion envenomation.

Management

First aid in scorpion: The victim should stay calm and bite site can be washed with clean water. The scorpion should not be touched, be it dead or alive.

Prazosin: The dose recommended for Prazosin (1 mg tablet) is 30 microgram/kg/dose. In case of vomiting, it can be administered through nasogastric tube. After giving prazosin, mother should be advised not to lift the child to prevent the effects of 'First dose phenomenon' due to prazosin. Oral hydration and milk feeds must be encouraged. If needed, intravenous maintenance fluids should be given to correct dehydration due to excessive sweating and vomiting. Prazosin can be given irrespective of blood pressure provided there is no hypovolemia. Blood pressure, pulse rate and respiration must be monitored every 30 minutes for 3 hrs, every hour for next 6 hrs and later every 4 hrs till improvement. Prazosin should be repeated in the same dose at the end of 3 hrs according to clinical response and later every 6 hrs till extremities are warm, dry and peripheral veins are visible easily. The time lapse between the sting and administration of prazosin for symptoms of autonomic storm determines the outcome fall in blood pressure. Children should not be lifted.

Treatment of pulmonary edema: In children with pulmonary edema with or without hypertension, management should be directed towards relieving after-load without compromising preload. The use of diuretics to minimize or reduce fluid overload seems a reasonable measure but only when renal water excretion is impaired. Otherwise, the best way to prevent fluid overload is to maintain an adequate cardiac output. Thus dobutamine support (5–15 mg/kg/min) with vasodilatation through sodium nitroprusside (0.3–5 mg/kg/min) or nitroglycerine (5 mg/min) infusate is preferred in this situation. Prazosin (30 microgram/kg/dose) is to be given one hour before termination of sodium nitroprusside

(SNP) drip. If SNP is not available, one can use isosorbide dinitrate 10 mg every 10 minutes sublingually as an emergency measure. Morphine, a standard therapy in pulmonary edema, should be avoided in scorpion sting, since narcotics worsen dysrrhythmias in these children. Occasionally, children with scorpion sting present with multi-organ failure. A systemic inflammatory response is presumably the cause; however, our knowledge on the pathogenesis of such a state is still incomplete. Presence of respiratory failure with or without CNS disturbances in the presence of hypertension or complicating those children with pulmonary edema should be aggressively treated with early ventilation, afterload reduction, careful sedation and acid-base correction.

Scorpion antivenom: Clinical evidence of its efficacy is lacking. Prazosin needs to be the standard therapy especially in resource restricted settings.

Prognosis: Cardiac dysfunction and pulmonary edema are the leading causes of death related to scorpion envenomation.

Bawaskar HS, Bawaskar PH. Indian red scorpion envenoming. *Indian J Pediatr* 1998;65:383–91.

Karnad DR, Deo AM, Apte N, et al. Captopril for correcting diuretic induced hypotension in pulmonary oedema after scorpion sting. *BMJ* 1989;298:1430–31.

Mahadevan S. Scorpion sting. Indian Pediatr 2000;27:504–14.

Narayanan P, Mahadevan S, Tiroumourougane Serane V. Nitroglycerine in Scorpion Sting with decompensated shock. *Ind Pediatr* 2006;43:613–17.

35.9 DISASTER MANAGEMENT

A disaster can be defined as "any occurrence that cause damage, ecological disruption, loss of human life or deterioration of health and health services on a scale sufficient to warrant an extraordinary response from outside the affected community or area".

Disasters are not confined to a particular part of the world; they can occur any where and at any time. Disasters can be natural such as earthquakes, cyclones, floods, land-slides, building collapse, volcanic eruptions, hurricanes, heat wave, snow-storms, severe air pollution (smog), famines, epidemics or man-made such as fire, mass transportation accidents, civil war, terrorist acts, toxins, chemical gas leaks, radiation leaks, etc. A disaster can be short lasting or may be slow and ongoing type like a civil war, famine, etc. A disaster may be followed by epidemics and malnutrition among the population, especially in children.

Extent of damage in disasters includes physical injury to people and loss of lives, damage to property, destruction of infrastructure of a locality (electricity,

---

Box 35.2: Ten key areas of medical preparedness and mass casualty management

1. Provision of Mobile hospitals at strategic locations earmarked by states/districts for on-site treatment of large number of casualties.
2. Development of Integrated Ambulance Network (IAN) of Ambulances, heli-ambulances, Accident Relief Medical Vans (ARMVs) of Railways, and boat/ship ambulances with inter-district evacuation services as a part of evacuation plan.
3. Development of new Research and Development models by adoption of global best practices after testing in the indigenous conditions.
4. Development of strategy to be adopted to integrate private health care sector for medical management of mass casualty events.
5. Development of specialized facilities like trauma centers, blood banks, poison information centers, burn centers, Biosafety laboratories, network of diagnostic, public health and DNA identification laboratories and mortuary facilities at all levels.
6. Preventive measures including strengthening of Integrated Disease Surveillance Programme, Epidemic control programmes, immunization, HIV control, etc. will be undertaken.
7. Development of provisions for emergency medical response at incident site and availability of trained Medical First Responders/Quick Response Medical Teams for triage, resuscitation and treatment at the incident site within golden hour.
8. Development of hospital disaster management plans at various levels with provisions for crisis expansion of beds, medical logistics including life saving drugs and equipment.
9. Development of specialized facilities including adequate personal protective gears, detection equipment, documentation facilities, decorporation agents, antidotes, essential medicine and specialized teams from NDRF and SDRFs.
10. Provide psycho-social support and mental health services integrated with general health care services.

water supply, roads, transportation, communication systems, health-services), disruption of business activity and services.

On the whole, morbidity which results from a disaster situation can be classified into four types: injuries, emotional stress, epidemic of disease, and increase in indigenous diseases. Government of India has taken initiatives in disaster management. The Parliament enacted the Disaster Management Act, 2005 (DM Act, 2005) on 23rd December 2005. The National Disaster Management Authority, Government of India (www.ndma.gov.in) has released Key Areas of Medical Preparedness and Mass Casualty Management (Box 35.2).

Bhave Swati, Tiwari Mukul. Pediatrician and Disaster. In: Mathur GP, Mathur Sarla (eds). *Current Trends in Pediatrics.* Vol 2. Delhi: Academa Publishers, 2006; 1–4.

The Pediatrician's role in Disaster Preparedness. American Academy of Pediatrics. *Pediatrics* 1997; 99 (1): 130.

Veenma TG, Schroeder-Bruce K. The aftermath of violence: Children, disaster and posttraumatic stress disorder. *J Pediatr Health Care* 2002; 16(5):235–244.

WHO strategy and approaches to humanitarian action. *Coping with major emergencies.* Geneva: World Health Organization, 1995.

36 ◆ Poisoning: Drugs and Chemicals

36.1 INTRODUCTION

Children are more exposed to poisoning exposures. More than 50% occurs in children in 5 yr or younger. Almost all of these exposures are unintentional and reflect the propensity for children in this age group to put virtually anything in their mouths. More than 90% of toxic exposures in children occur in the home and most involve only a single substance. Ingestion (GIT) is the most common route of poisoning exposure (76% of cases), with the dermal, ocular, and inhalation routes each occurring in about 6% of cases. About 60% of cases involve nondrug products, most commonly cosmetics, cleansing substances, plants, foreign bodies, and hydrocarbons, particularly kerosene oil. Pharmaceutical preparations comprise the remainder, with analgesics, cough and cold products, antimicrobial agents, iron and vitamins. Poisoning exposures in children 6–12 yr of age are less common (4%). Toxic exposures in adolescents are primarily intentional (suicide or abuse) or occupational. Poison prevention education should be an integral part when parents visit hospital for ailments of their children or during immunization. Poison tips for children to stay safe from poison are listed in Box 36.1.

36.2 MANAGEMENT PLAN FOR POISONING AND OVERDOSE

History: Take an accurate history, which is of paramount importance if a poisoning has occurred or is suspected. The following information should be obtained during the initial assessment.

Description of toxins: Product names (brand, generic, or chemical) and ingredients, along with their concentrations may be obtained from labels. Several characteristic toxic syndromes are described in Table 36.1. These may assist in identifying the offending agent.

Magnitude of exposure: Determine how much of the substance has been ingested. This can often be accomplished by counting the number of tablets or measuring the volume of liquid remaining. Because the toxicity of most agents is dose related, knowing

---

Box 36.1: Poison tips for children

1. If you don't know what something is, do not put it in your mouth. Always ask a grown-up first.
2. Never take medicine unless a grown-up gives it to you.
3. Some plants and berries are poisonous. Always ask a grown-up before you put them in your mouth.
4. Always let grown-ups use spray cans and bottles. You should not touch or play with them.
5. Stay away from things used to clean your house, clothes or car.

Table 36.1: Toxic syndromes

Syndrome	Symptoms	Causes
Anticholinergic	Exocrine gland hyposecretion, thirst, flushed skin, mydriasis, hyperthermia, urinary retention, delirium, hallucinations, tachycardia, respiratory insufficiency	Belladonna alkaloids, jimsonweed, some mushrooms, antihistamines, tricyclic antidepressants, scopolamine
Cholinergic (muscarinic and nicotinic)	Exocrine gland hypersecretion, urination, nausea, vomiting, diarrhea, muscle fasciculations, miosis, weakness or paralysis, bronchospasm, tachycardia, or bradycardia, convulsions, coma	Organophosphate and carbamate insecticides, some mushrooms, tobacco, black widow spider bites (severe)
Extrapyramidal	Tremor, rigidity, opisthotonos, torticollis, dysphonia, oculogyric crisis	Phenothiazines, haloperidol, metoclopramide
Hypermetabolic	Fever, tachycardia, hyperpnea, restlessness, convulsions, metabolic acidosis	Salicylates, some phenols, triethyltine, chlorophenoxy herbicides
Narcotic	Central nervous system depression, hypothermia, hypotension, hypoventilation, miosis	All narcotics, propoxyphene, heroin
Sympathomimetic	Excitation, psychosis, seizures, hypertension, tachypnea, hyperthermia, mydriasis	Amphetamines, phencyclidine, cocaine, crack cocaine, phenylpropanolamine, methylphenidate, theophylline, caffeine
Withdrawal	Abdominal cramps, diarrhea, lacrimation, sweating, "goose flesh", yawning, tachycardia, restlessness, hallucinations	Cessation of alcohol, barbiturates, benzodiazepines, narcotics

the age or weight of the child aids in assessment. For inhalation, ocular, or dermal exposures, the concentration of the offending agent and the length of contact time with the material should be determined.

Time of exposure: For some products toxic manifestations may be delayed for hours or days. This may influence therapeutic intervention.

Progression of symptoms: Knowing the nature and progression of symptoms is helpful for assessing the need for immediate life support, the prognosis, and the type of intervention needed.

Medical history: Underlying diseases may make the child more susceptible to the effects of a toxin. Pregnancy is a common precipitating factor in adolescent suicide attempts and influences the treatment plan.

Initial medical care: If you think you got into a poison, tell a grown-up right away. The patient may be treated at home. Patient with life-threatening symptoms should be immediately brought to hospital for the appropriate medical care. All product containers thought to be related to the exposure should be collected and transported with the patient. If the patient has vomited, the emesis should also be brought to the emergency department for toxicologic analysis. Once the patient has arrived, initial attention should focus on life support, with primary emphasis on

cardiorespiratory care. Initial treatment of shock, dysrhythmias, and seizures should be started. Antidotes exist for only a few patients (*see* Chapter 40).

Preventing absorption: Prompt action to remove the toxin and minimize contact with the absorptive surface is essential and may prevent the development of major toxicity. Dermal and ocular decontamination can be accomplished by flushing the affected area with tepid water. A minimum of 10 min is recommended for ocular exposures, although some chemicals, particularly alkaline corrosives, may require much longer periods of flushing. For dermal exposures, mild soap and water can be used. For inhaled toxins decontamination is generally accomplished by moving the patient to fresh air, or if necessary administrating oxygen. Several procedures are used to prevent absorption of a toxin from the stomach and gastrointestinal tract, and each has limitations and risks. In general, most liquid drug products are almost completely absorbed within 30 minutes of ingestion and most solid dosage forms within 1–2 hr. Gastrointestinal decontamination beyond this time is unlikely to be of value.

Emesis: The emetic used is syrup of ipecac. The onset of emesis is usually 20–30 min after dosing with vomiting occurring in 90–95% of patients. Several episodes of vomiting usually occur over a period of

1–2 hr. The recommended dose is 10 ml for infants 6–12 mo of age, 15 ml for children age 1–12 yr, and 30 mL for older children and adults. Ipecac should not be used in infants younger than 6 mo. Ipecac administration is followed by at least 500 ml of water. The use of ipecac syrup has declined.

Gastric lavage: This technique involves placing a tube into the stomach to aspirate contents, followed by flushing with normal saline. Lavage is time consuming and under the best circumstances, removes only a fraction of gastric contents. It should only be used in older children and only in select situations.

Activated charcoal: Oral administration of activated charcoal is an effective means to decrease or prevent the intestinal absorption of a few drugs and toxins as well as enhance the elimination of drugs already absorbed and present within the systemic circulation. Many, but not all toxins, are adsorbed onto its surface, preventing absorption from the gastrointestinal tract. Some toxins, including heavy metals, iron, lithium, hydrocarbons, cyanide, and low molecular weight alcohols are not significantly bound to charcoal. The usual dose is 10–50 g ($\approx$ 1g/kg) for a child and 50–100 g for an adolescent or adult. Airway reflexes must be preserved or the airway protected by endotracheal intubation. Activated charcoal is commonly mixed as a slurry in water or a solution of sorbitol, a cathartic. A cathartic should be used only with the 1st charcoal dose to prevent major fluid loss and dehydration. Approximately 25% of patients receiving activated charcoal experience 1st episode of vomiting. Aspiration of activated charcoal into the lungs occurs occasionally. Aspiration of activated charcoal is not more serious than aspiration of gastric contents alone. If charcoal is given through a gastric tube, placement of the tube should be carefully confirmed before activated charcoal is given because instillation of charcoal directly into the lungs has disastrous effects.

Some toxicologists recommend the use of repeat-dose activated charcoal (a dose every 2–4 hr) for the hospitalized patients at a dose of approximately 0.25–0.50g/kg every 2–4 hr or hourly at a rate of approximately 0.25 g/kg for 24 hr as long as bowel sounds are present due to the risk of constipation or intestinal impaction. The benefit of oral activated charcoal in the treatment of severe poisoning is its effect of increasing the body (systemic) clearance of toxins already present within the body.

Cathartics: Cathartics are commonly used in conjunction with activated charcoal to hasten the clearance of the charcoal-toxin complex, although no evidence shows their value. Cathartics should not be administered with each dose of activated charcoal, but used as needed. Commonly used cathartics are sorbitol (maximum dose, 1 g/kg), magnesium sulfate (maximum dose, 250 mg/kg), and magnesium citrate (maximum dose, 250 ml/kg). In young children, cathartics should be used with caution because of the risk of dehydration and electrolyte imbalance.

Whole bowel irrigation: In whole bowel irrigation (WBI) large volumes of a polyethylene glycol electrolyte solution are instilled into the stomach to cleanse the entire gastrointestinal tract. This technique has been successfully used to remove slowly absorbed products such as iron or sustained-release preparations. Whole bowel irrigation can be combined with the use of activated charcoal, if appropriate. In young children, cathartics should be used with care because of the risk of dehydration and electrolyte imbalance.

Enhancing elimination: Enhancing excretion is useful for only a few toxins; not useful for drugs that are either highly protein bound or have a large volume of distribution. These techniques are invasive and also associated with risk.

Diuresis: Diuresis alone does not increase elimination, but increasing the pH of the urine with intravenously administered bicarbonate increases the elimination of weak acids, such as salicylates and phenobarbital.

Dialysis: Hemodialysis, and peritoneal dialysis have been used successfully to treat poisoning. Examples of toxins for which dialysis may be useful include methanol, ethylene glycol, and large symptomatic ingestions of salicylate, theophylline or lithium.

Hemoperfusion: Hemoperfusion is a dialytic technique in which blood is passed through a column of activated charcoal or resin. It has been used to treat large ingestion of salicylate, theophylline, and a few other selected agents. It is rarely used in children.

Laboratory evaluation: For some intoxications (e.g. salicylates, acetaminophen, iron, menthol, ethylene glycol) blood levels are integral part of the treatment plan. For other intoxicants (e.g. opioid, cyanide), qualitative measurements may assist in establishing a diagnosis but is not likely to change treatment.

36.3 ACETAMINOPHEN (PARACETAMOL)

Acetaminophen is the most widely used analgesic and antipyretic. Consequently, acetaminophen is commonly available in the home, where it can be unintentionally ingested by young children or taken in an intentional overdose by adolescents. Acetaminophen toxicity results from the formation of a highly reactive inter-mediate metabolite, Nacetyl-p-benzoquinoneimine (NAPQI).

Toxic dose: The toxic dose for children younger than 12 yr is more than 200 mg/kg and for adolescents and adults ii is more than 7.5 g as a single dose.

Clinical manifestations: Untreated patients who have acutely overdosed pass through four stages of toxicity (Table 36.2). Because early symptoms are nonspecific, physicians may fail to diagnose the ingestion without a good history or high index of suspicion.

Laboratory findings: If a toxic ingestion is suspected, a plasma acetaminophen level should be measured 4 hr or more after ingestion. Measurement earlier than 4 hr after ingestion may be useful to determine if ingestion has occurred, but cannot be used to determine the severity of an overdose. Liver function tests including bilirubin, prothrombin time; hepatic enzymes are elevated and should be followed daily to every other day in all patients with acetaminophen levels falling.

Treatment: When treatment started within 1–2 hr of the ingestion, activated charcoal administration should be considered. The antidote for acetaminophen poisoning is N-acetylcysteine (NAC) [Mucomix tablet 600 mg; inj. 200 mg/ml]. NAC serves as a precursor for glutathione synthesis, thus replenishing glutathione stores and preventing the reaction of NAPQI with hepatocytes. NAC therapy should be initiated as soon as possible after ingestion but may be useful even if started 24–36 hr after ingestion in severe cases. Intravenous doses are administered initially, 150 mg/kg in 200 ml of 5% glucose given IV over 15–30 minutes; maintenance, IV 50 mg/kg in 500 mL of 5% glucose given over 4 hr, followed by 100 mg/kg in 1 liter of 5% glucose given over 16 hr (total dose 300 mg/kg over 21 hr). With established hepatotoxicity, begin as above then continue giving 50 mg/kg in 500 ml of 5% glucose over 8 hr until prothrombin time and liver enzymes begin to return to normal. NAC is equally effective per oral route (140 mg/kg loading, followed by 70 mg/kg every 4 hr for 17 doses), but is unpalatable and irritating to the gastrointestinal tract and should be diluted with fruit juice or a 5% solution with soda to minimize vomiting. Antiemetics may be used to control vomiting. *Adverse drug* reactions include flushing, urticaria, itch, stomatitis, nausea, vomiting, fever, rhinorrhea, drowsiness, chest tightness, bronchoconstriction, diarrhea, anaphylactoid reactions and rashes. Severely affected patients may require liver transplantation.

36.4 SALICYLATES (INCLUDE ASPIRIN, SALICYLAMIDE, SODIUM SALICYLATE)

Salicylates directly or indirectly affect most organ systems by uncoupling oxidative phosphorylation, inhibiting Krebs cycle enzymes, and inhibiting aminoacid synthesis. Salicylates also decrease platelet adhesiveness and increase pulmonary capillary permeability.

Toxic dose: The acute toxic dose of salicylates is generally considered to be more than 150 mg/kg.

Clinical manifestations: The signs and symptoms simulate as flu or other febrile illness. Seriously poisoned patients are more than 5–10% dehydrated. CNS changes include agitation, restlessness, confusion, and coma, which may develop secondary to cerebral edema. Death results from pulmonary edema and respiratory failure, cerebral edema, hemorrhage, severe electrolyte imbalance or cardiovascular collapse.

Laboratory findings: Serum electrolyte levels should be obtained every 2–3 hr to evaluate for either continued absorption or impairment of excretion. Serum salicylate levels >20 mg/dl should be monitored and levels > 70 mg/dl may produce life-threatening effects.

Treatment: Initial treatment should include gastric decontamination with activated charcoal. Urine pH should be raised at least 7–7.5 using intravenous bicarbonate which will convert salicylate to the ionized form, which is then excreted in the urine. Each one-unit increase in urine pH increases urinary salicylate clearance 4-fold. Potassium should also be administered, because it is not possible to alkaline the urine without adequately replenishing tissue stores of potassium. Dialysis may be required in severe cases. Hemodialysis is preferred over peritoneal or charcoal or hemoperfusion.

Stage	Time after ingestion	Characteristics
		Table 36.2: Stages in the clinical course of acetaminophen toxicity
I	½ – 24 hr	Anorexia, nausea, vomiting, malaise, pallor, diaphoresis
II	24 – 48 hr	Resolution of above; right upper quadrant abdominal pain; elevated bilirubin, prothrombin time, hepatic enzymes; oliguria
III	72 – 96 hr	Peak liver function abnormalities; anorexia, nausea, vomiting, malaise may reappear
IV	4 days – 2 wk	Resolution of hepatic dysfunction or complete liver failure

36.5 IBUPROFEN

Ibuprofen and other nonsteroidal anti-inflammatory drugs (NSAIDs) are often involved in unintentional and intentional overdoses, because of their wide distribution and their common use as analgesics; in particular, ibuprofen is used as an antipyretic. Ibuprofen inhibits prostaglandin synthesis, and this disruption produces the side effects reported with therapeutic use such as gastrointestinal irritation, reduced renal blood flow and platelet dysfunction.

Toxic dose: In children, doses less than 100 mg/kg of ibuprofen do not produce toxicity, whereas doses greater than 400 mg/kg produce more serious effects, including seizures and coma.

Clinical manifestations: Symptoms usually develop within 4 hr of ingestion and resolve within 24 hr. Common effects include nausea, vomiting, epigastric pain, drowsiness, lethargy, and ataxia. Anion gap metabolic acidosis, coma, transient apnea, renal failure, hypotension, nystagmus, diplopia, headache, tinnitus, transient deafness, and seizures are rare.

Laboratory findings: Renal function studies and acid-base balance should be monitored after ingestion of large doses.

Treatment: Good supportive care is essential; activated charcoal can be administered.

36.6 ANTIDEPRESSANTS

The tricyclic antidepressants (TCAs) and the selective serotonin reuptake inhibitors (SSRIs) represent the two most common classes of antidepressants of toxicologic significance.

Tricyclic Antidepressants (TCAs)

These agents block the neuronal reuptake of norepinephrine, serotonin, and dopamine, in both the central and peripheral nervous systems. They also produce varying degrees of sedation, α-blocking, and anticholinergic effects. Inhibition of fast sodium channels in the myocardium leads to the development of cardiac dysrhythmias and myocardial depression.

Toxic dose: The potentially toxic dose of these agents in children ranges from 5 to 20 mg/kg.

Clinical manifestations: TCAs include amitriptyline, nortriptyline, and sinequan. The primary organ systems affected are the CNS and cardiovascular systems; symptoms can develop as early as 30 min after ingestion, with serious symptoms developing within 6 hr of ingestion. Drowsiness, lethargy, coma or seizures have been reported. Tachycardia is the most common cardiovascular effect. Hypertension may occur soon after ingestion. Hypotension is uncommon. Other cardiac findings include myocardial dysrhythmias and myocardial depression. Other reported effects include hypoventilation with respiratory arrest, hyperthermia, choreiform movements, agitation, twitching, mydriasis, disorientation, hallucinations, urinary retention, and diminished bowel sounds.

Laboratory findings: The electrocardiogram (ECG) should be closely monitored for QRS widening and QT and QTc prolongation. ECG changes may not be useful predictors of toxicity in younger children because of normal variation. Blood levels of TCAs are not helpful in assessing or predicting the severity of the exposure but may aid in establishing a diagnosis.

Treatment: After general life support measures are instituted, including endotracheal intubation if indicated, efforts should be made to prevent absorption. Activated charcoal should be administered. Sodium bicarbonate in doses sufficient to achieve a serum pH of 7.45–7.55 should be administered to treat and prevent dysrhythmias. Lidocaine is used to treat dysrhythmias that are unresponsive to serum alkalization. Hypotension may respond to standard fluid therapy, although vasopressors such as norepinephrine may be required. Severe, unresponsive hypotension is a poor prognostic sign. Hypertension usually is transient and does not require treatment. Seizures, if they require treatment, usually respond to benzodiazepine therapy

Asymptomatic children should be observed and the ECG monitored for at least 6 hr after exposure. If any manifestations of toxicity (e.g. increased QRS interval) conduction defects, altered mental status, hypotension, or hypoventilation) develop, continue monitoring in an intensive care unit for 24 hr. Only completely asymptomatic children should be discharged after 6 hr of observation.

Selective Serotonin Reuptake Inhibitors (SSRIs)

SSRI agents include fluoxetine, sertraline, paroxetine, and citalopram. These agents differ from TCAs in that they specifically inhibit reuptake of serotonin in the CNS. They have a little or no effect on norepinephrine or dopamine reuptake and minimal, if any anticholinergic or α-blocking effects.

Clinical manifestations: The toxic effects are mild. The usual onset of symptoms is within 3 hr, with resolution of symptoms within 24 hr in treated patients. Drowsiness or hyperactivity, agitation, and tachycardia are the most common reported effects. Nausea, vomiting, tremor, dizziness, abdominal pain, life-threatening effects (reported after very large ingestions, such as seizures and coma) and cardiac conduction defects are rare.

A *serotonin syndrome* has been reported after accidental over-dose of SSRIs as well as therapeutic use. It is an idiosyncratic reaction that includes confusion and disorientation, agitation, coma, hyperthermia, myoclonus, hyperreflexia, tremor, and muscle rigidity.

Treatment: Gastrointestinal decontamination with activated charcoal is preferred. There is no specific therapy other than supportive care.

36.7 CLONIDINE

Clonidine is used in attention deficit/hyperactivity disorder (ADHD) and tic syndromes in children, although it was first introduced for use as an antihypertensive agent. The toxic effects of clonidine are a result of α_2-adrenergic receptor inhibition in the CNS.

Toxic dose: Children are very sensitive to the toxic effects of clonidine, with as little as 0.1 mg reported to produce significant toxicity.

Clinical manifestations: In children symptoms frequently develop within 1 hr of ingestion, thus rapid recognition and intervention is essential. Lethargy, miosis, bradycardia, and hypotension occur in all age groups. Apnea, respiratory depression, coma are common findings in younger children. Serious symptoms usually resolve within 24 hr of ingestion.

Treatment: Immediate recognition of an exposure with transfer to a health care centre is of paramount importance. Aggressive supportive care is essential. The ECG, vital signs and blood gases are monitored as symptoms appear. Naloxone has been used to reverse CNS and respiratory depression. Because the duration of effect of naloxone is shorter than that of clonidine, administration by continuous infusion may be necessary.

36.8 CALCIUM CHANNEL BLOCKERS

Calcium channel blockers (CCBs) produce various effects on the myocardium and the systemic vasculature. Specific agents include nifedipine, diltiazem, verapamil, amlodipine, and felodipine. They are available as regular-release and sustained release preparations as well as in combination with diuretic and other antihypertensive agents.

Clinical manifestations: The onset of symptoms may occur within minutes of the ingestion of a regular release product or may be delayed several hours after the ingestion of a sustained-release product. Bradycardia and varying degrees of atrioventricular block are common. Hypotension develops secondary to dilation of vascular smooth muscle. Myocardial depression may lead to shock in severe cases. Nausea and vomiting are common. Confusion, agitation, or lethargy and possible coma may occur.

Laboratory findings: Blood pressure and ECG monitoring is essential. Hyperglycemia is also common, so serial serum glucose measurements should be followed.

Treatment: After appropriate supportive care has been instituted absorption should be prevented using activated charcoal if appropriate. Whole bowel irrigation should be considered if a sustained-release product has been ingested. Bradycardia and conduction disturbances are frequently unresponsive to atropine and often require the placement of a pacemaker. Hypotension may be treated with fluids and vasopressors. Because the duration of action of calcium salts is much shorter than that of CCBs, administration of calcium chloride by continuous infusion may be necessary. Hypercalcemia does not produce clinical effects. High-dose infusion of regular insulin and glucose therapy has demonstrated some effectiveness. Glucagon improves cardiac conduction and contractility by promoting calcium ion influx through calcium channels indirectly. Its efficacy in the treatment of CCB overdose is not consistent.

36.9 IRON

Iron is one of the most common causes of childhood poisoning death. Iron-containing products are common in many homes and often resemble candy. The potential severity of exposure is based on the amount of elemental iron ingested. The amount of elemental iron ingested is calculated on the basis of the number of tablets ingested and the percentage of iron in the salt. Ferrous sulfate contains 20%, ferrous gluconate 12% and ferrous fumarate 33% of elemental iron. Iron is corrosive to the gastrointestinal mucosa. It also accumulates in the mitochondria and tissues to produce cellular damage and systemic toxicity. Iron causes venodilation and increased capillary permeability leading to hypotension. Reduced peripheral perfusion and mitochondrial damage result in lactic acid and citric acid accumulation, and causing metabolic acidosis. Hepatic necrosis develops after serious poisoning, resulting in abnormal liver function tests and coagulopathies.

Toxic dose: The toxic dose is more than 60 mg/kg of elemental iron.

Clinical manifestations: Nausea, vomiting, diarrhea and abdominal pain usually develop within 30 min to 6 hr after ingestion. Hemetemasis and bloody diarrhea may develop in more serious poisonings. The gastrointestinal signs may subside over 6–12 hr, but systemic toxicity may ensue early hypotension or drowsiness. Gastric scarring and pyloric stenosis can develop 2–4 wk after a large ingestion or when iron tablets remain in prolonged contact with the gastrointestinal mucosa.

Laboratory findings: Iron levels should be obtained about 4 hr after ingestion. Serum iron levels less than 500 g/dl measured 4–8 hr after ingestion, indicate a low risk of toxicity. A level greater than 500 g/dl indicate significant toxicity is likely. Abdominal radiograph may confirm the ingestion because iron is radiopaque. Repeated radiographs may help with assessment of the efficacy of gastric decontamination methods. A negative result does not rule out iron ingestion because only undissolved tablets can be seen.

Treatment: Good supportive and symptomatic care is needed in cases of iron poisoning. Deferoxamine is a specific chelator of iron and is the antidote for moderate to severe iron intoxication. Indications for deferoxamine include a serum iron level greater than 500 µg/dL. Deferoxamine is administered in infusion of 15 mg/kg/hr (maximum 6 g/24 hr by IV route). Hypotension is minimized by avoiding rapid infusion rates. It should be administered as a continuous intravenous infusion, continued until a patient is symptom free. The deferoxamine-iron complex may color the urine reddish (vin rosé). Pyloric stenosis may be symptomatic and occasionally requires surgical intervention.

36.10 CAUSTICS

Caustics include acids and alkalies as well as a few common oxidizing agents such as bleach. Acids coagulate proteins, causing tissue necrosis, whereas alkalies digest and dissolve proteins, producing liquefaction necrosis with the risk of perforation if the injury is located in the intestinal tract. The severity of the chemical burn produced depends on the pH, the concentration of the agent and the duration of the contact.

Toxic dose: Agents with a pH 2 or above 12 are most likely to produce significant injury.

Clinical manifestations: Ingestion of caustic materials may produce oral burns, which are visualized as reddened areas or whitish plaques. Symptoms include pain, drooling, vomiting or difficulty or refusal to swallow. Circumferential burns of the esophagus may cause strictures on healing. Strong acids may produce scarring around the pylorus, leading to delayed onset

of gastric obstruction. Caustics on the skin or in the eye can cause severe tissue damage.

Treatment: Initial treatment of caustic exposure includes thorough removal of the product from the skin or eye by flushing with water. Contaminated clothing should be removed. Ingested agents should be rinsed from the oral cavity. Emesis and lavage are contraindicated; activated charcoal should not be used. Patients should be evaluated for evidence of esophageal burns and, if symptoms are present, oral fluids or solids should be withheld. Endoscopy should be performed in symptomatic patients or those in whom injury is highly suspected on the basis of history. Esophageal strictures may require repeated dilation or surgical correction. Prophylactic antibiotics do not improve outcomes.

36.11 METHANOL AND ETHYLENE GLYCOL

Menthol is commonly found in windshield washer fluids, fuel additives, liquid fluid canisters and industrial solvents. Ethylene glycol is commonly found in car radiator antifreeze. Both solvents are well absorbed via inhalation or after skin contact; however, accidental ingestion is the most common route of exposure in children.

Menthol

Menthol is metabolized in the liver by alcohol dehydrogenase to formaldehyde, which is further metabolized to formic acid by aldehyde dehydrogenase. Formic acid is metabolized through folate-dependent pathways to carbon dioxide and water. Toxicity is primarily by formic acid, which inhibits mitochondrial respiration.

Clinical manifestations: Drowsiness, mild intoxication, and gastric irritation, including nausea and vomiting develop early after ingestion. The onset of serious effects, including profound metabolic acidosis and visual disturbances (blurred vision, constricted visual fields, and decreased acuity) is delayed up to 24 hr. Pupils may be dilated and unreactive to light and retinal edema and optic disc hyperemia may be noted. Visual disturbances are usually reversible, but in significant poisonings, blindness has occasionally been permanent.

Laboratory findings: An anion-gap metabolic acidosis develops; thus serum electrolytes, pH, and acid-base balance should be monitored. The osmolar gap can be used to estimate the serum methanol level using the following formula:

$$\text{Osmolar gap} \times 3.2 = \text{Estimated methanol level (in mg/dl)}.$$

Ethylene Glycol

Ethylene glycol is metabolized in the liver by alcohol dehydrogenase to glycoaldehyde, which is further metabolized to glycolic acid by aldehyde dehydrogenase. Glycolic acid is metabolized to glyoxylic acid and oxalic acid, which cause toxicity. The development of serious toxic effects is delayed while these acids are generated and accumulate in blood and tissues. Oxalic acid combines with serum and tissue calcium causing hypocalcemia and the formation of calcium oxalate crystals.

Clinical manifestations: Ethylene glycol toxicity occurs in three stages. Early symptoms occur 1–12 hr after ingestion and include gastric irritation, with nausea and vomiting and CNS effects, including drowsiness and inebriation. Metabolic acidosis begins to develop. From 12–24 hr after ingestion, cardiac dysrhythmias, muscle pain, and tetany due to hypocalcemia may occur. Later, cardiac failure, seizures, cerebral edema, and renal failure occur. Renal failure is caused by the deposition of calcium oxalate crystals in renal tubules.

Laboratory findings: Ethylene glycol levels can be estimated from an osmolar gap. The osmolar gap can be used to estimate the serum ethylene glycol level using the following formula: Osmolar gap × 3.2 = Estimated ethylene glycol level (in mg/dL). Calcium oxalate crystals are commonly seen in urine on microscopy. Electrolytes, including calcium, should be monitored, as well as the ECG and renal function studies.

Methanol and Ethylene glycol treatment: Gastric decontamination is usually not of value as methanol and ethylene glycol are rapidly absorbed. Metabolic acidosis is treated with intravenous sodium bicarbonate at doses of 1–2 mEq/kg. Ethanol is an antidote for both methanol and ethylene glycol poisoning, because it is preferentially metabolized over methanol and ethylene glycol by alcohol dehydrogenase, thus minimizing formation of toxic metabolites. The parent compounds are then excreted via the lungs and kidneys. Indications for ethanol therapy are a serum ethylene glycol level greater than 25 mg/dL or methanol level greater than 20 mg/dL, a significantly symptomatic patient or ingestion of more than 0.4 mL/kg of 100% ethylene glycol or methanol. Fomepizole is a potent competitive inhibitor of alcohol dehydrogenase that has been used in both methanol and ethylene glycol poisoning. Fomepizole (15 mg/kg load; 10 mg/kg q12 hr for 4 doses; 15 mg/kg q12 hr until level < 20 mg/dl) is infused slowly over 30 min, increase doses to q4hr if dialysis is concurrent.

Hemodialysis effectively removes ethylene glycol, methanol and their acid metabolites. It is also useful for correcting severe metabolic acidosis. The indications for hemodialysis are refractory metabolic acidosis, renal failure, or ethylene glycol or methanol blood levels exceeding 50 mg/dl.

36.12 HYDROCARBONS

Kerosene oil is one of the low viscosity hydrocarbons, which is the common cause of poisoning in children. The other low viscosity hydrocarbons are petrol (gasoline), mineral spirits, naphtha, and lamp oil.

Toxic dose: Ingestion of more than 30 ml (approximate volume of an adult swallow) of hydrocarbon is associated with an increased risk of severe pneumonitis. Small quantities (< 1 ml) of low viscosity hydrocarbons if aspirated produce significant injury.

Clinical manifestations: Aspiration is characterized by coughing. Fever may persist for as long as 10 days after aspiration. Pneumonic involvement is seen more frequently by X-ray chest than by physical findings. After a stormy clinical course, which averages 2–5 days, recovery occurs in most cases. Systemic symptoms of hydrocarbon ingestion include somnolence, convulsions, and coma.

Laboratory findings: Leucocytosis may be present, in most cases; no bacteria are present in the lungs. Chest X-rays may be normal 8–12 hr after aspiration. Chest X-rays may remain abnormal for a long time after a patient is clinically normal. Pneumatoceles may appear on the chest radiograph 2–3 wk after exposure.

Complications: Pneumothorax, subcutaneous emphysema of the chest wall, pleural effusion and empyema and after the first week, pneumatoceles may develop in areas of extensive consolidation. There may be secondary infection with bacteria and viruses.

Treatment: Do not treat with gastric lavage, emesis and activated charcoal and corticosteroids and prophylactic antibiotics. For dyspnea, cyanosis or chemical pneumonitis supportive measures, such as oxygen, physiotherapy and if necessary, continuous positive air pressure or other forms of ventilatory assistance are of paramount importance.

Prognosis: Some children survive without complications or sequelae, some progress rapidly to respiratory failure and death.

36.13 ORGANOPHOSPHATES

The most commonly used insecticides are either organophosphates or carbonates. Both are inhibitors of cholinesterase enzymes. Nerve agents used in warfare are organophosphates. Poisoning occurs in home or farm. Both organophosphates and carbonates bind to cholinesterase enzymes, preventing the degradation of acetylcholine, resulting in its accumulation at nerve synapses (nicotinic and muscarinic synapses). Symptoms caused by carbamate toxicity are usually less severe.

Clinical manifestations: Signs and symptoms of toxicity relates to muscarinic, nicotinic and CNS. Muscarinic signs and symptoms include diaphoresis, emesis, urinary and fecal incontinence, tearing, drooling, bronchorrhea (bronchitis with profuse expectoration) and bronchospasm, miosis, hypotension and bradycardia. Nicotinic signs and symptoms include muscle weakness, fasciculations, tremors, hypoventilation (diaphragm paralysis), hypertension, tachycardia, and dysrhythmias. CNS effects include malaise, confusion, delirium, seizures, and coma. A commonly used acronym for the most common symptoms is SLUDGE, which stands for salivation, lacrimation, urination, defecation, gastrointestinal cramps, and emesis.

Laboratory findings: Significant symptoms appear only when measured enzymes (red blood cell cholinesterase and pseudocholinesterase) levels fall below 25% of normal.

Treatment: Dermal and ocular decontamination is done to prevent absorption of a toxin. Basic supportive care includes fluid and electrolyte replacement and intubation with artificial ventilation. Two antidotes (atropine and pralidoxime [2-PAM]) are used. Atropine (0.05 mg/kg IV repeated q5–10 min as needed; dilute in 1–2 mL of NS for ET instillation) is useful for both organophosphates and carbamates. Pralidoxime (25–50 mg/kg over 5–10 min, maximum 200 mg/ min; repeated after 1–2 hr then q10–12 hr as needed) is useful in only organophosphates poisoning.

36.14 TOXIC GASES

Many industrial and naturally occurring gases pose a health risk by inhalation. Two toxic gases-carbon monoxide (CO) and hydrogen cyanide pose a health risk by inhalation. Chlorine, chloramine, and hydrogen chloride are severe lung irritants and may cause a chemical pneumonitis. Nitrogen, propane and methane are asphyxiants.

Carbon Monoxide

CO is a colorless, odorless gas, which is produced during the combustion of any carbon-containing fuel and poses a health risk by inhalation. CO toxicity develops through at least three mechanisms, and the net result is tissue hypoxia. First, CO binds to hemoglobin, displacing oxygen, with an affinity for hemoglobin that is about 250 times that of oxygen. Second, CO impairs the ability of hemoglobin to release oxygen to tissues. Third, CO also binds to cytochrome oxidase in tissue, impeding oxygen utilization.

Clinical manifestations: Early symptoms are nonspecific and include headache, malaise and nausea. At higher exposure levels headache becomes more severe and dizziness, visual changes, and weakness may be present. Children may experience syncopal episodes as a first symptom. At higher concentrations, coma, seizures, respiratory instability, and death may occur.

Laboratory findings: Carboxyhemoglobin levels in blood are useful in documenting an exposure and CO poisoning symptoms are proportionate to the concentration of carboxyhemoglobin levels in blood.

Treatment: First move the patient to fresh air, or if necessary administration of high concentration of oxygen along with general supportive care. High concentrations of oxygen shorten the half-life of CO to the blood and tissues. Severed poisoned patients benefit from hyperbaric oxygen therapy. Some patients after a significant exposure may experience delayed-onset neurotoxicity, which may be permanent.

36.15 HYDROGEN CYANIDE

Hydrogen cyanide and cyanide salts are used in many industrial processes. It is also produced during combustion of many plastics and fabrics and is released during the metabolism of some chemicals, including the solvent acetonitrile and the drug nitroprusside. Cyanide produces toxicity by interfering with oxygen use in the cytochrome oxygen system, resulting in cellular hypoxia.

Clinical manifestations: The clinical symptoms occur rapidly and include headache, agitation, and confusion, loss of consciousness, convulsions, and cardiac dysrhythmias. Severe metabolic acidosis occurs rapidly. Death may occur. Severe metabolic acidosis in a patient with suspected cyanide exposure (e.g. fire victims) should be assumed to be cyanide poisoning.

Laboratory findings: Cyanide levels can be measured in the blood but levels do not correspond well with symptoms.

Treatment: Rapid administration of high concentrations of oxygen together with two drugs (nitrites, sodium thiosulfate) is used in the treatment of hydrogen cyanide poisoning. Nitrites (amyl nitrite and sodium nitrite) used to produce methemoglobin, which reacts with cyanide, forming cyanmethemoglobin. Sodium thiosulfate is given to hasten the metabolism of cyanomethemoglobin to hemoglobin and the less toxic thiocyanate.

Anas N, Nanasonthi V, Ginsberg CM. Criteria for hospitalizing children who have ingested products containing hydrocarbons. *JAMA* 1981; 246:840–843.

Barbey JT, Roose SP. SSRI Safety in overdose. *J Clin Psychiatry* 1998; 59 (suppl 15): 42–48.

Barillo DJ, Goode R, Esch V. Cyanide poisoning in victims of fire: Analysis of 364 cases and review of the literature. *J Burn Care Rehabil* 1994; 15: 46–57.

Bates N, Edwards N, Roper J, Volan G (eds). Pediatric Toxicology: *Handbook of Poisoning in Children*. New York: Stockton Press, 1993.

Brenner BE, Simon RR. Management of salicylate intoxication. *Drugs* 1992; 24: 335–340.

Caravati EM. Unintentional acetaminophen ingestion in children and potential for hepatotoxicity. *J Toxicol Clin Toxicol* 1994; 32: 513–525.

Casavant MJ. Fomepizole in the treatment of poisoning. *Pediatrics* 2001; 107: 170.

Erickson SJ, Duncan A. Clonidine poisoning-an emerging problem: Epidemiology, clinical features, management and preventive strategies. *J Pediatr Child Health* 1998; 34: 280–282.

Gleyzer A. Traub S, Hoffman RS. Calcium channel blocker ingestions in children. *Am J Emerg Med* 2001; 19: 456–457.

Lifshitz M, Shahak E, Sofer S. Carbamate and organophosphate poisoning in young children. *Pediatr Emerg Care* 1999; 15: 102–103.

Rodgers GC Jr, Condurache T, Reed MD, Bestic M, Gal P. Poisonings. In: Kliegman RM, Behrman RE, Jenson HB, Stanton BF (eds). *Nelson Textbook of Pediatrics*. 18th edn. Vol. 1. Philadelphia: Saunders, 2007; 339–357.

Rumack BH, Peterson RG. Acetaminophen overdose: Incidence, diagnosis and management in 416 patients. *Pediatrics* 1978; 62: 898–903.

Spitz L, Lakhoo K. Caustic ingestion. *Arch Dis Child* 1993; 68: 157–158.

Weaver LK, Hopkins RO, Chan KJ, et al. Carbon monoxide poisoning. *N Engl J Med* 2002; 347: 1057–1067.

37 Health Programs

37.1 NATIONAL HEALTH PROGRAMMES IN INDIA

Under the Constitution, health is a State subject. Central government's intervention to assist the State governments is needed in the areas of control/ eradication of major communicable and non-communicable diseases, besides activities concerning the containment of population growth including child survival and safe motherhood (CSSM) and immunization programmes (Box 37.1).

Several National health programmes are being implemented as centrally sponsored schemes aimed mainly at reduction of mortality and morbidity caused by major diseases. The major health schemes include the national programmes for eradication of malaria, blindness, leprosy, tuberculosis, AIDS including blood safety measures and STD control, cancer control. Pilot projects have also been taken up in respect of diabetes, mental health and cancers, etc.

National Rural Health Mission (NRHM)

NRHM was launched to address infirmities and problems across primary health care and bring about improvement in the health system and the health status of those who live in the rural areas. The Mission aims to provide universal access to equitable, affordable, and quality health care that is accountable and at the same time responsive to the needs of the

---

Box 37.1: List of national health programmes

1. Revised National Tuberculosis Programme (RNTCP).
2. National Leprosy Eradication Programme.
3. The National Anti-Malaria Programme.
4. National AIDS Control Programme.
5. Reproductive and Child Health Programme.
6. The National Family Welfare Programme.
7. Pulse Polio Immunization Programme.
8. National Disease Surveillance Programme.
9. National Nutritional Anaemia Control Programme (NNACP).
10. National Iodine Deficiency Disorders Control Programme (NIDDCP) in India: Current status and future strategies.
11. Mid Day Meal Programme (MDM).
12. The National Filaria Control Programme.
13. The National Programme for Control of Blindness (NPCB).
14. The National Mental Health Programme.
15. National Programme for Prevention of Nutritional Blindness due to Vitamin A Deficiency.
16. National Diabetes Control Programme.
17. National Cancer Control Programme.
18. National Rural Health Mission.

people. The Mission is expected to achieve the goals set under the National Health Policy and the Millennium Development Goals (MDGs).

To achieve these goals, NRHM facilitates increased access and utilization of quality health services by all, forges a partnership between the Central, State, and the local governments, sets up a platform for involving the PRIs and the community in the management of primary health programmes and infrastructure, and provides an opportunity for promoting equity and social justice. The NRHM establishes a mechanism to provide flexibility to the States and the community to promote local initiatives and develop a framework for promoting intersectoral convergence for promotive and preventive health care. The Mission has also defined core and supplementary strategies.

Strategies of NRHM

Core Strategies

1. Train and enhance capacity of PRIs to supervise and manage public health services.
2. Promote access to improved health care at household level through the female health activist (Accredited Social Health Activist—ASHA).
3. Health Plan for each village through Village Health Committee of the Panchayat.
4. Strengthen SC through an untied fund to enable local planning and action and more Multipurpose Workers (MPWs).
5. Strengthen existing PHCs and CHCs and provide 30–50 bedded CHC per lakh population for improved curative care to a normative standard (Indian Public Health Service Standards [IPHS] defining personnel, equipment, and management standards).
6. Prepare and implement an intersectoral District Health Plan prepared by the District Health Mission, including drinking water, sanitation, hygiene, and nutrition.
7. Integrate vertical health and family welfare programmes at national, State, and district levels.
8. Technical Support to National, State, and District Health Missions for Public Health Management.
9. Strengthen capacities for data collection, assessment, and review for evidence-based planning, monitoring, and supervision.
10. Formulate transparent policies for deployment and career development of Human Resources for health.
11. Develop capacities for preventive health care at all levels for promoting healthy life styles, reduction in consumption of tobacco and alcohol, etc.
12. Promote non-profit sector particularly in underserved areas.
13. Supplementary strategies
14. Regulation of private sector including the informal rural practitioners to ensure availability of quality service to citizens at reasonable cost.

Five planks of the NRHM

i. The Mission is expected to address the gaps in the provision of effective health care to rural population with a special focus on 18 states, which have weak public health indicators and/or weak infrastructure.
ii. The Mission is a shift away from the vertical health and family welfare programmes to a new architecture of all inclusive health development in which societies under different programmes will be merged and resources pooled at the district level.
iii. The Mission aims at the effective integration of health concerns with determinants of health like safe drinking water, sanitation, and nutrition through integrated District Plans for Health. There is a provision for flexible funds so that the States can utilize them in the areas they feel are important.
iv. The Mission provides for appointment of ASHA in each village and strengthening of the public health infrastructure, including outreach through mobile clinics. It emphasizes involvement of the non-profit sector, especially in the under-served areas. It also aims at flexibility at the local level by providing for untied funds.
v. The Mission, in its supplementary strategies, aims at fostering PPPs; improving equity and reducing out of pocket expenses; introducing effective risk-pooling mechanisms and social health insurance; and taking advantage of local health tradition. Promotion of PPPs for achieving public health goals. Reorienting medical education to support health issues including regulation of Medical Care and Medical Ethics. Effective and viable risk-pooling and social health insurance to provide health security to the poor by ensuring accessible, affordable, accountable, and good quality health care.

The expected outcomes of NRHM are listed below:

1. IMR-reduced to 30/1000 live births by 2012.
2. Maternal Mortality—reduced to 100/100000 live births by 2012.
3. TFR-reduced to 2.1 by 2012.
4. Malaria Mortality Reduction—50% up to 2010, additional 10% by 2012.
5. Kala-azar Mortality Reduction—100% by 2010 and sustaining elimination until 2012.

6. Filaria/Microfilaria Reduction—70% by 2010, 80% by 2012, and elimination by 2015.

7. Dengue Mortality Reduction—50% by 2010 and sustaining at that level until 2012.

8. Cataract operations—increasing to 46 lakh until 2012.

9. Leprosy Prevalence Rate–reduce from1.8 per 10000 in 2005 to less that 1 per 10000 thereafter.

10. Tuberculosis DOTS-maintain 85% cure rate through entire Mission Period and also sustain planned case detection rate.

11. Upgrading all health establishments in the district to IPHS.

12. Increase utilization of First Referral Units (FRUs) from bed occupancy by referred cases of less than 20% to over 75%.

Under the NRHM, it was planned to have:

1. Over 5 lakh ASHAs, one for every 1000 population/large habitation, in 18 Special Focus States and in tribal pockets of all States by 2008.

2. All SCs (nearly 1.75 lakh) functional with two ANMs by 2010.

3. All PHCs (nearly 30000) with three staff nurses to provide 24 × 7 services by 2010.

4. 6500 CHCs strengthened/established with seven specialists and nine staff nurses by 2012.

5. 1800 Taluka/Sub Divisional Hospitals and 600 District Hospitals strengthened to provide quality health services by 2012.

6. Mobile Medical Units for each District by 2009.

7. Functional Hospital Development Committees in all CHCs, Sub Divisional Hospitals, and District Hospitals by 2009.

8. Untied grants and annual maintenance grants to every SC, PHC, and CHC released regularly and utilized for local health action by 2008.

In the Eleventh Five Year Plan, the emphasis under NRHM will not be on numerical achievements only but also on IPHS and enforcement of guidelines for improving the functioning of infrastructure being strengthened and created. It has been felt that the Mission Directors, both at the Centre and the States, should be officials with public health background, supported by the Civil Service cadres.

National Urban Health Mission (NUHM)

The NUHM will meet health needs of the urban poor, particularly the slum dwellers by making available to them essential primary health care services. This will be done by investing in high-caliber health professionals, appropriate technology through PPP, and health insurance for urban poor.

Recognizing the seriousness of the problem, urban health has been taken up as a thrust area for the Eleventh Five Year Plan. NUHM will be launched with focus on slums and other urban poor. At the State level, besides the State Health Mission and State Health Society and Directorate, there would be a State Urban Health Programme Committee. At the district level, similarly there would be a District Urban Health Committee and at the city level, a Health and Sanitation Planning Committee. At the ward slum level, there will be a Slum Cluster Health and Water and Sanitation Committee. For promoting public health and cleanliness in urban slums, the Eleventh Five Year Plan also encompass experiences of civil society organizations (CSO) working in urban slum clusters. It will seek to build a bridge of NGO-GO partnership and develop community level monitoring of resources and their rightful use. NUHM would ensure the following:

- Resources for addressing the health problems in urban areas, especially among urban poor.
- Need based city specific urban health care system to meet the diverse health needs of the urban poor and other vulnerable sections.
- Partnership with community for a more proactive involvement in planning, implementation, and monitoring of health activities.
- Institutional mechanism and management systems to meet the health-related challenges of a rapidly growing urban population.
- Framework for partnerships with NGOs, charitable hospitals, and other stakeholders.
- Two-tier system of risk pooling: (i) women's Mahila Arogya Samiti to fulfill urgent hard-cash needs for treatments; (ii) a Health Insurance Scheme for enabling urban poor to meet medical treatment needs.

NUHM will cover all cities with a population of more than 100000. It would cover slum dwellers; other marginalized urban dwellers like rickshaw pullers, street vendors, railway and bus station coolies, homeless people, street children, construction site workers, who may be in slums or on sites.

The existing Urban Health Posts and Urban Family Welfare Centres will continue under NUHM. They will be marked on a map and classified as the Urban Health Centres on the basis of their current population coverage. All the existing human resources will then be suitably reorganized and rationalized. These centres will also be considered for upgradation. Intersectoral coordination mechanism and convergence will be planned between the Jawaharlal Nehru National Urban Renewal Mission (JNNURM) and the NUHM.

Strengthening Existing Health System

There is a need to shift to decentralization of functions to hospital units/health centres and local bodies. The States need to move away from the narrow focus on the implementation of budgeted programmes and vertical schemes. They need to develop systems that comprehensively address the health needs of all citizens. Thus, in order to improve the health care services in the country, the Eleventh Five Year Plan will insist on Integrated District Health Plans and Block Specific Health Plans. It will mandate involvement of all health related sectors and emphasize partnership with PRIs, local bodies, communities, NGOs, Voluntary and Civil Society Organizations.

Janani Suraksha Yojana (JSY) *see* Section 37.3

Primary Health Care

During the Eleventh Five Year Plan, major focus will be on NRHM initiatives. Efforts will be made for restructuring and reorganizing all health facilities below district level into the Three Tier Rural Primary Health Care System. Under the NRHM, emphasis has been given to allocate 70% of the total financial resources to below district level (block level and below), 20% at district level, and 10% at State level. Efforts will be made to allocate funds under various schemes and programmes as per NRHM guidelines. Further, the requirements of funds for a fully functional primary health care system (defined as all services at block level and below, including field-based implementation of disease control and preventive activities, but not administration) will also be worked out.

Secondary and Tertiary Health Care

Secondary and Tertiary health care will receive attention. There is an urgent need to take a fresh look at how public and private sector can be better utilized during the Eleventh Five Year Plan. The NRHM addresses these issues through a few strategies. Priorities will be given to strategies involving PPPs, risk-pooling mechanisms, and cross subsidization.

Administration of the secondary and tertiary care hospitals will be professionalized and trained professionals posted as Medical Superintendents. Hospitals will be allowed to recruit various staff including junior doctors on adhoc and contract basis. Drugs purchase should be made through centralized rate contract and decentralized distribution with zero stock at headquarter level. Emergency and disaster stock should be located at each hospital. Drugs at all levels with minimum of one year shelf life should be supplied.

District hospitals, which play a key role in providing health services to the poor, need substantial improvement in infrastructure and other facilities to perform their role more effectively. This would also be a key intermediate step in the health strategy, till the vision of health care through PHCs and community health centres is fully realized. It is often observed that Government Medical Colleges and Hospitals are on the verge of de-recognition mainly because they fail to adhere to the infrastructure, equipment, and staff norms, as laid down by MCI. This is thought to be due to lack of funding. The Centre and States will have to make provisions for strengthening these institutions.

During the Eleventh Five Year Plan period, the following will receive priority:

- Establishment of Hospital Development Committees in all government hospitals.
- Improvement of infrastructure and facilities in district hospitals.
- Provision of high-quality secondary health care services for every block in the country.
- Creation of state-of-the-art medical education, research, and care institutions in all disciplines of medicine.
- Creation of new institutions and up gradation of existing tertiary care hospitals.
- Main streaming of AYUSH systems to actively supplement the efforts of the allopathic systems.

Access to Essential Drugs and Medicines

Drugs and medicines form a substantial portion of the out-of-pocket spending on health by households. The poor are the worst affected because they are frequently affected by diseases and are least able to purchase and utilize the health services, such as drugs. On the other hand, the component of drugs and medicines accounts for a mere 10% of the overall health budget of both the Central and State Governments. Timely supply of drugs of good quality that involves procurement as well as logistics management is of critical importance in any health system.

An essential component of strengthening primary health facilities will be a system of guaranteeing essential drugs. Standard treatment guidelines will be available for doctors at PHCs and CHCs. The Central Government will provide assistance to States for strengthening the drug regulatory system. During the Plan, the following will be emphasized:

i. Developing essential drug lists for all levels of institutions
ii. Making available essential drugs of good quality in adequate quantities in all government health facilities

iii. Increasing efficiency, economy, and transparency in drug procurement, warehousing, and distribution

iv. Initiating strategies in coordination with professional and consumer bodies to ensure safe drugs and rational use of drugs

v. Disseminating information on essential drugs to medical professionals, pharmacists, and to the people including all essential drugs under a system of price monitoring

vi. Implementing and reinforcing the concept of Standard Treatment Guidelines in the in-service and pre-service training programmes of the doctors and health workers.

Amdekar YK. DOTS Program in Children and Adolescents. In: Mathur GP, Mathur Sarla (eds). *Current Trends in Pediatrics.* Vol 2. Delhi: Academa Publishers, 2006; 216–219.

Kapil U. National Nutrition Programme in India. In: Mehta MN, Kulkarni M (eds). *Proceedings of National Symposium cum Workshop in Child Nutrition -The Indian Scene.* Bombay: Sai Creation and Advertising Co., 1991; 78–107.

Kapil U. Status of Nutrition Programme in India. *Report of National Seminar on Towards a National Nutritional policy.* New Delhi: National Institute of Public cooperation and Child Development, 1989.

Kapil U. Monitoring and continuing education system in ICDS scheme-A module for National Health Programmes. *Indian Pediatr* 1989; 26: 863–867.

Kapil U. Nutrition programme for mothers and children. *Journal of State Health Education Bureau* SEHAT 1990; 5: 2–4.

Kapil U, Sharma RP. Current status of integrated Child Development Services Programme and Future Strategies. In: Mathur GP, Mathur Sarla (eds). *Current Trends in Pediatrics.* Vol 2. Delhi: Academa Publishers, 2006; 13–19.

Kapil U. National Health Programmes in India. In: Mathur GP, Mathur Sarla (eds). *Current Trends in Pediatrics.* Vol 3. Delhi: Academa Publishers, 2007; 419–445.

Prevention and Treatment of Vitamin A Deficiency. Ministry of Health and Family welfare, Government of India. New Delhi: Government of India press, 1991.

Tandon BN. The Impact of ICDS on the status of child health in India towards the implementation of a National Nutrition policy in India, 1986. *Indian Council of Medical Research.* New Delhi: ICMR Press, 1986; 6–11.

37.2 CURRENT STATUS OF INTEGRATED CHILD DEVELOPMENT SERVICES PROGRAMME AND FUTURE STRATEGIES

1 Introduction

Government of India proclaimed a National Policy on Children in August 1974 declaring children as, "supremely important asset". The policy provided the required framework for assigning priority to different needs of the child. The programme of the Integrated Child Development Services (ICDS) was launched in 1975 seeking to provide an integrated package of services in a convergent manner for the holistic development of the child.

2 Integrated Child Development Scheme

Launched on *2nd October 1975 in 33 Community Development Blocks*, ICDS today represents one of the world's largest programmes for early childhood development. ICDS is the foremost symbol of India's commitment to her children—India's response to the challenge of providing pre-school education on one hand and breaking the vicious cycle of malnutrition, morbidity, reduced learning capacity and mortality, on the other.

It is an inter-sectoral programme which seeks to directly reach out to children, below six years, especially from vulnerable and remote areas and give them a head-start by providing an integrated programme of early childhood education, health and nutrition. No programme on Early Childhood Care and Education can succeed unless mothers are also brought within it ambit as it is in the lap of the mother that human beings learn the first lessons in life.

3 Objectives of ICDS

i. Lay the foundation for proper psychological development of the child

ii. Improve nutritional and health status of children 0–6 yrs

iii. Reduce incidence of mortality, morbidity, malnutrition and school drop-outs

iv. Enhance the capability of the mother and family to look after the health, nutritional and development needs of the child

v. Achieve effective coordination of policy and implementation among various departments to promote child development

4 Services

The Scheme provides an integrated approach for converging basic services through community-based workers and helpers. The services are provided at a centre called the 'Anganwadi'. The Anganwadi, literally a courtyard play centre, is a childcare centre, located within the village itself. A package of following six services is provided under the ICDS Scheme:

i. Supplementary nutrition
ii. Non-formal pre-school education
iii. Immunization
iv. Health Check-up
v. Referral services
vi. Nutrition and Health Education

The three services, namely immunization, health check-up and referral are delivered through public health infrastructure, viz. Health Sub Centres, Primary and Community Health Centers under the Ministry of Health and Family Welfare. Target groups and service providers are listed in Table 37.1.

4.1 *Supplementary nutrition:* This includes supplementary feeding and growth monitoring; and *prophylaxis against vitamin A deficiency and control of nutritional anaemia.* All families in the community are surveyed, to identify children below the age of six and pregnant and nursing mothers. They avail of supplementary feeding support for 300 days in a year. By providing supplementary feeding, the **Anganwadi attempts to bridge the protein energy gap between the recommended dietary allowance and average dietary intake of children and women.**

Growth Monitoring and nutrition surveillance are two important activities that are undertaken. Children below the age of three years of age are weighed once a month and children 3–6 yrs of age are weighed every quarter. Weight-for-age growth cards are maintained for all children below six years. This helps to detect growth faltering and helps in assessing nutritional status. Besides, severely malnourished children are given special supplementary feeding and referred to health sub-centres, Primary Health Centres as and when required.

Supplementary nutrition norms: The effort is to provide, on an average, daily nutritional supplements to the extent indicated in Table 37.2: **Revised vide letter No. 5–9/2005-ND-Tech Vol. II dated 24.2.2009.**

4.2 *Pre-school education:* This component for the three-to-six years old children in the anganwadi is directed towards providing and ensuring a natural, joyful and stimulating environment, with emphasis on necessary inputs for optimal growth and development. The early learning component of the ICDS is a significant input for providing a sound foundation for cumulative lifelong learning and development. It also contributes to the universalization of primary education, by providing to the child the necessary preparation for primary schooling and offering substitute care to younger siblings, thus freeing the older ones—especially girls—to attend school.

4.3 *Immunization:* Immunization of pregnant women and infants protects children from six vaccine preventable diseases—poliomyelitis, diphtheria, pertussis, tetanus, tuberculosis and measles (Table 37.3). These are major preventable causes of child mortality, disability, morbidity and related malnutrition. Immunization of pregnant women against tetanus also reduces maternal and neonatal mortality.

Table 37.1: Target groups and service provider		
Services	*Target group*	*Services provided by*
Supplementary Nutrition	Children below 6 years; pregnant and lactating mothers	Anganwadi Workers (AWW) and Anganwadi Helper (AWH)
Immunization*	Children below 6 years; pregnant and lactating mothers	ANM/MO
Health Check-ups*	Children below 6 years; pregnant and lactating mothers	ANM/MO/AWW
Referral	Children below 6 years; pregnant and lactating mothers	AWW/ANM/MO
Pre-School Education	Children 3–6 years	AWW
Nutrition and Health Education	Women (15–45 years)	AWW/ANM/MO

* AWW assists ANM in identifying and mobilizing the target group

Table 37.2: Supplementary nutrition norms				
Beneficiaries	*[Pre-revised]*		*[Revised]*	
			Per beneficiary per day	
	Calories (K cal)	**Protein (g)**	**Calories (K cal)**	**Protein (g)**
Children below 3 years*	300	8–10	500	12–15
Children 3–6 years	300	8–10	800	20–25
[Severely malnourished children on medical advice after health check-up)]	(double of above)		(double of above)	
Pregnant and lactating (P and L) mothers	500	20–25	600	18–20

* Provisions regarding promotion of breast-feeding as recommended in Infant and Child Feeding (IYCF) guidelines are relevant.

Vaccine	Age				
	Birth	6 wks	10 wks	14 wks	9 months
Primary Vaccination					
BCG	✓				
Oral Polio	✓[1]	✓	✓	✓	
DPT		✓	✓	✓	
Hepatitis B		✓	✓	✓	
Measles					✓
Booster Doses					
DPT + Oral Polio	18 to 24 mo				
DT	5 yrs				
Tetanus Toxoid	At 10 yrs and again at 16 yrs				
Vitamin A	9, 18, 24, 30 and 36 mo				

Table 37.3: Immunization status in infants and pregnant women

Tetanus Toxoid—Pregnant Women		
	1st Dose	As early as possible during pregnancy after 1st trimester
	2nd Dose	1 month after 1st Dose
	3rd Dose	If previously vaccinated within 3 years

1. In all institutional deliveries and in all endemic areas
2. In pilot areas. A dose at birth is recommended for babies born in health care institutions
3. Vaccination schedule may get modified if newer vaccine is introduced in future under National Immunization Programme

This service is delivered by the Ministry of Health and Family Welfare under its Reproductive Child Health (RCH) programme. In addition, the iron and vitamin "A" supplementation to children and pregnant women is done under the RCH Programme of the Ministry of Health and Family Welfare.

4.4 Health check-ups: This includes health care of children less than six years of age, antenatal care of expectant mothers and postnatal care of nursing mothers. These services are provided by the ANM, Medical Officers (MOs) incharge of Health Sub-Centres and Primary Health Centres under the RCH programme of the Ministry of Health and Family Welfare. The various health services include regular health check-ups, immunization, management of malnutrition, treatment of diarrhea, deworming and distribution of simple medicines, etc.

4.5 Referral services: During health check-ups and growth monitoring, sick or malnourished children, in need of prompt medical attention, are referred to the Primary Health Centre or its sub-centre. The Anganwadi worker has also been oriented to detect disabilities in young children. She enlists all such cases and refers them to the ANM and Medical Officer in charge of the Primary Health Centre/Sub-centre. These cases referred by the Anganwadi worker are to be attended by health functionaries on priority basis.

4.6 Nutrition and health education: Nutrition and Health Education (NHE) is a key element of the work of the Anganwadi worker. This forms part of BCC (Behavior Change Communication) strategy. This has the long term goal of capacity-building of women—especially in the age group of 15–45 yrs—so that they can look after their own health, nutrition and development needs as well as that of their children and families.

5. The ICDS Team: The ICDS team comprises the Anganwadi helpers, Anganwadi workers, supervisors, Child Development Project Officers (CDPOs) and District Programme Officers (DPOs). Anganwadi Worker, a lady selected from the local community, is a community based frontline voluntary worker of the ICDS Programme. She is also an agent of social change, mobilizing community support for better care of young children, girls and women. Besides, the medical officers, the lady health visitors (LHVs) and Auxiliary Nurse Midwife (ANM) and female health workers from nearby primary health centres (PHCs) and Health Sub-Centre form a team with the ICDS functionaries to achieve convergence of different services.

NIPCCD (National Institute of Public Cooperation and Child Development), 1992, National Evaluation of Integrated Child Development Services, New Delhi.

NFI (Nutrition Foundation of India) 1988. The Integrated Child Development Services (ICDS) Scheme, New Delhi.

NPAN (National Plan of Action on Nutrition), DWCD, GOI, 1995.

National Consultation on Benefits and Safety of Administration of vitamin A to Preschool Children and Pregnant and Lactating Women.

National Policy for Prevention and Control of Anaemia. MOHFW .1990

National Family Health Survey, IIPS, India 1992–93, Bombay.

Vir, Sheila C, and Nigam, A.K., Nutritional Status of Children in Uttar Pradesh. NFI Bulletin 22 Jan 2001.

National Family Health Survey, (NFHS-2), 1998–99, IIPS, Mumbai.

ICDS-III Project Tamil Nadu, October 2000, Project Coordinator, World Bank assisted ICDS-III Project, Chennai.

Agnihotri, Satish B., Removing Severe Malnutrition from Orissa by October 2001-personal communication.1999

Singh J.M., Singh Beena, Vir, Sheila, Social Mobilisation and Child Nutrition, personal communication.2001

WHO (1999) Management of Severe Malnutrition—A Manual for Physicians and Senior health workers.

37.3 JANANI SURAKSHA YOJANA PROGRAM

Janani Suraksha Yojana (JSY) is an Indian government-sponsored conditional cash transfer scheme to reduce the numbers of maternal and neonatal deaths and increase health facility deliveries in BPL families (Table 37.4). The objective is for increasing institutional delivery. The JSY covers all pregnant women belonging to households below the poverty line, above 19 yrs of age and up to two live births. The JSY integrates help in the form of cash with antenatal care during pregnancy period, institutional care during delivery as well as post-partum. This is provided by field level health workers through a system of coordinated care and health centers. Benefits for institutional delivery are more generous in rural areas and in low-performing states, ranging from ₹ 600 to ₹ 1,400. A subsidy is also available to private sector providers is emergency cesareans, on referral. An overview of this central government sponsored scheme is presented in Table 37.5. Login to Contact This Program website http://india.gov.in/citizen/health/janani_suraksha.php.

37.4 SCHOOL HEALTH SERVICES

A good primary health care is essential for the growth of a nation. The health of children is a good indicator of the health of a community. In Delhi, a large group of children exist who come from low socioeconomic status who have multitudes of health problems ranging from infections, infestations, nutritional imbalances, congenital anomalies to those of psycho social in origin. They are the children studying in MCD primary schools and are over 9 lakhs in number. To cater the health needs of MCD primary schools, school health services was established in 1952 by the great visionary of his times, Pt. Jawahar Lal Nehru. At school health services preventive, promotive, curative and rehabilitative services are provided to these children at their doorstep.

Table 37.4: Janani Suraksha Yojana Program	
Program Type	*Changing Behaviors > Health awareness/education* *Regulating Performance > Pay for performance*
Health Focus	Family Planning and Reproductive Health
Target Geography	Urban/Peri-Urban/Rural
Target Population	Children < 5 Children > 5 Women

Table 37.5: Overview of JYS program central government sponsored scheme in India	
Implementing organization:	*The World Bank* *Implementation Partner(s):* *Ministry of Health and Family Welfare*
Year Launched:	2005
Stage:	Existing/expansion stage
Funding:	Primary Source of Funding: Donor Additional Source(s) of Funding: Government
Funders:	**Bill and Melinda Gates Foundation**

Annual Report 2008–2009 Ministry of Health & Family Welfare, Government of India, New Delhi, India.
National Rural Health Mission, Ministry of Health and Family Welfare, Government of India, New Delhi, India.

A child who is coming to school is obviously not so sick as to render him incapable of carrying out daily activities but he may be suffering from morbidities which can be treated and make him healthier and better off. Also, he needs to know about healthy practices through which he can avoid ill health and mishaps in future. So, instead of patients driven to doctors for various illnesses, compelled by their symptoms, it is the doctor who is reaching out to children telling about various conditions they may be having and treating them.

Services Provided

1. *Immunisation:* i. DT and TT for classes 1st and 5th respectively. ii. Pulse polio programme
2. *Anaemia control programme:* Mass deworming by tablet Albendazole 200 mg. with a tablet. F.S. (Ferrous sulphate 200 mg.) and folic acid (5 mg.) every week along with mid day meal.
3. *Thalassemia control programme:* NESTROFT test (Naked Eye Single Tube Red Cell Osmotic Fragility Test) for screening of thalassaemia carriers is being done on all class 5th children and those found positive are put to genetic counselling The test is done by taking 2 ml 0.36% buffered saline in one tube and 2 ml distilled water in another. One drop blood is added to each tube and they are left for ½ hr at room temperature. The tubes are shaken and held against a white paper with a thin black line drawn on it. The line is clearly visible through the contents of tube with distilled water. If the line is also visible through the contents of tube with buffered saline, the test is negative. If it is not visible, it is positive.
4. *Xerophthalmia:* Full dose (6 lac I.U.) of oil soluble vitamin A to those with xerosis and Bitot spots.
5. *Health education:* Subjects covered in health education are listed in Box 37.2.

Box 37.2: Subjects covered in health education

1. Personal hygiene and cleanliness; 2. Mosquito breeding: Dengue and malaria; 3. Management of diarrhoea and preparation of ORS; 4. Healthy nutrition; 5. Eye care; 6. Dental care—proper tooth brushing; 7. Prevention of injuries and first aid.

---

6. *Health promotion:* Mid-day meal is being provided with 1/3rd of total calorie and ½ of total protein requirement.
7. *Curative services:* Regular school visits are made by medical officers and public health nurses where medical check up is done. Those who cannot be managed at primary level are referred to secondary or tertiary centres. According to prevalence, major diseases reported are listed in Box 37.3.

Box 37.3: Major diseases

1. Worm infestation and anemia; 2. URI and respiratory allergies; 3. Dental caries and tartar; 4. Conjunctivitis; 5. Refractive errors; 6. Injuries; 7. Pyoderma; 8. Growing pains; 9. Cervical lymphadenopathy; 10. Ear discharge; 11. Other diseases commonly seen are: i. Tuberculosis; ii. Malnutrition; iii. Heart diseases; iv. Epilepsy; v. Asthma; vi. Diarrhoea; vii. Xerosis; viii. Dermatophytosis; ix. Scabies; 12. Eye diseases: i. Corneal ulcers; ii. Squints; iii. Glaucoma; iv. Congenital cataract; 13. Dental diseases: i. Malocclusion; ii. Gingivitis; iii. Fluorosis

---

8. *Rehabilitation:* i. *Spectacles are provided free of cost to those with refractive errors after proper vision screening and refraction under pupillary dilatation. With the help of* autorefractometer, accuracy can be maintained. ii. Provision of **hearing aids** to children with impaired hearing. iii. Appliances and **mobility aids** for polio affected children.

Problems and Achievements

Working in school health services is not without obstacles. Due to large number of children complete coverage is at times not possible. Secondly there is a poor coordination between primary and tertiary levels. Patients referred to hospitals are generally lost to follow up. Laboratory facilities are practically not existing. Transportation and carrying out activities in far flung schools is at times difficult.

In spite of all difficulties there are certain achievements to cite: 1. 70% immunisation coverage; 2. Worm load has decreased from 50% to 10% as per survey carried out by National Institute of Communicable Diseases; 3. Prevalence of xerophthalmia has considerably decreased as published in Journal of Indian Medical Association.

Agarwal O P, Chaturvedi S. Structural and Organizational Features of School Health Schemes in Delhi. *Indian J Pediatr* 2000; 67: 185–188.

Chaturvedi S, Agarwal O P. Assessment of availability and working components of school Health services in Delhi. Indian J Pediatr 2000; 67: 179–184.

Park K. School health service. In: *Park's Textbook of Preventive and Social Medicine*. 19th edn. Jabalpur: M/s Banarsidas Bhanot, 2007; 463–466.

Sunder Lal. Health and development of school children. Indian J Community *Med* 1998; 23: 3–6.

37.5 IODINE DEFICIENCY DISORDERS

Iodine Deficiency Disorders (IDD) constitutes one of the major healthcare problems in India. It leads to serious consequences especially in the new born and growing child interfering with brain development. The term Iodine Deficiency Disorders (IDD) refers to all the effects of iodine deficiency on growth and development in a human and animal population, which can be prevented by correction of iodine deficiency. These include goiter, stillbirths, neonatal and other types of hypothyroidism but the most important effect is that of fetal brain damage. The term was first proposed in 1983 by Hetzel and is now widely accepted.

Pathophysiology: Iodine is an essential element required for the synthesis of thyroid hormones thyroxine (T4) and tri iodothyronine (T3). Dietary iodide is actively and efficiently absorbed by the gastrointestinal tract and actively taken up into thyroid cells. It subsequently gets incorporated into the thyroid hormones. Inadequate iodine intake results in inadequate thyroxine synthesis. The TSH concentration rises. TSH stimulates cell division of the thyroid follicular cells leading to goiter formation. There is more efficient use of iodine by the thyroid tissue with production of relatively more T3 (more potent with less iodine atoms) as compared to T4, and thus preventing metabolic effects of hypothyroidism. With more severe deficiency, hypothyroidism occurs.

Epidemiology: Iodine deficiency is considered the most common preventable cause of mental retardation. 130 countries in the world are affected by iodine deficiency. A total population in excess of 2 billion is at risk for the occurrence of varying degrees of brain damage. A recent WHO report suggested that nearly 2 billion individuals worldwide (35% of the world population) might be having iodine deficiency. 285 million children in a cross sectional analysis, were having inadequate iodine intake (dietary iodine intake

< 100 mcg/day). Thus IDD easily becomes the world's most prevalent thyroid disease. In India, no state is free from iodine deficiency and 200 million people are at risk of IDD. 13 million children born each year in India are in an environment unprotected from iodine deficiency disorders.

The problem occurs because the soil in iodine deficient areas has been leached of iodine due to flooding of river valleys or in hilly and mountainous areas by high rainfall or glaciations. The deficiency in the soil leads to deficiency in all forms of plant life including all cereals grown in the soil. Studies showing an inverse correlation between the iodine content of soil and water and prevalence of these disorders support the causative role of iodine deficiency in their occurrence. It is also supported by the iodine kinetic studies in patients with these disorders and a decrease in their incidence with iodine supplementation. The occurrence of these disorders may be exacerbated by the presence of environmental goitrogens that interfere with iodine utilization and thyroid hormone synthesis. The daily dietary requirement of iodine is shown in Table 37.6.

Clinical manifestations: Consequences of iodine deficiency are goiter, hypothyroidism, mental retardation, cretinism and increased perinatal and infant mortality. The effects may be classified by the age group of the patient population (Table 37.7, *see* Fig. 37.1 in CD).

Diffuse and nodular goiter: Goiter is the most obvious manifestation of iodine deficiency. It occurs as a compensatory response to decreased iodine. Decreased iodine leads to decreased t4 and an increase in TSH. TSH stimulates thyroid growth. Goiter is initially diffuse, but later tends to become nodular. Some

Table 37.6: Recommended daily intake of iodine in various age groups

Age group	Iodine requirement (mcg/day)
Infants (0–11m)	50
Children (1–5yr)	90
School children (6–12 yr)	120
Adults (above 12 yr)	150
Pregnant and lactating women	200

Table 37.7: Spectrum of iodine deficiency disorders

Fetus	Abortions, still births, congenital anomalies, neurologic cretinism myxedematous cretinism psychomotor defects
Neonate	Increased perinatal mortality, neonatal hypothyroidism, retarded mental and physical development
Child and adolescent	Increased infant mortality, retarded mental and physical development
Adult	Goitre and its complications, iodine induced hyperthyroidism
All ages	Goitre, hypothyroidism, impaired mental function, increased susceptibility to nuclear radiation

follicles proliferate more than others which results in nodularity. Some of the nodules may later become autonomous patient may become hyperthyroid especially when iodine is supplemented. Goiter is traditionally assessed by palpation. The size may be graded for epidemiological studies. Ultrasound is the preferred modality for accurately assessing the size of the thyroid gland. Goiter is usually a cosmetic problem. Patient is usually euthyroid unless the iodine deficiency is severe. Large goiters may produce local compression.

Hypothyroidism: Hypothyroidism occurs when iodine intake is very low. For growing fetus and infant, thyroid hormone is essential for normal development of CNS, especially myelination. Hypothyroidism in this stage leads to permanent mental retardation and cretinism. It is reported that 10% or more of new borns in goiter endemic areas are at risk of neonatal hypothyroidism and hence its neurological consequences. Adults will have typical symptoms of hypothyroidism.

Cretinism: Cretinism is the most severe form of hypothyroidism. Affected children have mental retardation, neurologic and somatic defects. Two types of cretinism are defined—neurologic and myxedematous. But there may be considerable overlap between the 2 and combined neurologic and myxedematous forms also exist. Both conditions are preventable with maternal and infant iodine supplementation.

a. Neurologic—results from hypothyroidism in the mother during early pregnancy. Mental retardation, deaf mutism, gait disturbance and spasticity are also present. There is no hypothyroidism.

b. Myxedematous—results from iodine deficiency and thyroid abnormality late in pregnancy and after birth. These children have mental retardation, hypothyroidism and short stature.

Some degree of mental retardation and lower IQ points in individuals from iodine deficient areas has been reported, when compared with populations in iodine sufficient areas. Mental retardation caused by the effect of iodine deficiency is not reversible. Iodine deficiency may also result in increased auditory threshold and increased perinatal and infant mortality. Based on median urinary iodine concentration in the population, severity of iodine deficiency in the community may be classified as in Table 37.8.

Diagnosis: **Iodine nutrition is assessed by 1. Urinary iodine levels, 2. Thyroid size and 3. Serum TSH and Thyroglobulin.** Iodine concentration in a random urinary sample is used in epidemiological studies to assessing adequacy of iodine levels. 90% or more of ingested iodine appear in urine eventually. Random urinary iodine concentration correlates well with urinary iodine/creatinine ratio and 24 hr urinary iodine. Elevated TSH in neonatal hypothyroidism screening correlates with severity of iodine deficiency. Serum thyroglobulin level is elevated in children with iodine deficiency. This is a sensitive but non-specific test. The values correlate with severity of iodine deficiency.

Thyroid size is a sensitive but non-specific marker for iodine deficiency. Ultrasound is helpful for quantification. Radioactive iodine uptake is increased in iodine deficiency, but the test is not routinely necessary. T3, T4 and TSH are usually within the normal ranges in most patients and are not sensitive in detecting iodine deficiency.

Prophylaxis and Treatment

Iodization of salt: Universal salt iodisation (USI) defined as iodisation of all salt used for human and animal consumption is the main strategy used to control iodine deficiency. It is an easy and effective way for iodine supplementation. 10–50 gm per kg of salt as potassium iodide or iodate is added. Adequately iodised salt contains 15 mg iodide per kg salt at the household level. For salt iodisation to have the desired impact and protect children from brain damage, adequately iodised salt should be accessible and used by at least by 90 percent of the households on a regular basis.

Alternatives to iodised salt are iodized oil (lipiodol), iodised water, iodine tablets or drops. Lipiodol contains 480 mg/ml of iodine and 0.5 –1 ml oral dose supplies enough iodine to last 6 mo to a year.

Table 37.8: Severity of IDD according to mean urinary iodine levels and iodine intake		
Median Urinary iodine (mcg/L)	*Corresponding iodine intake (mcg/day)*	*Severity*
<20	<30	Severe
20–49	30–74	Moderate
50–99	75–149	Mild
100–199	150–299	Optimal
200–299	300–499	More than adequate
>299	>499	Possible excess

Source ICCIDD

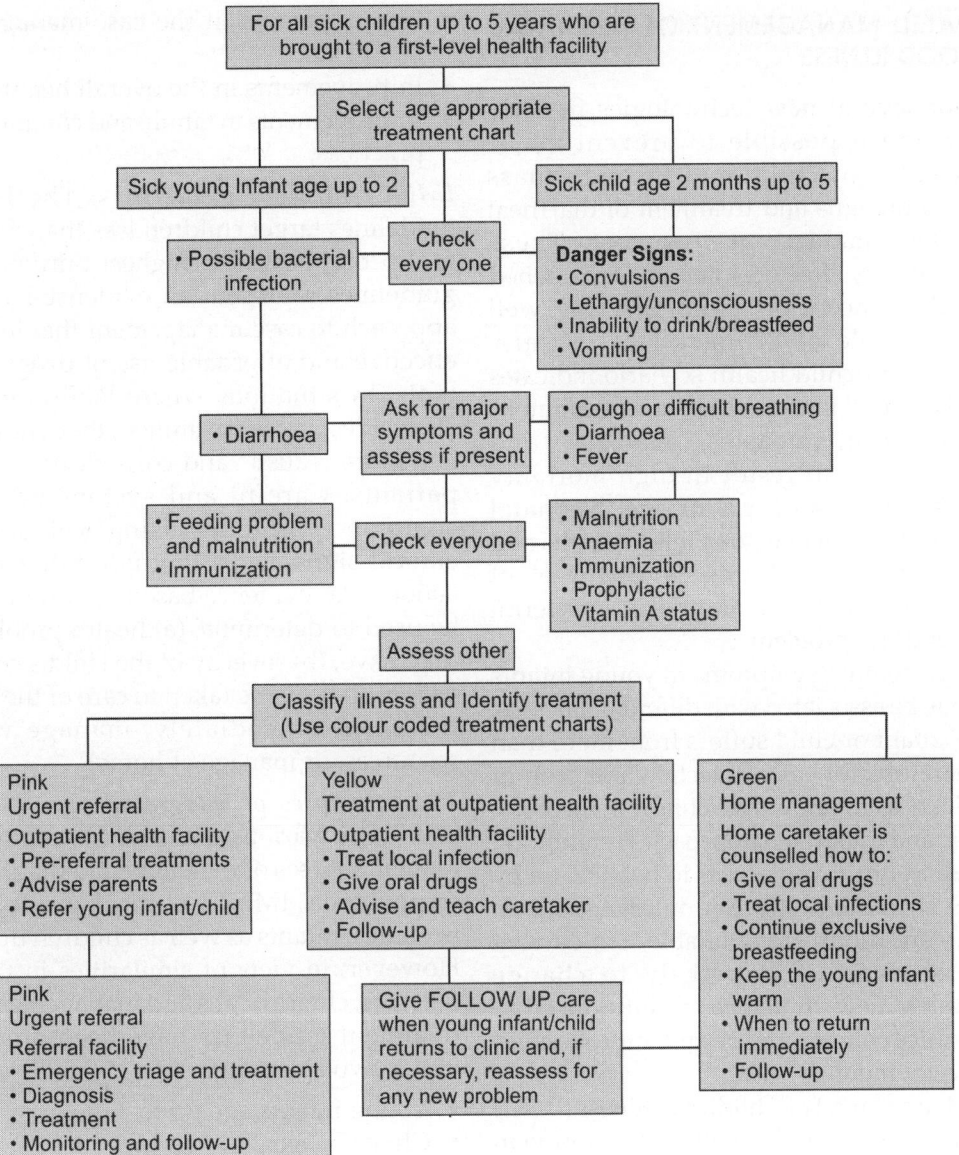

Fig. 37.1: IMNCI Case Management Process

Intramuscular injection of the same supplies enough iodine for 2–3 yrs.

Other options include tablets or solution of potassium iodide. For sustaining iodine sufficiency, regular monitoring of iodine nutrition essential.

Anderson M, Takkouche B, Egli I, Allen HE, de Benoist B. Current global iodine status and progress over the last decade towards the elimination of iodine deficiency. *Bull World Health Organ* 2005; 83(7): 518–525.

de Benoist B, Andersson M, Takkouche B, Egli I. Prevalence of iodine deficiency worldwide. *Lancet* 2003 Nov 29; 362(9398): 1859–1860.

Hetzel BS. Iodine Deficiency Disorders (IDD) and their eradication. *Lancet* 1983; 2 (8359): 1126–1129.

Sheila C Vir. Current Status of Iodine Deficiency Diseases and Strategy for Its control in *India Indian J Pediatr* 2002: 69 : 589–596.

Salt Department, Ministry of Industry. Universal Salt Iodisation (USI). India: progress and current status. New Delhi, 1996: 8.

WHO, UNICEF, ICCIDD. Recommended iodine levels in salt and guidelines for monitoring their adequacy and effectiveness. WHO/NUT/96.13. Geneva. 1996.

World Health Organization. Iodine and Health. A statement by the World Health Organization. WHO/NUT/94.4. Geneva, 1994.

WHO, UNICEF, ICCIDD. Recommended iodine levels in salt and guidelines for monitoring their adequacy and effectiveness. WHO/NUT/96.13. Geneva, 1996.

37.6 INTEGRATED MANAGEMENT OF NEONATAL AND CHILDHOOD ILLNESS

Introduction of several new technologies in early 1980's have made it possible to prevent major infectious diseases of childhood through mass immunization campaigns and treatment of diarrheal dehydration and malaria at low cost. These inexpensive and highly effective interventions opened our vision to the concept of 'Child Survival' well beyond the principle of Primary Health Care. However, the current child health scenario indicates that common childhood illnesses like acute respiratory infections, diarrhea, measles, malaria, and malnutrition continue to result in high mortality among children less than 5 yrs of age. Neonatal mortality contributes to over 64% of infant deaths and most of these deaths occur during the first week of life. Poor access to health care and delay in referral further compound the problem.

Most of the presenting symptoms in young infants and children may be associated with different illnesses. Often a young infant or child suffers from more than one illness. Therefore, for early detection and prompt treatment of sickness in under five children, there is a need for holistic and integrated approach to childhood illnesses as well as improved access to health care by community. Even though effective interventions to manage these conditions are available, the current child health scenario is not likely to change significantly unless new strategies are introduced to significantly reduce child mortality and improve child health and development.

Integrated Management of Childhood Illness (IMCI) strategy, developed by World Health Organization in collaboration with UNICEF and many other agencies in mid-1990s, combines improved management of common childhood illnesses as well as prevention of diseases and promotion of health by dealing with counselling on feeding, immunization and assessment of other problems. This strategy has been expanded in India to include neonatal care at home as well as in the health facilities and renamed *'Integrated Management of Neonatal and Childhood Illness (IMNCI)'*.

Essential components of IMNCI strategy: The IMNCI strategy includes both preventive and curative interventions that aim to improve practices in health facilities, the health system and at home. At the core of the strategy is integrated case management of the most common neonatal and childhood problems with a focus on the most common causes of death in under five children. The strategy includes three main components:

- Improvements in the case-management skills of health staff;
- Improvements in the overall health system;
- Improvements in family and community health care practices.

IMNCI clinical guidelines: The IMNCI clinical guidelines target children less than 5 yrs old, the age group that bears the highest burden of deaths. The guidelines represent an evidence-based, syndromic approach to case management that includes rational, effective and affordable use of drugs and diagnostic tools. In situations where laboratory support and clinical resources are limited, the syndromic approach is a more realistic and cost-effective way to manage patients. Careful and systematic assessment of common symptoms, using well-selected reliable clinical signs, helps to guide rational and effective actions. An evidence-based syndromic approach can be used to determine: (a) health problem(s) the child may have, (b) severity of the child's condition and (c) actions that can be taken to care of the child (e.g. refer the child immediately, manage with available resources, or manage at home).

The principles of integrated care: Depending on a child's age, various clinical signs and symptoms differ in their degrees of reliability and diagnostic value and importance. IMNCI clinical guidelines focus on neonates, infants as well as children up to 5 yrs of age. However, in view of similarities in the spectrum of illnesses, clinical signs and management protocols, the treatment guidelines have been broadly described under two age categories:

- Young infants age up to 2 mo
- Children age 2 mo up to 5 yrs

The IMNCI guidelines are based on the following principles:

- *All children* under 5 yrs of age must be examined for conditions which indicate *immediate referral*.
- Children must be *routinely assessed* for: Major symptoms, Nutritional and immunization status, Feeding problems and other problems.
- Only a limited number of carefully *selected clinical signs* are used for assessment.
- *'Classification'*—a combination of individual signs is used rather than a 'diagnosis'. Classifications are colour coded and suggest referral **(pink)**, treatment in health facility (yellow) or management at home **(green)**.
- IMNCI guidelines address *most common*, but not all pediatric problems.
- IMNCI management procedures use a limited number of *essential drugs*.
- Caretakers are *actively involved* in the treatment of children.

- Counselling of caretakers about *home care* including feeding, fluids and when to return to health facility is an essential component of IMCI.

IMNCI Case Management Process

Steps of Case Management Process (Fig.37.1) are:

- Assess the young infant/child
- Classify the illness
- Identify Treatment
- Treat the young infant/child
- Counsel the mother
- Follow up care

In the classification table (see IMNCI Chart), a young infant/child receives classifications in one colour only. If the young infant has signs from more than one row, always select the most severe **(pink)** classifications. However, if the classification table has *more than one arm* (Possible Bacterial Infection/Jaundice and Diarrhea in a young infant, and Diarrhea and Fever in a sick child), one can choose a classification from each arm. Classification tables are used starting with the **pink** rows. If the young infant does not have the severe classifications, look at the **yellow** rows. For the classification tables that have a **green** row, if the young infant does not have any of the signs in the pink or yellow rows, select the classification in the green row.

Effective Communication with the mother/care provider

It is critical to communicate effectively with the infant's mother or caretaker. Good communication techniques and an integrated assessment are required to ensure that common problems or signs of disease or malnutrition are not overlooked. Proper communication helps to reassure the mother or caretaker that the infant will receive appropriate care. In addition, the success of home treatment depends on how well the mother or caretaker knows about giving the treatment and understands its importance. Good communication skills based on principles of **APAC** (Ask and Listen, Praise, Advise and Check) are helpful for effective counseling.

Outpatient Management of Young Infants Age up to 2 Mo

Assess and Classify Sick Young Infants

Young infants have special characteristics that must be considered when classifying their illness. They can become sick and die very quickly from serious bacterial infections. They frequently have only general signs such as a few movements, fever or low body temperature. Mild chest indrawing is normal in young infants because their chest wall is soft. For these reasons, assessment, classification and treatment of young infant is somewhat different from an older infant or young child. The assessment procedure for this age group includes a number of important steps that must be followed by the health care provider, including: 1. history taking and communicating with the caretaker about the young infant's problem; 2. checking for possible bacterial infection/jaundice; 3. checking for diarrhea; 4. checking for feeding problem or malnutrition; 5. checking immunization status; and 6. assessing other problems (Tables 37.9 to 37.12).

Checking for Possible Bacterial Infection /Jaundice

All sick young infants must be assessed first for signs of possible bacterial infection and jaundice. A young infant can become sick and die very quickly from serious bacterial infections such as pneumonia, sepsis and meningitis. It is important to assess the signs in the order mentioned in the chart. The young infant *must be calm* and may be asleep while assessing the first five signs, that is, count breathing and looking for chest indrawing, nasal flaring, grunting and bulging fontanelle. To assess the next few signs, undress the young infant, look at the skin all over his body and measure his temperature.

Clinical Assessment

Many clinical signs point to possible bacterial infection in sick young infants. The most informative and easy to check signs are: *Convulsions* (as part of the current illness), Fast breathing (The cut-off rate to identify fast breathing in young infants is 60 breaths per minute or more. If the count is 60 breaths or more, the count should be repeated, because the breathing rate of a young infant is often irregular. If the second count is also 60 breaths or more, the young infant has fast breathing); *Severe chest indrawing; Nasal flaring; Grunting; Bulging fontanelle; Umbilicus red or draining pus ; Pus draining from the ear; Skin pustules; Temperature; Lethargy or unconsciousness; Less than normal movement; Jaundice.*

Classification of Possible Bacterial Infection/Jaundice

- *All sick young infants* are classified for Possible Bacterial Infection. There are only two classifications under this category. If any of the signs shown in the top (pink) row of the classification table are present, classify as **POSSIBLE SERIOUS BACTERIAL INFECTION**. If none of the signs in the pink row are present and any of the signs in the yellow box are present classify as **LOCAL BACTERIAL INFECTION**. If none of the signs in the pink or yellow row are present, there is **no classification** for Possible Bacterial Infection.

- **Additionally if the sick young infant has Jaundice**, classify as SEVERE JAUNDICE if any of the signs in pink row are present. If none of the signs in the pink row are present, classify as JAUNDICE.
- **Additionally, sick young infants who have axillary temperature between 35.5 amd 36.4°C (both inclusive)** should also be classified as 'Low Body Temperature'. Low body temperature in such cases could be the due to inadequate clothing in cold weather or be a sign of bacterial infection.

Checking for Diarrhea

A young infant is considered to have diarrhea if the stools have changed from usual pattern and are many and watery (more water than faecal matter). Babies who are exclusively breastfed often have stools that are soft; this is not diarrhea. Ask the mother/caretaker if young infant has diarrhea. If the answer is 'yes', assess for diarrhea. A young infant with diarrhea can be placed in one of the following 3 categories: 1. acute watery diarrhea; 2. dysentery (bloody diarrhea); and 3. persistent diarrhea (diarrhea that lasts more than 14 days).

Clinical Assessment

All infants with diarrhea should be assessed to determine the duration of diarrhea, if blood is present in the stool and if dehydration is present. A number of clinical signs are used to determine the level of dehydration: *Infant's general condition* (lethargic or unconscious or restless/irritable); *Sunken eyes* and *Elasticity of skin* (skin pinch goes back very slowly, slowly or immediately).

Classification of Dehydration

All young infants with diarrhea should be classified for dehydration based on a combination of clinical signs detected on assessment. Dehydration is classified into three categories: Young infants identified by any two of the signs in pink row are classified as **SEVERE DEHYDRATION**. Those who have any of the two signs in yellow row are classified as **SOME DEHYDRATION**. If enough signs to classify as severe or some dehydration are not present, the young infant is classified as **NO DEHYDRATION** (green row).

Classification of Persistent Diarrhea

Persistent diarrhea is an episode of diarrhea, with or without blood, which begins acutely and lasts at least 14 days. It accounts for up to 15% of all episodes of diarrhea but is associated with 30 to 50% of deaths. Persistent diarrhea is usually associated with weight loss and often with serious non-intestinal infections. Many infants and children who develop persistent diarrhea are malnourished, greatly increasing the risk of death. Persistent diarrhea is uncommon in infants who are exclusively breastfed. All young infants with diarrhea lasting for 14 days or more are considered 'severe' cases and these classified as **Severe Persistent Diarrhea**.

Classification of Dysentery

The mother or caretaker of a child with diarrhea should be asked if there is blood in the stool. All young infants with blood in the stools are considered 'severe' cases and therefore classified as **Severe Dysentery**. Blood in the stool in a young infant may often be due to systemic or surgical causes rather than gastro-intestinal infection.

Checking for Feeding Problems or Malnutrition

All sick young infants seen in outpatient health facilities should be assessed for weight and adequate feeding, as well as for breast-feeding technique (see IMNCI Chart-Council the mother about feeding problems).

Clinical Assessment

Assessment of feeding and malnutrition: In order to decide whether *Assessment of Breastfeeding* is necessary, ask questions to determine if the mother is having difficulty feeding the infant, and by determining weight for age.

a. *Ask:* Is there any feeding difficulty? Is the infant breastfed? If yes, how many times in 24 hrs? Does the infant usually receive any other foods or drinks? If yes, how often? What do you use to feed the infant?

b. *Determine weight for age:* Weight for age compares the young infant's weight with the infants of the same age in the reference population (*see* IMNCI Chart: WHO Child Growth Standards). The VERY LOW WEIGHT FOR AGE identifies children whose weight is −3 standard deviations below the mean weight of infants in the reference population (Z score <−3). The LOW WEIGHT FOR AGE identifies children whose weight is −2 standard deviations below the mean weight of infants in the reference population (Z score <−2). Infants who are Very Low Weight for Age should be referred to a hospital. Infants who are Low Weight for Age need special attention to how they are fed and on keeping them warm.

How to assess breastfeeding: If the mother complains of any feeding difficulty or the infant's weight is below the weight for age line, observe a breastfeed as descried below. Low weight for age is often due to low birth weight. Low birth weight infants are particularly likely to have a problem with breastfeeding. Assessing breastfeeding requires careful observation. If the infant has not been fed in the previous hour, he may be willing to breastfeed. Ask the mother to put her infant to the breast. Observe a whole breastfeed if possible, or observe for at least 4 minutes. Sit quietly and watch the infant breastfeed (*see* IMNCI Chart- counsel the mother about feeding problems).

Is the infant able to attach?: The four signs of good attachment are (If all of these four signs are present, the infant has good attachment: i. chin touching breast (or very close), ii. mouth wide open, iii. lower lip turned outward and iv. more areola visible above than below the mouth. If a very sick infant cannot take the nipple into his mouth and keep it there to suck, he has no attachment at all. He is not able to breastfeed at all. If an infant is not well attached, the results may be pain and damage to the nipples. Or the infant may not be able to remove breast milk effectively, which may cause engorgement of the breast. All these problems may improve if attachment can be improved.

Is the infant suckling effectively? (that is, slow deep sucks, sometimes pausing): The infant is suckling effectively if he suckles with slow deep sucks and sometimes pauses. You may see or hear the infant swallowing. An infant is not suckling effectively if he is taking only rapid, shallow sucks, and you do not see or hear swallowing. The infant is not satisfied at the end of the feed, and may be restless. He may cry or try to suckle again, or continue to breastfeed for a long time. An infant who is not suckling at all is not able to suck breast milk into his mouth and swallow. Therefore he is not able to breastfeed at all. If a blocked nose seems to interfere with breastfeeding, clear the infant's nose. Then check whether the infant can suckle more effectively. *Look for ulcers or white patches in the mouth (thrush).*

Classification of Feeding Problems and Malnutrition

Based on an assessment of feeding and weight, a sick young infant may be classified into one of the three categories. If any of the signs in the pink row are present classify as *not able to feed—possible serious bacterial infection or severe malnutrition.* If there are no signs in the pink row and any of the signs listed in yellow row are present classify as *feeding problems or low weight.* If there are no signs in pink or yellow row classify as *no feeding problem.*

Checking Immunization Status

Immunization status should be checked in *all sick young infants.* A young infant who is not sick enough to be referred to a hospital should be given the necessary immunizations before he is sent home.

Assessing other Problems

All sick young infants need to be assessed for other potential problems mentioned by the mother or observed during the examination. If a potentially serious problem is found or there is no means in the clinic to help the infant, he should be referred to hospital.

Treatment of Sick Young Infants

The first step is to *Identify Treatment* required for the young infant according to the classification. All the treatments required are listed in the "Identify Treatment" column of the *Assess* and *Classify the Sick Young Infant* chart. If a sick young infant has more than one classification, treatment required for all the classifications must be identified. For some young infants, the *Assess* and *Classify the Sick Young Infant* chart says "Refer *Urgently* to hospital." 'Hospital' pertains to a health facility with inpatient beds, supplies and expertise to treat a very sick young infant. Referral may mean admission to the inpatient department of the same facility where the young infant has been examined as an outpatient.

Referral of Sick Young Infants age up to 2 mo

All infants and children with a severe classification (pink) are referred to a hospital as soon as assessment is completed and necessary pre-referral treatment is administered. However, if an infant only has severe dehydration and no other severe classification, and IV infusion is available in the outpatient clinic, an attempt should be made to rehydrate the sick infant. Successful referral of severely ill infants to the hospital depends on effective counselling of the caretaker. The first step to give *Urgent Pre-referral Treatment(s). Possible Pre-referral Treatments* include:

- First dose of intramuscular ampicillin and gentamicin. (*If referral is not possible, give oral amoxicillin every 8 hrs and intramuscular gentamicin once daily*).
- If infant is convulsing, give diazepam IV or rectally.
- Treatment of severe dehydration according to Plan C of WHO Guidelines for treatment of dehydration.
- Keeping the infant warm on the way to the hospital.
- Prevention of hypoglycemia with breast milk or sugar water (4 level teaspoons of sugar in a 200 mL cup of clean water). If young infant is not able to swallow give expressed breast milk/appropriate animal milk with added sugar/sugar water by NG tube.
- In young infants with diarrhea, giving frequent sips of ORS solution on the way to the hospital.

Treatment in Outpatient Clinics

- Counselling a mother/caretaker is critical not only for successful referral of a severely ill young infant but also treatment in the outpatients clinic as well as for home care. Use good communication skills from the beginning of the visit particularly while counselling the mother/caretaker for treatment. Following principles are helpful for effective counselling: *Ask* and *Listen* to find out the infant's problems and what the mother is already doing for the infant; Praise the mother for what she has done well; *Advise* her how to care for her infant at home; and *Check* the mother's understanding before she leaves.

- Treat 'Some' and 'No' dehydration according to Plan B and Plan A respectively, as per WHO Guidelines for treatment of dehydration.

- Treat local bacterial infection with oral antibiotic (amooxycillin or cotrimoxazole) and administer the first dose in the clinic. In addition, the mother/caretaker should be taught how to give an oral antibiotic at home. Avoid cotrimoxazole in infants less than 1 month of age who are premature or jaundiced.

- *Teach* the mother to apply 0.5% gentian violet twice daily for umbilicus that is red or draining pus and skin pustules. For oral thrush use 0.25% gentian violet twice daily. *Show* the mother how to wick her child's ear dry. Advise her to dry the ear 3 times daily.

Teach correct positioning and attachment for breast-feeding: Positioning is important because poor positioning often results in poor attachment, especially in younger infants. If the infant is positioned well, the attachment is likely to be good. *Good positioning* is recognized by the following signs: infant's neck is straight or bent slightly back; infant's body is turned towards the mother; infant's body is close to the mother, and infant's whole body is supported, not just neck and shoulders. *Poor positioning* is recognized by any of the following signs: infant's neck is twisted or bent forward; infant's body is turned away from mother; infant's body is not close to mother or only the infant's head and neck are supported.

If in your assessment of breastfeeding you find any difficulty with attachment or suckling, help the mother position and attach her infant better. Make sure that the mother is comfortable and relaxed. Explain and demonstrate what you want her to do. Then let the mother position and attach the infant herself. Then look for signs of good attachment and effective suckling again. If the attachment or suckling is not good, ask the mother to remove the infant from her breast and to try again. When the infant is suckling well, explain to the mother that it is important to breastfeed long enough at each feed. She should not stop the breastfeeding before the infant wants to.

Teach the mother to manage breast and nipple problems: During the first few weeks after birth, breast and nipple problems can be important causes of feeding problems and poor growth in young infants. Some of the common problems are flat or inverted nipples, sore nipples or breast abscess in the mother. Reassure the mother, give appropriate advise, support and treatment if necessary.

Counselling about other Feeding Problems

- If a mother is breastfeeding her infant less than 8 times in 24 hrs, advise her to increase the frequency of breastfeeding. Breastfeed as often and for as long as the infant wants, day and night.

- If the infant receives other foods or drinks, counsel the mother about breastfeeding more, reducing the amount of the other foods or drinks, and if possible, stopping altogether. Advise her to feed the infant any other drinks from a cup, and not from a feeding bottle.

- If the mother does not breastfeed at all, consider referring her for breastfeeding counseling and possible re-lactation. If the mother is interested, a breastfeeding counselor may be able to help her to overcome difficulties and begin breastfeeding again. Advise a mother who does not breastfeed about choosing and correctly preparing dairy/locally appropriate animal milk. Also advise her to feed the young infant with a cup, and not from a feeding bottle.

Advise when to Return

- A mother is advised **return immediately** if the infant has any of these signs: *Breastfeeding or drinking poorly; Becomes sicker; Develops a fever or feels cold to touch; Fast breathing; Difficult breathing; Yellow palms and soles (if young infant has jaundice); Diarrhea with blood in stool.*

- A sick young Infant should be brought again for follow up after 2 days if he has *local bacterial infection, jaundice, diarrhea, any feeding problem or oral thrush. For low weight for age* advise follow up after 14 days.

- Next **Well-Child Visit** for the next immunization according to immunization schedule.

Follow-up Care

If the child *does not have a new* problem, use the IMNCI follow-up instructions for each specific problem. Assess the child according to the instructions; Use the information about the child's signs to select the appropriate treatment; give appropriate treatment.

Counsel the Mother about her own Health

During a sick infant visit, listen for any problems that the mother herself may be having. The mother may need treatment or referral for her own health problems. If the mother is sick, provide care for her, or refer her for help. Advise her to eat well to keep up her own strength and health. Check the mother's immunization status and give her tetanus toxoid if needed. Give the mother iron folic acid tablets if she is not already taken them. Make sure she has access to family planning and counselling on STD and AIDS prevention.

Outpatient Management of Sick Child age 2 mo up to 5 Yr

Assess and Classify Sick Child

The assessment procedure for this age group includes a number of important steps (*see* IMNCI Charts, Color Plates 4 to 8) that must be taken by the health care provider, including: (1) history taking and communicating with the caretaker about the child's problem; (2) checking for general danger signs; (3) checking main symptoms; (4) checking for malnutrition; (5) checking for anaemia; (6) assessing the child's feeding; (7) checking immunization status; and (8) assessing other problems.

Checking for General Danger Signs

A sick child brought to an outpatient facility may have signs that clearly indicate a specific problem. For example, a child may present with chest indrawing and cyanosis, which indicate severe pneumonia. However, some children may present with serious, non-specific signs called *"General Danger Signs"* that do not point to a particular diagnosis. For example, a child who is lethargic or unconscious may have meningitis, severe pneumonia, cerebral malaria or any other severe disease. Great care should be taken to ensure that these general danger signs are not overlooked because they suggest that a child is severely ill and needs urgent attention. The following *general danger signs* should be routinely checked in all children: i. History of convulsions during the present illness, ii. unconsciousness or lethargy, iii. inability to drink or breastfeed when mother tries to breastfeed or to give the child something to drink, and iv. child vomits everything.

If a child has *one or more* of these signs, he must be considered *seriously ill* and will almost always need referral. In order to start treatment for severe illnesses without delay, the child should be quickly assessed for the most important causes of serious illness and death—cough or difficult breathing (acute respiratory infection), diarrhea, and fever (especially associated

with malaria and measles). A rapid assessment of nutritional status is also essential, as malnutrition is another main cause of death in this age group.

Checking Main Symptoms

After checking for general danger signs, the health care provider must check for the following main symptoms: 1. cough or difficult breathing; 2. diarrhea; 3. fever; and 4. ear problems. The first three symptoms are included because they often result in death. Ear problems are included because they are considered one of the main causes of childhood disability.

a. Assess Cough or Difficult Breathing

A child with cough or difficult breathing may have pneumonia or severe respiratory infection. In developing countries, pneumonia is often due to bacterial infection. The most common are *Streptococcus pneumoniae* and *Hemophilus influenzae*. Children with bacterial pneumonia may die from hypoxia or sepsis. Many children are brought to the clinic with less serious respiratory infections. Most children with cough or difficult breathing have only a mild infection. They do not need treatment with antibiotics. Their families can manage them at home. Very sick children with cough or difficult breathing need to be identified as they require antibiotic therapy. Fortunately, one can identify almost all cases of pneumonia by checking for these two clinical signs: fast breathing and chest indrawing. Chest indrawing is a sign of severe pneumonia.

Clinical Assessment

A child presenting with cough or difficult breathing should first be assessed for general danger signs. This child may have pneumonia or another severe respiratory infection. Three key clinical signs are used to assess a sick child with cough or difficult breathing: Fast Breathing (Cut-off respiratory rate for Fast Breathing is 50 breaths per minute or more for a child 2 mo up to 12 mo, and 40 breaths per minute or more for 12 mo up to 5 yrs); Lower chest wall indrawing and Stridor in calm child.

Classification of Cough or Difficult Breathing

Based on a combination of the above clinical signs, children presenting with cough or difficult breathing can be classified into one of the three categories. If a child has any of the signs in the pink row classify as *severe pneumonia or very severe disease.* If there are no signs in pink row but fast breathing is present classify as *PNEUMONIA.* If there are no signs of very severe disease or pneumonia classify as *no pneumonia: cough or cold.* A child with cough or cold normally improves in one or two weeks. However, a child with chronic cough (more than 30 days) needs to be further assessed (and, if needed, referred) to exclude tuberculosis, asthma, whooping cough or any other problem.

b. Assess Diarrhea

Diarrhea occurs when stools contain more water than normal. It is common in children, especially those between 6 mo and 2 yrs of age. In many regions diarrhea is defined as three or more loose or watery stools in a 24-hr period. Frequent passing of normal stools in not diarrhea. Mothers usually know when their children have diarrhea. They may say that the child's stools are loose or watery. Mothers may use a local word for diarrhea. A child with diarrhea may have 1. acute watery diarrhea (including cholera); 2. dysentery (bloody diarrhea); and 3. persistent diarrhea (diarrhea that lasts 14 days or more).

Most diarrheal episodes are caused by agents for which antimicrobials are not effective and therefore antibiotics should not be used routinely for treatment of diarrhea. Anti-diarrheal drugs *do not* provide practical benefits for children with acute diarrhea, and some may have dangerous side effects. Therefore these drugs should never be given to children less than 5 yrs old.

Clinical Assessment

Ask the mother/caretaker if the child has diarrhea. If yes, check to determine the duration of diarrhea, presence of blood in the stool and signs of dehydration. All children with diarrhea should be assessed for dehydration based on the following clinical signs: *Child's general condition* (lethargic or unconscious or restless/irritable); *Sunken eyes; Child's response when offered to drink* (not able to drink or drinking poorly or drinking eagerly/thirsty or drinking normally) and elasticity of skin (skin pinch goes back very slowly, slowly or immediately). After the child is assessed for dehydration, the caretaker of a child with diarrhea should be asked how long the child has had diarrhea and if there is blood in the stool. This will allow identification of children with persistent diarrhea and dysentery.

Classification of Dehydration

Based on a combination of the above clinical signs, children presenting with diarrhea are classified into one of the three categories. A child is classified as *severe dehydration* if he has any combination of two signs in the pink row. If not, look at the yellow row. If he has any combination of two signs in the yellow row classify as some dehydration. If there are not enough

signs to classify severe or some dehydration, classify as no dehydration.

Classification of Persistent Diarrhea

Persistent diarrhea is usually associated with weight loss and often with serious non-intestinal infections. Many children who develop persistent diarrhea are malnourished, greatly increasing the risk of death. Persistent diarrhea is uncommon in infants who are exclusively breastfed. All children with diarrhea for 14 days or more should be classified based on the presence or absence of dehydration.

Classification of Dysentery

Bloody diarrhea in young children is usually a sign of invasive enteric infection that carries a substantial risk of serious morbidity and death. About 10% of all diarrhea episodes in children under 5 yrs old are dysenteric, but these cause up to 15% of all diarrheal deaths. Dysentery is especially severe in infants and in children who are undernourished, who develop clinically evident dehydration during their illness, or who are not breastfed. It also has a more harmful effect on nutritional status than acute watery diarrhea. Dysentery occurs with increased frequency and severity in children who have measles or have had measles in the preceding month. Diarrheal episodes that begin with dysentery are more likely to become persistent than those that start without blood in the stool. Ask the mother or caretaker of a child with diarrhea if there is blood in the stool. A child is classified as having dysentery if the mother or caretaker reports blood in the child's stool.

c. Assess Fever

Fever is a very common condition and is often the main reason for bringing children to the health centre. It may be caused by minor infections, but may also be the most obvious sign of a life-threatening illness, particularly malaria (especially lethal *P. falciparum* malaria), or other severe infections, including meningitis, typhoid fever, or measles. When diagnostic capacity is limited, it is important first to identify those children who need urgent referral with appropriate pre-referral treatment (antimalarial or antibacterial). All sick children should be checked for fever if there is history of fever, child feels hot or temperature is recorded 37.5°C or above.

Clinical Assessment

A child presenting with fever should be assessed for: Risk of malaria (high and low malaria risk); Duration of fever (history of fever more than seven days can mean that the child has a more severe disease such as typhoid fever. If the fever has been present for more than seven days, it is important to check whether the fever has been present every day); Bulging fontanelle; Stiff neck; Runny nose (when malaria risk is low, a child with fever and a runny nose does probably have a common cold); Measles (now or within the last three months). If the child has measles currently or within the last three months, he should be assessed for possible complications. Measles damages the epithelial surfaces and the immune system, and lowers vitamin A levels. It is important to check every child with recent or current measles for possible mouth or eye complications. Clouding of the cornea is a dangerous eye complication. It may be due to vitamin A deficiency that has been made worse by measles. If not treated, cornea can ulcerate and cause blindness. An infant with corneal clouding needs urgent treatment with vitamin A. Before classifying fever, check for other obvious causes of fever.

Classification of Fever

Children with fever and any general danger sign or stiff neck are classified as having *VERY SEVERE FEBRILE DISEASE*. Further classifications depend on the level of malaria risk in the area. In a high malaria risk area, children with fever and no general danger sign or stiff neck should be classified as having *MALARIA*. In a low malarial risk area, children with fever and no general danger sign or stiff neck are classified as having *MALARIA* but those with runny nose, measles or clinical signs of other possible infection are classified as having *FEVER-MALARIA UNLIKELY*.

Classification of Measles

All children with fever should be checked for signs of current or recent measles (within the last three months) and measles complications. A child is classified as *severe complicated measles* is if he has any of the signs in pink row. If there are no signs in the pink row but one of the signs in yellow row classify the child as *MEASLES with eye or mouth complications*. If none of the signs shown in pink or yellow row are present classify as *measles*.

d. Assess Ear Problems

A child with an ear problem may have otitis. It may be acute or chronic infection. If the infection is not treated, the eardrum may perforate. Although ear infections rarely cause death, they are the main cause of deafness in low-income areas, which in turn leads to learning problems. Sometimes the infection can spread from the ear and cause mastoiditis. Infection can also spread from the ear to the brain causing

meningitis. Ask the mother/caretaker if the child has any ear problem. If yes, assess the child for ear problem.

Clinical Assessment

Ask about history of ear pain and ear discharge or pus. Examine the ear with an otoscope if available. Also look for tender swelling behind the ear.

Classification of Ear Problems

A child is classified as *mastoiditis* if there is a tender swelling behind the ear. If pus is seen draining from the ear and discharge is reported for less than 14 days or he/she has ear pain classify as *acute ear infection*. If pus is seen draining from the ear and discharge is reported for 14 days or more classify as *chronic ear infection*. If *no* ear pain and *no* ear discharge seen draining from the ear classify as *no ear infection*.

Checking for Malnutrition

After assessing for general danger signs and the four main symptoms, **all children should be assessed for malnutrition**. There are two main reasons for routine assessment of nutritional status in sick children: 1. to identify children with severe malnutrition who are at increased risk of mortality and need urgent referral to provide active treatment; and 2. to identify children with sub-optimal growth (stunting) resulting from ongoing deficits in dietary intake plus repeated episodes of infection and who may benefit from nutritional counselling and resolution of feeding problems.

Clinical Assessment

Visible severe wasting: This is defined as severe wasting of the shoulders, arms, buttocks, and legs, with ribs easily seen, and indicates presence of marasmus. To look for visible severe wasting, remove the child's clothes. Look for severe wasting of the muscles of the shoulders, arms, buttocks and legs. Look to see if the outline of the child's ribs is easily seen. Look at the child's hips. They may look small when you compare them with the chest and abdomen. Look at the child from the side to see if the fat of the buttocks is missing. When wasting is extreme, there are many folds of skin on the buttocks and thigh. It looks as if the child is wearing baggy pants. The face of a child with visible severe wasting may still look normal. The child's abdomen may be large or distended.

Oedema of both feet: The presence of oedema in both feet may signal kwashiorkor.

Weight for age: Plotting weight for age in the growth chart, based on reference population (*see* IMNCI

Chart-WHO Child Growth Standards), helps to identify children with *low* (Z score less than -2) or *very low* (Z score less than-3) weight for age, those who are at increased risk of infection and poor growth and development.

Classification of Nutritional Status

Using a combination of the simple clinical signs above, children can be classified in one of the 3 categories. Children with visible severe wasting or oedema of both feet are classified as *severe malnutrition* (pink row). If there are no signs in pink row but the child has very low weight for age classify as *very low weight* (yellow row). If there are no signs in pink or yellow row classify as *not very low weight*.

Checking for Anaemia

All children also should be assessed for anaemia. The most common cause of anaemia in young children in developing countries is nutritional or because of parasitic or helminthic infections. However, there may be other more serious causes of anaemia such as haemolytic anaemia, aplastic anaemia or leukaemia.

Clinical Assessment

Palmar pallor: Palmar pallor can help to identify sick children with severe anaemia. Wherever feasible, diagnosis of anaemia can be supported by using a simple laboratory test for hemoglobin estimation. For clinical assessment of anaemia compare the colour of the child's palm with your own palm and with the palms of other children. If the skin of the child's palm is pale, the child has *some palmar pallor*. If the skin of the palm is very pale or so pale that it looks white, the child has *severe palmar pallor*.

Classification of Anaemia

Children can be classified in one of the following 3 categories. Children with severe palmar pallor are classified as *SEVERE ANAEMIA* (pink row), those with some pallor as *ANAEMIA* (yellow row) and those who don't have any palmar pallor as *NO ANAEMIA* (green row).

Assessing the Child's Feeding

All children *less than 2 yrs old* and *all children classified* as *anaemia or very low weight* need to be assessed for feeding even if they have a normal Z-score. Feeding assessment includes questioning the mother or caretaker about: 1. breastfeeding frequency and night feeds; 2. types of complementary foods or fluids, frequency of feeding and whether feeding is active; and 3. feeding patterns during the current illness. The mother or caretaker should be given

appropriate advice to help overcome any feeding problems found. However, if the mother has already received many treatment instructions and is overwhelmed, you may delay assessing feeding and counselling the mother about feeding until a later visit. When counseling a mother about feeding, one should use the same communication skills *(APAC)* described earlier. To assess feeding, ask the mother the questions detailed in Annex. I. One must listen for correct feeding practices as well as those that need to be changed that are appropriate for the child's age.

Identify feeding problems

It is important to complete the assessment of feeding and identify all the feeding problems before giving advice. Based on the mother's answers to the feeding questions, identify any differences between the child's actual feeding and the feeding recommendations. These differences are problems. In addition to differences from the feeding recommendations, some other problems may become apparent from the mother's answers. Other common feeding problems are: *Difficulty breastfeeding, use of feeding bottle, lack of active feeding and not feeding well during illness.*

Checking Immunization, Vitamin A and Folic Acid Supplementation Status

The immunization status of *every sick child* brought to a health facility should be checked. Illness is not a contraindication to immunization. In practice, sick children may be even more in need of protection provided by immunization than well children. A vaccine's ability to protect is not diminished in sick children. As a rule, there are only four common situations that are contraindications to immunization of sick children:

"Children who are *being referred* urgently to the hospital should not be immunized. There is no medical contraindication, but if the child dies, the vaccine may be incorrectly blamed for the death."

Live vaccines (BCG, measles, polio) should not be given to children with immunodeficiency diseases, or to children who are immunosuppressed due to malignant disease, therapy with immunosuppressive agents or irradiation. However, all the vaccines, including BCG and yellow fever, can be given to children who have, or are suspected of having, HIV infection but are not yet symptomatic.

- *DPT2/ DPT3* should not be given to children who have had convulsions or shock within three days of a previous dose of DPT. DT can be administered instead of DPT.
- *DPT* should not be given to children with recurrent convulsions or another active neurological disease

of the central nervous system. DT can be administered instead of DPT.

- *BCG*, if not given at birth, can be given in the next visit.

After checking immunization status, determine if the child needs vitamin A supplementation and/or prophylactic iron folic acid supplementation.

Assessing other Problems

The IMNCI clinical guidelines focus on five main symptoms. In addition, the assessment steps within each main symptom take into account several other common problems. For example, conditions such as meningitis, sepsis, tuberculosis, conjunctivitis, and different causes of fever such as ear infection and sore throat are routinely assessed within the IMNCI case management process. If the guidelines are correctly applied, children with these conditions will receive presumptive treatment or urgent referral. Nevertheless, health care providers still need to consider other causes of severe or acute illness. It is important to address the child's other complaints and to ask questions about the caretaker's health (usually, the mother's).

Treatment Procedures for Sick Children

IMNCI classifications are not necessarily specific diagnoses, but they indicate what action needs to be taken. In the IMNCI guidelines, all classifications are colour coded: pink calls for hospital referral or admission, yellow for initiation of treatment, and green means that the child can be sent home with careful advice on when to return. After completion of the assessment and classification procedure, the next step is to identify treatment.

Referral of children age 2 mo up to 5 yr

All sick children with a severe classification (pink) are referred to a hospital as soon as assessment is completed and necessary pre-referral treatment is administered. If a child only has severe dehydration and no other severe classification, and IV infusion is available in the outpatient clinic, an attempt should be made first to rehydrate the sick child.

The principles of referral of a sick child are similar to those described for a sick young infant. Possible Pre-referral treatment (s) include:

- For convulsions diazepam IV or rectally. If convulsions continue after 10 minutes, give a second dose.
- First dose of injectable Chloramphenicol (*if not possible give oral amoxicillin*) for Severe Pneumonia or Severe Disease, Very Severe Febrile Disease, Severe Complicated Measles and Mastoiditis.
- First dose of Quinine (for severe malaria) as per NAMP guidelines.
- Vitamin A (persistent diarrhea, measles, severe malnutrition).

- Prevention of hypoglycemia with breast milk or sugar water.
- Oral antimalarial as per NAMP guidelines.
- Paracetamol for high fever (38.5°C or above) or pain
- Tetracycline eye ointment (if clouding of the cornea or pus draining from eye).
- Frequent sips of ORS solution on the way to the hospital in sick children with diarrhea.

If a child does not need *urgent* referral, check to see if the child needs *non-urgent referral* for further assessment; for example, for a cough that has lasted more than 30 days, or for fever that has lasted seven days or more. These referrals are not as urgent, and other necessary treatments may be done before transporting for referral.

Treatment in Outpatient Clinics

- The treatment guidelines associated with each non-referral classification (*yellow and green*) are clearly spelled out in the IMNCI chart. Treatment uses a minimum of affordable essential drugs.
- Counselling a mother/caretaker for looking after the child at home is very important. Good communication skills based on principles of *APAC* are helpful for effective counselling.
- Give the first dose of the antibiotics (amoxicillin or cotrimoxazole for pneumonia and acute ear infection, *and amoxicillin in very severe disease if it is not possible to administer injectable chloramphenicol*) in the clinic and continue for 5 days, and antimalarials (as per NAMP guidelines). For Dysentery give ciprofloxacin for 3 days. Teach the mother how to give oral drugs at home. If a child 2 yrs or older has severe dehydration and there is cholera in the area, give a single dose of doxycycline.
- Treat' SOME' and 'NO' dehydration according to Plan B and Plan A respectively, as per WHO guidelines for treatment of dehydration. Give reduced osmolarity ORS (75 mEq/L of sodium, 75 mmol/L of glucose, osmolarity 245 mOsm/L) for prevention and treatment of dehydration.
- For 'Persistent Diarrhea', encourage the mother to continue breastfeeding and mange as per WHO guidelines.
- Give zinc supplements for 14 days for acute diarrhea, persistent diarrhea and dysentery.
- Give iron folic acid for treatment of anaemia.
- Use *Safe home remedies* for cough and cold. Breast milk alone is a good soothing remedy.
- For local infection, teach the mother or caretaker how to treat the infection at home. Instructions may be given about how to: Treat eye infection with tetracycline eye ointment; Dry the ear by wicking

to treat ear infection; Treat mouth ulcers with gentian violet.

Counselling A Mother or Caretaker

A child who is seen at the clinic needs to continue treatment, feeding and fluids at home. The child's mother or caretaker also needs to recognize when the child is not improving, or is becoming sicker. The success of home treatment depends on how well the mother or caretaker knows how to give treatment, understands its importance and knows when to return to a health care provider. Some advice is simple; other advice requires teaching the mother or caretaker how to do a task. When you teach a mother how to treat a child, use three basic teaching steps: *give information; show an example; let her practice.*

- Advise to continue feeding and increase fluids during illness;
- Teach how to give oral drugs or to treat local infection;
- Counsel to solve feeding problems (if any);
- Advise when to return. Every mother or caretaker who is taking a sick child home needs to be advised about when to return to a health facility. The health care provider should a. teach signs that mean to return immediately for further care (For any sick child—Not able to drink or drink or breastfeed, becomes sicker or develops a fever; If child has *no pneumonia: cough or cold*—also return if fast breathing, difficult breathing; if child has *diarrhea-* blood in stool, drinking poorly), b. advise when to return for a follow-up visit (After 2 days— pneumonia; *dysentery; malaria*, if fever persists; *fever malaria unlikely*, if fever persists; *measles with eye or mouth complications;* after 5 days—*diarrhea*, if not improving; *persistent diarrhea; acute ear infection; chronic ear infection; feeding problem; any other illness,* if not improving; After 14 days—*anaemia;* after 30 days—*very low weight for age;* and c. schedule the next well-child or immunization visit.

Gove S. For the WHO Working Group on Guidelines for Integrated Management of the Sick Child. *Bull WHO* 1997,75:7– 24.

Integrated Management of Neonatal and Childhood Illness. *Training Modules for Physicians*. Ministry of Health and Family Welfare, Govt. of India, 2003.

Integrated Management of Neonatal and Childhood Illness. *Physician Chart Booklet*. Ministry of Health and Family Welfare, Govt. of India, 2005.

Murray CJL, Lopez AD. *The global burden of disease : a comprehensive assessment of mortality and disability from diseases, injuries and risk factors in 1990 and projected to 2020.* In: Global Burden of Disease and Injury Series (vol. I), Cambridge, MA, Harvard School of Public Health,1996.

World Health Organization. Integrated Management of the Sick Child. *Bull* WHO 1995; 73:735–740.

World Health Organization. *Management of the Child with a Serious Infection or Severe Malnutrition : Guidelines for care at the first-referral level in developing countries.* WHO, Geneva, 2000.

World Health Organization. *Integrated Management of Childhood Illness.* WHO/CHD/97.3.A–3.G, WHO, Geneva, 1997.

ASSESS AND CLASSIFY THE SICK YOUNG INFANT AGE UP TO 2 MONTHS

ASSESS	CLASSIFY	IDENTIFY TREATMENT

Ask the mother what the young infant's problems are

- Determine if this is an initial or follow-up visit for this problem.
  - if follow-up visit, use the follow-up instructions on the bottom of this chart.
  - if initial visit, assess the young infant as follows:

A child with a pink classification needs **URGENT** attention, complete the assessment and pre-referral treatment immediately so referral is not delayed

USE ALL BOXES THAT MATCH INFANT'S SYMPTOMS AND PROBLEMS TO CLASSIFY THE ILLNESS.

CHECK FOR POSSIBLE BACTERIAL INFECTION/JAUNDICE

		SIGNS	CLASSIFY AS	IDENTIFY TREATMENT (Urgent pre-referral treatments are in bold print.)
ASK:	**LOOK, LISTEN, FEEL:**			
- Has the infant had convulsions?	- Count the breaths in one minute. Repeat the count if elevated. } YOUNG INFANT MUST BE CALM - Look for severe chest indrawing. - Look for nasal flaring. - Look and listen for grunting. - Look and feel for bulging fontanelle. - Look for pus draining from the ear. - Look at the umbilicus. Is it red or draining pus? - Look for skin pustules. Are there 10 or more skin pustules or a big boil? - Measure axillary temperature (if not possible, feel for fever or low body temperature). - See if the young infant is lethargic or unconscious. - Look at the young infant's movements. Are they less than normal? - Look for jaundice? - Are the palms and soles yellow?	**CLASSIFY ALL YOUNG INFANTS** - Convulsions or - Fast breathing (60 breaths per minute or more) or - Severe chest indrawing or - Nasal flaring or - Grunting or - Bulging fontanelle or - 10 or more skin pustules or a big boil or - If axillary temperature 37.5°C or above (or feels hot to touch) or temperature less than 35.5°C (or feels cold to touch) or - Lethargic or unconscious or - Less than normal movements.	**POSSIBLE SERIOUS BACTERIAL INFECTION**	**Give first dose of intramuscular ampicillin and gentamicin.** **Treat to prevent low blood sugar.** **Warm the young infant by skin to skin contact if temperature less than 36.5°C (or feels cold to touch) while arranging referral.** **Advise mother how to keep the young infant warm on the way to the hospital.** **Refer URGENTLY to hospital** *
		- Umbilicus red or draining pus or - Pus discharge from ear or - <10 skin pustules.	**LOCAL BACTERIAL INFECTION**	**Give oral amoxycillin for 5 days.** Teach mother to treat local infections at home. Follow up in 2 days.
		AND IF THE INFANT HAS JAUNDICE - Palms and soles yellow or - Age <24 hours or - Age 14 days or more	**SEVERE JAUNDICE**	**Treat to prevent low blood sugar.** **Warm the young infant by Skin to Skin contact if temperature less than 36.5°C (or feels cold to touch) while arranging referral.** **Advise mother how to keep the young infant warm on the way to the hospital.** **Refer URGENTLY to hospital.**
		- Palms and soles not yellow	**JAUNDICE**	Advise mother to give home care for the young infant. Advise mother when to return immediately. Follow up in 2 days.
		AND IF THE TEMP. IS BETWEEN 35.5 and 36.4°C - Temperature between 35.5 and 36.4°C	**LOW BODY TEMPERATURE**	Warm the young infant using Skin to Skin contact for one hour and REASSESS. If no improvement, refer Treat to prevent low blood sugar.

* If referral is not possible, see the section **Where Referral is Not Possible** in the module **Treat the Young Infant and Counsel the Mother.**

See Color Plate 1

THEN ASK:
Does the young infant have diarrhoea?*

IF YES, ASK:
- For how long?
- Is there blood in the stool?

LOOK AND FEEL:
- Look at the young infant's general condition.
  Is the infant:
  - Lethargic or unconscious?
  - Restless and irritable?
- Look for sunken eyes.
- Pinch the skin of the abdomen.
  Does it go back:
  - Very slowly (Longer than 2 seconds)?
  - Slowly?

CLASSIFY DIARRHOEA

FOR DEHYDRATION	Classification	Treatment
Two of the following signs: • Lethargic or unconscious • Sunken eyes • Skin pinch goes back very slowly	**SEVERE DEHYDRATION**	Give first dose of intramuscular ampicillin and gentamicin. If infant also has low weight or another severe classification: - Refer URGENTLY to hospital with mother giving frequent sips of ORS on the way. - Advise mother to continue breastfeeding. - Advise mother how to keep the young infant warm on the way to the hospital. **OR** If infant does not have low weight or any other severe classification: - Give fluid for severe dehydration (Plan C) and then refer to hospital after rehydration.
Two of the following signs: • Restless, irritable • Sunken eyes • Skin pinch goes back slowly	**SOME DEHYDRATION**	If infant also has low weight or another severe classification: - **Give first dose of intramuscular ampicillin and gentamicin** - **Refer URGENTLY to hospital with mother giving frequent sips of ORS on the way.** - **Advise mother to continue breastfeeding.** - **Advise mother how to keep the young infant warm on the way to the hospital.** If infant does not have low weight or another severe classification: - Give fluids for some dehydration (Plan B). - Advise mother when to return immediately. - Follow up in 2 days
• Not enough signs to classify as some or severe dehydration	**NO DEHYDRATION**	Give fluids to treat diarrhea at home (Plan A). Advise mother when to return immediately. Follow up in 5 days if not improving.

AND IF DIARRHOEA 14 DAYS OR MORE

	Classification	Treatment
• Diarrhoea lasting 14 days or more	**SEVERE PERSISTENT DIARRHOEA**	**Give first dose of intramuscular ampicillin and gentamicin if the young infant has low weight, dehydration or another severe classification.** **Treat to prevent low blood sugar.** Advise how to keep infant warm on the way to the hospital. Refer to hospital.#

AND IF BLOOD IN STOOL

	Classification	Treatment
• Blood in the stool	**SEVERE DYSENTERY**	Give first dose of intramuscular ampicillin and gentamicin if the young infant has low weight, dehydration or another severe classification. Treat to prevent low blood sugar. Advise how to keep infant warm on the way to the hospital. Refer to hospital.#

* **What is diarrhoea in a young infant?**
If the stools have changed from usual pattern and are many and watery (more water than fecal matter). The normally frequent or loose stools of a breastfed baby are not diarrhoea.

If referral is not possible, see the section **Where Referral Is Not Possible** in the module **Treat the Young Infant and Counsel the Mother.**

See Color Plate 2

THEN CHECK FOR FEEDING PROBLEM AND MALNUTRITION:

ASK:

- Is there any difficulty feeding?
- Is the infant breastfed? If yes, how many times in 24 hours?
- Does the infant usually receive any other foods or drinks? If yes, how often?
- What do you use to feed the infant?

LOOK, FEEL:

- Determine weight for age.

IF AN INFANT:

Has any difficulty feeding, or
Is breastfeeding less than 8 times in 24 hours, or
Is taking any other foods or drinks, or
Is low weight for age,
AND
Has no indications to refer urgently to hospital:

ASSESS BREASTFEEDING:

- Has the infant breastfed in the previous hour?

If the infant has not fed in the previous hour, ask the mother to put her infant to the breast. Observe the breastfeed for 4 minutes.

(If the infant was fed during the last hour, ask the mother if she can wait and tell you when the infant is willing to feed again.)

- Is the infant able to attach?

  no attachment at all   not well attached   good attachment

  TO CHECK ATTACHMENT, LOOK FOR:
  - Chin touching breast
  - Mouth wide open
  - Lower lip turned outward
  - More areola visible above than below the mouth

  (All of these signs should be present if the attachment is good)

- Is the infant suckling effectively (that is, slow deep sucks, sometimes pausing)?

  not suckling at all   not suckling effectively   suckling effectively

  Clear a blocked nose if it interferes with breastfeeding.

- Look for ulcers or white patches in the mouth (thrush).

- Does the mother have pain while breastfeeding? If yes, look and feel for:
  - Flat or inverted nipples, or sore nipples
  - Engorged breasts or breast abscess

CLASSIFY FEEDING

Signs	Classify as	Treatment
• Not able to feed or • No attachment at all or • Not suckling at all or • Severely Underweight (<-3 S.D)	**NOT ABLE TO FEED - POSSIBLE SERIOUS BACTERIAL INFECTION OR SEVERE MALNUTRITION**	**Give first dose of intramuscular ampicillin and gentamicin.** **Treat to prevent low blood sugar.** **Warm the young infant by skin to skin contact if temperature less than 36.5°C (or feels cold to touch) while arranging referral.** **Advise mother how to keep the young infant warm on the way to the hospital.** **Refer URGENTLY to hospital #**
• Not well attached to breast or • Not suckling effectively or • Less than 8 breastfeeds in 24 hours or • Receives other foods or drinks or • Thrush (ulcers or white patches in mouth) or • Moderately Underweight (<-2 to -3 S.D) or • Breast or nipple problems	**FEEDING PROBLEM OR LOW WEIGHT FOR AGE**	If not well attached or not suckling effectively, teach correct positioning and attachment. If breastfeeding less than 8 times in 24 hours, advise to increase frequency of feeding. If receiving other foods or drinks, counsel mother about breastfeeding more, reducing other foods or drinks, and using a cup and spoon. - If not breastfeeding at all, advise mother about giving locally appropriate animal milk and teach the mother to feed with a cup and spoon. If thrush, teach the mother to treat thrush at home. If low weight for age, teach the mother how to keep the young infant with low weight warm at home. If breast or nipple problem, teach the mother to treat breast or nipple problems. Advise mother to give home care for the young infant. Advise mother when to return immediately. Follow-up any feeding problem or thrush in 2 days. Follow-up low weight for age in 14 days.
• Not low weight for age (≥ -2SD) and no other signs of inadequate feeding	**NO FEEDING PROBLEM**	Advise mother to give home care for the young infant. Advise mother when to return immediately. Praise the mother for feeding the infant well.

If referral is not possible, see the section Where **Referral Is Not Possible** in the module **Treat the Young Infant and Counsel the Mother.**

See Color Plate 3

THEN CHECK THE YOUNG INFANT'S IMMUNIZATION STATUS

IMMUNIZATION SCHEDULE*:

AGE	VACCINE	
Birth	BCG	OPV 0
6 weeks	DPT I	OPV I HEP-B I

* **Hepatitis B** to be given wherever included in the immunization schedule

ASSESS OTHER PROBLEMS

ASSESS AND CLASSIFY THE SICK CHILD AGE 2 MONTHS UP TO 5 YEARS

ASSESS	CLASSIFY	IDENTIFY TREATMENT

ASK THE MOTHER WHAT THE CHILD'S PROBLEMS ARE

- Determine if this is an initial or follow-up visit for this problem.
  - if follow-up visit, use the follow-up instructions on *TREAT THE CHILD* chart.
  - if initial visit, assess the child as follows:

CHECK FOR GENERAL DANGER SIGNS

ASK:

- Is the child able to drink or breastfeed?
- Does the child vomit everything?
- Has the child had convulsions?

LOOK

- See if the child is lethargic or unconscious.

A child with any general danger sign needs URGENT attention; complete the assessment and any pre-referral treatment immediately so referral is not delayed.

THEN ASK ABOUT MAIN SYMPTOMS:
Does the child have cough or difficult breathing?

IF YES, ASK:	LOOK, LISTEN:
- For how long?	- Count the breaths in one minute. - Look for chest indrawing. - Look and listen for stridor.

CHILD MUST BE CALM

CLASSIFY COUGH OR DIFFICULT BREATHING

If the child is:	Fast breathing is:
2 months up to 12 months	50 breaths per minute or more
12 months up to 5 years	40 breaths per minute or more

USE ALL BOXES THAT MATCH THE CHILD'S SYMPTOMS AND PROBLEMS TO CLASSIFY THE ILLNESS.

SIGNS	CLASSIFY AS	IDENTIFY TREATMENT *(Urgent pre-referral treatments are in bold print.)*
- Any general danger sign or - Chest indrawing or - Stridor in calm child	SEVERE PNEUMONIA OR VERY SEVERE DISEASE	**Give first dose of injectable chloramphenicol (If not possible give oral amoxicillin).** **Refer URGENTLY to hospital.** #
- Fast breathing	PNEUMONIA	**Give Amoxicillin for 5 days.** Soothe the throat and relieve the cough with a safe remedy if child is 6 months or older. Advise mother when to return immediately. Follow-up in 2 days.
No signs of pneumonia or very severe disease	NO PNEUMONIA: COUGH OR COLD	If coughing more than 30 days, refer for assessment. Soothe the throat and relieve the cough with a safe home remedy if child is 6 months or older. Advise mother when to return immediately. Follow-up in 5 days if not improving.

If referral is not possible, see the section **Where Referral Is Not Possible** in the module **Treat the Child.**

See Color Plate 4

Does the child have diarrhoea?

IF YES, ASK:
- For how long?
- Is there blood in the stool?

LOOK AND FEEL:
- Look at the child's general condition. Is the child:
  - Lethargic or unconscious?
  - Restless and irritable?
- Look for sunken eyes.
- Offer the child fluid. Is the child:
  - Not able to drink or drinking poorly?
  - Drinking eagerly, thirsty?
- Pinch the skin of the abdomen. Does it go back:
  - Very slowly (longer than 2 seconds)?
  - Slowly?

CLASSIFY DIARRHOEA

FOR DEHYDRATION

Signs	Classification	Treatment
Two of the following signs: • Lethargic or unconscious • Sunken eyes • Not able to drink or drinking poorly • Skin pinch goes back very slowly	**SEVERE DEHYDRATION**	If child has no other severe classification: - Give fluid for severe dehydration (Plan C). **If child also has another severe classification:** **Refer URGENTLY to hospital * with mother giving frequent sips of ORS on the way.** **Advise the mother to continue breastfeeding.** **If child is 2 years or older and there is cholera in your area, give doxycycline for cholera.**
Two of the following signs: • Restless, irritable. • Sunken eyes. • Drinks eagerly, thirsty • Skin pinch goes back slowly	**SOME DEHYDRATION**	Give fluid, zinc supplements and food for some dehydration (Plan B). **If child also has a severe classification:** **Refer URGENTLY to hospital # with mother giving frequent sips of ORS on the way.** **Advise the mother to continue breastfeeding.** Advise mother when to return immediately. Follow-up in 5 days if not improving.
• Not enough signs to classify as some or severe dehydration	**NO DEHYDRATION**	Give fluid, zinc supplements and food to treat diarrhoea at home (Plan A). Advise mother when to return immediately. Follow-up in 5 days if not improving.

AND IF DIARRHOEA I= DAYS OR MORE

Signs	Classification	Treatment
• Dehydration present	**SEVERE PERSISTENT DIARRHOEA**	*Treat dehydration before referral unless the child has another severe classification.* *Refer to hospital.**
• No dehydration	**PERSISTENT DIARRHOEA**	Advise the mother on feeding a child who has PERSISTENT DIARRHOEA. **Give single dose of vitamin A.** Give zinc supplements daily for 14 days. Follow-up in 5 days.

AND IF BLOOD IN STOOL

Signs	Classification	Treatment
• Blood in the stool	**DYSENTERY**	**Treat for 3 days with ciprofloxacin.** **Treat dehydration** Give zinc supplements for 14 days Follow-up in 2 days.

If referral is not possible, see the section **Where Referral Is Not Possible** in the module **Treat the Child.**

See Color Plate 5

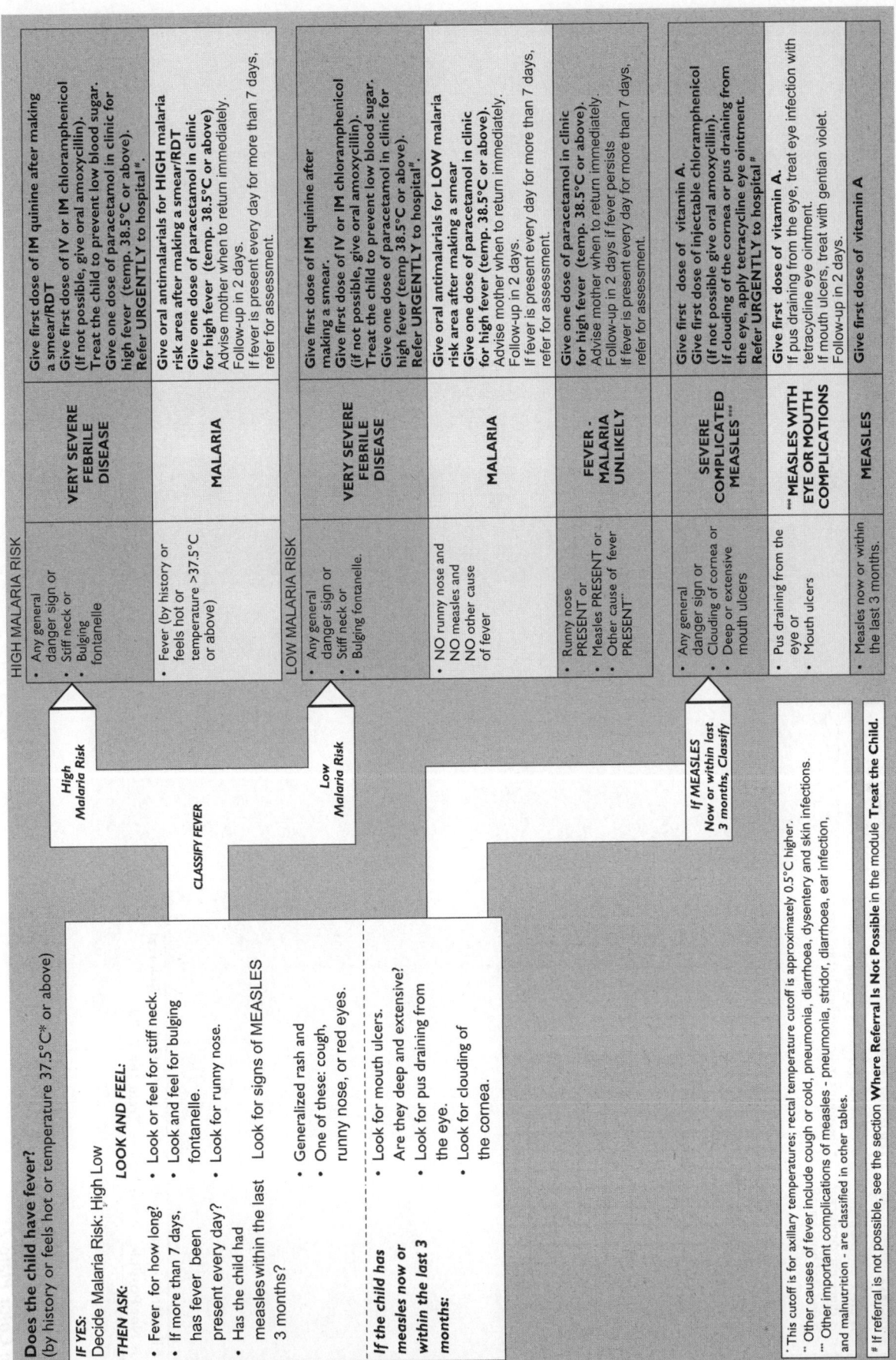

Does the child have fever?
(by history or feels hot or temperature 37.5°C* or above)

IF YES:
Decide Malaria Risk: High Low

THEN ASK:

- Fever for how long?
- If more than 7 days, has fever been present every day?
- Has the child had measles within the last 3 months?

LOOK AND FEEL:

- Look or feel for stiff neck.
- Look and feel for bulging fontanelle.
- Look for runny nose.

Look for signs of MEASLES

- Generalized rash and
- One of these: cough, runny nose, or red eyes.

If the child has measles now or within the last 3 months:

- Look for mouth ulcers. Are they deep and extensive?
- Look for pus draining from the eye.
- Look for clouding of the cornea.

CLASSIFY FEVER

High Malaria Risk

Low Malaria Risk

If MEASLES Now or within last 3 months, Classify

HIGH MALARIA RISK

Signs	Classification	Treatment
• Any general danger sign or • Stiff neck or • Bulging fontanelle	**VERY SEVERE FEBRILE DISEASE**	**Give first dose of IM quinine after making a smear/RDT** **Give first dose of IV or IM chloramphenicol** (If not possible, give oral amoxycillin). **Treat the child to prevent low blood sugar.** **Give one dose of paracetamol in clinic for high fever (temp. 38.5°C or above).** **Refer URGENTLY to hospital\#.**
• Fever (by history or feels hot or temperature >37.5°C or above)	**MALARIA**	**Give oral antimalarials for HIGH malaria risk area after making a smear/RDT** **Give one dose of paracetamol in clinic for high fever (temp. 38.5°C or above)** Advise mother when to return immediately. Follow-up in 2 days. If fever is present every day for more than 7 days, refer for assessment.

LOW MALARIA RISK

Signs	Classification	Treatment
• Any general danger sign or • Stiff neck or • Bulging fontanelle.	**VERY SEVERE FEBRILE DISEASE**	**Give first dose of IM quinine after making a smear.** **Give first dose of IV or IM chloramphenicol** (if not possible, give oral amoxycillin). **Give one dose of paracetamol in clinic for high fever (temp 38.5°C or above).** **Refer URGENTLY to hospital\#.**
• NO runny nose and NO measles and NO other cause of fever	**MALARIA**	**Give oral antimalarials for LOW malaria risk area after making a smear** **Give one dose of paracetamol in clinic for high fever (temp. 38.5°C or above).** Advise mother when to return immediately. Follow-up in 2 days. If fever is present every day for more than 7 days, refer for assessment.
• Runny nose PRESENT or • Measles PRESENT or • Other cause of fever PRESENT**	**FEVER - MALARIA UNLIKELY**	**Give one dose of paracetamol in clinic for high fever (temp. 38.5°C or above).** Advise mother when to return immediately. Follow-up in 2 days if fever persists If fever is present every day for more than 7 days, refer for assessment.

Signs	Classification	Treatment
• Any general danger sign or • Clouding of cornea or • Deep or extensive mouth ulcers	**SEVERE COMPLICATED MEASLES*****	**Give first dose of vitamin A.** **Give first dose of injectable chloramphenicol** (If not possible give oral amoxycillin). **If clouding of the cornea or pus draining from the eye, apply tetracycline eye ointment.** **Refer URGENTLY to hospital\#**
• Pus draining from the eye or • Mouth ulcers	**MEASLES WITH EYE OR MOUTH COMPLICATIONS*****	**Give first dose of vitamin A.** If pus draining from the eye, treat eye infection with tetracycline eye ointment. If mouth ulcers, treat with gentian violet. Follow-up in 2 days.
• Measles now or within the last 3 months.	**MEASLES**	**Give first dose of vitamin A**

---

* This cutoff is for axillary temperatures; rectal temperature cutoff is approximately 0.5°C higher.
** Other causes of fever include cough or cold, pneumonia, diarrhoea, dysentery and skin infections.
*** Other important complications of measles - pneumonia, stridor, diarrhoea, ear infection, and malnutrition - are classified in other tables.

\# If referral is not possible, see the section **Where Referral Is Not Possible** in the module **Treat the Child.**

See Color Plate 6

Does the child have an ear problem?

IF YES, ASK:
- Is there ear pain?
- Is there ear discharge? If yes, for how long?

LOOK AND FEEL:
- Look for pus draining from the ear.
- Feel for tender swelling behind the ear.

Classify EAR PROBLEM

Signs	Classify	Treatment
• Tender swelling behind the ear	**MASTOIDITIS**	**Give first dose of injectable chloramphenicol (If not possible give oral amoxycillin). Give first dose of paracetamol for pain. Refer URGENTLY to hospital#.**
• Pus is seen draining from the ear and discharge is reported for less than 14 days, or • Ear pain.	**ACUTE EAR INFECTION**	**Give Amoxycillin for 5 days.** Give paracetamol for pain. Dry the ear by wicking. Follow-up in 5 days.
• Pus is seen draining from the ear and discharge is reported for 14 days or more.	**CHRONIC EAR INFECTION**	Dry the ear by wicking. Topical ciprofloxacin ear drops for 2 weeks. Follow-up in 5 days.
• No ear pain and No pus seen draining from the ear.	**NO EAR INFECTION**	No additional treatment.

If referral is not possible, see the section **Where Referral Is Not Possible** in the module **Treat the Child.**

See Color Plate 7

THEN CHECK FOR MALNUTRITION

LOOK AND FEEL:
- Look for visible severe wasting.
- Look for oedema of both feet.
- Determine weight for age.

Classify
NUTRITIONAL STATUS

• Visible severe wasting or • Oedema of both feet.	**SEVERE MALNUTRITION**	**Give single dose of Vitamin A.** **Prevent low blood sugar.** **Refer URGENTLY to hospital #** *While referral is being organized, warm the child.* **Keep the child warm on the way to hospital.**
• Severely Underweight (≤ 3 SD)	**VERY LOW WEIGHT**	Assess and counsel for feeding - if feeding problem, follow-up in 5 days Advise mother when to return immediately. Follow-up in 30 days.
• Not Severely Underweight (≥3SD)	**NOT VERY LOW WEIGHT**	If child is less than 2 years old, assess the child's feeding and counsel the mother on feeding according to the FOOD box on the COUNSEL THE MOTHER chart. - If feeding problem, follow-up in 5 days. Advise mother when to return immediately.

THEN CHECK FOR ANAEMIA

LOOK
- Look for palmar pallor. Is it:
  Severe palmar pallor?
  Some palmar pallor?

Classify
ANAEMIA

• Severe palmar pallor • Some palmar pallor	**SEVERE ANAEMIA** **ANAEMIA**	Refer URGENTLY to hospital #. Give iron folic acid therapy for 14 days. Assess the child's feeding and counsel the mother on feeding according to the FOOD box on the *COUNSEL THE MOTHER chart.* - If feeding problem, follow-up in 5 days. Advise mother when to return immediately. Follow-up in 14 days.
• No palmar pallor	**NO ANAEMIA**	Give prophylactic iron folic acid if child 6 months or older.

THEN CHECK THE CHILD'S IMMUNIZATION *, PROPHYLACTIC VITAMIN A & IRON-FOLIC ACID SUPPLEMENTATION STATUS

	AGE	VACCINE
IMMUNIZATION SCHEDULE:	Birth	BCG + OPV-0
	6 weeks	DPT-1 + OPV-1(+ HepB-**1)
	10 weeks	DPT-2 + OPV-2(+ HepB-**2)
	14 weeks	DPT-3 + OPV-3(+ HepB-**3)
	9 months	Measles
	16–18 months	DPT Booster + OPV
	60 months	DT

* A child who needs to be immunized should be advised to go for immunization the day vaccines are available at AW/SC/PHC
** Hepatitis B to be given wherever included in the immunization schedule

PROPHYLACTIC VITAMIN A
Give a single dose of vitamin A:
*100,000 IU at 9 months with measles immunization
200,000 IU at 16–18 months with DPT Booster
200,000 IU at 24 months, 30 months, 36 months,
42 months, 48 months, 54 months and 60 months*

PROPHYLACTIC IFA
Give 20 mg elemental iron + 100 mcg folic acid (one tablet of Pediatric IFA or IFA syrup/IFA drops) for a total of 100 days in a year after the child has recovered from acute illness **if:**
The child is 6 months of age or older, and
Has not received Pediatric IFA Tablet/syrup/drops
for 100 days in last one year.

If referral is not possible, see the section **Where Referral Is Not Possible** in the module **Treat the Child.**

ASSESS OTHER PROBLEMS

MAKE SURE CHILD WITH ANY GENERAL DANGER SIGN IS REFERRED after first dose of an appropriate antibiotic and other urgent treatments.
Exception: Rehydration of the child according to Plan C may resolve danger signs so that referral is no longer needed.

See Color Plate 8

COUNSEL THE MOTHER

Feeding Recommendations During Sickness and Health

Up to 6 Months of Age

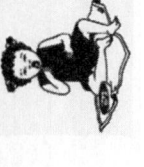

- Breastfeed as often as the child wants, day and night, at least 8 times in 24 hours.
- Do not give any other foods or fluids not even water.

Remember:
- Continue breastfeeding if the child is sick.

6 Months up to 12 Months

- Breastfeed as often as the child wants.
- Give at least one katori serving* at a time of:
  - Mashed roti/rice/bread/biscuit mixed in sweetened undiluted milk OR
  - Mashed roti/rice/bread mixed in thick dal with added ghee/ oil or khichri with added oil/ghee. Add cooked vegetables also in the servings OR
  - Sevian/dalia/halwa/kheer prepared in milk or any cereal porridge cooked in milk OR
  - Mashed boiled/fried potatoes
  - Offer banana/biscuit/cheeko/mango/papaya

*3 times per day if breastfed;
5 times per day if not breastfed.
Remember:
- Keep the child in your lap and feed with your own hands.
- Wash your own and child's hands with soap and water every time before feeding.

12 Months up to 2 Years

- Breastfeed as often as the child wants.
- Offer food from the family pot.
- Give at least 1½ katori serving* at a time of:
  - Mashed roti/rice/bread mixed in thick dal with added ghee/ oil or khichri with added oil/ghee.
  - Add cooked vegetables also in the servings OR
  - Mashed roti/rice/bread/biscuit mixed in sweetened undiluted milk OR
  - Sevian/dalia/halwa/kheer prepared in milk or any cereal porridge cooked in milk OR
  - Mashed boiled/fried potatoes
  - Offer banana/biscuit/cheeko/mango/papaya

* 5 times per day.
Remember:
- Sit by the side of child and help him to finish the serving.
- Wash your child's hands with soap and water every time before feeding.

2 Years and Older

- Give family foods at 3 meals each day.
- Also, twice daily, give nutritious food between meals, such as: banana/biscuit/ cheeko/mango/ papaya as snacks.

Remember:
- Ensure that the child finishes the serving.
- Teach your child wash his hands with soap and water every time before feeding.

Feeding Recommendations For a Child who Has PERSISTENT DIARRHOEA

- If still breastfeeding, give more frequent, longer breastfeeds, day and night.
- If taking other milk:
  - replace with increased breastfeeding OR
  - replace with fermented milk products, such as yoghurt OR
  - replace half the milk with nutrient-rich semisolid food.
  - Add cereals to milk (Rice, Wheat, Semolina).
- For other foods, follow feeding recommendations for the child's age.

➤ Counsel the Mother About Feeding Problems

If the child is not being fed as described in the above recommendations, counsel the mother accordingly. In addition:

➤ **If the mother reports difficulty with breastfeeding, assess breastfeeding:** (See YOUNG INFANT chart.)

As needed, show the mother correct positioning and attachment for breastfeeding.

➤ **If the child is less than 6 months old and is taking other milk or foods:**

- Build mother's confidence that she can produce all the breast milk that the child needs.
- Suggest giving more frequent, longer breastfeeds day or night, and gradually reducing other milk or foods.

If other milk needs to be continued, counsel the mother to:

- Breastfeed as much as possible, including at night.
- Make sure that other milk is a locally appropriate dairy/animal milk.
- Make sure other milk is correctly and hygienically prepared and given in adequate amounts.
- Finish prepared milk within an hour.

➤ **If the mother is using a bottle to feed the child:**

- Recommend substituting a cup for bottle.
- Show the mother how to feed the child with a cup.

➤ **If the child is not being fed actively, counsel the mother to:**

- Sit with the child and encourage eating.
- Give the child an adequate serving in a separate plate or bowl.

➤ **If the child is not feeding well during illness, counsel the mother to:**

- Breastfeed more frequently and for longer if possible.
- Use soft, varied, appetizing, favourite foods to encourage the child to eat as much as possible, and offer frequent small feedings.
- Clear a blocked nose if it interferes with feeding.
- Expect that appetite will improve as child gets better.

➤ **Follow-up any feeding problem in 5 days.**

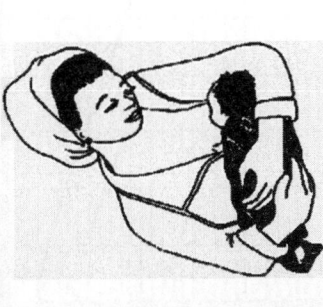
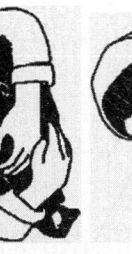
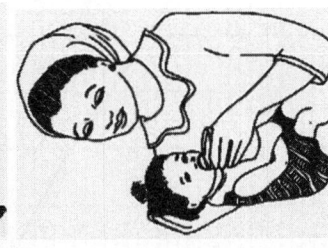
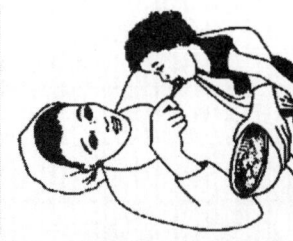

Weight-for-age GIRLS

Birth to 6 months (z-scores)

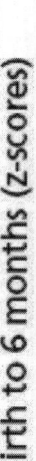

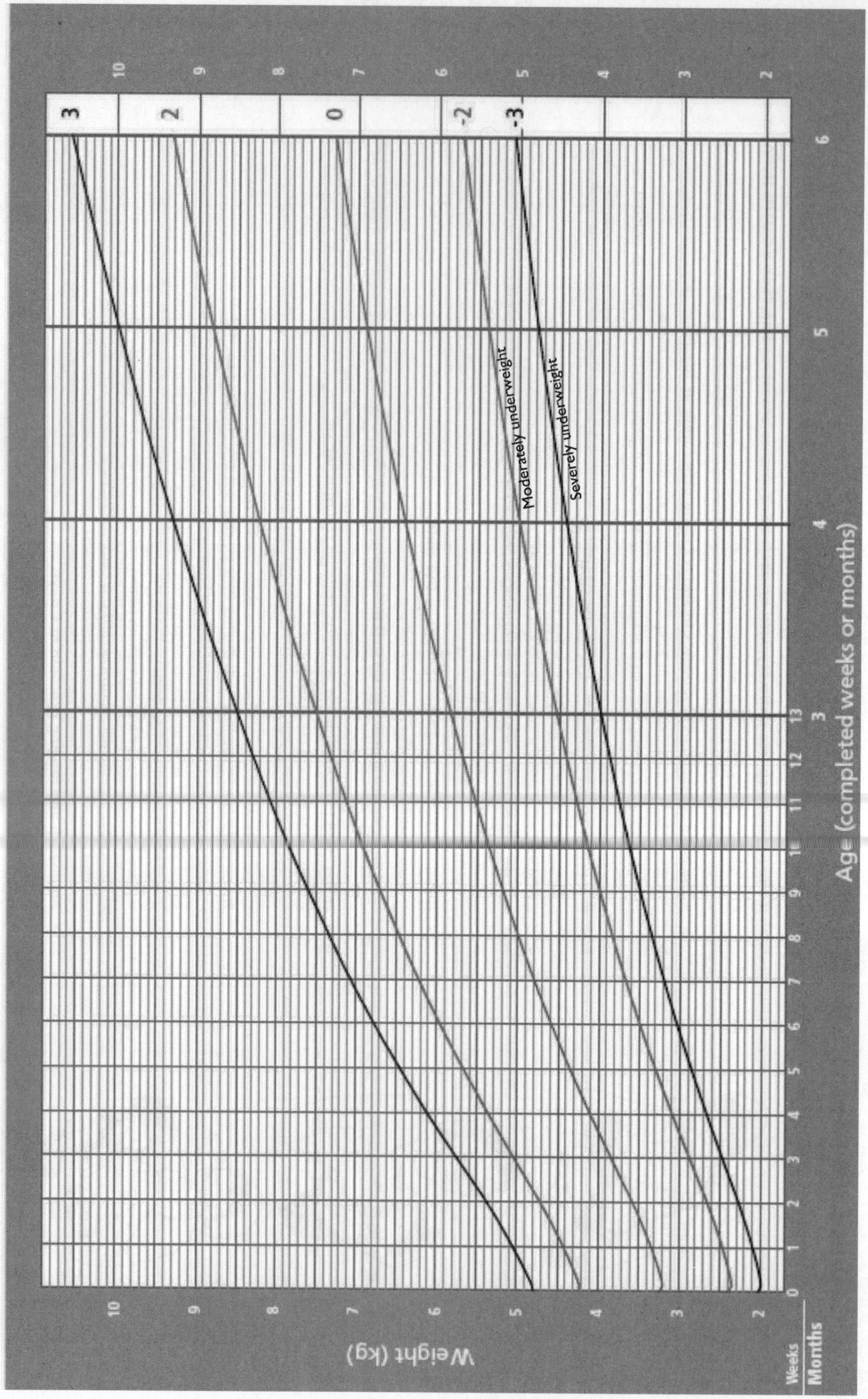

Weight (kg)
Age (completed weeks or months)
Weeks
Months
Moderately underweight
Severely underweight
3
2
0
-2
-3
0 1 2 3 4 5 6 7 8 9 10 11 12 13
3 4 5 6
2 3 4 5 6 7 8 9 10

Weight-for-age GIRLS

Birth to 5 years (z-scores)

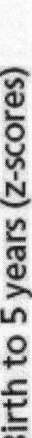

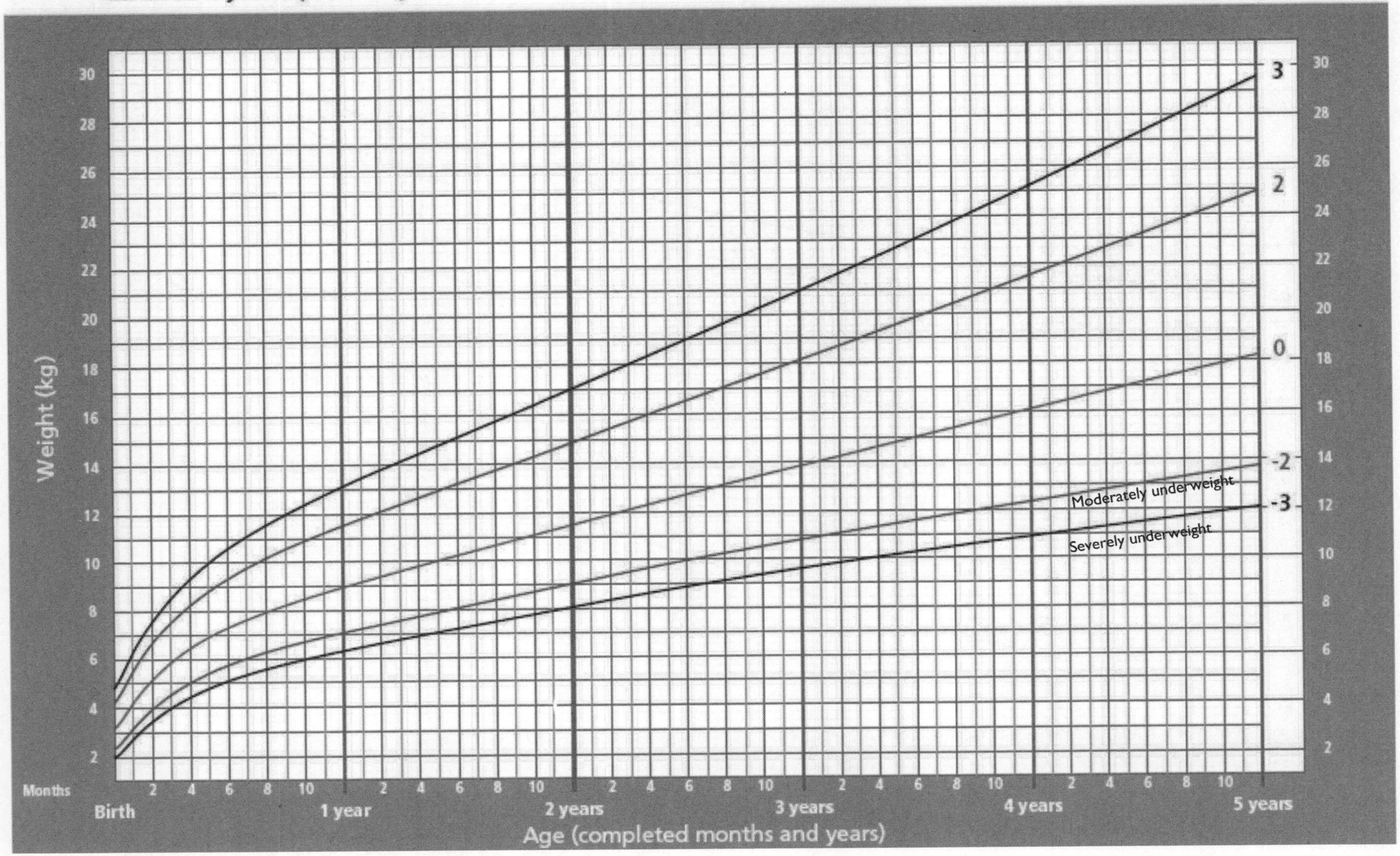
Weight (kg)
30
28
26
24
22
20
18
16
14
12
10
8
6
4
2
3
2
0
-2
-3
Moderately underweight
Severely underweight
Months
2 4 6 8 10
Birth
1 year
2 years
3 years
4 years
5 years
Age (completed months and years)

Weight-for-age BOYS

Birth to 6 months (z-scores)

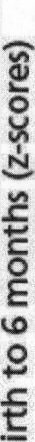

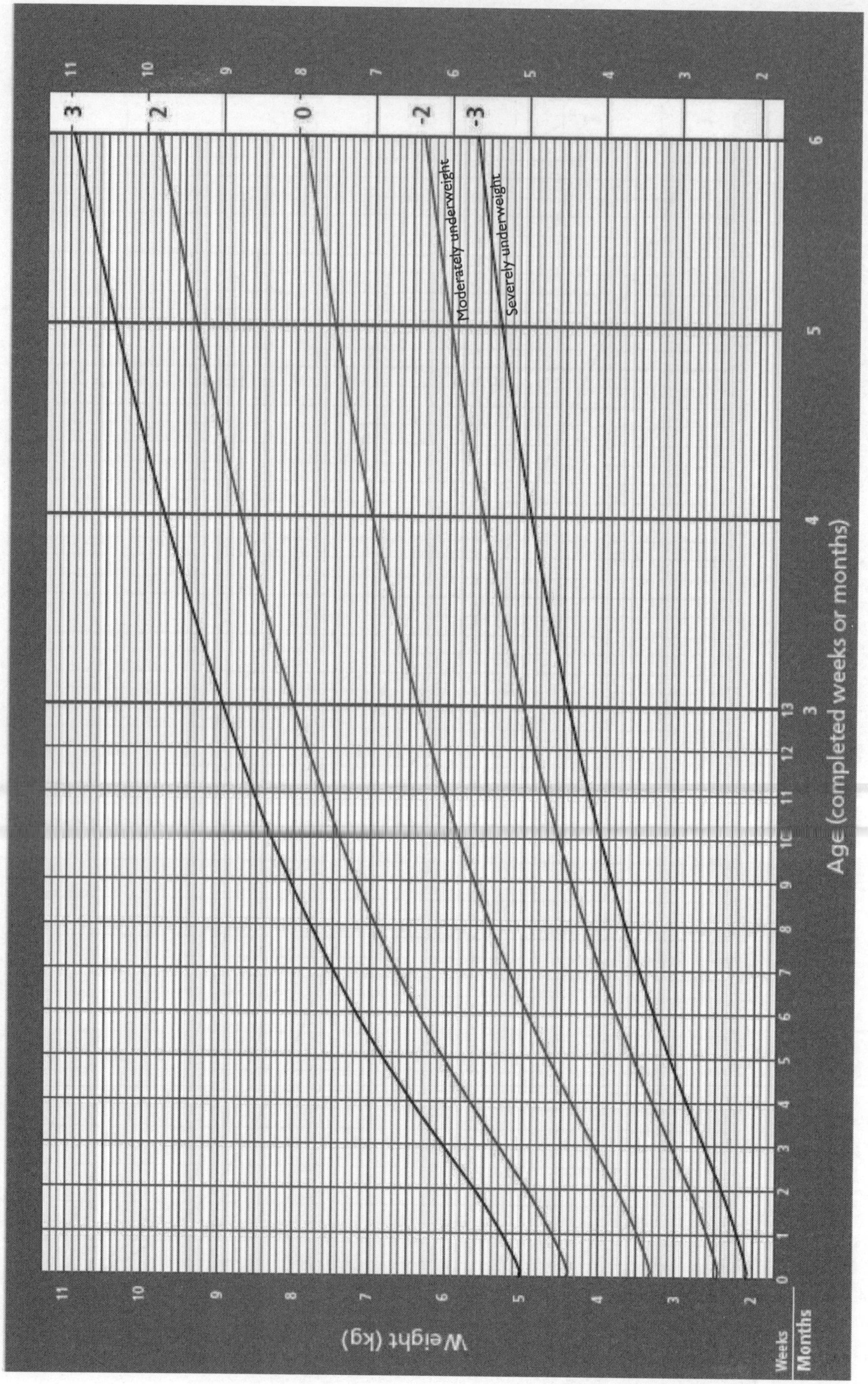
Weight (kg)
11
10
9
8
7
6
5
4
3
2
3
2
0
-2
-3
Moderately underweight
Severely underweight
Weeks
Months
0
1
2
3
4
5
6
7
8
9
10
11
12
13
3
4
5
6
Age (completed weeks or months)

Weight-for-age BOYS

Birth to 5 years (z-scores)

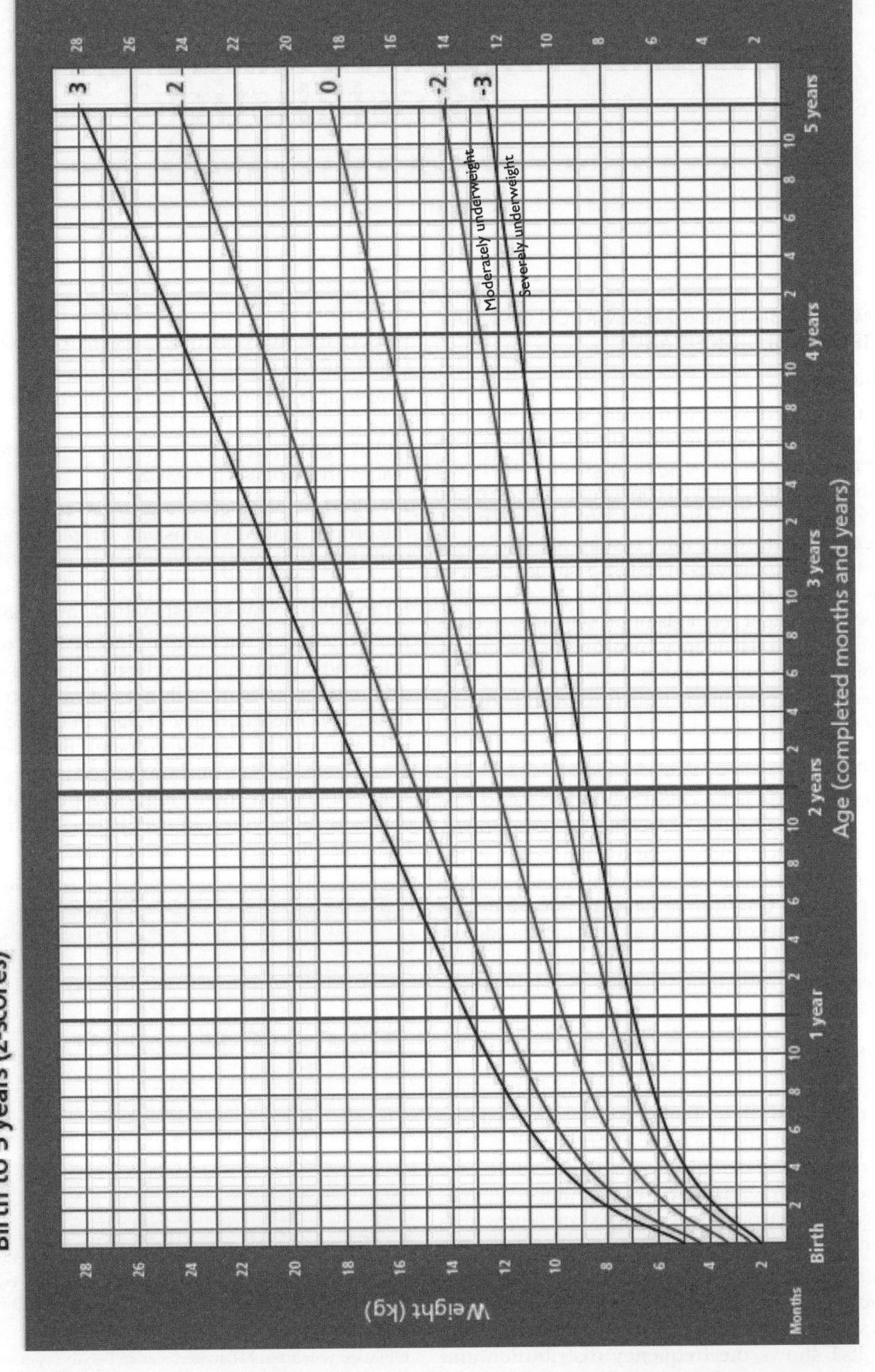

38.1 MEDICAL STATISTICS-PRESENTATION OF DATA AND TESTING OF SIGNIFICANCE

Introduction

Medical knowledge is continually getting updated with accumulation of more and more information. This information needs to be presented and analyzed scientifically so that rational conclusions can be made and evidence-based medicine can be practiced. Medical practitioners and researchers need to understand the principles of statistics so that they can utilize the vast medical information in a scientific manner. The salient methods of presentation of data, measures of central tendency, measures of dispersion, probability distributions and tests of significance are discussed. Non-parametric tests (except Chi Square) are not discussed.

Types of Data

Information comes in two most common types of data which can be quantitative or qualitative. *Quantitative* data are numerical and can be discrete, such as the number of days of illness; and continuous, such as blood pressure. *Qualitative* data are non-numerical or based on a categorical scale and can be: unordered, such as breastfeeding (exclusive, predominant, complementary); and ordered, such as height (short, medium, tall, etc.).

Presenting and Summarizing Statistical Data

The first part of any statistical analysis involves summarising and describing the data. This may be achieved through the use of tables and graphs.

A *Frequency distribution* shows the value of a variable, together with number of the number of times each value occurs. These counts are known as frequencies.

Frequency table: The information of a frequency distribution can be summarized in the form of a table which shows the number of data in a specific group. Table 38.1 shows the frequency distribution and cumulative frequency distribution of the age of 31 persons in a study on hypertension from Example 38.1 (Annexure 1).

Cross-tables are used to present the data variation of data over groups. From the information in Example 38.1 we can present the variation in hypertension for blacks and whites (Table38.2).

Pie chart: A pie chart is a pictorial representation of the proportional divisions of a sample or population, with the divisions represented as parts of a whole circle. Fig. 38.1 presents the occupation distribution for the data on hypertension in Example 38.1.

Bar diagram: A bar diagram is used for comparing categories of mutually exclusive discrete data. The different categories usually are indicated on the x-axis (abscissa). The frequency of data in each category is indicated on the y-axis (ordinate). Because the data are discrete, the bars can be arranged in any order with spaces between them. Fig. 38.2 presents the bar chart on distribution of occupation for the data in Example 38.1.

Table 38.1: Frequency table on age distribution.		
Age group	*Frequency*	*Cum. Frequency*
0–9	1	1
11–19	7	8
20–29	8	16
30–39	3	19
40–49	7	26
50–59	2	28
60+	3	31
All ages	31	31

Table 38.2: Race* HT cross tabulation				
Count				
		HT		
		0	1	Total
Race	b	7	7	14
	w	15	2	17
Total	22	9	31	

b-blacks; w-whites; HT-hypertension; 0–Nil; 1–yes

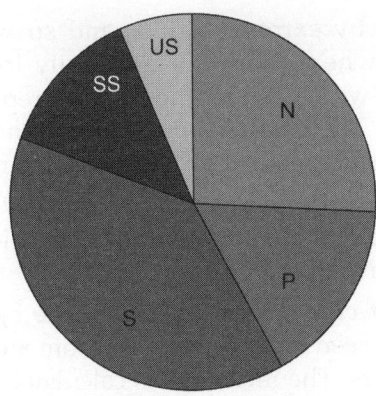

US: unskilled, SS: semiskilled, S: skilled, P: professional, N: unemployed.

Fig. 38.1: Pie diagram showing distribution of occupation

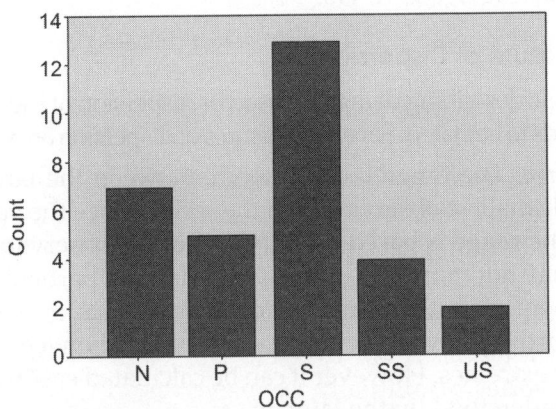

Fig. 38.2: Bar diagram depicting distribution of OCC

Histogram: A histogram represents categories of continuous and ordered data. The bars are adjacent to each other on the x-axis, and there is no intervening space. The frequency of data in each category is depicted on the y-axis, and the width of the bar represents the interval of each category. Fig. 38.3 presents the histogram for distribution of age for the data in Example 38.1.

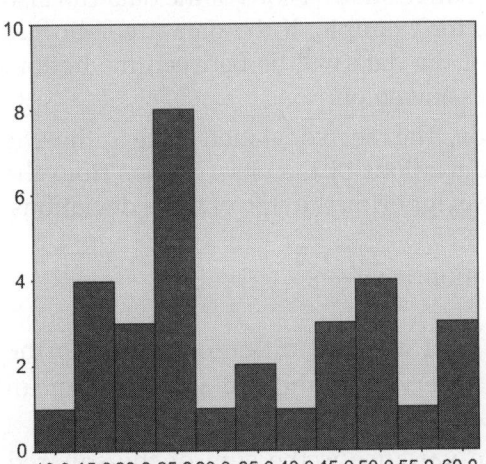

Std. Dev = 15.78
Mean = 33.4
N = 31.00

Fig. 38.3: Histogram showing age distribution

Frequency polygon: A frequency polygon represents the distribution of categories of continuous and ordered data. The x-axis presents the categories of data and the y-axis the frequency of data in each category. The frequency is plotted against the midpoint of each category, and a line is drawn through each of these plotted points. Fig. 38.4 presents the Frequency polygon for the distribution of age for the data in Example 38.1.

Cumulative frequency graph: A cumulative frequency graph is also a representation of the distribution of continuous and ordered data. Here, the frequency of data in each category represents the sum of the data from that category and from the preceding categories. The x-axis depicts the categories of data, and the y-axis is the cumulative frequency of data. The cumulative frequency graph is useful in calculating distributions by percentiles. Fig. 38.5 presents the Cumulative Frequency polygon for the distribution of age for the data in Example 38.1.

Scatter diagram: A scatter diagram shows the relationship between two variables. If the points in the graph are scattered randomly, absence of any relationship between the variables is suggested. If the points are clustered along a pattern, some relationship is suggested which can be further analyzed using correlation. Fig. 38.6 presents the Scatter Diagram for age and blood pressure for the data in Example 38.1. From the figure there appears to be a positive correlation between age and blood pressure.

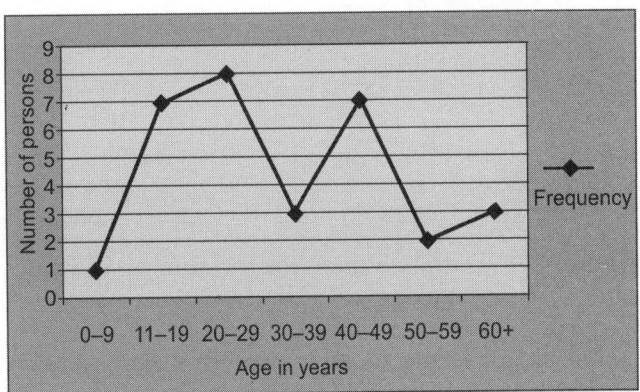

Fig. 38.4: Frequency polygon for age

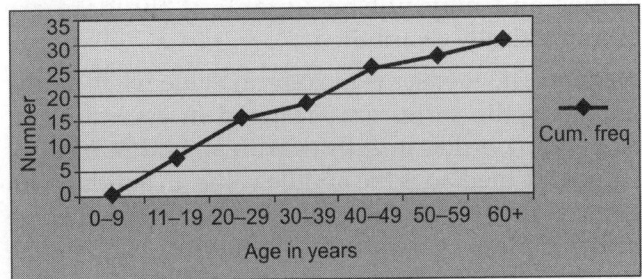

Fig. 38.5: Cumulative freq polygon for age

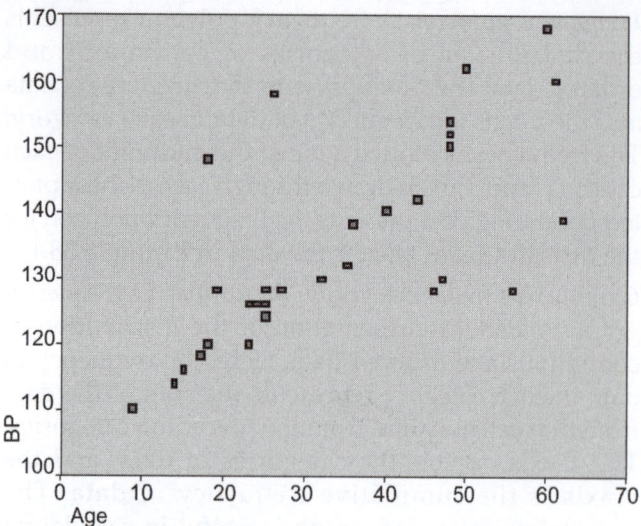

Fig. 38.6: Scatter plot for age and blood pressure

Tables and graphs provide a simple representation of a set of data but to further analyze the data, statistical estimates need to be calculated. The two most important elements of a dataset are its measures of central tendency and location (where on average the data lie) and its variability (the extent to which individual data values are spread out).

Measures of Central Tendency and Location

Arithmetic mean: The arithmetic mean which is also simply called the mean is the sum all of the values in a dataset divided by the total number of values.

For a set of n values ($X_1, X_2, ..., X_n$), the mean is:

$$\bar{X} = \frac{\sum_{i-1}^{n} X_i}{n} \qquad ...(1)$$

where $\dfrac{\sum_{i-1}^{n} X_i}{n}$ is the notation for the sum of all values ($X_1, X_2, ..., X_n$).

The mean is the most commonly used measure central tendency because it is easily understood and can be manipulated. However, it is sensitive to extreme values and may not be suitable if the data are asymmetrically distributed.

Median: The median is the central value when all the values in the series are arranged in ascending or descending order. In a series with an odd number of values the median is the middle value. In a series with an even number of values the median is the average of the middle two values. The median can also be estimated by determining the 50% value of a cumulative frequency curve. The median is not influenced by extreme values and so is useful in situations where there are unusually low or high values that would render the mean unrepresentative of the data. The median, however, does not have the beneficial mathematical properties of the mean.

Mode: The mode is the most commonly occurring value. It is not generally used because it is often not representative of the data.

Example of calculating location: The ages of five individuals seen in an emergency room are 17, 18, 18, 21 and 26 yrs. The mean age is calculated 100/5 =20 yrs , the median age is the age of the third individual when the individuals are arranged in ascending order which is 18 years and the mode, the most frequently occurring age is 18 yrs.

Measure of Dispersion

While describing data the spread or dispersion of the data needs to be stated. Several measures of dispersion are used.

Range: The range is the interval between the largest and smallest observation in the series. Since the value of the range is based on only two of the observations it may not represent of the whole dataset, particularly if there are outliers. In addition, it gives no information regarding how the data are distributed between the two extremes. However it can be calculated easily and is understood by the layman.

Interquartile range: The whole data series can be divided into different sections. While the median splits a dataset into two equally sized groups, quartiles splits a dataset into four equally sized groups. The interquartile range is the interval between the bottom and top quartiles of the series, and indicates where the middle 50% of the data lie. The interquartile range is not influenced by extremes of values and is suitable when data are not symmetrically distributed. Ranges based on alternative subdivisions of the data can also be calculated; for example, if the data are split into deciles, 80% of the data will lie between the bottom and top deciles and so on.

Mean deviation: The mean deviation is the arithmetic mean of the deviations of the observations from the arithmetic mean ignoring the sign of these deviations.

$$\text{Mean deviation} = \frac{\Sigma|X - \bar{x}|}{N}$$

Where $|X - \bar{x}|$ indicates the difference between the value of the observation and the arithmetic mean ignoring the sign of the difference.

Variance: The variance is the sum of the squared deviations from the mean divided by the number values the series −1.

$$\text{Variance} = \frac{\sum_{i=1}^{n}\left(X_i - \bar{X}\right)^2}{(n-1)}$$

Standard deviation: The standard deviation is a measure of the deviation of individual observations from the mean. It is calculated by taking the square root of the variance.

Algebraically the standard deviation for a set of n values $(X_1, X_2,..., X_n)$ is written as follows:

$$SD = \sqrt{\frac{\sum_{i=1}^{n}\left(X_i - \bar{X}\right)^2}{(n-1)}} \qquad ...(2)$$

where $\sum_{i=1}^{n}\left(X_i - \bar{X}\right)^2 = \left(X_1 - \bar{X}\right)^2 + \left(X_2 - \bar{X}\right)^2$

$$+ ... + \left(X_n - \bar{X}\right)^2$$

and $\bar{X}$ is the mean described above (Eqn 1). The standard deviation is the most useful measure of dispersion and, like the mean, has useful mathematical properties.

Coefficient of variation (CV): The standard deviation expressed as a percentage of the mean, known as the coefficient of variation. The CV is used to compare the relative variation of different samples or populations (Table 38.3).

The variance is the sum of the squared deviations from the mean (54) divided by the number values of the series minus 1 or 4 =13.5.

The SD is the square root of variance = 3.7 years.

Probability Distributions

When making inferences from data we need to know what kind of distribution the data belongs to and the probabilities associated with such distributions.

Normal distribution: A number of variables have distributions, which are bell-shaped unimodal and symmetrical about their mean, with a single peak in the middle and equal tails at either side and is called the normal or 'Gaussian'. distribution. The equation for the distribution is as follows.

$$f(x) = \frac{1}{\sqrt{2\pi\sigma}} e^{-\frac{1}{2}\left(\frac{x-\mu}{\sigma}\right)^2} = \text{for} -\infty < x < \infty$$

where μ = the mean and σ = the standard deviation of the distribution.

The Normal Distribution has many useful properties and is central to many statistical techniques. The normal curve is defined entirely by its mean and SD, and the following will always apply regardless of the specific values of these quantities: a. 68.3% of the distribution falls within 1 SD of the mean (i.e. between mean—SD and mean+SD); b. 95% of the distribution falls between mean – 1.96 SD and mean + 1.96 SD. c. 95.4% of the distribution falls between mean – 2 SD and mean + 2 SD; d. 99.7% of the distribution falls between mean –3 SD and mean + 3 SD. The proportion of the Normal curve that falls between other ranges be calculated from tabulated values. For distributions with small standard deviations the bell is tall and narrow, and for distributions with large standard deviations the bell is short and wide. As the sample size increases other distributions tends toward the normal distribution.

The standard normal distribution: As there can be an infinite number of normal curves depending on the mean and SD statisticians have devised one standard normal distribution from which the area between two any two ordinates under a normal curve can be estimated. The standard normal distribution has a mean of 0 and a standard deviation of 1 and the total area under the curve is 1. A suitable change of units can transform any other normal distribution to the standard normal distribution. This is done by subtracting the mean from each observation and then dividing by the standard deviation. The standard normal distribution (SND) is given as follows:

$$\text{SND,} \qquad z = \frac{x-\mu}{\sigma} \qquad \text{Eqn. (1)}$$

Table 38.3: Example of calculating variability				
Case No.	*Age*	*Mean age (Years)*	*Deviation from the mean*	*Deviation from the mean squared*
1	17	20	–3	9
2	18	20	–2	4
3	18	20	–2	4
4	21	20	+1	1
5	26	20	+6	36
Total	100	–	0	54

Where x is the original variable with mean μ and standard deviation and z is the new standard normal deviate (SND).

Tables of the standard normal distribution are available which give the area under the curve of the standard normal distribution. These can be used to determine the proportion of the population which has values in some specified range.

Student's T distribution: Often the population mean and standard deviation is not known and the sample standard deviation is used to estimate the population standard deviation. The statistic "t" is estimated

$$t = \frac{(\bar{x} - \mu)}{\frac{s}{\sqrt{n}}}$$

Where s = sample standard deviation
  n = sample size
  μ = population mean
  $\bar{x}$ = sample mean

This does not follow the standard normal distribution, but follow a similar symmetrical, bell shaped distribution called the t distribution with $(n-1)$ degrees of freedom. The t distribution also has a mean of 0, but the tails of the distribution are more spread out. The exact shape of the t distribution depends on the degrees of freedom (df). The df are equal to the sample size minus 1. The greater the sample size, and thus the degrees of freedom, then the narrower is the bell shape, until, the sample size is so large, the t distri-bution resembles the standard normal distribution.

Other probability distributions: There are several other probability distributions; –Binomial (data characterized by two mutually exclusive categories), Piosson (for rare events in a large population), Log–Normal (skewed when plotted in arithmetic scale but normal when plotted in Logarithmic scale) ; F, χ^2 distribution, etc. Each of them have mathematical formulae from which the probabilities are estimated. Tables which give these probabilities are available in standard textbooks of statistics.

Statistical Inference and Tests of Significance

In research we collect data from a sample and draw conclusions based on this data. This process of drawing conclusions from quantitative or qualitative information using methods of statistics to describe and arrange the data and to test hypotheses is called statistical inference.

Process of hypothesis testing: This involves making an assumption about a parameter and checking the plausibility of the assumption using sample data.

The types of situations encountered are:
• Comparison of sample data with population parameter. (Mean/Proportion)
• Comparison of two or more populations, e.g. patients using drug A vs patients using drug B. (Mean/Proportion)
• Relationship between two or more factors in a population, e.g. smoking vs cancer.

There are three basic steps in the **process of hypothesis testing:**

a. Asserting the null hypothesis (H_0). The null hypothesis states that there is no real difference between the populations or there is no real association between the two variables.
b. establishing the level.

When concluding from the data collected we can make two kinds of errors:
1. False positive error, i.e when H_0 is true but we reject it, also called error or type I error (there is no real difference/association but we conclude that there is a difference/association).
2. False negative error or Type II error or error when H_0 is false but we accept it (there is a real difference/association but we conclude that there is no difference/association).

By convention the error or Type I error is usually set at $P = 0.05$ (5%) which means that the investigator is willing to run a of 5% risk (but no more) of being in error in concluding that there is a real difference when actually there is no real difference/association.

c. Accepting the null hypothesis or the alternative hypothesis. If the null hypothesis is unlikely the alternative hypothesis which states that there is actually a real difference or association is accepted.

α level and p value: The value obtained by a statistical test is the probability that the observed difference could have been obtained by chance alone. Once the α level is established the p value for a given set of data has to be estimated by calculating the critical ratio (such as the $t, z, F\ X^2$) and consulting standard tables for the possible values of p at that critical ratio. If the p value obtained from the tables is < or the pre-selected α level (most often kept at 0.05) the null hypothesis is rejected and the alternative hypothesis is accepted.

p values do not give any indication as to the clinical importance of an observed effect. For example, if a new drug for lowering blood cholesterol is tested against standard treatment, and the resulting p value is extremely small, it indicates that the difference is unlikely to be due to chance, but decisions on whether to prescribe the new drug will depend on many other factors, including the cost of the new treatment, any potential contraindications or side effects, etc.

Standard Error (SE) and Confidence Intervals (CI)

The **Standard Error of mean** is the standard deviation of a population of sample means, rather than individual observations, and refers to the variability of means.

$$SE = \frac{SD}{\sqrt{N}}$$

The larger the sample size the smaller the *SE*. The *SE* helps us to estimate the amount of error and for performing tests of significance.

The mean ± 1.96 *SE* estimates the range in which 95% of the means of repeated samples would be expected to fall and gives the range of values in which the investigator can be 95% confident that the true mean of the underlying population will fall which is called the **95% confident intervals**. Other confidence intervals can also be calculated, for example, 99% CI is given by Mean 2.58SE.

Standard Error of Proportion is calculated by the formula: $\sqrt{\dfrac{pq}{N}}$.

(Where *p* is the measured proportion; *q* = (1 – *p*); *N* = sample size).

Tests of Significance

These tests are used to estimate the population parameters from sample statistics, compare two parameters such as means or proportions and to assess whether the difference between them is statistically significant. The most commonly applied tests are:

"t" Tests (Students t tests and paired t tests) which compare difference between two means.

"z" test which compares the difference between two proportions.

These tests

a. estimate a critical ratio (*CR*) which is
  CR = Parameter/*SE* of that Parameter
  t = difference between two means
    standard error of difference between two means
  Z = difference between two proportions
    standard error of difference between two proportions

b. Determine the *p* value for the observed critical ratio (*t*/*z*) by consulting standard tables. The larger the CR the more likely it is that the difference is not due to chance. Unless the total sample size is small (< 30) the finding of a *CR* > about 2 usually indicates that the difference is not due to chance and the null hypothesis is rejected. For small sample sizes the *p* value for the estimated degrees of freedom are taken.

Degrees of freedom (DF): This refers to the number of observations that are free to vary. In general df for any test is the total sample size minus 1 for each mean calculated. For the student's t test the formula for df is $N_1 + N_2 - 2$.

a. Comparison of sample mean with population mean
Problem: The normal mean serum hemoglobin value of children in a village is 10.0 gm%. A hemoglobin value of a group of 20 children receiving iron tablets was studied. The mean hemoglobin value for this group was 10.8 gm%, standard deviation σ = 0.56. Can we say that these children have different hemoglobin levels than the general population?

Solution:
a. *Question to be answered:*
Is the serum hemoglobin value for the children receiving iron tablets different from the serum hemoglobin of other children?

Get Data
  Sample size *n* = 20
  Mean of sample χ = 10.8 gm%, standard deviation σ = 0.56
  Population mean =10.0 gm%
b. *Null Hypothesis:* The serum hemoglobin value of the children receiving iron tablets is not different than that of the other children (i.e. the sample is taken from the population mean of 10.0 gm%)
c. *Standard error of mean*

$$= \frac{\sigma}{\sqrt{n}} = \frac{0.56}{\sqrt{20}} = 0.125$$

d. *Critical ratio:*

$$t = \frac{\text{difference in mean}}{\text{Estimate of standard error}}$$

  Estimate of standard error

$$= \frac{18.8 - 10.0}{0.125} = 6.4$$

e. *Comparison with theoretical value*
Value of t (critical ratio) at (*n* – 1) = 19 degrees of freedom from tables: for 5% level is 2.093, 1% level is 2.861 and 1-in –100 is 3.883. Observed value of t is 6.4 which is more than 3.883. Thus probability of a chance finding of difference is less than 1 in 100.
f. *Decision: Reject null hypothesis*
g. *Inference:* There is difference in the sample children's hemoglobin level from the general level.

b. Testing the equality of two means: independent samples
The unpaired *t* test (also referred to as the **student t test** or the **independent sample *t* test or pooled *t* test**) is used to assess the statistical significance of the

difference between two population means in a study based on data obtained from independent samples.

Example: From the data in Table 38.1 can we conclude that blacks have higher Blood Pressure than whites?

a. *Question to be answered:* Do blacks have higher Blood Pressure than whites?

b. *Null Hypothesis (H$_0$):* "Mean blood pressure levels are equal in both races (Table 38.4)".

Get data

Standard error of mean

a. The pooled variance, S_p^2, is computed using the formula:

$$S_p^2 = \frac{(n_1 - 1)s_1^2 + (n_2 - 1)s_2^2}{n_1 + n_2 - 2}$$

Thus, for this example, s_p^2 is

$$S_p^2 = \frac{(17 - 1)(11.3959)^2 + (14 - 1)(16.5828)^2}{17 + 14 - 2}$$

and the standard error of the mean is

$$SE = \frac{\sqrt{S_p^2}}{n_1} + \frac{s_p^2}{n_2}$$

$$= 5.0388$$

d. *Critical ratio:*

$$t = x_1 - x_2 / SE$$
$$= 142.2857 - 127.3529 / 5.0388$$
$$= 2.964$$

e. **Evaluate the evidence against H$_0$**

Comparison with theoretical value For $n_1 + n_2 - 2$ degrees of freedom (*df*) (in this example) from t tables it is verified that the 2 tailed **p-value is 0.006**.

f. *Decision: Reject null Hypothesis,* Since $p \leq 05$, H_0 is rejected

g. *Inference:* **Statistical conclusion:** The difference between the two population means is statistically significant. **Clinical interpretation:** Mean blood pressure is significantly higher in the blacks than in whites. ($p < 0.006$). **Chance of error:** The change that the statistical test had led to the conclusion that mean blood pressure is higher in the blacks than in whites when, in fact, the mean blood pressures are equal (i.e. H_0 is true) is 6 in 1000 or less.

d. Paired *t* test

The paired t test is used to assess the statistical significance of the difference between two population means in studies of paired or matched samples. In this design the subjects may be **self-paired**, that is, they serve as their own controls as in before- and - after trials or the subjects are **"artificially" matched** with respect to one or more factors.

Example: From Table 38.1 the effect of treatment (Example salt restriction) on the blood pressure is studied. BP1 shows the blood pressure of the subjects after treatment. Can we say that treatment has a significant impact on the blood pressure?

a. *Question to be answered:* Does treatment truly reduce blood pressure?

b. *Null Hypothesis (H$_0$):* "There is no difference in the mean blood pressure level of the population of individuals (Table 38.5) who take treatment and the population of individuals who do not," that is, H_0: $\mu = 0$.

Get data: From

BP = Blood Pressure before treatment, BP1 Blood Pressure after treatment (Table 38.6).

Standard Error of the mean of differences

The standard deviation of the differences (SD) is obtained using the formula

$$sd = \frac{\sqrt{\Sigma d_i^2 - (\Sigma d_i)^2 / n}}{n - 1}$$

Hence   sd = 7.9999

Standard Error = sd/n = 7.9999/30 = 1.4368

Table 38.4: Mean blood pressure levels are equal in both races				
RACE	*N*	*Mean BP*	*Std. Deviation*	*Std. Error Mean*
whites	17(n_1)	127.3529	11.3959	2.7639
blacks	14(n_2)	142.2857	16.5828	4.4319

Table 38.5: Paired samples statistics				
Paired samples statistics				
	Mean	*N*	*Std. Deviation*	*Std. Error Mean*
Pair 1 BP	134.0968	31	15.6681	2.8141
BP 1	128.8387	31	16.6195	2.9849

Table 38.6: Blood Pressure before treatment, BP1 Blood Pressure after treatment		
BP Before treatment (BP)	*BP After treatment (BP1)*	*Difference(BP–BP1)*
Y_{11}	Y_{21}	$D_1 = Y_{11} - Y_{21}$
Y_{12}	Y_{22}	$D_2 = Y_{12} - Y_{22}$
—	—	—
—	—	—
—	—	—
Y_{1n}	Y_{2n}	$D_n = Y_{1n} - Y_{2n}$
Mean $\hat{Y}_1 = Y_{1i}/n$	$Y_2 = \hat{Y}_{2i}/n$	$\hat{Y}_{2d} = di/n$
Exercise Group	**Control Group**	**Difference**
$\hat{Y}_1 = 134.096$	$\hat{Y}_2 = 128.838$	$\hat{Y}_d = 5.2581$
$S_1 = 15.668$	$S_2 = 16.619$	$Sd = 7.9999$
$n = 31$	$n = 31$	$n = 31$

d. *Critical ratio:*

Critical ratio

$$= \frac{\text{sample estimate} - \text{hypothesized polulation value}}{\text{Standard error of sample estimate}}$$

$$t = \frac{\hat{Y}_d - \mu_0}{sd/\sqrt{n}}$$

$$= \frac{5.2581 - 0}{1.4368}$$

$$= 3.660$$

e. *Comparison with theoretical value:* For $n-1$ degrees of freedom (*df*) (in this example) from t tables it is verified that the 2 tailed **p-value is 0.001**.

f. *Decision: Reject null Hypothesis,* Since p .05, HO is rejected

g. *Inference: **Statistical conclusion:*** The reduction of Mean blood pressure by taking treatment is statistically significant. Clinical interpretation: Mean blood pressure is significantly reduced by taking treatment. (p. 0.001).Chance of error: The chance that the statistical test had led to the conclusion that mean blood pressure is reduced by treatment when, in fact, the mean blood pressures does not change (i.e. H_0 is true) is 1 in 1000 or less.

d. Z TESTS

Z tests are used to estimate the population proportion from a sample proportion and compare two proportions.

The same procedure as uses for t test is used except that the formulae are different.

$$SE \text{ of proportion} = \sqrt{pq/N}$$

Where p = Observed proportion
$q = (1 - p)$
N = Sample siz.
95% CI = p 1.96 SE

Example: If 20% (0.20) of individuals in a sample of 100 individuals are ill at any point of time the calculation for *SE* and *CI* would be:

$$SE = 0.20 \times 0.80/100 = 0.04$$
$$95\% \ CI = 0.20 \ 1.96 \ (0.04)$$
$$= 0.2 - 0.078 \text{ to } 0.2 + 0.078$$
$$= \text{From } 0.122 \text{ to } 0.278$$

Thus in 95% of cases the true proportion of individuals ill at any point of time ranges from 12.2% to 27.8%.

i. Comparison of sample proportion with population proportion.

Problem: It is known that 20% of the children in a school are anaemic. It was found that 30 of a group of 200 children in the school receiving iron tablets were anaemic. Can we say that the proportion children having anaemia in this group is lesser than that in the general population of school children?

Solution:

a. *Question to be answered:*

Is the prevalence of anaemia among the children receiving iron tablets different from that in the general population of school children?

Get Data

Sample size $n = 200$
Sample proportion p = 30/200 * 100 = 15%
Population proportion $P = 20\%$

b. *Null Hypothesis:* The prevalence of anaemia among the children receiving iron tablets is the same as in the general population of school children.

c. *Standard error of proportion*

$$= \sqrt{pq/N} = 15* \ 85/200 = 2.5248$$

d. *Critical ratio:*

$$z = \frac{\text{difference in proportions}}{\text{Standard error of proportion}}$$

$$= \frac{20-15}{2.5248} = 1.98$$

e. *Comparison with theoretical value*
This critical ratio (z) follows a Normal Distribution whose 5% level is 1.96 and 1% level is 2.576. Observed value of z is 1.98 which is more than 1.96. Thus probability of a chance finding of difference is less than 5%.

f. *Decision: Reject null Hypothesis.*

g. *Inference:* The prevalence of anemia among the children receiving iron tablets is lesser than in the general population of school children.

ii. ***SE of difference between two proportions:***

Example: In a study it was found that 30 out of 200 whites had cancer stomach compared to 36 out of 300 blacks. Can we say that the occurrence of cancer is different in blacks compared to whites (Table 38.7)?

a. *Question to be answered:* Is occurrence of cancer different in blacks compared to whites?

Get data:

b. *Null Hypothesis:* Occurrence of cancer is the same in blacks and whites (Table 38.7).

c. *Standard error of* **proportion**
Standard error of proportion

$$= S\,(P_1 - P_2) = \sqrt{pq/n_1 + pq/n_2}$$

(where P = Pooled proportion q = (100 – P) (Table 38. 8)

d. *Critical ratio:* $z = \dfrac{P_1 - P_2}{S(P_1 - P_2)} = \dfrac{15-12}{2.96} = 1.01$

Table 38.7: Occurrence of cancer is different in blacks compared to whites	
Whites	Blacks
$n_1 = 200$	$n_2 = 300$
Number with cancer = 30	Number with cancer = 36

e. *Comparison with theoretical value*
This critical ratio (z) follows a Normal Distribution whose 5% level is 1.96 and 1% level is 2.576. Observed value of z is 1.01 which is less than 1.96. Thus probability of a chance finding of difference is more than 5%.

f. *Decision:* Accept null Hypothesis.

g. *Inference:* There is no statistically significant difference in the occurrence of cancer in blacks and in whites.

e. Chi Square Test

The chi-square test is a statistical test used to examine differences with categorical variables. The test is applied for estimating how closely an observed distribution matches an expected distribution—the *goodness-of-fit test* and estimating whether two random variables are independent.

This test was developed by Karl Pearson in 1889 and involves calculation of a quantity called chi square from the Greek letter chi (x) pronounced as "kye".

The formula for chi square: The deviation of the observed numbers from those specified by the hypothesis forms the basis of the chi square. Each deviation is squared, each square is divided by the hypothetical or expected numbers and the results are added. Thus $x^2 = \Sigma^{(0-E)^2/E}$ where O is the observed frequency, E the expected frequency and denotes summation.

Degrees of freedom: The term degrees of freedom refers to the number of observations that are free to vary. According to the null hypothesis, the best estimate of the expected distribution of counts in the cells of a contingency table is provided by row and column totals. Therefore, the row and column totals are considered to be fixed. An observed count can be entered freely into the of the cells of a $2x^2$ (e.g. The top left cell, devoted by). Once that count is entered none of the other cells are free to vary. This means that a

Table 38.8		
Proportion with cancer $P_1 = \dfrac{30 \times 100}{200} = 15\%$		
Proportion with cancer $P_2 = \dfrac{36 \times 100}{300} = 12\%$		
Pooled proportion with cancer $= P = \dfrac{n_1 P_1 + n_2 P_2}{n_1 + n_2} = \dfrac{30+36}{500} = 12.12\%$		
$S(P_1 - P_2) = \sqrt{pq/n_1 + pq/n_2}$		
(where $p = 12.12$, $q = (100 - P) = (100 - 12.12) = 87.88$)		
$S(P_1 - P_2) = \sqrt{8.8} = 2.96$		

$2x^2$ table has only one degree of freedom. The general formula for calculating the degree of freedom $=(R-1)(C-1)$ where R indicates Row and C indicates Column. The steps for finding statistical significance by conducting chi square test.

1. Fix the null hypothesis
2. Choose the alternative hypothesis
3. Find the value of the statistic
   a. Make the contingency table
   b. Determine the expected number in each group of the sample a cell of table on assumption of null hypothesis, i.e. no variation exists between the sample and the universe. Formula for calculating the expected count of cell 'y' is

$$E(y) = \frac{(\text{Total value of rows of } y)(\text{Total value of columns of } y)}{\text{Study total}}$$

   c. Find the difference between the observed and the expected frequencies in each cell ($0-E$)
   d. Calculated the x^2 value for each cell by the formula $X^2 = \dfrac{(O-E)^2}{E}$
   e. Sum up the x^2 values of all the cells to get the total chi square value $X^2 = (0-E)^2/E$
4. Find the degree of freedom by the formula $df = (R-1)(C-1)$.
5. Assess significance level: Find the tabulated value from the table of chi square distribution and compare value with tabulated value.
6. Draw conclusion

Example: In a study on breast cancer it was found that 35 out of 50 patients on Chemotherapy survived 5 years compared to 30 out of 55 on Radiotherapy. Does this prove that 5 year survival of the patients was dependent on the type of treatment received.

1. *Establish hypotheses:* The null hypothesis is that the method of treatment has no influence on the 5 year survival of breast cancer, i.e. two variables are independent and so the 5 year survival is the same for Chemotherapy and Radiotherapy.
2. *Alternative hypothesis* states that method of treatment influences the 5 year survival of breast cancer, i.e. two variables are dependent and so the 5 year survival is different Chemotherapy and Radiotherapy.
3. *Calculate Chi-square statistic*
   a. **Contingency Table 38.9.**
   b. **Calculate the expected value for each cell of the table.**
      The expected value for each cell of the table can be calculated using the following formula:

$$\frac{\text{Row total} \times \text{Column total}}{\text{Total } \eta \text{ for table}}$$

   c. **Calculate X Square: Table 38.10**
      Chi-square = Sum of

$$\frac{(\text{observed} \times \text{frequency} - \text{expected} \times \text{frequency})^2}{(\text{expected} \times \text{frequency})}$$

4. *Degree of freedom:* $df = (R-1)(C-1)$
   In this table, there were two rows and two columns. Therefore, the number of degrees of freedom is: $df = 1$.
5. *Assess significance level:* The tabulated value from the table of chi square distribution for df 1 and 0.05 level is 3.84. The calculated value is $= 2.63$ which is lesser than 3.84.

Draw conclusion: Since the calculated value is lesser than the tabulated value we accept the null hypothesis that the two variables are independent and method of treatment has no influence on the 5 year survival of breast cancer.

The expected counts in each cell of a $2X^2$ contingency table should be five or more or else the

Table 38.9: Contingency table

Treatment	Survived 5 years	Died	Total
Chemotherapy	35 (30.9)	15 (19.0)	50
Radiotherapy	30 (34.04)	25 (20.95)	50
Total	65	40	100

Values in parentheses indicate expected values.

Table 38.10: Calculate *X* Square

$$\frac{(35-30.9)^2}{30.9} + \frac{(15-19.0)^2}{19.0} + \frac{(30-34.04)^2}{34.04} + \frac{(20-20.95)^2}{20.95}$$
$$= 2.63$$

Serial number	Age	Occupation	BP	Race	Hypertension	BP1
1	9	*n*	110	*w*	0	110
2	23	*ss*	120	*w*	0	118
3	25	*s*	124	*w*	0	120
4	14	*n*	114	*w*	0	120
5	15	*n*	116	*w*	0	120
6	17	*n*	118	*w*	0	100
7	18	*n*	120	*w*	0	110
8	18	*n*	148	*w*	1	140
9	23	*us*	126	*w*	0	110
10	14	*n*	114	*b*	0	110
11	19		128	*w*	0	130
12	24	*ss*	126	*w*	0	130
13	25	*s*	128	*w*	0	120
14	25	*s*	126	*w*	0	120
15	26	*s*	158	*b*	1	158
16	27	*s*	128	*b*	0	120
17	32	*ss*	130	*b*	0	134
18	35	*p*	132	*w*	0	132
19	36	*s*	138	*b*	0	136
20	40	*p*	140	*w*	0	110
21	44	*p*	142	*b*	0	136
22	47	*ss*	130	*b*	0	120
23	48	*s*	150	*w*	1	130
24	48	*s*	152	*b*	1	148
25	46	*p*	128	*b*	1	128
26	48	*s*	154	*b*	1	150
27	50	*s*	162	*b*	1	168
28	56	*s*	128	*b*	0	120
29	60	*us*	168	*b*	1	160
30	62	*p*	139	*w*	0	136
31	61	*s*	160	*b*	1	150

Table 38.11: Data of 31 persons with hypertension and their occupation

w: white; *b*: black ; *us*: unskilled, *ss*: semiskilled, *s*: skilled, *p*: professional, *n*: unemployed.

assumptions and approximations of a Kye square test may break down. For small numbers the Yates correction for continuity can be used.

$$\text{Yates } X^2 = \Sigma \frac{(|O - E| - 0.5)^2}{E}$$

Drawing Conclusions from Results of Statistical Analysis

While interpreting statistical information, especially tests of significance, the strength of the study designs and methodology needs to be kept in mind and more importantly the biological plausibility of the associations to distinguish causal from spurious associations.

Annexure 1

Example 38.1: A study on hypertension was conducted where 31 persons were asked to take salt restricted diet to determine its efficacy on lowering blood pressure. The systolic Blood pressure was recorded at base line (BP) and repeated after 6 months of salt restricted diet (BP1). The data of Example 38.1 is presented in Table 38.11.

Armitage P, Berry G, Matthews JNS. *Statistical Methods in Medical Research*. 4th edn. Cornwall UK: Blackwell Science, 2002.

Jekel JF, Elmore JG, Katz DL. *Epidemiology, Biostatistics and Preventive Medicine*. Pennsylvania 19106. WB Saunders Company, 1996

Jerrold H Zar. *Bio-statistical analysis*. 4th edn. Delhi: Dorling Kinderslay (India) Pvt. Ltd. 2007.

Panneerselvam R. *Research methodology*. New Delhi: Prentice Hall of India Pvt. Ltd. 2004.

Peck R, Olsen C, Devore J. *Introduction to statistics and data analysis*. Duxbury, CA 93950 USA, 2001.

PSS Sundar Rao, Jesudan G, Richard J. *An introduction to biostatistics—A manual for students in Health Sciences*. 2nd edn. Vellore: CMC Vellore, 1983.

Rebecca G K, Miller MCIII. Clinical Epidemiology and Biostatistics, NMS Series. Pennsylvania: Harwal Publishing Company, 1992.

Triola MM, Triola MF. *Biostatistics for the biological and health sciences*. San Francisco NY: Addison Wesley, 2006.

39.1 DIAGNOSTIC MICROBIOLOGY

Infectious diseases can only be finally diagnosed with certainty by laboratory diagnosis. Laboratory diagnosis is based on one or more of the following investigations:

1. Direct examination of specimens by microscopic or antigenic techniques
2. Isolation of microorganisms in culture
3. Serologic testing for detection of antibodies (serological diagnosis)
4. Molecular detection of the pathogen's genome (DNA, RNA)
5. Testing for antimicrobial drug susceptibility, and
6. Detecting and clarifying the epidemiology of nosocomial infections. Clinicians must select the appropriate tests and specimens, and send them to the microbiologist for identifying the etiological agent.

Laboratory diagnosis of bacterial and fungal infections: Diagnosis of bacterial and fungal infections is possible mainly on direct demonstration of the microorganisms by microscopic examination or antigen detection and on growth of microorganisms on nutrient culture media. Molecular diagnostic methods for direct detection of certain pathogens are available for some pathogens.

Laboratory diagnosis of viral infections: Specimens for viral diagnosis should be collected early in the course of infection when viral shedding is maximal. Fluids and respiratory secretions should be collected in sterile containers and delivered to the laboratory promptly. Swabs should be rubbed vigorously against mucosal or skin surfaces to obtain as much cellular material as possible, and sent in viral transport media that contain antibiotics to inhibit bacterial growth. Rectal swabs should not be heavily covered with feces because the antibiotics present in viral transport media may be insufficient to kill a large inoculum of bacteria. All specimens should be transported on ice. Laboratory diagnosis of viral infections may be done by electron microscopy, antigen detection, virus isolation in culture, serologic testing or by detection of virus genomes by molecular biology techniques. Immunofluorescent-antibody (IFA) techniques or other methods such as enzyme immunoassay (EIA) that use antibodies to detect viral antigens directly in clinical specimens permit rapid identification of viruses. In addition to providing rapid diagnosis, antigen detection EIA tests are commonly used for the diagnosis of viruses that are difficult to culture, such as rotavirus, noroviruses, and hepatitis B viruses.

Laboratory diagnosis of parasitic infections: Most parasites are detected by microscopic examination of clinical specimens. *Plasmodium* and *Babesia* can be detected in stained blood smears, *Leishmania* in bone marrow smears, and helminth eggs, *Entamoeba histolytica*, *Giardia lamblia* cysts, and trophozoites in fecal smears. Ova and parasite examination of fecal specimens includes a wet mount (to detect motile organisms if fresh stool is received), concentration (to improve yield), and permanent staining, such as trichrome, for microscopic examination.

Serologic diagnosis: Serologic tests are primarily used in the diagnosis of infectious agents that are difficult to culture in vitro or detect by direct examination. Antibody test may be specific for immunoglobulin G (IgG) or M (IgM) or may measure antibody response regardless of immunoglobulin class. The IgM response occurs earlier in the illness, generally peaking at 7–10 days after infection, and usually disappears within a few weeks but for some infections (e.g. hepatitis A) may persist for months. The IgG response peaks at 4–6 wk and usually persists for life. Because the IgM response is transient, the presence of IgM antibody in most cases correlates with recent infection; therefore, a single positive serum specimen is considered diagnostic. The presence of IgG antibody may indicate new seroconversion or past exposure to the pathogen. To confirm a new infection using IgG testing, it is essential to demonstrate either seroconversion or a rising IgG titer. A four-fold increase in a convalescent titer obtained 2–3 wk after the acute titer is considered diagnostic in most situations.

Molecular diagnostic techniques: Molecular diagnostic techniques are most useful for detecting and identifying pathogens for which culture and serologic tests are difficult, slow or not available. Two of the widely used techniques in clinical microbiology are *DNA probes* for direct detection and *nucleic acid amplification* using polymerase chain reaction (PCR).

Ananthanarayan R, Paniker CKJ (eds). In: *Textbook of Microbiology.* 6th edn. Chennai: Orient Longman Pvt. Ltd., 2000.

Goldmann DA, Zaidi AKN. Diagnostic microbiology. In: Kliegman RM, Behrman RE, Jenson HB, Stanton BF (eds). *Nelson Textbook of Pediatrics.* 18th edn. Vol. 1. Philadelphia: Saunders, 2007; 1053–1057.

Greenwood D, Slack R, Peutherer J (eds). In: *Medical Microbiology A guide to microbial infections: Pathogenesis, Immunity, Laboratory Diagnosis and Control.* 15th edn. Edinburgh: Churchill Livingstone, 1997.

Lennette HE, Balows A, Hauser WJ et al (eds). Collection, Handling and processing of specimen. In: *Manual of Clinical Microbiology.* 4th edn. Washington DC: ASM, 1985;73–98.

Shrestha CD. Diagnostic microbiology in pediatric practice. In: Mathur GP, Mathur Sarla (eds). *Current Trends in Pediatrics.* Vol 1. Delhi: Academa Publishers, 2005;174–189.

Storch GA. Diagnostic virology. *Clin Infect Dis* 2000; 31: 739–751.

39.2 REFERENCE RANGES FOR LABORATORY TESTS AND PROCEDURES

In the following Tables 39.1–39.13C, the reference ranges apply to infants, children, and adolescents when possible. For many analyses, however separate reference ranges for children and adolescents are not well delineated. When interpreting a test result, reference range supplied by the laboratory interpreting a test result, the reference range supplied by the laboratory performing the test should always be used. Figures 39.1 and 39.2 for estimations related to dosages.

Table 39.1: Abbreviations

amp	Ampule, ampoule
bid (bis in die)	Twice a day (BD)
Cap	Capillary
caps	Capsule, capsules
CK	Creatine Kinase
Cr	Creatinine
CNS	Central nervous system
CSF	Cerebrospinal fluid
F	Female
g	Grams
g/mL	Gram per milliliter
GABA	Gamma-aminobutyric acid
hr	Hour, hours
Hb	Hemoglobin
hpf	High power field
Hs (hora sommi)	At bed time
IM	Intramuscular
inj	Injection, injections
IU	International unit of hormone activity
IV	Intravenous
kg	Kilogram, kilograms
L	Liter
M	Male
MB	Heart isoenzyme of creatine kinase
ml	Milliliter
mL	Milliliter
mg	Milligram
mg/l	Milligram per liter
mg/L	Milligram per liter
mEq/L	Milliequivalents per liter
mg/mL	Microgram per milliliter
mm³	Cubic millimeter, microliter (L)
mmHg	Millimeters of mercury
min	Minute, minutes
mo	Month, months
mol	Mole
mmol	Millimole
mOsm	Milliosmole
mmol/L	Micromole per liter
min	Minute, minutes
MW	Relative molecular weight
ND	Not detected
nm	Nanometer (wavelength)
Od (omni die)	Everyday
Pa	Pascal
pc	Postparandial
PO	Per oral
q	Quantity
qid (quarter in die)	Four times a day
RBC	Red blood cell (s), erythrocyte (s)
RT	Room temperature
s	Second, seconds
sec	Second, seconds
sc	Subcutaneous
SD	Standard deviation
SOS (si opus sit)	As and when required

Contd...

Table 39.1: Abbreviations (*Cotd...*)

susp	Suspension
syp	Syrup
tabs	Tablets
tid (ter in die)	Three times a day (TDS)
TR	Trace
U	Internationl unit of enzyme activity
V	Volume
WBC	White blood cell (s)
WHO	World Health Organization
wk	Week, weeks
yr	Year, years

Table 39.2: Symbols

>	Greater than
$\geq$	Greater than or equal to
<	Less than
$\leq$	Less than or equal to
$\pm$	Plus/minus
$\approx$	Almost equal to
~	Tide
μ	Micro sign
α	Alpha
β	Beta
γ	Gamma
δ	Delta
£	Pound
lb	Pounds

Table 39.3: Abbreviation for specimens

AM	Amniotic fluid
C	Citrate
CSF	Cerebrospinal fluid
EDTA	Ethylenediaminetetraacetic acid
F	Feces
H	Heparin
LH	Lithium heparin
NaC	Sodium citrate
NH_4H	Ammonium heparinate
O	Oxalate
P	Plasma
S	Serum
U	Urine
W	Whole blood

Table 39.4: International system of units (SI units)

Examples of basic SI units

Length	Meter	m
Mass	kilogram	kg
Amount of substance	mole	mol
Energy	joule	J
Pressure	pascal	Pa

Examples of decimal multiples and submultiples of SI units

Factor	Name	Symbol
10^6	mega-	M
10^3	kilo-	k
10^2	hecto-	h
10^1	deka-	da
10^{-1}	deci-	d
10^{-2}	centi-	c
10^{-3}	milli	m
10^{-6}	micro-	μ
10^{-9}	nano-	n
10^{-12}	pico-	p
10^{-15}	femto-	f

Table 39.5: Weights and measurements	
Liquid measurements	
Metric	Approx. Apothecary equivalents
1000 ml (1 liter)	1 quart (qt)
750 ml	1 1/2 pints
500 ml	1 pint
250 ml	8 fluid ounces
4 ml	1 fluid dram
1 ml	15 minims
Weight measurements	
30 g	1 ounce
15 g	4 drams
1 g	15 grains
60 mg	1 grain

Table 39.6: Measurement of length in centimetre and inches	
Centimetre (cm) (approx)	*Inch*
2.5	1
28	11
33	13
35.5	14
61	24
89	35
91.5	36
122	48
152	60

A milliliter (ml) is the approximate equivalent of a cubic centimeter (cc); 1 gallon = 4.55 liters
One Pound (lb) = 16 ounces (oz); 2.2 Pounds (lb) = 1 Kilogram (kg); 1,000 g = 1 kilo (gram); 1,000 kilogram = 1 tonne
Adapted by the latest Pharmacopeia, National Formulatory, and New and nonofficial Remedies, and approved by the Federal food and drug Administration
Dorland's Pocket medical Dictionary. 20th edn abridged from Dorland's Illustrated Medical Dictionary. Philadelphia: WB Saunders Co, 1959; W3-W10.

Table 39.7: Equivalent temperature readings (Celcius [C] and Fahrenheit [F])							
C	*F*	*C*	*F*	*C*	*F*	*C*	*F*
0	32.0	37.2	99.0	39.2	102.6	41.2	106.2
20	68.0	37.4	99.3	39.4	102.9	41.4	106.5
30	86.0	37.6	99.7	39.6	103.3	41.6	106.9
31	87.8	37.8	100.1	39.8	103.7	41.8	107.2
32	89.6	38.0	100.4	40.0	104	42	107.6
33	91.4	38.2	100.8	40.2	104.4	43	109.4
34	93.2	38.4	101.2	40.4	104.7	44	111.2
35	95.0	38.6	101.5	40.6	105.1	100	212
36	96.8	38.8	101.8	40.8	105.4	104.4	220
37	98.6	39.0	102.2	41.0	105.8	120	230

To convert Celsius (centigrade) readings to Fahrenheit (multiply by 1.8 and add 32). To convert Fahrenheit readings to Celsius, substract 32 and divide by 1.8. 0 centigrade is freezing; 100 centigrade is boiling point.

Table 39.8: Additive solutions	
50%	0.5 g/ml
Sodium chloride	2.5 and 5 mEq/ml
Sodium acetate	2 and 4 mEq/ml
Sodium lactate	5 mEq/ml
Sodium bicarbonate	0.5 (4.2%) mEq/ml and 0.9 (7.5%) mEq/ml
Potassium acetate	2 and 4 mEq/ml
Potassium chloride	2 and 3 mEq/ml
Potassium phosphate	4.4 mEq/ml of potassium and 3 mM/mL phosphate
Calcium gluconate 10%	9.3 mg (0.465 mEq/ml) elemental calcium
Calcium chloride 10%	27.3 mg (1.4 mEq/ml) elemental calcium
Ammonium chloride	5 mEq/ml
Magnesium sulfate	0.8 mEq/ml, 1 mEq/ml, and 4 mEq/ml available as the 10%, 12.5%, and 50% solutions

Table 39.9: Factors for conversion of concentration expressed in Milliequivalents per Liter to Milligrams per Deciliter (100 mL) and vice versa, for common ions that occur in physiologic solutions

Element or Radical	mEq/L to mg/dL		mg/dL to mEq/L	
Sodium	1	2.30	1	.4348
Potassium	1	3.91	1	.2558
Calcium	1	2.005	1	.4988
Magnesium	1	1.215	1	.8230
Chloride	1	3.55	1	.2817
Bicarbonate	1	6.1	1	.1639
Phosphorus valence 1	1	3.10	1	.3226
Phosphorus valence 1.8	1	1.72	1	.5814
Sulfur valence 2	1	1.60	1	.625

Table 39.10: Milliequivalents and milligrams of cations and anions present in one Millimole of salts commonly used in physiologic solutions

Salt	Salt (mg/ mmol)	Cation	Salt (mEq/ mmol)	Salt (mg/ mmol)	Anion	Salt (mEq/ mmol)	Salt (mg/ mmol)
Sodium chloride (NaCl)	58.5	Na^+	1	23.0	Cl^-	1	35.5
Potassium chloride (KCl)	74.6	K^+	1	39.1	Cl^-	1	35.5
Sodium bicarbonate (NaHCO$_3$)	84.0	Na^+	1	23.0	HCO_3^-	1	61.0
Sodium lactate (CH$_3$CHOHCOONA)	112.0	Na^+	1	23.0	CH_3CHOH COO^-	1	89.0
Potassium phosphate monobasic (K$_2$HPO$_4$)	174.2	K^+	1	78.2	HPO_4^{2-}	2	96.0
Potassium phosphate dibasic (KH$_2$PO$_4$)	136.1	K^+	1	39.1	$H_2PO_4^-$	1	97.0
Calcium chloride, anhydrous (CaCl$_2$)	111.0	Ca^{2+}	2	40.0	Cl_2^{2-}	2	71.0
Calcium chloride, dihydrae (CaCl$_2$ 2H$_2$0)	147.0	Ca^{2+}	2	40.0	Cl_2^{2-}	2	71.0
Magnesium chloride, anhydrous (MgCl$_2$)	95.2	Mg^{2+}	2	24.3	Cl_2^{2-}	2	71.0
Magnesium chloride, hexaydrate (MgCl$_2$-6H$_2$O)	203.33	Mg^{2+}	2	24.3	Cl_2^{2-}	2	71.0
Ammonium chloride (NH$_4$Cl)	53.5	NH_4^+	1	18.0	Cl^-	1	35.5

Table 39.11: Prefixes denoting decimal factors

Prefix	Symbol	Factor
Mega	M	10^6
Kilo	k	10^3
Hecto	h	10^2
Deka	da	10^1
Deci	d	10^{-1}
Centi	c	10^{-2}
Milli	m	10^{-3}
Micro	μ	10^{-6}
Nano	n	10^{-9}
Pico	P	10^{-12}
Femto	f	10^{-15}

Table 39.12: Key to Comments

30°, 37° Temperature of enzymatic analysis (Celsius)
- Values obtained are significantly method-dependent
- Values in older males are higher than those in older females
- Values in older females are higher than those in older males
- Atomic absorption
- Borate affinity chromatography
- Cation exchange chromatography
- Vitros, a proprietary analytic system of Ortho Clinical Diagnostics. Inc.
- Electrophoresis
- Enzymatic assay
- Enzyme-amplified immunoassay
- Fluorometric method
- Fluorescence-activated cell sorting (FACS)
- Fluorescence polarization
- Gas chromatography
- High performance liquid chromatography (HPLC)
- Indirect fluorescence antibody (IFA) assay
- Ion selective electrode
- Nephelometry
- Optical density
- Radial immunodiffusion (RID)
- Radioimmunoassay (RIA)
- Spectrophotometry

Table 39.13: Reference Ranges (Reference Values)

Table 39.13A: Coagulation factors

Analyte or procedure	Specimen	Reference values (USA)	Conversion factor	Values (SI)
Activated partial thromboplastin time (APTT)	P (C)	25–35s Infants <90s	× 1	25–35s Infants <90s
Clotting time Lee-White, 37°C	W	Glass tubes 5–8 min (5–15 min at RT) Silicone tubes about 30 min prolonged	× 1	Glass tubes 5–8 min (5–15 min at RT) Silicone tubes about 30 min prolonged
Factor I, see Fibrinogen	P (C)	0.5–1.5 U/ml or 60–150% of normal	× 1	0.5–1.5 U/ml or 60–150 AU
Factor II				
Factor IV, see Calcium	S	0.5–2U/ml or 60–150% of normal	× 1	0.5–2 U/ml or 60–150AU
Factor V		65–135% of normal	× 1	65–135 AU
Factor VII		60–135% of normal	× 1	60–135 AU
Factor VIII		60–145% of normal	× 1	60–145 AU
Factor VIII antigen		50–200% of normal	× 1	50–200 AUl
Factor IX		60–140% of normal	× 1	60–140 AU
Factor X		60–130% of normal	× 1	60–130 AIU
Factor XI		65–135% of normal	× 1	65–135 AU
Factor XII		65–150% of normal	× 1	65–150 AU
Factor XII (Fibrin stabilizing factor, FSF)	W (C,O)	Minimal hematostatic level 0.02–0.05U/mL1–2% of normal	× 1, 000 × 1	20–50 U/L or 1–2 AU
Fibrin degradation products (D-dimer)	P (C)	Adults: 68–494 µg/L Mean 207	× 1	Adults: 68–494 µg/L Mean 207
Fibrinogen	(NaC)	New born: 125–300 mg/dL Adult: 200–400	× 0.01	New born: 1.25–3.00 g/L Adult: 2.00–4.00

Table 39.13B: Complete blood count

Analyte or procedure	Specimen	Reference values (USA)	Conversion factor	Values (SI)
Hematocrit (HCT, Hct) Calculated from mean corpuscular volume (MCV) and RBC count (electronic displacement of laser)	W(E)	% of packed red cells (V red cells/V whole blood cells × 100)		Volume fraction (V red cells/ V whole blood)
		1 day (cap): 48–69%	× 0.01	1day (cap): 0.48–0.69
		2 days: 48–75%		2 days: 0.48–0.75
		3 days: 44–72%		3 days: 0.44–0.72
		2 mon: 28–42%		2 mon: 0.28–0.42
		6–12 yr: 35–45%		6–12 yr:0.35–0.45
		12–18 yr M: 37–49%		12–18 yr M: 0.37–0.49
		F: 36–46%		F: 0.36–0.46
		18–49 yr M: 41–53%		18–49 yr M: 41–53%
		F: 36–46%		F: 36–46%
Hemoglobin (Hb)	W(E)	g/dl	× 0.155	Mmol/L
		1–3 days (cap): 14.5–22.5		1–3 days (cap): 2.25–3.49
		2 mo: 9.0–14.0		2 mo: 1.40–2.17
		6–12 yr: 11.5–15.5		6–12 yr: 1.78–2.40

Contd...

Table 39.13B: Complete blood count (*Contd...*)

Analyte or procedure	Specimen	Reference values (USA)	Conversion factor	Values (SI)
		12–18 yr M: 13.0–16.0		12–18 yr M: 2.02–2.48
		F: 12.0–16.0		F: 1.86–2.48
		18–49 yr M: 13.5-17.5		18–49 yr M: 2.09–2.27
		F: 12.0–16.0		F: 1.86–2.48
Mean corpuscular hemoglobin (MCH)	W(E)	pg/cell	× 0.0155	fmol/cell
		Birth : 31–37		Birth : 0.48–0.57
		1–3 days (cap): 31–37		1-3 days (cap): 0.48–0.57
		1 wk–1 mo: 28–40		1 wk–1 mo: 0.43–0.62
		2 mo: 26–34		2 mo: 0.40–0.53
		3–6 mo: 25–35		3–6 mo: .39–.54
		0.5–2 yr: 23–31		0.5-2 yr: 0.36–48
		2–6 yr: 24–30		2-6 yr: 0.37–0.47
		6–12 yr: 25–33		6-12 yr: 0.39–0.51
		12–18 yr: 25–35		12–18 yr: 0.39–0.54
		18–49 yr: 26–34		18–49 yr: 0.40-0.53
Mean corpuscular hemoglobin concentration (MCHC)	W(E)	% Hg/cell or g Hb/dL RBC	× 0.155	mmol Hb/L RBC
		Birth: 30–36		Birth: 4.65–5.58
		1–3 days (cap): 29–37		1–3 days (cap): 4.50–5.74
		1–2 wk: 28–38		1–2 wk: 4.34–5.69
		1–2 mo: 29-37		1–2 mo: 4.50–5.74
		3 mo–2 yr: 30–36		3 mo-2 yr: 4.65–5.58
		2–18 yr: 31–37		2–18 yr: 4.81–5.74
		>18 yr: 31–37		>18 yr: 4.81–5.74
Mean corpuscular volume (MCV)	W(E)	μm^3	× 1	fL
		1–3 days (cap): 95–121		1–3 days (cap): 95–121
		0.5–2 yr:70-86		0.5–2 yr:70–86
		6–12 yr: 77–95		6–12 yr: 77–95
		12–18 yr M:78–98F: 78–102		12–18 yr M:78–98F: 78–102
		18–49 yr M: 80–100F: 80–100		18–49 yr M: 80–100F: 80–100
Leukocyte count (WBC count)	W(E)	× 1,000 cells/mm^3 (μL)	× 1	× 10^9 cells/L
		Birth: 9.0–30.0		Birth: 9.0–30.0
		24 hr: 9.4–34.0		24 hr: 9.4–34.0
		1 mo: 5.0–19.5		1 mo: 5.0–19.5
		1–3 yr: 6.0–17.5		1–3 yr: 6.0–17.5
		4–7 yr:5.5–15.5		4–7 yr: 5.5–15.5
		8–13 yr: 4.5–13.5		8–13 yr: 4.5–13.5
		Adult: 4.5–11.0		Adult: 4.5–11.0
Leukocyte differential	W(E)	%	× 0.01	Number fraction
Myelocyte		0%		0
Neutrophils ("bands")		3–5%		0.03–0.05
Neutrophils ("segs")		54–62%		0.54–0.62
Lymphocytes		25–33%		0.25–0.33
Monocytes		3–7%		0.03–0.07
Eosinophils		1–3%		0.01–0.03
Basophils		0–0.75%		0–0.0075
		Cells/mm^3 (μL)	× 1	× 10^6 cells/L
Myelocyte		0		0
Neutrophils ("bands")		150–400		150–400
Neutrophils ("segs")		3,000–5,800		3,000–5,800
Lymphocytes		1,500–3,000		1,500–3,000

Contd...

Table 39.13B: Complete blood count (*Contd...*)

Analyte or procedure	Specimen	Reference values (USA)	Conversion factor	Values (SI)
Monocytes		285–500		285–500
Eosinophils		50–250		50–250
Basophils		15–50		15–50
Platelet count (thrombocyte count)	W(E)	$\times 10^3/mm^3$ (µL) Newborn: 84–478 (after 1wk, same as adult) Adult: 150–400	$\times 10^6$	$\times 10^9/L$ Newborn:84–478 Adult: 150–400
Reticulocyte count	W (E,H,O)	Adults 0.5–1.5% of erythrocytes or 25,000–75,000/ mm³ (µL) %	$\times 0.01 \times 10^6$	0.005–0.015 (number fraction) or 25,000–75,000 $\times 10^6$/L Number fraction
	W(cap)	1 day: 0.4–6.0% 7 day: <0.1–1.3% 1–4 wk: <1.0–1.2% 5–6 wk: <0.1–2.4% 7–8 wk: 0.1–2.9% 9–10 wk: <0.1–2.6% 11–12 wk: 0.1–0.3%	$\times 0.01$	1 day: 0.004–0.060 7 day: <0.001–0.013 1–4 wk: <0.001–0.012 5–6 wk: <0.001–0.024 7–8 wk: 0.001–0.029 9–10 wk: <0.001–0.026 11–12 wk: 0.001–0.003

Table 39.13C: Other blood values

Analyte or procedure	Specimen	Reference values (USA)	Conversion factor	Values (SI)
Alanine amino-transferase (ALT, SGPT)	S	0–5 days: 6–50 U/L; 1–19 yr: 5–45 U/L	$\times 1$	0–5 days: 6–50 U/L; 1–19 yr: 5–45 U/L
Albumin	P	Premature 1 day: 1.8–3.0 g/dL; Full term <6 days: 2.5–3.4 g/dL; <5 yr: 3.9–5.0 g/dL; 5–19 yr: 4.0–5.3 g/dL	$\times 10$	Premature 1 day: 18–30 g/dL; Full term <6 days: 25–34 g/dL; <5 yr: 39–50 g/dL; 5–19 yr: 40–53 g/dL
Ammonia	W	<30 days: 21–95 µmol/L; 1–12 mo: 18–74 µmol/L; 1–14 yr: 17–68 µmol/L; >14 yr: 19–71 µmol/L	$\times 1$	<30 days: 21–95 µmol/L; 1–12 mo: 18–74 µmol/L; 1–12 mo: 18–74 µmol/L; 1–12 mo: 18–74 µmol/L; >14 yr: 19–71 µmol/L
Amylase	S,P	1–19 yr: 30–100 U/L	$\times 1$	1–19 yr: 30–100 U/L
Amylase isoenzymes	S,P(H)	% pancreatic fraction Cord-8 mo: 0–34%; 7 mo–4 yr: 5–56%; 5–19 yr: 23–59%	$\times 0.01$	% pancreatic fraction Cord-8 mo: 0–0.34%; 7 mo–4 yr:0.05–0.56%; 5–19 yr: 0.23–0.59%
Anion gap (sodium-[chloride + bicarbonate])	P(H)	7–16 mEq/L	$\times 1$	7–16 mEq/L
Anti-deoxyribo-nuclease B titer (anti-DNase B titer)	S	Age: Upper limit of normal 4–6 yr: 240–480 U; 7–12 yr: 480–800 U	$\times 1$	Age: Upper limit of normal 4–6 yr: 240–480 U; 7–12 yr: 480–800 U
Anti-diuretic hormone (hADH), vasopressin)	P(E)	Plasma osmolality (mOsm/kg)— Plasma ADH (pg/mL) 270–280 <1.5 280–285 <2.5 285–290 1–5 290–295 2–7 295–300 4–12	$\times 1$	Plasma ADH ng/L <1.5 <2.5 1–5 2–7 4–12

Contd...

Table 39.13C: Other blood values (*Contd...*)

Analyte or procedure	Specimen	Reference values (USA)		Conversion factor	Values (SI)	
Antistreptolysin-0 titer (ASO titer)	S	Age: Upper limit of normal 2–5 yr: 120–160 Todd units 6–9 yr: 240 Todd units 10–12 yr: 320 Todd units		× 1	Upper limit of normal 2–5 yr: 120–160 Todd units 6–9 yr: 240 Todd units 10–12 yr: 320 Todd units	
Aspartate amino-transferase (AST, SGOT)	S	U/L 0–5 days 35–140 1–9 Yr 15–55 10–19 yr 5–45		× 1	U/L 0–5 days 35–140 1–9 Yr 15–55 10–19 yr 5–45	
Base excess	W(H)	mmoL/L Newborn: (–10)–(–2) Infant: (–7)–(–1) Child: (–4)–(+2) Thereafter: (–3)–(+3)		× 1	mmoL/L Newborn: (–10)–(–2) Infant: (–7)–(–1) Child: (–4)–(+2) Thereafter: (–3)–(+3)	
Bicarbonate	S, P	mmoL/L Arterial 21–28 Venous 22–29			mmoL/L Arterial 21–28 Venous 22–29	
C-reactive protein (high sensitivity)	S	M (mg/dL) 0–90 days 0.08–1.58 91days–12 mo 0.08–1.12 13 mo–3 yr 0.08–1.12 4–10 yr 0.06–0.79 11–14 yr 0.08–0.76 15–18 yr 0.04–0.79	F (mg/dL) 0.09–1.58 0.05–0.79 0.08–0.79 0.5–1.0 0.06–0.81 0.06–0.79	F (mg/dL) × 10	M (mg/dL) 0.8–15.8 0.8–11.2 0.8–11.2 0.6–7.9 0.8–7.6 0.4–7.9	F 0.9–15.8 0.5–7.9 0.8–7.9 0.5–10.0 0.6–8.1 0.6–7.9
Calcium, ionized (Ca)	S,P(H), W(H)	mg/dL Cord blood 5.0–6.0 Newborn 3–24 hr 4.3–5.1 24–48 hr 4.0–4.7 Thereafter 4.8–4.92 Or 2.24–2.46 Eq/L		× 0.25 × 0.5	mmol/L 1.25–1.50 1.07–1.27 1.00–1.17 1.12–1.23 1.12–1.23	
Calcium, total	S	mg/dL Cord blood 9.0–11.5 Newborn 3–24 hr 9.0–10.6 24–48 hr 7.0–12.0 4–7 days 90–10.9 Child 8.8–10.8 Thereafter 8.4–10.2		× 0.25	mmol/L 2.25–2.88 2.3–2.65 1.75–3.00 2.25–2.73 2.20–2.70 2.10–2.25	
Carbon dioxide, partial pressure (PCO₂)	W(H)	mm Hg Newborn 27–40 Infant 27–41 Thereafter: M 35–48 F 32–45		× 0.1333	kPa 3.6–5.3 3.6–5.5 4.7–6.4 4.3–6.0	
Carbon monoxide (Carboxyhemoglobin)	W(E)	Nonsmoker <2% HbCo Smoker <10% Lethal >505		× 0.01	HbCO fraction <0.02 <0.10 >0.5	
Chloride	S,P(H)	Cord blood 96–104 mmol/L Newborn 97–110 Thereafter 98–106		× 1	96–104 mmol/L 97–110 98–106	
Cortisol	S,P(H)	µg/dL Newborn 1–24 Adults: 8:00 AM 5–23		× 27.59 × 0.01	nmol/L 28–662 138–635 82–413	

Contd...

Table 39.13C: Other blood values (*Contd...*)

Analyte or procedure	Specimen	Reference values (USA)		Conversion factor	Values (SI)	
Creatine kinase	S	4:00 PM 3–15 8:00 PM <50% of 8:00AM Cord blood 70–380 U/L 5–8 hr 214–1,175 24–33 hr 130–1, 200 72–100 hr 87–725 Adult 5–130		×1	Fraction of 8.00AM ≤ 0.50 70–380 U/L 214–1,175 130–1,200 87–725 5–130	
Creatine kinase isoenzyme	S	% MB Cord blood 0.3–3.1% 5–8 hr 1.7–7.9% 24–33 hr 1.6–5.0% 72–100 hr 1.4–5.4% Adult 0–2%	%BB 0.3–10.5% 3.6–13.4% 2.3–8.6% 5.1–13.3 0%			
Creatinine Jaffe, kinetic, enzymatic	S,P	mg/dL Cord blood 0.6–1.2 Newborn 0.3–1.0 Infant 0.2–0.4 Child 0.3–0.7 Adolescent 0.5–1.0 Adult M 0.6–1.2 F 0.5–1.1		× 88.4	µmol/L 53–106 27–88 18–35 27–62 44–88 53–106 44–97	
Creatinine clearance (endogenous)	S,P,U	Newborn 40–65 mL/min/1.73 m² <40 yr, M97–137 F 88–128 Decreases< 6.5 ml/min/decade				
Ferritin	S	ng/mL Newborn 25–200 1 mo 200–600 2–5 mo 50–200 6 mo–15 yr 7–140 Adult, M 15 200 F 12–150		× 1	µg/L 25–200 200–600 50–200 7–140 15–200 12–150	
Folate	S	Newborn 7.0–32 ng/ml Thereafter 1.8–9.0		× 2.265	15.9–72.4 nmol/L 4.1–20.4	
	W(E)	150–450 ng/mL RBCs			340–1,020 nmol/L cell	
Glucose	S	mg/mL Cord blood 45–96 Premature 20–60 Neonate 30–60 Newborn 1 day 40–60 >1 day 50–90 Child 60–100 Adult 70–105		× 0.0555	nmol/L 2.5–5.3 1.1–3.3 1.7–3.3 2.2–3.3 2.8–5.0 3.3–5.5 3.9–5.8	
	W(H)	Adult 65–95			3.6–5.3	
Glucose 2 hr post	S	<120 mg/dl			<6.7 mmol/L	
Glucose tolerance test GTT) Oral dose Adult: 75 g Child: 1.75 g/kg ideal weight, up to a maximum of 75 g	S	mg/dl Normal Diabetic Fasting 70–105 ≥126		× 0.0555	mmol/L Normal Diabetic 3.9-5.8 ≥7.0	

Contd...

Table 39.13C: Other blood values (*Contd...*)

Analyte or procedure	Specimen	Reference values (USA)		Conversion factor	Values (SI)	
		60 min	120–170 ≥ 200		6.7–9.4	≥11
		90 min	100–140 ≥ 200		5.6–7.8	≥11
		120 min	70–120 ≥ 200		3.9–6.7	≥11
Glucose-6-phosphate dehydrogenase (G6PD) In erythrocytes	W(E,H,C)	Adult			Adult	
		3.4–8.0 U/g Hb		× 0.0645	0.22–0.52 mu/mol Hb	
		98.6–232 U/10^{12} RBC		× 10^{-3}	0.10–0.23 nU/10^6 RBC	
		1.16–2.72 U/mL RBC		× 1	1.16–2.72 KU/L RBC	
Bishop modified		Newborn: 50% higher			Newborn: 50% higher	
γ-glutamyl transpeptidase (GGT, GGTP)	S	U/L		× 1	U/L	
		Cord blood	37–193		37–193	
		0–1 mo	13–147		13–147	
		1–2 mo	12–123		12–123	
		2–4 mo	8–90		8–90	
		4 mo–10 yr	5–32		5–32	
		10–15 yr	5–24		5–24	
Immunoglobulin A (IgA)	S	mg/dL			mg/dL	
		Cord blood	1.4–3.6	× 10	14–36	
		1–3 mo	1.3–53		13–530	
		4–6 mo	4.4–84		44–840	
		7 mo–1 yr	11–106		110–1,060	
		2–5 yr	14–159		140–1,590	
		6–10 yr	33–236		330–2,360	
		Adult	70–312		700–3,120	
Immunoglobulin D (IgD)	S	Newborn: none detected		× 10	None detected	
		Thereafter: 0–8 mg/dl			0–80 mg/L	
Immunoglobulin E (IgE)	S	M 0–230 IU/mL		× 1	0–230 KIU/L	
		F 0–170			0–170	
Immunoglobulin G (IgG)	S	mg/dL			g/L	
		Cord blood	636–1,606	× 0.01	6.36–16.06	
		1 mo	251–906		2.51–9.06	
		2–4 mo	176–601		1.76–6.01	
		5–12 mo	172–1,069		1.72–10.69	
		1–5 yr	345-1,236		3.45–12.36	
		6–10 yr	608–1,572		6.08–15.72	
		Adult	639–1,349		6.39–13.49	
Immunoglobulin M (IgM)	S	mg/dL			mg/L	
		Cord blood	6.3–25	× 10	63–250	
		1–4 mo	17–105		170–1,050	
		5–9 mo	33–126		330–1,260	
		10 mo–1yr	41–173		410–1,730	
		2–8 yr	43–207		430–2,070	
		9–10 yr	52–242		520–2,420	
		Adult	56–352		560–3,520	
Iron	S	All ages	22–184 µg/dL	× 0.1791	4–33 µmol/L	
Iron-binding capacity, total (TIBC)	S	Infant: 100–400 µg/dL		× 0.179	17.90–71.60 µmol/L	
		Thereafter 250–400			44.75–71.60	
L+ lactate	W	mmol/L			mmol/L	
		1–12 mo	1.1–2.3	× 1	1.1–2.3	
		1–7 yr	0.8–1.5		0.8–1.5	
		7–15 yr	0.6–0.9		0.6–0.9	
D-lactate	P (H)	mmol/L			mmol/L	
		6 mo–3 yr	0.0–0.3	× 1	0.0–0.3	

Contd...

Table 39.13C: Other blood values (*Contd...*)

Analyte or procedure	Specimen	Reference values (USA)	Conversion factor	Values (SI)
Lactate dehydrogenase	S	U/L <1 yr　170–580 1–9 yr　150–500 10–19 yr　120–330	× 1	U/L 170–580 150–500 120–330
Isoenzymes	S	% of total activity 　　　　　1–6 yr　7–19 yr LD1　20–38　20–35 LD2　27–38　31–38 LD3　16–26　19–28 LD4　5–16　7–13 LD5　3–13　5–12		
Lead	W(H)	μg/dL		mmol/L
Lipase	PS	Child　<10 Toxic　≥70 1–18 yr 145–216 U/L	× 0.0483 × 1	<0.48 ≥1.38 145–216 U/L
Magnesium	P(H)	mg/dL 0–6 days　1.2–2.6 7 days–2 yr　1.6–2.6 2–14 yr　1.5–2.3	× 0.411	mmol/L 0.48–1.05 0.65–1.05 0.60–0.95
Methemoglobin (MetHb)	W(E,H,C)	0.06–0.24 g/dL or 0.78±0.37% of total Hb	× 155 × 0.01	9.3–37.2 μmol/L 0.0078±0.0037 (mass fraction)
Osmolarity	S	Child, Adult 275–295 mOsmol/kg H_2O		
Phosphatase, alkaline	S	U/L 1–9 yr　　145–420 10–11 yr　130–560 M 12–13 yr M: 200–495 F:195–420 14–15 yr M: 130–525 F: 70–230 16–19 yr M: 65–260 F: 50–130	× 1	U/L 1–9 yr　　145–420 10–11 yr　130–560 M 12–13 yr　M: 200–495 F:195–420 14–15 yr M: 130–525 F: 70–230 16–19 yr M: 65–260 F: 50–130
Phosphorus, inorganic	S,P(H)	mg/dL 0–5 days　4.8–8.2 1–3 yr　3.8–6.5 4–11 yr　3.7–5.6 12–15 yr　2.9–5.4 16–19 yr　2.7–4.7	× 0.3229	mmol/L 1.55–2.65 1.25–2.10 1.20–1.80 0.95–1.75 0.90–1.50
Potassium	S	mmol/L <2 mo　3.0–7.0 2–12 mo　3.5–6.0 >12 mo　3.5–5.0	×	mmol/L 3.0–7.0 3.5–6.0 3.5–5.0
	P(H)	3.5–4.5 mmol/L		3.5–4.5 mmol/L
Prealbumin (transthyretin)	P	mg/L 2–6 mo　142–330 6–12 mo　120–274 1–3 yr　108–259	× 1	mg/L 142–330 120–274 108–259
Protein, total	S	g/dL Premature　4.3–7.6 Newborn　4.6–7.4 1–7 yr　6.7–7.9 8–12 yr　6.4–8.1 13–19 yr　6.6–8.2	× 10	g/dL 43–76 46–74 67–79 64–81 66–82

Contd...

Table 39.13C: Other blood values (*Contd...*)

Analyte or procedure	Specimen	Reference values (USA)	Conversion factor	Values (SI)
Pyruvate	W	7–17 yr 0.076; 0.826 mmol/L	× 1	0.076; 0.826 mmol/L
Sodium	S,P	mmol/L	× 1	mmol/L
		Newborn 134–146		134–146
		Infant 139–146		139–146
		Child 138–145		138–145
		Thereafter 136–146		136–146
Thyroid stimulating hormone	S	MlU/L	× 1	MlU/L
		Cord blood 2.3–13.2		2.3–13.2
		1–2 days 3.2–34.6		3.2–34.6
		3–4 days 0.7–15.4		0.7–15.4
		2–20 wk 1.7–9.1		1.7–9.1
		21 wk–20 yr 0.7–6.4		0.7–6.4
Thyroid uptake of radioactive iodine	Activity over thyroid gland	2 hr <6%	× 0.01	2 hr <0.06
		6 hr 3–20%		6 hr 0.03–0.20
		24 hr 8–30%		24 hr 0.08–0.30
Thyroid uptake of technetium 99m	Activity over thyroid gland	After 24 hr 0.43.0%	× 0.01	Fractional uptake 0.004–0.030
Thyrotropin releasing hormone (hTRH)	P	5–60 pg/ml	× 2.759	14–165 pmol/L
Thyroxine-binding globulin (TBG)	S	mg/dl	× 10	mg/L
		Cord blood 1.4–9.4		14–94
		1–4 wk 1.0–9.0		10–90
		1–12 mo 2.0–7.6		20–76
		1–5 yr 2.9–5.4		29–54
		5–10 yr 2.5–5.0		25–50
		10–15 yr 2.1–4.6		21–46
		Adult 1.5–3.4		15–34
Throxine, total	S	Full term infants μg/dl	× 12.9	Full term infants nmol/L
		1–3 days 8.2–19.9		1–3 days 106–256
		1 wk 6.0–15.9		1 wk 77–205
		1–12 mo 6.1–14.9		1–12 mo 79–192
		Prepubertal children		Prepubertal children
		1–3 yr 6.8–13.5		1–3 yr 88–124
		3–10 yr 5.5–12.8		3–10 yr 71–165
		Pubertal children and		Pubertal children and
		Adults 4.2–13.0		Adults 54–167
Throxine, free	S	Newborn infants ng/dl	× 12.9	Full term infants pmol/L
		3 days 2.0–4.9		3 days 26–63
		Infants 0.9–2.6		Infants 12–33
		Preubertal		Preubertal
		Children 0.8–2.2		Children 10–28
		Pubertal children and		Pubertal children and
		Adults 0.8–2.3		Adults 10–30
Throxine , total	W	Newborn screen (filter paper) 6.2–22.0 μg/dl	× 12.9	80–283 nmol/L
Triidothyronine, free	S	pg/dl	× 0.01536	pmol/L
		Cord blood 20–240		0.3–3.7
		1–3 days 200–610		3.1–9.4
		6 wk 240–650		3.7–8.6

Contd...

Table 39.13C: Other blood values (*Contd...*)

Analyte or procedure	Specimen	Referece values (USA)		Conversion factor	Values (SI)
Triidothyroxine, total	S	Adult (20–50 yr) 230–660 ng/dL		× 0.0154	3.5–10.0 nmol/L
		Cord blood	30–70		0.46–1.08
		New born	75–260		1.16–4.00
		1–5 yr	100–260		1.54–4.00
		5–10 yr	90–240		1.39–3.70
		10–15 yr	80–210		1.23–3.23
		Thereafter	115–190		1.77–2.93
Triidothyroxine resin uptake test (T,RU)	S			× 0.01	Fractional uptake
		New born	26–36%		0.26–0.36
		Thereafter	26–35%		0.26–0.35
Urea nitrogen	S,P	mg/dL		× 0.357	mmol urea/L
		Cord blood	21–40		7.5–14.3
		Premature (1wk) 3–25			1.1–9.0
		Newborn	3–12		1.1–4.3
		Infant or child	5–18		1.8–6.4
		Thereafter	7–18		2.5–6.4
Uric acid	S	mg/dL		× 59.48	μmol/L
		1–5 yr	1.7–5.8		100–350
		6–11 yr	2.2–6.6		130–390
		M 12–19 yr	3.0–7.7		180–460
		F 12–19 yr	2.7–5.7		160–340

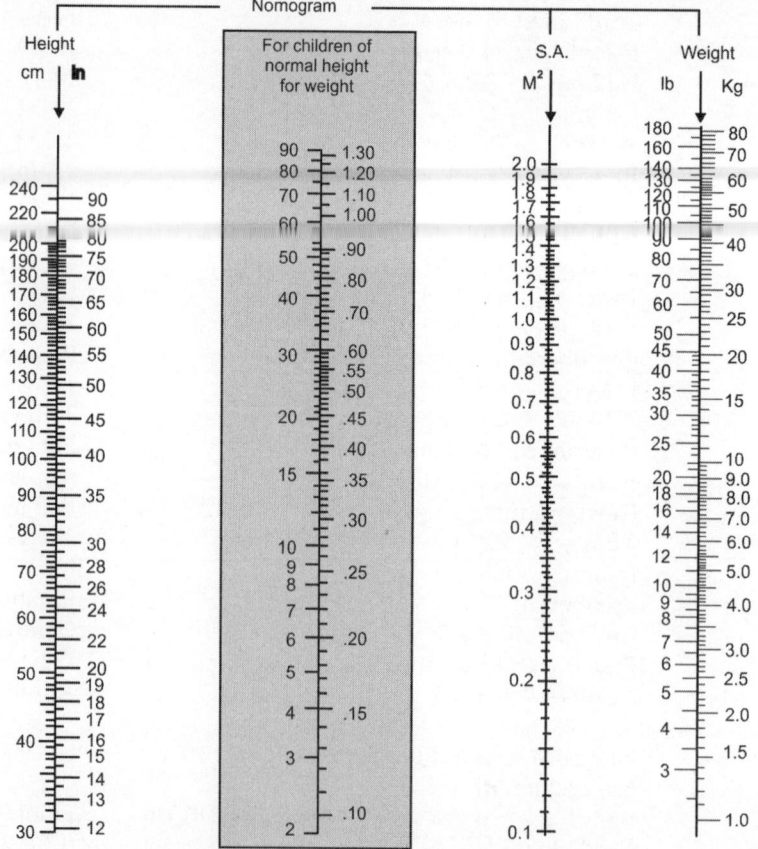

Fig. 39.1: Nomogram for the estimation of the surface area. The surface is indicated where a straight line that connects the height and weight levels intersects the surface area column, or if the patient is roughly of average size, from the weight alone (*enclosed area*). (Source: Nomogram modified from the data of E. Boyd by C.D. West. See also Briars GL, Bailey BJ: Surface area estimation; Pocket calculator v nomogram. *Arch Dis Child* 1994; 70: 246–247.)

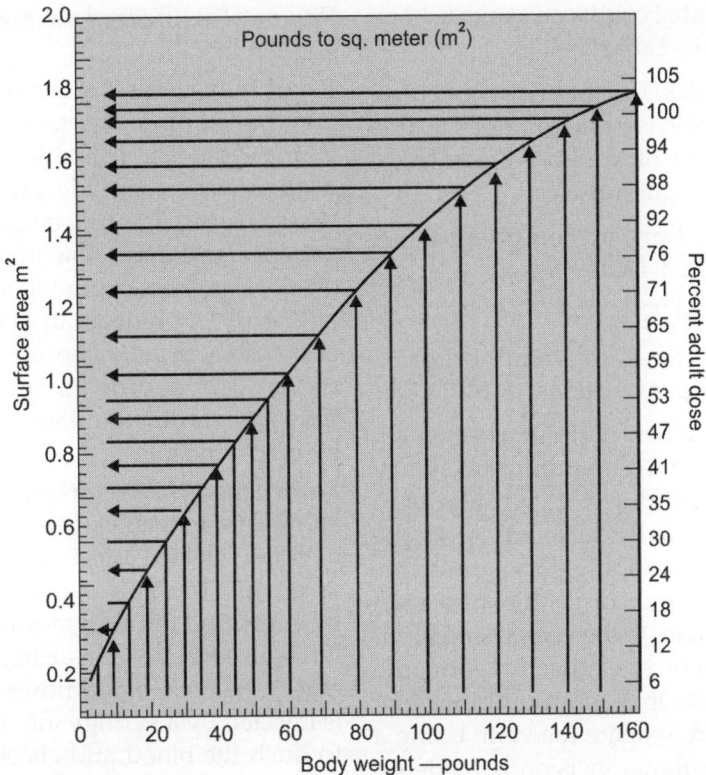

Fig. 39.2: Relationship among body weight (lb), body surface area, and adult dosage. The surface area values correspond with those set forth by Crawford JD, Terry ME, Rourke GM. Simplification of drug dosage calculation by application of the surface area principle. *Pediatrics* 1950;5: 783-790. Note that the 100% adult dose is for a patient weighing approximately 140 lb and having a surface area of approximately 1.7 M². (*Source:* Talbot NB, Richie RH, Crawford JH. *Metabolic Homeostasis: a syllabus for Those Concerned with the Care of Patients.* Cambridge: Harvard University Press, 1959.)

A more comprehensive list of reference ranges can be found on line at: *www.nelsonpediatrics.com*

Pesce MA. Reference ranges for Laboratory tests and procedures. In: Kliegman RM, Behrman RE, Jenson HB, Stanton BF (eds). *Nelson Textbook of Pediatrics.* 18th edn. Vol. 2. Philadelphia: Saunders, 2007; 2943–2951.

39.3 COMMON MEDICAL PROCEDURES

Common procedures should be conducted under aseptic precations. The operator should always wear the surgical gloves. The skin is cleaned, drapped and anesthetized.

To perform a procedure, clean the skin area with 70% alcohol (e.g., ethanol) or 0.5% chlorhexidine (5% dluted 1 in 10 in ethanol). Infiltrate the skin, subcutaneous tissue and periosteum or renal, abdomen over the selected site with a anesthetic such as 2.5 ml to 5 ml 2% lignocaine.

Abdominal paracentesis: For diagnostic and therapeutic purposes ascitic fluid is obtained via paracentesis. The child lies supine in bed. The lower quadrant on either side of abdomen or a site in the midline halfway between umbilicus and pubic symphysis are preferred sites for the tap. A wide gauge needle or trocar and cannula is used depending on the amount of fluid to be aspirated. The needle is inserted obliquely to prevent leaking of the fluid. After sufficient fluid is aspirated, the wound is sealed (*see* Section 16.17).

Arterial cannulation for continuous blood pressure and arterial blood gas monitoring is often required in critically ill infants and children. Sites available for arterial access include the radal, femoral, posterior tibial, and dorsalis pedis arteries. Radial artery is the most commonly used vessel for arterial puncture and cannulation. The skin is approached at a 30 to 45° angle to the horizontal aiming the needle towards the pulse slowly until arterial blood flows into the butterfly tubing or an arterial cannula/catheter.

Bone marrow aspiration and bone trephine biopsy: Samples of bone marrow are usually aspirated from the sternum, iliac crest or anterior superior spines by Salah and Klima needle. In children iliac puncture, particularly in the region of the posterior spine is preferred. Sternal puncture should be avoided.

Normal ranges for differential counts on aspirate bone marrow are documented in Table 20.3.

Capillary blood by heel prick: Do not prick the central portion of the heel. A needle is punctured at the side of the heel. The blood is obtained by alternate squeezing and releasing of calf muscles.

Cardiovascular support: Cardiac compression *see* Section 7.5 (Figs 7.8–7.10 and Table 7.7).

Catheterization: *See* section 22.1.

Closed thoracotomy: In cases of pneumothorax, pleural effusion, empyema, *see* Sections 18.16; 18.18.

Cut-Down (venesection): When peripheral veins are not available for giving an intravenous infusion, it may be necessary to perform a cut-down. A site anterior to the medial malleolus is usually selected. After the antiseptic precautions and drapping, local anesthetic is infiltrated into the skin and a full thickness skin incision is made at right angles to the vein. Using blunt mosquito forceps, the vein is exposed. Using the forceps, two silk sutures are looped around the vein; the distal one may be used to ligate the vein. Using a fine dissecting forceps, a smmal incision is made on the vein below the proximal loop of the thread, with tension being applied to the proximal suture loop. The catheter is slowly guided up the vein as the tension on the vein wall by thethread is slowly released. As the blood start flowing through the catheter, it is tied with catgut or thread loop to prevent seepage of blood around the catheter. The skin wound is closed with the silk sutures. The catheter is looped around the area under dressing to prevent its slipping due to inadvertent traction on the catheter.

Intraosseous infusion: Any intravenous drug or fluid required for resuscitation can be safely administered by this route. Site of cannulation is the anteromedial tibial surface, 1–3 cm below the tuberosity.

Insertion nasogastric tube: In children 10 F tube in 1 year old and incresing sizes upto 14–16 F in teenagers is used (See also Section 8.6).

Liver biopsy: Before biopsy, the degree of jaundice, prothrombine time, platelet count and blood group should be ascertained. The patient lies down supine on the edge of the bed with the arms behind his head. The liver is palpated in the midaxillary line. The upper border of liver dullness ia also percussed. The skin (usually at the 10th intercostals space) is cleaned, drapped and anesthetized. The skin is nicked with a scalpel blade. Liver tissue is biopsed by biopsy needle.

Lumbar puncture (LP) and CSF examination *see* Section 24.1.

Pericardiocentesis: See Section 19.14.

Removal aspirated foreign body (*see* Section 7.5, Figs 7.5 to 7.7).

Renal biopsy: Heavy sedation or general anesthesia may be required for kidney biopsy in infants and young children. The child is placed prone with his head turned to one side, arms abducted and forearms beside his head. A rolled up towel is placed under the patient's abdomen. The bony landmarks for this are the dosal process of lumbar spine and the lower border of 12th rib. A point about 2 cm below the lower border of the rib is usually chosen as the site for biopsy. The procedure should preferably be done under ultrasonographic guidance. Kidney tissue is biopsed by biopsy needle.

Scalp vein catheterization: The infant is restrained and an assistant steadies the head of the child. The skin over the selected area is shaved and cleaned with skin area with 70% alcohol (e.g. ethanol). The vein is fixed by stretching the skin taut with fingers. The needle is introduced in the vein at an angle of 30°. As the needle enters the vein, blood flows into the scalp vein. Fluid is injected by a syringe into the scalp vein set in order to flush the blood and check the patency. Scalp vein set is connected to the intravenous line. The needle is fixed at an angle of 30° with sticking plaster strips.

Subdural tap see Section 24.1

Ventricular tap see Section 24.1

Umbilical catheterization: Umbilical vein catheterization is done in a newborn infant for administering drugs during resuscitation or during exchange transfusions. When the catheter is withdrawn after the procedure its tip must be sent to the laboratory for microbial culture as it may be a focus for embolus formation and infection.

39.4 INFECTION CONTROL AND PROPHYLAXIS

Infection control is an extremely important part of child care system. Infection control is the responsibility of every health care provider. Such control measures include universal immunizations, optimal nutrition and prevention of transmission of infection from child to child, child to adult, and adult to child.

Factors responsible for infections: For an infection to occur in the hospital the prerequisites are: a. A susceptible host, b. A microbe capable of producing an infection, c. An environment that is congenial for the multiplication of the microbe.

A number of factors include prior invasive procedures, use of catheters and other devices, use of antibiotics, and exposure to other patients, visitors or health care providers with contagious diseases. Host factors that increase the risk for infection include anatomic abnormalities (dermoid sinuses, cleft palate, and obstructive uropathy), damage to skin, organ dysfunction, malnutrition, and underlying diseases or co-morbidities. Diseases and therapies that alter immunity are most likely to predispose to infection. Prior procedures may introduce pathogens and damage anatomic host defenses. Intravenous and other catheters bypass host defenses, provide direct access to sterile sites, provide adherence sites for microbes, and may occlude normal ostia such as the eustachian tubes. Antibiotics often alter normal bowel flora and encourage colonization by resistant flora, and they may suppress hematopoiesis. Exposure to adults or children with contagious diseases is a clear risk for nosocomial transmission of disease.

Source of the infecting organism may be *exogenous*—from another patient or a member of the hospital staff, or from the inanimate environment in the hospital; or it may be *endogenous* from the patients own flora which at the time of infection may include organisms brought into the hospital at admission and certain others acquired subsequently. The infecting organisms may spontaneously invade the tissues of the patient or may be introduced into them by surgical procedures, instrumental manipulation or nursing procedures.

The inanimate environment of the hospital that acts as an important source comprises of:
a. Contaminated air, water, food and medicaments
b. Used equipment and instruments
c. Soiled linen
d. Hospital waste (Bio-medical waste)

Transmission of infection: Transmission of infectious agents occurs by various routes, but by far the most common and important route is via the hands. Children are constantly touching things in the environment, touching each others, and placing their hands in their noses, eyes, and mouths. Child-to-child exchange secretions are common whenever children are together. Bacteria, fungi, viruses, and parasites often travel on hands from one person to another. Medical equipment, toys, and hospital and office furnishings can be contaminated and thus have a role as fomites for transmission of potential pathogens. Pagers, phones, and computer mouse are easily contaminated by health care personnel; these inanimate objects serve as reservoirs for bacteria. Thermometers and other equipment that come in contact with mucous membranes are social risks. Some agents are disseminated by airborne transmission, such as varicella virus, measles virus, and *M. tuberculosis*. Food and water can be contaminated and have been involved in hospital outbreaks.

Causes and sites of infection: Common causes of health care-associated infections in children are seasonal viruses, staphylococci and gram-negative bacilli. Fungi and resistant bacteria are frequent causes of infection in immunocompromised children and in those who require intensive care and prolonged hospitalization. Common sites of infection are the respiratory tract, gastrointestinal tract blood stream, skin, and urinary tract.

Hand hygiene: Hand washing is the single most important procedure for preventing the spread of biological contamination. Despite this fact many hospital personnel don't wash their hands properly. The important component of hand washing is placement of hands under water and use of friction with or without soap. A 15-second scrub removes the majority of transient flora but does not alter the permanent flora. A variety of hand gels and rubs can be used in place of hand washing. Waterless hand hygiene products increase compliance and save time; these agents are the preferred agents for routine hygiene. These products are effective in killing most microbes; they will not remove dirt or debris. Hands should be cleaned before and after every patient is examined. Hand washing with soap and water can be taught to families and children in child-care settings, homes, and schools and the rates of infection are decreased when children as well as caregivers regularly clean their hands.

There are five critical times in washing hands with soap and/or using of a hand antiseptic related to *fecal-oral transmission*: after using a bathroom (private or public), after changing a diaper, before feeding a child, before eating and before preparing food or handling raw meat, fish, or poultry, or any other situation leading to potential contamination and see below. To reduce the spread of germs, it is also better to wash the hands and/or use a hand antiseptic before and after tending to a sick person. If your hands are not visibly dirty or soiled, washing one's hands with a good hand antiseptic is the most effective overall way to prevent the spread of *infectious disease*. If your hands are dirty or soiled, washing your hands with soap and water followed by a good hand antiseptic is the most effective overall way to prevent the spread of *infectious disease*.

Here are some handwashing tips and procedures for your use (Box 39.1).

Standard precautions are intended to protect health care workers from blood and body fluids and should be used whenever providing care. Infected individuals are often contagious before symptoms of disease develop, and asymptomatic carriers are capable of transmitting agent. Standard precautions involve the use of barriers-gloves, gowns, masks, goggles, and face shields-as needed to prevent transmission of microbes associated with contact with blood or body fluids.

Isolation of patients infected with certain pathogens decreases the risk for nosocomial transmission. The type of isolation depends on the infecting agent and the route of transmission. 1. *Contact transmission* is the most common mode of transmission and involves direct contact or contact with a contaminated intermediate object. 2. *Droplet transmission* is by droplets propelled a short distance through the air and deposited on mucous membranes. 3. *Airborne transmission* occurs by dissemination of droplet nuclei (≤5 μm) of evaporated droplets or dust particles carrying the infectious agents. Contact precautions include gowns and gloves and single room isolation. Droplet precautions include masks for close contact (<3 feet) and single room isolation. For both contact and droplet precautions, a single room is preferred; cohorting of children infected with the same pathogen is acceptable. Airborne precautions include masks and single room isolation with negative pressure ventilation. Transmission based precautions are continued for as long as a patient is considered to be contagious.

In every office/outpatient department proper cleaning, disinfection and sterilization methods should be used. Many practices and clinics provide separate waiting areas for sick and well children. It is essential to ensure that contagious children or adults are not present in waiting areas. Toys and items that are shared between patients should be cleaned between uses; soap and water are sufficient to clean these items. More complete disinfection or sterilization is required for items that encounter mucous membranes and for all reusable items used for body fluid sampling.

Additional measures: Other preventive measures include aseptic technique, catheter care, prudent use of antibiotics, isolation of contagious patients, clearing of the environment, disinfection and sterilization of medical equipment, reporting of infections, safe handling of needles, and other sharp instruments, and establishment of employee health services. Aseptic technique must be used for all invasive procedures; this is especially important during catheter placement and manipulation. Catheter care also includes limiting the duration and number of catheters as much as possible and removing catheters as soon as they become unnecessary.

Box 39.1: Handwashing tips and procedures

1. Consider the sink, including the faucet controls, contaminated.
2. Avoid touching the sink.
3. Turn water on using a paper towel and then wet your hands and wrists.
4. Work soap into a lather. (removal of microorganisms from skin requires the addition of soap to water; warm, soapy water is more effective than cold, soapy water at removing the natural oils on your hands, which hold soils and bacteria). Solid *soap*, because of its reusable nature, may hold bacteria acquired from previous uses, so it's important to wash the soap itself before and after use. Hand washing with contaminated soap could colonize the hands with *Gram-negative bacteria*, which results in an increase in bacterial counts on the skin.
5. Vigorously rub together all surfaces of the lathered hands for 15 seconds. Friction helps remove dirt and microorganisms. Wash around and under rings, around cuticles, and under fingernails [*six steps-1 palms and fingers, 2 back of hands, 3 fingers and knuckles, 4 thumbs, 5 finger tips, 6 wrists*]. Nursery personnel should use chlorhexidine or iodophor-containing antiseptic soap for routine hand washing before caring each infant. Rigid enforcing hand-to-elbow washing for 2 min in the initial wash and 15–30 sec in the second wash is essential for staff and visitors entering the nursery. Equally thorough washes between handling infants are also required.
6. Rinse hands thoroughly under a stream of water. Running water carries away dirt and debris. Point fingers down so water and contamination won't drip toward elbows.
7. Dry hands completely with a clean dry paper towel. Effective drying of the hands is an essential part of the hand hygiene process, but there is some debate over the most effective form of drying in washrooms. A growing volume of research suggests paper towels are much more hygienic than the electric hand dryers found in many washrooms.
8. Use a dry paper towel to turn faucet off.
9. To keep soap from becoming a breeding place for microorganisms, thoroughly clean soap dispensers before refilling with fresh soap.
10. When hand washing facilities are not available at a remote work site, use appropriate antiseptic hand cleaner or antiseptic towelettes. As soon as possible, rewash hands with soap and running water. Enough *hand antiseptic* or *alcohol rub* must be used to thoroughly wet or cover both hands. The front and back of both hands and between and the ends of all fingers are rubbed for approximately 30 seconds until the liquid, foam or gel is dry. The use of a hand antiseptic or alcohol rub is much quicker and more effective than hand washing with soap and water. Hand antiseptics and alcohol rubs with moisturizers will also not dry out the skin on hands as much as soap and water.

Surgical prophylaxis must be appropriate when there is a high risk of postoperative infection or when the consequences of infection are catastrophic. The choice of antibiotic depends on the use and type of surgery. Four categories are recognized: clean wounds, clean contaminated wounds, contaminated wounds, and dirty infected wounds.

Employee health is important because employees are at risk for acquiring infection from patients and infected employees pose a risk to patients. This risk is minimized by use of standard precautions and hand hygiene before and after all patient contacts. New employees should be screened for the presence of infectious diseases. Their immunization history should be noted and necessary immunizations should be offered.

All health care workers (medical or nonmedical, paid or volunteer, full time or part time, student or nonstudent, with or without patient care responsibilities) who work in facilities that provide health care to patients (inpatient or outpatient, public or private) should be immune to measles, rubella, and varicella. All workers who might be exposed to blood or body fluids should be immunized against hepatitis B. Annual influenza immunizations are recommended for all health care workers who have contact with patients at risk for influenza or its complications. This program lessens staff illness and absenteeism during the influenza season and reduces health care-associated infections. All health care workers who have duties that have face-to-face contact with patients

with suspected or confirmed tuberculosis (including transport staff) should be included in a tuberculosis screening program. Regular educational sessions should be performed to ensure that the staff is aware of infection control methods and that they adhere to infection control policies.

Abrutyn E, Goldman DA, Schekler WE (eds). *Saunders Infection Control Reference Service: The Experts' Guide to the Guidelines.* 2nd edn. Philadelphia: WB Saunders, 2001.

Bennett JV, Brachmann PS (eds). *Hospital Infections.* 3rd edn. Boston: Little Brown, 1992.

Burke JP. Infection control- A problem for patient safety. *N Engl J Med* 2003; 348: 651–656.

Hota B. Contamination, disinfection, and cross-colonization: Are hospital surfaces reservoirs for nosocomial infection? *Clin Infect Dis* 2004; 39:702–709.

39.5 DOCTOR'S DECLARATION OF BREASTFEEDING

Despite the advantages of breastfeeding, the practice has declined with serious consequences for infant health.

Doctors have allowed the manufacturers of infant foods to influence the way in which they work and think. Thus, doctors have, themselves, unintentially contributed to the decline of breast feeding.

A group of concerned pediatricians and physicians meeting at the 10th anniversary of IBFAN, in Manila on October 12, 1989 reaffirmed the 20-point declaration which was drawn up in Thailand in October 1986 to guide the conduct and practice of any medical practitioner who wishes to promote and protect breast feeding.

We invite pediatricians and other concerned doctors to endorse this declaration. Under all ordinary circumstances, medical practioners who endorse the declaration shall:

1. Ensure that mothers in their care are informed about the unique qualities of human milk and about the risks to their infant's health of using any substitute. This information should be provided both before and after a baby is born.
2. Encourage and enable mothers to hold and suckle their babies immediately after birth, within, at most, 2 hours of delivery.
3. Ensure that babies stay with their mothers in the post-partum ward day and night from the time of delivery.
4. Encourage and enable mothers to feed their babies on demand with no restriction on either frequency or duration of feeds.
5. Ensure that mothers receive emotional support and skilled assistance to establish lactation; especially help in getting the baby to take enough of the breast into the mouth. This support and assistance should be given within 24 hours of delivery. Mothers should have access to further assistance to maintain lactation whenever they request it.
6. Ensure that mothers receive appropriate information about the physiology of lactation, especially:
   - That colostrums is beneficial;
   - That only small quantities of milk are produced and needed for the first few days after delivery;
   - That more sucking makes more milk;
   - That early supplements depress milk production.
7. Not allow newborn babies to receive any prelacteal feeds of formula, animal milk, glucose water, water, honey, or of any food substance other human milk.
8. Discourage use of any complementary or supplementary feeds for infants under the age of 4 months and, when possible, discourage them for infants under the age of 6 months.
9. Not permit the use of feeding bottles or teats in any hospital ward, nor the use of pacifiers.
10. Ensure that mothers delivered by Caesarean section receive the same lactation management and all necessary assistance from the time they regain consciousness from the anesthetic.

11. Ensure that mothers learn how to express their breast milk, and when this may be useful.
12. Ensure that low birth weight babies are fed exclusively on expressed breast milk by means other than bottles, until they are able to suck directly from the breast; and ensure that mothers have unrestricted access to their babies.
13. Support the continuation or re-establishment of lactation during or after illness in mother or baby; and try to make it possible for mothers to stay in hospital with their sick babies and babies to stay in hospital with their sick mothers.
14. Not accept free samples of formula, bottles, or teats directly or indirectly from industry.
15. Not give free samples of formula, bottles, or teats to a mother.
16. Not prescribe or recommend infant formula.
17. Not instruct mothers in the technicalities of bottle feeding, if necessary a cup should be used.
18. Not accept or display any promotional material or free gifts from any infant food company or their agents.
19. Not accept personnel funding from an infant food company or their agents for purposes such as travel, research, equipment, or teaching material.
20. Not give assistance to any infant food company with the production of promotional material.

Signed

1. *Dr. Prasong Tuchinda*
   Department of Paediatrics
   Faculty of Medicine, Siraraj Hospital
   Mahidol University, Bangkok, Thailand

2. *Dr. Felicity Savage King*
   Institute of Child Health
   30 Guilford Street
   London WCIN 1EH, UK

3. *Dr. GP Mathur*
   Professor of Paediatrics
   BRD Medical College
   Gorakhpur, Uttar Pradesh, India.

4. *Dr. Jayam*
   Consultant Paediatrician and
   Neonatologist, Public Health Centre
   Lake View Road
   West Mambalam
   Madras-600033, Tamil Nadu, India

5. *Dr. Paul Frans Matulesssy*
   Department of Nutrition
   Medical Faculty
   University of Indonesia
   Jalan Salemba 4
   Jakarta 10430, Indonesia

6. *Dr. Ching-Hwa Chiu*
   Associate Professor
   School of Public Health
   National Taiwan University Medical
   College, Taipei,
   Taiwan, ROC.

7. *Dr. Juan A. Perez*
   64 Lantana St.
   Cubao
   Quezon City, Philippines.

8. *Dr. Syed Rizwanuddin Ahmad*
   Civil Hospital
   Karachi, Pakistan.

Mathur GP. Doctor's Declaration of Breastfeeding. News from the Regions News from the Philippines. J Trop Pediatr 1990;36:199.

40 ◆ Rational Drug Therapy

40.1 PRINCIPLES OF PRESCRIBING DRUGS

Drugs should only be prescribed when they are necessary, and in all cases the benefit of administering the medicine should be considered in relation to the risks involved. Bad prescribing habits lead to ineffective and unsafe treatment, exacerbation or prolongation of illness, distress and harm to patient, and higher cost. Antimicrobial resistance (AMR) is a global problem. Preventing AMR involves encouraging rational antibiotic, therapy at individual, hospital and community level. Indian Academic of Pediatrics (IAP) has declared 26th september as the 'Rational antibiotic day, and plans to celebrate antibiotic awareness week. Rational prescribing of drugs depends on a fundamental understanding of the pharmacokinetic/pharmacodynamic dosing approaches have better respond rates and less toxicity. Pharmacokinetics is the quantitative evaluation of each component of disposition of a compound that is the process of absorption, distribution, metabolism, and excretion. Pharmacodynamics involves the correlation of pharmacologic response to a measured drug concentration in blood (or other body fluid).

Drug-drug interactions: When two or more drugs are administered to the same patient, the pharmacokinetic and pharmacodynamic properties of each agent may be modified by their combined interaction.

Maternal medication: Medications taken during pregnancy affect the fetus and taken by the lactating mother adversely affect her infant. All women should be specifically counseled to abstain from the use of alcohol, tobacco, and illicit drugs during pregnancy. In general, drug use should be as minimal as possible during lactation.

Adverse drug effects: Adverse effect is 'any undesirable or unintended consequence of drug administration'. It is a broad term, which includes all kinds of noxious effect-trivial, serious or even fatal.

Compliance with the prescribed regimen: Many patients frequently do not take medication consistently or in the manner intended or prescribed. A child's compliance with a prescribed treatment regimen depends on clearly understanding its importance by the parents. The compliance can be improved through patient education.

Bhatia Monica. CIMS. 113, India [Update-2]. UBM Medica India, Private Limited. Gurgaon (Haryana): Delhi-NCR Office, April–July2011.

Gal P, Reed MD. Medications. In: Kliegman RM, Behrman RE, Jenson HB, Stanton BF (eds). *Nelson Textbook of Pediatrics.* 18th edn. Vol. 2. Philadelphia: Saunders, 2007; 2955–2999.

General advice to prescribers. *WHO Model Formulary.* Geneva. World Health Organization, 2002; 1–15.

Gulhati CM (Ed). *Monthly Index of Medical Specialties (MIMS).* New Delhi: MIMS India, 2004 (Dec); 1–336.

Haslett C, Chilvers ER, Boon NA, Colledge NR, Hunter JAA (eds). *Davidson's Principles and Practice of Medicine.* 19th edn. Edinburgh: Churchill Livingstone, 2002.

Kasper DL, Braunwald E, Fauci AS, Hauser SL, Longo DL, Jameson JL (eds). *Harrison's Principles of Internal Medicine.* 16th edn. Vol I and Vol II. New York: McGraw-Hill, 2005.

Laurence DR, Bennett PN (eds): In: *Clinical Pharmacology.* 7th edn. Edinburgh: ELBS with Churchill Livingstone, 1992.

Tripathi KD (Ed). *Essentials of Medical Pharmacology*. 6th edn. New Delhi: Jaypee Brothers Medical Publishers (P) Ltd., 2008.

Yewale VN. Antimicrobial resistance–A ticking bomb. Indian Pediatr 2014;51:171–172.

40.2 Analgesic, Antipyretic and Nonsteroidal Anti-Inflammatory Drugs (NSAID)

Non-Narcotic Analgesics

Aspirin: (Acetylsalicylic acid) (NSAID): Pain, inflammation, fever: 10–15 mg/kg/dose PO q4–6 hr. Kawasaki disease (acute phase): 80–100 mg/kg/24 hr divided q6 hr. Rheumatic fever: 60–100 mg/kg/24 hr divided q6 hr. Caution: Contraindicated in children < 16 yr with chickenpox or flu-like symptoms due to risk of Reye syndrome. Discontinue if hearing loss or tinnitus occurs. *Side effects:* Bleeding from gums or from GIT, gastric ulcers, bronchospasm in asthmatics, hearing loss, and tinnitus.

Baclofen: Spasticity associated with multiple sclerosis or spinal cord lesions, trigeminal neuralgia. 2–7 yr: 10–15 mg/24 hr PO divided q8 hr and titrate quantity up to 3 days (max: 40 mg/24 hr PO). *Side effects:* Vertigo, psychiatric reactions, ataxia.

Colchicine: (Anti-inflammatory/anti-gout agent): Familial Mediterranean fever, acute and chronic gouty arthritis:< 5 yr: 0.5 mg/24 hr. > 5 yr: 1–1.5 mg/24 hr in 2–3 divided doses. *Side effects:* Abdominal pain.

Diclofenac sodium: (NSAID): PO: 2–3 mg/kg/24 hr in 2–4 divided doses. *Side effects:* Dizziness, headache.

Ibuprofen: (NSAID): Pain, fever: 5–10 mg/kg/dose q6–8 hr.Juvenile rheumatoid arthritis: 30–50 mg/24 hr in 4 divided doses. *Side effects:* Gastrointestinal bleeding.

Indomethacin: [NSAID]: Closure of the patent ductus arteriosus (PDA) in neonates: IV: 0.10–0.25 mg/kg/dose q12 hr for 3–6 doses. Rheumatoid disorders: Children: 1–2 mg/kg/24 hr PO in 2–4 doses (max: 4 mg/kg/24 hr). Do not use in premature neonates in necrotizing enterocolitis, poor renal function, or active bleeding.

Mefenamic acid: 8 mg/kg/dose 3 times a day.

Naproxen: [NSAID]: 5–7 mg/kg PO q8–12 hr.

Precaution: Do not administer to infants < 3 months of age. *Side effects:* Gastrointestinal upset/irritation.

Nimesulide: 5mg/kg/day q8–12 hr. Safety not established in children less than 6 months of age. *Side effects:* Hepatic enzyme elevation.

Paracetamol: (Acetaminophen) (NSAID): Infants and Children < 12 yr: 10–15 mg/kg/dose PO q4–6 hr. Children > 12 yr (max: 5 doses/24 hr) PO.

Piroxicam: (NSAID): Pain, rheumatoid disorders. 0.2–0.3 mg/kg q24 hr PO (max dose: 15 mg/kg/24 hr). *Side effects:* Gastrointestinal upset, decreased renal function.

Narcotic Analgesics

Codeine: (Narcotic analgesic): Pain: 0.5 mg/kg/dose q4–6 hr (max: 60 mg/dose). Cough: 1–1.5 mg/kg/24 hr divided q4–6 hr. Adverse events: Drowsiness, constipation, nausea.

Meperidine (Pethidine): [Narcotic analgesic]: Analgesic, adjunct to anesthesia. IM, IV, SC: 1–1.5 mg/kg/dose q3–4 hr. *Side effects:* Physical and psychological dependence.

Morphine: [Narcotic analgesic]: Neonates: IV, IM, SC: 0.05–0.2 mg/kg/dose q2–4 hr. Infants and Children: IV, IM, SC: 0.1–0.2 mg/kg/dose q2–4 hr; PO: 0.2–0.5 mg/kg/dose q4–6 hr. Adolescents >12 yr: IV: 3–4 mg; may repeat in 5 min if needed. *Side effects:* Hypotension, sedation, respiratory depression.

Pentazocine: [Opiate analgesic]: Children >14 yr of age PO q3–4 hr; titrate to effect to 100 mg dose not to exceed 600 mg/24 hr. May be given IM or IV reducing oral dose by one third. *Side effects:* CNS and respiratory depression.

40.3 Antibacterial Medications (Antibiotics)

Amikacin sulphate: [Aminoglycoside antibiotic active against gram-negative bacilli, especially *Escherichia coli, Klebsiella, Proteus, Entrobacter Serratia, and Pseudomonas*]: Neonates: Postnatal age ≤ 7 days 1,200–2,000 g: 7.5 mg/kg IV or IM q12–18 hr; >2,000 g: 10 mg/kg IV or IM q12 hr; Postnatal age >7 days 1,200–2,000 g: 7.5 g/kg IV or IM q8–12 hr; >2,000 g: 10 mg/kg IV or IM q8 hr. Children: 15–25 mg/kg/24 hr IV or IM divided q8–12 hr. Administered IV over 30–60 min. *Side effects:* Ototoxicity and nephrotoxicity.

Amoxicillin: [Penicillinase-susceptible β-Lactum: gram-positive pathogens except *Staphylococcus, Salmonella, Shigella, Neisseria, E. coli,* and *Proteus mirabilis*]: Children: 20–50 mg/kg/24 hr PO divided q8–12 hr; higher dose of 80–90 mg/kg/24 hr PO for otitis media. Uncomplicated gonorrhea: 3 g with 1 g probenecid PO. *Side effects:* Rash, diarrhea, abdominal cramping.

Amoxicillin-clavulanate: [β–Lactum (amoxicillin) and β-Lactamase inhibitor (clavulanate) enhances amoxicillin activity against penicillinase-producing bacteria: *S. aureus* (not methicillin-resistant organism), *Streptococcus, Haemophilus influenzae, Moraxella catarrhalis, E. coli, Klebsiella, Bacteroides fragilis*]:

Neonates: 30 mg/kg/24 hr PO divided q12 hr. Children: 20–45 mg/kg/24 hr PO divided q8–12 hr; higher dose of 80–90 mg/kg/24 hr PO for otitis media.

Amoxycillin-cloxacillin: See amoxicillin and cloxacillin.

Ampicillin: [β–Lactum with same spectrum of antibacterial activity as amoxicillin]: Neonates: Postnatal age ≤ 7 days ≤ 2,000 g: 50 mg/kg/24 hr IV or IM q12 hr (meningitis: 100 mg/kg/24 hr IV or IM divided q12 hr); >2,000 g: 75 mg/kg/24 hr IV or IM divided q8 hr (meningitis: 150 mg/kg/24 hr IV or IM divided q8 hr); Postnatal age >7 days 1,200 g: 50 mg/kg/24 hr IV or IM q12 hr (meningitis: 100 mg/kg/24 hr IV or IM divided q12 hr); 1,200–2,000 g: 75 mg/kg/24 hr IV or IM divided q8 hr (meningitis: 100 mg/kg/24 hr IV or IM divided q8 hr); >2,000 g: 100 mg/kg/24 hr IV or IM divided q6 hr (meningitis: 200 mg/kg/24 hr IV or IM divided q6 hr). Children: 100–200 mg/kg/24 hr IV or IM divided q6 hr (meningitis: 200–400 mg/kg/24 hr IV or IM divided q4–6 hr). *Side effects:* Rash and greater diarrhea than amoxicillin.

Ampicillin-cloxacillin: See ampicillin and cloxacillin.

Ampicillin-sulbactam: β-Lactum (ampicillin) and β-Lactamase inhibitor (sulbactam) enhances ampicillin activity against penicillinase-producing bacteria: *S. aureus , Streptococcus, Haemophilus influenzae, Moraxella catarrhalis, E. coli, Klebsiella, Bacteroides fragilis*]: Children: 100–200 mg/kg/24 hr IV or IM divided q4–8 hr (meningitis: 200–400 mg/kg/24 hr IV or IM divided q4–6 hr). Drug is dosed on ampicillin component. *Side effects:* Rash, diarrhea.

Azithromycin: [*Azilide antibiotic with activity against S. aureus, Streptococcus, H. influenzae, Mycoplasma, Legionella, Chlamydia trachomatis*]: 10 mg/kg PO on day 1 (max: 500 mg) followed by 5/kg PO q24 hr for 4 days. Group A *Streptococcus* pharyngitis: 12 mg/kg/24 hr PO (max : 500 mg) for 5 days. In uncomplicated *C. trachomatis* infection: single 1 g dose PO. *Side effects:* Gastrointestinal upset.

Carbenicillin: [Extended-spectrum penicillin (remains susceptible to penicillinase destruction) active against *Entrobacter, indole positive Proteus* and *Pseudomonas*]: Neonates: Postnatal age ≤ 7 days ≤ 2,000 g: 225 mg/kg/24 hr IV or IM divided q8 hr; >2,000 g: 300 mg/kg/24 hr IV or IM divided q6 hr; Postnatal age >7 days: 300–400 mg/kg/24 hr IV or IM divided q6 hr. Children: 400–600 mg/kg/24 hr IV or IM divided q4–6 hr. *Side effect:* Rash.

Cefaclor: [Second-generation cephalosporin active against *S. aureus, Streptococcus* including *S. pneumonia, H. influenzae, E. coli, Klebsiella and Proteus*]: Children: 20–40 mg/kg/24 hr PO divided q8–12 hr (max dose: 2 g). *Side effects:* β-lactum safety profile (rash,

eosinophilia) with high incidence of serum sickness reaction.

Cefadroxil: [First generation cephalosporin active against *S. sureus, Streptococcus, E. coli, Klebsiella,* and *Proteus*]: 30 mg/kg/24 hr PO divided q12 hr (max dose: 2 g).
Adverse events: See Cefaclor.

Cefazolin: [First-generation cephalosporin active against *S. aureus, Streptococcus, E. coli, Klebsiella and Proteus*]: Neonates: Postnatal age ≤ 7 days 40 mg/kg/24 hr IM, IV divided q12 hr; > 7 days 40–60 mg/kg/24 hr IM, IV divided q8 hr. Children: 50–100 mg/kg/24 hr IM, IV divided q8 hr. *Side effects:* See Cefaclor.

Cefdinir: [Extended spectrum, semi-synthetic cephalosporin]: Children 6 mo–12 yr: 14 mg/kg/24 hr PO in 1 or 2 doses (max: 600 mg/24 hr). Adverse events: See Cefaclor.

Cefepime: [Fourth-generation cephalosporin having expanded spectrum active against many gram-positive and negative pathogens including many drug-resistant pathogens]: 100–150 mg/kg/24 hr IV or IM q8–12 hr. *Side effects:* See Cefaclor.

Cefixime: [Third-generation cephalosporin active against *Streptococcus* including *S. pneumonia, H. influenzae, M. catarrhalis, N. gonorrhoeae, S. marcesens,* and *Proteus vulgaris*. No anti-staphylococcal or anti-pseudomonal activity]: 8 mg/kg/24 hr PO divided q12–24 hr. *Side effects:* see Cefaclor.

Cefoperazone sodium: [Third-generation cephalosporin active against gram-positive and negative pathogens]: Neonates: 100 mg/kg/day IM, IV, divided q12 hr. Children: 100–150 mg/kg/day IM, IV divided q8–12 hr. *Side effects:* see Cefaclor.

Cefotaxime sodium: [Third-generation cephalosporin active against gram-positive and negative pathogens. No antipseudomonal activity]: Neonates: Postnatal age ≤ 7 days 100 mg/kg/day IM, IV divided q12 hr; > 7 days, <1,200 g 100 mg/kg/day divided q12 hr; > 1200 g 150 mg/kg/day divided q8 hr. Children: 150 mg/kg/day IM, IV, divided q6–8 hr (meningitis 200 mg/kg/day IV, divided q6–8 hr). *Side effects:* See Cefaclor.

Cefotetan disodium: [Second-generation cephalosporin active against *S. aureus, Streptococcus* including *S. pneumonia, H. influenzae, E. coli, Klebsiella, Proteus,* and *Bacteroides*. Not active against *Enterobacter*]: 40–80 mg/kg/24 hr IV or IM q12hr. *Side effects:* See Cefaclor.

Cefoxitin sodium: [Second-generation cephalosporin active against *S. aureus, Streptococcus* including *S. pneumonia, H. influenzae, E. coli, Klebsiella, Proteus,* and *Bacteroides*. Not active against *Enterobacter*]: Neonates: 70–100 mg/kg/24 hr IV or IM divided q8–12 hr.

Children: 80–160 mg/kg/24 hr IV or IM divided q6–8 hr. *Side effects: see* Cefaclor.

Cefpodoxime proxetil: [Third-generation cephalosporin active against *S. aureus, Streptococcus, S. pneumonia, H. influenzae, M. catarrhalis, N. gonorrhoeae, E. coli, Klebsiella, and Proteus.* No antipseudomonal activity]: 10 mg/kg/day PO divided q12 hr. Uncomplicated gonorrhea 200 mg PO single dose therapy. *Side effects: see* Cefaclor.

Cefprozil: [Second-generation cephalosporin active against *S. aureus, Streptococcus, H. influenzae, M. catarrhalis, E. coli, Klebsiella, and Proteus*]: 30 mg/kg/day PO divided q8–12 hr. *Side effects: see* Cefaclor.

Ceftazidime: [Third-generation cephalosporin active against gram-positive and negative pathogens including *Pseudomonas aeruginosa*]: Neonates: Postnatal age ≤ 7 days 100 mg/kg/day IM, IV divided q12 hr; > 7 days, < 1,200 g 100 mg/kg/day divided q12 hr; > 1200 g 150 mg/kg/day divided q8 hr. Children: 150 mg/kg/day IM, IV, divided q8hr (meningitis 150 mg/kg/day IV, divided q8hr). *Side effects: see* Cefaclor.

Ceftibuten: [Semi-synthetic third generation cephalosporin for oral administration]: 9 mg/kg/24 hr as a single dose (max: 400 mg daily). *Side effects: see* Cefaclor.

Ceftizoxime: [Third-generation cephalosporin active against gram-positive and negative pathogens. No antipseudomonal activity]: 150 mg/kg/day IM, IV, divided q6–8 hr. *Side effects: see* Cefaclor.

Ceftriaxone sodium: [Third-generation cephalosporin active against gram-positive and negative pathogens. No antipseudomonal activity. Very potent and β-lactamase stable]: Neonates: 50–75 mg/kg IV or IM q24 hr. Children: 50–75 mg/kg IV or IM q24 hr (meningitis 75 mg/kg dose 1 then 80–100 mg/kg/24 hr divided q12–24 hr IV or IM).
Side effects: see Cefaclor.

Cefuroxime: [Second-generation cephalosporin active against *S. aureus, Streptococcus, H. influenzae, M. catarrhalis, E. coli, Klebsiella, and Proteus*]: Neonates: 40–100 mg/kg/24 hr IM, IV divided q12 hr. Children: 200–240 mg/kg/24 hr IM, IV q8 hr; 20–30 mg/kg/24 hr PO divided q8 hr. *Side effects: see* Cefaclor.

Cephalexin: [First-generation cephalosporin active against *S. aureus, Streptococcus, E. coli, Klebsiella, and Proteus*]: 25–100 mg/kg/24 hr PO divided q6–8 hr. *Side effects: see* Cefaclor.

Cephalexin-carbocisteine: *see* Cephalexin.

Cephradine: [First-generation cephalosporin active against *S. aureus, Streptococcus, E. coli, Klebsiella, and*

Proteus]: 50–100 mg/kg/24 hr PO divided q6–12 hr. *Side effects: see* Cefaclor.

Chloramphenicol: [Active against gram-positive and negative bacteria, *Rickettsia, Chlamydia, Mycoplasma, Salmonella, Bacteroides*; other anerobes, *Pseudomonas* usually resistant]: Neonates: Initial loading dose 20 mg/kg followed 12 hr later by: Postnatal age ≤ 7 days 25 mg/kg/day IV q24 hr; >7 days, ≤ 2,000 g 25 mg/kg/day IV q24 hr; > 2,000 g 50 mg/kg/day divided q12 hr. Children: 50–75 mg/kg/day IV, PO divided q6–8 hr (meningitis 75–100 mg/kg/day IV divided q6 hr). *Side effects:* Gray baby syndrome; bone marrow suppression, aplastic anemia.

Ciprofloxacin: [Quinolone antibiotic active against *Pseudomonas aeruginosa, Serratia, Enterobacter* spp., *Shigella, Salmonella, Compylobacter, H. influenzae, M. catarrhalis, N. gonorrhoeae,* some *S. aureus, Stertococcus spp.*]: Neonates: 10 mg/kg PO or IV q12 hr. Children: 15–30 mg/kg/24 hr PO or IV divided q12 hr; Cystic fibrosis: 20–40 mg/kg/24 hr PO or IV divided q8–12 hr. *Side effects:* Tendonitis, superinfection.

Clarithromycin: [Macrolide antibiotic active against *S. aureus, Streptococcus, H. influenzae, Mycoplasma, C. trachomatis, Legionella*]: 15 mg/kg/day PO, divided q12hr. *Side effects:* Less than erythromycin.

Clindamycin: [Protein synthesis inhibitor active against most gram-positive aerobic and anaerobic cocci (not *Enterococcus*]: Neonates: Postnatal age ≤ 7 days ≤ 2,000 g 10 mg/kg/day IM, IV divided q 12 hr; >2,000 g 15 mg/kg/day IM, IV divided q8 hr; > 7 days <1,200 g 10 mg/kg/day IM, IV divided q12 hr; 1,200–2,000 g 15 mg/kg/day divided q8 hr; >2,000 g 20 mg/kg/day divided q8 hr. Children: 10–40 mg/kg/day IM, IV, PO divided q6–8 hr. *Side effects:* Diarrhea, pseudomembranous colitis, rash.

Cloxacillin sodium: [Penicillinase-resistant penicillin effective against *S. aureus* and other gram-positive cocci except *Enterococcus* and coagulase-negative staphylococci]: 50–100 mg/kg/day PO divided q6 hr. *Side effects: see* Cefaclor.

Co-trimoxazole: (Trimethoprim [TMP]-sulfamethoxazole [SMZ]) [Active against: *Shigella, Pneumocystis carinii, Legionella, Nocardia, Chlamydia.* Dosage based on TMP component]: 6–20 mg TMP/kg/day PO, IV divided q12hr (Pneumocystitis: 15–20 mg TMP/kg/day PO, IV divided q12 hr (Pneumocystitis prophylaxis: 5 mg TMP/kg/day PO or 3 times/wk). *Side effects:* Sulfonamide skin reactions— rash, Stevens-Johnson syndrome, nausea, leukopenia; renal and hepatic elimination.

Demeclocycline: [Tetracycline active against most gram-positive cocci (except *Enterococcus*); many gram-negative bacilli, *Mycoplasma, Borrelia burgdorferi* (Lime disease), *Chlamydia,* anaerobes]: 6–12 mg / kg/day PO divided q6–12 hr.

Syndrome of inappropriate ADH secretion: 900–1,200 mg PO/day or 13–15 mg/kg/day PO divided q6–8 hr with dose reduction based on response to 600–900 mg/day. *Side effects:* Teeth staining, possibly permanent (<8 yr of age) with prolonged use; photosensitivity, diabetes insipidus, diarrhea, superinfections.

Dicloxacillin: [Penicillinase-resistant penicillin effective against *S. aureus* and other gram-positive cocci except *Enterococcus* and coagulase-negative staphylococci]: 12.5–100 mg/kg/day PO divided q6 hr. *Side effects: see* Cefaclor.

Doxycycline: [Tetracycline active against most gram-positive cocci (except *Enterococcus*); many gram-negative bacilli, *Mycoplasma, Borrelia burgdorferi* (Lime disease), *Chlamydia,* anaerobes]: 2–5 mg / kg/day PO divided q12–24 hr (maximum dose: 200 mg/day). *Side effects: see* Demeclocycline.

Erythromycin: [Macrolide antibiotic active against *S. aureus, Streptococcus, H. influenzae, Mycoplasma, C. trachomatis, Legionella*]: Neonates: Postnatal age ≤ 7 days 20 mg/kg/day PO divided q12 hr; > 7 days < 1,200 g: 20 mg/kg/day divided q12 hr; ≥ 1,200 g: 30 mg/kg/day PO q8 hr. Children: usual maximum dose 2 g/day: Base: 30–50 mg/kg/day PO divided q6–8 hr. Estolate: 30–50 mg/kg/day PO divided q8–12 hr. Stearate: 20–40 mg/kg/day PO divided q6 hr. Lactobionate: 20–40 mg/kg/day IV divided q6–8 hr. Gluceptate: 20–50 mg/kg/day IV divided q6–8 hr (usual maximum dose: IV 4 g/day). Topically effective as an acne treatment. *Side effects:* GI upset.

Gatifloxacin: [Quinolone antibiotic active against both gram negative and gram positive organisms, more effective against legionella, *Chlamydia, Mycoplasma* species and *M. tuberculosis*]: 10 mg/kg/24 hr PO single dose. Not recommended below 15 yr of age. *Side effects: see* Ciprofloxacin.

Gentamicin: [Aminoglycoside antibiotic effective against gram negative bacilli, especially *Pseudomonas, Proteus, E. coli, Klebsiella, Enterobacter, Serratia*]: Neonates: IM, IV (over 30–60 min): Postnatal age ≤ 7 days 1,200–2,000 g: 2.5 mg/kg q12–18 hr; >2,000 g: 2.5 mg/kg q12 hr; Postnatal age >7 days 1,200–2,000 g: 2.5 mg/kg q8–12 hr; > 2,000 g: 2.5 mg/kg q8 hr. Children: 2.5 mg/ kg/24 hr divided q8–12 hr IV or IM; alternatively may administer 5–7.5 mg/kg/day IV once daily. Intrathecal: Preservative-free preparation for intraventricular or intrathecal use: neonate: 1 mg/day; child: 1–2 mg/day. *Side effects: see* Amikacin sulphate.

Imipenem-cilastatin: [Carbapenem antibiotic active against broad spectrum gram-positive cocci and negative bacilli including *Pseudomonas aeruginosa* (not *Stenotrophomonas maltophilia*)]: Neonates: Postnatal age £7 days <1,200 g 20 mg/ kg IM, IV q18–24 hr; >1200 g 40 mg/kg divided q12 hr; >7 days 1, 200–2,000 g 40 mg/kg q12 hr; >2,000 g 60 mg/ kg q8hr. Children: 60–100 mg/ kg/day IM, IV divided q6–8 hr.

Side effects: see Cefaclor.

Kanamycin: [Aminoglycoside antibiotic used in combination with other agents]: 15 mg/kg/24 hr IM or IV divided q12hr. *Side effects: see* Amikacin sulphate.

Levofloxacin: [Quinolone antibiotic; active against *Streptococcus pneumoniae* and some other gram negative and gram positive organisms]: 250–500 mg once or twice daily for upto 14 days. Not recommended below 15 yr of age. *Side effects: see* ciprofloxacin.

Meropenem: [Carbapenem antibiotic active against broad spectrum gram-positive cocci and negative bacilli including *Pseudomonas aeruginosa* (not *Xanthomonas maltophilia*)]: 60 mg/kg/day IV divided q8 hr. *Meningitis:* 120 mg/kg/day IV divided q8hr (maximum dose: 6 g/day). *Side effects: see* Cefaclor.

Metronidazole: [*see* section 40.8 Antiparasitic medications]: Indication: Highly effective in the treatment of infections due to anaerobes. Neonates: 0–4 wk < 1,200 g 7.5 mg/ kg PO, IV q48 hr; postnatal age ≤ 1,200–2,000 g 7.5 mg/kg/day PO IV q24 hr; 2,000 g 15 mg/kg/day PO, IV divided q12 hr; > 7days 1,200–2,000 g 15 mg/kg/day PO, IV divided q12 hr; >2,000 g 30 mg/ kg/day PO, IV divided q12 hr. Children: 30 mg/kg/day PO, IV divided q6–8 hr. *Side effects:* Metallic taste, disulfiram-like reaction with alcohol.

Mupirocin: [Topical antibiotic effective against *staphylococci* and *streptococci*]: Topical application: nasal (eliminate nasal carriage) and to the skin 2–4 times per day.

Nafcillin sodium: [Penicillinase-resistant penicillin effective against *S. aureus* and other gram-positive cocci except *Enterococcus* and coagulase-negative staphylococci]: Neonates: Postnatal age ≤ 7 days 1,200–2,000 g 50 mg/kg/day IM, IV q12 hr; > 2,000 g 75 mg/kg/day divided q8hr; > 7 days 1,200–2,000 g 75 mg/kg/day q8 hr; > 2,000 g 100 mg/kg/day IV divided q6–8 hr (meningitis 200 mg/kg/day IV divided q6 hr). Children: 100–200 mg/kg/day PO divided q4–6 hr. *Side effects: see* Cefaclor.

Nalidixic acid: [First-generation quinolone effective for short-term treatment of lower urinary tract infections caused by *E. coli, Enterobacter, Klebsiella, proteus*]: 50–55 mg/kg/day PO divided q6 hr. *Side effects: see* Ciprofloxacin.

Neomycin sulfate: [Aminoglycoside antibiotic]: Infants: 50 mg/kg/day PO divided q6 hr. Children: 50–100 mg/kg/day PO divided q6–8 hr. *Side effects: see* Amikacin sulphate.

Netilmicin: [Aminoglycoside antibiotic; similar to gentamicin]: Neonates: IV, IM: < 1,200 g (age 0–4 wk) 2.5 mg/kg q18–24 hr; 1,200–2,000 g (age 0–7 days) 2.5 mg/kg q12–18 hr; 1,200–2,000 g (age > 7 days) 2.5 mg/kg q8–12 hr; > 2,000 g (age 0–7 days) 2.5 mg/kg q12 hr; >2,000 g (age > 7 days) 2.5 mg/kg q8 hr. *Side effects: see* Gentamicin.

Nitrofurantoin: [Treatment of lower urinary tract infections caused by gram-positive and gram-negative pathogens]: 5–7 mg/kg/day PO divided q6 hr (maximum dose: 400 mg/day); suppressive therapy 1–2.5 mg/kg/day PO divided q 12–24 hr (maximum dose: 100 mg/day). *Side effects:* Vertigo, jaundice, interstitial pneumonitis.

Ofloxacin: [Quinoline antibiotic]: Genitourinary, respiratory, gastrointestinal, skin, and soft tissue infections, peritonitis, gonorrhea. 15 mg/kg/day PO q12 hr; 5–10 mg/kg/day q12 hr IV. Children > 6 yr should be given in 2 divided doses (max: 800mg). Gonorrhea: 400 mg as a single dose. Not recommended for children below 16 yr. *Side effects: see* Suprafloxacin.

Penicillin G aqueous: [Active against most gram-positive cocci; *S pneumoniae*, group A *Streptococcus viridans* and some gram-negative bacteria (*N. gonorrhoeae, N. meningitidis*): Neonates: Postnatal age IM, IV ≤ 7 days 1,200–2,000 g 50,000 units/kg/day divided q12 hr (meningitis 100,000 units/kg/day divided q12 hr); > 2,000 g 75, 000 units/kg/day divided q8 hr (meningitis 150,000 units/kg/day divided q8 hr); > 7days ≤ 1,200 g 50,000 units/kg/day divided q12 hr (meningitis 100,000 units/kg/day divided q12 hr); 1,200–2,000 g 75, 000 units/kg/day divided q8 hr (meningitis 225,000 units/kg/day divided q8 hr); > 2,000 g 100, 000 units/kg/day divided q6 hr (meningitis 200,000 units/kg/day divided q6 hr). Children: 100,000 (60 mg)–250,000 units/kg/day IV, IM divided q4–6 hr (up to 400,000 units/kg/day). *Side effects:* β-lactam safety profile (rash, eosinophilia).

Penicillin G Benzathine: [long-acting (repository form) penicillin effective in the treatment of infections responsive to persistent, low penicillin concentrations (1–4 wk), e.g. *Streptococcus pharyngitis*, rheumatic fever prophylaxis]: Neonates: >1,200 g 50, 000 units/kg once IM. Children: 300,000–1.2 million units/kg IM once every 3–4 wk (maximum: 1.2–2.4 million units/dose). *Side effects: see* Penicillin G aqueous.

Penicillin G Procaine: [Repository form of penicillin providing low penicillin concentrations for 12 hr]:

Neonates: >1,200 g 50, 000 units/kg IM qid. Children: 25,000–50,000 units/kg IM qid for 10 days (maximum: 4.8 million units/dose). Gonorrhea: 100,000–50,000 units/kg IM qid for 10 days (maximum: 4.8 million units/day) once with probenecid 25 mg/kg (maximum dose: 1 g). *Side effects: see* Penicillin G aqueous.

Penicillin V: (phenoxymethyl penicillin) [Oral form of penicillin active against most gram-positive cocci and some gram-negative bacteria (*N. gonorrhoeae, N. meningitidis*): 25–50 mg/kg/day PO divided q 4–8 hr. *Side effects: see* Penicillin G aqueous.

Pentamidine isetionate: [Antiprotozoal agent effective to the prevention and treatment *Pneumonocystis carinii* infections]: *P. carinii* treatment 4 mg/kg/day IM, IV qid for 14 days. Prophylaxis: 4 mg/kg/day IM, IV every 2–4 wk; aerosol adjusted to minute ventilation (4–8 mg/kg/dose) up to 300 mg/dose. Visceral leishmaniasis: 4 mg/kg/day IM, IV qd for 14 days. *Side effects:* Hypotension, hypoglycemia, bronchospasm with aerosol.

Piperacillin: [Extended-spectrum penicillin active against *Enterobacter, Serratia, E. coli, Bactericides* spp., *P. aeruginosa*]: Neonates: Postnatal age ≤ 7 days 150 mg/kg/day IV q8–12 hr; >7days 200 mg/kg/day IV divided q 6–8 hr. Children: 200–300 mg/kg/day IV divided q 4–6 hr. *Cystic fibrosis:* 350–500 mg/kg/day IV divided q 4–6 hr. *Side effects: see* Cefaclor.

Piperacillin-tazobactam: [Extended-spectrum penicillin combined with a beta-lactamase inhibitor (tazobactam) active *against S. aureus, H. Influenzae, Enterobacter, Serratia, E. coli, Bactericides* spp., *Acinetobacter, P. aeruginosa*]: 300–400 mg/kg/day IM, IV divided q 6–8 hr. *Side effects: see* Cefaclor.

Roxithromycin: [Macrolide antibiotic with activity against *S. aureus, Streptococcus, H. influenzae, Mycoplasma, Legionella, Chlamydia trachomatis*]: 5–8 mg/kg daily bid for a maximum for a maximum of 10 days. *Side effects: see* Clarithromycin.

Sisomicin: [Aminoglycoside; similar to gentamicin but some what more potent on Pseudomonas]: 3 mg/kg in 3 divided doses. *Side effects: see* Gentamicin.

Spiramycin: [Macrolide antibiotic indicated primarily for the treatment of *Toxoplasma gondii*]: Toxoplasmosis: Pregnant women: 1 g every 8 hour given without food in the first trimester for prevention of congenital infection to fetus (lower doses are less effective). 6–9 MIU (4–6 tablets) daily in 2–4 divided doses for 3 wk repeated after 2 wk intervals till parturition. *Side effects:* Paresthesias, rash.

Sulfadiazine: [Sulfonamide antibiotic primarily indicated for the treatment of lower urinary tract infections due to *E. coli, P. mirabilis, Klebsiella* spp.,Toxoplasmosis]: Neonates: 100 mg/kg/day PO; Children: 120–200 mg/kg/day PO divided q6 hr. Rheumatic fever prophylaxis: ≤30 kg 500 mg/day; >30 kg 1 g/day PO qid. Avoid use with renal disease. Half life -10 hr. *Side effects:* Rash, Stevens-Johnson syndrome, leukopenia, crystalluria.

Tetracycline: [Active against most gram-positive cocci (except *Enterococcus*); many gram-negative bacilli, *Mycoplasma, Borrelia burgdorferi* (Lime disease), *Chlamydia*, anaerobes]: 20–40 mg/kg/day PO in 4 divided doses (max dose: 1000 mg/day). *Side effects: see* Demeclocycline.

Ticarcillin: [Extended-spectrum penicillin active *against Enterobacter, Serratia, E. coli, Bactericides* spp., *P. aeruginosa*]: Neonates: Postnatal age ≤7 days <2,000 g 150 mg/kg/day IV divided q8–12 hr; >2,000 g 225 mg/kg/day IV divided q8 hr; > 7 days < 1,200 g 150 mg/kg/day IV divided q12 hr; 1,200–2,000 g 225 mg/ kg/ day IV divided q8 hr; >2,000 g 300 mg/kg/day IV divided q6–8 hr. Children: 200–400 mg/kg/day IV divided q4–6 hr. *Cystic fibrosis:* 400–600 mg/kg/day IV divided q4–6 hr. *Side effects: see* Cefaclor.

Ticarcillin-clavulanate: [Extended-spectrum penicillin combined with a beta-lactamase inhibitor (clavulanate) active *against S. aureus, H. Influenzae, Enterobacter, Serratia, E. coli, Bactericides* spp., *Acinetobacter, P. aeruginosa*]: 280–400 mg/kg/day IM, IV divided q4–8 hr. *Side effects: see* Cefaclor.

Tobramycin: [Aminoglycoside antibiotic effective against gram negative bacilli, esp. *Pseudomonas, Proteus, Klebsiella, Enterobacter, Serratia, E. coli*]: Neonates: IM, IV (over 30–60 minutes) Postnatal age ≤7 days 1,200–2,000 g 2.5 mg/kg q12–18 hr; >2,000 g 2.5 mg/kg q12 hr; >7 days 1,200–2,000 g 2.5 mg/kg q8–12 hr; >2,000 g 2.5 mg/kg q8 hr.

Children: 2.5 mg/kg/day IM, IV divided q8–12 hr; alternatively may administer 5–7.5 mg/ kg/day IV qid. *Intrathecal/intraventricular:* Neonate 1 mg/24 hr; child 1–2 mg/day intrathecal; adult 4–8 mg/day intrathecal. *Side effects: see* Amikacin sulphate.

Trimethoprim: [Folinic acid antagonist effective in the prophylaxis and treatment of *E. coli, P. mirabilis, Klebsiella* and *Enterobacter* spp. urinary tract infections, *Pneumocystis carinii* pneumonia]: UTI: 4–6 mg /kg/ day PO divided q12 hr. >12 yr: 100–200 mg/dose PO q12 hr. *Pneumocystis carinii* pneumonia (with dapsone): 15–20 mg/kg/day PO divided q6hr for 21 days. *Side effects:* Megaloblastic anemia, bone marrow suppression.

Vancomycin: [Glycopeptide antibiotic effective against most gram-positive pathogens including *staphylococci* (methicillin-resistant *S. aureus* and cogulase-negative *staphylococci*) and *enterococci, clostridia, pneumococci* including penicillin-resistant strains]: Neonates: Postnatal age ≤ 7 days 1,200 g 15 mg/kg/day IV divided q24 hr; 1,200–2,000 g 15 mg/kg/day IV divided q12–18 hr; >2,000 g: 30 mg/kg/day IV divided q12 hr; >7 days <1,200 g 15 mg/kg/day IV divided q24 hr; 1,200–2,000 g 15 mg/kg/day IV divided q 8–12 hr; >2,000 g 45 mg/kg/day IV divided q8 hr. Children: 45–60 mg/kg/day IV divided q4–12 hr; oral dose for antibiotic-associated enterocolitis; 40–50 mg/kg/day PO divided q6–8 hr. *Side effects:* Ototoxicity, nephrotoxicity.

40.4 ANTIMYCOBACTERIAL MEDICATIONS

Antitubercular medications, see Section 14.3. Antileprotic medications, *see* Section 30.14.

40.5 ANTIFUNGAL MEDICATIONS

Amphotericin B: [*Candida, Aspergillus, Coccidioides, Histoplasma, Sporothrix, Blastomyces*]: Initial dose: 0.1–0.25 mg/ kg IV infused over 1–2 hr. Maintenance dose: 0.5–1 mg/ kg/24 hr infused IV over 4–6 hr quantity daily. Bladder irrigation: 5–15 mg amphotericin B/100 ml.

Amphotericin B Lipid complexes: Initial dose: 2.5–5 mg/ kg IV infused over 1–2 hr; may use higher doses of 7.5–10 mg/kg/24 hr if indicated and if tolerated. *Side effects:* Hypotension, fever, chills, flushing.

Amphotericin B Lipid complexes: Injection: 10 mg, 25 mg, 50 mg per unit.

Caspofungin: Aspergillus, Candida: 1–2 mg/kg/24 hr IVas single daily dose.

Clotrimazole: *Cryptococcus, Aspergillus, Candida,* and *Coccidioides* for the treatment of oropharyngeal, skin, vaginal infections: One troche dissolved 5–6 times daily. Vaginal cream/tablet: 2% cream or100 mg tablet (preferred) deeply into the vagina for six consecutive nights or 200 mg for three consecutive nights. Topical cream: Apply twice daily.

Econazole nitrate: Tinea corporis, cruris, pedis, and cutaneous candidiasis: Apply over affected areas once daily. Vulvovaginal candidiasis: Insert one tablet into the vagina for 3 consecutive days.

Fluconazole: *Cryptococcus* and *Candida* infections of the oropharynx, vagina, meningitis, *Tinea versicolor*: Neonates: Thrush 6 mg/kg IV or PO q24 hr for first day then 3 mg/kg/24 hr q24 hr for 14–21 days. Systemic infections: Postnatal age <14 days 6–12 mg/kg/day IV or PO q72 hr or once daily for postnatal age > 14 days. Children: 6–12 mg/kg/24 hr IV or PO q24 hr; Cryptococcal meningitis: 12 mg/kg/24 hr first day then 6–12 mg/kg/24 hr IV or PO q24 hr. Tinea versicolor: 400 mg repeated in 1 wk. Vaginal candidiasis: One capsule (150 mg) only, single oral dose. *Side effects:* Rash, elevated liver function tests.

Flucytosine [Used in combination with amphotericin B against *Candida, Cryptococcus,* and *Aspergillus* infections]: Neonates: 50–100 mg/ kg/24 hr PO divided q12–24 hr. Children: 100–150 mg/ kg/24 hr PO divided q6–8 hr. *Side effects:* Rash, bone marrow suppression.

Griseofulvin [Treatment of tinea infections of the hair, nails, and skin due to *Microsporum, Epidermophyton,* and *Trichophyton*]: Microsize 10–20 mg/kg/24 hr PO divided q12–24 hr; ultra-microsize 5–10 mg/kg/24 hr PO divided q12 hr. *Side effects:* Rash, photosensitivity.

Hamycin: Oral thrush due to *Candida albicans.* Topical: Apply 2 lac unit per ml suspension 2–4 times daily for 7–10 days. *Side effects:* Sensitization, irritation.

Itraconazole [*Candida, Aspergillus, Histoplasmosis, Cryptococci, Tinea versicolor*]: 3–5 mg/ kg/24 hr PO once daily (maximum dose: as high as 5–10 mg/ kg/24 hr). *Side effects:* Hypertension, rash, hepatitis.

Ketoconazole: Disseminated coccidioidomycosis: 3–10 mg/kg/24 hr. Familial male gonadotropin-independent precocious puberty/familial male precocious pseudopuberty: 600 mg/24 hr in 8 hr divided doses. Tinea versicolor: 400 mg repeated in 1 wk. *Side effects:* Hepatic dysfunction and inhibit testosterone synthesis; adrenal insufficiency by inhibiting adrenal enzymes.

Miconazole [*Cryptococcus, Candida, Coccidioides* and *Pseudallescheria boydii* for topical or IV use in superficial infections]: Neonates: 5–15 mg/kg/24 hr IV divided q8–24 hr. Children: 20–40 mg/kg/24 hr IV divided q8 hr; vaginal cream/tablet 100–200 mg qhs; topical cream: apply twice daily. Vulvovaginal candidiasis: Apply gel 5 g intravaginally, with additional cream smeared on to affected areas for 14 consecutive nights. *Side effects:* Hyperlipidemia, tremors.

Natamycin [Fungal eye infections caused by *Candida, Aspergillus, Cephalosporium, Fusarium,* and *Penicillium*)]: Keratitis: Instill 1 drop into conjunctival sac every 1–2 hr for 3–4 days, then may reduce to 6–8 doses/24 hr. Blepharitis and conjunctivitis: Instill 1 drop 4–6 times daily

Nystatin: Oral Candidiasis: Neonates: 100,000 units 4 times daily.
Infants: 200,000 units 4 times daily. Children: 400,000–600,000 units 4 times daily. Topical: Apply 2–4 times daily. Vaginal candidiasis: 1–2 tablets daily inserted high into the vagina; usual duration therapy is 2 weeks.

Terbinafine: Onychomycosis and tinea pedis: Children <20 kg: 62.5 mg PO q24 hr (fingernails for 6 wk; toenails for 12 wk, tinea for 2 wk). Children 20–40 kg: 125 mg PO q24 hr (fingernails for 6 wk; toenails for 12 wk, tinea for 2 wk). Children > 40 kg: 250 mg PO q24 hr (fingernails for 6 wk; toenails for 12 wk, tinea for 2 wk). Administer with food.

40.6 ANTIVIRAL MEDICATIONS

Acyclovir: Herpes simplex (HSV) encephalitis, mucosal, cutaneous, genital infections; herpes zoster, varicella-zoster, cytomegalovirus (CMV) prophylaxis. Neonate: HSV encephalitis: 30–40 mg/kg/day IV divided q8 hr. Children: 15 mg/kg/day IV divided q8–12 hr. HSV infection in immunocompromised host: Children: 15–30 mg/kg/day IV divided q8 hr. HSV encephalitis/varicella infection/CMV prophylaxis in immunocompromised host: Children: 30 mg/kg/day IV divided q8 hr. Oral dosing for HSV/zoster infection: Children: 1,200 mg/day PO divided q4–8 hr (maximum dose: 80 mg/kg/day). *Side effects:* Headache, rash, bone marrow suppression.

Amantadine: Prophylaxis and treatment of influenza A infections. Prophylaxis or treatment: Children: 1–9 yr or <40 kg: 5 mg/kg/day PO divided q12hr (maximum dose: 150 mg/day). Children >9 yr (and >40 kg): 200 mg/day PO divided q12 hr. *Side effects:* Drowsiness, hypotension, urinary retention.

Ganciclovir: CMV retinitis: Induction therapy: 10 mg/kg/day IV (over 1–2 hr) divided q12 hr for 14–21 days; maintenance therapy: 5–6 mg/kg/day IV once daily. CMV disease and prophylaxis (solid organ transplant): Induction therapy: 10 mg/kg/day IV divided q12 hr for 7–14 days; maintenance therapy: 5–6 mg/kg/day IV once daily. *Side effects:* Seizures, hypertension, bone marrow suppression.

Idoxuridine (IDU): Topical therapy for herpes simplex keratitis. Apply ointment 5 times daily and ophthalmic solution (1 drop) to affected eye (s) 7–10 times daily and at bedtime. *Side effects:* Local irritation, pruritus, ocular edema.

Oseltamivir: prophylaxis or treatment of influenza A and B infections. Children >1 yr: 30 mg q12 hr PO up to 15 kg; 45 mg q12 hr PO 16–23 kg; 60 mg q12 hr PO >23–40 kg and 75 mg q12 hr PO >40 kg. *Side effects:* Nausea, vomiting, diarrhea.

Ribavirin: Acute hepatitis, herpes virus infections, influenza and respiratory syncytial virus (RSV) infections. Aerosol therapy for RSV infections, particularly for patients with underlying conditions, including brochopulmonary dysplasia (BPD) and/or congenital heart diseases. 10 mg/kg/24 hr in divided doses 3–4 times. Use nebulizer at 20 mg/mL concentration for continuous aerosolization 12–18 hr per day. *Side effects:* Rash, irritation, hypotension.

Rimantadine: Prophylaxis and treatment (>13 yr) of influenza A infections. Prophylaxis only: Children: 1–9 yr or <40 kg: 5 mg/kg/day PO divided q12 hr (maximum dose: 150 mg/day). Children 10–13 yr: 100 mg/day PO divided q12 hr. Prophylaxis or treatment: Children >13 yr: 200 mg/day PO divided q12 hr. *Side effects:* Hypotension, urinary retention.

Trifluridine: Herpes simplex keratitis: Instill 1 drop into affected eye (s) q2 hr while awake and at bedtime for up to 21 days. *Side effects:* Local irritation, pruritus, ocular edema.

Valacyclovir: Herpes Zoster. Dose: 1,000 mg tid PO for 7 days.

Vidarabine (Ara-A): Herpes simplex (HSV), and Varicella-zoster infections. HSV infections: Neonate: 15–30 mg/kg/day IV infusion over 18–24 hr. Children: 15 mg/kg/day IV once daily over 12 hr. *Side effects:* Bone marrow suppression, ataxia, seizures, SIADH.

Zanamivir: Influenza infections type A and B. Children and Adolescents: $\geq$ 7 yr: 2 inhalations (10 mg) q12 hr for 5 days. Day 1 administer 2 doses provided dosing interval is > 2 hr. *Side effects:* Nasal symptoms and sinusitis.

40.7 ANTIRETROVIRAL–HIV MEDICATIONS

Abacavir: Children >3 mo and < 50 kg: 8 mg/kg q12 hr. Children > 50 kg: 20 mg/kg q12 hr or 15 mg/kg q8 hr. *Side effects:* GI upset, hypersensitivity reactions.

Amprenavir: Children 4–12 yr or < 50 kg: 20 mg/kg bid or 15 mg/kg tid (max daily dose: 2,400 mg; or 22.5 mg/kg bid or 17 mg/kg tid as oral solution). Adolescents 13–16 yr and > 50 kg: 1,200 mg bid. *Side effects:* May exacerbate diabetes mellitus.

Didanosine: Infants < 90 days: 100 mg/m^2/day PO divided q12 hr. Children: 180–300 mg/m^2/day PO divided q12 hr. Adolescents (>13 yr): <60 kg 125 mg PO divided q12 hr (buffered oral solution 167 mg PO q12 hr). Administer on an empty stomach 1 hr before or 2 hr after a meal to decrease food effect. *Side effects:* Peripheral neuropathy.

Efavirenz: Children $\geq$ 3 yr: 10- < 15 kg = 200 mg; 15- <20 kg = 250 mg; 20- < 25 kg = 300 mg; 25- <32.5 kg = 350 mg; 32.5- <40 kg = 400 mg; $\geq$ 40 kg = 600 mg (give all doses once daily). Adolescents: 600 mg/24 hr, at bedtime. *Side effects:* Psychiatric symptoms.

Indinavir: 1500 mg/m^2/day PO divided q8 hr (maximal single dose: 800 mg). Chemoprophylaxis after heavy risk-exposure: Given in combination with zidovudine and lamivudine. Administer on an empty stomach 1 hr before or 2 hr after a meal to decrease food effect. *Side effects:* Nephrolithiasis, hyperbilirubinemia, diabetes.

Lamivudine: Neonates: 4 mg/kg/day PO divided q12 hr. Children and Adolescents: 12 mg/kg/day PO divided q12 hr (maximum dose: 150 mg). *Side effects:* Psychomotor disorders, musculoskeletal pain.

Nelfinavir: Neonates: 30 mg/kg/day PO divided q8 hr. Children and Adolescents: 60–90 mg/kg/day PO divided q8 hr. Administer with a meal to optimize absorption. *Side effects:* Hypertension, anemia, leukopenia.

Nevirapine: Neonates: 5 mg/kg/day PO qd for 14 days then 240 mg/m^2/day PO divided q12 hr for 14 days, then 400 mg/m^2/day PO divided q12 hr. Children: 240 mg/m^2/day PO divided q12 hr for 14 days; if tolerated increase dose to maximum dose 400 mg/m^2/day PO divided q12 hr. Adolescents: 200 mg/day PO qd for 14 days if tolerated 200 mg/dose PO q12 hr. *Side effects:* Severe skin rash, Stevens-Johnson syndrome.

Ritonavir: Children: 500 mg/m^2/day PO divided q12hr, titrate upward in 50 mg/m^2 per dose increments to 800 mg/m^2/day PO q12 hr. Adolescents: 400–600 mg/dose PO q12 hr.

Administer dose with food to enhance bioavailability. *Side effects:* Taste aversion.

Saquinavir: 1,050–2,000 mg/m^2/day PO divided q8 hr. Administer dose with a high-fat food to enhance bioavailability. *Side effects:* Severe skin rash, Stevens-Johnson syndrome.

Stavudine: Children < 30 kg: 2 mg/kg/day PO divided q12 hr (maximum dose: 150 mg). Adolescents: 30–60 kg 30 mg/dose PO q12 hr; > 60 kg 40 mg/dose PO q12 hr. *Side effects:* Peripheral neuropathy, liver function tests, rash.

Zalcitabine: Children: 0.015–0.03 mg/kg/day PO divided q8 hr. Adolescents: 0.75 mg/dose PO q8 hr. *Side effects:* Peripheral neuropathy, pancreatitis, cardiac dysfunction.

Zidovudine: Neonates: 8 mg/kg/day PO divided q6–8 hr; 6 mg/kg/day IV divided q6 hr. Infants and Children: 270–540 mg/m^2/day PO divided q6–8 hr; 480 mg/m^2/day IV divided q6 hr; continuous infusion 20 mg/m^2/hr. Children >12 yr: 200 mg/dose PO 8 hr or 300 mg/dose q12 hr; 1–2 mg/kg per dose IV q4 hr. *Side effects:* Seizure, rash.

40.8 ANTIPARASITIC MEDICATIONS

Albendazole: Giardiasis: 400 mg PO once a day for 5 days, for all ages. Ascariasis, Hookworms, Trichuriasis: 400 mg PO once, for all ages. Cutaneous larva migrans, Trichuriasis (in heavy infections): 400 mg daily PO for 3 days, for all ages.
Cysticercosis: 15 mg/kg/24 hr divided bid PO for 28 days; maximum: 800 mg/24 hr. Echinococcosis: 15 mg/kg/24 hr divided bid PO for 28 days; maximum: 800 mg/24 hr. Enterobiasis, *Gnathostoma spinigerum*: 400 mg bid PO, for all ages for 3 weeks. Liver flukes-Clonorchiasis: 10 mg/kg once daily PO for 7 days. Loiasis: 400 mg PO once, for all ages for 3 weeks. Trichinosis: 400 mg bid PO for 8–14 days for all ages. Toxocariasis: 400 mg PO once for 5 days for all ages. *Caution:* Corticosteroids for 2–3 days before and during drug therapy can ameliorate worsening of symptoms that follow drug administration. Administer prednisolone (1 mg/kg/24 hr PO for 2–4 weeks) to suppress local inflammation. Absorption is improved if taken with a fatty meal.

Atovaquone: Treatment of *P. carinii* pneumonia: <13 yr: 40 mg/kg/24 hr PO q12 hr. Adolescents: 750 mg/dose PO q12 hr for 21 days. Prophylaxis of *P. carinii*: Children <13 yr: 40 mg/kg/24 hr PO q12hr. Adolescents: 1500 mg/dose PO qid. Toxoplasmosis prophylaxis: Adolescents: 1500 mg qid. Drug absorption is increased when co-administered with food. *Side effects:* Rash, neutropenia.

Bithionol: Liver flukes (Fascioliasis). 30–50 mg/kg once daily PO and then on alternate days for a total of 10–15 doses.

Chloroquine phosphate: Effective in suppression and treatment of malaria and extraintestinal amebiasis. (Dose drug on base equivalent). Extraintestinal amebiasis: 10 mg/kg PO daily for 2–3 wk (maximal daily dose: 300 mg). Administration with meals decreases GI upset. *Side effects:* Rash, peripheral neuropathy, blood dyscrasias, retinopathy, tinnitus.

Dehydroemetine: Fulminant cases of amebiasis. 1mg/kg/24 hr SC or IM. *Side effects:* GI upset, cardiac dysrhythmia, pain at the injection site.

Diethylcarbamazine: Lymphatic filariasis (Brugia malayi, Brugia timori, Wuchereria bancrofti): 1 mg/kg PO as a single dose on day I; 1 mg/kg tid PO on day 2; 1–2 mg/kg tid PO on day 3; and 6 mg/kg/24 hr divided tid PO on days 4–14. Caution: Dose should be increased gradually. For patients with no microfilaria in the blood the full dose (6 mg/kg/24 hr divided tid PO) can be given beginning on day 1. Tropical pulmonary eosinophilia: 5 mg/kg/24 hr PO for 10 days. Loiasis: 1 mg/kg PO as a single dose on day 1; 1 mg/kg tid PO on day 2; 1–2 mg/kg tid PO on day 3; and 9 mg/kg/24 hr divided tid PO on days 4–21. Caution: Dose should be increased gradually. For patients with no microfilaria in the blood the full dose (9 mg/kg/24 hr divided tid PO) can be given beginning on day 1. *Side effects:* Urticaria, hypotension.

Furazolidone: Treatment of protozoal diarrhea, enteritis. Infants >1 month and children: 5–9 mg/kg/24 hr (usual dose 6 mg/kg/24 hr) PO divided q6hr (maximal daily dose: 400 mg) for 10 days. *Side effects:* Hemolytic anemia in infants with G6PD deficiency, hypersensitivity reactions.

Ivermectin: Cutaneous larva migrans, Strongyloidiasis: 200 µg/kg daily PO for 1–2 days; (in cases of Strongyloidiasis with hyperinfection syndrome treat for 7–10 days). Onchocerciasis: 150 µg/kg PO, repeated after 3–6 months. *Side effects:* Nausea, vomiting, constipation, abdominal pain.

Levamisole: Round worms and hookworms. 50 mg single dose. Repeat dose after 1 month to prevent recurrence. *Side effects:* Altered taste, flu-like syndrome, dermatitis.

Lindane: Scabies: Apply thin layer to affected area, remove (by showering) in 6–8 hr in children and after 18–24 hr in adults. Pediculosis: Shampoo with adequate amount (15–30 ml) and lather for 5 minutes then rinse thoroughly and comb. *Side effects:* Dermal absorption may cause seizures, dizziness, hepatitis, blood dyscrasias.

Mebendazole: Ascariasis, Hookworms, Trichuriasis: 100 mg bid PO for 3 days or 500 mg PO once for all ages; 2nd course, if needed, in 3–4 wk. Enterobiasis: 100 mg PO for all ages, repeated in 2 week. Trichinosis: 200–400 mg tid PO for 3 days then 400–500 mg tid PO for 10 days for all ages. Toxocariasis: 100–200 mg bid PO for 5 days for all ages. *Side effects:* Leukopenia, transient elevation in liver function tests.

Metronidazole: Amebiasis: 30–50 mg/kg/day PO divided q8hr for 10 days (maximum: 500–750 mg/dose). Giardiasis: 15 mg/kg/24 hr PO divided q8 hr for 5 days (maximum: 750 mg/dose). Balantidiasis: 45 mg/kg/24 hr PO divided q8 hr for 5days (maximum: 750 mg/dose). Dracunculiasis: 25 mg/kg tid PO for 10 days (maximum dose: 750 mg). *Side effects: see* Section 40.3.

Metronidazole-diloxanide furoate: Amebiasis, giardiasis. Dose is the same as mentioned in metronidazole. *Side effects:* Same as mentioned in metronidazole.

Niclosamide: Beef and fish tapeworm: 40 mg/kg PO once (maximum dose: 2 g). Dwarf tapeworm: 40 mg/kg

PO qid for 7 days (maximum daily dose: 2 g). *Side effects:* Rash, alopecia, abdominal pain.

Ornidazole: Amebiasis, amebic dysentery, amebic liver abscess, giardiasis, trichomoniasis: 40 mg/kg once daily for 3 days. *Side effects:* Alopecia, seizures, unpleasant taste, leucocytosis, dark urine.

Pentamidine isetionate: Pneumocystis carinii pneumonia: 4 mg/kg/day IM, IV for 14–21 days. *Pneumocystis carinii* pneumonia prophylaxis: 4 mg/kg/dose IM, IV every 2–4 week. Aerosol once/month using nebulizer: Infant: Use dose formula (2.27 mg/kg pentamidine) × (nebulizer output (L/minute) × patient body weight (kg) divided by alveolar ventilation (L/min). Child >5 yr: 300 mg/dose every 4 wk. *Side effects:* Hypotension, hypoglycemia, nephrotoxicity.

Permethrin: Scabies: Apply leaving on for 8–16 hr before removing with water. Head lice: Wash areas, rinse, apply cream, rinse liberally, leave in hair for 10 minutes, rinse and comb; may repeat treatment in 7 days. Do not apply to denuded/inflamed skin; avoid contact to eyes/mucous membranes. *Side effects:* May cause rash.

Piperazine citrate: Pinworm: 65 mg/kg/day PO once daily for 7 days; may repeat course in 7 days. Roundworm: 75 mg/kg/day PO once daily for 2 days (maximum dose: 3.5 g/day); may repeat course in 7 days. *Side effects:* Neurotoxicity, seizures, tremor.

Praziquantel: Schistosomiasis: 20 mg/kg/dose PO q8hr for 1 day. Other trematodes: 75 mg/kg/24 hr divided tid PO for 1–2 days. Lung flukes: 75 mg/kg/24 hr divided tid PO for 2 days. Cysticercosis: 50–100 mg/kg/24 hr divided tid PO for thirty days. Corticosteroids for 2–3 days before and during drug therapy can ameliorate worsening of symptoms that follow anticysticercal drugs. Tapeworm: 5–10 mg/kg PO once (as a single dose). *Side effects:* CNS depression, rash, abdominal pain, eosinophilia.

Pyrantel pamoate: Roundworm, pinworm, trichostrongyliasis: 100 mg PO once; may repeat in 2 weeks. Roundworm/ hookworm/whipworm: 11 mg/kg PO single dose (maximum dose: 1 g); may repeat for 2 wk for pinworm infection. Hookworm: 11 mg/kg PO once daily for 3 consecutive days (max dose: 1 g/24 hr). *Side effects:* Rash, abdominal cramps.

Pyrimethamine: Malaria prophylaxis: (Begin drug 2 wk before entering in endemic areas) 0.5 mg/kg PO once wk (maximum dose: 25 mg). Chloroquine-resistant malaria (with quinine and sulfa). Toxoplasmosis (with sulfadiazine): 2 mg/kg/day PO divided q12 hr for 2–3 days then 1 mg/kg/day PO qid with sulfadiazine for 6 months then 1 mg/kg/day

PO qid 3 times/wk (maximum daily dose: 25 mg/day). *Toxoplasma gondii* prophylaxis: Infants>1 mo: 1 mg/kg/day PO q24 hr plus dapsone. Adolescents: 50 mg PO once weekly plus dapsone. *Pneumocystis carinii* prophylaxis: Adolescents: 50–75 mg PO once weekly plus dapsone. Administer folinic acid (5–10 mg/kg 3 times in a week) to prevent hematologic toxicity. *Side effects:* Seizures, folic acid deficiency, marrow suppression, tremor.

Sodium antimony gluconate: Kala-azar. 20 mg/kg/24 hr IV or IM for 20 days (LCL and DCL) or 28 days (for ML or DL); 4–6 g for full course. [LCL = Localized cutaneous leishmaniasis; DCL = Diffuse cutaneous leishmaniasis; ML = Mucosal leishmaniasis; VL = Visceral leishmaniasis]. *Side effects:* Abdominal pain, anaphylactic shock.

Thiabendazole: Strongyloidiasis. 50 mg/kg bid PO for 2 days; maximum: 3 g/24 hr. *Side effects:* Rash, leucopenia.

Tinidazole: Amebiasis: 50 mg/kg as single dose PO for 5 days in liver abscess, and for intestinal amebiasis for 3 days (maximum: 2 g). Giardiasis: 50 mg/kg PO once (maximum: 2g). Trichomoniasis: Drug doses are the same as mentioned for giardiasis. *Side effects:* Unpleasant taste, leucopenia, ulceration, CNS disturbances, dark urine.

Tinidazole-diloxanide furoate: Amebiasis, giardiasis. Dose is the same as mentioned in tinidazole. *Side effects:* Same as mentioned in tinidazole.

Antimalarial Drugs

Amodiaquine: Treatment of malaria. Partially immune subjects: 10 mg/kg as single dose. Non-immune subjects: 10 mg/kg initially followed by 5 mg/kg daily for 2 days. *Side effects:* Agranulocytosis, hepatitis, peripheral neuropathy.

Arteether: Severe and complicated malaria including cerebral malaria. 3 mg/kg IM daily for 3 consecutive days. *Side effects:* Nausea, headache, increase in eosinophil count.

Artesunate: Chloroquine resistant malaria; cerebral malaria. Adults: PO: 2 doses of 100 mg on the first day followed by 50 mg twice daily on the following 4 to 6 days. (Total dose: 10 mg/kg). IV or IM: 120 mg on day one followed by 60 mg once daily for next 4 days (total dose: 360–480 mg). Children: Half the adult dose. *Side effects:* Abdominal pain, reduction of neutrophil and reticulocytes. *Contraindication:* G6PD deficiency.

Chloroquine phosphate: (Dose of drug on base equivalent). Malaria prophylaxis: 5 mg/kg/wk PO (maximum dose: 300 mg/dose). Acute malaria treatment: 10 mg/kg PO initial dose (maximum dose:

600 mg); 5 mg/kg 6 hr later then 5 mg/kg PO once daily for 2 days. IM: 5 mg/kg initial dose, 5 mg/kg 6 hr later (maximum IM dose: 10 mg/kg/24 hr). *Side effects:* Hypotension, rash, peripheral neuropathy, blood dyscrasias, retinopathy, tinnitus. Administration with meals decreases GI upset.

Hydroxychloroquine: Suppression or chemoprophylaxis of malaria; treatment of systemic lupus erythematosus and rheumatoid arthritis. Children: Chemoprophylaxis of malaria: 5 mg/kg once wk (Begin 1–2 wk before exposure and continue for 4 wk after leaving high-risk area). Acute malarial attack: 10 mg/kg initial dose followed by 5 mg/kg in 6–8 hr on day 1, 400 mg once on day 2 and day 3. *Caution:* Avoid in porphyria or psoriasis. Tablet: 200 mg. *Side effects:* Visual field defects, retinitis, blindness, bone-marrow suppression, thrombocytopenia, liver failure, bleaching of hair, ototoxicity.

Mefloquine: Treatment of chloroquine-resistant malaria, severe malaria due to *P. falciparum* and *P. vivax* including cerebral malaria. 15 mg/kg followed by 10 mg/kg PO 8–12 hr later (maximum: 1, 250 mg) for 1 day. *Side effects:* Neuropsychiatric reactions.

Mepacrine HCl: Prophylaxis and treatment of Plasmodium falciparum. Prophylaxis: 600 mg/wk, may be given in divided doses. Treatment: 900 mg on the first day; 600 mg on 2nd and 3rd days and 300 mg on 4th, 5th, and 6th days in divided doses. *Side effects:* GI disturbances, yellow discoloration of skin and/or/ blue or black pigmentation of the nails may occur after prolonged usage.

Primaquine phosphate: Prevention and treatment of malaria (dose of drug on base equivalent). 0.3 mg base/kg/day PO once daily for 14 days [maximum daily dose: 15 mg base (26.3 mg salt)]. A G6PD screening test should be performed before initiating treatment because the drug can cause hemolytic anemia. Pregnant women should not be administered primaquine. *Side effects:* Pruritus, GI upset, anemia.

Proguanil HCl: Prevention and suppression of malaria. >14 yr: 200 mg daily. Children <1 yr: 25 mg; 1–4 yr: 50 mg; 5–8 yr: 100 mg; 9–14 yr: 150 mg. All daily during exposure and continued for 6 wk after exposure. *Side effects:* Mouth ulceration,

Quinine: Treatment of malaria and babesia. Chloroquine resistant malaria: 30 mg/kg/day PO divided q8 hr for 3–7 days, preferably for 7 days (maximum: 650 mg/dose) along with tetracycline 20 mg/kg/24 hr divided in 4 doses for 7 days (maximum: 250 mg/dose); weigh the benefits of tetracycline therapy against the possibility of dental staining in children younger than 8 yr of age. Quinine

dihydrochloride injection IV: 20 mg/kg over 4 hr, then 10 mg/kg over 2–4 hr q8 hr (max: 1,800 mg/24 hr) until oral therapy can be started. Babesiosis (Babesia): Combination of quinine (25 mg/kg/day divided tid PO), and clindamycin (20–40 mg/kg/day divided tid PO) for 7–10 days. *Side effects:* G6PD hemolysis, cinchonism (ringing in ears, nausea, vomiting, headache, mental confusion, vertigo, difficulty in hearing and visual defects; diarrhea, flushing and marked perspiration may also occur. The syndrome subsides completely if the drug is stopped).

Sulphadoxine-pyrimethamine: Chloroquine-resistant malaria. <1 yr: Single dose of ¼ tablet; 1–3 yr: Single dose of ½ tablet; 4–8 yr: Single dose of 1 tablet; 9–14 yr: Single dose of 2 tablets; >14 yr: Single dose of 3 tablets *Side effects:* Skin rash, pruritus, GI distress, blood dyscrasias.

40.9 ANTITOXINS AND IMMUNOGLOBULINS

Anti-human thymocyte immunoglobulin: [Lymphoglobuline, Thymoglobulin].

Lymphoglobuline (Equine anti-human thymocyte immunoglobulin): Indications: Treatment of severe aplastic anemia, GVHD and for prophylaxis and therapy of rejection episodes after kidney, heart, pancreas or liver transplantations. Injection: 100 mg/5 ml vial. Prophylaxis of rejection: 1 vial/10 kg body wt/ 24 hr for 1–3 wk. Treatment of rejection crisis and acute GVHD: 1–2 vials/10 kg body wt/ 24 hr until clinical and biological signs disappear. Treatment of aplastic anemia: 1–2 vials/10 kg body wt/ 24 hr during 5 days.

Antirabies serum: Dose: 40 iu/kg delivered in the same manner as for HRIG. Injection: 1,000 IU per 5 ml. *Caution:* Test for hypersensitivity before administration. Prefer HRIG. Sensitivity reactions, including anaphylaxis (treat with epinephrine and antihistamine and brief holding the dose). *Side effects:* Serum sickness, urticaria, skin eruptions, and allergic reactions.

Anti-snake venom: Used for the treatment of poisonous snake bite. Dose: Dosing depends on severity of bite. 1–2 vials initially, further depending upon persistency of envenomation. . Injection: 10 ml vial (1 ml of the reconstituted serum neutralizes 0.6 mg of dried Indian cobra (Naza Naza) venom, 0.45 mg of dried common Krait (Bungarus Caeruleus) venom, 0.6 mg of dried Russell's Viper (Vipera Russell) venom, 0.45 mg of dried saw scaled Viper (Echis Carinatus) venom, per 10 ml). *Side effects: see* Antirabies serum.

Anti-T lymphocytic globulin: Used for prophylaxis and therapy of rejection of transplanted organs and severe aplastic anemia. Dose: 200 mg/day IV between days 20–23 and 40–48 in post-transplant cases. Injection: 100 mg vial. Caution: Sensitivity reactions, including anaphylaxis (treat with epinephrine and antihistamine and brief holding the dose). *Side effects: see* Antirabies serum.

Antivenin (crotalidae) polyvalent: Indication: Antivenom for snake bite from North and South American crotalids, i.e. rattle snake, copperhead, cottonmouth, tropicalmoccasins, fer-de-lance, bushmaster. Dosing based on severity of bite-mild: 5 vials; moderate: 10 vials; severe: >15 vials. Injection: Lyophilized serum, diluent (10 ml); one vacuum vial to yield 10 ml of antivenom. Caution: Test for hypersensitivity before administration. Sensitivity reactions, including anaphylaxis (treat with epinephrine and antihistamine and brief holding of antivenom). *Side effects: see* Antirabies serum.

Diphtheria antitoxin: Indication: Antitoxin is administered as a single empirical dose of 20,000–120,000 units based on the degree of toxicity, site and size of membrane and duration of illness. Injection: 10,000 iu, 10 ml ampule. Caution: Test for hypersensitivity before administration. Sensitivity reactions, including anaphylaxis (treat with epinephrine and antihistamine and brief holding the dose). *Side effects: see* Antirabies serum.

Gas-gangrene Antitoxin: Indications: Prophylactic: 1000 units IM/IV; Therapeutic: Not more than 3000 units, IM/IV. Injection: 4,000, 10,000 iu. Caution: Test for hypersensitivity before administration. Sensitivity reactions, including anaphylaxis (treat with epinephrine and antihistamine and brief holding the dose). *Side effects: see* Antirabies serum.

Hepatitis B immunoglobulin: Indications: (i) For prophylaxis of hepatitis B after exposure to HbsAg; (ii) For prophylaxis of hepatitis B in neonates born to HbsAg positive mothers. Neonates: Initial dose 100–200 IU, IM administered with in 5 days after birth (preferably within 48 hr) and booster dose 38–48 iu/kg, administered between 2–3 months after the first dose. Children: 38-48 IU/kg, IM administered within 7 days (preferably within 48 hr) after exposure. Injection: 100 IU/0.5 ml, 200 IU/1 ml. Treat sensitivity reactions, including anaphylaxis with epinephrine and antihistamine and brief holding the dose.

Human anti-D immunoglobulin: Used for prevention of Rh sensitization in Rh-negative mother within 72 hr of delivery of an Rh-positive infant, ectopic pregnancy, abdominal trauma in pregnancy, amniocentesis, chorionic villus biopsy, or abortion.

Anti-D vaccine administered at 28–32 wk and again at birth (40 wk) is more effective than single dose. Dose: 300 mcg IM within 72 hr after delivery, abortion after 12 wk. Injection: 100 µg, 300 µg per 1 ml; 300 µg/1.5 ml, 300 µg/2 ml. Treat sensitivity reactions, including anaphylaxis with epinephrine and antihistamine and brief holding the dose.

Human rabies immunoglobulin (HRIG): Treaitment after suspected exposure to rabies. Dose: 20 iu/kg, (max: 1,500 µu), 50% of the dose to be injected locally around the wound and the balance to be given IM at a site distant from Vaccine inoculation. Injection: 150 iu/mL. Treat sensitivity reactions, including anaphylaxis with epinephrine and antihistamine and brief holding the dose.

Immune globulin intravenous (IVIG) (Human gamma globulin): Management of Immunodeficiency syndrome, Immunotherapy, acute bacterial or viral infections in immunocompromised or neutopenic patients, primary and secondary hypogammaglobulinemia, idiopathic thrombocytopenic purpura, Guillain-Barré syndrome, Kawasaki disease, neonatal sepsis, demyelinating polyneuropathy (replacement therapy or interference with Fc receptors in the reticuloendothelial system for autoimmune diseases). Neonates: 500–750 mg/kg once. Children and Adults: Immunodeiciency syndromes: 100–400 mg/kg/dose q2–4 wk. Chronic lymphocytic leukemia: 400 mg/kg/dose q3 wk. Idiopathic thrombocytopenic purpura: 1,000 mg/kg/dose for 2–5 consecutive days, then q3–6 wk. Kawasaki disease: 2 g/kg single dose. Cytomegalovirus infection: 500–1,000 mg/kg/dose every other day for 7 doses. Severe systemic infection: 500–1,000 mg/kg/wk. Polyneuropathy: 1 g/kg/24 hr for two consecutive days each month. Injection: 500 mg, 3 g, 6 g; Infusion 2.5 g, 5 g, 10 g; 10%, 16%. Caution: Doses should be based on ideal body weight (not total body weight). Sensitivity reactions, including anaphylaxis (treat with epinephrine and antihistamine and brief holding the dose). *Side effects:* Flushing, hypersensitivity reactions.

Scorpion venom antiserum: Dose: 1 vial initially, further depending upon persistency of envenomation. Injection: 1 mL of the reconstituted serum neutralizes, dried red scorpion 1 mg, vial (with 10 ml of water for inj). Caution: Test for hypersensitivity before administration. Sensitivity reactions, including anaphylaxis (treat with epinephrine and antihistamine and brief holding the dose). *Side effects: see* Antirabies serum.

Tetanus antitoxin: Used in the prevention or treatment of tetanus when human tetanus immunoglobulin is not available. Children: SC/IM: Prophylaxis: < 30 kg

1,500 units; > 30 kg 3,000–5.000 units. Treatment: Inject 10,000–40,000 units into wound and 40,000–100,000 units IV. Injection: 750 iu, 1,500 iu, 10,000 iu. Caution: Test for hypersensitivity before administration. *Side effects: see* Antirabies serum.

Tetanus immune globulin/Tetanus immunoglobulin (TIG) [Human tetanus immunoglobulin]: Used in prophylaxis and treatment of tetanus. Prophylaxis: Children: 4 units/kg, IM. Injuries (including dog/animal bites): IM 250–500 μu; Burns: IM 500 μu on day 1 and followed by 250 iu at the end of exudative phase.

Thymoglobulin: [Rabbit anti-human thymocyte immunoglobulin]. Treatment of severe aplastic anemia, GVHD and for prophylaxis and therapy of rejection episodes after kidney, heart, pancreas or liver transplantations. Prophylaxis of rejection: 1.25–2.5 mg/kg/day for 1–3 wk after transplant. Treatment of rejection crisis and acute GVHD: 2.5–5 mg/kg/24 hr until clinical and biological signs disappear. Treatment of aplastic anemia: 2.5–5 mg/kg / 24 hr during 5 days. Injection: 25 mg vial.

40.10 ANTIDOTES FOR POISONING

Atropine: Organophophate and carbamate poisoning; Bradycardia due to atrioventricular conduction defects. Dose: 0.05 mg/kg IV/ET, repeated q5–15 min as needed. Dilute in 1–2 ml of normal saline for ET (Endotracheal instillation). Injection: 0.6 mg/ml. *Side effects:* Tachycardia, dry mouth, blurred vision, urinary retention. BAL in oil (Dimercaprol) [2, 3-dimercaptopropanol or British antilewisite (BAL)]:

Heavy metals (Arsenic; mercury; lead) poisoning. Dose: 3–5 mg/kg/dose Deep IM q4hr, for the first day, subsequent dosing depends on toxin. A period of 5 days between courses of chelation is recommended. Injection: 50 mg/2 ml, 100 mg/2 ml. *Side effects:* Local injection site pain and sterile abscess, nausea, fever, salivation, nephrotoxicity.

Charcoal: Emergency treatment of poisoning by certain drugs and chemicals; gastrointestinal dialysis of certain to promote elimination of certain drugs and toxins; treat diarrhea. Gastric decontamination with activated charcoal of: Calcium channel blockers (nifedipine, diltiazem, verapamil, amlodipine, and felodipine); Salicylates (aspirin, methyl salicylates); Antidepressants (tricyclic antidepressants, TCAs: (amitryptiline, nortriptyline and sinequan); Selective serotonin reuptake inhibitors, SSRIs: (fluoxetine, sertraline, paroxetine and citalopram). Children: 1–2 g/kg or 5–10 times the weight of the ingested poison (limit sorbitol to 1–2 times daily); may repeat doses q2–6 hr. Tablet: Activated charcoal 400 mg with

simethicone 80 mg. *Side effects:* Constipation, black stools.

Cyanide antidote kit: Cyanide, hydrogen sulfide. ***Cyanide:*** Amyl nitrite: 1 crushable ampule, inhale 30 sec of each minute, inhalation. ***Hydrogen sulfide:*** Sodium nitrite: 0.33 ml/kg of 3% solution IV if hemoglobin level not known otherwise based on tables with product. Inhalation; Injection. *Side effects:* Methemoglobinuria.

Desferrioxamine (Deferoxamine): Treatment of acute iron intoxication or secondary chronic iron overload (hemochromatosis), aluminium overload in dialysis patients. Dose: Infusion of 15 mg/kg/hr (max: 6 g/24 hr) SC over 10–12 hr, 5–6 days a week. Oral administration has not been effective and may cause neutropenia, arthritis and hepatic fibrosis. Some prefer IV instead SC. Can be administered IM in the doses of 90 mg/kg/dose q8 h (maximum 6 g/24 hr). Injection: 500 mg vial. Caution: Contraindicated in patients with primary hemochromatosis. *Side effects:* Hypotension, ototoxicity, retinal changes, and bone dysplasia with truncal shortening.

Digoxin Immune Fab: Digoxin Immune Fab is used for the treatment of digitalis intoxication from digoxin or digitoxin administered (one vial binds 0.6 mg of digitalis glycoside). i). Dose of digoxin immune Fab (mg) = TBL digoxin x76; ii). Dose of digoxin immune Fab (no. of vials) = TBL/0.5.

Total body load (TBL) digoxin = concentration (ng/ml) × 0.56 × wt (kg)/1000

TBL digitoxin = mg ingested × 0.8.

Dose of digoxin immune Fab (mg) = TBL digoxin × 76.

Dimercaptosuccinic acid: [2,3-dimercaptosuccinic acid (DMSA)]: Lead and probably mercury, arsenic, and perhaps other metals. Dose: 10 mg/kg/dose PO q8 hr for 5 days, then 10 mg/kg PO q12 hr for 14 days (repeated courses may be needed. A period of 2 wk between courses of chelation is recommended). Capsule: 100 mg. *Side effects:* Flu-like symptoms.

Diphenhydramine: Extrapyramidal symptoms, acute dystonic reactions, allergic reactions. Dose: 5 mg/kg IV, PO divided q8 hr (max: 300 mg/hr). Capsule: 25 mg; Syrup: 12.5 mg/5 ml; Injection: 10 mg/ml, 50 mg/ml. *Side effects:* Sedation, ataxia.

Edetate disodium: Emergency treatment of hypercalcemia and digitalis-induced ventricular dysarrhythmias. Hypercalcemia Children: 40–70 mg/kg /24 hr slowly infusion over 3–4 hr; administer for 5 days then 5 days off drug. Digitalis arrhythmias Children: 15 mg/kg/hr continuous infusion (max: 60 mg/kg/hr). Injection: 150 mg/ml. *Side effects:* Hypotension, seizures, skin eruptions, nephrotoxicity.

EDTA, calcium: Lead, manganese, nickel, zinc, chromium poisoning. Dose: 1–1.5 g/m²/day IV in divided doses q12 hr for 5 days. *Side effects:* Hypertension, arthralgia, allergic reactions, local inflammation, nephrotoxicity.

Ethanol (Ethyl alcohol): Methanol; Ethylene glycol poisoning: Dose: 750 mg/kg IV/PO loading dose followed by 80–150 mg/kg/hr infusion of 5% or 10% ethanol. *Side effects:* Nausea, vomiting, sedation.

Flumazenil: [Benzodiazepines; *see* Central system medications]. Benzodiazepine antagonist to reverse sedative effects. Dose: 0.2 mg over 30 sec IV; if inadequate response, repeat q 1 min to 1 mg max. *Side effects:* Facial flushing, seizures.

Fomepizole: Ethylene glycol; Methanol poisoning. Dose: 15 mg/kg IV loading dose; 10 mg/kg IV q12 hr for 4 doses; 15 mg/kg IV q12 hr until level < 20 mg/dl. *Caution:* Infuse slowly over 30 min.

Glucagon: Beta-blockers (e.g. Propranolol), Calcium Channel Blockers poisoning; Hypoglycemic agents. Dose: 0.05 mg/kg bolus IV followed by infusion of 0.05 mg/kg/hr. Injection: 1 mg/mL. *Side effects:* Hyperglycemia, nausea, vomiting.

Ipecac syrup: Induces vomiting to treat certain toxic substances. Children: May repeat dose in 20 min one time. 6–12 mo: 5–10 ml followed by 20 ml/kg of water. 1–12 yr: 15 ml followed by 20 ml/kg of water. > 12 yr: 30 ml followed by 300 ml of water. Syrup: 70 mg/ml. *Side effects:* Lethargy, persistent vomiting, diarrhea.

Methylene blue: Cyanide poisoning and drug induced methemoglobinemia. Children: Methemoglobinemia: IV: 1–2 mg/kg; may repeat after 1 hr if needed; or 0.1–0.2 ml/kg IV of 1% solution, slow infusion, may be repeated q30–60 min. NADPH-methemoglobin reductase deficiency: PO: 1–1.5 mg/kg/24 hr (given with 5–8 mg/kg/24 hr of ascorbic acid. Injection: 10 mg/mL; Tablet: 65 mg. *Caution:* Avoid in G6PD deficiency and renal insufficiency. *Side effects:* Urine and faces turn blue–green, anemia.

N-Acetylcysteine: Acetaminophen; Carbon Tetrachloride; Chloroform (experimental). Dose: 140 mg/kg loading dose followed by 70 mg/kg PO q4 hr for 17 doses. Injection: 200 mg/ml; Tablet: 600 mg. *Side effects:* Nausea, vomiting.

Naloxone: Narcotics [Morphine, other opiates, semi and synthetic narcotics (heroin), meperidine, propoxyphene, lomotil (diphenoxylate hydrochloride)]; Clonidine. Neonates and Children: 0.1 mg/kg IV (max dose: 2 mg); if no effect, repeat q2–3 min until desired effect. Injection: 20 mcg/ml (0.02 mg/ml), 400 mcg/mL (0.4 mg/ml). *Side effects:* Acute withdrawal symptoms if given to addicted patients.

Penicillamine: Wilson disease, lead intoxication, rheumatoid arthritis. Wilson disease: Dose titrated to maintain >1 mg/24 hr urinary copper excretion. Infants and Children: 20 mg/kg/24 hr PO q6–12 hr (max: 1 g/24 hr). Lead intoxication: Infants and Children: 30–40 mg/kg/24 hr PO q8–12hr (max: 1.5 g/24 hr). Rheumatoid arthritis: Children: 3 mg/kg/24 hr PO q12hr, increasing by 3 mg/kg/24 hr q2–3 mo to max 10 mg/kg/24 hr. Capsule: 250 mg. Side effects: Bone marrow suppression, nephrotic syndrome, systemic lupus erythematosus-like syndrome.

Physostigmine: Used in the reversal of anticholinergic effects (anticholinergic agent). Children: 0.02 mg/kg IV/IM slowly push; may repeat q15–20 min to desired effect (max total dose: 2 mg). *Side effects:* Bradycardia, asystole, seizures, bronchospasm.

Pralidoxime: Organophosphorous poisoning (insecticides which are cholinesterase inhibitors-melathion, TEPP, parathion, dichlorvos, fenthion). Dose: 25–50 mg/kg IV 5–10 min (max: 200 mg/min); can be repeated after 1–2 hr, then q10–12 hr as needed. Injection: 500 mg, 1 g vial. *Side effects:* Nausea, tachycardia, muscle rigidity, and bronchospasm (if administered rapidly).

Protamine sulfate: Antidote for heparin. Dose: 1 mg protamine neutralizes 90 USP units of lung-derived heparin and 115 USP units of intestinal-derived heparin. Protamine dose calculated on duration of time since last heparin dose using heparin elimination half-life (~1 hr) to determine estimated heparin body stores. Injection: 10 mg/ml. *Side effects:* Hypotension, hypersensitivity.

Pyridoxine (vitamin B₆): Isoniazid; Gyromitra mushrooms; Ethylene glycol (investigational). Isoniazid: Dose= dose of isoniazid IV, uncommon adverse effect. Mushrooms: 25 mg/kg. Pyridoxine-dependent seizures: PO, IM, IV: 50–100 mg; maintenance dose 50–100 mg/24 hr

Sodium polystyrene sulfonate (Kayexalate): Treatment of hyperkalemia. Children: 4 g/kg/24 hr PO 48 hr delay. Rectal 4–12 g/kg/24 hr PR q2–6 hr. Adults: 15 g/dose PO q6–12 hr. Powder for suspension. *Side effects:* Hypokalemia.

Sodium thiosulfate: Cyanide (nitroprusside) and cisplatin antidote.

Nitroprusside: Children: 1 g sodium thiosulfate for every 100 mg nitroprusside administered. Injection: 100 mg/ml, 250 mg/ml. *Side effects:* Hypotension, local irritation at infusion site.

Trientine: Treatment of Wilson disease in patients intolerant to penicillamine. Children <12 yr: 500–

1500 mg/24 hr in 2–4 doses. Children >12 yr: 750–2,000 mg/24 hr in 2–4 doses. Comments: Take 1 hr before or 2 hr after meals. Capsule: 250 mg. *Side effects:* Iron-deficiency anemia, muscle cramps, systemic lupus erythematosus.

Vitamin K (Phytomenadione): [Neutralizes heparin anticogulant effect]. Warfarin. Dose: Oral administration of vitamin K, equal to the amount of the daily warfarin dose.

40.11 Vaccines

AIDS Vaccine: Dose: 6 vaccinations over 6 months–4 with ALVAC, 2 with AIDSVAX. Boost vaccine to protect at least 70 percent people immunized; will lower infection risk by 31.2 percent. Vaccine protects against HIV-1 subtypes E and B, predominant in US and Thailand, not against subtype C predominant in India.

BCG (Bacille Calmette-Guérin): [Live attenuated BCG vaccine (Bacillus Calmette–Guérin strain). Each 0.1 ml contains between: 1×10^5 and 33×10^5 CFU. Freeze-dried vaccine; store in dark between 2 and 8°C. Protect from light (ultraviolet rays in sunlight also kill the organisms rapidly)]: Dose: 0.05 ml ID for infants under 1 yr old. Comment: The vaccination causes the nodule at the site in about 4–6 wk. This nodule gradually settles down but sometimes forms a sore with some discharge, before it is healed. Formulation: Injection: Vial of 20 doses to be reconstituted with 1 ml of sodium chloride injection. [BCG (Serum Institute)].

DTP adsorbed: [Vaccine contains Diphtheria Toxoid ≥ 25 Lf (≥ 30 IU), Tetanus Toxoid ≥ 5 Lf (≥ 40 IU), B. Pertussis ≤ 16 OU (≥ 4 PU), per 0.5 mL IM injection. Adsorbed on aluminium phosphate $(AlPO_4) \geq 1.5$ mg. Preservative 0.01% Thiomersal. Shake well. Preserve 2–8°C]: Dose: Infants (6 weeks): 3 doses of 0.5 ml IM at 6, 10, 14 weeks interval and a booster dose at 18–24 months. Comment: Limit of flocculation (Lf) content is a measure of the quantity of toxoid. The pediatric preparation (i.e., DT, DTP) contains 25 Lf units of diphtheria toxoid per 0.5 ml dose; the adult preparation (i.e., dT) contains no more than 2 Lf units of toxoid per 0.5 ml dose, because the lower concentration of diphtheria toxoid is adequately immunogenic and because increasing the content of diphtheria toxoid heightens reactogenicity with increasing age. True contraindications: Encephalopathy (e.g. coma, decreased levels of consciousness, prolonged seizures) within 7 days of administration of previous dose of DTP; progressive neurologic disorder, including infantile spasms, uncontrolled epilepsy, and progressive encephalopathy. Precautions: Fever of > 40.5° C ≤ 48 hr after vaccination with a previous dose of DTP; collapse or shock-like state ≥ 48 hr after receiving a previous dose of DPT; seizure ≤ 3 days of receiving the previous dose of DTP; persistent inconsolable crying lasting ≥ 3 hours and ≤ 48 hr after receiving a previous dose of DPT. Untrue contraindications (Vaccines can be administered): Temperature of < 40.5°C, fussiness or mild drowsiness after a previous dose of DTP; family history of seizures; family history of sudden infant death syndrome, family history of adverse event after DTP administration; stable neurologic conditions (e.g., cerebral palsy, well-controlled seizures, developmental delay). Formulation: Injection: 0.5 ml, 5 ml (10 doses). [DTP (Serum Institute of India), Triple antigen].

DTP with Hepatitis B: [Contains diphtheria toxoid not less than 30 µu, tetanus toxoid not less than 60 µu, inactivated pertussis bacteria not less than 4 iu and recombinant HB_SAG protein 10 µg adsorbed on aluminium salts, per 0.5 ml]: Dose: 3 doses of 0.5 ml IM at 6, 10, 14 weeks interval and a booster dose at 18–24 months. Formulation: Injection: 10 µg/0.5 ml].

DTP with Haemophilus b conjugate: [Adsorbed diphtheria, tetanus, pertussis, and Haemophilus influenzae type b conjugate vaccine]: Dose: 3 injections at 6, 10, 14 wk and a booster dose at 18–24 months. Caution: The combination products should not be used for primary immunization in infants at ages 2, 4 or 6 months, but can be used as boosters following any Hib vaccine. Formulation: Injection: 0.5 ml.

DTP HB+ HiB: [Pentavalent vaccine, a combination of diphtheria, tetanus, pertussis, hepatitis B and Haemophilus influenzae type b conjugate vaccine]: Dose: 3 injections at 6, 10, 14 wk and a booster dose at 18–24 months. Formulation: Injection: 0.5 ml

DT: [Contains diphtheria toxoid 25 Lf (≥ 30 IU) and tetanus toxoid 5 Lf (≥ 40 IU)]:

Dose in children having contraindication to pertussis component or coming after 2 year of age: 3 doses of 0.5 ml IM at 6, 10, 14 weeks interval and a booster dose at 18–24 months. Dose in children who are immunized with DPT/DTP: 0.5 ml IM at 5 yr.

Dose in children >5 yr: 0.5 ml at 10 and 16 yr and then every 10 yr throughout life.

Precaution: Guillain-Barré syndrome ≤ 6 wk after previous dose of DT. Formulation: Injection: 0.5 ml.

Hepatitis A vaccine: [Hepatitis A virus HM175 strain 360 (pediatric) or 720 (junior) or 1440 (adult) ELISA unit per dose]: Dose: Children > 2 yr: 2 doses 0.5 ml IM at least 6–12 months apart. Precaution: Pregnancy. Formulation: Injection: 0.5 ml.

Hepatitis B vaccine, Recombinant. [Contains HB$_S$AG]: Indication: Prophylaxis against hepatitis B infection. Children below 10 yr: 10 µg IM 3 injections at 6, 10, 14 wk. Children above 10 yr: 20 µg IM 3 injections at 0, 1, 6 month after the first dose. Precaution: Infant weighing <2,000 grams. Formulation: Injection: 10 µg/ 0.5 ml, 20 µg/1 ml, 100 µg/5 ml.

HIB conjugate vaccine: [Capsular polysaccharide (10 µg) of *Haemophilus influenzae* type b conjugate vaccine]: Dose: 2 doses of 0.5 mL IM at ages 6 and 14 wk; booster dose at 15–18 months. Contraindication: Age <6 wk. Formulation: Injection: 10 µg/0.5 ml.

Easyfive: [DTwP-Hep B-Hib vaccine]: Easyfive is a sterile and uniform suspension of diphtheria toxoid, Tetanus toxoid, Whole cell B. pertussis, Hepatitis B surface Antigen (HB)and conjugated *Haemophilus influenzae* type b (Hib) vaccine adsorbed on aluminum phosphate gel and suspended in isotonic sodium chloride solution. Composition: one dose of 0.5 ml contains Diphtheria toxoid 20 (Lf), Tetanus typhoid (7.5 Lf), inactivated w; Bordetella pertussis (12 OU), Hepatitis B surface antigen (10 µg), Hib oligosaccharide (10 µg), Aluminum phosphate gel 0.25 mg, Thiomersal (as preservative) (0.025 mg), normal saline qs (0.5 ml). Vaccine should be stored at +2°C to +8°C. Do not freeze. Discard if the vaccine is frozen. Indications: For active immunization against diphtheria, tetanus, pertussis, Hib and Hb in infants from 6 weeks onwards. Three vaccine doses must be administered intramuscularly (IM) into the anterolateral aspect of the thigh region at intervals of at least 4–6 weeks (i.e. 6, 10, 14 weeks of age). A booster dose of DTwP and Hib can be given at the age of 15–18 months. A reinforcing injection of the 0.5 ml intramuscularly of the DTwP combination should be administered at 5 years of age (i.e. at the time of school entry). The injection should not be given in the intragluteal or deltoid region. Shake well before use. Contraindications: Should not be administered to subjects with known hypersensitivity to any component of the vaccine. Adverse effects: Mild reaction at the injection site, such as pain, local tenderness, warmth, edema, induration with or without tenderness. Formulation: Injection: 5 mL vial.

Five-in-one vaccine: [Vaccine for 5 diseases: Poliomyelitis, Pertussis, Diphtheria, Tetanus, *H. influenzae*; Contains IPV & acellular pertussis based pentavalent vaccine; Diphtheria, Tetanus, acellular pertussis, inactivated poliomyelitis vaccine, adsorbed and *H. influenzae* type b conjugate vaccine]: Dose: 3 doses at 6, 10, 14 weeks followed by a booster dose at 15–18 months.

Human Papillomavirus vaccine: [Quadrivalent human papillomavirus (Types 6, 11, 16, 18); Recombinant vaccine]: Dose: 3 separate intramuscular injections; individuals are encouraged to adhere to the 0-, 2-, and 6-month vaccine schedule. Gardasil is indicated 3 doses of HPV 6/11/16/18 in females 9 through 45 yr for prevention of cervical, vulvar, and vaginal cancer, precancerous or dysplastic lesions, genital warts, and infections caused by Human Papillomavirus (HPV) Types 6, 11, 16 and 18 (which are included in the vaccine). Syncope, sometimes associated with falling, has occurred after vaccination with Gardasil. Therefore, vaccines should be carefully observed for approximately 15 minutes after administration of Gardasil. Gardasil is contraindicated in individuals who are hypersensitive to the active substances or to any of the excipients of the vaccine. Individuals who develop symptoms indicative of hypersensitivity after receiving a dose of Gardasil should not receive further doses of Gardasil. Pregnancy should be avoided during the vaccination regimen for Gardasil. The vaccine-related adverse reactions at a frequency of at least 1% includes pain at the injection site, swelling, erythema, headache, pruritus, bruising, pin in extremity, fever, nauseas, and dizziness. [Gardasil (MSD)].

Inactivated Poliomyelitis Vaccine (IPV): Composition: One dose (0.5 ml) contains: Inactivated type 1 poliomyelitis virus antigen D 40 units, type 2 antigen D 8 units, and type 3 antigen D 40 units. Indication: For the prevention of polio in infants, children and adults both as primary vaccination and as a booster. Dose: 0.5 ml IM or SC; primary vaccination: from the age of 2 months, 3 successive doses of 0.5 mL should be given at intervals of one to two months. A 4th dose (1st booster) is administered one year after the 3rd injection. From 6 wk of age may be administered following the 6, 10, 14 weeks schedule, according to EPI recommendations. For subsequent boosters, an injection is given every 5 yr in children and adolescents and every 10 yr in adults. Vaccine may be prescribed any time during pregnancy if required; vaccination may be used during lactation. Contraindications: hypersensitivity to one of the active ingredients, to one of the excipients, to neomycin, to streptomycin and to polymyxin B or following a previous injection of this vaccine. Usual transient contraindications to all vaccinations: vaccination should be delayed in the case of fever, acute disease or progressive chronic disease. Patients receiving immunosuppressive therapy or suffering from immune deficiency disorders defer vaccination until the end of treatment or to ensure the subject is well protected; vaccination of subjects with chronic immunodeficiency such as HIV infection is recommended if the immune deficiency allows induction of an antibody response even limited. Adverse effects are rare; local reactions at the injection site: pain, erythema, induration, and edema may occur during the 48 hr following the injection and persist for one or two days. Shelf-life: 3 yr; store between +2°C and +8°C (in the refrigerator) protected from light. Do not freeze. The immediate use of the product is recommended after opening. Nature and contents of container: 0.5 ml of suspension for injection in a prefilled syringe (type 1 glass) with a plunger stopper (elastomer). [IMOVAX POLIO; Prefilled syringe presentation (sanofi pasteur)]

Influenza vaccine: [Inactivated vaccine]: Indication: Recommended annually for children age ≥ 6 months with certain risk factors (including asthma, cardiac disease, sickle cell disease, HIV, diabetes, and household members of persons in groups at high risk), and can be administered to all others wishing to obtain immunity; healthy children age 6–23 months; children aged ≤ 12 yr; children aged ≥ 8 yr not vaccinated previously, should receive 2 doses at 4 weeks apart. Dose: Two doses of vaccine at least 1 month apart is recommended for primary immunization of children < 9 yr of age. Children 6–35 months: 0.25 ml IM; Children aged 3–8 yr: 0.5 ml IM. Formulation: Injection: 0.5 ml.

Japanese encephalitis vaccine: [Inactivated vaccine for children 1 yr of age and older]:

Dose: 3 doses SC 0.5 ml for 1–3 yr of age; 1 ml for >3 yr of age; the first 2 doses are given 1 wk apart and the third dose 30 days later. Booster doses are given every 2 yr while risk of exposure continues. Caution: The vaccine has an a efficacy of more than 95%, but hypersensitivity reactions occur in up to 0.6% of vaccine recipients; 1 in 1,000 vaccines have urticarial reactions or facial or oropharyngeal angioedema that may occur within minutes or up to 2 wk after vaccination. The series should be completed 2 wk before travel so that any adverse reactions to the vaccine can be observed and treated.

Adverse events: Reactions to vaccination, including headache, malaise, myalgia, tenderness, redness, and swelling occurs in about 20% of vaccines. Serious generalized urticaria, facial angioedema, and respiratory distress have been observed in adults. Because vaccine is prepared in mouse brain, surveillance should be maintained for central nervous system disease after Japanese encephalitis vaccination. Formulation: Injection: 1 ml inj.

Measles vaccine: [Measles virus (live, attenuated; freeze-dried) Edmonston Zagreb strain containing at least 1000 CCID-50]: Dose: Children at 9 months: 0.5 ml SC but may be given for measles postexposure and outbreak prophylaxis as early as 6 months of age. Formulation: Injection: 0.5 ml.

Measles, mumps, rubella (MMR): [Live attenuated measles vaccine not less than 1,000 CCID-50, Live attenuated mumps vaccine not less than 5,000 CCID-50, Live attenuated rubella vaccine not less than 1,000 CCID-50 per 0.5 ml dose; Lyophilised live attenuated measles, mumps, rubella virus vaccine]: Dose: A single dose of 0.5 ml is injected SC or IM at the age of 12–15 months but may be given for measles post-exposure and outbreak prophylaxis as early as 6 months of age. The second dose of MMR is recommended routinely at age 4–6 yr but may be administered during any visit, provided at least 4 wk have elapsed since the first dose and that both doses are administered beginning at or after age 12 months. Those who have not previously received the second dose should complete the schedule by the 11–12 year old visit. Contraindications: Pregnancy; known severe immunodeficiency (e.g., hematologic and solid tumors, congenital immuno-deficiency, long term immunosuppressive therapy, or severely symptomatic human immunodeficiency virus (HIV) infection). Precautions: Recent (≤ 11 months) receipt of antibody-containing blood product; history of thrombocytopenia or thrombocytopenic purpura. Formulation: Injection: 0.5 ml.

Meningococcal A and C vaccine: [Groups A & C polysaccharide meningococcal vaccine (lyophilised preparation) 50 mcg from each group]: Dose: 0.5 ml SC in subjects over 2 yr of age. Formulation: Injection: 0.5 ml.

A quadrivalent (A,C,Y,W-135), conjugated vaccine (MCV-4) is recommended to 11–12 yr old adolescents, high risk children older than 2 yr (anatomic or functional asplenia or deficiencies of terminal complement protein), college freshmen.

Pneumococcal vaccine: [Pneumococcal Saccharide Conjugated Vaccine, Adsorbed; Pneumococcal 7-valent conjugate vaccine is a sterile solution of saccharides of the capsular antigens of *Streptococcus pneumoniae* serotypes 4, 6B, 9V, 14, 18C, 19F, and 23F; *(PCV7)*]: Indications: For active immunization of infants and toddlers. Adverse reactions: mild erythema, induration and tenderness. Warning: It will not protect against *Streptococcus pneumoniae* diseases other than caused by serotypes included in the vaccine. Dose: 4 doses IM or SC at 2, 4, 6 and 12–15 months of age; it can be given at 6 weeks of age. The recommended dosing interval is 4–8 weeks. The fourth dose should be administered at least 2 months after the third dose. Storage: Should not be freezed.

Store refrigerated away from freezer compartment at 2°C to 8°C (36°F to 46°F).
Formulation: Injection: 0.5 ml.

23-valent polysaccharide vaccine (PPV23): (Each dose contains purified polysaccharides of 23 serotypes of *Streptococcus pneumoniae*)]: High-risk children ≥2yr of age, such as those with asplenia, sickle cell disease, immune deficiency, HIV infection, or chronic lung, heart, or kidney disease (including nephrotic syndrome) may benefit from the vaccine administered IM or SC. After the initial immunization, a single supplemental dose may be used 3 yr after the first dose for children <10 yr of age at the time of revaccination, or it may be used at 5 yr after the first dose for children 10 yr of age or older at the time revaccination. Formulation: Injection: 0.5 mL. [Pneumo 23].

Polio vaccine (Oral) (OPV): [Stabilized suspension of type 1, 2, 3 live attenuated poliomyelitis virus (Sabin strains)]: Dose: 2 drops oral at 6, 10, 14 wk and a booster dose at 18–24 months. Formulation: Oral Drops.

Rabies vaccine: [Chicken fibroblast cell or duck embryo or human diploid cell or sheep brain suspension or Vero cells vaccine]: Dose: Children and Adults: Pre-exposure: IM: three 1 mL deltoid region on days 0, 7, and 21 or 28; Post-exposure: IM: five 1 mL deltoid region on days 0, 3, 7, 14, and 28. Children doses are same as that of adults.

Formulation: Injection: Not less than 2.5 IU/1 ml of inactivated rabies virus potency.

[Berirab, Berirab-P, MIRV-HDC Vaccine (human diploid cell vaccine), Rabies vaccine (human diploid cell vaccine), Rabies vaccine (Human) (sheep brain suspension vaccine), Rabipur (chicken fibroblast cell vaccine), Vaxirab (duck embryo vaccine), (chicken fibroblast cell vaccine), Verorab (Vero cells vaccine), Verovax-R (Vero cells vaccine)].

Rotavirus vaccines [Rotavirus vaccine (RIX-4414) Live attenuated human strain rotavirus]: Dose: 2 doses (one dose: 1 ml) 4 wk apart by oral route to infants from the age of 6 wk for prevention of gastroenteritis from rotavirus infection and the vaccination course should be completed by 24 wk. Composition: 1 dose (1 ml) contains live attenuated human rotavirus RIX-4414 strain. Lyophilized vaccine to be reconstituted with a liquid diluents before oral administration. Contraindications: Hypersensitivity after previous administration of vaccine; subjects with congenital anomalies, such as Meckel diverticulum and of the gastrointestinal tract that would predispose to intussusception and acute febrile illness. [Rotarix™ (GlaxoSmithKline)]

Rotavirus vaccine [Live, Oral, Pentavalent]: Dose: 3 doses series to infants between the ages of 6 to 32 weeks. RotaTeq is a live, oral pentavalent vaccine indicated for the prevention of rotavirus gastroenteritis in infants and children caused by the serotypes G1, G2, G3, G4 when administered a 3 dose series to infants between the ages of 6 to 32 weeks. Vaccination with RotaTeq may not result in complete protection in all recipients.
[RotaTeq (MSD)].

Rubella vaccine: [Live attenuated Rubella virus Wistar RA 27/3 strain 1,000 CCID-50, per 0.5 ml]: Dose: 12 months to puberty: SC or IM: 0.5 ml. Contraindication: Pregnancy. Formulation: Injection: 0.5 ml.

Tdap Vaccine: [Reduced antigen Tdap booster vaccine]: Dose: In children who have missed the 2nd booster of DTwP/DTaP and who are 7 yr of age or more, one injection. Formulation: Injection: 0.5 ml.

Tetanus toxoid (TT): [Tetanus toxoid 5 Lf (≥ 40 IU)]. Children: 2 injections 0.5 ml IM at 10 and 16 yr. Pregnant women: 2 injections at 4 weeks apart (20–24 wk and second dose at 4 wk apart). Tetanus prophylaxis in wound management: Clean, Minor wounds: Prior tetanus doses uncertain, or <3 give TT/DT, IM ; if prior doses 3 or more give TT/DT, IM only if the person has received the last dose ≥10 yr. Other wounds: Prior tetanus doses uncertain, or <3 give TT/DT, IM along with 250 U of TIG, IM, and 500 U, IM for highly tetanus-prone wounds (i.e., can not be debrided, with bacterial contamination, or >24 hr old); if prior doses 3 or more give TT/DT, only if the person has received the last dose ≥ 5 yr (more frequent doses are not needed and can accentuate adverse events). Formulation: Injection: 0.5 ml, 5 ml (10 doses).

Typhoid vaccine: Typhoid vaccine [Purified VI capsular polysaccharides of S. typhi 0.025 mg per 0.5 mL injection]: Children over 2 yr and Adults: SC or IM single dose inj 0.5 ml (inj 2.5 ml with TYVAX Vi-PLUS 150 MCG); ensures 3 yr protection. Formulation: Injection: 0.5 ml, 2.5 ml.

Typhoid oral vaccine: [Attenuated Salmonella strain Ty21a Bema not less than 10^9 capsule]: Children over 6 yr and Adults: One capsule orally on alternate days taken approximately 1 hr before meal with cold or lukewarm drink (water, milk), total dose 3 capsules. Formulation: Capsule.

Varicella vaccine: [Lyophilised vaccine containing live attenuated Oka strain of varicella-zoster 3.3^{10} plaque forming units (PFU) per vial]: Vaccine is recommended for administration in children at 12–18 months of age. Older children, adolescents and adults without a history of varicella-zoster virus (VZV) infection should also be immunized. Administration of varicella vaccine within

4 week of MMR vaccine has been associated with a higher risk of breakthrough disease; therefore, the vaccines either be administered simultaneously at different sites or be given at least 4 weeks apart. Dose: Children 12 months to 12 yr: S C, one dose (0.5 ml); Children >12 yr and Adults: 2 doses SC (0.5 ml) at dose interval of 8 weeks (not less than 6 weeks interval). Children with acute lymphoblastic leukemia and HIV-infected children with CD4% greater than 25%: 2 doses of vaccine, 3 months apart. Contraindications: Substantial suppression of cellular immunity; pregnancy. Precaution: Recent (≤ 11 months) receipt of antibody-containing blood product. Formulation: Injection: 0.5 ml.

Yellow fever vaccine: [17D is a live, attenuated vaccine]: Administered as a single 0.5 ml SC at least 10 days before arrival in a yellow fever endemic area. Residence or travel to known or anticipated yellow fever activity, which places an infant at high risk, warrants immunization of infant 4–9 months of age. Immunization of children ≥ 9 month of age is routinely recommended before entry into endemic areas. Caution: Vaccination should be avoided for persons with a history of egg allergy. A skin test can be performed to determine whether a serious allergy exists that would preclude vaccination. Formulation: Injection: 0.5 ml.

Index

PLATE 1

ASSESS AND CLASSIFY THE SICK YOUNG INFANT AGE UP TO 2 MONTHS

ASSESS

Ask the mother what the young infant's problems are

- Determine if this is an initial or follow-up visit for this problem.
  - if follow-up visit, use the follow-up instructions on the bottom of this chart.
  - if initial visit, assess the young infant as follows:

CLASSIFY

USE ALL BOXES THAT MATCH
INFANT'S SYMPTOMS AND PROBLEMS
TO CLASSIFY THE ILLNESS.

IDENTIFY TREATMENT

A child with a pink classification needs URGENT attention,
complete the assessment and pre-referral treatment
immediately so referral is not delayed

CHECK FOR POSSIBLE BACTERIAL INFECTION/JAUNDICE

ASK:

- Has the infant had convulsions?

LOOK, LISTEN, FEEL:

- Count the breaths in one minute.
  Repeat the count if elevated.
- Look for severe chest indrawing.
- Look for nasal flaring.
- Look and listen for grunting.
- Look and feel for bulging fontanelle.
- Look for pus draining from the ear.
- Look at the umbilicus. Is it red or draining pus?
- Look for skin pustules. Are there 10 or more skin pustules or a big boil?
- Measure axillary temperature (if not possible, feel for fever or low body temperature).
- See if the young infant is lethargic or unconscious.
- Look at the young infant's movements.
  Are they less than normal?
- Look for jaundice?
- Are the palms and soles yellow?

{ YOUNG INFANT MUST BE CALM }

CLASSIFY ALL YOUNG INFANTS

AND IF THE INFANT HAS JAUNDICE

AND IF THE TEMP. IS BETWEEN 35.5 and 36.4°C

SIGNS	CLASSIFY AS	IDENTIFY TREATMENT *(Urgent pre-referral treatments are in bold print.)*
• Convulsions or • Fast breathing (60 breaths per minute or more) or • Severe chest indrawing or • Nasal flaring or • Grunting or • Bulging fontanelle or • 10 or more skin pustules or a big boil or • If axillary temperature 37.5°C or above (or feels hot to touch) or temperature less than 35.5°C (or feels cold to touch) or • Lethargic or unconscious or • Less than normal movements.	**POSSIBLE SERIOUS BACTERIAL INFECTION**	**Give first dose of intramuscular ampicillin and gentamicin.** Treat to prevent low blood sugar. **Warm the young infant by skin to skin contact if temperature less than 36.5°C (or feels cold to touch) while arranging referral.** Advise mother how to keep the young infant warm on the way to the hospital. **Refer URGENTLY to hospital** *
• Umbilicus red or draining pus or • Pus discharge from ear or • <10 skin pustules.	**LOCAL BACTERIAL INFECTION**	**Give oral amoxycillin for 5 days.** Teach mother to treat local infections at home. Follow up in 2 days.
• Palms and soles yellow or • Age <24 hours or • Age 14 days or more	**SEVERE JAUNDICE**	Treat to prevent low blood sugar. **Warm the young infant by Skin to Skin contact if temperature less than 36.5°C (or feels cold to touch) while arranging referral.** Advise mother how to keep the young infant warm on the way to the hospital. **Refer URGENTLY to hospital.**
• Palms and soles not yellow	**JAUNDICE**	Advise mother to give home care for the young infant. Advise mother when to return immediately. Follow up in 2 days.
• Temperature between 35.5 and 36.4°C	**LOW BODY TEMPERATURE**	Warm the young infant using Skin to Skin contact for one hour and REASSESS. If no improvement, refer Treat to prevent low blood sugar.

\# If referral is not possible, see the section **Where Referral is Not Possible** in the module **Treat the Young Infant and Counsel the Mother.**

PLATE 2

THEN ASK:
Does the young infant have diarrhoea?*

IF YES, ASK:	LOOK AND FEEL:
• For how long?	• Look at the young infant's general condition. Is the infant:
• Is there blood in the stool?	–Lethargic or unconscious?
	–Restless and irritable?
	• Look for sunken eyes.
	• Pinch the skin of the abdomen. Does it go back:
	– Very slowly (Longer than 2 seconds)?
	– Slowly?

CLASSIFY DIARRHOEA

FOR DEHYDRATION

Signs	Classify	Treatment
Two of the following signs: • Lethargic or unconscious • Sunken eyes • Skin pinch goes back very slowly	SEVERE DEHYDRATION	Give first dose of intramuscular ampicillin and gentamicin. If infant also has low weight or another severe classification: - Refer URGENTLY to hospital with mother giving frequent sips of ORS on the way. - Advise mother to continue breastfeeding. - Advise mother how to keep the young infant warm on the way to the hospital. **OR** If infant does not have low weight or any other severe classification: - Give fluid for severe dehydration (Plan C) and then refer to hospital after rehydration.
Two of the following signs: • Restless, irritable • Sunken eyes • Skin pinch goes back slowly	SOME DEHYDRATION	If infant also has low weight or another severe classification: - Give first dose of intramuscular ampicillin and gentamicin - Refer URGENTLY to hospital with mother giving frequent sips of ORS on the way. - Advise mother to continue breastfeeding. - Advise mother how to keep the young infant warm on the way to the hospital. If infant does not have low weight or another severe classification: - Give fluids for some dehydration (Plan B). - Advise mother when to return immediately. - Follow up in 2 days
• Not enough signs to classify as some or severe dehydration	NO DEHYDRATION	Give fluids to treat diarrhea at home (Plan A). Advise mother when to return immediately. Follow up in 5 days if not improving.

AND IF DIARRHOEA 14 DAYS OR MORE

Signs	Classify	Treatment
• Diarrhoea lasting 14 days or more	SEVERE PERSISTENT DIARRHOEA	Give first dose of intramuscular ampicillin and gentamicin if the young infant has low weight, dehydration or another severe classification. Treat to prevent low blood sugar. Advise how to keep infant warm on the way to the hospital. Refer to hospital.#

AND IF BLOOD IN STOOL

Signs	Classify	Treatment
• Blood in the stool	SEVERE DYSENTERY	Give first dose of intramuscular ampicillin and gentamicin if the young infant has low weight, dehydration or another severe classification. Treat to prevent low blood sugar. Advise how to keep infant warm on the way to the hospital. Refer to hospital.#

* What is diarrhoea in a young infant?
If the stools have changed from usual pattern and are many and watery (more water than fecal matter). The normally frequent or loose stools of a breastfed baby are not diarrhoea.

If referral is not possible, see the section **Where Referral Is Not Possible** in the module **Treat the Young Infant and Counsel the Mother.**

PLATE 3

THEN CHECK FOR FEEDING PROBLEM AND MALNUTRITION:

ASK:

LOOK, FEEL:

- Is there any difficulty feeding?
- Is the infant breastfed? If yes, how many times in 24 hours?
- Does the infant usually receive any other foods or drinks? If yes, how often?
- What do you use to feed the infant?

- Determine weight for age.

IF AN INFANT:

Has any difficulty feeding, or
Is breastfeeding less than 8 times in 24 hours, or
Is taking any other foods or drinks, or
Is low weight for age,
AND
Has no indications to refer urgently to hospital:

ASSESS BREASTFEEDING:

- Has the infant breastfed in the previous hour?

If the infant has not fed in the previous hour, ask the mother to put her infant to the breast. Observe the breastfeed for 4 minutes.

(If the infant was fed during the last hour, ask the mother if she can wait and tell you when the infant is willing to feed again.)

- Is the infant able to attach?

  no attachment at all   not well attached   good attachment

  TO CHECK ATTACHMENT, LOOK FOR:
  - Chin touching breast
  - Mouth wide open
  - Lower lip turned outward
  - More areola visible above than below the mouth

  (All of these signs should be present if the attachment is good)

- Is the infant suckling effectively (that is, slow deep sucks, sometimes pausing)?

  not suckling at all   not suckling effectively   suckling effectively

  Clear a blocked nose if it interferes with breastfeeding.

- Look for ulcers or white patches in the mouth (thrush).

- Does the mother have pain while breastfeeding? If yes, look and feel for:
  - Flat or inverted nipples, or sore nipples
  - Engorged breasts or breast abscess

If referral is not possible, see the section Where **Referral Is Not Possible** in the module **Treat the Young Infant and Counsel the Mother.**

CLASSIFY FEEDING

Signs	Classify as	Treatment
• Not able to feed or • No attachment at all or • Not suckling at all or • Severely Underweight (<-3 S.D)	**NOT ABLE TO FEED - POSSIBLE SERIOUS BACTERIAL INFECTION OR SEVERE MALNUTRITION**	**Give first dose of intramuscular ampicillin and gentamicin.** **Treat to prevent low blood sugar.** **Warm the young infant by skin to skin contact if temperature less than 36.5°C (or feels cold to touch) while arranging referral.** **Advise mother how to keep the young infant warm on the way to the hospital.** **Refer URGENTLY to hospital"**
• Not well attached to breast or • Not suckling effectively or • Less than 8 breastfeeds in 24 hours or • Receives other foods or drinks or • Thrush (ulcers or white patches in mouth) or • Moderately Underweight (<-2 to -3 S.D) or • Breast or nipple problems	**FEEDING PROBLEM OR LOW WEIGHT FOR AGE**	If not well attached or not suckling effectively, teach correct positioning and attachment. If breastfeeding less than 8 times in 24 hours, advise to increase frequency of feeding. If receiving other foods or drinks, counsel mother about breastfeeding more, reducing other foods or drinks, and using a cup and spoon. - If not breastfeeding at all, advise mother about giving locally appropriate animal milk and teach the mother to feed with a cup and spoon. If thrush, teach the mother to treat thrush at home. If low weight for age, teach the mother how to keep the young infant with low weight warm at home. If breast or nipple problem, teach the mother to treat breast or nipple problems. Advise mother to give home care for the young infant. Advise mother when to return immediately. Follow-up any feeding problem or thrush in 2 days. Follow-up low weight for age in 14 days.
• Not low weight for age (≥-2SD) and no other signs of inadequate feeding	**NO FEEDING PROBLEM**	Advise mother to give home care for the young infant. Advise mother when to return immediately. Praise the mother for feeding the infant well.

PLATE 4

ASSESS AND CLASSIFY THE SICK CHILD AGE 2 MONTHS UP TO 5 YEARS

| ASSESS | CLASSIFY | IDENTIFY TREATMENT |

ASK THE MOTHER WHAT THE CHILD'S PROBLEMS ARE

- Determine if this is an initial or follow-up visit for this problem.
  - if follow-up visit, use the follow-up instructions on *TREAT THE CHILD* chart.
  - if initial visit, assess the child as follows:

CHECK FOR GENERAL DANGER SIGNS

ASK:

- Is the child able to drink or breastfeed?
- Does the child vomit everything?
- Has the child had convulsions?

LOOK

- See if the child is lethargic or unconscious.

A child with any general danger sign needs URGENT attention; complete the assessment and any pre-referral treatment immediately so referral is not delayed.

THEN ASK ABOUT MAIN SYMPTOMS:

Does the child have cough or difficult breathing?

IF YES, ASK:

- For how long?

LOOK, LISTEN:

- Count the breaths in one minute.
- Look for chest indrawing.
- Look and listen for stridor.

> *CLASSIFY COUGH OR DIFFICULT BREATHING*

CHILD MUST BE CALM

If the child is:	Fast breathing is:
2 months up to 12 months	**50** breaths per minute or more
12 months up to 5 years	**40** breaths per minute or more

USE ALL BOXES THAT MATCH THE CHILD'S SYMPTOMS AND PROBLEMS TO CLASSIFY THE ILLNESS.

SIGNS	CLASSIFY AS	IDENTIFY TREATMENT *(Urgent pre-referral treatments are in bold print.)*
- Any general danger sign or - Chest indrawing or - Stridor in calm child	SEVERE PNEUMONIA OR VERY SEVERE DISEASE	**Give first dose of injectable chloramphenicol (If not possible give oral amoxycillin).** **Refer URGENTLY to hospital.** #
- Fast breathing	PNEUMONIA	**Give Amoxicillin for 5 days.** Soothe the throat and relieve the cough with a safe remedy if child is 6 months or older. Advise mother when to return immediately. Follow-up in 2 days.
No signs of pneumonia or very severe disease	NO PNEUMONIA: COUGH OR COLD	If coughing more than 30 days, refer for assessment. Soothe the throat and relieve the cough with a safe home remedy if child is 6 months or older. Advise mother when to return immediately. Follow-up in 5 days if not improving.

If referral is not possible, see the section **Where Referral Is Not Possible** in the module **Treat the Child.**

PLATE 5

Does the child have diarrhoea?

IF YES, ASK:	LOOK AND FEEL:
• For how long?	• Look at the child's general condition. Is the child:
• Is there blood in the stool?	– Lethargic or unconscious?
	– Restless and irritable?
	• Look for sunken eyes.
	• Offer the child fluid. Is the child:
	– Not able to drink or drinking poorly?
	– Drinking eagerly, thirsty?
	• Pinch the skin of the abdomen. Does it go back:
	– Very slowly (longer than 2 seconds)?
	– Slowly?

CLASSIFY DIARRHOEA

FOR DEHYDRATION

Signs	Classify as	Treatment
Two of the following signs: • Lethargic or unconscious • Sunken eyes • Not able to drink or drinking poorly • Skin pinch goes back very slowly	**SEVERE DEHYDRATION**	If child has no other severe classification: - Give fluid for severe dehydration (Plan C). *If child also has another severe classification:* *Refer URGENTLY to hospital # with mother giving frequent sips of ORS on the way.* *Advise the mother to continue breastfeeding.* *If child is 2 years or older and there is cholera in your area, give doxycycline for cholera.*
Two of the following signs: • Restless, irritable. • Sunken eyes. • Drinks eagerly, thirsty • Skin pinch goes back slowly	**SOME DEHYDRATION**	Give fluid, zinc supplements and food for some dehydration (Plan B). *If child also has a severe classification:* *Refer URGENTLY to hospital # with mother giving frequent sips of ORS on the way.* *Advise the mother to continue breastfeeding.* Advise mother when to return immediately. Follow-up in 5 days if not improving.
• Not enough signs to classify as some or severe dehydration	**NO DEHYDRATION**	Give fluid, zinc supplements and food to treat diarrhoea at home (Plan A). Advise mother when to return immediately. Follow-up in 5 days if not improving.

AND IF DIARRHOEA 14 DAYS OR MORE

Signs	Classify as	Treatment
• Dehydration present	**SEVERE PERSISTENT DIARRHOEA**	*Treat dehydration before referral unless the child has another severe classification.* *Refer to hospital.#*
• No dehydration	**PERSISTENT DIARRHOEA**	Advise the mother on feeding a child who has PERSISTENT DIARRHOEA. **Give single dose of vitamin A.** Give zinc supplements daily for 14 days. Follow-up in 5 days.

AND IF BLOOD IN STOOL

Signs	Classify as	Treatment
• Blood in the stool	**DYSENTERY**	*Treat for 3 days with ciprofloxacin.* *Treat dehydration* Give zinc supplements for 14 days Follow-up in 2 days.

If referral is not possible, see the section **Where Referral Is Not Possible** in the module **Treat the Child.**

PLATE 6

Does the child have fever?
(by history or feels hot or temperature 37.5°C* or above)

IF YES:
Decide Malaria Risk: High Low

THEN ASK:	**LOOK AND FEEL:**
• Fever for how long?	• Look or feel for stiff neck.
• If more than 7 days, has fever been present every day?	• Look and feel for bulging fontanelle.
• Has the child had measles within the last 3 months?	• Look for runny nose.
	Look for signs of MEASLES
	• Generalized rash and
	• One of these: cough, runny nose, or red eyes.

If the child has measles now or within the last 3 months:

• Look for mouth ulcers.
  Are they deep and extensive?
• Look for pus draining from the eye.
• Look for clouding of the cornea.

CLASSIFY FEVER

HIGH MALARIA RISK

High Malaria Risk

Signs	Classification	Treatment
• Any general danger sign or • Stiff neck or • Bulging fontanelle	**VERY SEVERE FEBRILE DISEASE**	Give first dose of IM quinine after making a smear/RDT Give first dose of IV or IM chloramphenicol (If not possible, give oral amoxycillin). Treat the child to prevent low blood sugar. Give one dose of paracetamol in clinic for high fever (temp. 38.5°C or above). Refer URGENTLY to hospital.*
• Fever (by history or feels hot or temperature >37.5°C or above)	**MALARIA**	Give oral antimalarials for HIGH malaria risk area after making a smear/RDT Give one dose of paracetamol in clinic for high fever (temp. 38.5°C or above) Advise mother when to return immediately. Follow-up in 2 days. If fever is present every day for more than 7 days, refer for assessment.

LOW MALARIA RISK

Low Malaria Risk

Signs	Classification	Treatment
• Any general danger sign or • Stiff neck or • Bulging fontanelle.	**VERY SEVERE FEBRILE DISEASE**	Give first dose of IM quinine after making a smear. Give first dose of IV or IM chloramphenicol (if not possible, give oral amoxycillin). Treat the child to prevent low blood sugar. Give one dose of paracetamol in clinic for high fever (temp. 38.5°C or above). Refer URGENTLY to hospital.*
• NO runny nose and NO measles and NO other cause of fever	**MALARIA**	Give oral antimalarials for LOW malaria risk area after making a smear Give one dose of paracetamol in clinic for high fever (temp. 38.5°C or above). Advise mother when to return immediately. Follow-up in 2 days. If fever is present every day for more than 7 days, refer for assessment.
• Runny nose PRESENT or • Measles PRESENT or • Other cause of fever PRESENT**	**FEVER - MALARIA UNLIKELY**	Give one dose of paracetamol in clinic for high fever (temp. 38.5°C or above). Advise mother when to return immediately. Follow-up in 2 days if fever persists If fever is present every day for more than 7 days, refer for assessment.

If MEASLES Now or within last 3 months, Classify

Signs	Classification	Treatment
• Any general danger sign or • Clouding of cornea or • Deep or extensive mouth ulcers	**SEVERE COMPLICATED MEASLES *****	Give first dose of vitamin A. Give first dose of injectable chloramphenicol (If not possible give oral amoxycillin). If clouding of the cornea or pus draining from the eye, apply tetracycline eye ointment. Refer URGENTLY to hospital*
• Pus draining from the eye or • Mouth ulcers	***** MEASLES WITH EYE OR MOUTH COMPLICATIONS	Give first dose of vitamin A. If pus draining from the eye, treat eye infection with tetracycline eye ointment. If mouth ulcers, treat with gentian violet. Follow-up in 2 days.
• Measles now or within the last 3 months.	**MEASLES**	Give first dose of vitamin A

* This cutoff is for axillary temperatures; rectal temperature cutoff is approximately 0.5°C higher—
** Other causes of fever include cough or cold, pneumonia, diarrhoea, dysentery and skin infections.
*** Other important complications of measles - pneumonia, stridor, diarrhoea, ear infection and malnutrition - are classified in other tables.

* If referral is not possible, see the section **Where Referral Is Not Possible** in the module **Treat the Child.**

PLATE 7

Does the child have an ear problem?

IF YES, ASK:
- Is there ear pain?
- Is there ear discharge?
If yes, for how long?

LOOK AND FEEL:
- Look for pus draining from the ear.
- Feel for tender swelling behind the ear.

Classify
EAR PROBLEM

Signs	Classification	Treatment
• Tender swelling behind the ear	**MASTOIDITIS**	**Give first dose of injectable chloramphenicol (If not possible give oral amoxycillin).** Give first dose of paracetamol for pain. **Refer URGENTLY to hospital#.**
• Pus is seen draining from the ear and discharge is reported for less than 14 days, or • Ear pain.	**ACUTE EAR INFECTION**	**Give Amoxycillin for 5 days.** Give paracetamol for pain. Dry the ear by wicking. Follow-up in 5 days.
• Pus is seen draining from the ear and discharge is reported for 14 days or more.	**CHRONIC EAR INFECTION**	Dry the ear by wicking. Topical ciprofloxacin ear drops for 2 weeks. Follow-up in 5 days.
• No ear pain and No pus seen draining from the ear.	**NO EAR INFECTION**	No additional treatment.

If referral is not possible, see the section **Where Referral Is Not Possible** in the module **Treat the Child.**

PLATE 8

THEN CHECK FOR MALNUTRITION

LOOK AND FEEL:
- Look for visible severe wasting.
- Look for oedema of both feet.
- Determine weight for age.

Classify
NUTRITIONAL
STATUS

Signs	Classify	Treatment
• Visible severe wasting or • Oedema of both feet.	**SEVERE MALNUTRITION**	**Give single dose of *Vitamin A*.** **Prevent low blood sugar.** ***Refer URGENTLY to hospital #*** ***While referral is being organized, warm the child.*** ***Keep the child warm on the way to hospital.***
• Severely Underweight ≤ 3 SD	**VERY LOW WEIGHT**	Assess and counsel for feeding - if feeding problem, follow-up in 5 days Advise mother when to return immediately Follow-up in 30 days.
• Not Severely Underweight ≥ 3SD	**NOT VERY LOW WEIGHT**	If child is less than 2 years old, assess the child's feeding and counsel the mother on feeding according to the FOOD box on the COUNSEL THE MOTHER chart. - If feeding problem, follow-up in 5 days. Advise mother when to return immediately.

THEN CHECK FOR ANAEMIA

LOOK
- Look for palmar pallor. Is it:
  Severe palmar pallor?
  Some palmar pallor?

Classify
ANAEMIA

Signs	Classify	Treatment
• Severe palmar pallor	**SEVERE ANAEMIA**	Refer URGENTLY to hospital #.
• Some palmar pallor	**ANAEMIA**	Give iron folic acid therapy for 14 days. Assess the child's feeding and counsel the mother on feeding according to the FOOD box on the COUNSEL THE MOTHER chart. - If feeding problem, follow-up in 5 days. Advise mother when to return immediately. Follow-up in 14 days.
• No palmar pallor	**NO ANAEMIA**	Give prophylactic iron folic acid if child 6 months or older.

THEN CHECK THE CHILD'S IMMUNIZATION *, PROPHYLACTIC VITAMIN A & IRON-FOLIC ACID SUPPLEMENTATION STATUS

IMMUNIZATION SCHEDULE:	AGE	VACCINE
	Birth	BCG + OPV-0
	6 weeks	DPT-1 + OPV-1(+ HepB-**1)
	10 weeks	DPT-2 + OPV-2(+ HepB-*2)
	14 weeks	DPT-3 + OPV-3(+ HepB-*3)
	9 months	Measles
	16–18 months	DPT Booster + OPV
	60 months	DT

PROPHYLACTIC VITAMIN A
Give a single dose of vitamin A:
100,000 U at 9 months with measles immunization
200,000 U at 16–18 months with DPT Booster
200,000 U at 24 months, 30 months, 36 months,
42 months, 48 months, 54 months and 60 months

PROPHYLACTIC IFA
Give 20 mg elemental iron + 100 mcg folic acid (one tablet of Pediatric IFA or IFA syrup/IFA drops) for a total of 100 days in a year after the child has recovered from acute illness **if:**
- The child is 6 months of age or older, and
- Has not received Pediatric IFA Tablet/syrup/drops for 100 days in last one year.

* A child who needs to be immunized should be advised to go for immunization the day vaccines are available at AW/SC/PHC
** Hepatitis B to be given wherever included in the immunization schedule

ASSESS OTHER PROBLEMS

MAKE SURE CHILD WITH ANY GENERAL DANGER SIGN IS REFERRED after first dose of an appropriate antibiotic and other urgent treatments.
Exception: Rehydration of the child according to Plan C may resolve danger signs so that referral is no longer needed.

If referral is not possible, see the section **Where Referral Is Not Possible** in the module **Treat the Child.**